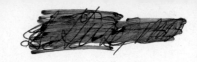

D0743670

THE BRIGHAM INTENSIVE REVIEW OF INTERNAL MEDICINE

THE BRIGHAM INTENSIVE REVIEW OF INTERNAL MEDICINE

EDITED BY

Ajay K. Singh, MBBS,
FRCP (UK), MBA

DIRECTOR, GLOBAL PROGRAMS
ASSOCIATE PROFESSOR OF MEDICINE
HARVARD MEDICAL SCHOOL
AND
PHYSICIAN, RENAL DIVISION
DIRECTOR, POSTGRADUATE MEDICAL
EDUCATION
DEPARTMENT OF MEDICINE
BRIGHAM AND WOMEN'S HOSPITAL
BOSTON, MASSACHUSETTS

EDITED BY

Joseph Loscalzo, MD, PhD

HERSEY PROFESSOR OF THE THEORY
AND PRACTICE OF PHYSIC
HARVARD MEDICAL SCHOOL
AND
CHAIRMAN, DEPARTMENT OF MEDICINE
PHYSICIAN-IN-CHIEF
BRIGHAM AND WOMEN'S HOSPITAL
BOSTON, MASSACHUSETTS

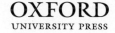

OXFORD
UNIVERSITY PRESS

OXFORD
UNIVERSITY PRESS

Oxford University Press, Inc., publishes works that further
Oxford University's objective of excellence
in research, scholarship, and education.

Oxford   New York
Auckland   Cape Town   Dar es Salaam   Hong Kong   Karachi
Kuala Lumpur   Madrid   Melbourne   Mexico City   Nairobi
New Delhi   Shanghai   Taipei   Toronto

With offices in
Argentina   Austria   Brazil   Chile   Czech Republic   France   Greece
Guatemala   Hungary   Italy   Japan   Poland   Portugal   Singapore
South Korea   Switzerland   Thailand   Turkey   Ukraine   Vietnam

Copyright © 2012 by Oxford University Press, Inc.

Published by Oxford University Press, Inc.
198 Madison Avenue, New York, New York 10016
www.oup.com

Oxford is a registered trademark of Oxford University Press

All rights reserved. No part of this publication may be reproduced,
stored in a retrieval system, or transmitted, in any form or by any means,
electronic, mechanical, photocopying, recording, or otherwise,
without the prior permission of Oxford University Press.

Library of Congress Cataloging-in-Publication Data

The Brigham intensive review of internal medicine / edited by Ajay K. Singh, Joseph Loscalzo.
    p. ; cm.
    Intensive review of internal medicine
    Includes bibliographical references and index.
    ISBN 978–0–19–536627–3 (North American ed. : pbk. : alk. paper)—
    ISBN 978–0–19–991787–7 (International ed. : pbk. : alk. paper)
    I. Singh, Ajay, M.D.   II. Loscalzo, Joseph.   III. Brigham and Women's Hospital.
    IV. Title: Intensive review of internal medicine.
    [DNLM: 1. Internal Medicine—methods.   2. Physical Examination—methods. WB 115]

This material is not intended to be, and should not be considered, a substitute for medical or other professional advice. Treatment for the conditions described in this material is highly dependent on the individual circumstances. And, although this material is designed to offer accurate information with respect to the subject matter covered and to be current as of the time it was written, research and knowledge about medical and health issues are constantly evolving, and dose schedules for medications are being revised continually, with new side effects recognized and accounted for regularly. Readers must therefore always check the product information and clinical procedures with the most up-to-date published product information and data sheets provided by the manufacturers and the most recent codes of conduct and safety regulation. The publisher and the authors make no representations or warranties to readers, express or implied, as to the accuracy or completeness of this material. Without limiting the foregoing, the publisher and the authors make no representations or warranties as to the accuracy or efficacy of the drug dosages mentioned in the material. The authors and the publisher do not accept, and expressly disclaim, any responsibility for any liability, loss, or risk that may be claimed or incurred as a consequence of the use and/or application of any of the contents of this material.

9 8 7 6 5 4 3 2
Printed in China
on acid-free paper

Ritu my wife, my children Anika, Vikrum, Nikita, and my parents Gita and JJ,
sister Anjali and brother Sanjay

Charlotte and Nicholas

FOREWORD

We are witnessing rapid change in all aspects of internal medicine. Within each specialty, there is a deeper understanding of the mechanism of disease, how it should be treated, and the consequences of treatment. This breathtaking progress has been spanned by a course at the Brigham and Women's Hospital and Harvard Medical School that I founded in 1977 entitled, "The Intensive Review of Internal Medicine." The objectives of the course were to provide an in-depth review of the major areas of internal medicine both for practicing internists and for physicians preparing for the certifying examination for the American Board in Internal Medicine. Of course, more recently, physicians are expected to recertify every 10 years to update their knowledge, and this course serves this purpose, as well. Our goal also included correlating pathophysiology with clinical presentation, something that I view as one of our strengths, because at Harvard Medical School we sit at the interface between practice and cutting-edge clinical science. Thirty-four years later, I could hardly have envisioned that the IRIM course, as our course affectionately became known, would still be going strong and that there would be demand for a companion text. Its success has much to do with the outstanding faculty and my successors as chairs in the Department of Medicine, Victor Dzau and Joseph Loscalzo, who have strongly supported it.

The Brigham Intensive Review of Internal Medicine is very capably edited by Drs. Singh and Loscalzo. They have selected outstanding authors, many drawn from the faculty at Harvard Medical School and its affiliated hospitals, in particular the Brigham and Women's Hospital. Each author is an authority in the particular area he or she covers. The book is superbly written and illustrated. It elegantly weaves together the many separate strands of internal medicine to provide a thorough understanding of the field. The editors have skillfully incorporated over 500 board-simulated questions and their answers into the book so that it is a "must have" for anyone preparing for board certification or recertification in internal medicine. In addition, the book will be a valuable resource for physicians who are in training and for practicing clinicians alike.

I am, therefore, very pleased to welcome *The Brigham Intensive Review of Internal Medicine* and anticipate that this text will become the standard in internal medicine board review.

Eugene Braunwald, MD

EUGENE BRAUNWALD, MD is the Distinguished Hersey Professor of Medicine at Harvard Medical School, and Founding Chairman of the TIMI Study Group at the Brigham and Women's Hospital.

CONTENTS

PREFACE

We are pleased to offer the first edition of The Brigham Intensive Review of Internal Medicine.

Dr. Soma Weiss, Physician-in-Chief at the Brigham in 1941, wrote in "Routine Practices," a manual for interns at the Peter Bent Brigham Hospital: "To become a good physician one must acquire the habit of caring for patients with a keen mind, and with good judgment, tact and sympathy. To these abilities must be added hard work and a willingness to give one's self. Without these attributes one cannot become a good physician; with them it is still difficult." This book provides the knowledge required to be the physician that Dr. Weiss idealized in his handbook, but it also reflects the evolving content required to prepare for the American Board of Internal Medicine. In addition to comprehensive sections in the specialties of internal medicine, we have included chapters on palliative care, occupational medicine, psychiatry, and geriatric medicine. We have emphasized board review by including hundreds of board-simulated questions featured both at the end of each chapter and as separate sections of the book. We have Board Review Practice examinations authored by former chief residents at the Brigham that span the content spectrum of all of internal medicine. Our overarching objective is to cover the broad base of knowledge that is now required both for practice and for success on the board examination.

Our book builds on the rich 34-year history of board review at the annual Intensive Review of Internal Medicine course. We have assimilated the collective feedback from many faculty who have taught in the course, to whom we are indebted for their years of outstanding service to the course; the course directors and section leaders, who have maintained the high quality over all of the many years of this course; and the many thousands of physicians who have participated as attendees. We are deeply indebted to our colleagues in the Department of Medicine at the Brigham and Women's Hospital and also to those across the Harvard Medical School community for their commitment to this project.

We would like to acknowledge the hard work and commitment of our administrative colleagues, Michelle Deraney and Christine Imperato at the Brigham, and Staci Hou and Andrea Seils at Oxford University Press, who have been magnificent in their support. We hope that you find the book useful and enriching.

Ajay K. Singh, MBBS, FRCP (UK), MBA
Joseph Loscalzo, MD, PhD

CONTRIBUTORS

Erik K. Alexander, MD
Endocrinology, Diabetes and Hypertension Division
Department of Medicine
Brigham and Women's Hospital
Associate Professor of Medicine
Harvard Medical School
Boston, MA

Mariam P. Alexander, MD
Department of Pathology
Brigham and Women's Hospital
Research Fellow in Pathology
Harvard Medical School
Boston, MA

Edwin P. Alyea III, MD
Medical Oncologist
Dana-Farber Cancer Institute
Department of Medicine
Brigham and Women's Hospital
Associate Professor of Medicine
Harvard Medical School
Boston, MA

Kenneth C. Anderson, MD
Program Director and Chief
Division of Hematologic Neoplasias
Dana-Farber Cancer Institute
Department of Medicine
Brigham and Women's Hospital
Kraft Family Professor of Medicine
Harvard Medical School
Boston, MA

Joseph H. Antin, MD
Medical Oncologist
Dana-Farber Cancer Institute
Department of Medicine
Brigham and Women's Hospital
Professor of Medicine
Harvard Medical School
Boston, MA

Elliott M. Antman, MD
Cardiovascular Medicine Division
Department of Medicine
Brigham and Women's Hospital
Professor of Medicine
Harvard Medical School
Boston, MA

C. Ryan Antolini, MD
Physician
Denver Arthritis Clinic
Denver, CO

Lindsey R. Baden, MD
Infectious Diseases Division
Department of Medicine
Brigham and Women's Hospital
Associate Professor of Medicine
Harvard Medical School
Boston, MA

Rebecca Marlene Baron, MD
Pulmonary and Critical Care Medicine Division
Department of Medicine
Brigham and Women's Hospital
Assistant Professor of Medicine
Harvard Medical School
Boston, MA

Kenneth Lee Baughman, MD*
Cardiovascular Medicine Division
Department of Medicine
Brigham and Women's Hospital
Boston, MA

Hasan Bazari, MD
Nephrology Division
Department of Medicine
Massachusetts General Hospital
Associate Professor of Medicine
Harvard Medical School
Boston, MA

Deceased.

Carolyn B. Becker, MD
Endocrinology, Diabetes and Hypertension Division
Department of Medicine
Brigham and Women's Hospital
Department of Medicine Associate Professor of Medicine
Harvard Medical School
Boston, MA

Rafael Bejar, MD, PhD
Hematology Division
Department of Medicine
Brigham and Women's Hospital
Instructor in Medicine
Harvard Medical School
Boston, MA

Rebecca A. Berman, MD
Department of Medicine
Massachusetts General Hospital
Instructor in Medicine
Harvard Medical School
Boston, MA

Bonnie L. Bermas, MD
Rheumatology and Allergy-Immunology Division
Department of Medicine
Brigham and Women's Hospital
Assistant Professor of Medicine
Harvard Medical School
Boston, MA

James D. Berry, MD
Department of Neurology
Massachusetts General Hospital
Instructor in Neurology
Harvard Medical School
Boston, MA

Tyler M. Berzin, MD, MS
Gastroenterology Division
Department of Medicine
Beth Israel Deaconess Medical Center
Instructor, Medicine
Harvard Medical School
Boston, MA

J. Andrew Billings, MD
Palliative Care Service
Department of Medicine
Massachusetts General Hospital
Associate Professor of Medicine
Harvard Medical School
Boston, MA

Alphonso Brown, MD
Gastroenterology Division
Department of Medicine
Beth Israel Deaconess Medical Center
Assistant Professor of Medicine
Harvard Medical School
Boston, MA

Jonathan D. Brown, MD
Cardiovascular Medicine Division
Department of Medicine
Brigham and Women's Hospital
Instructor, Medicine
Harvard Medical School
Boston, MA

Andrew E. Budson, MD
Department of Neurology
VA Boston Healthcare System
Professor of Neurology
Boston University School of Medicine
Department of Neurology
Brigham and Women's Hospital
Lecturer on Neurology
Harvard Medical School
Boston, MA

Robert S. Burakoff, MD, MPH
Gastroenterology, Hepatology and Endoscopy Division
Department of Medicine
Brigham and Women's Hospital
Associate Professor of Medicine
Harvard Medical School
Boston, MA

Julie E. Buring, ScD
Department of Population Medicine
Brigham and Women's Hospital
Professor of Population Medicine
Harvard Medical School
Boston, MA

Flavia V. Castelino, MD
Rheumatology Unit
Department of Medicine
Massachusetts General Hospital
Instructor in Medicine
Harvard Medical School
Boston, MA

Mariana C. Castells, MD, PhD
Rheumatology, Immunology, and Allergy Division
Department of Medicine
Brigham and Women's Hospital
Associate Professor of Medicine
Harvard Medical School
Boston, MA

Susan Cheng, MD
Cardiovascular Medicine Division
Department of Medicine
Brigham and Women's Hospital
Instructor in Medicine
Harvard Medical School

Murali Chiravuri, MD, PhD
Electrophysiologist/Cardiologist
Cardiac Specialists
Danbury, CT

Tracey A. Cho, MD
Department of Neurology
Massachusetts General Hospital
Assistant Professor of Neurology
Harvard Medical School
Boston, MA

Emily Choi, MD
Neurologist
Crozer-Chester Medical Center
Upland, PA

Sanjiv Chopra, MD
Gastroenterology Division
Department of Medicine
Beth Israel Deaconess Medical Center
Professor of Medicine
Harvard Medical School
Boston, MA

Jonathan S. Coblyn, MD
Rheumatology, Immunology, and Allergy Division
Department of Medicine
Brigham and Women's Hospital
Associate Professor of Medicine
Harvard Medical School
Boston, MA

Mark A. Creager, MD
Cardiovascular Medicine Division
Department of Medicine
Brigham and Women's Hospital
Professor of Medicine
Harvard Medical School
Boston, MA

Daniel J. DeAngelo, MD, PhD
Medical Oncologoist
Dana-Farber Cancer Institute
Department of Medicine
Brigham and Women's Hospital
Associate Professor of Medicine
Harvard Medical School
Boston, MA

Paul F. Dellaripa, MD
Rheumatology, Immunology, and Allergy Division
Department of Medicine
Brigham and Women's Hospital
Assistant Professor of Medicine
Harvard Medical School
Boston, MA

Bradley M. Denker, MD
Nephrology Division
Department of Medicine
Beth Israel Deaconess Medical Center
Associate Professor of Medicine
Harvard Medical School
Boston, MA

Robert G. Dluhy, MD
Endocrinology, Diabetes, and Hypertension Division
Department of Medicine
Brigham and Women's Hospital
Professor of Medicine
Harvard Medical School
Boston, MA

Benjamin L. Ebert, MD, PhD
Hematology Division
Department of Medicine
Brigham and Women's Hospital
Assistant Professor of Medicine
Harvard Medical School
Boston, MA

Aymen A. Elfiky, MD, MPH
Medical Oncologist
Dana-Farber Cancer Institute
Department of Medicine
Brigham and Women's Hospital
Instructor, Medicine
Harvard Medical School
Boston, MA

Joshua A. Englert, MD
Department of Medicine
Massachusetts General Hospital
Research Fellow in Medicine
Harvard Medical School
Boston, MA

Lawrence J. Epstein, MD
Sleep Medicine Division
Department of Medicine
Brigham and Women's Hospital
Clinical Instructor in Medicine
Harvard Medical School
Boston, MA

Kenneth R. Falchuk, MD
Gastroenterology Division
Department of Medicine
Beth Israel Deaconess Medical Center
Associate Clinical Professor of Medicine
Harvard Medical School
Boston, MA

Christopher H. Fanta, MD
Pulmonary and Critical Care Medicine Division
Department of Medicine
Brigham and Women's Hospital
Associate Professor of Medicine
Harvard Medical School
Boston, MA

Steven D. Freedman, MD, PhD
Division of Translational Research
Department of Medicine
Beth Israel Deaconess Medical Center
Professor of Medicine
Harvard Medical School
Boston, MA

Sonia Friedman, MD
Gastroenterology, Hepatology and Endoscopy Division
Department of Medicine
Brigham and Women's Hospital
Assistant Professor of Medicine
Harvard Medical School
Boston, MA

Rajesh K. Garg, MD
Endocrinology, Diabetes and Hypertension Division
Department of Medicine
Brigham and Women's Hospital
Assistant Professor of Medicine
Harvard Medical School
Boston, MA

Wolfram Goessling, MD, PhD
Divsion of Genetics
Department of Medicine
Brigham and Women's Hospital
Assistant Professor of Medicine
Harvard Medical School
Boston, MA

Samuel Z. Goldhaber, MD
Cardiovascular Medicine Division
Department of Medicine
Brigham and Women's Hospital
Professor of Medicine
Harvard Medical School,
Boston, MA

Norton J. Greenberger, MD
Gastroenterology, Hepatology and Endoscopy Division
Department of Medicine
Brigham and Women's Hospital
Clinical Professor of Medicine
Harvard Medical School
Boston, MA

Florencia Halperin, MD
Endocrinology, Diabetes, and Hypertension Division
Department of Medicine
Brigham and Women's Hospital
Instructor in Medicine
Harvard Medical School
Boston, MA

Robert I. Handin, MD
Hematology Division
Department of Medicine
Brigham and Women's Hospital
Professor of Medicine
Harvard Medical School
Boston, MA

Michael J. Hassett, MD, MPH
Medical Oncologist
Dana-Farber Cancer Institute
Department of Medicine
Brigham and Women's Hospital
Assistant Professor of Medicine
Harvard Medical School
Boston, MA

Simon M. Helfgott, MD
Rheumatology, Immunology, and Allergy Division
Department of Medicine
Brigham and Women's Hospital
Associate Professor of Medicine
Harvard Medical School
Boston, MA

Galen V. Henderson, MD
Department of Neurology
Brigham and Women's Hospital
Assistant Professor of Medicine
Harvard Medical School
Boston, MA

Li-Li Hsiao, MD, PhD
Renal Division
Department of Medicine
Brigham and Women's Hospital
Assistant Professor of Medicine
Harvard Medical School
Boston, MA

Brian Hyett, MD
Gastroenterology PA
Portsmouth, NH

Vicki A. Jackson, MD, MPH
Department of Medicine
Massachusetts General Hospital
Assistant Professor of Medicine
Harvard Medical School
Boston, MA

Jennifer A. Johnson, MD
Infectious Diseases Division
Department of Medicine
Brigham and Women's Hospital
Instructor in Medicine
Harvard Medical School
Boston, MA

Ursula B. Kaiser, MD
Endocrinology, Diabetes, and Hypertension Division
Department of Medicine
Brigham and Women's Hospital
Associate Professor of Medicine
Harvard Medical School
Boston, MA

Joel T. Katz, MD
Infectious Diseases Division
Department of Medicine
Brigham and Women's Hospital
Associate Professor of Medicine
Harvard Medical School
Boston, MA

Leah M. Katz
Lank Center for Genitourinary Oncology
Dana-Farber Cancer Institute
Boston, MA

Yuli Y. Kim, MD
Philadelphia Adult Congenital Heart Center
Assistant Professor of Medicine
Penn Medicine and the Children's
    Hospital of Philadelphia
Philadelphia, PA

Douglas B. Kirsch, MD
Sleep Medicine Division
Department of Medicine
Brigham and Women's Hospital
Clinical Instructor in Medicine
Harvard Medical School
Boston, MA

Michael Klompas, MD, MPH
Department of Population Medicine
Brigham and Women's Hospital
Assistant Professor of Population Medicine
Harvard Medical School
Boston, MA

Patricia A. Kritek, MD
Pulmonary and Critical Care Medicine Division
Associate Medical Director of Critical Care
University of Washington Medical Center
Seattle, WA

Ann S. LaCasce, MD
Hematologic Malignancies
Dana-Farber Cancer Institute Service
Department of Medicine
Brigham and Women's Hospital
Assistant Professor of Medicine
Harvard Medical School
Boston, MA

Michael J. Landzberg, MD
Cardiovascular Medicine Division
Children's Hospital Boston
Department of Medicine
Brigham and Women's Hospital
Assistant Professor of Medicine
Harvard Medical School
Boston, MA

Meryl S. LeBoff, MD
Endocrinology, Diabetes, and Hypertension Division
Department of Medicine
Brigham and Women's Hospital
Professor of Medicine
Harvard Medical School
Boston, MA

Alfred Ian Lee, MD, PhD
Assistant Professor of Medicine
Yale School of Medicine
New Haven, CT

I-Min Lee, MD, MPH, ScD
Division of Preventive Medicine
Department of Medicine
Brigham and Women's Hospital
Associate Professor of Medicine
Harvard Medical School
Boston, MA

Eldrin Foster Lewis, MD, MPH
Cardiovascular Medicine Division
Department of Medicine
Brigham and Women's Hospital
Assistant Professor of Medicine
Harvard Medical School
Boston, MA

Leonard S. Lilly, MD
Cardiovascular Medicine Division
Department of Medicine
Brigham and Women's Hospital
Professor of Medicine
Harvard Medical School
Boston, MA

Kenneth Lim, MB, ChB
Division of Renal Medicine
Department of Medicine
Brigham and Women's Hospital
Research Fellow in Medicine
Harvard Medical School
Boston, MA

Julie-Aurore Losman, MD
Medical Oncologist
Dana-Farber Cancer Institute
Department of Medicine
Brigham and Women's Hospital
Instructor in Medicine
Harvard Medical School
Boston, MA

Thomas J. Lynch, MD
Yale Comprehensive Cancer Center
Richard Sackler and Jonathan Sackler Professor of Medicine
Yale School of Medicine
Smilow Cancer Hospital at Yale-New Haven
New Haven, CT

James H. Maguire, MD, MPH
Infectious Diseases Division
Department of Medicine
Brigham and Women's Hospital
Professor of Medicine
Harvard Medical School
Boston, MA

Francisco M. Marty, MD
Infectious Diseases Division
Department of Medicine
Brigham and Women's Hospital
Assistant Professor of Medicine
Harvard Medical School
Boston, MA

Erica L. Mayer, MD, MPH
Medical Oncologist
Dana-Farber Cancer Institute
Department of Medicine
Brigham and Women's Hospital
Assistant Professor of Medicine
Harvard Medical School
Boston, MA

Robert J. Mayer, MD
Medical Oncologist
Dana-Farber Cancer Institute
Department of Medicine
Brigham and Women's Hospital
Stephen B. Kay Family Professor of Medicine
Harvard Medical School
Boston, MA

Sylvia C.W. McKean, MD
General Medicine Division
Department of Medicine
Brigham and Women's Hospital
Associate Professor of Medicine
Harvard Medical School
Boston, MA

Graham T. McMahon, MB, BCh
Endocrinology, Diabetes and Hypertension Division
Department of Medicine
Brigham and Women's Hospital
Associate Professor of Medicine
Harvard Medical School
Boston, MA

Jeffrey A. Meyerhardt, MD, MPH
Medical Oncologist
Dana-Farber Cancer Institute
Department of Medicine
Brigham and Women
Associate Professor of Medicine
Harvard Medical School
Boston, MA

Amy Leigh Miller, MD, PhD
Cardiovascular Medicine Division
Department of Medicine
Brigham and Women's Hospital
Instructor in Medicine
Harvard Medical School
Boston, MA

Constantine S. Mitsiades, MD
Medical Oncologist
Dana-Farber Cancer Institute
Department of Medicine
Brigham and Women's Hospital
Instructor in Medicine
Harvard Medical School
Boston, MA

Elinor A. Mody, MD
Rheumatology, Immunology, and Allergy Division
Department of Medicine
Brigham and Women's Hospital
Assistant Professor of Medicine
Harvard Medical School
Boston, MA

Charles A. Morris, MD, MPH
Department of Medicine
Brigham and Women's Hospital
Instructor in Medicine
Harvard Medical School
Boston, MA

David B. Mount, MD
Renal Division
Department of Medicine
Brigham and Women's Hospital
Assistant Professor of Medicine
Harvard Medical School
Boston, MA

Gilbert H. Mudge, Jr., MD
Cardiovascular Medicine Division
Department of Medicine
Brigham and Women's Hospital
Professor of Medicine
Harvard Medical School
Boston, MA

Stuart B. Mushlin, MD
Department of Medicine
Brigham and Women's Hospital
Assistant Professor of Medicine
Harvard Medical School
Boston, MA

Muthoka L. Mutinga, MD
Gastroenterology, Hepatology and Endoscopy Division
Department of Medicine
Brigham and Women's Hospital
Instructor in Medicine
Harvard Medical School
Boston, MA

David M. Nathan, MD
Department of Medicine
Massachusetts General Hospital
Professor of Medicine
Harvard Medical School
Boston, MA

Chiadi E. Ndumele, MD
Cardiology Division
Johns Hopkins Hospital
Baltimore, MD

Joel Neal, MD, PhD
Assistant Professor of Oncology
Stanford University School of Medicine
Stanford, CA

Anju Nohria, MD
Division of Cardiovascular Medicine
Department of Medicine
Brigham and Women's Hospital
Assistant Professor of Medicine
Harvard Medical School
Boston, MA

Patrick T. O'Gara, MD
Cardiovascular Medicine Division
Department of Medicine
Brigham and Women's Hospital
Professor of Medicine
Harvard Medical School
Boston, MA

William K. Oh, MD
Division of Hematology and Medical Oncology
Mount Sinai Medical Center
New York, NY

Maureen M. Okam, MD, MPH
Hematology Division
Department of Medicine
Brigham and Women's Hospital
Instructor in Medicine
Harvard Medical School
Boston, MA

Merri Pendergrass, MD, PhD
Medco Diabetes Therapeutic Resource Center
Medco Health Solutions, Inc.
Franklin Lakes, NJ

Molly L. Perencevich, MD
Department of Medicine
Brigham and Women's Hospital
Research Fellow in Medicine
Harvard Medical School
Boston, MA

Brijmohan K. Phull, MBBS
Assistant Professor of Psychiatry
Harvard University
University Heath Services
Cambridge, MA

Rattna K. Phull, MD
Department of Medicine
Brigham and Women's Hospital
Instructor in Medicine
Harvard Medical School
Boston, MA

Gregory Piazza, MD
Cardiovascular Medicine Division
Department of Medicine
Brigham and Women's Hospital
Clinical Fellow in Medicine
Harvard Medical School
Boston, MA

Mary L. Pisculli, MD, MPH
Infectious Diseases Division
Department of Medicine
Brigham and Women's Hospital
Instructor, Medicine
Harvard Medical School
Boston, MA

Rebeca M. Plank, MD
Infectious Diseases Division
Department of Medicine
Brigham and Women's Hospital
Instructor in Medicine
Harvard Medical School
Boston, MA

Jorge Plutzky, MD
Cardiovascular Medicine Division
Department of Medicine
Brigham and Women's Hospital
Associate Professor of Medicine
Harvard Medical School
Boston, MA

Mark M. Pomerantz, MD
Medical Oncologist
Dana-Farber Cancer Institute
Department of Medicine
Brigham and Women's Hospital
Assistant Professor of Medicine
Harvard Medical School
Boston, MA

Anthony M. Reginato, MD, PhD
Warren Alpert Medical School of Brown University
Providence, RI

John J. Reilly, MD
Department of Medicine
University of Pittsburgh
Pittsburgh, PA

Jeremy B. Richards, MD
Pulmonary, Critical Care and Sleep Medicine Division
Beth Israel Deaconess Medical Center
Instructor in Medicine
Harvard Medical School
Boston, MA

Paul G. Richardson, MD
Jerome Lipper Center for Multiple Myeloma
Dana-Farber Cancer Institute
Department of Medicine
Brigham and Women
Associate Professor of Medicine
Harvard Medical School
Boston, MA

David H. Roberts, MD
Pulmonary, Critical Care and Sleep Medicine Division
Department of Medicine
Beth Israel Deaconess Medical Center
Assistant Professor of Medicine
Harvard Medical School
Boston, MA

Christian T. Ruff, MD
Cardiovascular Medicine Division
Department of Medicine
Brigham and Women's Hospital
Instructor in Medicine
Harvard Medical School
Boston, MA

Marc S. Sabatine, MD, MPH
Cardiovascular Medicine Division
Department of Medicine
Brigham and Women's Hospital
Associate Professor of Medicine
Harvard Medical School
Boston, MA

Daniel C. Sacchetti, MA
Department of Psychology
Harvard University
Cambridge, MA

Suzanne E. Salamon, MD
Gerontology Division
Department of Medicine
Beth Israel Deaconess Medical Center
Instructor in Medicine
Harvard Medical School
Boston, MA

Fidencio Saldana, MD, MPH
Cardiovascular Medicine Division
Department of Medicine
Brigham and Women's Hospital
Instructor in Medicine
Harvard Medical School
Boston, MA

John R. Saltzman, MD
Gastroenterology, Hepatology and Endoscopy Division
Department of Medicine
Brigham and Women's Hospital
Associate Professor of Medicine
Harvard Medical School
Boston, MA

Paul E. Sax, MD
Infectious Diseases Division
Department of Medicine
Brigham and Women's Hospital
Associate Professor of Medicine
Harvard Medical School
Boston, MA

Adam C. Schaffer, MD
Department of Medicine
Brigham and Women's Hospital
Instructor in Medicine
Harvard Medical School
Boston, MA

Peter C. Schalock, MD
Rheumatology, Immunology, and Allergy Division
Department of Dermatology
Massachusetts General Hospital
Assistant Professor of Dermatology
Harvard Medical School
Boston, MA

Peter H. Schur, MD
Division of Rheumatology
Department of Medicine
Brigham and Women's Hospital
Professor of Medicine
Harvard Medical School
Boston, MA

Julian L. Seifter, MD
Renal Division
Department of Medicine
Brigham and Women's Hospital
Associate Professor of Medicine
Harvard Medical School
Boston, MA

Lawrence N. Shulman, MD
Medical Oncologist
Dana-Farber Cancer Institute
Department of Medicine
Brigham and Women's Hospital
Associate Professor of Medicine
Harvard Medical School
Boston, MA

Jane S. Sillman, MD
Division of General Medicine
Department of Medicine
Brigham and Women's Hospital
Assistant Professor of Medicine
Harvard Medical School
Boston, MA

Mark J. Simone-Skidmore, MD
Division of Aging
Department of Medicine
Brigham and Women's Hospital
Instructor in Medicine
Harvard Medical School
Boston, MA

Aneesh B. Singhal, MD, MBBS
Department of Neurology
Massachusetts General Hospital
Associate Professor of Neurology
Harvard Medical School
Boston, MA

Arthur J. Sober, MD
Department of Dermatology
Massachusetts General Hospital
Professor of Dermatology
Harvard Medical School
Boston, MA

Caren G. Solomon, MD
Department of Medicine
Brigham and Women's Hospital
Associate Professor of Medicine
Harvard Medical School
Boston, MA

Theodore I. Steinman, MD
Renal Division
Department of Medicine
Beth Israel Deaconess Medical Center
Clinical Professor of Medicine
Harvard Medical School
Boston, MA

Garrick C. Stewart, MD
Cardiovascular Medicine Division
Department of Medicine
Brigham and Women's Hospital
Instructor in Medicine
Harvard Medical School
Boston, MA

Kuyilan Karai Subramanian, MD
Research Fellow
Renal Division
Brigham and Women's Hospital
Boston, MA

Usha B. Tedrow, MD
Cardiovascular Medicine Division
Department of Medicine
Brigham and Women's Hospital
Assistant Professor of Medicine
Harvard Medical School
Boston, MA

Lori Wiviott Tishler, MD
Department of Medicine
Brigham and Women's Hospital
Assistant Professor of Medicine
Harvard Medical School
Boston, MA

Derrick J. Todd, MD, PhD
Division of Rheumatology
Department of Medicine
Brigham and Women's Hospital
Instructor in Medicine
Harvard Medical School
Boston, MA

Subbulaxmi Trikudanathan, MBBS
Endocrinology, Diabetes and Hypertension Division
Brigham and Women's Hospital
Research Fellow in Medicine
Harvard Medical School
Boston, MA

J. Kevin Tucker, MD
Renal Division
Department of Medicine
Brigham and Women's Hospital
Assistant Professor of Medicine
Harvard Medical School
Boston, MA

Alexander Turchin, MD, MS
Endocrinology, Diabetes and Hypertension Division
Department of Medicine
Brigham and Women's Hospital
Assistant Professor of Medicine
Harvard Medical School
Boston, MA

Chinweike Ukomadu, MD, PhD
Gastroenterology, Hepatology and Endoscopy Division
Department of Medicine
Brigham and Women's Hospital
Assistant Professor of Medicine
Harvard Medical School
Boston, MA

Anne Marie Valente, MD
Cardiovascular Medicine Division
Department of Pediatrics
Children's Hospital Boston
Assistant Professor of Medicine
Harvard Medical School
Boston, MA

Deborah J. Wexler, MD
Department of Medicine
Massachusetts General Hospital
Assistant Professor of Medicine
Harvard Medical School
Boston, MA

Mark E. Williams, MD
Renal Division
Department of Medicine
Beth Israel Deaconess Medical Center
Associate Professor of Medicine
Harvard Medical School
Boston, MA

Sigal Yawetz, MD
Infectious Diseases Division
Department of Medicne
Brigham and Women's Hospital
Assistant Professor of Medicine
Harvard Medical School
Boston, MA

Maria A. Yialamas, MD
Endocrinology, Diabetes and Hypertension Division
Department of Medicine
Brigham and Women's Hospital
Instructor, Medicine
Harvard Medical School
Boston, MA

SECTION 1

INFECTIOUS DISEASE

1.

PNEUMONIA AND RESPIRATORY INFECTIONS

Joel T. Katz

Respiratory symptoms are among the most frequent reasons for patients to seek medical attention. Seventy percent of patients presenting with a new cough will be diagnosed with acute bronchitis. Other common causes of a new cough include pneumonia, cough-variant asthma, congestive heart failure, rhinosinusitis, and aspiration of oral contents. Among patients presenting to their primary care provider with a cough, clinical predictors of the 10–15% who will have pneumonia are advanced patient age (OR 4.6), shortness of breath (2.4), fever (5.5), tachycardia (3.8), and localizing chest auscultation findings such as focal respiratory crackles (23.8) or rhonchi (14.6). The etiology, prognosis, and treatment of these major respiratory tract infections are vastly different and are reviewed in this chapter.

ACUTE BRONCHITIS

Acute bronchitis (AB) is a common seasonal (winter peak) infection of the upper respiratory tract that is generally viral in origin and does not require antibiotic therapy. The incidence of AB is 30–170 cases/100,000 per year. The most common causes are rhinoviruses, respiratory syncytial virus, influenza, parainfluenza, and adenovirus. These are highly contagious pathogens that spread rapidly through exposure to respiratory secretions or indirectly through shared environmental fomites. AB is generally a self-limited condition that lasts no more than 1–2 weeks. When symptoms last more than 2 weeks, one should consider "atypical" bacteria, such as *B. pertussis* or *M. pneumoniae* infections, or alternative diagnoses such as postnasal-drip syndrome from conditions of the nose and sinuses, asthma, gastroesophageal reflux disease, chronic bronchitis caused by cigarette smoking or other irritants, bronchiectasis, eosinophilic bronchitis, or the use of an angiotensin-converting–enzyme inhibitor. At least nine randomized trials and a number of subsequent meta-analyses have addressed the benefit of antibiotics in AB. There is modest or no benefit to prescribing antibiotics in AB, and this must be weighed against the significant cost and adverse consequences of these medications. Overtreatment of AB leads directly to increasing rates of antimicrobial resistance in the general population, and it is estimated to be responsible for spending in excess of $300 million on unnecessary antibiotics on a yearly basis.

A small subset of patients with AB merit treatment, including those with episodes that occur during documented *B. pertussis* outbreaks, chronic bronchitis (lasting more than 2 weeks), or individuals with underlying lung disease (chronic obstructive pulmonary disease, asthma, or heavy tobacco use). In such settings, a second-generation macrolide, such as clarithromycin or azithromycin, is the ideal agent.

COMMUNITY-ACQUIRED PNEUMONIA

Despite major advances in understanding its pathophysiology and management over the century since Sir William Osler declared it the "[c]aptain of the men of death," pneumonia remains the leading infectious cause of death in the United States and in the world. Three major incremental reductions in community-acquired pneumonia (CAP) mortality have resulted from the introduction of antipneumococcal serum therapy (discovered 1895, widely adopted by the 1920s), antibiotics (discovered 1928, widely adopted by the 1940s), and mechanical ventilation (discovered in 1952, widely adopted in the 1960s). Pneumococcal vaccination has added only marginal survival benefit compared to these other advances. Annually, about 4 million cases of CAP are reported in the United States, leading to 1 million hospitalizations and 45,000–50,000 deaths. Mortality in all hospitalized patients with CAP ranges from 2% to 30%, and those patients who are assigned to the intensive care unit for their initial care have a mortality as high as 40%. In contrast, mortality in outpatients ranges from <1% to 3%.

CAP is defined as an acute infection of the lung parenchyma accompanied by a new infiltrate on chest radiography or compatible auscultatory findings in a patient who is not hospitalized or living in a long-term facility for at least

3

Table 1.1 ETIOLOGY OF CAP (%), BY SITE OF INITIAL TRIAGE

	OUTPATIENT (N = 457)	INPATIENT (N = 6152)	INTENSIVE CARE (N = 1415)
Unknown	64.4	48.3	39.7
S. pneumoniae	4	20.3	22.5
H. influenzae	4	6	5.3
M. pneumoniae	15.3	3.9	1.9
C. pneumoniae	4.5		
Legionella spp.	0.9	3.4	5.9
S. aureus		1.8	2.5
GNR		3.2	10
P. jiroveci		1.3	1.6
Influenza	3.5	2.8	
Polymicrobial	1.5	8.6	5.4

2 weeks prior to the onset of symptoms. CAP symptoms usually include at least two of the following features: fever or hypothermia, sweats, rigors, pleurisy, and new cough with or without sputum production or change in color of respiratory secretions. The absence of mucoid sputum production is associated with "atypical" pathogens (*M. pneumoniae, C. pneumoniae, Legionella* species, *B. pertussis*).

As was the case in Osler's day, *Streptococcus pneumoniae* is the leading identifiable cause of CAP (table 1.1). "Atypical" pathogens are increasingly recognized as the cause of both outpatient and inpatient CAP, and these pathogens should be covered with empirical antibiotics in all cases. Despite thorough investigation, the etiological cause of CAP cannot be identified in half of all cases. The high rate of culture-negative CAP may be attributed to antibiotic pretreatment, inability to produce sputum for analysis, viral causes, or emerging pathogens that remain to be elucidated.

Table 1.2 MORTALITY AND ICU ADMISSION, BASED ON CURB-65 SCORE

POINTS	MORTALITY/ICU
0	0.7
1	3.2
2	13
3	17
4	41.5
5	57

Table 1.3 PNEUMONIA SEVERITY INDEX POINT ASSIGNMENTS

CHARACTERISTIC OR DEMOGRAPHIC FACTOR	POINTS ASSIGNED
Age	
Men	Age (yr)
Women	Age (yr) − 10
Nursing home resident	10
Coexisting illness	
Cancer	30
Liver disease	20
Congestive heart failure	10
Cerebrovascular disease	10
Renal disease	10
Physical examination findings	
Altered mental status	20
Respiratory rate >30	20
Systolic blood pressure <90 mm Hg	20
Temperature <35 or ≥40°C	15
Pulse >125	10
Laboratory and radiographic findings	
Arterial pH <7.35	30
BUN >30 mg/dL	20
Sodium <130 mmol/L	30
Glucose >250 mg/dL	10
Hemocrit <30%	10
Partial pressure of arterial oxygen < 60 mm Hg	10
Pleural effusion	10

In the appropriate clinical situation, the diagnosis of CAP is established by demonstration of focal pulmonary findings, either by lung auscultation or chest radiograph. Chest radiographs should be done in all patients with suspected CAP because this test is useful in excluding complications (e.g., pleural effusions), associated findings that may predict the pathogen (e.g., lymphadenopathy), or alternative diagnoses (e.g., lung mass, lung abscess). When examined in a blinded fashion, the radiographic pattern does not reliably differentiate specific pathogens. This is particularly true among the elderly and immunocompromised patients,

Table 1.4 PSI RISK CLASSIFICATION AND RECOMMENDATION

CLASS	POINTS	MORTALITY (%)	RECOMMENDATION*
I	**	0.1	Home antibiotics
II	<70	0.6	Home antibiotics
III	71–90	0.9	Consider short hospitalization
IV	91–130	9.3	Hospitalize
V	>130	27	Hospitalize

* If the patient can be cared for at home (social).
** Risk class I requires age < 50, lacking PSI comorbidities and abnormal vital signs (table 1.3).

who may have unusual or no infiltrate in the setting of CAP. Radiographic improvement lags behind clinical response, and routine serial chest radiographs are not recommended unless the patient is not improving; however, all tobacco smokers and patients over the age of 65 should have follow-up chest radiographs 3–6 months after an episode of pneumonia in order to exclude an occult lung nodule.

Various risk-stratification methods have been developed and validated to predict which patients are at sufficiently low mortality risk to justify home therapy, which costs 20-fold less than an inpatient stay. The easy-to-use CURB-65 risk score can be calculated on the basis of five simple features, including the presence of confusion (1 point), blood urea nitrogen > 30 mmol/dL (1 point), respiratory rate ≥ 30 (1 point), systolic blood pressure < 90 mm Hg or diastolic blood pressure < 60 mm Hg (1 point), and patient age 65 or older (1 point). The risk of death or ICU admission increases with increasing CURB-65 scores (table 1.2).

The Pneumonia Severity Index (PSI) is a validated risk stratification method that considers the risk contributions of patient demographic features (age having the greatest influence) and key physical examination and laboratory findings (table 1.3). Of note, other than a measurement of arterial oxygenation, all laboratory testing is left up to the discretion of the healthcare provider. Patients in risk class I or II can be safely cared for at home. Risk class III can generally be cared for at home, but an inpatient observation is reasonable. Patients in risk classes IV and V should be admitted to the hospital (table 1.4). All CAP patients with unexplained or a high degree of hypoxemia should be admitted to the hospital. Clinical judgment should supersede the recommendations of clinical prediction rules.

Key principles of pharmacotherapy for CAP include these: (1) once the diagnosis is established, delays in administering antibiotics are associated with increased mortality; (2) all patients with CAP should be covered for "atypical" pathogens; and (3) recent antibiotic exposure should be considered when choosing empirical antibiotics. Clinicians should seek specific environmental exposures that may suggest an unusual pathogen (table 1.5).

Table 1.5 EPIDEMIOLOGICAL CONDITIONS RELATED TO SPECIFIC PATHOGENS IN PATIENTS WITH SELECTED CAP

CONDITION	COMMONLY ENCOUNTERED PATHOGEN(S)
Alcoholism	*Streptococcus pneumoniae* and anaerobes
COPD and/or smoking	*S. pneumoniae, Haemophilus influenzae, Moraxella catarrhalis,* and *Legionella* species
Nursing home residency	*S. pneumoniae,* Gram-negative bacilli, *H. influenzae, Staphylococcus aureus,* anaerobes, and *Chlamydia pneumoniae*
Poor dental hygiene	Anaerobes
Epidemic Legionnaires' disease	*Legionella* species
Exposure to bats or soil enriched with bird droppings	*Histoplasma capsulatum*
Exposure to birds	*Chlamydia psittaci*
Exposure to rabbits	*Francisella tularensis*
HIV infection (early stage)	*S. pneumoniae, H. influenzae,* and *Mycobacterium tuberculosis*
HIV infection (late stage)	Above plus *P. carinii, Cryptococcus,* and *Histoplasma* species
Travel to southwestern United States	*Coccidioides* species
Exposure to farm animals or parturient cats	*Coxiella burnetii* (Q fever)
Influenza active in community	Influenza, *S. pneumoniae, S. aureus, Streptococcus pyogenes,* and *H. influenzae*
Suspected large-volume aspiration	Anaerobes (chemical pneumonitis, obstruction)
Structural disease of lung (bronchiectasis, cystic fibrosis, etc.)	*Pseudomonas aeruginosa, Burkholderia (Pseudomonas) cepacia,* and *S. aureus*
Injection drug use	*S. aureus,* anaerobes, *M. tuberculosis,* and *S. pneumoniae*
Airway obstruction	Anaerobes, *S. pneumoniae, H. influenzae,* and *S. aureus*

Table 1.6 IDSA/ATS TREATMENT GUIDELINES FOR CAP

INITIAL TRIAGE	TREATMENT
Outpatients	Macrolides or doxycycline Fluoroquinolones may be preferred for older patients or in individuals with underlying chronic illnesses (heart, liver, renal, diabetes, alcoholism, malignancy, immunosuppressive medications) Generally avoid antibiotic classes that have been administered in the past 3 months
Hospitalized (general medical ward)	Extended-spectrum cephalosporin or beta-lactam/beta-lactamase inhibitor plus a macrolide; or fluoroquinolone (alone)
Hospitalized (ICU)	Extended-spectrum cephalosporin or a beta-lactam/beta-lactamase inhibitor plus either a macrolide or fluoroquinolone
Special considerations	
Individuals with structural lung disease	Antipseudomonal agents (piperacillin, piperacillin-tazobactam, carbapenem, or cefepime) plus a fluoroquinolone
Beta-lactam allergy	Fluoroquinolone +/− clindamycin
Suspected ca-MRSA	Add vancomycin or linezolid
Suspected aspiration	Fluoroquinolone +/− clindamycin, metronidazole, or a beta-lactam/beta lactamase inhibitor

SOURCE: Mandell LA, Wunderink RG, Anzueto A, et al. Infectious Diseases Society of America/American Thoracic Society consensus guidelines on the management of community-acquired pneumonia in adults. *Clin Infect Dis.* 2007;44:S27–72.

A summary of the Infectious Diseases Society of America (IDSA) and American Thoracic Society (ATS) combined recommendations is given in table 1.6. Once a specific organism has been identified, antibiotics should be narrowed to cover this agent with the least overlap in spectrum and additional cost. Indications for transition to oral antibiotics and for hospital discharge are reviewed by File (2003).

Increasingly, healthcare providers and facilities are being graded publicly by their adherence to established quality measures. The current Agency for Healthcare Research and Quality CAP quality measures are:

1. Measurement of oxygen saturation on admission

2. Blood cultures before antibiotics

3. Appropriate antibiotics within 6 hours of presentation

4. Tobacco cessation counseling if appropriate

5. Documentation of pneumococcal vaccine before discharge

Finally, a number of vaccines are available for the prevention of *S. pneumoniae* and influenza virus infections. Hospitalization for other problems should not be overlooked as an opportunity to protect unvaccinated patients by administering these vaccines. Updated adult vaccine recommendations are available at http://www.cdc.gov/vaccines/recs/schedules/adult-schedule.htm.

ADDITIONAL READING

Carratalà J, Garcia-Vidal C. An update on *Legionella*. *Curr Opin Infect Dis.* 2010;23(2):152–7.

File TM. Community-acquired pneumonia. *Lancet.* 2003;362(9400): 1991–2001.

File TM Jr. Case studies of lower respiratory tract infections: Community-acquired pneumonia. *Am J Med.* 2010;123(4 Suppl):S4–15.

Fine MJ, Auble TE, Yealy DM, et al. A prediction rule to identify low-risk patients with community-acquired pneumonia. *N Engl J Med.* 1997;336(4):243–50.

Gharib AM, Stern EJ. Radiology of pneumonia. *Med Clin North Am.* 2001;85:146–92.

Gupta SK, Sarosi GA. The role of atypical pathogens in community-acquired pneumonia. *Med Clin North Am.* 2001;85:1349–65.

Hoare Z, Lim WS. Pneumonia: Update on diagnosis and management. *BMJ.* 2006;332:1077–9.

Irwin RS, Madison JM. The diagnosis and treatment of cough. *N Engl J Med.* 2000;343:1715–21.

Kabra SK, Lodha R, Pandey RM. Antibiotics for community-acquired pneumonia in children. *Cochrane Database Syst Rev.* 2010;3: CD004874.

Mandell LA, Wunderink RG, Anzueto A, et al. Infectious Diseases Society of America/American Thoracic Society consensus guidelines on the management of community-acquired pneumonia in adults. *Clin Infect Dis.* 2007;44:S27–72.

Neuhaus T, Ewig S. Defining severe community-acquired pneumonia. *Med Clin North Am.* 2001;85:1413–25.

Smith PR. What diagnostic tests are needed for community-acquired pneumonia? *Med Clin North Am.* 2001;85:1367–79.

Smucny J, Fahey T, Becker L, Glazier R. Antibiotics for acute bronchitis. *Cochrane Database Syst Rev.* 2004;4:CD000245.

Talwar A, Lee H, Fein A. Community-acquired pneumonia: What is relevant and what is not? *Curr Opin Pulm Med.* 2007;13(3):177–85.

Torres A, Rello J. Update in community-acquired and nosocomial pneumonia 2009. *Am J Respir Crit Care Med.* 2010;181(8):782–7.

QUESTIONS

QUESTION 1. A 77-year-old man with well-controlled diabetes mellitus and chronic renal failure (creatinine baseline 1.6) presents with 3 days of fevers, chills, and a cough productive of green sputum. Physical examination reveals temperature 102.9°F, respiratory rate 16, and focal crackles in the right lung base. Initial laboratory evaluation should include all of the following *except*:

A. Measurement of arterial oxygen saturation by pulse oximetry
B. Pneumococcal urinary antigen
C. Blood cultures
D. Serum electrolytes
E. Chest radiograph

QUESTION 2. Which of the following oral antibiotics should NOT be used as a single agent in the empirical coverage of outpatient community-acquired pneumonia?

A. Levofloxacin
B. Amoxicillin-clavulanic acid
C. Clarithromycin
D. Doxycycline
E. Azithromycin

QUESTION 3. A 32-year-old woman presents to the emergency department with fever, chills, progressive and a persistent dry cough. She tells you that she had been seen approximately 1 week earlier in an emergency room while on her vacation in Florida with fever, chills, and a dry cough. She says that she was told that the chest x-ray was normal. She was prescribed amoxicillin and was sent home. She has a past medical history of lupus nephritis and is being treated with mycophenolate mofetil (MMF) at a dose of 1 g twice daily for the past 2 years. On physical examination, she is in moderate distress with a respiratory rate of 34, using accessory muscles. Blood pressure is 142/74 mm Hg, heart rate 110 beats per minute. Lung examination reveals moist crackles at the right base. Arterial blood gases: pH 7.48, pCO_2 28 mm Hg, pO_2 62 mm Hg on 100% FIO_2 with a nonrebreather mask. Chest x-ray shows a lobar infiltrate at the right base. Blood and sputum cultures are sent.

Which of the following is the most appropriate initial management for this patient?

A. Switch antibiotic treatment to ceftriaxone
B. Switch antibiotic treatment to azithromycin and ceftriaxone
C. Withhold antibiotics pending sputum culture results
D. Switch antibiotic treatment to vancomycin, ciprofloxacin, and Zosyn (piperacillin and tazobactam injection)

ANSWERS

1. B
2. B
3. D

2.

HIV INFECTION AND AIDS

Rebeca M. Plank and Paul E. Sax

Internists often provide medical care both to patients with as yet undiagnosed human immunodeficiency virus (HIV) infection and to those with known infection. Through early diagnosis and management of patients with HIV infection, physicians can significantly impact both individual patient health and public health. Early diagnosis and appropriate management of patients with HIV are crucial for the health of the individual and for the public's health, as those with known HIV infection can take measures to avoid transmitting the virus to others.

According to CDC estimates at the end of 2006, approximately 1.1 million persons with HIV infection were estimated to be living in the United States. It is estimated that approximately 56,300 new infections occurred in the United States in 2006 and that almost 25% of people living with HIV infection in the United States are unaware of the diagnosis. Because those aware of their HIV infection may be less likely than those who do not know they are HIV-infected to engage in high-risk behavior, the need to identify undiagnosed individuals is critical. Additionally, patients with primary HIV are especially infectious due to high virus load in the blood (typically >100,000 to 1 million copies/mL), and identifying acute HIV infection allows for timely counseling regarding the reduction of risky behaviors. Furthermore, early diagnosis of HIV infection prior to the onset of opportunistic infections improves prognosis. Internists have a critical role in diagnosing new infection, preventing transmission, and providing appropriate care for HIV-infected patients in the internal medicine setting.

HISTORY AND EPIDEMIOLOGY

HIV and AIDS first entered public consciousness with the CDC's *Morbidity and Mortality Weekly Report* (MMWR) published on June 5, 1981, discussing five cases of *Pneumocystis carinii* (now known as *P. jirovecii*) pneumonia (PCP) among previously healthy gay men living in Los Angeles.

By the late 1980s it appeared that the initial education efforts and activism focusing on disease awareness among men who have sex with men (MSM) to curb the epidemic were having an appreciable impact on AIDS incidence within this high-risk group. By the end of the 1990s, however, the trend toward decreasing incidence among MSM had reversed and has since been steadily rising. Between 2001 and 2006 the highest HIV transmission rate in the United States was among MSM, and it was the only category for which numbers were increasing. Nonetheless several other groups are disproportionately infected: in 2007 the largest percentage of AIDS cases in men were among black/African-American men (40%), followed by white men (31%), and Hispanic/Latino men (21%), while of the new cases in women, 64% were among black/African-American women, 18% among Hispanic/Latino women, and 17% among white women.

SIGNS AND SYMPTOMS

The presenting signs and symptoms of primary HIV infection can be protean, resembling many other common infections: simply considering the diagnosis may be the key to recognizing new cases. Primary HIV infection typically presents as a mononucleosis-like syndrome and, in fact, is on the differential for EBV-negative mononucleosis. In one series approximately 75% of persons acutely infected with HIV experienced symptoms attributable to an acute retroviral syndrome. Symptoms can occur from a few days to 10 weeks after exposure. The severity of the illness can range from a mild flu-like illness that resolves promptly to a severe multisystem disease requiring hospitalization. The most common symptoms of acute HIV infection include fever, maculopapular rash (fig. 2.1), mucocutaneous ulcers, lymphadenopathy, arthralgias, pharyngitis, malaise, weight loss, aseptic meningitis, and myalgias (see table 2.1). The symptoms of fever and rash (especially in combination), followed by oral ulcers and pharyngitis, had the highest positive predictive value for diagnosis of acute HIV infection.

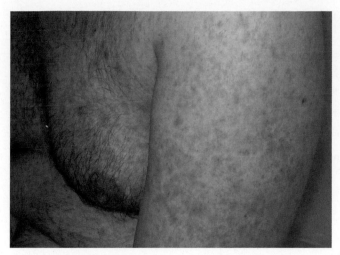

Figure 2.1. Rash in Acute HIV.

Because of a precipitous drop in CD4 lymphocytes that can be seen during acute HIV infection, some individuals can present during this phase with opportunistic infections, such as PCP or thrush.

Patients with chronic HIV infection may present with myriad symptoms depending on disease stage and degree of immunologic dysfunction. Conditions seen with significant immune suppression and that are clinically AIDS-defining include those that are shown in table 2.2.

Conditions commonly seen by internists in the outpatient setting that are not AIDS-defining conditions but

Table 2.1 SIGNS AND SYMPTOMS OF ACUTE HIV RETROVIRAL SYNDROME

SIGN/SYMPTOM	FREQUENCY (IN 209 CASES)
Fever	96%
Adenopathy	74%
Pharyngitis	70%
Rash	70%
Myalgia/Arthralgia	54%
Thrombocytopenia	45%
Leukopenia	38%
Diarrhea	32%
Headache	32%
Nausea/Vomiting	27%
Transaminitis	~20%
Thrush	12%
Neuropathy	6%
Encephalitis/meningitis	6%

should prompt consideration of HIV testing include *Herpes zoster*, seborrheic dermatitis, thrush, or recurrent vaginal candidiasis—all occur commonly in those without HIV infection, but the incidence and severity in patients with HIV tends to be greater. Furthermore, for those seeking care for a sexually transmitted infection, HIV testing should be offered during each visit for a new complaint because the mode of transmission is the same. Tuberculosis can present in HIV-infected individuals even with a relatively high CD4 count, and all persons initiating treatment for TB should be tested for HIV. Many HIV-infected persons will be asymptomatic, however, underscoring the need for routine screening.

ESTABLISHING THE DIAGNOSIS

The CDC guidelines for HIV testing published in the September 2006 MMWR recommend one-time routine opt-out testing for patients aged 13–64 years in all healthcare settings unless the patient declines and annual testing among those who engage in high-risk behavior. It is important to recognize that the notion of high-risk groups has been replaced by that of high-risk behavior and that many people who engage in high-risk behaviors do not disclose these. A recent study of MSM in New York City found that about 40% of those engaging in high-risk behaviors had not disclosed attraction to or having had sex with other men to their health care providers.

To diagnose established infection, HIV antibody testing should be performed. If the initial enzyme-linked immunosorbent assay (ELISA) is positive, a confirmatory Western blot assay is performed. A Western blot is interpreted as positive if at least two of three viral antigens (p24, gp41, gp120/160) are present and negative if no bands are present (fig. 2.2). An "indeterminate" result (any positive band or bands but not meeting criteria for positive) usually indicates either a false-positive ELISA (can be caused by pregnancy, autoimmune disease, lymphoma, and recent influenza vaccination, to name a few), or seroconversion in progress. In cases of seroconversion in progress, the follow-up Western blot will generally be fully positive within 1 month, and HIV RNA (viral load) will typically be detectable at very high levels (>100,000 copies/mL). Viral loads should not be sent as routine screening tests for established HIV infection since false positives at low levels (such as <1000 copies/mL) are not uncommon and can lead to unnecessary repeat testing and anxiety. In cases where acute HIV infection is suspected, however, a viral load should be performed because seroconversion may take several weeks (the "window period").

Rapid HIV testing is becoming increasingly utilized owing to its convenience, low cost, and accuracy. The rapid HIV test can be done on both blood specimens and oral secretions, and a negative test carries the same implications as a negative ELISA; a positive rapid test needs to be confirmed with standard ELISA/Western blot testing. Providers

Table 2.2 AIDS-DEFINING CONDITIONS IN HIV-INFECTED PERSONS

INFECTIOUS	ONCOLOGIC	OTHER
Candidiasis of bronchi, trachea, lungs, esophagus	Cervical cancer, invasive	Encephalopathy, HIV-related
Coccidioidomycosis, disseminated or extrapulmonary	Kaposi sarcoma	HIV-attributed wasting syndrome
Cryptococcosis, extrapulmonary	Lymphoma, Burkitt (or equivalent)	
Cryptosporidiosis, chronic intestinal (>1 month)	Lymphoma, immunoblastic (or equivalent)	
Cytomegalovirus other than liver, spleen, or nodes including retinitis	Lymphoma, primary, of brain	
Herpes: chronic ulcers (>1 month) or bronchitis, pneumonitis, esophagitis		
Histoplasmosis, disseminated or extrapulmonary		
Isosporiasis, chronic intestinal (>1 month)		
Mycobacterium spp. (*M. avium* complex or *M. kansasii,* *M. tuberculosis,* or other) disseminated or extrapulmonary		
Pneumocystis jirovecii pneumonia (PCP)		
Pneumonia, recurrent		
Progressive multifocal leukoencephalopathy		
Salmonella septicemia, recurrent		
Brain toxoplasmosis		

should note that rapid testing has been associated with a relatively high number of false-positive results when done in low-prevalence settings; hence, reactive results should be communicated as "preliminary" or "inconclusive," with need for confirmatory testing. This disadvantage notwithstanding, the CDC continues to recommend its use as this type of test increases the number of persons tested and the number of persons who actually receive their test results.

The CDC recommends that opt-out HIV screening (a special written consent should not be required) should be part of the routine panel of prenatal screening tests for all pregnant women. Repeat screening in the third trimester

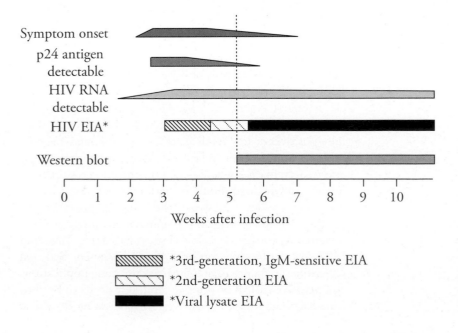

Figure 2.2. Time to HIV detection for various generations of diagnostic tests, relative to times of symptom onset and detection of p24 antigen and HIV RNA. Reprinted with permission from Branson BM. State of the art for diagnosis of HIV infection. *Clin Infect Dis.* 2007; 45(Suppl 4): S221–S225. Copyright 2007 by the Infectious Diseases Society of America. Data taken from Fiebig EW, Wright DJ, Rawal BD, et al. Dynamics of HIV viremia and antibody seroconversion in plasma donors: implications for diagnosis and staging of primary HIV infection. *AIDS.* 2003;17:1871–9.

should be performed in states with elevated HIV incidence rates (≥17 per 100,000 person years in women aged 15–45, in 2004: the states of Alabama, Connecticut, Delaware, the District of Columbia, Florida, Georgia, Illinois, Louisiana, Maryland, Massachusetts, Mississippi, Nevada, New Jersey, New York, North Carolina, Pennsylvania, Puerto Rico, Rhode Island, South Carolina, Tennessee, Texas, and Virginia).

INITIAL EVALUATION

The initial evaluation of an individual with HIV infection should include a complete medical and social history, physical examination, and laboratory evaluation. Of particular importance, the stage of HIV illness should be determined, and the presence of other possible concurrent infections should be evaluated.

Initial laboratory evaluation should include confirmation of the HIV antibody (if the original laboratory test is not available for review), CD4 count, and HIV RNA (viral load). To evaluate for bone marrow suppression as well as underlying liver or kidney disease, complete blood counts, chemistry, and liver function tests should be obtained. A urinalysis should be obtained to evaluate for HIV-associated nephropathy, which would be an indication for early initiation of therapy. In addition, a fasting lipid panel and glucose measurement are included in the initial evaluation. Laboratory findings, such as hyperlipidemia, renal or liver dysfunction, or presence of anemia or thrombocytopenia, could potentially alter the selection of an antiretroviral regimen.

Initial evaluation should also include a screening test for syphilis, (rapid plasma reagin [RPR] or treponemal IgG), toxoplasmosis IgG, cytomegalovirus (CMV) IgG, and hepatitis serologies (including hepatitis A antibody, hepatitis B surface antigen and antibody, hepatitis B core antibody, and hepatitis C antibody). In addition, a tuberculin skin test (TST) or interferon-γ release assay (IGRA) (unless there is a history of prior tuberculosis or positive TST or IGRA) should be obtained. If a TST is performed and the patient's CD4 is <200 cells/mm³ at the time, it should be repeated when the CD4 rises to >200 cells/mm³ on treatment. If the TST or IGRA is positive or there are pulmonary symptoms, a chest x-ray should be obtained. Women should undergo a Papanicolaou (Pap) smear, and one should consider baseline testing for gonorrhea and chlamydia. Although there are no formal recommendations for performing annual anal Pap smears for MSM, many experts in the field support this practice. Finally, recommendations from the DHHS suggest obtaining baseline genotypic resistance testing (a test that requires an HIV RNA >1000 copies/mL to be run). Laboratory tests recommended for initial assessment and for ongoing care of HIV-infected patients are found in table 2.3.

Social issues can powerfully affect the outcome of treatment by influencing adherence and access to care: substance use, mental illness, social support, economic stressors, ongoing high-risk behaviors, and family-planning issues should all be assessed. Given the stigma that still surrounds the diagnosis of HIV, it is worth exploring with patients whether they have disclosed the diagnosis to anyone else and, if so, to whom. Education about HIV risk behaviors and prevention of HIV transmission to others should be provided at each patient visit.

INITIATION OF THERAPY

The optimal time to start antiretrovirals (ARVs), the medications directly targeting the replication of HIV, remains uncertain. Although potent and well-tolerated medications are available, concerns remain about long-term side effects, selection of drug-resistant virus, and costs. For many years the guidelines suggested starting therapy for all those with symptomatic HIV disease or a CD4 count <200 cells/mm³ and considering therapy for those with a CD4 count <350 cells/mm³ or viral load >100,000 copies/mL. Now the guidelines are to start therapy for:

- Those with CD4 <500 cells/mm³
  - Therapy could be considered for those with CD4 >500 cells/mm³ (which reduces the rate of sexual transmission of HIV)

- Those with a history of AIDS-defining condition (see table 2.2)

- Pregnant women (regardless of CD4 count, with the goal of preventing perinatal transmission)

- Those with HIV-associated nephropathy

- Those with hepatitis B virus (HBV) and HIV co-infection requiring treatment for HBV (see co-infections below)

The risks and benefits of starting ARVs for those with CD4 ≥ 500 cells/mm³ are listed in table 2.4. The need for long-term adherence and identifying and addressing barriers to adherence should be emphasized at each visit, as poor adherence is associated with the development of ARV-resistant virus.

CO-INFECTIONS

Those at risk for HIV infection are also at risk for other chronic infections with similar modes of transmission. Co-infections of particular clinical interest in the HIV-infected person include HBV, hepatitis C (HCV), and syphilis.

Chronic HBV infection develops more frequently in HIV co-infected patients than in those with HBV alone. Although HIV infection affects the natural course of HBV infection, HBV co-infection does not appear to have an effect on CD4 depletion or progression to AIDS. Many agents used to treat HBV are also active against HIV. Treating only HBV may lead to drug-resistant HIV. For

Table 2.3 LABORATORY MONITORING FOR PATIENTS PRIOR TO AND AFTER INITIATION OF ANTIRETROVIRALS

	ENTRY INTO CARE	FOLLOW-UP BEFORE ARVS	ARV INITIATION OR SWITCH	2-8 WEEKS AFTER ARV INITIATION	EVERY 3-6 MONTHS	EVERY 6 MONTHS	YEARLY	TREATMENT FAILURE	CLINICAL INDICATION
CD4	X	Every 3–6 months	X		X	In clinically stable patients with suppressed viral load, CD4 count can be monitored every 6–12 months		X	
HIV RNA (viral load)*	X	Every 3–6 months	X	X	X			X	X
Drug-resistance testing	X							X	X
HLA-B*5701			If considering abacavir						
CCR5 tropism testing			If considering a CCR5 antagonist					If considering a CCR5 antagonist or for failure of CCR5 antagonist-based regimen	
Chemistries and liver enzymes	X	Every 6–12 months	X	X	X				X
CBC	X	Every 3–6 months	X	X	X				X
Fasting lipids	X	If normal: annually	X	Consider 4–8 weeks after starting new ART		Borderline or abnormal at last measurement	If normal at last measurement		X
Fasting glucose	X	If normal: annually	X		Borderline or abnormal at last measurement	If normal at last measurement			X
Urinalysis	X		X			If on tenofovir			X
Pregnancy test	X		If considering efavirenz						X

* If HIV RNA is detectable at 2–8 weeks, repeat every 4–8 weeks until suppression to <200 copies/mL, then every 3–6 months. For adherent patients with suppressed viral load and stable clinical and immunologic status for >2–3 years, some experts may extend the interval for HIV RNA monitoring to every 6 months.

this reason, those requiring treatment for HBV should be started on a standard HIV ARV regimen with two agents active against both HIV and HBV (such as tenofovir and emtricitabine).

HIV and HCV co-infection can accelerate the clinical course of both infections. Although immunologic decline from HIV disease may be more rapid and CD4 responses blunted, HCV RNA levels are increased in these patients, and they are more likely to develop cirrhosis or decompensated liver disease. Patients co-infected with HIV and HBV/HCV would benefit from expert consultation from providers experienced in assessment and management of both these infections.

Although the rate of syphilis was at an all-time low in 2000, cases in the United States have been increasing in number since then, particularly among MSM. Those with HIV

Table 2.4 POTENTIAL RISKS AND BENEFITS OF INITIATING ANTIRETROVIRALS IN ASYMPTOMATIC
HIV-INFECTED PERSONS WITH CD4 COUNT ≥350 CELLS/MM³

POTENTIAL BENEFITS	POTENTIAL RISKS
Maintenance of a higher CD4 count and prevention of potentially irreversible damage to the immune system	Development of treatment-related side effects and toxicities
Decreased risk for HIV-associated complications that can sometimes occur at CD4 counts >350 cells/mm³, including tuberculosis, non-Hodgkin lymphoma, Kaposi sarcoma, peripheral neuropathy, HPV-associated malignancies, and HIV-associated cognitive impairment	Development of drug resistance because of incomplete viral suppression, resulting in loss of future treatment options and possible subsequent transmission of drug-resistant virus in patients who do not maintain full virologic suppression
Decreased risk of nonopportunistic conditions, including cardiovascular disease, renal disease, liver disease, and non-AIDS–associated malignancies and infections	Less time for the patient to learn about HIV and its treatment and less time to prepare for the need for adherence to therapy
Decreased risk of HIV transmission to others, which will have positive public health implications	Increased total time on medication, with greater chance of treatment fatigue
	Premature use of therapy before the development of more effective, less toxic, and/or better-studied combinations of antiretroviral drugs

are especially susceptible to neurosyphilis if the CD4 count is <350 cells/mm³ and the RPR titer is ≥1:128. Cerebral spinal fluid (CSF) abnormalities may be common in patients with early syphilis and in persons with HIV infection. Because of this, some specialists recommend CSF examination before treatment of HIV-infected persons with early syphilis, with follow-up CSF examination conducted after treatment. Serologic follow-up should be done at 6, 12, 18, and 24 months to ensure a decline in the RPR titers. Furthermore, syphilitic ulcers can facilitate transmission or acquisition of HIV, and all those who engage in high-risk behaviors should be counseled in avoiding or promptly treating infection.

ANTIRETROVIRAL REGIMENS

ARVs are now available that target multiple stages of the HIV life cycle: (1) viral entry (cell fusion inhibitors and co-receptor antagonists), (2) transcription of viral RNA to DNA (nucleoside/nucleotide reverse transcriptase inhibitors and non-nucleoside reverse transcriptase inhibitors), (3) integration into host DNA (integrase strand transfer inhibitors), and, (4) viral protein assembly (protease inhibitors). At least three active agents should be administered. Standard regimens for initial therapy include two nucleoside/nucleotide reverse transcriptase inhibitors (NRTIs) plus one of the following: a non-nucleoside reverse transcriptase inhibitor (NNRTI), a protease inhibitor (PI) that is frequently a "boosted PI," or an integrase strand transfer inhibitor (INSTI) Cell fusion inhibitors and co-receptor antagonists are generally reserved for those with multidrug-resistant virus or have limited options for treatment for other reasons. Recommended combinations are found in table 2.5.

There are seven NRTIs available for use in the United States: zidovudine (AZT), lamivudine (3TC),

emtricitabine (FTC), stavudine (d4T), didanosine (ddI), abacavir (ABC), and tenofovir (TDF). The choice of which to use may depend on pre-existing conditions (such as renal dysfunction or anemia) and ease of use (such as once-daily dosing and co-formulation). In general, the preferred NRTI combination is tenofovir co-formulated with emtricitabine, available in a one-pill daily tablet.

- Zidovudine is associated with macrocytic anemia and gastrointestinal side effects.

- All NRTIs, but in particular stavudine, zidovudine, and didanosine, may cause lactic acidosis through inhibition of mitochondrial DNA; as such, these agents are rarely used as first-line treatments in the United States, although zidovudine is still used for pregnant women (along with other antiretroviral agents) for its established efficacy in preventing mother-to-child transmission.

- Abacavir may cause life-threatening hypersensitivity, an adverse reaction strongly associated with the presence of the HLA-B*5701 allele; as such, all patients should be tested for HLA-B*5701 prior to receiving this medication, and abacavir allergy should be listed in a patient's medical record if he or she tests positive.

- Tenofovir can cause renal dysfunction and should be avoided if possible in patients with renal dysfunction.

The most commonly used NNRTI in the United States is efavirenz. Some potential side effects include rash and central nervous system symptoms such as dizziness, somnolence, and vivid dreams. Efavirenz is a teratogen and should not be given to women who are pregnant or who are planning on becoming pregnant. Efavirenz is

Table 2.5 RECOMMENDED ANTIRETROVIRAL COMBINATION THERAPY FOR TREATMENT-NAIVE PATIENTS

RECOMMENDATION	AGENT	POPULATION IN WHICH TO AVOID OR USE WITH CAUTION
Dual NRTI "backbone" combination		
Preferred NRTI combination	Tenofovir + emtricitabine	*Do not use* in combination with unboosted atazanavir *Use with caution* in patients with underlying renal insufficiency or in those initiating nevirapine due to reports of early virologic failure
Alternative NRTI combination	Abacavir + lamivudine	*Do not use* in patients who test positive for HLA-B*5701 *Use with caution if:* HIV RNA >100,000 copies/mL (high rate of virologic failure) or high risk for cardiovascular disease
	Zidovudine + lamivudine	*Use with caution* in the presence of pretreatment anemia and/or neutropenia (may improve or worsen with zidovudine). Generally reserved for use in pregnancy.
NNRTI-based regimen		
Preferred NNRTI	Efavirenz	*Do not use* during first trimester of pregnancy or in those with high pregnancy potential *Use with caution* if unstable psychiatric disease
Alternative NNRTI	Nevirapine	*Do not use* in patients with moderate to severe hepatic impairment (Child-Pugh score B or C) *Do not use* in women with pre-ARV CD4 >250 cells/mm^3 or in men with pre-ARV CD4 >400 cells/mm^3 *Use with caution in* patients on tenofovir/emtricitabine (or lamivudine)—early virologic failure reported
	Rilpivirine	*Use with caution* in patients with pretreatment HIV RNA >100,000 copies/mL *Use of proton* pump inhibitors is contraindicated with rilpivirine
Integrase inhibitor-based regimen	Raltegravir twice daily	Raltegravir with tenofovir + emtricitabine is one of the preferred first line regimens for therapy naive patients
PI-based regimen		
Preferred PIs	Atazanavir + ritonavir once daily	*Do not use* in those who require >20 mg omeprazole equivalent/day proton pump inhibitors (PPI) *Use with caution* in patients on PPIs (any dose), H$_2$ blockers, or antacids
	Darunavir + ritonavir once daily	
Alternative PIs	Fosamprenavir + ritonavir twice daily	
	Lopinavir/ritonavir once or twice daily	*Do not use* once-daily dosing in pregnant women
Preferred regimen for pregnant women	Zidovudine + lamivudine + lopinavir/ritonavir twice daily	

co-formulated with the NRTIs tenofovir and emtricitabine, providing a fully active combination regimen as a single once-daily pill. Nevirapine is an alternative NNRTI that may cause liver and skin hypersensitivity, including Stevens-Johnson syndrome and fulminant hepatitis; because the risk of these severe side effects is greater for men with CD4 cell counts >250 and women >400, it should be avoided in these populations. Rilpivirine is another alternative NNRTI that also comes co-formulated with the NRTIs tenofovir and emtricitabine in a once-daily pill. It should not be used in those with a baseline viral load >100,000 copies/mL due to higher rates of virologic failure compared with efavirenz. There are numerous PIs available. Guidelines list atazanavir and darunavir (both boosted with ritonavir) as preferred PIs for first-line regimens. Although ritonavir is also a PI, its side effects are dose-limiting, and it is now used exclusively as a "booster" for other PIs. The boosting effect comes from ritonavir's inhibitory effect on the P450 system—advantageous for increasing the levels of other PIs but a potential problem for the dosing of other, some very common, medications. For this reason, providers must be very careful about drug–drug interactions with ritonavir, including seemingly benign agents such as inhaled corticosteroids, which have caused hypercortisolism (see table 2.6). Besides drug–drug interactions, the main side effects of the PIs include dyslipidemia and gastrointestinal side effects. Currently there is one only

Table 2.6 IMPORTANT RITONAVIR DRUG–DRUG INTERACTIONS (NOT EXHAUSTIVE: PLEASE CHECK DRUG–DRUG INTERACTIONS FOR ALL MEDICATIONS ON PATIENT-TO-PATIENT BASIS)

Antimicrobials

  Antifungal agents
  Atovaquone
  Clarithromycin
  Fusidic acid
  Halofantrine
  Peginterferon Alfa-2b
  Rifamycin derivatives (rifabutin, rifampin)

Antineoplastics

  Everolimus
  Ixabepilone
  Sorafenib
  Nilotinib
  Tamoxifen
  Topotecan

Cardiac agents

  Alpha$_1$ blockers (alfuzosin, silodosin)
  Amiodarone
  Calcium channel blockers (dihydropyridine and nondihydropyridine)
  Digoxin
  Flecainide
  Lipid-lowering agents (HMG-CoA reductase inhibitors)
  Nebivolol
  Propafenone
  Quinidine
  Ranolazine
  Warfarin

Antihistamine

  Astemizole
  Terfenadine

Gastrointestinal

  Alosetron (selective 5-HT$_3$ receptor antagonist)
  Cisapride

Immunosuppressants

  Cyclosporine
  Pimecrolimus

Neuroleptics

  Carbamazepine
  Lamotrigine
  Pimozide
  Phenytoin
  Valproic acid

Psychotropics

  Atomoxetine (norepinephrine reuptake inhibitor)
  Benzodiazepines
  Bupropion
  Codeine
  Disulfiram
  Fentanyl
  Meperidine
  Methadone
  Nefazodone
  Tetrabenazine
  Thioridazine
  Tramadol
  Trazodone
  Tricyclic antidepressants

Pulmonary

  Bosentan
  Salmeterol
  Theophylline derivatives

Ergot-alkaloids

  Dihydroergotamine (DHE 45)
  Ergotamine (various forms)
  Ergonovine methylergonovine

Corticosteroids

  Ciclesonide
  Fluticasone

Others

  Dabigatran etexilate (thrombin inhibitor)
  Deferasirox (chelating agent)
  Dronabinol (antiemetic/appetite stimulant)
  Eplerenone (aldosterone blocker)
  Fesoterodine (anticholinergic)
  Oral contraceptive (estrogens)
  P-Glycoprotein inducers/inhibitors/substrates
  Phosphodiesterase 5 inhibitors (tadalafil, sildenafil, vardenafil)
  Rivaroxaban (factor Xa inhibitor)

Herbs

  St. John's wort
  Garlic

integrase inhibitor available: raltegravir. It is well tolerated and has few drug-grug interactions but must be administered twice daily.

GOALS OF THERAPY

The goal of HIV therapy should be to suppress the replication of HIV as demonstrated by an undetectable viral load from serum. CD4 cell count recovery will be variable and dependent on many factors. Once begun, treatment should not be interrupted without a compelling reason because those on intermittent therapy have been shown to have a poorer prognosis. Frequency of monitoring (CD4 and HIV viral load) depends in part on the clinical course, but generally it is performed every 3–4 months, and every 6 months in stable patients with long term virologic suppression. Patients reporting therapy adherence with a detectable viral load should have testing for drug-resistant virus (see table 2.3).

ADDITIONAL READING

Aberg JA, Kaplan JE, Libman H, et al. Primary care guidelines for the management of persons infected with human immunodeficiency virus: 2009 update by the HIV Medicine Association of the Infectious Diseases Society of America. *Clin Infect Dis.* 2009;49(5):651–81.

Bucher HC, Wolbers M, Porter K. 2010 guidelines for antiretroviral treatment of HIV from the International AIDS Society–USA Panel. *JAMA*. 2010;304(17):1897.

CDC: Division of HIV/AIDS Prevention NCfHA, Viral Hepatitis, STD, and TB Prevention. *HIV Prevalence Estimates—United States, 2006*. Atlanta, GA: CDC; 2006:1073–6.

CDC: National Center for HIV/AIDS VH, STD, and TB Prevention. *Revised Recommendations for HIV Testing of Adults, Adolescents, and Pregnant Women in Health-Care Settings*. Atlanta, GA: CDC; 2006:1–17.

CDC. *AIDS-Defining Conditions*. Atlanta, GA: CDC; 2008.

Cohen MS, Chen YQ, McCauley M, et al. Prevention of HIV-1 infection with early antiretroviral therapy. *N Engl J Med*. 2011;365:493–505.

El-Sadr WM, Lundgren JD, Neaton JD, et al. CD4+ count-guided interruption of antiretroviral treatment. *N Engl J Med*. 2006 Nov 30;355(22):2283–96.

Hecht FM, Busch MP, Rawal B, et al. Use of laboratory tests and clinical symptoms for identification of primary HIV infection. *AIDS*. 2002;16(8):1119–29.

Kahn JO, Walker BD. Acute human immunodeficiency virus type 1 infection. *N Engl J Med*. 1998;339(1):33–9.

Niu MT, Stein DS, Schnittman SM. Primary human immunodeficiency virus type 1 infection: Review of pathogenesis and early treatment intervention in humans and animal retrovirus infections. *J Infect Dis*. 1993;168(6):1490–1501.

Panel on Antiretroviral Guidelines for Adults and Adolescents. *Guidelines for the Use of Antiretroviral Agents in HIV-1-Infected Adults and Adolescents*. Washington, DC: Department of Health and Human Services; 2011:1–166.

QUESTIONS

QUESTION 1. A 61-year-old man complains of headache, fever, and diarrhea for approximately 3 days. His past medical history includes hyperlipidemia (LDL 205 mg/dL, HDL 30 mg/dL) and hypertension. His current medications include hydrochlorothiazide and atorvastatin 10 mg PO daily. He has no recent travel and no animal exposure. He reports inconsistent condom use with his male partner. On exam a maculopapular rash is seen over the torso, and diffuse lymphadenopathy is detected. Leukocyte count is 3.8, hematocrit is 36%, and platelet count is 88,000. Test for HIV antibodies is negative. The diagnostic test of choice for acute HIV infection would be:

A. CD4 cell count
B. HIV RNA (viral load)
C. HIV drug resistance test

QUESTION 2. The HIV viral load in the patient is >500,000 copies/mL, and the diagnosis of acute HIV retroviral syndrome is made. A CD4 count is 520 cells/mm³. The patient is very anxious to begin treatment right away. All of the following are benefits of early initiation of ARVs EXCEPT:

A. Maintenance of a higher CD4 count and prevention of potentially irreversible damage to the immune system
B. Decreased risk for HIV-associated complications that can sometimes occur at CD4 counts >350

cells/mm³, including tuberculosis, non-Hodgkin lymphoma, Kaposi sarcoma, peripheral neuropathy, HPV-associated malignancies, and HIV-associated cognitive impairment
C. Decreased risk of nonopportunistic conditions, including cardiovascular disease, renal disease, liver disease, and non-AIDS–associated malignancies and infections
D. Increased risk of HIV transmission to others

QUESTION 3. Before beginning therapy, a test for HLA-B*5701 is sent and is positive. This means that the patient is NOT a candidate for which antiretroviral because of high risk of hypersensitivity reaction?

A. Abacavir
B. Efavirenz
C. Nevirapine
D. Ritonavir
E. Tenofovir

QUESTION 4. Which initial ARV combination would be indicated in this patient?

A. Tenofovir + emtricitabine + nevirapine
B. Tenofovir + emtricitabine + zidovudine
C. Tenofovir + emtricitabine + atazanavir
D. Tenofovir + emtricitabine + atazanavir + ritonavir

QUESTION 5. Because this patient will be taking ritonavir and you are concerned about drug–drug interactions, what should be done about his hyperlipidemia?

A. Start simvastatin at highest possible dose
B. Continue atorvastatin at lowest possible dose and monitor lipid profile, increasing dose slowly if needed
C. Increase atorvastatin to highest possible dose
D. Start gemfibrozil

ANSWERS

1. B
2. D
3. A
4. D
5. B

Note: The statins are the only class of lipid-lowering drugs to demonstrate clear improvements in overall mortality. Fibrates such as gemfibrozil have a major role in treatment of hypertriglyceridemia, which this patient does not have. Serum concentrations of statins may be increased by ritonavir, increasing the risk of myopathy/rhabdomyolysis. Lovastatin or simvastatin should never be used with ritonavir (30-fold increase in plasma simvastatin). Use pravastatin or lowest possible dose of atorvastatin (74% increase in total active atorvastatin exposure).

3.

INFECTIVE ENDOCARDITIS

Ajay K. Singh and Anju Nohria

OVERVIEW

Infective endocarditis (IE) is an infection of the endocardial surface of the heart. It is characterized by one or more vegetations, which comprise a mass of platelets, fibrin, microorganisms, and inflammatory cells. IE primarily involves the heart valves (native or prosthetic). Other structures may also be involved, including the interventricular septum, the chordae tendineae, the mural endocardium, or intracardiac devices such as a pacemaker. The most common infective causes are bacterial; however, fungal endocarditis can be seen in patients who are immunocompromised. There is controversy about the existence of viral endocarditis. Valvular involvement in IE may lead to congestive heart failure, conduction abnormalities, and myocardial abscesses. Systemic complications in IE include embolization of both sterile and infected emboli, abscess formation, and mycotic aneurysms.

IE should be distinguished from nonbacterial endocarditis or marantic endocarditis. The latter is most commonly found on previously undamaged valves, and, unlike IE, the vegetations are usually small and sterile. Nonbacterial endocarditis does not cause a systemic illness, but systemic embolization may occur. Causes of nonbacterial endocarditis include a hypercoagulable state, cancer (usually mucinous adenocarcinoma), Libman-Sacks endocarditis, or pregnancy.

The incidence of IE in the United States is approximately 2–4 cases per 100,000 persons per year, and this is similar in other countries around the world. This rate has not changed in the past 50 years. IE is three times more common in males than in females. There is no racial predilection. IE may occur at any age but is more frequent in the elderly. Untreated, IE has a very high morbidity and mortality. Antibiotic therapy is the mainstay of treatment. Surgery may be required under certain circumstances.

PATHOPHYSIOLOGY

IE develops as a result of local adherence and invasion of bacteria onto the valvular leaflet. Various procedures are associated with bacteremia (table 3.1); however, there are other potential causes for bacteremia, including the presence of colon cancer, urinary tract infections, and intravenous drug abuse (IVDA).

Invasion results in the formation of a sterile fibrin-platelet vegetation. In acute IE the thrombus may be produced by the invading organism (i.e., *Staph. aureus*) or by valvular trauma from intravenous catheters or pacing wires. *S. aureus* can invade the endothelial cells (endotheliosis) and increase the expression of adhesion molecules and of procoagulant activity on the cellular surface. The pathogenesis of pacemaker IE is similar: shortly after implantation, the development of a fibrin-platelet thrombus involves the generator box and conducting leads. After approximately 1 week, the connective tissue proliferates, partially embedding the leads in the wall of the vein and endocardium.

IE develops most commonly on the mitral valve, closely followed in descending order of frequency by the aortic valve, the combined mitral and aortic valve, the tricuspid valve, and, rarely, the pulmonic valve. Mechanical prosthetic and bioprosthetic valves exhibit equal rates of infection.

CAUSES OF INFECTIVE ENDOCARDITIS

The causes of IE are shown in table 3.2. Whereas in the past rheumatic fever was the most common underlying valvular abnormality predisposing to infective endocarditis, mitral valve prolapse (MVP) currently represents the most common underlying cardiac abnormality in IE and is the predisposing condition in 30% of cases of native valve endocarditis (NVE) in young adults. Among adults age <20 years with MVP, there is a female predilection; however, among adults with MVP age >20 males have a greater risk for developing IE. Rheumatic heart disease currently accounts for fewer than 20% of cases, and 6% of patients with rheumatic heart disease eventually develop IE. Approximately 50% of elderly patients have calcific aortic stenosis as the underlying pathology. Other contributing congenital abnormalities

Table 3.1 LIKELIHOOD OF BACTEREMIA WITH VARIOUS PROCEDURES AND ORGANISMS INVOLVED

PROCEDURE	BACTEREMIA RATE (%)	PREDOMINANT ORGANISMS
Endoscopy	0–20	CoNS, streptococci, diphtheroids
Colonoscopy	0–20	*Escherichia coli*, *Bacteroides* species
Barium enema	0–20	Enterococci, aerobic and anaerobic *GNR*
Dental extractions	40–100	*S. viridans*
Transurethral resection of the prostate	20–40	Coliforms, enterococci, *S. aureus*
Transesophageal echocardiography	0–20	*S. viridans*, anaerobic organisms, streptococci

include ventricular septal defect, patent ductus arteriosus, and tetralogy of Fallot. Atrial septal defect (secundum variety) is rarely associated with IE. Congenital heart disease accounts for 15% of cases, with the bicuspid aortic valve being most common.

Nosocomial causes (nosocomial infective endocarditis [NIE]), IVDA IE, and prosthetic valve endocarditis (PVE) are becoming increasingly common. In 75% of cases of IVDA IE, no underlying valvular abnormalities are noted, and 50% of these infections involve the tricuspid valve.

PVE accounts for 10–20% of cases of IE. Eventually, 5% of mechanical and bioprosthetic valves become infected. Mechanical valves are more likely to be infected within the first 3 months of implantation, and, after 1 year, bioprosthetic valves are more likely to be infected. Valves in the mitral valve position are more susceptible than those in the aortic position.

Pacemaker endocarditis (and endocarditis with cardioverter-defibrillators) is also quite common. Devices may become infected within a few months of implantation. Infection of pacemakers includes that of the generator pocket (the most common), infection of the proximal leads, and infection of the portions of the leads in direct contact with the endocardium. Of pacemaker infections, 75% are produced by staphylococci, both coagulase-negative and coagulase-positive.

CLINICAL FEATURES

IE presents either acutely or subacutely. Risk factors for IE are shown in table 3.3.

ACUTE IE

Acute IE frequently involves normal valves. It is a rapidly progressive illness. Clinical features include acute onset of high-grade fevers and chills and a rapid onset of congestive heart failure. There is rapid destruction of the valvular leaflets by bacteria that multiply rapidly within the

Table 3.2 IE SYNDROMES

ORGANISM	EPIDEMIOLOGY	SPECIAL FEATURES
S. aureus	Most common cause of IE, including PVE, acute IE, and IVDA IE 35–60.5% of staphylococcal bacteremias are complicated by IE 7.8% *S. aureus* bacteremias per year associated with intravascular catheters Mortality rate of *S. aureus* IE is 40–50%	Incidence of methicillin-resistant *S. aureus* (MRSA) infections, both the hospital- and community-acquired varieties, has dramatically increased (50% of isolates) Primary risk factor for *S. aureus* is presence of intravascular lines Other risk factors include cancer, diabetes, corticosteroid use, IVDA, alcoholism, and renal failure
Streptococcus viridans	50–60% of cases of subacute disease	Most common cause of community acquired NVE in non-IVDA cases
Abiotrophia defectiva	1–2% of cases of subacute disease	May be misdiagnosed as culture negative endocarditis They require metabolically active forms of vitamin B-6 for growth This type of IE is associated with large vegetations that lead to embolization and a high rate of posttreatment relapse
Streptococcus intermedius group	Infections may be acute or subacute	These *S. intermedius* infections account for 15% of streptococcal IE cases. *S. intermedius* is unique among the streptococci; it can actively invade tissue and can cause abscesses
Group D streptococci (*Enterococci* or *S. bovis*)	Third most common cause of IE	Most cases are subacute; source is the gastrointestinal or genitourinary tract *S. bovis* may be associated with colon cancer

Table 3.2 (Continued)

ORGANISM	EPIDEMIOLOGY	SPECIAL FEATURES
Group B streptococci	Mortality rate is 40%	Acute disease develops in pregnant patients and older patients with underlying diseases (e.g., cancer, diabetes, alcoholism) Complications include metastatic infection, arterial thrombi, and congestive heart failure It often requires valve replacement for cure
Group A, C, and G streptococci	30–70% mortality rate	Acute disease resembles that of *S. aureus* IE with suppurative complications Group A organisms respond to penicillin alone Group C and G organisms require a combination of synergistic antibiotics (as with enterococci)
Coagulase-negative *S. aureus*	It accounts for approximately 30% of PVE cases and <5% of NVE cases	Can produce native-valve endocarditis in MVP Usually subacute, difficult to diagnose, and disregarded as a contaminant Delay in diagnosis and treatment may account for the severe complications: myocardial abscess formation, valvular insufficiency requiring valve surgery, death
Pseudomonas aeruginosa		This is usually acute, except when it involves the right side of the heart in IVDA IE Surgery is commonly required for cure
HACEK organisms (i.e., *Haemophilus aphrophilus, Actinobacillus actinomycetemcomitans, Cardiobacterium hominis, Eikenella corrodens, Kingella kingae*)	These account for approximately 5% of IE cases	These organisms usually cause subacute disease They are the most common Gram-negative organisms isolated from patients with IE Complications may include massive arterial emboli and congestive heart failure Cure requires ampicillin, gentamicin, and surgery
Fungi		These usually cause subacute disease The most common organism of both fungal NVE and fungal PVE is *Candida albicans* Fungal IVDA IE is usually caused by *C. parapsilosis* or *C. tropicalis* *Aspergillus* species are observed in fungal PVE and NIE
Polymicrobial IE		IV drug use is the predominant risk factor Younger age (mean 36.5 years) Two-thirds were male Right-sided cardiac involvement in >60% Streptococci more frequent than *S. aureus* One-third of patients died Mortality rate is 4× higher for pure left-sided vs. pure right-sided endocarditis

Culture-negative endocarditis		Occurs in 2.5–31% of cases of infective endocarditis
		Causes:
		  1. Prior antibiotic administration
		  2. Infection with:
		    Bartonella quintana
		    Brucella
		    Legionella
		    Mycobacteria
		    Nocardia
		    Coxiella burnetii
		    Tropheryma whipplei
		    Fungi (*H. capsulatum* and *C. neoformans*)

ever-growing friable vegetations. Murmurs are absent in approximately one-third of patients with acute IE. The most common type is an aortic regurgitation murmur. Owing to the suddenness of onset, the left ventricle does not have a chance to dilate. In this situation, the classic finding of increased pulse pressure in significant aortic valvular insufficiency, for example, is absent. Fever is always present and is usually high. Complications include severe congestive heart failure and a wide spectrum of neuropsychiatric complications resulting from CNS involvement. Patients with

Table 3.3 RISK STRATIFICATION OF IE

High Risk
Prosthetic cardiac valve
Prior episodes of endocarditis
Complex congenital cardiac defect
Surgically constructed systemic-pulmonary shunts or conduits

Moderate Risk
Patent ductus arteriosus
VSD, primum ASD
Coarctation of the aorta
Bicuspid aortic valve
Hypertrophic cardiomyopathy
Acquired valvular dysfunction
MVP with mitral regurgitation

Low Risk
Isolated secundum atrial septal defect
ASD, VSD, or PDA >6 months past repair
"Innocent" heart murmur by auscultation in the pediatric population
"Innocent" heart murmur by echocardiography in adult patients

right-sided IVDA IE (53% of cases) frequently present with pleuropulmonary (pneumonia and/or empyema) manifestations. Symptoms due to metastatic infection develop early in *S. aureus* infections. Infection with *P. aeruginosa* has a high rate of neurological involvement, with two distinctive features: (1) mycotic aneurysms with a higher-than-average rate of rupture, and (2) panophthalmitis (10% of patients). The course of infection with *P. aeruginosa* is much slower than that of *S. aureus*. Right-sided disease is associated with a low rate of congestive heart failure and valvular perforation. The course of left-sided IVDA IE is similar to that of non-IVDA disease.

Janeway lesions are irregular erythematosus and painless macules (1–4 mm in diameter). They most often are located on the thenar and hypothenar eminences of the hands and feet. They usually represent an infectious vasculitis of acute IE resulting from *S. aureus* infection. Acute septic monoarticular arthritis in patients with acute IE most often is caused by *S. aureus* infection. Purulent meningitis may be observed in patients with acute IE.

SUBACUTE IE

Subacute IE typically affects only abnormal valves. Clinical features include malaise, fever, fatigue, anorexia, back pain, weight loss, flu-like symptoms, polymyalgia-like syndromes, pleuritic pain, syndromes similar to rheumatic fever (e.g., fever, dulled sensorium as in typhoid, headaches), and abdominal symptoms (e.g., right upper-quadrant pain, vomiting, postprandial distress, appendicitis-like symptoms). The vast majority of patients have detectable heart murmurs. The presence of a murmur is so common (99% of cases) that its absence should cause clinicians to reconsider

the diagnosis of IE. The major exception is right-sided IE, in which only one-third of patients have a detectable murmur. Because many of these murmurs are hemodynamically insignificant and have been present for years, their role in the patient's illness may be underestimated. The saying "a changing murmur is extremely helpful in diagnosing subacute IE" is a myth, as only 15% do so early in the course of infection.

Systemic Stigmata of Subacute IE

These embolic stigmata of subacute IE are observed in only approximately 20% of patients, compared with 85% in the pre-antibiotic era.

1. Petechiae: These may occur on the palpebral conjunctivae, the dorsa of the hands, feet, and toes, the anterior chest and abdominal walls, the oral mucosa, and the soft palate.

Subungual hemorrhages (i.e., splinter hemorrhages) are linear and red. Hemorrhages that do not extend for the entire length of the nail are more likely the result of infection rather than trauma.

2. Osler nodes: These are tender nodules that range from red to purple and are located primarily in the pulp spaces of the terminal phalanges of the fingers and toes, soles of the feet, and the thenar and hypothenar eminences of the hands. Their appearance is often preceded by neuropathic pain. They last from hours to several days. They remain tender for a maximum of 2 days. The underlying mechanism is probably the circulating immunocomplexes of subacute IE. They have also been described in various noninfectious vasculitides.

3. Clubbing of fingers and toes: Observed in <10% of patients, it primarily occurs in those patients who have an extended course of untreated IE.

4. Arthritis: This is associated with subacute IE, is asymmetrical, and is limited to one to three joints. Clinically, it resembles the joint changes found in patients with rheumatoid arthritis, Reiter syndrome, or Lyme disease. The fluid is usually sterile.

5. Splenomegaly: This is observed more commonly in patients with long-standing subacute disease. It may persist long after successful therapy. Splenic infarcts can also be a manifestation of embolization.

6. Roth spots: These are retinal hemorrhages with pale centers. The Litten sign represents cotton-wool exudates. Roth spots arise from immune-mediated vasculitis.

7. Neurological: Acute meningitis with sterile spinal fluid and stroke in the distribution of the middle cerebral artery. Cerebral emboli occur in 33% of patients. In 50% of patients with cerebral emboli, this event is the first manifestation of IE and is associated with a two- to four-times higher mortality rate. Other neurological embolic damage includes cranial nerve palsies, cerebritis, and mycotic aneurysms caused by weakening of the vessel walls and produced by embolization to the vasa vasorum.

8. *Renal:* Regional infarcts in the kidney from peripheral embolization cause painless hematuria and infarction of the kidney. (Patients with subacute IE may also develop a postinfectious glomerulonephritis.)

9. *Cardiac:* Myocardial infarction is due to embolization of a coronary artery in IE.

10. *Pulmonary:* Embolization from right-sided IE commonly produces pulmonary infarcts.

FACTORS INFLUENCING EMBOLIZATION

The rate of embolization is related to the organism, the size of the vegetation and its rate of growth or resolution, and its location. The vegetations of *S. aureus, Haemophilus influenzae, H. parainfluenzae,* and the fungi are much more likely to embolize than those of *S. viridans.* Vegetations >10 mm in diameter that grow in size and are mobile or prolapsing have a high rate of embolization. Mitral valve vegetations are much more likely to embolize than those in any other location. The risk of embolization markedly decreases after 1 week of appropriate antibiotic therapy.

CLINICAL IE SYNDROMES

IVDA IE

The incidence of IE in IVDAs is 2–5% per year with an overall death rate of 5–10%. IVDAs often develop recurrent IE (recurrence rate of ~40%). The prevalence of HIV infection among IVDAs with IE ranges between 30% and 70% in urban areas in developed countries. Approximately 5% to 8% of febrile individuals who abuse intravenous drugs have underlying IE. Overall, *S. aureus* is the most common etiological agent and in most geographical areas is sensitive to methicillin. The remainder of cases is caused by streptococci, enterococci, Gram-negative rod (GNR), *Candida* spp., and other less common organisms. Polymicrobial infection occurs in 2% to 5% of cases. The tricuspid valve is the most frequently affected (60–70%), followed by the mitral and aortic valves (20–30%); pulmonic valve infection is rare (<1%). More than one valve is infected in 5% to 10% of cases. Many users of illicit drugs may lose their fever within a few hours of hospitalization. This phenomenon, termed cotton-wool fever, is probably caused by the presence of adulterants contained within the injected drugs. The prognosis of right-sided endocarditis is generally good; overall mortality is <5%, and with surgery, <2%. In contrast, the prognosis of left-sided IE is less favorable; mortality is 20–30%, and even with surgery it is 15%–25%. IE caused by Gram-negative organisms or fungi has the worst prognosis.

This can occur early—defined as infection within 60 days of valve implantation. Late PVE occurs after this period. For valvular infection with coagulase-negative staphylococci (CoNS), this division should be extended to 12 months. Clinical features of PVE closely resemble those of NVE. Congestive heart failure occurs earlier and is more severe in persons with PVE. The patient may present with symptoms of myocarditis or pericarditis. The rate of embolic stroke is high in the first 3 days of PVE. Patients with PVE must be monitored carefully for signs of valve dysfunction, congestive heart failure, and heart block. They should also be monitored for clinical response to therapy, conversion of positive blood culture results, renal function status, and serum blood levels of vancomycin and aminoglycosides. There are important differences between the organisms that cause early versus late PVE. The causative organisms for early PVE tend to be CoNS, Gram-negative bacilli, and *Candida* species, whereas late PVE tends to have staphylococci, alphahemolytic streptococci, and enterococci as the common causative organisms. Of note, some have suggested that *S. aureus* is the most common infecting organism in both early and late PVE.[1]

Clinical features depend on the site of infection (e.g., generator pocket vs. intravascular leads or epicardial leads), the type of organism, and the origin of the infection (e.g., pocket erosion, localized infection of the generator pocket, bacteremia from a remote site). Infections may be early or late.

Early infections, within a few months of implantation, present as acute or subacute infections of the pulse-generator pocket. Bacteremia may be present even in the absence of clinical signs and symptoms. Fever is the most common finding and may be the only finding in approximately 33% of patients.

Late infections of the pocket may be due to erosion of the overlying skin without systemic involvement. Such erosions always indicate infection of the underlying device. The most significant late infections involve the transvenous or epicardial leads. With epicardial infection, signs and symptoms of pericarditis or mediastinitis may be present along with bacteremia. Infection of the transvenous electrode produces signs and symptoms of right-sided endocarditis. Those that occur early after implantation (33% of cases) show prominent systemic signs of infection, often with obvious localization to the pacemaker pocket. Late infections have much more subtle manifestations, and may occur up to several years after implantation or reimplantation. Signs of right-sided endocarditis (i.e., pneumonia, septic emboli) are observed in up to 50% of patients.

DIAGNOSIS AND WORKUP OF IE

The Duke criteria list is generally used for the diagnosis of IE. To make a diagnosis of IE either two major criteria, or one major and three minor, or five minor criteria are required (see table 3.4). A diagnosis of possible IE is made when findings consistent with IE fall short of the criteria for definite IE but do not meet the criteria for rejection. Rejection criteria for the diagnosis of IE are as follows:

• The presence of a firm alternative diagnosis of the manifestations of endocarditis

• Resolution of manifestations of endocarditis after 4 or fewer days of antimicrobial therapy

• No pathologic evidence of IE at surgery or autopsy after 4 or fewer days of antimicrobial therapy

These criteria may, at times, overdiagnose IE and may not be as applicable in patients with subacute disease.

Blood cultures are key in making the diagnosis of IE; however, echocardiography has become essential for the workup and diagnosis of IE and should be performed in all cases of suspected IE. Echocardiographic evidence of an oscillating intracardiac mass or vegetation, an annular

Table 3.4 **DUKE CRITERIA FOR IE**

Definite Infective Endocarditis
Pathologic criteria
Microorganisms: demonstrated by culture or histology in a vegetation, or in a vegetation that has embolized, or in an intracardiac abscess, or Pathological lesions: vegetation or intracardiac abscess present, confirmed by histology showing active endocarditis
Clinical criteria, using specific definitions listed below:

2 major criteria, or
  1 major criterion and 3 minor criteria, or
  5 minor criteria

Possible Infective Endocarditis
Findings consistent with infective endocarditis that fall short of "definite," but not "rejected" Rejected

Firm alternate diagnosis for manifestations of endocarditis, or
  Resolution of manifestations of endocarditis, with antibiotic therapy for 4 days or less, or
  No pathogenic evidence of endocarditis at surgery or autopsy, after antibiotic therapy for 4 days or less.

Major Criteria

Positive blood culture for infective endocarditis
  Typical microorganisms for infective endocarditis from two separate blood cultures:
    *Viridans streptococci,** *Streptococcus bovis*, HACEK group, *S. aureus,* or
    Community-acquired *enterococci*, in the absence of a primary focus, or
  Persistently positive blood culture, defined as recovery of a microorganism consistent with infective endocarditis from:
    i. Blood cultures drawn more than 12 hours apart, or
    ii. All of three or majority of four or more separate blood cultures, with first and last drawn at least 1 hour apart.
    iii. Single positive blood culture for Coxiella burnetti or serology showing phase I antibody >1:800

Evidence of endocardial involvement
Positive echocardiogram for infective endocarditis

i. Oscillating intracardiac mass on valve or supporting structures or in the path of regurgitant jets or on implanted material in the absence of an anatomic explanation, or
    ii. Abscess, or
    iii. New partial dehiscence of prosthetic valve, or
  New valvular regurgitation (increase or change in pre-existing murmur not sufficient)

Minor Criteria
Predisposition: predisposing heart condition or intravenous drug use Fever ≥38.0°C (100.4°F) Vascular phenomena: major arterial emboli, septic pulmonary infracts, mycotic aneurysm, intracranial hemorrhage, conjunctival hemorrhages, Janeway lesions Immunologic phenomena: glomerulonephritis, Osler nodes, Roth spots, rheumatoid factor Microbiologic evidence: positive blood culture but not meeting major criterion as noted previously[†] or serologic evidence of active infection with organism consistent with infective endocarditis Echocardiogram: consistent with infective endocarditis but not meeting major criterion as noted previously

HACEK = *Haemophilus* spp., *Actinobacillus actinomycetemcomitans, Cardiobacterium hominis, Eikenelle* spp., and *Kingella kingae.*
* Including nutritional variant strains.
[†] Excluding single positive cultures for coagulase-negative staphylococci and organisms that do not cause endocarditis.
SOURCE: Reprinted from Durack DT, Lukes AS, Bright DK. New criteria for diagnosis of infective endocarditis: Utilization of specific echocardiographic findings. Duke Endocarditis Service. *Am J Med.* 1994;96(3):200–9, with permission from Elsevier.

abscess, prosthetic valve partial dehiscence, and new valvular regurgitation are major criteria in the diagnosis of IE.

Echocardiography is useful for predicting the potential complications of IE, especially those that are embolic in nature. By contrast, the diagnosis of IE can never be excluded based on negative echocardiogram findings, either transthoracic or transesophageal (TEE).

Transthoracic echocardiography (TTE) can detect vegetations in approximately 60% of patients with NVE but in only 20% of patients with PVE. The sensitivity of TEE in detecting the vegetations of NVE is 90–100%. In patients with PVE, the sensitivity of TEE under optimal circumstances is >90%. TEE is far more sensitive than TTE for detecting myocardial abscesses (95% vs. 28%). TEE successfully visualizes vegetations of the leads or of the tricuspid valve in more than 90% of cases of pacemaker IE, compared with less than the 50% achieved by TTE. Figure 3.1 depicts an algorithm for deciding whether to opt for a TTE or a TEE. Twenty-five percent of patients with staphylococcal bacteremia and 23% of those with catheters as the primary focus have evidence of IE based on TEE findings, in the absence of clinical and TTE findings.

Echocardiographic predictors of systemic embolization in patients with IE are shown in table 3.5.

Radionuclide scans, such as gallium Ga-67–tagged white cells and indium In-111–tagged white cells, are of marginal use in diagnosing IE. Catheterization of the heart is rarely required for the diagnosis of IE or any of its complications. A CT scan of the head should be obtained in patients who exhibit CNS symptoms or findings consistent with a mass effect (e.g., macroabscess of the brain).

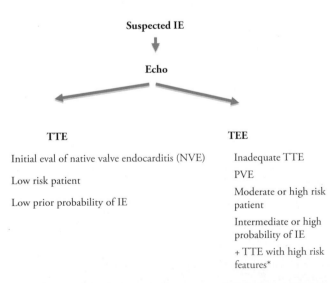

Figure 3.1 Algorithm for TTE vs. TEE in Patients with IE. *Large/mobile vegetation, valvular insufficiency, suggestion of paravalvular extension, or secondary valve dysfunction.

Table 3.5 ECHOCARDIOGRAPHIC PREDICTORS OF SYSTEMIC EMBOLIZATION IN PATIENTS WITH IE

Large valvular vegetations (>10 mm in diameter)
Multiple vegetations
Mobile but pedunculated vegetations
Noncalcified vegetations
Vegetations that are increasing in size
Prolapsing vegetations

TREATMENT OF IE

Treatment of IE comprises antimicrobial therapy to address the bacterial infection and medical and surgical strategies to deal with complications. In patients at high risk of endocarditis, based on either the clinical picture or the patient's risk factor profile, such as injection drug use or a history of previous endocarditis, the presumption of endocarditis often is made before blood culture results are available.

ANTIMICROBIAL THERAPY

Antibiotic therapy as soon as possible after taking multiple sets of blood cultures (usually three to five sets). Antibiotics remain the mainstay of treatment for IE. Initial antibiotic choice is empiric and intravenous until culture and sensitivity data become available. Patients should generally be hospitalized for treatment. The antibiotic regimen depends very much on the identified organism(s) (see table 3.6).

Empirical therapy of IVDA IE should be aimed at *S. aureus*. Whether to use vancomycin or oxacillin/nafcillin depends on the incidence of MRSA in the community. Generally, Gram-negative organisms occur infrequently, and delay in covering them initially is acceptable.

Relapse of IE usually occurs within 2 months of finishing clinically effective therapy. Infection with *S. aureus*, enterococci, and Gram-negative organisms (especially *P. aeruginosa*) is associated with a high rate of relapse. Those with pretreatment symptoms of IE of more than 3 months' duration are at greater risk for relapse. Enterococcal infection of the mitral valve has the greatest potential for relapse. Other significant risk factors for recurrence include a previous episode of IE, the presence of a prosthetic valve, and congenital heart disease.

MEDICAL TREATMENT OF IE COMPLICATIONS

Complications of IE are listed in table 3.7.

Mild congestive heart failure resulting from valvular insufficiency or myocarditis may be managed with

Table 3.6 RECOMMENDED ANTIMICROBIAL THERAPY FOR COMMON IE INFECTION

ORGANISM	RECOMMENDED TREATMENT
Adult native valve endocarditis (NVE) caused by penicillin-susceptible *S. viridans, S. bovis,* and other streptococci	Penicillin G at 12–18 million U/d intravenously or ceftriaxone or penicillin G and gentamicin In patients who are allergic to penicillin, use vancomycin
For NVE caused by relatively resistant streptococci	Penicillin G at 18 million U/d IV or cefazolin or pen G/cefazolin combined with gentamicin In patients who are allergic to penicillin, use vancomycin
IE caused by nonresistant enterococci, resistant *S. viridans* (MICs of penicillin G of >0.5 μg/mL), or nutritionally variant *S. viridans* and PVE caused by penicillin-G–susceptible *S. viridans* or *S. bovis*	Penicillin G at 18–30 million U/d IV, combined with gentamicin at 1 mg/kg every 8 hours for 4–6 weeks In patients who are allergic to penicillin, use vancomycin
NVE caused by methicillin-sensitive *S. aureus*	Administer nafcillin or oxacillin at 2 g IV every 4 hours for 4–6 weeks. Administer cefazolin at 2 g IV every 8 hours for 4–6 weeks For patients who are allergic to penicillin, administer vancomycin
HACEK	Administer ceftriaxone at 2 g/d IV for 4 weeks Alternatively, ampicillin at 12 g/d +/− gentamicin at 1 mg/kg IV every 8 hours for 4 weeks

standard medical therapy. Often, this is progressive and, despite achieving a microbiological cure, requires valvular surgery.

Anticoagulation is controversial, despite the embolic complications encountered with IE. Patients who are anticoagulated have a higher rate of intracerebral bleeding.

SURGICAL CARE

Approximately 15% to 25% of patients with IE eventually require surgery. Indications for surgery for NVE are depicted in table 3.8. The indications for surgery in patients with PVE are shown in table 3.9.

Removal of a pacemaker and its wires is usually required for treatment of pacemaker endocarditis. Occasionally, local debridement and the administration of appropriate antibiotics may be sufficient to cure an uncomplicated pacemaker pocket infection. After removal of the infected device, placing a temporary transvenous pacer is best. Immediate insertion of a permanent pacemaker at a new site can be safely accomplished.

Table 3.7 COMPLICATIONS OF IE

Valvular dysfunction, usually insufficiency of the mitral or aortic valves

Myocardial or septal abscesses

Congestive heart failure

Metastatic infection

Embolic phenomenon

Immune complex-mediated glomerulonephritis

ANTIBIOTIC PROPHYLAXIS FOR IE

The American Heart Association's (see Additional Reading) recommendation that prophylaxis be provided for patients at high risk for IE rests on three principles: (1) certain underlying cardiac conditions predispose patients to IE; (2) because bacteremia with organisms known to cause IE occurs commonly in association with invasive dental, GI, or GU tract procedures; and (3) antimicrobial prophylaxis is thought to be effective in IE associated with dental, GI, or GU tract procedures.

Table 3.8 INDICATIONS FOR SURGERY WITH NATIVE VALVE ENDOCARDITIS (NVE)

Congestive heart failure refractory to standard medical therapy

Fungal IE (except that caused by *Histoplasma capsulatum*)

Persistent infection after 1 week of appropriate antibiotic treatment

Recurrent septic emboli, especially after 2 weeks of antibiotic treatment

Rupture of an aneurysm of the sinus of Valsalva

Conduction disturbances caused by a septal abscess

Kissing infection of the anterior mitral leaflet in patients with IE of the aortic valve

Congestive heart failure

Paravalvular abscess and intracardiac fistula

Persistent hypermobile vegetations, especially those with a history of embolization beyond 7 days of antibiotic therapy

Multiresistant organisms (e.g., gram negative bacteria, Pseudomonas)

Metastatic infections (e.g., cerebral and other types of aneurysms and macroabscesses of the brain and spleen)

Table 3.9 INDICATIONS FOR VALVE REPLACEMENT SURGERY IN PROSTHETIC VALVE ENDOCARDITIS (PVE)

Moderate to severe congestive heart failure

Valve dysfunction

Perivalvular or myocardial abscess formation

Presence of unstable valve that is becoming detached from the valve ring

More than one embolic episode with persistent vegetations observed on transtracheal echocardiogram

Vegetations larger than 1 cm in diameter

PVE with fungus, *S. aureus*, or multi-resistant organisms

Table 3.11 SUGGESTED REGIMENS FOR A DENTAL PROCEDURE

SITUATION	AGENT	ADULT DOSE
Oral medication	Amoxicillin	2 g 30 to 60 min before procedure
Allergic to penicillin	Cephalexin	2 g 30 to 60 min before procedure

The administration of prophylactic antibiotics solely to prevent endocarditis is now not recommended for patients who undergo GU or GI tract procedures, including diagnostic esophagogastroduodenoscopy or colonoscopy.

ADDITIONAL READING

Baddour LM, Wilson WR, Bayer AS, et al. Infective Endocarditis: Diagnosis, Antimicrobial Therapy and Management of Complications: A Statement for Healthcare Professionals from the Committee on Rheumatic Fever, Endocarditis, and Kawasaki Disease, Council on cardiovascular Disease in the Young, and the Councils on Clinical Cardiology, Stroke, and Cardiovascular Surgery and Anesthesia, American Heart Association: Endorsed by the Infectious Diseases Society of America. *Circulation*. 2005;111(23):e394–434.

Miró JM, del Río A, Mestres CA. Infective endocarditis in intravenous drug abusers and HIV-1 infected patients. *Infect Dis Clin North Am*. 2002;16(2):273–95, vii–viii.

Wilson W, Taubert KA, Gewitz M, et al. Prevention of infective endocarditis: guidelines from the American Heart Association: a guideline from the American Heart Association Rheumatic Fever, Endocarditis, and Kawasaki Disease Committee, Council on Cardiovascular Disease in the Young, and the Council on Clinical Cardiology, Council on Cardiovascular Surgery and Anesthesia, and the Quality of Care and Outcomes Research Interdisciplinary Working Group. *Circulation*. 2007;116:1736–54.

www.emedicine.medscape.com/article/216650-overview. Accessed March 20, 2010.

The cardiac conditions deemed at highest risk are listed in table 3.10. The AHA no longer recommends IE prophylaxis based solely on an increased lifetime risk of acquisition of IE. In particular, this applies to mitral valve prolapse (MVP). The AHA no longer recommends routine prophylaxis for MVP because IE is extremely rare with MVP, and the consequences of IE in these patients who often do not have associated comorbidities are generally mild. All patients deemed of high IE risk undergoing dental procedures that involve manipulation of gingival tissue or the periapical region of teeth or perforation of the oral mucosa should be treated with a prophylactic antibiotic regimen. A suggested antibiotic regimen is shown in table 3.11. The antibiotic dose should be administered in a single dose before the procedure. If the dosage of antibiotic is *inadvertently* not administered before the procedure, the dosage may be administered up to 2 hours after the procedure. However, administration of the dosage after the procedure should be considered only when the patient did not receive the preprocedure dose.

QUESTIONS

QUESTION 1. Infective endocarditis prophylaxis is only routinely recommended for which of the following procedures:

A. Cystoscopy
B. Vaginal hysterectomy
C. Esophageal dilatation
D. Flexible bronchoscopy with biopsy
E. Tooth extraction in a patient with a prosthetic heart valve

QUESTION 2. Which of the following statements regarding endocarditis in intravenous drug abusers (IVDAs) is FALSE?

A. Right-sided (tricuspid valve) endocarditis is most common.
B. Polymicrobial infections are observed most commonly

Table 3.10 CARDIAC CONDITIONS AT HIGH RISK OF IE FOR WHICH PROPHYLAXIS SHOULD BE ADMINISTERED

Prosthetic cardiac valve or prosthetic material used for cardiac valve repair

Previous IE

Unrepaired cyanotic CHD, including palliative shunts and conduits

Completely repaired congenital heart defect with prosthetic material or device, whether placed by surgery or by catheter intervention, during the first 6 months after the procedure*

Repaired CHD with residual defects at the site or adjacent to the site of a prosthetic patch or prosthetic device (which inhibit endothelialization)

Cardiac transplantation recipients who develop cardiac valvulopathy

*When endothelialization occurs

C. Data support the use of short-course (2-week) therapy for right-sided endocarditis caused by methicillin-sensitive *Staphylococcus aureus* in IVDAs.
D. Fungi account for approximately 5% of cases of endocarditis in IVDAs.
E. *Candida albicans* is the most common fungal organism causing endocarditis in IVDAs.

QUESTION 3. Clinical features that should raise the suspicion of infective endocarditis include all of the following, EXCEPT:

A. A new regurgitant murmur
B. Embolic events of unknown origin
C. Fever
D. Hematuria
E. Erythema marginatum

ANSWERS

1. E
2. E
3. E

4.

IMMUNIZATIONS

Mary L. Pisculli and Lindsey R. Baden

Childhood immunizations are responsible for the control of many infectious diseases once common in the United States including polio, measles, mumps, rubella, diphtheria, pertussis, and *Haemophilus influenzae* type b. Vaccine-induced immunity, however, may decrease with time, and adult immunization recommendations take into account both waning immunity and age-related risks of exposure and infection. Benefits of immunization are not limited to the vaccinated individual but also include promotion of herd immunity for the population at large, including nonimmunized persons and those with waning immunity or who may not have fully responded to prior vaccination. Immunizations, however, also carry risks that can range from common minor local skin reactions to rare, life-threatening adverse reactions. These risks are carefully weighed in the creation of immunization schedule recommendations, balancing the individual's risk of exposure with the earliest timing that immunizations can be safely and effectively administered.

This chapter reviews the recommendations for adult immunizations in the United States as promoted by the Centers for Disease Control and Prevention (CDC) and the Advisory Committee on Immunization Practices (ACIP) and provides information regarding the basic principles underlying immunization and specific contraindications to vaccination. Immunization recommendations for travelers to other parts of the world require specific information regarding the infectious risks endemic to each area and are beyond the scope of this chapter. Further detailed information for both recommended immunizations in the United States and travel vaccines can be obtained from the CDC website: http://www.cdc.gov/vaccines.

BASIC PRINCIPLES OF IMMUNIZATIONS

Protection against infectious organisms may be via induction of either passive or active immunity. Passive immunity results from the transfer of preformed antibodies, whereas active immunity requires the generation of an antigen-specific cellular and/or humoral immune response. Although passive immunity provides immediate protection, the effects are short-lived (usually 3–6 months). Conversely, active vaccination strategies provide long-lasting immunity through the induction of a memory response, although this response may wane with age and require intermittent vaccination "boosters." Halting community spread of wild-type infections may decrease natural boosting. This poses a potential challenge to successful vaccination strategies and highlights the importance of maintaining up-to-date booster schedules.

A variety of different types of antigens or immunogens have been used as vaccines to induce active immunity. Vaccines comprised of live attenuated infectious agents are generally the most efficacious in stimulating long-lasting immunity, although their use is contraindicated in certain populations, such as individuals with severe immune impairment and pregnant women. Polysaccharide vaccines generate a T-cell–independent immune response, and their immunogenicity is generally poor in infants and children younger than 2 years of age. Polysaccharides conjugated to protein carriers increase their overall antigenicity and elicit T-cell help, thus facilitating the induction of a memory response. Toxoid vaccines typically consist of deactivated toxins and may be used to generate immunity against specific toxins produced by infectious agents rather than against the causative organism.

Passive immunization is produced through the administration of specific or pooled immunoglobulins (IG). These preformed antibodies are typically administered following recent exposure to an infectious agent or just prior to possible exposure. In the United States only plasma that has tested negative for hepatitis B surface antigen, HIV antibody, and HCV antibody is used to produce IG. Available specific IG products include tetanus IG, rabies IG, hepatitis A IG, and hepatitis B IG. Passive and active immunizations may be combined to provide both immediate and sustained protection. For example, following a bite from an animal potentially infected with rabies, both rabies IG and the rabies vaccine should be given. When this type of combined strategy is employed, the preformed immunoglobulins and the active vaccine must be administered at separate sites.

PRECAUTIONS AND CONTRADICTIONS

In general, severely immunocompromised individuals should not receive live vaccines because of the theoretical concern for infection despite the agent's attenuated status (see table 4.1). Owing to the theoretical risk to the fetus, pregnant women should also not receive live vaccines. The only contraindication applicable to all vaccines is a history of a severe allergic reaction following a previous dose of the vaccine or a known allergy against a vaccine constituent. For example, persons with an anaphylactoid reaction to eggs should not receive influenza vaccine, as the vaccine is grown in eggs. Patients with severe allergies to certain antibiotics also require careful consideration prior to receiving vaccinations that contain that antibiotic. Both available polio vaccines contain neomycin, streptomycin, and polymyxin, whereas the mumps, measles, rubella (MMR) and varicella vaccines contain trace amounts of neomycin. Anaphylactoid reactions to these antibiotics are considered a contraindication to vaccination, whereas milder reactions such as rash are not. No currently available vaccine contains penicillin or penicillin products, and allergy to this antibiotic is not a contraindication to vaccination. The CDC provides a vaccine information sheet called a VIS for each vaccine, containing information on individual vaccine constituents, and they should be reviewed prior to administration.

Vaccination should be postponed in the setting of moderate or severe acute illness with or without fever. Although a common misconception, vaccination does not need to be deferred in patients with a mild illness or low-grade fever. Concurrent treatment with antibiotics also does not represent a contraindication to vaccination with the single exception of the oral typhoid vaccine, as certain antibiotics may interfere with the effectiveness of this live attenuated bacterial vaccine. Similarly, the live attenuated influenza vaccine should not be administered in conjunction with antiviral chemoprophylaxis.

Table 4.1 LIVE VACCINES

LIVE VIRAL ATTENUATED VACCINES	LIVE BACTERIAL VACCINES
MMR	Typhoid (Ty21a)
VZV	Bacille Calmette-Guérin (BCG)
Live attenuated influenza vaccine	
Oral polio virus	
Yellow fever	

Patients with immunoglobulin A deficiency should not receive immunoglobulin preparations unless the risk of illness outweighs the risk of anaphylaxis.

ADULT IMMUNIZATION RECOMMENDATIONS

The CDC's National Center for Immunization and Respiratory Diseases maintains annual updates of recommended childhood, adolescent, and adult immunization schedules. Table 4.2 demonstrates the most recent recommended adult immunization schedule. For newer vaccines, future surveillance efforts of the durability of vaccine-associated immunity help to determine the optimal booster interval.

INFLUENZA

The influenza vaccine is administered annually in the fall or winter (influenza season in the United States). Two available formulations of the influenza vaccine exist—a trivalent inactivated influenza preparation administered intramuscularly (IM) and a live attenuated virus vaccine (LAIV) administered via a nasal spray. The vaccine contains two influenza A viruses (H2N3 and H1N1) and one B virus. Seasonal influenza epidemics occur as a result of antigenic drift prompting the need for annual reassessment of circulating strains and formulation of the vaccine. Antigenic shifts occur less frequently; however, they can result in novel influenza A subtypes and pandemics because of lack of pre-existing immunity. Although the vaccine does not provide complete protection against all influenza strains, both the LAIV and trivalent inactivated vaccine are efficacious in preventing influenza corresponding to the strains they contain.

The inactivated influenza vaccine is specifically recommended for all adults aged 50 years or older or persons with chronic medical problems (e.g., diabetes, renal dysfunction, cardiac disease, hemoglobinopathy). Patients with compromised respiratory function or increased risk of aspiration (e.g., seizure disorder, spinal cord injury, cognitive impairment) should also receive the vaccine. Additionally, persons living in chronic care facilities or who work or live with high-risk people should be vaccinated, including all healthcare personnel. Vaccination of close contacts of vulnerable individuals is an effective infection control measure, as it provides a ring of protection. The vaccine may also be considered for any adult interested in decreasing his or her risk of becoming ill with influenza or spreading it to others.

Contraindications to receiving LAIV are similar to those of other live attenuated vaccines. The following groups should not receive the LAIV: persons younger than 5 or older than 50 years of age, persons with chronic medical illnesses or with known or suspected immunosuppressed states, and pregnant women. This vaccine also carries a

Table 4.2 RECOMMENDED VACCINES BY AGE GROUP

VACCINE	AGE GROUP		
	19–49 YEARS	50–64 YEARS	≥65 YEARS
Influenza		1 dose annually	
Pneumococcal (polysaccharide)	1–2 doses		1 dose
Meningococcal		1 or more doses	
Tetanus, diphtheria, pertussis (Td/Tdap)	Substitute 1 dose of Tdap for Td	1 dose of Td	Booster every 10 years
Measles, mumps, rubella (MMR)	1 or 2 doses	1 dose	
Varicella		2 doses (0, 4–8 weeks)	
Zoster			1 dose annually
Hepatitis A		2 doses (0, 6–12 month or 0, 6–18 months)	
Hepatitis B		3 doses (0, 1–2 months, 4–6 months)	
Human papillomavirus (HPV)	3 doses for women aged ≤26 (0, 2, 6 months)		

YELLOW indicates for all persons in this category who meet the age requirements and lack evidence of immunity.
Gray indicates recommended if a risk factor is present.
SOURCE: Centers for Disease Control and Prevention. Recommended adult immunization schedule—United States, October 2007–September 2008. *MMWR.* 2007;56 (No. RR41):1–4.

theoretical risk of person-to-person transmission, and the inactivated form of the vaccine is preferred for vaccinating household members, healthcare workers, and others who have close contact with immunosuppressed persons.

Administration of either vaccine is contraindicated in a person with a history of previous anaphylaxis to this vaccine or any of its components, or to eggs. Vaccination may also be deferred during moderate or severe acute illness and in any patient with a history of Guillain-Barré syndrome occurring within 6 weeks of prior influenza vaccination. As above, the live attenuated influenza vaccine is contraindicated in unvaccinated persons receiving antiviral chemoprophylaxis. In an influenza outbreak setting, these unvaccinated persons should be offered the trivalent inactivated influenza vaccine.

PNEUMOCOCCUS

Streptococcus pneumoniae is an encapsulated Gram-positive bacterium that remains a leading cause of pneumonia, otitis media, bacterial meningitis, and bacteremia. It is also an important cause of other invasive bacterial infections including acute sinusitis, brain abscess, osteomyelitis, septic arthritis, peritonitis, endocarditis, and pericarditis. The pneumococcal polysaccharide vaccine (Pneumovax) contains 23 serotypes of pneumococcal capsular polysaccharide corresponding to 85–90% of all pneumococcal disease. This vaccine is specifically recommended for all persons aged 65 years or older and persons older than age 2 at high risk of complication from pneumococcal infection, namely persons with chronic cardiac or pulmonary disease, chronic liver disease, diabetes, alcoholism, or cerebrospinal fluid leak. Certain populations are also

at higher risk for invasive pneumococcal infection, including Alaska Natives and Navajo. Groups at the highest risk of fatal pneumococcal infection include patients with anatomic or functional asplenia or sickle cell disease; immunocompromised patients including persons with HIV infection, leukemia, lymphoma, multiple myeloma, other malignancy, chronic renal failure or nephritic syndrome; persons receiving immunosuppressive therapy or who have received or are candidates for an organ or bone marrow transplant; and candidates for or recipients of cochlear implants.

A one-time booster is administered at least 5 years after the initial dose in patients who are older than 65 and who received the first dose prior to age 65 years, and to those at highest risk of fatal pneumococcal infection. A conjugated polysaccharide vaccine (Prevnar) containing seven serotypes of pneumococcal capsular polysaccharide is available for administration to infants and young children.

MENINGOCOCCUS

Neisseria meningitidis is a leading cause of bacterial meningitis in the United States, in large part due to the successful vaccination campaigns and protection against *Streptococcus pneumoniae* and *Haemophilus influenzae* type B (administered in childhood). *N. meningitidis* is spread through direct contact with respiratory secretions from either infected patients or asymptomatic carriers, and disease is associated with a high fatality and morbidity rate. In the United States most cases are sporadic, although localized outbreaks have occurred. Postexposure antibiotic prophylaxis for close contacts, ideally within 24 hours after identification of the index patient, is effective in reducing nasopharyngeal carriage of *N. meningitidis*. Acceptable and recommended antimicrobial agents include rifampin, ciprofloxacin, and ceftriaxone; azithromycin also has activity against *N. meningitidis* and is approved for use among children. Meningococcal vaccination is also an important control measure in outbreak settings.

The meningococcal vaccine is currently available in two formulations in the United States—a polysaccharide vaccine (MPSV4 or Menomune) and a polysaccharide conjugate vaccine (MCV4 or MenactraT)—and both contain purified meningococcal polysaccharides of groups A, C, Y, and W-135. Neither vaccine provides protection against all serogroups of *N. meningitidis*, most notably serogroup B, which is responsible for over 50% of cases among infants in the United States; however, 75% of cases of meningococcal disease among persons aged ≥11 years were caused by serogroups C, Y, or W-135.

N. meningitidis is an encapsulated organism, and meningococcal vaccination is recommended for all adults with anatomic or functional asplenia or terminal complement component deficiencies. Vaccination is also recommended for college freshmen living in a dormitory, microbiologists who are routinely exposed to isolates of *N. meningitidis,* military recruits, and travelers to endemic areas such as the "meningitis belt" of sub-Saharan Africa. The government of Saudi Arabia also requires vaccination for all travelers to Mecca during the annual Hajj. The polysaccharide conjugate vaccine (MCV4) is the preferred vaccine among persons aged 11–55, although if unavailable, MPSV4 is an acceptable alternative. The unconjugated vaccine, MPSV4, is recommended among children aged 2–10 years and persons aged >55 years. Both vaccines are administered as a single dose, and revaccination after 5 years can be considered in adults who previously received MPSV4 and remain at increased risk. There are insufficient data at this time to recommend a revaccination strategy for adults who previously received MCV4.

HAEMOPHILUS INFLUENAZE B

Haemophilus influenzae b (Hib) can cause severe bacterial infections primarily in infants and children under 5 years of age, and vaccination against this infectious agent is routinely administered to infants. Owing to a paucity of data, there are currently no formal recommendations for vaccination of adults; however, this polysaccharide vaccine may be considered in persons who have chronic conditions associated with an increased risk for Hib disease including patients with sickle cell disease, asplenia or hyposplenia, HIV/AIDS, or other immunosuppressed states.

TETANUS–DIPTHERIA–PERTUSSIS

Tetanus, although not a communicable disease, is preventable with vaccination. Adult disease is generally contracted via wound contamination with toxin-producing *Clostridium tetani*. Diphtheria is an acute infectious respiratory illness primarily caused by strains of *Corynebacterium diphtheriae* and is characterized by a grayish adherent membrane in the pharynx, palate or nasal mucosa, larynx, or trachea and can lead to airway obstruction. Diphtheria toxin can also cause systemic complications, most notably cardiac and neurologic. Immunization strategies in the United States have made both tetanus and respiratory diphtheria a rare occurrence; however, exposure to diphtheria is possible during travel to endemic areas. Due to waning immunity, adult booster immunizations with Td (adult tetanus and diphtheria toxoids) are recommended every 10 years.

Pertussis, an acute respiratory infection caused by *Bordetella pertussis,* remains endemic in the United States in large part due to waning immunity 5–10 years after childhood vaccination. Compared with older age groups, infants less than 12 months old are at the greatest risk for pertussis-related complications and hospitalizations, and adult close contacts have been implicated in pertussis transmission. Whereas adults are more likely to have asymptomatic infection, pertussis can cause pneumonia. In addition, prolonged paroxysmal cough is common and can lead to multiple physician visits and extensive medical evaluation when the etiology is unrecognized. Clinical complications of paroxysmal cough include rib fracture, cough syncope, urinary incontinence, as well as aspiration, pneumothorax, inguinal hernia, lumbar disc herniation, and subconjunctival hemorrhages.

In 2005, Tdap, consisting of tetanus toxoid, reduced diphtheria toxoid, and acellular pertussis vaccine (marketed as Adacel and Boostrix), was licensed in the United States for use in persons 11–64 years of age. To promote herd immunity, routine Tdap vaccination is recommended as a single replacement dose of a Td booster for adults aged 19–64 if their last dose of Td was more than 10 years ago. Adults under the age of 65 in close contact with infants should receive Tdap, and an interval as short as 2 years between Td and Tdap is acceptable.

Appropriate tetanus prophylaxis in the management of a contaminated wound depends on the patient's prior tetanus vaccination history. Injuries that are associated with a risk of tetanus include wounds contaminated with dirt, feces, soil, or saliva. Puncture wounds, avulsions, or other injuries occurring as a result of frostbite, burns, crush, or missiles are also considered at increased risk for tetanus. Adults who completed the three-dose primary tetanus vaccination series and have received a tetanus-toxoid–containing vaccine (Td or Tdap) less than 5 years prior to the wound are considered protected and do not require further specific tetanus prophylaxis. Adults vaccinated ≥5 years earlier who have not received Tdap should receive Tdap rather than Td if possible. For adults vaccinated with Tdap in the past, Td should be used. Patients with unknown or uncertain previous tetanus vaccination histories may require both tetanus toxoid and passive immunization with tetanus immune globulin (TIG) for full protection.

Clean, minor wounds do not require tetanus prophylaxis but provide an opportunity to complete the primary tetanus vaccination series. Adults with incomplete or unknown history of vaccination should receive the three-dose primary series. The preferred schedule is a single dose of Tdap, followed by Td at ≥4 weeks and another Td dose 6–12 months later. Tdap can substitute for any of the Td doses.

MEASELS, MUMPS, RUBELLA

The MMR vaccine contains three live attenuated viruses, measles, mumps, and rubella, and is generally administered to children around age 1 and again at school entry (around 4–6 years of age). The second immunization is not a booster; rather, the objective of the second dose is to promote immunity in the small proportion of persons who do not respond to one dose. Any adult born after 1956 without serologic evidence of immunity should receive at least one dose of MMR. A second dose of MMR is recommended for (1) adults who have recently been exposed to measles or mumps or are in an outbreak setting, (2) adults previously immunized with an unknown type of measles vaccine between 1963 and 1967 or a killed measles vaccine, (3) students in postsecondary educational institutions, (4) healthcare workers, and (5) persons planning international travel. Women of childbearing age with unknown rubella vaccination history or who lack serologic evidence of immunity should also receive one dose of MMR. Women should be counseled to delay pregnancy at least 4 weeks after receiving MMR.

Serious adverse events with MMR vaccination include encephalitis, pneumonia, epididymo-orchitis, and arthropathy (rubella), particularly in postpartum women. These adverse events, however, are quite rare and are outweighed by the risks of naturally acquired measles, mumps, or rubella disease.

VARICELLA ZOSTER VIRUS

The varicella zoster virus (VZV) can cause both primary infection (varicella, chicken pox) and recurrent, or reactivated, infection (herpes zoster, shingles). Infection with varicella carries the highest hospitalization rates among adults older than 19 years and infants less than 1 year (in comparison to children aged 5–9 years). Complications leading to hospitalization include skin and soft tissue infection, particularly invasive group A streptococcal infection, pneumonia, dehydration, and encephalitis. In the prevaccine era prenatal infection was uncommon as the majority of women of childbearing age had acquired natural immunity to VZV through childhood infection; however, prenatal maternal infection can have adverse outcomes for the fetus and infant.

Three vaccines are currently available in the United States, each containing increasing concentrations of the live-attenuated (Oka strain) varicella virus. The varicella vaccine Varivax contains 1440 pfu and is recommended for children older than 12 months and any adult who does not have evidence of immunity to VZV. Evidence of immunity to varicella in adults includes any of the following: (1) U.S. born prior to 1980 (although this does not suffice as evidence for healthcare personnel and pregnant women), (2) documentation of two doses of varicella vaccine administered at least 4–8 weeks apart, (3) history of varicella based on diagnosis or verification by a healthcare provider, (4) history of herpes zoster based on healthcare provider diagnosis, or (5) laboratory evidence of immunity or confirmation of disease.

Adolescents (aged 13 years and older) and adults without evidence of varicella immunity should receive two doses of Varivax spaced 4–8 weeks apart. Special consideration should be given to at-risk groups including school-aged children, members of households with children, college students, employees, residents and staff of institutional settings, and nonpregnant women of childbearing age. Breakthrough varicella disease post-vaccination has been documented but is usually mild (CDC, 2005).

The varicella vaccine Proquad has 9800 pfu of the live varicella vaccine (seven times Varivax) as well as MMR and is approved only for children ages 12 months through 12 years old.

A third varicella vaccine, Zostavax, contains 14 times the amount of live attenuated (Oka strain) varicella vaccine as the varicella vaccine and is FDA approved for adults older than 60 years of age, whether or not they report a prior episode of shingles (CDC, 2008b). For persons aged 60 and older who anticipate immunosuppressive therapy, zoster vaccine should be administered at least 14 days prior to the start of therapy. Persons taking antiviral medications active against herpes viruses (e.g., acyclovir, famciclovir, or valacyclovir) should discontinue these medications 24 hours before receiving the zoster vaccine and not resume therapy for at least 14 days after immunization. Zoster vaccine should not be administered to any person with a primary or acquired immunodeficiency including leukemia, lymphoma, and HIV infection complicated by AIDS (CD4 count <200).

HUMAN PAPILLOMA VIRUS

Genital human papilloma virus (HPV) is the most common sexually transmitted infection in the United States. Most HPV infections are transient and asymptomatic; however, persistent infection can result in cervical cancer in women as well as anogenital cancers and warts in both men and women. There are over 100 types of HPV, and about 40 are mucosal types that can infect the anogenital area. "High-risk" types (types 16, 18, 31, 33, 35, 39, 45, 51, 52, 56, 58, 59, 68, 69, 73, and 82) have been linked with low- and high-grade cervix cell changes, precancers as well as anogenital cancers. Nearly all cases of cervical cancer are related to HPV, and about 70% are caused by HPV types 16 or 18. Genital warts, or condyloma acuminata, are associated with "low-risk" types, with approximately 90% of cases due to types 6 and 11. Low-risk types can also cause cervical cellular changes that do not develop into cancer.

A quadrivalent HPV vaccine, Gardasil, targeting types 6, 11, 16, and 18, is licensed for use in the United States among women aged 9 through 26 years old; efficacy studies are ongoing in men. A second vaccine, Cervarix, is pending FDA approval and targets HPV types 16 and 18 only. Neither vaccine provides protection against persistent infection, development of genital warts, or precursor cancer lesions for an HPV type that a woman is infected with at the time of vaccination. HPV vaccination does protect, however, against disease caused by other not-yet acquired vaccine HPV types. Ideally vaccination should occur before the onset of sexual activity and potential exposure to HPV, and the recommended age for vaccination is 11–12 years. Catch-up vaccination is recommended for women aged 13–26 years who have not yet been vaccinated. The recommended schedule is three doses administered at 0, 2, and 6 months, and it can be simultaneously administered with other vaccines.

Side effects include local reactions, most commonly pain, as well as swelling and erythema at the injection site. Vasovagal syncope has been observed after vaccination, especially among adolescents and young adults, and patients receiving this vaccine should be observed for 15 minutes after administration. The HPV vaccine is a recombinant vaccine produced with *Saccharomyces cerevisiae* (baker's yeast) and is contraindicated for any person with a history of immediate hypersensitivity to yeast (or any vaccine component). Owing to limited data, this vaccine is not recommended for use in pregnancy.

Vaccination with the HPV vaccine does not replace routine cervical cancer screening.

HEPATITIS A VIRUS

Hepatitis A virus (HAV) can cause either asymptomatic or symptomatic infection. Infection is typically asymptomatic in children under the age of 6 years and symptomatic among older children and adults. The majority of clinical syndromes last less than 2 months (although approximately 10–15% experience a prolonged or relapsing course lasting up to 6 months). Persons with chronic liver disease, especially due to HCV, are at increased risk for fulminant hepatitis A and death. In the United States, transmission is primarily via a fecal–oral route, and young asymptomatic children can act as sources of infection for others. Persons at increased risk of HAV infection include travelers to endemic areas, men who have sex with men, users of injection and noninjection drugs (suggesting infection via both percutaneous and fecal–oral routes), persons with clotting factor disorders, and persons working with nonhuman primates susceptible to HAV infection. Improvements in viral inactivation procedures, donor screening, and vaccination strategies have decreased the risk of transmission from clotting factors.

Hepatitis A vaccination is recommended routinely for children, for persons at increased risk of infection or at high risk of complications of infection (persons with chronic liver disease), and for anyone interested in obtaining immunity. During community outbreak settings, hepatitis A vaccination should be considered. Routine vaccination of all food handlers is not recommended, primarily due to cost, but may be considered. Proper hygiene to reduce the risk of fecal contamination of food and awareness of the signs and symptoms of hepatitis A remain the mainstay of food preparation safety.

Hepatitis A vaccines currently licensed in the United States are made from inactivated HAV: two types of single-antigen vaccines (Havrix and Vaqta) and a combination vaccine containing both HAV and HBV antigens (Twinrix). Havrix and Vaqta are both available in two formulations that differ according to the patient's age (pediatric vs. adult). In adults, Havrix is administered in two doses scheduled at 0 and 6–12 months; Vaqta is administered in two doses scheduled at 0 and 6–18 months.

After hepatitis A exposure in nonvaccinated persons, either administration of the single-antigen hepatitis A vaccine or hepatitis A immunoglobulin (IG) is recommended for postexposure prophylaxis and should be administered as soon as possible (within 2 weeks). Hepatitis A IG is 80–90% effective in preventing hepatitis A when administered within 2 weeks postexposure. A single dose of 0.02 mL/kg of IG provides effective protection for 3 months, and a dose of 0.06 mL/kg provides protection for 3–5 months (CDC, 2006c). Hepatitis A vaccine administration in exposed persons younger than 40 years of age appears to be as efficacious as IG in preventing disease. Owing to a paucity of data, hepatitis A IG is preferred among exposed persons older than 40 years or those with underlying medical illnesses, including chronic liver disease. In these groups, while hepatitis A IG is preferred, vaccine can be used if hepatitis A IG is unavailable. Persons who receive hepatitis A IG and who meet criteria for routine hepatitis A vaccination should initiate the vaccine series simultaneously with IG (at separate sites). Household and sexual contacts of, as well as people who have shared illicit drugs with, a person with serologically confirmed hepatitis A should receive postexposure prophylaxis.

Hepatitis A vaccine can be administered as pre-exposure prophylaxis to travelers to endemic areas. Persons who are either allergic to a vaccine component or elect not to receive the vaccine should receive a single dose of hepatitis A IG. Persons who are older than 40 years of age, immunocompromised, or have chronic liver disease should receive IG in addition to the vaccine if they plan to travel to a high-risk area within the next 2 weeks (prior to the development of optimal protection from vaccination).

HEPATITIS B VIRUS

Hepatitis B virus (HBV) can cause both acute and chronic hepatitis with viral transmission occurring via percutaneous or mucosal exposure to infectious blood or body fluids (e.g., saliva, semen). Prior to routine hepatitis B vaccination in the United States, 30–40% of chronic infections were attributable to perinatal or early childhood transmission. Chronic hepatitis B infection carries an increased risk of cirrhosis and hepatocellular carcinoma as well as liver failure and death, thus making the hepatitis B vaccine the first vaccine effective in preventing the development of a cancer. Routine screening of pregnant women for chronic infection and universal immunization of newborns and previously unvaccinated children have greatly reduced the incidence rate of acute hepatitis B in the United States. Additionally, vaccination of healthcare workers and adherence to universal precautions have also significantly decreased the occupational hazard of HBV infection. Adult groups at increased risk for infection in the United States include injection drug users, household contacts of persons with chronic HBV infection, developmentally disabled persons in long-term care facilities, hemodialysis patients, and persons with chronic liver disease or HIV infection. Persons engaging in higher-risk sexual behaviors, such as men who have sex with men, are also more likely to contract HBV infection. Travelers to HBV-endemic areas may also be at risk if they are involved in disaster relief activities, receive medical care, or partake in drug use or sexual activity. Vaccination for hepatitis B is recommended for long-term travelers. Pregnancy is not a contraindication to vaccination.

Available hepatitis B vaccine formulations in the United States contain recombinant hepatitis B surface antigen (HBsAg) and are available both as a single-antigen and combination formulations. The licensed single-antigen vaccines for adults are Recombivax HB and Engerix-B, both produced using recombinant HBsAg. The recommended dosing schedule is three injections at 0, 1, and 6 months, and the different formulations of the vaccine may be interchanged. Twinrix, a combination formulation of recombinant HBsAg and inactivated HAV, is also licensed for adult administration.

The response rate in adults less than 40 years of age is greater than 90% after the complete three-dose series. The protective antibody response diminishes in the elderly (only 75% of persons ≥ 60 develop protective antibody). Smoking, obesity, and immune suppression are also associated with lower response rates. Serologic testing for immunity is not necessary after routine vaccination of adults; however, it is recommended for healthcare workers and public safety workers, chronic hemodialysis patients, HIV-infected persons and other immune-compromised patients, and sex partners of HBsAg-positive persons. Testing should be performed 1–2 months after the completion of the series, and those with low anti-HBs concentrations (<10 mIU/mL) should be revaccinated with the three-dose series.

Hepatitis B immune globulin (HBIG) may be administered along with hepatitis B vaccine for postexposure prophylaxis or administered alone following exposure for nonresponders to prior hepatitis B vaccination. Postexposure prophylaxis with HBIG plus hepatitis B vaccine, hepatitis B vaccine alone, and HBIG alone have all been demonstrated to be effective in preventing HBV transmission. The effectiveness of HBIG postexposure decreases with delayed administration, and the recommended interval for administration is less than 7 days after a needle stick and less than 14 days for sexual exposures.

FURTHER CONSIDERATIONS

SPACING OF MULTIPLE IMMUNIZATIONS

Inactivated vaccines may be effectively administered either simultaneously or at any time before or after another vaccine. Nonsimultaneous administration of live vaccines, however, may lead to interference in the immune response and impaired protective effect. If live vaccines are not administered on the same day, their administration should be separated in time by at least 4 weeks. Exceptions to this rule are the live oral typhoid and yellow fever vaccines.

Blood and other antibody-containing blood products (e.g., intravenous immune globulin) may inhibit the response to live vaccines with the inhibition potentially lasting for greater than 3 months. The measles and rubella vaccines are particularly impaired in the setting of blood product administration; data regarding the mumps and varicella vaccines are more limited. No interference between blood products and Ty21a typhoid, yellow fever, or the live attenuated influenza vaccine has been observed, and with the exception of these three vaccines, the administration of a live vaccine should be delayed for at least 3 months after receipt of an antibody-containing blood product to allow sufficient degradation of the passive antibody (Ada, 2001).

SPECIAL RISK GROUPS

Timing of Vaccines for Persons with Immunosuppression

Immunosuppressed adults are at increased risk for severe infection with several vaccine-preventable infections. However, as discussed above, live vaccines should be deferred until immune function improves. Inactivated vaccines administered during periods of severe immunosuppression may have to be repeated after immune function has improved.

Although corticosteroid therapy alters immune competence, it is not a contraindication to vaccination with a live virus. Persons who may safely receive live virus vaccines include those receiving short-term oral corticosteroid

Table 4.3 INDICATIONS FOR VACCINES BY KEY RISK GROUPS

INDICATION

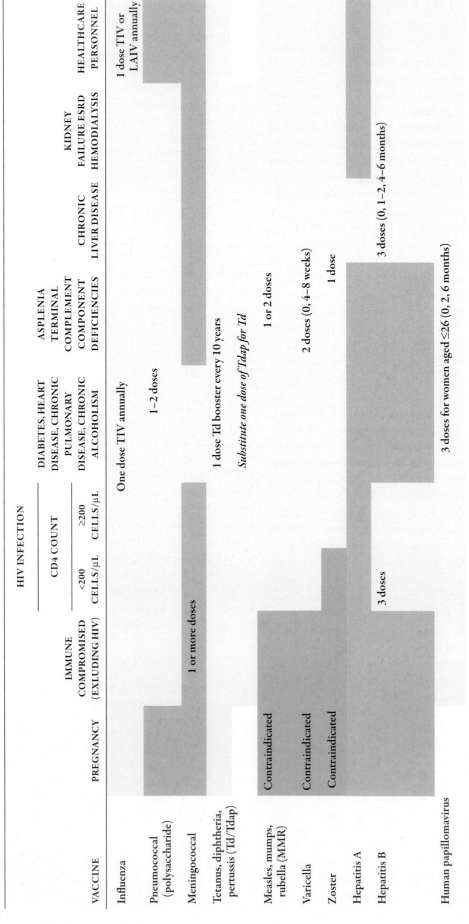

VACCINE	PREGNANCY	IMMUNE COMPROMISED (EXLUDING HIV)	HIV INFECTION CD4 COUNT <200 CELLS/µL	HIV INFECTION CD4 COUNT ≥200 CELLS/µL	DIABETES, HEART DISEASE, CHRONIC PULMONARY DISEASE, CHRONIC ALCOHOLISM	ASPLENIA TERMINAL COMPLEMENT COMPONENT DEFICIENCIES	CHRONIC LIVER DISEASE	KIDNEY FAILURE ESRD HEMODIALYSIS	HEALTHCARE PERSONNEL
Influenza					One dose TIV annually				1 dose TIV or LAIV annually
Pneumococcal (polysaccharide)					1–2 doses				
Meningococcal		1 or more doses							
Tetanus, diphtheria, pertussis (Td/Tdap)					1 dose Td booster every 10 years — Substitute one dose of Tdap for Td				
Measles, mumps, rubella (MMR)	Contraindicated					1 or 2 doses			
Varicella	Contraindicated					2 doses (0, 4–8 weeks)			
Zoster	Contraindicated					1 dose			
Hepatitis A							3 doses (0, 1–2, 4–6 months)		
Hepatitis B			3 doses				3 doses (0, 1–2, 4–6 months)		
Human papillomavirus					3 doses for women aged ≤26 (0, 2, 6 months)				

Yellow indicates for all persons in this category who meet the age requirements and lack evidence of immunity.
Gray indicates recommended if a risk factor is present.
Red indicates contraindicated

SOURCES: Patja A, Davidkin I, Kurki T, Kallio MJ, Valle M, Peltola H. Serious adverse events after measles-mumps-rubella vaccination during a 14-year prospective follow-up. Pediatr Infect Dis J. 2000;19:1127–34; Centers for Disease Control and Prevention. Recommendations of the Advisory Committee on Immunization Practices (ACIP). MMWR. 2008;57(early release):1–40; Centers for Disease Control and Prevention. Prevention of Herpes Zoster: recommendations of the Advisory Committee on Immunization Practices (ACIP). MMWR. 2008;57(early release):1–40; Centers for Disease Control and Prevention. Prevention of hepatitis A through passive or active immunization: Recommendations of the Advisory Committee on Immunization Practices (ACIP). MMWR. 2006;55(No. RR07):1–23. Adapted from the CDC guidelines for vaccines that may be indicated for adults based on medical conditions and other indications.

therapy (<2 weeks) or low- to moderate-dose therapy (<20 mg of prednisone daily) or are on replacement therapy.

Adults with anatomic or functional asplenia are at increased risk of infection by encapsulated bacteria, namely *S. pneumococcus, N. meningitides,* and *H. influenzae b.* If splenectomy is elective, vaccines against these agents should be administered at least 2 weeks prior to surgery. If not, they should be administered as soon as clinically possible. See table 4.3 for additional immunization recommendations for special risk groups.

Close Contacts of Immunocompromised Persons

Close contacts (including household members and care providers) of immunocompromised persons should receive all age-appropriate vaccines, including an annual influenza vaccine. Owing to the potential for shedding of live virus, household contacts of immunosuppressed persons should not receive the live oral polio virus; however, MMR and varicella virus vaccines are reasonably safe. As stated above, the trivalent influenza vaccine is preferred over the live attenuated virus vaccine.

on Immunization Practices (ACIP). *MMWR.* 2007c;56(No. RR02):1–23.

Centers for Disease Control and Prevention. Update: Prevention of hepatitis A after exposure to hepatitis A virus and in international travelers. Updated recommendations of the Advisory Committee on Immunization Practices (ACIP). *MMWR.* 2007d;56(41):1080–4.

Centers for Disease Control and Prevention. Recommended adult immunization schedule—United States, October 2007–September 2008. *MMWR.* 2007e;56(No. RR41):1–4.

Centers for Disease Control and Prevention. Prevention and control of influenza: Recommendations of the Advisory Committee on Immunization Practices (ACIP), 2008. *MMWR.* 2008a;57(early release):1–60.

Centers for Disease Control and Prevention. Prevention of herpes zoster: Recommendations of the Advisory Committee on Immunization Practices (ACIP). *MMWR.* 2008b;57(early release): 1–40.

Marin M, Broder KR, Temte JL, Snider DE, Seward JF, Centers for Disease Control and Prevention (CDC). Use of combination measles, mumps, rubella, and varicella vaccine: Recommendations of the Advisory Committee on Immunization Practices (ACIP). *MMWR.* 2010;59(RR-3):1–12.

Orenstein WA, Wharton M, Bart KJ, Hinman AR. Immunization. In: Mandell GL, Bennett JE, Dolin R, eds. *Principles and Practice of Infectious Diseases.* Philadelphia, PA: Elsevier; 2005:3557–89.

Patja A, Davidkin I, Kurki T, Kallio MJ, Valle M, Peltola H. Serious adverse events after measles-mumps-rubella vaccination during a 14-year prospective follow-up. *Pediatr Infect Dis J.* 2000;19:1127–34.

ADDITIONAL READINGS

Ada G. Vaccines and vaccination. *N Engl J Med.* 2001;345:1042–53.

Centers for Disease Control and Prevention. Prevention and control of meningococcal disease: Recommendations of the advisory committee on immunization practices (ACIP). *MMWR.* 2005;54(No. RR07):1–28.

Centers for Disease Control and Prevention. General recommendations on immunization: Recommendations of the Advisory Committee on Immunization Practices (ACIP). MMWR 2006a;55(No. RR15):1–48.

Centers for Disease Control and Prevention. Prevention of tetanus, diphtheria, and pertussis among adults: Use of tetanus toxoid, reduced diphtheria toxoid and acellular pertussis vaccine: Recommendations of the Advisory Committee on Immunization Practices (ACIP) and recommendation of ACIP, supported by the Healthcare Infection Control Practices Advisory Committee (HICPAC) for use of Tdap among health-care personnel. *MMWR.* 2006b;55(No. RR17):1–44.

Centers for Disease Control and Prevention. Prevention of hepatitis A through passive or active immunization: Recommendations of the advisory committee on immunization practices (ACIP). *MMWR.* 2006c;55(No. RR07):1–23.

Centers for Disease Control and Prevention. A comprehensive immunization strategy to eliminate transmission of hepatitis B virus infection in the United States: Recommendations of the advisory committee on immunization practices (ACIP) part II: Appendix A: Immunization management issues. *MMWR.* 2006d;55(No. RR16):25–29.

Centers for Disease Control and Prevention. A comprehensive immunization strategy to eliminate transmission of hepatitis B virus infection in the United States: Recommendations of the advisory committee on immunization practices (ACIP) part II. *MMWR.* 2006e;55(No. RR16):1–25.

Centers for Disease Control and Prevention. Recommended adult immunization schedule—United States, October 2007–September 2008. *MMWR.* 2007a;56 (No. RR41):1–4.

Centers for Disease Control and Prevention. Prevention of varicella: Recommendations of the Advisory Committee on Immunization Practices (ACIP). *MMWR.* 2007b;56(No. RR04):1–48.

Centers for Disease Control and Prevention. Quadrivalent human papillomavirus vaccine: Recommendations of the Advisory Committee

QUESTIONS

QUESTION 1. A 63-year-old man with rheumatoid arthritis begins therapy with a TNF-alpha inhibitor. Which vaccines should he receive as part of his routine primary care?

A. Trivalent inactivated influenza, pneumococcal polysaccharide vaccine, varicella zoster vaccine

B. Trivalent inactivated influenza, pneumococcal conjugated vaccine, varicella vaccine

C. Live attenuated influenza vaccine, pneumococcal conjugated vaccine, Tdap

D. Trivalent inactivated influenza, pneumococcal polysaccharide vaccine, Tdap

QUESTION 2. Which of the following adults should not receive Tdap?

A. A child daycare worker who last received Td 4 years ago

B. A 47-year-old man status post a gunshot wound to the leg who last received Td 7 years ago

C. A 27-year-old woman who is 1 week postpartum and last received Td 3 years ago

D. A 70-year-old man who last received Td 10 years ago and who has close contact with his 5-month-old grandson

QUESTION 3. A 28-year-old man undergoes splenectomy after a traumatic motor vehicle collision. Which of the following vaccines should he receive once his clinical condition stabilizes?

A. Pneumococcal conjugated vaccine, polysaccharide meningococcal vaccine (MPSV4, Menomune)

B. Pneumococcal polysaccharide vaccine, Hib, conjugate meningococcal vaccine (MenactraT)
C. Pneumococcal conjugated vaccine, Hib, conjugate meningococcal vaccine (MenactraT)
D. Pneumococcal polysaccharide vaccine, varicella zoster vaccine, Td

QUESTION 4. A 22-year-old woman presents for prenatal care prior to conception. She has not attended college and does not recall immunization with MMR (or any other immunizations) since childhood. On laboratory evaluation you find she has undetectable titers of varicella IgG. She does not want to receive more than two injections at a time. Which of the following vaccination schedules would be acceptable?

A. MMR and the trivalent inactivated influenza virus vaccine at the first visit, followed by the VZV vaccine 2 weeks later
B. Tdap and VZV vaccines at the first visit, followed by MMR and intranasal live attenuated influenza virus in 2 weeks
C. MMR and Tdap at the first visit, followed by the VZV vaccine in 4 weeks

QUESTION 5. Which of the following scenarios would be considered a contraindication to vaccination with the MMR vaccine?

A. A 23-year-old man with allergies to penicillin and sulfa who previously experienced an anaphylactic reaction to the influenza vaccine
B. A 45-year-old woman experiencing low-grade fevers and upper respiratory symptoms
C. A 37-year-old woman undergoing in vitro fertilization
D. A 45-year-old man whose wife underwent kidney transplantation

ANSWERS

1. D
2. D
3. B
4. C
5. C

5.

TROPICAL INFECTIONS

James H. Maguire

Diseases endemic to the tropics and subtropics remain major causes of morbidity and mortality in resource-poor areas of the world and are a challenge for practitioners in industrialized countries who care for returning travelers and immigrants. As a rule, the infectious diseases of travelers are different from or present differently than those of persons who have lived for long periods of time in endemic areas. For example, hepatitis A is rare among immigrants arriving from the tropics, who typically acquired infection and lasting immunity early in life, whereas travelers from industrialized countries lack immunity unless vaccinated and are at high risk of becoming infected during travel. In this review several of the most common clinical syndromes and the tropical infectious diseases that cause them are discussed.

FEVER

Fever following travel requires prompt attention because infections such as falciparum malaria, typhoid fever, and meningococcemia can be rapidly fatal. Prompt recognition of other illnesses such as hepatitis A, measles, viral hemorrhagic fevers, and pulmonary tuberculosis is necessary for timely implementation of infection control measures to prevent transmission to others. Leading causes of febrile illness in travelers who seek medical attention in travel clinics are listed in table 5.1.

MALARIA

Anopheles mosquitoes transmit malaria to several hundred million persons in the tropics and subtropics, of whom nearly 1 million die each year. Approximately 1500 cases of malaria are imported into the United States annually, and several persons die because of missed diagnosis or delay in diagnosis and failure to administer appropriate treatment in a timely fashion. The risk of malaria to travelers is highest in sub-Saharan Africa, Papua New Guinea, and several islands in the south

Pacific; lower in the Indian subcontinent; and lowest in Latin America and Southeast Asia. In the United States, more than half of the imported cases of malaria occur among persons who visit friends and relatives in their countries of origin and do not take proper chemoprophylaxis.

Clinical Features

Fever, rigors, headache, nausea, vomiting, myalgia, anemia, and thrombocytopenia occur in infections due to all species of *Plasmodium. P. falciparum* accounts for nearly all of the deaths from malaria because of its ability to infect erythrocytes of all ages and attain high parasitemias. It also expresses antigens on the surface of infected red blood cells that cause the cells to adhere to the endothelium of small blood vessels and block flow of blood; and it elicits production of high levels of tumor-necrosis factor and other cytokines. As a result, falciparum malaria progresses rapidly, and its various complications can mimic other infectious processes such as meningitis, encephalitis, pneumonia, hepatitis, and sepsis (table 5.2). In contrast, *P. vivax, malariae,* and *ovale*, are rarely fatal. Vivax and ovale malaria can relapse up to 4 years later or longer if treatment does not include primaquine, which eliminates persistent parasites in the liver. *Plasmodium knowlesi,* a parasite of rhesus monkeys, is responsible for a growing number of human infections, including fatal cases, in persons living in or traveling from forested areas of southeastern Asia.

Diagnosis, Treatment, and Prevention

Malaria should be considered in all persons who develop fever 1 week or longer after travel or residence in an endemic area, and thin and thick Giemsa-stained smears of peripheral blood should be examined by a skilled microscopist. Rapid tests that detect malaria antigens in the blood can be used to screen persons with fever, but microscopic examination of blood is necessary for confirmation of both negative and positive tests.

Table 5.1 COMMON CAUSES OF FEVER IN PERSONS ARRIVING FROM THE TROPICS

DISEASE	PERCENTAGE OF FEBRILE TRAVELERS WITH DISEASE
Malaria	25%
Dengue	6%
Rickettsial disease	2%
Enteric fever	2%
Diarrheal disease	15%
Respiratory illness	14%
Hepatitis	1%

SOURCE: Wilson ME, Weld LH, Boggild A, et al. *Clin Infect Dis.* 2007;44:1654.

Chloroquine is the drug of choice for infections due to *P. malariae* and *ovale* and chloroquine-sensitive strains of *P. vivax*, and can be used to treat chloroquine-sensitive strains of *P. falciparum*. After G6PD deficiency has been ruled out, primaquine should also be given to persons with *vivax* or *ovale* malaria to prevent relapses. *P. falciparum* should be considered chloroquine-resistant unless acquired in the Caribbean, Central America, parts of the Middle East, and North Africa. Drugs for treating falciparum malaria are listed in table 5.3. Two artemisin derivatives have become the drugs of choice: oral artemether-lumefantrine and, for severe cases, intravenous artesunate. Artemether and artesunate are faster acting and better tolerated than other antimalarials. They are always given with a second agent, such as lumefantrine, mefloquine, or atovaquone-proguanil to prevent recrudescences. Monotherapy with artemisinin derivatives has led to drug resistance in parts of Southeast Asia.

Chemoprophylaxis, as outlined in table 5.4, should be given to all travelers to malarious areas. Travelers should avoid mosquito bites by using repellents, protective clothing, insecticide-impregnated nets, and screens on windows.

Table 5.2 COMPLICATIONS OF FALCIPARUM MALARIA

Cerebral malaria (alterations of consciousness including coma)

Hypoglycemia

Noncardiac pulmonary edema, acute respiratory failure

Renal failure, including blackwater fever (hemoglobinuria)

Severe anemia

Lactic acidosis and shock

Jaundice, tender hepatomegaly

Diarrhea, dysentery, malabsorption

Placental dysfunction

Table 5.3 TREATMENT OF FALCIPARUM MALARIA

Mild to Moderate Cases	
Chloroquine-sensitive strains	Oral artemether-lumefantrine Oral chloroquine
Chloroquine-resistant strains	Oral artemether-lumefantrine or Oral atovaquone-proguanil or Oral quinine and either doxycycline or clindamycin

Severe Cases or Persons Unable to Take Oral Medications	
All strains	Intravenous artesunate (available through CDC in the United States) Intravenous quinidine gluconate and either doxycycline or clindamycin
Life-threatening cases	Exchange transfusion

BABESIOSIS

Babesiosis, a tick-borne protozoan disease, is rarely reported from tropical areas, but it is a life-threatening problem for residents of or travelers to endemic areas in the northeastern United States, Minnesota, Wisconsin, California, and Washington state. *Babesia microti* and other species of *Babesia* cause malaria-like illness with fever, splenomegaly, anemia, and thrombocytopenia. Asplenic persons, the elderly, and persons with debilitating diseases are at risk for high parasitemias, respiratory failure, and death. Mild to moderate illness is treated with atovaquone-proguanil; the combination of quinine and clindamycin is indicated for severe illnesses. Because the tick vector of *B. microti* may be co-infected with other pathogens, Lyme disease and anaplasmosis (ehrlichiosis) should be considered in persons who remain ill after appropriate treatment of babesiosis.

DENGUE

Dengue virus, transmitted primarily by daytime-biting *Aedes aegypti* mosquitoes in urban areas, infects more than 100 million persons a year in the Caribbean, Latin America, sub-Saharan Africa, tropical Asia, Australia, and the Pacific

Table 5.4 CHEMOPROPHYLAXIS OF MALARIA

Areas without chloroquine resistance	Chloroquine
Areas with chloroquine resistance	Doxycycline or Atovaquone-proguanil or Mefloquine (not certain border areas in Southeast Asia)
Terminal prophylaxis for vivax, ovale malaria	Primaquine (G-6-PD screen)

Islands. Increasing numbers of cases among tourists and other returning travelers have paralleled the global resurgence and rapid spread of dengue. After an incubation period of 3–7 days and occasionally longer, there is an abrupt onset of fever, chills, headache, myalgia, arthralgia, diffuse lymphadenopathy, neutropenia, and thrombocytopenia. An erythematous macular rash occurs in about 50% of cases. Life-threatening dengue hemorrhagic fever and dengue shock syndrome from capillary leak occur among persons who experience a second infection but with a different serotype.

A clinical diagnosis of dengue is confirmed by serological tests. Viral isolation or PCR-based assays to detect virus are not widely available. Treatment is supportive because no antiviral therapy is available. Currently there is no dengue vaccine, and infection is avoided by prevention of mosquito bites.

RICKETTSIAL INFECTIONS

Rickettsia africae, the agent of African tick typhus, has become a common cause of fever among travelers returning from safaris or other outdoor activities in sub-Saharan Africa, especially in southern Africa. Patients present with fever, headache, myalgia, regional lymphadenopathy, leukopenia, and thrombocytopenia and an erythematous lesion with a black necrotic center at the site of the tick bite (figure 5.1). Rashes are usually absent. The diagnosis is confirmed by serological tests, and the illness responds quickly to doxycycline. Travelers may encounter other tickborne rickettsial infections in different parts of the world. The spotted fever group includes Rocky Mountain spotted fever due to *Rickettsia rickettsii* in the Americas and Mediterranean spotted fever (boutonneuse fever) due to *Rickettsia conorii* in southern Europe, northern Africa, and western Asia. Scrub typhus (tsutsugamushi fever) is caused by *Orienta tsutsugamushi*, which is transmitted by the bite of larval mites in the Far East, South Pacific, and Australia.

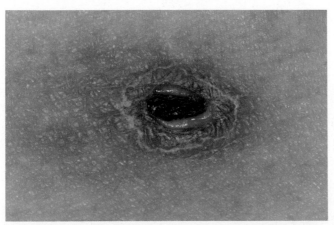

Figure 5.1. Ulcerative lesion with eschar in a traveler with African tick bite fever.

TYPHOID

Salmonella enterica serotype Typhi (*S. typhi*) and serotype Paratyphi (*S. paratyphi*) cause enteric fever in persons who ingest fecally contaminated food or water. The risk is highest for travelers to the Indian subcontinent, Southeast Asia, Africa, and Latin America.

Clinical Features

Typhoid fever is characterized by the gradual onset of rising temperatures, rigors, and headache followed by sustained high fevers (often with a comparatively slow pulse), abdominal pain, and hepatosplenomegaly. Constipation is frequent, but up to 50% of patients have diarrhea. Complications include bowel perforation, intestinal bleeding, and shock.

Diagnosis, Treatment, and Prevention

Diagnosis is made by culture of blood, stool, urine, or bone marrow. Ciprofloxacin, other fluoroquinolones, and ceftriaxone are active against most isolates, but increasing resistance to fluoroquinolones and cephalosporins has made azithromycin the drug of choice in some areas of India.

Prevention of typhoid fever includes avoidance of contaminated food and water and vaccination, either with a single dose of polysaccharide vaccine (Vi) or four doses of oral attenuated live Ty21a vaccine. Neither vaccine is 100% protective, and neither prevents infection with *S. paratyphi*.

MENINGOCOCCAL INFECTION

Meningococcal meningitis and meningococcemia occur throughout the world, but risk is high in the "meningitis belt" of sub-Saharan Africa, which extends from Senegal to Ethiopia during outbreaks in the dry months of November to June. Outbreaks also have occurred during the Hajj. Prompt diagnosis and treatment with ceftriaxone, cefotaxime, or chloramphenicol, which is still used in developing areas, are essential for preventing fatalities, neurological deficits, and gangrene. Quadrivalent vaccine should be administered to travelers to high-risk destinations.

LEPTOSPIROSIS

Transmission of *Leptospira interrogans* occurs by contact of skin or mucous membranes with fresh water or moist soil contaminated with the urine of rodents and other mammals. Infection of animals occurs worldwide, and outbreaks have been associated with flooding, military operations, ecotourism, white-water rafting, and other water sports.

Leptospirosis presents with fever, headache, myalgia, conjunctival suffusion, and often hepatosplenomegaly or rash. Complications include aseptic meningitis and Weil syndrome with hepatitis, intense jaundice, renal insufficiency, and hemorrhage. The diagnosis is usually made with serological tests, although the organism can be identified by dark field microscopy or culture on special media. Doxycycline, penicillins, or ceftriaxone are equally effective for treatment, and weekly doxycycline can prevent infections in persons with unavoidable exposures.

DIARRHEA

Diarrhea is the most common health problem of travelers to the tropics and developing countries. Bacterial infections are the most frequent cause of travelers' diarrhea, and most cases present acutely and resolve within a week. The most common pathogens, enterotoxigenic *Escherichia coli*, *Salmonella*, *Campylobacter*, and *Shigella* respond to short courses of fluoroquinolones or azithromycin; the latter is active against fluoroquinolone-resistant Campylobacter, which is becoming more prevalent in parts of the world. Persistent diarrhea, that is, lasting at least 2–3 weeks, is a common problem that prompts returning travelers to seek health care. Table 5.5 lists the principal causes of persistent diarrhea.

INTESTINAL PROTOZOA

Intestinal protozoan infections, including giardiasis, amebiasis, cryptosporidiosis, and cyclosporiasis account for many cases of persistent diarrhea in returning travelers. All are transmitted by ingestion of fecally contaminated drink or water containing the cyst stage and, with the exception of *Cyclospora cayetanensis*, can be transmitted by direct person-to-person contact. *Giardia*, *Cryptosporidium*, and *Cyclospora* infect the small bowel and cause voluminous watery stool, often with nausea, vomiting, or malabsorption. *Entamoeba histolytica* infects the colon and causes dysentery with cramping and frequent, bloody, small-volume stools. Amebiasis may also cause episodes of nondysenteric diarrhea that may alternate with periods of constipation.

Evaluation of persistent diarrhea should include three stool examinations for ova and parasites in a qualified laboratory. Antigen tests of stool are available for individual pathogens (*Giardia*, *Cryptosporidium*, *E. histolytica*), but these will miss less common protozoa that cause diarrhea, such as *C. cayetanensis*, *Isospora belli*, and *Dientamoeba fragilis*, and intestinal helminths. *E. histolytica* cannot be differentiated from the nonpathogenic *E. dispar* by microscopy, and specific diagnosis may require a special stool antigen tests or PCR-based technique.

Treatment depends on the pathogen: metronidazole or tinidazole for giardiasis; metronidazole or tinidazole plus an agent effective in the lumen of the bowel such as paromomycin or iodoquinol for amebiasis; trimethoprim-sulfamethoxazole for cyclosporiasis and *I. belli* infection; and nitazoxanide for cryptosporidiosis.

SKIN DISEASES

Common dermatological problems among persons returning from warm tropical areas include sunburn, insect bites, dermatophyte infections, superficial streptococcal and staphylococcal infections, scabies, and sexually transmitted diseases such as herpes simplex and syphilis. The most common cause of fever and maculopapular rash among travelers is dengue. Because some of the causes of fever and maculopapular rash can be life threatening, patients with these symptoms deserve immediate attention (see table 5.6).

Table 5.5 CAUSES OF PERSISTENT DIARRHEA IN TRAVELERS RETURNING FROM THE TROPICS

Infections
Intestinal protozoan infections (giardiasis, amebiasis, cryptosporidiosis, cyclosporiasis, and isosporiasis)
Intestinal helminth infections (schistosomiasis, strongyloidiasis)
Infection with enteroadherent *Escherichia coli*, *Plesiomonas*, *Aeromonas*
Clostridium difficile colitis
Prolonged episodes of common enteric bacterial infections (salmonellosis, shigellosis, *Campylobacter* infection)
Tropical sprue (infectious agent not identified)
Underlying Gastrointestinal Unmasked by Enteric Infections
Inflammatory bowel disease
Celiac sprue
Colonic malignancies
Postinfectious Processes
Lactase deficiency
Bacterial overgrowth with malabsorption
Irritable bowel syndrome

Table 5.6 DIFFERENTIAL DIAGNOSIS: FEVER AND DIFFUSE MACULAR RASH IN TRAVELERS RETURNING FROM TROPICS AND SUBTROPICS

Dengue
Enterovirus infection
Acute EBV or HIV infection
Measles
Chikungunya
Lassa fever, Marburg virus infection
Syphilis
Rickettsial infections
Leptospirosis
Drug reaction
Others

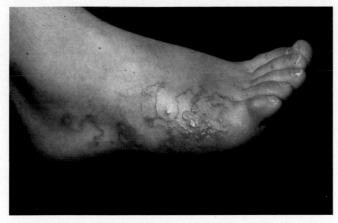

Figure 5.2. Cutaneous larva migrans.

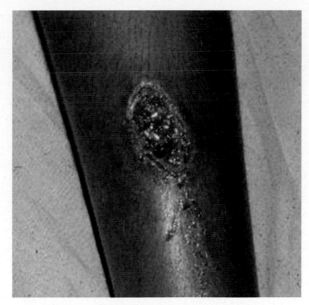

Figure 5.3. Cutaneous leishmaniasis.

Persons with exposure to beaches and other sandy areas may present with cutaneous *larva migrans,* and travelers to nature parks and persons with exposure to rural and forested areas may return with myiasis or cutaneous leishmaniasis.

CUTANEOUS LARVA MIGRANS (CREEPING ERUPTION)

Cutaneous larva migrans occurs when larval forms of the dog or cat hookworm penetrate bare skin following contact with moist, sandy soil contaminated with animal feces in tropical and subtropical climates. Larvae migrate through the skin a rate of 2 to 4 cm/day and produce a pruritic, elevated, erythematous, serpiginous rash, often with vesicles (see figure 5.2). The diagnosis is made by inspection, and treatment is with either a 3-day course of albendazole or a single dose of ivermectin.

FURUNCULAR MYIASIS

Larvae (maggots) of the human botfly, *Dermatobium hominis,* in Latin America and the tumbu fly, *Cordylobia anthropophaga,* in Africa penetrate human skin and produce boil-like lesions, in which they develop and grow until they emerge spontaneously several weeks later. Patients complain of pain and a sensation of movement within the lesions, and close examination reveals a central punctum through which the organism breathes. The maggots can be extracted by occluding the punctum with petrolatum jelly and squeezing the boil or making a small incision in the skin.

CUTANEOUS LEISHMANIASIS

Tiny phlebotomine sand flies transmit over 20 different species of the protozoan *Leishmania* in warm climates throughout the world except in Australia, Southeast Asia, and the South Pacific. Parasites replicate at the site of the insect bite and produce slow- or nonhealing, painless nodules or more commonly, ulcers with heaped-up edges (see figure 5.3).

The diagnosis is made by identifying parasites by culture, smears, or histopathology of specimens taken by biopsy, needle aspirate, or scrapings of the ulcer base. Treatment, which may be topical or systemic, is based on the site of the lesion, species of parasite, and geographic origin. Drugs of choice include antimonials such as sodium stibogluconate, amphotericin-containing compounds, topical paromomycin, and others. Adequate treatment of lesions caused by *Leishmania braziliensis* in Latin America is necessary to prevent mucosal leishmaniasis, which causes destructive and disfiguring lesions of the upper airways.

COMMON CHRONIC INFECTIONS OF IMMIGRANTS

Immigrants may harbor chronic infections that place them at risk for serious complications in the future. Although latent tuberculosis is the most common, clinicians should consider parasitic diseases such as strongyloidiasis, schistosomiasis, Chagas disease, cysticercosis, filariasis, echinococcosis, and other infections when evaluating immigrants, including those who left their native countries years or decades ago. Peripheral blood eosinophilia may be the first indication of a number of infectious and noninfectious conditions associated with travel (table 5.6).

AMERICAN TRYPANOSOMIASIS (CHAGAS DISEASE)

Trypanosoma cruzi, the agent of American trypanosomiasis or Chagas disease, infects approximately 8–10 million persons in Mexico and Central and South America and perhaps as many as 300,000 immigrants living in the United States. Most infected persons acquired their infection while living in poorly constructed houses in rural areas infested by the vector triatomine bug (kissing bug, reduviid bug). Infection also occurs via blood transfusion, organ transplantation from infected donors, from an infected mother to the fetus in utero, and occasionally by ingestion of soups or juices contaminated with triatomine bugs or their parasite-laden feces. Screening of blood donors since 2007 in over 75% of blood banks in the United States has identified nearly 1500 infected donors, nearly all immigrants from endemic areas, but also a small number of persons who acquired infection from the insect vector in the southern United States. Several Latin American countries have eliminated both insect-borne and transfusion-associated transmission to human beings, and control programs in the other endemic countries are making progress towards interruption of transmission.

Clinical Features

Infection is lifelong and, in most cases, asymptomatic. Acute infection may present with a mononucleosis-like illness or acute myocarditis or meningoencephalitis, but it is usually not recognized. Only 20–30% of persons with chronic infection develop symptoms, which appear after a latent period of two or more decades. Chronic Chagas heart disease is a progressive cardiomyopathy that causes congestive heart failure, sudden cardiac death, arrhythmias, and heart block; right bundle branch block is present in most persons who become ill. Denervation of the esophagus or colon leads to megaesophagus or megacolon and difficulty swallowing or defecating, respectively. Persons with advanced HIV infection or receiving immunosuppressing medications may experience reactivation of infection with fever, acute myocarditis, and focal lesions of the brain or skin.

Diagnosis and Treatment

The diagnosis of acute or reactivated infection is made by visualizing parasites in the blood or tissues. The diagnosis of chronic infections requires identification of specific antibodies by at least two different types of serological test (e.g., immunoflourescent antibody and enzyme-linked immunosorbent assay (ELISA)). Treatment is with either nifurtimox or benzimidazole, oral medications available in the United States from the Centers for Disease Control (CDC). Treatment is indicated for all acute or reactivated infections, chronic infections in all persons 18 years old or younger, and in selected cases of chronic infection in older persons. Supportive measures include cardiac medications or cardiac transplant for cardiomyopathy and dietary modification and surgery for megaesophagus or megacolon.

INTESTINAL ROUNDWORM INFECTIONS

Clinical Features

The roundworms *Ascaris lumbricoides,* the whipworm *Trichuris trichiura,* and the hookworms *Necator americanus* and *Ancylostoma duodenale* infect greater than 1 billion persons in warm climates where sanitation is inadequate. Infection with adult worms lasts about 1 year for persons with ascariasis, 4 to 7 years for those with trichuriasis, and occasionally longer for persons with hookworm infection.

Most infected persons are infected with a small number of worms and have no symptoms. Peripheral blood eosinophilia is prominent during larval migration during the first several months of infection and then subsides to low levels or, in the case of *Ascaris,* subsides altogether. Moderately heavy infection with adult worms in children can impair growth and cognitive development. Heavy infection can lead to intestinal obstruction due to a bolus of adult *Ascaris* in the lumen of the small bowel, iron deficiency anemia from hookworms attaching to small bowel mucosa and feeding on blood, and dysentery or rectal prolapse from whipworms embedded in colonic mucosa. Obstruction of the biliary or pancreatic ducts by a single or few adult *Ascaris* can cause biliary colic, cholangitis, or pancreatitis.

Diagnosis, Treatment, and Prevention

Diagnosis is made by microscopic identification of eggs in stool or occasionally by identification of adult worms passed in feces. Depending on the infection, treatment is with one to three doses of oral albendazole, mebendazole, pyrantel pamoate, or ivermectin. Infection is prevented by avoiding eating uncooked vegetables or other foods that may be contaminated, hand washing before meals, drinking clean water, and wearing shoes to prevent contact of bare skin with contaminated soil.

SCHISTOSOMIASIS (BILHARZIA)

Clinical Features

Approximately 200 million persons in South America, the Caribbean, Africa, the Middle East, the People's Republic of China, Southeast Asia, and the Philippines suffer from infection with schistosomes, flukes that live in the lumen of veins that drain the intestines or lower urinary tract. Infection is acquired when cercariae (larval parasites) penetrate skin during contact with fresh water containing the snail intermediate host. Acute schistosomiasis occurs 2–8 weeks after infection in previously uninfected persons and is an important cause of fever and eosinophilia, typically in returning travelers but not immigrants.

Chronic schistosomiasis is seen more commonly among immigrants from endemic areas than in short-term travelers.

Adult worms live about 3–5 years but can persist for as long as 30 years. Schistome eggs that are trapped in tissue elicit an immune response with granulomas and fibrosis, which are responsible for the disease. Chronic infections are usually light and asymptomatic, and eosinophilia is present in fewer than half of infected persons. Heavy infections can cause chronic diarrhea, hepatic fibrosis, and portal hypertension with splenomegaly and esophageal varices (*Schistosoma mansoni, japonicum*), or hematuria, bladder polyps, urinary tract infections, obstructive uropathy, and bladder cancer (*S. hematobium*). Aberrant deposition of eggs in the brain or spinal cord can lead to cerebral mass lesions, seizures, focal neurological signs, and transverse myelitis.

Diagnosis, Treatment, and Prevention

All persons with a history of fresh water contact in an endemic area should be evaluated for schistosomiasis. Serological tests are more sensitive than microscopic examination of urine or stool for eggs. Praziquantel is the drug of choice. Infection is prevented by avoiding snail-infested fresh water bodies in endemic countries.

STRONGYLOIDIASIS

Infection with the intestinal roundworm *Strongyloides stercoralis* occurs worldwide, but it is most common in developing areas with poor sanitation, where infection results from contact of bare skin with larvae on fecally contaminated soil. Because *Strongyloides* can complete its life cycle within its host, infection persists for decades. Direct person-to-person transmission can occur because infective larvae are shed in the stool.

Clinical Features

Asymptomatic infections are common, but 75% of persons have peripheral blood eosinophilia. When present, symptoms of chronic strongyloidiasis include abdominal pain and intermittent diarrhea and pruritic rashes, including urticaria and a migrating rash called *larva currens*. Persons with HTLV-1 infection (but not HIV infection) and immunosuppressed persons, especially those receiving corticosteroids, may develop highly lethal hyperinfection with dissemination of larvae throughout the body.

Diagnosis, Treatment, and Prevention

Strongyloidiasis should be ruled out in any person who may have been exposed to infection and is receiving or about to receive immunosuppressive therapy. Serology is more sensitive than microscopic examination of stool, which requires special techniques and multiple specimens because the number of larvae shed in the stool is small. The drug of choice is one or two doses of ivermectin for chronic infection and

longer courses for hyperinfection. The alternative, albendazole, is less effective even when given for 10 days or longer. Treatment of hyperinfection or disseminated strongyloidiasis requires longer courses of ivermectin, and a successful outcome may require reversal of immunosuppression.

CYSTICERCOSIS

Cysticercosis, infection with the larval stage of the pork tapeworm, *Taenia solium,* is acquired by ingestion of eggs shed in the stool of a person harboring an adult tapeworm in the intestinal tract. Infection with the adult tapeworm, which can live for several decades, develops when pork containing cysticerci is ingested without proper cooking. Pork tapeworms are transmitted in developing areas with poor sanitation and inadequate inspection of meat. Mexico, Central America, northern South America, Haiti, Dominican Republic, Cape Verdes, India, and the Philippines are areas with a high prevalence of infection. Transmission of cysticercosis can occur wherever there is an adult tapeworm carrier, including in the United States and other nonendemic countries.

Clinical Features

Most persons harboring an adult tapeworm have no symptoms other than passing egg-laden tapeworm segments in the stool. Cysticerci, fluid-filled cysts containing the tapeworm scolex, typically cause no symptoms while they are alive and able to evade the host immune response. Symptoms occur on average 2 to 5 years after infection, when degenerating cysts provoke an inflammatory response. Cysts in the central nervous system cause seizures, hydrocephalus,

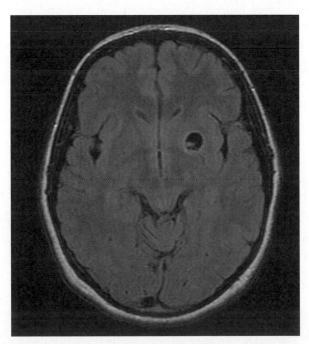

Figure 5.4. Cysticercosis: MR showing fluid-filled cyst with scolex.

aseptic meningitis, increased intracranial pressure, and other complications.

Diagnosis, Treatment, and Prevention

MR or CT scans identify cysticerci in the brain and spinal cord (figure 5.4). Serologic tests confirm the clinical suspicion of cysticercosis, but these may be negative in persons infected with one or a few cysts that have not begun to degenerate. Microscopic examination of stool identifies only about 30% of adult tapeworm carriers. Segments of tapeworms passed in the stool need to be distinguished from segments of the beef tapeworm, *T. saginata*. Treatment of cysticercosis is with oral albendazole or praziquantel. Corticosteroids and anticonvulsants may be needed to prevent seizures and other complications resulting from the inflammatory response to degenerating cysts. Adult tapeworm carriers respond to single doses of either niclosamide or praziquantel. Cysticercosis is prevented by identifying and treating persons harboring an adult tapeworm. In endemic areas, handwashing and avoiding food or water potentially contaminated with *T. solium* eggs are important as well. Prevention of infection with the adult tapeworm requires proper cooking of pork.

SUMMARY

- Potentially life-threatening infections such as falciparum malaria, typhoid fever, and meningococcal infection should always be considered in travelers returning from the tropics.

- Falciparum malaria can present with neurological, pulmonary, gastrointestinal, and other complications and can be rapidly fatal if not treated promptly.

- Important viral causes of fever and macular rashes in travelers include dengue, enteroviral infection, measles, acute HIV infection, and others.

- Ulcerative lesions covered with an eschar in travelers with fever suggest rickettsial infection; painless ulcers in travelers without fever suggest cutaneous leishmaniasis; and boil-like lesions with a sensation of movement within suggest myiasis (infestation with a fly larva).

- Travelers with more than 2 weeks of diarrhea should be evaluated for protozoan, helminthic, and bacterial infections; underlying gastrointestinal diseases unmasked by diarrhea; and postinfectious conditions that cause malabsorption.

- Asymptomatic immigrants from endemic areas should be evaluated for infections that put them at risk for severe complications in the future. Examples include latent tuberculosis, American trypanosomiasis,

strongyloidiasis and other intestinal roundworm infections, schistosomiasis, cysticercosis, and others.

ADDITIONAL READING

CDC, USPHHS, PHS. *Health Information for International Travel 2012*. Atlanta, GA: CDC. http://wwwn.cdc.gov/travel/content/yellowbook/home-2012.aspx.

Drugs for Parasitic Infections. *The Medical Letter*. www.medletter.com.

Guerrant RL, Walker DH, Weller PF, eds. *Tropical Infectious Diseases: Principles, Pathogens and Practices*. 3d ed. Edinburgh: Elsevier; 2011.

Keystone JS, Kozarsky PE, Freedman DO, Nothdurft HD. eds. *Travel Medicine*. 2nd ed. Philadelphia, PA: Mosby; 2008.

Strickland GT, ed. *Hunter's Tropical Medicine and Emerging Infectious Diseases*. 9th ed. Philadelphia, PA: W. B. Saunders; 2000.

Walker P, Barnett ED, eds. *Immigrant Medicine*. Philadelphia, PA: Saunders Elsevier; 2007.

QUESTIONS

QUESTION 1. Which of the following is a complication of chronic Chagas disease (American trypanosomiasis)?

    A. Hydrocephalus
    B. Esophageal varices
    C. Rectal prolapse
    D. Sudden death
    E. Megaloblastic anemia

QUESTION 2. A 42-year-old woman returning from a 3 day business trip to India presents to the emergency department, 3 days after her return home, with an abrupt onset of fever, chills, headache, myalgia, and arthralgia, She also describes pain behind her eyes. On physical examination, her vital signs are normal with a blood pressure of 132/60 mm Hg and a heart rate of 88 beats per min. Her temperature is 38.2°C. She has diffuse lymphadenopathy and an erythematous macular rash that blanches under pressure.

Which of the following statements is FALSE?

    A. The presence of an eschar (erythematous lesion with black necrotic center) on physical examination would point to rickettsial infection.
    B. The most likely diagnosis is dengue fever; however, workup for malaria is essential.
    C. Thick and thin blood films for malaria parasites should be performed.
    D. A macular rash on the abdomen or chest suggests the possibility of rose spots from typhoid fever.
    E. Cutaneous leishmaniasis is the most likely diagnosis because of the skin lesions and the lymphadenopathy.

QUESTION 3. Which one of the following statements about malaria is correct?

    A. Malaria is naturally transmitted by the bite of a female *Aedes aegypti* mosquito.

B. *Plasmodium vivax* is the most dangerous form of malaria.

C. Evidence shows that mosquito nets are not useful in reducing infection and transmission of malaria.

D. *P. falciparum* is responsible for about 90% of the deaths from malaria.

E. Primaquine is necessary to prevent relapses of falciparum malaria.

1. A
2. E
3. D

6.

SEXUALLY TRANSMITTED DISEASES

Sigal Yawetz and Jennifer A. Johnson

A wide variety of infectious agents are sexually transmitted (see table 6.1), causing an array of disease manifestations that are frequently not confined to the genital tract. According to the most recent Centers for Disease Control (CDC) surveillance data from 2009, the most common reportable sexually transmitted diseases (STDs) in the United States are chlamydia, gonorrhea, and primary and secondary syphilis, respectively, and the annual incidence of chlamydia and early syphilis is still increasing. Case reporting for more common STDs, such as genital *herpes simplex* virus (HSV), trichomonas, and human papilloma virus (HPV) infections is not required. In this chapter several of the most common ulcerative and nonulcerative STDs are discussed. The viral hepatitides (A, B, and C) and HIV merit individual attention and are not addressed in this chapter. Vaginitis and HPV are also not discussed here.

THE ULCERATIVE STDs

In the United States, HSV and syphilis are the most common causes of genital ulcers, with chancroid occurring infrequently and other ulcerative STDs occurring only rarely. For evaluating a patient with genital ulcers, the history and physical (table 6.2) are essential but often misleading, and diagnostic testing is important. All patients presenting with genital ulcers should undergo testing for herpes and syphilis, whereas testing for chancroid (*H. ducreyi* culture of the leading edge of the lesion) and lymphogranuloma venereum should be reserved for individuals at increased risk. However, given limitations of testing modalities, providers should consider empirical treatment of the most likely diagnosis while awaiting laboratory test results; despite comprehensive evaluation, it is estimated that at least 25% of patients with genital ulcers never have a laboratory-confirmed diagnosis. Ulcerative STDs are also co-factors for HIV transmission. Routine HIV screening is now recommended for all adult and sexually active adolescent patients; however, regardless of prior testing,

all patients newly diagnosed with syphilis or chancroid should undergo HIV testing, and HIV testing should also be strongly considered for those diagnosed with genital herpes infections.

GENITAL HSV

Epidemiology

It is estimated that in 2007, 50 million adolescents and adults in the United States were infected with HSV-2, the most common cause of genital herpes infections: approximately 16.2% of all US residents 14–49 years of age. These estimates are based on serologic testing for HSV-2 and do not include genital HSV-1 infections. Large epidemiologic surveys suggest that as many as 70–90% of HSV-2–seropositive individuals are not aware of their infection yet may still transmit the infection to others. Risk factors for HSV-2 infections in the United States include female gender, duration of sexual experience, African-American ethnicity, and history of prior genital infections. Other risk factors may include number of sex partners and socioeconomic status. A previous HSV-1 infection in an individual does not affect the likelihood of HSV-2 acquisition, but it does decrease the likelihood of developing a symptomatic infection with HSV-2.

Etiology and Pathogenesis

HSV is a double-stranded DNA virus. There are two human HSV types, which are distinguished based on their envelope glycoproteins: HSV-1 (glycoprotein G1) and HSV-2 (glycoprotein G2). Most genital HSV infections are caused by HSV-2, although the proportion of HSV-1 as the cause for genital HSV among adolescents and young women is increasing over time, and in young American women HSV-1 may now account for the majority of newly acquired genital HSV infections.

Initial genital HSV infection occurs through direct contact of the virus with the genital mucosa or nonintact skin in

Table 6.1 MAJOR CAUSATIVE AGENTS IN STDs

Viruses: HSV-1 and -2, HPV, Molluscum contagiosum, Hepatitis (A, B, C), CMV, HIV, HTLV

Bacteria: *N. gonorrhoeae, H. ducreyi* (chancroid), *Klebsiella granulomatis* (granuloma inguinale), *G. vaginalis* and other mixed flora (BV, PID), Spirochetes (*T. pallidum*/syphilis), *Chlamydia trachomatis, Mycoplasma hominis, Mycoplasma genitalium,* and *Ureaplasma urealyticum* (NGU, PID)

Protozoa: *Trichomonas vaginalis, Entamoeba histolytica, Giardia lamblia*

Ectoparasites: *Phthirius pubis* (crab louse), *Sarcoptes scabei* (scabies)

the genital area. *Primary infection* occurs when an individual acquires HSV-1 or HSV-2 without previously having antibodies to either viral type. A *nonprimary first episode* occurs when an individual who has antibodies to one viral type (e.g., HSV-1) acquires the other viral type (e.g., HSV-2) for the first time. During primary infection HSV infects cells in the epidermis and dermis and then becomes latent in the sensory neuron. Reactivation of viral replication in the sensory ganglia may result in subclinical viral shedding or in symptomatic outbreaks. A *recurrent infection* occurs when an HSV-1 or HSV-2 lesion develops in an individual with pre-existing antibodies to the same HSV type. *Subclinical shedding* occurs when HSV can be isolated from a patient without symptoms. Recurrence and subclinical shedding are more common with HSV-2 than HSV-1 genital infection and in immunocompromised hosts. In patients with HSV-2 infection, viral shedding occurs at roughly the same rate for those who are symptomatic as for those who are asymptomatic.

Clinical Manifestations

The classic presentation of genital herpes, present in about 60–70% of patients is painful, clustered vesicular lesions. However, symptoms of primary genital HSV infections may range from asymptomatic infection to a severe systemic illness. Severe illness presents with multiple, bilateral, painful, or pruritic genital lesions. The lesions are vesicular, pustular, or ulcerated. Common associated symptoms include fever, myalgias, malaise, headache, dysuria, and inguinal lymphadenopathy. Nonprimary first episodes are more likely to have less severe symptoms or be asymptomatic.

Symptoms of recurrent HSV infections are less severe than primary or nonprimary first episodes, and the duration of symptoms and viral shedding are typically shorter. Lesions of recurrent HSV are usually unilateral and systemic symptoms are infrequent. Approximately 50% of patients with recurrent episodes describe a typical prodrome of neuropathic symptoms in the nerve distribution of the skin lesions, such as pruritus, tingling, or shooting pains. Recurrent genital herpes episodes are more common with HSV-2 than HSV-1, although the frequency is variable for both. Recurrences are earlier and more frequent in patients with more severe primary infection and in immunocompromised hosts.

Atypical presentations of genital HSV include vulvovaginitis or proctitis, often with fissures, urethritis, and cervicitis. HSV-2, the major cause of genital HSV, may also cause extragenital syndromes. These may include other skin or mucosal sites (e.g., erythema multiforme, herpes labialis), meningitis (often recurrent), hepatitis, and disseminated skin and visceral infections (which are more common in the immunocompromised host).

Diagnosis

Viral culture of the lesion remains the preferred diagnostic method for HSV disease, but the sensitivity of this method varies by the features of the disease. Rates of isolation of HSV are higher for primary lesions as compared to those of recurrent disease and decline as lesions begin to heal and crust over. More rapid testing for viral antigen by direct fluorescent antibody (DFA) may be performed within several hours. Polymerase chain reaction (PCR) testing for HSV DNA is the preferred test for diagnosis of HSV in the

Table 6.2 FEATURES OF GENITAL ULCERS BY ETIOLOGY

	HSV	SYPHILIS	CHANCROID	LGV	DONOVANOSIS (GRANULOMA INGUINALE)
Ulcer	Painful, often many, papules	Painless	Painful, purulent, irregular, deep	Small, painless, heals before lymph nodes	Large, irregular, bleeding
Lymph nodes	Rare in primary infection	Small	1–2 weeks later	Large draining nodes	None, hypertrophied tissue
Comments	Common	Must test for and treat	Unusual in the U.S.	At risk populations	Rare in the U.S.

Table 6.3 TREATMENT OF GENITAL HSV DISEASE

TREATMENT OF PRIMARY EPISODE	TREATMENT OF RECURRENT EPISODES	DAILY SUPPRESSIVE THERAPY
Acyclovir, 400 mg orally tid for 7–10 days, or 200 mg orally 5 times daily for 7–10 days, OR	Acyclovir, 400 mg orally tid for 5 days, or 800 mg orally bid for 5 days, or 800 mg tid for 2 days, OR	Acyclovir, 400 mg orally bid, OR
Famciclovir, 250 mg orally tid for 7–10 days, OR	Famciclovir, 125 mg orally bid for 5 days, or 1 g orally bid for 1 day, OR	Famciclovir, 250 mg orally bid, OR
Valacyclovir, 1 g orally bid for 7–10 days	Valacyclovir, 500 mg orally bid for 3 days, or 1 g orally once daily for 5 days	Valacyclovir, 500 mg orally once daily, OR Valacyclovir, 1 g orally once daily

cerebrospinal fluid (CSF); it is currently not approved for testing of genital specimens.

Serologic testing for antibodies to HSV type-specific gly-coproteins (GP-G1 and G2 for HSV-1 or -2) has a sensitivity of 80–98% and specificity of >96%. Serologic testing may be helpful in evaluating culture-negative ulcers and is potentially helpful in identifying asymptomatic carriers, assessing and counseling partners of infected individuals, and STD screening. However, serologic testing is limited by a lag time to the development of antibodies after initial exposure, and the fact that a positive result only indicates a previous exposure and may not be diagnostic of concurrent lesions.

Treatment

Treatment of genital HSV disease is usually aimed at control of symptoms, prevention of symptomatic outbreaks, and prevention of shedding and transmission. Treatment does not eradicate the latent virus. Systemic antiviral agents are the treatment of choice; topical therapy has minimal effect on shedding and symptoms. Specific regimens, based on the clinical syndrome, are outlined in table 6.3. Treatment of a first episode decreases symptom duration and shedding. Episodic therapy for outbreaks will decrease symptoms if administered during the prodrome, at the onset of an outbreak, or within 1 day of the appearance of a lesion. Daily suppressive therapy may reduce the frequency of outbreaks by 70–80% for patients who experience frequent (e.g., more than six annually) anogenital HSV outbreaks. Abstinence during outbreaks and routine condom use should be discussed as measures to reduce transmission to others, although condoms provide incomplete protection against transmission of HSV. Suppressive therapy may be given to HSV-2–infected individuals to reduce transmission to sero-negative partners.

Pregnancy

Genital HSV infection during pregnancy poses a risk to both the developing fetus and the newborn. Approximately 10% of HSV-2–seronegative pregnant women have partners who are HSV-2 seropositive. The overall rate of HSV-1 or HSV-2 sero-conversion during pregnancy in the United States is about 2%. Most new infections in pregnant women are asymptomatic, and most neonatal HSV disease is in infants born to asymptomatic mothers. The risk of transmission is highest during primary infection (30–50%), followed by nonprimary first episode, and then recurrent disease (<1%). Pregnant women should be treated with systemic antiviral medications for active outbreaks. Cesarean section is offered to women with symptoms of genital HSV or visible lesions at the time of delivery in order to reduce the risk of neonatal HSV disease.

Immunocompromised Hosts

Atypical clinical presentations of anogenital HSV including more severe and prolonged symptoms are more common in immunocompromised patients, and HSV viral shedding is more common in HIV-infected individuals. The treatment of HSV in immunocompromised patients is outlined in table 6.4. For severe HSV disease in immunocompromised patients, acyclovir, 5 mg/kg intravenously every 8 hours, should be considered. HSV acyclovir resistance is rare. However, in immunocompromised hosts HSV resistance to acyclovir may be seen, and foscarnet should be considered in the treatment of acyclovir-resistant HSV disease.

SYPHILIS
Background and Epidemiology

Syphilis is caused by the spirochete bacteria *Treponema pallidum*. Between 1990 and 2000 rates of early syphilis in the

Table 6.4 TREATMENT OF HSV INFECTION IN HIV-INFECTED PATIENTS

REGIMENS FOR DAILY SUPPRESSIVE THERAPY FOR HSV IN HIV-INFECTED PATIENTS	REGIMENS FOR EPISODIC HSV INFECTION IN HIV-INFECTED PATIENTS
Acyclovir 400–800 mg orally twice or three times daily, OR	Acyclovir 400 mg orally three times daily for 5–10 days, OR
Famciclovir 500 mg orally twice daily, OR	Famciclovir 500 mg orally twice daily for 5–10 days, OR
Valacyclovir 500 mg orally twice daily	Valacyclovir 1 g orally twice daily for 5–10 days

United States had declined, but since 2001 rates have been increasing. The rising incidence of syphilis is primarily due to outbreaks in large cities among men who have sex with men (MSM). Until 2009, rates among women have been increasing as well, but rates of congenital syphilis continue to decline.

Transmission and Clinical Manifestations

Early syphilis includes all stages of syphilis within the first year after infection. This includes primary infection, secondary infection, and early latent infection. *Late syphilis* includes all stages of syphilis after the first year since acquisition. This includes late latent infection and tertiary syphilis. *Latent syphilis* includes any case of asymptomatic syphilis infection: early within the first year of acquisition and late thereafter.

Sexual transmission of *T. pallidum* occurs through direct exposure to an open lesion during primary and secondary infection. The incubation period before the development of primary syphilis is up to 90 days. *Primary infection* is characterized by a painless ulcer, or chancre, at the site of inoculation. The painless nature of the lesion often helps to distinguish it from the lesions of chancroid and genital herpes; however, the painless chancre often goes unnoticed. *Secondary infection* results from systemic dissemination and occurs 2 to 8 weeks after the appearance of the chancre in about 25% of untreated patients. Rarely, the primary chancre is still present when secondary infection develops. The most common presentation is a generalized skin rash. Lesions are usually discrete pink or red macules or pustules, beginning on the trunk and bilateral proximal extremities. Any surface of the body may be involved, and, although their involvement suggests the diagnosis, the palms (see figure 6.1) and soles are not always involved. Systemic symptoms of fever, headache, myalgia, malaise, and lymphadenopathy are common. Other common skin manifestations include mucocutaneous lesions, condylomata lata, and alopecia. Other organ involvement may lead to hepatitis, ulcerative gastroenteritis, synovitis, immune-mediated glomerulonephritis, and nephrotic syndrome. *Tertiary infection* may involve any organ system, but the most common form in the United States is neurosyphilis followed by cardiac manifestations and gummatous lesions. *Neurosyphilis* can occur at any stage of infection. When symptomatic, symptoms may include cognitive, motor, or sensory deficits, ophthalmic disease (e.g., uveitis or optic neuritis), auditory symptoms, cranial nerve palsies, or symptoms of meningitis. Tabes dorsalis is the slow degeneration and demyelination of the dorsal column of the spinal cord associated with neurosyphilis, leading to a variety of deficits including weakness, diminished reflexes, gait disturbances, and paresthesias (e.g., formication).

Diagnosis

The definitive diagnostic tests for early syphilis are direct visualization of the spirochete by dark field microscopy or DFA testing of exudate from a lesion. However, these require expertise and are often not attainable. The most commonly used diagnostic tool for syphilis is serology, with tests falling into two categories: the nontreponemal tests and the treponemal tests (see table 6.5). The nontreponemal tests are the Venereal Disease Research Lab (VDRL) and the rapid plasma reagin (RPR). They are used primarily as screening tools, and their titers are used to follow response to therapy. The two tests are equally valid, but the results of both tests cannot be directly compared, so only one should be followed over time in a single patient. Nontreponemal tests may be negative in 20–30% of patients with a primary chancre. The tests may also be negative in approximately 2% of patients with secondary syphilis due to a prozone phenomenon, in which a high antigen burden in undiluted serum leads to an a false positive result. In this case, dilution

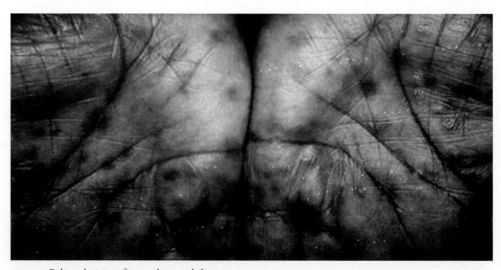

Figure 6.1 Palmar lesions of secondary syphilis

Table 6.5 SEROLOGIC TESTS FOR SYPHILIS

	TEST FEATURES	CLINICAL UTILITY	COMMENTS
Nontreponemal tests: RPR VDRL	Quantitative tests, high sensitivity (lower in HIV patients), poor specificity	Often screening tests, titers important to guide treatment for every patient	RPR false negatives with prozone phenomenon—dilute the sample
Treponemal tests: FTA-abs TP-PA EIA	Qualitative tests, high sensitivity and specificity (some false positive with EIA)	Used for confirmation of nontreponemal tests (only EIA used in screening)	Remain positive for life in most patients, despite treatment

of the sample will correct the results. Negative results are also seen in a proportion of patients with late untreated or previously treated syphilis. The treponemal tests are qualitative assays using *T. pallidum* antigens; they include the fluorescent treponemal antibody absorbed (FTA-abs) and the *T. pallidum* particle agglutination (TP-PA). These tests are more specific and are used to confirm infection. The treponemal tests may be negative in a proportion of patients with primary syphilis but remain positive for life, despite treatment, in >90% of patients. Several newer tests are available including the *T. pallidum* enzyme immunoassays (CAPTIA, using native *T. pallidum* antigens, and ICE, using recombinant *T. pallidum* antigens) and the *T. pallidum* Western blot. The *T. pallidum* enzyme immunoassays (EIA) tests have a high sensitivity and may be automated, so are useful for high-volume screening but are not widely used at present. All patients diagnosed with syphilis should also be tested for HIV.

Nontreponemal serologic tests may be negative in as many as 25% of patients with neurosyphilis. The diagnosis of neurosyphilis is made by CSF analysis. CSF analysis is recommended for patients with suspected neurosyphilis, patients with known syphilis and neurologic, ophthalmic, or otic symptoms, patients with active tertiary disease, and patients with treatment failure. Many authorities recommend CSF examination for all HIV-infected patients with latent syphilis or syphilis of unknown duration. It remains

controversial whether CSF analysis should be performed for all patients with latent syphilis and a nontreponemal titer of 1:32 or greater. CSF analysis should include a cell count, protein level, and CSF-VDRL titer. The CSF protein and CSF white blood cell (WBC) count are usually elevated, but these finding are nonspecific. The CSF-VDRL is specific but not sensitive for diagnosing neurosyphilis. When positive, titers are used for follow-up. When neurosyphilis is suspected clinically, empirical treatment should be strongly considered even when the CSF-VRDL is negative.

Treatment

The preferred treatment for syphilis, at any stage of disease, is parenterally administered penicillin G (benzathine, aqueous procaine, or aqueous crystalline, but not combination benzathine-procaine). For nonpregnant patients who are allergic to penicillin, alternative therapy may include doxycycline and tetracycline. Ceftriaxone may also be considered, but the data to support its use are lacking. Pregnant women with syphilis should always be treated with penicillin-based regimens, even if this requires desensitization in the case of a penicillin allergy. Penicillin-based therapies are the only regimens that have clearly been shown to be effective during pregnancy, including prevention of transmission to the fetus. Treatment regimens depend on the stage of infection (see table 6.6).

Table 6.6 TREATMENT OF SYPHILIS

STAGE OF INFECTION	PREFERRED REGIMEN	ALTERNATIVE REGIMEN*
Primary, secondary, or early latent syphilis	Benzathine penicillin G, 2.4 million units as a single intramuscular injection	Doxycycline, 100 mg orally twice daily (or tetracycline, 500 mg orally four times daily) for 14 days
Late latent syphilis, latent syphilis of unknown duration, or tertiary syphilis	Benzathine penicillin G, 2.4 million units intramuscularly once weekly for 3 weeks	Doxycycline, 100 mg orally twice daily (or tetracycline 500 mg orally four times daily for 28 days)
Neurosyphilis	Aqueous crystalline penicillin G, 18–24 million units intravenously per day, as continuous infusion or divided doses every 4 hours, for 10–14 days	Procaine penicillin, 2.4 million units intramuscularly once daily PLUS Probenecid, 500 mg orally four times daily, both for 10–14 days

NOTE: *Alternative regimens should not be used for pregnant patients. Pregnant women with penicillin allergies should be desensitized in order to receive penicillin-based treatment.

Follow-up After Treatment

After treatment of syphilis all patients should be followed clinically and by nontreponemal test titer (RPR or VDRL). There are no definitive criteria for cure or treatment failure, but the primary goals of treatment are resolution of symptoms and a sustained decrease in titer of fourfold or greater (e.g., 1:32 decreases to 1:8). Such response is expected by 6–12 months in patients with early treatment and 12–24 months in patients with late treatment. Titers are checked at months 6 and 12 for all patients; in addition they are checked at months 18 and 24 for patients with neurosyphilis and at month 24 for patients with late syphilis. RPR titers in HIV-infected patients are followed more closely with testing at 3, 6, 9, 12, and 24 months after treatment. Patients with neurosyphilis should have a repeat CSF analysis at 6 months to follow up VDRL titers. Before treatment is considered a failure, patients with persistent signs or symptoms of active disease and those who fail to achieve a fourfold decrease in RPR or VDRL (or have an increase in RPR or VDRL titer) should be evaluated for reinfection. If treatment failure is still suspected, CSF analysis should be performed. If the CSF analysis is normal, these patients receive an additional course of benzathine penicillin G 2.4 million units intramuscularly once weekly for 3 weeks, and follow-up testing is resumed. All patients with treatment failure should be screened for HIV.

Management of Sex Partners

Individuals who report sexual contact with persons with any stage of syphilis should be evaluated and tested, and treatment should be considered. Contacts with positive serologic tests for syphilis after exposure should be treated according to the stage of their disease. Contacts who are seronegative after exposure to a sex partner with syphilis should be empirically treated for primary syphilis if the exposure occurred within 90 days prior to the partner's diagnosis of primary, secondary, or early latent syphilis or if patient follow-up for repeat testing and treatment is uncertain.

LYMPHOGRANULOMA VENEREUM

Lymphogranuloma venereum (LGV) is a relatively infrequent genital ulcerative disease in the United States, caused by three serovars (L1, L2, and L3) of *Chlamydia trachomatis*. However, recent outbreaks have been reported in large U.S. cities in MSM. The primary lesion of LGV, a small papule or ulcer that is often painless, usually presents 3–30 days following exposure and often goes unnoticed by the patient. Patients more commonly present for medical attention after developing unilateral painful lymphadenopathy, characteristic of the secondary stage of infection, which occurs approximately 2–6 weeks after exposure.

Clinical manifestations at this stage may also include systemic symptoms, local cellulitis, buboes, and proctocolitis (purulent, mucoid, or bloody) in the case of anal exposure. Late manifestations are the result of fibrosis and scarring and may include chronic ulceration, anal fistulae and strictures, genital elephantiasis, and male and female infertility. Diagnostic testing is not well standardized, and providers must often rely on clinical suspicion to guide treatment. Culture of genital or lymph node specimens has a poor sensitivity for diagnosis of LGV. Nucleic acid amplification tests (NAAT) for *C. trachomatis* may be helpful for genital samples, but further testing to distinguish LGV subtypes is not always available, and this testing is not widely available for rectal samples. Chlamydia serologies by complement fixation (CF; positive titer is 1:64 or greater) or microimmunofluorescence (MIF; positive titer is 1:128 or greater) may be useful to support a clinical diagnosis where testing is available, but the interpretation of results has not been well standardized. The preferred regimen for treatment of LGV is doxycycline, 100 mg orally twice daily for 21 days. Alternative regimens, with less supporting data, are erythromycin, 500 mg orally four times per day for 21 days, or azithromycin, 1 g orally once weekly for 3 weeks. Treatment of local complications of LGV (e.g., drainage of buboes) may also be necessary. Asymptomatic sex partners of patients with LGV should be treated with doxycycline 100 mg orally twice daily for 7 days or azithromycin 1 g orally as a single dose.

GRANULOMA INGUINALE

Granuloma inguinale or donovanosis is rare in the United States but endemic in some tropical areas and developing nations. This ulcerative disease is caused by *Klebsiella granulomatis*, formerly known as *Calymmatobacterium granulomatis*, which is an intracellular pathogen and therefore difficult to culture. Clinically this disease usually manifests as progressive, painless, highly vascular ulcerative lesions, which may bleed easily. Lymphadenopathy is usually not present. Diagnosis is usually by identification of dark-staining Donovan bodies within a tissue crush preparation or biopsy sample. There are no serologic or PCR-based assays available for this disease. The preferred treatment for granuloma inguinale is doxycycline, 100 mg orally twice daily for at least 21 days. Alternative regimens for treatment are azithromycin, 1 g orally once weekly, ciprofloxacin, 750 mg orally twice daily, erythromycin, 500 mg orally four times per day, or trimethoprim-sulfamethoxazole, 160 mg/800 mg (one double-strength tablet) orally twice daily, each for at least 21 days. If lesions persist at the end of the 21-day treatment course, treatment should be continued until all lesions are completely healed. Parenteral aminoglycosides may be added in the event of treatment failure or for pregnant women because other recommended regimens may not be safe for the fetus.

CHANCROID

Chancroid is also rare in the United States, occurring primarily in discrete outbreaks in endemic areas, most often among patients who are also infected with HIV or other ulcerative STDs. The disease is caused by *Haemophilus ducreyi* and usually manifests as a painful genital ulcer with tender suppurative inguinal lymphadenopathy. The painful and irregular nature of the ulcer distinguishes it from the syphilitic chancre. Definitive diagnostic testing by culture of *H. ducreyi* from the leading edge of the lesion carries a sensitivity of <80% and can be performed only at the limited number of sites with access to the required special culture media. Because diagnostic testing is limited, clinical diagnosis is often important for the purposes of treatment and surveillance. A probable clinical diagnosis of chancroid rests on four criteria: (1) presence of one or more painful genital ulcers; (2) absence of evidence of syphilis, either by dark field examination of the ulcer exudate or by serologic testing performed more than 7 days after the appearance of the ulcer; (3) clinical appearance of the ulcer and lymphadenopathy consistent with chancroid; and (4) negative tests for HSV of the ulcer exudate. The preferred treatment regimens for chancroid are azithromycin 1 g orally in a single dose or ceftriaxone 250 mg intramuscularly in a single dose. Ciprofloxacin and erythromycin may also be used in 3-day courses, but resistance to these medications has been reported.

THE NONULCERATIVE STDS

GENITAL *CHLAMYDIA TRACHOMATIS* INFECTIONS

Epidemiology

Genital chlamydia is the most commonly reported infectious disease in the United States. It is caused by serovars D-K of the intracellular bacterium *C. trachomatis*. The highest infection rate is among women younger than 25 years of age. Asymptomatic infection is common, accounting for 50–75% of cases in women and up to 50% of cases in men. Risk factors among women include age, unmarried status, multiple sex partners, a recent new sex partner, inconsistent use of condoms, mucopurulent cervicitis and cervical ectopy, prior STD, and lower socioeconomic status.

Clinical Manifestations

When symptomatic, *C. trachomatis* may cause a urethritis, prostatitis, epididymitis, and proctitis in men, and cervicitis, urethritis, pelvic inflammatory disease, and perihepatitis (Fitz-Hugh-Curtis syndrome) in women. Patients may also develop *reactive arthritis*, formerly known as Reiter syndrome, more commonly in men but also in women. If left untreated, up to 40% of women with chlamydia will develop pelvic inflammatory disease (PID) and be at risk for further complications of PID such as ectopic pregnancy, chronic pelvic pain, and infertility. *C. trachomatis* may also be transmitted to the neonate from exposure to a mother's infected cervix during delivery. Neonatal chlamydial infections may have ophthalmic, pulmonary, or urogenital manifestations, often with sustained sequelae, so screening and treatment of pregnant women are particularly important.

Diagnosis

Cell culture techniques for *C. trachomatis* have a very low sensitivity. Therefore, nucleic acid amplification tests (NAAT), which are highly sensitive and specific, have replaced cell culture in the diagnosis of chlamydial infections. These tests are the most sensitive when performed on endocervical or urethral specimens but can also be performed on urine. Rectal swabs are not well standardized. Antigen testing (DFA) and nucleic probe assays are also available, but they require an endocervical or urethral specimen.

Screening programs for *C. trachomatis* infections in young women have been shown to reduce the rates of lower genital tract infections and their long-term complications, as well as associated medical costs. For this reason some practice guidelines and state health departments strongly recommend routine screening for chlamydia for all pregnant women, women younger than 25 years of age, and women 25 or older with risk factors. There is no evidence to support routine screening for men at this time, except in high-risk populations such as MSM, adolescents, patients at STD clinics, and incarcerated patients in correctional facilities.

Treatment and Follow-up

Treatment of genital *C. trachomatis* infection is aimed not only at resolution of symptoms but also prevention of complications of infection and prevention of transmission to sexual partners and neonates. Treatment options for both pregnant and nonpregnant patients are described in table 6.7. Single-dose azithromycin may be given as directly observed therapy on site and thus is particularly recommended for patients with poor treatment compliance or unreliable follow-up. Azithromycin has recently replaced erythromycin as the preferred therapy for pregnant patients. Patients diagnosed with gonococcal infections should also be empirically treated for *C. trachomatis* because co-infection is common. Patients undergoing treatment should be instructed to abstain from sexual intercourse for 7 days and until all sex partners have been treated; sex partners should be treated even if asymptomatic. Patient-delivered partner therapy may be considered if the sex partner is unlikely to seek evaluation and treatment; however, this is not

Table 6.7 TREATMENT OF GENITAL *C. TRACHOMATIS* INFECTIONS

	PREFERRED REGIMEN	ALTERNATIVE REGIMEN
Nonpregnant patients	Azithromycin, 1 g orally as a single dose, OR Doxycycline, 100 mg orally bid for 7 days	Erythromycin base, 500 mg orally four times daily for 7 days, OR Erythromycin ethylsuccinate, 800 mg orally four times daily for 7 days, OR Ofloxacin, 300 mg orally bid for 7 days, OR Levofloxacin, 500 mg orally once daily for 7 days
Pregnant patients	Azithromycin, 1 g orally as a single dose, OR Amoxicillin, 500 mg orally tid for 7 days	Erythromycin base, 500 mg orally four times daily for 7 days, or 250 mg orally four times daily for 14 days, OR Erythromycin ethylsuccinate, 800 mg orally four times daily for 7 days, or 400 mg orally four times daily for 14 days

recommended for MSM because of the high prevalence of other STDs that require more thorough evaluation.

Unless poor treatment adherence is suspected or symptoms persist, test of cure (repeat testing 3–4 weeks after treatment) of *C. trachomatis* infection is not recommended except for pregnant patients. However, repeated infections are common and are usually due to reacquisition after treatment rather than to antibiotic resistance. Women should therefore be rescreened for *C. trachomatis* infection 3–4 months after treatment or when they next present for care. In order to ensure prevention of transmission to the neonate, all pregnant women should have a test of cure approximately 3 weeks after completing therapy.

GONORRHEA

Background

Gonorrhea is the second most commonly reported STD in the United States. It is caused by *Neisseria gonorrhoeae*, a Gram-negative diplococcus. Co-infection with *C. trachomatis* is common.

Clinical Manifestations

Asymptomatic infection may occur in both men and women but is much less common in men. An asymptomatic lower-tract infection in a woman may still lead to upper-tract infection (PID) with complications such as infertility, chronic pelvic pain, and ectopic pregnancy. When symptomatic, genital manifestations include urethritis, epididymitis, prostatitis, cervicitis, and PID. Extragenital manifestations may include pharyngitis, proctitis, conjunctivitis, or disseminated gonococcal infection (DGI) from gonococcal bacteremia. DGI commonly causes acral skin lesions (petechiae or raised pustules on a red base; see figure 6.2A,B), unilateral tenosynovitis, and polyarticular septic arthritis. Less commonly, DGI may cause hepatitis, meningitis, or endocarditis. Neonates may acquire *N. gonorrhoeae* infection from cervical exudates during delivery. Manifestations of neonatal disease may include ophthalmic complications, arthritis, meningitis, or frank sepsis.

Diagnosis

Available diagnostic tests for gonorrhea include Gram stain, culture, DNA probes, and nucleic acid amplification techniques. A Gram stain of urethral smear exudate from symptomatic men, looking for intracellular Gram-negative diplococci, has a high sensitivity and specificity, but this test performs poorly in asymptomatic men and women. When a specimen is collected for culture, viability of the fastidious organism on a cotton swab is limited, and therefore the exudate must be quickly transferred to an appropriate culture medium, such as a modified Thayer-Martin medium. Culture remains the gold standard for diagnosis and the test of choice for diagnosis of *N. gonorrhoeae* infection of nongenital sites (e.g., pharynx, rectum). Culture is also useful for antimicrobial susceptibility testing in cases of suspected treatment failure. For genital disease, testing by nonculture assays is rapid and reliable. DNA probes have a high sensitivity and specificity for cervical and urethral specimens, and NAATs have a high sensitivity and specificity for cervical, urethral, and urine samples. Screening for gonorrhea is suggested for women at risk, including pregnant women at risk and women younger than 25 years of age. Testing for other STDs, including HIV, syphilis, and chlamydia, should be strongly considered for all patients diagnosed with gonorrhea.

Treatment

Since the incidence of quinolone-resistant *N. gonorrhoeae* (QRNG) infection is significant and increasing, the preferred treatment for gonococcal infections is with cephalosporin-based regimens (see table 6.8). All patients who are being treated for gonorrhea should also be empirically treated for chlamydia unless infection is ruled out. All sex partners of patients diagnosed with gonorrhea should be referred for evaluation and treatment. Patient-delivered partner therapy may be considered if the sex partner is unlikely to seek evaluation and treatment; however, this is not recommended for MSM because of the high prevalence of other STDs requiring more thorough evaluation. Patients undergoing treatment should be instructed to

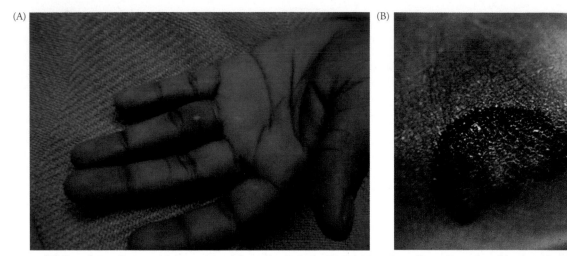

Figure 6.2. (A) *Pustule in a Patient with Disseminated Gonorrhea Infection (DGI).* Note the red base. Contributed by Anna R. Thorner, MD. Published on the Partners Infectious Disease Images website, www.idimages.org. Copyright Partners Healthcare System, Inc. (B) *Petechial Lesion in a Patient with Disseminated Gonorrhea Infection (DGI).* Note the red base. Contributed by Arnold N. Weinberg, MD. Published on the Partners Infectious Disease Images website, www.idimages.org. Copyright Partners Healthcare System, Inc.

abstain from sexual intercourse until both they and their partners have completed treatment and are no longer symptomatic. Because spectinomycin is not available in the U.S., azithromycin 2 g orally may be considered for pregnant women who cannot tolerate a cephalosporin.

NON-GONOCCOCAL URETHRITIS AND EPIDIDYMITIS

Etiologies and Clinical Manifestations

Non-gonococcal urethritis (NGU) may result from a variety of pathogens, and the etiology is often unknown. The most common cause of NGU is *C. trachomatis* infection, but *Ureaplasma urealyticum*, *Mycoplasma genitalium*, *Trichomonas vaginalis*, enteric bacteria, HSV, and adenovirus may also cause NGU. By definition, urethritis must be present to support the diagnosis of NGU. Urethritis may present with symptoms of dysuria, urethral discharge, or pelvic pain.

Diagnosis

All patients with urethritis, or suspected urethritis, should be tested for chlamydia and gonorrhea. NGU is defined as urethritis with negative testing for gonorrhea. Urethritis is diagnosed by the presence of a mucopurulent urethral discharge or smear of urethral discharge showing at least 5 WBC per high-power field or a positive leukocyte esterase test or >10 WBC per high-power field in a first-void urine specimen. Detection of other pathogens causing NGU may be difficult, so empirical treatment is often recommended.

Treatment

The preferred treatment regimens for NGU are azithromycin, 1 g orally as a single dose, or doxycycline, 100 mg orally twice daily for 7 days. Azithromycin may be more advantageous, with slightly increased efficacy for treatment of

Table 6.8 TREATMENT OF GONORRHEA

	PREFERRED REGIMEN	ALTERNATIVE REGIMEN*
Uncomplicated infections of the cervix, urethra or rectum	*Ceftriaxone* 250 mg IM in a single dose OR, IF NOT AN OPTION *Cefixime* 400 mg orally in a single dose PLUS Treatment for Chlamydia	
Uncomplicated pharyngeal infections	Ceftriaxone 250 mg IM in a single dose PLUS Treatment for Chlamydia	
Disseminated infection	*Ceftriaxone* 1 g intramuscularly or intravenously every 24 hours	*Cefotaxime* 1 g intravenously every 8 hours OR *Ceftizoxime* 1 g intravenously every 8 hours

* If severe cephalosporin allergy, azithromycin 2 g orally is effective against uncomplicated gonococcal infection. Due to concerns over emerging resistance cephalosporin following desensitization is favored especially in complicated cases.

U. urealyticum, M. hominis, and M. genitalium and because the single dose may be given on site as directly observed therapy. Erythromycin, ofloxacin, and levofloxacin may also be used as alternative treatment regimens. Sex partners should be referred for evaluation and treatment, and patients should abstain from sexual intercourse until they and their partners have been treated and symptoms have resolved.

Follow-up

Patients with persistent symptoms after treatment should be tested for *T. vaginalis* by culture of urethral swab or first-void urine specimen. Repeat testing for *C. trachomatis* and *N. gonorrhoeae* should be considered when reinfection may have occurred. Empirical retreatment with azithromycin should also be considered if initial treatment was with doxycycline, given the difference in efficacy for some causative agents. Empirical additional treatment with a single 2-g oral dose of metronidazole or tinidazole should be administered to patients with persistent urethral inflammation without an identifiable pathogen.

PELVIC INFLAMMATORY DISEASE

Etiology

PID is a general term for inflammation of the female upper genital tract involving any combination of the reproductive pelvic organs (uterus, ovaries, fallopian tubes) and surrounding peritoneum. Infections are often polymicrobial. The sexually transmitted pathogens *N. gonorrhoeae* and *C. trachomatis* are frequently involved. Other associated pathogens include *G. vaginalis*, enteric Gram-negative rods, anaerobes, *H. influenzae*, *M. hominis*, *U. urealyticum*, *M. genitalium*, and cytomegalovirus (CMV). In women with a retained intrauterine device (IUD), *Actinomyces istarlii* may be involved. PID caused by *Mycobacterium tuberculosis* infections is seen in endemic areas. Fitz-Hugh Curtis syndrome, or perihepatitis, is the extension of gonococcal or chlamydial PID to the liver capsule without significant parenchymal involvement.

Complications

Early diagnosis and initiation of therapy for PID are essential because the long-term sequelae can be devastating and costly. PID may lead to ectopic pregnancies, chronic pelvic pain, and infertility. Sex partners of patients with PID should be tested for STDs and treated appropriately to reduce the risk of reinfection. There is an increased risk of PID during the first few weeks after IUD insertion.

Diagnosis

PID is a clinical diagnosis that may be challenging because of the broad spectrum of manifestations of the disease. PID is often associated with only mild symptoms, resulting in a

Table 6.9 **TREATMENT OF PID**

	PREFERRED REGIMEN	ALTERNATIVE REGIMEN
Oral therapy (for outpatients)	*Ceftriaxone* 250 mg IM in a single dose PLUS *Doxycycline* 100 mg orally twice a day for 14 days **WITH or WITHOUT** *Metronidazole* 500 mg orally twice a day for 14 days **OR** *Cefoxitin* 2 g IM in a single dose and Probenecid, 1 g orally in a single dose PLUS *Doxycycline* 100 mg orally twice a day for 14 days **WITH or WITHOUT** *Metronidazole* 500 mg orally twice a day for 14 days **OR** Other parenteral third-generation cephalosporin (e.g., ceftizoxime or cefotaxime) **PLUS** *Doxycycline* 100 mg orally twice a day for 14 days **WITH or WITHOUT** Metronidazole 500 mg orally twice a day for 14 days	
Parenteral therapy (for patients requiring hospitalization)	*Cefotetan* 2 g intravenously every 12 hrs, or *Cefoxitin* 2 g intravenously every 6 hours **PLUS** *Doxycycline* 100 mg orally or intravenously every 12 hours **OR** *Clindamycin* 900 mg intravenously every 8 hours, **PLUS** *Gentamicin* intravenously	*Ampicillin/sulbactam* 3 g intravenously every 6 hours, **PLUS** *Doxycycline* 100 mg orally or intravenously every 12 hours

delay in diagnosis. A diagnosis of PID is presumed in sexually active young women experiencing pelvic or lower-abdominal pain, without another identified cause, who have cervical motion or uterine or adnexal tenderness. Additional features to support the diagnosis of PID include fever, purulent cervical or vaginal discharge, abundant WBC on wet preparation of vaginal secretions, elevated erythrocyte sedimentation rate (ESR) or C-reactive protein (CRP), and diagnosis of *C. trachomatis* or *N. gonorrhoeae* genital infection. Diagnosis may be confirmed by endometrial biopsy, transvaginal ultrasound, MRI, or laparoscopic examination, but these tests are not frequently utilized. All patients with PID should be also be evaluated for pregnancy.

Treatment

Even when endocervical testing is negative, treatment of PID must include therapy for both *C. trachomatis* and *N. gonorrhoeae* (see table 6.9). It remains unclear whether the addition of treatment for anaerobic pathogens is of added clinical benefit. PID is often treated with outpatient oral therapy, but hospitalization is appropriate for severe disease. Indications for hospitalization for PID may include pregnant patients, patients clinically not responding to oral therapy, patients unable to tolerate outpatient regimens, patients with severe symptoms such as nausea and vomiting, patients in whom surgical diagnoses (e.g., appendicitis) have not been excluded, and patients with tubo-ovarian abscess.

BACTERIAL VAGINOSIS

Bacterial vaginosis (BV) is the most common cause of vaginal discharge or malodor. It is caused by the replacement of normal vaginal flora (*Lactobacillus* species) with other bacteria (*Gardnerella vaginalis*, *Mycoplasma hominis*, *Prevotella* sp., and *Mobiluncus* sp.). Although the development of BV seems to be related to sexual activity, the pathogenesis is poorly understood, and it is unclear whether the pathogens are actually sexually transmitted. BV is most frequently diagnosed by clinical criteria including a thin white vaginal discharge with a fishy odor (whiff test), the presence of clue cells (vaginal epithelial cells with a stippled appearance) on wet-prep examination, and a vaginal fluid pH > 4.5. Gram stain, used to identify the relative concentrations of vaginal bacteria, may be useful, but culture of *G. vaginalis* is not recommended because of low specificity. One rapid antigen detection test (AFFIRM) is currently approved for diagnosis of *G. vaginalis* infection. All symptomatic women should be treated with metronidazole, 500 mg orally twice daily for 7 days, or metronidazole gel (0.75%), 5 g intravaginally once daily for 5 days, or clindamycin cream (2%), 5 g intravaginally once daily for 7 days. Oral tinidazole, oral clindamycin, or clindamycin ovules may be used as alternative treatment regimens. Oral single-dose 2-g metronidazole is not recommended

because of poor efficacy. All symptomatic pregnant women and those asymptomatic pregnant women who are already at increased risk for preterm labor should be evaluated and treated. Pregnant women should be treated with systemic (oral) regimens. Routine treatment of sex partners has not been shown to decrease incidence of recurrence and is not recommended. BV may be associated with PID and endometritis, particularly in patients who have recently had invasive genital procedures such as abortions.

TRICHOMONIASIS

Trichomoniasis is caused by the protozoan *Trichomonas vaginalis*. Infected men and women are often asymptomatic. When symptomatic, men may develop urethritis, and women may develop a malodorous yellow-green vaginal discharge or vulvar irritation. Diagnosis by microscopic evaluation of an immediately inspected wet preparation of vaginal secretions has a sensitivity of only 60–70%. Cultures of vaginal secretions, urethral swab, urine, or semen are the most sensitive and specific methods for diagnosis of trichomoniasis. Point-of-care rapid antigen detection tests are now available with sensitivity of approximately 83% and specificity of approximately 97%. Current preferred treatment regimens are oral single-dose metronidazole (2 g) or oral single-dose tinidazole (2 g). Metronidazole may also be given as 500 mg orally twice daily for 7 days as an alternative treatment regimen. Sex partners should also be treated to reduce the risk of recurrence. Treatment failure is rare, and follow-up examination or testing is not necessary unless symptoms persist after treatment.

ADDITIONAL READING

Anderson MR, Klink K, Cohrssen A. Evaluation of vaginal complaints. *JAMA.* 2004;291(11):1368–79.

Centers for Disease Control and Prevention. Sexually Transmitted Diseases Treatment Guidelines, 2010. *MMWR.* 2010;59(1–114).

Centers for Disease Control and Prevention. Update to CDC's Sexually Transmitted Diseases Treatment Guidelines, 2006: Fluoroquinolones no longer recommended for treatment of gonococcal infections. *MMWR.* 2007;56(14):332–6.

Centers for Disease Control and Prevention. Sexually transmitted disease surveillance, 2009. Atlanta, GA: U.S. Department of Health and Human Services; 2010.

Corey L, Adams HG, Brown ZA, Holmes KK. Genital herpes simplex virus infections: Clinical manifestations, course, and complications. *Ann Intern Med.* 1983;98(6):958–72.

Hart G. Syphilis tests in diagnostic and therapeutic decision making. *Ann Intern Med.* 1986;104(3):368–76.

Marra CM, Maxwell CL, Smith SL, et al. Cerebrospinal fluid abnormalities in patients with syphilis: association with clinical and laboratory features. *J Infect Dis.* 2004;189(3):369–76.

Meyers DS, Halvorson H, Luckhaupt S. Screening for chlamydial infection: An evidence update for the U.S. Preventive Services Task Force. *Ann Intern Med.* 2007;147(2):135–42.

Ness RB, Soper DE, Holley RL, et al. Effectiveness of inpatient and outpatient treatment strategies for women with pelvic inflammatory disease: results from the Pelvic Inflammatory Disease Evaluation and

Clinical Health (PEACH) Randomized Trial. *Am J Obstet Gynecol.* 2002;186(5):929–37.

Wald A, Zeh, J, Selke S, et al. Reactivation of Genital Herpes Simplex Virus Type 2 Infection in Asymptomatic Seropositive Persons. *N Engl J Med.* 2000;342(12):844–50.

QUESTIONS

QUESTION 1. All of the following statements about genital herpes are correct, EXCEPT:

A. Genital herpes is caused by simplex viruses type 1 (HSV-1) or type 2 (HSV-2).
B. Most genital herpes is caused by HSV-1.
C. Most individuals have no or only minimal signs or symptoms from HSV-1 or HSV-2 infection.
D. Genital HSV-2 infection is more common in women than in men.
E. Cong HSV can lead to potentially fatal infections in neonates.

QUESTION 2. A 22-year-old male presents to the STD clinic complaining of a sore on his penis for 1 week. His last sexual exposure was approximately 3 weeks previously and was without a condom. He indicates that he has predominantly female partners although he has occasionally had sexual relations with a male partner. His HIV test 6 months ago was negative. Physical examination was unremarkable except for a genital exam that showed an uncircumcised penis with a red, indurated, clean-based, and nontender lesion on the ventral side near the frenulum. He also had two enlarged tender right inguinal nodes.

The most likely diagnosis is:

A. Primary syphilis
B. HSV
C. Chancroid
D. LGV

QUESTION 3. Risk factors for pelvic inflammatory disease include all of the following EXCEPT:

A. Douching
B. Presence of an intrauterine device
C. More than one sexual partner
D. Past history of a sexually transmitted infection
E. Over the age of 40 and being sexually active

ANSWERS

1. B
2. A
3. E

7.

DERMATOLOGIC MANIFESTATIONS OF INFECTIOUS DISEASE

Peter C. Schalock and Arthur J. Sober

Infections are a leading cause of death globally. Skin lesions can be a primary location for infection or can manifest as an outward sign of a systemic infection. This chapter aims to review the common fungal, bacterial, and viral skin infections, as well as skin manifestations of sexually transmitted diseases and of bugs and bites of medical importance.

CUTANEOUS FUNGAL INFECTIONS

SUPERFICIAL FUNGAL INFECTIONS

Fungal infections of the skin are extremely common. The two most often seen infections are dermatophytes and yeasts. A dermatophyte is a fungus that infects and digests the keratin of the stratum corneum of the epidermis. Common fungi include members of *Trichophyton*, *Epidermophyton*, or *Microsporum* species. The typical lesion seen is an oval scaling plaque, sometimes colloquially called "ring worm," although a vesicular or bullous variant can also be present, especially on the feet. These bullous lesions are often multiloculated and multifocal. The various names of tinea infections are defined by the location of infection. Tinea capitis is an extremely common infection of inner-city children, caused by *T. tonsurans*. A deep boggy inflammatory plaque may be seen on the scalp is a termed kerion. Tinea faciei is infection of the face, tinea corporis is of the body, tinea cruris is of the groin, and infection of the feet is tinea pedis (figure 7.1). Majocchi's granulomas are deep tinea infections usually within hair follicles on steroid-treated areas, commonly the lower legs/shins of women.

Infection (onychomycosis) of the keratin of the nails, toenails, or fingernails, also occurs. Subtypes of onychomycosis include distal lateral subungual onychomycosis (note distal lateral onychomycosis (DLSO) on great toenail in figure 7.1) and proximal subungual (most commonly caused by *T. rubrum*), white superficial (*T. mentagrophytes* or nondermato-

phytic molds), endonyx (white lines without onycholysis or subungual hyperkeratosis), and candidal. Proximal white subungual onychomycosis is a frequent sign of HIV infection. Tinea versicolor is a very common superficial infection by *Malassezia* spp. of yeasts. Typical lesions are hypopigmented subtle scaling patches most often on the trunk. The decrease in pigment is due to fungal inhibition of tyrosinase in the melanocyte and the presence of the fungus blocking UV reaching the skin below and thus preventing tanning. Treatment is usually topical; selenium sulfide lotions/shampoos or azole antifungals are often successful. The pigment changes will take several months to resolve even after the infection is treated.

Definitive diagnosis of a fungal or yeast infection is made by performing a potassium hydroxide (KOH) wet mount and seeing characteristic hyphae or pseudohyphae in the scale. Alternately, a fungal culture can be sent, but it can take 3–4 weeks for definitive results. Diagnosis of onychomycosis also can be done by sending nail clippings for periodic acid Schiff staining and histopathology. Treatment for limited cutaneous infection is topical. Use of topical steroids will worsen infection, although it mitigates associated pruritus in many cases. For extensive surface involvement, tinea capitis, or nail infections a systemic agent should be considered. The most common oral therapies consist of terbinafine, which inhibits fungal production of ergosterol. Fluconazole also can successfully treat dermatophyte infections, both of the nail and the skin, but is not FDA approved for these indications and should be used for candidal infections. Topical therapies include terbinafine, azole derivatives (i.e., ketoconazole), and ciclopirox.

SYSTEMIC FUNGAL INFECTIONS

There are multiple invasive fungi that can infect the skin. Infection is through local trauma to the skin, through IV catheters, or by inhalation. In the United States, coccidioidomycosis, histoplasmosis, and blastomycosis are the most likely infections to be seen, although rarely are they causes of

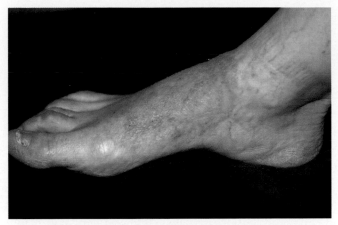

Figure 7.1. Leading Scale and Scaly Surface of Tinea Pedis. Also note distal lateral subungual onychomycosis on the great toe.

dermatologic disease. In immunosuppressed individuals cryptococcal infections of the skin may occur. Coccidioidomycosis is caused by the dimorphic fungi *Coccidioides immitis* (limited geographically to the San Joaquin Valley in California) and *C. posadasii* (in the desert Southwest of the United States, Mexico, and Central/South America).

Symptoms are similar for both species. Infection is by the respiratory route with skin manifestations being rare, usually limited to reactive findings such as erythema nodosum or erythema multiforme. *Histoplasma capsulatum* is another dimorphic fungus endemic to the central United States (Ohio, Missouri, and Mississippi River valleys) that causes respiratory infections and rare skin infections. North American blastomycosis is caused by *Blastomyces dermatitidis* and is found in similar distributions to *Histoplasma*. Both *Histoplasma* and *Blastomyces* rarely cause skin findings in immunocompetent individuals, but in HIV-infected patients, cutaneous infection can be found. Cutaneous histoplasmosis may present as erythematous papules, ulcerations, or acneiform or molluscum-like lesions, whereas blastomycosis presents as a disseminated morbilliform eruption. Cutaneous cryptococcosis *(Cryptococcus neoformans)* also may occur in HIV-infected individuals with multiple presentations including cellulitis, papules/plaques/ulcerations, or lesions similar to molluscum contagiosum. Diagnosis is established by tissue biopsy and/or culture.

CUTANEOUS DEEP FUNGAL INFECTIONS

Chronic fungal infection of the skin caused by direct infection of the skin can occur due to a variety of organisms. *Sporothrix schenckii* lives on decaying organic material and is implanted most often in the skin of an extremity (characteristically by prick from a rosebush thorn). Fungal infection develops and spreads along lymphatic channels, causing erythematous nodules in a linear lymphatic distribution. Mycetoma is caused by a wide variety of fungal species including *Nocardia* spp., *Pseudallescheria boydii* (the most common cause worldwide), *Acremonium* spp., and *Madurella*

spp. Men are more affected than women, and presentation is usually on the foot, caused by traumatic inoculation. This is rarely seen in the United States. Diagnosis is by KOH, fungal culture, and/or biopsy as well as examination of the type of "grains" produced by the infection. Black grains suggest a common fungal infection such as *Madurella*; small white grains suggest *Nocardia*. Grains with red coloration are due to *Acrinomadurapelletieri*. Larger yellow-white to white grains are either fungal or actinomycotic. Other fungal infections to consider include zygomycetes (such as *Mucor*) or chromoblastomycosis caused by multiple organisms including *Phialophora verrucosa*, *Cladosporium carrionii*, *Rhinocladiella aquaspersa*, and *Fonsecaea* spp.

CUTANEOUS BACTERIAL INFECTIONS

Bacterial infection of the skin can present in a variety of ways. Superficial infection in the epidermis by Gram-positive organisms, usually staphylococcal or streptococcal, causes impetigo. The primary lesion is a superficial pustule that rapidly is traumatized/erupts, and a honey-colored crust forms (figure 7.2). When this crust is removed, the base is glistening and moist. A bullous variant also exists, most often caused by staphylococci. Deeper infection, usually ulcerated lesions on the lower extremities, is called ecthyma. Treatments for both types of infection are gentle local debridement and cleansing, topical antibiotics such as mupirocin, and appropriate oral antibiotics.

Cellulitis and erysipelas are bacterial infections with deeper cutaneous involvement. Cellulitis is infection of the dermis and subcutaneous tissues. It presents as spreading, erythematous, tender and hot patches and plaques (figure 7.3). Men have infections more often than women, and the lower extremity is frequently involved. Streaking along lymphatics is called lymphangitis. Cellulitis with a violaceous color and bullae suggest infection by *Streptococcus pneumoniae*. Erysipelas is more superficial than cellulitis and is usually caused by group A beta-hemolytic streptococci.

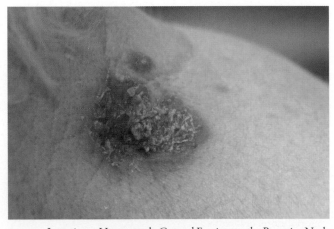

Figure 7.2. Impetigo—Honeycomb-Crusted Erosion on the Posterior Neck.

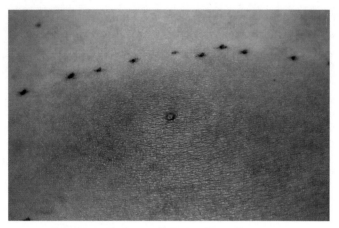

Figure 7.3. Cellulitis on the Lower Abdomen due to *S. aureus*.

It involves the local lymphatics and is characterized by the induration and sharp cutoff notable on palpation. It is found most commonly on the lower extremities followed by the face.

Staphylococcal scalded skin syndrome (SSSS) is caused by phage group 2 *Staphylococcus aureus* toxin production. Toxin production (A and B toxin) cause cleavage of desmoglein 1 in epidermal desmosomes, resulting in superficial cleavage of the epidermis at the granular cell layer and below. This results in skin desquamation, bullae formation, and erosions. This must be differentiated expeditiously from

Stevens-Johnson syndrome or toxic epidermal necrolysis, usually by a skin biopsy, which should be processed by frozen section that allows for immediate pathologic examination. SSSS is common in infants and children (98% of cases are <6 years old) and has a lower mortality (1–5%) in this age group. In adults, it is an uncommon finding associated with a much higher mortality (up to 50%) (Amagai, 2001). Adults with SSSS may be immunosuppressed.

CUTANEOUS VIRAL INFECTIONS

Many viral infections cause skin manifestations. Diseases of childhood and occasionally adulthood with skin manifestations are summarized in table 7.1. Human herpes viruses, frequent causes of human disease, are summarized in table 7.2. Nonspecific morbilliform exanthems are associated with many viral infections, although the most common cause is enteroviruses. Whereas many of these are considered diseases of childhood, it is important to consider the cause of a morbilliform eruption because many of these also affect adults.

HPV—WARTS/CONDYLOMA

Human papillomavirus (HPV) infection causes warts. The main types that are commonly seen are verruca vulgaris on the hands/feet, condyloma acuminatum in genital area,

Table 7.1 **COMMON VIRAL CAUSES OF SKIN RASH**

DISEASE	CAUSE	NOTES
Hand–foot–mouth	Coxsackie virus A16 and Enterovirus 71	Usually children
Gianotti-Crosti syndrome	United States and Europe: Epstein-Barr virus (EBV), otherwise hepatitis B	Syn: Papulovesicular acrodermatitis of childhood
Measles (rubeola)	Paramyxovirus of genus *Morbilli*	Rare in the United States
German measles (rubella)	Togavirus of genus *Rubella*	Infection in pregnancy can cause fetal infection and congenital rubella syndrome
Chickenpox	Varicella virus	Reactivation causes shingles (herpes zoster)
Erythema infectiosum	Parvovirus B19	Fifth disease; Three phases: begins with slapped-cheek appearance, followed by morbilliform eruption, and finally a lacy reticular dermatitis
Papular-purpuric gloves and socks syndrome	Parvovirus B19	Reaction to viral infection: Symmetric erythema/edema of hands and feet, progress to petechial and purpuric macules, papules, and patches, followed by fine desquamation. Sharp demarcation at the wrists and ankles
Roseola (erythema subitum)	Human herpes virus 6	Sixth disease
Nonspecific exanthems	Echovirus, adenovirus, many others	
Infectious mononucleosis	EBV	Amoxicillin or ampicillin causes rash during infection
Transient generalized morbilliform dermatitis	Human immunodeficiency virus	Associated with primary infection

Table 7.2 HUMAN HERPESVIRUSES

TYPE	DISEASE/CONDITION	TRANSMISSION	NOTES
Herpes simplex virus type 1 (HSV-1)	Oral herpes simplex	Close contact	~10% of cases of genital HSV are caused by type 1
Herpes simplex virus type 2 (HSV-2)	Genital herpes simplex	Close contact, usually sexual	Can occur on oral mucosa or away from the genitals
Varicella zoster virus (VZV)	Shingles/herpes zoster/ chickenpox	Contact or respiratory	Primary infection is chickenpox Reactivation causes shingles (herpes zoster)
Epstein-Barr virus (EBV)	Infectious mononucleosis, oral hairy leukoplakia, Burkitt lymphoma, nasopharyngeal carcinoma	Saliva	No good therapy EBV lacks thymidine kinase
Cytomegalovirus (CMV)	Maternal-fetal transmission → congenital CMV, retinitis, and pneumonia problematic in AIDS	Contact, blood transfusions, transplantation, congenital, transplacental	Infection rate rises with age → 50% by age 35
Human herpes virus 6/7	Exanthem subitum/roseola infantum	Contact or respiratory	Infection >90% after age 2
Human herpes virus 8 (Kaposi sarcoma–associated herpes virus)	Kaposi sarcoma—4 subtypes: classic, immunocompromised, endemic African, and AIDS-related	Unknown	Other HIV-associated disease: primary effusion lymphoma and multicentric Castleman disease
Herpes B	Humans can have localized disease	Bites/trauma from infected monkeys	Infects primarily monkeys; no human-to-human transmission

SOURCE: Hunt, R. Microbiology and immunology online. Virology chapter 11: Herpes viruses. http://pathmicro.med.sc.edu/virol/herpes.htm.

and flat warts on the face/arms. There are multiple subtypes of HPV that are responsible for the different types and morphologies seen. The typical verruca vulgaris (VV) is a discreet, well-demarcated, exophytic verrucous papule, often found on the digits. VV on the feet can be exophytic (figure 7.4) or endophytic. A characteristic finding on exam is small red/black flecks on the surface, which are thrombosed capillary loops. Genital warts (condyloma acuminatum) range from subtle thin papules and plaques to large, exophytic plaques. Ninety percent of all genital warts are caused by HPV 6 and HPV 11. Some subtypes of HPV are carcinogenic and are associated with cervical cancer and dysplasia. The most common oncogenic types are HPV 16, 18, 31, and 33, which can also cause genital warts. Diseases and HPV types are reviewed in table 7.3. Treatments are destructive in nature. The most common and successful therapy is superficial application of liquid nitrogen (LN_2). Multiple visits are often necessary to achieve complete removal. There are a myriad of other options including electrocautery, surgical removal, CO_2 laser destruction, and topical immunomodulators (imiquimod).

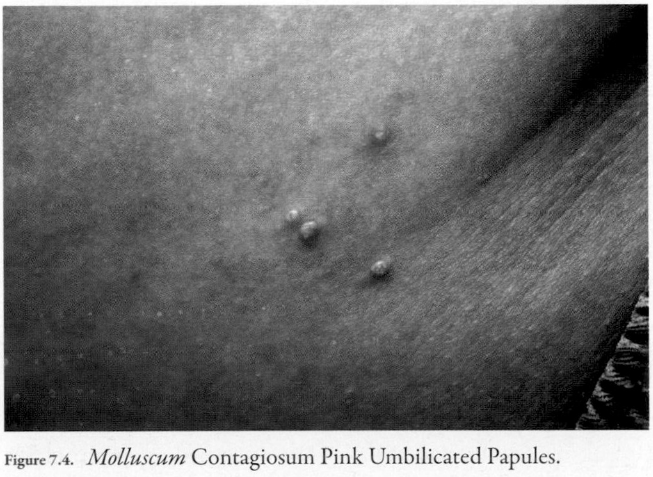

MOLLUSCUM CONTAGIOSUM

Discrete flesh-colored papules with a central umbilication caused by a poxvirus infection are molluscum contagiosum (figure 7.5). In children, they are a common finding, passed by fomites, and are seen at increased rates in those using public swimming pools. Sexual transmission is frequent in adults. Treatment is removal by destruction (LN_2), topical imiquimod, or curettage. These lesions will spontaneously resolve at times, although they are communicable while present.

HIV INFECTION-RELATED SKIN FINDINGS

Individuals infected with human immunodeficiency virus (HIV) show a variety of skin manifestations of their infection. With initial infection, a transient morbilliform eruption may occur. Kaposi sarcoma, a vascular

Figure 7.4. *Molluscum* Contagiosum Pink Umbilicated Papules.

Table 7.3 VERRUCA AND CONDYLOMA

VERRUCA TYPE	HPV TYPE
Anogenital warts	6, 11, 42, 43, 44, 55, and others
Bowenoid papulosis	16, 18, 34, 39, 42, 45
Butcher's warts (meat, poultry, and fish handlers)	7
Common warts (verruca vulgaris)	1, 2, 4, 26, 27, 29, 41, 57, 65
Epidermodysplasia verruciformis	5, 8, though more than 15 types
Flat cutaneous warts (verruca plana)	3, 10, 27, 28, 38, 41, 49
Focal oral epithelial hyperplasia (Heck)	13, 32
Genital cancers	16, 18, 31, 33, 35, 39, 45, 51
Oral papillomas	6, 7, 11, 16, 32
Plantar warts (verruca plantaris)	1, 2, 4, 63

neoplasm related to infection with human herpes virus 8, can present with violaceous patches and papules/nodules at any point in the course of HIV infection. Later manifestations, usually related to immunosuppression, include verruca vulgaris, condyloma acuminatum, mucocutaneous candidal infection, recurrent herpes zoster and herpes simplex virus infections, recalcitrant seborrheic dermatitis, psoriasis, and oral hairy leukoplakia (caused by Epstein-Barr virus).

BUGS AND BITES: TICK-BORNE

Bacteria of the genus *Rickettsia* and *Borrelia* are responsible for most infections related to tick bites. The typical presentation of the rickettsioses consists of a triad of fever, headache, and rash. The Weil-Felix reaction tests for agglutinating antibody to antigens of Proteus Ox-2, Ox-19, and Ox-K. The reaction is not specific, but it is positive in many

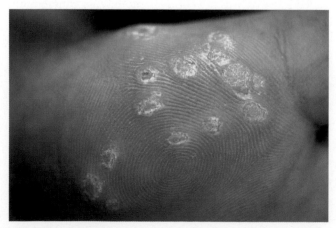

Figure 7.5. Verruca Plantaris.

rickettsioses. Complement fixation and immunofluorescence tests are more specific. These conditions are summarized in table 7.4.

PEDICULOSIS

Pediculus humanus mites infect the scalp (*capitis*) and body (*corporis*), whereas pubic lice (*Phthirus pubis*) are common parasites on the hairs in the genital region. Head lice are passed by close contact or fomites. Pubic lice are passed by sexual contact in most cases. Treatments are generally topical with permethrin or lindane. Neither of these external parasite infections is known to be a vector of internal disease, as opposed to the body louse. *P. humanis* var. *corporis* mites live on clothing and not on the human body. Often those with infections live in close contact with others and have poor hygiene. Trench fever, caused by *Bartonella quintana* and epidemic typhus caused by *Rickettsia prowazekii* are both spread by the body louse vector.

FLIES, FLEAS, AND MOSQUITOS

Bites of various flying and jumping insects cause skin disease. Bites of the blackfly *Simulium* transmit *Onchocerca volvulus,* the cause of various types of onchocerciasis. Filariasis (tropical elephantiasis) is transmitted by mosquitoes of the genus *Anopheles, Culex, Aedes,* and *Mansonia.* African sleeping sickness is caused by the tsetse fly of genus *Glossina.* Tungiasis is caused by sand flea (or chigger) *Tunga penetrans* larvae living in the skin of the human host. It is rarely seen in North America, but it is seen in travelers returning from endemic areas. The rat flea, *Xenopsylla cheopis,* transmits infection with *Rickettsia typhi* causing endemic typhus as well as *Yersinia pestis* causing bubonic plague.

SCABIES

Sarcoptes scabiei var. *hominis* mites are human epidermal parasites that live in the stratum corneum. Infection is passed by close contact and rarely by fomites. Skin findings are superficial linear burrows, excoriations, and in some cases nonspecific dermatitis. Pruritus is exceedingly common, often worst in the evening or after bedtime. Web spaces of the fingers, arms, waistline, and genitalia are common locations. The skin reactions and pruritus are not caused by the mite itself but are allergic reactions to the scabies feces. Crusted, thickened plaques with hundreds of scabies mites called "Norwegian" scabies may present in immunosuppressed/immunocompromised or institutionalized individuals. In common cases of scabies infections, only a few mites will be present on the body.

First-line therapy is topical. Permethrin cream applied from the neck down and left on overnight, then repeated in 1 week, is usually successful. Other topical agents include

Table 7.4 INFECTIONS CAUSED BY ARTHROPOD OR INSECT BITES

DISEASE	AGENT/WEIL-FELIX TEST	VECTOR	HOST/NOTES
Rocky Mountain spotted fever	R. rickettsii/(+)	Dermacentor andersoni (wood tick) Dermacentor variabilis (brown dog tick) Lone star tick	Dogs, small animals
Boutonneuse fever	R. conorri/(+)	Ixodes tick Rhipicephalus sanguineus tick	Wild rodents and dogs
Rickettsialpox	R. akari/(−)	Allodermanyssus sanguineus (house mouse mite)	House mouse
Epidemic typhus	R. prowazekii/(+)	Pediculosis corporis var. humanus	Flying squirrel and humans
Endemic typhus	R. typhi/(+)	Xenopsylla cheopis (rat flea)	Rats
Scrub typhus	R. tsutsugamushi/(+)	Trombiculid mite (chigger) (Leptotrobidium spp.)	Rodents
Lyme disease	Borrelia burgdorferi	Ixodes tick	Deer
Cat scratch fever	Bartonella henselae	Cat bite/scratch, fleas	Cats
Bacillary angiomatosis	B. henselae, B. quintana (Gram-neg rod)	Cat flea/Pediculosis corporis var. humanus	Cats
Trench fever	B. quintana	Pediculosis corporis var. humanus	Humans
Carrion disease (Oroya fever), (Bartonellosis), verruga peruana	B. bacilliformis	Sandfly (Lutzomyia verrucarum)	Frequent co-infection with Salmonella
Ehrlichiosis	Ehrlichia chaffenis, E sennetsu	Amblyomma americanum (lone star tick)	Dogs
Q fever	Coxiella burnettii	Various tick species, though transmission respiratory route not bite	Cattle, sheep, goats, cats
Leishmaniasis	Leishmania spp.	Sandfly (various species)	Humans, rodents, hyrax, dogs

crotamiton, lindane, and malathion. A 10% sulfur ointment can also be used safely for infants under 2 months of age (who may also have face/scalp involvement) or pregnant women. Alternately, oral therapy with ivermectin is effective in most cases. For everyone, cleaning of all bedding, clothing, and other areas of frequent contact is essential.

BITES

Arthropod bite reactions are type IV delayed-type hypersensitivity reactions. Findings are typically linear or grouped papules/wheals, sometimes with a small central punctum. Pruritus is nearly universal. In general, these reactions are self-limited, although a persistent bite reaction, most often to mosquito bites, can be seen in those with chronic lymphocytic leukemia. Leukemia patients can also have persistent bite-like reactions that are not clearly temporally linked to bites. The most common biting insects are mosquitos (various genus and species), bedbugs (Cimex lectularius), fleas (various genera and species; Pulex irrilans is the human flea), ticks, and various species of flies. Treatment is symptomatic, including topical steroids or in extensive cases oral corticosteroids.

SEXUALLY TRANSMITTED DISEASES

Sexually transmitted diseases (STDs) are commonly presenting problems in the outpatient setting. The most common STDs, such as chlamydia and gonorrhea, rarely have skin findings. Chlamydia, caused by Chlamydia trachomatis, does not have skin ulceration or lymphadenopathy (other than in lymphogranuloma venereum [LGV]). There can be a thin urethral discharge in males, but the symptoms are generally nondermatologic. Gonorrhea is caused by the Gram-negative diplococcus Neisseria gonorrhoeae. Gonorrhea has dermatologic findings in 25% of cases, including morbilliform, pustular, necrotic, or vesicular eruptions. These commonly present below the neck. A characteristic finding is pustules over a joint. Other less common findings include erythema nodosum, urticaria, hemorrhagic lesions, or erythema multiforme. Skin lesions often present in different stages of development. Syphilis is again increasing in prevalence in the United States and has both common and rare skin findings that will be discussed below. Other less common STDs include granuloma inguinale, chancroid, and lymphogranuloma venereum. These conditions are summarized in table 7.5.

Table 7.5 SEXUALLY TRANSMITTED DISEASES

DISEASE	CAUSE	SKIN FINDINGS	ULCER	LYMPHADENOPATHY
Chlamydia	*C. trachomatis*	None	n/a	n/a
Chancroid	*H. ducreyi* "school of fish" on pathological exam	Tender papule initially, then ulceration	Painful ulcer (3 mm–5 cm)	Painful
Gonorrhea	Gram-negative diplococci: *Neisseria gonorrhoeae*	See text	n/a	n/a
Granuloma inguinale	*Calymmatobacterium granulomatis*	Nontender papules, subsequently ulcerate	Painless	None
LGV	*Chlamydia trachomatis* types L1–L3	Genital papules/ulcers, also rectal ulcers	Painless	Painful
Syphilis	*Treponema pallidum*	See text	Painless	Painless

Granuloma inguinale is rarely diagnosed in the United States. Otherwise known as Donovanosis, this is a common STD in the developing world. The bacteria *Calymmatobacterium granulomatis* causes this condition. Infection presents as nontender papules or nodules after 10–40 days of incubation. After some time, the nodules will break down, creating oozing nontender ulcers. Tissue destruction and spread will not cease until the disease is treated. Typical locations are at the base of the penis, labia, or perianal region. Rarely vaginal or cervical disease can occur. Standard therapy is with oral erythromycin, streptomycin, tetracycline, or ampicillin.

Chancroid is found more frequently in developing countries in commercial sex workers and their contacts. It is caused by an infection by *Haemophilus ducreyi* and is more common in uncircumcised men. Presentation is with a tender papule that rapidly ulcerates, causing a painful ulceration and lymphadenopathy. This combination is suggestive of chancroid, but syphilis and herpes simplex must first be ruled out. Treatment is with azithromycin, ceftriaxone, or erythromycin.

LGV is caused by three serotypes of *Chlamydia trachomatis*, L1–L3. Presentation on the genitals is with painless papules, which subsequently ulcerate. Compared to chancroid, the lymphadenopathy is painless. LGV may also produce rectal ulcers, bleeding, pain, and discharge, especially among those who practice receptive anal intercourse.

SYPHILIS

Skin findings can occur in each of the stages of syphilis (primary, secondary, or tertiary), as well as in congenital syphilis infections. Findings of primary syphilis are painless (Hunterian) chancre, dory flop (chancre on prepuce), phagedenic chancre (combination of syphilitic chancre and contaminating bacteria), edema indurativum (marked solid edema with chancre), and chancre redux (relapse due to insufficient treatment associated with lymphadenopathy). Cutaneous manifestations in secondary syphilis are called

syphilids. The many findings include macular eruptions, livedo reticularis, papular eruptions, papulosquamous eruptions, and follicular lichenoid eruptions. Alopecia with moth-eaten appearance may occur. Color of the eruption may be that of a copper penny. Itch is typically absent. Palms and soles may be involved. The prozone phenomenon may occur when very high antibody titers produce a false-negative result. Finding of tertiary syphilis include noduloulcerative gummas, most commonly on the legs. The tongue is the most common location in the oral cavity, and a smooth atrophy with superficial glossitis causing ulcers, atrophy of papillae, and smooth shiny scarring may also occur in the mouth. Osseous syphilids are gummatous osteoarthritis, osteocope-bone pain, and Charcot joint. Signs of neurosyphilis are Argyll Robertson pupils, tabes dorsalis, and a positive Romberg sign. Aortic aneurysm may also occur.

Diagnosis is by the nontreponemal antigen tests rapid plasma reagin [RPR], Venereal Disease Research Laboratory [VDRL]. These will be positive within 6 weeks after infection and strongly positive throughout the secondary phase. The tests become negative again during therapy and in late syphilis. These tests may become negative after a few decades of infection, even without treatment. False positives may occur with Lyme disease and borreliosis. The specific treponemal tests are the microhemagglutination assay for T. pallidum (MHA-TP) and fluorescent treponemal antibody absorbed (FTA-ABS). These tests become positive early, before nontreponemal tests, and usually remain positive for life. False positives may occur from lupus, scleroderma, rheumatoid arthritis (RA), smallpox vaccination (rarely performed), pregnancy, genital herpes, and HIV.

ADDITIONAL READING

Amagai M, Matsuyoshi N, Wang ZH, Andl C, Stanley JR. Toxin in bullous impetigo and staphylococcal scalded-skin syndrome targets desmoglein 1. *Nat Med.* 2000 Nov;6(11):1275–7.

Dana AN. Diagnosis and treatment of tick infestation and tick-borne diseases with cutaneous manifestations. *Dermatol Ther.* 2009;22(4): 293–326.

Farhi D, Dupin N. Management of syphilis in the HIV-infected patient: Facts and controversies. *Clin Dermatol.* 2010;28(5):539–45.

Elston DM. Update on cutaneous manifestations of infectious diseases. *Med Clin North Am.* 2009;93(6):1283–90.

Wilson M, Lountzis N, Ferringer T. Zoonoses of dermatologic interest. *Dermatol Ther.* 2009;22(4):367–78.

QUESTIONS

QUESTION 1. A 45-year-old monogamous homosexual male presents with a 1-month history of a spreading asymptomatic morbilliform dermatitis with pityriasiform scale on his trunk and arms. He is in a stable relationship and reports no new exposures/partners or medications. He is in excellent health otherwise. What is the most likely diagnosis?

A. Pityriasis rosea
B. Secondary syphilis
C. Psoriasis
D. Medication hypersensitivity dermatitis
E. Atopic dermatitis

QUESTION 2. A patient presents in the office with an itchy rash on the forearm. You suspect that the patient may have scabies. The tell-tale lesion pathognomonic for scabies that you would look for would be:

A. Raised, tender, boggy plaques with pustules simulating an abscess
B. Sharply circumscribed single or multiple skin-colored, dome-shaped papules with waxy surface
C. Linear burrows
D. Mild erythema and scaling of the skin
E. Flaky, macular itchy rash

QUESTION 3. All of the following are true about nongenital warts EXCEPT:

A. Warts are caused by HPV.
B. Common warts or verruca vulgari are most commonly seen on the hands and knees.
C. 65% of warts may regress spontaneously within 2 years.
D. Salicylic acid is a first-line therapy used to treat warts.
E. There is a high risk of nongenital warts progressing to verrucous carcinoma in elderly patients.

ANSWERS

1. B
2. C
3. E

8.

INFECTIOUS DISEASE BOARD REVIEW QUESTIONS

Francisco M. Marty

QUESTION 1. A 62-year-old man with history of hypertension and diabetes mellitus presents with acute appendicitis. On laparotomy, he is found to have perforated. The appendix is removed, and the patient is started on ampicillin and gentamicin. Two hours after surgery the patient develops fever and hypotension. Electrocardiogram (EKG) demonstrated 4-mm ST depression in V4–V6 and troponin I returns positive. A multilumen catheter is inserted in the right internal jugular vein. His blood cultures are obtained and grow Gram-negative anaerobes, eventually identified as *Bacteroides fragilis*. Metronidazole is added to the antimicrobial regimen empirically. He is transferred to the cardiac care unit for further care. Once admitted, his course is complicated by a non-Q-wave acute myocardial infarction, acute renal failure (creatinine peaked at 3.2 mg/dL), and hypotension from acute gastrointestinal bleeding (peptic ulcer). IV heparin is stopped, gentamicin is switched to levofloxacin, and the patient required two therapeutic endoscopies to stop the bleeding. He required 4 units of packed red blood cells. The patient is placed on high-dose proton pump inhibitor and fluconazole prophylaxis. Eight days after admission he is transferred to the step-down unit. Two days later, he spikes to 102°F. You notice the central line insertion site is erythematous, so you draw two sets of blood cultures, remove the line, and switch the patient from ampicillin to vancomycin. The next day his temperature is down to 100.5°F, and the microbiology lab reports yeast cells growing on one of four blood culture bottles.

What do you do now?

A. Dismiss culture, likely a contaminant.
B. Culture is real, but line has been removed. Nothing to do.
C. Culture is real, patient already on fluconazole. Nothing to do.
D. Start amphotericin B, discontinue fluconazole.
E. Start caspofungin, discontinue fluconazole.

QUESTION 2. A 35-year-old male truck driver is admitted with a week-long history of cough, fevers and chills, and right-sided chest pain. He reports a 30-lb weight loss over the previous 3 months as well as fatigue and occasional headaches he treats with over-the-counter (OTC) ibuprofen. He appears emaciated, blood pressure (BP) 80/40, heart rate (HR) 140, 101°F. Exam reveals oral hairy leukoplakia, and chest radiographs confirm your diagnosis of right lower-lobe pneumonia with a small effusion. Blood pressure normalizes with IV fluids after placing of a central line, and you start treatment with IV ceftriaxone and oral azithromycin after obtaining initial labs, sputum, and blood cultures. Sputum culture reveals *Streptococcus pneumoniae*, which is pansusceptible. Blood cultures are negative. He is leukopenic and lymphopenic. He is anemic with a hemoglobin of 10 g/dL, with a normochromic normocytic pattern. The patient admits to multiple female sexual partners and former IV drug use. He agrees to be HIV tested. You stop the azithromycin. Three days later the patient remains febrile and continues to experience daily headaches, so you redraw blood cultures and do a thoracentesis, which reveals a noncomplicated parapneumonic exudate. HIV enzyme-linked immunosorbent assay (ELISA) returns positive. CD4 count is 30 cells/μL. Two days later the microbiology lab reports yeast cells growing in one of four bottles from your last cultures.

What do you do now?

A. Dismiss culture, likely a contaminant.
B. Removing line should be enough.
C. Start fluconazole 400 mg/day.
D. Start amphotericin B 0.7 mg/kg.
E. Start caspofungin 70 mg/day, followed by 50 mg/day.

QUESTION 3. A 60-year-old woman with chronic obstructive pulmonary disease, chronic renal insufficiency (baseline creatinine of 1.8 mg/dL), and osteoarthritis presents with a day history of cough, rigors, and progressive dyspnea. On exam in the emergency room her blood pressure is 75/40 mm Hg, heart rate 135 per minute, respiratory rate 34 per minute, SpO$_2$ 81%. She appears cyanotic, and there are signs of consolidation in her right lower chest, which are confirmed on a chest x-ray. Blood cultures are drawn, and she is started on cefotaxime and levofloxacin together with a 2-liter NS bolus and supplemental oxygen. Initial labs reveal a white blood cell (WBC) of 2K/μL, 25% bands, creatinine of 2.7 mg/dL, HCO$_3$ of 12 mmol/L, and an arterial blood gas reveals a pH of 7.25. She remains hypotensive, so vasopressors and mechanical ventilation are initiated. Your intern calls you with this history, and your medical student has calculated an APACHE II score of 26 for the patient. Blood cultures grow Gram-positive diplococci in pairs.

What do you do next?

A. Add vancomycin
B. Add gentamicin
C. Add drotrecogin alpha
D. Add low-molecular-weight heparin
E. Add nitric oxide

QUESTION 4. You want to transfer a 76-year-old woman to a skilled nursing facility after she suffered a stroke. She has residual right hemiplegia, aphasia, and got a G-tube for swallowing dysfunction. The facility requires a urinalysis (straight catheterization): it demonstrated 15–20 WBC, 10^5 CFU of *Escherichia coli*, resistant only to trimethoprim/sulfamethoxazole. She is otherwise afebrile and asymptomatic. You start ciprofloxacin via G-tube, and the patient is accepted to the skilled nursing facility. Other medications are aspirin, atenolol, sucralfate, and pravastatin. The patient is transferred back to your hospital 5 days later with fever and decreased sensorium. Workup reveals a clear chest x-ray, sodium of 148, creatinine of 1.5, and a cloudy urine with 100 WBC; Gram stain demonstrates Gram-negative rods.

What happened?

A. SNF did not read order to continue ciprofloxacin.
B. *E. coli* became resistant to ciprofloxacin.
C. Patient is infected with second pathogen.
D. There is a drug interaction.
E. Patient developed poststroke malabsorption.

QUESTION 5. Three days after sustaining hand and arm lacerations when his motorcycle spun off the road into the dirt, a 17-year-old man presents with fever, severe arm pain, and malaise. Examination reveals a temperature of 101.8°F, blood pressure 90/50 mm Hg, and dusky blue fingers with erythema extending to the elbow. Radiograph of the arm reveals subcutaneous gas in the hand, below an area of healing laceration.

The antimicrobial regimen that has the most activity against the most likely pathogen is:

A. Ceftriaxone
B. Vancomycin and gentamicin

C. Penicillin
D. Cefazolin and metronidazole
E. Clindamycin and penicillin

QUESTION 6. An elderly man with long-standing aortic stenosis presents with persistent *Enterococcus faecalis* bacteremia and new aortic insufficiency. The organism is susceptible to penicillin, ampicillin, vancomycin, and ciprofloxacin by in vitro susceptibility testing but shows high-level resistance to gentamicin. The patient has no known drug allergies. The patient develops interstitial nephritis while receiving ampicillin and is given vancomycin. During infusion of the first dose of vancomycin he becomes flushed, and his systolic blood pressure drops to 70 mm Hg and quickly recovers.

It would be most appropriate to continue therapy with which of the following?

A. Quinupristin/Dalfopristin
B. Vancomycin
C. Ciprofloxacin
D. Linezolid
E. Daptomycin

QUESTION 7. A 32-year-old man is admitted for further treatment of acute myelogenous leukemia. He is undergoing myeloablative allogeneic hematopoietic stem cell transplantation. His absolute neutrophil count is 0. He develops persistent febrile neutropenia despite ceftazidime treatment. His blood cultures remain negative. A chest computed tomography (CT) is done demonstrating a nodular infiltrate 3 cm in diameter with surrounding ground glass on the right lower lobe. Galactomannan EIA index is 1.2 (normal <0.5).

What additional treatment is the most appropriate?

A. Amphotericin B, lipid formulation
B. Caspofungin
C. Posaconazole
D. Voriconazole
E. Any combination of the above

QUESTION 8. Which of the following patients does not need prophylaxis to prevent endocarditis?

A. A 58-year-old woman with a urinary tract infection and prosthetic aortic valve for Foley catheter placement
B. A 35-year-old woman with mitral valve prolapse with regurgitation who is undergoing dental extraction
C. A 50-year-old man with a history of prior endocarditis, undergoing suturing of a finger laceration from clean razor injury
D. A 58-year-old woman with a history of rheumatic heart disease undergoing incision and drainage of an abscess

QUESTION 9. An elderly diabetic presents with a 3-week history of earache. On examination there is purulent drainage and granulation tissue in the right external auditory canal and a facial nerve palsy on that side. There is no fever, and the peripheral white blood cell count is normal.

Appropriate initial therapy includes which of the following agents?

A. Topical ciprofloxacin
B. Amphotericin B
C. Ceftazidime
D. Isoniazid and rifampin
E. Vancomycin

QUESTION 10. Ingestion of or contact with fresh water is an important route of transmission of all of the following except:

A. Cryptosporidiosis
B. Cercarial dermatitis
C. Leptospirosis
D. Ehrlichiosis
E. Legionellosis

QUESTION 11. A patient with adenocarcinoma of the colon develops an abrupt and excruciating pain in the thigh and fever to 39.3° C. On examination of the painful area, there is marked tenderness and nondependent edema. There is no history of trauma, and the overlying skin and perineum are intact.

The most likely cause of this infection is:

A. *Clostridium septicum*
B. *Aeromonas hydrophila*
C. Group A *Streptococcus*
D. Mixed infection (e.g., *Escherichia coli* and *Bacteroides fragilis*)
E. *Bacillus anthracis*

QUESTION 12. Appropriate management of household contacts of a person with pertussis includes:

A. Identification of carriers
B. Treatment only in the presence of symptoms
C. Antibiotic prophylaxis
D. Booster vaccination
E. Do nothing

QUESTION 13. A patient experiences a third episode of pneumococcal meningitis in the past 10 months. Which of the following underlying conditions is most likely?

A. Deficiency of terminal components of complement
B. Neutrophil dysfunction
C. Dural epidermoid cyst
D. Cerebrospinal fluid leak
E. Mollaret meningitis

QUESTION 14. A 76-year-old female with a history of chronic obstructive pulmonary disease and dementia is seen in clinic in December with 1 day of fever, malaise, cough, and myalgias. On exam, temp 38.5°C, HR 96. Otherwise normal. Chest x-ray normal. Rapid influenza EIA of nasopharyngeal secretions returns positive for influenza B.

What would you do next?

A. Start amantadine
B. Start azithromycin
C. Start oseltamivir
D. Start rimantadine
E. Start zanamivir

QUESTION 15. A 35-year-old Brazilian man is admitted to the hospital following a generalized seizure. A CT scan of the head shows a ring-enhancing lesion in the right parietal lobe. All of the following could be the responsible pathogen except:

A. *Streptococcus milleri*
B. *Mycobacterium tuberculosis*
C. *Taenia solium*
D. *Borrelia burgdorferi*
E. *Toxoplasma gondii*

QUESTION 16. A 40-year-old man with Hodgkin disease has pain in the right flank and upper abdomen. He has just completed his fourth course of methotrexate, vincristine, procarbazine, and prednisone chemotherapy. Physical examination shows several coalscent vesicular lesions, which begin under the right costal margin and extend from the flank to the midline anteriorly in two distinct (noncontiguous) dermatomes.

The most appropriate therapy would be:

A. Analgesics for pain
B. Prednisone
C. Intravenous antiviral chemotherapy with acyclovir
D. Zoster immune globulin
E. Immune serum globulin

QUESTION 17. A 38-year-old man from Oregon had diarrhea consisting of four to five loose stools per day, abdominal cramps, bloating, and nausea while on a business trip in South America. The symptoms began on the fifth day of the trip, lasted for 3 days, and were partially relieved by an antimotility agent. The most likely cause of this illness was:

A. Enteroinvasive *Escherichia coli*
B. Enterotoxigenic *E. coli*
C. *Salmonella* species
D. *Campylobacter jejuni*
E. *Shigella* species

QUESTION 18. The combination of amoxicillin and clavulanic acid (Augmentin) is more active than ampicillin against some strains of each of the following bacteria EXCEPT:

   A. *Staphylococcus aureus*
   B. *Neisseria gonorrhoeae*
   C. *Streptococcus pyogenes*
   D. *Haemophilus influenzae*
   E. *Branhamella catarrhalis*

QUESTION 19. A 35-year-old man who is the captain of a fishing boat has fever, chills, and several hemorrhagic bullae on the left wrist and dorsal surface of the hand. Lymphangitis and left epitrochlear and axillary lymphadenopathy are present. The captain harvested shrimp 4 days ago.

The most likely causative organism is:

   A. *Staphylococcus aureus*
   B. *Haemophilus influenzae*
   C. *Clostridium perfringens*
   D. *Vibrio vulnificus*
   E. *Pseudomonas aeruginosa*

QUESTION 20. An elderly man has bacteremia with *Salmonella typhimurium* that has relapsed three times after 28-day courses of ciprofloxacin, to which the organism is susceptible. The most likely site of infection is the:

   A. Gallbladder
   B. Colon
   C. Aorta
   D. Spine

QUESTION 21. A young man with chronic sinusitis presents with fever, headache, mild confusion, and a mildly stiff neck. Over the next 24 hours, he develops neurological deficits that rapidly progress to hemiparesis, hemisensory defects, and hemianopsia. He has several focal seizures, and signs of increased intracranial pressure appear.

The most likely diagnosis is:

   A. Bacterial meningitis
   B. Cavernous sinus thrombosis
   C. Brain abscess
   D. Subdural empyema

QUESTION 22. A person who underwent splenectomy in the past following trauma experiences the sudden onset of high fever, rigors, and hypotension. By the time he reaches the hospital he has multiple petechiae and purpura over his face, arms, and legs. Acute renal failure and disseminated intravascular coagulation are demonstrated. He gives a history of frequent bites and scratches from a new pet dog.

The Gram-negative bacillus isolated from the patient's blood is most likely:

   A. *Pasteurella multocida*
   B. *Fusobacterium necrophorum*

   C. *Capnocytophaga canimorsus*
   D. *Ehrlichia canis*

QUESTION 23. A hand infection following a human bite progresses despite treatment with clindamycin. In the absence of a process that requires surgical debridement, which of the following organisms is most likely to be the cause of treatment failure in this case?

   A. *Streptococcus milleri*
   B. *Prevotella melaninogenica*
   C. *Eikenella corrodens*
   D. *Staphylococcus epidermidis*

QUESTION 24. A 68-year-old woman with history of chronic obstructive pulmonary disease (COPD) is admitted. She presented 2 weeks prior to admission with COPD exacerbation during an upper respiratory infection. She was admitted for observation overnight, improved with inhalers, prednisone, and levofloxacin. She now presents with a 3-day history of progressive watery diarrhea, abdominal pain, and new fever to 38.8°C. On exam she appears ill, BP 100/60, HR 128/min, RR 22/min. Abdomen is slightly distended with pain in both lower quadrants. Abdominal CT scan demonstrates diffuse colonic thickening, no diverticulitis. *Clostridium difficile* toxin EIA is positive.

Appropriate infection control measures in this case include all of the following EXCEPT:

   A. Isolation (single room use)
   B. Contact precautions (use of gloves and gowns)
   C. Hand hygiene with alcohol-based solution
   D. Hand washing with soap and water
   E. Discontinuation of unnecessary antibacterials

QUESTION 25. Which of the following infectious diseases agents is not transmitted by blood transfusions:

   A. West Nile virus
   B. *Trypanosoma cruzi*
   C. Cytomegalovirus
   D. *Babesia microti*
   E. None of the above

QUESTION 26. A 46-year-old woman reports erythema, mild pain, and cloudy discharge from her lower abdomen for 3 weeks. She reports undergoing a "tummy tuck" a month prior during a visit to a Caribbean island. The most likely organism causing this infection is:

   A. *Staphylococcus aureus*
   B. *Mycobacterium abscessus*
   C. *Aeromonas* sp.
   D. *Ancylostoma braziliensis*
   E. *Leishmania major*

QUESTION 27. A 56-year-old man, JFK airport employee (Long Island, NY), presents with fever to 39.5°C, malaise,

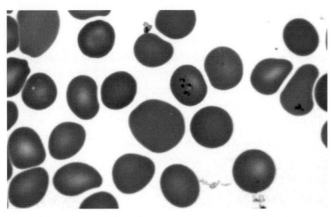

Figure 8.1 Giemsa-stained blood smear demonstrating a tetrad of intra-erythrocytic merozoites of Babesia microti.

fatigue and myalgias for 1 week in September. Initial blood work demonstrates new onset of anemia (Hb 11.3 g/L), mild leukopenia, and thrombocytopenia. Reticulocyte count is 6%, low-density lipoprotein (LDL) is elevated, and Coombs tests are negative. Blood smear results are shown in figure 8.1.

This infection was most likely transmitted by:

A. *Anopheles quadrimaculatus*
B. *Aedes aegypti*
C. *Culex pipiens*
D. *Ixodes scapularis*
E. None of the above

ANSWERS

1. E. The patient developed candidemia in the setting of gastrointestinal perforation and prolonged intensive care unit stay. *Candida* blood isolates cannot be dismissed as contaminants, and in current practice all patients with candidemia should be treated. Blood cultures should be repeated until persistently negative, and treatment should continue for at least 2 weeks following the last positive blood isolate. Given the risk factors of the patient, his doctors elected to use fluconazole prophylaxis. Although not routinely recommended, this increases the risk of fluconazole-resistant *Candida* infections. For someone who develops candidemia during fluconazole administration, azole resistance should be assumed and other treatments used while the isolate is identified and susceptibility testing is performed. The options for this patient include amphotericin B or one of its lipid formulations or any of the echinocandins (caspofungin, micafungin, or anidulafungin). As the patient has already acute renal dysfunction, the best option for the patient is to start an echinocandin. Echinocandins are fungicidal against *Candida* sp. by disrupting fungal cell wall synthesis

by inhibiting 1,3-β-D-glucan synthase. They are as effective as amphotericin B with a better safety profile (Mora-Duarte et al. *N Engl J Med.* 2002;347:2020–9). *Candida* has a high tendency to form biofilms; thus, removal and replacement of all intravenous access is recommended routinely if feasible. An ophthalmologic exam is frequently recommended to exclude endophthalmitis. It is an infrequent complication but one that can require a different management (Rodríguez-Adrián et al. *Medicine.* 2003;82:187–202). We favor routine identification of *Candida* species and susceptibility testing of all invasive infections. Patients with fluconazole or voriconazole susceptible isolates can be safely switched to oral azole treatment after susceptibility testing results become available. New *Candida* treatment guidelines (Pappas et al. *Clin Infect Dis.* 2009;48:503–35, are available at www.idsociety.org.).

2. D. Not all yeasts isolated from blood are *Candida* sp. This patient is at increased risk of cryptococcosis given new diagnosis of AIDS and history of headaches. AIDS patients often present with more than one synchronous problem. Patient was also at risk of candidemia given central venous access placed under urgent conditions. Removing central access is reasonable given data, but patient needs antifungal therapy. Fluconazole is a reasonable initial treatment for candidemia but not for cryptococcosis, especially when there is concern for disseminated or central nervous system involvement; it is associated with treatment failures and emergence of resistance in that setting. Caspofungin and other echinocandins are not active against *Cryptococcus neoformans*, so they are not a good option if cryptococcosis is in the differential.

Best empirical treatment in this case is amphotericin B. If cryptococcemia is confirmed by identification of the yeast or by determination of a serum cryptococcal antigen, the patient should undergo examination of his cerebrospinal fluid to exclude or confirm presence of cryptococcal meningitis. If cryptococcal meningitis is confirmed, flucytosine at 100 mg/kg per day can be added to the initial regimen for induction treatment for cryptococcal meningitis. (For further details, please see Perfect et al. *Clin Infect Dis.* 2010;50:291–322, available at www.idsociety.org.)

3. C. Patient has pneumonia and septic shock due to *Streptococcus pneumoniae*. Although vancomycin should be used empirically for the treatment of pneumococcal meningitis until antimicrobial susceptibilities are back, vancomycin is not usually indicated for treatment of pneumococcal pneumonia or bacteremia. The combination of third-generation cephalosporins and quinolones provides excellent empirical treatment for pneumonia for severely ill patients. Gentamicin adds little to the regimen chosen in the emergency room given your clinical impression; the patient is already in renal failure (gentamicin is not a pressor drug). This patient should be screened and started on drotrecogin alpha if she meets criteria, as it is the only additional

intervention that may reduce her chance of dying (Bernard et al. *N Engl J Med.* 2001;344:699–709; Mandell et al. *Clin Infect Dis.* 2007;44:S27–S72).

4. D. Antacids containing magnesium or aluminum salts, including sucralfate, will bind quinolones efficiently and impede their absorption. Quinolones should be administered at least 2 hours apart from antacids (Davies, Maesen. *Rev Infect Dis.* 1989;11 Suppl 5:S1083–90).

5. E. Although broad-spectrum antibiotic treatment is appropriate in a patient with evidence of cellulitis and sepsis, this patient has the classical presentation of clostridial myonecrosis (gas gangrene) caused by traumatic exposure to *C. perfringens.* Features include soft tissue trauma followed in 1–4 days by the sudden onset of unrelenting pain at the wound site with evidence of gas in the underlying tissue. Optimal management includes rapid surgical debridement and antibacterial administration. Penicillin G in combination with clindamycin is considered the treatment of choice. Other agents with activity are considered second-line agents, including chloramphenicol, metronidazole, imipenem, and combination beta-lactam/beta-lactamase inhibitors. Hyperbaric oxygen could be considered but without delay to surgical intervention (Stevens et al. *Clin Infect Dis.* 2005;41:1373–406, available at www.idsociety.org).

6. B. The treatment of choice for enterococcal endocarditis is the combination of a cell-wall-active drug (ampicillin, penicillin, or vancomycin) and an aminoglycoside (gentamicin or streptomycin). When used alone, cell-wall-active drugs are bacteriostatic against enterococci. The combination, however, is bactericidal because of synergy between the two classes of drugs. Synergy is most commonly achieved when gentamicin is the antibiotic used, but about 10–25% of enterococci that are resistant to gentamicin are susceptible to streptomycin (when used with a cell-wall-active drug). Because the organism in this case is susceptible to ampicillin and does not produce a beta-lactamase, sulbactam, a beta-lactamase inhibitor, has no additional effect.

Quinupristin/dalfopristin is a combination of two streptogramin antibiotics. It has bacteriostatic activity against Gram-positive organisms including vancomycin-resistant (VRE) *Enterococcus faecium* (not active against *E. faecalis*) and methicillin-resistant *Staphylococcus aureus* (MRSA). It is used for treatment of VRE and MRSA but not for vancomycin- or ampicillin-susceptible enterococci or methicillin-sensitive staphylococci. Enterococci susceptible to ampicillin may be susceptible to imipenem, but ampicillin is preferred for treating these strains. Linezolid and daptomycin have good activity against enterococci, but the data on non-VRE enterococcal endocarditis are lacking.

The reaction described is an example of the "red man" syndrome that occurs when vancomycin is administered rapidly or in high concentrations. It is not an allergy but is caused by the release of histamine from mast cells. By slowing the infusion rate and/or diluting the concentration of vancomycin, recurrence of this reaction can be avoided.

Ciprofloxacin is active in vitro against this patient's isolate but is less effective than ampicillin or vancomycin and is not considered first- or second-line therapy for enterococcal infections (Baddour et al. *Circulation.* 2005;111:e394–e433).

7. D. The chest CT image describes a lung nodule with a halo sign. The presence of a halo sign is highly suggestive of invasive aspergillosis in patients with prolonged neutropenia during induction chemotherapy for acute leukemia or myeloablative allogeneic stem cell transplantation. Other angioinvasive molds and hematogenous seeding of the lung from septic emboli can have the same radiologic appearance. The presence of elevated circulating serum levels of galactomannan, a carbohydrate present in the cell wall of *Aspergillus* and *Penicillium* species, increases the certainty that the infection is indeed invasive aspergillosis to probable. Although a definitive diagnosis of invasive aspergillosis requires biopsy of the affected site and growth in culture of the mold, the clinical scenario, the presence of the halo sign, and an elevated galactomannan make a diagnosis of invasive aspergillosis likely.

The standard treatment of probable or proven invasive aspergillosis since its FDA approval in 2002 is voriconazole, which demonstrated improved successful treatment and survival when compared to initial use of amphotericin B. Lipid formulations of amphotericin B are approved for patients who are intolerant or develop toxicity to amphotericin B deoxycholate. Caspofungin is approved for salvage, but not for initial, treatment of invasive aspergillosis in patients intolerant or refractory to standard treatment. Posaconazole was recently approved for prophylaxis of invasive fungal infections, including *Aspergillus* infections, but is not approved for treatment of invasive aspergillosis. Although some authors have suggested use of combination treatment for invasive aspergillosis, especially of the combination of an echinocandin such as caspofungin and voriconazole, properly conducted clinical trials are not available to address whether this strategy is associated with improved outcomes when compared to voriconazole alone and cannot be recommended at this time (Walsh et al. *Clin Infect Dis.* 2008;46:327–60, available at www.idsociety.org).

8. C. Prophylaxis for endocarditis is recommended for individuals with high and moderate risk underlying conditions undergoing certain high-risk procedures (Wilson et al. *Circulation.* 2007;116:1736–54, available at www.idsociety.org). Conditions that raise the risk of developing endocarditis and whose outcomes are bad enough to warrant routine prophylaxis include prosthetic valves, previous

bacterial endocarditis, complex congenital heart diseases, and rheumatic heart disease. Although mitral valve prolapse with regurgitation increases the lifetime risk of endocarditis, the absolute increase in risk does not warrant routine antibacterial prophylaxis, and it is no longer recommended (Wilson et al. *Circulation.* 2007;116:1736–54). Procedures requiring prophylaxis in this group include dental extractions and periodontal work, teeth cleaning if bleeding is anticipated, surgery on respiratory mucosa, gastrointestinal surgery, Foley catheter placement with infected urine, and drainage of an abscess. Prophylaxis is not recommended for suturing clean lacerations or for procedures performed under sterile conditions, such as central venous catheter placement.

9. C. The clinical syndrome of otalgia, otorrhea, and granulation tissue visible in the external auditory canal is typical of malignant otitis externa, a severe necrotizing infection that involves soft tissue, cartilage, and bone. The disease occurs almost exclusively in diabetics and is nearly always caused by *Pseudomonas aeruginosa.* Involvement of cranial nerves, especially the facial nerve, is common as infection spreads. Although treatment with ciprofloxacin has been reported to be highly successful, initiating treatment with ceftazidime is preferable given its good tissue penetration and lower risk of resistance. Uncomplicated otitis externa or swimmer's ear is a benign and self-limiting process that responds to topical antibiotics and corticosteroids; *Pseudomonas aeruginosa* is often the predominant organism. Fungi such as *Aspergillus* also may be isolated in cases of benign otitis externa; topical therapy is sufficient in such cases. Tuberculous otitis media can lead to a chronically draining ear.

10. D. Contamination of drinking water has been the cause of sporadic cases and city-wide episodes of diarrheal illness caused by the protozoan parasite *Cryptosporidium parvum.* Infection by avian schistosomes causes a pruritic rash in previously sensitized persons who have contact with infected fresh water in lakes and ponds in the United States and elsewhere. Leptospirosis usually results from contact with fresh water contaminated by the urine of infected animals. *Legionella* species frequently can be isolated from shower heads, faucets, cooling systems, and other common water sources. Ehrlichiosis is a tick-borne disease that causes a febrile illness in infected persons.

11. A. The finding of crepitus in an area of intense tenderness and tense edema of overlying skin suggests a necrotizing soft tissue infection with a gas-forming organism or combination of organisms, although crepitus is not always found. Although group A *Streptococcus* by itself may produce necrotizing fasciitis or a rare fulminating myositis in the absence of an obvious portal of entry, it does not produce gas. *Aeromonas* causes necrotizing cellulitis and myositis following injuries associated with water but also does not produce gas. Gas production is commonly seen in necrotizing cellulitis and fasciitis due to synergistic infections involving anaerobes and facultative organisms; such infections commonly are the result of contamination of a wound with bowel flora or a complication of diabetes (as in diabetic foot infections). Clostridial myonecrosis or gas gangrene may involve healthy soft tissues even at a distance from the portal of entry, which is often the bowel or a wound. When *Clostridium septicum* is the offending organism, there is frequently an underlying malignancy.

12. C. Because the efficacy of the pertussis vaccine wanes with time, many persons, especially adolescents and adults, are susceptible to infection. Erythromycin has been shown to decrease the risk of infection following exposure to *Bordetella pertussis*, and prophylaxis of all directly exposed individuals without prior testing for infection is recommended. Azithromycin could also be used for this indication. A booster vaccination with acellular pertussis vaccine for adults is now recommended [Centers for Disease Control and Prevention. Recommended adult immunization schedule—United States, 2009. *MMWR.* 2008;57(53)]. Certainly, persons who acquire pertussis should be treated.

13. D. Recurrent meningococcal meningitis occurs in persons with deficiencies in the terminal components of complement. Persons with neutrophil dysfunction are especially susceptible to infection with staphylococci. Dural epidermoid cysts can be the source of recurrent episodes of aseptic meningitis and is in the differential diagnosis of recurrent aseptic meningitis, also called Mollaret meningitis. The most common cause of Mollaret meningitis is recurrent herpes simplex II infection. The most common cause of bacterial meningitis in persons with chronic leakage of cerebrospinal fluid is *Streptococcus pneumoniae.*

14. C. The patient has the clinical diagnosis of influenza B based on her presentation and test result. There is no evidence of influenza or secondary bacterial pneumonia. As the patient is presenting within 72 hours of symptoms and is at risk of complications of influenza given her age and history of COPD and dementia, she should receive treatment for influenza B. Amantadine and rimantadine bind to the M2 nucleocapsid protein of influenza A but not of influenza B. Azithromycin is prescribed frequently for patients with bacterial respiratory infections, but it is of no value for treating influenza B. Both zanamivir and oseltamivir are active against both influenza A and B, as well as against avian strains such as H5N1. Zanamivir is only available in inhaled form and can cause bronchospasm; thus it may not be the optimal choice for a patient with COPD and dementia.

15. D. *Streptococcus milleri* is a viridans streptococcus that is often isolated from brain abscesses originating from a focus of infection in the sinuses or oropharynx. Brain

abscesses may result from *S. aureus* bacteremia or endocarditis. *Mycobacterium tuberculosis* may cause focal lesions in the brain (tuberculomas) as well as a subacute meningitis. Cysticercosis, due to the larval form of the pig tapeworm, *Tenia solium*, is a common cause of seizures in persons in many developing countries. *Toxoplasma gondii* produces necrotizing lesions of the brain in persons with the acquired immunodeficiency syndrome. Localized central nervous system lesions of this type are not seen with *B. burgdorferi*, the cause of Lyme disease. Neurological manifestations of chronic Lyme disease include aseptic meningitis, cranial nerve palsies, motor and sensory radiculoneuropathy, and meningoencephalitis.

16. C. The clinical presentation of radicular pain and vesicular rash with a dermatomal distribution is highly suggestive of herpes zoster infection. The diagnosis can be confirmed by finding of multinucleated giant cells on a Tzanck (Giemsa) smear, immunostaining, or virus culture. In about one-fourth of patients with Hodgkin disease complicated by herpes zoster, generalized (disseminated) cutaneous or visceral dissemination will develop. Herpes zoster is associated with prolonged lesions in immunosuppressed patients. This patient's lesions will probably continue to progress during the next 3 to 4 days. Prednisone has been shown to prolong the course of herpes zoster in immunosuppressed patients and is not recommended in this setting. Several studies have shown that systemic antiviral treatment (acyclovir, valacyclovir, famciclovir) decreases the frequency of dissemination and the morbidity in patients with malignancies. The presence of varicella zoster virus (VZV) in two noncontiguous dermatomes suggests dissemination, and treatment should be initiated promptly. Intravenous acyclovir has been used initially in these cases, but it may not be necessary in most cases with the availability of valacyclovir and famciclovir, which have good bioavailability.

Post-herpetic neuralgia occurs after herpes zoster. Because herpes zoster is caused by reactivation of a latent varicella-zoster infection, circulating antibodies to varicella-zoster antigens already are present. Immunoglobulins (immune serum globulin or zoster immune globulin) have not been shown to affect herpes lesions or to reduce complications.

17. B. This patient had traveler's diarrhea, which occurs in approximately one-third of travelers from industrialized countries to developing countries in Latin America, Africa, the Middle East, and Asia. Although the spectrum of clinical illness varies considerably, four to five loose or watery stools per day is characteristic.

Various infectious agents that are acquired through ingestion of fecal-contaminated food and water may cause traveler's diarrhea. In all countries, enterotoxigenic *Escherichia coli* is the commonest cause. Other organisms that cause traveler's diarrhea less commonly include viruses, enteroinvasive *E. coli*, *Salmonella* species, *Shigella* species, *Campylobacter jejuni*, *Giardia lamblia*, *Cryptosporidium*, and *Entamoeba histolytica*.

Antimotility drugs such as loperamide or diphenoxylate, or absorbents such as bismuth subsalicylate, are usually effective treatment for milder forms of traveler's diarrhea. Antimicrobial agents such as quinolones, trimethoprim-sulfamethoxazole, doxycycline, or rifaximin have been shown to shorten the duration of illness.

18. C. Beta-lactamases are enzymes that cleave the beta-lactam ring of beta-lactam antibiotics, such as penicillins and cephalosporins. Clavulanic acid, sulbactam, and tazobactam are currently available beta-lactamase inhibitors. Clavulanic acid is available with ticarcillin as Timentin® and with amoxicillin as Augmentin®, and sulbactam is available with ampicillin as Unasyn®, and tazobactam is available with piperacillin as Zosyn®. *Streptococcus pyogenes* is the only one of the organisms listed that has not been shown to produce penicillinase; thus, ampicillin is as effective as amoxicillin and clavulanic acid or ampicillin and sulbactam. Although staphylococci were initially (in the 1940s) susceptible to penicillin and ampicillin, they rapidly acquired penicillinase. Today most isolates, whether acquired in the community or in the hospital, are resistant to penicillin and ampicillin. *Neisseria gonorrhoeae* and *Haemophilus influenzae* have acquired penicillinases, and up to 20%–30% of strains of these species in some areas are now resistant to penicillin and ampicillin, and an even higher percentage are resistant in some other countries. Resistance to ampicillin caused by production of penicillinase is also commonly found in *Branhamella catarrhalis*. For these strains that produce penicillinase as well as for *Bacteroides fragilis* and for several Enterobacteriaceae with plasmid-mediated resistance, amoxicillin and clavulanic acid and ampicillin and sulbactam are superior in vitro to ampicillin alone. The beta-lactamase inhibitors, however, have little or no activity against the cephalosporinases characteristic of *Enterobacter cloacae* and several other species.

19. D. The epidemiologic and clinical features of this patient strongly suggest wound infection caused by *Vibrio vulnificus*, an organism that lives in coastal waters. Infection is usually associated with exposure to brackish or salt water or to shellfish harvested from these waters. Cellulitis, bullae, necrosis, lymphangitis, and lymphadenopathy are characteristic. Myositis occasionally may develop. Therapy should consist of vigorous surgical debridement and antibiotics. Although *Staphylococcus aureus* and *Haemophilus influenzae* may cause wound infection similar to that occurring in this patient, neither pathogen is associated with handling of shellfish. *Clostridium perfringens* causes gas gangrene or cellulitis, usually occurring after trauma or vascular compromise. Ecthyma gangrenosum (characteristic ulcerative skin lesion surrounded by an erythematous

halo) typically occurs in leukopenic patients with cancer and *Pseudomonas aeruginosa* bacteremia. Another cause of cellulitis that may follow handling of raw seafood is *Erysipelothrix rhusiopathiae.*

20. C. Although the gallbladder is a common site of *Salmonella* carriage, it is rarely the source of bacteremia. Persons who chronically carry *Salmonella* in the gallbladder shed the organism in the stool. Prolonged colonic carriage also occurs following *Salmonella* gastroenteritis, especially after treatment with antibiotics. *Salmonella* may cause chronic osteomyelitis of the spine and other bones, but the associated bacteremia is usually transient. Persistent bacteremia is characteristic of endovascular infections with *Salmonella.* Infected aneurysms and large atherosclerotic plaques give rise to high-grade bacteremias that recur following antibiotic therapy unless the vascular lesion is excised. Other conditions associated with prolonged *Salmonella* bacteremia include HIV infection, other immunodeficiency states, and chronic hepatosplenic schistosomiasis.

21. D. Catastrophic neurological complications such as those described in this case can occur with bacterial meningitis, cavernous sinus thrombosis, and brain abscesses, all of which may be sequelae of chronic sinusitis. However, the rapid development of defects involving one entire hemisphere and progression to increased intracranial pressure are characteristic of subdural empyema, a condition that occurs most commonly in persons with frontal sinusitis.

22. C. Splenectomized persons are at risk for overwhelming infection with a variety of organisms, including encapsulated bacteria (especially *Pneumococcus*), *Babesia,* and malaria parasites. There have been a number of cases of overwhelming sepsis following dog bites or licks due to *Capnocytophaga canimorsus* (formerly known as DF-2), an organism found in the oral cavity of healthy dogs. *Pasteurella multocida,* a Gram-negative bacillus, is part of the normal oral flora of cats (and to a lesser extent, dogs); it is responsible for cellulitis, tenosynovitis, septic arthritis, osteomyelitis, sepsis, and a variety of other syndromes, but infections are not more severe in persons without spleens. *Ehrlichia canis,* a rickettsia transmitted by ticks, causes pancytopenia in dogs; ehrlichiosis in human beings is also tick-borne; the organism cannot be cultivated in routine blood cultures. *Fusobacterium necrophorum* is a Gram-negative anaerobic bacillus that is part of the normal flora of the human oral cavity. It is associated with aggressive infections such as necrotizing pneumonia and postanginal sepsis (septic thrombophlebitis of the internal jugular vein due to parapharyngeal space infection, also known as Lemierre disease).

23. C. Clindamycin is active against most isolates of *Prevotella* (formerly *Bacteroides*) *melaninogenica* and *Streptococcus milleri,* organisms found in the oropharynx of healthy persons. Although strains of coagulase-negative staphylococci can be resistant to clindamycin, they are unlikely to be the cause of an aggressive hand infection. *Eikenella corrodens,* a small Gram-negative bacillus also found in the human mouth, is characteristically resistant to clindamycin. It may cause necrotizing soft tissue infections, and it is one of the HACEK group of fastidious bacteria that cause subacute bacterial endocarditis. Penicillin, ampicillin, and cephalosporins are active against this organism.

24. C. Hand hygiene with alcohol-based rub solutions has had an important role in the reduction of health care-associated infections by facilitating hand cleaning in busy wards. Although they are bactericidal against most bacteria and yeasts, they are not active against the spore forms of *C. difficile.* Thus, hand washing with soap and water is still required before and after contact with patients with *C. difficile.* As *C. difficile* spores are present in the environment surrounding the infected patient, use of single rooms and contact precautions by use of gowns and gloves are advisable. Decreasing the antimicrobial pressure by stopping unnecessary antibacterials is also a recommended strategy hospital-wide.

25. E. All of the microorganisms listed can be transmitted by red blood cell transfusion. In the United States, West Nile virus is now screened by nucleic acid amplification, which has reduced, but not completely eliminated, transmission. CMV can be transmitted from latently infected leukocytes, and the risk of transmission can be reduced by leukocyte filtration. Other countries in the Americas have screened blood donors for Chagas disease for years; this has finally become practice in the United States. Babesiosis has been transmitted by blood transfusion and is not currently systematically screened for.

26. B. Multiple outbreaks of subcutaneous and other surgical-site infections caused by rapidly growing nontuberculous mycobacteria have been described and reported. The infections are subacute and have been associated with contaminated surgical solutions and nonoptimal equipment sterilization techniques. These bacteria can grow on usual culture systems or on special mycobacterial media. Sometimes tissue biopsy is required for definitive diagnosis. *M. cheloneae, M. fortuitum,* and *M. abscessus* are the most common isolates. Treatment requires prolonged antimicrobial treatment.

S. aureus is a very common cause of surgical-site infections, although subacute, indolent presentations are rare. *Aeromonas* cellulitis can occur in patients who are exposed to water sources. Cutaneous larva migrans occurs with skin contact with soil/sand infested with animal hookworm larvae (cats, dogs), but it is usually a nonsuppurative process. Cutaneous leishmaniasis can present with single or multiple ulcerative lesions, papules, or nodules but is usually not a suppurative process.

27. D. The smear demonstrates intraerythrocytic merozoites of *Babesia microti*, a zoonosis endemic in the northeastern United States and areas of the Midwest. It is transmitted by the deer tick, *Ixodes scapularis*. The patient is at some risk of malaria given his work at the airport where cases have been described from infected *Anopheles* sp. mosquitoes that travel inside airplanes and then go on to infect people in the surrounding areas ("airport malaria"), but the intraerythrocytic forms do not resemble ring forms or merozoites of *Plasmodium* species. *Culex pipiens* is the main vector of West Nile virus, and *Aedes aegypti* is the main vector of dengue fever, but neither of them is known to transmit babesiosis.

9.

INFECTIOUS DISEASE SUMMARY

Michael Klompas and Paul E. Sax

STAPHYLOCOCCUS AUREUS INFECTION

*S*taphylococcus aureus is the most frequent cause of severe infections in the inpatient setting. There have been four major trends in *S. aureus* infections over the past two decades:

1. **A sustained rise in the incidence of *S. aureus* bacteremia.** This is likely attributable to the rising prevalence of immunocompromised hosts and long-term indwelling devices such as percutaneous catheters.

2. **A dramatic increase in the prevalence of healthcare-associated methicillin-resistant *S. aureus* (MRSA).** Risk factors for MRSA infection include MRSA colonization, prolonged hospitalization, intensive care, hemodialysis, and antibiotic use. Healthcare providers face a major challenge containing the spread of this organism from patient to patient within their premises. One of the most potent measures to prevent spread of MRSA is fastidious handwashing with soap and water or an alcohol-based hand rub before and after every patient contact.

3. **The appearance and ascendance of community-acquired methicillin-resistant *S. aureus* (CA-MR-SA).** These now account for the majority of skin and soft tissue infections seen in emergency departments. There have been highly publicized outbreaks of CA-MRSA among sports teams, prisoners, and men who have sex with men. Risk factors for CA-MRSA include skin trauma, incarceration, and close contact with people colonized or infected with the organism. However, CA-MRSA now occurs commonly in healthy individuals with none of the above risk factors.

4. **The increasing availability of novel antibiotics to treat methicillin-resistant** infections including linezolid, daptomycin, tigecycline, and ceftaroline. These agents tend to be reserved for severe infections; hence,

clinicians have also come to recognize the value of older oral agents to treat minor MRSA skin infections. These include trimethoprim-sulfamethoxazole, doxycycline, and clindamycin. Importantly, CA-MRSA isolates that are resistant to erythromycin tend to have inducible resistance to clindamycin; hence, clindamycin should not be used to treat CA-MRSA if erythromycin resistance is present.

CLINICAL PRESENTATION

Common clinical manifestations of *S. aureus* include skin and soft tissue infections, necrotizing pneumonia, endocarditis, and bacteremia. Skin and soft tissue infections can run the gamut from postsurgical infections to necrotizing fasciitis and the staphylococcal toxic shock syndrome. Necrotizing *S. aureus* pneumonia can be a complication of influenza. These patients present with a biphasic illness that begins with a classic influenza-like syndrome that transiently improves and then dramatically worsens with severe respiratory compromise. *S. aureus* pneumonia is often caused by methicillin-resistant strains.

EVALUATION

Evaluation of patients with *S. aureus* endocarditis and bacteremia should focus on locating the source of infection (most frequently indwelling lines or devices) and identifying all distant sites that might have been seeded with infection (typical destinations include heart valves, vertebrae, brain, and joints).

TREATMENT

Treatment success critically depends on removal of indwelling devices, particularly venous catheters, and drainage of abscesses seeded by the infection. Antimicrobial therapy should be promptly instituted and continued for *at least* 4 to 6 weeks even in patients without identified metastatic foci of infection because these can often be subclinical. Patients with methicillin-susceptible strains should preferentially be treated with nafcillin rather than vancomycin because nafcillin is a much more potent agent.

INFECTIVE ENDOCARDITIS

EPIDEMIOLOGY AND MICROBIOLOGY

Patients with abnormal heart valves are at greatest risk for endocarditis. In the developing world, the most frequent underlying lesion is rheumatic heart disease. In the developed world, the majority of patients have prosthetic valves or mitral valve prolapse associated with valve thickening and mitral regurgitation.

The microbiology of endocarditis is usefully considered in two categories: native valve infections and prosthetic valve disease (see table 9.1). Native valves tend to be infected by *Streptococcus* species, *Staphylococcus aureus,* and *Enterococcus.* The microbiology of prosthetic valve infections varies with proximity to surgery: patients with recently implanted valves tend to get infected with skin organisms such as coagulase-negative *Staphylococci* or *Propionibacterium acnes* and nosocomial pathogens such as methicillin-resistant *Staphylococcus aureus* or vancomycin-resistant enterococci. Patients with valves in place for more than a year tend to be infected with the same pathogens as patients with native valves. The mitral valve and aortic valve are the most common sites of infection. Tricuspid valve disease is usually only seen in intravenous drug users and patients with long-term indwelling venous catheters.

DIAGNOSIS

The typical symptoms of endocarditis are prolonged fever, fatigue, weight loss, and back pain. Patients with this constellation of symptoms should be closely evaluated for cardiac murmurs. Additional findings on physical examination include Roth spots, Osler nodes, Janeway lesions, splinter hemorrhages, and conjunctival petechiae. These findings are typically only present, however, in patients with subacute disease who have been infected for weeks to months. Patients should be carefully examined for metastatic sites of infection—typical destinations include the vertebrae, joints, liver, spleen, and eye. Draw at least two sets of blood cultures before beginning any empirical antibiotics.

Echocardiography is the test of choice for patients with suspected endocarditis. A transthoracic echocardiogram is a reasonable place to start because it is noninvasive, but endocarditis cannot be excluded until the patient gets a transesophageal echocardiogram. Transthoracic studies are only about 50–60% sensitive compared to transesophageal imaging.

TREATMENT

Consultation with an infectious disease specialist is recommended for all patients with proven endocarditis to help guide management. In general terms, however, treatment is tailored to the antimicrobial susceptibility of the specific pathogen isolated from the patient's blood or resected valve. Typical agents include penicillin or ceftriaxone for streptococci, with the addition of gentamicin for isolates with partial resistance to penicillin; nafcillin for methicillin-susceptible *S. aureus* or vancomycin for methicillin-resistant organisms; and a combination of penicillin or vancomycin and gentamicin for enterococcal infections. Patients should get two sets of blood cultures daily until bacteremia has cleared. Length of treatment varies between 4 and 6 weeks depending on the specific pathogen. The duration of therapy is counted from the first day of negative blood cultures rather than from the first day antibiotics were administered. Some patients require surgical therapy in addition to antibiotics. Indications for surgery include hemodynamic compromise, significant valvular dysfunction, myocardial abscess, and persistently positive blood cultures despite appropriate therapy. In the case of hemodynamic compromise or congestive heart failure, surgery should not be delayed even when signs and symptoms suggest ongoing active infection.

PROPHYLAXIS

The most recent recommendations for antibiotic prophylaxis against endocarditis dramatically reduced the population of eligible patients. Currently, only patients with cardiac conditions associated with a high risk of adverse outcomes from endocarditis are targeted for antibiotic prophylaxis. These include patients with prosthetic valves or prosthetic cardiac repair materials, previous endocarditis, unrepaired or incompletely repaired congenital cyanotic heart disease, and cardiac transplant patients with valve disease. These patients should receive 2 g of amoxicillin 30–60 minutes prior to dental work, respiratory tract procedures that include incision or biopsy, and surgery on infected skin, muscle,

Table 9.1 MICROBIOLOGY OF ENDOCARDITIS

NATIVE VALVE (COMMUNITY ACQUIRED)	NATIVE VALVE (HOSPITAL ACQUIRED)	PROSTHETIC VALVE <30 DAYS POST-IMPLANTATION*
Streptococcus viridans	*Staphylococcus aureus*	Coagulase-negative staphylococci
Streptococcus pneumoniae	*Enterococcus* sp.	*Propionibacterium acnes*
	Gram-negative aerobes	*Staphylococcus aureus*
	Candida sp.	*Enterococcus* sp.

NOTE: *After 30 days postimplantation, the microbiology of prosthetic valve endocarditis increasingly resembles that of community-acquired native valve endocarditis.

or bones. Antibiotic prophylaxis is *not* recommended for patients with other cardiac conditions (such as mitral valve prolapse) or for any patient undergoing gastrointestinal or genitourinary procedures.

CLOSTRIDIUM DIFFICILE

EPIDEMIOLOGY AND RISK FACTORS

Clostridium difficile is the most frequent pathogen associated with nosocomial diarrhea. The disease has taken on new importance in the past few years as a result of the emergence of a hypervirulent strain associated with a substantially increased risk of colectomy and death. Evaluation of every hospitalized patient with diarrhea should include testing for *C. difficile*. The major risk factors for *C. difficile* are antibiotic exposure and hospitalization. Any antibiotic can precipitate *C. difficile* including quinolones, cephalosporins, and penicillins, as well as clindamycin. Rarely, *C. difficile* can occur after cancer chemotherapy due to the antimicrobial activity of chemotherapeutic agents.

NOSOCOMIAL TRANSMISSION

Nosocomial transmission of *C. difficile* is distressingly common because the organism forms spores that are resistant to conventional hospital cleaning agents. Bleach is the only common cleaning agent that kills *C. difficile* spores. In a similar vein, alcohol-based hand washes are also ineffective against *C. difficile* spores. Clinicians need to wash their hands with soap and water for at least 2 minutes to mechanically rid their hands of *C. difficile* after touching a contaminated patient or environment. Patients with *C. difficile* should be isolated from uninfected patients to prevent the spread of infection.

CLINICAL PRESENTATION

The clinical manifestations of *C. difficile* infection include fever, abdominal cramping or bloating, severe diarrhea, and leukocytosis. Computed tomography findings can include colonic dilatation and colonic wall thickening (figure 9.1). The organism is difficult to culture; hence, diagnosis is accomplished by assaying stool for *C. difficile* toxins using an enzyme immunoassay. The immunoassay has variable sensitivity; thus, a negative test in a patient with a high clinical probability of disease should prompt repeat testing up to three times total. A cytotoxicity assay is more sensitive, but the slower turnaround time of this test has led most clinical laboratories to switch to the enzyme immunoassay method.

TREATMENT

The treatment strategy for *C. difficile* depends on the severity of the infection. Patients with relatively mild disease (diarrhea but minimal abdominal pain, fever, or leukocytosis)

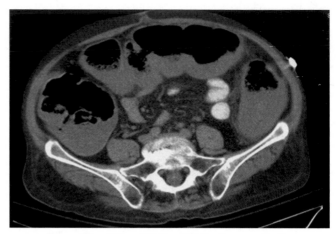

Figure 9.1 Severe Clostridium difficile colitis (toxic megacolon).

can be treated with oral metronidazole. Patients with refractory or severe disease (septic physiology, high fever, severe abdominal pain, marked leukocytosis) should be treated with oral vancomycin along with intravenous metronidazole. A recently-added option for treatment is fidaxomicin; it is as effective as vancomycin, but much more expensive. A surgeon should be consulted in all patients with severe infection because early colectomy is sometimes the only way to save the life of someone infected with a hypervirulent strain. Consultation with an infectious disease specialist is also advised to guide the management of severe infections.

TRAVEL MEDICINE

PREVENTION

Pretrip counseling and vaccination form the keystones of travel medicine. Advice and immunizations ought to be tailored to the traveler's destination, duration of time abroad, and planned activities. First ensure that the patient is up to date in routine immunizations such as measles-mumps-rubella, tetanus-diphtheria-acellular pertussis, *Haemophilus influenzae, Streptococcus pneumoniae,* and influenza. Depending on destination and activities, the patient might also merit vaccines against hepatitis A and B, *Neisseria meningitidis,* polio, typhoid fever, yellow fever, rabies, and Japanese encephalitis. Travelers to malaria-endemic regions should be offered malaria prophylaxis tailored to the resistance profile of parasites in the traveler's destination. Clinicians are advised to check the website of the Centers for Disease Control and Prevention (www.cdc.gov/travel) for specific recommendations on vaccines and malaria prophylaxis.

TRAVELER'S DIARRHEA

Diarrhea is the most common illness afflicting travelers to developing countries. Half or more of travelers to developing countries for 2–3 weeks develop diarrhea. The management of diarrhea begins with prevention. Advise travelers to avoid drinking untreated water and eating uncooked produce or vegetables that have come into contact with untreated water. The catch phrase is "peel it, boil it, or don't eat it."

Should diarrhea develop, travelers should focus on aggressive self-hydration followed by empiric therapy with a quinolone [for example, ciprofloxacin, 250 mg twice daily for 1–3 days or a single dose of azithromycin (1 g)]. Patients can also take loperamide for symptom relief so long as they are not experiencing fever or hematochezia.

Persistent diarrhea in a returning traveler can be divided into bloody and nonbloody categories. Bloody diarrhea is usually caused by enteroinvasive strains of *E. coli, Salmonella, Shigella, Campylobacter, Yersinia,* and *Entamoeba histolytica.* The stool of patients with acute bloody diarrhea should be cultured for these pathogens to confirm diagnosis and determine antibiotic susceptibility. Empiric treatment with a quinolone or azithromycin is reasonable after a specimen has been taken. Patients with subacute, nonbloody diarrhea more typically have parasitic infections with organisms such as *Giardia lamblia* or *Cryptosporidium* sp. These can be diagnosed with stool antigen detection assays or microscopic examination for ova and parasites. In the case of *Cryptosporidium* sp., laboratories will need to utilize special stains to visualize the organism, and the clinician should alert the lab that this diagnosis is being considered. Some travelers with persistent symptoms despite negative stool studies have developed a postinfectious irritable bowel syndrome rather than active, ongoing infection.

FEVER IN THE RETURNING TRAVELER

The first priority in a returning traveler with fever is evaluation for malaria. A delay in the diagnosis or treatment of malaria can lead to substantial morbidity and death. Returning travelers with fever should have thin and thick blood smears sent to assess for malaria. Antigen detection assays can supplement visual examination. A diagnosis of malaria should prompt rapid consultation with an infectious disease expert or a malaria clinician at the Centers for Disease Control and Prevention (Malaria Hotline: 770-488-7788).

Other causes of fever in returning travelers include enteric fever caused by *Salmonella typhi* or *paratyphi,* dengue, viral hepatitis, acute HIV, leptospirosis, schistosomiasis, tick-bite fever, and tuberculosis (see table 9.2). Of note, dengue fever has become a more common cause of fever in the returning traveler in more recent series.

LYME DISEASE

EPIDEMIOLOGY

Lyme disease is the most common tick-borne illness in the United States and Europe. The causative pathogen is the spirochete *Borrelia burgdorferi. Borrelia* is transmitted to humans by the deer tick *Ixodes scapularis* or *Ixodes pacificus.*

Table 9.2 SOURCES OF FEVER IN THE RETURNING TRAVELER

Malaria	35%
Viral hepatitis	5%
Respiratory tract infections	5%
Dysentery	5%
Dengue fever	5%
Urinary tract infections	3%
Typhoid fever	2%
Tuberculosis	1%
Rickettsial infection	1%
Acute HIV infection	1%
Amebic liver abscess	0.5%

Lyme disease is found throughout the United States, but it is most commonly reported in the U.S. Northeast and in northwest California. Most cases occur during the summer months. People with dogs and those living in or visiting wooded areas are at greatest risk.

CLINICAL PRESENTATION

The clinical presentation of Lyme occurs in three stages (table 9.3). The disease begins at the site of a tick bite with an erythema migrans rash (figure 9.2). In order for disease transmission to occur, an infected tick must feed on its human host for at least 36 hours. Nonetheless, many patients do not recall the precipitating tick bite. The appearance of an erythema migrans rash is diagnostic of Lyme disease. Patients with an erythema migrans rash ought to be treated without further investigation because up to 60% of patients with primary disease will have negative Lyme enzyme-linked immunosorbent assays (ELISA). Since ticks often bite in areas that are not easily visualized (such as in the gluteal folds or back of the neck), patients may not be aware that they have erythema migrans and therefore do not present for medical care.

Within days to weeks of inoculation, the *Borrelia* spirochetes disseminate through the body. Patients at this second stage of infection can present with multiple erythema migrans rashes spread over the body and with systemic symptoms such as fever, chills, headache, myalgias, and fatigue (figure 9.3). A small subset of patients go on to develop transient focal disease in just about any organ of the body including meningitis, facial palsy, neuritis, conjunctivitis, atrioventricular heart block, myocarditis, migratory joint pains, and mild hepatitis. Patients at this stage of infection typically have positive Lyme ELISA tests.

Table 9.3 LYME DISEASE: STAGES, PRESENTATION, TREATMENTS

STAGE	CLINICAL PRESENTATION	TREATMENT	DURATION
Stage 1	Erythema migrans	Doxycycline	14 days
Stage 2 (early)	Fever, headache, fatigue, adenopathy Disseminated erythema migrans lesions	Doxycycline	14 days
Stage 2 (late)	Cardiac: first degree atrioventricular block	Doxycycline	14 days
	Cardiac: complete heart block	Ceftriaxone	14–21 days
	Musculoskeletal: migratory joint pains, transient arthritis	Doxycycline	28 days
	Neuro: meningitis, encephalitis, facial palsy, radiculitis, mononeuritis multiplex	Ceftriaxone	14–28 days
Stage 3	Chronic encephalomyelitis Chronic arthritis Chronic axonal radiculopathy	Ceftriaxone	28 days

NOTE: *Alternatives: amoxicillin, 500 mg PO tid, or cefuroxime, 500 mg PO bid.

Months to years later, a further subset of patients manifest with symptoms and signs of tertiary persistent infection. These patients can have intermittent pain and swelling of large joints (especially the knees) or neurological complaints such as encephalomyelitis or multiple axonal radiculopathies. These patients also have persistently positive Lyme ELISAs.

LABORATORY DIAGNOSIS

The Lyme ELISA test is sensitive in the second and third stages of infection. By 1 month after inoculation almost all patients have positive Lyme ELISA tests. The ELISA is prone, however, to false-positive results, and hence the Centers for Disease Control and Prevention (CDC) recommend follow-up testing of all positive ELISA tests with a Western blot assay to increase specificity. The CDC has established criteria for interpretation of Western blots by designating certain bands as potentially significant. A Western blot is considered positive for IgM if a patient has at least two out of three designated bands present, and the IgG is considered positive if a patient has at least 5 out of 10 designated bands present. ELISA and Western blots can remain positive for many years, even with treatment; hence, the diagnosis of repeat infections must be made on clinical rather than laboratory grounds. Typically, only patients with early infections aborted by rapid therapy are susceptible to reinfection.

Some clinicians and patients maintain that negative Lyme testing in the face of symptoms such as fatigue and myalgia do not exclude the diagnosis of Lyme. Although it

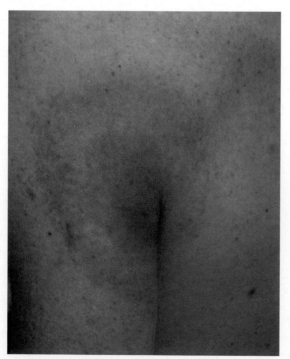

Figure 9.2. Erythema migrans rash of early lyme disease.

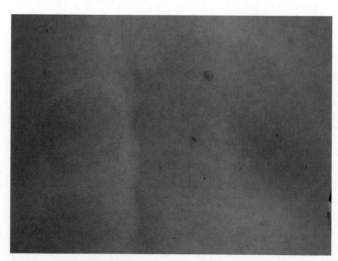

Figure 9.3. Disseminated lyme disease.

is well described that patients with early Lyme disease can have negative antibody tests, there is a substantial body of scientific evidence supporting the high sensitivity of Lyme antibody testing for patients with manifestations of late disease. Consequently, clinical guidelines published by the Infectious Diseases Society of America do not recommend antibiotic treatment for patients with nonspecific symptoms and negative Lyme antibody tests.

Patients suspected of Lyme disease should also be tested for ehrlichiosis and babesiosis because these diseases often co-occur with Lyme.

TREATMENT

Patients who meet clinical diagnostic criteria (an erythema migrans rash) or laboratory diagnostic criteria (a positive ELISA followed by a positive Western blot) ought to be treated (see table 9.3). Stage 1 and stage 2 disease including first-degree atrioventricular block can be treated with doxycycline, 100 mg PO bid for 14 to 21 days. An alternative agent is amoxicillin, 500 mg PO tid. Patients with arthritis should be treated with an oral agent for 28 days. Facial palsies can also be treated with an oral regimen, but patients with other neurological manifestations or high-degree atrioventricular block merit intravenous penicillin or ceftriaxone for 14–28 days.

POST–LYME DISEASE SYNDROME

A small percentage of patients have persistent myalgias, arthralgias, impaired cognition, and fatigue despite appropriate treatment. This appears to be a postinfectious syndrome. Randomized trials of prolonged intravenous and oral antibiotics versus placebo do not show any benefit of antimicrobial therapy for this population.

HIV INFECTION AND THE ACQUIRED IMMUNODEFICIENCY SYNDROME

EPIDEMIOLOGY

The incidence of HIV in the United States has been steady over the past few years at approximately 55,000 new infections per year. Among men, approximately 75% acquire HIV through contact with other men; among women, a similar proportion contract it from a man infected with HIV. The major risk factor for HIV transmission in the United States is unprotected sexual intercourse with an infected partner or, to a lesser extent, intravenous drug use. A large driver for the persistently high number of new infections is felt to be a large reservoir of people unaware of their serostatus; in response, the CDC is encouraging more widespread testing: every adult patient seen in any kind of healthcare facility ought to be tested at least once for HIV. Patients at high risk for HIV infection should be tested annually, and pregnant patients should be tested as part of their routine prenatal evaluation. The CDC advocates replacing opt-in testing (where providers seek written consent prior to testing) with opt-out testing (where patients are tested without written consent unless they explicitly refuse). Testing legislation varies by state, however, and many do not currently permit testing without prior written consent.

NATURAL HISTORY

Acute infection with HIV is often symptomatic. Days to weeks after virus acquisition patients experience an acute mononucleosis-like syndrome characterized by fever, headache, sore throat, rash, myalgias, and fatigue. The syndrome typically resolves after a few days or weeks, and infected patients become asymptomatic. This seroconversion syndrome may be highly symptomatic at one extreme (requiring hospitalization) and completely asymptomatic at the other. People with HIV can subsequently remain asymptomatic for anywhere from a few years to 20 years or more. During this period, the HIV virus is actively replicating within the body, but new virions are destroyed by the immune system at the same rate as they are produced. HIV tends to harness the immune system's CD4 cells for viral replication, killing the cells in the process. Eventually, the number of CD4 cells in the body declines, viral replication exceeds immune destruction, and the viral load begins to rise. Decreasing CD4 cell counts lead to progressively more immune dysfunction and increasing susceptibility to opportunistic infections. Untreated patients typically succumb to opportunistic infections or neoplasms rather than directly to HIV itself.

OPPORTUNISTIC INFECTIONS

Patients become susceptible to different opportunistic infections at characteristic levels of CD4 counts (see table 9.4). HIV patients with relatively preserved CD4 counts (>350 cells/mm^3) are at increased risk of invasive pneumococcal infections, tuberculosis, and herpes zoster. When the CD4 count drops below 200 cells/mm^3, patients become susceptible to oral thrush, esophageal candidiasis, and *Pneumocystis jiroveci* pneumonia (PCP). Below 50–100 CD4 cells/mm^3, *Mycobacterium avium* complex, cryptococcal meningitis, and invasive cytomegalovirus (CMV) infections are possible. Importantly, these CD4 cell count thresholds are generalizations, and some individuals with HIV have opportunistic infections at higher levels, whereas others with severely depleted counts remain without infection for months or even years.

TREATMENT

The decision to initiate treatment is a shared decision between patient and provider. Parties need to balance the inconvenience and potential toxicity of antiretroviral therapy on the one hand against the risk of opportunistic

Table 9.4 OPPORTUNISTIC INFECTIONS IN HIV-INFECTED PATIENTS

CD4 COUNT (CELLS/MM^3)	DISEASE	FIRST-LINE TREATMENT
>350	*Mycobacterium tuberculosis*	Isoniazid + rifampicin + ethambutol + pyrazinamide
	Streptococcus pneumoniae pneumonia	Ceftriaxone
	Herpes zoster shingles	Valacyclovir, famciclovir, or acyclovir
<200	*Pneumocystis jiroveci* (PCP) pneumonia	Trimethoprim-sulfamethoxazole
	Candida sp. pharyngitis or esophagitis	Fluconazole
<100	*Toxoplasma gondii* encephalitis	Pyrimethamine + sulfadiazine + leucovorin
	Cryptococcus neoformans meningitis	Amphotericin B lipid formulation + flucytosine
<50	*Mycobacterium avium* complex	Clarithromycin + ethambutol ± rifabutin
	Cytomegalovirus retinitis, myelitis, or esophagitis	Valganciclovir PO or ganciclovir IV
	JC virus progressive multifocal leukoencephalopathy	HIV antiretrovirals to reconstitute the immune system

infections and irreversible damage to the immune system on the other hand. Over the past few years the trend has been toward offering patients treatment at earlier stages of infection in light of dramatic advances in HIV therapeutics including the availability of more potent agents with low pill burdens and few adverse effects. It is now possible to treat patients with a highly efficacious regimen requiring only a single pill (containing three different active antiviral medications) once a day. There is also increasing evidence that delayed institution of therapy increases the risk for impaired immune reconstitution.

Current recommendations advise initiating therapy in any patient who has suffered an opportunistic infection, patients with CD4 counts below 500 cells/mm^3, all pregnant women, patients with HIV-associated nephropathy, and in patients with hepatitis B co-infection who require hepatitis B treatment.

Initial therapy should be with a combination of three active agents from two or more antiretroviral classes. The particular choice of agents should be guided by viral resistance testing, prior antiretroviral exposure, comorbidities, and pregnancy status. Currently available antiretroviral classes include nucleoside reverse transcriptase inhibitors, non-nucleoside reverse transcriptase inhibitors, protease inhibitors, fusion inhibitors, CCR5 antagonists, and integrase inhibitors. Typical first-line therapies include the non-nucleoside reverse transcriptase inhibitor efavirenz and two nucleoside reverse transcriptase inhibitors such as tenofovir and emtricitabine. The ritonavir-boosted protease inhibitors atazanavir or darunavir can be substituted for efavirenz; another option is the integrase inhibitor raltegravir.

Prior to prescribing abacavir, clinicians should test patients for the presence of the multihistocompatibility complex class I allele HLA-B*5701. The presence of this allele is highly correlated with hypersensitivity to abacavir, causing a multiorgan syndrome with fatigue, myalgias and fever, rash, diarrhea, or dyspnea. The absence of HLA-B*5701 appears to reliably exclude the possibility of a severe hypersensitivity reaction to abacavir.

MONITORING

HIV-infected patients should see a physician and have serial evaluation of their CD4 count and viral load every 3–4 months. Patients recently started on therapy or switched to a novel therapy should be seen more often and have viral-load testing within 2–8 weeks of the new prescription.

SEXUALLY TRANSMITTED INFECTIONS

CHLAMYDIA

Chlamydia trachomatis is the most common sexually transmitted bacterial infection. The disease can present with symptoms of cervicitis or urethritis but frequently is asymptomatic in both men and women. Untreated infection can lead to pelvic inflammatory disease, ectopic pregnancy, infertility, and chronic pelvic pain. Chlamydia infection during pregnancy is also associated with poor outcomes including miscarriage and premature birth. Consequently, the United States Preventative Task Force recommends screening all sexually active women age 24 or younger for occult infection as well as all older women with risk factors (history of sexually transmitted infections, new or multiple sex partners, inconsistent condom use, and exchanging sex for money or drugs). The most sensitive diagnostic test is a nucleic acid amplification test. Infected patients can be treated with azithromycin, 1 g PO × 1, or doxycycline, 100 mg PO bid × 7 days. Test of cure is recommended only for pregnant women.

GONNORHEA

Gonorrhea is the second most common sexually transmitted bacterial infection. *Neisseria gonorrhoeae* infection presents

Table 9.5 SYPHILIS: STAGES, PRESENTATION, TREATMENTS

STAGE	CLINICAL PRESENTATION	TESTS	TREATMENT	DURATION
Primary	Chancre (painless)	RPR + FTA-Abs ± TP-PA±	Penicillin G, 2.4 million units IM	1 dose
Secondary	Fever, generalized rash involving palms and soles, mucous patches, diffuse lymphadenopathy	RPR + FTA-Abs ± TP-PA+	Penicillin G, 2.4 million units IM	1 dose
Latent	Asymptomatic	RPR ± FTA-Abs + TP-PA+	Penicillin G, 2.4 million units IM	1 dose per week × 3 weeks
Tertiary	Aortitis (aneurysms, aortic regurgitation) Encephalitis (dementia, tabes dorsalis) Ophthalmic disease Deafness	RPR ± FTA-Abs + TP-PA+	Penicillin G, 18–24 million units IV per day	10–14 days

with cervicitis and urethritis. Depending on patients' sexual practices, however, gonorrhea can also manifest as pharyngitis and proctitis. A small proportion of untreated local infections can disseminate to cause a syndrome of fever and arthritis accompanied by a small number of scattered pustules. Some patients, however, especially women, suffer no symptoms at all. The United States Preventative Task Force therefore recommends routine gonorrhea screening for all high-risk women (same risk factors as described above for chlamydia). Diagnosis is based on nucleic acid amplification testing of urine or swabs from the urethra, mouth, and cervix or anus. Localized infection should be treated with ceftriaxone, 125 mg TM × 1, or cefixime, 400 mg PO × 1. Quinolones are no longer recommended to treat this disease because of increasing resistance. Patients with gonorrhea should be empirically treated for concurrent chlamydia unless formal testing rules out co-infection.

SYPHILIS

Syphilis infection proceeds in three stages (table 9.5). About 3 weeks after inoculation patients develop primary infection characterized by a painless ulcer called a *chancre* at the site of inoculation. The chancre spontaneously clears after 2–8 weeks. About 6 weeks after inoculation, a dramatic secondary stage develops characterized by fever, malaise, pharyngitis, diffuse lymphadenopathy, generalized rash involving the palms and soles, and mucous patches on the tongue. This phase can also spontaneously resolve, leading the patient to a period of asymptomatic latent infection. A small subset of patients go on to develop tertiary syphilis characterized principally by aortic disease (dilatation, aneurysm, aortic regurgitation) and neurological disease (tabes dorsalis, ocular lesions, deafness, dementia).

Syphilis can be diagnosed by direct visualization of spirochetes under dark field microscopy. Suitable specimens for microscopy include swabs of chancres from patients with primary infection and swabs of oral mucous patches from patients with secondary infection. More commonly,

serologic tests are used. There are two kinds of serologic tests available: (1) nonspecific, nontreponemal tests such as the RPR (rapid plasma reagin) and VDRL (Venereal Diseases Research Laboratory); and (2) specific treponemal antibody tests directed against different treponemal antigens such the fluorescent treponemal antibody absorption (FTA-ABS) test, the *Treponema pallidum* particle agglutination (TP-PA) test, or the microhemagglutination–*Treponema pallidum* (MHA-TP) test. The nonspecific, nontreponemal tests are useful as rapid, inexpensive screening tests and to monitor patients' response to therapy. The specific treponemal tests are useful to confirm diagnosis in patients with positive nontreponemal tests or compatible clinical syndromes.

Primary, secondary, and early latent (<1 year since infection) syphilis can be treated with a single dose of benzathine penicillin, 2.4 million units IM. Late latent or syphilis of unknown duration should be treated with benzathine

Table 9.6 COMMON CAUSES OF MENINGITIS AND THEIR TREATMENT

Streptococcus pneumoniae	
Penicillin MIC < 0.1 µg/mL	Penicillin G, 18–24 million units per day, or ampicillin, 2 g IV q4h
Penicillin MIC 0.1–1.0 µg/mL	Ceftriaxone, 2 g IV q12h
Penicillin MIC > 1.0 µg/mL	Vancomycin, 1 g IV q 12h, plus ceftriaxone, 2 g IV q12h
Haemophilus influenzae	
Beta-lactamase negative	Ampicillin, 2 g IV q4h
Beta-lactamase positive	Ceftriaxone, 2 g IV q12h
Neisseria meningitidis	
Penicillin MIC < 0.1 µg/mL	Penicillin G, 18–24 million units per day, or ampicillin, 2 g IV q4h
Penicillin MIC 0.1–1.0 µg/mL	Ceftriaxone, 2 g IV q12h
Listeria monocytogenes	Ampicillin, 2 g IV q4h, or penicillin G, 18–24 million units per day

penicillin 2.4 million units IM once weekly × 3 weeks. Neurosyphilis is treated with aqueous penicillin 18–24 million units IV daily × 10–14 days administered as continuous infusion or divided into six doses per day.

BACTERIAL MENINGITIS

EPIDEMIOLOGY AND RISK FACTORS

Despite widespread immunization against pneumococcus and meningococcus, acute bacterial meningitis continues to claim the lives of young, otherwise healthy people. Young people living in close quarters such as college dormitories or military barracks are at particular risk for meningococcal meningitis. Many cases begin with a prodrome of upper respiratory tract infection, otitis media, or sinusitis that subsequently spreads to the central nervous system.

CLINICAL PRESENTATION

The classic presentation of bacterial meningitis is fever, headache, and neck stiffness. Ongoing illness can lead to impaired consciousness and progressive neurological deficits. Kernig's sign (patient resists passive extension of the knee when hip is flexed), Brudzinski's sign (passive flexion of the neck precipitates flexion of the hip and knees), and nuchal rigidity may be found on physical examination.

DIAGNOSIS

Patients with suspected meningitis should be evaluated and treated as expeditiously as possible. Treatment should not be delayed awaiting the execution or results of diagnostic tests. If possible, draw blood cultures prior to administering antibiotics. Patients with papilledema or focal neurological deficits should get immediate empirical dexamethasone and antibiotics and then proceed to head CT to assess for space-occupying lesions prior to lumbar puncture. Patients without papilledema or focal neurological deficits can proceed directly to lumbar puncture followed by empirical therapy with dexamethasone and antibiotics.

Cerebrospinal fluid from patients with bacterial meningitis typically has >1000 white blood cells/mm³ with a neutrophil predominance, elevated protein, and low glucose. Less-marked pleocytosis suggests viral meningitis or other nonbacterial etiology. The most common pathogens responsible for community-acquired meningitis are listed in table 9.6.

TREATMENT

Empirical therapy should include vancomycin, 1 g IV q12h, ceftriaxone, 2 g IV q12h, and dexamethasone, 10 mg IV q6h. The purpose of the vancomycin is to provide coverage for pneumococcal infections that are highly resistant to beta-lactam antibiotics. Early administration of dexamethasone has been shown to decrease mortality and morbidity, particularly in cases caused by *Streptococcus pneumoniae*. Add ampicillin, 2 g IV q4h, when treating elderly, alcoholic, and immunocompromised patients to cover *Listeria monocytogenes*. Add acyclovir, 10 mg/kg IV q8h, if there is a clinical suspicion of *Herpes simplex* virus encephalitis. Once an etiologic pathogen has been identified, tailor antibiotic therapy accordingly (see table 9.6).

PROPHYLAXIS

Close contacts of patients with proven *Neisseria meningitidis* meningitis should receive antibiotic prophylaxis to eradicate possible colonization with invasive *N. meningitidis*. Close contacts are defined as household members (including roommates), day-care center contacts, and people directly exposed to the patient's oral secretions (e.g., kissing, mouth-to-mouth resuscitation, endotracheal intubation, or endotracheal tube management), but not school or office contacts. Acceptable agents to eradicate *N. meningitidis* include rifampin, 600 mg PO bid × 2 days, ceftriaxone, 250 mg IM × 1, and azithromycin 500 mg PO × 1. Ciprofloxacin should be used with caution due to emerging reports of quinolone-resistant *N. meningitidis* in Minnesota and North Dakota.

ADDITIONAL READING

Bamberger DM, Boyd SE. Management of *Staphylococcus aureus* infections. *Am Fam Physician.* 2005;72:2474–81.

Bartlett JG. Narrative review: The new epidemic of *Clostridium difficile*-associated enteric disease. *Ann Intern Med.* 2006;145:758–64.

Bratton RL, Whiteside JW, Hovan MJ, Engle RL, Edwards FD. Diagnosis and treatment of Lyme disease. *Mayo Clin Proc.* 2008;83:566–71.

Mylonakis E, Calderwood SB. Infective endocarditis in adults. *N Engl J Med.* 2001;345(13):18–30.

Panel on Antiretroviral Guidelines for Adults and Adolescents. Guidelines for the use of antiretroviral agents in HIV-1-infected adults and adolescents. Department of Health and Human Services. January 10, 2011;1–166. Available at http://www.aidsinfo.nih.gov/ContentFiles/AdultandAdolescentGL.pdf.

Ryan ET, Wilson ME, Kain KC. Illness after international travel. *N Engl J Med.* 2002;347:505–16.

van de Beek D, de Gans J, Tunkel AR, Wijdicks EF. Community-acquired bacterial meningitis in adults. *N Engl J Med.* 2006;354:44–53.

Wilson W, Taubert KA, Gewitz M, et al. Prevention of infective endocarditis: Guidelines from the American Heart Association: A guideline from the American Heart Association Rheumatic Fever, Endocarditis, and Kawasaki Disease Committee, Council on Cardiovascular Disease in the Young, and the Council on Clinical Cardiology, Council on Cardiovascular Surgery and Anesthesia, and the Quality of Care and Outcomes Research Interdisciplinary Working Group. *Circulation.* 2007;16:1736–54.

Workowski KA, Berman SM. Sexually transmitted diseases treatment guidelines, 2006. *MMWR Recom Rep.* 2006;55:1–94.

Wormser GP, Dattwyler RJ, Shapiro ED, et al. The clinical assessment, treatment, and prevention of Lyme disease, human granulocytic anaplasmosis, and babesiosis: Clinical practice guidelines by the Infectious Diseases Society of America. *Clin Infect Dis.* 2006;43:1089–134.

SECTION 2

HEMATOLOGY AND ONCOLOGY

10.

BREAST CANCER

Michael J. Hassett and Lawrence N. Shulman

EPIDEMIOLOGY

Among women in the United States, breast cancer is the most common cancer and the second most common cause of cancer mortality (excluding basal and squamous cell skin cancer). In 2010 it will account for approximately 209,060 new cancers (28% of all new cancers among women) and 40,230 cancer deaths (15% of cancer deaths in women). The incidence and mortality of breast cancer peaked around 1998 at 145 cases and 32 deaths per 100,000 women. Since then, improvements in screening, prevention, and risk factor modification have led to a modest reduction in breast cancer incidence to approximately 122 cases per 100,000 women; and earlier diagnosis combined with improvements in treatments have led to a modest reduction in breast cancer mortality to 23 cases per 100,000 women. Whereas breast cancer is more common among white women (124 cases/100,000 women) compared to African-American women (113 cases/100,000 women), breast cancer deaths are more common among African-American women (33 deaths/100,000 women) compared to white women (24 deaths/100,000 women).

Risk factors for breast cancer include female sex, age, personal history of breast cancer or benign breast disease, exposure to ionizing radiation, family history of breast cancer, inherited genetic factors, race/ethnicity, diet, alcohol, and estrogen exposure (see table 10.1). Smoking does not appear to be a risk factor for breast cancer. Older age and gender are the strongest risk factors for breast cancer. The odds of developing breast cancer are approximately 1:2525 by age 30, 1:50 by age 50, 1:14 by age 70, and 1:8 over a women's lifetime. Half of all breast cancers occur in women 61 and older. Although breast cancer can develop in men, it is approximately 100 times more frequent among women. Exposure to ionizing chest radiation at a young age, such as that administered for the treatment of lymphoma, is associated with an increased risk of breast cancer and has become an indication for early screening.

Family history is a heterogeneous risk factor. A woman's risk of developing breast cancer is 1.8-fold greater if she has one affected first-degree relative; the magnitude of this risk increases as the age at diagnosis of the affected relative decreases and as the number of affected first-degree relatives increases. Only 15% to 20% of all women who develop breast cancer report a family history of breast cancer. Approximately 5% to 7% of all breast cancer cases are attributable to an inherited breast cancer susceptibility gene, such as BRCA1, BRCA2, p53, PTEN, and ATM (ataxia-telangiectasia). BRCA carriers have a lifetime breast cancer risk that varies from family to family but approaches 80%, and they are at increased risk for ovarian and other cancers as well.

Higher weight/body mass index (BMI) is associated with a higher risk of postmenopausal breast cancer and may be associated with a lower risk of premenopausal breast cancer. Moderate alcohol intake confers a higher risk of hormone-receptor positive breast cancer. Longer exposure to and higher concentrations of endogenous estrogen—as manifest by early menarche, nulliparity, older age at first birth, older age at menopause, and possibly not breast-feeding—is associated with a higher risk of breast cancer. Although oral contraceptives do not increase breast cancer risk, prolonged postmenopausal hormone replacement therapy (HRT), especially formulations that combine estrogen and progesterone, does do so (1.24-fold increase in the relative risk). The reduction in HRT use that followed the Nurses Health Study report that identified this association may partly explain the fall in breast cancer incidence observed over the past decade. Short-term postmenopausal hormone replacement therapy does not significantly increase breast cancer risk and may help abate perimenopausal symptoms.

PREVENTION

Factors that may reduce the risk of developing breast cancer include minimizing the duration of postmenopausal HRT, avoiding weight gain as an adult, engaging in regular physical activity, limiting alcohol consumption, having

Table 10.1 RISK FACTORS FOR DEVELOPMENT OF BREAST CANCER

INCREASE IN RISK	DECREASE IN RISK	UNCERTAIN EFFECT ON RISK

Lifestyle factors
  Higher weight/BMI (in postmenopausal women)
  Alcohol consumption (together with folate deficiency)
	Lifestyle factors
	  Breast-feeding > 6 months
	  Vigorous exercise, especially in postmenopausal women
	  Higher weight/BMT in premenopausal women
		Fat consumption
		Red meat consumption
		Calcium/vitamin D
		Phytoestrogens (e.g., soy)
		Antioxidant use (e.g., selenium; vitamins C, E, beta-carotene)
		Caffeine
		Smoking
		Abortion
		Diabetes
		Oral contraceptive use
		Infertility treatment
		NSAID use

Demographics
  Gender (female)
  Age
  Caucasian		

Estrogen exposure
  Early menarche
  Late menopause
  Nulliparity
  Older age at first birth
  Hormone replacement therapy (combination estrogen/progesterone)		

Family history and genetics
  Family history
  Germline mutations (BRCA 1/2, p53, and others)		

Other Radiation exposure before the age of 30		

a first child at an earlier age, and breast-feeding for at least 6 months. Among women who carry mutations of either BRCA1 or BRCA2, prophylactic mastectomy and prophylactic oophorectomy appear to reduce the risk of developing breast cancer. Tamoxifen (20 mg/day × 5 years) and raloxifene (60 mg/day × 5 years), two selective estrogen receptor modulators, both reduce the risk of developing invasive breast cancer by 50%. Among post-menopausal women, aromatase inhibitors also appear to reduce the risk of developing invasive breast cancer. Neither medication, when given for the purpose of preventing breast cancer, has been shown to improve overall survival; tamoxifen is associated with a modest increase in the risk of developing uterine cancer and having a thromboembolic event; aromatase inhibitors are associated with an increased risk of osteoporosis, among other side effects.

Screening

Mammography screening conducted yearly or biyearly can detect asymptomatic early-stage breast cancers. A systematic review conducted for the United States Preventive Services Task Force found that mammography reduces the relative risk of breast cancer mortality by 0.78 among women ≥50 years of age and by 0.85 among women 40 to 49 years of age. Most expert groups recommend initiating mammography screening at age 40 (American Cancer Society, American Medical Association, National Cancer Institute), although some recommend individualized risk assessment for women 40–49 (United States Preventive Services Task Force and American College of Physicians). Women 40 to 49 years old have a lower risk of developing breast cancer and denser breast tissue, so mammography is less sensitive and less specific in this subgroup. One study found that only 12% of biopsies done on women 40 to 49 years old identified malignancy, whereas 43% of biopsies done on women 60 to 69 years old identified malignancy. Although few studies of screening mammography included women older than 70 years of age, experts tend to recommend continued screening so long as a woman's life expectancy is >10 years. It is important to remember that mammography is unremarkable in approximately 10% of breast cancers, so a suspicious lump should not be disregarded simply because the mammogram is negative (i.e., an ultrasound, breast MRI, or biopsy may still be required). Breast self-examination has not been shown to increase the rate of breast cancer diagnosis, to change the stage at diagnosis, or to reduce the risk of death from breast cancer. Clinical breast examination may modestly improve early detection.

Magnetic resonance imaging (MRI) detects more cancers (i.e., is more sensitive) than mammography, but it results in more false positives and, therefore, more biopsies of non-malignant lesions. It does not detect all cancers and notably misses some cases of ductal carcinoma-in-situ (DCIS). Therefore, it does not replace mammography. In 2007 the American Cancer Society recommended including MRI as one of the regular, annual screening tests for women who have had chest radiation for Hodgkin lymphoma, carry a BRCA mutation, or have multiple first-degree relatives with breast and/or ovarian cancer. Regardless of how a suspicious breast abnormality is identified (via palpation, mammography, ultrasound, or MRI), core biopsy has supplanted excisional biopsy as the standard diagnostic procedure.

PATHOLOGY AND STAGING

Normal breast tissue contains epithelial elements (branching ducts that connect lobules to the nipple) and stromal elements (adipose and fibrous connective tissue). The vast majority (>95%) of breast cancers arise from epithelial cells and are, therefore, classified as carcinomas. These carcinomas can be divided into two distinct groups: (1) in situ carcinomas—where cancer cells are confined inside ducts or lobules and do not invade into the surrounding stroma; and (2) invasive or infiltrating carcinomas—where cancer cells invade into the breast stroma and consequently have the potential to metastasize. There are two major histologic types of in situ carcinoma, referred to as ductal carcinoma in situ (DCIS) and lobular carcinoma in situ (LCIS). There are several different histologic types of invasive breast cancer, including invasive ductal carcinoma (IDC), invasive lobular carcinoma (ILC), mixed ductal/lobular carcinoma, mucinous (colloid) carcinoma, tubular carcinoma, medullary carcinoma, and papillary carcinoma. IDC is the most common histologic subtype, accounting for approximately 75% of all invasive breast cancers. Although most histology types are thought to behave similarly, small studies suggest that tubular and colloid cancers may have a lower risk of recurrence and are generally considered favorable histology types.

Several factors affect the prognosis and influence the treatment of breast cancer, including grade, stage, hormone receptor status, and HER2 status. Grade, a description of the architectural and cytologic features of an invasive cancer, is usually classified as well differentiated (grade 1), moderately differentiated (grade 2), or poorly differentiated (grade 3). Stage ranges from 0 to IV, and, as with grade, a higher stage is associated with a higher risk of recurrence. Invasive carcinomas are classified as stage I–IV based on the size of the tumor (T), the extent to which lymph nodes in the axilla, internal mammary, or supraclavicular areas are involved by cancer (N), and the presence or absence of metastases beyond the breast and local lymph nodes (M). In situ carcinomas are classified as stage zero (T0, N0, M0).

Two-thirds of all invasive breast cancers are hormone-receptor positive, meaning at least 10% of the cancer cells express either the estrogen receptor (ER) or the progesterone receptor (PR). In one-fifth of invasive breast cancers, the human epidermal growth factor cell surface receptor 2 (HER2) is overexpressed; of these, approximately half are hormone-receptor positive and half are hormone-receptor negative. The risk of recurrence is higher for hormone-receptor–negative compared to hormone-receptor–positive breast cancer, and for HER2-positive compared to HER2-negative breast cancer. Invasive breast cancers that express none of these three receptors (approximately 10% of all invasive breast cancers) are called "triple negative" breast cancers. Inflammatory breast cancer is a unique, uncommon clinical presentation of breast cancer in which the skin overlying the breast is warm, thickened, and has a "peau d'orange" (or orange peel) appearance. It can have variable ER, PR and HER2 status; a palpable breast mass usually cannot be found. This is a particularly aggressive form of breast cancer with a relatively high risk of recurrence.

STAGE 0 BREAST CANCER (CARCINOMA IN SITU)

LCIS is a noninvasive form of breast cancer that arises from the lobules and terminal ducts. Because it usually cannot be identified by physical examination, mammogram, or gross pathologic examination, it is most frequently identified incidentally on microscopic pathologic examination. The presence of LCIS serves as a marker for an increased risk of developing invasive breast cancer (7- to 18-fold greater relative risk compared to the general population). After an LCIS diagnosis, the risk of developing a subsequent invasive breast cancer, in either breast, is approximately 1% per year and persists indefinitely. Excision of breast tissue to achieve negative margins and radiation therapy are not indicated. Management options include careful observation or primary prevention with a selective estrogen-receptor modulatory, an aromatase inhibitor, or prophylactic bilateral mastectomy (none of these has been showed to confer an overall survival advantage).

DCIS is a noninvasive form of breast cancer that is entirely confined within the duct system of the breast. Historically, DCIS was uncommon, representing <2% of breast cancers diagnosed in 1980. Now, DCIS is the most rapidly growing subgroup of breast cancer, accounting for approximately 20% of all new cases diagnosed each year in the United States. This change is due in large part to the increasing use of screening mammography, which detects microcalcifications that can be associated with DCIS. More than 90% of DCIS cases are detected by mammography alone (i.e., are not palpable). DCIS actually encompasses a heterogeneous group of proliferative lesions that exhibit diverse malignant potential. In other words, some forms of DCIS are very likely to develop into invasive cancer, whereas others rarely do. Because it is not possible to characterize the malignant potential of any particular DCIS, in general treatment for all types of DCIS is the same. DCIS is present in conjunction with nearly all cases of invasive ductal cancer.

Unlike LCIS, excision of breast tissue to achieve negative margins is routinely recommended for DCIS. Management options include mastectomy or lumpectomy (breast-conserving therapy) with complete removal of the tumor. Lumpectomy is only an option if there has been no previous radiation therapy to the breast and the DCIS is not sufficiently extensive as to preclude a complete and cosmetically acceptable resection. Radiation therapy to the breast follows lumpectomy and reduces the risk of local recurrence. Sampling of the axillary lymph nodes is not indicated for cases of pure DCIS (i.e., no evidence of invasive cancer). Both mastectomy and lumpectomy followed by radiation therapy confer a high likelihood of survival (>98%). Compared with mastectomy, lumpectomy followed by radiation therapy is associated with a higher risk of in-breast recurrence. It is hard to generate an accurate estimate of this risk because it is difficult to distinguish between true local recurrence and new primary breast cancer. Regardless, with routine surveillance these local, ipsilateral recurrences are usually found early and are nearly always curable. Several studies have explored the use of tamoxifen (20 mg/day × 5 years) after the DCIS has been removed to reduce the risk of developing DCIS or invasive breast cancer in the future; the results have been mixed, and a clear consensus has not emerged.

STAGE I, II, AND III BREAST CANCER (NONMETASTATIC)

Nonmetastatic invasive breast cancer is confined to the breast and/or ipsilateral local (predominantly axillary) lymph nodes. Cure is the goal of therapy. Surgery, either mastectomy or lumpectomy, is recommended to remove the primary cancer. A lumpectomy allows a woman to retain normal breast tissue but is contraindicated if there is cancer in more than one quadrant (multicentric), the woman has received breast radiation therapy or is pregnant, the resection margins are persistently positive after reasonable attempts at reexcision, or there are signs of inflammatory breast cancer. Breast reconstruction, either implant or autogenous tissue (e.g., TRAM flap), is an option following mastectomy. To reduce the risk of local cancer recurrence after surgery and to improve overall survival, radiation therapy to the breast following lumpectomy is required. Radiation therapy to the chest wall following mastectomy is occasionally recommended (e.g., if the tumor is >5 cm or multiple axillary lymph nodes are involved). Radiation therapy sometimes also involves the regional lymph nodes, such as the axillary and supraclavicular areas. Radiation treatments are usually given 5 days per week over 6–7 weeks, although a shorter

course may be an option for some women. The likelihood of survival after mastectomy compared with lumpectomy followed by radiation therapy is the same. The risk of local recurrence after lumpectomy and radiation therapy is low—approximately 5% or less at 5 years.

Sampling of the axillary lymph nodes is required in most patients to determine prognosis, define optimal treatment, and reduce the likelihood of a recurrence in the axilla. If the axilla is negative on clinical exam, a sentinel node biopsy can be performed. Using a blue dye or radioactive tracer injected into the breast at the time of surgery, it is usually possible to identify one or a few lymph nodes to which the cancer is most likely to spread. If the sentinel lymph nodes contain no cancer deposits >0.01 cm in diameter, then it is highly unlikely that any other lymph nodes will be involved with cancer, and a complete axillary lymph node dissection, together with the associated risks, can be avoided. If the sentinel lymph node is involved with cancer, then a complete dissection and removal of the level 1 and 2 ipsilateral axillary lymph nodes is usually recommended to reduce the risk of local cancer recurrence and gather prognostic information. However, some women treated with lumpectomy who have involved sentinel lymph nodes and are going to receive post-lumpectomy radiation therapy may be able to forgo completion axillary dissection and not experience any difference in overall survival. Serious complications following completion dissection are uncommon, but approximately 10% to 20% of women will experience chronic edema of the ipsilateral arm.

Patients with cancer confined to the breast and/or axilla are often cured by local therapy (surgery and radiation if indicated), but many are still at risk for developing metastatic disease. Hormone-receptor–negative breast cancers tend to recur within 5 years of diagnosis, whereas hormone-receptor–positive breast cancers can recur within 10 years of diagnosis. The goal of adjuvant therapy is to reduce the risk of cancer recurrence; it involves the administration of medications systemically to kill microscopic foci of cancer that were not removed by surgery or killed by radiation. Deciding whether to administer adjuvant therapy, and if so then what type to administer, depends on the risk of recurrence and the type of cancer. The higher the risk of recurrence the greater the potential absolute benefit of adjuvant therapy. Risk factors for the development of metastatic breast cancer include larger tumor size, higher tumor grade, presence of lymphovascular invasion in the breast, hormone-receptor–negative disease, presence of HER2 overexpression, and involvement of the axillary lymph nodes. For women with newly diagnosed, ER-positive, node-negative breast cancer who receive anti-estrogen therapy, a multiparameter gene expression analysis (i.e., the OncotypeDX assay) may also help estimate the risk of cancer recurrence and predict the benefit from adjuvant chemotherapy.

Determining what type of adjuvant therapy to administer also depends on the type of cancer because some

Table 10.2 BENEFITS AND HARMS OF MAMMOGRAM SCREENING

BENEFITS AND HARMS	AGE	
	40–49 YEARS OLD	50–59 YEARS OLD
10-year chance of dying from breast cancer		
• No screening	3.5/1000	5.3/1000
• Screening	3.0/1000	4.6/1000
• Deaths avoided because of screening	0.5/1000	0.7/1000
False-positive screening tests requiring a biopsy	60–200/1000	50–200/1000
Overdiagnosis and treatment (of cancers that would not have caused symptoms or led to premature death)	1–5/1000	1–7/1000

Reprinted with permission from Woloshin & Schwartz. The benefits and harms of mammography screening: Understanding the trade-offs. *JAMA*. 2010;303(2):164-5. Copyright © 2010 American Medical Association. All rights reserved.

therapies help treat only certain types of breast cancer. We now think of breast cancer as four different biological diseases: hormone-receptor–positive/HER2-positive, hormone-receptor–positive/HER2-negative, hormone-receptor–negative/HER2-positive, and hormone-receptor–negative/HER2-negative (see table 10.2). Women with hormone-receptor–positive breast cancer (either estrogen- or progesterone-receptor–positive) are eligible to receive adjuvant anti-estrogen therapy. The standard treatment for premenopausal women is tamoxifen daily for 5 years starting after the completion of surgery and chemotherapy, when administered. The standard treatment for postmenopausal women is either tamoxifen daily for 2–3 years followed by an aromatase inhibitor or an aromatase inhibitor alone for 5 years. Adjuvant anti-estrogen therapy reduces the risk of death by approximately one-third (Early Breast Cancer Trialists' Collaborative, 2005). However, these medications have side effects; both types of anti-estrogen medications can cause hot flashes; tamoxifen can cause thromboembolic disease, uterine cancer, and irregular menses; aromatase inhibitors can cause fatigue, aches, and osteoporosis.

Adjuvant chemotherapy can reduce the risk of recurrence for all types of breast cancer. It reduces the relative risk of relapse and death by 37% and 30% for women <50 years old and by 19% and 12% for women 50–69 years; the benefits of chemotherapy for women >70 years old have not been clearly established (Early Breast Cancer Trialists' Collaborative, 2005). Adjuvant chemotherapy usually involves the administration of two or three medications with nonoverlapping toxicity profiles; commonly used medications include cyclophosphamide, methotrexate, 5-fluorouracil, doxorubicin, epirubicin, paclitaxel, and docetaxel. Potential side effects/risks from chemotherapy include fatigue, hair loss, nausea, fever, infection, neuropathy, infusion reaction, heart failure, and leukemia (see Table 10.4). Chemotherapy is a standard recommendation for women with hormone-receptor–negative cancer measuring >1 cm and for hormone-receptor–positive cancer involving the axillary lymph nodes. The use of chemotherapy for hormone-receptor–positive, HER2-negative cancer not involving the axillary lymph nodes is more controversial.

Approximately 20% of breast cancers overexpress the HER2 cell surface signal-transduction protein. Patients with HER2-positive breast cancer experience a higher risk of recurrence compared to patients with HER2-negative breast cancer. Trastuzumab is a humanized monoclonal antibody designed to target HER2-positive cancer cells. When given in conjunction with adjuvant chemotherapy, trastuzumab reduces the relative risk of recurrence and death by 50% and 33%, respectively. Professional organizations recommend administering trastuzumab in conjunction with chemotherapy for patients with HER2-positive node-positive cancer or node-negative cancer measuring >1 cm. Approximately 2% to 3% of patients who receive trastuzumab develop symptomatic congestive heart failure. Consequently, this medication is contraindicated in patients with pre-existing heart failure. For those patients who receive trastuzumab, monitoring of left ventricular ejection fraction periodically throughout treatment is recommended.

STAGE IV BREAST CANCER (METASTATIC)

Approximately 15% to 20% of women diagnosed with breast cancer have stage IV (metastatic) disease, and approximately 20% of women diagnosed with nonmetastatic breast cancer eventually develop recurrent, metastatic disease. Common sites of metastatic breast cancer include the bone, distant lymph nodes, lungs, liver, pleura, brain, and other sites. The diagnosis is confirmed through the biopsy of a suspicious mass outside the ipsilateral breast or axilla. Occasionally, a confirmatory biopsy is not performed if the clinical scenario is fully consistent with metastatic breast cancer and/or the suspicious mass is not easily accessible to biopsy. Metastatic breast cancer is not curable. The median survival is approximately 2 to 2½ years. A small fraction of patients, perhaps 5% to 10%, survive 5 or more years. Women are likely to experience a slower rate of cancer progression and a better survival if they have a hormone-receptor–positive or low-grade cancer, are more fit (have a good performance status), have fewer sites of metastatic disease, have little visceral organ involvement, or if there was a long interval between their original cancer diagnosis and their recurrence. The primary goal of therapy is to maximize quality of life by reducing or preventing symptoms caused by the cancer without precipitating therapy-related side effects. Studies suggest that systemic treatments (chemotherapy and/or hormonal therapy) may also prolong survival, although any survival benefits that do exist are likely modest.

The initial management of hormone-receptor–positive metastatic breast cancer most commonly involves the administration of an anti-estrogen medication. Approximately 75% of cancers respond to initial hormonal therapy. Hormonal treatment options include tamoxifen with or without a gonadotropin-releasing hormone (GnRH) agonist for premenopausal women and a selective aromatase inhibitor (e.g., anastrozole, letrozole, or exemestane) for postmenopausal women. The initial management of hormone-receptor–negative metastatic breast cancer typically involves the administration of systemic chemotherapy. Chemotherapy is also a reasonable treatment option for any woman who has extensive or symptomatic metastatic disease, regardless of the cancer's hormone-receptor status. Approximately 50–75% of cancers experience clinical benefit from initial chemotherapy (i.e., the cancer shrinks or remains stable). A number of chemotherapy medications and one monoclonal antibody, trastuzumab, have been approved to treat metastatic breast cancer. Trastuzumab targets the HER2 receptor, so it can only be used to treat women with HER2-positive breast cancer. When used in combination with chemotherapy, trastuzumab improves overall survival by approximately 5 months. Much of the current research into new breast cancer treatments involves the development of targeted therapies. One such therapy, lapatinib, blocks the HER2 receptor and, when given together with the chemotherapy medication capecitabine,

improves time to tumor progression by approximately 4 months. Other targeted therapies currently under development include inhibitors of the PI3 kinase signal transduction pathway. Once started, a systemic treatment is usually continued until the cancer grows/progresses or the patient experiences intolerable side effects.

Targeted local therapies, such as surgical excision, radiation therapy, or radio-frequency ablation, are sometimes indicated to palliate symptomatic metastatic deposits. Treating pain, anxiety, depression, and other symptoms commonly experienced by women with metastatic breast cancer is an integral aspect of cancer care as well. For women who have metastatic bony deposits, the regular administration of an intravenous bisphosphonate (e.g., pamidronate or zoledronic acid) or the subcutaneous medication denosumab (a RANK ligand inhibitor) helps prevent/delay the development of skeletal complications and palliates bone pain. Finally, providing optimal palliative care often requires the collaboration of multiple specialists, including the oncologist, psychiatrist, social worker, and the hospice service.

SUMMARY OF BREAST CANCER TREATMENT

With nonmetastatic breast cancer (stage 0–III; see table 10.3), cure is the goal of therapy, and surgery is the primary treatment used to achieve this goal (table 10.4). Even with optimal surgical resection, there is still a risk that breast cancer can recur. Radiation therapy (to the breast, chest wall, and/or surrounding lymph nodes) is sometimes used to reduce the risk of local recurrence, and medications (anti-estrogen, HER2-directed, and/or cytotoxic chemotherapy) are sometime used to reduce the risk of local (in the breast and local axillary lymph nodes) and distant (beyond the breast and local lymph nodes) recurrence. Reducing the risk of recurrence helps to increase the chance of cure. The major factors to consider when deciding which treatments to recommend and how to sequence the therapies include stage, biological subtype

Table 10.3 BIOLOGIC SUBTYPES OF BREAST CANCER AND TREATMENT OPTIONS

	BIOLOGICAL SUBTYPE			
TREATMENT	ER-POSITIVE HER2-NEGATIVE	ER-POSITIVE HER2-POSITIVE	ER-NEGATIVE HER2-POSITIVE	ER-NEGATIVE HER2-NEGATIVE (TRIPLE NEGATIVE)
Hormonal	Yes	Yes	No	No
HER2-targeted therapy	No	Yes	Yes	No
Chemotherapy	Sometimes	Usually	Usually	Usually

NOTES: ER = estrogen receptor; HER2 = human epidermal growth factor receptor-2.

Table 10.4 MEDICATIONS USED TO TREAT BREAST CANCER

DRUG CLASS	MEDICATION NAME	POSSIBLE ADVERSE EFFECTS	NOTES
Anti-estrogen: selective estrogen receptor modulator (SERM)	Tamoxifen Raloxifene	Hot flashes/sweats Vaginal spotting Vaginal discharge Irregular menses Endometrial cancer (only tamoxifen) Nausea Leg cramps Blood clots	Raloxifene only approved for prevention. Tamoxifen used for prevention and treatment of breast cancer.
Anti-estrogen: aromatase inhibitor (AI)	Anastrozole Letrozole Exemestane	Hot flashes/sweats Vaginal dryness Nausea Headache Joint/muscle aches Fatigue Osteoporosis/fractures	Only effective among postmenopausal women.
Anti-estrogen: ovarian suppression	Goserelin Leuprolide	Hot flashes/sweats Absence of menses Vaginal dryness Osteoporosis/fractures Changes in mood	An injection, usually given monthly. Only effective among premenopausal women.
Anti-estrogen: other	Fulvestrant	Hot flushes/sweats Nausea/emesis Diarrhea Fatigue/weakness Headaches Aches	An intramuscular injection given monthly. Only for postmenopausal women. Only approved for recurrent/metastatic disease.
Anti-HER2	Trastuzumab Lapatinib	Heart failure Infusion reaction Rash Nausea Diarrhea	Trastuzumab is a monoclonal antibody administered intravenously. Lapatinib is a small-molecule tyrosine kinase inhibitor administered orally; it is only approved for recurrent/metastatic disease.
Cytotoxic chemotherapy	Doxorubicin Cyclophosphamide Paclitaxel Docetaxel 5-Fluorouracil Methotrexate Capecitabine Vinorelbine Gemcitabine Others	Fatigue Hair loss Nausea/emesis Diarrhea Mouth sores Fever and Infection Anemia Heart failure Neuropathy Myelodysplasia Leukemia	Chemotherapy medications can be used alone, in combination with each other, or in combination with anti-HER2 therapy. They are not used with anti-estrogen medications. Except for capecitabine, these medications are usually given intravenously.

(hormone receptor status, HER-2 status, and grade), age, menopausal status, comorbid medical conditions/general health, and patient preference. Metastatic breast cancer (either stage IV at diagnosis or distant recurrence some time after diagnosis of an earlier-stage breast cancer) is not curable. The goals of therapy are to reduce/alleviate symptoms from cancer and possibly prolong survival. Treatment usually involves medications; surgery and radiation are sometimes used to help control symptoms.

ADDITIONAL READING

Chlebowski RT, Hendrix SL, Langer RD, et al. Influence of estrogen plus progestin on breast cancer and mammography in healthy postmenopausal women: The Women's Health Initiative Randomized Trial. *JAMA.* 2003;289(24):3243–53.

Clarke N, Collins R, Darby S, et al. Early Breast Cancer Trialists' Collaborative. Effects of radiotherapy and of differences in the extent of surgery for early breast cancer on local recurrence and 15-year survival: An overview of the randomised trials. *Lancet.* 2005;366(9503):2087–106.

Drews RE, Shulman LN. Update in hematology and oncology. *Ann Intern Med.* 2010;152(10):655–62.

Early Breast Cancer Trialists' Collaborative. Effects of chemotherapy and hormonal therapy for early breast cancer on recurrence and 15-year survival: An overview of the randomised trials [see comment]. *Lancet.* 2005;365(9472):1687–717.

Fisher B, Costantino J, Redmond C, et al. Lumpectomy compared with lumpectomy and radiation therapy for the treatment of intraductal breast cancer. [see comment]. *N Engl J Med.* 1993;328(22):1581–6.

Humphrey LL, Helfand M, Chan BK, Woolf SH. Breast cancer screening: A summary of the evidence for the U.S. Preventive Services Task Force. *Ann Intern Med.* 2002;137(5 Part 1):347–60. [Summary for patients 2002;137(5 Part 1):147.

Jemal A, Siegel R, Xu J, Ward FL. 2010. Cancer statistics, 2010. *CA* 2010;60(5):277–300.

Kooistra B, Wauters C, Strobbe L, Wobbes T. Preoperative cytological and histological diagnosis of breast lesions: A critical review. *Eur J Surg Oncol.* 2010;36(10):934–40.

Meyer JE, Smith DN, Lester SC, et al. Large-core needle biopsy of non-palpable breast lesions. *JAMA.* 1999;281(17):1638–41.

Owusu C. Clinical management update: Evaluation and management of older patients with breast cancer. *J Am Geriatr Soc.* 2009;57(Suppl 2):S250–2.

Smith RA, Cokkinides V, Brawley OW. Cancer screening in the United States, 2009: A review of current American Cancer Society guidelines and issues in cancer screening. *CA.* 2009;59(1):27–41.

QUESTIONS

QUESTION 1. A 63-year-old woman is 8 years status post-lumpectomy and radiation therapy for a 1.5-cm, estrogen-receptor–positive, node-negative breast cancer for which she had received 5 years of tamoxifen, stopped 3 years ago. She presents to your office with severe, localized back pain. Physical examination is normal including the neurological exam. The alkaline phosphatase is 330 (elevated) and the CA27.29 is 156 (elevated). A bone scan is positive in several areas of the thoracic and lumbar spine as well as in several ribs. The course of action at this point should be:

A. Combination chemotherapy
B. Tamoxifen therapy
C. MRI scan of the spine
D. Radiation therapy to areas of localized disease
E. Stem cell transplantation

QUESTION 2. A 46-year-old woman presents to your office for routine health care. She is concerned about the possibility of developing breast cancer and asks you about her risk factors. Which statement is most correct?

A. A previous biopsy which revealed LCIS does not substantially increase her risk of developing breast cancer.

B. Presence of a BRCA-1 germ line mutation will substantially increase her risk of developing breast cancer.

C. A maternal aunt with postmenopausal breast cancer will substantially increase her risk of developing breast cancer.

D. The majority of women with breast cancer have identifiable risk factors for the development of breast cancer.

E. Duration and degree of estrogen (endogenous and exogenous) exposure is not associated with increased risk of developing breast cancer.

QUESTION 3. In regard to potential effects of tamoxifen and raloxifene, the following is most true:

A. Raloxifene is a bone-strengthening agent but tamoxifen is not.

B. Both increase the risk of endometrial cancer.

C. Both decrease the risk of developing a future breast cancer.

D. Tamoxifen increases risk of hot flashes, but raloxifene does not.

QUESTION 4. A 42-year-old woman is diagnosed with a 3-cm poorly differentiated breast cancer with five involved axillary lymph nodes. The cancer is negative for estrogen receptors and positive for HER2. Which of the following is most true?

A. The presence of HER2 on breast cancer cells does not affect prognosis.

B. Adjuvant chemotherapy is not effective in reducing the risk of her subsequently developing metastatic breast cancer.

C. Trastuzumab, when added to chemotherapy, substantially reduces the risk of developing metastatic disease in the future.

D. Letrozole, an aromatase inhibitor, would further improve the cure rate for this patient.

E. The addition of trastuzumab to chemotherapy is not associated with additional short- and long-term complications.

ANSWERS

1. C
2. B
3. C
4. C

11.

LUNG CANCER

Joel Neal and Thomas J. Lynch

OVERVIEW

Cancer of the lung is a group of heterogeneous malignant disorders composed of small cell lung cancer (13%), non-small cell lung cancer (NSCLC) (86%), and rare thoracic malignancies such as mesothelioma and carcinoid tumors. In 2008 the American Cancer Society estimated that 215,020 people in the United States would develop lung cancer, and 161,840 people would die of their disease. In men the age-adjusted cancer death rate for lung cancer peaked in 1990 at approximately 90 deaths per 100,000 and has since decreased to 70 per 100,000. In women, the incidence reached a plateau in 1990 at 40 per 100,000. These changes are in part due to alterations in smoking patterns, but the overall incidence of lung cancer continues to increase with the aging population. Despite the trend of decreased smoking rates in industrialized countries, lung cancer remains the leading cause of cancer death in both men and women in the United States (American Cancer Society, 2008). Lung cancer is also the leading cause of cancer death worldwide.

RISK FACTORS

A number of environmental factors are causally related to the development of lung cancer. In contrast, no simple genetic association has been identified. The single most important risk factor, smoking, accounts for approximately 85% of all lung cancers. Other associated factors include exposure to radon, asbestos, and heavy metals.

SMOKING

Before 1900, lung cancer was considered a relatively unusual malignancy. As tobacco smoking became more popular throughout the 20th century, the incidence of lung cancer increased. Worldwide, over 1 billion people smoke, which makes lung cancer an epidemic of global proportions.

The epidemiologic relationship between tobacco smoke and lung cancer was demonstrated in the 1950s. Both amount and duration of smoking appear to increase the risk of developing lung cancer (Bartecchi, MacKenzie, et al., 1994; MacKenzie, Bartecchi, et al., 1994; Hecht, 1999). People who smoke one to nine cigarettes daily, or have smoked over 15 years, have a fourfold increase in the risk of lung cancer. Smoking >20 cigarettes daily or for >40 years further raises the risk by 15- to 20-fold over nonsmokers. This results in a cumulative lifetime risk for smokers of up to 30% (Samet, 1991). "Second-hand" household smoke, which is associated with a reduced intensity but earlier and chronic exposure to tobacco smoke, appears to double the risk of developing lung cancer. The effect of workplace and other second-hand smoke is also beginning to be appreciated (U.S. Department of Health and Human Services, 2006).

Smoking cessation is the single most effective way to reduce mortality from lung cancer. After quitting, the risk of developing lung cancer appears to transiently rise in epidemiological studies, possibly from the subsequent diagnosis in people who quit due to pre-existing symptoms of cancer. However, the risk of lung cancer starts to fall 5 years after quitting. After 10 years it is only fourfold above never-smokers, and at 25 years it is less than twofold above never-smokers (Samet, 1991). Therefore, physicians who assist their patients with smoking cessation can make a tremendous impact in reducing morbidity and mortality from lung cancer as well as other tobacco-related diseases.

RADON

Radon is a colorless, odorless, radioactive gas resulting from the decay of radioactive metals in the soil. It can accumulate in poorly ventilated homes in certain geographic areas. Radon exposure appears to result in significant risk of developing lung cancer in miners and a small but linear risk of lung cancer in others. An analysis of multiple case-control studies suggests that 10% or more of lung cancers in both smokers and nonsmokers may be attributable to radon exposure in the home (Darby, Hill, et al., 2005).

ASBESTOS

Asbestos is the term for a group of naturally occurring silicate fibers whose heat-resisting properties made them historically useful in construction and industrial applications. Asbestos fiber exposure has been strongly correlated with mesothelioma risk. However, exposed workers have a higher overall chance of developing adenocarcinoma of the lung than mesothelioma. Unlike the relationship between smoking and lung cancer, the risk of mesothelioma following asbestos exposure increases with time even after exposure has stopped, peaking at around 20 to 40 years (Berry and Gibbs, 2008).

OTHER EXPOSURES

Lung cancer has also been associated with exposure to wood smoke, previous chest radiotherapy, and a number of metals including arsenic, chromium, nickel, beryllium, and cadmium. However, the total fraction of lung cancers attributable to these factors is likely small.

CLINICAL DETECTION OF LUNG CANCER

SYMPTOMS

In a patient population that smokes heavily, the respiratory symptoms of lung cancer often mimic the effects of chronic tobacco use. Many patients present with cough, worsening dyspnea, or hemoptysis, which can also be symptoms of bronchitis or pneumonia. Symptoms such as weight loss, chest pain, bone pain, hoarseness, or neurological symptoms should prompt a more extensive workup but often correspond to invasive or metastatic disease, which tends to have a minimal chance of cure.

PARANEOPLASTIC SYNDROMES

Paraneoplastic syndromes more commonly manifest in patients with SCLC, but they can be seen in either type of lung cancer.

Hematologic Abnormalities

Leukocytosis has been observed in up to 15% of patients with NSCLC and may be due to tumor secretion of granulocyte colony-stimulating factor (G-CSF). This can result in white blood cell counts over three times the upper limit of normal with a marked left shift, known as a *leukemoid reaction*.

Anemia may be observed in up to 40% of patients presenting with NSCLC, and thrombocytosis in up to 15%.

Syndrome of Inappropriate Antidiuretic Hormone secretion (SIADH)

Up to 10% of SCLC may secrete ADH, resulting in profound hyponatremia. This syndrome responds to chemotherapy within a few weeks, but patients can be managed in the interim with free water restriction and vasopressor receptor antagonists such as demeclocycline.

Hypercalcemia

Hypercalcemia in malignancy may result from direct bone invasion or secretion of osteoclast-activating factors. In particular, high levels of parathyroid hormone-related peptide (PTHrP) may cause hypercalcemia and is associated with NSCLC of squamous histology.

Cushing Syndrome

Excess production of ACTH by tumor tissue can lead to Cushing syndrome: truncal obesity, hypertension, hyperglycemia, hypokalemic alkalosis, and osteoporosis. Most often seen in patients with SCLC, cortisol excess correlates with a poor prognosis.

Pancoast Syndrome

Lung tumors that arise in the superior sulcus of either lung can cause damage to the brachial plexus and the sympathetic ganglia. This results in a syndrome of shoulder/arm pain, ipsilateral Horner syndrome, bone destruction, and atrophy of the hand muscles. Typically, superior sulcus tumors arise from NSCLC of squamous histology.

Thrombosis

All patients with cancer are predisposed to develop disorders of hypercoagulability, including deep vein thrombosis and pulmonary embolism. Patients who develop spontaneous clots without a clear predisposing factor should undergo screening for malignancy and be treated with low-molecular-weight heparin instead of warfarin (Lee, Levine, et al., 2003).

DIAGNOSIS

A nodule on a chest x-ray or computed tomography (CT) scan often leads to the diagnosis of lung cancer. A CT of the chest with IV contrast gives an overview of the extent parenchymal disease and regional nodal involvement and can also demonstrate metastatic disease to the bones, liver, or adrenal glands. Positron emission tomography (PET) scans and combined PET/CT scans are used to further evaluate the extent of regional or metastatic disease. With the exception of small NSCLC <1 cm in diameter, most patients with lung cancer should have brain imaging at the time of staging with a brain magnetic resonance imaging

(MRI), but a head CT scan with contrast can be done if an MRI is contraindicated.

Establishing the diagnosis of NSCLC involves obtaining tissue for histopathologic analysis. Generally, the initial diagnosis should be made via the least invasive means to obtain the highest pathologic stage. Therefore, patients with a potential metastasis should have that site biopsied for staging. Patients with possible mediastinal lymph node involvement can undergo diagnostic mediastinoscopy. CT-guided fine needle biopsy of the lung is often used to establish the diagnosis but does carry a risk of pneumothorax and severe pulmonary hemorrhage. Bronchoscopy, increasingly in combination with endobronchial ultrasound (EBUS), is most useful for proximal tumors and can yield information about a primary tumor and lymph node staging. Although the diagnosis can be made from fine-needle aspiration alone, advanced molecular testing requires more tissue in the form of a core biopsy or surgical sample.

SCREENING

Owing to the high mortality associated with advanced lung cancer, as well as the strong association with smoking, there are a number of trials that have attempted to screen for lung cancer. Although radiologic imaging can detect malignant lung nodules, these tumors tend to be less aggressive than lung cancers detected by clinical criteria.

Four large early randomized trials, together including >30,000 patients, have been conducted using various combinations of chest x-ray (CXR) and sputum cytology. However, none of these compare screening with a completely unscreened group of patients. Instead, they have tested the effect of adding sputum cytology to CXR screening, or test annual versus more-frequent CXR screening. These studies generally demonstrate an increased detection of early-stage lung cancer but no difference in survival. The Mayo Lung Project, which randomized almost 11,000 male smokers to sputum cytology plus CXR every 4 months versus "usual care" with an annual CXR, actually demonstrated significantly more lung cancer-related deaths in the screened group at 20-year follow-up (Marcus, Bergstralh, et al., 2000).

The ongoing Prostate, Lung, Colorectal, and Ovarian (PLCO) clinical trial has randomized over 150,000 patients, of any smoking status, to screening with an initial CXR versus no screening. Although mortality data are not yet available, 9% of screening chest x-rays were suspicious for lung cancer. After confirmatory CT scanning, 1 out of 30 patients required biopsy, of which about half were positive for lung cancer. These lung cancers were mostly early stage, and data on disease-specific mortality are awaited (Oken, Marcus, et al., 2005).

The lack of positive results using CXR screening has led to an increased interest in screening with modern CT scanning techniques. Observational cohort studies demonstrate that CT scanning can identify more early-stage lung cancers than CXR, but CT scans also lead to more false-positive scans resulting in biopsy. These also tend to identify very early-stage tumors that may have a more favorable natural history than tumors identified clinically. Recently, the results from the National Lung Screening Trial were released (Aberle et al., 2011). Over 50,000 asymptomatic moderate to heavy prior and current smokers were randomized to undergo either annual CXR or low-dose CT screening exams. While 95% of the results were false positive, there was a 20% relative reduction in lung cancer specific mortality with CT screening as compared with CXR. Based on these results, centers are beginning to offer low dose CT screenings for lung cancer. The previous recommendation by the United States Preventive Services Task Force, that there was insufficient evidence to recommend screening for lung cancer, is currently under review. As lung biopsies and surgery are relatively invasive and carry a risk of morbidity and mortality, there is interest in less-invasive techniques to help further stratify patients with potentially benign lung nodules.

NON-SMALL CELL LUNG CANCER

PATHOLOGY

Histology

NSCLC accounts for approximately 86% of primary lung tumors. The diagnosis includes a variety of morphologic subtypes that fall primarily into the categories of adenocarcinoma and squamous cell carcinoma (table 11.1). Historically, the histologic subtype has not influenced treatment decisions. However, newer therapies, such as erlotinib, bevacizumab, and pemetrexed, appear to be safer and more effective in adenocarcinoma, whereas experimental drugs that target the IGF-1 receptor appear to be more effective in squamous cell carcinoma. This may reflect different underlying molecular changes in these tumors.

Molecular Changes in NSCLC

A variety of DNA changes have been identified in NSCLC, including genetic alterations in a number of oncogenes and tumor suppressors: epidermal growth factor receptor (EGFR), KRAS, EML4-ALK, HER2, BRAF, C-MYC, and TP53. Of these, EGFR mutations have been the best characterized.

Mutations in the tyrosine kinase domain of EGFR are seen in 10% of NSCLC in the United States and in 40% of lung cancers in Asian countries. They are more prevalent in never-smokers, women, and people of Asian descent, and they are virtually always associated with adenocarcinoma histology. These mutations cause constitutive activation of the EGFR signaling pathway, which drives tumor proliferation and prevents apoptosis. The small-molecule tyrosine kinase inhibitors gefitinib and erlotinib potently

Table 11.1 SELECTED NSCLC HISTOLOGIC SUBTYPES

I. Squamous cell carcinoma
  A. Variants: papillary, clear cell, small cell, basaloid

II. Adenocarcinoma
  Preinvasive lesions
    Atypical adenomatous hyperplasia
    Adenocarcinoma in situ (≤3 cm formerly
    (bronchioloalveolar carcinoma [BAC])
      Nonmucinous
      Mucinous
      Mixed mucinous/nonmucinous
  Minimally invasive adenocarcinoma (≤3 cm lepidic
  predominant tumor with ≤5 mm invasion)
    Nonmucinous
    Mucinous
    Mixed mucinous/nonmucinous
  Invasive adenocarcinoma
    Lepidic predominant (formerly nonmucinous BAC
    pattern, with >5 mm invasion)
    Acinar predominant
    Papillary predominant
    Micropapillary predominant
    Solid predominant with mucin production
  Variants of invasive adenocarcinoma
    Invasive mucinous adenocarcinoma (formerly mucinous BAC)
    Colloid
    Fetal (low and high grade)
    Enteric

III. Large cell carcinoma

  Variants: large cell neuroendocrine carcinoma, combined
  large cell neuroendocrine carcinoma, basaloid carcinoma,
  lymphoepithelioma-like carcinoma, clear cell carcinoma, large
  cell carcinoma with rhabdoid phenotype

IV. Adenosquamous carcinoma
 V. Carcinomas with pleomorphic, sarcomatoid, or sarcomatous
    elements
VI. Unclassified carcinoma (i.e., poorly differentiated)

SOURCES: Reproduced with permission of the European Respiratory Society
© 2001. Brambilla E, Travis WD, Colby TV, et al. The new World Health
Organization classification of lung tumours. *Eur Respir J.* 2001;18:1059–68.
II. Adenocarcimona section reprinted with permission from Travis WD,
Brambilla E, Noguchi M, et al. International Association for the Study of Lung
Cancer/American Thoracic Society/European Respiratory Society International
multidisciplinary classification of lung adenocarcinoma. *J Thorac Oncol.*
2011;6(2):244–85.

inhibit many mutant forms of EGFR, resulting in profound responses in patients with exon 19 deletions or the L858R point mutation (Sequist and Lynch, 2008)

STAGING OF NSCLC

Lung cancer has been staged using the AJCC sixth edition staging system, but the proposed seventh edition staging system was incorporated by 2010 (see table 11.2). Changes include further subdivision of tumor categories by size, downstaging of "satellite" pulmonary nodules, and upstaging of malignant effusions to metastatic disease to better reflect survival patterns.

In the workup of patients with suspected lung cancer, the extent of the workup is determined by the patient's presentation, performance status, and treatment preferences. The goal of the staging is to determine the extent of disease. If metastatic disease is confirmed, curative treatment is generally not possible.

Owing to the high frequency of metastatic disease in 25–30% of patients with lung cancer, even those with small tumors, most patients with suspected lung cancer should have the following workup:

- Chest CT (often used during diagnosis)

- PET or combined PET/CT

- Head MRI with contrast or head CT with contrast

- Bone scan if PET is not available

- Pulmonary function testing (for possible operative candidates)

- Laboratory workup to rule out hematologic, electrolyte, renal, or hepatic abnormalities

Many patients who are considered surgical candidates have historically undergone mediastinoscopy to rule out the possibility of mediastinal nodal involvement. PET scanning and co-registered PET/CT scanning helps to identify the extent of lymph node involvement or can identify metastatic disease, which helps patients avoid unnecessary surgery. A combined PET/CT that demonstrates neither enlarged mediastinal lymph nodes nor PET activity in the mediastinum has only a 5% false-negative rate (Pieterman, van Putten, et al., 2000).

TREATMENT

Stage I–II NSCLC

Even very early-stage NSCLC only has a 50–70% 5-year survival (table 11.1). Therefore, an aggressive and often combined-modality approach to treatment is essential to maximize the chance of cure.

Initial treatment for stage I (small tumor without lymph node involvement) and stage II (larger and more invasive tumors or hilar lymph node involvement) consists of surgical resection, which can be achieved through several different procedures. The choice of the optimal surgical procedure depends on the extent of primary tumor, nodal involvement, and underlying pulmonary function of the patient. Wedge resection (removal of a section of lung without respect to anatomic borders) can result in a higher local failure rate. For patients with impaired pulmonary function, this may be a reasonable option in order to preserve lung function. Segmentectomy (removal of a defined anatomic segment) is slightly better than wedge resection when feasible. Lobectomy (removal of the entire lobe including hilar nodes) is the procedure of choice for early-stage NSCLC because it has a lower recurrence risk than wedge resection or segmentectomy.

Table 11.2 SEVENTH EDITION NSCLC STAGING

STAGE	TUMOR	NODES	MET	MEDIAN SURVIVAL TIME (MONTHS)*	5-YEAR SURVIVAL*
Stage IA	T1a,b	N0	M0	60–119	50–73%
Stage IB	T2a	N0	M0	43–81	43–58%
Stage IIA	T1a,b	N1	M0	34–49	36–46%
	T2a	N1	M0		
	T2b	N0	M0		
Stage IIB	T2b	N1	M0	18–31	25–36%
	T3	N0	M0		
Stage IIIA	T1, T2	N2	M0	14–22	19–24%
	T3	N1, N2	M0		
	T4	N0, N1	M0		
Stage IIIB	T4	N2	M0	10–13	7–9%
	Any T	Any N	M0		
Stage IV	Any T	Any N	M1a,b	8–12	<2%

NOTES: *First number in range denotes survival by clinical stage, second number by pathologic stage.
DEFINITION of TNM:

Primary tumor (T)

- TX: Primary tumor cannot be assessed, or tumor proven by the presence of malignant cells in sputum or bronchial washings but not visualized by imaging or bronchoscopy
- T0: No evidence of primary tumor
- Tis: Carcinoma in situ
- T1: Tumor ≤3 cm in greatest dimension, surrounded by lung or visceral pleura, without bronchoscopic evidence of invasion more proximal than the lobar bronchus (i.e., not in the main bronchus). The uncommon superficial spreading tumor of any size is classified as T1 even when extending to the main bronchus, as long as the invasive component is limited to the bronchial wall.
  - T1a: Tumor ≤2 cm in greatest dimension
  - T1b: Tumor >2 cm but ≤3 cm in greatest dimension
  - T2: Tumor >3 cm but ≤7 cm or tumor with any of the following features (T2 tumors with these features are classified T2a if ≤5 cm)
- Involves the main bronchus, ≥2 cm or more distal to the carina
- Invades the visceral pleura
- Associated with atelectasis or obstructive pneumonitis that extends to the hilar region but does not involve the entire lung
  - T2a: Tumor >3 cm but ≤5 cm in greatest dimension
  - T2b: Tumor >5 cm but ≤7 cm in greatest dimension
- T3: >7 cm or one that directly invades any of the following: chest wall (including superior sulcus tumors), diaphragm, phrenic nerve, mediastinal pleura, parietal pericardium; or tumor in the main bronchus <2 cm distal to the carina but without involvement of the carina; or associated atelectasis or obstructive pneumonitis of the entire lung or separate tumor nodule(s) in the same lobe
- A tumor of any size that directly invades any of the following: chest wall (including superior sulcus tumors), diaphragm, mediastinal pleura, parietal pericardium; or tumor in the main bronchus <2 cm distal to the carina but without involvement of the carina; or associated atelectasis or obstructive pneumonitis of the entire lung
- T4: Tumor of any size that invades any of the following: mediastinum, heart, great vessels, trachea, recurrent laryngeal nerve, esophagus, vertebral body, carina; separate tumor nodule(s) in a different ipsilateral lobe

Regional lymph nodes (N)

- NX: Regional lymph nodes cannot be assessed
- N0: No regional lymph node metastasis
- N1: Metastasis to ipsilateral peribronchial and/or ipsilateral hilar lymph nodes and intrapulmonary nodes including involvement by direct extension of the primary tumor
- N2: Metastasis to ipsilateral mediastinal and/or subcarinal lymph node(s)
- N3: Metastasis to contralateral mediastinal, contralateral hilar, ipsilateral or contralateral scalene, or supraclavicular lymph node(s)

Distant metastasis (M)

- MX: Distant metastasis cannot be assessed
- M0: No distant metastasis
- M1a: Separate tumor nodule(s) in a contralateral lobe, tumor with pleural nodules or malignant pleural or pericardial effusion
- M1b: Distant metastasis

SOURCE: Reprinted with permission from Goldstraw P, Crowley J, Chansky K, et al. The IASLC Lung Cancer Staging Project: Proposals for the revision of the TNM stage groupings in the forthcoming (seventh) edition of the *TNM Classification of Malignant Tumours*. *J Thorac Oncol.* 2007;2(8):706–14.

Pneumonectomy (resection of an entire lung with associated nodes) may be necessary for many large tumors or tumors with proximal airway invasion, but the procedure may result in a higher rate of postoperative complications. For proximal tumors, sleeve resection allows sparing of distal lung tissue via construction of an airway anastomosis. Performing these procedures via video-assisted thoracoscopic surgery (VATS) is gaining acceptance, but comparing outcomes after standard or VATS approaches is an area of investigation.

For large stage Ib tumors, and for all stage II tumors, it is estimated that patients have approximately a 5% overall survival benefit to cisplatin-based doublet adjuvant chemotherapy (Pignon, Tribodet, et al., 2008). For small stage I tumors, there is no evidence of benefit from adjuvant chemotherapy, so current practice guidelines recommend close monitoring of these patients after resection. There is no role for adjuvant radiation therapy in completely resected NSCLC.

Stage III NSCLC

Stage III NSCLC encompasses a heterogeneous spectrum of disease, ranging from large superior sulcus tumors without lymphadenopathy and a 5-year survival rate of 40% to tumors with extensive mediastinal nodal involvement and a 5-year survival <5% (see table 11.1).

The treatment strategy for stage III NSCLC involves a combination of chemotherapy, radiation, and sometimes surgical resection. Stage IIIB disease is generally considered surgically unresectable and is treated with concurrent chemotherapy and high-dose radiation with curative intent ("definitive" treatment). Sometimes additional cycles of chemotherapy are given, either before or after chemoradiation.

The treatment of stage IIIA disease is less standardized and often includes surgery. One treatment strategy utilizes neoadjuvant concurrent chemotherapy with preoperative doses of radiation, followed by surgical resection, then chemotherapy. Patients may also have initial surgical resection followed by chemotherapy, or pre-operative chemotherapy followed by surgery, with radiation depending on the operative results. Finally, definitive chemoradiotherapy without surgery is reasonable for nonoperative candidates. The chance of cure likely depends more on the pre-existing extent of disease than the particular treatment strategy.

Stage IV NSCLC

Stage IV NSCLC has a median survival of 8–12 months (see table 11.1), and these patients are generally not considered curable. However, rare patients with oligometastatic disease, consisting of a single resectable lung primary and a solitary brain or adrenal metastasis, may have up to a 10% 5-year survival following definitive treatment of both sites of disease. For stage IV NSLCL, the goals of treatment are to prolong survival while minimizing side effects and morbidity. Radiation is often used for control of symptomatic lesions, and palliative care is a paramount part of the treatment of metastatic NSCLC.

Systemic chemotherapy is the cornerstone of the treatment of stage IV NSCLC of patients with good performance status, that is, those who are minimally symptomatic from their disease and out of bed most of the time. Standard first-line chemotherapy consists of platinum-based doublet chemotherapy. Most platinum-based doublets (carboplatin or cisplatin, in combination with paclitaxel, docetaxel, gemcitabine, vinorelbine, or pemetrexed) generally have equivalent impacts on survival. In a large trial comparing four different platinum-based chemotherapy doublets, all regimens appeared equivalent, with response rates of 19%, median survival of 8 months, 1-year survival of 33%, and 2-year survival of 11%.

Treatment with platinum-based doublets continues for four to six total cycles of therapy (Schiller, Harrington, et al., 2002). Following treatment, patients who respond are monitored with periodic CT scans and symptom screening for signs of disease recurrence, but mounting evidence may suggest a role for early second-line or maintenance therapy with non-platinum-based chemotherapy.

A number of novel agents have been investigated for advanced disease, but most have failed to improve outcome. Bevacizumab, an anti-angiogenic monoclonal antibody against vascular endothelial growth factor, was the first agent to improve median survival in NSCLC to over 1 year when administered in combination with chemotherapy in a large clinical trial (Sandler, Gray, et al., 2006); however, patients with squamous cell histology, untreated brain metastasis, recent surgical procedures, and necrotic tumors are at higher risk for bleeding complications from this agent. Cetuximab, a monoclonal antibody to EGFR, also appears to provide modest benefit when combined with chemotherapy.

There is mounting support for molecular-directed therapy in NSCLC. The presence of EGFR mutations in the tumor correlate strongly with clinical response to the EGFR tyrosine kinase inhibitors erlotinib and gefitinib in a number of retrospective clinical trials (Sequist and Lynch, 2008). A recent large randomized study that included never-smokers and light smokers from Asia demonstrated that patients with EGFR mutations treated with first-line gefitinib had a response rate of 70% and progression-free survival of 9 months, compared with a response rate of 1% and progression-free survival of 2 months in patients without an EGFR mutation (Mok, Wu, et al., 2008). Therefore, prospective identification of patients harboring tumors with EGFR mutations may influence first-line treatment decisions. Unfortunately, many patients eventually develop resistance to these tyrosine kinase inhibitors. Mechanisms of resistance include secondary mutations in the EGFR gene (such as the point mutation T790M, which impairs binding of erlotinib and gefitinib) and activation of alternate signaling pathways (such as amplification of the MET oncogene)

(Kobayashi, Boggon, et al., 2005; Engelman, Zejnullahu, et al., 2007).

The EML4-ALK genetic translocation has also been identified as a driver oncogene in about 4% of NSCLC adenocarcinomas. In heavily pretreated patients with ALK-positive NSCLC, the ALK tyrosine kinase inhibitor crizotinib was FDA approved in 2011 based on a 57% response rate and progression-free survival of 9.2 months in a phase I/II study, and a confirmatory phase III study is currently ongoing (Kwak et al., 2010). Research is currently ongoing to identify ways to overcome resistance to these agents as well as to identify molecular targeted treatments in NSCLC for tumors that contain alterations in KRAS.

At the time of disease progression, subsequent treatment can consist of single-agent non-platinum chemotherapy, clinical trials, or supportive care. The expected response rate to chemotherapy is lower with each successive round of chemotherapy.

SMALL CELL LUNG CANCER

PATHOLOGY OF SCLC

SCLC is a high-grade neuroendocrine tumor arising from the lungs. Development of SCLC is strongly associated with smoking and can be distinguished from NSCLC due to the small cell size as well as expression of the neuroendocrine immunohistochemical markers chromogranin A and synaptophysin.

DIAGNOSIS AND STAGING OF SCLC

Staging of SCLC utilizes CT scans of the chest, abdomen, and pelvis; cranial imaging; and bone scan or PET scan. Staging is broken into two categories: limited stage and extensive stage. Limited-stage disease fits within a single radiation field (one side of the chest including associated lymph nodes), whereas extensive-stage disease is more widespread and often involves metastases to the lungs, liver, adrenal glands, bones, or brain. SCLC is frequently associated with paraneoplastic syndromes such as SIADH and Cushing syndrome (see discussion above).

TREATMENT

Limited-Stage SCLC

The standard of care for treatment of limited-stage SCLC involves concurrent radiotherapy and concurrent full-dose chemotherapy with cisplatin and etoposide, followed by chemotherapy alone. This treatment can result in a response rate of over 80% and median survival of 14–20 months. At 5 years, 15–20% of patients may still be alive without disease. Surgery has not been shown to improve survival in patients with SCLC, and even small localized tumors have a high likelihood of recurrence after surgical resection.

Following chemotherapy and radiation, patients with controlled disease should undergo prophylactic cranial irradiation, which has been shown to improve overall survival.

Extensive-Stage SCLC

Extensive-stage SCLC is incurable, with a median survival between 9 and 11 months. Like stage IV NSCLC, it is initially treated with platinum-based doublet chemotherapy, but the expected response rate is much higher at 70–80%. Patients who respond to initial therapy also have a survival benefit from prophylactic cranial irradiation. Second-line therapy is more successful in patients with a disease-free interval longer than 3 months after initial therapy ("relapsed" disease) than patients with a disease-free interval of <3 months ("refractory" disease). Supportive care also plays an essential role in the management of SCLC.

ADDITIONAL READING

Aberle DR, Adams AM, Berg CD, et al. Reduced lung-cancer mortality with low-dose computed tomographic screening. N Engl J Med. 2011 Aug 4;365(5):395–409.

American Cancer Society: Cancer Facts and Figures, 2008. http://www.cancer.org/downloads/STT/2008CAFFfinalsecured.pdf, 2008.

Bartecchi CE, MacKenzie TD, Schrier RW. The human costs of tobacco use (1). N Engl J Med. 1994;330:907–12.

Berry G, Gibbs GW. An overview of the risk of lung cancer in relation to exposure to asbestos and of taconite miners. Regul Toxicol Pharmacol. 2008;52:S218–22.

Darby S, Hill D, Auvinen A, et al. Radon in homes and risk of lung cancer: collaborative analysis of individual data from 13 European case-control studies. BMJ. 2005;330:223.

Engelman JA, Zejnullahu K, Mitsudomi T, et al. MET Amplification Leads to Gefitinib Resistance in Lung Cancer by Activating ERBB3 Signaling. Science. 2007;316:1039–43.

Goldstraw P, Crowley J, Chansky K, et al. The IASLC Lung Cancer Staging Project: proposals for the revision of the TNM stage groupings in the forthcoming (seventh) edition of the TNM Classification of malignant tumours. J Thorac Oncol. 2007;2:706–14.

Gordon IO, Sitterding S, Mackinnon AC, Husain AN. Update in neoplastic lung diseases and mesothelioma. Arch Pathol Lab Med. 2009;133(7):1106–15. Erratum in Arch Pathol Lab Med. 2009; 133(11):1733.

Hecht SS. Tobacco smoke carcinogens and lung cancer. J Natl Cancer Inst. 1999;91:1194–210.

Jones KD. An update on lung cancer staging. Adv Anat Pathol. 2010; 17(1):33–7.

Kobayashi S, Boggon TJ, Dayaram T, et al. EGFR mutation and resistance of non-small-cell lung cancer to gefitinib. N Engl J Med. 2005;352:786–92.

Kwak EL, Bang YJ, Camidge DR, et al. Anaplastic lymphoma kinase inhibition in non-small-cell lung cancer. N Engl J Med. 2010;363: 1693–703.

Lee AY, Levine MN, Baker RI, et al. Low-molecular-weight heparin versus a coumarin for the prevention of recurrent venous thromboembolism in patients with cancer. N Engl J Med. 2003;349:146–53.

MacKenzie TD, Bartecchi CE, Schrier RW. The human costs of tobacco use (2). N Engl J Med. 1994;330:975–80.

Marcus PM, Bergstralh EJ, Fagerstrom RM, et al. Lung cancer mortality in the Mayo Lung Project: impact of extended follow-up. *J Natl Cancer Inst*. 2000;92:1308–16.

Mazzone PJ. Lung cancer screening: An update, discussion, and look ahead. *Curr Oncol Rep*. 2010;12(4):226–34.

Mok T, Wu Y-L, Thongprasert S, et al. Phase III, randomised, open-label, first-line study of gefitinib (G) vs carboplatin/paclitaxel (C/P) in clinically selected patients (Pts) with advanced non-small-cell lung cancer (NSCLC) (IPASS). *Ann Oncol*. 19:Abstract #LBA2, 2008.

Oken MM, Marcus PM, Hu P, et al. Baseline chest radiograph for lung cancer detection in the randomized prostate, lung, colorectal and ovarian cancer screening trial. *J Natl Cancer Inst*. 2005;97:1832–9.

Pieterman RM, van Putten JW, Meuzelaar JJ, et al. Preoperative staging of non-small-cell lung cancer with positron-emission tomography. *N Engl J Med*. 2000;343:254–61.

Pignon JP, Tribodet H, Scagliotti GV, et al. Lung adjuvant cisplatin evaluation: a pooled analysis by the LACE Collaborative Group. *J Clin Oncol*. 2008;26:3552–9.

Samet JM. Health benefits of smoking cessation. *Clin Chest Med*. 1991;12:669–79.

Sandler A, Gray R, Perry MC, et al. Paclitaxel-carboplatin alone or with bevacizumab for non-small-cell lung cancer. *N Engl J Med*. 2006;355:2542–50.

Schiller JH, Harrington D, Belani CP, et al. Comparison of four chemotherapy regimens for advanced non-small-cell lung cancer. *N Engl J Med*. 2002;346:92–8.

Sculier JP, Berghmans T, Meert AP. Update in lung cancer and mesothelioma 2009. *Am J Respir Crit Care Med*. 2010 Apr 15;181(8):773–81.

Sequist LV, Lynch TJ. EGFR tyrosine kinase inhibitors in lung cancer: an evolving story. *Annu Rev Med*. 2008;59:429–42.

Thiessen NR, Bremner R. The solitary pulmonary nodule: Approach for a general surgeon. *Surg Clin North Am*. 2010;90(5):1003–18.

U.S. Department of Health and Human Services: The Health Consequences of Involuntary Exposure to Tobacco Smoke: A Report of the Surgeon General. Atlanta, GA, U.S. Department of Health and Human Services, Centers for Disease Control and Prevention, Coordinating Center for Health Promotion, National Center for Chronic Disease Prevention and Health Promotion, Office on Smoking and Health, 2006.

QUESTIONS

QUESTION 1. A 60-year-old man with a 50-pack-year history of smoking, who still smokes 1 pack per day, presents to the clinic. He is currently asymptomatic. Following the United States Preventive Services Task Force (USPSTF) 2004 guidelines, what is your recommendation for his care?

A. Provide smoking cessation management and other age-appropriate cancer screening but recommend against low-dose chest computerized tomography (LDCT), chest x-ray (CXR), sputum cytology, or a combination of these tests.

B. Provide smoking cessation management and other age-appropriate cancer screening but discuss that there is insufficient evident to recommend chest CT, CXR, sputum cytology, or a combination of these tests.

C. Provide smoking cessation management and other age-appropriate cancer screening and recommend screening chest CT.

D. Provide smoking cessation management and other age-appropriate cancer screening and recommend CXR plus sputum cytology.

QUESTION 2. A 45-year-old woman who has never smoked develops a cough. Three weeks after antibiotic treatment, the cough persists. CXR demonstrates a 4-cm mass in the left lung. Chest CT scan confirms a mass in the left upper lobe and demonstrates a 2-cm left adrenal mass and numerous hypodense 1- to 2-cm lesions in the liver. These are all F-18 FDG PET positive. Brain MRI shows no abnormalities. What is the best way to establish a diagnosis?

A. Bronchoscopy to evaluate for endobronchial lesions
B. Video-assisted thorascopic surgery (VATS) and mediastinoscopy to evaluate extent of disease
C. Biopsy of the primary lung mass via CT-guided needle biopsy
D. Biopsy of the adrenal gland or the liver nodules via CT-guided or ultrasound-guided needle biopsy

QUESTION 3. Biopsy of the patient in question 2 reveals that she has metastatic adenocarcinoma, consistent with NSCLC. She is initially treated with six cycles of carboplatin, paclitaxel, and bevacizumab, but 3 months after finishing treatment she develops new brain metastases. After completing whole-brain radiation, she is generally feeling well and is returning to work part time. Molecular testing of her initial core biopsy demonstrates an exon 19 deletion in the EGFR gene. Which second-line option offers the highest likelihood of a response?

A. Erlotinib
B. Pemetrexed, docetaxel, or vinorelbine
C. Pemetrexed, docetaxel, or vinorelbine plus cisplatin
D. Best supportive care

ANSWERS

1. B
2. D
3. A

12.

GASTROINTESTINAL CANCERS

Jeffrey A. Meyerhardt

In the United States there will be an estimated 270,000 cases of gastrointestinal malignancies leading to 124,000 deaths annually (table 12.1). Gastrointestinal cancers are the second most common cancers behind those of the genital system (inclusive of gynecological, prostate, and testicular cancer). Worldwide, an estimated 6 million new cases of gastrointestinal cancers are diagnosed annually, accounting for 2.5 million deaths. The most common gastrointestinal cancers in the United States are esophageal, gastric, pancreatic, and colorectal, and these are the focus of this review.

ESOPHAGEAL CANCER

Esophageal cancer is diagnosed in approximately 16,000 individuals in the United States annually, leading to nearly 14,000 deaths. There are two major histology types, squamous cell carcinoma and adenocarcinoma, although rarely melanomas, carcinoids, lymphomas, and sarcomas can arise from the esophagus. Squamous cell carcinomas develop in the upper third and middle third of the esophagus and have relatively decreased in incidence over time. In contrast, adenocarcinomas primarily develop in the lower third of the esophagus and, particularly cancers at the gastroesophageal junction, have increased in the past several decades. The shift in incidence of each histology is reflective of changes of likelihood of exposure to associated risk factors.

RISK FACTORS FOR ESOPHAGEAL CANCER

The primary risk factors for squamous cell carcinomas are tobacco and alcohol (table 12.2). Risk is correlated with duration of smoking and number of cigarettes. There is a synergistic effect of tobacco and alcohol leading to chronic irritation and inflammation of the esophageal mucosa. As these factors are also strongly associated with risk of head and neck cancers, a prior history of head and neck is associated with risk of squamous cell of the esophagus, and about 2% of patients with newly diagnosed head and neck cancer will have a synchronous esophageal cancer. Cessation of smoking will decrease one's risk of esophageal squamous cell carcinoma, particularly after 10 years.

Other conditions that lead to irritation of the esophageal mucosa and increase the risk of squamous cell carcinoma are achalasia, caustic injury to the esophagus, and esophageal diverticuli. Rare conditions that carry a very high risk of squamous cell carcinoma are nonepidermolytic palmoplantar keratoderma (tylosis), a rare autosomal dominant disorder characterized by hyperkeratosis of the palms and soles and thickening of the oral mucosa, and Plummer-Vinson syndrome, a nutritional deficiency characterized by dysphagia, iron-deficiency anemia, and esophageal webs.

Adenocarcinomas of the esophagus principally develop in the setting of Barrett's esophagitis (table 12.2). Risk factors associated with Barrett's, including gastroesophageal reflux disease (GERD) and obesity, are thus associated with lower-esophageal cancers. Approximately one in seven Americans has GERD. Reflux can cause the normal squamous epithelium of the esophagus to develop metaplasia. Approximately 5% to 8% of those with GERD will develop metaplasia (Barrett's) of the esophagus. Of those with metaplasia, 4% per year will evolve into low-grade dysplasia, and 1% per year will evolve into high-grade dysplasia. Once patients have high-grade dysplasia, the rate of development of adenocarcinoma is 5% per year. Overall, the risk of esophageal adenocarcinoma is 0.5% per year for patients with metaplasia and 0.05% for those with GERD. Patients with Barrett's esophagitis require intermittent endoscopic surveillance for dysplasia, although the optimal timing of surveillance and management for both low- and high-grade dysplasia remains uncertain. Additional risk factors for adenocarcinoma of the esophagus are tobacco smoking (although smokers have a relatively higher risk of squamous cell histology) and prior radiation exposure to the esophagus (principally related to treatment of breast cancer). As opposed to squamous cell carcinoma, smokers who quit do not lower their associated risk of adenocarcinoma even decades after cessation.

Table 12.1 ESTIMATED INCIDENCE AND MORTALITY ASSOCIATED WITH GASTROINTESTINAL MALIGNANCIES IN THE UNITED STATES IN 2008

DISEASE	NEW CASES	DEATHS
Esophageal	16,470	14,280
Stomach	21,500	10,880
Small intestine	6,110	1,110
Colorectal	148,810	49,960
Anal cancer	5,070	680
Liver and intrahepatic bile duct	21,370	8,410
Gallbladder and other biliary	9,520	3,340
Pancreas	37,680	34,290
Other digestive organs	4,760	2,180

SOURCE: Jemal A, Siegel R, Ward E, et al. Cancer statistics, 2008. *CA.* 2008;58:71-96.

Table 12.2 RISK FACTORS FOR ESOPHAGEAL CANCER

SQUAMOUS CELL HISTOLOGY	ADENOCARCINOMA HISTOLOGY
Tobacco usage	Barrett's esophagitis
Alcohol usage	Gastroesophageal reflux
Prior history of head and neck cancer	Obesity
Caustic injury to esophagus	Tobacco usage
Achalasia	Prior radiation for breast cancer
Tylosis	
Plummer-Vinson syndrome	
Prior radiation for breast cancer	

CLINICAL PRESENTATION AND MANAGEMENT OF ESOPHAGEAL CANCER

Patients with esophageal cancer most commonly present with symptoms of difficulty swallowing (dysphagia) and, less commonly, pain with swallowing (odynophagia). Initially, patients will have dysphagia to certain solids, then most solids, and eventually liquids if undiagnosed. They may also present with hematemesis, unexpected weight loss, cough, hoarseness, or symptoms related to areas of metastases.

Treatment and prognosis of esophageal cancer are strongly associated with stage of disease at diagnosis. For the most part, squamous cell carcinomas and adenocarcinomas have a similar workup and treatment strategy (figure 12.1). Patients who are diagnosed with esophageal cancer by upper endoscopy should undergo staging workup. Computed tomography of the chest, abdomen, and pelvis would be standard (CT) to assess for metastases. The most common sites of metastases are liver, lung, lymph nodes, and bone. Brain imaging is warranted only if the patient has neurological symptoms. Up to 50% of patients will have metastatic disease at presentation, and initial scanning will diagnose most such cases. For patients without metastatic disease, further workup for resectability is warranted. Patients should undergo an endoscopic ultrasound to determine the extent of invasion of the tumor through the wall of the esophagus and whether any localized lymph nodes are involved. In addition, positron emission tomography (PET) scans have been shown to be beneficial in evaluating for resectability to further evaluate for metastatic disease and evaluate suspicious regional or distant lymph nodes that may have been detected on CT scans or endoscopic ultrasound. For patients with tumors in the upper third of the esophagus, brochoscopy is recommended to rule out a fistula between the esophagus and trachea.

For patients with disease that does not extend beyond the muscle layer of the esophageal wall and without evidence of lymph node involvement, immediate surgery is recommended. For those with disease that extends beyond the muscle layer or with locoregional lymph nodes, neoadjuvant therapy with chemotherapy and radiation should be considered prior to surgery. Chemoradiation therapy is given over 5 to 6 weeks with daily radiation and various acceptable combinations of chemotherapy agents. The

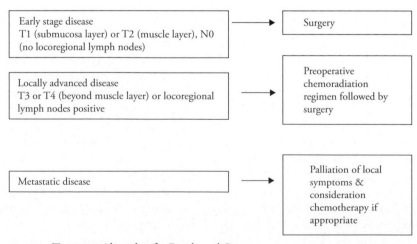

Figure 12.1. Treatment Algorithm for Esophageal Cancer.

data for neoadjuvant therapy are mixed, with a few trials demonstrating a survival benefit and multiple trials not. Nonetheless, despite uncertainty in benefit of preoperative therapy, most thoracic surgeons, medical oncologists, and radiation oncologists favor such an approach for localized advanced disease prior to surgery. Following the completion of neoadjuvant therapy, restaging is recommended followed by surgery approximately 6 weeks after the last dose of radiation. In contrast, studies for adjuvant chemotherapy or radiation after surgery have not shown a benefit (except for patients with tumors at the gastroesophageal junction, who can be treated similarly to those with gastric cancer).

For patients with localized disease who are not surgical candidates because of concurrent medical conditions or who refuse surgery, a randomized trial of chemoradiation versus radiation alone demonstrated a survival advantage to combined modality therapy. Further, there does seem to be a definitive long-term recurrence-free rate (up to 25%) in patients treated with chemoradiation alone.

Patients with metastatic disease should be considered for palliative therapy. Chemotherapy can palliate symptoms relating to swallowing and prolong overall survival. There is no single optimal first-line chemotherapy regimen, although in general patients are offered combination regimens that include a platinum agent. Other options for relief of dysphagia in patients with metastatic disease include radiation (either alone or with chemotherapy) or endoscopically placed esophageal stenting.

The prognosis of patients with esophageal cancer is stage dependent. Patients diagnosed with disease limited to the submucosal layer of the esophageal wall and no lymph node involvement experience 50% to 80% 5-year survival. If the disease is more extensive within the wall but not involving lymph nodes, 5-year survival is 30% to 40%. Patients with nonmetastatic disease but positive locoregional lymph nodes have a 10% to 30% 5-year survival. Patients with beyond locoregional lymph nodes or distant metastases have a 5-year survival of <5%. The median survival with metastatic esophageal cancer treated with palliative chemotherapy is 8 months.

GASTRIC CANCER

An estimated 21,500 new cases of gastric cancer and 11,000 related deaths occur in the United States annually. The incidence of gastric cancer in the United States has markedly decreased over decades, likely related to near elimination of certain risk factors for the disease. In 1930, there were 33 new cases of gastric cancer per 100,000 men and 30 new cases per 100,000 women; in 1990, incidence rates dropped to 10 and 5 per 100,000 men and women, respectively. However, gastric cancer remains the fourth most commonly diagnosed cancer (estimated 934,000 new cases annually) and the second leading cause of cancer-related death (700,000 deaths annually).

HISTOLOGY TYPES OF GASTRIC CANCER

The vast majority of tumors in the stomach are adenocarcinomas. Other markedly less frequent histologies are lymphomas, carcinoids, leiomyosarcomas, and gastrointestinal stromal tumors (GISTs). There are two subtypes of gastric adenocarcinomas, an intestinal type with cohesive neoplastic cells forming gland-like tubular structures and a diffuse type in which individual cells infiltrate and thicken the stomach wall. Intestinal-type lesions occur in the distal stomach more often than the diffuse type and are often preceded by a prolonged precancerous phase. Diffuse carcinomas are detected more often in young patients, develop throughout the stomach, particularly the cardia, and are associated with a worse prognosis.

RISK FACTORS FOR GASTRIC CANCER

Multiple factors have been associated with the risk of developing gastric cancer (table 12.3). Chronic atrophic gastritis and its associated condition, intestinal metaplasia, can result in reduced gastric acid production and progression to metaplasia, dysplasia, and, eventually, adenocarcinoma. Infection with *Helicobacter pylori* has been associated with gastric cancer. Prospective studies have demonstrated between three- and sixfold increased risk of gastric cancer in patients serologically positive for *H. pylori*. Nonetheless the majority of patients who are *H. pylori* positive will not develop gastric cancer.

Table 12.3 **RISK FACTORS FOR THE GASTRIC CANCER**

Nutritional
Low fat or protein consumption
Salted meat or fish
High nitrate consumption
Environmental
Poor food preparation (smoked)
Lack of refrigeration
Poor drinking water (well water)
Occupation (Rubber, Coal Workers)
Smoking
Low social class
Medical
Gastric atrophy and gastritis
Helicobacter pylori infection
Pernicious anemia
Prior gastric surgery
Hereditary
E cadherin mutation families

The marked decline in gastric cancer in the United States is presumed to be related to dietary and environmental exposure. The introduction of refrigeration has led to reduced use of salting, smoking, and pickling of food and to improved food preservation, factors that have been associated with atrophic gastritis. Before refrigeration, nitrates and nitrites were used to preserve meat, fish, and vegetables. Foods rich in nitrates, nitrites, and secondary amines can form N-nitroso compounds that have been associated with gastric tumors in animal models. Further, anaerobic bacteria, which colonize in areas with atrophic gastritis or intestinal metaplasia, can convert nitrates and nitrites to carcinogenic nitroso compounds.

CLINICAL PRESENTATION AND MANAGEMENT OF GASTRIC CANCER

Early detection of gastric cancer is difficult because most early-stage lesions do not cause symptoms. In the United States most patients are diagnosed with locally advanced or metastatic disease. In contrast, given the higher incidence rates of gastric cancer in Asia, screening endoscopy programs lead to more frequent detection of localized disease. The most common symptoms leading to medical attention are unexplained weight loss, abdominal pain, fatigue, nausea, anorexia, dysphagia, early satiety, and melena. Initial evaluation of symptoms suspicious for gastric cancer includes barium swallow and/or upper endoscopy. Once a diagnostic biopsy demonstrates adenocarcinoma, staging with CT is recommended. However, imaging is limited in detecting peritoneal metastases, which can be present in up to 10–30% of patients who appear to have localized disease. At the time of surgery, an initial exploratory laparotomy is necessary, and detection of peritoneal disease or distant metastases should lead to either a palliative resection or bypass gastrojejunostomy.

The pathological stage is the most important determinant of prognosis and determines treatment strategy. Those patients with metastatic disease should be considered for palliative chemotherapy. Multiple randomized trials have shown that chemotherapy prolongs survival and maintains or improves quality of life compared to best supportive care only in patients with metastases. No single regimen is considered standard. For patients with a good performance status, combination regimens that include a platinum agent are reasonable first-line choices.

For the patient with nonmetastatic disease, surgery can be curative. Cancers in the proximal and distal stomach are surgically approached differently, but both have the principle of wide margins and adequate lymph node dissection. The extensiveness of lymph node dissection remains controversial. In general, patients in Asia undergo considerably more extensive removal of lymph nodes than those in the United States and Europe. Randomized trials in Western populations have not demonstrated a survival benefit to

removing lymph nodes beyond 3 cm from the tumor. The more problematic controversy is that many surgeries in the United States have an inadequate nodal resection, which likely impacts on outcomes.

Following surgical resection, nonmetastatic patients whose disease extended beyond the muscle layer of the gastric wall or with positive lymph nodes should be considered for adjuvant chemoradiotherapy. A large, randomized North American trial demonstrates a survival advantage to a program of chemotherapy and combined chemotherapy and radiation lasting approximately 5 months after surgery. Most trials for adjuvant chemotherapy alone have not demonstrated a statistically significant advantage, although meta-analyses of these trials suggest some modest benefit. Although combined modality adjuvant therapy is considered preferable after surgery, for patients who have a contraindication to radiation (most commonly due to radiation for a different cancer that included some of the stomach field) or who refuse radiation, adjuvant chemotherapy alone is an alternative.

An alternative approach for nonmetastatic gastric cancer has been validated in Europe. Patients deemed surgically resectable are treated with 3 months of combination chemotherapy followed by surgery followed by further chemotherapy. This schema showed a statistically significant survival advantage over surgery alone. Survival rates from these two approaches (surgery followed by adjuvant chemoradiotherapy and neoadjuvant/adjuvant chemotherapy) are not comparable given the difference in timing of when the survival clock starts as well as the bias inherent in selecting out patients with peritoneal or other undetected metastases who underwent upfront surgery.

Survival is dependent on stage. Five-year survival is 65–80% for patients with disease with either T1 N0-1 disease (limited to submucosa and either no positive lymph nodes or fewer than seven positive nodes) or T2 N0 disease (disease into the muscularis propria but node negative). Patients with more advanced but nonmetastatic disease have considerably worse outcome, with 5-year survival ranging from 10% to 40%. Metastatic disease is not considered curable, and median survival with chemotherapy is 8–10 months.

PANCREAS CANCER

Pancreas cancer is one of the most fatal cancers because it is rarely detected at an early stage. Although it is the 10th most common cancer in incidence in the United States, it is the fourth most common cause of cancer-related deaths (behind lung, colorectal, and breast cancer). An estimated 37,000 new cases and 33,000 deaths occur annually in the United States. Despite much research in pancreatic cancer, outcomes have not dramatically changed in the last several decades.

Table 12.4 RISK FACTORS FOR PANCREATIC CANCER

Convincing evidence for risk

Hereditary syndromes (hereditary nonpolyposis colorectal cancer, Peutz-Jeghers, hereditary BRCA2 mutations, p16 syndrome, ataxia-telangiectasia, hereditary pancreatitis)
Tobacco
Diabetes mellitus

Likely risk

Chronic pancreatitis
Cystic fibrosis
Pernicious anemia
Obesity

RISK FACTORS FOR PANCREATIC CANCER

Pancreatic adenocarcinoma has been associated with various hereditary syndromes (table 12.4). Hereditary nonpolyposis colorectal cancer (HNPCC) results from mutations of mismatch repair genes and is most commonly associated with colorectal and gynecological cancers, although there is an increased risk of pancreatic cancer. Inherited mutations of p16 result in familial atypical multiple-mole melanoma syndrome associated with melanomas and pancreatic cancer. Other syndromes in which the risk of pancreatic cancer is increased are BRCA2, ataxia-telangiectasia, Peutz-Jeghers syndrome, and hereditary pancreatitis.

Diabetics appear to have an increased risk of pancreatic cancer. Initially, the association was primarily reported for recently diagnosed diabetics, which is likely more a reflection of a symptom of pancreatic cancer rather than a cause. However, more recent observational studies have shown that long-time diabetics have a modestly increased risk of pancreatic cancer compared to nondiabetics. Tobacco is the one modifiable risk factor most consistently associated with development of pancreatic cancer; however, obesity and certain dietary factors may increase the risk as well.

CLINICAL PRESENTATION AND MANAGEMENT OF PANCREATIC CANCER

Nearly three-quarters of pancreatic cancers derive from the exocrine pancreas ductal system and are adenocarcinomas. The other histologies are neuroendocrine tumors that arise in the islets of Langerhans, lymphomas, or metastatic disease. Adenocarcinomas most commonly arise in the head of the pancreas (65%) and less commonly are restricted to the body or tail (15%) or appear diffusely throughout the pancreas (20%). Whereas treatment strategies are similar regardless of origin (although surgical approach is different), the likelihood of curing patients with body or tail lesions is nearly 0%.

Although painless jaundice is a classical presentation of pancreatic cancer, patients more commonly present with unexpected weight loss, back pain wrapping to the right upper quadrant, anorexia, and nausea. Laboratory tests may show elevated levels of total bilirubin and other liver-function tests (alkaline phosphatase more than transaminases). Patients with suspicious symptoms are usually evaluated by CT when a pancreatic mass is detected. For patients with metastatic disease at presentation, the liver is the most common site of metastases, although distant lymph nodes, peritoneum, and lungs are frequent areas of spread. Patients who present with jaundice should have an endoscopic retrograde cholangiopancreatography (ERCP) with stent placement and cytology by brushings and/or biopsy. Alternatively, percutaneous biopsy of the primary pancreatic mass or metastases can be done with the assistance of ultrasound or CT.

Although a TNM (tumor, node, metastases) system that is utilized for solid organ tumors exists for pancreatic cancer, the more practical classification of pancreatic cancers divides them into three stages—local disease, locally advanced, and metastatic (figure 12.2). Local disease implies surgically resectable and is the only potentially curable stage of pancreatic cancer. Unfortunately, only 15% of patients have local disease at diagnosis. For surgery to be considered, preservation of fat planes around the major blood vessels in the area is required, including the superior mesenteric artery, celiac axis vessels, superior mesenteric vein, and portal vein. Typically, either pancreatic protocol CT or magnetic resonance imaging (MRI) can determine the status of these vessels. However, ultimately the determination of resectability is based on a surgeon's judgment at the time of laparotomy. For head of the pancreas lesions, a pancreaticoduodenectomy (Whipple) operation is performed, with resection of part of the pancreas and duodenum, common bile duct, gallbladder, and distal stomach (figure 12.3). For body or tail of the pancreas lesions, a distal pancreatectomy with or without splenectomy is performed. Resection of body or tail lesions is considerably less common since most such cancers are metastatic at time of diagnosis. Following resection, adjuvant therapy is considered with either chemotherapy alone or combination of chemotherapy and radiation. Only 15–20% of patients who undergo surgical resection will not have recurrences; most recurrences will be detected within the first 2 years after surgery.

Patients who are not surgically curable because of invasion of at least one major blood vessel but do not have evidence of distant metastases are staged as locally advanced. Randomized clinical trials have demonstrated a survival benefit to combined-modality chemotherapy and radiation compared to radiation alone. Alternatively, patients with locally advanced pancreatic cancer can be treated with chemotherapy alone, as nonrandomized comparison of chemotherapy versus chemoradiation suggests similar

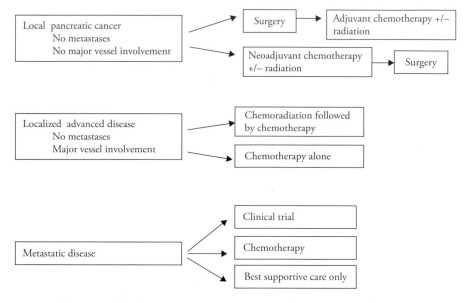

Figure 12.2. Treatment Algorithm for Pancreatic Cancer.

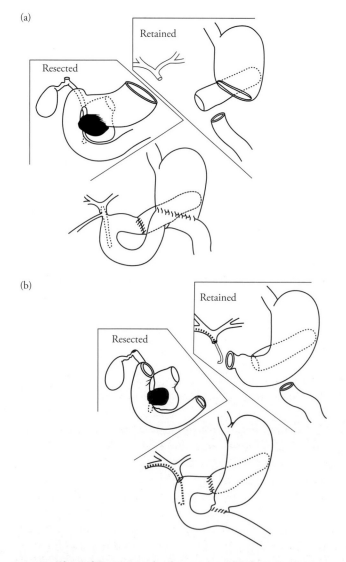

(a)

Retained

Resected

(b)

Retained

Resected

Figure 12.3. Classical Pancreaticoduodenectomy and Pylorus-Sparing Pancreaticoduodenectomy.

survival outcomes. Ultimately, patients with locally advanced disease will develop metastatic disease.

Chemotherapy has provided limited benefit to patients with metastatic disease. Median survival without therapy ranges from 3 to 6 months and with palliative chemotherapy from 6 to 8 months. The first step in approaching patients with metastatic pancreatic cancer is palliation of symptoms (either with surgery or nonoperative interventions) and determination of overall performance status to determine suitability for palliative chemotherapy. Gemcitabine, a deoxycytidine analogue that inhibits DNA replication and repair, is considered a first-line agent for metastatic pancreatic cancer. Various gemcitabine combination regimens have been tested and generally have minimal to no additional benefit compared to gemcitabine alone. Recently, a randomized trial in good performance status patients founds a superior survival benefit to a 4 drug regimen (5-fluorouracil, irinotecan, oxaliplatin, and leucovorin) compared to gemcitabine alone, though at the potential risk for greater toxicity. Most treatment guidelines suggest that clinical trials should be considered for patients with metastatic pancreatic cancer, even in the first-line setting.

COLORECTAL CANCER

Colorectal cancer is the third most common cancer diagnosed in men and women in the United States, and the fourth most common cancer overall. Approximately 148,000 people in the United States are diagnosed annually with colorectal cancer. It is the second most common cause of cancer-related death in the United States, with an estimated 50,000 deaths each year. Worldwide, over 1 million people are diagnosed annually and one-half million die from colorectal cancer. Colorectal cancer is probably the cancer

Table 12.5 RISK FACTORS ASSOCIATED WITH
COLORECTAL CANCER DEVELOPMENT

DECREASE RISK	INCREASE RISK	UNCERTAIN IMPACT
Screening	Family history	Folic acid
Exercise	Obesity	Fiber
Vitamin D/calcium	Diabetes	Fruits/Vegetables
Postmenopausal estrogen	Inflammatory bowel disease	Cholesterol-lowering agents
Aspirin	Red meat	Glycemic index
	Alcohol	
	Smoking	
	Acromegaly	

with the most consistent research implicating modifiable risk factors associated with its development (table 12.5) as well as effective screening techniques for precursor lesions, albeit underutilized.

RISK FACTORS FOR COLORECTAL CANCER

Up to 25% of patients with colorectal cancer have a family history of the disease. Multiple hereditary syndromes carry a markedly increased risk of colorectal cancer. Familial adenomatous polyposis (FAP) results from truncating mutations of the adenomatous polyposis coli (APC) gene. Afflicted individuals develop hundreds to thousands of polyps by their second decade of life and, if untreated, will develop colorectal cancer by age 40. Patients should have a total colectomy by age 20. Variants of FAP include Gardner syndrome (in which prominent extraintestinal lesions such as desmoid tumors and sebaceous or epidermoid cysts are seen in addition to extensive polyposis) and Turcot syndrome (brain tumors, particularly medulloblastomas, in addition to colonic tumors).

Hereditary nonpolyposis colon cancer (HNPCC), or Lynch syndrome, is characterized by the early onset of colorectal cancer, often involving the right side of the colon and typically occurring in the absence of numerous colonic polyps. Several germline defects responsible for HNPCC have been identified; the most common of these are mutations in hMLH1 and hMSH2. These genes are essential components of a nucleotide mismatch repair system. HNPCC is also associated with the development of extracolonic tumors, including malignancies of the endometrium, ovary, stomach, and small bowel. Genetic screening for individuals at risk for HNPCC is available.

In addition to familial syndromes, a family or personal history of colorectal cancer increases one's risk of developing colorectal cancer. This risk is modified by number of family members affected and age of diagnosis of family members, particularly first-degree relatives. Importantly, this risk is similar for individuals with a family history of adenomatous polyps, likely because such polyps may have evolved to cancer if untreated.

Patients with inflammatory bowel disease (IBD) have an increased risk of colorectal cancer that can be three- to fivefold higher than that of the general population. The risk is associated with both ulcerative colitis and Crohn disease, particular for patients with Crohn disease affecting the large bowel. Extent of disease involvement of the colon and rectum and duration of disease are the main determinants of the increased risk. In general, patients with ulcerative colitis do not have an appreciable increase in risk until about 8 to 10 years from time of diagnosis.

Two other medical conditions associated with higher risk of colorectal cancer are diabetes mellitus and acromegaly. Case-control and cohort studies have suggested that diabetic patients have a 1.3- to 1.5-fold increased risk of colorectal cancer, compared to nondiabetics. Given the prevalence of diabetes, such a relative risk is clinically significant. Individuals with acromegaly have a 2.5-fold increased risk of colorectal cancer.

Obesity and physical activity have consistently been shown to influence the risk of colorectal cancer. Greater body-mass index and lower levels of physical activity increase the risk of developing colorectal cancer, with relative risks ranging from 1.4 to 2.0 in most studies. Recent hypotheses have linked physical activity, obesity, and adipose distribution to circulating insulin and free insulin-like growth factor 1 (IGF-1).

Studies of diet and colorectal cancer have led to mixed results. The most consistent results show an increased risk of colorectal cancer with higher intakes of red meat. Fiber, fruit, and vegetables have been studied extensively as risk factors, although the majority of studies show little or no association except in the case of very low intake of these dietary factors.

There is emerging evidence consistently demonstrating that individuals with lower serum levels of vitamin D have an increased risk of colorectal cancer. Because the minority of vitamin D is obtained from diet, supplementation and/or sunlight exposure may be protective. Folic acid was considered to have consistent evidence of a protective effect against colorectal cancer, although a recent intervention trial of folic acid supplementation in patients with prior history of adenomatous polyps has challenged prior evidence; further studies are required to determine if there is an association between folic acid and colorectal cancer.

An association between alcohol consumption and an increased risk of colorectal cancer has been observed in several studies. A pooled analysis of eight cohort studies estimated a 40% increased risk of colorectal cancer in those whose alcohol consumption exceeded 45 g per day. Cigarette smoking has been associated both with increased incidence and mortality from colorectal cancer.

Preclinical, epidemiologic, and intervention studies support a protective effect of aspirin, nonsteroidal anti-inflammatory medications, and selective cyclooxygenase-2 inhibitors on the risk of colorectal cancer and adenomas. However, the risks of bleeding and renal dysfunction associated with these agents may outweigh the benefit if universally adopted in normal-risk individuals.

The most protective factor against colorectal cancer is screening. A recent revision of guidelines from the American Cancer Society recommended every 5 years flexible sigmoidoscopy, every 10 years colonoscopy, every 5 years double contrast barium enema or every 5 years CT colonography (virtual colonoscopy) as screening options to detect polyps or cancer. Further, annual guaiac-based fecal occult blood testing (FOBT), annual fecal immunochemical test (FIT), or intermittent stool DNA testing are options to screen for cancer. The method with the strongest evidence of protection from colorectal cancer mortality is FOBT; four randomized trials have demonstrated statistically significant benefits to FOBT screening. However, colonoscopies are the most sensitive and specific screening test and have the advantage of intervening on precursor lesions as well as biopsying malignant lesions at the time of screening. Patients without a family history of IBD should initiate screening at age 50. Those with a family history should initiate screening at least 10 years prior to their family member's diagnosis or at age 40, whichever is earlier.

PATHOLOGICAL FEATURES AND PRESENTATION OF COLORECTAL CANCER

Over 98% of large intestine cancers are adenocarcinomas. Most colorectal carcinomas originate from adenomatous polyps. Progression from early adenomatous proliferations through adenomatous polyp, high-grade dysplasia, and, ultimately, invasive carcinoma occurs as a continuum. This progression coincides with the accumulation of genetic alterations within the neoplasm, including mutations of tumor suppressor genes, for example p53 and APC, as well as activation and/or overexpression of oncogenes, for example c-myc and k-ras. Although the order of occurrence of these genetic changes may vary, the quantitative accumulation of defects correlates with biological and histologic parameters of neoplastic progression, suggesting a multistep model of tumorigenesis. The remaining 2% of colorectal cancers consist of lymphomas, leiomyosarcomas, and miscellaneous tumors.

Patients with cancer of the cecum and ascending colon usually present with anemia caused by intermittent gastrointestinal bleeding. Obstruction is rare because the bowel wall is more distensible and has a greater circumference than the descending colon. These cancers are often large and may be fungating or friable. Carcinomas of the transverse colon and either the hepatic or the splenic flexure, which account for about 10% of total cases, are somewhat less common than cecal neoplasms and much less common than rectosigmoid tumors. They frequently cause cramping pain, bleeding, and sometimes obstruction or perforation. Large bowel obstruction is the most common complication of colon carcinoma and may lead to proximal ulceration or perforation. Other complications include iron deficiency anemia, hypokalemia (particularly associated with large villous rectal lesions), and intussusception in adults. Tumors of the sigmoid colon and rectum cancers usually cause changes in normal bowel habits with tenesmus, decrease in stool caliber, secretion of mucus, and hematochezia.

MANAGEMENT OF COLORECTAL CANCER

Colorectal cancers are generally staged at the time of surgery. Computed tomography scans of the abdomen and pelvis and chest radiographs are usually performed to evaluate for metastatic disease. Bone scans are not routinely carried out in the absence of bone pain because of the low incidence of bone metastases. Extension of primary rectal cancers into adjacent soft tissues can often be assessed by endorectal coil MRI or endoscopic ultrasound. The commonly employed staging system is the TNM (tumor, node, metastases) staging classification (figure 12.4). In stage I and II disease, disease is localized to the bowel wall without involvement of regional lymph nodes or presence of distant metastases. Patients with stage III disease have involvement of regional lymph nodes but no distant metastases, whereas those with stage IV disease have distant metastases (most commonly liver, lung, distant lymph nodes, and peritoneum).

Colorectal cancers spread by direct invasion, through lymphatic channels, along hematogenous routes, and by implantation. Spread of colon cancers through the portal venous circulation leads to liver metastases. Cancers that originate below the peritoneal reflection (12–15 cm from the anal verge) are considered rectal cancers. The location of these lesions and the lymphatic drainage of this area necessitate special management decisions. Rectal cancers situated below the peritoneal reflection have a high rate of local recurrence. Cancers of the lower rectum may metastasize via the paravertebral plexus to supraclavicular nodes, lungs, bone, and brain, without liver involvement. Initial staging remains the most predictive prognostic factor for overall survival.

Patients with stage I disease have >90% 5-year survival with surgery. Patients with stage II disease have 70–85% 5-year survival (dependent on extent of disease through bowel wall and existence of other prognostic features—clinical bowel obstruction, bowel perforation, poor differentiation lead to higher risk for recurrence). Patients with stage III disease have a 5-year survival ranging from 35% to 70% (depending on number of positive lymph nodes and presence of other high-risk features). Finally, patients with stage IV disease (metastatic) have <5% long-term survival.

Treatment for colorectal cancer depends on stage of disease (table 12.6). The bases of the treatment algorithm are both the potential curability of the disease and likelihood of recurrence. The principal treatment modalities utilized are surgery, chemotherapy, and radiation therapy.

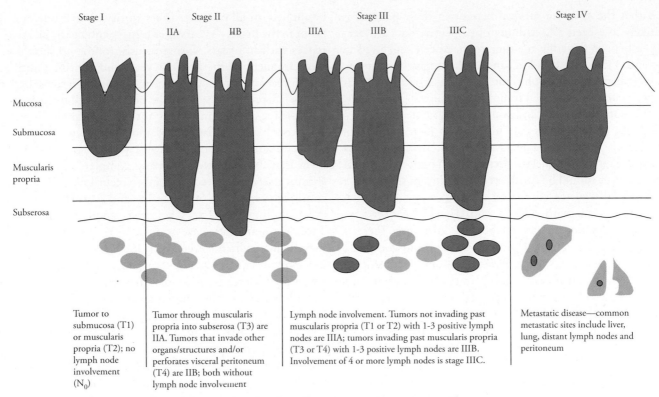

| | Stage I | Stage II | | Stage III | | | Stage IV |

| Mucosa | | IIA | IIB | IIIA | IIIB | IIIC | |

Muscularis propria

Subserosa

| Tumor to submucosa (T1) or muscularis propria (T2); no lymph node involvement (N₀) | Tumor through muscularis propria into subserosa (T3) are IIA. Tumors that invade other organs/structures and/or perforates visceral peritoneum (T4) are IIB; both without lymph node involvement | Lymph node involvement. Tumors not invading past muscularis propria (T1 or T2) with 1-3 positive lymph nodes are IIIA; tumors invading past muscularis propria (T3 or T4) with 1-3 positive lymph nodes are IIIB. Involvement of 4 or more lymph nodes is stage IIIC. | Metastatic disease—common metastatic sites include liver, lung, distant lymph nodes and peritoneum |

Figure 12.4. TMN Staging of Colorectal Cancer. (American Joint Commission on Cancer Version 6.)

Surgery is considered the only curative therapy for colorectal cancers. Although other modalities, including chemotherapy and radiation, are critical components of many patients' treatment, a critical step in approaching patients is determining the suitability and timing of surgery. Eighty percent of patients will present without detectable metastases. For such patients with colon cancer, surgery is usually the first step in treatment. For patients with rectal cancer, preoperative staging with either pelvis MRI or endorectal ultrasound is required to determine whether the patient has clinically stage II or III disease; in most patients with stage II or III disease, neoadjuvant combined chemotherapy and radiation should be offered. Alternatively, for patients with metastatic disease, removal of the primary tumor still remains an important consideration to palliate and prevent symptoms due to the colorectal lesion (including bleeding and obstruction). A limited number of patients with metastatic disease may be appropriate for consideration of curative-intent surgery of the primary tumor and metastatectomies.

Multiple clinical trials have demonstrated a survival benefit for adjuvant chemotherapy in stage III (lymph node–positive) colon cancer patients following surgery. In 1990, a National Cancer Institute consensus conference recommended fluorouracil-based adjuvant therapy as standard of care for patients with resected stage III colon cancer. No single randomized clinical trial has demonstrated a survival benefit for adjuvant therapy in patients with stage II colon cancer. In addition, subset analyses of trials that included patients with stage II and III disease have repeatedly failed to demonstrate a statistically significant survival benefit for stage II patients. An expert panel convened by the American Society of Clinical Oncology (ASCO) concluded that direct evidence from clinical trials does not support the routine use of adjuvant therapy in patients with stage II colon cancer

Table 12.6 TREATMENT ALGORITHM FOR COLORECTAL CANCER

STAGE	COLON	RECTAL
I	Surgery only	Surgery only
II	Surgery +/− adjuvant chemotherapy	Surgery, radiation, chemotherapy (either neoadjuvant chemoradiation followed by surgery followed by chemotherapy OR surgery followed by adjuvant chemotherapy and radiation)
III	Surgery and adjuvant chemotherapy	Surgery, radiation, chemotherapy (either neoadjuvant chemoradiation followed by surgery followed by chemotherapy OR surgery followed by adjuvant chemotherapy and radiation)
IV	Chemotherapy (consider surgery for primary tumor and whether metastases are resectable)	

and that the absolute survival benefit in these patients is unlikely to exceed 5%. Although prospective data are lacking, a benefit for adjuvant therapy has been suggested in patients with stage II colon cancer with high-risk features, such as inadequate lymph node sampling, lymphovascular or perineural invasion, T4 tumor stage, clinical colonic perforation or obstruction, and poorly differentiated histology. Although these features may indicate an increased risk of recurrence, they do not necessarily predict for efficacy of chemotherapy. Nonetheless, patients with high-risk stage II colon cancer should be considered for adjuvant therapy.

Clinical trials of combined chemotherapy and radiation for patients with stage II and III rectal cancer have also demonstrated a survival benefit. Although there is some controversy on the benefit of radiation in good-risk, T3 N0 rectal cancers, such patients should be considered for therapy in addition to surgery. In the past several years neoadjuvant chemoradiotherapy followed by surgery followed by further adjuvant chemotherapy has become the standard approach in the United States for patients whose tumor extends at least through the muscle layer or who are lymph node positive by endoscopic ultrasound or endorectal coil MRI. Radiation is employed with rectal cancer and not colon cancer because the bony constraints of the pelvis limit surgical access to the rectum, leading to a lower likelihood of achieving widely negative margins and a higher risk of local recurrence.

Chemotherapy is an important component of the treatment of patients with metastatic disease as well as many patients with surgically resected tumors. The backbone of colorectal cancer treatment for the past four decades is the fluorinated pyrimidine 5-fluorouracil (5-FU). Recently, multiple new agents have been added to the treatment armamentarium for colorectal cancer. In addition to intravenous fluorouracil, oral derivatives of fluorouracil include capecitabine and uracil plus tegafur (UFT). Two other traditional cytotoxic therapies that have definitive activity against colorectal cancer include irinotecan and oxaliplatin. Finally, more specific targeted therapies against the vascular endothelial growth factor (bevacizumab) and epidermal growth factor receptor (cetuximab and panitumumab) are having an expanding role against colorectal cancer. For patients with metastatic colorectal cancer, the expansion of agents has led to multiple viable combinations and lines of therapy to palliate symptoms and prolong survival. Whereas in the era of only 5-FU the median survival of patients with metastatic colorectal cancer was 12 months, patients able to receive all of the available agents in some sequencing experience a median survival of over 2 years.

Following surgical resection plus or minus adjuvant therapy, patients with nonmetastatic colorectal cancer should have regular follow-ups with their treating physicians. Despite multiple attempts at addressing the question of optimal follow-up strategies, no single trial has adequately determined which tests and what frequency of tests should

be applied for all patients. The majority of recurrences will occur in the first 2–3 years after surgery and nearly all recurrences within 5 years. Consequently, follow-up should be more frequent in the first few years and continue until at least 5 years post-resection. The most common surveillance tools that are recommended and being utilized include physician visits, carcinoembryonic antigen (CEA) monitoring, colonoscopic surveillance, and additional sigmoidoscopies for rectal cancer patients. Conversely, there is general agreement that liver function tests and complete blood counts are not useful in detecting cancer recurrences. The main controversy has been on the utility and frequency of imaging, including chest x-rays, CT scans, and liver ultrasound. Three meta-analyses have concluded that more intensive surveillance (which has generally included radiology imaging) provides a modest but statistically significant survival advantage to less-intensive surveillance. As a result, ASCO recently updated their guidelines for surveillance of stage II or III colon and rectal cancer patients. An expert panel recommended history and physical examination every 3 to 6 months for the first 3 years, every 6 months during years 4 and 5, and subsequently at the discretion of the physician. Carcinoembryonic antigen (CEA) should be tested every 3 months postoperatively for at least 3 years after diagnosis (usually continued through 5 years with less frequency). In addition, for patients who would undergo surgery for a metastasis, the panel recommended annual CT of the chest and abdomen for 3 years and pelvic CT scan for patients with rectal cancer. The group suggested a colonoscopy 3 years after resection and, if normal, every 5 years thereafter. For patients with rectal cancer who underwent a low anterior resection and did not undergo radiation, more frequent sigmoidoscopies (every 6 months for 5 years) should be considered. It should be noted that an initial colonoscopy is often recommended by other organizations sooner than 3 years because there is a definitive, albeit low, risk of an adenoma or second colorectal cancer missed at the time of diagnosis before surgery.

ADDITIONAL READING

Alberts SR, Cervantes A, van de Velde CJ. Gastric cancer: Epidemiology, pathology and treatment. *Ann Oncol.* 2003;14 Suppl 2:ii-31–6.

Anandasabapathy S. Endoscopic imaging: Emerging optical techniques for the detection of colorectal neoplasia. *Curr Opin Gastroenterol.* 2008;24(1):64–9.

Desch CE, Benson AB 3rd, Somerfield MR, et al. Colorectal cancer surveillance: 2005 update of an American Society of Clinical Oncology practice guideline. *J Clin Oncol.* 2005;23:8512–9.

D'souza MA, Singh K, Shrikhande SV. Surgery for gastric cancer: An evidence-based perspective. *J Cancer Res Ther.* 2009;5(4):225–31.

Enzinger PC, Mayer RJ. Esophageal cancer. *N Engl J Med.* 2003;349(23):2241–52.

Giovannucci E. Modifiable risk factors for colon cancer. *Gastroenterol Clin North Am.* 2002;31(4):925–43.

Gollub MJ, Schwartz LH, Akhurst T. Update on colorectal cancer imaging. *Radiol Clin North Am.* 2007;45(1):85–118.

Holt PR, Kozuch P, Mewar S. Colon cancer and the elderly: From screening to treatment in management of GI disease in the elderly. *Best Pract Res Clin Gastroenterol.* 2009;23(6):889–907.

Ko AH, Tempero MA. Systemic therapy for pancreatic cancer. *Semin Radiat Oncol.* 2005;15(4):245–53.

Konner J, O'Reilly E. Pancreatic cancer: Epidemiology, genetics, and approaches to screening. *Oncology (Williston Park).* 2002;16(12):1615–22, 1631–2; discussion 1632–3, 1637–8.

Levin B, Lieberman DA, McFarland B, et al.; American Cancer Society Colorectal Cancer Advisory Group; US Multi-Society Task Force; American College of Radiology Colon Cancer Committee. Screening and surveillance for the early detection of colorectal cancer and adenomatous polyps, 2008: A joint guideline from the American Cancer Society, the US Multi-Society Task Force on Colorectal Cancer, and the American College of Radiology. *Gastroenterology.* 2008;134(5):1570–95.

Meyerhardt JA, Mayer RJ. Systemic therapy for colorectal cancer. *N Engl J Med.* 2005;352(5):476–87.

QUESTIONS

QUESTION 1. Your patient is a 72-year-old carpenter who presents with a several-month history of difficulty swallowing, primarily just certain foods. He has lost approximately 10 lb in the past month, but he claims that he was trying to diet. You order an EGD, and there is a mass in his midesophagus. Biopsies demonstrate squamous cell carcinoma. He consults a thoracic surgeon, who performs an esophagectomy, and final pathology reveals invasion through the muscle to subserosa (T3) and two positive lymph nodes. Margins were all negative. You now recommend:

A. Adjuvant chemotherapy
B. Adjuvant radiation
C. Combined chemotherapy and radiation
D. Observation and intermittent surveillance

QUESTION 2. Your patient is a 68-year-old former smoker who presented over Memorial Day weekend to an outside hospital's emergency department with new-onset jaundice. Computed tomography revealed a lesion at the head of her pancreas with intrahepatic biliary dilation. She underwent an ERCP, and a plastic stent was placed, which improved her bilirubin back to normal range. She was evaluated by a surgical oncologist and was determined to have resectable disease. She is scheduled to undergo a Whipple operation. All of the following would have been contraindications to Whipple surgery EXCEPT:

A. Circumferential invasion of the superior mesenteric artery
B. Two liver metastases
C. Three subcentimeter peripancreatic lymph nodes
D. Evidence of peritoneal disease at time of laparotomy

QUESTION 3. A patient presents to her gastroenterologist. She has had a long-standing history of irritable bowel syndrome. However, her sister recently was diagnosed with stage II colon cancer, and she is distraught because her mother also had colon cancer at age 48. Her sister's oncologist recommended testing for a hereditary syndrome, and she was found to have a deletion of *MLH1* (a mismatch repair gene). The patient requests testing. The gastroenterologist sends the test and the patient, who is 38, has the same genetic mutation. Recommendations for this patient include all of the following EXCEPT:

A. Total colectomy
B. Yearly colonoscopy
C. Screening for gynecological cancers
D. Discussion of testing of the patient's children by age 20

QUESTION 4. Your patient is a 56-year-old school teacher who presented with about 2 months of intermittent blood in the toilet bowl with bowel movements. A colonoscopy is performed that demonstrates a mass in the midsigmoid, and biopsy confirms adenocarcinoma. He undergoes laparoscopic hemicolectomy, and final pathology reveals a 3-cm, moderately differentiated adenocarcinoma through the muscle layer into the serosa with two of nine lymph nodes positive. The next step would be:

A. Reoperate for more complete lymph node dissection
B. Referral to medical oncologist for consideration of chemotherapy
C. Follow-up colonoscopy in 1 year
D. Referral to radiation oncologist for postoperative radiation

QUESTION 5. A new patient presents to your primary care clinic after relocating from Memphis to San Francisco because of work. He is a 58-year-old with history of type II diabetes mellitus and stage III colon cancer. You review records related to his colon cancer. The cancer was resected 4 years ago. He received adjuvant chemotherapy. He has not had a colonoscopy since prior to his surgery. He wants to avoid having to establish care with a new oncologist unless necessary. At this point, 4 years from his operation, surveillance testing should include all of the following EXCEPT:

A. Colonoscopy in near future and then every 3–5 years thereafter
B. Carcinoembryonic antigen testing every 6 months until full 5 years from surgery
C. Liver function testing every 6 months until 5 years from surgery
D. Physical exam every 6 months until 5 years from surgery

ANSWERS

1. D
2. C
3. A
4. B
5. C

13.

GENITOURINARY CANCERS
PROSTATE, KIDNEY, BLADDER, AND TESTIS

Mark M. Pomerantz, Aymen A. Elfiky, Leah M. Katz, and William K. Oh

PROSTATE CANCER

OVERVIEW

Since the introduction of widespread prostate cancer screening in the United States in the early 1990s, the incidence of prostate cancer has increased substantially. After skin cancer, prostate cancer is the most commonly diagnosed cancer in American men. In the prostate cancer-screening era, the majority of newly diagnosed cases are localized (i.e., tumor is confined to the prostate gland). Therefore, most patients have the opportunity for curative therapy. Yet, the benefits of population-wide screening and optimal treatment remain controversial. This section reviews the epidemiology, risk factors, and screening of prostate cancer, as well as treatment options at different stages of disease.

EPIDEMIOLOGY

Prostate cancer represents approximately 25% of all cancers diagnosed in men each year. In the United States approximately 186,000 cases are diagnosed, and approximately 29,000 deaths occur annually. The lifetime risk of prostate cancer for an American man is approximately one in six over the course of his lifetime. It is the second leading cause of cancer death in American men.

Prostate cancer incidence differs significantly around the world. The disease is generally more common in the United States. Although it is the leading cause of non-skin cancers among American men, the disease is the sixth most common worldwide. The differences in rates of prostate cancer across different world populations are due, in part, to environmental and genetic factors, and the ubiquity of prostate cancer screening in the United States undoubtedly accounts for much of the discrepancy. Increased screening leads to more biopsies that, in turn, lead to more diagnoses. Whether this is associated with improved mortality is a subject of much debate and discussed in detail below.

RISK FACTORS

Of several known prostate cancer risk factors, the most important are age and genetic factors, such as family history and ethnicity. Diet may also play a role in disease risk. The correlation between age and prostate cancer is remarkably strong. Prostate cancer is exceedingly rare in young men and data from the Surveillance Epidemiology and End Results (SEER) database in 1995 showed that the incidence of prostate cancer in American men of European ancestry was approximately 100, 600, and 1000 per 100,000 in men in their early 50s, 60s, and 70s, respectively.

A positive family history has been recognized as a strong risk factor for the development of prostate cancer. A meta-analysis of 33 epidemiologic studies reported a relative risk of 2.53 for subjects with a first-degree relative with prostate cancer, and the risk increases as the number of affected relatives increases. Similar trends are seen when comparing ethnic or racial groups. African Americans have the highest known incidence of prostate cancer in the world. When controlling for socioeconomic, clinical, and pathologic factors, African Americans also present with higher-stage disease compared with other groups. These trends suggest a strong genetic component to prostate carcinogenesis.

Studies of male twins lend further support to genetics playing a key role in the development of disease. In 2000 an analysis of 44,788 pairs of twins in Scandinavia revealed a 21.1% concordance rate for monozygotic twins and 6.4% rate for dizygotic twins. Heritable factors were estimated to account for 42% of prostate cancer risk, greater than the other 10 cancers analyzed, including breast and colorectal.

Until recently, the exact causal factors within the genome were unknown. Taking advantage of profound developments, such as the sequencing of the human genome and the mapping of common variants, several genome-wide association studies of prostate cancer have been conducted. To date, over 40 independent genetic polymorphisms throughout the human genome have been identified as markers of prostate cancer risk. These studies provide compelling evidence for the first bona fide genetic risk factors responsible for an appreciable fraction of risk in the general population. Because many of these markers reside in areas of unknown significance, further work is necessary to define their function.

Dietary intake and prostate cancer risk have been widely studied, although most results are equivocal or complicated by conflicting results in other studies. For instance, data suggest that a diet high in certain fats, particularly those high in alpha-linoleic acids (common in red meats and some dairy products), is associated with prostate cancer risk. Some, but not all, studies have demonstrated that diets rich in lycopene, found in tomato-based products, and phytoestrogens, found in soy products, decrease prostate cancer risk. Early studies showed a profound benefit to selenium and vitamin E supplementation, leading to a large, prospective randomized trial called SELECT. This trial was recently reported to be negative for any benefit, and, thus, neither selenium nor vitamin E should be recommended to patients to prevent prostate cancer.

The influence of hormonal factors on prostate cancer risk is unclear. While depleting circulating testosterone is highly effective in reducing prostate tumor burden in men diagnosed with the disease, there is no convincing evidence that hormone levels affect risk of disease development.

SCREENING AND DIAGNOSIS

Most prostate cancer diagnoses in the United States are made through prostate-specific antigen (PSA) screening. Although prostate cancer incidence in the United States has increased dramatically in the PSA era, prostate cancer-specific mortality has decreased. Screening may be partly or largely responsible for the decline, although this remains controversial.

Observational studies in Europe and the United States have compared outcome in the pre- and post-PSA eras and estimated that PSA screening has led to a threefold decline in prostate cancer-associated mortality. In the PSA era, the incidence of high-grade, more aggressive prostate cancer is less common in screened populations and the proportion of patients diagnosed with metastatic disease has also declined. On the other hand, the lifetime risk of death from prostate cancer is only 3% for U.S. males, suggesting that a high proportion of men with prostate cancer will

die with the disease but not from it. PSA screening may uncover clinically insignificant cancers, exposing patients to unnecessary treatment with significant morbidity as well as to the psychological distress associated with a cancer diagnosis.

In addition, it is well accepted that the PSA test is imperfect. PSA is made by normal as well as tumor cells; benign prostatic hypertrophy (BPH) and prostatitis commonly can cause elevations in PSA. At the traditional cutoff for "normal" (4.0 ng/mL), the positive predictive value for PSA—that is, the proportion of men with a PSA >4.0 ng/mL who have prostate cancer—is approximately 30%. It is only 25% for the majority of men whose elevated PSA is between 4 and 10 ng/mL. In one series, PSA levels between 2 and 9 ng/mL had less association with prostate cancer than with BPH. Two large, randomized controlled trials involving thousands of patients in Europe and the United States have not definitively determined that prostate cancer screening improves mortality at 10 years.

Nonetheless, given the data supporting screening, PSA testing has become a standard of care in many U.S. primary care practices even though there are no universally accepted screening guidelines. The American Urologic Association, as well as the American Cancer Society, recommend initiating screening at age 50 and continuing until age 70, or as long as life expectancy is > 10 years. The recommended age is lowered in higher-risk groups such as African-American men or men with a family history of prostate cancer. The United States Preventive Services Task Force argues that there is a lack of evidence justifying screening and, as such, recommends discussing with patients whether or not to check PSA levels. They recently recommended against screening men over the age of 75 years. The American College of Physicians (ACP) encourages physicians to heed patient preferences prior to routine screening of all men over age 50 and recommends discussion of this option for men with life expectancy over 10 years. The ACP argues against earlier screening in African-American men or in men with a family history because of a paucity of data showing benefit (table 13.1).

Although a PSA <4 ng/mL has commonly been considered "normal range," the optimal cutoff for referral for biopsy is unclear. In the placebo arm of the Prostate Cancer Prevention Trial (PCPT), a large randomized trial that included 18,000 healthy men over age 55, 26.9% of those with a PSA ranging from 3.1 to 4.0 ng/mL were diagnosed with prostate cancer on biopsy. Alarmingly, approximately 15% of these cancers were high grade. Thus, there is debate as to whether the benefits of lowering the PSA threshold and diagnosing this subset of men with high-grade disease outweigh costs of diagnosing more cancers likely to remain indolent if left undiscovered.

Many have focused on improving the precision of the PSA test. The digital rectal exam, for example, when positive,

Table 13.1 GUIDELINES FOR PROSTATE CANCER SCREENING

AGENCY	RECOMMENDATIONS
American Cancer Society (ACS)	Annual PSA and DRE beginning at age 50 for men with ≥10-year life expectancy (if PSA <2.5 ng/ml, screening every two years is acceptable) Earlier screening (age 40–45) for high-risk groups (African-American men and men with a family history of prostate cancer) Information should be provided on the potential risks and benefits of screening
American Urologic Association (AUA)	Combined annual PSA and DRE in men age ≥50 and with ≥10-year life expectancy Annual screening starting at age ≥40 in men with family history of prostate cancer or men of African decent
United States Preventive Services Task Force (USPSTF)	PSA and DRE not recommended for asymptomatic men and men age ≥75 For men age <75, the benefits of screening for prostate cancer are uncertain and the balance of benefits and harms cannot be determined
American Academy of Family Physicians	No recommendation for PSA and DRE based on insufficient evidence

adds significantly to the positive predictive value of PSA and should be part of routine patient screening. Other attempts at improving PSA screening, such as PSA density and free PSA, have not consistently outperformed PSA alone when compared in retrospective series. PSA velocity and doubling time have also been examined. PSA velocity has proven the most useful in determining prognosis once a prostate cancer diagnosis has been established. A rise in PSA >2.0 ng/mL in the year prior to diagnosis is associated with an increased risk of death due to prostate cancer.

The prostate biopsy is performed using a transrectal 18-gauge-core needle under ultrasound guidance. Twelve to 14 core needle biopsies are the current standard of care. A substantial proportion of patients report pain and discomfort with the procedure and, in one series, over 50% developed hematospermia, and 22.6% developed hematuria following the biopsy.

When invasive cancer is identified in one or more core biopsies, the pathologist assigns a Gleason score. The Gleason score is a measure of the glandular architecture. Tumor cells with a lower score are more capable of forming glandular-appearing tissue than cells with a higher score. The pathologist grades the most prevalent cells in a tumor on a scale of 1 to 5, with 1 generally being the most and 5 being the least differentiated. The second most prevalent type of cell is similarly graded, and the two scores are added together to give an overall Gleason score. A score of 6 (Gleason 3+3) or below is considered low grade, 7 (Gleason 3+4 or 4+3) is considered intermediate grade, and 8 (Gleason 4+4) or above is considered high-grade disease.

When Gleason score, PSA level, and clinical stage are used in combination they are powerful predictors of outcome. A PSA <10 ng/mL and Gleason score ≤6, and T2a (tumor confined to less than one-half of one lobe of the gland) or T1c (no palpable tumor) is considered low risk. PSA levels between 10 and 20 ng/mL or Gleason 7 or T2b disease (tumor comprising more than one-half of one lobe) is considered intermediate risk. PSA >20 ng/mL or Gleason 8–10, or T2c disease (tumor in both lobes) or higher stage is considered high risk. In one

large series, 10-year disease-free survival after surgery in the three risk groups was 83%, 46%, and 29%, respectively.

Further staging via bone scan and/or computed tomography (CT) scan is not necessary in all newly diagnosed patients. Although bone is the most common site of distant prostate metastases, only 1% of patients with Gleason score <7, a PSA <50 ng/mL, and tumor confined to one lobe of the prostate will have an abnormal bone scan. For patients with higher-grade and/or higher-stage disease, these tests, and others such as endorectal coil magnetic resonance imaging (MRI), may be indicated and may provide guidance for further management.

TREATMENT OF LOCALIZED PROSTATE CANCER

Several treatments exist for those with low to intermediate risk localized prostate cancer: radical prostatectomy (RP) using both open and robot-assisted laparoscopic techniques, external beam radiation therapy, or brachytherapy (radiation seed implants). Watchful waiting—close surveillance without treatment—is an additional, and often preferable, option for low-risk patients. Once the decision is made to treat, each method offers a good chance for a positive outcome; however, head-to-head data definitively comparing one modality to another do not exist. Historically surgical and radiation approaches compare favorably in terms of prostate cancer-specific survival for patients with low- to intermediate-risk disease. A patient with a Gleason 6, low-volume prostate cancer with a PSA <10 ng/mL (a common scenario in the PSA era) has a greater than 90% chance of remaining disease-free at 5 years. The major long-term complications from local treatment are erectile and urinary dysfunction. In a recent prospective analysis of over 1200 patients, satisfaction with erectile and urinary function worsened over 24 months following either RP or radiation therapy but was similar across treatment groups. Of note, RP patients who did not receive nerve sparing surgery—a technically challenging attempt to preserve the nerves associated with erectile function—had appreciably worse sexual and urinary outcomes.

For patients with localized prostate cancer with high-risk features, emerging data suggest that adjuvant treatments improve outcomes. In particular, adding androgen-deprivation therapy (ADT), usually a leuteinizing hormone-releasing hormone (LHRH) agonist, to standard radiation therapy consistently proves superior to radiation alone in randomized trials. Side effects associated with ADT include hot flashes, erectile dysfunction, loss of libido, fatigue, decreased bone density, and increased risk of cardiovascular events. These effects largely resolve on discontinuation of treatment, but quality of life (QOL) is diminished during therapy. There is also some risk among older patients of permanent testosterone suppression. Although hormonal treatment clearly augments external beam radiation therapy, it has not been shown to have a similar effect in the setting of RP or brachytherapy.

As mentioned above, most men harboring prostate cancer do not die of their disease. Indeed, several recent studies confirm that expectant management, often called watchful waiting or active surveillance, is a reasonable choice for a large proportion of men with low-risk prostate cancers. Perhaps the most important study examining the relative benefits and risks of watchful waiting is the Scandinavian Prostate Cancer Group Study 4. This trial randomized 695 men diagnosed with prostate cancer to watchful waiting or radical prostatectomy. Approximately two-thirds of the cancers were Gleason 6 or below. The absolute risk reduction for death from prostate cancer was 5.4% in favor of the RP arm. Those receiving RP also had a 10% absolute risk reduction in incidence of metastases and an improvement in 10-year survival (73% vs. 68%). RP appeared to benefit primarily those less than 65 years old, with no advantage detected for patients older than 65. The results suggest that radical treatment should be considered for men with localized disease diagnosed by age 65. Several factors, however, must be considered. First, the side effects from RP are considerable. Rates of erectile dysfunction and urinary leakage in RP patients were 35% and 28% higher, respectively, in the RP group compared to the watchful-waiting group. Moreover, given an absolute risk reduction of disease progression of 10% means that the majority of RPs were performed without benefit, at least at the current endpoint. Almost 20 RPs would need to be performed to prevent one death in 10 years. Many men with low-risk disease may, therefore, favor a watchful-waiting approach. A reasonable surveillance protocol would include PSA checks every 3 months and repeat biopsies every 12–24 months. A significant change in either test should elicit some form of treatment.

TREATMENT OF RECURRENCE AFTER LOCAL TREATMENT AND ADVANCED DISEASE

Despite definitive local treatment, prostate cancer often recurs. Recurrence may be local or distant. The distinction is important because the site of recurrence can dictate the next step in treatment. Local recurrences after RP, for example, may be successfully salvaged with radiation therapy. Patients with distantly recurrent disease, on the other hand, are unlikely to benefit from postsurgical radiation to the pelvis. However, owing to the sensitivity of the PSA test, prostate cancer recurrences can be detected quite early, well before there is clinical evidence of disease. Clinical parameters have therefore been established to identify those patients most likely to recur locally and therefore most likely to benefit from salvage radiation therapy: less advanced disease at initial presentation (low PSA, low Gleason score, and early stage), positive surgical margins, and favorable PSA kinetics (low PSA nadir after surgery, PSA doubling time >12 months).

Many men who receive salvage treatment may still have recurrences. Others are not candidates for salvage treatment at all because of unfavorable clinical parameters such as a rapid PSA doubling time or the presence of overt metastases. Some men present with metastatic disease and are not candidates for any localized therapies. These scenarios each represent advanced disease, and for these patients, ADT remains the standard of care. Though ADT is not curative, over 90% of men respond with a decrease in PSA and alleviation of prostate cancer-related symptoms.

The timing of initiation of ADT is an area of controversy. Randomized data for early versus delayed treatment for men with rising PSA are lacking. Some treat immediately on suspicion of progressive disease, and, at the opposite extreme, others wait until the onset of symptoms from metastatic disease, sparing patients the side effects associated with ADT for as long as possible. Some data suggest that early treatment (e.g., when PSA reaches 10 ng/mL) delays the onset of metastases, particularly for patients whose disease has aggressive features.

In light of the morbidity associated with hormonal therapy and the prospect of long-term treatment for those with biochemically recurrent disease, many physicians have considered treating patients with intermittent androgen deprivation (IAD). Cycling ADT provides patients with a short-term respite from side effects and delays onset of long-term side effects such as osteopenia. Physicians typically treat for 12–24 months and then monitor expectantly. Treatment is usually reinitiated when PSA reaches 5–10 ng/mL. Patients on intermittent treatment appear to fare no worse than those on continuous treatment in terms of long-term outcome.

Despite the initial effectiveness of hormonal therapy in almost all patients, progressive disease ultimately develops. When this occurs, patients are considered to have castration-resistant prostate cancer (CRPC). Among patients who have metastatic disease at the time of ADT initiation, the average time to CRPC is approximately 2 years. The natural history of men treated with ADT for a rising PSA only (i.e., no metastases) is less well established. It appears that these men respond to ADT by PSA criteria for a longer period of time, but whether early treatment with ADT is associated with a survival advantage is unknown.

Despite developing resistance to ADT, patients with CRPC may still respond to further hormonal manipulation. Drugs in the antiandrogen class (such as bicalutamide and nilutamide); ketoconazole, which inhibits the adrenal androgen pathway; and estrogens may be effectively added to ADT, lowering PSA levels and inducing radiographic responses. Eventually, however, these secondary hormone therapies also fail, and patients are considered truly "hormone refractory."

Until recently, chemotherapy offered, at best, palliation for morbidity, primarily bone pain, associated with HRPC. The Food and Drug Administration (FDA) approved the regimen mitoxantrone/prednisone for advanced prostate cancer for this reason. Based on promising phase II data, two pivotal phase III trials using the microtubule inhibitor docetaxel were published in 2004. These trials provide the first definitive evidence of an approximately 25% survival benefit for chemotherapy in prostate cancer. Moreover, this benefit is comparable to that seen in other solid tumors such as breast cancer. As a result of these landmark studies, docetaxel every 3 weeks with prednisone was approved by the FDA for metastatic CRPC and is now the standard of care in this setting.

RENAL CELL CARCINOMA

OVERVIEW

Renal cell carcinoma (RCC) accounts for approximately 3% of adult malignancies and over 90% of neoplasms arising from the kidney. RCC has five distinct histologic subtypes, although the most common is clear cell carcinoma (75%). RCC is characterized by a lack of early warning signs, diverse clinical manifestations, relative resistance to radiation and chemotherapy, and infrequent responses to immunotherapy agents such as interferon-alpha and interleukin (IL)-2. Newer targeted anti-angiogenic agents that target multiple receptor kinases, such as sorafenib and sunitinib, have demonstrated major activity in these patients and have become first-line treatment in metastatic disease.

EPIDEMIOLOGY

RCC is among the 10 most common cancers in both men and women, with a lifetime risk of about 1 in 75 (1.34%). The age-adjusted incidence of renal cell carcinoma has been rising by about 3% per year. According to the American Cancer Society, in 2008 there were 54,390 cases (33,130 in males and 21,260 in females) of malignant kidney tumors diagnosed in the United States with 13,010 deaths (8,100 in males and 4,910 in females); renal cell cancer accounted for

80% of this incidence and mortality. The 5-year survival rates initially reported by Robson in 1969 were 66% for stage I renal carcinoma, 64% for stage II, 42% for stage III, and only 11% for stage IV (see figure 13.1). Except for stage I, these survival statistics have remained essentially unchanged for several decades. The greatest increase in incidence currently is observed in African Americans. Most people with this cancer are older, with the average age at diagnosis being 65 years. It has a low incidence below age 45 except in those people with hereditary risk factors.

RISK FACTORS

The tissue of origin for renal cell carcinoma is the proximal renal tubular epithelium. Renal cancer occurs in both sporadic (nonhereditary) and hereditary forms, although both forms are associated with structural alterations of the short arm of chromosome 3 (3p). Genetic studies of families at high risk for developing renal cancer led to the cloning of genes whose alteration results in tumor formation. These genes are either tumor suppressor genes (*VHL, TSC*) or oncogenes (*MET*). At least four hereditary syndromes associated with renal cell carcinoma have been identified, including von Hippel-Lindau (VHL) syndrome, hereditary papillary renal carcinoma (HPRC), familial renal oncocytoma (FRO) associated with Birt-Hogg-Dube syndrome (BHDS), and hereditary renal carcinoma (HRC).

Lifestyle-related risk factors such as cigarette smoking double the risk of RCC and contribute to as many as one-third of all cases. The risk appears to increase with the amount of cigarette smoking in a dose-dependent fashion. Obesity is another risk factor, particularly in women; increasing body weight has a linear relationship with

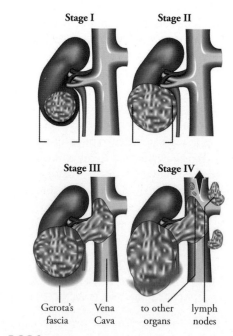

Figure 13.1. RCC Staging.

increasing risk. Hypertension may be associated with an increased incidence of RCC. There is an increased incidence of acquired cystic kidney cancer in patients undergoing long-term renal dialysis as well as in the native kidney of renal transplant recipients. Epidemiologic studies have suggested that certain workplace exposures also increase the risk of RCC, including asbestos, cadmium, pesticides, benzene, and certain organic solvents.

CLINICAL PRESENTATION AND DIAGNOSIS

RCC may remain clinically occult for most of its course. At least 30% of patients are asymptomatic, with their cancers found on incidental radiologic study. The most common presentations include hematuria (40%), flank pain (40%), and a palpable mass in the flank or abdomen (25%); however, the classic triad of all three findings is uncommon (10%) and indicative of advanced disease. Common nonspecific constitutional symptoms include weight loss (33%), fever (20%), and hypertension (20%).

Renal cell carcinoma is also a unique tumor because of the occurrence of paraneoplastic syndromes, including hypercalcemia, erythrocytosis, and nonmetastatic hepatic dysfunction. Polyneuromyopathy, amyloidosis, anemia, fever, cachexia, dermatomyositis, and increased erythrocyte sedimentation rates also are associated with RCC.

TREATMENT

More than 50% of patients with renal cell carcinoma are cured in early stages, but the outcome for metastatic (stage IV) disease is poor. About 25–30% of patients have metastatic disease at diagnosis, and fewer than 5% have a solitary metastasis. The probability of cure is related directly to the stage or degree of tumor dissemination, so the approach is curative for early-stage disease. The treatment options for renal cell cancer include surgery, radiation therapy, chemotherapy, immunotherapy, targeted biological therapy, or combinations of these. Outcomes for patients with metastatic disease have been positively affected by the recent advent of novel pathway-targeted agents that affect multiple signal

Table 13.2 **MEDICAL THERAPIES FOR ADVANCED RENAL CANCER**

Targeted biological therapy (now considered first line):
  Sunitinib malate—VEGF receptor and multitargeted kinase inhibitor
  Sorafenib tosylate—VEGF receptor and multitargeted kinase inhibitor
  Temsirolimus—inhibitor of the mammalian target of rapamycin
  Bevacizumab—humanized VEGF-neutralizing antibody

Immunotherapy
  Interleukin-2 (IL-2)—FDA-approved when used in high doses
  Interferon (IFN)-alpha

Traditional cytotoxic chemotherapy—minimal activity

---

transduction pathways related to angiogenesis and cell proliferation (table 13.2).

Surgery

Surgical resection remains the only known effective treatment for localized renal cell carcinoma, and it also is used as palliation in metastatic disease. Radical nephrectomy, which remains the most commonly performed standard surgical procedure today for treatment of localized renal carcinoma, involves complete removal of Gerota's fascia and its contents, including a resection of kidney, perirenal fat, and ipsilateral adrenal gland, with or without ipsilateral lymph node dissection. Laparoscopic nephrectomy is a less invasive procedure; however, given concerns about spillage and technical difficulties in defining surgical margins, it should be considered at centers with experience in this procedure.

In the setting of metastatic disease, a randomized trial demonstrated a modest survival benefit to palliative nephrectomy when combined with immunotherapy, compared with immunotherapy alone, particularly in patients with an excellent performance status. In addition, nephrectomy can be performed to alleviate symptoms such as pain, hemorrhage, and hypercalcemia.

Radiation

Renal cell carcinoma is generally considered radioresistant. However, palliative radiation is often used for symptomatic metastatic disease, such as painful osseous lesions or brain metastasis to halt potential neurological progression.

Chemotherapy

Options for chemotherapy are limited, with no regimens being accepted as a standard of care, given objective response rates lower than 15%.

Immunotherapy

Because RCC is an immunogenic tumor, immune modulators have been evaluated including interferon-alpha (IFN), IL-2, lymphokine-activated killer (LAK) cells plus IL-2, tumor-infiltrating lymphocytes, and nonmyeloablative allogeneic peripheral blood stem-cell transplantation. Until recently, IFN and high-dose IL-2 had represented the mainstay of treatment for advanced RCC. However, the range of toxicities associated with these treatments precludes their use in the majority of patients, and the few responses that are seen are often not durable, with fewer than 10% of patients remaining progression-free at 3 years.

Targeted Systemic Agents

A growing understanding of the underlying molecular biology of RCC has led to the development of drugs designed to disrupt fundamental biological pathways that are active in RCC pathogenesis. Specifically, vascular-endothelial growth factor (VEGF), its related receptor VEGFR, and the mTOR signal transduction pathway have been exploited through the use of sunitinib malate, sorafenib tosylate, temsirolimus, and bevacizumab, which have each demonstrated significant improvements in response rates, PFS, and overall survival (in the case of temsirolimus) with manageable side effects. Importantly, these agents represent the first new drug approvals for treatment of advanced RCC in almost two decades, which in turn has brought about a major shift in treatment paradigm. A variety of other novel targeted agents are currently under development for the treatment of metastatic RCC, including other mTOR inhibitors (everolimus), VEGF ligand inhibitors (VEGF Trap), and additional tyrosine kinase inhibitors (axitinib and pazopanib).

BLADDER CANCER

OVERVIEW

Transitional cell carcinoma (TCC) of the bladder arises from urothelial cells and comprises 90% of all bladder neoplasms. The remaining 10% of bladder cancers are squamous cell carcinomas, adenocarcinomas, small cell carcinomas, and sarcomas. The prognosis and treatment of bladder cancer rest on the stage of disease and the overall health of the affected individual (see figure 13.2).

EPIDEMIOLOGY

Bladder cancer is the fourth most common cancer in men and the ninth in women. Eighty percent of all bladder cancer patients are over the age of 60, and it is the second most prevalent disease among men in this age group. It is estimated that 50,000 males and 17,500 females develop cancer of the bladder annually in the United States, and 9950 males and 4150 females would die from the disease in 2008. The higher incidence in men is likely due to higher rates of smoking and occupational exposures. Yet, women have a disproportionately higher death rate from bladder cancer, possibly due to delayed diagnosis.

RISK FACTORS

Bladder cancer was among the first cancers whose etiology was linked to environmental exposure when factory workers exposed to aniline dye were increasingly diagnosed with the disease. Other aromatic amines such as aryl amines are also linked to disease risk. In the present era, cigarette smoking is by far the leading underlying cause of bladder cancer. Smokers are 6- to 10-fold more likely to develop bladder cancer compared with nonsmokers. Other etiologies have been proposed, some with compelling data, such as exposure to arsenic or chronic cystitis. Though bladder cancer risk is largely derived from environmental factors, genome-wide analysis has also uncovered inherited markers associated with disease (table 13.3).

CLINICAL PRESENTATION AND DIAGNOSIS

The diagnosis of bladder cancer is often complicated by the tendency for patients with cancer to remain asymptomatic until disease is advanced or to present with symptoms that mimic benign disorders such as urinary tract infections. The most common presenting symptom is gross, painless hematuria. Patients may present with microhematuria, although this is uncommon. In one large series, 13% of healthy adult men and women presented with microscopic hematuria, and 0.4% of these cases represented bladder cancer.

Urinary voiding symptoms such as new onset of increased frequency, urgency, or dysuria are seen in up to one-third of bladder cancer patients. Obstructive symptoms are less common and often reflect clot formation in the setting of hematuria. Patients may present with flank, suprapubic, or bony pain, which are usually associated with metastatic disease. Patients may present with nonspecific constitutional symptoms, also reflective of advanced disease.

Until proven otherwise, the presence of hematuria in an individual over the age of 40 represents a possible cancer. Urinalysis should be obtained to help assess etiology. Red cell casts, for example, may suggest glomerular disease rather than tumor or infection. Urine should also be collected for cytology. Cytology is >90% sensitive for detecting higher-grade bladder cancer and considerably less sensitive for detecting lower-grade disease or disease in the upper tracts. Several newer molecular tests of the urine may offer increased sensitivity.

Cystoscopy is the critical procedure in establishing the diagnosis of bladder cancer. The cystoscope allows visual inspection of the bladder and identifies sites for biopsy and transurethral resection of bladder tumor (TURBT). In addition to lesions suspicious for tumor, normal-appearing

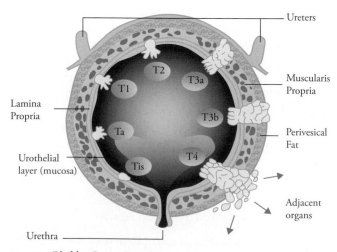

Figure 13.2. Bladder Cancer Staging.

tissue must be sampled in order to assess for diffuse carcinoma in situ, a condition that influences treatment options. In addition, if upper urinary tract disease is suspected—if, for example, cytology is positive but no disease is seen in the bladder—catheterization of the ureters is required. Retrograde intravenous pyelogram (IVP) may be used as part of the workup because it is capable of identifying large tumors in the ureter and renal pelvis as well as the bladder.

After the diagnosis of bladder cancer is made, CT is often used to detect extravesical involvement, pelvic or retroperitoneal lymph node involvement, or overt metastases. However, sensitivity of the CT scan is often not adequate to definitively rule out advanced disease or nodal involvement, particularly after cystoscopy when the bladder is irritated.

Stage and grade of disease are the most important variables in determining outcome. In particular, invasion into muscle (muscularis propria) of the bladder wall is the key determinant in assessing prognosis. If tumor does not invade muscularis propria, the disease is considered superficial. Involvement into the muscularis propria is considered invasive, and aggressive treatment is warranted.

TREATMENT

Superficial Bladder Cancer

The initial treatment for superficial bladder cancer is TURBT—surgical removal of all tumors visualized by cystoscopy. Even when complete transurethral resection is achieved, most superficial bladder cancers will recur,

Table 13.3 **BLADDER CANCER RISK FACTORS**

Smoking—2 × greater risk

Workplace/industrial exposures—dye, rubber, leather, textiles, paint, printing, machinists

Race—Caucasians have 2 × greater risk compared to African Americans and Hispanics

Age—increased risk with aging

Gender—men have 4 × greater risk

Chronic bladder inflammation—infections (schistosomiasis), kidney and bladder stones, etc.

Personal history of bladder cancer

Bladder birth defects—urachal presence at birth, exstrophy

Genetics—Rb1, PTEN mutations, HNPCC syndrome, GST and NAT genes (have slower rate of chemical and toxin breakdown)

Chemotherapy—cyclophosphamide, ifosfamide; mesna can be combined with these drugs to help protect the bladder

Radiation therapy to the pelvis

Arsenic—i.e., drinking water contamination

Low fluid consumption

and more than 10% of patients will ultimately develop advanced, muscle-invasive disease. The risk of developing invasion into the muscularis propria is associated with degree of superficial invasion, the grade of disease, extent of disease within the bladder, and time to recurrence after resection. Multifocal, bulky, high-grade disease; invasion into the lamina propria; and disease recurring twice per year are poor prognostic signs. Patients with very few or no risk factors may be treated with TURBT alone. For higher-risk patients, a more aggressive approach is often indicated.

Intravesicular treatment is typically recommended for high-risk superficial disease after all tumor has been removed by TURBT. The most commonly used and effective intravesical agent is bacillus Calmette-Guérin (BCG). BCG therapy delays progression to a more advanced stage, forestalling, and sometimes preventing, the need for definitive treatment with cystectomy. The exact mechanism of BCG's activity remains unknown, but it is assumed to serve as a form of immunotherapy. Those with more robust immune responses on the introduction of BCG have superior antitumor responses.

BCG is administered directly into the bladder weekly for 6 weeks. Several trials have assessed the efficacy of longer courses of treatment. Most show increased toxicity but few show improved outcomes, such as delay in tumor progression. The most common toxicities associated with BCG include increased urinary frequency, cystitis, hematuria, and fever. Close follow-up is important, with repeat cystoscopy and cytology performed every 3–6 months. Careful attention must also be paid to the upper tracts, which are not exposed to BCG. If residual tumor is discovered, a repeat course of BCG may be indicated. Cystectomy may be recommended for patients who repeatedly fail local therapy or otherwise have high-risk features that predict future invasive cancer.

Invasive Bladder Cancer

Radical cystectomy with bilateral lymph node dissection is the standard treatment for patients with muscle-invasive TCC of the bladder. The procedure involves resection of multiple structures: the bladder, prostate, seminal vesicles, proximal urethra, and a considerable volume of pelvic adipose tissue, and peritoneum. Urinary flow must be redirected, either through an ileal conduit to an external reservoir at the skin surface or to a neobladder made from a segment of bowel that is in turn anastomosed to a urethral remnant. The latter option has gained popularity, as it avoids the need for an external appliance. Many patients undergoing urinary diversion experience a relatively good quality of life, although most men suffer loss of sexual function after the procedure. Bladder-sparing alternatives to radical cystectomy have been investigated, with multimodality approaches, such as chemoradiotherapy, a consideration in the treatment of selected patients.

The prognosis after radical cystectomy is closely tied to pathologic stage of disease. In one large series of over 1000 patients with TCC of the bladder treated with radical cystectomy, 5-year overall survival was 78% for those with organ-confined, lymph node–negative disease but only 31% for those with lymph-node involvement.

The addition of systemic chemotherapy before (neoadjuvant) or after (adjuvant) cystectomy is regularly used in an attempt to improve outcome for those with locally advanced disease. Several underpowered randomized studies assessing adjuvant treatment did not show a survival benefit, although adjuvant treatment delayed tumor progression and prevented recurrence. However, two randomized trials examining the use of neoadjuvant chemotherapy demonstrated a survival advantage for those receiving treatment prior to cystectomy. Neoadjuvant treatment also allows for a detailed assessment of response to chemotherapy. Evidence of a complete response in the pathology specimen from cystectomy has important prognostic significance.

For patients who are progressing to or presenting with metastatic disease, the overall prognosis is poor. Median survival rates range from 6 to 9 months, and few survive 5 years. Combination chemotherapy significantly increases life expectancy, although even with aggressive chemotherapy treatments, overall survival is poor. Median survival for patients receiving supportive care alone is 4 to 6 months, and chemotherapy improves survival to 12 to 14 months. Three-year survival is approximately 20%.

TESTICULAR CANCER

OVERVIEW

Testicular cancers are most commonly germ cell tumors (GCT) and are classified as either seminomas or nonseminomas, based on their histology. Other uncommon testicular malignancies include sex cord-stromal tumors, including Leydig and Sertoli cell tumors, gonadoblastoma, and tumors of other cell types presenting in the testes such as lymphoma, carcinoid tumors, and metastatic carcinoma.

EPIDEMIOLOGY OF GCTS

Testicular GCTs are rare, occurring in only 1–2% of all male malignancies and occurring in 1 of 250 men by age 65 years. However, testicular GCTs are the most common malignancy in men aged 15–35 years. Incidence rates are 3.7 and 0.9 cases per 100,000 persons per year for Caucasian and African-American males, respectively.

RISK FACTORS

Studies of GCTs have suggested that cyclin D2 is overexpressed in malignant germ cells and is oncogenic. GCT differentiation may be influenced by several interacting pathways, such as regulators of germ-cell totipotentiality, embryonic development, and genomic imprinting. Sensitivity and resistance to chemotherapy may be based in part on a p53-dependent apoptotic pathway. Almost 100% of tumors show increased copy numbers of 12p (i12p). This chromosomal marker has been noted in carcinoma in situ (CIS), suggesting that it is one of the early changes associated with the origin of GCT. CIS is considered to be a precursor of all GCTs.

There are a number of known risk factors for testicular cancer, including cryptorchidism and a personal or family history of testicular cancer. These risk factors predispose to the development of carcinoma in situ and invasive testicular cancer. Other disorders such as Klinefelter syndrome have been associated with mediastinal extragonadal GCTs, whereas Down syndrome has been associated with testicular cancer, although these are rare associations.

CLINICAL PRESENTATION AND DIAGNOSIS

Testicular tumors usually present as a nodule or painless swelling of one testicle, which may be noted incidentally by the patient or by his sexual partner. Approximately 30–40% of patients complain of a dull ache or heavy sensation in the lower abdomen, perianal area, or scrotum, and acute pain is the presenting symptom in 10%. In another 10%, the presenting manifestations of testicular cancer are attributable to metastatic disease; symptoms vary with the site of metastasis. Approximately 5% may have gynecomastia.

TREATMENT

Nearly all GCTs are potentially curable. The likelihood of cure is dependent on clinical stage. Stage I disease is limited to the testicles, stage II to the abdomen, and stage III anywhere else.

Stage I Disease Management

Seminoma
Surgical care of seminomas consists of inguinal orchiectomy. Adjuvant radiotherapy to para-aortic and ipsilateral pelvic lymph nodes was the historical treatment of choice for stage I and nonbulky stage II seminoma. Recent studies have shown that about 15% of patients with clinical stage I disease have occult retroperitoneal disease, and 3–6% of patients relapse after radiation therapy, usually outside the radiation therapy field. As an alternative to radiotherapy, single-agent carboplatin has been shown to be an alternative. The Medical Research Council compared adjuvant carboplatin with radiotherapy and found equivalent relapse rates after a median follow-up period of 4 years. A third option would be active surveillance with radiographic monitoring.

Nonseminoma

Surgical care consists of inguinal orchiectomy alone and is curative in 70% of patients. Retroperitoneal lymph node dissection (RPLND) has diagnostic as well as therapeutic utility. Occult metastases can be found in about 30% of patients with clinical stage I disease and are classified as pathologic stage IIA. Some patients choose surveillance over RPLND, with chemotherapy used at the time of recurrence. Patient compliance is absolutely vital for a surveillance strategy, and patients must be made aware of the 30% rate of disease relapse. Intense monitoring with physical examinations, radiographic imaging, and tumor markers occurs with decreasing frequency from monthly in the first year to annually by the fifth year.

Patients with high-risk stage I nonseminomas include those with lymphovascular invasion and/or embryonal-predominant histologies. For such patients, use of two cycles of adjuvant cisplatin-based multiagent chemotherapy has been investigated.

Stage II Disease Management

Seminoma

Radiation is considered the treatment of choice for patients with nonbulky stage II disease, with a relapse rate of less than 5%. Primary chemotherapy can be considered an alternative to radiation therapy, especially in patients with extensive, bulky, retroperitoneal, visceral metastases or supradiaphragmatic nodal disease. Cisplatin-based systemic chemotherapy cures over 80–90% of stage II seminoma patients.

Nonseminoma

RPLND is an option in patients with clinical stage II disease, but in most patients, systemic chemotherapy with multiagent cisplatin-based therapy is indicated. Radiation is used in patients with metastatic nonseminomas to the brain. Postchemotherapy resection is performed on patients with persistent radiographic abnormalities following chemotherapy.

Stage III Disease Management

Patients with stage III diseases are assessed according to the International Germ Cell Cancer Consensus Group (IGCCCG) system to good-, intermediate-, or poor-risk disease. Treatment consists of three to four cycles of multiagent cisplatin-based chemotherapy. Prognosis is based on factors such as whether the GCT is extragonadal or testicular in origination, sites of metastases, and level of tumor markers (AFP, beta-HCG). Sperm banking should be offered to all patients prior to chemotherapy because therapy for GCTs results in sterility in approximately 35% of patients.

Table 13.4 **INCIDENCE OF TUMOR MARKERS IN TESTICULAR CANCERS**

	PROPORTION OF CASES (%)	
NEOPLASM	BETA-HCG[a]	ALPHA-FETOPROTEIN[b]
Seminoma	10	<1
Embryonal carcinomas with or without teratomas	65	>70
Choriocarcinoma	100	<1

NOTES: [a]Normal levels of beta-HCG = 0 ng/mL. [b]Normal levels of alpha-Fetoprotein <40 μg/mL.

Management of Relapse After Chemotherapy

About 25% of patients relapse or do not achieve a complete response to cisplatin-based chemotherapy. The response rate for salvage chemotherapy is as high as 50% or more, including autologous stem cell transplants. Some responses are durable. In contrast, late relapsed (>2 years following initial therapy) GCT is associated with a poor prognosis because of high resistance to chemotherapy. Median survival in this setting has been reported to be approximately 2 years, and fewer than 50% of patients experience a complete response to chemotherapy.

ADDITIONAL READING

Andriole GL, Levin DL, Crawford ED, et al. Prostate Cancer Screening in the Prostate, Lung, Colorectal and Ovarian (PLCO) Cancer Screening Trial: Findings from the initial screening round of a randomized trial. *J Natl Cancer Inst.* 2005;97(6):433–8.

Bosl GJ, Motzer RJ. Testicular germ-cell cancer. *N Engl J Med.* 1997;337(4):242–53.

Chou R, Dana T. *Screening Adults for Bladder Cancer: Update of the 2004 Evidence Review for the US Preventive Services Task Force* [Internet]. Rockville, MD: Agency for Healthcare Research and Quality; 2010.

Chu D, Wu S. Novel therapies in genitourinary cancer: An update. *J Hematol Oncol.* 2008;1:11.

Kohli M, Tindall DJ. New developments in the medical management of prostate cancer. *Mayo Clin Proc.* 2010;85(1):77–86.

Lin K, Lipsitz R, Janakiraman S. *Benefits and Harms of Prostate-Specific Antigen Screening for Prostate Cancer: An Evidence Update for the U.S. Preventive Services Task Force [Internet].* Rockville, MD: Agency for Healthcare Research and Quality; 2008. Available from http://www.ncbi.nlm.nih.gov/bookshelf/br.fcgi?book=es63.

Mohr DN, Offord KP, Owen RA, Melton LJ 3rd. Asymptomatic microhematuria and urologic disease. A population-based study. *JAMA.* 1986;256(2):224–9.

Motzer RJ, Bander NH, Nanus DM. Renal-cell carcinoma. *N Engl J Med.* 1996;335(12):865–75.

Trottier G, Lawrentschuk N, Fleshner NE. Prevention strategies in prostate cancer. *Curr Oncol.* 2010;17(Suppl 2):S4–S10.

U.S. Preventive Services Task Force. Screening for prostate cancer: U.S. Preventive Services Task Force recommendation statement. *Ann Intern Med.* 2008;149(3):185–91.

Wolf AM, Wender RC, Etzioni RB, et al.; American Cancer Society Prostate Cancer Advisory Committee. American Cancer Society guideline for the early detection of prostate cancer: update 2010. *CA.* 2010;60(2):70–98.

QUESTIONS

QUESTION 1. A 55-year-old female teacher presents who 4 years earlier underwent radical nephrectomy for a 5-cm clear cell RCC confined to the kidney with no evidence of recurrence on surveillance scans. On chest CT, she is now noted to have multiple new pulmonary nodules bilaterally, biopsy proven to be metastatic RCC. Clinically she is asymptomatic with no findings on physical examination. What is the next appropriate course of action?

    A. Observation
    B. Interferon-alpha
    C. Sunitinib
    D. Surgical resection
    E. Bevacizumab

QUESTION 2. A 63-year-old male insurance broker with a PSA 11 ng/mL, clinical stage T2, biopsy Gleason 7 adenocarcinoma of the prostate in 8/8 cores with no metastases on staging workup undergoes radical prostatectomy. Findings on pathology include Gleason 8, extracapsular extension, seminal vesicle involvement, LN (–), margin (+). He is referred for radiation therapy to the prostate bed. Within 18 months, his PSA is rapidly rising, and a bone scan shows new metastases in multiple areas without symptoms. What is your next choice of intervention?

    A. Observation
    B. LHRH agonist
    C. Referral to radiation oncology for more prostate radiation
    D. Surgery to the bone lesions
    E. Docetaxel chemotherapy

QUESTION 3. A 60-year-old man with newly diagnosed high-grade superficial TCC of the bladder presents for a second opinion. One week ago, the patient underwent transurethral resection of the bladder tumor (TURBT) with multiple random biopsies, which revealed superficial TCC associated with several areas of carcinoma in situ, invasion into lamina propria but not into the muscle, and vascular invasion. He was told by another physician that his only option is a radical cystectomy. He would like to preserve his bladder but is worried about the possible spread of the cancer. What should be recommended to this patient?

    A. Combined chemoradiotherapy
    B. Radical cystectomy
    C. Repeat TURBT and close surveillance
    D. Repeat TURBT followed by intravesical bacillus Calmette-Guérin (BCG) therapy

QUESTION 4. A 22-year-old man presents with a left testicular mass, serum beta-HCG of 8200 ng/mL, alpha-fetoprotein of 12,200 μg/mL, and an elevated LDH level. Radical orchiectomy reveals a mixed nonseminomatous germ cell tumor. Staging CT scan reveals an 8-cm conglomeration of nodes in the para-aortic region. CXR demonstrates multiple bilateral pulmonary nodules, and a mass lesion in the frontal lobe is detected on CT scan of the brain. What is the best next step to treat this patient?

    A. Radiation to testicles
    B. Multiagent cisplatin-based chemotherapy × 4 cycles
    C. Carboplatin chemotherapy × 1 cycle
    D. Surgical resection of all brain and lung lesions
    E. Immediate stem cell transplant

ANSWERS

1. C
2. B
3. D
4. B

14.

LEUKEMIA

Joseph H. Antin

A lifetime of sustained lymphohematopoiesis requires a stem cell compartment that produces maturing progeny with immaculate fidelity over almost a century. The stem cell gives rise to progenitor cells that are committed to either lymphoid or myeloid development. A variety of mutations can occur in either the stem cell or in a more committed cell that result in excessive proliferation, failure of differentiation, or both. The genes that are affected determine whether the leukemia is myeloid or lymphoid, whether acute or chronic, response to therapy, and, ultimately, prognosis.

CHRONIC MYELOGENOUS LEUKEMIA

The hallmark of chronic myelogenous leukemia (CML) is a balanced translocation of chromosomes 9 and 22 [t(9;22)] or Philadelphia chromosome. This anomaly was first observed in the 1960s by Nowell and Hungerford. The translocation links the ABL oncogene to BCR, an unrelated gene. A new fusion peptide is transcribed called BCR/ABL. The BCR component causes BCR/ABL to tetramerize, which allows the ABL component of the fusion peptide to function as an autonomous tyrosine kinase with transforming ability. The resulting leukemic cells grow without regulation and are resistant to apoptosis, resulting in accumulation of cells in the marrow and blood. In contrast to acute leukemia, there is no defect in maturation, so the cells mature normally and carry on their specific functions without compromise. This is a genetically unstable condition. If untreated, new mutations will be acquired that result in failure of differentiation and transformation into acute leukemia. The latter acute phase is called blast transformation or blast crisis.

CML is an uncommon disease. It affects all races equally at an incidence of about 1 case per 100,000 per year. The median age is 67 years and the gender ratio is 1:1. There are no geographic or exposure associations with the possible exception of nuclear weapon survivors.

DIAGNOSIS AND STAGING

There are three phases to the disease: chronic, accelerated, and blast phase. Typically the onset is insidious. Clinical manifestations are summarized in table 14.1. The generally preserved ability of the hematopoietic cells to mature and function results in long asymptomatic periods.

Presentation in accelerated phase (AP) may occur, although it is unusual. Most patients with symptoms are not in AP, and symptoms will resolve with control of counts. AP is associated with weight loss, fever, bone pain, extramedullary disease, increased drug requirements, increasing blasts, increasing basophils, anemia or thrombocytopenia, marrow fibrosis, and additional chromosomal abnormalities, especially a second Philadelphia chromosome or iso(17). AP portends a poor prognosis and evolution into blast transformation.

Blast transformation is a form of acute leukemia and manifests with weight loss, manifestations of anemia and thrombocytopenia, fevers, bruising, and abdominal pain. When blast crisis occurs, approximately two-thirds of the time the leukemic blasts are myeloid (AML) and one-third of the time they are lymphoid (ALL). This is an ominous event with a median survival of 6 months.

THERAPY AND PROGNOSIS

Historically the two principal treatments were oral busulfan and hydroxyurea. Busulfan is almost never used any more. Hydroxyurea is not a remission-inducing agent, and it is now primarily used to control the white blood count rapidly. On the other hand interferon-α is a remission-inducing agent, although only a minority of patients enter remission. In 20% of patients the number of Philadelphia chromosome-positive metaphases in the marrow declines to <35%, and when these good responses are observed, there may be a survival advantage. The responders have a median survival of 7–10 years compared with 3–5 years in nonresponders. Interferon toxicity is substantial. Flu-like syndrome, insomnia, autoimmune manifestations, depression, alopecia, and

Table 14.1 CLINICAL MANIFESTATIONS OF CML

CLINICAL OR LABORATORY FINDING	FREQUENCY
Diagnosis in chronic phase	85–90%
Asymptomatic	50%
Symptoms are often nonspecific	
-Fatigue	80%
-Weight loss	60%
-Abdominal discomfort	40%
-Easy bruising	35%
-Leukostasis, priapism, thrombosis	Unusual
Laboratory	
-WBC > 100,000/mL	~30%
-Left shift. Presence of basophilia is very helpful	100%
-Philadelphia chromosome, t(9;22)	100%
-Mild anemia (Hb<12 g/dL)	65%
-Platelets	
> 700,000/mL	25%
< 150,000/mL	5%
-Increased vitamin B-12, B-12 binding capacity	100%

neurotoxicity limit its use, and 20% of patients are intolerant. It is used rarely in current management.

Recognition of the dysregulated tyrosine kinase activity of the fusion BCR/ABL protein led to the development of imatinib (Gleevec) as the principal therapy for CML. This is a remission-inducing tyrosine kinase inhibitor with an excellent toxicity profile. It is administered orally and may be associated with fluid retention, rash, or nausea, but most people tolerate it very well. Most responses occur within 30 days of starting therapy, and 95% of patients in chronic phase will have a clinical response. It appears that suppression of the BCR/ABL mRNA by 3 logs (measured by quantitative polymerase chain reaction) results in more than 83% progression-free survival at more than 5 years. These patients are not cured, but the relapse rate is extremely small on continued therapy. Major cytogenetic responses are more likely to occur in patients with less-advanced disease. In accelerated and blast phase, higher doses are necessary, but ultimately patients relapse. In advanced disease the imatinib is a bridge to allogeneic hematopoietic stem cell transplantation (HSCT). Some patients develop resistance to imatinib. Newer agents such as dasatinib (Sprycel) and nilotinib (Tasigna) may be useful in many instances, but usually HSCT is required in eligible individuals.

HSCT remains the only curative therapy (60–80% long-term disease-free survival in chronic phase), but the success of imatinib has relegated HSCT to a secondary role. It is used primarily in patients with resistant or advanced disease or who are intolerant to tyrosine kinase inhibitors. HSCT is also the only own curative therapy in AP and BC CML, although the outcomes are less encouraging. Matched sibling HSCT outcomes are dependent on age, cytomegalovirus (CMV) status, disease stage, and the presence of comorbidities. Young patients (<50 years) with fully matched donors transplanted in stable phase generally do the best. Unrelated donor HSCT outcome data are asymptotically approaching matched sibling donor HSCT outcomes as HLA technology has improved.

ACUTE MYELOGENOUS LEUKEMIA

Acute myelogenous leukemia (AML) is *rare*, with an incidence of approximately two to five cases per 100,000 per year. It is a disease of aging, and the incidence increases in individuals over 65 to as much as 50 cases per 100,000 per year.

Most cases of AML are sporadic and occur without known predisposing cause, but there are well-established factors or conditions that increase the risk of AML: exposure to benzene, ionizing radiation, chemotherapy (especially alkylating agents); congenital disorders such as Down syndrome; and pre-existent hematologic disorders such as polycythemia vera or myelodysplastic syndrome.

In contrast to CML, in which cellular maturation is normal but proliferation is excessive, AML requires two defects: (1) a proliferation signal (as in CML) and (2) failure of cellular maturation. Specific genetic abnormalities are associated with specific disease phenotypes. For example, acute promyelocytic leukemia (APML) is known to involve a balanced translocation involving the retinoic acid receptor alpha and a partner gene called PML [t(15;17)]. This translocation is definitive for APML, and it results in a maturation block—locking the myeloid cells into the promyelocyte stage of differentiation; however, a second mutation is necessary that provides the proliferative thrust in order for APML to develop. In some cases this is due to a mutation in the gene FLT3, which is a tyrosine kinase involved in cellular proliferation. Thus, all-*trans* retinoic acid (ATRA) is an extremely useful therapy for APML, a disease that not coincidently involves the retinoic acid receptor.

Other subclasses of AML have similar defects involving other genes. Using molecular analysis, additional genetic defects can be detected that are not observed in conventional cytogenetics. More than 100 mutations have been described in AML. These provide a more precise prognosis and open the door to gene-specific therapies (table 14.2).

DIAGNOSIS AND STAGING

Usually signs and symptoms are associated with bone marrow failure: pallor, fatigue, mucosal bleeding, bruising, or fever and infection. Leukemic infiltrates of the skin, mucous membranes, and meninges are common. Very high blast counts are associated with cerebral or pulmonary leukostasis. Hyperuricemia may cause renal failure. Disseminated intravascular coagulation (DIC) can occur with any of the subsets of AML, but it is most prominent in APML.

The diagnosis is made on examination of the peripheral blood smear and/or bone marrow. Typical leukemic blast morphology is supplemented by flow cytometry,

Table 14.2 AML PROGNOSTIC FACTORS

GOOD PROGNOSIS	POOR PROGNOSIS
Age < 60 years	Age >60 years
De novo AML	Secondary to underlying hematologic disorder
	Secondary to prior therapy
Cytogenetics and mutations	
NPM1 nucleolar transport protein t(15;17)	FLT3 tyrosine kinase c-KIT
t(8;21)	Monosomy 7 or monosomy 5
inv(16)	Complex cytogenetics
Failure to achieve an initial complete remission	
African-American men have a lower remission rate and overall survival when other prognostic factors are considered	
Less important: high WBC or LDH at diagnosis	

cytogenetics, and molecular analysis. Morphology and cytochemistries were the principal criteria to distinguish subtypes of AML in the past. For instance, the French-American-British (FAB) classification distinguished APML (M3) from conventional AML (Ml or M2). This schema had modest prognostic value and gave no insight into AML biology. AML is now classified based on molecular defects—a much more useful approach.

THERAPY

Standard therapy for remission induction in patients under age 60 (excluding APML) is a combination of an anthracycline (e.g., idarubicin) and cytarabine (Ara-C). This is an intensive regimen and typically requires a prolonged hospital stay to deal with complications of cell lysis syndrome, DIC, severe cytopenias, and infections. Approximately 70% of younger patients will enter remission. The results are much less favorable in patients >60 years of age, where toxicity tends to be higher, remissions less frequent (45%), and long-term outcome poorer. In the elderly, intensive regimens are not typically used. Once remission is achieved, consolidation therapy is administered. In good-risk disease [e.g., t(8;2l) or inv(16)] the therapy is four courses of high-dose cytarabine. In poor-risk disease, eligible patients typically undergo allogeneic HSCT or clinical trials. APML is a special case where therapy consists of an anthracycline and all-trans retinoic acid, followed by maintenance therapy with ATRA, and a regimen of antimetabolites.

PROGNOSIS

There are well-defined factors that contribute to prognosis in AML (table 14.2). A principal factor is age. The outcome for older adults (generally greater than age 60) is markedly inferior to that in younger adults with the same disease. Reasons for the poor results in the older cohort include poor stem-cell reserve, comorbid disease, and intrinsic resistance to chemotherapy. For patients <60 years the complete remission rate is approximately 70% with an overall survival of about 30%. However, for patients >60 years the remission rate is only 45% and the survival is 10%.

Cytogenetics and molecular markers are critical determinants of outcome in younger patients. For instance, in the presence of t(15:17) or t(8:2l) there is a 60–80% long-term disease-free survival, whereas monosomy 7 results in a <10% long-term disease-free survival.

ACUTE LYMPHOBLASTIC LEUKEMIA

Acute lymphoblastic leukemia (ALL) is primarily a disease of childhood; however, one-third of cases occur in adults. There are approximately 1000 cases per year in adults with a slight increase in incidence over the age of 50. Males are slightly more affected than females, and African Americans have a 60% lower risk. Exposure associations are less clear than in AML. There does seem to be an increased risk in industrialized countries.

ALL can derive from primitive lymphoid cells of either B-cell or T-cell lineage, although B-lineage disease is more common. ALL is divided into pre–B-cell, T-cell, and B-cell disease. Pre–B-cell ALL is the most frequent form of ALL, representing malignant transformation of a lymphoid progenitor that has undergone incomplete maturation along the B-cell lineage. T-cell ALL has similarly become transformed before full T-cell maturation has occurred. In contrast, B-cell ALL, the least common type of ALL, is the leukemic phase of Burkitt lymphoma. In contrast to pre-B ALL, the cells have matured adequately to express cell surface immunoglobulins.

DIAGNOSIS AND STAGING

Usually signs and symptoms are associated with bone marrow failure: pallor, fatigue, mucosal bleeding, bruising, or fever and infection. Leukemic infiltrates of the meninges are common, although usually later in the course. T-cell ALL presents with the highest white blood counts and has a specific association with mediastinal masses.

The diagnosis is made on examination of the peripheral blood smear and/or bone marrow. Typical leukemic blast morphology is supplemented by flow cytometry, cytogenetics, and molecular analysis. Morphologically they appear somewhat different from AML, having fewer granules and less cytoplasm. Pre–B-cell ALL is characterized by cell surface CD10, CD19, and cytoplasmic terminal deoxynucleotidyl transferase (TdT), and immunoglobulin gene rearrangements. Chromosome abnormalities include hyper- and hypodiploidy as well as specific translocations. In 30% of adults there is a variant of the Philadelphia chromosome that produces a smaller BCR/ABL fusion peptide than occurs in CML. Many of the other chromosomal abnormalities use translocations that involve the immunoglobulin gene locus, or the MLL gene. T-cell ALL expresses TdT and cell surface T-cell markers such as CD7, has rearranged T-cell receptor genes, and chromosomal abnormalities involve the T-cell receptor rather than immunoglobulin genes. In contrast to pre-B ALL, B-cell ALL expresses surface immunoglobulin and has translocations involving one of the immunoglobulin gene loci and the MYC oncogene on chromosome 8.

THERAPY

In general, principles of therapy are similar to those for AML, except that risk of central nervous system (CNS) relapse is much higher and requires specific prophylaxis. Typically, induction therapy consists of a combination of anthracycline, vincristine, prednisone, cyclophosphamide, and L-asparaginase. Induction is followed by a complex series of treatments including CNS prophylaxis, intensified postremission therapy, and 1–2 years of maintenance chemotherapy. Alternative multiagent regimens (e.g., hyper-CVAD) are similarly effective. Patients who have t(9;22) are treated with imatinib or dasatinib in addition to intensive chemotherapy. Allogeneic HSCT plays an important role in the management of ALL. A recent international collaboration of the Eastern Cooperative Oncology Group and the Medical Research Council of Great Britain demonstrated that allogeneic HSCT improves outcome in patients with standard risk disease. All patients with t(9;22) should be offered HSCT if feasible.

PROGNOSIS

The prognosis of adult ALL has not yet approached the high cure rates observed in childhood ALL. This reflects in part a higher prevalence of high-risk cytogenetic variants in adults as well as reluctance or inability on the part of adult hematologist-oncologists to use L-asparaginase intensively. Intensive chemotherapy combined with allogeneic HSCT results in long-term disease-free survival of >50% in adults with pre-B ALL. If the Philadelphia chromosome is present, outcomes are less favorable. The recent addition of imatinib or dasatinib to conventional therapy is promising, although results are less mature.

CHRONIC LYMPHOCYTIC LEUKEMIA

Chronic lymphocytic leukemia (CLL) originates from antigen-stimulated mature B lymphocytes, which either avoid apoptotic death or undergo apoptosis, followed by replacement from a pool of precursor cells. CLL is the most

frequent and prevalent leukemia. There are more than 15,000 new cases per year in the United States. There are no known etiologic factors, although there is a tendency for patients to have a family history of a hematologic malignancy. CLL is a disease of aging—the median age is >60 years and only 10–15% of patients are <50 years of age.

DIAGNOSIS AND STAGING

The diagnosis of CLL is commonly incidental, and approximately half of patients are asymptomatic. Other patients may have some combination of lymphadenopathy, splenomegaly, anemia, thrombocytopenia, and hypogammaglobulinemia. Examination of the blood reveals mature-appearing lymphocytes, although some cells will be damaged in processing the slide resulting in "smudge cells." Immunophenotyping is normally used to differentiate CLL from other lymphoid malignancies in a leukemic phase. CLL typically expresses the B-cell antigens CD5, CD19, and CD20, as well as clonal immunoglobulin light chains. The two common staging systems are Rai (stage 0–4) and Binet (stage A, B, C) as shown in table 14.3.

THERAPY

Those patients who are asymptomatic and who have better prognosis disease (e.g., 13q-) may be safely followed without therapy. Typically treatment is begun when disease-related symptoms, progressive lymphadenopathy or hepatosplenomegaly, autoimmune hemolytic anemia, or thrombocytopenia unresponsive to corticosteroids supervene. Lymphocytosis per se is not a criterion for treatment.

Fludarabine-based therapy has largely replaced chlorambucil (Leukeran) as the mainstay of treatment. Fludarabine is often used in combination with rituximab (anti-CD20 monoclonal antibody). However, chlorambucil is inexpensive, nontoxic, and easy to administer, making it appealing for some elderly patients. In addition to rituximab, the monoclonal antibody alemtuzumab (Campath, anti-CD52) may be used in fludarabine-refractory CLL. This drug is highly immunosuppressive, and its use mandates *pneumocystis* prophylaxis and close monitoring for CMV reactivation. Newer agents in development include lenalidomide (Revlimid), an immunomodulatory agent used in myelodysplasia, and flavopiridol, a cyclin-dependent kinase inhibitor that is under development. The only curative therapy for CLL is allogeneic HSCT. There are increasing data that reduced-intensity regimens that are tolerable to older people control the disease immunologically via a graft-versus-leukemia (GVL) effect, although opportunistic infections and graft-versus-host disease remain concerns. Patient selection must be undertaken carefully.

PROGNOSIS

Younger patients with stage 0 disease or good prognosis chromosomes often have a survival that is similar to an

Table 14.3 STAGING OF CHRONIC LYMPHOCYTIC LEUKEMIA

	LYMPHOCYTOSIS	LYMPHADENOPATHY	SPLENOMEGALY + HEPATOMEGALY	ANEMIA*	THROMBOCYTOPENIA*
Rai					
0	x	–	–	–	–
1	x	x	–	–	–
2	x		x	–	–
3	x			x	–
4	x				x
Binet					
A		<3 nodal areas	–		
B		≥3 nodal areas	–		
C		–	–	either	

Cytogenetics	Prognosis (median survival)
13q-	10–12 years
Trisomy 12 or normal	9–10 years
11g-	6–7 years
17p-	2–3 years

NOTE: *Anemia and thrombocytopenia are not immune mediated.

age-matched population. Older patients particularly with more indolent disease tend to die of causes independent of CLL. Patients with more advanced disease may have a median survival of 6–7 years, while patients with the most aggressive forms have a median survival of 1–3 years. Prognosis is related to staging, but cytogenetic abnormalities as established by fluorescence in situ hybridization (FISH) have proven to be more helpful. The most common abnormality is deletion of 13q. It is observed in about 40% of patients, and it is the most favorable. Normal karyotypes and trisomy 12 are the next most common and have intermediate outcomes. Deletions of 17p or of 11q as well as complex abnormalities have the worst outcome but fortunately are least common as well (table 14.3).

A frequent cause of morbidity and mortality are infections related to hypogammaglobulinemia. The most common bacterial pathogens are *Streptococcus pneumoniae*, *Staphylococcus aureus*, and *Haemophilus influenzae*; however, particularly after chemotherapy there is an increased risk of candidiasis, listeriosis, *Pneumocystis jiroveci*, and herpes virus infections such as CMV and HSV. All fevers must be taken seriously with appropriate diagnostic testing. Patients receiving highly immunosuppressive regimens should be monitored for CMV reactivation, but prophylactic intravenous immunoglobulins are reserved for patients with recurrent bacterial infections.

Coombs' positive hemolytic anemia and/or immune thrombocytopenia occur in about 20% of patients. These sometimes develop after the initiation of therapy and reflect immunologic dysregulation since the clone does not produce the antibodies. Failure of immune surveillance results in an increased risk of solid tumors such as skin and colon cancers. Moreover, transformation to large-cell lymphoma (so-called Richter transformation) occurs in 15% of patients. It is heralded by increasing lymphadenopathy, hepatosplenomegaly, fever, abdominal pain, weight loss, anemia, and thrombocytopenia with a rapid rise in lactate dehydrogenase (LDH), and it has a poor prognosis.

RELATED B-CELL LEUKEMIAS

Two additional B-cell leukemias—prolymphocytic leukemia and hairy cell leukemia—although rare, should be considered in the differential diagnosis of CLL.

Prolymphocytic leukemia may be of either B-cell or T-cell lineage. It occurs in somewhat older patients than CLL and tends to be more advanced at presentation. Symptoms include weight loss, fevers, and abdominal pain from splenomegaly. The white count tends to be quite high, and the smear is characteristically different from CLL— the cells are larger with a more prominent nucleolus. The immunophenotype distinguishes it from CLL by virtue of stronger expression of surface immunoglobulins, and they are less likely to express CD5. This disease responds poorly to therapy with a median survival of 1–3 years.

Hairy cell leukemia is rarer than CLL and has a strong male predominance. Patients often have symptoms related to marrow depression with little in the way of leukocytosis, although characteristic hairy cells are usually seen in the blood. Like CLL, the cells express the B-cell antigens CD19, CD20, but also the monocyte antigen CD11c, and characteristically CD103. Treatment is indicated in the setting of massive or progressive splenomegaly, serious cytopenias, recurrent infections, or bulky lymphadenopathy. The purine analogues cladribine (Leukostatin) and pentostatin (Nipent) are extremely effective, resulting in long-term remissions in 70–80% of patients with little disease-related mortality.

ADDITIONAL READING

Auer RL, Gribben J, Cotter FE. Emerging therapy for chronic lymphocytic leukaemia. *Br J Haematol.* 2007;139:635–44.

Betz BL, Hess JL. Acute myeloid leukemia diagnosis in the 21st century. *Arch Pathol Lab Med.* 2010;134(10):1427–33.

Estey E. Acute myeloid leukemia and myelodysplastic syndromes in older patients. *J Clin Oncol.* 2007;25:1908–15.

Goldman JM. How I treat chronic myeloid leukemia in the imatinib era. *Blood.* 2007;110:2828–37.

Hamadani M, Awan FT, Copelan EA. Hematopoietic stem cell transplantation in adults with acute myeloid leukemia. *Biol Blood Marrow Transplant.* 2008;14:556–67.

Hehlmann R, Hochhaus A, Baccarani M; European LeukemiaNet. Chronic myeloid leukaemia. *Lancet.* 2007;370:342–50.

Jabbour E, Cortes JE, Giles FJ, O'Brien S, Kantarjian HM. Current and emerging treatment options in chronic myeloid leukemia. *Cancer.* 2007;109:2171–81.

Nabhan C, Shanafelt TD, Kay NE. Controversies in the front-line management of chronic lymphocytic leukemia. *Leuk Res.* 2008;32:679–88.

Pui CH, Robison LL, Look AT. Acute lymphoblastic leukaemia. *Lancet.* 2008;371:1030–43.

Ravandi F, Burnett AK, Agura ED, Kantarjian HM. Progress in the treatment of acute myeloid leukemia. *Cancer.* 2007;110:1900–10.

Rubnitz JE, Gibson B, Smith FO. Acute myeloid leukemia. *Hematol Oncol Clin North Am.* 2010;24(1):35–63.

Shanafelt TD, Kay NE. Comprehensive management of the CLL patient: A holistic approach. *Hematology Am Soc Hematol Educ Program.* 2007:324–31.

Stein A, Forman SJ. Allogeneic transplantation for ALL in adults. *Bone Marrow Transplant.* 2008;41:439–46.

Tallman MS, Gilliland DG, Rowe JM. Drug therapy for acute myeloid leukemia. *Blood.* 2005;106(4):1154–63. Erratum in *Blood.* 2005;106(7):2243.

Wang ZY, Chen Z. Acute promyelocytic leukemia: From highly fatal to highly curable. Blood. 2008;lll:2505–15.

QUESTIONS

QUESTION 1. A 35-year-old man calls because he noted large bruises on his arms and legs. He had been playing touch football but felt that the bruising was unexpectedly severe. He had no fevers or weight loss. Physical exam confirmed several 5- to 10-cm ecchymoses on the arms and legs including bruises on the medial surfaces. Exam was otherwise normal. White blood count was 1300/dL with 25% PMN, 55% lymphocytes, and 20% atypical cells. Hb 13.6, platelets 22,000/dL, INR 2.2, PTT 50, D-dimer is elevated. Which of the following is true?

A. Postviral ITP is the most likely diagnosis, and a course of prednisone is warranted.

B. The low white blood count precludes the diagnosis of AML.

C. Pancytopenia plus evidence of DIC are suspicious for promyelocytic leukemia.

D. HLA typing should be obtained immediately in anticipation of stem cell transplantation.

E. Cytogenetics is likely to show evidence of a translocation involving the MYC oncogene.

QUESTION 2. All of the following are true EXCEPT:

A. CLL uniformly requires therapy.

B. Staging of CLL does not require a bone marrow aspirate.

C. Chromosomal abnormalities provide critical prognostic information in CLL.

D. White blood count elevation in excess of 100,000 cells/dL does not require emergency therapy.

E. CLL is typically a disease of antigen-stimulated B cells.

QUESTION 3. A 70-year-old man is found to have an enlarged spleen (5 cm below the costal margin) on routine annual evaluation. He has been feeling well, although on close questioning may have lost 5 pounds in the last 6 months, and he has had a few episodes of night sweats. Laboratory studies show WBC 56,000/dL, with 50% PMN, 15% bands, 10% lymphocytes, 5% monocytes, 5% basophils, 3% metamyelocytes, 5% myelocytes, 2% promyelocytes, 5% blasts. Hb 13.8, platelets 1,250,000/dL. Which of the following statements is true?

A. Prognosis is grim with 2-year survival of 10%.

B. The most appropriate therapy is lifetime daily interferon-alpha.

C. Cytogenetic analysis of the bone marrow is unlikely to provide useful information.

D. Imatinib therapy has a 95% chance of normalizing hematopoiesis within 3 months.

E. DIC is a common complication of therapy.

ANSWERS

1. C
2. A
3. D

15.

NON-HODGKIN AND HODGKIN LYMPHOMA

Alfred Ian Lee and Ann S. LaCasce

Lymphomas are malignancies of lymphoid cells. These neoplasms originate from cells in the B lymphocyte and T lymphocyte/natural killer (NK) cell lineages. Broadly they are categorized into non-Hodgkin (NHL) and Hodgkin lymphomas (HL). The World Health Organization (WHO) recognizes over 40 major types of NHL and five major types of HL.

OVERVIEW OF THE LYMPHATIC SYSTEM AND LYMPHOCYTE IMMUNOLOGY

The lymphatic system is composed of central and peripheral lymphoid organs (see figure 15.1). Central lymphoid organs are the sites where immature lymphoid cells develop into mature B and T cells; these sites are the bone marrow (for B-cell development) and the thymus (for T-cell development). Peripheral lymphoid organs are sites where mature lymphoid cells aggregate into functioning units; these sites are the lymph nodes, spleen, and mucosa-associated lymphoid tissues (MALT).

Immature lymphoid cells in the bone marrow differentiate into pro-B and pro-T cells. The former complete development into mature B cells in the bone marrow, whereas the latter undergo subsequent maturation in the thymus. Mature B and T cells exit the bone marrow and thymus, respectively, and migrate to the peripheral lymphoid organs. Mature B and T cells bear cell surface immunoglobulins (Ig, containing heavy- and light-chain proteins) and T-cell receptors (TCR, containing alpha and beta, or delta and gamma, subunits), respectively, that en masse possess an infinite repertoire of antigenic specificities. The molecular basis for Ig and TCR antigenic diversity is the process of V(D)J recombination that occurs during B- and T-cell development, whereby variable (V), diversity (D), and joining (J) gene segments of Ig and TCR genes are assembled together in semirandom fashion to generate the mature genes. Somatic hypermutation of mature rearranged Ig genes further modifies the repertoire of antigenic specificities in activated B cells.

Within each lymph node, a fibrous capsule surrounds a central parenchyma, which is divided into an outer cortex, a paracortex, and an inner medulla. The cortex contains primary follicles with mostly unstimulated B cells and secondary follicles with antigen-stimulated, activated B cells. Secondary follicles are further partitioned into a germinal center containing activated B cells, surrounded by a mantle zone of mostly unstimulated B cells and a few T cells. The lymph node paracortex contains mostly T cells. The medulla contains mostly macrophages and Ig-secreting plasma cells.

NON-HODGKIN LYMPHOMA

NHL is the fifth most common cancer and the most common hematologic malignancy in the United States, with approximately 65,000 new cases diagnosed each year. NHL is also the sixth most common cause of cancer-related deaths in the United States, accounting for approximately 19,000 deaths per year.

CLINICAL PRESENTATION NHL

- *Lymphadenopathy* is present in over two-thirds of patients with NHL, with the rapidity of lymph node enlargement reflecting the aggressiveness of the underlying lymphoma.

- *B symptoms* are defined as fever greater than 38°C (100.4°F), drenching night sweats requiring a change of clothes, and weight loss of at least 10 pounds or 5% baseline body weight over a 6- to 12-month period. B symptoms are observed in about 45% of aggressive or highly aggressive NHL, and in less than 25% of indolent NHL; when present in the setting of an indolent NHL, B symptoms tend to indicate a large burden of disease or transformation into aggressive lymphoma.

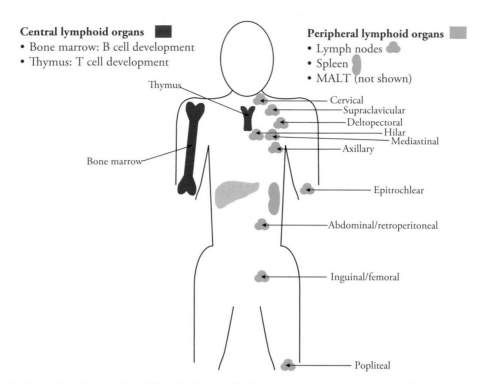

Central lymphoid organs ▮
- Bone marrow: B cell development
- Thymus: T cell development

Peripheral lymphoid organs ▮
- Lymph nodes ♣
- Spleen
- MALT (not shown)

Thymus

Bone marrow

Cervical
Supraclavicular
Deltopectoral
Hilar
Mediastinal
Axillary

Epitrochlear

Abdominal/retroperitoneal

Inguinal/femoral

Popliteal

Figure 15.1. Overview of the Lymphatic System. Central lymphoid organs (red) are the bone marrow, where B-cell development occurs, and the thymus, where T-cell development occurs. Peripheral lymphoid organs (green) are the lymph nodes, spleen, and mucosa-associated lymphoid tissues (MALT). The major lymph node regions are shown (green clover).

- *Local symptoms* reflect the degree to which a lymphoma impairs the function of involved or adjacent tissues, with different NHLs displaying varying degrees of extranodal (i.e., external to the lymph nodes) involvement. Common sites of extranodal disease include the liver, spleen, gastrointestinal tract, skin, bone marrow, and central nervous system (CNS); rare sites include the kidneys, bladder, adrenals, heart (particularly the pericardial space), lungs, breast, testes, and thyroid.

EVALUATION OF NHL

Evaluation of a new or suspected diagnosis of NHL requires a thorough history, physical examination, laboratory evaluation, imaging analysis, and tissue sampling for pathology review (see figure 15.2).

History

A comprehensive history in the evaluation of a new or suspected diagnosis of NHL should assess for B symptoms and for factors known to be associated with NHL, including:

- *Autoimmune and inflammatory diseases.* Examples are systemic lupus erythematosus, rheumatoid arthritis, inflammatory bowel disease, dermatomyositis, and Sjögren syndrome, all of which may be associated with NHL and, occasionally, HL. Celiac disease is associated with enteropathy-associated T-cell lymphoma, autoimmune thyroiditis

with extranodal marginal zone lymphoma, and cryoglobulinemia with NHL. Sarcoidosis is both associated with and may mimic NHL by virtue of lymphadenopathy.

- *Viral infections.* Examples include human immunodeficiency virus (HIV), associated with diffuse large B-cell lymphoma, Burkitt lymphoma, primary CNS lymphoma, primary effusion lymphoma, plasmablastic lymphoma, and HL; Epstein-Barr virus (EBV), associated with diffuse large B-cell lymphoma, Burkitt lymphoma, NK- and T-cell lymphomas, and HL; human T lymphotropic virus type I (HTLV-l), associated with adult T-cell lymphoma/leukemia; human herpesvirus 8 (HHV-8), associated with HIV+ primary effusion lymphoma and with HIV+ plasmablastic lymphoma; and hepatitis C virus (HCV), associated with splenic and extranodal marginal zone lymphomas.

- *Bacterial infections.* The major association of bacterial infections is with extranodal marginal zone lymphomas in various organs. The most common infections are *Helicobacter pylori* (stomach, a.k.a. gastric MALToma), *Borrelia burgdorferi* (skin), *Campylobacter jejuni* (small intestine), and *Chlamydophila psittaci* (eye).

- *Medications.* The most important medications associated with NHL are immunosuppressive agents (e.g., methotrexate, infliximab, 6-mercaptopurine, azathioprine, tacrolimus, cyclosporine, and mycophenolate) and targeted therapies against tumor necrosis factor (TNF)-alpha [e.g., infliximab (Remicade), adalimumab (HUMIRA), and etanercept (Enbrel)].

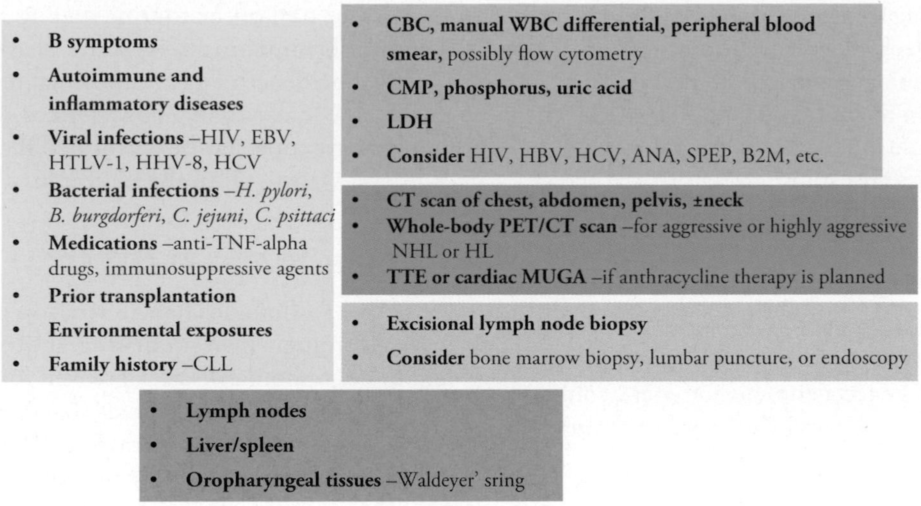

- **B symptoms**
- **Autoimmune and inflammatory diseases**
- **Viral infections** –HIV, EBV, HTLV-1, HHV-8, HCV
- **Bacterial infections** –*H. pylori, B. burgdorferi, C. jejuni, C. psittaci*
- **Medications** –anti-TNF-alpha drugs, immunosuppressive agents
- **Prior transplantation**
- **Environmental exposures**
- **Family history** –CLL

- **CBC, manual WBC differential, peripheral blood smear,** possibly flow cytometry
- **CMP, phosphorus, uric acid**
- **LDH**
- **Consider** HIV, HBV, HCV, ANA, SPEP, B2M, etc.

- **CT scan of chest, abdomen, pelvis, ±neck**
- **Whole-body PET/CT scan** –for aggressive or highly aggressive NHL or HL
- **TTE or cardiac MUGA** –if anthracycline therapy is planned

- **Excisional lymph node biopsy**
- **Consider** bone marrow biopsy, lumbar puncture, or endoscopy

- **Lymph nodes**
- **Liver/spleen**
- **Oropharyngeal tissues** –Waldeyer' sring

Figure 15.2. Evaluation of NHL. Shown are components of history (yellow), physical exam (purple/pink), laboratory investigation (orange), imaging (green), and tissue analysis (blue) that should be explored in evaluation of new cases of NHL.

- *History of prior transplantation*, associated with B- or T-cell posttransplant lymphoproliferative disease.

- *Environmental exposure* to pesticides, solvents, chemicals, or chemotherapy.

- *Family history* of lymphoma (particularly chronic lymphocytic leukemia), leukemia, or other hematologic diseases.

Physical Examination

- *Lymph node examination.* The major peripheral lymph node groups are the cervical (anterior and posterior), supraclavicular, axillary, epitrochlear, inguinal, and popliteal nodes. Features suggestive of malignancy include nodes that are >1 cm in diameter; have a firm, rubbery consistency; are fixed or immobile; are nontender to palpation; are located in the posterior cervical, supraclavicular, or epitrochlear chains; or are diffusely distributed.

- *Liver and spleen examination.* Every patient with a new or suspected diagnosis of NHL or HL should be evaluated for hepatomegaly or splenomegaly, as the liver and spleen are common sites of extranodal involvement.

- *Oropharyngeal examination.* Waldeyer's ring, a region of lymphoid tissue encompassing the tonsils, base of tongue, and nasopharynx, may be involved by various lymphomas, particularly mantle cell lymphoma. Aphthous ulcers may rarely be manifestations of oral lymphoma. Oral petechiae may indicate thrombocytopenia or disseminated intravascular coagulation.

Laboratory Evaluation

- *Complete blood count (CBC).* Anemia or thrombocytopenia may reflect marrow infiltration or an associated autoimmune process such as autoimmune hemolytic anemia

(AIHA) or immune thrombocytopenia (ITP), both of which may be seen with chronic lymphocytic leukemia. The white blood cell (WBC) differential should be manually counted to assess for lymphocytosis. Peripheral blood smear should be examined for unusual lymphoid cell morphologies. In select cases, flow cytometry may be performed to evaluate for circulating monoclonal lymphoid populations.

- *Comprehensive metabolic panel* (CMP), phosphorus, and uric acid. Creatinine and liver function tests assess for end-organ damage due to lymphomatous infiltration. Calcium, potassium, phosphorus, and uric acid assess for tumor lysis, which may be seen with aggressive or highly aggressive lymphomas.

- *Lactate dehydrogenase (LDH).* The serum LDH level is a marker of tumor lysis in aggressive or highly aggressive NHL and serves as an important prognostic factor in many NHL subtypes. It may also be an indicator of transformation from indolent into aggressive NHL.

- *Additional laboratory tests* may include specific serologic, polymerase chain reaction (PCR), and culture studies for infectious or autoimmune processes, as indicated by the clinical scenario. Examples are HIV, EBV, HTLV-l, hepatitis B virus (HBV), HCV, *H. pylori*, antinuclear antibody (ANA), rheumatoid factor (RF), serum protein electrophoresis (SPEP), beta-2 microglobulin (B2M), cryoglobulin, and Coombs' testing.

Imaging Evaluation

The imaging study of choice in the evaluation of NHL is a computed tomography (CT) scan of the chest, abdomen, and pelvis. CT scan of the neck may be performed if there is suspicion for cervical or upper oropharyngeal disease.

- For aggressive and highly aggressive NHL (and HL), whole-body fluorodeoxyglucose positron emission tomography, in combination with CT (PET/CT), is routinely obtained in the initial staging and subsequent evaluation of response to therapy. In general, rapidly growing malignancies are exquisitely sensitive to detection on PET imaging due to robust uptake of fluorodeoxyglucose. The role of PET/CT in evaluation of indolent NHL is less clear.

- Transthoracic echocardiogram (TTE) or cardiac multigated acquisition (MUGA) scan should be performed in all patients who will be receiving chemotherapy containing anthracyclines (e.g., doxorubicin or Adriamycin).

Tissue Evaluation

- Full excisional biopsy of an involved lymph node is the preferred procedure for obtaining tissue for pathologic review in evaluation of lymphoma. In patients with multiple enlarged peripheral lymph nodes, supraclavicular nodes have the highest diagnostic yield, followed by cervical or axillary nodes. Inguinal nodes are of low diagnostic utility, as their enlargement is often reactive.

- CT-guided core needle biopsy may be performed in cases where excisional lymph node biopsy is not feasible. Due to the small size of tissue obtained, diagnostic ability is reduced with core needle biopsy as compared to excisional biopsy.

- Fine needle aspiration of an involved lymph node is not recommended in evaluation of lymphoma, as cytology samples do not allow for evaluation of lymph node architecture.

- Bone marrow biopsy is performed in the majority of patients with aggressive or highly aggressive NHL and in some patients with indolent NHL.

- Lumbar puncture may be performed in patients with highly aggressive NHL who have suspicious neurologic manifestations or risk factors for CNS involvement (e.g., elevated LDH at initial presentation, involvement of more than one extranodal site, or infiltration of bone marrow, testes, or paranasal sinuses). In cases where the suspicion for CNS involvement is high, or where there may be concern for possible hematogenous seeding of the CNS by circulating lymphoma cells during lumbar puncture, intrathecal chemotherapy may be administered.

- Endoscopic evaluation of the gastrointestinal tract may be performed if there are suspicious gastrointestinal symptoms (e.g., dysphagia, abdominal pain, diarrhea, or constipation). At many academic centers, endoscopy has become part of the routine staging evaluation of mantle cell lymphoma irrespective of symptoms, due to the high incidence of gastrointestinal involvement with this disease (Salar et al., 2006). Direct visualization and laryngoscopy may be performed if examination of Waldeyer's ring is clinically indicated.

PATHOLOGIC CHARACTERIZATION OF NHL

- *Histology.* Pathologic characterization of NHL begins with a histologic review of tissue. Individual lymphoid and nonlymphoid cells are observed for malignant characteristics such as irregular shape, uniform or monotonous appearance, or nucleoli. Global lymphoid architecture is also evaluated, as normal follicular lymph node architecture is often preserved in follicular lymphoma and other indolent NHL subtypes but may be disrupted in diffuse large B-cell lymphoma, Burkitt lymphoma, and other aggressive or highly aggressive NHLs.

- *Immunophenotyping* (figure 15.3). The immunophenotype is the unique signature of cell surface proteins displayed by each type of NHL. Immunophenotyping may be performed by immunohistochemistry or flow cytometry; these techniques measure binding of antibodies directed against specific molecular targets. For B-cell NHL, the most important cell surface marker is CD20, which serves as the molecular target of the anti-CD20 antibody rituximab (Rituxan), used in treatment of a variety of B-cell NHLs.

- *Cytogenetic analysis* (figure 15.3). Specific cytogenetic abnormalities, particularly translocations, are associated with different NHLs. Cytogenetic analysis is performed by karyotyping or FISH.

- *Ki-67 or MIB-1 fraction.* Staining for Ki-67 or MIB-1 identifies actively dividing cells. The Ki-67 index or MIB-1 fraction may help distinguish the clinical aggressiveness of different NHL subtypes and may have prognostic significance in specific NHLs (e.g., mantle cell lymphoma).

STAGING OF NHL

Staging for NHL (table 15.1) utilizes the Ann Arbor Staging System, originally devised for HL.

CLASSIFICATION OF NHL

The WHO classifies NHL according to the parental cell type of origin and recognizes four broad categories of NHL: precursor lymphoid neoplasms, mature B-cell neoplasms, mature T-cell and NK-cell neoplasms, and

- **B-cell markers**: CD19, CD20, CD22, CD79a. *The most important B-cell marker is CD20, the molecular target of rituximab.*

- **T-cell markers**: CD3, CD4, CD5, CD8, CD5. *The most important T-cell marker is CD5, as CD5 positivity in a B-cell NHL restricts the differential diagnosis to CLL and MCL*

- **Surface Ig expression**: IgG, IgM, IgA, IgD, κ light chain, λ light chain.

- **CD52**: all mature B and T cells. *CD52 is the molecular target of alemtuzumab, used in the treatment of CLL.*

- **CD138**: plasma cells (*myeloma*), lymphoplasmacytic cells (*Waldenstrom's macroglobulinemia*).

- **CD10**: germinal center-derived B cells (*Burkitt's lymphoma, B lymphoblastic lymphoma/leukemia, FL subset of DLBCL*).

- **CD30/CD15**: *either marker may be expressed in some subsets of peripheral T cell lymphoma. CD30 is expressed in anaplastic large cell lymphoma. Both are expressed in classical HL.* ·

- **TdT (terminal deoxynucleotidyl transferase)**: *B lymphoblastic lymphoma/leukemia, T lymphoblastic leukemia/lymphoma.*

- **cyclin D1**: *MCL.*

- **t(8;14), t(2;8), or t(8;22)**: *BL. These translocations place c-myc proto-oncogene (chromosome 8) next to the enhancer elements of the Ig heavy chain (chromosome 14), κ light chain (chromosome 8), or λ light chain (chromosome 22).*

- **t(14;18)**: *FL. This places bcl-2 (chromosome 18) next to the Ig heavy chain enhancer.*

- **t(11;14)**: *MCL. This positions cyclin D1 (chromosome 11) next to the Ig heavy chain enhancer.*

- **t(9;22), "Philadelphia chromosome"**: *subset of B-lymphoblastic lymphoma/leukemia. This generates a tyrosine kinase that is the molecular target of imatinib(Gleevec).*

Figure 15.3. Major Immunophenotypic (yellow) and Cytogenetic (pink) Markers in NHL.

posttransplant lymphoproliferative disorders (Swerdlow, 2008). For practical reasons, and from the perspective of the general internist, the different NHL subtypes may be classified as indolent, aggressive, or highly aggressive (see figure 15.4). Survival of untreated indolent NHL is generally on the order of years; aggressive NHL, months; and highly aggressive NHL, weeks. Major NHL subtypes are presented below.

Highly Aggressive NHL

B Lymphoblastic Leukemia/Lymphoma

B lymphoblastic leukemia/lymphoma is the lymphomatous counterpart of pre-B acute lymphoblastic leukemia (pre-B ALL) and is evaluated and treated similarly. The disease is defined as leukemia if the bone marrow is more than 25% involved. B lymphoblastic leukemia/lymphoma is more common in children but may present in older adults. Both B lymphoblastic leukemia/lymphoma and pre-B ALL express terminal deoxynucleotidyl transferase (TdT), which is unique to these diseases and to T lymphoblastic leukemia/lymphoma, distinguishing these disorders from mature B- and T-cell lymphomas. B lymphoblastic leukemia/lymphoma and pre-B ALL are also associated with a number of translocations, the most important being the t(9;22) translocation (Philadelphia chromosome). Whereas pediatric cases have a favorable prognosis, the clinical course in adult patients is generally unfavorable, particularly for t(9;22)+ disease. First-line treatment is a combined approach incorporating intensive chemotherapy, prophylactic CNS therapy, and

allogeneic stem cell transplant; the tyrosine kinase inhibitor imatinib (Gleevec) is added in t(9;22)+ cases.

T Lymphoblastic Leukemia/Lymphoma

T lymphoblastic leukemia/lymphoma is the T-cell counterpart to B lymphoblastic leukemia/lymphoma and is

Table 15.1 ANN ARBOR STAGING SYSTEM FOR NHL AND HL

ANN ARBOR STAGING SYSTEM

STAGE	CLINICAL FEATURES
I	Single lymph node or lymph node area on one side of diaphragm
II	Two or more involved lymph node areas on same side of diaphragm
III	Disease on both sides of diaphragm, contained within nodal tissues (including spleen)
IV	Extranodal involvement (marrow, liver, lung)

NOTES: For NHL and HL, the following subscripts are commonly used:
A: absence of B symptoms
B: presence of B symptoms
E: involvement of one extranodal site

For HL, two additional subscripts are used:
X: bulky disease, defined as a nodal mass >10 cm in greatest transverse diameter, or a mediastinal mass whose maximum width is more than one-third the thoracic diameter at the level of the T5-T6 intercostal space
S: splenic involvement

SOURCE: Rosenberg SA. Validity of the Ann Arbor staging classification for the non-Hodgkin's lymphomas. *Cancer Treat Rep.* 1977;61(6):1023–7.

treated similarly. It presents in young males with a mediastinal mass.

Adult T-Cell Leukemia/Lymphoma

Adult T-cell leukemia/lymphoma (ATLL) is caused by the HTLV-l virus, endemic to southern Japan and the Caribbean, and also found in Africa, Latin America, and the Middle East. About 5% of HTLV-1+ patients develop ATLL, usually following a latency period of over 30 years. Although there are indolent and smoldering subsets, the majority of patients present with aggressive disease and have a poor prognosis. Treatment approaches include intensive chemotherapy, allogeneic stem cell transplant, and in some cases, antiviral agents such as interferon-alpha or zidovudine.

Burkitt Lymphoma

Burkitt lymphoma (BL) represents more than half of pediatric NHL and less than 5% of all adult NHL in the United States (Blum et al., 2004).

Pathologic features: BL is characterized by medium-sized B cells with round nuclei containing multiple nucleoli and cytoplasmic vacuoles. Owing to a high proliferative rate, spontaneous cell destruction and necrosis are common, with macrophages recruited to remove cellular debris; the overall appearance is of sheets of lymphoma cells perpetrated by gaps of macrophages, forming a "starry sky" pattern (figure 15.5). By definition, BL cells harbor translocations involving the *c-myc* proto-oncogene on chromosome 8, the most common being the t(8;14) translocation, which positions *c-myc* close to the Ig heavy chain enhancer on chromosome 14, leading to c-myc overexpression. t(8;14) accounts in part for the very high proliferative index of BL cells, with Ki-67 staining 100% of cells.

Clinical presentation: The three major subtypes of BL are endemic, sporadic (nonendemic), and immunodeficiency-associated BL. Endemic BL is found in Africa, is strongly associated with EBV infection, and presents as a jaw tumor with bone marrow, CNS, and other multi-organ involvement. Sporadic BL is found throughout the world, is associated with EBV in 30% of cases, and presents as disseminated disease with abdominal lymphadenopathy, ascites, and often bone marrow and/or CNS involvement. Immunodeficiency-associated BL occurs primarily in association with HIV, with only a subset being EBV+.

Prognosis: BL is potentially curable, although bone marrow and CNS involvement at presentation are adverse features and predict a higher risk of relapse. Response rates to chemotherapy are very high, in part reflecting the high proliferative rate of BL cells. Children with BL have an excellent prognosis with high rates of durable remission, whereas adults have a less favorable course due to an increased risk of relapsed disease.

Treatment: First-line treatment is intensive combination chemotherapy. Two commonly used chemotherapy regimens are hyper-CVAD (cyclophosphamide, vincristine, doxorubicin, dexamethasone) and the modified Magrath regimen ("CODOX-M/IVAC"; cyclophosphamide, vincristine, doxorubicin, high-dose methotrexate, ifosfamide, cytarabine, etoposide), both of which incorporate prophylactic CNS therapy. Rituximab has recently been combined with both regimens, with encouraging results.

Aggressive NHL

Diffuse Large B-Cell Lymphoma

Diffuse large B-cell lymphoma (DLBCL) is the most common subtype of NHL, accounting for approximately 30% of all NHLs (Swerdlow et al., 2008).

Pathologic features: DLBCL is characterized by heterogeneous large B cells that proliferate in a diffuse pattern, disrupting normal lymph-node architecture. The Ki-67 index is typically around 70%; cases with a Ki-67 index

---

Indolent: median survival of several years (untreated)
  Follicular lymphoma (FL)
  Chronic lymphocytic leukemia/small lymphocytic lymphoma (CLL/SLL)
  Marginal zone lymphoma (MZL)
  *Mantle cell lymphoma (MCL)**
  Lymphoplasmacytic lymphoma/Waldenstrom's macroglobulinemia (LPL/WM)

* *MCL is classified as indolent but behaves as aggressive NHL*

Aggressive: median survival of a few to several months (untreated)
  Diffuse large B cell lymphoma (DLBCL)
  Peripheral T and NK cell lymphoma
  Anaplastic large cell lymphoma

Highly aggressive: median survival of a few weeks (untreated)
  B lymphoblastic leukemia/lymphoma
  T lymphoblastic leukemia/lymphoma
  Adult T cell leukemia/lymphoma
  Burkitt lymphoma

Figure 15.4. Major NHL Subtypes, Classified by Clinical Aggressivenes.

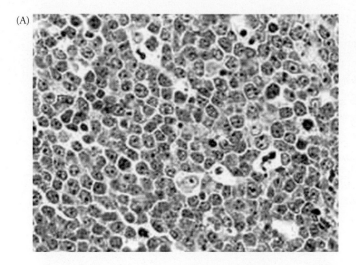

(A)

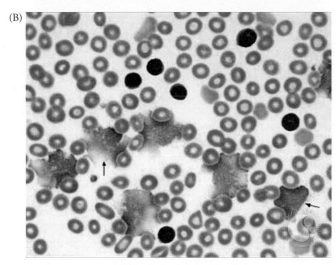

(B)

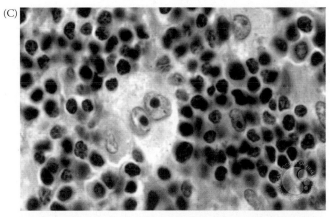

(C)

Figure 15.5. Histologies of Select NHL and HL Subtypes. (A) The starry sky pattern of BL. Hematoxylin and eosin stain. Reprinted from Harris NL, Horning SJ. Burkitt's lymphoma. The message from microarrays. *N Engl J Med*. 2006;354(23):2495–8. Copyright © 2006 Massachusetts Medical Society. All rights reserved. (B) Peripheral blood smear of CLL, showing lymphocytes, thrombocytopenia, and smudge cells (arrows). This image was originally published in ASH Image Bank. Lazarchick J (2001). Chronic lymphocytic leukemia: thrombocytopenia. Image #00001359 © the American Society of Hematology. (C) Owl's eye nuclei of RS cell in classical HL, nodular sclerosis subtype. This image was originally published in ASH Image Bank. Kadin M (2002). Hodgkin lymphoma. Image #00001741 © the American Society of Hematology.

higher than 90% may occur, particularly in association with translocations involving or overexpression of c-myc, which can cloud histologic distinction from BL. About one-third of DLBCL cases bear the t(14;18) translocation of follicular lymphoma (FL), which may indicate transformation from an earlier FL.

Clinical course: The median age of DLBCL is 64. The majority of patients present with advanced-stage (III or IV) disease. About 40% have extranodal involvement at the time of initial presentation, including gastrointestinal, skin, bone, CNS, thyroid, or testicular infiltration. Another 10–20% have bone marrow involvement. B symptoms and elevated LDH are common. In some cases, DLBCL may arise from a prior indolent NHL such as FL or CLL; the latter is known as Richter transformation and has an aggressive clinical course. Intravascular large B-cell lymphoma (ILCL) is a rare subtype of DLBCL in which the malignant cells infiltrate small blood vessels distributed across multiple organs; the classic presentation is of a "vasculitic disease without vasculitis," with neurologic symptoms being common, and prognosis is poor, in part because the disease is often not suspected until late in the course.

Prognosis: Prognosis of DLBCL is determined by the International Prognostic Index (IPI) (table 15.2) (International Non-Hodgkin's Lymphoma Prognostic Factors Project, 1993). Prior to the introduction of rituximab into standard therapy for DLBCL, 5-year overall survival of DLBCL ranged from 26% to 73%, depending on the number of IPI risk factors. Both disease-free and overall survival have increased by 10–15% with the addition of rituximab to standard therapy for DLBCL (Sehn et al., 2007).

Treatment: The prognosis of treated DLBCL is favorable, with a high rate of durable responses after chemotherapy, reflecting, in part, the high proliferative rate of DLBCL cells. Treatment of DLBCL depends on disease stage (figure 15.6) (National Comprehensive Cancer Network, 2011). For advanced-stage (III or IV) DLBCL, first-line treatment is combination chemotherapy with addition of rituximab. An early phase III study of advanced-stage DLBCL compared combination CHOP chemotherapy (cyclophosphamide, doxorubicin, vincristine, prednisone) with more intensive regimens and found decreased toxicity of CHOP without differences in efficacy. A landmark study from the French GELA group compared CHOP with or without rituximab in treatment of advanced-stage DLBCL and found an increase in overall survival with CHOP plus rituximab (RCHOP) without a significant increase in toxicity. RCHOP is therefore first-line therapy for advanced-stage DLBCL, with a typical course being six cycles administered every 3 weeks, or, in elderly patients, six cycles administered every 2 weeks. DLBCL patients with risk factors for CNS disease (discussed above; see Evaluation of NHL, section on Tissue Evaluation) may benefit from prophylactic CNS therapy using intrathecal chemotherapy or high-dose systemic methotrexate. For limited stage (I or II) DLBCL, first-line treatment is abbreviated chemotherapy with

Table 15.2 INTERNATIONAL PROGNOSTIC INDEX FOR DLBCL

INTERNATIONAL PROGNOSTIC INDEX (IPI) FOR DLBCL

Adverse prognostic factors ("APLES"):	Advanced age Poor performance status Elevated LDH Extranodal disease Stage III or IV disease

Treatment without rituximab:

NO. OF RISK FACTORS	COMPLETE REMISSION	5-YEAR RELAPSE-FREE SURVIVAL	5-YEAR OVERALL SURVIVAL
0–1 Low risk	87%	70%	73%
2 Low-intermediate risk	67%	50%	51%
3 High-intermediate risk	55%	49%	43%
4–5 High risk	44%	40%	26%

SOURCE: Reprinted with permission from The International Non-Hodgkin's Lymphoma Prognostic Factors Project. A Predictive Model for Aggressive Non-Hodgkin's Lymphoma. *N Engl J Med.* 1993;329(14):987–94. Copyright © 1993 Massachusetts Medical Society. All rights reserved.

Treatment with rituximab:

NO. OF RISK FACTORS	4-YEAR PROGRESSION-FREE SURVIVAL	4-YEAR OVERALL SURVIVAL
0 Very good risk	94%	94%
1–2 Good risk	80%	79%
3–5 Poor risk	53%	55%

SOURCE: Reprinted with permission from Sehn et al. The Revised International Prognostic Index (R-IPI) is a better predictor of outcome than the standard IPI for patients with diffuse large B-cell lymphoma treated with R-CHOP. *Blood.* 2007;109(5):1857–61.

radiation; alternately, rituximab-containing chemotherapy without radiotherapy may be an appropriate option in certain circumstances (Armitage, 2007). Following completion of first-line therapy, a post-treatment PET/CT scan is performed, with complete remission defined as reduction in the size of the initial lesions on CT and absence of fluorodeoxyglucose uptake on PET. For patients who attain complete remission, routine surveillance CT or PET/CT scans may be performed every 6 to 12 months for the first few years to monitor for relapsed disease. Notably, the efficacy of surveillance radiography of DLBCL in first remission in the absence of symptoms is uncertain and is increasingly being challenged by concerns regarding radiation exposure from excessive radiographic imaging. Patients who fail first-line treatment with RCHOP, or who develop relapsed DLBCL within 1 year after therapy, have a poor prognosis. For relapsed or treatment-refractory DLBCL, the standard approach is salvage chemotherapy, followed by high-dose chemotherapy and autologous stem cell transplant for patients with chemosensitive disease, based on a seminal randomized clinical trial from the Parma study group; alternately, such patients may be evaluated for clinical trials.

Peripheral T- and NK-Cell Lymphomas

Peripheral T- and NK-cell lymphomas comprise a heterogeneous collection of malignancies that include peripheral T-cell lymphoma, angioimmunoblastic T-cell lymphoma (AITL), extranodal NK/T-cell lymphoma of nasal type, subcutaneous panniculitis-like T-cell lymphoma, enteropathy-associated T-cell lymphoma, hepatosplenic gamma/delta T-cell lymphoma, cutaneous T-cell lymphoma, and anaplastic large cell lymphoma. In general, CHOP is used as first-line chemotherapy for peripheral T- and NK-cell lymphomas, although the efficacy is significantly lower than in the B-cell lymphomas. The role of stem cell transplantation in first remission is under investigation.

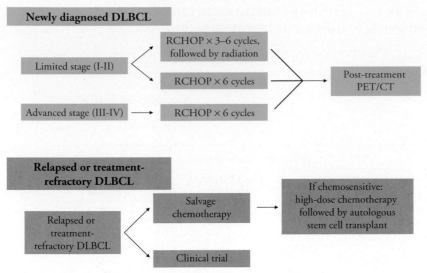

Figure 15.6. Treatment of DLBCL From the National Comprehensive Cancer Network (2011); www.nccn.org.

Angioimmunoblastic T cell lymphoma presents with fever, generalized lymphadenopathy, hepatosplenomegaly, B symptoms, marrow involvement, and a vasculitic rash. It is associated with HIV, EBV, polyclonal gammopathy, and AIHA. Prognosis is poor, although high-dose chemotherapy with autologous stem cell transplant may offer long-term disease control.

Cutaneous T-cell lymphoma manifests as a plaque-like rash with associated erythroderma. It represents a spectrum of disease, ranging from mycosis fungoides, an indolent disease mostly (but not exclusively) limited to the skin, to Sézary syndrome, an aggressive malignancy with circulating lymphoma cells. Multiple skin biopsies may be required to establish a definitive diagnosis. Treatment approaches include radiation, topical chemotherapy, systemic retinoids, systemic phototherapy, and chemotherapy, depending on the extent and responsiveness of disease.

Anaplastic large cell lymphoma (ALCL) has cutaneous and systemic subtypes. Systemic ALCL may be further classified according to ALK expression, with ALK-positive ALCL showing a more favorable prognosis than ALK-negative ALCL. Standard treatment is anthracycline-containing combination chemotherapy (e.g., CHOP), which yields a high overall survival in patients with ALK+ disease.

Indolent NHL

Follicular Lymphoma

Follicular lymphoma (FL) is the second most common subtype of NHL, accounting for 20% of all NHLs (Swerdlow et al., 2008).

Pathologic features: FL cells are small B cells with cleaved nuclei ("butt cells") that in aggregate preserve the follicular architecture of involved lymph nodes. FL is categorized into three different histologic grades (I–III), with grade III FL demonstrating an aggressive clinical course similar to DLBCL. Ninety percent of FL cases carry the t(14;18) translocation,

which positions the antiapoptotic bcl-2 gene on chromosome 18 near the Ig heavy-chain enhancer element.

Clinical presentation: The median age of FL is in the late 50s. Seventy to 80% have advanced-stage (III–IV) disease at the time of initial presentation; 40–70% have bone marrow involvement (Solal-Celigny, 2004; Swerdlow et al., 2008; Federico et al., 2009). Lymphadenopathy may wax and wane. Median survival from the time of diagnosis is over 10 years; most patients die from FL even after appropriate therapy because of decreased chemoresponsiveness and reduced durable remission rates following treatment. Spontaneous remissions may occasionally occur. One-third of patients transform into an aggressive disease NHL, such as DLBCL.

Prognosis: Prognosis of FL is gauged by the Follicular Lymphoma International Prognostic Index (FLIPI) (table 15.3). The original prognostic index (FLIPI-1), performed in the pre-rituximab era, identified age, stage III or IV disease, a large number of involved nodes, anemia, and high LDH as the most important prognostic factors, with 10-year median survivals ranging from 36% to 71% (Solal-Celigny et al., 2004). Following the introduction of rituximab to standard therapy, an updated prognostic index (FLIPI-2) identified age, anemia, B2M, size of the largest involved lymph node, and presence of bone marrow involvement as the factors with greatest prognostic significance in FL, with 5-year progression-free survival ranging from 19% to 80% (Federico et al., 2009).

Treatment: For asymptomatic patients with advanced-stage (III–IV) FL, early initiation of therapy has not been conclusively shown to improve outcomes compared to observation. Asymptomatic advanced-stage FL may be managed expectantly with observation until patients become symptomatic or show evidence of end-organ compromise, at which point a variety of treatment options may be used, including chemoimmunotherapy with CHOP, CVP(cyclophosphamide, vincristine, and prednisone), or bendamustine in combination with rituximab (Gribben, 2007). Although it is unclear which chemotherapy regimen

Table 15.3 FOLLICULAR LYMPHOMA INTERNATIONAL PROGNOSTIC INDEX-1 (FLIPI-1) AND FLIPI-2

FL INTERNATIONAL PROGNOSTIC INDEX (FLIPI)-1

Adverse prognostic factors:	Advanced age Stage III or IV More than four nodal areas Anemia Elevated LDH

Treatment without rituximab:

NO. OF RISK FACTORS	5-YEAR OVERALL SURVIVAL	10-YEAR OVERALL SURVIVAL
0–1 Low risk	91%	71%
2 Intermediate risk	78%	51%
3–5 High risk	53%	36%

SOURCE: Reprinted with permission from Solal-Celigny P, Roy P, Colombat P, et al. Follicular lymphoma international prognostic index. *Blood.* 2004;104(5):1258–65.

FL INTERNATIONAL PROGNOSTIC INDEX (FLIPI)-2

Adverse prognostic factors:	Advanced age Anemia B2M Size of largest involved lymph node Bone marrow involvement

Treatment with rituximab:

NO. OF RISK FACTORS	3-YEAR PROGRESSION-FREE SURVIVAL	5-YEAR PROGRESSION-FREE SURVIVAL
0 Low risk	91%	80%
1–2 Intermediate risk	69%	51%
3–5 High risk	51%	19%

SOURCE: From Federico M, Bellei M, Marcheselli L, et al. Follicular Lymphoma International Prognostic Index 2: A new prognostic index for follicular lymphoma developed by the International Follicular Lymphoma Prognostic Factor Project. *J Clin Oncol.* 2009;27(27):4555–62. Reprinted with permission. © 2009 American Society of Clinical Oncology. All rights reserved.

is optimal in treatment of FL, the addition of rituximab to front-line chemotherapy appears to improve response rates, remission duration, progression-free survival, and overall survival compared to treatment regimens without rituximab, and addition of rituximab as "maintenance" therapy after initial front-line chemoimmunotherapy improves progressive free survival. Limited stage (I–II) FL is treated with radiotherapy. Alternative approaches include radiolabeled anti-CD20 antibodies (e.g., ibritumomab conjugated to Yttrium-90 or tositumomab conjugated to Iodine-131), high-dose chemotherapy followed by autologous stem cell transplant, and nonmyeloablative allogeneic stem cell transplant, all of which have been used effectively in relapsed, treatment-refractory, or previously untreated FL (Gribben, 2007). Autologous and allogeneic stem cell transplantation has also been implemented as consolidative therapy for patients in first remission after front-line therapy. Notably, treatment practices for FL vary considerably among clinicians across the United States, reflecting regional and institutional variation, along with patient preferences.

B-cell Small Lymphocytic Lymphoma

B-cell small lymphocytic lymphoma (B-SLL) is the lymphomatous counterpart of chronic lymphocytic leukemia (CLL). CLL is the most common adult leukemia in the Western world (Swerdlow et al., 2008).

Pathologic features: CLL/B-SLL is characterized by a monomorphic population of small round lymphocytes that invade multiple tissues, including peripheral blood, lymph nodes, and bone marrow. The malignant cells have a unique immunophenotype (CD5+ CD23+ CD19+ CD20^{weak} surface Ig+) requiring that flow cytometry or other immunohistochemical studies be used to establish the diagnosis. Of the various cell surface markers, CD5 positivity is conceptually important as it necessitates distinction between CLL (CD5+ CD23+) and mantle cell lymphoma (CD5+ CD23–). CLL is defined by a malignant population of CLL cells with a circulating absolute lymphocyte count of at least 5000/mL. B-SLL is diagnosed when there is lymph node involvement by CLL cells with a circulating absolute lymphocyte count of <5000/mL. The premalignant condition of monoclonal B cell lymphocytosis is defined by the presence of circulating CLL cells with an absolute lymphocyte count of 4000–5000/mL and no evidence of lymph node or other organ involvement. Examination of the peripheral blood smear characteristically shows an increased number of lymphocytes; smudge cells, representing lymphocytes smashed in the smear-making process (figure 15.5); and in some cases, a small population of large, irregularly shaped precursor prolymphocytes.

Clinical course: The median age of CLL/B-SLL is 65. There is a strong correlation with family history; no known environmental, radiation, or drug associations have been definitively demonstrated. The most commonly used staging system is the Rai staging system, with stage 0 disease defined by lymphocytosis; stage I, lymphadenopathy; stage II, hepatosplenomegaly; stage III, anemia; and stage IV, thrombocytopenia. Median survival ranges from 19 to 150 months, depending on Rai stage. High-risk clinical features, in addition to advanced Rai stage, include systemic symptoms, progressive lymphadenopathy or splenomegaly, a 50% increase in circulating lymphocyte count over a 2-month period, and a doubling of absolute lymphocyte count in less than 6–12 months. High-risk molecular markers include absence of somatic hypermutation in the Ig heavy-chain variable region; deletion of 11q23; deletion of 17p or mutation of the p53 gene located on chromosome 17p; CD38 positivity; increased expression of thymidine kinase; and expression of ZAP-70. The most significant favorable molecular prognostic feature is the presence of a deletion in 13q as the sole chromosomal abnormality.

Three clinical features specific to CLL/B-SLL merit discussion. First, patients with CLL/B-SLL may develop AIHA or ITP. (Of note, only nonimmune anemia or thrombocytopenia meets criteria for stage III or IV disease in the Rai staging system.) Purine analogs, used as therapy in CLL/B-SLL, further increase the risk of these phenomena (see Treatment, below) (Weiss et al., 1998). AIHA in CLL is predominantly a warm agglutinin (IgG-mediated) disease, although cold agglutinin (IgM-mediated) disease can occur. Second, patients with CLL/B-SLL have an increased risk of infection due to hypogammaglobulinemia, CLL/B-SLL-mediated immune dysfunction, and the immunosuppressive effects of purine analog treatment. Prophylactic intravenous immune globulin (IVIG) decreases the infectious rate in CLL/B-SLL patients with recurrent bacterial infections. Third, roughly 5% of CLL/B-SLL patients develop a Richter transformation into DLBCL, which carries a poor prognosis

(see DLBCL discussion above, section on Clinical Course). A smaller percentage transform into HL.

Treatment: Treatment of CLL/B-SLL is indicated for Rai stage III or IV disease; symptoms related to disease, including painful lymphadenopathy or B symptoms; high-risk clinical features (enumerated above); recurrent infections; AIHA; or ITP. High-risk molecular features alone are not an indication for treatment. Similarly, asymptomatic patients with Rai stage I or II disease do not require treatment. Historically, chlorambucil, an alkylating agent, was the standard of care for treatment of CLL/B-SLL. In the past decade, the purine analog fludarabine and fludarabine-containing therapies (e.g., FCR (fludarabine, cyclophosphamide, rituximab)) have emerged as first-line therapy for CLL/B-SLL; bendamustine with or without rituximab is another widely-used first-line therapy. Purine analogs exhibit a number of specific side effects, including persistent neutropenia, CD4+ T cell lymphopenia, and an increased risk of infections; AIHA and, rarely, ITP, may also be associated. These same regimens may also be used for relapsed or treatment-refractory disease (Gribben, 2007). Alemtuzumab (Campath), a monoclonal antibody against the CD52 antigen expressed on the surfaces of all mature lymphocytes, has favorable activity in first-line treatment of CLL/B-SLL, particularly in cases with unfavorable cytogenetic abnormalities (i.e., deletions of 11q23 or 17p), although its efficacy is limited in nodal disease; the major side effect of alemtuzumab is infection, with a 50% rate of CMV reactivation. The second-generation, humanized, anti-CD20 monoclonal antibody ofatumumab is another option for CLL that is refractory to fludarabine and alemtuzumab. Nonmyeloablative allogeneic stem cell transplant may be effective in patients with treatment-refractory disease and is the only effective cure for CLL (Gribben, 2007).

Lymphoplasmacytic Lymphoma

Lymphoplasmacytic lymphoma (LPL), more commonly referred to as Waldenstrom macroglobulinemia (WM), is a B-cell lymphoproliferative disease in which the malignant cells are morphologically and immunophenotypically intermediate between lymphocytes and plasma cells. LPL/WM cells secrete IgM, which forms pentavalent aggregates that cause hyperviscosity symptoms, including bleeding (particularly epistaxis), ocular abnormalities (e.g., blurring, retinal hemorrhages, retinal vein thrombosis, and tortuous retinal vessels), cryoglobulinemia, and cold agglutinin AIHA. LPL/WM may also be associated with amyloidosis, peripheral demyelinating neuropathy, and an increased risk of infections. All patients have marrow involvement; 20–30% have lymphadenopathy and/or hepatosplenomegaly. As with FL, CLL, and other indolent lymphomas, treatment of LPL/WM is deferred for asymptomatic patients. For those with symptomatic or progressive LPL/WM, plasmapheresis is used for control of hyperviscosity symptoms; rituximab, fludarabine, steroids, the nuclear factor kappa-B inhibitor bortezomib (Velcade), and combinations of these with other chemotherapy agents (e.g., fludarabine/rituximab with or without cyclophosphamide, RCVP, RCHOP, bortezomib/rituximab, bortezomib/dexamethasone/rituximab) have all been successfully used (Treon, 2009). Of note, treatment with rituximab-containing regimens may precipitate an IgM flare, particularly if single-agent rituximab is used (Treon, 2009).

Mantle Cell Lymphoma

Mantle cell lymphoma (MCL) comprises 3–10% of all NHLs (Swerdlow et al., 2008). It has an aggressive clinical course despite its classification as an indolent NHL.

Pathologic features: MCL consists of small- or medium-sized B cells that resemble CLL, FL, or marginal zone lymphoma. Immunophenotypically, MCL cells express CD5, necessitating distinction from CLL/B-SLL (see CLL/B-SLL above, in section on Pathologic Features). The most important molecular feature of MCL is translocation t(11;14), which positions the cell cycle gene cyclin D1 on chromosome 11 next to the Ig heavy chain locus, leading to overproduction of cyclin D1.

Clinical course: MCL is a disease of older men, with a median age of 63. Roughly 70% present with stage IV disease, including over 60% with bone marrow infiltration. A substantial proportion of patients have gastrointestinal involvement, some with intestinal polyposis, prompting routine endoscopy of such patients at many academic centers (Salar et al., 2006). Historical studies showed median survivals on the order of 3 to 4 years; prognosis has improved with newer therapies, particularly with incorporation of high-dose chemotherapy and autologous stem cell transplant. A high Ki-67 index in MCL is a prognostic marker of aggressive disease. A minority of patients may develop an aggressive variant known as blastoid MCL characterized by a high proliferative index and circulating MCL cells with a blast-like appearance.

Treatment: Standard treatment for MCL is either intensive chemotherapy (e.g., hyper-CVAD), or combination chemotherapy with rituximab (e.g., RCHOP) followed by high-dose chemotherapy and autologous stem cell transplant. Bortezomib, inhibitors of the mammalian target of rapamycin (mTOR) pathway (e.g., temsirolimus), and allogeneic stem cell transplant have also been used, particularly in relapsed or treatment-refractory disease.

Marginal Zone Lymphomas

The marginal zone lymphomas (MZL) include splenic MZL with or without villous lymphocytes, extranodal MZL of MALT type, and nodal MZL. The classic pathologic description of MZL is of malignant B cells with lymphoplasmacytic differentiation (similar to LPL/WM) that are immunophenotypically negative for multiple cell-surface markers (e.g., CD5– CD10– CD23–), except for major B-cell markers such as CD20+ and CD79a+.

Splenic MZL is a disease of older men. Patients present with massive splenomegaly; 40% have hepatomegaly. Most patients have bone marrow involvement. Lymphadenopathy is rare. The disease is associated with HCV infection. Median survival is greater than 10 years. First-line treatment is splenectomy, which is beneficial in relieving abdominal symptoms and cytopenias; single agent rituximab may be used in patients not appropriate for splenectomy.

Extranodal MALT lymphoma consists of a heterogeneous population of B lymphocytes and plasma cells occupying MALT sites distributed throughout the body. Anatomic involvement is varied and is frequently associated with local inflammation or infection. The most common site of disease is the gastrointestinal tract (a.k.a. "gastric MALToma"), particularly the stomach in association with *H. pylori* infection. Other sites include the thyroid, ocular adnexa, lungs, salivary gland, and breast. Local lymph node involvement is common; one-third of patients have monoclonal gammopathy. First-line treatment of *H. pylori* + gastric MALToma is antibiotics, which induces remission in the majority of cases. For other disease sites, chemotherapy or local radiation may be used.

Nodal MZL is similar to extranodal MALToma except that the disease is restricted to lymph nodes and, in many cases, the bone marrow, without other extranodal involvement. Management is similar to that of FL.

HODGKIN LYMPHOMA

Compared to NHL, HL is a far less common disease, with over 8000 new cases and approximately 1300 deaths in the United States each year.

CLINICAL PRESENTATION OF HL

Epidemiology

HL has a bimodal age distribution, with one peak presenting between the ages of 15 and 34, another peak over age 50, and a median age in the mid-20s (Swerdlow et al., 2008). An increased incidence is observed in industrialized countries and among persons of increasing socioeconomic status. A minority of cases are associated with EBV or with HIV. Correlations with family history and HLA genotype have also been reported.

Systemic Symptoms

As with NHL, the most important systemic symptoms in HL are B symptoms. The classic B symptom is Pel-Ebstein fever, a cyclic fever occurring in intervals of 1 to 2 weeks. Two additional, albeit uncommon, symptoms characteristic of HL are pruritus without rash and pain after alcohol consumption, the latter localized to sites of disease.

Patterns of Lymph Node Involvement

The most common presentation of HL is of a young person with painless lymphadenopathy in the neck. Cervical or supraclavicular lymph nodes are involved in 75% of cases, followed by mediastinal, paraaortic, axillary, and inguinal nodes (in order of decreasing frequency). HL spreads anatomically through contiguous lymph nodes, infiltrating the spleen before spreading systemically and invading the bone marrow, as reflected by the Ann Arbor staging system.

EVALUATION OF HL

The evaluation of HL is similar to that of NHL and includes physical examination, with careful attention to peripheral lymph nodes and hepatosplenic enlargement, laboratory evaluation, radiographic imaging, and tissue analysis. All patients with HL should have a comprehensive metabolic panel, a complete blood count with a peripheral blood differential, and erythrocyte sedimentation rate, the latter of which is prognostic in early stage (I–IIA) HL. HL may be associated with a number of laboratory abnormalities, including anemia, leukocytosis, lymphopenia, monocytosis, and hypoalbuminemia. LDH is rarely elevated in advanced-stage HL and is therefore not routinely checked in the evaluation of HL. The imaging study of choice in the workup of HL is a whole-body PET/CT scan, which is integral in initial staging and response assessment in HL. An excisional biopsy of an involved lymph node is the gold standard for tissue evaluation. Bone marrow biopsy may be performed under certain circumstances.

STAGING OF HL

Staging of HL uses the Ann Arbor staging system (table 15.1).

CLASSIFICATIONS OF HL

The WHO recognizes two distinct disease entities of HL: classical HL and nodular lymphocyte-predominant HL (NLPHL). The former includes the histologic subtypes of nodular sclerosis, lymphocyte-rich, mixed cellularity, and lymphocyte-depleted HL.

PATHOLOGY OF HL

The neoplastic cell in classical HL is the Reed-Sternberg (RS) cell, characterized by a bilobed ("owl's eyes") nucleus (see figure 15.5). RS cells are of B-cell origin but have an unusual immunophenotype (CD20+/− CD15+ CD30+). Histologically, RS cells occupy only a very small fraction of the total cellularity of an involved lymph node, rendering full excisional lymph node biopsy essential in diagnostic evaluation. In nodular sclerosis HL, RS cells are scattered among a fibrous nodular architectural pattern, whereas in the other histologic subtypes of classical HL, varying degrees of infiltration by other lymphocytes are seen. The neoplastic cell in NLPHL is a variant of the RS cell known as the popcorn or lymphocyte predominant (LP) cell, with an immunophenotype (CD20+ CD15− CD30−) that differs from classical RS cells (Lee and LaCasce, 2009).

TREATMENT OF CLASSICAL HL

In the modern era treatment of classical HL utilizes a combination of chemotherapy and limited radiation fields (figure 15.7) (Borchmann and Angert, 2010; National Comprehensive Cancer Network, 2011). Advanced-stage (IIB–IV) classical HL is treated with chemotherapy alone; radiation may be added to sites of bulky disease or in cases where a partial rather than complete remission is achieved. Prognosis in advanced HL is gauged by the International Prognostic Score (IPS), comprising seven factors that predict poor prognosis (see table 15.4) (Hasenclever and Diehl, 1998). Forty to 85% of patients with advanced-stage classical HL achieve long-term disease control with standard chemotherapy, depending on IPS risk factors. Early stage (I–IIA) classical HL is typically treated with a combination of chemotherapy and radiation; chemotherapy alone may alternately be used in many centers (Borchmann and Angert, 2010). More than 85% of patients with early stage classical HL will be cured following initial therapy. PET/CT scans are performed in the middle of therapy to assess the interim response (which may have prognostic value, although this is controversial) and at the end of therapy. The use of interim PET/CT scans to guide decisions regarding therapy is presently under investigation (Borchmann and Angert, 2010). Complete remission is gauged by the end-of-treatment PET/CT scan, using the same criteria as for DLBCL (see DLBCL above, in section on Treatment). HL patients in first remission are frequently subjected to routine surveillance CT scans, although surveillance radiography in HL is costly and is associated with significant radiation exposures. Relapsed or treatment-refractory classical HL is treated with a combined approach of salvage chemotherapy followed by high-dose chemotherapy, autologous stem cell transplant, and radiation therapy; alternately, such patients may be evaluated for clinical trials.

Chemotherapy Regimens

The first successful combination chemotherapy regimen in classical HL was MOPP (nitrogen mustard, vincristine, procarbazine, and prednisone), which cured approximately half of patients with advanced disease. Long-term toxicities, including infertility and secondary leukemia, eventually led to the replacement of MOPP by the more effective and less toxic regimen of ABVD (doxorubicin, bleomycin, vinblastine, and dacarbazine). Two other, more intensive

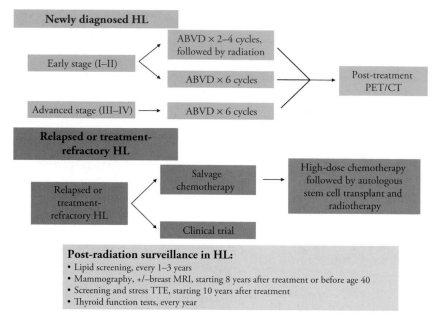

Figure 15.7. Treatment of Hodgkin's Lymphoma (HL). From National Comprehensive Cancer Network (2011), www.nccn.org; Ng et al. (2010).

chemotherapy regimens currently in use are BEACOPP (bleomycin, etoposide, Adriamycin, cyclophosphamide, vincristine, procarbazine, and prednisone), used in Germany; and the Stanford V regimen (doxorubicin, vinblastine, mechlorethamine, vincristine, bleomycin, etoposide, and prednisone), used at Stanford University. Both regimens incorporate radiation therapy for bulky disease (Borchmann and Angert, 2010). Recent clinical trials have found no difference in outcomes of patients with early- or advanced-stage HL treated with either Stanford V or ABVD.

LONG-TERM CONSEQUENCES OF RADIATION THERAPY

Radiation therapy to the chest, particularly when administered in a "mantle distribution" encompassing the mediastinum and thorax, has been associated with extensive long-term toxicities, including secondary malignancies (e.g., leukemia and cancers of the breast, lung, and thyroid), cardiac disease (congestive heart failure, early coronary artery disease, valvular heart disease, arrhythmias, and pericarditis), hypothyroidism, and lung disease (radiation pneumonitis and pulmonary fibrosis) (Ng et al., 2010). The importance of long-term complications from thoracic radiation is underscored by the observation that deaths from radiotherapy-related complications ultimately exceed those from relapsed HL in recipients of mantle radiation. Significant efforts have been made in the modern era to limit radiation fields in HL patients who require radiotherapy. Recipients of mantle or other thoracic radiation are advised to undergo comprehensive surveillance for secondary malignancies and for cardiovascular and pulmonary disease (figure 15.7) (Ng et al., 2010).

TREATMENT OF NLPHL

For NLPHL, early-stage (I–IIA) disease is treated with radiation, whereas advanced-stage (IIB–IV) disease is treated with chemotherapy with or without radiation. Rituximab may have a therapeutic role, owing to CD20 expression by LP cells. The

Table 15.4 INTERNATIONAL PROGNOSTIC SCORE FOR ADVANCED (STAGE IIB–IV) HODGKIN LYMPHOMA

INTERNATIONAL PROGNOSTIC SCORE FOR ADVANCED HL

Adverse factors (WALMASH):	Elevated WBC Young age Lymphopenia Male gender Low albumin Stage IV disease Low hemoglobin

Treatment with combination chemotherapy, with or without radiation:

NO. OF RISK FACTORS	5-YEAR FREEDOM FROM PROGRESSION	5-YEAR OVERALL SURVIVAL
0	84%	89%
1	77%	90%
2	67%	81%
3	60%	78%
4	51%	61%
5 or more	42%	56%

SOURCE: Reprinted with permission from Hasenclever D, Diehl V. A prognostic score for advanced Hodgkin's disease. International Prognostic Factors Project on Advanced Hodgkin's Disease. *N Engl J Med.* 1998;339(21):1506–14. Copyright © 1998 Massachusetts Medical Society. All rights reserved.

clinical course of NLPHL is generally favorable, particularly for early stage disease (Lee and LaCasce, 2009).

ADDITIONAL READING

Armitage JO. How I treat patients with diffuse large B cell lymphoma. *Blood.* 2007;110(1):29–36.

Blum KA, Lozanski G, Byrd JC. Adult Burkitt leukemia and lymphoma. *Blood.* 2004;104(10):3009–20.

Borchmann P, Engert A. Clinical advances in Hodgkin lymphoma. The past: What we have learned in the last decade. *Hematology Am Soc Hematol Educ Program.* 2010;101–7.

Federico M, Bellei M, Marcheslli L, et al. Follicular lymphoma international prognostic index 2: A new prognostic index for follicular lymphoma developed by the International Follicular Lymphoma Prognostic Factor Project. *J Clin Oncol.* 2009;27:4555–62.

Gribben JG. How I treat indolent lymphoma. *Blood.* 2007;109(11): 4617–26.

Hasenclever D, Diehl V. A prognostic score for advanced Hodgkin's disease. International Prognostic Factors Project on Advanced Hodgkin's Disease. *N Engl J Med.* 1998;339(21):1506–14.

International Non-Hodgkin's Lymphoma Prognostic Factors Project. A predictive model for aggressive non-Hodgkin's lymphoma. *N Engl J Med.* 1993;329(14):987–94.

Kadin M. Hodgkin lymphoma. *ASH Image Bank,* 2002; Image 100484.

Lazarchick J. Chronic lymphocytic leukemia: Thrombocytopenia. *ASH Image Bank,* 2001; Image 100175.

Lee AI, LaCasce AS. Nodular lymphocyte predominant Hodgkin lymphoma. *Oncologist.* 2009;14(7):739–51.

National Comprehensive Cancer Network. Clinical practice guidelines in oncology: Non-Hodgkin's lymphomas, Version 1.2011. Available at www.nccn.org.

Ng AK, Abramson JS, Digumarthy SR, et al. A 56 year-old woman with a history of Hodgkin's lymphoma and sudden onset of dyspnea and shock. *N Engl J Med.* 2010;363:664–75.

Salar A, Juanpere N, Bellosillo B, et al. Gastrointestinal involvement in mantle cell lymphoma: a prospective clinic, endoscopic, and pathologic study. *Am J Surg Pathol.* 2006;30(10):1274–80.

Sehn LH, Berry B, Chhanabhai M, et al. The revised International Prognostic Index (R-IPI) is a better predictor of outcome than the standard IPI for patients with diffuse large B cell lymphoma treated with R-CHOP. *Blood.* 2007;109(5):1857–61.

Solal-Celigny P, Roy P, Colombat P, et al. Follicular lymphoma international prognostic index. *Blood.* 2004;104(5):1258–65.

Swerdlow SH, Campo E, Harris NL, et al. *WHO Classification of Tumours of Haematopoietic and Lymphoid Tissues.* 4th ed. Lyon, France: WHO; 2008.

Treon SP. How I treat Waldenstrom's macroglobulinemia. *Blood.* 2009;114(12):2375–85.

Weiss RB, Freiman J, Kweder SL, et al. Hemolytic anemia after fludarabine for chronic lymphocytic leukemia. *J Clin Oncol.* 1998;16(5):1885–9.

QUESTIONS

QUESTION 1. Which one of the following statements about Hodgkin lymphoma (HL) is correct?

A. Nodular lymphocyte-predominant Hodgkin lymphoma (NLPHL) is characterized by large numbers of Reed-Sternberg cells.

B. Axillary lymphadenopathy is present in 75% of classical HL cases.

C. First-line treatment of advanced-stage (IIB–IV) classical HL is usually combination chemotherapy with ABVD, followed by radiation to involved nodes.

D. CT scan of the neck, chest, abdomen, and pelvis is preferred over combination whole-body PET/CT in the end-of-treatment evaluation of HL patients who complete first-line therapy due to concerns regarding excessive radiation exposures with PET/CT scans.

E. For female HL patients who receive thoracic radiation, screening mammography should begin no later than 8 years after completion of therapy.

QUESTION 2. Which one of the following statements about non-Hodgkin lymphomas (NHL) is correct?

A. Most patients with diffuse large B-cell lymphoma (DLBCL) have limited-stage (I–II) disease.

B. Patients with follicular lymphoma (FL) have a protracted clinical course, with most dying from causes other than lymphoma.

C. Mantle cell lymphoma (MCL) rarely involves the gastrointestinal tract.

D. Prophylactic intravenous immune globulin (IVIG) may decrease the risk of recurrent infections in patients with chronic lymphocytic leukemia (CLL).

E. For patients with relapsed diffuse large B-cell lymphoma (DLBCL), allogeneic stem cell transplantation is the preferred therapy.

QUESTION 3. An 80-year-old female presents with a history of a rapidly growing swelling on the left lateral border of the tongue of 1 month's duration. She reports unintentional weight loss of 15 lb in the preceding month but denies fever or drenching night sweats. Local examination shows a 4 cm × 3 cm firm nodular lesion involving the lateral margin of the left half of the tongue. Other parts of the oral cavity, oropharynx, and neck are normal, as are examinations of the lungs, heart, abdomen, and nervous system. Biopsy of the tongue lesion shows NHL. All of the following are acceptable next steps in the evaluation, EXCEPT:

A. Bone marrow aspirate and biopsy

B. Whole-body PET scan

C. CT scan of the neck, chest, abdomen, and pelvis

D. Erythrocyte sedimentation rate

E. Serum lactate dehydrogenase level

ANSWERS

1. E
2. D
3. D

16.

MULTIPLE MYELOMA

Constantine S. Mitsiades, Kenneth C. Anderson, and Paul G. Richardson

DEFINITION AND EPIDEMIOLOGY

Multiple myeloma (MM) is a clonal accumulation of malignant plasma cells (PCs) that typically produce a monoclonal immunoglobulin (Ig) (or fragment thereof), termed M-protein, detectable in the serum or urine. Despite recent advances in its treatment (median overall survival is now 5–7 years, compared to 2–3 years for patients diagnosed 10 or more years ago), MM remains incurable. Monoclonal gammopathy of undetermined significance (MGUS) is a premalignant condition in which a clonal population of plasma cells accumulates in the bone marrow (BM). MGUS is asymptomatic and does not otherwise meet diagnostic criteria for MM, but it can develop into MM, other plasma cell dyscrasia, or lymphoproliferative disease with a transformation rate of approximately 2% per year.

EPIDEMIOLOGY

MM is the second most commonly diagnosed hematologic malignancy in the Western world (with >19,000 new cases annually in the United States compared to 5000 per annum for either CLL or CML). MM represents approximately 1% of all cases of malignancy, 2% of cancer deaths, and approximately 10% of all hematologic malignancies in the United States, with a prevalence of about 60,000. The annual incidence of MM is currently approximately 4/100,000, and some data suggest a recent increase in incidence rates. This may reflect increased access and use of medical services, improved diagnostic testing, and awareness of the disease and its management rather than a true increase in incidence, as suggested by studies from Olmsted County, Minnesota. However, more recent studies from Taiwan point to a five-fold increase in the last 25 years. The median age at diagnosis is 65 years—and although patients <40 years are estimated to be about 2% of the MM patient population, MM is not exclusively a disease of the elderly in that a sizable proportion of patients are between 40 and 60. There are reports of higher incidence of MM in African Americans, Afro-Caribbeans, and Pacific Islanders compared to Caucasians, as well as higher incidence in certain other populations, and a greater age-adjusted incidence in men versus women (4% vs. 2.7%). Occupational and lifestyle-related risk factors include agricultural work, exposure to pesticides, herbicides (e.g., Agent Orange), petroleum products, wood workers, paper producers, furniture manufacturers, and healthcare workers. Families with multiple affected members have also been reported, but familial MM appears rare.

DIAGNOSTIC CRITERIA—CLINICAL PRESENTATION

A key goal in the diagnostic evaluation of a patient with possible MM is to distinguish the presence of MM (which can have nonspecific symptoms in its early stages) from other symptoms of advancing age in an otherwise healthy individual. It is also important to distinguish MM from other gammopathies and dysproteinemias (e.g., MGUS, Waldenstrom macroglobulinemia, primary amyloidosis, heavy chain disease, cryoglobulinemia, idiopathic cold agglutinin disease) or B-cell neoplasias (e.g., non-Hodgkin lymphoma). The formal diagnosis of MM (and whether it is active or smoldering) versus MGUS is based on criteria (table 16.1) related to histologic evidence of plasma cell accumulation (as PC infiltration in the BM or plasmacytomas), detection of monoclonal immunoglobulin (Ig), and the presence or absence of end-organ damage. The older Durie-Salmon classification has now been simplified by the introduction of International Myeloma Working Group criteria, which are based on the original system but easier to apply and now widely used (table 16.2).

When serologic and histologic criteria for MM are met, but a patient has no evidence of end-organ damage (hypercalcemia, renal insufficiency, anemia, or skeletal lesions) and/or symptoms attributable to MM, then the condition is defined as smoldering MM (SMM) or asymptomatic MM. SMM has a 10–20%/year risk of progression to symptomatic MM.

Table 16.1 CRITERIA FOR MM DIAGNOSIS

MAJOR CRITERIA	MINOR CRITERIA
1. Plasmacytomas on tissue biopsy	a. BM plasmacytosis (10–30% PCs)
2. BM plasmacytosis (>30% PCs)	b. Monoclonal immunoglobulin (Ig) spike present, but of lesser magnitude than for Major Criterion 1.
3. Monoclonal immunoglobulin (Ig) spike on serum electrophoresis: IgG > 3.5 g/dL or IgA > 2.0 g/dL, kappa or lamda light chain excretion > 1.0 g/day on 24-hour urine electrophoresis	c. Lytic bone lesions
	d. Suppressed normal uninvolved immunoglobulins (i.e., IgM, IgA, or IgG <50, <100, or <600 mg/dL, respectively)

MM diagnosis is confirmed by any of the following:
* Any two major criteria
* Major criterion 1 + minor criteria b, c, or d
* Minor criteria a, b, and c, OR a, b, and d

SOURCE: Reprinted with permission from Durie BG. Staging and kinetics of multiple myeloma. *Semin Oncol.* 1986;13(3):300–9.

CLINICAL PRESENTATION

The diagnosis of MM should be considered in patients who present with a constellation of fatigue, bone pain, recurrent infections, and symptoms compatible with renal impairment and/or hypercalcemia (table 16.3). In the past, retrospective analyses of case series of MM patients indicated that at the time of diagnosis, 98% of patients were over 40 years old, 88% had dysproteinemia, 79% had skeletal abnormalities on x-rays, 49% had Bence Jones proteinuria, 68% reported bone pain, 62% had anemia, 55% had renal insufficiency, 30% had hypercalcemia, 21% had hepatomegaly on examination, and 5% were found to have splenomegaly. More recent studies indicate that about 70% of MM patients have anemia, and 97% have detectable M protein in the serum or urine at the time of diagnosis, with lytic lesions, osteoporosis, or fractures present in 80%. It should be noted, however, that the precise percentage of some of the presenting features may change considerably in the coming years with increased awareness about MM diagnosis and treatment as well as the trend for more widespread use of serum protein electrophoresis in routine workups that may significantly increase the proportion of patients diagnosed earlier in the course of the disease and, thus, without many of these presenting features. Conversely, the absence of these presenting symptoms does not preclude the diagnosis of MM.

STAGING SYSTEMS

The most commonly used staging systems for MM are the Durie-Salmon (D-S) system (table 16.4) and the recently developed International Staging System (ISS; table 16.5). The D-S system classifies patients according to a series of parameters that reflect tumor volume (e.g., M-protein levels, lytic bone lesions) or indirectly (impact of disease on Hb, Ca^{2+}, and renal function), whereas the ISS applies specific cutoff points to baseline albumin and beta-2-microglobulin values that identified, in retrospective evaluation of a large series of patients, three subgroups of patients with favorable (stage I), less favorable (stage III), and intermediate (stage II) prognosis in terms of their overall survival.

A large variety of candidate prognostic factors have been proposed for MM. These include plasmablastic morphology; high serum levels of beta-2-microglobulin, interleukin-6

Table 16.2 CRITERIA FOR THE CLASSIFICATION OF MONOCLONAL GAMMOPATHIES, MULTIPLE MYELOMA, AND RELATED DISORDERS: A REPORT OF THE INTERNATIONAL MYELOMA WORKING GROUP

MGUS:
    M-protein in serum <30 g/L
    Bone marrow clonal plasma cells <10% and low level of plasma cell infiltration in a trephine biopsy (if done)
    No evidence of other B-cell proliferative disorders
    No related organ or tissue impairment (no end organ damage, including bone lesions)

Myeloma-related organ or tissue impairment (end-organ damage) due to the plasma cell proliferative process
    Calcium levels increased: serum calcium >0.25 mmol/L above the upper limit of normal or > 2.75 mmol/L
    Renal insufficiency: creatinine >173 mmol/L
    Anemia: hemoglobin 2 g/dL below the lower limit of normal or hemoglobin <10 g/dL
    Bone lesions: lytic lesions or osteoporosis with compression fractures (MRI or CT may clarify)
    Other: symptomatic hyperviscosity, amyloidosis, recurrent bacterial infections (>2 episodes in 12 months)
    CRAB (calcium, renal insufficiency, anemia, or bone lesions).

Asymptomatic myeloma (smouldering myeloma)
    M-protein in serum ≥ 30 g/L and/or bone marrow clonal plasma cells ≥10%*
    No related organ or tissue impairment (no end organ damage, including bone lesions) or symptoms

(continued)

Table 16.2 (Continued)

Symptomatic multiple myeloma
  M-protein in serum and/or urine
  Bone marrow (clonal) plasma cells* or plasmacytoma
  Related organ or tissue impairment (end organ damage, including bone lesions)

Nonsecretory myeloma
  No M-protein in serum and/or urine with immunofixation
  Bone marrow clonal plasmacytosis ≥10% or plasmacytoma
  Related organ or tissue impairment (end-organ damage, including bone lesions)

Solitary plasmacytoma of bone
  No M-protein in serum and/or urine*
  Single area of bone destruction due to clonal plasma cells
  Bone marrow not consistent with multiple myeloma
  Normal skeletal survey (and MRI of spine and pelvis if done)
  No related organ or tissue impairment (no end organ damage other than solitary bone lesion)*
NOTE: *A small M-component may sometimes be present.

Extramedullary plasmacytoma
  No M-protein in serum and/or urine*
  Extramedullary tumor of clonal plasma cells
  Normal bone marrow
  Normal skeletal survey
  No related organ or tissue impairment (end organ damage including bone lesions)
NOTE: *A small M-component may sometimes be present.

Multiple solitary plasmacytomas (± recurrent)
  No M-protein in serum and/or urine*
  More than one localized area of bone destruction or extramedullary tumor of clonal plasma cells, which may be recurrent
  Normal bone marrow
  Normal skeletal survey and MRI of spine and pelvis if done
  No related organ or tissue impairment (no end organ damage other than the localized bone lesions)
NOTE: *A small M-component may sometimes be present.

Plasma cell leukemia (PCL)
  Peripheral blood absolute plasma cell count of at least $2.0 \times 10^9/L$ and >20% plasma cells in the peripheral blood differential
    white cell count
  PCL may be primary (when it presents in the leukemic phase) or secondary (leukemic transformation of a previously recognized MM);
    approximately 60% of patients with PCL have the primary type

(IL-6), lactate dehydrogenase (LDH), or C-reactive protein (CRP); increased plasma cell labeling index (PCLI); abnormal karyotype of MM cells in metaphase, such as chromosome 13 deletion; cell surface markers on MM cells (e.g., CD56); serum levels of cytokines such as HGF, soluble IL-6 receptor (sIL-6R), and syndecan-1 (CD138), as well as low serum hyaluronate levels; presence of Ras or p53 mutations in MM cells; detection of malignant plasma cells in the peripheral blood (especially when the absolute count is ≥2000, which defines plasma cell leukemia); as well as various sets of transcripts identified by oligonucleotide microarray analysis of MM cells—all of these have been previously proposed in at least one study to correlate with inferior clinical outcome in MM and/or to have significant differences between MM patients with early-stage disease versus advanced MM.

Although some of these parameters (such as beta-2-microglobulin, cytogenetics, and, in some centers, PCLI) are routinely used in the workup of MM patients, the optimal set of markers for prognostication in MM patients remains to be defined not only because of the continuum of change in the methods for evaluation of these markers but also

because of the evolution in the paradigm of MM therapy. For instance, chromosome 13 deletion, which is associated with inferior outcome to conventional anti-MM treatments

Table 16.3 DIAGNOSTIC WORKUP IN PATIENTS WITH SUSPECTED MM

History and physical examination
Hb, WBC with differential count, platelets
Serum creatinine, Ca^{2+}, uric acid, beta-2-microglobulin, albumin
Serum C-reactive protein, lactate dehydrogenase values (useful but not required for formal diagnosis)
Radiographic skeletal survey (including humeri and femurs)
MRI of the thoracolumbar spine (especially in the presence of symptoms, such as back pain)
CT imaging of the chest and abdomen (including PET/CT if appropriate)
Serum protein electrophoresis with immunofixation
Quantification of immunoglobulins
Serum free light-chain (sFLC) determination
BM aspirate and biopsy
Urinalysis
Electrophoresis and immunofixation of an adequately concentrated aliquot from a 24-hour urine specimen
If available, cytogenetics, FISH of BM

Table 16.4 DURIE-SALMON MYELOMA STAGING SYSTEM CRITERIA

STAGE I	STAGE II	STAGE III
All of the following: • Hb >10 g/L • Serum Ca²⁺ normal(<12 mg/dL) • X-rays: normal bone structure or solitary bone plasmacytoma only • Low M-component production rates IgG value <5 g/dL IgA value <3 g/dL Urine light chain M-component on electrophoresis <4 g/24 hours	Overall data are minimally abnormal as shown for stage I and no single value as abnormal as defined for stage III	One or more of the following: • Hb <8.5 g/L • Serum Ca²⁺ >12 g/dL • Advanced lytic bone lesions (scale 3) • High-M-component production rates IgG value >7 g/dL IgA value >5 g/dL Urine light-chain M-component on electrophoresis >12 g/24 hours

Subclassification:
A = relatively normal renal function (serum creatinine value <2.0 mg/dL).
B = abnormal renal function (serum creatinine >2.0 mg/dL).

such as glucocorticoids and standard or high-dose cytotoxic chemotherapy, does not confer an adverse prognostic role in patients treated with bortezomib. This further supports the concept that the association of a potential prognostic marker with a clinical outcome is dependent on the treatment that is being administered. As the therapeutic algorithm for MM continues to evolve with the introduction of new drug classes (for example, thalidomide, its analogues, and proteasome inhibitors such as bortezomib), the role of various prognostic markers will have to be evaluated in prospective studies of patients homogeneously treated with regimens that include these new forms of treatment.

GENERAL ALGORITHM FOR THERAPEUTIC MANAGEMENT

Patients with MGUS or asymptomatic (smoldering) myeloma can be observed, often for years, without need for treatment, although it is important to note that the latter group are at a significantly higher risk of progression to symptomatic disease. There are no data thus far to indicate that early treatment of asymptomatic MM patients can prolong overall survival, but some studies have suggested clinical benefit from the use of bisphosphonates, especially in patients with very early bone disease and/or osteopenia.

Table 16.5 INTERNATIONAL STAGING SYSTEM STAGE CRITERIA

STAGE	BETA-2-M AND ALBUMIN LEVELS	MEDIAN SURVIVAL (MONTHS)
I	Beta-2-M <3.5 mg/L Albumin ≥3.5 g/dL	62
II	Neither stage I nor III*	44
III	Beta-2-M ≥5.5 mg/L	29

NOTES: * There are two subcategories for stage II: serum beta-2-microglobulin <3.5 mg/L but serum albumin <3.5 g/dL; and serum beta-2-microglobulin 3.5 to <5.5 mg/L irrespective of the serum albumin level.

A key question in the therapeutic management of a newly diagnosed symptomatic MM patient pertains to his/her eligibility for autologous stem cell transplant (auto-SCT).

Transplant-eligible patients can be treated with a variety of regimens, the choice of which is dictated by the goal of decreasing the pretransplant tumor burden so that the steep dose-response curve of myeloablative doses of alkylation in the transplant's conditioning regimen can maximize the depth and durability of disease control. Patients' recovery from the transplant depends on the rapid reengraftment of reinfused autologous stem cells, which in turn depends on their quantity and quality at their pretransplant collection. Consequently, the induction treatment for a transplant-eligible patient should be conducted with agents that impose the minimum damage to hematopoietic stem cells. This is not a requirement for patients ineligible for transplant, and, depending on the patient's hematopoietic reserve, stem-cell-targeting drugs such as melphalan can be an important part of treatment.

Eligibility for auto-SCT is determined in many institutions by an age cutoff of 65 years or above, especially in Europe. However, this limit can seem arbitrary because patients in their late 60s or older may also be transplant-eligible if they are relatively healthy. Insufficient functional reserve for the liver (e.g., direct bilirubin >2.0 mg/dL) or kidneys (e.g., serum creatinine >3.0 mg/dL), pulmonary insufficiency, or Eastern Cooperative Oncology Group (ECOG) performance status 3 or 4 (unless due to bone pain), or New York Heart Association functional status class III or IV confer a high risk of complications with transplant and are usually considered not compatible with successful SCT, although younger and otherwise well dialysis-dependent patients can be transplanted at selected SCT centers where the requisite expertise may reside.

RESPONSE CRITERIA

The response of MM patients to a given therapy is assessed on the basis of decrease in the serum and/or urine levels of M-protein produced by the MM cells. The two main systems of criteria used for evaluation of response are the Blade criteria (table 16.6) and the recently developed International Myeloma Working Group uniform response criteria (table 16.7).

KEY DRUG CLASSES USED FOR MM THERAPY

Established Conventional Agents (Glucocorticoids, Alkylators, Anthracyclines)

Until the late 1990s, MM treatment, at all stages of the disease, was based on combinations of glucocorticoids and DNA-damaging chemotherapy, specifically alkylators (such as melphalan, cyclophosphamide) and anthracyclines (doxorubicin/adriamycin). Melphalan-prednisone was shown to be as active and effective as the more complex combinations of multiple chemotherapeutics with glucocorticoids that were becoming the mainstay for transplant-ineligible patients. The VAD combination (vincristine, adriamycin, dexamethasone [Dex]) was also used, primarily as induction therapy for the transplant-eligible patient and to achieve more rapid reduction of tumor burden when deemed clinically necessary. The biggest proportion of the tumor-debulking properties of these regimens was attributed

Table 16.6 **CRITERIA FOR RESPONSE**

RESPONSE	CRITERIA FOR RESPONSE
Complete response (CR)	Requires all of the following: Disappearance of the original monoclonal protein from the blood and urine on at least two determinations for a minimum of 6 weeks by immunofixation studies <5% plasma cells in the bone marrow on at least two determinations for a minimum of 6 weeks. No increase in the size or number of lytic bone lesions (development of a compression fracture does not exclude response). Disappearance of soft tissue plasmacytomas for at least 6 weeks.
Partial response (PR)	PR includes patients in whom some, but not all, criteria for CR are fulfilled providing the remaining criteria satisfy the requirements for PR. Requires all of the following: 50% reduction in the level of serum M-protein for at least two determinations 6 weeks apart If present, reduction in 24-hour urinary light-chain excretion by either >90% or to <200 mg for at least two determinations 6 weeks apart. ≥50% reduction in the size of soft tissue plasmacytomas (by clinical or applicable radiographic examination, i.e., two-dimensional magnetic resonance imaging or CT scan) No increase in size or number of lytic bone lesions (development of compression fracture does not exclude response)
Minimal Response (MR)	MR includes patients in whom some, but not all, criteria for PR are fulfilled providing the remaining criteria satisfy the requirement for MR. Requires all of the following: ≥25% to <50% reduction in the level of serum monoclonal protein for at least two determinations If present a 50%–89% reduction in 24-hour light-chain excretion, which still exceeds 200 mg/24 hours for at least two determination 6 weeks apart 25–49% reduction in the size of plasmacytomas (by clinical or applicable radiographic examination, i.e., two-dimensional magnetic resonance imaging or CT scan) No increase in size or number of lytic bone lesions (development of compression fracture does not exclude response)
No change (NC)	Not meeting the criteria for MR or PD.
Progressive disease (PD) for patients not in CR	Requires one or more of the following: >25% increase in the level of monoclonal paraprotein, which must also be an absolute increase of at least 5 g/L and confirmed on repeat investigation 1 to 3 weeks later >25% increase in 24-hour urinary light chain excretion, which must also be an absolute increase of at least 200 mg/24 hours and confirmed on a repeat investigation in 1–3 weeks >25% increase in plasma cells in a bone marrow aspiration or on trephine biopsy, which must also be an absolute increase of at least 10% Definite increase in the size of existing lytic bone lesions or soft tissue plasmacytomas Development of new bone lesions or soft tissue plasmacytomas (not including compression fractures) Development of hypercalcemia (corrected serum Ca^{2+} >11.5 mg/dL or 2.8 mmol/L, not attributable to other causes)
Relapse from CR	Requires at least one of the following: Reappearance of monoclonal paraprotein on immunofixation or routine electrophoresis to an absolute value >5 g/L confirmed by at least one follow-up 6 weeks later and excluding oligoclonal immune reconstitution; >5% plasma cells in a bone marrow aspirate or biopsy Development of new lytic bone lesions or soft tissue plasmacytomas, or definite increase in the size of residual bone lesions (not including compression fractures) Development of hypercalcemia (corrected serum Ca^{2+} > 11.5 mg/dL or 2.8 mmol/L, not attributable to other causes)

SOURCE: Reprinted with permission from Blade J, Samson D, Reece D, et al. Criteria for evaluating disease response and progression in patients with multiple myeloma treated by high-dose therapy and haemopoietic stem cell transplantation. Myeloma Subcommittee of the EBMT. European Group for Blood and Marrow Transplant. *Br J Haematol.* 1998;102(5):1115–23.

Table 16.7 INTERNATIONAL MYELOMA WORKING GROUP UNIFORM RESPONSE CRITERIA: CR AND OTHER RESPONSE CATEGORIES

RESPONSE SUBCATEGORY	RESPONSE CRITERIA[a]
CR	Negative immunofixation on the serum and urine and Disappearance of any soft tissue plasmacytomas and ≤5% plasma cells in bone marrow[b]
sCR	CR as defined above plus Normal FLC ratio and Absence of clonal cells in bone marrow[b] by immunohistochemistry or immunofluorescence[c]
VGPR	Serum and urine M-component detectable by immunofixation but not on electrophoresis or 90 or greater reduction in serum M-component plus urine M-component <100 mg per 24 hours
PR	≥50% reduction of serum M-protein and reduction in 24-hour urinary M-protein by ≥90% or to <200 mg per 24 hours If the serum and urine M-protein are unmeasurable, a ≥50% decrease in the difference between involved and uninvolved FLC levels is required in place of the M-protein criteria If serum and urine M-protein are unmeasurable, and serum free light assay is also unmeasurable, ≥50% reduction in plasma cells is required in place of M-protein, provided baseline bone marrow plasma cell percentage was ≥30% In addition to the above listed criteria, if present at baseline, a ≥50% reduction in the size of soft tissue plasmacytomas is also required
SD	Not meeting criteria for CR, VGPR, PR or progressive disease

NOTES: Abbreviations: CR, complete response; FLC, free light chain; PR, partial response; SD, stable disease; sCR, stringent complete response; VGPR, very good partial response.

[a] All response categories require two consecutive assessments made at any time before the institution of any new therapy; complete and PR and SD categories also require no known evidence of progressive or new bone lesions if radiographic studies were performed. Radiographic studies are not required to satisfy these response requirements.

[b] Confirmation with repeat bone marrow biopsy not needed.

[c] Presence/absence of clonal cells is based upon the k/ratio. An abnormal k/ratio by immunohistochemistry and/or immunofluorescence requires a minimum of 100 plasma cells for analysis. An abnormal ratio reflecting presence of an abnormal clone is k/of >4:1 or <1;2. Alternatively, the absence of clonal plasma cells can be defined based on the investigation of phenotypically aberrant PC. The sensitivity level is 10⁻³ (less than one phenotypically aberrant PC within a total of 1000 Pc). Examples of aberrant phenotypes include (1) CD38+dim and CD56+strong and CD19– and CD45–; (2) CD38+dim and CD138+ and CD56++ and CD28+; (3) CD138+, CD19– CD56++, CD117+.

SOURCE: Reprinted from Rajkumar SV, Buadi F. Multiple myeloma: New staging systems for diagnosis, prognosis and response evaluation. *Best Pract Res Clin Haematol.* 2007;20(4):665–80, with permission from Elsevier.

to the glucocorticoid component. Melphalan (typically at 200 mg/m²) has also become a standard conditioning regimen for auto-SCT. Side effects were consistent with those of glucocorticoids and DNA-damaging chemotherapy with some important distinctions: melphalan is more stem-cell toxic than cyclophosphamide or Adriamycin, Adriamycin (and less so cyclophosphamide) can be cardiotoxic, and vincristine can cause significant peripheral neuropathy. Most patients would generally respond at least to some extent to these regimens, but resistance would invariably eventually develop. The lack of other non-cross-resistant drug classes until recently for the therapy of MM meant that regimens used at relapse were again based on steroids plus DNA-damaging agents, which resulted in a progressive decrease in the rate, depth, and durability of response seen with each successive round of salvage treatment attempted.

Novel Agents (Bortezomib, Thalidomide, Lenalidomide)

The landscape of MM treatment changed radically with the development of thalidomide (first used in the late 1990s,

and FDA approved in 2006), bortezomib (FDA approved in 2003), and lenalidomide (FDA approved in 2006). All of these drug classes not only target MM tumor cells (although with mechanisms different from classical DNA-damaging chemotherapy or from glucocorticoids) but also target the critical interaction of MM cells with the local microenvironment of the BM milieu. Thalidomide and lenalidomide have anti-angiogenic and immunomodulatory properties, although incompletely understood targeting of multiple molecular pathways. Bortezomib (formerly known as PS-341) binds to the beta5 subunit of the 20S core of the proteasome and blocks one (specifically the chymotryptic-like activity) of the three proteolytic activities of the proteasome. This activity regulates the expression and function of many regulators of tumor cell proliferation, survival, and drug resistance, and its inhibition by bortezomib kills MM cells both potently and rapidly.

Thalidomide, lenalidomide, and bortezomib share several pharmacologic features that clearly set these novel agents apart from conventional therapies:

- All three novel anti-MM agents can induce, as single agents, objective clinical responses in large proportions of patients resistant or even refractory to conventional treatment (including high-dose therapy with auto-SCT).

- When combined with conventional agents, these novel agents further improve the rates, depth, and durability of clinical responses.

- Either as single agents (bortezomib) or when combined with conventional agents (e.g., thalidomide + Dex, lenalidomide + Dex, bortezomib + melphalan-prednisone, bortezomib + liposomal doxorubicin), the novel agents offer improved rates, depth, and durability of clinical responses and, importantly, prolong overall survival of patients compared to conventional agents in randomized phase III clinical trials

- The side-effect profiles of the novel agents are distinct from those of conventional chemotherapy: Nausea, vomiting, and alopecia are typically absent, and diarrhea, although sometimes present with bortezomib (or with lenalidomide), is usually manageable. Lenalidomide can cause neutropenia/thrombocytopenia, and bortezomib can cause thrombocytopenia, but these are usually not associated with significant increase in infectious risk or clinically significant bleeding, and typically respond favorably to dose/schedule modifications, transfusion, and/or myeloid growth factor support.

Bortezomib and thalidomide use does not compromise stem cell collection, thereby allowing their use in induction regimens for transplant-eligible patients. Lenalidomide is not considered toxic to hematopoietic stem cells per se, but there are early data suggesting that its ability to modulate adhesion of hematopoietic cells in the BM could influence the yield of stem cell collection, making early stem cell collection and the use of cyclophosphamide-based mobilization (versus growth factor alone) potentially important.

Importantly, these novel agents cause certain side effects not typically associated with the conventional anti-MM agents. Thalidomide and bortezomib can both cause a significant peripheral sensory neuropathy (PN), though with some difference in their clinical features; for example, PN that is more polymorphic (with occasional facial and truncal involvement) with thalidomide, compared to the involvement of feet and then hands with centripetal progression using bortezomib.

Thalidomide also causes somnolence and constipation. Although structurally related to thalidomide, lenalidomide is devoid of significant PN, somnolence, or constipation. On the other hand, combinations of either thalidomide or lenalidomide with glucocorticoids are associated with increased risk for thromboembolic events.

Thalidomide and lenalidomide are oral agents administered typically once daily (thalidomide typically is administered at night before sleep, given its sedative properties),

whereas bortezomib is given intravenously typically twice weekly (72 hours must elapse between successive doses).

It should be noted that some of these agents (e.g., lenalidomide or bortezomib) are not available in all countries outside the United States. For instance, lenalidomide is not yet approved for use in Australia, and some restrictions exist for the use of both bortezomib and lenalidomide in the United Kingdom.

Management of Transplant-Eligible Patients in the Era of Novel Agents

For newly diagnosed MM patients <65 years who have normal renal function and are fit to undergo autologous-SCT, the procedure-related mortality is <5% and usually of the order of 1–2%. In this group of patients randomized studies have confirmed that auto-SCT offers superior clinical outcome to conventional-dose combination chemotherapy, with longer progression-free survival as well as a significant increase in median overall survival by approximately 1–2 years.

The introduction of novel agents for MM therapy has led to more available options for pretransplant induction regimens: currently available first-line therapeutic options include thalidomide plus Dex, lenalidomide plus Dex, bortezomib plus Dex, or the triple combination of bortezomib, thalidomide, and Dex (VTD), and most recently lenalidomide, bortezomib, and Dex (RVD), with response rates of PR or better in all patients (100%) treated at maximal doses.

The precise choice of regimen is determined by a series of considerations that include the extent and clinical aggressiveness of the disease (as determined by Durie-Salmon and/or ISS staging, cytogenetics, and other clinical features associated with worse outcome); the extent of bone disease (which, if pronounced, merits consideration for use of a bortezomib-based regimen); the status of concomitant end-organ dysfunction (e.g., renal insufficiency, neuropathy), and risk factors for side effects to each of the potential anti-MM agents, including thromboembolism; regional differences in practice patterns and approval status of a particular agent; as well as patient's preference for oral therapy versus regimens with infusional components. Importantly, recent randomized trials have supported the role of bortezomib therapy in any patient going forward to auto-SCT.

The role of allogeneic SCT in MM remains the topic of intense research. Allogeneic SCT following myeloablative conditioning regimens can induce molecular remissions, and, in some studies, about one-third of MM patients remain disease free for 6 years. These cases of long-term remission are attributed to the immune response of donor's lymphoid cells against the host's MM cells, termed graft-versus-myeloma (GVM) effect, and have supported the notion that allogeneic SCT, in at least a subset of patients, may have the potential to cure MM or at least provide a platform for the long-term control of the disease. However, the toxicity of fully ablative allogeneic SCT is very high, with treatment-related mortality, mostly related to infections and GVHD-related complications, of up to 50% in some studies of previously treated MM patients. As a result, allogeneic SCT is not proposed for patients older than 50–55 years. Reduced-intensity conditioning (RIC) allogeneic SCT has been developed with the goal to reduce transplant-related mortality while sustaining a GVM effect. However, RIC regimens that induce less GVHD are associated with higher rates of relapse, suggesting that the relationship between GVM and GVHD is very close and difficult to manipulate therapeutically at this point.

Management of Patients Not Eligible for Transplant

The fundamental difference in the management of transplant-ineligible MM patients, compared to those eligible for the auto-SCT procedure is that the former do not have to receive extensive alkylator-free first-line therapy. Therefore, in addition to all other possible treatment induction regimens that are applicable to transplant-eligible patients, the noneligible patients can also receive melphalan-containing combinations, such as melphalan-prednisone (MP), melphalan-prednisone-thalidomide (MPT), melphalan-prednisone-bortezomib (MPV), or melphalan-prednisone-lenalidomide (MPR). Again, the precise choice of regimen is determined by a series of considerations including: the extent and clinical aggressiveness of the disease (as determined by Durie-Salmon and/or ISS staging, cytogenetics, etc.); the extent of bone disease (which, if pronounced, merits consideration for use of a bortezomib-based regimen); the status of concomitant end-organ dysfunction (e.g., renal insufficiency where bortezomib-based therapy is currently preferred, underlying neuropathy, such that lenalidomide may be preferred) and other risk factors for side effects to each of the potential anti-MM agents; regional differences in practice patterns and approval status of a particular agent; as well as patient's preference for oral therapy versus regimens with infusional components. Again, response rates have proven dramatic with overall response rates of 90% now being reported.

Relapsed and Refractory MM

The term *relapsed myeloma* refers to patients who have initially responded to a treatment and then have disease progression. In those patients, their disease may be sensitive to a rechallenge with their last treatment, but this usually requires additional agents. Relapsed patients who develop resistance while on treatment with an active regimen (or within 60 days of completion of their last treatment) are classified as having "relapsed and refractory" or "refractory" myeloma. In the pre-thalidomide era this latter group of patients had a uniformly unfavorable outcome with short overall survival. However, with the development of novel anti-MM agents, such as thalidomide, lenalidomide, and bortezomib, the management of relapsed and refractory

MM has improved dramatically: studies of single-agent treatment with either of these three novel agents have shown that they can be active in patients with disease refractory to conventional or high-dose chemotherapy. Therefore, as the use of these newly established agents has shaped a new paradigm in the management of MM, the significance of the term "relapsed and refractory MM" also changes, because it directly depends on the specific agents to which the term applies: patients with refractoriness to conventional or high-dose chemotherapy often respond to bortezomib-, thalidomide- or lenalidomide-based therapies. Patients refractory to one of these new drug classes may still respond to one of the others, while patients refractory to multiple new agents may still respond to combinations of new and conventional agents (e.g., lenalidomide-bortezomib-dexamethasone, often called RVD, or bortezomib-thalidomide-dexamethasone, also known as VTD). Refractoriness to combinations of proteasome inhibitors and glucocorticoids with thalidomide or lenalidomide (especially if a patient is also refractory to alkylator/anthracycline treatment) now represents the most challenging clinical setting for which new treatment approaches are urgently needed.

Recent Developments and Future Perspectives from Investigational Agents

The therapeutic management of MM represents a rapidly changing field. During the span of a decade, three new agents (bortezomib, thalidomide, and lenalidomide) and two combination regimens (bortezomib plus liposomal doxorubicin, and bortezomib with melphalan and prednisone) have received FDA approval. Intensive basic and clinical research efforts are taking place to further expand the therapeutic armamentarium for this disease. Some of the many options currently explored in the clinical trial setting have yielded encouraging early results and may perhaps soon be added to the rapidly evolving standard of care. It is not possible to specifically predict which of these encouraging leads will successfully translate to FDA approval sooner and to what extent they may transform the MM field. However, some interesting themes have evolved and are likely to be central to the management of MM in the coming years: recent results from the IFM group suggest that bortezomib as part of the pre-auto-SCT regimen plays an important role in improving the auto-SCT outcome, with Italian data similarly strongly supporting its role.

Furthermore, results from the VISTA study support the use of bortezomib plus melphalan-prednisone as a major option for upfront therapy of nontransplant candidates. An ECOG trial showed that lenalidomide plus low-dose Dex is better tolerated and has better overall survival than lenalidomide combination with high-dose Dex indicating that combinations of conventional or novel agents with lenalidomide should incorporate low-dose Dex in an effort to improve response rates without conferring increased treatment-related mortality and/or morbidity. Finally, the early results from clinical trials of the triplet lenalidomide-bortezomib-Dex (RVD) indicate encouraging tolerability, high response rates, and favorable duration of responses in both the relapsed/refractory and the newly diagnosed setting, suggesting that the RVD combination may become the therapeutic backbone for other more complex combination regimens designed to improve the depth and durability of clinical responses in MM patients.

GENERAL MANAGEMENT AND SUPPORTIVE CARE

SUPPORTIVE MANAGEMENT

Anemia

Low hemoglobin (Hb) is a frequent feature at presentation but can also develop eventually during the course of the disease. The etiology can be multifactorial (BM infiltration by MM cells; anemia of chronic disease, sometimes further complicated by anemia related to MM-associated renal dysfunction). Erythropoietin (Epogen, Procrit) decreases transfusion requirements and increases Hb levels in over half of MM patients, with the higher probability of response among MM patients with low baseline serum erythropoietin levels. Most physicians proceed with a trial of erythropoietin (Epogen, Procrit), 150 U/kg three times weekly, or 40,000 U once a week. Darbepoetin, a long-lasting erythropoietin (Aranesp), may be given weekly or biweekly. Epo should be used with caution not only because of its association with increased risk for cardiovascular events in other settings, but also because its administration in thalidomide/lenalidomide patients increases the risk of thromboembolism.

It is also worth noting that monoclonal M-protein exerts an osmotic effect that (especially at high M-protein levels) tends to increase plasma volume and spuriously lower both Hb and Hct levels.

Skeletal Lesions

Bone lesions with pain and fractures (spontaneous or trauma-induced fractures) are frequently the first manifestation of MM and can also become a major problem during the disease course. MM can cause not only discrete lytic lesions but also diffuse osteopenia in areas of the skeleton macroscopically unaffected by tumor cells. The management of bone disease in MM involves skeletal radiographic surveys that should be performed at least at yearly intervals (or earlier, if new pain develops), and, for all MM patients with lytic lesions, pathologic fractures, or severe osteopenia, bisphosphonate therapy is recommended. In the United States the bisphosphonates typically chosen for MM treatment are zoledronate (zoledronic acid or Zometa, 4 mg IV over 15 minutes every 4 weeks) or pamidronate (Aredia, 90 mg IV over 2 hours

every 4 weeks). These regimens have comparable efficacy, but the shorter duration of infusion is a potential advantage of zoledronate. Bisphosphonates can cause renal dysfunction and even nephritic-range proteinuria. Therefore, the monitoring of serum creatinine and 24-hour urine protein is necessary, and the drug dose should be reduced or omitted according to the level of renal insufficiency. As MM patients now survive longer, the issue of osteonecrosis of the jaw has been recognized, making the duration and frequency of longer-term bisphosphonate therapy a matter of ongoing debate. It has been proposed that after 2 years of IV bisphosphonate, if there is no evidence of progressive skeletal disease, the frequency of doses should be adjusted to every 3 months. Moreover, once in CR, additional bisphosphonate can be deferred as long as the patient's bone disease is quiescent.

The novel agents for MM treatment (thalidomide, lenalidomide, and bortezomib) conceivably help MM bone disease by suppressing the tumor clone that triggers it as well as inhibiting osteoclast activation directly. Interestingly, bortezomib appears to have, independent of its effect on the tumor, the potent ability to suppress bone resorption (by affecting osteoclast maturation) and trigger new bone formation (by stimulating osteoblast function). As a result of these considerations, bortezomib is a reasonable option for treatment of any patient with extensive bone lesions.

In terms of other measures, vertebroplasty and/or kyphoplasty may be helpful for patients with compression fracture of the spine. Patients should be encouraged to be as active as possible because confinement to bed increases demineralization of the skeleton. Trauma must be avoided because even mild stress may result in a fracture. Fixation of long bone fractures or impending fractures with an intramedullary rod and methyl methacrylate can give excellent results.

Osteonecrosis of the Jaw

Osteonecrosis of the jaw has been reported in patients receiving bisphosphonates for MM or other cancers (incidence estimated between 1.5% among patients treated for 4–12 months to 7.7% for treatment of 37–48 months). Etiology is unclear. Complete dental evaluation and preventive dental treatments should take place before onset of bisphosphonate therapy. During bisphosphonate treatment, careful oral hygiene should be practiced, and invasive procedures, particularly dental extractions, are not recommended. Osteonecrosis of the jaw should be managed conservatively.

Renal Insufficiency

Up to 20% of MM patients have serum Cr levels >2.0 mg/dL at diagnosis. Myeloma M-protein itself (particularly light chains) and MM-related hypercalcemia are two major causes of renal impairment in this setting. Other contributing factors include dehydration (e.g., in relationship to hypercalcemia or independently of it), infection, nonsteroidal anti-inflammatory drug (NSAID) use (e.g., for relief of MM bone pain), contrast for radiographic studies, hyperuricemia, or amyloid deposition. Acute (or subacute) renal failure in MM requires prompt fluid and electrolyte replacement as well as active anti-MM treatment to decrease the tumor burden, the release of M-protein, and their impact on renal function. Although Dex, thalidomide, their combination (or even VAD, in the pre-thalidomide era) have been used for cytoreduction in the context of renal impairment, a bortezomib-containing regimen (e.g., bortezomib-Dex or bortezomib-thal-Dex) has emerged recently as a reasonable and very active option for such settings because bortezomib is not excreted renally and does not further compromise renal function as well, it exerts a rapid cytotoxic effect on MM cells, thus being more conducive to the goal for rapid cytoreduction and light chain removal. A direct protective effect of bortezomib has been hypothesized but has not yet been formally proven. The use of plasmapheresis can be attempted to prevent the need for chronic dialysis, but randomized data are conflicting in terms of benefit. Patients with symptomatic azotemia or other indications for renal replacement therapy can receive either hemodialysis or peritoneal dialysis, which have comparable efficacy in this setting. Kidney transplantation for renal failure in the context of MM has been followed by prolonged survival, but the decision to perform the procedure has to take into account the probability for long-term control as limited data so far suggest the procedure can be challenging.

In general, MM patients, and in particular those with Bence Jones proteinuria, need to maintain high fluid intake to prevent renal failure. A reasonable target for fluid intake leads to 24-hr urine volume of approximately 3 L in patients with Bence Jones proteinuria. In the event of hyperuricemia, allopurinol (at a dose of up to 300 mg daily) is an effective therapy. Computed tomography (CT) with IV contrast should be avoided.

Hypercalcemia

Hypercalcemia must be suspected in cases of MM patients with anorexia, nausea, vomiting, polyuria, constipation, weakness, confusion, stupor, or coma. If left untreated, hypercalcemia in MM patients can precipitate serious renal insufficiency. Therefore, hydration with isotonic saline and prednisone (e.g., at a dose of 25 mg orally four times daily) is effective in most patients. The dosage of prednisone must be reduced and discontinued as soon as possible. After hydration has been achieved, furosemide may be helpful, and a bisphosphonate such as zoledronic acid or pamidronate constitutes a standard of care in this setting.

Infections

Compared to the general population, MM patients are at higher risk for bacterial infections, and such infections remain the most common direct cause of death in MM patients overall.

This risk has multifactorial etiology: suppression of uninvolved immunoglobulins by high levels of M-protein, neutropenia due to BM infiltration and/or therapy, and defects in antigen-presenting function of dendritic cells (DCs). This infection risk is higher during the first 2 months after initiation of induction chemotherapy. Sinopulmonary bacterial infections are among the most common infections in MM patients.

Even if MM can be associated with suboptimal antibody response to antigen challenge, pneumococcal and influenza immunization should be given to all MM patients.

Prophylactic antibiotics may be useful, and commonly used agents include trimethoprim-sulfamethoxazole (Bactrim, Septra) or prophylactic daily oral penicillin (which may benefit patients with recurrent pneumococcal infections). Prophylactic levofloxacin has good bioavailability in sinopulmonary tissues, where infections commonly occur in MM patients, but this advantage has to be carefully weighed against the risk for emergence of fluoroquinolone resistance. Intravenous immunoglobulin (IVIG) administration may be useful for short-term treatment of recurrent infections, especially in the context of selective IgG subclass deficiency. Appropriate cultures, chest x-rays, and empirical antibiotic therapy are warranted not only for febrile MM patients but also for nonfebrile MM patients with pronounced neutropenia.

Fungal infections, particularly in the context of prolonged steroid use, are an important consideration. Finally, herpes zoster virus (HZV) has been shown to occur in MM patients receiving the agent bortezomib, possibly through effects on the immunoproteasome. Viral prophylaxis with acyclovir or its equivalent is therefore recommended.

Radiation Therapy

Palliative radiation (XRT) is used for patients with significant pain due to well-defined focal involvement of MM that does not respond to systemic pharmacological treatment. The combination of analgesics with specific therapy directed against the MM itself can also provide pain control, which may not be limited to one particular site, therefore providing an advantage over radiation therapy. The cumulative myelosuppression by radiotherapy and chemotherapy should be taken into account when considering palliative radiotherapy, but XRT can often be safely combined with thalidomide, glucocorticoids, and bortezomib.

Thromboembolic Complications

Malignancies in general can be associated with increased risk for thromboembolic events. In the setting of MM in particular these complications have been mostly treatment emergent in association with combinations of dexamethasone with thalidomide or lenalidomide. Reports suggest that this risk is increased in patients receiving erythropoietin. Conversely, the risk appears to be lower in bortezomib-containing regimens. Patients should receive low-molecular-weight heparin or warfarin in therapeutic doses. Aspirin may reduce the risk of thromboembolic complications and is an alternative in patients who cannot or do not want to receive anticoagulation.

Hyperviscosity Syndrome

Hyperviscosity syndrome can be manifested as oronasal or gastrointestinal bleeding, blurred vision, neurologic symptoms, or congestive heart failure, and it is more common with the rare form of IgM myeloma, less common with IgA myeloma, and even less common in IgG myeloma. The clinical manifestations are not directly proportional to serum viscosity measurement, but symptoms are more likely to appear when serum viscosity reaches values of >4 cP. It is important to note that in general the decision to perform plasmapheresis, which promptly relieves the symptoms of hyperviscosity, should be made on clinical grounds rather than serum viscosity level alone.

Spinal Cord Compression

This important complication should always be suspected and ruled out in MM patients with lower extremity weakness, difficulty in urinary voiding or defecation, or sudden onset of severe radicular or severe back pain. Workup must include magnetic resonance imaging (MRI) or CT, and, if diagnosis of spinal cord compression is confirmed, radiation therapy, with dexamethasone to decrease edema, is appropriate.

Emotional Support

MM patients must receive continuing emotional support. It is important to inform patients and family members of the major progress achieved in the field in recent years and the fact that there has been a consistent trend for improved survival since the introduction of new drugs and supportive measures. An increasing proportion of MM patients survive for 10 years or more. However, it is also important to remember that the disease unfortunately remains incurable. Therefore, it is necessary to establish with patients and family members an appropriate and not unrealistic level of expectation about long-term outcome, based on the clinical and laboratory evidence for each patient, as well as the responsiveness seen to therapy used. The support of medical social workers and experienced psychiatrists is invaluable, especially given the complexity of an incurable malignancy combined with the profound psychotropic effects of steroid-based therapy.

SOME CLINICAL PEARLS IN MANAGEMENT OF MM PATIENTS

- The advent of novel therapies, specifically bortezomib, lenalidomide, and thalidomide, which target the myeloma and its microenvironment, has transformed the management of this disease (see figure 16.1).

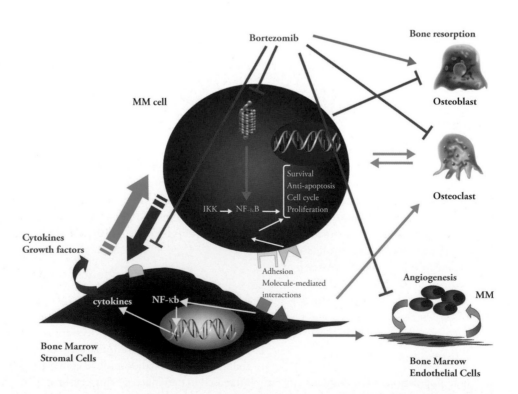

Figure 16.1. Schematic representation of how the proteasome inhibitor bortezomib, as an example of a novel anti-MM agent, influences key molecular pathways in MM cells, as well as how they interact with nonmalignant cells of the bone marrow microenvironment.

- The choice of thalidomide versus lenalidomide use in diabetics, and in other patients with neuropathy, should take into account the lack of significant neuropathy with lenalidomide use.

- Epo in MM patients may increase the risk of thromboembolic events when used with thalidomide or lenalidomide, especially when combined with steroids.

- Patients with light chain disease can be especially responsive to bortezomib and are more likely to achieve CR compared to bortezomib responders with intact monoclonal immunoglobulin.

- Serum free-light-chain (sFLC) measurement is a useful tool if careful serial measurements are followed up over time, and the test is used in patients with oligosecretory or hyposecretory disease. Sometimes it can detect a relapse earlier than conventional measurements; however, results can fluctuate considerably. Thus, it is important to interpret cautiously "spot" measurements.

- Rechallenge with novel and conventional agents (including Dex, alkylating agents, and anthracyclines) is feasible and can often be effective, especially when using combinations with a therapeutic "backbone" of proteasome inhibition (bortezomib) with thalidomide or its derivative lenalidomide (see figure 16.2.)

- It is sometimes advisable not to change treatments too rapidly in the face of mild to moderate treatment-emergent side effects: managing toxicities proactively and facilitating patients remaining on a particular regimen can be important, since duration of therapy correlates with clinical benefit, including improved response rate and increased time to disease progression.

- The use of amino-bisphosphonates in the management of myeloma-related bone involvement and hypercalcemia remains a cornerstone of disease management, but it is important to be aware of potential side effects, both short and long term.

FUTURE DIRECTIONS

The management of MM has undergone radical changes in the last 10 years, and, based on the pace of preclinical and translational research in the field, it seems very likely that more important changes will also occur over the next 5 to 10 years. Current studies with combinations of lenalidomide-bortezomib-Dex (RVD) in relapsed/refractory and up-front populations suggest that this triplet could become a backbone for treatment. The development of more complex combinations with other agents is under way, including not only established anti-MM drugs (such as alklyators and/or anthracyclines) but also other novel agents that are beginning to emerge in both the MM field and other tumor types. Examples of such newer novel agents include histone deacetylase inhibitors, second-generation proteasome inhibitors, a monoclonal antibodies, and perifosine, many of which have already shown encouraging early results when combined with backbone agents such as lenalidomide and bortezomib in advanced MM.

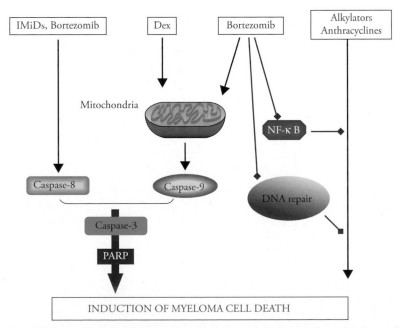

Figure 16.2. Schematic representation of how the proteasome inhibitor bortezomib can complement the molecular mechanisms of action of other anti-MM agents.

ADDITIONAL READING

Arellano-Rodrigo E. Case 23–2010: Unusual paraprotein effects in MGUS—treat or not? *N Engl J Med.* 2010;363(19):1874.

Criteria for the classification of monoclonal gammopathies, multiple myeloma and related disorders: a report of the International Myeloma Working Group. *Br J Haematol.* 2003;121(5):749–57.

Dimopoulos MA, Terpos E, Chanan-Khan A, et al. Renal impairment in patients with multiple myeloma: A consensus statement on behalf of the International Myeloma Working Group. *J Clin Oncol.* 2010;28(33):4976–84.

Kyle BA. Multiple myeloma: Review of 869 cases. *Mayo Clin Proc.* 1975;50(1):29–40.

Kyle RA, Remstein ED, Themeau TM, et al. Clinical course and prognosis of smoldering (asymptomatic) multiple myeloma. *N Engl J Med.* 2007;356(25):2582–90.

Laubach JP, Richardson PG, Anderson KC. The evolution and impact of therapy in multiple myeloma. *Med Oncol.* 2010;27(Suppl 1):S1–6.

Lin P. Plasma cell myeloma. *Hematol Oncol Clin North Am.* 2009;23(4):709–27.

Lynch HT, Ferrara K, Barlogie B, et al. Familial myeloma. *N Engl J Med.* 2008;359(2):152–7.

Mitsiades CS, Hayden PJ, Anderson KC, Richardson PG. From the bench to the bedside: Emerging new treatments in multiple myeloma. *Best Pract Res Clin Haematol.* 2007;20(4):797–816.

Mitsiades CS, Hideshima T, Chauhan D, et al. Emerging treatments for multiple myeloma: Beyond immunomodulatory drugs and bortezomib. *Semin Hematol.* 2009;46(2):166–75.

Podar K, Tai YT, Hideshima T, Vallet S, Richardson PG, Anderson KC. Emerging therapies for multiple myeloma. *Expert Opin Emerg Drugs.* 2009;14(1):99–127.

Raab MS, Podar K, Breitkreutz I, Richardson PG, Anderson KC. Multiple myeloma. *Lancet.* 2009;374(9686):324–39.

Richards T, Weber D. Advances in treatment for relapses and refractory multiple myeloma. *Med Oncol.* 2010;27(Suppl 1):S25–42.

Richardson PG, Weller E, Jagannath S, et al. Multicenter, phase I, dose-escalation trial of lenalidomide plus bortezomib for relapsed and relapsed/refractory multiple myeloma. *J Clin Oncol.* 2009;27(34):5713–9.

Richardson PG, Weller E, Lonial S, et al. Lenalidomide, bortezomib, and dexamethasone combination therapy in patients with newly diagnosed multiple myeloma. *Blood.* 2010;116(5):679–86.

QUESTIONS

QUESTION 1. All of the following are recognized side effects observed with thalidomide, EXCEPT:

A. Peripheral sensory neuropathy
B. Somnolence
C. Constipation
D. Acute kidney injury
E. Venous thromboembolic disease

QUESTION 2. All of the following statements regarding multiple myeloma are correct, EXCEPT:

A. Pathologic fractures are very common in multiple myeloma.
B. Spinal cord compression is observed in approximately one in five patients.
C. Bone marrow aspirate in MM is characterized by a lymphoplasmacytic infiltration.
D. Plasma cells in the bone marrow aspirate in patients with multiple myeloma are characterized by eccentric nuclei with clumped chromatin and a perinuclear halo.
E. Plain radiography remains a standard imaging modality procedure for staging newly diagnosed and relapsed myeloma.

QUESTION 3. Adjunctive therapy for multiple myeloma includes all of the following, EXCEPT:

A. Radiation therapy to areas of pain, impending pathologic fracture, or existing pathologic fracture
B. Bisphosphonate therapy
C. Anticoagulation in patients being treated with thalidomide
D. Prophylaxis with low-dose fluconazole to prevent fungemia
E. Vaccinations against pneumococcal organisms and influenza

ANSWERS

1. D
2. C
3. D

Thalidomide also causes somnolence and constipation. Although structurally related to thalidomide, lenalidomide is devoid of significant peripheral neuropathy, somnolence, or constipation. On the other hand, combinations of either thalidomide or lenalidomide with glucocorticoids are associated with increased risk for thromboembolic events. Lymphoplasmacytic infiltrate is a feature of Waldenstrom's macroglobulinemia, not myeloma. Fluconazole as fungal prophylaxis may be useful in patients receiving regimens containing high-dose steroids, but is not required in steroid-sparing regimens. In contrast, regimens containing bortezomib require antiviral prophylaxis against herpes zoster (e.g., acyclovir 400 mg tid).

17.

ONCOLOGIC EMERGENCIES

Edwin P. Alyea III and Daniel J. DeAngelo

Medical emergencies related to cancer are often related to: (1) the anatomic localization of the tumor resulting in obstruction or mass effect, (2) metabolic or hormonal derangements, or (3) complications of cancer therapy. Common presentations of severe oncologic complications and their treatment are discussed in this chapter.

SUPERIOR VENA CAVA SYNDROME

Superior vena cava (SVC) syndrome results from reduction in venous blood flow from the head, neck, and upper extremities caused by extrinsic compression of the venous system by a mass. The most common tumors associated with superior vena cava syndrome are lung cancer, lymphoma, and metastatic tumors. Lung cancer accounts for approximately 85% of all cases. Less common etiologies include benign tumors, thyroid enlargement, vascular abnormalities such as aneurysms and thrombosis or fibrosing mediastinitis. Rarely, vascular thrombosis due to a central line may result in an SVC-like syndrome.

Swelling of the head and neck is the most common presenting symptom in patients with SVC syndrome. Other symptoms may include cough, dyspnea, headache, pain, dizziness, nightmares, and syncope. Symptoms are often made worse by either bending forward or lying down. On examination, in addition to the facial and neck fullness, the neck veins may be dilated, and collateral vessels covering the anterior chest may be noted. In severe cases, the patient may present with tracheal or bronchial obstruction, vascular collapse, or obtundation.

Diagnosis of SVC syndrome is made on a clinical basis. Radiologic imaging of the chest may demonstrate widening of the mediastinum. Pleural effusions are present in about 25% of cases. A computed tomography (CT) scan provides the best imaging and can help define the anatomy of the obstructing lesion. In patients without a diagnosis of cancer, a biopsy is mandatory to establish a diagnosis. If the only site of disease is the mediastinal mass, a needle biopsy or preferentially a surgical

biopsy should be obtained by skilled providers. In patients with a known history of cancer, appropriate treatment may be initiated without a need for a biopsy.

Emergent treatment includes stabilization of the cardiopulmonary system. The primary treatment modality depends on the tumor histology. For patients with lung cancer, radiation therapy is the treatment of choice. In patients with lymphoma, a combination of steroids and radiation may be used. Depending on the tumor type, chemotherapy may be indicated following initial stabilization.

SPINAL CORD COMPRESSION

Prompt recognition of the signs and symptoms associated with spinal cord compression and the initiation of urgent therapy can in some cases prevent catastrophic complications such as paralysis. Epidural compression of the spinal cord resulting in cord injury is the most common etiology. Less commonly, direct extension through the foramen may occur. Metastatic tumors involving the vertebral bodies are often responsible. Common cancers with metastasis to the bone include lung, prostate, and breast cancer, as well as multiple myeloma. Compression can occur at any point along the spinal cord. The thoracic spine is the most common site, representing 70% of lesions, followed by the lumbosacral spine at 20% and the cervical spine at 10%. It is important to recognize that multiple sites of compression may be present at the same time.

The most common presenting symptom of spinal cord compression is pain. The pain may be either localized back pain or, in some cases, radicular pain caused by compression of a nerve root. Pain is usually present for days or even months prior to the development of neurologic symptoms. The importance of recognizing pain as the presenting symptom of cord compression cannot be overemphasized since the development of neurologic symptoms is ominous, and the outcome for patients with neurologic impairment is poor. Signs of cord compression on physical exam include numbness, weakness in the extremities, or loss of bladder or bowel function. Motor weakness or numbness with loss of sense to pinprick may be present. The upper limit of the sensory loss is often one or two vertebrae below the site of cord compression. Deep tendon reflexes may be brisk. In advanced cases of cord compression, an extensor plantar reflex may be present. Loss of motor and sensory function often precedes sphincter dysfunction.

If cord compression is suspected a magnetic resonance imaging (MRI) of the spine should be performed immediately to confirm or exclude the diagnosis (table 17.1). An MRI of the entire spine should be performed if possible to ascertain if there are multiple sites of disease. Myelography in addition to CT scanning may also be used when an MRI cannot be obtained. In patients with a known diagnosis of cancer, treatment should be initiated immediately. For patients without a diagnosis, a biopsy should be performed while initiating therapy.

The goals of treatment are the relief of pain and preservation of neurologic function. Most commonly, treatment of cord compression includes the administration of steroids in addition to radiation therapy. Prompt therapy is critical because outcome for patients who are ambulatory at the time of diagnosis is good. Unfortunately, for patients who have already developed paralysis at the time of diagnosis, only 10% of these patients will resume ambulation. The role of surgical intervention in the treatment of spinal cord compression has evolved over the last several years. Early studies did not demonstrate a benefit of decompressive laminectomy compared with radiation therapy alone. More recently, a randomized trial demonstrated an improved outcome for patients receiving resection and radiation therapy compared with radiation therapy alone in terms of regaining and maintaining ambulation. Given the significant complications of the surgery, careful selection of patients with a good performance status and adequate life expectancy is needed. For patients with recurrent spinal cord compression, surgery and chemotherapy may be considered. Chemotherapy is often useful only in patients with tumors that respond well to chemotherapy. The need for immediate treatment must be emphasized because pretreatment neurologic status is the most important predictor for response to therapy.

BRAIN METASTASIS

Central nervous system involvement by cancer can be found in 25% of patients. Cancers that most commonly metastasize to the brain are lung cancer, breast cancer, and melanoma. Brain metastasis often occurs in the presence of systemic disease. Brain metastasis results in significant morbidity.

Presenting signs of central nervous system involvement include headache, nausea, vomiting, seizures, and focal neurologic deficits. Behavioral changes may also be noted in some patients. Abrupt presentations resembling a stroke may occur in the setting of hemorrhage associated with metastasis. This is most common in melanoma or hypervascular tumors such as germ cell tumors and renal cell cancers. Edema resulting from metastatic lesion results in increased intracranial pressure. On exam, patients may demonstrate decreased mental alertness. They may have papilledema and neck stiffness or cranial nerve findings. Muscular weakness is also common, depending on the location of the lesion.

CT with contrast or MRI is effective in diagnosing brain metastasis. MRI is more sensitive than CT scan at identifying small lesions as well as leptomeningeal disease. Emergent treatment includes steroid administration. Steroids lead to a reduction in edema associated with the metastatic lesion and improvement in the patient's condition. In patients with multiple brain metastases, whole-brain radiation therapy should be initiated. For patients with a single brain metastasis and controlled systemic disease, surgical excision followed by radiation therapy may be considered for younger individuals. Tumors that are not responsive to radiation therapy should also be considered for resection. Stereotactic radiosurgery may be used in treating tumors that have recurred or are in an anatomically sensitive location.

PERICARDIAL EFFUSION AND TAMPONADE

The most common cancers associated with pericardial involvement include lung cancer, breast cancer, leukemia, and

Table 17.1 CORD COMPRESSION

Tumors Commonly Associated With Cord Compression
Lung
Prostate
Breast cancer
Multiple myeloma
Melanoma
Symptoms
Pain, either back pain or radicular pain
Weakness
Sensory changes
Loss of bowel or bladder function
Evaluation
Progressive pain or pain associated with neurologic symptoms → immediate MRI
Radicular pain or stable pain → MRI within 24 hours
Treatment
Steroids
Radiation therapy
Surgery in selected cases

lymphoma. Malignant pericardial disease is common and may be present at autopsy in up to 10% of patients with cancer. The patient with symptomatic pericardial disease or tamponade may present with complaints of dyspnea, cough, or orthopnea. Other signs include sinus tachycardia, jugular venous distention, hepatomegaly, and peripheral edema. Chest radiograph often demonstrates an enlarged cardiac silhouette. The electrocardiogram (EKG) may demonstrate abnormalities such as low voltage or electrical alternans. Echocardiography should be performed to confirm the diagnosis. Treatment is pericardiocentesis. Placement of a pericardial window and, in some cases, pericardial stripping may be required. Acute pericardial tamponade with hemodynamic instability is a medical emergency and requires immediate drainage.

INTESTINAL OR URINARY TRACT OBSTRUCTION

Intestinal obstruction may be a complication associated with advanced cancers, particularly colorectal, gastric, and ovarian carcinoma. Other cancers such as melanoma, breast cancer, and lung cancer that have metastasized to the abdomen can also be associated with obstruction. There are often multiple sites of obstruction present simultaneously. Symptoms of obstruction typically include pain, which is colicky in nature, or abdominal distension. Physical exam may be notable for a palpable tumor mass or distension. Treatment includes decompression. Conservative management may be used in patients with advanced cancer. In other cases, surgical correction or stent placement may be used.

Urinary tract obstruction occurs most commonly in patients with either prostate, bladder, or gynecologic cancers. Other etiologies include extrinsic compression from lymphoma and from sarcoma in the retroperitoneum. Less commonly, radiation therapy to the pelvis or retroperitoneum may result in fibrosis leading to obstruction. The most common symptom is flank pain. Patients with bilateral obstruction may develop renal failure. Treatment includes internal stent placement or percutaneous nephrostomy. In cases of bladder outlet obstruction, a suprapubic cystostomy tube may be needed for urinary drainage.

TUMOR LYSIS SYNDROME

Tumor lysis syndrome (TLS) is the collection of electrolyte abnormalities that occur as a result of the rapid release of intracellular contents into the bloodstream. TLS is characterized by hyperuricemia, hyperkalemia, hyperphosphatemia, and hypocalcemia, which may result in metabolic acidosis and acute renal failure. The release of intracellular potassium and organic as well as inorganic phosphate into the bloodstream from cells undergoing apoptosis results in the development of hyperkalemia and hyperphosphatemia,

respectively. Prolonged and severe hyperphosphatemia may result in a marked decrease of the serum calcium concentration, but symptomatic hypocalcemia rarely develops. However, hypocalcemia may develop from overzealous alkalinization, and thus one needs to exercise caution when using IV fluids with bicarbonate.

Patients with large tumor burdens are at an increased risk for TLS, especially if the tumor is chemotherapy sensitive. These disorders include acute myelogenous and lymphoblastic leukemias, especially those with high circulating blast counts, Burkitt lymphomas, and other high-grade lymphoproliferative disorders. Large bulky solid tumors that undergo rapid cellular destruction also place patients at a significant risk for the development of TLS. TLS is more common in patients with elevated LDH levels. Although extremely rare, TLS has also been described after the use of nonchemotherapy agents such as interferon-α or with hormonal therapy for breast cancer. Older patients with poor renal function are at an increased risk of developing TLS. These patients have a lower glomerular filtration rate and are more susceptible to electrolyte disturbances as compared to patients with normal renal function.

HYPERURICEMIA

Xanthine oxidase catalyzes the breakdown of hypoxanthine and xanthine to uric acid. Purine nucleotides and deoxynucleotides are broken down within the liver. The pK_a of uric acid is approximately 5.75 at 37°C. Therefore, in the serum, uric acid is present in the acid-soluble form. However, within the acidic environment of the renal tubules, uric acid may be present in the nonionized less-soluble form. Renal insufficiency may develop due to the development of uric acid crystals in the renal tubules as well as the distal renal collecting system. Nephrolithiasis due to the development of uric acid stones is uncommon and usually develops only in patients with chronic hyperuricemia. Many medications, especially diuretics such as thiazides, as well as antituberculous drugs, IV contrast dye, and certain cytotoxic agents can aggravate hyperuricemia.

The most important factor to prevent hyperuricemia is to recognize patients who are most at risk for its development and then initiate appropriate prophylactic measures (table 17.2). Drugs that elevate serum uric acid levels should be discontinued if at all possible, and intravenous hydration should be initiated, preferably prior to the start of chemotherapy. Any pre-existing intravascular volume deficits must be corrected. The main focus in the treatment of hyperuricemia is to maintain adequate urinary volume. Alkalinization of the urine will further decrease uric acid solubility, which is usually achieved by the addition of sodium bicarbonate (50–100 mmol/L) to the intravenous fluids. The admixture should be adjusted so that the urine pH is maintained above 7.0 without over alkalinizing the serum, as this will lead to hypocalcemia. The most important factor in

Table 17.2 SIGNS AND SYMPTOMS OF TUMOR LYSIS SYNDROME

LABORATORY ABNORMALITY	CLINICAL SYMPTOMS
Hyperuricemia	Nausea, vomiting, diarrhea, joint pain, oliguria, anuria, azotemia, flank pain, hematuria, crystalluria
Hyperkalemia	Muscle cramps, nausea, weakness, paresthesias, paralysis, EKG changes, bradyarrhythmias, tachyarrhythmias, cardiac arrest
Hyperphosphatemia	Oliguria, anuria, azotemia, renal failure
Hypocalcemia	Muscle twitching, tetany, laryngospasm, paresthesias, hypotension, ventricular arrhythmias, heart block

decreasing uric acid levels is the maintenance of adequate urine output; alkalinization is a secondary factor. Although furosemide increases the renal tubular reabsorption of uric acid, this is offset by the preservation of increased urinary flow rates. Therefore, furosemide can be safely used in order to maintain a proper total body fluid balance.

Allopurinol is the standard treatment for both the prevention and treatment of hyperuricemia. Allopurinol is an inhibitor of xanthine oxidase and is extremely well tolerated. The most common adverse reaction is an erythematous skin rash due to a hypersensitivity reaction. There have also been rare reports of interstitial nephritis developing after the administration of allopurinol. Allopurinol is usually administered orally at a dose of 200–300 mg/m² per day with typical doses of 300–600 mg/day with a maximum oral dose of 800 mg/day. Allopurinol is cleared renally, and the dose should be adjusted in older patients or patients with chronic renal failure. Allopurinol is also available intravenously, and the typical dose is 200–400 mg/m² per day with a maximum adult dose of 600 mg/day. Both azathioprine and 6-mercaptopurine are metabolized by xanthine oxidase; therefore, use of these agents should be avoided.

Rasburicase is a recombinant urate oxidase enzyme that catalyzes the enzymatic oxidation of uric acid into its inactive, water-soluble metabolite, allantoin. The approved dose of rasburicase is 0.15 to 0.2 mg/kg IV over 30 minutes daily for 5 days; however, lower doses of rasburicase such as a fixed dose of 6 mg have been used with excellent efficacy. Data from preclinical studies suggested that rasburicase remains active ex vivo, leading to spuriously low uric acid levels in the absence of specialized handling: sample collection in prechilled heparin tubes, transportation to the laboratory, and centrifugation at 4°C, and testing within 30 minutes. These studies were conducted using healthy donor samples spiked with rasburicase in vitro. However, an independent study of these requirements in treated patient samples has not been well established. Alkalinization is not necessary with recombinant urate oxidase therapy. Rapid and early consultation of the nephrology team should be initiated if the renal function starts to deteriorate or in the case of severe hypervolemia that is not responsive to loop diuretics.

HYPERKALEMIA

Hyperkalemia is the most important, life-threatening electrolyte abnormality that develops during tumor lysis syndrome. Hyperkalemia results from the release of large intracellular stores due to cell lysis. Pseudohyperkalemia may result from poor phlebotomy technique, hemolysis, or due to marked leukocytosis or thrombocytosis. Measuring the plasma potassium using a heparinized tube may be required in the setting of a markedly elevated platelet count.

The intracellular and extracellular potassium ion concentrations maintain the resting membrane potential. Hyperkalemia leads to the partial depolarization of the resting cell membrane potential, and prolonged depolarization will eventually lead to impaired excitability resulting in muscular weakness, which may progress to flaccid paralysis. The most serious, life-threatening manifestation of hyperkalemia is ventricular arrhythmia. Unfortunately, cardiac toxicity does not correlate with the degree of hyperkalemia. The initial EKG abnormalities include increased amplitude of the T waves, which are often referred to as "peaked" T waves. Subsequent EKG changes include prolongation of the PR and QRS intervals, A-V conduction blocks, and flattening of the P waves. Eventually the QRS complex will merge with the T wave resulting in a sine wave pattern, which will often terminate in ventricular fibrillation or asystole. Fatal hyperkalemia rarely occurs at a plasma potassium concentration <7.5 mmol/L.

The treatment of hyperkalemia largely depends on the potassium serum concentration (see figure 17.1). All patients with hyperkalemia regardless of the degree of elevation require EKG. Furthermore, medications that interfere with potassium metabolism such as nonsteroidal anti-inflammatory drugs (NSAIDs) and angiotensin-converting enzyme (ACE) inhibitors should be discontinued. Oral cation-exchange resins promote the exchange of potassium and sodium ions within the lumen of the GI tract. This is an easy and effective initial strategy for patients with mild asymptomatic hyperkalemia. A dose of 15–30 g of sodium polystyrene sulfonate will generally lower the serum potassium concentration by 0.5 to 1.0 mmol/L within 1 to 2 hours and last for about 4 hours. Severe hyperkalemia requires more emergent treatment. Calcium gluconate should be given to decrease cellular membrane excitability. The usual dose is 10 mL of a 10% solution administered over 1–3 minutes. The effect, which can be seen in minutes, is unfortunately short lived. The administration of insulin with glucose will cause potassium to shift into cells. The usual combination is 10–20 units of regular insulin with 25–50 g of glucose. Glucose should be avoided if the patient is already severely hyperglycemic. This method will typically result

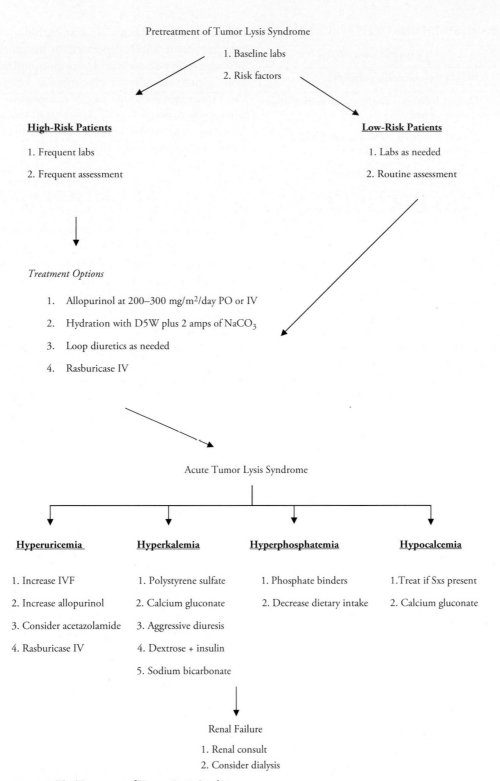

Pretreatment of Tumor Lysis Syndrome

1. Baseline labs

2. Risk factors

High-Risk Patients

1. Frequent labs

2. Frequent assessment

Low-Risk Patients

1. Labs as needed

2. Routine assessment

Treatment Options

1. Allopurinol at 200–300 mg/m²/day PO or IV

2. Hydration with D5W plus 2 amps of $NaCO_3$

3. Loop diuretics as needed

4. Rasburicase IV

Acute Tumor Lysis Syndrome

Hyperuricemia

1. Increase IVF

2. Increase allopurinol

3. Consider acetazolamide

4. Rasburicase IV

Hyperkalemia

1. Polystyrene sulfate

2. Calcium gluconate

3. Aggressive diuresis

4. Dextrose + insulin

5. Sodium bicarbonate

Hyperphosphatemia

1. Phosphate binders

2. Decrease dietary intake

Hypocalcemia

1. Treat if Sxs present

2. Calcium gluconate

Renal Failure

1. Renal consult

2. Consider dialysis

Figure 17.1. The Treatment of Tumor Lysis Syndrome.

in the lowering of the serum potassium concentration by 0.5–1.5 mmol/L and will last for several hours. Alkalinization of the serum with bicarbonate will also lead to a shift of potassium into cells. Hemodialysis and continuous venous-venous hemofiltration (CVVH) are the most effective methods for effectively lowering the serum potassium levels especially in patients with either pre-existing or acute renal failure. Peritoneal dialysis is not as effective as hemodialysis

in lowering the serum potassium level, and its initiation should be avoided in patients receiving chemotherapy.

HYPERPHOSPHATEMIA

Hyperphosphatemia results from the release of intracellular phosphate stores into the serum as a result of cell lysis and

Table 17.3 SIGNS AND SYMPTOMS OF HYPERCALCEMIA

CATEGORY	CLINICAL SYMPTOMS
Constitutional	Weight loss, anorexia, polydipsia
Neurological	Fatigue, lethargy, muscle weakness, confusion, seizure, coma
Gastrointestinal	Nausea, vomiting, constipation, ileus, abdominal pain, obstipation
Renal	Polyuria, azotemia, renal failure
Cardiac	Bradycardia, prolonged PR interval, shortened QT interval, wide T wave, arrhythmias

is defined as a serum phosphate level above 1.67 mmol/L (5.0 mg/dL). Spurious hyperphosphatemia may be seen in patients with a marked paraprotein level. Hyperphosphatemia is a potentially dangerous condition because of extraosseous calcification. Although it should only serve as guideline, a calcium-phosphorus product [serum Ca (mg/dL) × serum P (mg/dL)] >70 suggests a potential risk of metastatic calcification. Prolonged hyperphosphatemia may result in lowering the serum calcium levels. Except in those patients with renal failure, the initial treatment of hyperphosphatemia includes volume expansion (figure 17.1). This will effectively result in the increase of the fractional clearance of phosphorus by the kidney. Aluminum-based antacids bind to phosphorus in the gut and prevent further absorption. Although the chronic use of these agents may lead to aluminum toxicity, they are safe and effective for short-term use. Other phosphate binders such as calcium acetate or sevelamer may also be used. Calcium acetate is dispensed as two tablets or gelcaps (667 mg) with each meal, and the dose can be increased as long as hypercalcemia does not develop. Sevelamer, a cross-linked polyallylamine hydrochloride, is a cationic polymer that binds intestinal phosphate. The treatment of hyperphosphatemia in the setting of renal failure often requires hemodialysis.

HYPOCALCEMIA

Unlike the other metabolic alterations resulting from TLS, hypocalcemia is a direct manifestation of hyperphosphatemia. Many oncology patients will have hypocalcemia, with hypoalbuminemia as the principal cause in severely ill patients. Overalkalinization of the serum will increase the binding of calcium to proteins and result in a further reduction of the serum calcium level. In these cases, an ionized calcium level should be measured. Transient hypocalcemia may also arise from repeated transfusions of blood products due to the use of citrate as an anticoagulant. Transient hypocalcemia is seldom clinically significant, but if long-standing it can lead to several serious clinical manifestations. The QT interval on the EKG can become prolonged, which

may lead to serious ventricular arrhythmias. Rarely, patients may become irritable, depressed, or psychotic due to severe prolonged hypocalcemia. Calcium supplementation with oral calcium or calcium gluconate in severe symptomatic cases must be taken with caution, especially if the calcium-phosphate product is >70. In general, calcium should not be given in asymptomatic patients, as this may precipitate calcium phosphate deposition.

HYPERCALCEMIA

Hypercalcemia is the single most common metabolic disorder in patients with cancer. Hypercalcemia due to an underlying malignancy must be differentiated from hypercalcemia as a result of primary hyperparathyroidism. The association of elevated serum calcium with a low or normal parathyroid hormone (PTH) level excludes the diagnosis of primary hyperparathyroidism.

Serum calcium is highly bound to albumin; therefore, the total serum concentration will vary depending on serum protein concentrations. Measurement of the ionized calcium level can often assist in sorting out difficult cases. An adjustment for the total serum calcium concentration based on the serum albumin concentration can be made as follows: Corrected Calcium = Serum Calcium + 0.8 × [normal albumin − patient albumin].

Clinical symptoms that arise from hypercalcemia are as a direct result of both the rate of rise and the absolute serum calcium level (table 17.3). The most common constitutional symptoms include weight loss, anorexia, polydipsia, which may progress into nausea, vomiting, polyuria, azotemia, renal failure, constipation, ileus, abdominal pain, and even obstipation. With continued rise, patients may begin to experience neurologic symptoms such as fatigue, lethargy, muscle weakness, confusion, seizure, and even coma. Cardiac symptoms are rare, but when they occur can lead to fatal arrhythmias. The initial electrocardiographic changes include bradycardia, prolonged PR interval, shortened QT interval, and widening of the T wave.

The treatment of cancer-related hypercalcemia should be directed at the underlying malignancy. Hypercalcemia most commonly affects patients with underlying renal insufficiency. Immobilization can exacerbate hypercalcemia, and it is important to review the patient's medication list in order to avoid drugs that inhibit ordinary calcium excretion such as thiazide diuretics, nonsteroidal anti-inflammatory agents, as well as histamine receptor antagonists.

Most patients with hypercalcemia present with marked dehydration as a result of anorexia, nausea, and vomiting as well as polyuria due to kaliuresis. Therefore, aggressive fluid repletion with normal saline is the first line of therapy. Appropriate volume expansion will not only increase renal blood flow but also improve calcium excretion. Once euvolemia has been established, forced diuresis with furosemide can be initiated. The bisphosphonates pamidronate and zoledronic acid are most commonly used in the treatment of cancer-related hypercalcemia. The typical onset of action is within 24–48 hours. Bisphosphonates adsorb to the surface of hydroxyapatite and inhibit the release of calcium from bone. Bisphosphonates also interfere with the metabolic activity of osteoclasts.

Pamidronate is typically infused at a dose of 60–90 mg over 2–4 hours, and zoledronic acid is administered at a dose of 4 mg in patients with normal renal function. Peak levels of both pamidronate and zoledronic acid have been associated with renal tubular dysfunction. Zoledronic acid was initially infused over 15 minutes. However, infusion rates of 30 to 45 minutes are now recommended, and the dose should be reduced in patients with renal insufficiency. The use of steroids is most useful in patients with malignancies that are steroid responsive, such as multiple myeloma, lymphoma, and acute lymphoblastic leukemia.

SYNDROME OF INAPPROPRIATE ANTIDIURETIC HORMONE

Hyponatremia is a potentially life-threatening abnormality that has many causes, but first one must exclude pseudo-hyponatremia. The most common causes of pseudohyponatremia are hyperproteinemia, hyperlipidemia, and hyperglycemia. The differential diagnosis of hyponatremia cannot be made until the patient's volume status is accurately determined. Hypotonic hyponatremia is the result of primary water gain or sodium loss. In order to determine the cause of hyponatremia, it is important to measure plasma osmolality, urine osmolality, and urine sodium concentration, as well as urine potassium concentration. In patients with hypervolemia hyponatremia, the expanded extracellular fluid (ECF) status is due to a decrease in the effective circulating volume. This can be seen in patients with congestive heart failure, hepatic cirrhosis, or nephrotic syndrome.

The syndrome of inappropriate antidiuretic hormone secretion (SIADH) is the most common cause of hyponatremia that occurs in the euvolemic state. SIADH is a result of the nonphysiological release of arginine vasopressin (AVP) secreted from either the posterior pituitary or an ectopic source. SIADH is usually caused by the production of an ADH-like substance through ectopic production, although nonmalignant causes must be excluded. Approximately 10–15% of patients with small cell lung cancer will present with SIADH. SIADH can be caused by a variety of other tumors including non-small cell lung cancer, head and neck tumors, brain tumors, and, rarely, hematologic malignancies such as leukemia and lymphoma. There are several nonmalignant causes of SIADH such as central nervous system infections, vasculitis, and pulmonary infections, as well as a wide variety of drugs. Tumor-associated SIADH remains a diagnosis of exclusion; however, the treatment of both tumor-related SIADH and SIADH from other causes is similar.

The clinical manifestations of hyponatremia show a direct relationship to the rate of change in the serum plasma sodium concentration. Plasma sodium concentrations that fall slowly over long periods of time are often well tolerated, and patients usually remain asymptomatic. As the plasma sodium concentration falls to below 120 mmol/L, patients may develop neurologic symptoms, which include headache, lethargy, and confusion and, if left uncorrected, may develop into seizures and coma. The goal of therapy is to slowly increase the serum sodium concentration. In patients with mild to moderate hyponatremia, this can be efficiently corrected by restricting the patient's free water intake. In the event that free water restriction is ineffective, demeclocycline can be used. Demeclocycline inhibits the effect of AVP on the kidneys. The typical dose of demeclocycline is 600 mg/day. In patients with severe hyponatremia with the development of neurologic symptoms, it may be necessary to administer hypertonic saline. One must be extremely careful with the administration of hypertonic saline in order to avoid central pontine myelinolysis. This devastating neurologic syndrome can be avoided by ensuring that the plasma sodium concentration is raised by no more than 1–2 mmol/L per hour.

COMPLICATIONS RELATED TO CANCER TREATMENT

NEUTROPENIA AND INFECTION

Infections occurring in the setting of neutropenia are one of the most common complications of cancer therapy. The degree and duration of neutropenia are directly related to the incidence of febrile neutropenia. Normal barriers to infections such as mucosal surfaces and luminal epithelial cells in the gastrointestinal tract may be disrupted by chemotherapy and provide a portal of entry for bacteria. Development of fever in a neutropenic patient is a medical emergency requiring hospitalization and prompt administration of broad-spectrum antibiotics.

Patients may be infected with multiple organisms simultaneously. The epidemiology and antibiotic resistance pattern in the hospital should direct initial antibiotic coverage. Gram-negative rod infections are of most concern; therefore, antibiotics with antipseudomonal coverage should be used. A third-generation cephalosporin is often appropriate in this situation. Alternatives include a semisynthetic penicillin in combination with an aminoglycoside. If a skin source or line-associated source is suspected, administration of antibiotics with Gram-positive coverage, such as vancomycin, should also be considered. The patient should remain on broad-spectrum antibiotics until resolution of the neutropenia. If an organism is identified, antibiotics should be altered to assure activity against this organism, but broad-spectrum antibiotics should be continued because other pathogens not identified may also be present. For patients with prolonged neutropenia and persistent fever, the addition of antifungal agents should be considered. The most common fungal infections in this setting include *Candida albicans* and *Aspergillus*.

TYPHLITIS

Neutropenic enterocolitis, or typhlitis, is the necrosis of the cecum and adjacent colon. This condition is most commonly identified in patients undergoing chemotherapy for acute leukemia. Patients often present with right lower-quadrant abdominal pain that may progress to rebound tenderness and abdominal distension. Patients also commonly have diarrhea, which may be bloody. CT scanning demonstrates bowel wall thickening in the area of the cecum. Treatment includes the administration of broad-spectrum antibiotics and bowel rest. Surgical intervention may be required if there is no improvement or in cases of perforation.

PULMONARY COMPLICATIONS

Pneumonia is the most common cause of pulmonary complication in patients receiving treatment for cancer. In patients with lung cancer or other cancers involving the mediastinum and lung, postobstructive pneumonia may develop. Broad-spectrum antibiotics including treatment of anaerobic organisms are often needed in these situations. Relief of the obstruction by the use of either chemotherapy, radiation therapy, or stenting may be required. In severely immune-suppressed patients, such as those receiving high-dose corticosteroids or those who have undergone stem cell transplantation, *Pseudomonas carinii* infection should be considered. Diagnostic bronchoscopy may be required to establish a diagnosis.

Noninfectious pulmonary complications include radiation pneumonitis and drug toxicity. Radiation pneumonitis usually develops within 2–6 months after the completion of radiation therapy. Patients may present with dyspnea, cough, and low-grade fever. Chest x-ray often demonstrates an infiltrate confined to the radiation field. Bronchoscopy or lung biopsy may be needed to exclude other diagnoses. Steroids are the treatment for radiation pneumonitis.

A number of chemotherapeutic agents are associated with pulmonary toxicity. These agents can include bleomycin, methotrexate, and busulfan. Symptoms may include dyspnea and cough, and fever may also be present. Physical exam may demonstrate diffuse crackles. Chest x-ray often demonstrates an interstitial infiltrate. As with radiation pneumonitis, bronchoscopy may be required to exclude

infectious etiologies. Steroids may be helpful in the treatment of some patients.

ADDITIONAL READING

Arrambide K, Toto R. Tumor lysis syndrome. *Semin Nephrol.* 1993;13:273–80.

Bach F, Larsen BH, Rohde K, et al. Metastatic spinal cord compression. Occurrence, symptoms, clinical presentations and prognosis in 398 patients with spinal cord compression. *Acta Neurochir (Wien).* 1990;107(1–2):37–43.

Cairo MS, Coiffier B, Reiter A, Younes A; TLS Expert Panel. Recommendations for the evaluation of risk and prophylaxis of tumour lysis syndrome (TLS) in adults and children with malignant diseases: An expert TLS panel consensus. *Br J Haematol.* 2010;149(4):578–86.

Conger JD. Acute uric acid nephropathy. *Med Clin North Am.* 1990;74(4):859–71.

Giglio P, Gilbert MR. Neurologic complications of cancer and its treatment. *Curr Oncol Rep.* 2010;12(1):50–9.

Hughes WT, Armstrong D, Bodey GP, et al. 2002 guidelines for the use of antimicrobial agents in neutropenic patients with cancer. *Clin Infect Dis.* 2002;34(6):730–51.

Pelosof LC, Gerber DE. Paraneoplastic syndromes: An approach to diagnosis and treatment. *Mayo Clin Proc.* 2010;85(9):838–54.

Rice TW, Rodriguez RM, Light RW. The superior vena cava syndrome: Clinical characteristics and evolving etiology. *Medicine (Baltimore).* 2006;85(1):37–42.

Santarpia L, Koch CA, Sarlis NJ. Hypercalcemia in cancer patients: Pathobiology and management. *Horm Metab Res.* 2010;42(3):153–64.

Schnoll-Sussman F, Kurtz RC. Gastrointestinal emergencies in the critically ill cancer patient. *Semin Oncol.* 2000;27(3):270–83.

Stewart AF. Clinical practice. Hypercalcemia associated with cancer. *N Engl J Med.* 2005;352(4):373–9.

Taylor JW, Schiff D. Metastatic epidural spinal cord compression. *Semin Neurol.* 2010;30(3):245–53.

Verbalis JG. Hyponatremia: Epidemiology, pathophysiology, and therapy. *Curr Opin Nephrol Hypertens.* 1993;2(4):636–52.

Wilson D, Stewart A, Szwed J, and Einhorn, L.H. Cardiac arrest due to hyperkalemia following therapy for acute lymphoblastic leukemia. *Cancer.* 1977;39(5):2290–3.

QUESTIONS

QUESTION 1. A 19-year-old woman with metastatic medulloblastoma (metastases to the liver, mediastinal lymph nodes, and bone marrow) develops tumor-lysis syndrome on the second day following chemotherapy with cisplatin and etoposide. The next steps in management should include all of the following EXCEPT:

A. Use of intravenous isotonic sodium bicarbonate therapy

B. Consideration for early initiation of dialysis

C. Rasburicase (recombinant urate oxidase) to treat a high uric acid level

D. Calcitonin for the severe hypercalcemia

E. Phosphate binders for hyperphosphatemia

QUESTION 2. A 62-year-old patient is admitted to the hospital for evaluation of hemoptysis of 2 weeks' duration. He gives a history of gradually worsening dyspnea over the past 10 years. He has a cough productive of copious sputum during winter months and several prior lung infections during the winter months. He has noticed some general malaise, loss of appetite, and tiredness, worse recently. Social history is remarkable for a heavy smoking history 20–30 cigarettes/day for 40 years. Examination shows that he is tachypneic at rest. He is confused and agitated. Not cooperative. Blood pressure on admission is 168/92 mm Hg without orthostasis. HR 84 bpm. Lung exam shows that he has scattered rhonchi, reduced right base air entry, and dullness on percussion. He has no peripheral edema.

- Urinalysis: SG 1010, pH 5.0; rest negative

- Urine sodium 42 mEq/L

- Urine osmolality 615 mOsm

- Electrolytes: Na 100, K 3.5, CO_2 30, Cl 72, BUN 5.0, creatinine 0.6, glucose 108, uric acid 2.6

All of the following statements are true EXCEPT:

A. The patient's total body sodium is normal.
B. The calculated serum osmolality is approximately 208 mOs/kg.
C. The patient has evidence of either inappropriate or appropriate ADH secretion.
D. The urine sodium value seen in this patient is atypical of a patient with SIADH.
E. Use of 3% hypertonic saline would be the best treatment at this point in this patient.

QUESTION 3. All of the following are correct statements regarding typhlitis EXCEPT:

A. The typical presentation mimics acute appendicitis.
B. Symptoms of neutropenic enterocolitis (typhlitis) usually occur within 10–14 days after initiation of cytotoxic chemotherapy.
C. The cecum may be palpated as a boggy mass.
D. Abdominal ultrasonography should be performed and is preferable to contrast enemas.
E. Obtaining plain abdominal radiographs is usually critical to making the diagnosis.

ANSWERS

1. D
2. D
3. E

18.

DISORDERS OF PLATELETS AND COAGULATION

Robert I. Handin

The blood platelet, interacting with a complex network of coagulation proteins, makes up the hemostatic system, which provides the major body defense against excess bleeding after injury, surgery, or other invasive episodes. Disorders of the hemostatic system are a mixture of common and rare, inherited and acquired, mild or life-threatening illnesses. Furthermore, although excess bleeding is caused by a failure in the hemostatic system, patients who present with thrombosis and embolism may have a defect in the regulatory mechanisms that normally limit the hemostatic response. There has been substantial progress in both the diagnosis and treatment of hemostatic disorders. In addition, highly effective antiplatelet and anticoagulant drugs have been developed for treating patients with venous and arterial thromboembolism including coronary artery and cerebrovascular disease.

This chapter begins with an outline of the process of normal hemostasis and reviews the laboratory tests used to assess hemostasis. It then reviews the pathophysiology, clinical presentation, diagnosis, and treatment of the most important hemostatic disorders. Although diagnosis and treatment rely heavily on laboratory tests, it is crucial to emphasize the critical importance of the history and physical examination in assessing patients suspected of having a hemostatic disorder. A careful history will provide an assessment of the likelihood of a disorder and is sometimes positive even when initial screening tests are normal. In addition, the history can help focus the workup on platelets or coagulation proteins. The physical exam can provide important clues to the nature of the bleeding disorder and should not be overlooked.

NORMAL HEMOSTASIS

The process of normal hemostasis is initiated when there is disruption of the normal endothelial cell barrier that lines all blood vessels. When endothelial cells are detached, following vascular injury, flowing blood is exposed to vascular subendothelial proteins, principally collagen. Circulating platelets promptly (1) adhere to exposed collagen; (2) become activated and undergo dramatic change in shape and secrete their granule contents; and (3) recruit additional platelets to the site of injury, forming a platelet aggregate or hemostatic plug that temporarily stops the flow of blood out of the damaged vessel. This process is often referred to as *primary hemostasis* and is initiated within a few seconds of injury.

At the same time, the coagulation system is activated, leading to the formation of a fibrin meshwork that engulfs and stabilizes the platelet plug. Blood coagulation is initiated by the interaction of flowing blood with tissue factor and involves a series of linked proteolytic reactions. The final coagulation event is the generation of sufficient thrombin to convert plasma fibrinogen to fibrin. This process has been called *secondary hemostasis* and is complete several minutes after injury. Hours to days later, the definitive fibrin/platelet plug is slowly dissolved by the fibrinolytic pathway so that blood flow can be reestablished in the newly endothelialized vessel.

Thrombosis is the pathologic equivalent of normal hemostasis and has been called hemostasis at the wrong time or in the wrong place. Just as it is impossible to develop immunosuppressive drugs that do not perturb the normal immune and inflammatory process, drugs designed to prevent or limit thrombus formation inevitably increase the risk of bleeding. In arterial thrombosis, the triggering event, rather than vascular injury, is pathology within the vascular endothelium or subendothelium. The rupture of an atherosclerotic plaque is the most common arterial pathology. In venous thrombosis there may be a combination of excess thrombin generation and more subtle endothelial injury.

Platelets are critically important for hemostasis in the microvasculature and in skin and mucous membranes. Hence, platelet disorders tend to cause bleeding primarily in these areas. In contrast, the coagulation pathway is needed for optimal hemostasis in larger vessels and in joints and muscle, so that deficiencies lead to characteristic deep delayed bleeding and hemarthroses.

Coagulation was initially divided into intrinsic or contact-dependent and extrinsic or tissue-factor-dependent limbs. It is now clear that this separation is artificial and does not reflect how the reactions proceed in vivo. At present, there is a consensus that basal coagulation is driven by the formation of a tissue factor-VIIa complex, which activates factors IX and X with equal efficiency. In addition, traces of thrombin generated from these reactions can feed back and activate factor XI. The role of contact activation via actor XII (Hageman factor) in normal coagulation is now less clear.

CLINICAL EVALUATION AND COAGULATION TESTS

The key points to cover in the history of any patient suspected of having a hemostatic disorder can be summarized in these seven questions:

1. Has the patient bled on multiple occasions and from multiple sites?

2. Has any of the bleeding been severe enough to require blood transfusion?

3. What types of surgery or trauma precipitated the bleeding?

4. How long after injury did the bleeding occur?

5. Is there a pattern or specific location of the bleeding?

6. Is there a family history of abnormal bleeding, and what is the pattern of inheritance?

7. What, if any, medication does the patient take?

Key elements of the physical examination include these:

1. Any evidence of skin or mucous membrane bleeding—petechiae, ecchymoses

2. Evidence of either swelling, fluid accumulation, limited range of motion, or synovial thickening of a joint—hips, knees, ankles, shoulders, elbows are most often affected in hemophilia A and B (factors VIIII and IX deficiency)

3. Hematomas in deep subcutaneous tissues or muscle as well as bleeding into the head, airways, retroperitoneum that is out of proportion to known trauma or pathology

4. Vascular lesions like the nasal and lip hemangiomas seen in Osler-Weber-Rendu disease or abnormal skin laxity and joint hyperextensibility seen in Ehlers-Danlos syndrome.

SCREENING TESTS OF HEMOSTASIS

Basic screening tests should include the following:

1. Complete blood count (CBC)

2. Prothrombin time (PT), partial thromboplastin time (PTT)

3. Mixing studies to rule out an inhibitor and/or identify factor abnormalities if either PT or PTT is prolonged

4. von Willebrand factor level/activity in patients with suspected primary hemostatic defect by history

5. Platelet aggregation in patients with suspected inherited, acquired, or drug-induced primary hemostatic defect.

SPECIFIC DISORDERS

VON WILLEBRAND DISEASE

Von Willebrand disease (vWD) is one of the most common inherited disorders, affecting an estimate of 1 in 100 individuals. Many patients are minimally affected and may live their entire lives without untoward bleeding. vWD is an autosomal dominant disorder, affecting males and females with equal frequency, presenting as bleeding after surgery or dental procedures, menorrhagia, or easy bruising.

The von Willebrand factor (vWF) is a very large, heterogeneous plasma protein synthesized in endothelial cells and megakaryocytes and secreted into plasma as well as the vascular subendothelium. It is stored in unique endothelial organelles called Weibel-Palade bodies or in platelet alpha granules. vWF has two major functions—to stabilize platelet adhesion to the vessel wall under high-flow/high-shear conditions by binding to collagen and the platelet GpIb/IX/V complex and to serve as an intravascular carrier for the antihemophilic protein factor VIII.

The vast majority (85%) of patients with vWD have type 1 disease caused by missense mutations that perturb multimer assembly. They have a parallel decrease in vWF antigen, vWF activity measured as Ristocetin cofactor activity, and factor VIII. vWF levels are influenced by a number of physiological/pathologic states or additional genes. For example, acute or chronic inflammation can raise the vWF level, whereas hypothyroidism lowers the vWF level. The unique hormonal milieu present during pregnancy can completely normalize the vWF level, allowing for easy labor and delivery. vWF protein contains ABO blood group molecules that influence the rate of vWF clearance from plasma. Type O vWF is cleared most rapidly, types A and B less so, and type AB the slowest. Thus, type O patients have the lowest plasma levels of vWF and are more likely to have bleeding when they have inherited a mutant vWD allele.

Most of the remaining patients have type 2 vWD characterized by specific mutations in the vWF A1 domain that make the molecule abnormally sensitive to proteolytic degradation (type 2a disease) or partially activated and continually binding to circulating platelets (type 2b). There are some rare patients with mutations that inactivate the site in the A1 domain that binds to GpIb (type 2M disease). Some patients have a disorder that has been called autosomal hemophilia and have a mutation in the region of vWF that binds to and stabilizes factor VIII (type 2N disease). When a type 2N allele is combined with a type 1 mutant allele, the resulting double heterozygote patient can have very low VIII levels and present with hemarthroses that mimic classic hemophilia. Because the platelet adhesive function of vWF is preserved, there is no mucosal bleeding. An autosomal inheritance pattern can provide the clue to diagnosis and distinguish this condition from classic hemophilia A. There are a small number of patients with type 3 disease, which is due to large deletions in the vWF gene. The patients have inherited two abnormal alleles and have severe lifelong bleeding with no detectable vWF in their plasma.

QUALITATIVE PLATELET DISORDERS

The qualitative platelet disorders are a heterogeneous group of abnormalities that affect many different steps in platelet adhesion, signaling, granule packaging, and secretion and aggregation. Some disorders are quite common, whereas others are exceedingly rare, and one may spend an entire career in a primary-care or subspecialty practice without seeing a patient with one of these disorders. Some abnormalities occur in isolation, whereas others are a manifestation of a multiorgan systemic disorder. It is convenient to link the disorders to specific steps in platelet function as shown in figure 18.1.

Platelet membrane disorders affecting adhesion or aggregation, two critical steps in platelet function, are the result of cooperative activity between a membrane glycoprotein and a plasma glycoprotein. The interaction of vWF with the GpIb/IX/V complex facilitates platelet adhesion, while the binding of fibrinogen to GpIIb/IIIa regulates platelet aggregation. Rare patients with mutations in GpIb a or b polypeptides or GpIX fail to synthesize the GpIb/IX/V complex, a condition called the Bernard-Soulier syndrome.

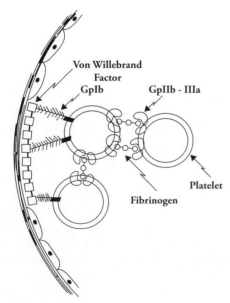

Figure 18.1. Platelet Function.

It is characterized by abnormally large platelets, mild to moderate thrombocytopenia, and an inability to support vWF-dependent adhesion. It is an autosomal recessive trait and causes lifelong bleeding. In a similar vein, patients with mutations in the GpIIb or GpIIIa polypeptides fail to synthesize the platelet GpIIb/IIIa complex and have platelets that cannot bind fibrinogen or aggregate. This disorder, called Glanzmann thrombasthenia, is also an autosomal recessive trait. It differs from Bernard-Soulier in that patients have a normal platelet count and normal-sized platelets. Like Bernard-Soulier patients, they also have severe, recurrent lifelong hemorrhage. In both cases, repeated platelet transfusions can lead to alloimmunization well as antibodies directed against the missing proteins, which can both limit the effectiveness of platelet transfusions.

Patients have been identified with selective defects in the transport and packaging of materials in platelet granules. Patients with dense body or delta storage pool disease have low levels of granule ATP, ADP, calcium, and serotonin and have defective secondary platelet aggregation. In contrast, patients with alpha granule or alpha-storage-pool disease have normal or near-normal aggregation. Patients with combined alpha/delta disease have platelets that have the appearance of Swiss cheese with multiple holes representing the limiting membrane of empty granules. They have a hemostatic defect and can also develop marrow fibrosis as proteins like the platelet-derived growth factor leak from megakaryocytes and stimulate the growth of marrow fibroblasts.

Patients with oculocutaneous albinism and patients with the Chediak-Higashi syndrome, who may also be partial albinos, have a generalized granule packaging defect that extends to the platelet and presents as delta-storage-pool disease. Patients with the Hermansky-Pudlak syndrome have delta-storage-pool disease and often develop severe pulmonary fibrosis. Many of these patients end up requiring continuous oxygen therapy and eventual lung transplants.

Patients have been identified with mutations in the P_2Y_{12} ADP receptor and in some of the important intraplatelet signaling molecules. A mutation in a myosin isoform, MyH9, causes the May-Hegglin anomaly, which is characterized by very large platelets, moderate thrombocytopenia, Dohle bodies in their leukocytes, but no hemostatic defect.

In clinical practice the most common platelet abnormalities are those caused by the administration of antithrombotic medications. Aspirin is far and away the most commonly administered drug and induces a mild hemostatic defect. Since it irreversibly inactivates platelet cyclo-oxygenase, a single dose can perturb hemostasis for 5–7 days. Other nonsteroidal anti-inflammatory drugs (NSAIDs) such as naproxen or ibuprofen are transient reversible cyclo-oxygenase inhibitors and rarely cause clinical bleeding. Of far more importance is their competition with aspirin for cyclo-oxygenase binding. Simultaneous ingestion of sodium naproxen or ibuprofen and aspirin will block the desired cardiovascular effect of aspirin and is one of the leading causes of "aspirin resistance." Patients need to be instructed to take aspirin first and to wait at least 30 minutes before taking another NSAID.

Clopidogrel and prasugrel are both P_2Y_{12} inhibitors that block ADP-induced aggregation. They are *prodrugs* whose active metabolites are irreversible inhibitors, so their effect is also prolonged. Two other popular drugs, Integrelin and abciximab (Rheo Pro), bind to the GpII/IIIa complex and block platelet fibrinogen binding and platelet aggregation. Integrelin has a short biological half-life and can be rapidly reversed by stopping its infusion. The effect of abciximab can persist for several days.

HEMOPHILIA A

Although patients have been described with deficits in each of the known coagulation proteins, three diseases predominate and account for well over 90% of patients with inherited coagulation disorders—deficiencies in factors VIII, IX, and XI. They are also known as hemophilias A, B, and C. Factors VIII and IX deficiency are X-linked disorders affecting primarily males, whereas factor XI deficiency is an autosomal recessive disorder that can affect both males and females.

Factor VIII deficiency occurs in 1 in 10,000 male births and causes lifelong, recurrent soft tissue, muscle, and, most importantly, joint bleeding or hemarthroses. There is a close relationship between factor VIII level and severity of bleeding. Patients with <1% activity have severe disease with frequent, life-threatening bleeding. Patients with 1–5% activity have moderate disease with bleeding weekly or even monthly. Patients with levels over 5% have milder disease with infrequent bleeding.

Treatment of hemophiliacs has steadily improved. At present, (1) many children and adolescents receive prophylactic therapy several times a week and have few major bleeds; (2) almost all children and adults self-administer coagulation factor concentrates at home on demand with minimal medical supervision; (3) most patients utilize highly purified recombinant factor concentrates that are free of all known viruses.

Although the life expectancy of a hemophilia patient is near normal and many patients have few damaged joints, there are unresolved health issues such as the increased incidence of hypertension and the enormous expense of optimal therapy. Perhaps the most dreaded complication of hemophilia at present is the development of an inhibitor to factor VIII. This occurs in 15–20% of patients and both complicates therapy and reduces the patient's quality of life.

HEMOPHILIA B AND C

Almost everything written above about factor VIII deficiency holds true for factor IX deficiency. It is less common, appearing in 1 in 50,000 births, and the protein has a longer plasma half-life so infusions are less frequent. Otherwise the diseases are nearly identical.

Factor XI deficiency is, however, quite distinct. First, it is autosomal recessive and usually presents as postoperative bleeding. It is more common in Ashkenazic Jewish populations. Also, the correlation between factor level and bleeding is not very strong for unknown reasons. Finally, the only available treatment is infusion with fresh frozen plasma because there is no approved factor XI concentrate.

ACQUIRED HEMOPHILIA AND VON WILLEBRAND DISEASE

Rarely, patients with perfectly normal hemostasis for their entire lives can develop a severe hemostatic defect due to acquisition of an antibody inhibitor to a particular coagulation factor, the adsorption of a coagulation factor onto a tumor surface, or an abnormal protein. These disorders present particular challenges and can, at times, cause very severe, sometimes lethal bleeding.

Acquired hemophilia is usually due to an antibody to factor VIII. It is seen as a reaction to drugs in patients with an autoimmune disorder such as systemic lupus, in pregnant women, and in otherwise healthy elderly individuals. The presentation in otherwise healthy older patients is the most common event. Patients require intensive support with factor VIII concentrates and, more recently, recombinant factor VIIa. With immunosuppressive therapy using agents like Rituxan along with the passage of time, most of these inhibitors will disappear, and patients make a complete recovery.

The first example of coagulation factor adsorption causing an acquired deficiency is the interaction of factor X with amyloid protein in patients with primary light-chain amyloidosis. Subsequently various groups have noted acquired von Willebrand disease due to adsorption of vWF onto tumor surfaces. This is particularly common in patients with lymphoproliferative disorders. Effective therapy requires reduction of the tumor mass.

Patients with monoclonal gammopathy of uncertain significance (MGUS) may have antibodies against the vWF protein and significant bleeding. A substantial number of patients with Waldenstrom macroglobulinemia, myeloma, and other lymphoproliferative disorders will develop anti-vWF antibodies and acquired vWD.

Finally, patients with aortic stenosis, patients with ventricular assist devices, and patients with myeloproliferative disorders may unfold and then proteolyze vWF and develop mild to moderate vWD.

IMMUNE THROMBOCYTOPENIA

Immune thrombocytopenia, formerly called idiopathic thrombocytopenic purpura (ITP), is the most common autoimmune disorder. In young children, it is a transient disorder that follows a viral infection. In adults, ITP is usually a chronic problem, affecting otherwise healthy women three times as often as men. Patients may, rarely, have other autoimmune phenomena. For example, the simultaneous or sequential appearance of autoimmune hemolytic anemia and thrombocytopenia is referred to as Evan syndrome. Although ITP is rarely fatal, it can cause recurrent and sometimes serious mucocutaneous and occasional intracerebral bleeding.

The most frequent target antigen is the platelet GpIIb/IIIa complex. A small number of patients have antibodies to the GpIb/IX/V complex or other platelet cell-surface proteins. In most cases the antibodies act as opsonins and increase the clearance of platelets from the circulation without perturbing platelet function. Occasionally, the antibody may perturb fibrinogen binding, and patients will have both thrombocytopenia and platelet dysfunction that mimics Glanzmann disease. There have been multiple attempts to develop laboratory tests for platelet autoantibodies in ITP patients. None of the tests has been successful for myriad reasons, including a high level of background IgG on the platelet surface and the presence of Fc receptors, which may bind immunoglobulins or immune complexes in a nonspecific manner.

The typical patient with ITP presents with a history of easy bruising, mucocutaneous bleeding, and, if the platelet count is sufficiently low—petechiae, which arise from the movement of red cells through leaky capillaries into the skin. Most patients have no pathognomonic physical findings or laboratory tests, and ITP remains a diagnosis of exclusion. In contrast with patients who have autoimmune hemolytic anemia, ITP patients have a normal-sized spleen. Typically, other than thrombocytopenia, the blood count is normal, although some patients may have atypical lymphocytes suggesting a recent viral infection. There is debate about what constitutes an adequate workup for ITP. Most hematologists have stopped performing bone marrow examinations in ITP patients unless a more global hematologic abnormality is suspected. The workup usually includes an antinuclear antibodies (ANA), which is usually normal. Many practitioners routinely order HIV testing in all sexually active patients, whereas others order it only if the patient has engaged in a high-risk behavior. Serologic panels for toxoplasmosis, cytomegalovirus (CMV) and other viral disorders are rarely positive and not recommended. Chronic ITP is defined as thrombocytopenia that has been present for at least 3 months. The likelihood of a viral etiology or a spontaneous remission is extremely low after 3 months.

For many years the standard initial therapy has been administration of large doses of glucocorticoids, usually 50 mg of prednisone or equivalent daily. In most patients, the platelet count will return to normal after several doses of prednisone, but it falls to pretreatment values as the steroid dose is reduced. If the count remains low after several months of prednisone therapy, the well-established second-line therapy is splenectomy. In most large centers, this is a laparoscopic procedure with minimal morbidity and mortality. Patients are immunized against encapsulated organisms such as pneumococcus, meningococcus, and *Haemophilus. influenzae* that are cleared primarily in the spleen. The only remaining infection that is worsened by splenectomy is babesiosis. In adults, the spleen seems to be dispensable, and immune function is largely preserved. Splenectomy raises the platelet count to normal in approximately 70% of ITP patients.

Patients who fail splenectomy and have dangerously low platelet counts ($<50,000/\mu L$) are usually given the immunosuppressive medications Imuran or oral cyclophosphamide. Recently, the favored drug is the anti-CD20 monoclonal antibody rituximab (Ritoxin). It will induce a remission in 70% of patients who have failed corticosteroids and splenectomy, but may require a second course of treatment within a year in 25% of initial responders. Although the complication rate is low, opportunistic infections are a potential problem, and several patients have developed progressive multifocal leukoencephalopathy after Rituxan treatment, so caution is advised.

There is a great desire among patients and treating physicians to avoid splenectomy. One new approach is the administration of pulses of very high-dose dexamethasone given for 4 days a month. After several months of therapy, a small percentage of patients go into remission. The remission rate may increase when patients are given both dexamethasone pulses and four doses of Rituxan as initial therapy. Although this regimen may induce remissions in 70% of patients, the ability to spare patients from splenectomy needs to be balanced against the known and unknown risks of these potent medications. Although not all my colleagues concur, my own approach is to use prednisone followed by splenectomy and to use Rituxan only in the small number of patients who fail these two standard therapies.

For patients who cannot be put into remission, there are several drugs that can transiently raise the platelet count. Large doses of intravenous immunoglobulin (IVIG) or the anti-RhD immunoglobulin RhoGam have both been used for many years. They both appear to reduce the clearance of antibody-coated platelets. RhoGam is not effective after splenectomy. Because of their expense, the need to administer them intravenously, and their short duration of action, they are recommended only for emergency use or to prepare patients for surgery. Recently, two thrombopoietin mimetics, romiplostim and eltrombopag, have received FDA approval. Both drugs will stimulate marrow production of megakaryocytes, which is suboptimal in many ITP patients, and thereby raise the platelet count. Romiplostim is a novel peptibody TPO mimetic, given as a weekly subcutaneous injection, that binds to the same site on the TPO receptor as native TPO. Eltrombopag is a small molecule, administered orally, that binds to the transmembrane domain of the TPO receptor.

These drugs may be useful as substitutes for IVIG and RhoGam or for the small number of ITP patients who cannot be put into remission with splenectomy and immunosuppressive medication. The drugs may cause a reversible increase in marrow reticulin and collagen with prolonged use, and there are reports of thrombotic events in association with their use.

HEPARIN-INDUCED THROMBOCYTOPENIA

Heparin is the most common cause of thrombocytopenia in hospitalized patients, affecting 15–20% of patients receiving unfractionated heparin. Heparin-induced thrombocytopenia (HIT) is caused by an antibody directed against a complex of heparin and the heparin-neutralizing protein, platelet factor 4. The heparin-PF4-antibody complex binds to the platelet Fc receptor, which induces both platelet activation and secretion and thrombocytopenia. The spectrum of HIT ranges from patients with mild nonprogressive thrombocytopenia to patients who develop profound thrombocytopenia and to an occasional patient who develops life-threatening thrombosis despite being fully anticoagulated. There is an increased risk of thrombus formation in all HIT patients, which persists for several months after heparin is discontinued.

HIT is diagnosed by a combination of clinical observation and judicious laboratory testing. The four key features are (1) the degree of thrombocytopenia; (2) the timing of thrombocytopenia; (3) the presence of concomitant thrombosis; and (4) the absence of other obvious causes of thrombocytopenia. A fall of over 50% of the platelet count since starting heparin with a nadir > 20,000/μL; onset of thrombocytopenia 5–14 days after starting heparin, 48 hours if previously exposed to heparin within 30 days; and new thrombosis, skin necrosis, or anaphylactic reaction to heparin infusion are all considered strong predictors of HIT. If HIT is suspected, a heparin-PF-4 enzyme-linked immunosorbent assay (ELISA) test should be ordered. The test has a reported sensitivity of 95% and thus a high negative predictive value. The limitation of the test is that it does not distinguish between IgM and IgA antibodies or the IgG antibodies that cause platelet activation. The reported specificity of 50% can be improved by looking at the optical density of the ELISA test. An OD > 1.00 is more likely to be due to a pathologic IgG antibody. Newer tests are being introduced using IgG-specific antisera that should increase the specificity of the test. A second set of tests that measure platelet activation, such as the serotonin release assay, can identify those antibodies that are most likely to cause HIT and are said to have >90% sensitivity and specificity. The test is quite specialized, not widely available, and may only be run once or twice a week even in large reference laboratories.

Once HIT is identified, heparin infusion should be immediately discontinued and patients switched to a direct thrombin inhibitor. The two drugs most often used to treat HIT are argatroban, a small-molecule derivative of L-arginine with a plasma half-life of 45 minutes and lepirudin

(recombinant hirudin), which has a half-life of 2 hours. Both drugs are given by intravenous infusion and monitored by measuring the PTT. When the platelet count has returned to >150,000/μL, patients are bridged to warfarin, which is continued for 30 days in patients with no thrombosis and 3–6 months in patients with HITT.

The incidence of HIT should decrease and eventually disappear as newer forms of heparin are introduced that are less immunogenic. For example, the incidence of HIT is <1% for low-Mr heparins like enoxaparin (Lovenox) or dalteparin (Fragmin). Only a handful of HIT cases have been reported in patients receiving the synthetic pentasaccharide fondaparinux (Arixtra). Given the efficacy and safety of the new heparins, unfractionated heparin should probably be reserved for patients who require minute-to-minute titration of heparin dose and prompt reversibility. Unfractionated heparin should only be needed for cardiac catheterization, cardiopulmonary bypass, in intensive care units, and, perhaps, in patients with impaired renal function. There is great interest in the pharmaceutical industry in the design and manufacture of reversible low-Mr heparins, and some are in clinical trials. Given the morbidity and mortality of HIT and, especially, HITT, one hopes that the new designer heparins reach the market soon.

THROMBOTIC THROMBOCYTOPENIC PURPURA

Thrombotic thrombocytopenic purpura (TTP) is a relatively rare disorder characterized by thrombocytopenia, microangiopathic hemolytic anemia, varying degrees of renal failure, and fluctuating neurologic symptoms. A majority of patients with sporadic TTP have an acquired deficiency in ADAMTS13, a plasma metalloprotease enzyme that remodels the vWF secreted by endothelial cells. In the absence of this enzyme, superlarge vWF multimers interact with circulating platelets and form the hyaline thrombi characteristic of TTP. Although there are rare patients who have a congenital deficiency in ADAMTS13, most patients with acquired deficiency have an autoantibody inhibitor. Patients who develop TTP after stem cell transplantation or drug ingestion have normal levels of ADAMTS13 and may have endothelial damage or dysfunction that induces the release of large quantities of large multimers.

Patients with the abrupt onset of thrombocytopenia, anemia, elevated blood urea nitrogen (BUN) and creatinine, and neurologic abnormalities, usually fluctuating levels of consciousness or fluctuating focal findings, are good candidates for TTP. The blood smear should show the presence of schistocytes, while coagulation parameters including PT, PTT, fibrinogen, and D dimer levels are normal. Elevated lactate dehydrogenase (LDH) is a cardinal feature. Blood should be sent to a reference laboratory for ADAMTS13 activity and inhibitor levels, although the results may not be available for several days or a week.

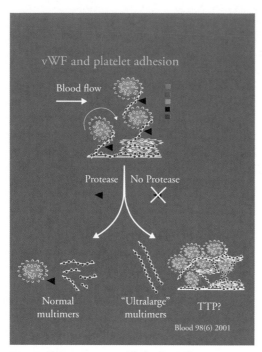

Figure 18.2. Von Willebrand Factor and Platelet Adhesion.

The best therapy for TTP is intensive plasmapheresis accompanied by infusion of fresh frozen plasma. Although the therapy was derived empirically, it is rational. Plasmapheresis may remove antibody or antibody-enzyme complexes, while plasma infusion replaces ADAMTS13. Once initiated, daily plasmapheresis should be continued until neurologic symptoms have abated and the creatinine returns to normal along with the platelet count and LDH. Approximately 20% of patients may relapse immediately after plasmapheresis is stopped and may require retreatment. Within a year of initial treatment, 20% of patients may relapse and require additional plasmapheresis. Before the advent of plasmapheresis and plasma replacement, the mortality of TTP was close to 100%. Now it is down to 10–15%

There is a long list of therapies that have *not* been effective in TTP. They include antiplatelet drugs, splenectomy, and some of the older immunosuppressive medications such as prednisone and azathioprine. There are small case series suggesting that the anti-CD20 monoclonal antibody rituximab (Rituxan) may be beneficial in TTP and certainly should be tried in patients with relapsing forms of the disorder.

The most common drugs causing TTP are the thienopyrimidines ticlopidine and its close derivative clopidogrel, which bind to the platelet P_2Y_{12} (ADP) receptor. Although they are very effective antithrombotic agents, the incidence of TTP following administration of ticlopidine was so high that the drug was taken off the market. TTP has been described after the administration of clopidogrel, but, given the widespread use of this drug, the incidence is quite low. The mortality in patients with drug-induced TTP is higher than in sporadic cases and approaches 50%. Although

plasmapheresis is prescribed, it is less clear that it is effective in this subset of TTP.

DISSEMINATED INTRAVASCULAR COAGULATION

Disseminated intravascular coagulation (DIC) is caused by the unregulated activation of the coagulation pathway. It is most commonly seen during labor and delivery and in patients with sepsis or malignancy. The trigger for DIC can be endotoxin from bacteria, a tissue factor, or other activators of coagulation and contact of blood with incompatible surfaces or membranes. Unregulated coagulation leads to excess thrombin generation, which causes the rapid conversion of plasma fibrinogen to fibrin. Platelets become trapped in the fibrin thrombi and red blood cells become skewered on fibrin strands. The fibrinolytic response to massive fibrin deposition in the microcirculation leads to additional coagulation abnormalities.

Classic laboratory findings include thrombocytopenia, anemia with schistocytes on the blood smear, a prolonged PT and PTT, and a low fibrinogen. Patients also have elevated fibrinogen/fibrin degradation products. The most common assay in use today is the D-dimer assay, which uses a fibrin-specific monoclonal antibody to detect cross-linked fibrin degradation products.

DIC is easily differentiated from TTP, but it may be more difficult to distinguish DIC from a primary fibrinolytic state. Primary fibrinolysis is a rare event seen with some malignancies that have high concentrations of fibrinolytic activators such as carcinoma of the prostate or in patients with advanced cirrhosis who fail to clear fibrinolytic activators from their blood. Although, in theory, patients with fibrinolysis should have normal platelet counts, no schistocytes, and normal D-dimer assays, in clinical situations these distinctions may get blurred perhaps due to a combination of DIC and primary fibrinolysis, limitations in the D-dimer assay, or the effects of plasmin on platelets.

Patients with DIC may present with small vessel thrombosis, often in digits, extremities, skin, or genitalia, with fulminant hemorrhage from multiple sites or with some combination of bleeding and thrombosis. Patients with DIC secondary to sepsis seem to have more prominent thrombosis, whereas patients with obstetrical DIC tend to have massive uncontrollable bleeding. Many patients with cancer have low-grade chronic DIC but may develop more active disease if they undergo tumor resection or other surgery. Patients with epithelial tumors that have metastasized to blood vessels can develop fulminant, intractable DIC.

The treatment of DIC varies with the clinical manifestation. Patients who have thrombosis are best treated with heparin. Prompt heparinization can be life saving and prevent subsequent tissue necrosis and amputation. Patients with bleeding are usually treated with platelets, red cells, and fresh frozen plasma to replace depleted coagulation factors. After this initial resuscitation, the most important next step is to try to treat the underlying pathology that is inducing DIC. In pregnant women the causes are placenta previa, premature placental separation with retroplacental clot, severe eclampsia, or retained products of conception. With delivery of the fetus and the placenta, DIC can disappear quite rapidly. Treatment of Gram-negative or other forms of sepsis can help to reverse DIC and stop bleeding. Although this should be attempted, there is no evidence that treatment of DIC per se improves the prognosis in septic patients. Patients with metastatic tumor provide the greatest challenge, as there may be no effective therapy for the underlying tumor. If the patient develops acute DIC in association with surgery, replacement therapy may help to stop bleeding, although low-grade DIC may persist. Heparin can be used as an adjunct to replacement therapy if fibrinogen and platelets are persistently low despite adequate replacement. Patients with DIC should be followed closely with serial measurements of fibrinogen level, D-dimer, or any other measure of fibrinogen/fibrin degradation products. The platelet count may lag behind these other parameters.

HYPERCOAGUABLE STATES

Patients with cancer, congestive heart failure, prolonged immobility, or patients undergoing surgical procedures have an increased risk of thrombosis. The mechanisms are not well understood and multifactorial. There is increasing use of prophylactic anticoagulation with heparin and/or warfarin in these patients. Most notable are the marked reductions in postoperative venous thromboembolism in orthopedic patients with hip fracture or hip or knee replacement following the universal use of warfarin in the perioperative period.

A group of genetic traits has been identified that increase the risk of venous thromboembolism and, collectively, may account for up to 70% of patients with recurrent deep vein thrombosis (DVT) or pulmonary emboli (PE). These mutations also heighten the risk of thrombosis in patients who are pregnant, use oral contraceptives, have malignancy, or are taking certain medications. In addition, the mutations are sufficiently common that patients often co-inherit two of the defects heightening their risk of thrombosis. Each of these disorders, reviewed below, has its own unique natural history, pathophysiology, and response to therapy.

1. *Antithrombin deficiency* was the first of this group of disorders to be identified. It is an autosomal dominant trait and occurs in approximately 1 in 2000 individuals. Because patients only have one affected allele (gene), they have only a modest deficiency in antithrombin. Because no patients have been identified with two defective alleles, we believe that homozygosity is an embryonic lethal condition. Most patients with antithrombin deficiency will develop symptoms of DVT or PE before they are 30. Although there are antithrombin concentrates available for "replacement" therapy, most patients have only a modest decrease in AT level and respond normally to heparin. The rare patient with a missense mutation that perturbs heparin binding or heparin-induced AT activation or a mutation in the AT active site will require replacement therapy. Since the risk of recurrence is quite high, patients who have an initial thrombotic event should be on lifelong oral anticoagulation with warfarin or its equivalent. Relatives of a patient with known AT deficiency should be tested, and, if they carry the mutation, should avoid oral contraceptives and receive prophylaxis with elective surgery.

2. *Protein S and C deficiency.* These two proteins, like coagulation factors II, VII, IX, and X, are synthesized in the liver and require a posttranslational modification, gamma carboxylation of specific glutamic acids, for biological activity. Anything that perturbs gamma carboxylation such as liver disease, vitamin K deficiency, or oral anticoagulants of the warfarin class, will reduce the levels of proteins C and S. Protein C binds to the endothelial cell surface protein thrombomodulin where it is activated by thrombin. Activated protein C (aPC) catalyzes the inactivation of factors V and VIII, two critical cofactors in the coagulation pathway, in concert with protein S and the endothelial surface protein thrombomodulin. Deficiencies in proteins C and S are very common, with estimates for protein C as common as 1 in 200 individuals. Most affected individuals are asymptomatic or minimally affected and may never develop venous thrombosis or embolism. However, the disorders do increase the lifetime risk of DVT/PE severalfold. Babies with homozygous protein C or S deficiency develop fulminant DIC just after birth and require lifelong plasma infusions to replace protein C or S. Parents of these severely affected children are often completely asymptomatic and have only a mild decrease in protein C or S. Protein C levels are reduced in patients taking warfarin. Because protein C has a short plasma half-life, during the initiation of warfarin therapy, its level drops before factors II, VII, IX, or X, creating a transient prothrombotic state. It is especially pronounced in patients who are started on warfarin and have protein C deficiency. This prothrombotic state is thought to cause the rare complication of warfarin-induced skin necrosis. This serious complication is, fortunately, very rare because most patients starting on warfarin are on heparin and, thus, protected.

Protein S acts as a high-molecular-weight cofactor and forms a complex with protein C and thrombomodulin to facilitate the inactivation of factors V and VIII. It exists in two forms—an active fraction that is "free" in plasma and an inactive fraction bound to a steroid-binding globulin. Pregnancy and the use of oral contraceptives can increase the level of this protein and, thereby, induce or exacerbate protein S deficiency. This reduction in protein S, when combined with another mild defect such as the factor V Leiden or prothrombin gene mutation, may account for the increase in DVT/PE in pregnancy and users of oral contraceptives who were previously asymptomatic.

3. *Factor V Leiden.* This mutation R506Q is present in 5% of the Caucasian population but is uncommon in Africans, Asians, and Latinos. The mutation modifies one of the two protease-sensitive sites in factor V that are cleaved by activated protein C and thereby results in excess thrombin generation. Despite a lot of speculation, we do not know how this invariant mutation arose and was propagated. Carrying the mutation increases the lifetime risk of DVT/PE approximately threefold—from 1 in 1000 individuals to 1 in 250 individuals. In case-control studies, patients who present with DVT/PE on oral contraceptives or during pregnancy often have this mutation. Homozygosity at this locus (inheritance of two defective genes) increases the risk of DVT/PE 30- to 80-fold—to 1 in 12 individuals.

The prothrombin gene mutation G20210A occurs in the 3' untranslated region of the gene rather than in the coding sequence. It stabilizes prothrombin mRNA levels and thereby increases the steady-state level of prothrombin in plasma by 25–30%. This results in increased thrombin generation. The clinical course is quite similar to factor V Leiden. It is a second example of an invariant mutation that has become common in the Caucasian population. Again, the possible advantage of carrying this mutation and maintaining it in the population is unknown. There are a few reports that patients with the prothrombin gene mutation may have a higher incidence of PE than those with the factor V Leiden defect.

ANTIPHOSPHOLIPID ANTIBODY

The antiphospholipid antibody syndrome, also called the anticardiolipin antibody or lupus/lupus-like anticoagulant syndrome, is an autoimmune disorder that increases patient risk of both venous and arterial thrombosis. The mechanism of induction of a hypercoagulable state remains speculative, and many patients have antibody but remain asymptomatic. The two most commonly ordered tests are measurement of anticardiolipin antibody and screening for a lupus-like inhibitor. If the screening test is positive, a confirmatory test using hexagonal phase phospholipid is performed. Anti-B2GPI and antiprothrombin antibody tests are available in research laboratories. There is some evidence that patients with anticardiolipin antibodies that also react with B2GPI are more prone to thrombosis. The serology is complicated, although most but not all patients are positive in both the LA and anticardiolipin tests.

Once a patient has an initial thrombotic event, the risk of recurrence is sufficiently high that patients are usually placed on indefinite/lifelong anticoagulation. Most patients have DVT or PE, a stroke, or a coronary arterial event. Rare patients may develop a more aggressive disorder—the catastrophic antiphospholipid antibody syndrome, with life-threatening thrombosis at multiple sites. Plasmapheresis is

Table 18.1 RELATIONSHIP BETWEEN THROMBOPHILIC STATUS AND RISK OF VENOUS THROMBOEMBOLISM

THROMBOPHILIC STATUS	RELATIVE RISK OF VENOUS THROMBOSIS
Normal	1
Oral contraceptive (OCP) use	4
Factor V Leiden, heterozygous	5 to 7
Factor V Leiden, heterozygous + OCP	30 to 35
Factor V Leiden, homozygous	80
Factor V Leiden, homozygous + OCP	??? >100
Prothrombin Gene Mutation, heterozygous	3
Prothrombin Gene Mutation, homozygous	??? possible risk of arterial thrombosis
Prothrombin Gene Mutation, heterozygous + OCP	16
Protein C deficiency, heterozygous	7
Protein C deficiency, homozygous	Severe thrombosis at birth
Protein S deficiency, heterozygous	6
Protein S deficiency, homozygous	Severe thrombosis at birth
Antithrombin deficiency, heterozygous	5
Antithrombin deficiency, homozygous	Thought to be lethal prior to birth

recommended, in addition to vigorous anticoagulation, for these patients.

Although the standard therapy for a thrombotic event is heparin followed by maintenance on a warfarin anticoagulant, there is some evidence that a course of the anti-CD20 antibody Rituxan may reduce or eliminate anticardiolipin antibodies and reduce the risk of thromboembolism. In some small, published series, approximately 50% of treated patients responded and were able to discontinue anticoagulant therapy.

ADDITIONAL READING

Bauer KA. Thrombophilia evaluation: The value of testing relatives. *Clin Adv Hematol Oncol.* 2010;8:229–31.

Drews RE, Shulman LN. Update in hematology and oncology. *Ann Intern Med.* 2010;152(10):655–62.

George JN. How I treat patients with thrombotic thrombocytopenic purpura: 2010. *Blood.* 2011;117:5551.

Goodeve AC. The genetic basis of von Willebrand disease. *Blood.* 2010;24:123–34.

Kelton JG, Warkentin TE. Heparin-induced thrombocytopenia: A historical perspective. *Blood.* 2008;112:2607–16.

Zaja F, Baccarani M, Mazza P, et al. Dexamethasone plus rituximab yields higher sustained response rates than dexamethasone monotherapy in adults with primary immune thrombocytopenia. *Blood.* 2010, 115:2755–62.

QUESTIONS

QUESTION 1. A 25-year-old woman comes for her first clinic visit after a recent flu-like illness. Her past medical history is only remarkable for occasional migraine headaches that usually occur around the time of her menstrual period. These are generally relieved by ibuprofen. She takes no other medications. On review of systems she notes that her last menstrual period was heavier than usual. Physical examination is unremarkable.

Laboratory studies reveal:

White blood cell count	7400/mm³	(4,000–10,000)
Hematocrit	36%	(36–48)
Platelets	23,000/mm³	(150,000–450,000)
Creatinine	0.7 mg/dL	(0.7–1.3)
LDH	176 IU/L	(107–231)

Peripheral blood smear reveals normal red and white cell morphology and decreased platelets.

The most appropriate next step should be:

A. Immediate hospitalization for intravenous gammaglobulin
B. Send HIV test, advise the patient to discontinue ibuprofen, treat with dexamethasone, 40 mg for 4 days
C. Obtain surgical consultation for splenectomy
D. Observation

QUESTION 2. A 76-year-old woman on warfarin for chronic atrial fibrillation normally anticoagulated to an INR of 2.5 is found to have an INR of 5.8 on routine testing. She is otherwise asymptomatic. The most appropriate next step is:

A. Decrease dose of warfarin by 50%
B. Hold warfarin, administer 1 mg vitamin K subcutaneously
C. Hold warfarin, administer 2.5 mg vitamin K orally
D. Hold warfarin for 1 day, restart at 50% of previous dose the next day
E. Hold warfarin, recheck INR in 1 to 2 days prior to restarting therapy

QUESTION 3. A 32-year-old Caucasian male is found to have a right popliteal deep venous thrombosis after injuring his leg playing football. Of the following heritable conditions, which is most likely to be found on diagnostic evaluation?

A. Antithrombin III deficiency
B. Protein C deficiency
C. Homocystinemia
D. Factor V Leiden
E. Prothrombin gene mutation (G20210A)

QUESTION 4. Which of the following statements is true regarding low-molecular-weight heparins (LMWHs)?

A. They should never be used for the management of pulmonary embolus.
B. The incidence of treatment failure for deep venous thrombosis is higher with LMWH.
C. All of the available preparations have similar pharmacologic properties.
D. The incidence of heparin-associated thrombocytopenia in previously untreated patients is <1%.
E. They can be used in any patient regardless of other underlying conditions.

QUESTION 5. A 28-year-old woman is seen for evaluation in the clinic. Her past medical history is notable for significant bleeding after extraction of her wisdom teeth, such that additional sutures were required. She takes no medications regularly and does not smoke cigarettes or drink alcohol. Her family history is notable for the fact that her mother required blood transfusions several days after the birth of each of her two children. Her sister also had major bleeding several days after the birth of her child. The patient wants to become pregnant, but she is concerned because of her family history.

An appropriate evaluation at this time would include:
A. PT, PTT, and fibrinogen assays
B. No evaluation necessary, perform testing for von Willebrand disease if patient becomes pregnant
C. von Willebrand antigen level, ristocetin cofactor level, and factor VIII level
D. Urea clot solubility test

ANSWERS

1. B
2. E
3. D
4. D
5. C

19.

ANEMIA AND HEMOGLOBINOPATHIES

Maureen M. Okam

ANEMIA

Anemia is defined as a hemoglobin (or hematocrit) below the lower limit of the normal range for age and sex of an individual. About 40 years ago, a World Health Organization expert committee suggested 12 g/dL as the lower limit of normal for nonpregnant women and 13 g/dL as the lower limit for adult men, values that have been used in many studies as the definition of normal. The "right" values for the upper and lower limits of normal remain a subject of intense debate, but they certainly vary according to age, race, and gender.

Erythrocyte development starts in the bone marrow where the earliest erythroid precursor, the pronormoblast, develops through a series of steps and extrudes its nucleus to become a reticulocyte. The reticulocyte then enters the bloodstream, loses its remaining RNA, and in 1–2 days becomes a mature red blood cell (RBC). The life span of the RBC in circulation is approximately 120 days, after which it is cleared by the reticuloendothelial system, primarily in the spleen. Hemoglobin, which is made up of two alpha chains and two beta chains, makes up 90% of the protein in the red blood cell and is responsible for the most important function of the RBC, oxygen delivery. In the absence of blood loss, the number of RBCs and amount of hemoglobin in circulation are functions of the rate of production of RBCs (and incorporation of hemoglobin) in the bone marrow and the rate of destruction or clearing by the spleen.

EVALUATION OF ANEMIA

An organized approach to the evaluation of anemia is essential to reaching an accurate diagnosis. Every case of anemia has an underlying cause that should be sought and identified. The evaluation of anemia should start with a focused history and physical exam, an exclusion of blood loss, a determination of the reticulocyte index (RI), and examination of the blood smear (see figure 19.1). Regardless of the cause of anemia, patients present with symptoms due to reduced oxygen delivery to tissues—dizziness, dyspnea on exertion, palpitations, headaches, nausea, and presyncope or syncope.

The RI is the reticulocyte count corrected for the degree of anemia in an individual. It is calculated as follows:

$$\text{Reticulocyte index (RI)} = \text{Reticulocyte count} \times \text{patient's hct}/40$$

where 40 is a normal hematocrit (hct).

The reticulocyte index broadly divides anemias into two categories:

1. *Hypoproliferative anemias:* those due to inadequate production of RBCs by the bone marrow; associated with a low RI, and

2. *Hyperproliferative anemias:* those due to increased clearing of RBCs by the spleen or frank blood loss, associated with a high RI. The RT in the normal healthy adult is between 1 and 2 (see figure 19.2).

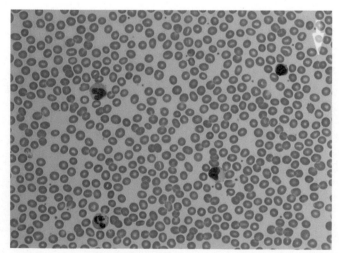

Figure 19.1. Normal Blood Smear.

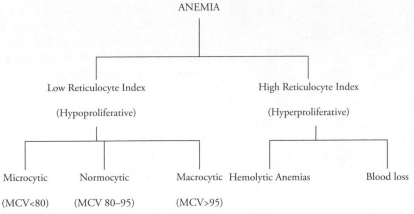

Figure 19.2. Initial Evaluation of Anemia. MCV, mean corpuscular volume.

The treatment of anemias in general is to treat the underlying cause and provide supportive care including administration of blood transfusions in unstable or high-risk patients.

HYPOPROLIFERATIVE ANEMIAS

The hypoproliferative anemias result from the inadequate production of RBCs by the bone marrow. This may be the result of a primary bone marrow pathology such as red cell aplasia, aplastic anemia, or Fanconi anemia, or from an inadequate supply of the ingredients needed by the bone marrow to produce RBCs, principally iron, vitamin B-12, folate, and erythropoietin, or from a dysregulation of cytokines that influence the bone marrow to make RBCs. The RI in these instances is < 1. These anemias can be classified based on the average size of the cells, the mean corpuscular volume (MCV), into microcytic, macrocytic, and normocytic anemias (see figure 19.3).

MICROCYTIC HYPOCHROMIC ANEMIAS

Microcytosis refers to the size of the RBC being small relative to the nucleus of a normal mature lymphocyte, and hypochromia refers to the central pallor of the RBC being greater than one-third the diameter of the RBC. The differential diagnosis of microcytic anemia includes iron deficiency, thalassemias, and other hemoglobinopathies, anemia of chronic disease, sideroblastic anemia, and lead poisoning.

IRON DEFICIENCY ANEMIA

Iron deficiency anemia is the most common hematologic problem encountered in general practice. The causes of iron deficiency include blood loss, decreased gastrointestinal absorption (after bariatric surgery or celiac disease), or increased iron requirements (during pregnancy or with exogenous erythropoietin use). In addition to the general clinical features of all anemias, iron deficiency is associated

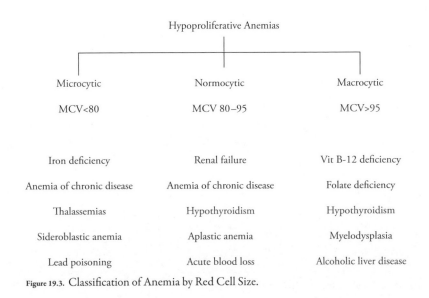

Figure 19.3. Classification of Anemia by Red Cell Size.

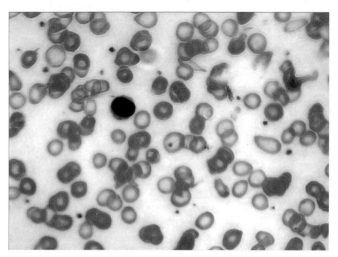

Figure 19.4. Iron Deficiency.

with symptoms in rapidly proliferating tissues: glossitis, angular stomatitis, gastric atrophy, koilonychia (spoon-shaped nails), and pica. The blood smear in iron deficiency shows microcytic hypochromic RBCs as well as pencil (shaped) cells and cells of all sizes and shapes (anisopoikilocytosis) (see figure 19.4). The best single test for making a diagnosis of iron deficiency is the ferritin level (the storage form of iron). A ferritin level <30 μg/mL is generally diagnostic. Other indices that aid a diagnosis are a low serum iron and a high total iron binding capacity (TIBC). The TIBC is a reflection of transferrin, the protein that transports iron in the plasma. Iron deficiency is also associated with a high RBC distribution width (RDW), which is a quantitative measure of the variation in RBC size and a high serum soluble transferrin receptor level. Anemia is a late feature of iron deficiency, and although iron deficiency is very often a hypochromic microcytic anemia, it may present as a normocytic anemia. Figure 19.5 shows the stages of iron deficiency. Once a diagnosis of iron deficiency has been made, a thorough search for the underlying cause should be undertaken, and blood loss must be ruled out.

First-line treatment for iron deficiency is oral replacement with iron sulfate, iron gluconate, or iron lactate. Ferrous sulfate, 325 mg twice daily, is the standard dose. Intravenous repletion should be used only if the patient is unable to absorb iron (malabsorption, celiac disease, etc.), unable to tolerate oral iron (severe constipation or other gastrointestinal upset), or under exceptional circumstances

such as in patients on renal dialysis. The American Society of Hematology recommends ferric gluconate for intravenous replacement, 125 mg per dose for a total dose of 1 to 1.5 g. Oral repletion usually takes 4–6 months to return ferritin to midnormal range.

NORMOCYTIC NORMOCHROMIC ANEMIAS

The differential diagnosis of normocytic anemias includes acute blood loss, anemia of chronic disease, anemia of renal failure, hypothyroidism, aplastic anemia, and hemolysis.

Anemia of Chronic Disease

Anemia of chronic disease (ACD) is the second most common form of anemia. ACD is characterized by impaired absorption of iron from the GI tract and iron trapping in macrophages preventing the utilization of iron by the body. The features that define ACD are mediated by the iron regulatory hormone, hepcidin, which is a 21-peptide hormone produced by the liver that is responsible for iron homeostasis. Hepcidin production is also stimulated by inflammation and binds to and causes the degradation of ferroportin. Ferroportin is the channel through which iron transverses to go from the enterocyte into the bloodstream and from the interior to the exterior of macrophages. Hepcidin, in inhibiting the function of ferroportin, blocks iron transportation across these membranes. Because ACD results in iron-deficient erythropoiesis, various laboratory features are similar to those seen in iron deficiency. ACD and iron deficiency can be differentiated by the ferritin, TIBC, and soluble transferrin receptor. Efforts are under way to develop a hepcidin assay. Medical conditions commonly associated with ACD include infective endocarditis, osteomyelitis, rheumatoid arthritis, tuberculosis, systemic lupus erythematosus, and vasculitides, although no conditions are exempt. Treatment of ACD involves treating the underlying disease and exogenous erythropoietin administration to a goal hemoglobin of about 11.5 g/dL.

MACROCYTIC ANEMIAS

The differential diagnoses of macrocytic anemias include vitamin B-12 and folate deficiency, myelodysplasia, alcoholic liver disease, reticulocytosis, hypothyroidism, and drugs that block folate metabolism (zidovudine, phenytoin, oral contraceptives, sulfasalazine, hydroxyurea).

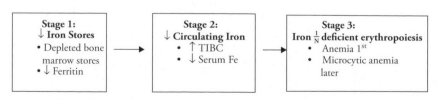

Figure 19.5. Stages of Iron Deficiency.

Folate and Vitamin B-12 Deficiency

Folate and vitamin B-12 deficiency are the two most important causes of macrocytic anemia. Folate and B-12 deficiencies cause impaired DNA synthesis that results in macrocytic and megaloblastic RBCs as well as white blood cells (WBC) with hypersegmented (>5 lobes) nuclei.

B-12 is found exclusively in animal proteins. On ingestion, B-12 is bound to intrinsic factor produced by the parietal cells in the stomach and then passes to the distal ileum where it is actively absorbed. It is then transported in the blood by transcobalamin for use in erythropoiesis. Dietary deficiency is rare except in the case of a strict vegan diet. Most causes of B-12 deficiency are related to ineffective absorption and include pernicious anemia (autoimmune destruction of parietal cells), partial gastrectomy, blind loop syndromes, fish tapeworm, pancreatic insufficiency, ileal resection, Crohn disease, and radiation enteritis. In addition to the general features of anemia, patients with deficiency can have GI symptoms such as diarrhea and glossitis and neurological deficits ranging from paresthesias and loss of vibration and position sense, gait disturbances, to psychosis or dementia—"megaloblastic madness." Neurological deficits from B-12 deficiency that go untreated for long durations may cause irreversible damage.

The Schilling test, which distinguishes among pernicious anemia, nutritional deficiency, and malabsorption, is no longer routinely used in clinical practice. The diagnosis of B-12 deficiency is made by the findings of low to low-normal levels of serum B-12 (lower limit of normal B-12 is 200 pg/mL) and elevated homocysteine and methylmalonic acid levels. An elevated lactate dehydrogenase (LDH) is also seen due to ineffective erythropoiesis. Vitamin B-12 levels are falsely low in pregnancy and oral contraceptive use. Treatment deficiency is traditionally with a loading dose of 1000 μg intramuscularly every week for 4 weeks followed by monthly injections at 1000 μg per month. In cases caused by nutritional deficiency, oral repletion is also an option at a dose of 1000 μg daily.

Folate is found exclusively in plant sources, and folate bodily stores are minimal. Unlike B-12 deficiency, which takes 1–2 years to develop, in the absence of intake, folate deficiency may develop in 1–3 months. Deficiency results from poor dietary intake and increased bodily demands (pregnancy and hemolysis). Patients with folate deficiency have similar symptoms to B-12 deficiency besides the neurological features. Folate is not involved in myelin synthesis and so does not affect the neurological system. Likewise, folate replacement may correct anemia due to B-12 deficiency but will not affect the neurological abnormalities. It is therefore important to differentiate B-12 deficiency from folate deficiency before treating with folate supplementation (see table 19.1).

HYPERPROLIFERATIVE ANEMIAS

These are anemias caused by inappropriate loss or premature destruction (hemolysis) of RBCs with an appropriate attempt by the bone marrow to compensate. The reticulocyte count and index are therefore high. Hyperproliferative anemias are either of hereditary or acquired causes. The hereditary causes include:

1. Defects in the RBC membrane

2. Defects of RBC metabolism

3. Defects in hemoglobin

The acquired causes include:

1. Immune etiology

2. Non-immune etiology (see table 19.2)

Table 19.1 LABORATORY FEATURES OF IRON DEFICIENCY, ANEMIA OF CHRONIC DISEASE, AND THALASSEMIA MINOR

	FE DEFICIENCY	ANEMIA OF CHRONIC DISEASE	THALASSEMIA MINOR
MCV	Low (70–80)	Normal or Low	Low (<70)
RBC count	$<5 \times 10^{12}/L$	$<5 \times 10^{12}/L$	$>5 \times 10^{12}/L$
RDW	High (>15)	High (>15)	Normal
Serum Fe	Low	Low	Normal
Total iron binding capacity (TIBC)	High	Low	Normal
Transferrin saturation (FE/TIBC)	Low (<9%)	Low or Normal	Normal (>15%)
Ferritin	Very low	Normal or High	Normal or High
Soluble transferrin receptor	High	Normal	Normal

Partially adapted from Internal Medicine Board Review Core Curriculum, 12th Edition, MedStudy Corporation, © 2007.

Table 19.2 HYPERPROLIFERATIVE ANEMIAS

GENETIC	ACQUIRED

Genetic conditions of RBC membranes
    Hereditary spherocytosis
    Hereditary elliptocytosis
Genetic conditions of RBC metabolism (enzyme defects)
    G6PD deficiency (or favism)
    Pyruvate kinase deficiency
Genetic conditions of hemoglobin
    Sickle cell disease
    Thalassemia
    Unstable hemoglobins
	Immune-mediated hemolytic anemia (direct Coombs' +)
	    Autoimmune hemolytic anemia
	    Idiopathic
	    SLE
	    Evan syndrome
	    Cold hemagglutinin syndrome
	    Paroxysmal cold hemoglobinuria
	    Alloimmune hemolytic anemi
	    Hemolytic disease of the newborn (HDN)
	    Other minor blood group incompatibility
	    Drug induced immune hemolytic anemia
	Non-immune-mediated hemolytic anemia (direct Coombs' negative)
	    Drugs/toxins
	    Trauma
	    Mechanical heart valves
	    MAHA: TTP, HUS, DIC, and HELLP syndrome
	    Malaria/babesiosis/other infections
	    PNH
	    Liver disease

ACQUIRED HYPERPROLIFERATIVE ANEMIAS

Acquired causes of hyperproliferative anemias are distinguished from hereditary causes by the time of onset and lack of a family history. Clinically, in addition to the general signs and symptoms of anemia, patients have indirect hyperbilirubinemia, an elevated LDH, low haptoglobin, and reticulocytosis. The two most important tests in the evaluation of acquired hyperproliferative anemias are (1) a direct Coombs' test (also known as the direct antiglobulin test), which detects the presence of antibodies or complement proteins bound to the RBC surface, and (2) an examination of the peripheral smear for the morphology of the RBCs (see table 19.3). The direct Coombs' test differentiates immune from non-immune causes.

IMMUNE HEMOLYTIC ANEMIAS (COOMBS' POSITIVE)

Autoimmune Hemolytic Anemia

Autoimmune hemolytic anemia (AIHA) is defined as a Coombs'-positive hemolytic anemia. In AIHA the patient produces antibodies against his or her RBC surface antigens. The antigen is most often IgG and less frequently IgM. Hemolysis in AIHA is due to premature clearing of spherocytes by the spleen or complement-mediated hemolysis. For unclear reasons, over 90% of all hospitalized patients may have a positive Coombs' test of unknown significance.

IgG Immune Hemolytic Anemia

IgG antibodies are called *warm antibodies* because they react with RBCs best at body temperature. The antigen–antibody complexes formed on the RBC membranes are nicked away in the spleen, producing the typical cells in AIHA, the spherocytes, which are then prematurely cleared by the spleen. Other conditions associated with spherocytes are hereditary spherocytosis, drug-induced hemolytic anemia, and hypophosphatemia. IgG also causes complement fixation, but this is usually inadequate to cause intravascular hemolysis. Most cases of warm AIHA are idiopathic, but AIHA can be secondary to lymphoproliferative diseases, ovarian cancer, viral infections, and other autoimmune disorders. The first-line treatment of choice is with corticosteroids starting at high doses of prednisone 1 mg/kg per day, which reduces the antibody production, and blood transfusions as needed for symptoms. Splenectomy is reserved for patients who fail steroid treatment. Immunosuppressive and cytotoxic drugs (azathioprine, cyclophosphamide, cyclosporine) also reduce the production of antibody and are used in cases of steroid failure. There are also case reports of success with the anti CD-20 monoclonal antibody, rituximab in AIHA.

Table 19.3 TYPICAL PERIPHERAL SMEAR FINDINGS

Schistocytes	Microangiopathies such as TTP, HELLP syndrome, mechanical heart valves, preeclampsia, etc.
Sickle cells	Sickle cell syndromes - HbSS, HbSC, HbSD, HbSE, etc.
Bite cells	Hemolytic anemias due to oxidant damage such as G6PD deficiency
Spherocytes	Autoimmune hemolytic anemia
Target cells	Thalassemias, iron deficiency anemia
Agglutination rouleaux	Cold agglutinin disease

IgM Immune Hemolytic Anemia (Cold Agglutinin Disease)

IgM antibodies are called *cold antibodies* because they typically react at room temperature. IgM is frequently directed against the "I" antigen on the RBC membrane causing complement activation. Because this happens at temperatures lower than body temperature, they are often clinically insignificant. Occasionally, these antibodies have a wide thermal amplitude of activity and may then be clinically relevant. Beside the typical features of anemia, patients present with a dusky appearance to the skin and acrocyanosis of fingers, toes, ears, and nose tip. The direct Coombs' test identifies complement (C3) binding on the RBC, which is induced by IgM. The peripheral smear in cold agglutinin disease is classic (see figure 19.6), and the agglutination disappears on warming. Cold agglutinins are associated with *Mycoplasma pneumoniae* (anti-I), infectious mononucleosis (anti-i), lymphoproliferative disorders, and connective tissue diseases. Treatment includes keeping the patient warm and treating the underlying disease or infection. In severe cases, plasmapheresis may reduce the titer of the antibody, since IgM remains in the plasma.

Drug-Induced Immune Hemolytic Anemia

Drugs can cause immune hemolysis in four ways: autoantibody type, hapten (drug-absorption) type, immune-complex type (innocent bystander), and nonspecific reactions. The diagnosis is made by careful history and exam, and treatment is by removal of the offending drug (see table 19.4).

Paroxysmal Cold Hemoglobinuria

This is a much less common, self-limited, autoimmune hemolytic anemia in which there is IgG-activated complement-mediated lysis. It is either idiopathic or secondary to infection, most commonly measles. Other infectious causes include mumps, chickenpox, and syphilis. Mainstay of treatment is keeping the patient warm and treating the underlying cause.

NON-IMMUNE HEMOLYTIC ANEMIAS

Paroxysmal Nocturnal Hemoglobinuria

Paroxysmal nocturnal hemoglobinuria (PNH) is an acquired clonal hematopoietic stem-cell disorder caused by a defective PIG-A gene that results in the loss of glycosylphosphatidyl inositol (GPI) anchors on RBCs, WBCs, and platelets and a loss of the protective proteins usually carried by these anchors. CD-55 (decay-accelerating factor) and CD-59 (membrane inhibitor of reactive lysis) are two of these GPI-anchored proteins usually used in diagnosis. Other GPI anchor proteins include CD-14 and CD-16. Loss of the GPI-anchored proteins leaves RBCs unusually sensitive to complement-mediated lysis. Patients present with hemolysis, hemoglobinemia, hemoglobinuria (particularly in the morning because plasma is most acidotic at night), dysphagia, abdominal pain, iron deficiency, thrombocytopenia, and a predisposition to thrombosis in unusual sites. PNH may be accompanied by a bone marrow failure syndrome, myelodysplasia, or aplastic anemia, in which case pancytopenia accompanies the symptoms. Morbidity is from severe anemia, and mortality is primarily from thrombotic complications in the cerebral and abdominal veins that are present in up to 50% of cases for unclear reasons. The median survival of patients with PNH is 10 years. Diagnosis is by flow cytometry to detect a lack of cell surface markers CD-55 and CD-59. Treatment includes the use of steroids when there is brisk hemolysis that may inhibit activation of complement by the alternate pathway, cyclosporine, and a new monoclonal antibody eculizumab (Soliris) that prevents the formation of the membrane attack complex of the complement system C5b-9. Blood transfusions are given as dictated by symptoms. The only treatment with a chance of cure is bone marrow transplant.

Thrombotic Thrombocytopenic Purpura

Thrombotic thrombocytopenic purpura (TTP) is a microangiopathic process in which uncleaved ultralarge von Willebrand factor (vWF) multimers aggressively bind platelets, causing profound thrombocytopenia and thrombotic complications. The pathogenesis centers around a reduction or absence of the vWF-cleaving protease (ADAMTS13), which typically limits the formation of very large vWF multimers. There are acquired and familial forms of TTP both defined by the same final mechanism of limited ADAMTS13 activity. The classic pentad of TTP includes thrombocytopenia, renal failure, fever, neurological changes, and microangiopathic hemolytic anemia (MAHA) with schistocytes. Figure 19.7 shows the smear of a patient with TTP; notice the fragmented and distorted

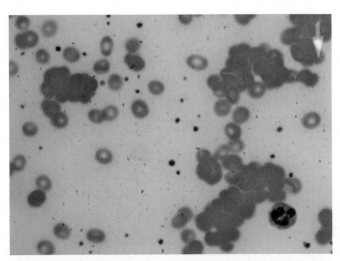

Figure 19.6. Cold Agglutinin Disease.

Table 19.4 MECHANISMS OF ACTION IN DRUG-INDUCED IMMUNE HEMOLYTIC ANEMIA

TYPE	MOA	ONSET AFTER INGESTION	DRUG EXAMPLES
Autoantibody type (Aldomet)	Similar to idiopathic warm AIHA. 25% patients develop IgG against RBC Rh Ags, <5% patients develop hemolysis. The drug itself is not involved in the Ag–Ab reaction.	18 weeks to 4 years	α-Methyl dopa, procainamide, ibuprofen, cimetidine
Hapten type (drug-adsorption; high-dose PCN)	The drug or drug metabolite binds to the RBC and forms a RBC Ag–drug complex, which induces an immune response only to RBCs with drug coating.	7–10 days	High-dose penicillin, cephalosporins, tetracycline, cisplatin, quinidine,
Immune-complex type; innocent bystander (quinidine)	This is an IgM Ab reaction. The drug binds to plasma proteins to form an immune complex. The complex then attaches to and cross-reacts with RBC Ags and activates complement causing intravascular hemolysis, hemoglobinemia, and hemoglobinuria.		Quinidine, quinine, acetaminophen, phenacetin, isoniazid, melphalan, sulfonylureas, insulin, rifampin, HCTZ, sulfa drugs
Nonspecific reactions	Some drugs induce immune hemolytic reactions by more than one of the mechanisms above or other mechanisms.		

RBCs, some shaped like helmets, the absence of platelets, and the polychromatophilic cells. The diagnosis should be suspected in patients with thrombocytopenia and hemolytic anemia (dyad) as patients infrequently have all five features at presentation. The diagnosis is clinical, and therefore TTP must be differentiated from other causes of MAHA (table 19.5). Without treatment over 90% of patients with TTP die of multiorgan failure. The standard of care for treatment is urgent plasmapheresis, which has the advantage of potentially removing ADAMTS13 antibodies and replacing ADAMTS13 (from the donor plasma). Plasma infusions, which are thought to be less effective, replace missing ADAMT13 and may be given while plasmapheresis is being arranged. Platelet transfusions can worsen the thrombosis and are contraindicated in TTP unless absolutely necessary.

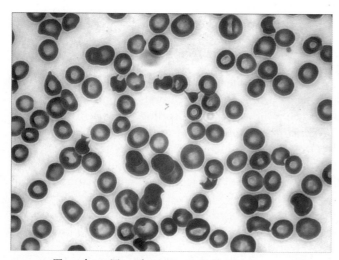

Figure 19.7. Thrombotic Thrombocytopenic Purpura.

HEREDITARY HEMOLYTIC ANEMIAS
Hereditary Conditions of the RBC Membrane
Hereditary Spherocytosis

Hereditary spherocytosis (HS) is a hemolytic condition caused by defects in the red cell membrane proteins, ankyrin, spectrin, band 3, and protein 4.2 that cause abnormal interactions between the RBC cytoskeleton and bilipid membrane. The most frequent mutation causing this is in the ankyrin gene, a mutation that causes a deficiency as well as spectrin. This leads to fragility of the RBC membrane. Most cases (75%) are autosomal dominant, so there is often a family his-

Table 19.5 MAJOR DIFFERENTIAL DIAGNOSIS OF MICROANGIPATHIC HEMOLYTIC ANEMIA

- Thrombotic thrombocytopenic purpura
- Hemolytic uremic syndrome
- HELLP (hypertension, elevated liver enzymes, and low platelets)
- Eclampsia/pre-eclampsia
- Malignant hypertension
- Disseminated intravascular coagulopathy
- Post bone marrow transplantation
- Metastatic cancer
- Prosthetic heart valves
- Collagen vascular disease
- Autoimmune disease
- HIV/AIDS
- Drugs—quinine, ticlopidine, etc.

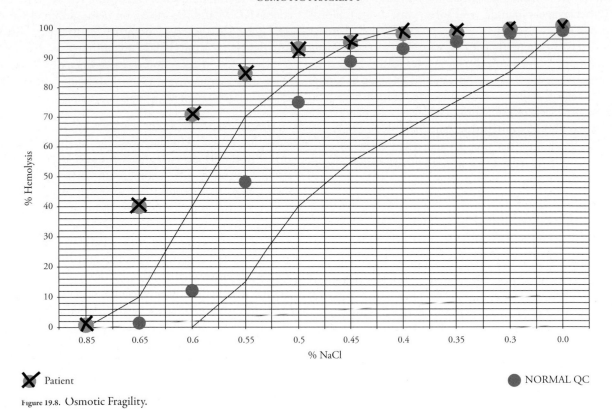

Figure 19.8. Osmotic Fragility.

tory. It is particularly common among Northern Europeans. Patients have chronic hemolysis, splenomegaly, bilirubin gall stones, and spherocytic RBCs on peripheral film causing an elevated mean corpuscular hemoglobin concentration (MCHC). Diagnosis is made by demonstrating increased osmotic fragility of RBCs when subjected to decreasing concentrations of saline (see figure 19.8: the black lines are the limits of normal, the gray dots show the control sample, and the crossed-out gray dots show the patient), and confirmation is by membrane studies. Figure 19.9 is the smear of a patient with HS. Although there are spherocytes pres-

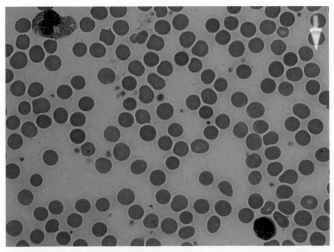

Figure 19.9. Hereditary Spherocytosis.

ent, some RBCs maintain normal biconcavity. Treatment includes folic acid daily to aid erythropoiesis and splenectomy, which decreases the rate of hemolysis. Asymptomatic patients with compensated hemolysis need no treatment.

Hereditary Conditions of RBC Metabolism (Enzymopathies)

Glucose-6-Phosphate Dehydrogenase (G6PD) Deficiency
G6PD deficiency is the most common RBC enzyme deficiency. There are over 300 variants of deficiency, all inherited in an X-linked fashion. The variants lead to levels of activity of the enzyme varying from normal to severely deficient activity. Males are more typically affected, but heterozygous females may also show hemolysis. The hemolysis is due to the inability of G6PD-deficient RBCS to produce enough NADPH to reduce glutathione and prevent oxidation and denaturation of hemoglobin by oxidant radicals. Denatured hemoglobin forms cytoplasmic inclusions (Heinz bodies), which are pitted in the spleen, leading to bite-cell formation and hemolysis. Severity of the disease depends on the level of enzyme activity and the degree of oxidant stress. G6PD deficiency confers some protection against malaria. The increased oxidant stress is thought to be unfavorable to *Plasmodium falciparum*. Patients present with severe hemolytic anemia, hyperbilirubinemia, methemoglobinemia, and/or hemoglobinuria during an episode of hemolysis. The most common trigger of hemolysis is infection,

commonly by *Pneumococcus, Salmonella,* and *Escherichia coli.* Other triggers include viral infections, drugs (chloroquine, primaquine, sulfonamides, aspirin, dapsone), ketoacidosis, liver disease, or kidney disease. Diagnosis is made by quantitative biochemical assays for G6PD. Note that false-negative results may be obtained if checked at a time of acute hemolysis because reticulocytes, which have relatively higher levels of G6PD than older RBCs, may be the predominant population during acute hemolysis. Diagnosis should be made months after an acute hemolytic episode. Management involves treating underlying infection/disease and/or withdrawing offending drugs.

Hemoglobinopathies (Hereditary Conditions of Abnormal Hemoglobin)

The hemoglobinopathies refer to abnormalities in hemoglobin that are of clinical consequence. The hemoglobinopathies are the most common heritable hematologic disease affecting mankind. The vast majority are due to point mutations leading to amino acid substitutions. Over 500 structurally abnormal hemoglobins have been discovered. Hemoglobinopathies can result from one of the following:

1. Qualitative abnormalities, as in the sickle cell syndromes

2. Quantitative abnormalities, as in the thalassemias

3. Abnormalities of hemoglobin causing instability (to heat and alcohol in the lab), unstable hemoglobins

Thalassemias

These are the most common hemoglobinopathies. Thalassemias are due to a quantitative deficiency or absence of alpha or beta chains of hemoglobin referred to as α-thalassemia and ß-thalassemia, respectively. Decreased production of globin chains results in decreased normal hemoglobin production and the formation of homotetramers of the excess globin chains that precipitate in the erythroid precursors causing hemolysis and ineffective erythropoiesis that worsen the anemia. Rarer forms of thalassemia include δß-thalassemia and εγδß-thalassemia.

ß-Thalassemia

ß-Thalassemia results from mutations of the beta-globin gene complex located on chromosome 11. The mutations may be nonsense mutations in which no beta-globin is produced or mutations that alter splicing and cause decreased production of beta-globin. The clinical manifestations depend on the number and severity of the abnormal beta-globin gene(s) inherited. The peripheral smear in ß-thalassemia characteristically shows hypochromic microcytic RBCs and target cells (see figure 19.10) and therefore is in the differential in cases of iron deficiency. Thalassemia

minor and iron deficiency can be differentiated by the RBC count, RDW, and the HbA2 on hemoglobin electrophoresis. Figure 19.10 shows laboratory features that distinguish iron deficiency from thalassemia minor.

There are three clinical categories of ß-thalassemia: (1) ß-thalassemia minor, (2) ß-thalassemia intermedia, and (3) ß-thalassemia major (Cooley's anemia).

1. ß-Thalassemia minor: Patients are asymptomatic and have no clinical sequelae. Patients do have microcytosis (MCV usually below 70) but with only mild or no anemia at all. Diagnosis is by hemoglobin electrophoresis, which shows two- to threefold elevations in levels of hemoglobin A_2 (HbA$_2$) and mild elevations of fetal hemoglobin (HbF).

2. ß-Thalassemia intermedia: Patients are severely anemic but are not chronically transfusion dependent. Patients inheriting homozygous ß0 alleles may present with thalassemia intermedia if modulating factors such as co-inheritance of α-thalassemia trait exist. Patients have ineffective erythropoiesis and so hyperabsorb iron, resulting in problems of iron overload. They often also have splenomegaly and bony expansion. Hemoglobin electrophoresis shows elevations of HbF and HbA$_2$. Patients often need iron chelation, which is now available as an oral formulation deferasirox (Exjade), 20–30 mg/kg per day. Prior to deferasirox the only formulation available was deferoxamine (Desferal) given intravenously or subcutaneously as a continuous nightly infusion.

3. ß-Thalassemia major (Cooley's anemia): Patients have essentially no production of beta-globin chains. Severe anemia is seen early in life due to alpha-chain homotetramer formation, which is toxic to erythroid precursors and causes ineffective erythropoiesis in the bone marrow and clearance of peripheral red cells by the spleen. Without RBC transfusions, patients show marked bone marrow expansion of the skull and long bones producing a "chipmunk" facies,

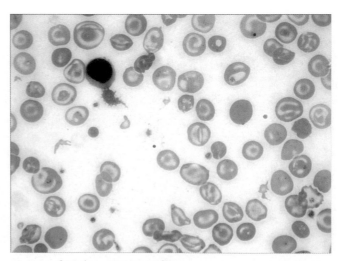

Figure 19.10. ß-Thalassemia Intermedia.

predisposition to fractures, growth retardation, and hepatosplenomegaly. Red cell transfusions suppress ineffective erythropoiesis and treat the anemia. Iron overload inevitably results from avid intestinal absorption of iron as well as from transfusions. Hemoglobin electrophoresis shows no HbA. Treatment is mainly supportive. Bone marrow transplant is the only curative approach.

α-Thalassemia

α-Thalassemia results from defects of the *alpha* genes located on chromosome 16. Human beings have duplicate copies of the alpha-gene on each chromosome; therefore, the clinical manifestations of α-thalassemia are more varied than those of ß-thalassemia. Just as in ß-thalassemia, the imbalance in globin chains leads to decreased hemoglobin and microcytosis. Although α-thalassemia is associated with hemolysis, there is no significant ineffective erythropoiesis because homotetramers $ß_4$ and $γ_4$ (seen in α-thalassemia) are more soluble than $α_4$ (seen in ß-thalassemia). Hemoglobin electrophoresis is normal in α-thalassemia, and DNA analysis is required to make a diagnosis. The clinical syndromes of α-thalassemia depend on the number of alpha-chains missing.

−α+-Thalassemia trait (-α/αα): These patients are heterozygous for an α+-thalassemia gene and have one of four alleles absent. These patients are called silent carriers and are clinically normal.

−α Thalassemia trait (−/αα): These patients are heterozygous for an α0-thalassemia gene and have two of four alleles missing. Patients are asymptomatic but have microcytosis and little or no anemia.

Hemoglobin H (−/-α): These patients are doubly heterozygous for α0-thalassemia and α+-thalassemia and have varied presentations. All patients are anemic; in severe forms patients exhibit transfusion dependence early in life, whereas other patients with milder disease are virtually asymptomatic until late adulthood.

Hemoglobin Bart's (−/−): Patients who are homozygous for α0-thalassemia have an absolute absence of alpha genes. Instead, homotetramers of $γ_4$ form and are able to carry oxygen but have such high oxygen affinity that oxygen is not delivered to tissues. This causes severe in utero hypoxia, hydrops fetalis, and death between 30 and 40 weeks or soon after birth. Hemoglobin Bart's is incompatible with life.

SICKLE CELL SYNDROMES

The sickle cell gene results from a mutation at the sixth amino acid position of the ß-globin gene of hemoglobin. The central abnormality in sickle hemoglobin is the tendency to polymerize in conditions of deoxygenation. Polymerized sickle hemoglobin causes RBC membrane stiffness, change in RBC shape to a crescent, abnormal RBC membrane permeability causing RBC dehydration, tissue ischemia, and tissue infarction. Patients with one of the sickle cell diseases frequently present with excruciating episodes of pain often precipitated by infection, dehydration, acidosis, or other stressors. There is wide clinical variability in patients with sickle cell disease, with some patients living fairly asymptomatic lives. The reason for this variability is the subject of ongoing research.

SICKLE CELL ANEMIA

Sickle cell anemia refers to the homozygous inheritance of the sickle cell gene. It is in general the most severe form of the sickle cell syndromes. The peripheral smear shows numerous sickle (shaped) cells. See figure 19.11. Patients present with severe anemia and jaundice from chronic hemolysis, hyposthenuria from renal microinfarctions, and leg ulcers. Splenic atrophy from chronic infarction causes predisposition to encapsulated organisms such as *Streptococcus pneumoniae*, *Klebsiella*, and *Neisseria meningitidis*. Every organ system is affected in the long run by chronic hypoxia, some of which include the following:

- *Central nervous system:* Strokes, transient ischemic attack (TIA), cognitive impairment, proliferative and nonproliferative retinopathy, retinal detachment
- *Cardiovascular system:* Cardiomegaly, high-output failure
- *Respiratory system:* Acute chest syndrome, pulmonary hypertension
- *Gastrointestinal system:* Bile gall stones, hepatic crisis
- *Genitourinary system:* Isosthenuria, renal papillary necrosis, nephrotic syndrome, hematuria, glomerulonephritis, priapism
- *Musculoskeletal system:* Avascular necrosis of long bones, "fish-mouthed" vertebrae

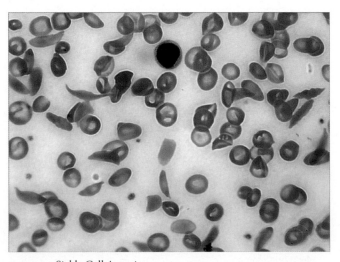

Figure 19.11. Sickle Cell Anemia.

- *Skin:* Chronic leg ulcers
- *Bone marrow:* Aplastic anemia (precipitated by parvovirus B 19)

Acute chest syndrome is a constellation of hypoxia, dyspnea, tachycardia, and a new infiltrate on chest x-ray in a patient with sickle cell disease. It is a frequent cause of mortality and an indication for urgent exchange blood transfusion to a goal HbS level of 30% and a hematocrit of 30%. Laboratory diagnosis is by hemoglobin electrophoresis, which in the absence of recent RBC transfusion shows no HbA, 80–95% HbS, and varying quantities of HbF and HbA2. The primary treatment modality is prevention of fever, dehydration, acidosis, high altitudes, extreme temperatures, and infections. The treatment of acute pain episodes is supportive, with administration of intravenous fluids, intravenous pain medication, blood transfusions, and oxygen when indicated by symptoms. The indications for an exchange blood transfusion are (1) acute chest syndrome and (2) cerebrovascular accidents (strokes and TIAs). The goal is to reduce HbS to 30% and maintain hematocrit close to 30%. Hydroxyurea is the only FDA-approved medication for sickle cell disease. It is used in the chronic setting. Hydroxyurea's main mechanism of action in sickle cell disease is in the induction of fetal hemoglobin (HbF), which interferes with the polymerization of HbS, ameliorating the disease.

HEMOGLOBIN SC DISEASE

This is the most common of the double heterozygous sickle cell diseases. Hemoglobin SC is due to the co-inheritance of HbS (ß6Glu→Val) and HbC (ß6Glu→Lys). Symptoms tend to be milder than in HbSS anemia, but patients have particular predisposition to sickle retinopathy and avascular necrosis. Both HbS and HbC are seen on hemoglobin electrophoresis to make a diagnosis. Other double heterozygous states include HbS/ß-thalassemia, HbSD, HbSE, and others. The clinical severity of each of these depends on the extent to which the other abnormal hemoglobin interferes with the polymerization of hemoglobin S. Treatment is supportive.

SICKLE CELL TRAIT

This is not one of the sickle cell syndromes. Sickle cell trait refers to the heterozygous inheritance of HbS with HbA and is not thought to be a disease state. Patients are asymptomatic, although a few may have hematuria, isosthenuria, and renal papillary necrosis.

ADDITIONAL READING

Bain BJ. Diagnosis from the blood smear. *N Engl J Med.* 2005; 353:498–507.

Cunningham MJ. Update on thalassemia: Clinical care and complications. *Hematol Oncol Clin North Am.* 2010;24(1):215–27.

Janus J, Moerschel SK. Evaluation of anemia in children. *Am Fam Physician.* 2010;81(12):1462–71.

Kaferle J, Strzoda CE. Evaluation of macrocytosis. *Am Fam Physician.* 2009;79(3):203–8.

Lechner K, Jäger U. How I treat autoimmune hemolytic anemias in adults. *Blood.* 2010;116(11):1831–8.

Rosse WF, Hillmen P, Schreiber AD. Immune-mediated hemolytic anemia. American Society of Hematology Education Book. Washington, DC: American Society of Hematology; 2004.

The Management of Sickle Cell Disease. NIH publication No. 02–2117 (4th ed). Bethesda, MD: NHLBI; 2002.

Weiss G, Goodnought LT. Anemia of chronic disease. *N Engl J Med.* 2005;352:1011–23.

Young, N. Acquired aplastic anemia. *JAMA.* 1999;282(3):271–8.

QUESTIONS

QUESTION 1. A 40-year-old man who refurbishes old city buildings presents for a routine physical. He is pale, has a discolored gum-tooth line, and has neuropathy.
Labs: WBC 6.2, hemoglobin 10.3 g/dL, platelets 232,000
Smear: microcytic hypochromic cells with basophilic stippling
Bone marrow: ringed sideroblasts
How would you manage this patient?

A. Ferrous sulfate, 325 mg bid, to replete ferritin
B. Vitamin B-12 shots and folic acid orally
C. Erythropoietin, 40,000 units SQ weekly to a goal hematocrit of 35%
D. Eliminate exposure, then give DMSA (oral chelator) to decrease lead levels <25 µg/dL

QUESTION 2. A 70-year-old woman develops tingling in her hands over 8 months. She is evaluated by a neurologist. Labs were normal. She is then lost to follow-up until 2 years later, when she has increasing fatigue and incoordination. Exam reveals a positive Romberg and absent position and vibration sense.

Labs: WBC 2.3, hemoglobin 7.3 g/dL, hematocrit 20%, platelet count is 35,000, reticulocyte count is 0.4%. B-12 is 220 pg/mL (normal 200–800), methylmalonic acid level is 0.51 micromol/L (normal < 0.4). The most likely diagnosis is which of the following?

A. Vitamin B-12 deficiency
B. Aplastic anemia
C. Anemia of chronic disease
D. Folic acid deficiency

QUESTION 3. A 60-year-old woman with rheumatoid arthritis presents with a 2-week history of worsening weakness and dizziness.
Labs: WBC 4.7, hemoglobin 5.3, hematocrit 15%, MCV 92, MCHC 39, platelet count 177,000. Total bilirubin 3.1, direct bilirubin 0.2, reticulocyte count 23%, LDH

936, haptoglobin <8, direct Coombs' positive for IgG and complement.

You would expect which of the following?

A. Osmotic fragility to be abnormal
B. Treatment with steroids to be beneficial
C. Thrombosis in unusual sites
D. Schistocytes on her peripheral smear
E. None of the above

QUESTION 4. A 39-year-old man is brought to the emergency room for acute onset of confusion. On physical exam he is afebrile, pale, and has an altered mental status.

Labs: WBC 7.1, hemoglobin 8, hematocrit 26%, platelets 21,000, BUN 30, creatinine 2.1, LDH 1040, reticulocyte count 12%. Lab data were normal during an annual physical 1 week earlier. How would you treat?

A. Steroids alone
B. Steroids followed by splenectomy
C. Platelet transfusion
D. Plasmapheresis
E. None of the above

QUESTION 5. A 32-year-old woman presents with 3-day history of colicky abdominal pain and fatigue.

Labs: hemoglobin 7.9, hematocrit 22%, MCV 78, platelets 60,000, reticulocyte count 9%, direct and indirect Coombs' negative, ferritin 10. Abdominal ultrasound scan shows portal vein thrombosis. Urinalysis shows hemosiderin.

The most likely diagnosis is:

A. Factor V Leiden mutation
B. Paroxysmal cold hemoglobinuria
C. Warm autoimmune hemolytic anemia
D. Paroxysmal nocturnal hemoglobinuria
E. Iron deficiency anemia

ANSWERS

1. D
2. A
3. B
4. D
5. D

20.

BOARD REVIEW IN HEMATOLOGY

Julie-Aurore Losman and Benjamin L. Ebert

QUESTIONS

QUESTION 1. A 28-year-old woman is seen in clinic for evaluation. Her past medical history is notable only for an episode of prolonged bleeding after extraction of her wisdom teeth. She takes no medications regularly and does not smoke cigarettes or drink alcohol. Her family history is notable for the fact that her father has an "allergy" to aspirin, characterized by extensive bruising, and her sister developed postpartum bleeding requiring a blood transfusion several days after the birth of each of her two children. The patient wants to become pregnant but is concerned because of her family history of bleeding.

An appropriate evaluation at this time would include:

A. Prothrombin time (PT), partial thromboplastin time (PTT) and fibrinogen assays
B. Factor VIII and factor IX levels
C. Von Willebrand antigen, ristocetin cofactor, and factor VIII levels
D. No evaluation necessary; perform testing for von Willebrand disease if patient becomes pregnant

QUESTION 2. A healthy, fit 25-year-old Caucasian woman with no significant past medical history develops a right popliteal deep venous thrombosis (DVT) several months after starting on oral contraception. She has no family history of spontaneous thrombosis, but her father did develop a pulmonary embolism (PE) after fracturing his leg in a motor vehicle accident several years ago. Of the following heritable conditions, which is most likely to have predisposed her to develop venous thrombosis:

A. Antithrombin III deficiency
B. Protein C deficiency
C. Hyperhomocysteinemia
D. Factor V Leiden
E. Prothrombin gene mutation (G20210A)

QUESTION 3. A 29-year-old African-American woman presents to the emergency room in acute respiratory distress and is found to have an oxygen saturation of 86% on room air. She undergoes a chest computed tomography (CT) scan and is found to have bilateral pulmonary emboli. She is immediately started on low-molecular-weight heparin and is admitted to the hospital. She reports that she has never been ill and takes no medications. Her only past medical history is a first-trimester spontaneous abortion several years ago. She has no family history of venous thromboembolic disease.

On the morning after admission her laboratory studies are as follows:

White blood cell count	12,600/mm³	(4000–10,000)
Hematocrit	34%	(36–48)
MCV	76 fL	(80–95)
Platelets	116,000/mm³	(150,000–450,000)
PT	11.6 sec	(11–13)
PTT	44 sec	(22–34)
Fibrinogen	230 mg/dL	(200–400)
LDH	260	(107–231)
Haptoglobin	96 mg/dL	(40–180)

An appropriate workup at this time would include:

A. Serologic testing for HIT antibodies
B. Peripheral blood flow cytometry for CD55 and CD59
C. Serologic testing for antibodies to ADAMTS13
D. A lupus anticoagulant test and serologic testing for anticardiolipin and beta-2-glycoprotein antibodies

QUESTION 4. A 43-year-old woman comes to the emergency room complaining of fatigue, shortness of breath with exertion over the past 3 days, and a mild headache for the past several hours. She denies any other systemic symptoms. Her past medical history is unremarkable, and she takes no medications. She is afebrile, and her vital signs are stable. Her physical examination is entirely unremarkable, and she looks well.

Laboratory studies reveal:

White blood cell count	8200/mm³	(4000–10,000)
Hematocrit	26%	(36–48)
Platelets	31,000/mm³	(150,000–450,000)
PT	12 sec	(11–13)
PTT	29 sec	(22–34)
Fibrinogen	320 mg/dL	(200–400)

Creatinine	0.9 mg/dL	(0.7–1.3)
LDH	652	(107–231)

Peripheral blood smear reveals decreased platelets and a moderate number of schistocytes.

The most appropriate initial therapy is:

A. Administer intravenous fluids and send stool studies for *Escherichia. coli* 0157:H7.

B. Observe for now. Initiate plasmapheresis if the patient's platelet count falls below 20,000/mm³.

C. Observe for now. Initiate plasmapheresis if the patient clinically worsens or her creatinine rises.

D. Initiate plasmapheresis with plasma exchange as soon as possible.

QUESTION 5. A 19-year-old female college student comes for her first clinic visit after a recent flu-like illness. Her past medical history is remarkable only for occasional menstrual cramps that are relieved by ibuprofen. She takes no other medications. On review of systems she notes that her last menstrual period was heavier than usual, but she is currently not menstruating. Her physical examination is unremarkable, and she looks well.

Laboratory studies reveal:

White blood cell count	6200/mm³	(4000–10,000)
Hematocrit	34%	(36–48)
Platelets	19,000/mm³	(150,000–450,000)
Creatinine	0.8 mg/dL	(0.7–1.3)
LDH	159 IU/L	(107–231)

Peripheral blood smear reveals normal red cell and white cell morphology, decreased platelets that appear somewhat larger than normal, and no schistocytes.

The most appropriate next steps are:

A. Observe. Repeat platelet count in 3–5 days.

B. Request an HIV test. Advise patient to discontinue ibuprofen. Treat patient with dexamethasone 40 mg daily for 4 days as an outpatient with close follow-up.

C. Obtain a surgical consultation for consideration of splenectomy.

D. Hospitalize the patient and treat her with intravenous gamma-globulin infusion.

QUESTION 6. A 71-year-old woman who recently underwent total hip replacement surgery is readmitted to the hospital with chest pain and acute-onset shortness of breath. She is found to have bilateral pulmonary emboli and is started on unfractionated heparin. Her complete blood count is normal on admission, but by hospital day 5 her platelet count is noted to have drifted down to 80,000/mm³. An enzyme-linked immunosorbent assay (ELISA) assay for antibodies to the heparin-PF4 complex is sent and is pending.

Which of the following management decisions is appropriate:

A. Unfractionated heparin may be continued pending results of the heparin-PF4 antibody assay, and a search for other causes of thrombocytopenia should be initiated.

B. Unfractionated heparin should be discontinued immediately, and the patient should be started on anticoagulation with low-molecular-weight heparin.

C. Unfractionated heparin should be discontinued immediately, and the patient should be started on anticoagulation with warfarin.

D. Unfractionated heparin should be discontinued immediately, and the patient should be started on anticoagulation with a direct thrombin inhibitor.

QUESTION 7. A 74-year-old man comes to the emergency room complaining of 6 hours of fever, rigors, severe abdominal pain, and nausea and vomiting. His past medical history is remarkable for a myocardial infarction 3 years ago that required coronary artery bypass grafting as well as peripheral vascular disease that required femoral-popliteal bypass surgery 2 years ago. He is somewhat delirious and cannot provide a history, but his wife reports that he was "fine" when he was seen by his primary care physician 6 months ago and that he has lost 25 pounds in the last 2 months due to severe postprandial "heartburn pain." He takes several blood pressure and cholesterol-lowering medications, but she cannot recall their names. He is febrile, tachycardic, and hypotensive, and his physical examination is remarkable for moderate abdominal distension, severe abdominal pain with mild palpation, and diminished bowel sounds.

Laboratory studies reveal:

White blood cell count	14,300/mm³	(4000–10,000)
Hematocrit	37%	(36–48)
Platelets	78,000/mm³	(150,000–450,000)
PT	24 sec	(11–13)
PTT	49 sec	(22–34)
Fibrinogen	210 mg/dL	(200–400)
Creatinine	1.8 mg/dL	(0.7–1.3)
LDH	426	(107–231)
AST	634	(10–50 U/L)
ALT	786	(10–50 U/L)
Lactate	19	(0.5–2.2 mmol/L)

Peripheral blood smear reveals neutrophils with toxic granulations and numerous bands, decreased platelets, and a moderate number of schistocytes.

His thrombocytopenia is most likely due to:

A. Drug-induced thrombocytopenia

B. Immune thrombocytopenic purpura

C. Thrombotic thrombocytopenic purpura

D. Disseminated intravascular coagulation

E. Splenic platelet sequestration secondary to liver disease

Question 8. An asymptomatic 43-year-old woman is noted on routine laboratory testing to have the following complete blood count:

White blood cell count	8200/mm³	(4000–10,000)
Hematocrit	38%	(36–48)
Platelets	863,000/mm³	(150,000–450,000)

The most appropriate next step is:

A. Low-dose aspirin therapy should be started as soon as possible to prevent thrombotic complications.

B. Warfarin therapy should be started as soon as possible to prevent thrombotic complications.

C. Hydroxyurea therapy should be started to lower the platelet count to within the normal range.

D. The patient should be evaluated for the presence of iron deficiency, an inflammatory state, or a chronic myeloproliferative disorder.

E. The patient should be counseled about her risk of developing acute leukemia.

QUESTION 9. A 46-year-old African-American man is seen for follow-up 4 days after completing a course of trimethoprim/sulfamethoxazole for an episode of bacterial sinusitis. On review of systems he notes that his sinus congestion has improved but that, during the past week, he has felt somewhat more short of breath with exertion and more fatigued than prior to starting his course of antibiotics.

Laboratory studies reveal:

White blood cell count	4100/mm³	(4000–10,000)
Hematocrit	26%	(36–48)
MCV	102 fL	(80–95)
Platelets	163,000/mm³	(150,000–450,000)

The most appropriate course of action at this time is:

A. Observe and have the patient return in a few weeks for further laboratory tests.

B. Send a dye decolorization test for glucose-6-phosphate dehydrogenase deficiency.

C. Inquire with patient about any recent history of heavy alcohol use.

D. Obtain patient's folate and vitamin B-12 levels.

QUESTION 10. A 39-year-old woman originally from the Dominican Republic comes to the clinic for her first visit. Her only past medical history is a diagnosis of iron deficiency anemia that was made 5 years ago, at the birth of her second child. At the time she was told to take iron tablets twice daily. This is her only medication.

Laboratory studies reveal:

White blood cell count	4600/mm³	(4000–10,000)
Hematocrit	35%	(36–48)
MCV	66 fL	(80–95)
Platelets	256,000/mm3	(150,000–450,000)
Fe	142 μg/dL	(40–159)
TIBC	320 μg/dL	(250–400)
Ferritin	220 ng/mL	(20–300)
Creatinine	0.7 mg/dL	(0.5–1.1)

The most appropriate management of this patient is to:

A. Discontinue her iron replacement therapy and initiate phlebotomy to reverse her hemochromatosis.

B. Discontinue her iron replacement therapy and start her on erythropoietin therapy.

C. Discontinue her iron replacement therapy and send a hemoglobin electrophoresis.

D. Switch her from oral to intravenous iron replacement therapy and work her up for occult blood loss.

QUESTION 11. A 43-year-old man who underwent gastric bypass surgery for morbid obesity 2 years ago presents to clinic for the first time since recovering from his surgery. He is very happy about the fact that he has lost 150 pounds and reports that he has generally felt well since his surgery, but recently he has noticed that he is more fatigued and irritable than usual. He was finally prompted to come in for a checkup when, a few weeks ago, he began experiencing numbness and tingling in his fingers and toes.

Laboratory studies reveal:

White blood cell count	3900/mm³	(4000–10,000)
Hematocrit	32%	(36–48)
MCV	116 fL	(80–95)
Platelets	156,000/mm3	(150,000–450,000)

The most appropriate course of action at this time is:

A. Check a hemoglobin A1c and counsel the patient on management of diabetic peripheral neuropathy.

B. Check a peripheral blood smear and reticulocyte count and order folate, vitamin B-12 levels.

C. Check a peripheral blood smear and reticulocyte count and order folate, vitamin B-12 levels, and start empirical treatment with folate.

D. Recommend that the patient undergo screening tests for an occult malignancy.

QUESTION 12. A 61-year-old man with benign prostatic hypertrophy, diabetes mellitus, and poorly controlled hypertension presents to clinic after a recent hospitalization for new-onset heart failure. He was switched from his oral diabetes medications to insulin and was started on several new blood pressure-lowering agents as well as Lasix. Review of his records reveals that his hematocrit has been gradually declining over the past 3 years.

Laboratory studies today reveal:

Hematocrit	29%	(36–48)
MCV	86 fL	(80–95)
RDW	14.1	(10–14.5)
Platelets	280,000/mm³	(150,000–450,000)
BUN	31 mg/dL	(9–25)
Creatinine	1.8 mg/dL	(0.7–1.3)
LDH	221	(107–231)

Peripheral blood smear reveals normochromic, normocytic red blood cells, few reticulocytes, and normal-appearing platelets, lymphocytes, and neutrophils.

The most likely etiology of his anemia is:
   A. Medication effect of Lasix
   B. Erythropoietin deficiency
   C. Combined iron and vitamin B-12 deficiency
   D. Replacement of his bone marrow by metastatic prostate cancer

QUESTION 13. A 21-year-old man with sickle-cell disease who frequently comes to the emergency department with simple pain crises presents 1 week after his last ED visit reporting that his pain has returned. He reports that he is having his typical symptoms of back, hip, and thigh pain and reports that he has been unable to eat or drink very much for the past 2 days. In the past day he has developed fevers and shortness of breath. In the emergency department he is noted to have a temperature of 101.9°, and his oxygen saturation is 94% on room air. On chest x-ray he has a right lower-lobe infiltrate that was not present 1 week ago.

Laboratory studies reveal:

White blood cell count	18,000/mm³	(4000–10,000)
Hematocrit	27%	(36–48)
Platelets	283,000/mm3	(150,000–450,000)

Appropriate management of this patient should include:

   A. Intravenous fluids and pain medication in the ED until his pain has improved, and then discharge home with oral pain medication and a prescription for antibiotics for community-acquired pneumonia.
   B. Intravenous fluids, oxygen supplementation, and intravenous pain medication, and admission to the hospital for pain control.
   C. Intravenous fluids, oxygen supplementation, antibiotics, and intravenous pain medication, and admission to the hospital for monitoring and initiation of hydroxyurea.
   D. Intravenous fluids, oxygen supplementation, antibiotics, and intravenous pain medication, and admission to the hospital for monitoring and exchange transfusion.

QUESTION 14. A 57-year-old woman with no significant past medical history presents to clinic after 4 days of worsening fatigue, dyspnea on exertion, and palpitations. She initially attributed her symptoms to being "out of shape," but she noticed this morning that her eyes looked yellowish. She is on no medications and has no family history of hematologic diseases. Her mother and sister both had Graves' disease.

Laboratory studies reveal:

White blood cell count	10,400/mm³	(4000–10,000)
Hematocrit	16%	(36–48)
MCV	101 fL	(80–95)
Platelets	242,000/mm³	(150,000–450,000)
Coombs' test		Positive

Peripheral blood smear reveals a predominance of microspherocytes and increased numbers of reticulocytes but is otherwise normal.

Appropriate management of this patient involves:
   A. Initiation of high-dose oral steroids with follow-up the next day for a recheck of her hematocrit
   B. Admission to the hospital for initiation of high-dose steroids
   C. Admission to the hospital for initiation of rituximab therapy
   D. Immediate blood transfusion and admission to the hospital for high-dose steroids
   E. Immediate blood transfusion and admission to the hospital for initiation of rituximab therapy

ANSWERS

1. C. This patient's personal and family histories are consistent with the diagnosis of von Willebrand disease (vWD), which is caused by defects in the activity of von Willebrand factor (vWF), a central mediator of hemostasis. The vWF protein is synthesized by megakaryocytes and endothelial cells as a dimeric protein that then multimerizes, resulting in the formation of very large vWF proteins that are highly prothrombotic. When released into the circulation, these long vWF multimers are cleaved by the ADAMTS13 metalloprotease into smaller, less prothrombotic polypeptides. These polypeptides bind to platelets and the subendothelium, serving as a tether between platelets and sites of endothelial damage during platelet plug formation. vWF also contributes to fibrin clot formation by binding to and stabilizing factor VIII, a critical coagulation factor that has a very short half-life in the circulation when not bound to vWF.

vWD, which is caused by mutations in the vWF gene, is the most common inherited disorder of hemostasis. There are three types of VWD as listed below:

- Type I is an autosomal dominant condition caused by mutations that impair the synthesis of vWF, resulting in a partial deficiency of the vWF protein. Bleeding is typically mild to moderate.

- Type II is a (usually) autosomal dominant condition caused by mutations that result in impaired function of vWF. Bleeding is typically moderate to severe.

- IIA is caused by mutations that disrupt normal intracellular processing of vWF, resulting in a relative deficiency of high- and intermediate-molecular-weight vWF multimers.

- IIB is caused by mutations that increase binding of vWF to platelets. vWF-platelet aggregates are cleared, resulting in low circulating vWF levels and thrombocytopenia.

- IIM is caused by mutations that decrease the affinity of vWF for platelets.

- IIN is caused by mutations in vWF that decrease the affinity of vWF for factor VIII.

• Type III is an autosomal recessive condition caused by mutations that result in complete deficiency of the vWF protein. These patients typically have severe bleeding.

vWD can also be an acquired disorder. Mechanisms of acquired vWD include development of autoantibodies to vWF in autoimmune and lymphoproliferative disorders, impaired vWF synthesis in hypothyroidism, aberrant vWF proteolysis in disseminated intravascular coagulation, and sequestration of vWF by binding to tumors cells.

The diagnosis of vWD, especially mild cases, can be difficult to make. The range of normal vWF levels is wide, and normal individuals who are blood type O have 25–30% lower vWF levels compared to type AB individuals. In addition many factors can influence vWF levels in normal individuals. Hypothyroidism decreases and exogenous estrogen increases vWF synthesis. More significantly, vWF and factor VIII are both acute-phase reactants, and their levels can vary widely during periods of physiological stress, including strenuous exercise, inflammatory conditions, and pregnancy. vWF levels increase throughout pregnancy and decline rapidly postpartum, resulting in bleeding several days after delivery in patients with vWD.

Testing for vWD involves assessing both vWF levels and vWF function (see table 20.1).

• The vWF antigen assay determines the amount of vWF protein present.

• The ristocetin cofactor assay tests the ability of vWF to agglutinate platelets, thereby assessing the integrity of the platelet-dependent activity of vWF.

• The ratio of vWF antigen to vWF activity (vWF:RCo) can distinguish the different types of vWD.

• vWF multimer analysis can also help differentiate the different subtypes of type II VWD.

• The factor VIII antigen assay tests the integrity of the factor VIII-stabilizing function of vWF.

• The aPTT will be prolonged in cases of VWD where factor VIII levels are significantly decreased.

In the above question, the patient's family history is suggestive of an autosomally inherited bleeding disorder.

vWD is epidemiologically the most likely diagnosis. The PT and fibrinogen levels are normal in patients with vWD and the PTT is only affected in cases where the defect in vWF function is severe. These are therefore not effective screening tests for vWD, and answer A is incorrect. Given that the patient's sister is affected, the diagnosis of hemophilia A or B, which are X-linked deficiencies in factors VIII and IX, respectively, is unlikely. Answer B is therefore incorrect. Because vWF levels increase during pregnancy, testing for vWD during pregnancy can give falsely normal results. Women with suspected vWD should therefore be tested before they become pregnant. Answer D is therefore incorrect.

2. D. Venous thromboembolism (VTE), which manifests clinically as deep vein thrombosis and pulmonary embolism, typically occurs in patients with risk factors for thrombosis. In most patients with VTE, one or more of Virchow's triad of thrombotic risk factors (venous stasis, endothelial injury, hypercoagulability) can be identified. Causes of venous stasis include prolonged immobilization, extended air travel, pregnancy, and obesity. Causes of vascular endothelial injury include trauma, surgery, intravenous drug use, vasculitis, and sickle-cell anemia. Hypercoagulable states can be acquired or inherited. Acquired hypercoagulable states include pregnancy, oral contraceptive use, hormone replacement therapy, nephrotic syndrome, malignancy, clonal hematologic disorders (including polycythemia vera, essential thrombocythemia, and paroxysmal nocturnal hemoglobinuria), heparin-induced thrombocytopenia (HIT), inflammatory conditions, and antiphospholipid syndrome. Inherited hypercoagulable conditions include mutations in factor V, prothrombin, methyltetrahydrofolate reductase, protein C and S, fibrinogen, and antithrombin III. This patient does not appear to have venous stasis or a recent vascular injury. Her VTE is therefore likely the result of her oral contraceptive use in addition to, possibly, an inherited hypercoagulable condition.

The factor V Leiden (FVL) mutation is the most common familial thrombophilia. FVL is present in 4.8% of Caucasians and in 0.05% of Africans and Asians, and the frequency of FVL in patients under 50 years of age with a family history of thrombosis or a history of recurrent thrombotic events and no acquired risk factors for thrombosis

Table 20.1 VON WILLEBRAND DISEASE ASSAY

VWD TYPE	VWF AG	RCO	VWF:RCO	FVIII	LARGE MULTIMERS
I	Low	Low	Normal	Proportional to vWF Ag	Proportional
IIA	Low	Lower	Low	Proportional to vWF Ag	Very low
IIB	Low	Lower	Low/normal	Proportional to vWF Ag	Low
IIM	Low/normal	Lower	Low	Proportional to vWF Ag	Proportional
IIN	Normal	Normal	Normal	Disproportionately low	Normal
III	Undetectable	Undetectable	-	Very low	Undetectable

except pregnancy or oral contraceptive use is 40%. FVL is the result of a missense mutation that changes the arginine at position 506 of factor V to glutamine, which prevents the inactivation of factor V by activated protein C and prevents termination of activation of the coagulation cascade.

The second most common familial thrombophilia is the prothrombin G20210A mutation, which is a mutation in the 3'-untranslated region of prothrombin that results in elevated levels of circulating prothrombin. The prothrombin G20210A mutation is present in 2.7% of Caucasians and 0.06% of Africans and Asians, and the frequency of the prothrombin gene mutation in patients less than 50 years of age with a family history of thrombosis or a history of recurrent thrombotic events and no acquired risk factors for thrombosis except pregnancy or oral contraceptive use is 16%.

Less common familial thrombophilias include antithrombin III deficiency, protein C deficiency, and protein S deficiency, which have a combined frequency of 13% in patients less than 50 years of age with a family history of thrombosis or a history of recurrent thrombotic events and no acquired risk factors for thrombosis except pregnancy or oral contraceptive use. Other, very rare, familial thrombophilias include homozygosity for the C677T mutation in the methylenetetrahydrofolate reductase gene that results in elevated levels of homocysteine, and mutations in fibrinogen that result in dysfibrinogenemia.

3. D. The patient's history is highly suggestive of antiphospholipid syndrome (APLS). APLS is an acquired hypercoagulable state that is characterized by the presence of autoantibodies to phospholipid-binding proteins and by recurrent thrombosis. The thrombotic complications of APLS include venous thrombosis (deep vein thrombosis, pulmonary embolism, portal vein thrombosis), arterial thrombosis (myocardial infarction, limb necrosis), and spontaneous pregnancy loss. APLS can occur in the context of systemic lupus erythematosus, but it can also occur in isolation.

The patient's prolonged PTT is an additional clue to her diagnosis of APLS. She was treated with low-molecular-weight heparin, which does not affect the PTT. Her prolonged PTT is therefore not due to her therapeutic anticoagulation. Rather, it is due to the presence of antiphospholipid antibodies in her blood. The PTT test requires phospholipid as a cofactor. The antiphospholipid antibodies in patients with APLS bind to and interfere with the in vitro aPTT reaction, resulting in prolongation of the activated PTT (aPTT) in some patients. As her PTT is prolonged due to the presence of an inhibitor and not a factor deficiency, her PTT would not correct upon mixing with normal plasma. Additional testing, including the lupus anticoagulant test and the dRVVT (dilute Russell viper venom time) test as well as direct serologic testing for the presence of antiphospholipid antibodies (anticardiolipin and anti-beta-2-glycoprotein) would help confirm the diagnosis.

In this patient the diagnosis of HIT is not consistent with her presentation or with the time course of her mild thrombocytopenia. HIT is a highly prothrombotic state that presents 5–10 days after initiation of heparin therapy in patients who develop autoantibodies to platelet factor 4–heparin complexes. The patient was on heparin for only 1 day when her blood tests were done, which is insufficient time for her to have developed HIT antibodies. Answer A is therefore incorrect. Peripheral blood flow cytometry for CD55 and CD59 is done to evaluate patients with suspected paroxysmal nocturnal hemoglobinuria (PNH). PNH is an acquired clonal disorder of red cell membranes in which red cells lack surface expression of GPI-anchored proteins, including proteins that protect red cells from complement-mediated lysis. Patients with PNH have recurrent episodes of intravascular hemolysis and, for unclear reasons, are predisposed to venous thrombosis, in particular Budd-Chiari syndrome (hepatic vein thrombosis). The patient's normal haptoglobin level argues against the presence of any significant intravascular hemolysis, and the diagnosis of PNH would not explain her prolonged PTT or her history of spontaneous pregnancy loss. Answer B is therefore incorrect. Serologic testing for autoantibodies to ADAMTS13 is done in patients with suspected thrombotic thrombocytopenic purpura (TTP) to confirm the diagnosis, although ADAMTS13 serologic testing is not a sensitive test for TTP. TTP is classically characterized by a pentad of signs and symptoms—fever, neurological changes, renal insufficiency, microangiopathic hemolytic anemia, and thrombocytopenia. Patients with TTP typically present with severe thrombocytopenia and very elevated LDH levels. This patient's mild thrombocytopenia, mildly elevated LDH, and normal haptoglobin are not consistent with the extensive platelet destruction and intravascular hemolysis that are hallmarks of TTP. In addition, TTP typically causes microvascular, not macrovascular, thrombosis, and the diagnosis of TTP would not explain her prolonged PTT or her history of spontaneous pregnancy loss. Answer C is therefore incorrect.

4. D. This patient meets the clinical criteria for thrombotic thrombocytopenia purpura (TTP). TTP is classically characterized by a pentad of signs and symptoms—fever, neurologic changes, renal insufficiency, microangiopathic hemolytic anemia, and thrombocytopenia, although, in the appropriate clinical context, only microangiopathic hemolytic anemia and thrombocytopenia are required to make the diagnosis.

Under normal physiological conditions, endothelial cells secrete unusually large multimers of von Willebrand factor (vWF), which are tethered to the endothelial cell surface. These large multimers are cleaved into smaller fragments by the von Willebrand factor–cleaving metalloprotease ADAMTS13. Cleavage releases the small vWF fragments into the circulation, where they help mediate platelet aggregation and clotting. In TTP, the activity of

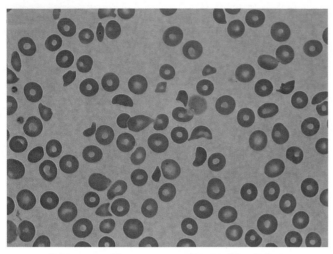

Figure 20.1. Schistocytes. Photo courtesy of Dr. Lindsley Coleman.

ADAMTS13 is impaired by the presence of autoantibodies to the metalloprotease. The lack of ADAMTS13 activity results in the accumulation of membrane-bound, unusually large vWF multimers. These large multimers inappropriately bind to and activate circulating platelets, resulting in in situ microvascular thrombus formation and tissue ischemia. If left untreated TTP can cause irreversible kidney damage and stroke. The primary treatment for TTP is plasmapheresis, which is thought to work both by removing anti-ADAMTS13 antibodies as well as by providing a large infusion of active ADAMTS13 enzyme. Ninety percent of cases of TTP improve with plasmapheresis, although about 30% of patients will subsequently relapse and require additional courses of plasmapheresis. About 10% of patients have refractory disease and require additional therapeutic interventions, which may include splenectomy, cytotoxic agents, and/or rituximab (anti-B-cell therapy).

Without immediate treatment, the morbidity and mortality of TTP is very high, and it is important to initiate therapy before permanent tissue damage occurs. Answers B and C are therefore incorrect. Answer A incorrectly presumes that the patient has hemolytic uremic syndrome. Hemolytic uremic syndrome (HUS) is another thrombotic microangiopathy that is characterized by renal failure, microangiopathic hemolytic anemia, and thrombocytopenia, but it is caused by a strain of *E. coli*, *E. coli* 0157, that produces shiga toxin, a toxin that interferes with ADAMTS13 activity. HUS is classically a disease of childhood and is rare in adults, and it is a self-limited condition for which plasmapheresis is not required. The age of the patient and the fact that she did not present with an antecedent diarrheal illness makes HUS unlikely. Given the high morbidity and mortality of TTP and the lack of a rapid diagnostic test to differentiate HUS from TTP, adult patients who present with microangiopathic hemolytic anemia and thrombocytopenia should be presumed to have TTP and should be treated accordingly.

Other causes of microangiopathic hemolytic anemia and thrombocytopenia that should be considered in the differential diagnosis of this patient include DIC (disseminated intravascular coagulation), HELLP syndrome of pregnancy (hemolysis, elevated liver enzymes, and low platelets), systemic vasculitides, malignant hypertension, advanced cancer, and drug effects. The patient is not on any medications and does not appear ill, and these conditions are therefore all less likely than TTP.

5. B. Immune thrombocytopenic purpura (ITP) is an acquired disorder in which platelets are destroyed in the peripheral circulation, presumably by an autoimmune mechanism. ITP is characterized by isolated thrombocytopenia with otherwise normal blood counts, no other abnormalities on peripheral blood smear, and the absence of an identifiable alternative cause for the low platelet count. ITP is commonly associated with autoimmune diseases as well as with HIV infection, although the majority of cases are idiopathic. Patients with ITP can also present with Evans syndrome, in which ITP and Coombs'-positive autoimmune hemolytic anemia occur concomitantly. ITP is a diagnosis of exclusion; there are no laboratory tests that can reliably confirm or rule out the diagnosis of ITP. Although antiplatelet antibody levels can be measured, the antibodies are neither sensitive nor highly specific for the diagnosis of ITP and are therefore of limited clinical utility.

The differential diagnosis of thrombocytopenia in ITP includes TTP (although microangiopathic hemolytic anemia is not present in ITP), DIC (although patients with DIC are typically ill-appearing and have abnormalities of coagulation, which are not present in ITP), drug-associated thrombocytopenia (commonly implicated drugs include alcohol, anticonvulsants, sulfonamides, quinine, penicillins), HIT, acute viral infections (HIV, Epstein-Barr virus [EBV], cytomegalovirus [CMV] hepatitis), hypersplenism, and primary bone marrow disorders (although other hematologic abnormalities are typically present).

The choice of first-line treatment for ITP depends primarily on the presence or absence of active bleeding. In ITP, megakaryocytes respond to thrombocytopenia by producing larger-than-normal platelets that have enhanced function, and spontaneous bleeding is therefore rare at platelet counts above 10,000/mm³. However, when thrombocytopenia is very severe (platelet counts <7000/mm³) and/or when patients with ITP are taking medications that interfere with platelet function (aspirin, nonsteroidal anti-inflammatory drugs (NSAIDs), clopidogrel), they can be at risk for spontaneous and even life-threatening bleeding. In patients who are not bleeding, ITP can be treated with dexamethasone, 40 mg by mouth for 4 days, or with prednisone, 1 mg/kg followed by a slow taper. Splenectomy, intravenous immunoglobulin, $Rh_o(D)$ immune globulin, cytotoxic agents (cyclophosphamide, vincristine), and rituximab are reserved for second-line treatment of refractory ITP. In patients who are actively bleeding, intravenous immunoglobulin in combination with steroids is a highly effective first-line treatment, although intravenous immunoglobulin is contraindicated in patients with renal insufficiency. $Rh_o(D)$ immune globulin can also be used to treat ITP in Rh+ patients, but as $Rh_o(D)$ immune globulin binds the patients' red blood cells, it can precipitate an autoimmune hemolytic episode and is therefore contraindicated in Rh+ ITP patients with anemia. Platelet transfusions are typically not effective at raising the platelet count of patients with ITP and should therefore be reserved for cases of life-threatening hemorrhage.

ITP rarely resolves spontaneously, and, without treatment, patients can be at risk for severe, even life-threatening bleeding. Answer A is therefore incorrect. As this patient has not failed primary therapy with steroids and is not actively bleeding, answers C and D are incorrect as well.

6. D. This patient meets the clinical criteria for heparin-induced thrombocytopenia (HIT). HIT is characterized clinically by the development of thrombocytopenia in patients on heparin, and the diagnosis should be considered in any patient whose platelet count drops by 50% or more within 5–10 days of initiation of heparin. HIT occurs in 1–10% of patients exposed to unfractionated heparin and in 0.1–0.5% of patients exposed to low-molecular-weight heparin. The incidence of HIT is highest in surgical patients undergoing cardiac and orthopedic procedures and lowest in obstetric patients.

HIT is an immune-mediated disorder in which autoantibodies develop to complexes of heparin and platelet factor 4, a factor secreted by activated platelets. The antibodies bind to the heparin-PF4 complexes and bind to the Fc receptors on the surface of platelets, which causes activation of the platelets and uncontrolled release by the platelets of procoagulant platelet microparticles. The activated platelets are cleared from the circulation by the spleen, resulting in thrombocytopenia, and the released procoagulant platelet microparticles bind to sites of endothelial injury and initiate uncontrolled thrombosis. The morbidity and mortality associated with HIT are not consequences of thrombocytopenia, which is rarely severe, but consequences of arterial and venous thrombosis, which occurs in as many as 50% of patients with HIT. Common thrombotic complications of HIT include DVT/PE, cerebral vein thrombosis, lower-limb ischemia and limb loss, stroke, and myocardial infarction. Untreated HIT has a mortality of 20–30%.

There are two diagnostic tests for HIT. The immunoassay that detects the presence of antibodies to the heparin-PF4 complex is highly sensitive but only moderately specific, whereas the platelet activation assay that detects the presence of heparin-PF4 antibodies that can bind to platelets and cause platelet degranulation is both highly sensitive and highly specific. However, despite the availability of laboratory tests, HIT remains a clinical diagnosis, and appropriate management of patients suspected of having HIT should never await results of laboratory tests.

Management of suspected HIT consists of immediate cessation of all heparin products and immediate initiation of alternative anticoagulants. Alternative anticoagulants that are FDA-approved for the treatment of HIT include the direct thrombin inhibitors argatroban and lepirudin. Simple cessation of heparin is not adequate intervention in patients suspected of having HIT because patients continue to be significantly hypercoagulable after discontinuation of heparin and are at continued risk for catastrophic thrombosis. Although low-molecular-weight heparin has a lower incidence of causing HIT than unfractionated heparin, it is absolutely contraindicated in patients with HIT. Answers A and B are therefore incorrect. Anticoagulation with warfarin should not be started in patients with HIT unless they are fully anticoagulated with a direct thrombin inhibitor, and warfarin should not be started until their platelet count has recovered. Premature initiation of anticoagulation with warfarin can result in the development of venous gangrene. Answer C is therefore incorrect.

7. D. The patient's clinical presentation is consistent with DIC, likely secondary to acute mesenteric ischemia. DIC is a condition in which uncontrolled activation of the coagulation cascade in response to severe physiological stress results in intravascular fibrin deposition and microvascular thrombosis as well as consumption of platelets and clotting factors. DIC can occur in a number of different clinical settings in which large amounts of tissue factor are released into the circulation, including sepsis, obstetric complications, malignancy, and trauma. Patients with DIC typically have prolonged clotting times (PT and PTT), inappropriately low/normal fibrinogen levels (fibrinogen, as an acute phase reactant, should be elevated in acute illness), and elevated D-dimer levels. Clinically, patients with DIC present with varying degrees of intravascular hemolysis, bleeding, tissue ischemia, and end-organ damage including renal failure, hepatic dysfunction, acute respiratory distress syndrome (ARDS) stroke, and shock. Treatment of DIC is supportive and involves maintaining organ perfusion and, in patients who are bleeding, transfusing blood products (red blood cells, platelets, fresh frozen plasma, cryoprecipitate) until the underlying cause of the DIC can be treated and reversed.

The morbidity and mortality of DIC are high, and resolution of DIC requires treatment of the underlying condition. It is therefore important to distinguish DIC from other thrombotic microangiopathies and from other causes of coagulopathy and thrombocytopenia that might need different specific treatments. The principal conditions that DIC must be distinguished from are TTP and the coagulopathy of liver failure. In differentiating DIC from TTP, it is important to remember that, whereas DIC results from the dysregulated activation and depletion of both platelets and clotting factors, TTP results from the inappropriate activation of platelets by uncleaved von Willebrand factor without perturbation of the coagulation cascade. Clotting times as well as fibrinogen and D-dimer levels should therefore be normal in TTP. In addition, TTP is a primary autoimmune disorder that typically occurs in patients who are otherwise well, whereas DIC occurs as a consequence of severe underlying physiological stress, and patients are typically ill. Differentiating DIC from severe liver failure may be more difficult and frequently relies largely on patient history and patient presentation. Liver failure, like DIC, is frequently associated with thrombocytopenia, due in the case of liver failure to portal hypertension, splenomegaly, and splenic sequestration of platelets. Also, as the liver synthesizes most coagulation factors, patients with severe liver disease frequently have elevated clotting times. Moderate elevations in D-dimer levels are also frequently seen in patients with liver cirrhosis because D-dimer products are cleared principally by the liver, and clearance is impaired in the setting of liver failure. Of note, although the liver does synthesize fibrinogen, fibrinogen levels are typically maintained within the normal range in patients with liver disease until their liver failure becomes extremely severe, and a low fibrinogen level should therefore raise the suspicion for DIC even in patients with hepatic synthetic dysfunction.

In the above question, although it is not clear from the patient's history whether he might be taking medications that are associated with drug-induced thrombocytopenia, a drug effect would not explain his overall presentation. Similarly, the diagnosis of ITP would not explain most of his laboratory findings or the severity of his presentation. Answers A and B are therefore incorrect. And although fever, acute renal failure, mental status changes, peripheral blood schistocytosis and thrombocytopenia are all features of TTP, the diagnosis of TTP would not explain his abnormal coagulation studies, and the patient is too acutely ill for TTP to be the underlying cause of his presentation. Answer C is therefore incorrect. The patient does have elevated liver enzymes, but this is likely due to hepatic hypoperfusion, and there is nothing in his history to suggest that he has underlying liver cirrhosis, portal hypertension, or splenomegaly. Answer E is therefore incorrect.

8. D. Even in people who have no apparent medical problems, the majority of cases of thrombocytosis are reactive, where the elevated platelet count is secondary to an underlying medical condition. Common causes of reactive thrombocytosis include iron deficiency, acute and chronic infections, inflammatory conditions, allergic reactions, occult malignancies, hyposplenism, recent trauma or surgery, and count recovery after episodes of thrombocytopenia (such as post-chemotherapy, post–vitamin B-12/folate repletion, and post–alcohol cessation). Reactive thrombocytosis is rarely, even at very elevated platelet counts, associated with thrombosis or bleeding, and appropriate therapy for reactive thrombocytosis consists of treating the underlying medical condition, not the platelet count.

The initial workup of an elevated platelet count should include a careful patient history, measurement of iron saturation levels to rule out iron deficiency (which is very common in premenopausal women), and measurement of markers of inflammation such as the erythrocyte sedimentation rate and ferritin and C-reactive protein levels. In patients who have sustained elevated platelet counts and none of the above-mentioned medical conditions, a workup for primary causes of thrombocytosis is indicated. Causes of autonomous platelet production include the chronic myeloproliferative disorders (chronic myelogenous leukemia, polycythemia vera, essential thrombocythemia, and idiopathic myelofibrosis), the 5q- myelodysplastic syndrome, and hereditary thrombocythemias (which are caused by activating mutations in thrombopoietin and the thrombopoietin receptor). Many of these thrombocythemias are associated with varying degrees of risk of thrombotic complications, including DVT/PEs and the Budd-Chiari syndrome and varying degrees of risk of progression to acute leukemia.

Essential thrombocythemia (ET) is one of the Philadelphia chromosome-negative chronic myeloproliferative disorders. It is characterized by a sustained elevated platelet count in the absence of evidence of reactive thrombocytosis or other causes of primary thrombocytosis. There is no single diagnostic laboratory test for ET. Although 30–50% of patients with ET test positive for the presence of the JAK2V617F mutation, the mutation is found in over 90% of patients with polycythemia vera and 30–50% of patients with idiopathic myelofibrosis and is therefore not diagnostic of ET. ET is associated with a low risk of thrombosis and bleeding and a very low risk of progression to marrow failure or acute leukemia, and the median survival of patients with ET approaches that of normal subjects. Many patients with ET do not require treatment, although elderly patients and patients who have risk factors for vascular disease are typically treated with low-dose aspirin even if asymptomatic. Indications for treatment with platelet-lowering agents include a platelet count <1,500,000/mm^3, symptoms of vasomotor instability (headaches, flushing), bleeding, arterial, venous and/or microvascular thrombosis, and recurrent fetal loss. The most commonly used platelet-lowering agent in ET is hydroxyurea, which effectively lowers the platelet count and the risk of thrombosis in the majority of ET patients. The principal dose-limiting toxicity of hydroxyurea is leukopenia, and anagrelide is frequently used to treat symptomatic patients who cannot tolerate hydroxyurea.

In the above question, until reactive thrombocytosis is ruled out, initiation of any antiplatelet therapy would be premature. Answers A and C are therefore incorrect. The thrombosis in ET and the other primary thrombocythemias are platelet-mediated, and warfarin, which targets the coagulation cascade, is therefore not an effective drug to decrease the risk of ET-associated thrombosis. Answer B is therefore incorrect. Finally, given the lack of a clear etiology for the patient's thrombocytosis, any discussion of her risk of developing leukemia would be premature. Answer E is therefore incorrect.

9. A. This patient has glucose-6-phosphate dehydrogenase (G6PD) deficiency. G6PD deficiency is an X-linked enzymatic disorder of red blood cells that results in a decreased ability of red blood cells to generate NADPH, a metabolic intermediate that is essential for the conversion of oxidized intracellular proteins to their reduced forms. When G6PD-deficient red blood cells are exposed to oxidative stress, the hemoglobin in the cells denatures and precipitates, resulting in the formation of Heinz bodies, which can be detected on peripheral blood smear. The oxidized red blood cells become rigid and nondeformable and are destroyed by the reticuloendothelial system of the liver, spleen, and bone marrow.

There are more than 100 mutations that are associated with G6PD deficiency, but the two most common mutations are the A-variant, which is present in 10% of African Americans, and the Mediterranean variant, which is present in 5% of people of Mediterranean descent. The A-variant has normal enzymatic activity but is unstable and has a shorter half-life than the wild-type enzyme. When A-variant red blood cells are exposed to oxidative stress, only the older cells have insufficient G6PD and preferentially undergo hemolysis, while reticulocytes and newly generated mature red blood cells survive. The A-variant is therefore generally associated with a mild, self-limited hemolysis. The Mediterranean variant has a mutation that results in very low baseline G6PD enzymatic activity and is associated with more severe hemolysis.

There are several diagnostic tests that quantify, with varying degrees of sensitivity, the amount of G6PD activity in red blood cells. These include the dye decolorization test, the rapid fluorescence screening test, the G6PD-tetrazolium cytochemical test, and spectrophotometric tests that determine the rate of NADPH production by red blood cells. The ability of all of these tests to diagnose A-variant G6PD deficiency during or immediately after an acute hemolytic episode is limited due to the preferential hemolysis of older, G6PD deficient, red blood cells, with relative preservation of the younger cells that have near-normal levels of G6PD activity. These diagnostic tests should therefore be performed in patients with suspected G6PD deficiency only after they have recovered from their hemolytic episode, when the hematocrit and reticulocyte count have normalized. The red blood cells of patients with the Mediterranean variant of G6PD, on the other hand, will have abnormal G6PD activity throughout the red blood cell lifespan and will test positive even during an acute hemolytic episode.

Common oxidative stresses that have been associated with hemolytic crises in patients with G6PD deficiency include the following:

Antibacterial	Antimalarials	Misc. agents/ foods	Misc. drugs
Dapsone	Primaquine	Fava beans	Doxorubicin
Nalidixic acid	Pamaquine	Naphthalene (mothballs)	Methylene blue
Nitrofurantoin		Toluene	Pyridium
Sulfamethoxazole			Phenylhydrazine
Sulfapyridine			Probenecid

This patient likely has the A-variant of G6PD deficiency given his ethnicity. Sending a diagnostic test while he is still recovering from his acute hemolytic episode is likely to give a false-negative result. Answer B is therefore incorrect. Answers C and D refer to the fact that the patient's red blood cell mean corpuscular volume (MCV) is slightly elevated, which can be seen with folate and vitamin B-12 deficiency and with chronic alcohol use—all causes of chronic anemia. However, the clinical scenario suggests none of these conditions. The patient's elevated MCV more likely reflects the fact that his bone marrow is responding to the acute drop in his hematocrit by producing increased numbers of reticulocytes, which have an MCV of 100 to 130.

10. C. This patient has a microcytic anemia in the presence of normal iron stores, which is highly suggestive of thalassemia. The thalassemias are a group of inherited disorders of hemoglobin production that are prevalent in people of Mediterranean, Asian, Middle Eastern, and Latin American descent. The thalassemias are caused by mutations in the regulatory elements of the globin genes that result in decreased synthesis of either the alpha or the beta chain of hemoglobin. Microcytic anemia results from both lack of normal $\alpha_2\beta_2$ hemoglobin complexes as well as from precipitation of the excess, unaffected subunit, which targets red blood cells for clearance by the reticuloendothelial system of the liver and spleen. The thalassemias are diagnosed by hemoglobin electrophoresis, which determines the relative abundance of the different hemoglobin complexes. β-Thalassemia can be distinguished from α-thalassemia by the presence of increased levels of hemoglobin A_2 ($\alpha_2\delta_2$) in β-thalassemia.

In patients with suspected iron deficiency it is important to correctly interpret the results of iron studies before starting patients on iron replacement therapy. In patients who are otherwise well, the diagnosis of iron deficiency can be confidently made when the transferrin saturation (iron:TIBC

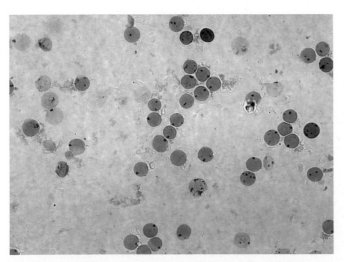

Figure 20.2. Heinz Bodies. Photo courtesy of Dr. Lindsley Coleman.

ratio) is <15%. A ferritin level of <20 ng/dL confirms the diagnosis of iron deficiency. However, in patients who are chronically ill, especially those with chronic inflammatory conditions, serum iron levels can be low in the absence of iron deficiency. However, in such patients, both serum iron and TIBC levels are proportionally decreased, and the transferrin saturation is therefore typically normal or near normal. Ferritin is an acute-phase reactant, and in inflammatory states the ferritin level may rise as high as 200 ng/dL in the presence of iron deficiency. Ferritin levels are therefore not an accurate measure of iron stores in patients with chronic inflammatory conditions. However, a ferritin level of <50 ng/dL in a patient with a chronic inflammatory condition is highly suggestive of iron deficiency.

If and when the diagnosis of iron deficiency is confirmed, it is important to investigate why the patient has low iron stores. Iron deficiency in men and in women who are not menstruating is usually indicative of an underlying medical condition. There are no physiological mechanisms other than bleeding that remove significant amounts of iron from the circulation, and a diagnosis of iron deficiency should therefore prompt a workup for impaired iron absorption and for occult blood loss. Impaired iron absorption most commonly occurs in the setting of celiac disease and atrophic gastritis. Patients with impaired iron absorption when given a therapeutic trial of oral iron are unable to absorb the iron, and their iron levels do not increase. Such patients require intravenous iron replacement therapy. In patients with iron deficiency due to occult blood loss, however, iron levels typically do increase after oral iron administration. Occult blood loss most commonly occurs via the GI tract and can be the presenting sign of an occult GI malignancy or occult inflammatory bowel disease.

This patient's presentation is consistent with thalassemia. Because her anemia is due to inefficient red cell production, she would be unable to respond to erythropoietin by increasing her red cell production. Answer B is therefore incorrect. Her iron stores are not low, and continued iron replacement therapy would eventually result in her developing iron overload, especially if she were to stop menstruating. Answer D is therefore incorrect. Although her iron levels are somewhat high, she is not, at present, iron overloaded. Iron overload is associated with an iron:TIBC ratio of over 50%. Discontinuing her iron replacement therapy may be sufficient to prevent her from developing iron overload. Phlebotomy is not an appropriate approach to removing excessive iron in patients with abnormal hematopoiesis and who are anemic at baseline. Answer A is therefore incorrect.

11. B. This patient presents with megaloblastic anemia due to severe vitamin B-12 deficiency. Vitamin B-12 (cobalamin) and folate are two nutrients that are essential cofactors in DNA synthesis. They are required for conversion of deoxyuridate to thymidylate, and nutritional deficiency in either cofactor causes a block in nuclear maturation, nuclear–cytoplasmic asynchrony, and impaired cell division. Cobalamin and folate deficiencies primarily impact rapidly dividing tissues, most notably the hematopoietic system and the gastrointestinal tract. The hematologic manifestations of cobalamin and folate deficiency include macrocytic anemia, hypersegmented (5+ lobes) neutrophils (figure 20.3), and, in severe cases, pancytopenia. Intestinal involvement results in glossitis and megaloblastic changes in the gut epithelium. In addition to its role in DNA synthesis, cobalamin, but not folate, plays a role in maintenance of neuronal myelination. Cobalamin deficiency can cause a myriad of neurologic problems including peripheral neuropathy, ataxia, personality changes, memory loss, and, in severe cases, dementia.

It is important to consider the possible presence of cobalamin and folate deficiency even in patients without overt macrocytic anemia. A normal hematocrit and MCV do not exclude the presence of clinically significant vitamin deficiencies. In patients with concurrent iron deficiency and/ or thalassemia, for example, the macrocytosis of cobalamin and folate deficiency can be masked, and patients with cobalamin deficiency can develop neurological complications prior to the development of anemia. Diagnosing cobalamin and folate deficiency is further complicated by the fact that blood cobalamin and folate levels have to be interpreted carefully. Folate levels fluctuate significantly and do not necessarily accurately reflect total body folate levels, and what constitutes a "normal" cobalamin level is not clearly defined. Cobalamin levels below 200 pg/mL are clearly low, and levels over 300 pg/mL are unlikely to be associated with deficiency, but borderline levels between 200 and 300 pg/mL can be associated with clinically significant deficiency in some patients but not others.

In patients with borderline vitamin B-12 levels and patients suspected of having folate deficiency but who have normal serum folate levels, measurement of methylmalonic acid (MMA) and homocysteine levels can be helpful. Vitamin B-12 deficiency results in high levels of both MMA

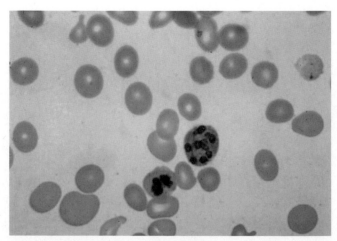

Figure 20.3. Hypersegmented Neutrophil. Photo courtesy of Dr. Franklin Bunn.

and homocysteine, whereas folate deficiency results in high levels of homocysteine alone. Although MMA and homocysteine are very sensitive tests for folate and cobalamin deficiency, they are not entirely specific. Elevated homocysteine levels are present in familial hyperhomocysteinemia, and elevated levels of MMA are present in methylmalonic aciduria, hypovolemia, and renal failure.

The principal causes of folate and vitamin B-12 deficiencies differ. The body does not store folate to any significant degree, and inadequate dietary intake is the most common cause of folate deficiency, which can develop quickly in malnourished patients, particularly people with poor dietary intake associated with alcoholism. Other causes of folate deficiency include gut malabsorption syndromes (celiac sprue, inflammatory bowel disease) and conditions associated with increased folate requirements, including hematologic recovery from severe anemia, growth spurts during infancy and adolescence, pregnancy, lactation, and exfoliative skin diseases. Certain drugs can also interfere with folate metabolism, most notably methotrexate, phenytoin, and nitrous oxide. Vitamin B-12, on the other hand, is extensively stored by the liver, and vitamin B-12 deficiency takes years to develop. Vitamin B-12 deficiency due to inadequate dietary intake is uncommon except in strict vegans and in patients who are severely malnourished for prolonged periods of time. The most common cause of vitamin B-12 deficiency is malabsorption. B-12-containing proteins must be adequately cleaved in the acidic environment of the stomach. B-12 must then bind to intrinsic factor (IF), a protein released by the parietal cells of the gastric mucosa, and then the IF–B-12 complexes must be taken up by IF-receptor-expressing cells in ileum. Perturbation of any step in cobalamin absorption can result in deficiency. Gastrectomy, atrophic gastritis, pancreatic insufficiency, and chronic use of proton pump inhibitors can inhibit the release of cobalamin from foods. Pernicious anemia, the autoimmune destruction of gastric parietal cells, results in a lack of intrinsic factor. And Crohn disease, celiac sprue, ileitis, blind loop syndrome, and ileal resection can all interfere with the uptake of IF–B-12 complexes by the small intestine. In addition, bacterial overgrowth and infection with fish tapeworms can result in depletion of nutritional cobalamin.

Vitamin B-12 and folate deficiency are treated by supplementation of dietary intake. Daily oral folate supplementation is generally sufficient to correct folate deficiency. Vitamin B-12 supplementation can be administered orally or by intramuscular injection. Even patients with impaired vitamin B-12 absorption will generally respond to high-dose oral vitamin B-12 because, in addition to specific intrinsic factor-mediated vitamin B-12 uptake, high levels of vitamin B-12 in the diet can also be absorbed by mass action.

This patient has a history of obesity, and, although diabetes could cause a peripheral neuropathy, diabetes would not explain his macrocytic anemia. Answer A is therefore incorrect. Whereas dramatic weight loss often prompts evaluation for occult malignancy, his weight loss occurred after gastric bypass surgery and is likely not pathologic. He should undergo age-appropriate routine cancer screening, but this is not a priority in light of his more urgent neurological issues. Answer D is therefore incorrect. The patient's macrocytic anemia and neurological complaints are most likely due to vitamin B-12 deficiency. Empirical treatment with folate may improve the macrocytic anemia somewhat, but it will not ameliorate the neurological symptoms, which may not be reversible. Answer C is therefore incorrect.

12. B. This patient has a normocytic anemia due to his chronic kidney disease. Erythropoietin is produced primarily by the kidneys in response to anemia and tissue hypoxia. The most common cause of erythropoietin deficiency is kidney failure. When renal function declines, there is a concomitant decrease in erythropoietin production. Patients with diabetes mellitus and even modestly abnormal renal function are often found to be erythropoietin deficient and anemic.

The other common cause of normocytic anemia is anemia secondary to chronic inflammatory conditions, which is characterized by underproduction of red blood cells (low reticulocyte count) and low circulating levels of iron (low serum iron) despite the presence of high iron stores (high ferritin levels) in the setting of chronic inflammation. Causes of chronic inflammation associated with anemia of chronic disease include connective tissue disorders (lupus, rheumatoid arthritis, inflammatory bowel diseases), chronic infections (osteomyelitis, tuberculosis, HIV, hepatitis), and metabolic disorders (uremia, cirrhosis, hypothyroidism). The cause of the anemia in chronic inflammatory states is not entirely clear, but it does appear to be mediated at least in part by hepcidin, a small polypeptide produced by the liver in response to cytokine (particularly interleukin-6) release. Hepcidin binds to and inhibits the activity of ferroportin, an iron-transport protein on macrophages, thereby inhibiting the release of iron from body iron stores. Lack of available iron inhibits erythropoiesis in the bone marrow.

Other less common causes of normocytic anemia include these:

- Acute and chronic hemolytic anemias, including autoimmune hemolytic anemia, microangiopathic hemolytic anemias, sickle cell anemia, hereditary spherocytosis, glucose-6-phosphate dehydrogenase deficiency, and drug-induced hemolysis.

- Primary bone marrow failure syndromes, including aplastic anemia.

- Myelophthisic anemias, which are characterized by the presence of abnormally shaped red blood cells and nucleated red blood cells in the peripheral blood caused by replacement of the bone marrow by fibrosis and foreign cells. The cells can be malignant (leukemia, lymphoma, solid tumors) or reactive (sarcoidosis, tuberculosis, myelofibrosis).

Although many medications, including Lasix, can cause bone-marrow suppression, the patient's anemia has been developing over several years, and he was only recently started on Lasix. Answer A is therefore incorrect. And although the concomitant presence of a microcytic and a macrocytic anemia can result in an apparent normocytic anemia with a normal mean corpuscular hemoglobin concentration (MCV), this patient has a normal red cell distribution width (RDW), which reflects the fact that his red blood cells are uniform in size. Answer C is therefore incorrect. Finally, the patient's relatively unremarkable peripheral blood smear strongly argues against marrow replacement as the etiology of his anemia. Answer D is therefore incorrect.

13. D. This patient is presenting with evolving acute chest syndrome (ACS), a potentially fatal manifestation of sickle cell disease. ACS is a relatively common and potentially life-threatening complication of SCD. It is characterized by the presence of fever, hypoxia, and new pulmonary infiltrates, although all three of these findings are not always apparent at the time of presentation. Distinguishing ACS from simple pneumonia can be difficult. Although patients with ACS do not always have a bacterial pneumonia, the syndrome is often associated with infection with atypical organisms such as *Chlamydia* or *Mycoplasma*, and patients with suspected ACS should, in addition to oxygen, intravenous fluids, and pain medications, receive antibiotics. Patients with ACS also frequently require simple or exchange blood transfusions.

The decision of whether to administer simple transfusions or to do an exchange transfusion in patients with SCD can be difficult. Frequent simple transfusions can result in iron overload and secondary hemochromatosis. In addition, increasing the hematocrit and blood viscosity of patients with SCD in crisis, all of whom have some degree of underlying microvascular disease, can worsen a pain crisis and precipitate strokes. Exchange transfusions, on the other hand, result in less iron overload and do not cause hyperviscosity, but exposure of SCD patients to multiple units of blood and large numbers of alloantigens can result in alloimmunization, which can complicate management of future crises. Exchange transfusions in adults with sickle cell disease are therefore typically reserved for patients with life-threatening crises, including strokes in evolution and patients with respiratory compromise from acute chest syndrome.

This patient is presenting with fever, hypoxia, and a new pulmonary infiltrate. Given the fact that he is having a complicated sickle cell crisis, outpatient management and management of only his pain would be inappropriate. Answers A and B are therefore incorrect. And although hydroxyurea can be very effective in preventing future crises, the medication takes weeks to months to have an effect and does not have any role in the acute management of sickle crises. Answer C is therefore incorrect.

14. D. This patient is presenting with severe autoimmune hemolytic anemia (AIHA). In AIHA, patients develop autoantibodies to antigens on the surface of their own red blood cells. These autoantibodies bind the red blood cells, and the cells are then cleared from the circulation by the reticuloendothelial system of the liver and spleen. This is a process referred to as *extravascular hemolysis*. Incomplete phagocytosis of red blood cells by macrophages results in the "pinching off" of portions of the red cell membranes, which disrupts the normal biconcave disc architecture of the red cells and leads to the formation of spherocytes. The diagnosis of AIHA is strongly suggested by the presence of microspherocytes on peripheral blood smear and is confirmed by the direct Coombs' test, which detects the presence in vitro of antibodies on the surface of the patient's red blood cells.

AIHA is commonly idiopathic, although it is frequently associated with other autoimmune conditions, including lupus, rheumatoid arthritis, Graves' disease and Hashimoto thyroiditis, and ITP. The concomitant presence of AIHA and ITP is referred to as Evans syndrome. AIHA can also be associated with lymphoproliferative disorders, especially chronic lymphocytic leukemia (CLL). Although AIHA is frequently idiopathic, Coombs'-positive immune hemolysis can also be associated with exposure to certain drugs, including cephalosporins, penicillins, quinine, and methyldopa. The precise mechanisms by which these drugs induce AIHA is not entirely clear, but it is believed that these drugs bind to and alter proteins on the surface of red blood cells, resulting in the formation of cryptic antigens that stimulate an immune response.

Most other conditions that cause hemolysis result in intravascular hemolysis and do not give rise to spherocytes. They include the following:

- *Severe liver disease*—which is characterized by target cells, spur cells, and burr cells on peripheral blood smear.

- *Microangiopathic processes*—DIC, TTP, HUS, malignant hypertension.

- *Infections*—parasites (malaria, babesiosis), *Clostridium perfringens*.

- *Intrinsic red cell defects*—G6PD deficiency, paroxysmal nocturnal hemoglobinuria.

- *Cold agglutinin disease*—which is mediated by IgM autoantibodies that fix complement.

The treatment of AIHA is aimed at suppressing autoantibody production, and the mainstay of treatment is high-dose steroids. Responses to steroids are typically seen in 1–3 weeks, although some patients respond to steroids in just a few days. Treatment response is measured by an increase in the hemoglobin concentration and hematocrit and a drop in the reticulocyte count. Once the hematocrit has recovered and is stable, steroids can gradually be tapered.

In this patient's case, her low hematocrit and her symptoms make outpatient management of her AIHA unsafe. Answer A is therefore incorrect. Answer B would be correct if the patient's hematocrit were not critically low and if she were minimally symptomatic from her anemia. However, steroids will take at least a few days to have an effect, and, in the meantime, she will continue to hemolyze her red blood cells. Although she will also hemolyze some of the transfused red cells she receives, she should receive blood transfusions to maintain her hematocrit in a safe range until her hemolysis slows down. Answer B is therefore incorrect. Finally, although other immunosuppressive drugs, including rituximab, cyclophosphamide, and azathioprine, can be effective in the treatment of AIHA, they are not used as first-line treatment but are reserved for patients with steroid-refractory disease and for patients who persistently relapse with withdrawal of steroids. Answers C and E are therefore incorrect.

21.

BOARD SIMULATION: MEDICAL ONCOLOGY

Lawrence N. Shulman

QUESTIONS

QUESTION 1. A 63-year-old woman is 8 years status post-lumpectomy and radiation therapy for a 1.5-cm, estrogen-receptor–positive, node-negative breast cancer for which she had received 5 years of tamoxifen, stopped 3 years ago. She presents to your office with severe, localized back pain. Physical examination is normal including the neurological exam. The alkaline phosphatase is 330 (elevated), and the CA27.29 is 156 (elevated). A bone scan is positive in several areas of the thoracic and lumbar spine as well as in several ribs. The course of action at this point should be:

A. Combination chemotherapy
B. Tamoxifen therapy
C. Magnetic resonance imaging (MRI) scan of the spine
D. Radiation therapy to areas of localized disease
E. Stem cell supported transplantation

QUESTION 2. A 68-year-old man presents with back pain, anemia, and fevers. The patient has no lymphadenopathy or splenomegaly. Laboratory evaluation reveals Hct = 34%, platelet count = 89,000/mm³, and a total protein of 9.8 g/dL. The serum creatinine is 3.2 mg/dL, and the serum calcium is 12.3 mg/dL. Plain x-rays of the spine show generalized osteoporosis without focal defects. The following best explains the situation:

A. Fever is a worrisome sign, and infection is a life-threatening risk for patients with this diagnosis.
B. Renal failure is uncommon and not likely to worsen.
C. Myeloma cannot be the diagnosis because lytic bone lesions are not seen.
D. Waldenstrom macroglobulinemia is never associated with lymphadenopathy and/or splenomegaly.
E. IgA and IgG paraproteins have similar serum viscosities and do not cause hyperviscosity syndrome.

QUESTION 3. A 46-year-old woman presents to your office for routine health care. She is concerned about the possibility of developing breast cancer and asks you about her risk factors. Which statement is most correct?

A. A previous biopsy that reveals lobular carcinoma in situ (LCIS) does not substantially increase her risk of developing breast cancer.
B. Presence of a BRCA-1 germ line mutation will substantially increase her risk of developing breast cancer.
C. A maternal aunt with postmenopausal breast cancer will substantially increase her risk of developing breast cancer.
D. The majority of women with breast cancer have identifiable risk factors for developing breast cancer.
E. Duration and degree of estrogen (endogenous and exogenous) exposure are not associated with increased risk of developing breast cancer.

QUESTION 4. A 67-year-old man brought to the emergency room by his family is complaining of headaches, forgetfulness, and poor coordination. Several times over the past few weeks he has had periods of confusion and urinary incontinence. He has a history of heavy smoking and hypertension for which he takes atenolol.

You perform an emergency computed tomography (CT) scan of the head, which reveals multiple round, enhancing lesions. Chest x-ray shows a 2-cm lesion in the right midlung field. The most likely diagnosis is:

A. Prostate cancer metastatic to lung and brain
B. Pneumonia with brain abscesses
C. Colon cancer with lung and brain metastases
D. Adenocarcinoma of the lung with brain metastases
E. Gastric cancer with lung and brain metastases

QUESTION 5. A 26-year-old woman with Hodgkin lymphoma and a large mediastinal mass is treated with ABVD (doxorubicin, bleomycin, vinblastine, dacarbazine) and radiation to the mediastinum. Which of the following is true?

A. She is more likely to die of causes other than Hodgkin lymphoma.
B. She is not at increased risk of developing breast cancer.

C. She has an increased risk of developing leukemia.

D. She is not likely to remain fertile after treatment.

E. She is not at increased risk for heart disease.

QUESTION 6. A 46-year-old woman who never smoked is diagnosed with stage IV non-small cell lung cancer, metastatic to liver and bone. Which of the following is most correct?

A. She is potentially curable with intensive modern chemotherapy.

B. The likelihood of responding to an epidermal growth factor receptor (EGFR) kinase inhibitor is related to the presence of a gene mutation in the intracellular portion of the kinase region.

C. The likelihood of having a mutation in the kinase region of EGFR is random and not related to gender or ethnic background.

D. Cytotoxic chemotherapy is the only potentially beneficial treatment.

E. Tumors initially sensitive to kinase inhibitors do not develop resistance to these kinase inhibitors.

QUESTION 7. A 22-year-old man, previously well, is found to have a left supraclavicular mass and an otherwise normal physical examination. Chest x-ray shows bilateral paratracheal adenopathy. Fine-needle aspiration cytology of the supraclavicular mass demonstrates undifferentiated carcinoma. The next clinical action should be:

A. Institution of multi-agent chemotherapy

B. MRI scan of the chest

C. Mediastinoscopy and biopsy of the paratracheal nodes

D. Testicular ultrasound

E. Institution of radiation therapy to the mediastinum and supraclavicular areas

QUESTION 8. The following is most true about the epidemiology of lung cancer:

A. Adenocarcinoma has become the most common histologic subtype of lung cancer.

B. Women who smoke develop lung cancer with a similar incidence and at a similar age as do men.

C. Asbestos does not add to the risk of developing lung cancer in smokers.

D. Cigarette filters reduce the carcinogenic effect of cigarettes.

E. 90% of patients with stage I non-small cell lung cancer will survive their cancer.

QUESTION 9. A 28-year-old man is admitted to the hospital with newly diagnosed acute lymphoblastic leukemia. Which of the following clinical characteristics would convey the worst prognosis?

A. Peripheral blood blast count of 200,000/mm^3

B. T-cell phenotype

C. Mediastinal mass

D. Philadelphia chromosome (t9;22)

E. Thrombocytopenia

QUESTION 10. A 51-year-old man is discovered to have a rectal cancer, which is then surgically resected. On pathology evaluation the tumor penetrates the serosa of the bowel, and one regional lymph node shows involvement with metastatic carcinoma. There is no evidence of distant metastases. Optimal therapy should include:

A. No postoperative therapy

B. Reresection of pelvic tissue surrounding the area of the original tumor

C. Radiation therapy to the pelvis

D. Systemic chemotherapy

E. Both radiation to the pelvis and chemotherapy

QUESTION 11. A 46-year-old woman is found to have epithelial ovarian cancer and is taken to the operating room for surgical debulking. At the time of surgery, a 6-cm left ovarian mass and a 3-cm right ovarian mass are found. Multiple peritoneal nodules and omental nodules are seen, as well as ascitic fluid. All tumor that can be removed is removed, but tumor masses of 2–3 cm remain. There is no evidence of disease outside the peritoneal cavity. Postoperatively, the patient is treated with paclitaxel and carboplatin for six cycles of therapy. Which best describes the probable outcome?

A. A very low chance of response to chemotherapy and a very low chance of cure

B. A high chance of complete clinical response, but a low chance for cure

C. A high chance of response and a high chance for cure

D. The need for radiation therapy delivered to the whole abdomen

E. The need for localized radiation therapy to the pelvis

QUESTION 12. A 72-year-old man presents with hematuria. Cystoscopy reveals multiple bladder nodules that are biopsied and reveal transitional cell carcinoma. The likelihood of developing metastatic bladder cancer is most closely related to:

A. The size of the tumors in the bladder

B. The number of tumors in the bladder

C. History of smoking

D. Family history

E. Bladder wall muscle invasion by the tumor

QUESTION 13. A 32-year-old man presents with acute myelogenous leukemia. Allogeneic bone marrow transplantation will most likely be recommended if a suitable donor can be found and if:

A. His initial blast count is >100,000/mm^3.

B. He is septic at presentation.

C. He has M3/acute promyelocytic leukemia and has disseminated intravascular coagulation (DIC).

D. His leukemic blasts have a 7q- chromosomal deletion.

E. His leukemic blasts have a t(8;21) chromosomal translocation.

QUESTION 14. You are evaluating a 52-year-old man with newly diagnosed non-small cell carcinoma of the right lung. Which of the following findings would NOT make him unresectable?

A. Contralateral (N3) mediastinal adenopathy
B. Enlarged (4-cm) left adrenal gland
C. Ipsilateral pleural effusion
D. Ipsilateral (N2) mediastinal adenopathy
E. Enlarged supraclavicular lymph nodes

QUESTION 15. In regard to effects of tamoxifen and raloxifene, the following is most true:

A. Raloxifene is a bone-strengthening agent, but tamoxifen is not.
B. Both increase the risk of endometrial cancer.
C. Both decrease the risk of developing a future breast cancer in women.
D. Tamoxifen increases the rate of hot flashes, but raloxifene does not.

QUESTION 16. A 42-year-old woman is diagnosed with a 3-cm poorly differentiated breast cancer with five involved axillary lymph nodes. The cancer is negative for estrogen receptors and positive for HER2. Which of the following is most true?

A. The presence of HER2 on breast cancer cells does not affect prognosis.
B. Adjuvant chemotherapy in not effective in reducing the risk of developing metastatic cancer for women with this type of breast cancer.
C. Trastuzumab, when added to chemotherapy, substantially reduces the risk of developing metastatic disease in the future.
D. Letrozole, an aromatase inhibitor, would further improve the cure rate for this patient.
E. The addition of trastuzumab to chemotherapy is safe, without short- or long-term complications.

QUESTION 17. A 56-year-old woman with a history of primary node-positive breast cancer 4 years ago, comes in with right upper quadrant pain and is found to have liver metastases from her breast cancer. Her tumor was estrogen- and progesterone-receptor negative and HER2/neu negative (so-called triple-negative breast cancer). Which of the following is most correct?

A. Because this patient's cancer is negative for HER2, her prognosis is excellent.
B. No therapy is effective or warranted, and the patient should be placed in hospice care.
C. The addition of bevacizumab to paclitaxel improves response rate and disease-free survival but does not extend overall survival.

D. Because bevacizumab, a humanized monoclonal antibody against VEGF, is not a cytotoxic chemotherapy agent, it has no significant toxicity.

QUESTION 18. A 64-year-old woman has a routine CBC showing a WBC = 14,500/mm^3 with 75% mature-appearing lymphocytes, Hct 41%, and Plt Ct = 180,000/mm^3. She has no adenopathy or splenomegaly and feels well. Which of the following is most correct?

A. The diagnosis of chronic lymphocytic leukemia (CLL) can only be made on a bone marrow aspirate and biopsy.
B. She is at increased risk for infection.
C. She is in need of urgent chemotherapy.
D. She is likely to die before her 70th birthday.
E. Splenomegaly is rare in patients such as this one.

ANSWERS

1. C. In a woman with localized back pain and suspected metastatic breast cancer involving the spine, compression of the spinal cord should always be a major consideration. Even if neurological symptoms are not present, impending spinal cord compression could be present, and the likelihood of a good neurological outcome is related to the absence of neurological findings at the time of diagnosis and institution of therapy. If spinal cord compression is present, emergent radiation to the involved area is the first treatment of choice. Systemic therapy, such as chemotherapy or hormonal therapy, may be indicated after radiation. Stem cell transplantation is not indicated for patients with breast cancer.

2. A. The most common cause of death for patients with multiple myeloma is infection, often with encapsulated organisms, but any bacterial organism is a threat. This is due to poor antigen-specific immunoglobulin production as well as neutropenia secondary to bone-marrow infiltration or chemotherapy treatment. The most common bone finding in patients with myeloma is osteoporosis, not lytic bone lesions. Patients with myeloma are at risk for renal failure due to increased serum viscosity, amyloid kidney, absorption of light chains in renal tubular cells, and hypercalcemia. Dehydration can exacerbate any of these and rapidly and irreversibly worsen renal failure. Patients with Waldenstrom macroglobulinemia frequently have lymphadenopathy and splenomegaly. IgA is variably hyperviscous, usually greater than IgG. IgA tends to form either doublets or multimers, making the aggregates more viscous than single antibodies.

3. B. Risk factors for breast cancer include germline genetic mutations such as BRCA-1 and BRCA-2, previous biopsy with lobular carcinoma in situ, which is a "field defect" marker, and duration and degree of estrogen exposure. First-degree relatives with breast cancer substantially increase the risk for the patient, but second- and third-degree relatives add little risk, especially if the relative developed

breast cancer at an older age. Most patients presenting with breast cancer have no identifiable risk factors.

4. D. The patient has metastatic disease in the brain and a lung nodule. Adenocarcinoma of the lung has now become the most common histologic type of lung cancer, and 40–50% of these patients will at some time in the course of their disease develop brain metastases; often they present with them at the time of initial diagnosis. Prostate cancer rarely metastasizes to the brain. Pneumonia with brain abscess is rare. Colon and gastric cancers metastasize to brain far less frequently than adenocarcinoma of the lung.

5. A. Current treatment for Hodgkin lymphoma results in a very high cure rate, but complications from treatment are not insignificant. Therefore, patients treated for Hodgkin lymphoma are more likely to die of other causes. In addition, patients who receive mantle radiation (radiation to the mediastinum) have an increased risk of developing breast cancer if the radiation is delivered before they are 30 years old. The risk increases after 8–10 years following radiation. Treatment with ABVD and radiation does not significantly increase the risk of the patient developing acute leukemia. ABVD and radiation to the mediastinum do not cause infertility in women or men, and babies born to parents who are treated for Hodgkin lymphoma do not have an increased rate of birth defects. Both doxorubicin and mediastinal radiation are associated with an increased risk of developing heart disease, either from damage to the proximal coronary arteries from radiation, or cardiomyopathy, short- and long-term, from administration of doxorubicin.

6. B. Unfortunately patients with stage IV metastatic non-small cell lung cancer are incurable. Some will benefit from inhibition of the epidermal growth factor receptor (EGFR) with small molecules that interact with the kinase region of that receptor. The likelihood of having a response is related to the presence of mutations in the kinase portion of the receptor, and those mutations are more common in women, those who never smoked, and Japanese, for reasons we do not understand. When tumors develop resistance to kinase inhibitors, there is often an additional acquired mutation of the kinase region of the receptor (cancer is unfortunately very adaptable). Cytotoxic chemotherapy is a reasonable therapeutic choice, but not the only one, if her tumor has mutations in the EGFR receptor.

7. D. A 22-year-old man with an undifferentiated tumor in the supraclavicular area should be considered as having primary testicular cancer until proven otherwise. Testicular cancers are sometimes not palpable and can be detected on ultrasound. Differentiation between seminoma and nonseminoma is important, and a radical orchiectomy is also an important part of the treatment both to confirm the diagnosis and as a therapeutic modality, because the testicle is a sanctuary site for chemotherapy. You NEVER want to miss diagnosing a cancer that is potentially curable, and appropriate histologic evaluation and staging are critical before the initiation of treatment.

8. A. Cigarette filters do not reduce the risk of developing lung cancer, but they appear to change the epidemiology, making adenocarcinomas more frequent than squamous cell cancers, possibly because smokers inhale more deeply when smoking filtered cigarettes, affecting more peripheral lung tissue. Asbestos and smoking are co-carcinogens, and they are additive in increasing the risk of developing lung cancer. Women appear to have a shorter latency period between smoking and the development of lung cancer than men do; they may be more sensitive to the carcinogenic effects of smoking, and, therefore, develop lung cancer statistically at an earlier age than men do. The reasons for this are unclear. Even when lung cancer is diagnosed at its earliest stages, almost half the patients will die of their lung cancer.

9. D. The Philadelphia chromosome is now known to be an extremely dire prognostic sign for patients with acute lymphoblastic leukemia. Essentially all patients treated with conventional chemotherapy will relapse and die within 3 years of diagnosis. They should all be offered allogeneic bone marrow transplantation if they have an appropriate donor. For adults, a high blast count, T-cell phenotype, or the presence of a mediastinal mass do not convey a bad prognosis.

10. E. It is now shown that the combination of pelvic radiation and systemic chemotherapy improves the rate of local tumor control, decreases the likelihood of developing distant metastatic disease, and improves overall survival for patients with B2 and C rectal carcinoma.

11. B. Stage III ovarian cancer that is incompletely surgically resected is very responsive to chemotherapy, particularly to regimens that include a platinum agent and a taxane. High response rates are attained, but almost all patients experience a relapse in their disease, and very few patients are ultimately cured. Radiation therapy does not play a role in the treatment of advanced ovarian cancer.

12. E. The presence or absence of muscle invasion in the bladder wall by transitional cell carcinomas of the bladder is the best predictive feature as to which tumors are likely to metastasize to regional nodes and distant sites. These are most often poorly differentiated tumors. Tumors that are superficial without muscle invasion are more often low-grade tumors and can often be treated with local therapies and have a low incidence of developing metastatic disease.

13. D. Height of the blast count at presentation may affect early morbidity with hyperviscosity syndrome but will not significantly influence ultimate prognosis. Likewise, sepsis at presentation will affect early but not ultimate prognosis. Acute promyelocytic leukemia (APML) has a good long-term prognosis if the early complications of DIC can be successfully managed. Early morbidity is higher due to DIC, but overall prognosis is excellent, particularly with the addition of all-*trans* retinoic acid to chemotherapy. Patients whose leukemic blasts contain deletions of the long arm or all of chromosome 7 have a poor ultimate prognosis and should undergo allogeneic bone marrow transplantation if they are of appropriate age and have a suitable donor.

Patients whose leukemic blasts contain t(8;21) have an excellent prognosis with standard chemotherapy without bone marrow transplantation.

14. D. Although the cure rate for patients with ipsilateral (N2) lymph node involvement is low, combining chemotherapy and radiation prior to surgical resection can result in long-term remission in a significant number of patients. Contralateral mediastinal adenopathy is a direct contraindication for surgical resection because these patients are almost never cured of their disease, as is the case with the presence of either a pleural effusion or supraclavicular adenopathy. Adrenal metastases are common, and an adrenal gland of 4 cm is not likely to represent a benign adrenal adenoma. Patients with metastatic disease in the adrenal gland are not curable.

15. C. Raloxifene is a new "designer" or selective estrogen receptor modulator (SERM). Raloxifene is approved to increase bone density in postmenopausal women, but tamoxifen has a similar effect. Tamoxifen stimulates the endometrium and is associated with an increased risk of developing endometrial cancers, and those cancers can be life-threatening. Raloxifene does not appear to stimulate the endometrium and does not appear to increase the risk of endometrial cancer. Both tamoxifen and raloxifene can increase the rates of vasomotor symptoms, including hot flashes.

16. C. Patients with primary, newly diagnosed breast cancers whose cancers overexpress HER-2 have an inherently worse prognosis. Administration of adjuvant chemotherapy will reduce the risk of recurrence and death for these patients, but the addition of trastuzumab (a humanized monoclonal antibody directed against HER2) to chemotherapy will further substantially reduce the risk of cancer recurrence. When trastuzumab is administered after doxorubicin, there is an increased risk of heart failure, and the long-term cardiac ramifications are not known. Aromatase inhibitors are ineffective against breast cancers whose estrogen receptors are negative.

17. C. Patients with breast cancers negative for estrogen and progesterone receptors, and for HER2 (so called triple-negative cancers) have a particularly poor prognosis, particularly when metastatic disease is present. Hormone therapy and trastuzumab have no benefit for these women. The addition of bevacizumab to paclitaxel has been shown to increase response rate and duration of response but not overall survival for patients with this subset of breast cancer. Hypertension and proteinuria are the two major side effects of bevacizumab.

18. B. The patient has CLL. The diagnosis can usually be made on flow cytometric analysis of the peripheral blood. The circulating lymphocytes can be demonstrated to be B cells, expressing the B-cell antigen CD20, but they also co-express the T-cell antigen CD5. Patients with CLL are at risk for infection, even early in the course of their disease, because of depressed antibody formation in response to specific antigen challenge. Because of this they are specifically at risk for infection with encapsulated bacteria as well as viral infections. She has early-stage CLL, and no treatment is required. Early therapy does not improve outcome in any way, including overall survival. Treatment is indicated when a patient has progressive and significant splenomegaly, lymphadenopathy, symptoms, or suppression of her normal blood counts. The median survival for patients with early-stage CLL, as is the case with this patient, is >15 years.

22.

ONCOLOGY SUMMARY

Erica L. Mayer and Robert J. Mayer

Much progress has been made in understanding the mechanisms of cancer cell growth, identifying specific "targets" unique to the cancer cell, and optimizing cancer treatment. Outcomes have improved for both rare and common cancers.

SELECTED CANCERS

BREAST CANCER

Breast cancer is the most common cancer in American women and the second most common cause of cancer mortality (excluding basal and squamous cell skin cancer). Risk factors for breast cancer are shown in table 22.1. Mammography can detect asymptomatic early-stage breast cancers. Most expert groups recommend initiating mammography screening at age 40, although expert groups differ in their recommendations (table 22.2). Mammography does not identify approximately 10% of breast cancers; therefore, biopsy is recommended for any suspicious lesion, even if mammographically undetectable. Breast self-examination has not been shown to increase the rate of breast cancer diagnosis, to change the stage at diagnosis, or to reduce the risk of death from breast cancer. Clinical breast examination may modestly improve early detection. Magnetic resonance imaging (MRI) detects more cancers (i.e., is more sensitive) than mammography but results in more false positives and therefore more biopsies of nonmalignant lesions. It does not detect all cancers, and notably misses some cases of ductal carcinoma in situ (DCIS). Therefore, screening breast MRI may complement, but not replace, screening mammography and is typically reserved for individuals at very high risk of cancer incidence such as BRCA1/2 mutation carriers. Regardless of how a suspicious breast mass is identified, a core biopsy has supplanted excisional biopsy as the standard diagnostic procedure.

The vast majority (>95%) of breast cancers are epithelial in origin and are classified as carcinomas. Breast carcinomas can be divided into two distinct groups: (1) in situ carcinomas, where cancer cells are confined inside ducts or lobules and do not invade into the surrounding stroma, and (2) invasive or infiltrating carcinomas, where cancer cells invade into the breast stroma and consequently have the potential to metastasize. There are two major histologic types of in situ carcinomas, referred to as ductal carcinoma in situ (DCIS) and lobular carcinoma in situ (LCIS). There are several different histologic types of invasive breast cancer, including invasive ductal carcinoma (IDC), invasive lobular carcinoma (ILC), mixed ductal/lobular carcinoma, mucinous (colloid) carcinoma, tubular carcinoma, medullary carcinoma, and papillary carcinoma. IDC is the most common histologic subtype, accounting for approximately 75% of all invasive breast cancers.

Two thirds of all invasive breast cancers are hormone receptor positive; that is, >10% of the cancer cells express either the estrogen receptor (ER) or the progesterone receptor (PR). In 20% of invasive breast cancers, the human epidermal growth factor cell surface receptor 2 (HER2) is overexpressed. The risk of recurrence is higher for hormone-receptor-negative compared to hormone-receptor-positive breast cancer, and for HER2-positive compared to HER2-negative breast cancer. Invasive breast cancers that express none of these three receptors (approximately 15% of all invasive breast cancers) are called "triple negative" breast cancers and carry a poor prognosis. Inflammatory breast cancer can be of any subtype and represents a particularly aggressive locally advanced form of breast cancer.

Management options are summarized in table 22.3.

LUNG CANCER

Lung cancer is a heterogeneous group of malignancies comprising small cell lung cancer (SCLC) (13%) and non-small cell lung cancer (NSCLC) (86%); additional rare thoracic malignancies include mesothelioma and carcinoid tumors. The single most important risk factor, smoking, accounts for approximately 85% of all lung cancers. Other associated factors include exposure to radon, asbestos, and heavy

Table 22.1 RISK FACTORS FOR BREAST CANCER

Gender

Age

Higher weight/BMI

Personal history of breast cancer or benign breast disease

Exposure to ionizing radiation

Family history of breast cancer

Race/ethnicity

Diet

Alcohol

Prolonged postmenopausal hormone replacement therapy (HRT)

Longer exposure to and higher concentrations of endogenous estrogen (early menarche, nulliparity, older age at first birth, later menopause)

Inherited breast cancer susceptibility gene; BRCA1/2, p53, etc.

metals. Other causative exposures include wood smoke, previous chest radiotherapy, and heavy metals such as arsenic, chromium, nickel, beryllium, and cadmium. Clinically, the respiratory symptoms of lung cancer often mimic the effects of chronic tobacco use. Many patients present with cough, worsening dyspnea, or hemoptysis, which can also be symptoms of bronchitis or pneumonia. Systemic symptoms include weight loss, chest pain, bone pain, hoarseness, or neurologic symptoms.

Paraneoplastic syndromes are most frequently seen in patients with small cell lung cancer, but can be seen in either type of lung cancer.

- *Hematologic abnormalities:* Leukocytosis (likely from tumor secretion of granulocyte colony-stimulating factor [G-CSF]), anemia, and thrombocytosis.

- *Syndrome of inappropriate antidiuretic hormone secretion* (SIADH): Up to 10% of SCLC may secrete ADH, resulting in profound hyponatremia.

- *Hypercalcemia:* Hypercalcemia in malignancy may result from direct bone invasion or secretion of osteoclast-activating factors and occurs most commonly in squamous cell cancers.

- *Cushing syndrome:* Excess production of adrenocorticotropic hormone (ACTH) by tumor tissue can lead to Cushing syndrome: truncal obesity, hypertension, hyperglycemia, hypokalemic alkalosis, and osteoporosis.

- *Pancoast syndrome:* Lung tumors that arise in the superior sulcus of either lung can cause damage to the brachial plexus and the sympathetic ganglia. This results in a syndrome of shoulder/arm pain, ipsilateral Horner syndrome, bone destruction, and atrophy of the hand muscles.

- *Neurological abnormalities:* Eaton-Lambert syndrome (a myasthenia-like neuropathy) and anti-neuronal antibodies (e.g. "anti-Hu").

- *Thrombosis:* Presenting with deep vein thrombosis and/ or pulmonary embolism.

Diagnostic evaluation should include a chest radiograph—a nodule on a chest x-ray or computed tomography (CT) scan may lead to the diagnosis of lung cancer. A CT of the chest with IV contrast gives an overview of the extent of parenchymal disease and regional nodal involvement and can also demonstrate metastatic disease to the bones, liver, or adrenal glands. PET/CT scans are used to further evaluate the extent of regional or metastatic disease. Bronchoscopy, increasingly in combination with endobronchial ultrasound, is most useful for proximal tumors and can yield information about a primary tumor and lymph node staging. Although the diagnosis can be made from fine-needle aspiration alone, advanced molecular testing requires more tissue in the form of a core biopsy or surgical sample. Chest radiographs have repeatedly been shown to be ineffective as a means of screening for lung cancers; recent observations have suggested a role for spiral CT scans as a screening approach for high-risk individuals with a heavy smoking history.

Management options are summarized in table 22.4.

Table 22.2 MAMMOGRAM GUIDELINES, U.S. PREVENTIVE SERVICES TASK FORCE (USPSTF) 2009

1. Screening mammograms should be done every 2 years beginning at age 50 for women at average risk of breast cancer.

2. Screening mammograms before age 50 should not be done routinely and should be based on a woman's values regarding the risks and benefits of mammography.

3. Doctors should not teach women to do breast self-exams.

4. There is insufficient evidence that mammogram screening is effective for women age 75 and older, so specific recommendations for this age group were not included.

NOTE: USPSTF guidelines differ from those of the American Cancer Society (ACS). The ACS mammogram guidelines recommend yearly mammogram screening beginning at age 40 for women at average risk of breast cancer. ACS guidelines indicate that the breast self-exam is optional in breast cancer screening.

Table 22.3 MANAGEMENT OPTIONS FOR BREAST CANCER

STAGES OF BREAST CANCER	MANAGEMENT OPTIONS
Stage 0 breast cancer (carcinoma in situ)	
LCIS	Consider preventative tamoxifen or raloxifene. Excision of breast tissue to achieve negative margins and radiation therapy are not indicated.
DCIS	Mastectomy, or lumpectomy (breast-conserving therapy) with complete removal of the tumor to achieve negative margins. Radiation therapy to the breast follows lumpectomy and reduces the risk of local recurrence. Sampling of the axillary lymph nodes is not indicated for cases of pure DCIS (i.e., no evidence of invasive cancer). Both mastectomy and lumpectomy followed by radiation therapy confer a high likelihood of survival (>98%). Tamoxifen is recommended after lumpectomy to reduce risk of local recurrence.
Stage I, II, and III breast cancer (nonmetastatic)	Cure is the goal of therapy. Surgical resection includes either mastectomy or lumpectomy with axillary nodal sampling to remove the primary cancer. Radiation therapy to the breast traditionally follows lumpectomy, and radiation therapy to the chest wall following mastectomy is occasionally recommended in higher-risk situations (e.g., if the tumor is >5 cm or more than four axillary lymph nodes are involved). Hormone-receptor–negative breast cancers tend to recur earlier, whereas hormone-receptor–positive breast cancers can recur 10 or more years after diagnosis. The choice of adjuvant systemic therapy depends on the risk of recurrence and the subtype of breast cancer. The higher the risk of recurrence the greater the potential benefit of adjuvant therapy. Adjuvant endocrine therapy is specifically indicated if a tumor is hormone-receptor positive. Adjuvant chemotherapy is typically indicated for women with hormone-receptor–negative cancers and selected higher-risk hormone-receptor–positive cancers. Gene expression analysis, e.g., Onco*type*DX®, can be used to determine if the addition of chemotherapy would provide reduction in the risk of recurrence. Chemotherapy for breast cancer usually involves the administration of two or three medications with nonoverlapping toxicity profiles; commonly used medications include cyclophosphamide, methotrexate, 5-fluorouracil, doxorubicin, epirubicin, paclitaxel, and docetaxel. The addition of adjuvant trastuzumab to chemotherapy is indicated for most HER2+ cancers that are at least 1.0 cm in size.
Stage IV breast cancer (metastatic)	The primary goals of treatment for incurable metastatic breast cancer include prolongation of survival and palliation of symptoms. Selection of systemic therapy is tailored for tumor subtype. Initial management of hormone-receptor–positive metastatic breast cancer most commonly involves the administration of an antiestrogen hormonal medication. Hormonal treatment options can include tamoxifen, a selective aromatase inhibitor (e.g., anastrozole, letrozole, or exemestane), fulvestrant, or a gonadotropin-releasing hormone (GnRH) agonist for premenopausal women. For endocrine-refractory/hormone-receptor–negative metastatic breast cancer or symptomatic metastatic disease, systemic chemotherapy is typically administered. Multiple chemotherapy medications have activity in advanced breast cancer. Anti-HER2-directed therapy, including trastuzumab and lapatinib, is indicated in the treatment of advanced HER2+ disease. For women who have metastatic bony deposits, the regular administration of an intravenous bisphosphonate (e.g., pamidronate or zoledronic acid) helps prevent/delay the development of skeletal complications and palliates bone pain. Targeted local therapies, such as surgical excision, radiation therapy, or radio-frequency ablation, are sometimes indicated.

GI MALIGNANCIES

The most common gastrointestinal cancers in the United States are esophageal, gastric, pancreatic, and colorectal.

Esophageal Cancer

Esophageal cancer is diagnosed in approximately 16,000 individuals in the United States annually, leading to nearly 14,000 deaths. There are two major histology types, squamous cell carcinoma and adenocarcinoma. Other histologic types, such as melanomas, carcinoids, lymphomas, and sarcomas are rare.

Squamous cell carcinomas develop in the upper third and middle third of the esophagus. Adenocarcinomas primarily develop in the lower third of the esophagus and, particularly in cancers at the gastroesophageal junction, have markedly increased in frequency during the past several decades. The primary risk factors for squamous cell carcinomas are tobacco and alcohol. Other conditions that lead to irritation of the esophageal mucosa and increase the risk of squamous

cell carcinoma include achalasia, caustic injury to the esophagus, and esophageal diverticuli. Rare conditions that carry a very high risk of squamous cell carcinoma include nonepidermolytic palmoplantar keratoderma (tylosis), a rare autosomal dominant disorder characterized by hyperkeratosis of the palms and soles and thickening of the oral mucosa, and Plummer–Vinson syndrome, a nutritional deficiency characterized by dysphagia, iron-deficiency anemia, and esophageal webs. Adenocarcinomas of the esophagus principally develop in the setting of Barrett's esophagitis. Risk factors associated with the development of Barrett's esophagitis include gastroesophageal reflux disease and obesity.

Patients with esophageal cancer more commonly present with symptoms of difficulty swallowing (dysphagia) and, less commonly, with pain with swallowing (odynophagia). Prior to diagnosis, patients may have dysphagia for certain solids, then for most solids, and eventually for liquids. Patients may also present with hematemesis, unexpected weight loss, cough, aspiration pneumonia, hoarseness, or symptoms related to areas of metastases.

Table 22.4 MANAGEMENT OPTIONS FOR LUNG CANCER

TYPE OF LUNG CANCER	MANAGEMENT OPTIONS
Stage I–II NSCLC	Initial treatment for stage I (small tumor without lymph node involvement) and stage II (larger and more invasive tumors or hilar lymph node involvement) consists of surgical resection. For large stage Ib tumors, and for all stage II tumors, it is estimated that patients have approximately a 5% overall survival benefit to cisplatin-based doublet adjuvant chemotherapy. For small stage I tumors, there is no evidence of benefit from adjuvant chemotherapy. There is no role for adjuvant radiation therapy in completely resected NSCLC.
Stage III NSCLC	Therapy for stage III NSCLC includes a combination of chemotherapy, radiation, and sometimes surgical resection. Stage IIIB disease is generally considered surgically unresectable, and is treated with concurrent chemotherapy and high-dose radiation with curative intent ("definitive" treatment). The treatment of stage IIIA disease is less standardized and often includes surgery, pre- and/or postoperative chemotherapy, and consideration of radiotherapy.
Stage IV NSCLC	The backbone of therapy for stage IV NSCLC is systemic chemotherapy. Standard first-line chemotherapy consists of platinum-based doublet chemotherapy. Most platinum-based doublets (carboplatin or cisplatin, in combination with paclitaxel, docetaxel, gemcitabine, vinorelbine, or pemetrexed) generally have equivalent impacts on survival. A number of novel agents are considered for advanced disease, including inhibitors of VEGF, EGFR, and EML4-ALK.
Limited-stage SCLC	Concurrent radiotherapy and concurrent full-dose chemotherapy with cisplatin and etoposide, followed by chemotherapy alone. Following chemotherapy and radiation, prophylactic cranial irradiation.
Extensive-stage SCLC	Extensive-stage small cell lung cancer is incurable. Patients who respond to initial therapy also have a survival benefit from prophylactic cranial irradiation. Second-line therapy is more successful in patients with a disease-free interval longer than 3 months after initial therapy ("relapsed" disease) than patients with a disease-free interval of less than 3 months ("refractory" disease). Supportive care also plays an essential role in the management of SCLC.

The treatment and prognosis of esophageal cancer reflect the stage of disease at diagnosis (table 22.5) Squamous cell carcinomas and adenocarcinomas are radiologically indistinguishable and are approached diagnostically and therapeutically in a similar fashion. Patients who are diagnosed with esophageal cancer by upper endoscopy should undergo staging evaluation including CT of the chest, abdomen, and pelvis to assess for metastases. PET/CT scans have been shown to be particularly effective in identifying spread to regional lymph nodes in such patients. The most common sites of metastases are liver, lung, lymph nodes, and bone.

Gastric Cancer

An estimated 21,500 new cases of gastric cancer and 11,000 related deaths occur in the United States annually. The vast majority of gastric tumors in the stomach are adenocarcinomas. Other markedly less frequent histologies are lymphomas, carcinoids, leiomyosarcomas, and gastrointestinal stromal tumors (GISTs). There are two subtypes of gastric adenocarcinomas, an intestinal-type with cohesive neoplastic cells forming gland-like tubular structures and a diffuse type in which individual cells infiltrate and thicken the stomach wall. Intestinal-type lesions occur in the distal stomach more often than the diffuse type and are often preceded by a prolonged precancerous phase associated with *Helicobacter pylori* infection. Diffuse carcinomas are detected more often in younger patients, develop throughout the stomach, particularly the cardia, and are associated with a worse prognosis.

The most common symptoms at presentation are unexplained weight loss, abdominal pain, fatigue, nausea, anorexia,

dysphagia, early satiety, and melena. Initial evaluation of symptoms suspicious for gastric cancer includes barium swallow and/or upper endoscopy. Once a diagnostic biopsy demonstrates adenocarcinoma, staging with CT is recommended. However, such imaging is limited in its ability to detect peritoneal metastases, which can be present in up in 10–30% of patients who appear to have localized disease. At the time of surgery, an initial exploratory laparoscopy is necessary, and detection of peritoneal disease or distant metastases should lead to either a palliative resection or bypass gastrojejunostomy.

The pathological stage is the most important determinant of prognosis and determines treatment strategy. Treatment is summarized in table 22.5. Those patients with metastatic disease should be considered for palliative chemotherapy.

Pancreas Cancer

Pancreas cancer carries a high risk of fatality as a result of the inability to detect such tumors at an early stage. It is the 10th most common cancer in incidence in the United States but the fourth most common cause of cancer-related deaths (after lung, colorectal, and breast cancer).

Pancreatic cancer has been associated with various hereditary syndromes. Hereditary nonpolyposis colorectal cancer (HNPCC) results from mutations of the mismatch repair genes, and although it is most commonly associated with colorectal and gynecological cancers, it also carries an increased risk of pancreatic cancer. Inherited mutations of p16 result in familial atypical multiple mole-melanoma syndrome associated with melanomas and pancreatic cancer. Other syndromes in which the risk of pancreatic cancer

Table 22.5 MANAGEMENT OPTIONS FOR GI CANCERS

GI CANCER	MANAGEMENT OPTIONS
Esophageal cancer	For patients with disease that does not extend beyond the muscle layer of the esophageal wall and without evidence of lymph node involvement, immediate surgery is recommended. For those with disease that extends beyond the muscle layer or with locoregional lymph nodes, neoadjuvant therapy with chemotherapy and radiation should be considered prior to surgery. Chemoradiation therapy is given over 5–6 weeks with daily radiation and various combinations of chemotherapy agents. Following the completion of neoadjuvant therapy, restaging is recommended, followed by surgery approximately 6 weeks after the last dose of radiation. For patients with localized disease who are not surgical candidates due to concurrent medical conditions or who refuse surgery, disease is treated with chemoradiation. Patients with metastatic disease should be considered for palliative therapy. Chemotherapy can palliate symptoms relating to swallowing and prolong overall survival.
Gastric cancer	For patients with nonmetastatic disease, the primary treatment modality is surgery. Following surgical resection, nonmetastatic patients whose disease extend's beyond the muscle layer of the gastric wall or with positive lymph nodes should be considered for adjuvant chemoradiotherapy. For patients with metastatic disease, palliative chemotherapy is the primary treatment modality. No single regimen is considered standard. For patients with a good performance status, combination regimens that include a platinum agent are reasonable first-line choices.
Pancreatic cancer	For head of the pancreas lesions, a pancreaticoduodenectomy (Whipple) operation is performed, with resection of part of the pancreas and duodenum, common bile duct, gallbladder, and distal stomach. For body or tail of the pancreas lesions, a distal pancreatectomy with or without splenectomy is performed. Resection of body or tail lesions is considerably less common because most such cancers are metastatic at time of diagnosis. Following resection, adjuvant therapy with chemotherapy alone or a combination of chemotherapy and radiation is recommended. Combined-modality chemotherapy and radiation is typically pursued for locally advanced pancreatic cancer. Palliative chemotherapy is utilized for metastatic pancreatic cancer; however, benefit tends to be limited.
Colorectal cancer	Treatment for colorectal cancer depends on stage of disease. Surgery is considered the only curative therapy for colorectal cancers. Multiple clinical trials have demonstrated a survival benefit for adjuvant chemotherapy in stage III (lymph node–positive) colon cancer patients following surgery. For patients with metastatic disease, removal of the primary tumor still remains an important consideration to palliate and prevent symptoms due to the colorectal lesion (including bleeding and obstruction). Chemotherapy is an important component of the treatment of patients with metastatic disease as well as many patients with surgically resected tumors. The backbone of colorectal cancer treatment for the past four decades is the fluorinated pyrimidine, 5-fluorouracil (5-FU). Newer regimens can also include oxaliplatin, irinotecan, and/or targeted biological therapy.

is increased include BRCA2, ataxia-telangiectasia, Peutz-Jeghers, and hereditary pancreatitis.

Tobacco is the most common modifiable risk factor most consistently associated with development of pancreatic cancer; however, obesity and certain dietary factors may increase risk as well.

Approximately 85% of pancreatic cancers are adenocarcinomas. The other histologies are neuroendocrine tumors arising from the islets of Langerhans, lymphomas, or metastatic disease. Adenocarcinomas most commonly arise in the head of the pancreas (65%) and less commonly are restricted to the body or tail (15%), or present diffusely throughout the pancreas (20%).

A classical presentation of pancreatic cancer is the acute onset of jaundice, occasionally unaccompanied by pain but more frequently associated with localized discomfort. Other presenting features include unexpected weight loss, pain radiating to the midback, anorexia, and nausea. Laboratory testing may show elevation of total bilirubin and other liver function tests (alkaline phosphatase more than transaminases). Occasionally, the new development of diabetes may herald the appearance of a pancreatic cancer.

Workup should include CT looking for a pancreatic mass. For patients with metastatic disease at presentation, the liver is the most common site of metastases, although distant lymph nodes, peritoneum, and lungs are frequent areas of spread. For patients who present with jaundice, endoscopic retrograde cholangiopancreatography (ERCP) with stent placement and cytology by brushings and/or biopsy are appropriate diagnostic-therapeutic maneuvers. Alternatively, percutaneous biopsy of the primary pancreatic mass or metastases guided by CT or ultrasound can be pursued.

Although a TNM (tumor, node, metastases) system that is utilized for solid organ tumors exists for pancreatic cancer, the more practical classification of pancreatic cancer describes three stages of disease: local, locally advanced, and metastatic. Local disease implies surgical resectability and is the only potentially curable stage of pancreatic cancer. Treatment options are listed in (table 22.5).

Colorectal Cancer

Colorectal cancer is the third most common cancer diagnosed in men, the third most common cancer diagnosed in women in the United States, and the fourth most common cancer overall. It is the second most common cause of cancer-related death in the United States, with an estimated 50,000 deaths each year.

Up to 25% of patients with colorectal cancer have a family history of the disease. Multiple hereditary syndromes carry a markedly increased risk of colorectal cancer. Familial adenomatous polyposis (FAP) results from truncating mutations in the adenomatous polyposis coli (APC) gene on chromosome 5. Afflicted individuals develop hundreds to thousands of polyps by their second decade of life and, if untreated, can develop colorectal cancer by age 40. It is recommended that patients with FAP pursue total colectomy by age 20. Variants of FAP include Gardner's syndrome (in which prominent extraintestinal lesions such as desmoid tumors and sebaceous or epidermoid cysts are seen in addition to extensive polyposis) and Turcot syndrome (brain tumors, particularly medulloblastomas, in addition to colonic tumors). Hereditary nonpolyposis colon cancer (HNPCC), or Lynch syndrome, is characterized by the early onset of colorectal cancer, often involving the right side of the colon, and typically occurs in the absence of numerous colonic polyps. The condition is associated with germline mutations in DNA repair genes, leading to mismatch repair defects and microsatellite instability. The presence of these DNA repair defects in colorectal tumors, interestingly, is associated with a more favorable prognosis. In addition to familial syndromes, a family or personal history of colorectal cancer increases one's risk of developing colorectal cancer. This risk is modified by number of family members affected and age of diagnosis of family members, particularly first-degree relatives. Importantly, this risk is similar for individuals with a family history of adenomatous polyps, likely because such polyps may have evolved to cancer if untreated.

Patients with inflammatory bowel disease have an increased risk of colorectal cancer that can be three- to five-fold higher than that in the general population. The risk is associated with both ulcerative colitis and Crohn disease, particular for patients with Crohn disease affecting the large bowel. Extent of disease involvement of the colon and rectum and duration of disease are the main determinants of the increased risk.

Screening for colorectal cancer is key. The 2008 American College of Gastroenterology Guidelines for Colorectal Cancer Screening are summarized in table 22.6.

Over 98% of large intestine cancers are adenocarcinomas. Most colorectal carcinomas originate from adenomatous polyps. Progression from early adenomatous proliferations through adenomatous polyp, high-grade dysplasia, and, ultimately, invasive carcinoma occurs as a continuum.

Patients with cancer of the cecum and ascending colon can present with anemia caused by intermittent gastrointestinal bleeding. Obstruction is rare because the bowel wall is more distensible and the stool is more liquid (i.e., less formed) than in the descending colon. These cancers are often large and may be fungating or friable. Carcinomas of the transverse colon and either the hepatic or the splenic flexure, which account for about 10% of total cases, are somewhat less common than cecal neoplasms and much less common than rectosigmoid tumors. They frequently

Table 22.6 KEY ELEMENTS OF 2008 CRC SCREENING GUIDELINES

1. Colonoscopy is the preferred CRC prevention test. Colonoscopy is recommended every 10 years beginning at age 50. Alternatives for patients who decline colonoscopy are flexible sigmoidoscopy or computed tomography (CT) colonography.

2. Screening for African-American persons should begin at age 45 due to the high incidence of CRC and a greater prevalence of proximal or right-sided polyps and cancerous lesions in this population.

3. CT colonography (also known as virtual colonoscopy) can be performed every 5 years as an alternative to colonoscopy every 10 years in patients who decline the traditional modality. CT colonography has a 90% sensitivity for colon polyps ≥1 cm; however, it is not considered to be equivalent to colonoscopy because of its inability to detect polyps ≤5 mm, which constitute 80% of colorectal neoplasms, and because false positives are common with CT colonography.

4. Barium enema is not recommended for CRC screening/prevention due to variability in quality of performance.

5. Fecal testing is a cancer detection test, not a cancer prevention test. Fecal immunohistochemical testing (FIT) is recommended over the older guaiac-based fecal occult blood test and is the preferred cancer detection test (performed annually).

6. Screening recommendations related to family history.
   - An increased level of screening is no longer recommended for those with a history of adenomas in a first-degree relative or in patients ≥60 years of age with colon cancer or advanced adenomas.
   - Single first-degree relative with CRC or advanced adenoma (adenoma ≥1 cm in size, or with high dysplasia or villous elements) diagnosed at age ≥60 years: Recommended screening is the same as for those at *average risk* (colonoscopy every 10 years beginning at age 50 years).
   - Single first-degree relative with CRC or advanced adenoma diagnosed at age <60 years *or* two first-degree relatives with CRC or advanced adenomas: Recommended screening is colonoscopy every 5 years beginning at age 40 or at 10 years younger than age at diagnosis of the youngest affected relative.
   - Single first-degree relative with only small tubular adenoma is not considered to increase the risk for CRC, and no changes beyond average-risk screening are needed.

cause cramping pain bleeding, and sometimes obstruction or perforation. Large bowel obstruction is the most common complication of colon carcinoma and may lead to proximal ulceration or perforation. Other complications include iron deficiency anemia, hypokalemia (particularly associated with large villous rectal lesions), and intussusception in adults. Tumors of the sigmoid colon and rectal cancers usually cause changes in normal bowel habits, with tenesmus, decrease in stool caliber, secretion of mucus, and hematochezia.

Management options are summarized in table 22.5.

GU MALIGNANCIES

Prostate Cancer

Prostate cancer is the most commonly diagnosed cancer in American men, representing approximately 25% of all cancers diagnosed each year, and is the second leading cause of cancer death in American men. The most relevant risk factors for prostate cancer include age and genetic factors, such as family history and ethnicity. Most prostate cancer diagnoses in the United States are made through prostate-specific antigen (PSA) screening; however, there is currently no definitive evidence that PSA screening improves mortality. Nonetheless, given the data supporting screening, PSA testing has become a standard of care in many U.S. primary care practices. When prostate cancer is identified, PSA level, clinical stage, and pathologic results from biopsy are powerful predictors of clinical outcome.

Multiple treatment options exist for the management of low-risk localized prostate cancer, including radical prostatectomy, external beam radiation therapy, or brachytherapy (radiation seed implants). Watchful waiting—close surveillance without treatment—is an additional, and often preferable, option for low-risk patients. For patients with high-risk features, emerging data suggest that adjuvant treatment, including the addition of androgen-deprivation therapy, improves outcomes.

Despite definitive local treatment, prostate cancer can recur. Patients with local recurrence may be successfully salvaged with radiation therapy. However, for those who cannot be salvaged or those with overt metastatic disease, androgen-deprivation therapy remains the standard of care, and over 90% of men respond to therapy. Disease eventually progresses, and further palliative therapy includes subsequent antiandrogen therapy and/or transition to chemotherapy.

Renal Cell Carcinoma

Renal cell carcinoma (RCC) accounts for approximately 3% of adult malignancies and over 90% of neoplasms arising from the kidney. RCC is characterized by a lack of early warning signs, diverse clinical manifestations, relative resistance to radiation and chemotherapy, and infrequent responses to immunotherapy agents such as interferon-α and interleukin (IL)-2. Although >50% of patients with RCC are cured in early stages, the outcome for metastatic disease is poor. Newer targeted anti-angiogenic agents, which target multiple receptor kinases, such as sorafenib and sunitinib, have demonstrated major activity in these patients and have become first-line treatment in metastatic disease.

Bladder Cancer

Bladder cancer is the fourth most common cancer in men and the ninth in women; the higher incidence in men is likely related to higher rates of smoking and occupational exposures. Presenting symptoms include hematuria as well as urinary voiding symptoms. The primary diagnostic maneuver is cystoscopy, which not only allows visual inspection of the bladder but also identifies sites for biopsy and transurethral resection of bladder tumor. Stage and grade of disease are the most important variables in determining outcome, with invasion into muscle of the bladder wall considered higher risk and warranting aggressive treatment.

Treatment for superficial disease consists of complete transurethral resection; in the setting of higher-risk superficial disease, intravesical bacillus Calmette-Guerin (BCG) may be utilized. Standard initial therapy for invasive bladder cancer is radical cystectomy with bilateral lymph node dissection, which may be accompanied by pre- or postoperative chemotherapy. Metastatic disease carriers a poor prognosis and is treated with combination chemotherapy.

Testicular Cancer

Testicular cancers are most commonly germ cell tumors (GCT) and are classified as either seminomas or non-seminomas, based on their histology. Testicular GCTs are the most common malignancy in men aged 15–35 years but occur rarely in the population in general. The classic presentation of testicular cancer is detection of a nodule or painless swelling of one testicle. Nearly all GCTs are potentially curable, with the likelihood of cure dependent on clinical stage. Treatment of early-stage disease can include surgery and/or chemotherapy. Advanced disease may require multimodality therapy.

Non-Hodgkin and Hodgkin Lymphoma

Lymphomas are malignancies of lymphoid cells. These neoplasms originate from cells in the B-lymphocyte and T-lymphocyte/natural killer (NK) cell lineages, and are categorized into Hodgkin and non-Hodgkin lymphomas. The World Health Organization (WHO) recognizes five major types of Hodgkin lymphomas and at least 40 major types of non-Hodgkin lymphomas. Non-Hodgkin lymphoma (NHL) represents the fifth most common cancer in the United States and is the most common hematologic malignancy.

Presenting symptoms for NHL include lymphadenopathy, constitutional symptoms, and local symptoms. Lymphadenopathy is present in over two-thirds of patients with NHL, with the rapidity of lymph node enlargement reflecting the aggressiveness of the disease. The most clinically significant constitutional symptoms are B symptoms, defined as fever >38°C (100.4°F), weight loss >10% of body weight over a 6-month period, or drenching night sweats. B symptoms are seen in about 45% of aggressive or highly aggressive NHLs and in <25% of indolent NHLs; when present in the setting of an indolent NHL, B symptoms tend to indicate a large burden of disease. Additional constitutional symptoms include fatigue and malaise.

Local symptoms reflect the degree to which a lymphoma impairs functioning of involved or adjacent tissues, with different NHLs displaying varying degrees of marrow, splenic, and extranodal (i.e., external to the lymphatic system) involvement. Common sites of extranodal involvement include the gastrointestinal tract, skin, and bone; rare sites include the kidneys, bladder, adrenals, heart, lungs, breast, testes, and thyroid. In addition, the central nervous system (CNS) may be infiltrated either in the form of a primary CNS lymphoma (i.e., a lymphoma that predominates in the CNS), a condition occurring particularly frequently in immunocompromised individuals, such as patients with HIV/AIDS, or a secondary CNS lymphoma (i.e., a lymphoma with predominantly systemic disease that spreads into the CNS).

The workup of a suspected NHL requires a thorough history, physical examination, laboratory evaluation, imaging, and tissue sampling for pathology review.

The treatment of Hodgkin disease (Hodgkin lymphoma) for most patients is combination radiation therapy and chemotherapy. In patients with advanced Hodgkin disease, involved-field XRT can be used for sites of persistent disease following chemotherapy. The treatment of NHL varies greatly depending on tumor stage, phenotype (B-, T- or NK/null-cell), histology (i.e., whether low-, intermediate-, or high-grade), symptoms, performance status, patient's age, and comorbidities.

The Identification of Cancer Subsets

The identification of subsets of cancers provides both prognostic (i.e., disease natural history) and predictive (likelihood of response to a given treatment) information highly relevant for clinical practice. Traditional pathologic analyses can discriminate cancer subgroups; for example, immunohistochemistry can identify cellular receptors, such as the human epidermal growth factor (HER2), in the setting of breast cancer, and cytogenetic analyses can detect specific chromosomal anomalies in acute myeloid leukemia. Contemporary molecular diagnostic testing

techniques, including polymerase chain reaction (PCR), reverse transcriptase-polymerase chain reaction (RT-PCR), RNA/DNA microarray analysis, and proteomics, have allowed the emergence of a far more specific description of DNA, RNA, or protein expression patterns in individual tumors. These "tumor fingerprints" provide an otherwise undetectable portrait of tumor behavior, growth potential, and sensitivity to treatment. Analyses can be performed on a variety of tissue sources, including fresh tumor obtained at the time of biopsy, tumor cells obtained from circulating blood, or paraffin-embedded tumor tissue from prior procedures. The accessibility of archival paraffin-embedded tissue provides the most ease in performing genomic analyses, although testing may be limited to a small collection of genes. A significantly broader panel of genetic material can be evaluated from fresh tissue, and a management strategy involving multidisciplinary input at the time of diagnosis and initial treatment may increase the likelihood that such fresh tissue specimens can be retrieved, thereby improving the utilization of advanced genomic techniques.

Clinical Importance of Genomic Predictors

Evaluations for both individual gene products and multigene arrays have gained utility as predictive tools in the selection of therapy. Such assays can focus on the overexpression or mutation of a given, gene which may affect protein function. The identification of such genetic changes enables more precision in the selection of targeted therapy. Additionally, subgrouping cancers by their molecular portrait has emerged as a relevant tool in clinical decision making as well.

Mutation in the Epidermal Growth Factor Receptor

The epidermal growth factor receptor (EGFR) is a member of the HER family of receptors. Multiple solid tumors overexpress EGFR, and the activation of the EGFR signaling cascade leads to cellular proliferation and subsequent tumor invasion. Both small-molecule tyrosine kinase inhibitors, administered orally, and monoclonal antibodies, administered parenterally, have been developed to target this receptor. Clinical trials in lung cancer patients treated with EGFR inhibitors demonstrate that only 15–20% of all patients with NSCLC respond to such therapy. The majority of those patients who responded to EGFR inhibition were found to have specific EGFR gene mutations, the presence of which significantly increased tumor sensitivity to EGFR-directed therapies. Treatment of NSCLC populations having EGFR mutations with EGFR inhibitor monotherapy is remarkably effective, with reported response rates of 55% and a median duration of control of metastatic disease of 9 months.

EML4-ALK Translocation

The EML4-ALK fusion oncogene has been identified in several cancers, specifically NSCLC, and less commonly anaplastic large cell lymphoma, inflammatory myofibroblastic tumors, and neuroblastomas. The presence of the fusion protein leads to ligand-independent activation of the ALK receptor tyrosine kinase and subsequent oncogenic transformation and cellular proliferation. EML4-ALK–positive NSCLC typically occurs in younger patients without a history of tobacco exposure and classically presents as an adenocarcinoma. It is estimated that the frequency of EML4-ALK–positive NSCLC ranges from 10% to 20% depending on the smoking history in the population. Early studies have suggested significant benefit from the use of an inhibitor specific for the EML4-ALK translocation, with response rates of >50% seen in pretreated metastatic patients.

Mutations in the Gene for KRAS

KRAS is a downstream target in the EGFR signaling cascade. The presence of mutations in the *KRAS* gene contributes important information for the selection of therapies in both colon and lung cancers. Approximately 30–40% of colon cancers have an activating *KRAS* mutation; the presence of such a mutation predicts a significantly lower likelihood of benefit from treatment with EGFR-targeting antibodies such as cetuximab and panitumumab. *KRAS* mutations occur in 10–30% of lung cancers and predict a diminished likelihood of response in patients treated with EGFR inhibitors.

Microsatellite Instability

Microsatellite instability (MSI), a pathologic footprint of defective DNA mismatch repair genes, occurs in 15–20% of colon cancers and can be detected by either immunohistochemical or PCR techniques. MSI has both prognostic and predictive value in that patients with MSI tend to experience less likelihood of disease recurrence but also appear to derive less benefit from 5-flourouracil (5-FU)-based chemotherapy programs. The presence of MSI can thus be utilized to optimize treatment for this subset of colon cancers.

Multiplex Genomic Analysis

In breast cancer, the use of multigene analyses has identified distinct tumor subgroups, including luminal A and B (typically hormone-receptor positive), HER2 positive, and basal-like (typically negative for both hormone receptors and HER2 ["triple negative"]). These classifications provide independent prognostic information corresponding to differential clinical outcomes. A more favorable prognosis is observed with luminal A breast tumors, and significantly inferior outcomes are observed in the basal-like subgroup.

Commercially available techniques evaluating smaller subsets of genes provide both prognostic and predictive information.

- Onco*type* DX® is an RT-PCR assessment of a 21-gene panel performed on paraffin-fixed tissue. The Onco*type* DX® result, called the Recurrence Score, provides a more precise estimate of the risk of recurrence in hormone-receptor–positive patients treated with standard endocrine therapy beyond that achieved with traditional anatomic and biological features. The Recurrence Score can also predict potential benefits from chemotherapy and help guide the selection of patients for adjuvant treatment. Scores are divided into three risk categories: low, intermediate, and high. Benefit from the addition of adjuvant cytotoxic chemotherapy to endocrine treatment appears to be limited to tumors that score in the high-risk range. The greatest benefit from the test lies in the ability to identify breast cancer patients with hormone-receptor–positive disease and with low or intermediate scores for whom limited benefit is to be expected from chemotherapy, and who can thus be spared exposure to the physical and economic costs of treatment. Guidelines from the National Comprehensive Cancer Network recommend the addition of Onco*type* DX® testing in the management of hormone-receptor–positive breast cancer.

- MammoPrint®, a similar test with regulatory approval in the United States, discriminates between tumors at low and high risk of recurrence through examination of a 70-gene profile; its clinical use is limited by the requirement for fresh tissue, as opposed to paraffin-embedded material.

TARGETED THERAPY

Targeted forms of treatment interact with a specific genetic site or protein that is unique to the cancer cell and on which cell survival and propagation are dependent. The development of targeted therapies has focused on identifying critical molecular sites within a cancer cell essential for tumor survival and growth, the classic "hallmarks of cancer." Creating a therapeutic strategy focusing directly on these sites may lead to cancer regression with minimal systemic toxicity. Two types of targeted therapy have been introduced: *monoclonal antibodies* that bind to unique protein receptors on the tumor cell surface, and *inhibitors of tyrosine kinases* within the cell itself that are essential for the signal transduction processes required for tumor cell growth. The monoclonal antibodies are administered intravenously, whereas the tyrosine kinase inhibitors are typically given orally. Toxicity profiles of these agents tend to be favorable when compared to chemotherapy, although specific dermatologic, cardiovascular, and immune effects may arise. Examples of monoclonal antibodies and tyrosine kinases, as well as their clinical indications, are shown in table 22.7.

Monoclonal Antibodies

Monoclonal antibodies have been developed to block ligand activation of tumor-specific cell surface proteins in patients

Table 22.7 COMMONLY USED TARGETED THERAPIES IN CLINICAL ONCOLOGY

AGENT	TARGET	DISEASE
Monoclonal Antibodies		
Trastuzumab	HER2	Breast cancer
Rituximab	CD-20	B-cell lymphoma
Cetuximab	EGFR	Colon cancer, head and neck cancer
Panitumumab	EGFR	Colon cancer
Bevacizumab	VEGF	Colon cancer, NSCLC, renal cell cancer, glioma
Alemtuzumab	CD-52	CLL
Tyrosine Kinase Inhibitors		
Imatinib	BCR-abl, c-kit	CML, GIST
Dasatinib	BCR-abl, c-kit	CML
Nilotinib	BCR-abl, c-kit	CML
Erlotinib	EGFR	NSCLC
Gefinitib	EGFR	NSCLC
Sunitinib	VEGFR, PDGFR, c-kit	Renal cell cancer, GIST
Sorafenib	VEGFR, PDGFR, Raf kinase, c-kit	HCC, renal cell cancer
Lapatinib	HER2, EGFR	Breast cancer
Motesanib	VEGFR, PDGFR, c-kit	Thyroid cancer

NOTE: Abbreviations: HER2, human epidermal growth factor receptor 2; EGFR, epidermal growth factor receptor; VEGF or VEGFR, vascular endothelial growth factor receptor; PDGFR, platelet-derived growth factor receptor; CML, chronic myelogenous leukemia; NSCLC, non-small cell lung cancer; GIST, gastrointestinal stromal cell tumor; CLL, chronic lymphocytic leukemia; HCC, hepatocellular carcinoma

with lymphoma (CD20, rituximab [Rituxan]), breast cancer (HER2, trastuzumab [Herceptin™]), and both colorectal and head and neck cancers (EGFR receptors, cetuximab [Erbitux™] and panitumimab [Vectibix™]). The anti-CD20 monoclonal antibody rituximab initially was proven to be effective in prolonging survival when administered with chemotherapy to patients with diffuse B-cell lymphomas, as demonstrated in figure 22.1, and subsequently has been shown to be beneficial in follicular lymphomas, chronic lymphocytic leukemia, and Waldenstrom macroglobulinemia. Rituximab also has an expanding role in management of such autoimmune disorders as rheumatoid arthritis and hemolytic anemias. The use of trastuzumab, a monoclonal antibody directed against the HER2 protein on the surface of breast cancer cells, has enhanced the efficacy of chemotherapy in patients with metastatic disease whose tumors overexpress HER2 and has significantly prolonged survival when administered with chemotherapy as adjuvant therapy (figure 22.2). Trastuzumab therapy is associated with a rare risk of cardiotoxicity and is typically not administered concomitantly with other cardiotoxic antineoplastic compounds, such as anthracyclines.

Bevacizumab (Avastin™) is a monoclonal antibody directed against the vascular endothelial growth factor (VEGF) receptor and is thought to act in large part through an anti-angiogenic mechanism, blocking the ability

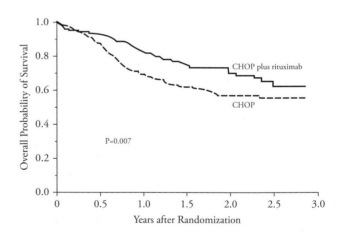

Figure 22.1. Chemotherapy for B-Cell Lymphoma. Overall survival among patients treated with chemotherapy alone versus chemotherapy plus rituximab for B-cell lymphoma. Kaplan-Meier plot describing overall survival for 399 patients (median age 69) with diffuse large B-cell lymphoma randomized to standard chemotherapy alone (CHOP: cyclophosphamide, doxorubicin, vincristine, prednisone) or with the addition of rituximab. The addition of rituximab resulted in a significant prolongation in overall survival ($p = 0.007$).
Source: Reprinted with permission from Coiffier B, Lepage E, Briere J, et al. CHOP chemotherapy plus rituximab compared with CHOP alone in elderly patients with diffuse large-B-cell lymphoma. N Engl J Med. 2002;346(4):235–42. Copyright © 2002 Massachusetts Medical Society. All rights reserved.

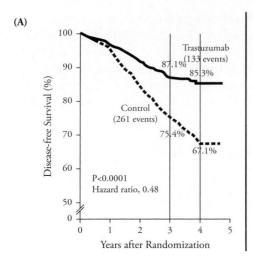

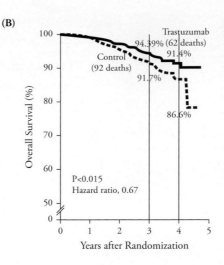

(A)

(B)

Figure 22.2. Trastuzumab Outcomes. Survival outcomes from the combined analysis of the North American Intergroup adjuvant trastuzumab trials. Progression-free (A) and overall survival (B) were improved with the addition of trastuzumab for 3351 women evaluated in the combined analysis of National Surgical Adjuvant Breast and Bowel Project trial B-31 and the North Central Cancer Treatment Group trial 9831. *Source*: Reprinted with permission from Romond EH, Perez EA, Bryant J, et al. Trastuzumab plus adjuvant chemotherapy for operable HER2-positive breast cancer. *N Engl J Med*. 2005;353(16):1673–84. Copyright © 2005 Massachusetts Medical Society. All rights reserved.

of tumors to elaborate new blood vessels essential for their survival. Bevacizumab has proven to be effective when administered alone in the treatment of renal cell cancer and when combined with chemotherapy in the management of advanced colorectal and lung cancers.

Tyrosine Kinase Inhibitors

The most dramatic example of the impact of targeted therapy has been imatinib mesylate (Gleevec™), a tyrosine kinase inhibitor that has proven to be amazingly effective through different molecular mechanisms in the management of chronic myelogenous leukemia (CML) by inhibiting the bcr-abl gene, gastrointestinal stromal cell tumors (GIST) by blocking c-kit gene function, and the hypereosinophilic syndrome through inhibition of the platelet-derived growth factor.

Chronic myelogenous leukemia is characterized by a balanced translocation between chromosomes 9 and 22 (i.e.,

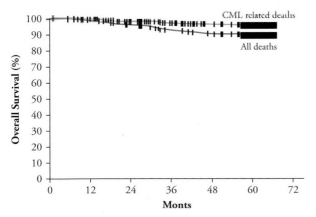

Figure 22.3. Imatinib Outcomes in CML. Overall survival among patients treated with imatinib as initial therapy for chronic phase of chronic myelogenous leukemia (CML). Overall survival at 5 years for 553 patients treated with imatinib demonstrates an overall survival rate of 89%, improving to 95% with censoring of non-CML-related deaths. *Source*: Reprinted with permission from Druker BJ, Guilhot F, O'Brien SG, et al. Five-year follow-up of patients receiving imatinib for chronic myeloid leukemia. N Engl J Med. 2006;355(23):2408–17. Copyright © 2006 Massachusetts Medical Society. All rights reserved.

the Philadelphia chromosome) in which the *ABL* oncogene from chromosome 9 adheres at the "break cluster region" (*BCR*) site on chromosome 22 to create the novel *BCR-ABL* fusion gene. This *BCR-ABL* gene product utilizes a specific tyrosine kinase to stimulate the production of a unique "fusion" protein, which has been shown to be instrumental in the pathogenesis of CML. Imatinib mesylate precisely blocks the action of the *BCR-ABL* tyrosine kinase, thereby targeting the specific molecular cause of CML. CML usually progresses from a chronic, myeloproliferative phase to an accelerated or leukemic phase that is highly resistant to therapy within 4 years after the time of diagnosis, leading shortly thereafter to death. Allogeneic bone marrow transplantation performed early during the chronic phase had been thought to be the only curative treatment for this hematologic malignancy. The use of imatinib mesylate as the only form of treatment in close to 500 newly diagnosed patients with CML who participated in a pivotal prospective clinical trial demonstrated a remarkable 5-year survival likelihood of 90%, as demonstrated in figure 22.3.

Imatinib mesylate is also effective in the management of GIST, a rare cancer arising in the abdomen which is resistant to cytotoxic chemotherapy and is characterized by mutations in the c-kit gene. Imatinib mesylate had been shown in the laboratory to arrest the growth of GIST cells and to induce apoptosis. When given to patients with GIST, imatinib mesylate therapy results in a PET scan–documented reduction in metabolic activity in tumor tissue (as well as a marked reduction in symptoms) within days to weeks (figure 22.4) and substantial improvement in overall survival compared to historic controls. This survival benefit has been achieved in many patients without objective shrinkage of measurable tumor masses, suggesting that the inhibition of the c-kit gene does not necessarily lead to cell death but rather to a reduction in proliferative capacity, making the tumor quiescent and prolonging patient survival.

Approximately 40–60% of melanomas have an activating mutation in the gene for the protein kinase B-RAF, leading to constitutive activation and stimulation of cancer cell

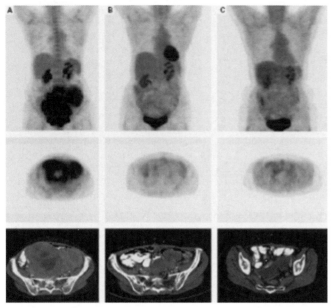

Figure 22.4. Imatinib Outcomes in GIST. Effect of imatinib on a pelvic gastrointestinal stromal cell tumor (GIST). Serial position emission scans obtained in a patient with a GIST tumor at baseline (A), after 1 month of imatinib (B), and after 16 months of continuous imatinib treatment (C). Images include a two-dimensional PET image (top), an axial PET image at the level of the pelvic tumor (middle), and a CT scan image corresponding to the same level (bottom).
Source: Reprinted with permission from Demetri GD, von Mehren M, Blanke CD, et al. Efficacy and safety of imatinib mesylate in advanced gastrointestinal stromal tumors. *N Engl J Med*. 2002;347(7):472–80. Copyright © 2002 Massachusetts Medical Society. All rights reserved.

growth. Inhibitors of B-RAF have been developed and are under study in advanced melanoma. One agent, PLX4032, specifically inhibits B-RAF activation related to the V600E mutation. In a large phase 1 trial, patients with a V600E mutation treated at the target drug dose had a response rate of 81%, a remarkable finding in an otherwise refractory disease.

Multiple other tyrosine kinase inhibitors are in development targeting a wide range of biological targets, including EGFR, EML4-ALK, HER2, VEGFR, and many others.

ADDITONAL READING

Bevers TB, Anderson BO, Bonaccio E, et al.; National Comprehensive Cancer Network. NCCN clinical practice guidelines in oncology: Breast cancer screening and diagnosis. *J Natl Compr Cancer Netw.* 2009;7(10):1060–96.

Burstein HJ, Prestrud AA, Seidenfeld J, et al.; American Society of Clinical Oncology. American Society of Clinical Oncology clinical practice guideline: Update on adjuvant endocrine therapy for women with hormone receptor-positive breast cancer. *J Clin Oncol.* 2010;28(23):3784–96.

Cunningham D, Atkin W, Lenz HJ, et al. Colorectal cancer. *Lancet.* 2010;375(9719):1030–47.

Drews RE, Shulman LN. Update in hematology and oncology. *Ann Intern Med.* 2010;152(10):655–62.

Ettinger DS, Akerley W, Bepler G, et al.; NCCN Non-Small Cell Lung Cancer Panel Members. Non-small cell lung cancer. *J Natl Compr Cancer Netw.* 2010;8(7):740–801.

Jiang Y, Ajani JA. Multidisciplinary management of gastric cancer. *Curr Opin Gastroenterol.* 2010;26(6):640–6.

National Comprehensive Cancer Network. *Clinical Practice Guideline in Oncology: Breast Cancer.* 2.2011.http://www.nccn.org/professionals/physician_gls/pdf/breast.pdf

Smith RA, Cokkinides V, Brooks D, Saslow D, Brawley OW. Cancer screening in the United States, 2010: A review of current American Cancer Society guidelines and issues in cancer screening. *CA.* 2010;60(2):99–119.

U.S. Preventive Services Task Force. Screening for breast cancer: U.S. Preventive Services Task Force recommendation statement. *Ann Intern Med.* 2009;151(10):716–26, W-236. Erratum *Ann Intern Med.* 2010;152(10):688. *Ann Intern Med.* 2010;152(3):199–200.

SECTION 3

RHEUMATOLOGY

23.

RHEUMATOID ARTHRITIS

Derrick J. Todd and Jonathan S. Coblyn

Rheumatoid arthritis (RA) is an idiopathic systemic autoimmune disorder that primarily involves the joints. It causes inflammation of the synovium (synovitis) that can lead to cartilage destruction and bone erosions. Extra-articular manifestations may also occur. The diagnosis of RA is based on a combination of clinical features, laboratory tests, and imaging studies. In recent years, great strides have been made in the pharmacologic treatment of RA, which consists primarily of immunosuppressive or immunomodulatory therapy with disease-modifying antirheumatic drugs (DMARDs). It is important to understand that RA is a heterogeneous disorder: some patients may have a severe, rapidly progressive disease with life-threatening extra-articular symptoms, whereas other patients may have indolent symptoms with little if any joint destruction over time. This point is important when making a diagnosis of RA, and especially when considering treatment options.

EPIDEMIOLOGY

RA is present in approximately 0.5–1% of the U.S. adult population and afflicts patients of all genders, ages, and races. Women are affected three to four times more frequently than men, and peak incidence occurs at 25–50 years of age. Patients of northern European ancestry are at increased risk for RA, in part because the identified genetic loci associated with disease are more common in this population. According to 1994 statistics, direct costs of RA care accounted for $4–5 billion in the United States for health care and indirect costs but approach $20 billion annually because of lost wages and productivity.

The risk of developing RA is influenced by both genetic and environmental factors. The strongest genetic risk is conferred by the "shared epitope" found in close association with the class II major histocompatibility complex (MHC) gene, human leukocyte antigen (HLA) DR4 (specifically DRB1*0401 and DRB1*0404). Other gene associations have been identified, but the odds ratio for these are small. Cigarette smoking is one environmental factor clearly associated with the development of RA. The risk of other environmental factors, such as stress and infection, is less clear.

PATHOLOGY AND PATHOGENESIS

The characteristic pathologic lesion in RA is proliferative synovitis in which the normally lace-like synovium is infiltrated by inflammatory cells to form inflammation and, with time, a thickened "pannus." The cellular infiltrate is comprised mostly of chronic inflammatory cells such as lymphocytes, macrophages, and plasma cells. Over time, pannus invades and destroys cartilage and eventually leads to bone erosions. Similar synovial proliferation can also be found in other synovial tissues, such as the lining of tendons and bursae, which explains why patients with RA can also experience inflammatory tenosynovitis.

The molecular and cellular processes leading to autoimmunity in human RA have yet to be fully established. Animal models of RA, including collagen-induced arthritis, have shed some light on the pathogenesis of synovitis. Cellular components of both innate and acquired immunity appear to contribute, as do tissue-resident synovial fibroblasts and lining cells. In years past, autoimmunity in RA was thought to be mediated by interferon-γ–secreting Th1 T helper cells. However, recent studies have discovered an alternative T helper cell population that may actually drive the autoimmunity in RA. These cells, termed Th17 cells, secrete the proinflammatory cytokine interleukin-17 (IL-17). Additional contributions to autoimmunity may come from effector T-cell populations, B cells, tissue-resident macrophages, dendritic cells, and mast cells. These cells secrete proinflammatory cytokines (e.g., IL-1, IL-6, and TNF-α) and chemokines to fuel inflammation. Infiltrating cells also produce collagenases and metalloproteinases to cause cartilage destruction and, eventually, bone erosion.

DIAGNOSIS

RA can cause irreversible joint damage. It is imperative to make a timely diagnosis in order to initiate DMARD therapy, ideally within the first 3 months of disease onset. However, there is no single test or study that can be used exclusively to diagnose RA. Rather, a combination of factors, including presenting symptoms, physical findings, laboratory data, and imaging studies, need to be considered. Table 23.1 lists the stringent 1987 American College of Rheumatology (ACR) classification criteria for the diagnosis of RA. Patients meeting these criteria almost certainly have RA.

In 2010, new RA classification criteria were published, representing the culmination of a collaborative multinational effort between the ACR and European League Against Rheumatism (table 23.2). These new criteria stress the presence of inflammatory arthritis and de-emphasize late changes of RA (e.g., erosions and rheumatoid nodules). Thus, they permit an earlier diagnosis of RA, allowing for earlier aggressive DMARD therapy in an effort to preserve joint structure and function. It should be emphasized that, strictly speaking, classification criteria are designed for the purposes of clinical research studies and not for day-to-day office practice; some patients with RA may not meet established criteria.

CLINICAL MANIFESTATIONS OF RA

RA most commonly presents as a symmetric inflammatory arthritis of the small joints of the upper and lower extremities. The presentation may be of an acute polyarthritis but it can also present as an indolent process. Patients with RA experience painful, swollen, red joints, usually with a morning stiffness that exceeds 30 minutes upon awakening and improves with physical activity. Tendons and bursae may also be involved because the lining of these structures is similar to synovial tissue. Tenosynovitis in the wrist can cause median nerve impingement and carpal tunnel syndrome (CTS), which manifests as numbness and paresthesia of the volar surface of the first through third fingers. An analogous process can occur in the ankle to cause tarsal tunnel syndrome.

The distribution of involved joints is useful in the differential of polyarthritis. RA can affect almost any joint in the body, often in a symmetric fashion but not exclusively so. Hands, wrists, and feet are most commonly involved, whereas the lumbar spine is rarely if ever affected. In the hands, RA tends to affect the proximal interphalangeal (PIP) joints, metacarpal intraphalangeal (MCP) joints, and wrists. It typically spares the distal interphalangeal (DIP) joints. Low back or DIP disease suggests a condition other than RA, such as osteoarthritis (OA) or spondylarthritis (SpA). In less than 10% of patients with RA, arthritis may manifest as a chronic, sterile, inflammatory monoarthritis. Table 23.3 lists the differential diagnosis of RA. The other inflammatory disorders that need to be distinguished from RA include psoriatic arthritis, microcrystalline disorders (e.g., gout and pseudogout), and polymyalgia rheumatica.

Hallmarks of RA upon physical examination include the presence of erythema, warmth, and swelling of the involved joints. Chronic RA can lead to specific deformities in the hand, such as wrist fusion and the classic swan neck and boutonniere deformities that occur upon joint subluxation at the MCPs and PIPs. The symptoms of CTS can be reproduced by forced flexion of the wrist (Phalen's sign) or by sharply percussing the volar wrist (Tinel's sign). Focal posterior knee swelling, calf swelling, or a dependent ecchymosis in the ankle may be indicative of a Baker's cyst (or rupture), which can occur in patients with RA and large knee effusions. Notably, patients may misinterpret their disability as weakness, which can confound the diagnostic workup. Hoarseness and odynophagia can indicate cricoarytenoid arthritis, which can cause laryngeal obstruction in patients following extubation.

LABORATORY TESTING

No single laboratory test can be used to diagnose RA in the absence of clinical findings. Laboratory studies are used to support the diagnosis of RA in a patient with suggestive symptoms, to monitor RA disease activity, and to rule out other possible causes of arthritis.

Serum rheumatoid factor (RF) testing provides some assistance in the diagnostic workup of patients with polyarthritis, as approximately 80% of patients with RA

Table 23.1 AMERICAN COLLEGE OF RHEUMATOLOGY 1987 CLASSIFICATION CRITERIA FOR RHEUMATOID ARTHRITIS

1. Morning stiffness >1 hour duration

2. Soft-tissue swelling or fluid in three or more joints simultaneously

3. Swelling involving wrists, MCPs, or PIPs

4. Symmetric arthritis

5. Rheumatoid nodules

6. Elevated rheumatoid factor

7. Radiographic erosion in the hand or wrist

   Must meet four of seven criteria.

   Criteria 1–4 must be present for >6 weeks

   Criteria 2–4 must be witnessed by a physician

   Exclude other diagnoses as deemed appropriate

NOTES: MCPs, metacarpal phalangeal joints; PIPs, proximal interphalangeal joints
SOURCE: Reprinted with permission from Arnett FC, Edworthy SM, Bloch DA, et al. The American Rheumatism Association 1987 revised criteria for the classification of rheumatoid arthritis. *Arthritis Rheum.* 1988;31:315–24.

Table 23.2 NEW 2010 AMERICAN COLLEGE OF RHEUMATOLOGY/EUROPEAN LEAGUE AGAINST RHEUMATISM CLASSIFICATION CRITERIA FOR RHEUMATOID ARTHRITIS

DESCRIPTOR	SCORE
Who should be tested? Patients with definite clinical synovitis of at least one joint not better explained by another disease process. Score-based algorithm: add scores of A-D; a score of ≥6/10 is needed for classification of a patient as having definite RA.	
A. Joint involvement (use highest applicable category)	
1 large joint	0
2–10 large joints	1
1–3 small joints (with or without large joint involvement)	2
4–10 small joints (with or without large joint involvement)	3
>10 joints (at least 1 small joint)	5
B. Serology (high-positive: ≥3× upper limit normal for the test)	
Negative RF and negative ACPA	0
Low-positive RF or low-positive ACPA	2
High-positive RF or high-positive ACPA	3
C. Acute-phase reactants	
Normal CRP and ESR	0
Abnormally elevated CRP or ESR	1
D. Duration of symptoms	
<6 weeks	0
≥6 weeks	1

NOTES: ACPA, anticitrullinated peptide antibodies; CRP, C-reactive protein; ESR, erythrocyte sedimentation rate; RA, rheumatoid arthritis.
SOURCE: Reproduced from Aletaha D, Neogi T, Silman AJ, et al. 2010 Rheumatoid arthritis classification criteria: an American College of Rheumatology/European League against Rheumatism collaborative initiative. *Ann Rheum Dis.* 2010;69:1580–8, with permission from BMJ Publishing Group, Ltd.

have RF detectable in the serum (termed "seropositive"). The remaining 20% of RA patients never develop detectable RF levels (termed "seronegative"), and thus, *the absence of RF does not rule out the presence of RA.* Routine RF analysis tests for IgM antibodies that have specificity directed against the constant (Fc) region of other antibodies. Many other medical conditions can cause an elevated RF (table 23.4), thereby limiting the test's specificity and utility.

More recently, RA has been associated with the presence of anti–citrullinated peptide antibodies (ACPAs), a subset of which are the more commonly termed anti-cyclic citrullinated peptide (anti-CCP) antibodies. Like RF, these ACPAs are present in the serum of 70–80% of patients with RA. When they are present, the specificity of ACPAs in RA approaches 95%. Importantly, ACPAs are rarely found in the conditions listed in table 23.4. Thus, a diagnosis of RA in a patient with ACPAs can be made with greater certainty. As with RF, 20–30% of patients with RA will never develop ACPAs, so the absence of these antibodies again does not rule out the presence of RA.

It is unclear whether RF complexes or ACPAs play a directly pathogenic role in RA. Seropositive RA patients tend to have more aggressive disease and greater numbers of extra-articular manifestations than do seronegative patients. However, serum RF and ACPA levels do not correlate with disease activity and, therefore, cannot be used to monitor

Table 23.3 DIFFERENTIAL DIAGNOSIS OF RHEUMATOID ARTHRITIS

Polymyalgia rheumatica
Other connective tissue disorders
    Systemic lupus erythematosus
    Sjögren syndrome
    Mixed connective tissue disease
    Polymyositis/dermatomyositis

Spondylarthritis disorders
    Psoriatic arthritis
    Reactive arthritis
    IBD-associated arthropathy
    Ankylosing spondylitis

Microcrystalline arthritis
    Gouty arthritis
    Pseudorheumatoid CPPD disease

Infectious arthritis
    Septic bacterial arthritis
    Viral arthritis
    Mycobacterium tuberculosis arthritis
    Lyme arthritis

Osteoarthritis
Vasculitis
Sarcoid arthritis

NOTES: CPPD, calcium pyrophosphate dihydrate; IBD, inflammatory bowel disease.

Table 23.4 CONDITIONS ASSOCIATED WITH AN ELEVATED SERUM RHEUMATOID FACTOR

Rheumatoid arthritis
Other connective tissue disorders
   Sjögren syndrome
   Systemic lupus erythematosus

Type II cryoglobulinemia (chronic viral hepatitis C)

Chronic bacterial infection
   Subacute bacterial endocarditis
   Osteomyelitis
   Leprosy

Malignancies and lymphoproliferative disorders
Elderly patients
Variant of normal

response to therapy. Instead, this is accomplished by measuring nonspecific markers of systemic inflammation, such as the erythrocyte sedimentation rate (ESR) and C-reactive protein (CRP). Improvement in these markers suggests an overall decrease in RA disease activity. Additional nonspecific markers of inflammation include a peripheral blood leukocytosis, thrombocytosis, anemia of chronic disease, and elevated acute-phase proteins (e.g., ferritin, haptoglobin, and complements).

Arthrocentesis of synovial fluid is used to rule out other potential causes of arthritis such as septic arthritis or microcrystalline diseases (e.g., gout and pseudogout). Synovial fluid analysis is also the most important way to differentiate inflammatory disorders from mechanical disorders such as OA. Rheumatoid synovial fluid is inflammatory, with white blood cell (WBC) counts typically ranging >1500–2000 WBC/mm³. One can feel assured that the condition is not inflammatory if the cell count is <1500 WBC/mm³, and infection should be considered if the cell count is >50,000 WBC/mm³. Neutrophils are often a dominant cell type in RA synovial fluid, but they rarely comprise >90% of WBCs. Although it is rarely done, synovial biopsy may be carried out to confirm inflammatory features or rule out atypical crystal disease, occult infection, or malignancy in clinically appropriate situations.

MUSCULOSKELETAL IMAGING

Similar to laboratory tests, imaging studies aid in the diagnostic workup of RA and can be used to monitor disease progression. Plain film radiographs have been the staple of imaging for decades, although other techniques have an ever-increasing role.

The plain film radiographic changes of RA tend to follow a uniform sequence of events, with the pace of radiographic progression depending primarily on severity and duration of disease activity. The earliest radiographic findings are periarticular soft tissue swelling and osteopenia. These are followed by joint space narrowing and marginal erosions. Joint ankylosis (fusion) can occur after long-standing inflammatory damage. Interestingly, seropositive patients are more likely to develop joint erosions. Effective DMARD therapy slows radiographic joint progression.

Magnetic resonance imaging (MRI), computed tomography (CT) scan, ultrasound, and bone scan are all imaging techniques that can provide additional anatomic definition in patients with RA. MRI allows visualization of preradiographic erosions, bone marrow edema, soft tissue swelling, synovitis, and tenosynovitis with much greater sensitivity than plain film radiography. Gadolinium-containing contrast agents are often used to enhance MR quality. These can be given intravascularly or intra-articularly (MR arthrogram) for definition of intra-articular structures such as ligaments and menisci. CT scan is most useful in the assessment of boney structures, especially when MRI may be contraindicated. Musculoskeletal power Doppler ultrasound has an emerging role in identifying bone erosions and synovitis. Bone scan is a fading technology that still has limited diagnostic utility in the patient with polyarthralgias but few objective findings of RA.

SPECIAL CONSIDERATIONS

RA involvement of the cervical spine deserves special mention because of its potentially devastating consequences if unrecognized. The articulation between C1 and C2 is a synovial joint and, thus, can be affected by synovitis. Patients need not have long-standing RA to have cervical spine disease. They may not complain of neck pain but may instead present with neurologic symptoms and signs to suggest a myelopathy. Paresthesias or weakness in a RA patient with brisk reflexes, clonus, or upgoing toes on Babinski's maneuver should prompt an immediate assessment for cervical spine disease. Flexion and extension films of the cervical spine are the most useful and readily available initial imaging study. CT scan and MRI provide additional anatomic definition of the neck. Consultation with a spine surgeon is warranted for any patient with evidence of C1–C2 instability because fusion may be required to avoid damage to the spinal cord or brainstem.

Although RA primarily afflicts the joints, extra-articular manifestations can occur. These processes can affect almost any organ or tissue in the body and are listed in table 23.5. Constitutional symptoms of fatigue and malaise occur commonly, whereas fever, anorexia, and weight loss are less frequently present. Pulmonary and hematologic complications deserve special mention. Pulmonary complications include pleural effusions whose hallmark is a strikingly low pleural fluid glucose. The effusion is often exudative, making the differentiation between RA and empyema of importance. The hematologic complications include anemia of chronic disease, thrombocytosis, and leukopenia associated with Felty syndrome or large granular lymphocyte (LGL) syndrome.

Table 23.5 EXTRA-ARTICULAR MANIFESTATIONS OF RHEUMATOID ARTHRITIS (DOES NOT INCLUDE POTENTIAL MEDICATION TOXICITIES)

INVOLVEMENT	POSSIBLE MANIFESTATIONS
Systemic	Constitutional symptoms Rheumatoid nodules (skin, tendons, and lungs commonly) Vasculitis (skin, kidneys, and peripheral nerves) Secondary amyloidosis (heart and kidneys)
Pulmonary	Pleural effusion Interstitial lung disease Bronchiectasis BOOP Pulmonary artery hypertension
Cardiovascular	Raynaud phenomenon Pericardial effusion Increased cardiovascular disease risk
Neurological	Compressive neuropathies (carpal tunnel syndrome) Myelopathy (cervical spine disease) Mononeuritis multiplex (rheumatoid vasculitis)
Hematologic	Generalized lymphadenopathy Felty and LGL syndromes Macrophage activation syndrome Increased lymphoma risk
Cutaneous	Petechiae and purpura (rheumatoid vasculitis) Pyoderma gangrenosum
Salivary/lacrimal Ocular	Keratoconjunctivitis sicca Episcleritis Scleritis Scleromalacia perforans Corneal ulceration Uveitis (JRA patients)
Overlap syndromes	Systemic lupus erythematosus Sjögren syndrome Polymyositis/dermatomyositis Scleroderma Mixed connective tissue disease

NOTES: BOOP, bronchiolitis obliterans, organizing pneumonia; JRA, juvenile rheumatoid arthritis; LGL, large granular lymphocyte.

Other extra-articular manifestations tend to occur in patients with clinically apparent arthritis, and a disproportionate number of patients are "seropositive" for RF or ACPAs. In addition, there is growing evidence that patients with RA are at increased risk of developing cardiovascular disease and lymphomas. It remains to be proven whether aggressive control of RA activity normalizes these risks.

Finally, it is worth emphasizing that patients with RA are at particular risk for septic arthritis, usually via hematogenous seeding of the joint. Contributing factors include a hypervascular synovium, the abnormal joint surface itself, any iatrogenic immunosuppression from DMARDs, and the possible presence of prosthetic joints. Septic arthritis should be strongly considered in the RA patient who presents with one joint swelling vastly out of proportion to the others. In this setting, arthrocentesis is warranted to assess for septic arthritis.

TREATMENT

The last 10–15 years have witnessed tremendous strides in the pharmacologic treatment of RA (table 23.6). Although corticosteroids and nonsteroidal anti-inflammatory drugs (NSAIDs) continue to play important roles in symptomatic relief of RA, the advent of DMARDs has radically changed patient long-term outcomes. Small-molecule DMARDs, such as methotrexate, are orally bioavailable, whereas biological DMARDs, such as antagonists of tumor necrosis factor-α (TNF-α), are administered parenterally. The goals of DMARD therapy are to interrupt the inflammatory process, to reduce pain, to improve function, to slow radiographic joint destruction, and to restore a patient's overall quality of life. Most DMARDs act by suppressing or modulating the immune system to dampen synovitis. Accordingly, one potentially serious side effect of many DMARDs is the increased risk of infection by common bacterial organisms and also opportunistic pathogens. Finally, nonpharmacologic interventions continue to be important for the treatment of RA as well. These include patient education, physical therapy, occupational therapy, assist devices, lifestyle modifications, and orthopedic surgery. Surgery is indicated in patients with destructive changes in a joint associated with refractory pain and functional disability.

TRADITIONAL PHARMACOTHERAPY

Aspirin, acetaminophen, other NSAIDs, corticosteroids, and opiate analgesics have been used to treat RA for decades. These drugs, especially corticosteroids, remain effective in reducing the joint symptoms of RA. However, except for steroids, they have little if any disease-modifying activity and carry potentially serious risks with chronic usage, especially at high doses. High-dose ASA (3–4 g/day) or NSAID therapy is associated with a very high risk of gastrointestinal (GI) hemorrhage from peptic ulcer disease as well as worsening of any pre-existing renal impairment. Cyclo-oxygenase (COX-2) inhibitors are presumably safer if the patient does not concomitantly use aspirin. In addition, emerging research has associated some and perhaps all NSAIDs with increased risk of cardiovascular events.

Relatively low doses of systemic corticosteroids (<15 mg prednisone daily) can control the synovitis of RA in most patients. Some studies have suggested low-dose daily corticosteroids may even have DMARD activity. However, chronic corticosteroid usage even at low doses is associated

Table 23.6 LIST OF PHARMACOLOGIC AGENTS COMMONLY USED FOR THE TREATMENT OF RHEUMATOID ARTHRITIS

AGENT OR DRUG CLASS	MECHANISM OF ACTION	COMMON OR SERIOUS ADVERSE EFFECTS
NSAIDs	Inhibit PG synthesis	Peptic ulcer disease Renal impairment Hepatotoxicity Cardiovascular risk
Corticosteroids	Immunosuppressant	Immunosuppression Hypertension Diabetes mellitus Weight gain Cushingoid habitus Osteoporosis Cataracts Avascular necrosis
Methotrexate	Inhibits DHFR Increases extracellular adenosine	Nausea, diarrhea Rash, alopecia Immunosuppression Hepatotoxicity Bone marrow toxicity Pulmonary hypersensitivity Teratogenic
Leflunomide	Inhibits DHOD	Similar to MTX but includes weight loss and excludes pulmonary hypersensitivity
Azathioprine	Purine antagonist	Nausea, diarrhea Immunosuppression Hepatotoxicity Bone marrow toxicity Pancreatitis
Sulfasalazine		Nausea, diarrhea Rash Hepatotoxicity Bone marrow toxicity Azospermia
Hydroxychloroquine		Retina pigmentation Myopathy Neuropathy
Gold		Nausea, diarrhea Rash, chrysiasis Proteinuria
TNF-α antagonist	Inhibits TNF-α	Immunosuppression Drug induced lupus Demyelination? Cancer?
Anakinra	Soluble IL1RA	Immunosuppression Injection reaction
Abatacept	Blocks T-cell costimulation	Immunosuppression
Rituximab	B-cell depletion	Immunosuppression Infusion reaction Serum sickness
Tocilizumab	IL6 receptor blocker	Immunosuppression Dyslipidemia Transaminitis Cytopenias Infusion reaction

NOTES: DHFR, dihydrofolate reductase; DHOD, dihydroorotate dehydrogenase; IL1RA, interleukin-1 receptor antagonist; MTX, methotrexate; NSAIDs, nonsteroidal anti-inflammatory drugs; PG, prostaglandin; TNF, tumor necrosis factor with many side effects: hypertension, diabetes mellitus, weight gain, cushingoid habitus, osteoporosis, avascular necrosis of bone, cataracts, and, perhaps most importantly, worsened cardiovascular outcomes. Intra-articular injections remain a suitable modality for the delivery of directed corticosteroids in a patient with only one or two persistently swollen joints.

With modern DMARD options, opiate analgesics play only a limited role in the control of RA pain. They are best reserved for patients who have contraindications to all other DMARDs, have postoperative joint pain, or have end-stage "bone-on-bone" secondary osteoarthritis as a complication of RA.

SMALL-MOLECULE DMARDs

There are many orally available small-molecule DMARDs that have been used to treat RA, sometimes with great effectiveness. The antimetabolite drugs methotrexate, leflunomide, and, to a lesser extent, azathioprine remain effective options and an anchor for any treatment regimen. Sulfasalazine and hydroxychloroquine are less potent but relatively safe DMARDs, making them good options for those with mild disease. Many other therapies have fallen out of favor because of ineffectiveness or excessive toxicity. These agents include gold salts, cyclophosphamide, cyclosporine, and D-penicillamine. Minocycline is rarely used as a DMARD and may take up to 1 year to be effective.

Methotrexate, the most commonly used DMARD in the treatment of RA, is a folic acid analogue that inhibits dihydrofolate reductase (DHFR), the enzyme that synthesizes folic acid. At low doses, methotrexate may also raise extracellular adenosine levels, which may be the mechanism for its anti-inflammatory activity in RA. Methotrexate has been used for over 30 years to treat RA, and it remains highly effective and safe in patients who are monitored closely. Indeed, methotrexate remains at the foundation of most DMARD therapy regimens. The benefits of methotrexate cannot be overstated, and even patients on other oral DMARDs or biological agents can benefit from combination therapy with methotrexate.

When used to treat RA, methotrexate is administered only once weekly, in doses up to 25 mg weekly. The once-weekly dosing markedly limits the potentially severe hepatic and bone marrow toxicities that occur with daily dosing, which should be avoided. The active metabolite is excreted primarily by the kidneys, and moderately impaired renal function is a contraindication to its use. Daily folic acid or weekly leucovorin administration can limit the drug's hepatic and hematologic toxicity as well as the other common side effects of rash, alopecia, and GI intolerance. Subcutaneous administration is sometimes performed to improve bioavailability and GI tolerance of the drug.

Patients prescribed methotrexate should be monitored at least every 6–8 weeks for renal function, liver toxicity,

and bone marrow suppression. They should also be advised to restrict alcohol consumption because of enhanced hepatotoxicity. Allergic interstitial pneumonitis is a rare, idiosyncratic, but potentially life-threatening reaction to methotrexate that precludes a rechallenge. Pulmonary toxicity may occur at any time in the course of therapy but tends to occur in the first 1–2 years. It is characterized by fever, cough, dyspnea, eosinophilia, and chest infiltrates. Symptoms are difficult to distinguish from opportunistic pneumonia, so patients often require bronchoscopy and sometimes lung biopsy for diagnosis. Finally, methotrexate is a potent teratogen and an abortifacient at high doses. Men and women both should be advised of this and use appropriate contraception.

Leflunomide inhibits dihydroorotate dehydrogenase, the enzyme responsible for the rate-limiting step in pyrimidine metabolism. It shares many features in common with methotrexate with regard to efficacy and toxicity profile. It may be combined with methotrexate or used in combination with other DMARDs. Notably, leflunomide is administered daily as opposed to weekly, and folic acid supplementation is unnecessary. Its most common side effects include anorexia, diarrhea, and weight loss. Leflunomide can cause hepatic and bone marrow toxicity, rare pulmonary toxicity, and is highly teratogenic. Therefore, as with methotrexate, patients should receive regular laboratory analysis for toxicity and use contraception as appropriate. Importantly, leflunomide has a half-life of at least 2 weeks due to extensive enterohepatic recirculation of drug. For this reason, its use in patients of childbearing age must be carefully considered, and simply discontinuing the drug for acute toxicity or pregnancy is ineffective; enteric binding therapy with cholestyramine is recommended. Finally, leflunomide can cause significant idiopathic weight loss correctable only by discontinuation of the drug.

Sulfasalazine and hydroxychloroquine have only modest activity in RA. They are often used in combination with other DMARDs (or each other) in patients with low disease activity or in those too frail or ill to take more effective DMARDs. Sulfasalazine is a sulfa-class agent that is administered in doses up to 3 g daily, split over the course of the day. It can cause nausea, diarrhea, and rash commonly. More serious side effects include hepatotoxicity and idiosyncratic severe pancytopenia, the latter of which requires cessation of drug. Reversible azospermia can also occur. Hydroxychloroquine is normally well tolerated, but can cause nausea or diarrhea; toxicity is dose related. Patients should not receive more than 6.5 mg/kg per day because higher doses over extended periods of time can lead to myopathy and the most serious potential adverse reaction, retinal pigmentation that can cause irreversible blindness. Regular ophthalmologic examinations are prudent in these patients.

Emerging small-molecule DMARDs are in the therapeutic pipeline. Unlike biological agents, new small-molecule drugs have the advantage of being orally administered. Intracellular kinase inhibitors represent one of the more exciting classes of small-molecule DMARDs. These agents block intracellular signaling cascades and display remarkable efficacy and tolerability in clinical trials.

BIOLOGICAL DMARDs

The advent of biological agents in the last decade has revolutionized the treatment of RA. Although methotrexate is an effective therapy for many RA patients, many more RA patients continue to experience active synovitis despite combination small-molecule DMARD therapy. Our growing understanding of RA disease pathogenesis has led to several new biological DMARDs. Currently, nine of these agents have been approved for use in the United States, and they fall into five categories: five TNF-α antagonists (adalimumab, certolizumab, golimumab, etanercept, and infliximab); an IL-1 antagonist (anakinra); an inhibitor of T-cell costimulation (abatacept); a B-cell-depleting antibody (rituximab); and an IL-6 receptor antagonist (tocilizumab). Of these agents, the TNF-α antagonists have had the most extensive and proven track record in the treatment of RA. All biological agents are expensive, costing approximately $20,000 for 1 year of therapy.

All biological agents are immunosuppressive drugs that convey a significantly increased risk of bacterial infection and sepsis (1–3% per year). Vaccination against pneumococcus is prudent. In addition, opportunistic infections can occur. Most importantly, patients must be assessed for latent or active infection with *Mycobacterium tuberculosis* because fatal outcomes have been associated with this pathogen in patients receiving biological drugs. Patients on any of the biological agents should not receive live vaccines because of the risk of disseminated infection. There appears to be an increased risk of nonmelanoma skin cancers in these patients, but the risk of hematologic or solid-tumor cancers is unclear. Even prior to the emergence of biological DMARDs, patients with RA were found to have an increased risk for the development of lymphomas and some solid tumors compared to control patients without RA. A history of cancer or active malignancy will warrant special consideration prior to the initiation of biological therapy.

The TNF-α antagonists all inhibit the proinflammatory cytokine TNF-α, which is present in rheumatoid synovium. These agents all reduce signs and symptoms of RA, slow radiographic joint changes, and improve patients' physical function. A substantial number of patients treated with these agents will have significant suppression of disease activity. Combination therapy with methotrexate can potentiate the effectiveness of these agents. There are subtle differences in the molecules and their route of administration, but effectiveness is believed to be similar. Infliximab is a chimeric mouse and human anti-TNF-α monoclonal antibody administered by intravenous infusion. Adalimumab and golimumab are fully human anti-TNF-α monoclonal antibodies that are given by subcutaneous injection. Etanercept is a fusion protein of soluble TNF-α receptor and the constant region of the immunoglobulin heavy chain. It is administered by subcutaneous injection. Certolizumab is a polyethylene glycol–conjugated (PEGylated) anti-TNF-α Fab fragment, administered by subcutaneous injection. Patients who do not respond to or lose response to one agent may benefit from a trial of another drug from this same class.

Anti-TNF-α agents are remarkably well tolerated. The principal toxicity is immunosuppression, as discussed above. Infusion or injection reactions are rare and generally well tolerated. A reversible drug-induced lupus reaction has been described. There may be a risk for unmasking a propensity for demyelinating disorders such as multiple sclerosis (MS), especially in a patient with a personal or family history of MS. In addition these therapies should be suspended in the face of an active infection or class III–IV heart failure.

Anakinra is a recombinant soluble IL-1 receptor antagonist that blocks the proinflammatory cytokine IL-1. It is of only modest efficacy in RA. Further, patients often develop an urticarial reaction to the daily subcutaneous injection, which decreases tolerability. Anakinra is particularly useful in febrile adult Still disease and the cryopyrin-associated diseases such as Muckle-Wells syndrome.

Abatacept is a recombinant fusion protein of cytotoxic T-lymphocyte-associated antigen-4 (CTLA4) and the constant region of the immunoglobulin heavy chain. It acts to impair costimulation of T cells, which is required for optimal T-cell activation. It is administered by intravenous infusion and generally well tolerated. It may not be as potent an agent as the anti-TNF-α agents, but head-to-head trials are lacking.

Rituximab is a chimeric mouse and human anti-CD20 monoclonal antibody that leads to depletion of B cells. It is also administered by intravenous infusion and is generally well tolerated, although potentially severe infusion reactions and serum sickness have been described with rituximab.

Tocilizumab is a relatively new fully human anti-IL-6 receptor antibody administered by intravenous infusion. IL-6 is a proinflammatory cytokine that contributes to synovial inflammation and systemic features of RA. Patients exhibit responses similar to those in patients treated with anti-TNF-α agents. Unlike other biological drugs, tocilizumab is associated with dyslipidemia and commonly causes transaminitis and significant cytopenias, which may limit its use.

SUMMARY

Rheumatoid arthritis is one of the most common systemic autoimmune disorders and is characterized by joint inflammation, cartilage destruction, and bone erosion. Patients typically present with signs and symptoms of synovitis:

tender, red, swollen, warm joints with effusions and a preponderance of morning stiffness. RF assay, ACPA testing, and various imaging studies can aid in the diagnosis. ESR and CRP assist in the measurement of disease activity and response to drug therapy. Cervical symptoms, extra-articular involvement, and the possibility of concurrent septic arthritis are all special considerations. Many treatment options exist for the patient with RA, and great strides have been made in DMARD therapies. Methotrexate forms the foundation of therapy for most patients with RA. Biological agents are emerging therapies that target inflammatory cytokines, B cells, or T-cell costimulation. They have revolutionized the treatment of RA, and the goal of therapy should now be to arrest disease activity with the least toxic medication(s) available.

ADDITIONAL READING

Aletaha D, Neogi T, Silman AJ, et al. 2010 Rheumatoid Arthritis Classification Criteria. *Arthritis Rheum.* 2010;62(9):2569–81.

Firestein GS. Evolving concepts of rheumatoid arthritis. *Nature.* 2003;423(6937):356–61.

Firestein GS. Inhibiting inflammation in rheumatoid arthritis. *N Engl J Med.* 2006;354(1):80–2.

Huizinga TW, Pincus T. In the clinic. Rheumatoid arthritis. *Ann Intern Med.* 2010;153(1):ITC1-1–ITC1-15; quiz ITC1-16.

McInnes IB, O'Dell JR. State-of-the-art: Rheumatoid arthritis. *Ann Rheum Dis.* 2010;69(11):1898–906.

O'Dell JR. Therapeutic strategies for rheumatoid arthritis. *N Engl J Med.* 2004;350(25):2591–602.

Olsen NJ, Stein CM. New drugs for rheumatoid arthritis. *N Engl J Med.* 2004;350(21):2167–79.

Rindfleish JA, Muller D. Diagnosis and management of rheumatoid arthritis. *Am Fam Physician.* 2005;72(6):1037–47.

Scott DL, Wolfe F, Huizinga TW. Rheumatoid arthritis. *Lancet.* 2010;376(9746):1094–108.

QUESTIONS

QUESTION 1. A 58-year-old woman with long-standing RA presents to your office with 3 days of accelerating pain and swelling in her left knee. Her other joints are asymptomatic. She has had fatigue for 1 week but denies fevers, chills, or night sweats. The remainder of her review of systems is unremarkable. Her medical history is notable only for her RA and a prosthetic right hip. Her last flare of RA was 5 months ago and responded to treatment with corticosteroids. Her current medications include prednisone, 5 mg daily, methotrexate, 20 mg weekly, and etanercept, 50 mg weekly. She has a life-threatening allergy to penicillin. Examination reveals a generally well-appearing woman of average stature with an antalgic gait. Vital signs reveal a temperature 37.2°C, blood pressure 98/70, heart rate 110, and respiratory rate 14 breaths per minute. She has a slightly warm and markedly swollen left knee; it is only mildly tender to palpation. However, on either active or passive range

of motion, severe pain is elicited with flexion greater than 30° or near full extension. The remainder of her musculoskeletal examination reveals mild deformities from RA but is otherwise unremarkable.

Which of the following is the most appropriate measure to do next?

A. Increase steroid dose to prednisone, 60 mg daily.
B. Initiate intravenous vancomycin and levofloxacin.
C. Perform arthrocentesis of her left knee.
D. Arrange for interventional radiology to perform arthrocentesis of her right hip.
E. Check Lyme serology and initiate doxycycline.

QUESTION 2. An 82-year-old woman suffered a large right hemispheric stroke and has been admitted to a nursing home after a 2-week hospitalization that was otherwise uncomplicated. She had been previously healthy except for a recent diagnosis of RA made 3 months prior to the stroke. At the time of her stroke, her only medications were methotrexate, 17.5 mg (7 × 2.5 mg tablets) by mouth once weekly, and folic acid, 1 mg daily. While in the hospital, she had also been prescribed aspirin, 325 mg daily, atenolol, 25 mg daily, and atorvastatin, 20 mg nightly. Four weeks after being admitted to the nursing home, she developed intense nausea, vomiting, and diarrhea. Her abdominal exam is unrevealing, and she has guaiac-negative stool. She is given intravenous fluids, and laboratory testing reveals the following:

WBC: 0.3×10^3 cells per mm^3
Hematocrit: 25.5%
Platelet count: 70×10^3 cells per mm^3
MCV: 110 fL

Which of the following would most like reveal the cause of her blood count abnormalities?

A. Bone marrow aspirate and biopsy
B. Serum testing for antineutrophil and antiplatelet antibodies
C. Abdominal ultrasound to measure spleen size
D. Review of daily medication administration sheets
E. Colonoscopy

QUESTION 3. A 30-year-old woman with RA of 10 months' duration visits your office for a scheduled follow-up visit. She continues to have 2 hours of morning stiffness and multiple swollen and tender joints despite being on subcutaneous methotrexate, 25 mg weekly. She receives her methotrexate injections in your clinic and has tolerated the drug. She has had to go on disability from her job as a security guard because of persistent joint pains. Her medical history is otherwise unremarkable, and her only other medications are folic acid, 1 mg daily, and naproxen, 500 mg bid. You note that she has had a nonreactive PPD test within the past 12 months and is up to date with immunizations. Physical examination demonstrates erythema, warmth, and swelling at her wrists, knees, ankles, and all metacarpal phalangeal, and proximal interphalangeal joints. Laboratory analysis reveals ESR 90 mm/hr.

Which of the following is the most appropriate next measure?

A. Initiate subcutaneous etanercept, 50 mg once weekly
B. Perform arthrocentesis of her left knee and, if no signs of septic arthritis, then inject corticosteroids
C. Change naproxen to celecoxib, 200 mg daily, and see her in follow-up in 3 months
D. Check antinuclear antibody titer
E. Initiate prednisone, 40 mg daily

QUESTION 4. A 42-year-old Hispanic man presents with 3 months of bilateral pain and swelling in his knees, elbows, wrists, and six metacarpal phalangeal joints. He has had 2 hours of morning stiffness and been fatigued. He has been out of work in construction for 3 weeks because of symptoms. The review of systems is otherwise negative, and he has never had problems with joint pain before. Ibuprofen, 800 mg tid, has provided only minor relief. He takes no other medications and is otherwise healthy. He drinks 8–10 beers per day and has done so for many years. Physical examination demonstrates swelling and limited range of motion of involved joints. Knee effusions are present bilaterally. Arthrocentesis of the right knee reveals 30 mL of nonbloody fluid with 8000 WBC/mm³ and 72% PMNs. Gram stain and crystal analysis of the fluid are negative. Additional laboratory tests show WBC normal, hematocrit 35%, platelet count 650 × 10³ cells per mm³, RF negative, ACPA negative, ANA negative, uric acid 8.0 mg/dL, and ESR 76 mm/hr. Radiographic imaging demonstrates periarticular soft tissue swelling but no osteopenia, joint space narrowing, or marginal erosions.

Which of the following is the most likely diagnosis?

A. Rheumatoid arthritis
B. Polyarticular gouty arthritis
C. Osteoarthritis
D. Polymyalgia rheumatica
E. Septic arthritis from *Neisseria gonorrhea*

QUESTION 5. A 38-year-old woman presents with 2 months of fever, abdominal pain, weight loss, generalized achiness, and rash on her lower extremities. She has noticed dyspnea on exertion and a 10-lb weight gain in the past 2 weeks. She is otherwise asymptomatic. She takes no medications. Medical history is notable only for a motor vehicle accident as a teen for which she received multiple blood transfusions. She does not smoke, use illicit drugs, or drink alcohol excessively. Physical examination demonstrates a thin woman in no acute distress. Vital signs are within normal limits. Oxygen saturation is 93% on room air. She has innumerable 1- to 2-mm nonblanching nontender erythematous lesions on her feet and calves bilaterally with pitting lower extremity edema to her thighs. Her jugular venous pressure is 10 cm, and she has rales discernible at the bilateral lung bases. She has a nontender abdomen with no hepatosplenomegaly or masses. Rectal exam reveals guaiac-positive brown stool. Musculoskeletal examination is notable for periarticular tenderness but no erythema or swelling. Laboratory analysis shows:

BUN 75 mg/dL, creatinine 4.1 mg/dL, electrolytes normal

Albumin 2.8 g/dL; total bilirubin 3.1 mg/dL, direct bilirubin 2.1 mg/dL; AST, ALT, and alk phos normal

WBC 7.6 × 10³ cells/mm³, Hct 32.4%, platelets 60 × 10³ cells/mm³, INR 1.8, PTT 31 sec

Urinalysis: 3 + protein, 20–40 RBC per high-powered field with dysmorphic RBC and one RBC cast

ESR 55 mm/hr, RF 280 IU/mL (normal <10), ACPA negative, ANA negative

C3 110 mg/dL (normal 90–180), C4 2 mg/dL (normal 10–40)

Blood cultures show no growth after 48 hours (3 sets)

Which of the following is the most likely diagnosis?

A. Rheumatoid vasculitis
B. Cryoglobulinemic vasculitis
C. Bacterial endocarditis
D. Systemic lupus erythematosus
E. Hemochromatosis

ANSWERS

1. C
2. D
3. A
4. A
5. B

24.

ACUTE MONOARTICULAR ARTHRITIS

C. Ryan Antolini, Flavia V. Castelino, and Anthony M. Reginato

Acute monoarticular arthritis represents one of the few rheumatologic emergencies that internists, emergency room physicians, and rheumatologists will encounter in their clinical practice. The possibility of joint infection leading to the loss of joint function is a serious potential consequence in delayed diagnosis of a septic joint. Despite advances in diagnosis and treatment, the morbidity and mortality from septic arthritis remains high; therefore, timely recognition of an infected joint is imperative for a favorable outcome. The differential diagnosis of acute monoarticular arthritis is broad and includes septic arthritis, crystalline disorders, inflammatory disorders, and mechanical problems with the joint (table 24.1).

EVALUATION OF A PATIENT WITH ACUTE MONOARTICULAR ARTHRITIS

HISTORY AND PHYSICAL EXAM

Any acute inflammatory process that develops in a single joint over a few days (<2 weeks) is considered acute monoarticular arthritis. A careful history with emphasis on the chronology of symptoms may help in assessing the diagnosis of acute monoarticular arthritis. Historical features that should be sought include fever, rigors, recent sexual activity, gastrointestinal or genitourinary symptoms, recent illnesses, tick exposure, travel to an endemic area, past history of recurrent attacks, renal insufficiency, and a family history of gout or other arthritic conditions. Patients may note concurrent or pre-existing involvement of other joints. Special attention should be paid to patients with rheumatoid arthritis (RA) who present with one joint that is significantly more painful and swollen than the rest of the other affected joints and those with a prosthetic joint, as these groups represent a high risk for septic arthritis.

The physical examination should focus on determining whether the source of pain is in the true joint or periarticular soft-tissues such as tendon or bursae. Asking the patient to point to the exact site of tenderness may be helpful. The joint should carefully be examined for warmth, erythema, and a possible effusion. Intra-articular involvement causes restriction of active and passive range of motion. Stress pain, maximum pain at limits of joint motion, is characteristic of true arthritis. Patients with a septic or crystalline arthritis will be exquisitely tender on examination of the joint. Specific maneuvers should assist in distinguishing true inflammatory arthritis from soft-tissue periarthritis or pain syndromes such as medial epicondylitis, bicipital or rotator cuff tendinopathy, trochanteric bursitis, and prepatellar and anserine bursitis. Joint effusion may not be readily visible on physical exam. In the knee joint, the "bulge sign" can signal a small effusion. The physical examination should focus not only on inspection of the involved joint but on other joints, as well as signs of an underlying systemic disorder. Subclinical involvement of fewer than four joints (oligoarticular) or more (polyarticular) would away toward crystal arthritis or seronegative or seropositive RA rather than septic arthritis or portend a worst prognosis for a patient with polyarticular septic arthritis.

DIAGNOSTIC STUDIES

The diagnostic test for acute monoarticular arthritis is arthrocentesis of the affected joint for analysis of cell count, polarized microscopy, and culture of the synovial fluid. Diagnostic arthrocentesis is required in most patients presenting with a monoarthritis and a suspicion of infectious arthritis. Superimposed cellulitis is a relative contraindication to arthrocentesis. The procedure can safely be performed in patients who are anticoagulated (Coumadin) by using the smallest possible needle size. In some instances, as little as one or two drops of synovial fluid may be aspirated in an initially presumed "dry tap," with a priority placed in obtaining a Gram stain culture and crystal analysis.

Normal synovial fluid is colorless, and the gross appearance of the fluid can provide a clue to a possible

Table 24.1 ETIOLOGY OF ACUTE MONOARTICULAR ARTHRITIS

COMMON	LESS COMMON	RARE CAUSES
Infectious arthritis	Reactive arthritis	Foreign body synovitis
Bacteria	Juvenile rheumatoid arthritis	Amyloidosis
Lyme disease	Rheumatoid arthritis	Behçet syndrome
Fungi	Seronegative arthritis	Familial Mediterranean fever (FMF)
Mycobacteria	Bowel-disease-associated arthritis	Hypertrophic pulmonary
Viruses	Psoriatic arthritis	osteoarthropathy
Crystals	Bone malignancies	Intermittent hydrarthrosis
Monosodium urate (MSU)	Loose bodies	Pigmented villonodular synovitis
Calcium pyrophosphate dihydrate (CPPD)	Sarcoidosis	Relapsing polychondritis
Basic calcium phosphate (BCP)	Hemoglobinopathies	Adult onset Still disease (AOSD)
Calcium oxalate (CaOx)		Synovial tumors
Internal derangement		Synovial metastasis
Trauma/overuse		
Hemarthrosis		
Osteoarthritis		
Osteomyelitis		

noninflammatory versus inflammatory joint process as shown in figure 24.1. Synovial fluid that is cloudy or purulent represents an inflammatory joint effusion. The presence of a bloody synovial effusion may represent a traumatic injury.

Analysis of the cell count of synovial fluid will give more information about an inflammatory versus noninflammatory effusion and the likelihood of a septic joint (table 24.2). Noninflammatory effusions have a white blood cell (WBC) count <2000 per cubic millimeter. An inflammatory synovial effusion will have a leukocyte count over 2000. WBC counts over 100,000 are generally associated with a septic arthritis until proved otherwise but can be seen with a variety of inflammatory disorders (i.e., gout, pseudogout, RA, and other inflammatory arthritis). Conversely, lower cell counts can be seen in patients with septic arthritis, especially with chronic atypical infections such as *Mycobacterium* or with partially treated infections. Although the cell count is useful in determining whether or not an effusion is inflammatory, a Gram stain and culture are required in all patients in whom a septic arthritis is suspected.

IMAGING STUDIES

Radiographs are of initial value if significant trauma or focal bone pain is present to exclude fracture, tumor, or osteomyelitis. However, they play no role in the initial distinction between acute crystal-induced or septic arthritis. Radiographs may confirm the presence of a joint effusion in joints where effusions are difficult to ascertain by physical exam (i.e., elbow, ankle, and hip). The presence of tophaceous erosions, chondrocalcinosis, and joint space narrowing does not exclude the possibility of infection as an etiology of acute monoarthritis. Musculoskeletal ultrasound may provide a simple technique to assess small effusion and aspiration of the affected joint. Computed tomography (CT) scans should be reserved to detect effusions and needle placement for joint aspirations of

difficult to assess joints such as the hip, sacroiliac (SI), or sternoclavicular joints. Magnetic resonance imaging (MRI) demonstrates adjacent soft tissue edema or abscess and may be helpful in detecting septic sacroiliitis.

SYNOVIAL BIOPSY AND ARTHROSCOPY

Needle biopsy of the synovial membrane under ultrasound or biopsy obtained during arthroscopy is seldom performed as initial evaluation of monoarticular arthritis. In rare instances, synovial biopsy may assist in the diagnosis of refractory monoarthritis such as seen with atypical infections agents such as tuberculosis or fungal infections, infiltrative diseases such as amyloidosis, sarcoidosis, pigmented villonodular synovitis, or intra-articular tumors.

DIFFERENTIAL DIAGNOSIS

Acute monoarthritis can have many causes (table 24.1), but crystals, trauma, and infection are most common. Prompt diagnosis of joint infection is critical because of its destructive nature, with a suggestive algorithm for evaluation of patients who present with acute monoarticular arthritis as outlined in figure 24.2. The crystal-induced arthritides are the most important forms of acute arthritis that are difficult to differentiate from acute monoarticular septic arthritis on clinical exam. Any form of chronic inflammatory joint disease such as a reactive arthritis (ReA), psoriatic arthritis (PsA), spondyloarthropathy (SpA), and arthritis associated with inflammatory bowel disease (IBD) can present with a swollen joint that simulates septic arthritis. Most patients with these conditions have extra-articular manifestations of their disease such as recent genitourinary or gastrointestinal symptoms, conjunctivitis or uveitis, enthesopathy, skin or mucous membrane lesions with a predilection for lower back pain, and stiffness or sacroiliac joint involvement. Another rheumatic disease that is important to

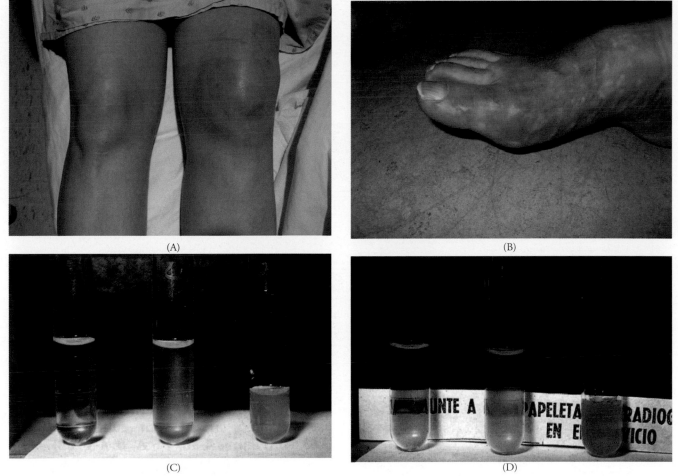

Figure 24.1. Joint Effusion and Gross Synovial Fluid Appearance from Diagnostic Arthrocentesis. (A) Right knee effusion, (B) First MTP synovitis, (C) Appearance of synovial fluid from monoarticular arthrocentesis: 1. Normal transparent synovial fluid. 2. Turbid inflammatory synovial fluid. 3. Opaque, nontransparent inflammatory pyogenic synovial fluid. (D) Opacity of synovial fluid from arthrocentesis: 1. Normal transparent synovial fluid. 2. Turbid inflammatory synovial fluid. 3. Opaque, nontransparent inflammatory pyogenic synovial fluid.

differentiate from septic arthritis is RA. Although the clinical presentation of RA is a symmetric, chronic polyarticular joint disorder, some patients may present with an acute or subacute exacerbation of one or few of their joints. One-third of the patients with RA may present with monoarticular arthritis as their initial presentation. They may present with a pseudo–septic arthritis picture including an explosive synovitis with marked synovial fluid leukocytosis; therefore, Gram stain and culture of synovial fluid are essential when evaluating new onset of synovitis in these patients. Other mimickers of septic arthritis include subacute bacterial endocarditis and any periarticular inflammation.

Table 24.2 SYNOVIAL FLUID AND ASSOCIATED CONDITIONS

NONINFLAMMATORY: <2000 WBC/MM³ (2 × 10⁹ PER L)	INFLAMMATORY: >2000 WBC/MM³ (2 × 10⁹ PER L)
Trauma	Septic arthritis
Osteoarthritis	Crystal-induced monoarthritis
Avascular necrosis (AVN)	Monosodium urate (MSU)
Charcot arthropathy	Calcium pyrophosphate dihydrate (CPPD)
Hemochromatosis	Basic calcium phosphate (BCP)
Pigmented villonodular synovitis	Calcium oxalate (CaOx)
	Rheumatoid arthritis (RA)
	Psoriatic arthritis (PsA)
	Spondyloarthropathy (SpA)
	Systemic lupus erythematosus (SLE)
	Juvenile rheumatoid arthritis (JRA)
	Lyme disease

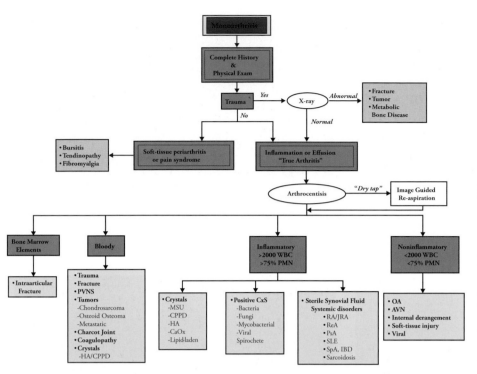

Figure 24.2. Algorithm for Evaluation of Patients with Monoarticular Arthritis. (WBCs: white blood cells; PMNs: polymorphonuclear neutrophils; HA: hydroxyapatite; CPPD: calcium pyrophosphate dihydrate; MSU: monosodium urate; CaOx: calcium oxalate; RA: rheumatoid arthritis; JRA: juvenile rheumatoid arthritis; ReA: reactive arthritis: SLE: systemic lupus erythematosus; SpA: spondyloarthropathy; IBD: inflammatory bowel disease; PsA: psoriatic arthritis; OA: osteoarthritis; and AVN: avascular necrosis).

SEPTIC ARTHRITIS

Normal, diseased, and prosthetic joints are all vulnerable to bacterial infection (table 24.3). Acute bacterial arthritis remains a medical emergency with significant morbidity and mortality even when proper antibiotic therapy is instituted; therefore, timely recognition is imperative for a favorable outcome. There are two peaks of incidence that seem to be age-dependent: one under the age of 15 and the other over the age of 55 years. The mortality rates in adults ranges from 10% to >50%. More than 30% of patients will be left with some irreversible residual joint damage. As with any monoarticular arthritis, a thorough history remains a key element in diagnosing septic arthritis.

PATHOGENESIS

The synovium is highly vascular and contains no limiting basement membrane, promoting easy access of blood contents to the synovial space. Most acute septic arthritis results from seeding of the joint through four possible entry routes: most commonly through hematogenous or contiguous spread of the organism and sometimes by penetrating trauma or, rarely, by iatrogenic joint injection. Any infection that affects the skin, soft tissues, or mucous membranes (respiratory, gastrointestinal, or genitourinary tracts) can seed a joint through the bloodstream. Localized infections from an adjacent focus can also spread contiguously into the joint space. Direct inoculation can occur with any penetrating trauma or any procedural invasion of the joint space, such as with an arthrocentesis or arthroscopy. Once the bacteria enter the closed joint space, they

Table 24.3 THE INFECTING BACTERIA IN NORMAL, DISEASED, AND PROSTHETIC JOINTS

Gram-positive cocci	*Staphylococci: aureus, epidermis* *Streptococci: pyogenes* (beta-hemolytic group A), other beta-hemolytic groups (esp B,G), *pneumoniae*, viridans group
Gram-negative cocci	*Neisseria gonorrhoeae* *Neisseria meningitides* Other: *Moraxella, Kingella, Branhamella*
Gram-positive bacilli	*Corynebacterium pyogenes* *Listeria monocytogenes*
Gram-negative bacilli	*Brucella* species *Campylobacter* species *Chryseobacterium meningosepticum* *E. coli* *H. influenzae* *K. kingae* *Klebsiella pneumonia* *Pasteurella multocida* *Proteus mirabilis* *Pseudomonas aeruginosa* *Salmonella* species *Serratia marcescens*
Anaerobes	*Bacteroides fragilis* *Clostridium* species *Fusobacterium necrophorum* *Peptococcus* and *Peptostreptococcus* species
Spirochetes	*Borrelia burgdorferi* *Treponema pallidum*
Mycoplasma	*Mycoplasma hominis* *Mycoplasma pneumoniae* *Ureaplasma urealyticum*

Table 24.4 PREDISPOSING FACTORS IN BACTERIAL ARTHRITIS

AGE	LOCAL FACTORS	SYSTEMIC FACTORS

Newborns and elderly old age	Direct joint trauma
	Recent joint surgery
	Open reduction fractures
	Arthroscopy
	Pre-existing joint disease: rheumatoid arthritis, crystal disease, osteoarthritis, hemophiliac arthropathy
	Prosthetic joint
		Rheumatoid arthritis
		Diabetes mellitus
		Psoriasis
		Comorbidities: cancer, diabetes, chronic renal failure, chronic liver disease
		Concomitant infection, e.g., skin
		Malignancies
		IVDA, alcoholism
		Hemodialysis
		Hemophilia
		Immunosuppression
		    Congenital: hypogammaglobulinemia, complement deficiency
		    Acquired: AIDS, organ transplantation, immunosuppressant medication (steroids, anti-TNF-α)

can trigger an acute inflammatory response within a few hours. The synovial membrane reacts with proliferative hyperplasia and an influx of acute and chronic inflammatory cells, creating the characteristic acute purulent joint inflammation. In a few days, the inflammatory cells release various cytokines and proteases, leading to cartilage damage, inhibition of cartilage synthesis, irreversible bone loss, and joint damage.

MICROBIOLOGY

Septic joint effusions may be due to bacteria, mycobacteria, or fungi. The most common etiology for joint infection is the Gram-positive cocci—either staphylococci or streptococci. *Staphylococcus aureus* is the most frequent cause in joint infection, including both native and prosthetic joints, although *Staphylococcus epidermidis* occurs more commonly in prosthetic joints. Gram-negative bacilli are seen in 5–20% of patients and usually occur in elderly adults, those with comorbidities, and intravenous drug abusers. Anaerobic organisms rarely cause septic arthritis; however, they can be seen in any penetrating trauma. *Neisseria gonorrhoeae* is the most common sexually transmitted organism causing infectious arthritis, and although it used to be a common cause for infectious arthritis in the 1970s and 1980s, the incidence has now decreased significantly.

RISK FACTORS

Experimental evidence suggests that normal joints are very resistant to infection compared with diseased or prosthetic joints. Systemic, local, and social factors are important risk factors that contribute to the risk of developing bacteremias and reduce the body's capacity to eliminate organisms from the joint (table 24.4). Systemic disorders affect the host's response through an impaired immune system. Local factors, such as damage to a specific joint from earlier trauma, recent joint surgery, or arthroscopy, and the presence of a prosthetic joint are important predisposing factors for septic arthritis. Social factors include occupational exposure to animals (e.g., brucellosis), exposure to tuberculosis, mass emigration from endemic areas of the world, and factors that lead to an immunocompromised state (AIDS, intravenous drug abuse [IVDA] homelessness, therapeutic noncompliance, and emergence of drug-resistant mycobacteria). In some cases, the risk factors are compounded by medications (e.g., patients with RA or inflammatory arthritis treated with immunosuppressant, anti-tumor necrosis factor-α [TNF-α] therapy, and steroids). Furthermore, it may also be difficult to distinguish an infectious etiology in patients receiving immunosuppressive therapy. The causes of increased risk factors for mortality in septic arthritis include age >65, mental status changes at presentation, multiple joint involvement, and systemic symptoms (suggesting a higher bacterial load).

CLINICAL FEATURES

The acute onset of monoarticular pain with increasing severity, tenderness, heat, and swelling is the classical presentation for septic arthritis. Although septic arthritis is most often monoarticular, polyarticular septic arthritis occurs in 15% of cases, usually with asymmetric involvement of three or four joints. The larger joints are more commonly involved, with the knee reported in more than 60% of cases. Hip infections are common in younger children. The hip may be held in a flexed and externally rotated position, and there is extreme pain on hip motion. It is often difficult to detect an effusion of the shoulder or the hip, although the joint is frequently warm and tender. The SI joint is involved in 10% of infections. These joints are difficult to evaluate by physical exam and may require imaging studies such as radiographs, CT scan, or MRI. Polyarticular septic arthritis is most likely to occur in patients with RA, systemic connective tissue disease, or in patients with overwhelming sepsis. Gonococcal and meningococcal infections present most commonly with migratory polyarticular arthritis.

Fewer than 50% of patients with gonococcal arthritis present with a purulent joint infection of the knee or wrist. The most common extra-articular manifestations of gonococcal arthritis include fever, tenosynovitis, and dermatitis with a characteristic erythematous papular or petechial rash; however, these features are seen in the disseminated form.

DIAGNOSTIC WORKUP

The key to the diagnosis of septic arthritis is the identification of bacteria in the synovial fluid by Gram stain or culture, thus making arthrocentesis the cornerstone for diagnosing septic arthritis. As previously stated, the synovial fluid is sent for cell count with differential, Gram stain, and culture. If the white blood cell count is extremely high (usually > 100,000), a presumed diagnosis of septic arthritis is made until cultures come back positive. However, cell counts can also range from 50,000 to 100,000 in patients with septic arthritis; therefore, Gram stain and cultures are imperative. Gram stains are positive only 60–80% of the time. For patients in whom gonococcal arthritis is suspected, the yield of culture can be higher if plated of chocolate agar or Thayer-Martin media are inoculated with synovial fluid. If there is a specific history of tuberculosis exposure or endemic exposure to Lyme disease or fungal organisms, then the appropriate cultures need to be ordered. Other laboratory studies such as peripheral WBC count can be normal in 30% of patients, and an elevated erythrocyte sedimentation rate (ESR) and/or C-reactive protein (CRP) may be nonspecific. In children, an elevated ESR and/or CRP may be more helpful in patients with possible septic monoarthritis of the hips. Blood cultures are positive in about half of the patients with nongonococcal septic arthritis and should be obtained in any patient with suspected bacterial arthritis. Negative cultures may occur in those who have received recent antimicrobial therapy or those who are infected with fastidious organisms, such as *Mycoplasma* or streptococci. The coexistence of crystal-induced arthritis and bacterial infection must not be overlooked, and a wet preparation for examination under compensated polarized light microscopy is an essential test in evaluating monoarticular arthritis due to crystal deposition diseases.

THERAPY

Immediate treatment with empirical antibiotic therapy (once arthrocentesis is complete) along with removal of any purulent material from the joint space is the mainstay of therapy. A typical antibiotic regimen is based on risk factors and shown in table 24.5. Once culture results and susceptibilities are available, the antibiotic therapy can then be modified; duration of therapy is usually 4 weeks or longer, and daily aspiration or lavage (arthroscopy or surgical drainage) results in removal of inflammatory products and yields a better outcome.

Table 24.5 EMPIRICAL ANTIBIOTIC TREATMENTS FOR SEPTIC ARTHRITIS

RISK FACTORS	ANTIBIOTIC SELECTION
No risk factors	Nafcillin or oxacillin, 2 g IV q4h
Risk for Gram-negative organisms	Ceftriaxone, 2 g IV q24h, or cefotaxime, 2 g IV q8h; if *Pseudomonas* is a concern, then cefepime, 2 g IV q12h
Methicillin-resistant *Staphylococcus aureus* (MRSA)	Vancomycin, 1 g IV q12h, or clindamycin, 900 mg IV q8h, or linezolid, 600 mg IV q12h
Suspected gonococcal or meningococcal infection	Ceftriaxone, 2 g IV q24h, or cefotaxime, 2 g IV q8h

LYME DISEASE

Lyme disease results from a tick-transmitted infection by the spirochete *Borrelia burgdorferi*. Patients with Lyme disease may present with an acute or chronic monoarthritis, especially of the knee. Early symptoms include erythema chronicum migrans, transient polyarthralgias with viral-like symptoms, and symptoms of aseptic meningitis. Chronic persistent synovitis develops in 20% of patients with untreated Lyme diseases. Monoarthritis occurs during the late infectious stage of Lyme disease or as an autoimmune arthritis or antibiotic-refractory arthritis with persistent joint swelling despite 2–3 months of oral or intravenous antibiotics in some patients.

VIRAL

Viral arthritis has also been associated with acute monoarthritis. Most viral arthritides present with an acute polyarthritis, fever, characteristic rash (parvovirus, hepatitis B and C, rubella) and are often associated with a pseudorheumatoid joint distribution. However, varicella zoster virus, cytomegalovirus, herpes simplex type 1, and HIV have been associated with monoarthritis or oligoarthritis. HIV infections may be associated with a wide variety of rheumatic disorders including reactive arthritis, psoriatic arthritis, vasculitis, and Sjögren syndrome. A subacute monoarthritis or oligoarthritis that mimics infection or gout has been described in HIV patients. HIV is an important risk factor for infectious arthritis including atypical bacterial as well as gonococcal and mycobacterial arthritis.

MYCOBACTERIAL AND FUNGAL

Mycobacterial and fungal arthritides both present with an insidious onset, have an indolent course, and create diagnostic difficulties because of lack of clinical findings. Joint swelling is marked, but signs of acute joint inflammation are absent or mild.

Osteoarticular involvement occurs in 1–5% of individuals with tuberculosis. Osseous infection occurs during hematogenous spread, either with primary infection or after late reactivation. Tuberculous arthritis affects mainly the hips, knees, and other joints with characteristic radiographic features including juxta-articular osteoporosis, marginal erosions, and gradual joint space narrowing (Phemister's triad). Additional findings include soft-tissue swelling, subchondral cysts, bony sclerosis, periostitis, and calcification. Synovial cultures are positive in 80–90% of tuberculous arthritis, and culture of synovial tissue in 94%. Caseating and noncaseating granulomas are present in 90% of synovial biopsies. Atypical mycobacterial monoarthritis, especially with *M marinum, M. Kansasii, or M. avium intracellulare,* show predominance of arthritis and tendinitis of the hands and wrist. *M. marinum* is acquired through exposure to fresh water, salt water, or marine life (fish tanks, swimming pools). Monoarticular involvement of the metacarpophalangeal and proximal interphalangeal joints is most frequently reported and is often only mildly painful without systemic symptoms. Patients with *M. marinum* and other atypical mycobacterial monoarthritides can test positive for PPD for *M. tuberculosis.*

Fungal arthritis may present as a self-limiting acute polyarthritis in the normal host with recent exposure to fungal infection. The chronic monoarthritis is seen primarily in immunocompromised hosts. When present, associated fungal skin lesions are a clue to diagnosis. Fungal arthritis occurs by direct inoculation or hematogenous spread in IVDA, critically ill hospitalized patients with indwelling lines, immunosuppressed patients, or patients with prosthetic joints, or via cutaneous inoculation by plant material, for example, with rose thorns. *Candida* infection causes a monoarthritis, whereas other fungal infections may cause an oligoarthritis in addition to monoarthritis. Other fungal etiologies such as coccidioidomycosis, sporotrichosis, blastomycosis, cryptococcosis, and histoplasmosis can cause arthritis (monoarthritis involving the knee or oligoarthritis), and their presentation is related to their geographic distribution, occupational exposure, and skin and lung involvement. Staining and culture of synovial fluid are critical for the diagnosis. Therapy for mycobacterial and fungal arthritis usually consists of appropriate pharmacologic and surgical debridement.

GONOCOCCAL ARTHRITIS

The most common complication from acute gonorrhea is disseminated gonococcal infection (DGI). Gonococcal arthritis mainly affects young adults, with a threefold higher incidence in women. It results from dissemination of *Neisseria gonorrhoeae* in the bloodstream from primary sexual contact. In patients younger than 30 years old, it is the most common cause of septic arthritis. Disseminated gonococcal infection can present as either an arthritis-dermatitis syndrome (more commonly) or as a localized septic arthritis. The disseminated infection is usually associated with the classic triad of dermatitis (papules, pustules with an erythematous base), tenosynovitis, and a migratory asymmetric polyarthritis. The recommended initial treatment is with 1 g/day of parenteral ceftriaxone for 24–48 hours followed by oral cefixime or ciprofloxacin to complete a 7- to 10-day course.

CRYSTAL-INDUCED MONOARTICULAR ARTHRITIS

A variety of crystal disorders can lead to acute and chronic inflammatory arthritides. Calcium-containing crystals such as basic calcium phosphate (BC), hydroxyapatite (HA), calcium pyrophosphate dihydrate (CPPD), calcium oxalate (CaOx), and monosodium urate (MSU) are deposited around the joint and soft tissue, leading to bursitis, tenosynovitis, synovitis, and acute monoarthritis. Their clinical presentations are often similar, requiring diagnostic arthrocentesis with examination of synovial fluid for crystals under compensated polarized light microscopy and sometimes the additional use of special stains for their identification (figure 24.3).

GOUT

The most common crystal-induced arthritis is gout. The underlying etiology in gout is MSU crystal deposition secondary to hyperuricemia. Patients initially develop acute attacks most commonly involving the lower extremities below the knee. Over time, these attacks become more frequent and occur on a background of chronic joint pain. Eventually, patients progress toward the formation of chronic tophaceous deposits.

EPIDEMIOLOGY AND RISK FACTORS

The epidemiology of gout has changed over time. Recent evidence shows an increasing incidence and prevalence of gout over the past two decades. A recent report of U.S. medical database claims showed an increase in gout prevalence from 2.9/1000 in 1990 to 5.2/1000 in 1999. Gout occurs more frequently in men than women due to the uricosuric effect of estrogen. It is very rare for a premenopausal woman to present with an attack of gout.

The main risk factor for the development of gout is hyperuricemia. Approximately 90% of hyperuricemic patients have underexcretion of uric acid as the underlying disorder due to renal insufficiency. Besides renal impairment, other risk factors for gout include alcohol consumption,

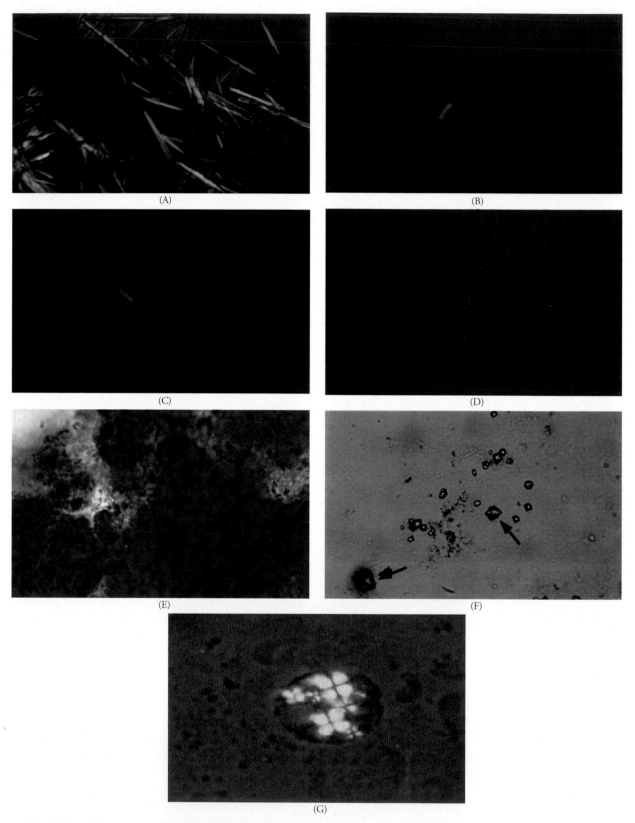

Figure 24.3. Morphology under Compensated Polarized Light Microscopy and Special Stain of Crystal-Associated Arthritis. A. Neddle-shaped MSU crystal with intense negative birefringent as seen under compensated polarized light microscopy; 400×. B. Rectangular, rhomboid shape CPPD crystal with weakly positive birefringent crystal when the crystal is parallel to the axis of compensator (arrow) adopts a blue color under compensated polarized light microscopy; 400×. C. CPPD crystal is rotated perpendicular to the axis of the compensator; it adopts a yellow color under compensated polarized light microscopy; 400×. D. HA and BCP crystals present with amorphic features and show no birefringence under compensated polarized microscopy; 400×. E. Alizarin red stain of HA staining orange-red color (400×). F. Bipyramidal and small polymorphic and small polymorphic CaOx crystals (ordinary light microscopy; 400×). G. Intracellular-cytoplasmic spherules with a birefringent Maltese cross-like appearance. *Negative birefringence—yellow when parallel to direction of the light (arrow), and blue when perpendicular. Positive birefringence—blue when is parallel to direction of the light (arrow), and yellow when perpendicular.*

the metabolic syndrome, hypertension, and diuretic use. Additionally, the consumption of meat and seafood can increase the purine load in patients and lead to an increase in serum uric acid (sUA) levels.

CLINICAL PRESENTATIONS

The clinical presentation of gout occurs in stages: asymptomatic hyperuricemia, acute intermittent gout, and chronic tophaceous gout. Initially, patients will have asymptomatic hyperuricemia for several years. Patients will then present with the sudden onset of an acute, painful, swollen joint. The joint will be warm, erythematous, and extremely painful to palpation or movement. Often, patients will have an acute development of pain that wakes them from sleep or is apparent when they first arise in the morning. The first acute attack will generally be monoarticular with a predilection for the big toe (podagra). Other commonly involved joints in acute attacks include the ankle, midfoot, and knee. Atypically, patients will present with the involvement of a joint in the finger, wrist, elbow, or bursa. There may be more than one joint involved in the early-phase acute attacks, but it is uncommon to have more than three joints involved in an early presentation. Women tend to have more atypical presentations and will present more often with the involvement of gout in the hand or wrist. These acute attacks generally resolve spontaneously within 7 to 14 days. In this acute intermittent state, attacks may occur infrequently and be separated by years. Over time and with increasing hyperuricemia, these attacks become more frequent and involve more joints with longer duration of attacks.

If left untreated, patients will go on to develop chronic tophaceous gout. Patients often develop a background of chronic pain from gout with superimposed acute, painful attacks. Patients may develop polyarticular arthritis at this stage. Tophi may or may not be apparent on clinical examination and can occur anywhere on the body, in particular at areas of pressure points. Clinically apparent tophi are found most commonly on the pinnae, olecranon bursa, at sites of nodal osteoarthritis (i.e., Heberden nodes), and Achilles tendon. Tophi can lead to bony destruction and chronic bone deformities, which at times may resemble RA.

DIAGNOSTIC WORKUP

The gold standard procedure for diagnosis of gout involves aspiration of the involved joint and visualization of MSU crystals under compensated polarized light microscopy. In addition, patients should have evaluation of their sUA levels. The solubility of uric acid is 6.7 mg/dL, and any level above this should be considered hyperuricemia. However, an elevated uric acid alone can only help in making a presumptive and not definitive diagnosis of gout. Serum uric acid level may drop and be within normal range during an acute flare of the gout. Other helpful laboratory evaluation should include a Gram stain and culture, as there can be coexistence of gout and septic arthritis, and assessment of renal function. Urinary quantification of uric acid excretion is only necessary in patients who are being considered for treatment with uricosuric agents (probenecid, sulfinpyrazone, or benzbromarone).

TREATMENT

The treatment of gout can be broken up into two separate management strategies: treatment of acute attacks and long-term management of hyperuricemia. For acute gouty attacks, treatment should be directed at pain relief and reduction of inflammation. First-line therapy for these attacks should be nonsteroidal anti-inflammatory drug (NSAID) therapy. The classic agent prescribed has been indomethacin, but any NSAID agent should improve pain and inflammation. In patients with contraindications to NSAID therapy, other options include colchicine or prednisone. Colcrys (colchicine) is another alternative therapy that interrupts the response of neutrophils by inhibiting neutrophil chemotaxis, activating the inflammasome, and producing IL-β in response to MSU crystals. The new recommendations for the treatment of gout flare consist of two tablets of Colcrys (1.2 mg) at the first sign of gout flare followed by one tablet (0.6 mg) 1 hour later for total dose of 1.8 mg/day during the acute flare followed by 0.6 mg once or twice a day for prophylaxis. The low-dose Colcrys was as effective as high-dose Colcrys but offers a greater margin of tolrability and safety than the high-dose Colcrys (1.2 mg followed by 0.6 mg every hour for 6 hours, a 4.8-mg total) in treating the acute gout flares. The use of Colcrys, 0.6 mg PO twice a day in conjunction with a serum uric acid–lowering agent is recommended during the first 6 months as gout prophylaxis to prevent mobilization flares while achieving the sUA target of <6.0 mg/dL with antihyperuricemic agents. Colcrys is contraindicated in patients with renal and hepatic impairment who are concurrently prescribed P-gp inhibitors or strong inhibitors of CYP3A4, as life-threatening and fatal toxicity has been reported. Dose adjustment of Colcrys may be required when it is coadministered with P-gp or CYP3A4 inhibitors. The most common adverse effects of colchicine include gastrointestinal symptoms and, rarely, myelosuppression, thrombocytopenia, leucopenia, and a myopathy that is characterized by an elevated creatine kinase (CK) level and proximal muscle weakness.

The first component of the long-term management of gout is mainly lifestyle changes, especially weight loss; avoiding fructose-rich soft drinks and diets with excess purines, such as meats and shellfish; and limiting alcohol consumption, particularly beer. Both essential hypertension and diuretic use are independently associated with hyperuricemia and gout. Given the benefits of thiazide diuretics in patients with hypertension and their low cost, we suggest switching to another antihypertensive drug to control the hypertension. Losartan has uricosuric effects and may be a good alternative agent, although in patients already taking a uric acid–lowering agent, the benefits are likely to be minimal. We recommend the use of uric acid–lowering agents in patients with history of frequent and disabling attacks of gouty arthritis, clinical or radiographic signs of chronic gout joint disease, tophi, otherwise unexplained renal insufficiency, recurrent nephrolithiasis, or urinary uric acid excretion >1100 mg/day.

Allopurinol and febuxostat are the only readily available xanthine oxidase inhibitors. In contrast to probenecid, which is primarily indicated in patients who have impaired renal excretion of uric acid, xanthine oxidase inhibitors are effective in virtually all circumstances warranting urate-lowering therapy for gout. The starting dose of allopurinol for patients with normal renal function should be 300 mg daily. In patients with chronic renal insufficiency, a starting dose of 100 mg daily may be more appropriate in patients with weight-adjusted creatinine clearance >40 mL/min and titrate the dose according to the antihyperuricemic effect achieved. The half-life of oxypurinol, an active metabolite of allopurinol, is prolonged in renal functional impairment, so caution is recommended during allopurinol up-titration with careful observation for adverse effects. In either setting, patients should be titrated to reach a uric acid level of <6 mg/dL. In certain individuals, doses of up to 800 mg and 900 mg daily are safe and may be required to reach serum uric acid level of <6 mg/dL. Once initiated, therapy with allopurinol should not be interrupted for any reason to avoid precipitation of an acute attack of gout. This includes patients who have a flare of gout while on allopurinol, as any adjustments to their normal allopurinol dosage can worsen a flare. Low-dose colchicine should be started 2 weeks prior to initiation of serum uric acid–lowering agent (0.6 mg twice a day for patients with normal renal and hepatic function) to prevent mobilization flares. A nonsteroidal antinflammatory drug may be used as an alternative option. We suggest that colchicine be continued for 6 months for prophylaxis after normal serum uric acid have been obtained in patients without tophi. Although the duration of prophylactic therapy is uncertain in patients with tophi, we suggest continuing colchicine until resolution of the tophi or until it becomes obvious that the tophaceous deposits will not resolve despite persistent normouricemia.

The most common adverse effects of allopurinol are minor abdominal pain, nausea, or vomiting. However, a very uncommon but potentially life-threatening reaction can occur with allopurinol. Patients should be counseled to immediately discontinue therapy if they develop a rash to allopurinol. Severe hypersensitivity reactions to allopurinol may involve rash, fever, acute interstitial nephritis, and hepatitis. Fatal accounts of Stevens-Johnson syndrome have been reported. For patients who are intolerant to allopurinol or develop a hypersensitivity reaction, other agents such as febuxostat or probenecid may be employed. Febuxostat is a thiazolecarboxylic acid derivative that, unlike allopurinol, is a non-purine-selective inhibitor of xanthine oxidase; it is administered orally and undergoes hepatic metabolism. Febuxostat given at 40 mg/day is the recommended starting dose; if a serum uric acid level of <6.0 mg/dL is not achieved after 2 weeks, the dose is increased to 80 mg/day. Febuxostat, 80 mg/day, was superior to allopurinol, 300 mg/day, in reducing serum uric acid levels to lower than 6 mg/dL in mildly to moderately renally impaired study participants. Mobilization flares were very common, and mild transaminase elevations greater than three times the normal limit were observed in the febuxostat group. The major clinical niche for febuxostat is patients for whom uricosuric therapy is contraindicated or ineffective when they are also intolerant of, or allergic to, allopurinol, and/or with mild to moderate chronic kidney disease.

Uricosuric agents (probenecid, sulfinpyrazone, and benzbromarone) represent another class of serum uric acid–lowering medications. They act by inhibiting the urate transporter URAT1 at the tubules, thus raising the renal excretion of urate. In patients with renal calculi, uricosuric drugs need to be used with caution. Alkalization of urine and high urine volumes are required. Benzbromarone has been removed from the U.S. and some European markets because of concerns about hepatotoxicity, but it is available in some countries with restricted use.

If available, uricases (rasburicase or pegloticase, its PEGylated form) provide an option for patients whose gout is actively symptomatic and refractory to or contraindicated to other urate-lowering therapies. Uricase mediates the conversion of uric acid into a more soluble molecule, allantoin. Uricase is present in most mammals but absent in humans because of mutation inactivation of the uricase gene. Pegloticase is contraindicated in patients with glucose-6-phosphate dehydrogenase (G6PD) deficiency, in whom it is associated with increased hypersensitivity reactions. Uricase is very effective in preventing and managing tumor lysis syndrome. Both forms of uricase have lowered serum uric acid levels in clinical trials, but the need for parenteral administration and development of antiuricase antibodies may limit their repetitive use in selected cases of severe gout.

CALCIUM PYROPHOSPHATE CRYSTAL DEPOSITION DISEASE (PSEUDOGOUT)

Calcium pyrophosphate (CPP) crystals can lead to several findings in patients. The most common finding is the report of chondrocalcinosis on radiographs of the knee or wrist. Chondrocalcinosis represents the calcification of articular cartilage and may be associated with the development of early osteoarthritis but is generally asymptomatic. Acute monoarticular attacks of pseudogout occur when CPP crystals are shed from the hyaline cartilage and fibrocartilage into the joint, inducing a sterile inflammatory response. CPP crystal-induced arthritis affects medium-large joints, including knees, wrists, hips, and shoulders, although small joints can be involved. Acute CPP crystal arthritis closely resembles gout with acute onset of pain, swelling, and erythema. The diagnosis of acute-onset, self-limiting synovitis with CPP crystal arthritis is established by arthrocentesis and visualization of CPP crystals under compensated polarized microscopy.

CPP deposition disease (CPPD) is a common incidental finding in elderly patients. However, the discovery of calcium pyrophosphate disease in younger patients, especially those <55 years, should prompt a workup for metabolic or genetic diseases. Diseases associated with calcium pyrophosphate disease include hemochromatosis, hyperparathyroidism, hypophosphatasia, hypomagnesemia, acromegaly, hypophosphatemic rickets (X-linked), Wilson disease, and hypomagnesemia-related kidney diseases such as Bartter syndrome and Gitelman disease. Specific laboratory tests to consider are calcium, alkaline phosphatase, magnesium, ferritin, liver function tests, and parathyroid hormone (PTH).

Guidelines for the treatment of CPP crystal deposition disease generally follow those for gout. Often, aspiration of the joint will improve the patient's condition. Due to the high rate of reaccumulation of joint effusions during an acute attack, intra-articular corticosteroids are injected to provide relief. Corticosteroids are the preferred therapeutic agents for this condition, although colchicine may be effective. Alternative or adjuvant therapies include NSAIDs therapy. Chronic CPPD disease is difficult to manage and often refractory to medical treatment. The use of antirheumatic disease-modifying agents (DMARDs) such as hydroxychloroquine or methotrexate has been found to be effective in reducing the frequency of flares in refractory cases.

BASIC CALCIUM PHOSPHATE DEPOSITION DISEASE

Basic calcium phosphate (BCP) crystal disease represents several different crystal types. The most common of these crystals are hydroxyapatite (HA) containing but can include crystals with octacalcium phosphate or tricalcium phosphate. These latter crystals are rarely encountered in clinical practice. HA deposition disease leads to a variety of musculoskeletal presentations including that of acute monoarticular arthritis, acute calcific periarthritis, soft tissue calcifications, and early osteoarthritis. HA may deposit in the small joints of the hands, wrists, elbows, hips, and ankles, but the shoulder joints are more commonly affected, leading to a rare destructive arthropathy, Milwaukee shoulder syndrome. Milwaukee shoulder generally occurs in elderly women who present with a large shoulder effusion associated with pain. Arthrocentesis of the shoulder effusion yields large volumes of synovial fluid. Basic calcium phosphate crystals are more difficult to detect in synovial fluid than MSU or CPP crystals and may appear as amorphous material under compensated polarized light microscopy. If BCP crystals are suspected, alizarin red staining can be performed on synovial fluid to demonstrate their presence. There is no clear treatment that will reduce the burden of BCP, and acute attacks should be treated with NSAIDs, analgesics, and/or intra-articular steroid injection similar to other crystalline disorders in the acute phase.

CALCIUM OXALATE

Oxalate is a metabolic product of glycine, serine, and other amino acids, and ascorbic acid. Oxalate is readily absorbed after ingestion and almost entirely cleared by renal excretion. Secondary oxalosis complicating stage 5 chronic kidney disease (CKD), which results from inefficient removal of oxalate by hemodialysis or peritoneal dialysis, has been reported infrequently. The associated clinical manifestations are similar to CPPD or MSU deposition. Radiographic manifestations of oxalosis resemble those of CPPD with chondrocalcinosis in the hands and knees. Therefore, diagnostic arthrocentesis and examination under compensated polarized microscopy is required for proper identification of calcium oxalate (CaOx) crystals. Diagnosis is made by visualization of the crystals, which have characteristic bipyramidal or envelope-shaped crystals. Cell counts from arthrocentesis of effusion related to CaOx crystals are generally <2000. Treatment generally follows those of other crystal arthropathies but with avoidance of vitamin C as contained in renal multivitamins because it contributes to the developing of secondary oxalosis.

LIPID-LADEN CRYSTALS

Rarely, crystals related to cholesterol may lead to a monoarticular presentation. Demonstration of "Maltese cross" particles that are frequently seen intracellularly in synovial fluid help to confirm this diagnosis. However, a few sparse "Maltese cross" crystals may be commonly seen and not the cause of a monoarticular arthritis.

OSTEOARTHRITIS

Osteoarthritis of a single joint, although usually associated with mild symptoms and a noninflammatory synovial fluid (WBC < 2000 cells/mm^3), can present as an acute monoarticular arthritis mimicking infection.

HEMARTHROSIS

Hemarthrosis, or bleeding into the joint, is common in patients with acquired or congenital clotting abnormalities, such as those on anticoagulation therapy or with hemophilia or other clotting deficiencies. Fractures should be considered in patients with hemarthrosis and trauma, especially if synovial fluid is bloody and contains fat.

REACTIVE ARTHRITIS

Monoarticular arthritis in reactive arthritis (ReA) is generally a diagnosis of exclusion. The pattern of involvement is often that of a large joint (knee) with lower extremity predominance. The monoarthritis is presumably reactive to an infection elsewhere in the body. Although the bacteria may have been cleared, systemic immune complex response can cause acute monoarthritis or oligoarticular aseptic synovitis and also lead to a predilection for spondylitis (vertebral inflammation) and sacroiliitis. The presence of extra-articular manifestations associated with HLA-B27 alleles such as mild conjunctivitis or uveitis, infectious urethritis, balanitis, psoriasiform skin lesions, oral ulcers, sausage digit, and enthesitis may assist in the clinical diagnosis. Primary organisms associated with reactive arthritis include *Chlamydia* sp., *Salmonella, Clostridium difficile, Campylobacter,* and *Yersinia* (table 24.6).

SYSTEMIC DISEASES

Many systemic diseases may present with an acute monoarthritis. This is true for a variety of rheumatic diseases such as the seronegative spondyloarthropathies (psoriatic arthritis, reactive arthritis, and inflammatory bowel disease), which can present with a monoarthritis of the lower extremities. Sarcoid periarthritis typically presents with pain around the ankle joints with or without erythema nodosum (EN) over the distal tibial region. Monoarthritis can be seen in early stages of RA. Myelodysplastic or leukemic disorders may cause arthralgias or acute monoarthritis. Septic monoarthritis may be the first clue to bacterial endocarditis, pneumonia, hypogammaglobulinemia, or AIDS. Serum sickness, hepatitis, and hyperlipidemias may occasionally present with an acute monoarthritis.

SUMMARY

Acute monoarticular arthritis is a common presenting complaint with a wide differential diagnosis. A directed history can help rule out trauma or overuse syndrome as the cause of the patient's symptoms. Clinicians should focus on excluding a septic arthritis because of the high morbidity and mortality from this condition. The identification of crystalline arthritis is critical in the prevention of future attacks and improves long-term patient outcomes. Additionally, one must be aware of monoarticular arthritis as the initial presentation of a wide array of systemic disorders.

ADDITIONAL READING

Courtney P, Doherty M. Joint aspiration and injection and synovial fluid analysis. *Best Pract Res Clin Rheumatol.* 2009;23:161–92.

Gardam M, Lim S. Mycobacterial osteomyelitis and arthritis. *Infect Dis Clin North Am.* 2005;19:819–30.

Goldenberg DL. Septic arthritis. *Lancet.* 1998;351:197–202.

Hu L. Lyme arthritis. *Infect Dis Clin North Am.* 2005;19:947–61.

Maldonado I, Prasad V, Reginato AJ. Oxalate crystal deposition disease. *Curr Rheumatol Rep.* 2002;4:257–64.

Mathews CJ, Kingsley G, Field M, et al. Management of septic arthritis: A systematic review. *Ann Rheum Dis.* 2007;66;440–5.

Petersel DL, Sigal LH. Reactive arthritis. *Infect Dis Clin North Am.* 2005;19:863–83.

Pioro MH, Mandell BF. Septic arthritis. *Rheum Dis Clin North Am.* 1997;23:239–58.

Rice PA. Gonococcal arthritis (disseminated gonococcal infection). *Infect Dis Clin North Am.* 2005;19:853–61.

Ross JJ. Septic arthritis. *Infect Dis Clin North Am.* 2005;19:799–817.

Terkeltaub R. Update on gout: New therapeutic strategies and options. *Nat Rev Rheumatol.* 2010;6:30–8.

Zhang W, Doherty M, Pascual E, et al.; EULAR Standing Committee for International Clinical Studies Including Therapeutics. EULAR evidence based recommendations for gout. Part I: Diagnosis. Report of a task force of the Standing Committee for International Clinical Studies Including Therapeutics (ESCISIT). *Ann Rheum Dis.* 2006;65:1301–11.

Zhang W, Doherty M, Bardin T, et al.; EULAR Standing Committee for International Clinical Studies Including Therapeutics. EULAR evidence based recommendations for gout. Part II: Management. Report of a task force of the EULAR Standing Committee for International Clinical Studies Including Therapeutics (ESCISIT). *Ann Rheum Dis.* 2006;65:1312–24.

Zhang W, Doherty M, Bardin T, et al. European League against Rheumatism recommendations for calcium pyrophosphate deposition. Part I: Terminology and diagnosis. *Ann Rheum Dis.* 2011;70:563–70.

Zhang W, Doherty M, Pascual E, et al. EULAR recommendations for calcium pyrophosphate deposition. Part II: Management. *Ann Rheum Dis.* 2011;70:571–5.

Table 24.6 **BACTERIA ASSOCIATED WITH REACTIVE ARTHRITIS (ReA)**

GENITOURINARY	GASTROINTESTINAL
Chlamydia trachomatis	*Shigella flexneri*
Chlamydia psittaci	*Campylobacter jejuni*
Possible: *Ureaplasma*	*Campylobacter fetus*
urealyticum	*Salmonella typhimurium*
	Salmonella enteritis (less common: *S. heidelberg, S. choleraesuis, S. paratyphi B*)
	Shigella sonnei
	Yersinia pseudotuberculosis
	Yersinia enterocolitica O:3 or O:9 (less common: *Y. enterocolitica O:8*)
	Clostridium difficile

QUESTIONS

QUESTION 1. A 65-year-old fireman with a history of gout presented to his primary physician with left first MTP pain, swelling, and erythema. He was treated with oral colchicine, 0.6 mg bid, and prednisone, 40 mg QD for 4 days. However, the patient calls you back complaining that his left first MTP has not improved and has actually gotten worse. The most useful diagnostic test in this patient includes:

A. Radiography of the right first MTP
B. Serum uric acid level
C. Complete blood cell count with differential, ESR, and CRP
D. Increase prednisone to 80 mg every day
E. Diagnostic arthrocentesis

QUESTION 2. In the same patient as Question 1, negatively birefringent needle-shaped crystals were seen under compensated polarized light microscopy of fluid obtained on aspiration of the left first MTP joint. Next, you should:

A. Increase oral colchicine to 1.2 mg bid
B. Perform depot corticosteroid injection of the joint
C. Wait for Gram stain and culture results to determine therapy
D. Start allopurinol, 300 mg PO qday

QUESTION 3. A 59-year-old male presents with serum uric acid level of 9.5 mg/dL. Clear-cut indications for treatment with allopurinol include:

A. A creatine value of 3.0 mg/dL
B. A history of two gout flares in the past 2 years
C. Presence of a small tophi on his right ear and tophaceous radiographic changes of MTPs
D. Patient being on chronic hydrochlorothiazide
E. A 24-hour urinary excretion of >1000 mg

QUESTION 4. An 18-year-old sexually active male is seen in the emergency room with right ankle joint swelling. He is afebrile. Physical exam demonstrates right ankle arthritis with an effusion. Diagnostic arthrocentesis showed an inflammatory fluid with white cell count of 35,000/mm³ and 87% neutrophils on differential. Examination of synovial fluid under compensated polarized light microscopy demonstrated no crystals. He is treated with broad-spectrum antibiotics. Gonorrhea and Chlamydia cultures are negative. Synovial fluid cultures after 48 hours are negative. The presumptive diagnosis is:

A. Gout
B. Avascular necrosis (AVN)
C. Tuberculous arthritis
D. Gonococcal arthritis
E. Reactive arthritis (ReA)

QUESTION 5. A 45-year-old male presents with acute monoarticular arthritis of the left knee. He is afebrile and symptom-free. Radiographs of the left knee showed mild chondrocalcinosis. Diagnostic arthrocentesis showed an inflammatory fluid with white cell count of 25,000/mm³ and 85% neutrophils on differential. Examination of synovial fluid under compensated polarized light microscopy demonstrated the presence of negative birefringent crystals consistent with CPPD. Gram stain and cultures were negative. On further examination he is noted to have some synovitis of the second and third metacarpophalangeal joints (MCPs) with radiographs of the hands showing osteoarthritis-like changes in the second and third MCPs. Further metabolic workup should include:

A. TSH
B. Ca, phosphate, and PTH
C. ACTH
D. Iron, transferrin/IBC, ferritin and liver biopsy
E. Magnesium

QUESTION 6. A 21-year-old female with a h/o SLE nephritis treated with high-dose steroids and Cytoxan in the past presents with acute-onset right hip pain. She is afebrile and symptom-free. Her SLE has been well controlled on Plaquenil, 200 mg PO bid, CellCept, 1000 mg PO qday, and prednisone, 5 mg PO qday. Laboratory studies showed a normal ESR and CRP. CBC, renal function, dsDNA, and complement levels were unremarkable. Radiograph of the right hip was also unremarkable. Diagnostic arthrocentesis was performed given the concern of septic arthritis. A small amount of fluid was obtained with synovial fluid white count of 2,000/mm³ and subsequent negative Gram stain and cultures. The most useful next diagnostic tests in this patient should include:

A. Pulse dose steroids and monitor response
B. CT scan
C. MRI
D. Synovial biopsy

ANSWERS

1. F
2. C
3. C
4. E
5. D
6. C

25.

SYSTEMIC LUPUS ERYTHEMATOSUS AND RELATED DISORDERS

Bonnie L. Bermas

SYSTEMIC LUPUS ERYTHEMATOSUS

Systemic lupus erythematosus (SLE) is a multisystem disease that preferentially affects women of childbearing age. This disorder is both more common and more severe in individuals of African and Asian ancestry. The etiology of SLE is not well understood, although genetics and environmental stimuli clearly are involved. Whether this disease is caused by a T-cell, B-cell, or other immunologic malfunction is debated, but all would agree that clearly autoantibodies such as antinuclear antibodies and anti–double-stranded DNA contribute to the pathophysiology of this disorder. This multisystem disease can affect the skin, joints, lungs, heart, kidneys, and central nervous system. Most of the morbidity and mortality is from renal and central nervous system (CNS) involvement, although accelerated atherosclerosis has recently been appreciated as a major contributor to disease burden. The treatment of SLE has improved over the past decade with less reliance on high-dose corticosteroids and more emphasis on immunosuppressive agents. It is our hope that future research into the pathophysiology of this disorder and the development of more specific therapy, such as biologics, will improve the outcome of this disease.

HISTORY AND EPIDEMIOLOGY

Systemic lupus erythematosus was named for the classic rash that occurs over the bridge of the nose and face. These lesions were thought to resemble "wolf bites," although the image of the butterfly is likewise used to depict "lupus." SLE can occur throughout one's lifetime, although the peak incidence is in the second to the fourth decade of life. The female-to-male ratio is 9:1, although in the older age groups this gender skewing becomes less pronounced. In the United States the overall prevalence of this disorder is 40–150 per 100,000. The prevalence in the African-American population is two to three times higher than in the Caucasian population.

GENETICS AND PATHOPHYSIOLOGY

There is a genetic contribution to the development of SLE. Twin studies have shown a concordance rate ranging from 24% to 60% for monozygotic twins and 2% to 5% for dizygotic twins. Genes that may contribute increased risk for the development of SLE include certain HLA haplotypes (HLA DR2 and HLA DR3) and genes that encode for a wide variety of immunologic factors. Current thinking is that the environment and possibly infectious exposures contribute to the development of this disorder on a susceptible genetic substrate.

Autoantibody production and deposition in specific organs and associated damage are the hallmark of this disease. However, the cause of this autoantibody production is unknown. Dysregulation of T and B cells may contribute to autoantibody production. Poor clearance of nuclear debris mediated by toll-like receptors may also play a role. Abnormal interferon gene expression, called the interferon "signature," has been found in persons with SLE and may correlate with disease activity. Other markers for this disease include low complement levels that are often found during periods of disease activation. Moreover, complement deficiencies such as C4 are found in greater frequency in patients with SLE. Nonetheless, the precise mechanism and pathway that lead to SLE has not been worked out, and it is plausible that there are several different breakdowns of the immune system that may lead to the different phenotypes of SLE. Clearly there is a genetic susceptibility, and most likely there is a subsequent environmental or infectious trigger that then contributes to disease development by disrupting the immune system.

CLINICAL MANIFESTATIONS

Skin

Cutaneous manifestations of SLE can be subdivided into subacute and acute findings. Some of the subacute and chronic conditions such as subacute cutaneous lupus erythematosus and discoid lesions can be entities unto themselves with no systemic involvement. Discoid and subacute cutaneous lupus lesions can be seen in full-blown lupus as well (table 25.1).

Subacute Cutaneous Lupus Erythematosus

Subacute cutaneous lupus erythematosus (SCLE) can be seen as an isolated disorder and also associated with systemic disorder. (Fifty percent of patients with SCLE will go on to develop full-blown SLE.) These individuals develop a rash that occurs in sun-exposed areas, mainly arms, trunk, and the neck. Although the face and lower extremities can be involved, it is less common. There are two types of rashes that can be seen: annular, in which ring-like lesions are seen, and papulosquamous (psoriasiform-like lesions). When the rash is severe, it may become superinfected. Involvement in the scalp can lead to hair loss.

Biopsy of these skin lesions can show hyperkeratosis and a mononuclear cell infiltrate in the dermal-epidermal junction. The majority of these patients have anti-Ro (SSA) and anti-La (SSB) antibodies. Some of these patients will have systemic symptoms, but it is rare to have significant organ involvement such as renal or CNS disease.

The first part of treatment is focused on behavioral therapy. Limiting sun exposure to nonpeak hours, wearing sun-protective clothing, and using sunscreen are important features of the treatment. Discontinuation of cigarette smoking may be helpful as well, and patients should be counseled accordingly. Medicines such as antimalarials and topical steroids can be used. Less frequently, systemic immunosuppression with steroids, azathioprine, or mycophenolate mofetil is used. Rarely thalidomide is employed for refractory cases. Current research into biologics as a treatment for the skin is also being done.

Chronic Cutaneous Lupus Erythematosus

Chronic cutaneous lupus erythematosus includes discoid lupus, lupus profundus, and other types of disorders. Discoid lesions are the most common and occur in up to 15–20% of patients with SLE. Like SCLE, these lesions occur in sun-exposed areas; however, the scalp, face, upper arms, and ears are more commonly involved than is usually seen in SCLE. These lesions can cause scarring that can be disfiguring. Follicular plugging with central atrophy is found on biopsy of lesions. Treatment is similar to the treatment for SCLE and includes sun avoidance and sun protection, antimalarial agents, and immunosuppressive agents.

Lupus profundus is a rare skin finding that occurs in the absence of systemic symptoms. Deep dermal layers and subcutaneous fat can be destroyed. As a result scarring, sunken lesions that can be disfiguring can occur. Treatment includes antimalarials, steroids, and dapsone. In some cases, plastic surgery is necessary to reconstruct the tissue.

Acute Cutaneous Lupus Erythematosus

The most common skin lesion found in acute cutaneous lupus is the malar rash. The malar rash is a reddish raised rash over the bridge of the nose and cheeks that can be pruritic. It is thought to be secondary to immune deposition at the dermal-epidermal junction. Often the rash appears after sunlight exposure. Acne rosacea is the rash most commonly confused with a malar rash and is more common in Caucasian women in their fourth and fifth decades of life. The latter is more likely to have an oily texture and scaling. Photosensitivity reaction is a skin rash that occurs after sun exposure in sun-exposed areas. This reddish rash mainly occurs over the face and neck and other sun-exposed areas. Blistering and superinfection can occur, and often patients will feel ill in conjunction with the skin rash.

Other

Aphthous ulcers can be painless or painful. They can occur nasally, vaginally, and orally on the soft or the hard palate. Bullous lesions can rarely occur in individuals with SLE. Other skin findings include small-vessel vasculitis (palpable purpura, petechiae, splinter hemorrhages) and panniculitis. Alopecia is also seen in SLE. In particular lesions are seen around the temporal region, or patches of hair loss leading to "bald spots" can occur. Urticarial lesions, more commonly urticarial vasculitis, is also found in SLE patients. Raynaud phenomenon (see below) is found in over half of lupus patients.

Pulmonary

The lungs are commonly involved in SLE. Pleural involvement, as manifested by pleuritis, is seen in up to 30–60% of patients with SLE. The most common symptom is inspiratory chest pain and associated shortness of breath. On physical exam a rub can be heard, but not always, and

Table 25.1 SKIN DISORDERS IN SYSTEMIC LUPUS ERYTHEMATOSUS

Subacute cutaneous lupus erythematosus	Subacute cutaneous lupus erythematosus Annular Papulosquamous
Chronic cutaneous lupus	Discoid lupus* Lupus profundus
Acute cutaneous lupus	Malar rash* Photosensitivity*
Other	Aphthous ulcers:* oral, nasal, vaginal Alopecia Bullous lupus Panniculitis Urticaria Vasculitis

NOTE: *Part of the diagnostic classification.

likewise radiographic evaluation is often negative. Thus, the diagnosis of pleuritis is often a clinical one. Treatment with NSAIDs (nonsteroidal anti-inflammatory drugs) and corticosteroids is generally effective.

An inflammatory interstitial lung disease can occur in SLE. Patients present with dyspnea and a dry nonproductive cough. On exam, dry crackles are heard, and a reduced single-breath diffusing capacity of the lung (DLCO) can be demonstrated. The most effective way of making a diagnosis is by high-resolution computed tomography (CT). Chronic interstitial lung disease can progress to fibrosis, causing permanent lung damage.

Pulmonary hemorrhage is a rare but devastating finding in SLE patients. Mortality from this disorder approaches 50%. Patients present with hemoptysis and dyspnea. A high percentage of these patients have associated antiphospholipid antibodies.

Shrinking lung syndrome is another rare manifestation of SLE. On radiographs, elevated diaphragms are found, and patients are dyspneic. Pathology is thought to be secondary to muscle weakness of the diaphragms and intercostal muscles, and interstitial lung disease can contribute to poor inspiratory effort as well.

Cardiac Involvement

Pericarditis is the most common cardiac manifestation of SLE. Patients present with chest pain and shortness of breath. Hemodynamic compromise in the setting of pericardial tamponade is rare but can occur. Diagnosis is suggested by flattened T-waves on electrocardiogram but is confirmed by echocardiogram. Treatment with NSAIDs and steroids is generally effective for small pericardial effusions. Larger effusions and situations in which hemodynamic compromise occurs may require pericardial drainage.

Coronary artery vasculitis and myositis are extremely rare manifestations of SLE. Leibman-Sacks endocarditis presents with microthrombi on the valves and subsequent impairment of valvular function. The vast majority of patients who have this disorder also have the presence of antiphospholipid antibodies. The vast majority of patients with Leibman-Sacks endocarditis have the presence of antiphospholipid antibodies.

Persons with SLE have higher incidences of coronary artery disease. Whether this is the result of the disease or the treatment is unclear, but it appears to be a combination of both risk factors. Some rheumatologists believe that lupus should be considered a cardiac risk factor, along with diabetes mellitus and hypertension. Certainly, patients who have lupus should have other risk factors such as hypertension, diabetes mellitus, and hypercholesterolemia well controlled. Early intervention with statins is being explored as potentially lowering the risk of accelerated atherosclerosis. Careful attention to lifestyle changes and maintaining a healthy weight, exercising, and smoking cessation are important measures as well.

Joint Symptoms

Ninety-five percent of people who have SLE will have joint symptoms at some time. Arthritis and arthropathy are the most common. Some patients may just experience joint achiness. Other patients developed a tendinopathy that leads to laxity that causes a particular type of deforming arthropathy called Jaccoud arthropathy. Still others will develop an arthritis that is indistinguishable from an inflammatory arthritis such as rheumatoid arthritis. This subgroup may have the presence of a positive rheumatoid factor or anticitrulline antibody (anti-CCP).

Osteonecrosis has been reported in patients with SLE. Most often the osteonecrosis occurs in individuals who are on steroids at doses greater than the equivalent of 20 mg of prednisone a day. Septic arthritis in particular can occur in individuals who have had prior damage to a joint and are on immunosuppressive agents.

Myositis can occur in patients with SLE, particularly those who have the presence of a ribonucleoprotein (RNP) antibody. Presentation includes muscle weakness and pain, and biopsy shows muscle inflammation. This inflammatory condition must be differentiated from steroid myopathy, which likewise presents with proximal muscle weakness, and from myopathies that are due to medication use such as antimalarials or statins.

Hematologic Disorders

Leukopenia and lymphopenia are found in individuals with SLE. An absolute white blood cell (WBC) count of <4000 and an absolute lymphocyte count of 1500 are part of the diagnostic criteria for classification of this disorder. Thrombocytopenia, defined as a platelet count of <100,000, is also found in systemic lupus. Anemia of chronic disease, as well as a Coombs-positive hemolytic anemia are likewise found in SLE patients.

Renal Disease

Over half of persons with SLE will develop renal disease. Clinically, patients will present with hypertension, edema, and proteinuria, although they may be asymptomatic. For classification purposes proteinuria and hematuria are used, although most would advocate obtaining a renal biopsy so that the renal disease can be categorized using the World Health Organization (WHO) classification. Renal disease is categorized into one of six classes of renal disease (table 25.2). In addition to these categories, pathology specimens are given an activity—chronicity rating that reflects the degree of inflammation occurring in the kidney. Most of the morbidity and mortality from renal disease occurs in those who have either focal or diffuse glomerulonephritis. In addition, a high degree of chronicity in the renal biopsy portends a poor prognosis, as these lesions tend to

Table 25.2 REVISED CLASSIFICATION OF GLOMERU-LONEPHRITIS IS SYSTEMIC LUPUS ERYTHEMATOSUS

Class I. Minimal change disease
Class II. Mesangial disease
ªClass III. Focal lupus nephritis
ᵇClass IV. Diffuse segmental (IV-S) or global (IV-G) lupus nephritis
Class V. Diffuse membranous glomerulonephritis
Class VI. Advanced sclerosing glomerulonephritis

ªFurther classified by active and sclerotic lesions
ᵇFurther classified by necrosis and cresents
SOURCE: Adapted from The Classification of Glomerulonephritis in SLE Revisited JASN, 2004, 15(2), 241–250.

be refractory to therapy. In the past, mortality from renal disease was quite high; however, due to newer treatments, this rate has drastically diminished.

Neurological Disease

Nineteen neurological syndromes have been reported to be part of neuropsychiatric lupus, although only two are listed among the classification criteria (table 25.3). Some of these disorders are thought to be due to focal lesions often associated with focal clotting events in the presence of antiphospholipid antibodies Transverse myelitis, focal seizures, stroke, and cognitive impairment are a few of these disorders. More global organic findings such as generalized seizures and psychosis are not associated with these antibodies. Some findings such as depression, migraines, and certain types of cognitive difficulties are found in many disorders, and it can become difficult to ascertain whether disorders

are purely associated with SLE. For example, although headaches are frequently described in individuals with SLE, the actual frequency of headaches may not be higher than what is found in the general population. For classification purposes, only seizures and psychosis are included as part of the criteria for SLE.

DRUG-INDUCED SLE

Drug-induced SLE can occur after the initiation of almost any medications. Isoniazid and procainamide are the most common offending agents, but many more medications can cause this entity. In most affected individuals, symptoms are limited to skin rashes, arthralgias, and fatigue. It is rare to have renal or CNS involvement. Over 95% of these individuals will have the presence of an antihistone antibody. In many cases, the symptoms will resolve once the medication is removed, but occasionally treatment with NSAIDs and low-dose steroids is needed. It is rare that more potent immunosuppressive or cytotoxic therapy is needed.

AUTOANTIBODIES

Autoantibodies are found in the vast majority of individuals with SLE (table 25.4). The most common, the antinuclear antibody (ANA), is found in 93–95% of individuals with the diagnosis of SLE. Antinuclear antibodies and precipitins have been found in individuals several years prior to the diagnosis of SLE. However, it is important to remember that low titers of these antibodies can be seen in up to 5% of the general population, in particular in those who are on certain

Table 25.3 NEUROLOGICAL MANIFESTATIONS OF SYSTEMIC LUPUS ERYTHEMATOSUS

CENTRAL	PERIPHERAL
Aseptic meningitis	Guillain-Barré syndrome
Cerebrovascular disease	Autonomic neuropathy
Demyelinating syndrome	Mononeuropathy
Headache	Myasthenia gravis
Movement disorder	Cranial neuropathy
Seizure disorder	Plexopathy
Myelopathy	Polyneuropathy
Acute confusional state	
Anxiety disorder	
Cognitive dysfunction	
Mood disorder	
Psychosis	

Table 25.4. AUTOANTIBODIES IN SLE AND OTHER COLLAGEN VASCULAR DISEASE

ANA	SLE, progressive systemic sclerosis, Sjögren, dermatomyositis/polymyositis
Anti-dsDNA	SLE, renal disease
Anti-Sm	SLE, renal disease
Anti-RNP	SLE, MCTD
Antihistone antibody	Drug-induced SLE
Anti-Ro (SSA), anti-La (SSB)	SLE, SCLE, Sjögren disease
Anti-SCL-70	Progressive systemic sclerosis (especially diffuse)
Anticentromere antibody	Progressive systemic sclerosis (especially limited)
Anti-Jo-1 antibody	Dermatomyositis/polymyositis (especially with lung involvement)

types of medications, postvirally, the elderly, and those who have other autoimmune conditions. Therefore, ANA alone can not be used to make the diagnosis of SLE. The higher the titer of antibody, the more likely it is to be a true positive and not a false positive. Other antibodies are more specific, such as the anti-dsDNA antibody, which is found in 75% of individuals with SLE, and the anti-Sm antibody, found in 25% of all individuals with SLE. The latter two are associated with renal disease. Anti-Ro (SSA) and anti-La (SSB) antibodies are seen in individuals who have SCLE as well as SLE and are the pathologic agents in neonatal lupus and congenital complete heart block. Anti-RNP antibodies are seen in higher frequency in those who have mixed connective tissue disease. Antihistone antibodies are associated with drug-induced SLE, although 60% of those with SLE have these antibodies as well.

DIAGNOSIS

Diagnosis of this disorder can be challenging. Given the myriad of combinations of clinical manifestations that individuals can present with it, is no wonder that SLE is called one of the great imitators. Individuals may present to clinicians with symptoms suggestive of SLE, and it is important to be rigorous in making the diagnosis. Although the diagnostic classification criteria were developed as a research tool, they do provide a useful guideline with which to make the diagnosis. Technically, individuals require 4 of 11 classification criteria to be diagnosed with SLE (table 25.5). However, if the clinical circumstance is highly suggestive of SLE, the clinician should use his or her judgment in making the diagnosis. Given that 93–95% of individuals will have the presence of an ANA and the majority of those who do not have an ANA will have the presence of another autoantibody seen in SLE, this author believes that antibody-negative SLE is extremely rare.

TREATMENT OF SYSTEMIC LUPUS ERYTHEMATOSUS

The treatment of SLE is aimed at two goals-disease control and prevention of long-term sequelae. Therapy is often targeted to specific organs. For many years only three medications—aspirin, corticosteroids, and hydroxychloroquine—were approved by the FDA for the treatment of SLE. Recently, belimumab, therapy that targets B cells was also approve for use in SLE patients.

Antimalarials

Hydroxychloroquine and chloroquine are the mainstays of therapy in the treatment of SLE. These medications were first used in the early 20th century for malarial treatment but were found to be effective in treating inflammatory arthritis. More recently, it has been found that antimalarials may interfere with the expression of toll-like receptors, and thus, this may be the mechanism of action of these drugs.

The major toxicity of hydroxychloroquine is retinal. This medication can cause pigment deposition in the retina and interfere with color vision first and then ultimately visual acuity. Dosing regimens that maintain a daily dose of under 6.5 mg/kg minimize this risk, and current recommendations are for ophthalmologic exams with visual field testing by an experienced ophthalmologist or optometrist twice a year. Chloroquine has increased potential for ocular toxicity. Other side effects include pigment deposition in the skin, leaving a grayish-blue hue, and, on very rare occasions, bone marrow suppression. Rarely antimalarials may induce a hemolytic anemia in individuals with a G6PD deficiency.

Evidence suggests that antimalarials are particularly effective in the treatment of skin disease, joint symptoms, and serositis. In addition, they may help some of the more protean systemic symptoms such as fatigue, fever, and malaise. In the long term, antimalarials may prevent renal disease and CNS manifestations. Many rheumatologists will advocate long-term maintenance therapy with antimalarials in lupus patients.

Corticosteroids

Corticosteroids are the most common immunosuppressive agent used in systemic lupus. Prednisone and methylprednisolone are the most commonly used of these agents. In low doses (<10 mg/day), these agents can be helpful for controlling systemic symptoms, joint symptoms, skin disease, and serositis. In higher doses, 0.5 mg/kg per day, they are effective in the management of severe serositis, skin disease, and CNS findings.

Methotrexate and Leflunomide

Methotrexate is used to control the joint symptoms of SLE. True inflammation and synovitis are rare but can be seen in some patients. Methotrexate can be an effective therapy for this disorder. Leflunomide has been used for the treatment of joint symptoms as well.

Azathioprine

Azathioprine can be used as a steroid-sparing agent in individuals who have a refractory skin disease, serositis. It is also used as maintenance therapy for individuals who have lupus nephritis and have received immunosuppressive therapy.

Cyclosporine

Cyclosporine has been used to treat renal disease and skin disease, although is less likely to be used than azathioprine.

Table 25.5 THE 1997 REVISED ACR CRITERIA FOR THE CLASSIFICATION OF SLE

Malar rash	Fixed erythema, flat or raised, over the malar eminences, sparing the nasolabial folds
Discoid rash	Erythematous raised patches with adherent keratotic scaling and follicular plugging: atrophic scarring may occur in older lesions
Photosensitivity	Skin rash as a result of unusual reaction to sunlight, by patient history or physician observation
Oral ulcers	Oral or nasopharyngeal ulceration, usually painless, observed by a physician
Nonerosive arthritis	Involving two or more peripheral joints, characterized by tenderness, swelling, or effusion
Pleuritis or pericarditis	Pleuritis: convincing history of pleuritic pain or rub heard by a physician or evidence of pleural effusion, or Pericarditis: documented by electrocardiogram (EKG) or rub or evidence of pericardial effusion
Renal disorder	Persistent proteinuria >0.5 g per day or greater than 3+ if quantitative not performed, or Cellular casts—may be red cell, hemoglobin, granular, tubular, or mixed
Seizures or psychosis	Seizures: in the absence of offending drugs or known metabolic derangement Psychosis: in the absence of offending drugs or known metabolic derangement
Hematologic disorder	Hemolytic anemia with reticulocytosis, or Leukopenia—<4000/mm^3 on two occasions, or Lymphopenia—<1500/mm^3 on two occasions, or Thrombocytopenia—<100,000/mm^3 in the absence of offending drugs
Immunologic disorder	Anti-DNA; antibody to native DNA in abnormal titer, or Anti-Sm: presence of antibody to Sm nuclear antigen, or positive finding of antiphospholipid antibodies based on: (1) an abnormal serum level of IgG or IgM anticardiolipin antibodies or (2) positive test for lupus anticoagulant using a standard method or (3) a false-positive test for at least 6 months and confirmed by *Treponema pallidum* immobilization or fluorescent treponemal antibody absorption test
Positive antinuclear antibody	An abnormal titer of antinuclear antibody by immunofluorescence or an equivalent assay at any point in time in the absence of drug

SOURCE: Reprinted with permission from Tan EM, Cohen AS, Fries JF, et al. The 1982 revised criteria for the classification of systemic lupus erythematosus. *Arthritis Rheum.* 1982;25:1271–7 and Hochberg MC. Updating the American College of Rheumatology revised criteria for the classification of systemic lupus erythematosus [letter]. *Arthritis Rheum.* 1997;40:1725.

Lupus Nephritis

Early studies at the National Institutes of Health (NIH) showed that lupus nephritis was better treated with a regimen of cyclophosphamide and steroids than steroids alone. For the ensuing 20 years, this regimen of monthly pulse cyclophosphamide at doses of 500 mg to 1 g/m^2 of cyclophosphamide for 6 months and then every 3 months for a period of 2 years in combination with glucocorticoid therapy has been the mainstay of therapy for this disorder. However, concern about the toxicities have made clinicians eager to look for alternative treatment regimens. These toxicities include secondary carcinomas, hemorrhagic cystitis with risk for bladder cancer, and reproductive failure—an issue particularly problematic in a patient population of young women. Over the past 5 years, alternative therapies have been explored.

Cyclosporine has been used in some cases to treat lupus nephritis. It's main benefit may be in membranous disease with resultant nephrotic syndrome. Although no large-scale head-to-head study has been done, this medication has been used with marginal success in individuals with renal disease. This medication has the side effect of hypertension.

Recently, mycophenolate mofetil has been used to treat renal disease both to induce remission and as maintenance therapy. In comparison to cyclophosphamide there is significantly less toxicity, although whether it is truly as effective as cyclophosphamide in the long run is unclear. There is also a newer European protocol for cyclophosphamide use that uses 500 mg of IV cyclophosphamide every 2 weeks for six total treatments as effective as the original NIH protocol and had the advantage of lower toxicity.

The initial data on the use of biologics in lupus nephritis have been disappointing. Recently, a B cell blocker, belimumab has been shown in clinical trials to improve nonrenal disease activity and enable small reductions in prednisone doses in SLE patients. Other experimental therapy has included immunoablative therapy and autologous stem cell transplantation for severe cases of SLE.

Other Severe Manifestations

Severe CNS disease and vasculitis are treated with either high doses of corticosteroids or immunosuppressive regimens.

CONCLUSION

Systemic lupus erythematosus is a multisystem disorder impacting women of childbearing age with an increased disease burden in those of African and Asian ancestry. This disorder can present with a variety of manifestations, but renal disease, CNS disease, and cardiovascular disease cause the most disease morbidity. Maintenance therapy with antimalarials is often used, but more potent treatment with glucocorticoids, immunosuppressive agents, and, in the future, possibly biologic agents can be used for their more significant findings.

ANTIPHOSPHOLIPID SYNDROME

The antiphospholipid syndrome is seen in association with SLE and other collagen vascular diseases or as its own entity. Roughly 40% of individuals with SLE will have the presence of these antibodies, although many fewer will have the actual disease. In this disorder, individuals make antibodies that react with phospholipids and have venous and arterial thrombotic events or obstetrical complications. Interestingly, recurrent events tend to be similar to the initial event. Thus, those who first present with an arterial clotting event are likely to have a subsequent arterial event and those who initially present with a venous event are likely to have a subsequent renal event.

CLINICAL FEATURES

Venous thrombotic events are found in this disorder. Deep vein thrombosis, superficial thrombophlebitis, renal vein thrombosis, and pulmonary emboli have all been described. Arterial clotting events are found as well. Myocardial infarctions, strokes, and clots involving major vessels have all been described in individuals with these antibodies. The obstetrical complications include recurrent miscarriages, intrauterine fetal demise in the second and third trimesters, intrauterine growth retardation, and pre-eclampsia.

Raynaud's is frequently seen in association with this syndrome. If one takes the subset of individuals with SLE who have Raynaud's, the many of these patients will have the presence of antiphospholipid antibodies. Migraine headaches are also described in this entity. Livedo reticularis, also seen in Sneddon syndrome, is also described. Hemolytic anemia and thrombocytopenia, also known as Evans syndrome, can be found in persons who have these antibodies. Rarely, widespread thrombotic events can occur that lead to multiple organ failure and a high incidence of death. This manifestation, the catastrophic antiphospholipid syndrome, is highly refractory to treatment.

Antibodies

Three general categories of antibodies have been described in this disorder: false-positive Venereal Disease Research Laboratory (VDRL) anticardiolipin antibodies including an anti-beta-2-glycoprotein I, and circulating lupus anticoagulant. The false-positive VDRL was the first to be described and was used for many years as part of the diagnostic criteria for the diagnosis of SLE. This test is really of historical significance but has little utility in the diagnosis of this disorder and is no longer included in the diagnostic criteria for this syndrome. In the early 1980s an enzyme-linked immunosorbent assay (ELISA) was developed to assess for the presence of cardiolipin antibodies. Currently, most laboratories will use internationally standardized sera to report results. Although there have been descriptions of other isotypes such IgA and IgD antibodies being associated with disease, the IgG and IgM antibodies are thought to be the most clinically relevant and are used in the diagnosis of this disorder. The binding of these antibodies to the phospholipid in the assay is mediated through beta-2-glycoprotein I. Direct measurements of anti-beta-2-glycoprotein I antibodies can be used to diagnose this disorder as well.

The term "circulating anticoagulant" is a misnomer. Initially described in lupus patients half a century ago, this abnormality is a prolongation of the commonly used clotting tests in the lab. However, the patients are predisposed to clotting events. Although many standard clotting tests such as an activated partial thromboplastin time, Russell viper venom time, and kaolin clotting time can all be used as a first screen for the presence of a circulating anticoagulant, it is important to remember that one ought to have a confirmatory test to verify the presence of a lupus anticoagulant. To confirm a positive screen, normal serum is added back to make certain that a factor deficiency is ruled out. If the clotting abnormality is still present after the addition of normal serum, phospholipids are added back to assess whether the clotting prolongation normalizes. This confirms that the antibody prolonging the agent is one that reacts with a phospholipid. It is important that one uses a laboratory that does confirmatory testing and not just an initial screen.

DIAGNOSIS

Diagnosis of the disorder is based on the presence of these antibodies on two separate occasions a minimum of 6 weeks apart, although recent recommendations are to test for these antibodies 12 weeks apart. In cases of high clinical suspicion it is important to test for both the lupus anticoagulant and the anticardiolipin antibody, as many patients will have the presence of only one of these categories of antibodies. In addition to the laboratory criteria one of the following clinical criteria must be met: (1) a venous or arterial thrombotic event or (2) poor pregnancy outcome as defined by three or more first-trimester spontaneous abortions, unexplained death at ≥10 weeks of gestation or one or more premature births before 34 weeks.

TREATMENT

Treatment of the nonobstetrical clotting complications includes lifelong anticoagulation. (The treatment of the obstetrical complications are beyond the scope of this chapter.) The International Normalized Ratio (INR) should be maintained between 2.5 and 3.5 in order to circumvent bleeding while minimizing the risk of recurrent thrombotic events.

SJÖGREN SYNDROME

Sjögren syndrome is a disorder in which damage done to the lacrimal ducts and the salivary glands results in dry eyes and dry mouth. This disorder can be seen alone (primary) or in conjunction with other rheumatologic disorders, rheumatoid arthritis being the most common. The disorder is more common in women, in particular during the fourth and fifth decades of life. The pathophysiology of Sjögren syndrome is that lymphocytic infiltrates of the lacrimal and salivary glands result in damage. The parotid glands can be involved as well, and approximately 60% of patients may present with parotid gland or salivary gland swelling. This damage causes the decrease of tear production and salivary production and associated clinical findings. Most of the clinical findings can be traced to the glandular damage, but extraglandular involvement can also occur.

CLINICAL

Keratoconjunctivitis Sicca

The damage to the lacrimal ducts causes decreased tear formation. As a result, the eyes are not as well lubricated. Usually patients will present with symptoms of dry and gritty eyes. Burning, blurriness, and photosensitivity can likewise occur. Later on, severe dryness can cause corneal epithelial damage. On exam, the eyes may appear injected, and the lacrimal glands enlarged. Testing for tear formation in a designated period of time (Schirmer test) can be used to confirm poor tear formation. Rose Bengal staining with slit lamp examination is also helpful for evaluating damage to the corneal epithelium

Xerostomia

Lymphocytic infiltration of the salivary glands with resultant damage leads to decreased salivary production in Sjögren syndrome. As a result, patients will suffer from mouth dryness. In addition to mouth dryness, patients complain of difficulty swallowing food or difficulty talking for long periods of time. Over time, the poor salivary production contributes to dental caries. Persistent dryness can also predispose to *Candida* infections in these patients. On exam, poor salivary pooling and dry mucosa are seen. In addition, poor dentition may also be present. Objective testing of salivary flow can be helpful.

Vaginal Dryness

Women with Sjögren syndrome can develop vaginal dryness as a result of decreased vaginal secretions. Increased urinary tract infections, local irritation, and dyspareunia can occur.

DIAGNOSIS

The diagnosis of Sjögren's syndrome is suggested by the clinical presentation of ocular and oral cavity dryness. In individuals who have ocular dryness a Schirmer's test may be positive. The definitive way to make the diagnosis is by salivary gland biopsy most often vis-à-vis a lip biopsy. Pathology reveals a CD4 T cell predominant lymphocytic infiltrate. About half of individuals with Sjögren's syndrome will have positive anti-Ro and anti-La antibodies. Treatment is symptomatic with lubricating and cholinergic agents and is often initiated in the absence of a biopsy.

About half of individuals with Sjögren syndrome will have positive anti-Ro and anti-La antibodies.

OTHER CLINICAL FINDINGS

Individuals with Sjögren syndrome can report systemic symptoms such as fatigue, myalgias, low-grade temperatures, and arthralgias. Dryness in the upper respiratory tract can predispose to recurrent infections and pneumonitis. Small-vessel and medium-vessel vasculitis have been reported in individuals who have Sjögren syndrome. This presentation is not specific to Sjögren as individuals will present with classic findings of small-vessel vasculitis such as palpable purpura and skin ulcerations. Rarely mononeuritis multiplex can occur. Peripheral neuropathies have been seen in individuals with Sjögren. It is unusual for individuals with Sjögren syndrome to develop erosive arthritis without the presence of a coexisting disease such as rheumatoid arthritis. Nonetheless, close to half of patients with Sjögren syndrome will present with joint pain and in some cases synovitis. Upper gastrointestinal tract dryness can lead to difficulty in swallowing. Rarely, lymphocytic infiltration in the stomach can lead to atrophic gastritis. Glomerulonephritis and interstitial nephritis are rare manifestations of Sjögren syndrome. However, up to one-third of patients can have tubular disease including renal tubular acidosis. Non-Hodgkin lymphoma is found in about 2.5% of patients with Sjögren disease, a rate that is significantly higher than that in the rest of the population.

Treatment for the disorder is primarily directed at symptom control as up until this time there has not been any approved medication for disease prevention. Avoidance of medications that may have anticholinergic effects is important. For the eyes, lubricating eye drops are used. In cases in which that is insufficient, immunosuppressive eye drops containing cyclosporine may be used. If these measures do not work, then plugs for the tear ducts can be placed to maintain moisture formation. For the mouth, trying to encourage saliva production by sucking on with sugar-free candies and chewing gum can help. Most patients will take frequent sips of water or other liquids to keep the mouth moist as well. In addition, it appears to delay the onset of dental caries. Cholinergic agents such as pilocarpine can help in more severe cases. Cevimeline may also help; however, in both medications, treatment is usually limited by side effects of flushing and sweating. Whether some of the newer B-cell therapies will have a role in Sjögren disease is unclear.

PROGRESSIVE SYSTEMIC SCLEROSIS (LIMITED AND DIFFUSE)

Progressive systemic sclerosis, limited and diffuse, or scleroderma, are relatively rare diseases characterized by skin thickening and vascular abnormalities. One to two individuals per 100,000 are impacted with this disorder, and there is an increased incidence in women in their fifth to seventh decades of life. Vasospasm and hypertrophy of blood vessels can occur that can lead to organ damage. Fibrotic changes of the skin lead to thickening of the cutaneous tissue. Pulmonary disease is seen in both limited and diffuse systemic sclerosis, whereas renal disease is limited to the diffuse form. How the immune system mediates these changes is not well understood.

Systemic sclerosis can occur in three major forms. Limited progressive systemic sclerosis, also referred to as CREST, diffuse progressive systemic sclerosis, and rarely scleroderma sine scleroderma in which individuals may get the systemic symptoms of systemic sclerosis without the skin findings. The latter finding is beyond the scope of this chapter.

LIMITED SYSTEMIC SCLEROSIS (CREST)

In limited systemic sclerosis, the skin findings are limited to the hands and the face. Patients will have features of CREST syndrome (calcinosis, Raynaud's, esophageal dysmotility, sclerodactyly, and telangiectasias). Most often, patients will have some but not all components of this disorder. Calcinosis is the deposition of calcium deposits under the skin. It is more commonly seen in the pediatric rather than the adult population. In Raynaud's phenomenon, the primary lesion is vascular spasm in response to cold or emotion. Typically the findings occur in the hands and the feet. At first, digits can have a bluish or white discoloration, often with a sharp demarcation dividing involved and uninvolved regions; the digits will then turn red on reperfusion. Esophageal dysmotility occurs when the distal esophagus becomes fibrosed and normal peristalsis can not occur. Manifestations include severe reflux, heartburn, and cough. Eventually esophageal strictures and swallowing difficulties may happen. Sclerodactyly refers to the thickening of the skin of the digits. The fingers will appear thickened and waxy. Examination of the capillaries of the fingers will reveal capillary dilatation.

Telangiectasias are small dilatations of vessels that mainly occur on the face and chest. Roughly 10% of individuals with limited systemic sclerosis can develop pulmonary hypertension. Mortality among this subgroup is quite high, although the prognosis among individuals without pulmonary involvement is excellent.

PROGRESSIVE SYSTEMIC SCLEROSIS

Individuals with progressive systemic sclerosis will have more widespread skin involvement that includes the arms, trunk, chest, and legs. These patients are more likely to have internal organ involvement including renal disease, pulmonary disease, and cardiac disease. Morbidity and mortality is quite high.

On physical exam, skin tightening and thickening can occur over the face arms trunk and lower extremities. In both limited and diffuse systemic sclerosis, narrowing of the oral aperture can occur. Individuals who have Raynaud's can have digital ulcers, and the skin involvement of the hands itself can cause bone reabsorption and autoamputation.

Diagnosis is made by clinical findings. Laboratory testing should include an ANA. Anticentromere antibodies are more likely to be positive in limited systemic sclerosis, whereas anti-Scl-70 (topoisomerase I) is more likely to be positive in those with diffuse systemic sclerosis.

ORGAN INVOLVEMENT

Cutaneous

Initially the skin appears swollen and inflamed, and eventually thickening with fibrosis occurs. The hands, arms, chest, and abdomen are most common, although the thighs, legs, and feet are involved. By definition, those with limited disease have skin changes only on the face, neck, and hands up to the wrist. Pigment changes can occur as well. Severe tightening of the skin of the hands can contribute to acrolysis of the distal digits and fixed deformities.

Pulmonary Disease

Pulmonary disease is the major cause of mortality in individuals with both limited and diffuse progressive systemic sclerosis. Close to one-third of individuals with diffuse disease have involvement of the lungs, whereas about 10% of individuals with limited disease will develop pulmonary hypertension. Restrictive lung disease and interstitial fibrosis can occur. Patients present with shortness of breath and fatigue. On exam dry bibasilar crackles are seen, and often elevated right-sided cardiac pressures suggestive of pulmonary hypertension can be found. Often the diagnosis needs to be made by high-resolution CT scan, as a plain radiograph can underestimate disease involvement.

Although individuals with CREST syndrome do not progress in terms of the skin involvement other than that seen on the face and on the hands, they remain at risk for pulmonary disease. Pulmonary fibrosis and pulmonary hypertension can be long-term sequelae. Patients will present with a dry cough, shortness of breath, and exertional limitations. There is a significant mortality with this manifestation.

Renal Disease

Roughly one-half of patients with progressive systemic sclerosis will have involvement of their kidneys. Patients will present with hypertension and proteinuria but a surprisingly bland urinary sediment. Scleroderma renal crisis is a rare finding in which sudden elevated blood pressure, hemolytic anemia, and renal insufficiency can occur. There are some suggestions that steroid therapy increases the risk of renal crisis in these patients. Other risk factors include diffuse disease. The use of angiotensin-converting enzyme (ACE) inhibitors has greatly reduced the onset of scleroderma renal crisis.

Cardiac Disease

Cardiac disease secondary to pulmonary hypertension and systemic hypertension is found in individuals with systemic sclerosis. This can lead to congestive heart failure. Pericarditis and pericardial effusions can occur, with fibrosis of the pericardium noted. In diffuse systemic sclerosis, myocardial fibrosis and vasospasm of the small vessels can lead to ventricular dysfunction. Fibrotic depositions in the conduction system can cause arrhythmias.

Gastrointestinal Disease

Esophageal dysmotility occurs in most patient with progressive and limited systemic sclerosis. Chronic reflux, aspiration, and esophageal strictures can occur. The stomach can be involved in systemic sclerosis. Gastritis can occur. The small and large intestines can be involved as well with poor motility leading to bacterial overgrowth.

Musculoskeletal Involvement

Rarely patients develop an inflammatory arthritis; however, sclerodactyly can lead to contractions and limited mobility. Myositis can also be seen.

TREATMENT

Unfortunately, there has been no proven therapy for systemic sclerosis. For many years, penicillamine was used with the hope of arresting the skin involvement, but its high toxicity and limited efficacy have decreased its use. Other studies have looked at methotrexate and cyclosporine, but the results are disappointing. The data on mycophenolate mofetil and cyclophosphamide are equivocal but some clinicians will use these medications in persons with systemic sclerosis in particular if there is lung involvement. The biggest improvement in treatment has been in the use of ACE inhibitors for the management of renal disease. Calcium channel blockers are used for the management of Raynaud's. Several trials evaluating cyclophosphamide for the management of pulmonary disease have shown a modest improvement in symptoms. Other agents such as bosentan and sildenafil citrate have likewise been employed with some modest benefits.

OVERLAP SYNDROMES AND MIXED CONNECTIVE TISSUE DISEASE

Some individuals will clearly present with features that are suggestive of a collagen vascular disease, yet they may not neatly fit into a clear diagnostic category. For example, an individual may present with arthritis, Raynaud's, sclerodactyly, and myositis, thereby not clearly fitting into the category of either SLE or progressive systemic sclerosis. Alternatively, patients may present with polymyositis and interstitial lung disease. The most common disorder that falls into this category is mixed connective tissue disease (MCTD).

MCTD is a sister disorder to SLE. Like SLE, this disorder is most frequently found in women of childbearing age; however, it does not have a predilection for those of African ancestry. These individuals are often initially diagnosed as having SLE because there are many features in common. In general, Raynaud's phenomenon and synovitis are more common findings. Renal disease is rare. These patients are more likely to have lung disease than lupus patients, and the lung involvement can lead to pulmonary hypertension. In addition, they may have myositis. Changes of the hands from chronic vasospasm of Raynaud's can occur. Many of these patients have a very high-titer ANA, and the anti-RNP antibody is often positive. Treatment is similar to that for SLE with the use of antimalarials and nonsteroidal anti-inflammatory medications. Corticosteroids can be used for more significant manifestations such as myositis or pulmonary involvement. Immunosuppression with azathioprine and methotrexate can help. Occasionally, cytotoxic therapy is used for severe lung disease and other systemic involvement.

IDIOPATHIC INFLAMMATORY MYOPATHIES: POLYMYOSITIS, DERMATOMYOSITIS, AND INCLUSION-BODY MYOSITIS

Idiopathic inflammatory myopathies are rare disorders. Polymyositis and dermatomyositis have an increased incidence in women. There is a bimodal distribution of disease onset with the peak incidence of these diseases occurring in early childhood and then again in the fourth and fifth decades of life. In polymyositis, the involvement is restricted to the muscles and occasionally the lungs, whereas in dermatomyositis, the skin can be involved as well. Inclusion-body myositis is rarer still, more likely affecting middle-aged men.

CLINICAL SYMPTOMS

Individuals with polymyositis and dermatomyositis present with weakness in the proximal muscles. Activities such as combing one's hair, reaching, lifting, getting out of a chair, and walking up and down stairs are difficult. In general, weakness in the lower extremities is noticed first. In more pronounced disease difficulty swallowing and breathing can be problematic, as individuals may have esophageal muscle weakness and respiratory muscle weakness. Some patients may present with muscle achiness and pain on palpation, especially during the acute phase. For those with inclusion-body myositis, symptoms have a slower onset, and more distal muscles are involved. Profound loss of muscle mass can occur prior to presenting to a physician. On physical exam proximal muscle weakness is found in particular in the neck flexors, upper arms, and hip flexors in individuals with polymyositis and dermatomyositis. For those with inclusion-body myositis, distal involvement can occur.

Skin

Those individuals with dermatomyositis may have distinct skin findings. Gottron papules are reddish scaly patches that appear over the knuckles of the hands and may occur over the extensor surfaces of the elbows as well. Individuals with dermatomyositis may also have a reddish purplish rash around the eyes and on the eyelids, referred to as a heliotropic rash. A rash over the neck and trunk in a distribution that looks like a shawl is also found. In dermatomyositis, nail bed changes with overgrowth of the cuticle can be seen. In both polymyositis and dermatomyositis patients may present with rough skin and cracking skin on the fingers, which is referred to as "mechanic's hands."

Pulmonary

In addition to muscle weakness leading to shortness of breath, interstitial lung disease occurs in up to 10% of all myositis patients and 50% of patients who have the anti-Jo-1 antibody. Individuals will present with dyspnea on exertion and a nonproductive cough, and they may be hypoxemic. Muscle weakness can cause a restrictive picture on pulmonary function tests. Swallowing difficulties can lead to chronic aspiration and resultant pulmonary disease.

On exam, dry crackles are heard, and decreased diffusion capacity is found on pulmonary function tests.

Cardiac

Rarely patients will have involvement of the cardiac conduction system that can lead to either heart block or arrhythmias. Global cardiomyopathy is very unusual.

Gastrointestinal

Most of the gastrointestinal abnormalities seen in the inflammatory myopathies are due to muscle dysfunction along the gastrointestinal tract. Reflux, abnormal peristalsis, and delayed gastric emptying have all been described.

LABORATORY ABNORMALITIES

Elevation of the creatinine kinase is found. Aldolase, another muscle enzyme, is often increased. Serum aspartate aminotransferase (AST), and alanine aminotransferase (ALT) are also often elevated. Many of these patients will have the presence of antinuclear antibodies. Anti-Jo1 antibodies are thought to be associated with pulmonary disease and suggest a worse prognosis.

DIFFERENTIAL DIAGNOSIS

Other clinical presentations that can mimic those of idiopathic inflammatory muscle disease include thyroid disease, toxic metabolic syndromes, drug reactions, steroid myopathy, and some infectious diseases. Fixed errors of metabolism that lead to elevations of creatinine kinase and weakness, in particular after exercise, can be difficult to distinguish from idiopathic inflammatory myopathies.

DIAGNOSIS

The diagnosis of an inflammatory muscle disease is first based on a high clinical suspicion. Laboratory testing is helpful as the majority of these individuals will have significant elevations in their muscle enzymes such as creatinine kinase levels and aldolase levels. In addition, elevated liver function tests can occur. Electromyography (EMG) findings are characteristic of these disorders and can be helpful in determining the diagnosis. There was some initial excitement for the use of magnetic resonance scanning for the diagnosis of inflammatory muscle disease; however, it has not been as helpful as initially anticipated. Magnetic resonance imaging (MRI) scanning can be useful to identify an area of inflammation that is likely to yield a good biopsy specimen. The gold standard for diagnosis remains the muscle biopsy. In dermatomyositis, perivascular inflammation around the muscle fibers is found, whereas in polymyositis, the inflammation is found within the muscle fibers. Special staining and electron microscopy are necessary to make the diagnosis of inclusion-body myositis. Findings in this disorder include eosinophilic and basophilic granules in the vacuoles. There are also abnormal tubular filaments of unknown significance.

MALIGNANCY ASSOCIATION

Both polymyositis and dermatomyositis are associated with a higher incidence of malignancies, dermatomyositis even more so than polymyositis. In cases of associated malignancies, most malignancies are diagnosed within 2 years of the initial diagnosis of muscle disease. Because of the increased risk for cancer in individuals who present with these disorders, it is recommended that an age-appropriate malignancy screening be performed (mammograms, colonoscopy, PSA, chest radiographs).

TREATMENT

The treatment of polymyositis/dermatomyositis is focused on rapid reduction of muscle inflammation. High-dose steroids (1 mg/kg of prednisone equivalent) are generally given for the first 6 weeks of therapy. After that time period, and depending on the individual's response to treatment, this medication may be tapered. Azathioprine or methotrexate up to 25 mg a week can be added both to hasten disease improvement and also as a steroid-sparing agent. In cases refractory to these measures, intravenous immunoglobulin (IVIG) has been used successfully. More recently, clinicians have been evaluating the tumor necrosis factor (TNF-α)blockers as therapeutic agents for this disorder. Anti-B-cell therapy such as rituximab for the treatment of inflammatory myositis has been studied. The initial data using this drug were not encouraging. For all treatments, the physical exam for muscle strength and measuring muscle enzymes such as creatinine kinase and aldolase are useful ways to monitor response to therapy. Once the active phase of inflammation has been controlled, physical rehabilitation to regain strength is important. Speech and swallowing therapy can be employed to improve swallowing. The treatment options for inclusion-body myositis are more limited, as there has been no proven therapy for this disorder.

SUMMARY

SLE, antiphospholipid syndrome, progressive systemic sclerosis, connective tissue disease, and the inflammatory myopathies are systemic diseases that often affect multiple organ systems. These disorders can be challenging to diagnose because there is not a laboratory test that by itself makes the diagnosis; rather, the correct clinical presentation in conjunction with laboratory testing are required. Previously, diseases such as SLE, progressive systemic sclerosis, and

inflammatory myopathies had a grim prognosis but now with improved recognition and earlier initiation of therapy the outcome is significantly better. It is our hope that, with better understanding of the pathophysiology of these disorders and the development of newer therapies, our treatment of these disorders will continue to improve.

ADDITIONAL READING

Asherson RA, Khamashta MA, Ordi-Ros J, et al. The "primary" antiphospholipid syndrome: Major clinical and serological features. *Medicine (Baltimore).* 1989;68:366–74.

Bitali C, Bombardieri S, Moutsopoulos HM, et al. Preliminary criteria for the classification of Sjogren's syndrome. Results of a prospective concerted action supported by the European community. *Arthritis Rheum.* 1992;36:340–8

Black CM. Scleroderma—clinical aspects. *J Intern Med.* 1993;234:115–118

Brandt JT, Triplett DA, Alving B, Scharrer I; on behalf of the Subcommittee on Lupus Anticoagulant/Antiphospholipid Antibody of the Scientific and Standardisation Committee of the ISTH. Criteria for the diagnosis of lupus anticoagulants: An update. *Thromb Haemostas.* 1995;74:1185–1190.

Cervera R, Piette JC, Font J, et al. Antiphospholipid syndrome: Clinical and immunologic manifestations and patterns of disease expression in a cohort of 1,000 patients. *Arthritis Rheum.* 2002;46:1019–27.

Chifflot H, Fautrel B, Sordet C, et al. Incidence and prevalence of systemic sclerosis: A systematic literature review. *Semin Arthritis Rheum.* 2008;37:223–35.

Cruz DPD, Khamashta MA, Hughes GRV. Systemic lupus erythematosus. *Lancet.* 2007;369:587–96.

Dalakas MC, Hohlfeld R. Polymyositis and dermatomyositis. *Lancet.* 2003;362:971.

Dooley MA, Ginzler EM. Newer therapeutic approaches for systemic lupus erythematosus: Immunosuppressive agents. *Rheum Dis Clin North Am.* 2006;32:91–102.

Ermann J, Bermas BL. The biology behind the new therapies for SLE. *Int J Clin Pract.* 2007;61:2113–9.

LeRoy EC, Black CM, Fleischmajer R, et al. Scleroderma (systemic sclerosis): Classification, subsets and pathogenesis. *J Rheumatol.* 1988;15:202–05.

Rothfield N, Sontheimer RD, Bernstein M. Lupus erythematosus: Systemic and cutaneous manifestations. *Clin Dermatol.* 2006;24:348–62.

Swanton J, Isenberg D. Mixed connective tissue disease: Still crazy after all these years. *Rheum Dis Clin North Am.* 2005;31:421–36.

Von Muhlen CA, Tan EM. Autoantibodies in the diagnosis of systemic rheumatic diseases. *Semin Arthritis Rheum.* 1995;24:323–58.

QUESTIONS

QUESTION 1. A 21-year-old female presents to the emergency department with an 8-day history of fever, chills, malaise, nausea, and dark urine. She complains of a malar rash and pain in her wrists and finger joints. On examination her heart rate is 94 beats per minute, blood pressure is 130/70 mm Hg, temperature is 38.2°C, and oxygen saturation on room air is 97%. The remainder of the examination is unremarkable. Laboratory data show a urinalysis with 3+ blood, 2+ protein, and a urine sediment showing multiple RBCs (some dysmorphic) but no casts.

BUN 32 mg/dL, Cr 1.2 mg/dL. CBC showed a hemoglobin of 11.2 g/dL, white blood count of $9 \times 10^3/mm^3$ with a normal differential. Complements are pending, ANA was 1:160, anti-dsDNA level 640 U/L. The next step should be:

A. Admit the patient for 3 consecutive days of methylprednisolone and arrange a renal biopsy
B. Treat the patient with Plaquenil, 200 mg bid, and arrange follow-up in rheumatology clinic
C. Admit the patient and arrange for emergency plasmapheresis for presumed cryoglobulinemia
D. Start the patient on ceftriaxone, 500 mg tid, and arrange for a renal biopsy for presumed postinfectious glomerulonephritis.

QUESTION 2. All of the following statements about mixed connective disease (MCTD) are correct EXCEPT:

A. Raynaud's phenomenon and synovitis are common findings.
B. Renal disease is rare.
C. ANA is usually positive.
D. Anti-Sm antibody is positive.
E. Initial treatment is usually with plaquenil and NSAIDs.

QUESTION 3. Systemic sclerosis (scleroderma) is characterized by all of the following, EXCEPT:

A. Skin tightening
B. Raynaud's phenomenon
C. Healed pitting ulcers in fingertips
D. Telangiectasias in the perioral area, hands, and anterior chest
E. Saddle nose deformity

ANSWERS

1. A
2. D
3. E

26.

SYSTEMIC VASCULITIS

Paul F. Dellaripa

The vasculitides are a group of disorders that are characterized by the presence of inflammation in vessel walls, which leads to vascular occlusion and tissue necrosis. Systemic vasculitic syndromes can present clinically in protean fashion and may be due to a variety of mechanisms involving immune dysregulation that leads to endovascular inflammation. However, these immune mechanisms are still not well understood, and thus, one must rely on clinical, descriptive parameters for classification and treatment. This chapter focuses on well-recognized patterns of presentation, treatment guidelines, and emerging insights on pathogenic mechanisms and implications for future treatment options.

Classification of systemic vasculitides (SV) has traditionally involved dividing them along the lines of vessel size, for example, giant-cell arteritis representing large-vessel disease and hypersensitivity vasculitis representing small-vessel disease, though in reality there is significant overlap in terms of size of vessels, and such a classification offers no information on pathogenesis or unique characteristics of different vasculitic syndromes. For this discussion, we focus on disease patterns most often associated with antineutrophil cytoplasmic autoantibody (ANCA), Wegener granulomatosis, which is now known as granulomatosis with ployangiitis (GPA), microscopic polyangiitis (MPA), Churg Strauss syndrome (CSS), and other vasculitides including polyarteritis nodosa, drug-induced and cryoglobulinemic vasculitis, Takayasu arteritis, giant-cell arteritis, and Behçet disease.

CLINICAL PRESENTATION

SV should be suspected in patients who present with systemic clinical findings or symptoms for which there is no readily identifiable source of infection or malignancy. For example, unexplained persistent fever will typically be investigated for underlying infection or lymphoma but can be a prominent feature of patients with giant-cell arteritis. Other signs and symptoms, such as weight loss, night sweats, rash, mononeuritis, arthritis, and malaise without identifiable etiology can represent clinical features of an underlying vasculitis. Sometimes these findings may be embedded within a pattern that fits into a well-described syndrome, but often they do not. Clinical syndromes that can mimic vasculitis include endocarditis, atrial myxoma, and hypercoagulable states such as antiphospholipid syndrome and atheroembolism.

ANTINEUTROPHIL CYTOPLASMIC AUTOANTIBODY VASCULITIS

Generally granulomatosis with polyangiitis (GPA) Churg Strauss syndrome, and microscopic polyangiitis are often considered together as a group of similar diseases because they have shared clinical features and are associated with ANCA in most cases. All three can frequently present with a pauciimmune necrotizing glomerulonephritis (GN) and pulmonary involvement. ANCA is detected by indirect immunofluorescence on ethanol-fixed neutrophils and can exhibit a cytoplasmic pattern (cANCA) or a perinuclear pattern (pANCA). If the immunofluorescence test is positive, then an enzyme-linked immunosorbent assay (ELISA) specific for proteinase 3 (PR-3) or myeloperoxidase (MPO) is performed. Most patients with GPA are PR-3 positive (up to 80%) and rarely MPO positive, and in microscopic polyangiitis up to 79–80% of cases are MPO positive and rarely PR-3 positive. In some cases, patients with GPA may be ANCA negative. Generally speaking, patients with PR3-positive ANCA-associated disease have a greater degree of multiorgan involvement, more frequent granulomatous disease, and a higher frequency of relapse. ANCA-MPO positive may also be seen in systemic lupus erythematosus (SLE), rheumatoid arthritis (RA), scleroderma, and inflammatory bowel disease and in certain drug-induced vasculitic syndromes (such as with propylthiouracil and allopurinol).

It is thought that the pathogenesis of ANCA-associated vasculitis involves cytokines and other factors that cause the expression of ANCA antigens onto cell surfaces of neutrophils, which can then bind to existing circulating ANCA. This results in activated neutrophils, which can interact with endothelial cells via adhesion molecules and release reactive oxygen species and toxic granular enzymes, which can result in tissue necrosis. Activated neutrophils may also activate complement such as C5a and C3a, which results in inflammation and disruption of endothelial surfaces of blood vessels. Recently, direct in vivo evidence has linked myeloperoxidase to pathogenesis in a murine model that developed necrotizing and crescentic GN after injection of mouse anti-MPO IgG.

WEGENER GRANULOMATOSIS

Wegener Granulomatosis is now known as Granulomatosis with polyangiitis (GPA). GPA is a systemic vasculitis characterized by granulomatous vasculitis of the upper and lower respiratory tract, and segmental necrotizing GN that involves small blood vessels. Some patients with GPA have what is termed "limited GPA," which is confined to the upper respiratory tract.

Findings often include the following:

- Rhinitis, epistaxis, otitis media

- Hearing loss, chondritis of the ears and nose

- Cough, dyspnea, hemoptysis, subglottic stenosis

- Hematuria related to GN, progressive renal insufficiency

- Mononeuritis multiplex, central nervous system (CNS) vasculitis

- Scleritis, conjunctivitis

- Palpable purpura, granulomatous skin lesions

- Arthritis, arthralgias

One of the more common clinical patterns that can present in GPA is lower respiratory tract symptoms with active GN, referred to as the pulmonary renal syndrome. In patients who present with GN and active pulmonary symptoms, especially alveolar hemorrhage, the differential diagnosis includes GPA, microscopic polyangiitis, SLE, cryoglobulinemia, and Goodpasture disease.

Pathologically, the vessels involved in GPA include small arteries and veins. The pathology of vasculitis includes fibrinoid necrosis with inflammatory mononuclear cell infiltrates of vessel walls, focal destruction of the elastic lamina, and narrowing or obliteration of the vessel lumen. Granulomatous vasculitis may involve the lung, skin, CNS, peripheral nerves, heart, kidney and other organs.

Most patients with GPA present with symptoms referable to the upper respiratory tract, including sinusitis, nasal obstruction, rhinitis, otitis media, hearing loss, ear pain, gingival inflammation, oral and nasal ulcers, epistaxis, sore throat, laryngitis, and nasal septal deformity. Upper respiratory tract involvement may lead to damage to nasal cartilage, resulting in the "saddle-nose" deformity.

Lower respiratory tract involvement occurs in most patients, although it is seen less frequently as a presenting symptom; it may include cough, sputum production, dyspnea, chest pain, hemoptysis, and life-threatening pulmonary hemorrhage. GPA may also be associated with inflammation and subsequent scarring/stenosis of the subglottic region.

Radiographic findings include multiple, nodular, often bilateral cavitary infiltrates, but infiltrates with less well-defined margins occur as well. Other less common chest radiographic abnormalities include paratracheal masses, large cavitary lesions, and massive pleural effusion. Computed tomography (CT) of the chest may reveal pulmonary lesions that are not well demonstrated on plain radiographs.

Urinalysis reveals renal involvement in approximately 80% of patients at presentation. The typical renal lesion is segmental necrotizing glomerulonephritis. Functional renal impairment may progress rapidly if appropriate therapy is not instituted promptly.

Diagnosis

Diagnosis can be based on the clinical findings of upper and lower respiratory tract noninfectious inflammation with glomerulonephritis and positive anti-PR3 ANCA without necessarily proceeding with a biopsy, although this is the subject of some debate. In cases with more limited involvement or where ANCA titers are negative or show the less typical MPO specificity, tissue diagnosis may be necessary and can be sought at sites of active disease including nasal biopsy, lung biopsy, kidney biopsy, nerve, and even conjunctival biopsy.

Treatment

Therapy is typically based on establishment of remission with a combination of corticosteroids and cyclophosphamide and then, once remission is achieved, usually within 3–6 months, step-down therapy utilizing agents such as azathioprine, methotrexate, or mycophenolate. Trimethoprim sulfamethoxazole may limit flares of upper respiratory symptoms and is also indicated as a prophylactic agent against *Pneumocystis pneumonia* (PCP). Initial treatment with corticosteroids is generally given as prednisone, 1 mg/kg per day orally. In a critically ill patient with severe systemic involvement, pulse corticosteroid with IV methylprednisolone, 1 g per day for 3 days, is advocated, transitioning to prednisone, 1 mg/kg per day orally or its IV equivalent. Cyclophosphamide can be administered as monthly intravenous boluses or as a daily oral dose. The risks associated with cyclophosphamide include hemorrhagic cystitis, opportunistic infections such as PCP and fungal infection, and the long-term, lifelong risk of bladder cancer, lymphoma, and leukemia. Emerging data suggest a role for B-cell–deleting therapy such as rituximab in patients with persistent ANCA positivity and recurrent disease.

MICROSCOPIC POLYANGIITIS

Microscopic polyangiitis is a necrotizing vasculitis that involves small vessels, capillaries, and venules, and presents predominately with segmental necrotizing glomerulonephritis. The patient may have concomitant evidence of alveolar hemorrhage in about a third of cases, which sometimes makes it difficult to distinguish between GPA and MPA and pathologically the lesions may be indistinguishable. Neuropathy and cutaneous vasculitis may also occur with microscopic polyangiitis, and, as noted previously, ANCA expression occurs in up to 80% of cases and nearly always specific for MPO. Treatment is similar to that for GPA.

In some cases of patients who present with severe manifestations of the pulmonary renal syndrome, the precise diagnosis may not be apparent and may include ANCA-associated disease, lupus and antiglomerular basement disease. In such cases where end organ failure is imminent and life-threatening, therapy with high-dose steroids, cytotoxic therapy, and plasmapheresis may be considered a clear diagnosis is evident.

CHURG STRAUSS SYNDROME

Churg Strauss syndrome is a disease characterized by the presence of eosinophilic infiltrates, granulomas in the respiratory tract, and necrotizing vasculitis in the setting of asthma and peripheral eosinophilia. The disease typically affects small to medium-sized muscular arteries, most frequently of the upper respiratory tract and the lungs. Patients with CSS present most often with a background history of asthma, in some cases lasting for many years, and then develop constitutional symptoms of weight loss followed by various forms of organ involvement including pulmonary infiltrates, mononeuritis, cardiomyopathy, cutaneous vasculitis, and GI tract involvement. Renal involvement is less frequent than in GPA or MPA, occurring in up to 40% of patients. Clinical manifestations of disease may become evident in some patients who are treated with leukotriene inhibitors and undergo steroid taper, though it is not believed that leukotriene inhibitors are themselves causative of CSS. ANCA to myeloperoxidase is positive in up to 40–60% of cases and seems to be positive in those patients with mononeuritis, cutaneous vasculitis, and glomerulonephritis.

Treatment

Treatment in CSS is high-dose corticosteroids. In patients with more than one of five prognostic factors (the Five Factor Score which includes proteinuria greater than 1 g, azotemia, cardiomyopathy, and GI and CNS involvement), therapy with cytotoxic agents may be warranted.

POLYARTERITIS NODOSA

Polyarteritis nodosa (PAN) is a rare disorder that involves small and medium-sized arteries. The GI tract, skin (often ulcers), and nerves with are most commonly affected, although virtually any organ can be affected. Patients may complain of weight loss, fatigue, fevers, and abdominal pain, and they may develop hypertension and azotemia with proteinuria as well as cardiac and CNS involvement. Glomerulonephritis and lung disease are rare. GI involvement is an important source of morbidity, which may be due to acute GI bleeding, perforation, and mesenteric thrombosis.

The pathogenesis of PAN is unknown. Hepatitis B surface antigen is noted in a small number (<10%) of patients, suggesting a role for circulating immune complexes in some cases of PAN. Pathology shows fibrinoid necrosis and pleomorphic cellular infiltration of lymphocytes, macrophages, and polymorphonuclear leukocytes involving the entire wall of blood vessel.

Diagnosis

Patients with PAN often have elevated markers of inflammation such as C-reactive protein (CRP) and erythrocyte sedimentation rate (ESR), although antinuclear antibodies (ANA), rheumatoid factor (RF), and ANCA are not typically present. Diagnosis is made either by biopsy of specific organs affected (such as sural nerve, skin, or muscle) or identification of characteristic aneurysms of the renal, hepatic, or mesenteric vessels on mesenteric angiogram, recalling, however, that microaneurysms can be seen in other conditions such as atrial myxoma, Ehlers-Danlos, and endocarditis, among other conditions.

Treatment

Corticosteroids are the treatment for PAN, in high doses, and in severe cases IV methylprednisolone, 1 g for several days, is reasonable. The use of a cytotoxic agent such as cyclophosphamide is guided by severity of illness and the Five Factor Score mentioned previously. Where PAN is associated with hepatitis B, concomitant use of immunosuppressive therapy and antiviral therapy directed against hepatitis B may be useful.

DRUG-INDUCED VASCULITIS

Certain drugs and vaccines can cause vasculitis through a variety of mechanisms. These have often been termed hypersensitivity vasculitides. For example, leukocytoclastic vasculitis (leukocytoclasis meaning nuclear fragmentation) involving small vessels might occur because of an antibiotic that results in the deposition of immune complexes within vessel walls, whereas another drug (such as propylthiouracil) may cause a systemic vasculitis that is related to the production of ANCA. In general, cases of drug-induced vasculitis can cause a self-limiting illness that resolves with discontinuation of the offending agent or can lead to multiorgan involvement. However, more severe cases can present with severe ulcerative skin lesions or renal, GI, or neurological involvement that may require corticosteroids or, rarely, other immunosuppressive agents.

Some commonly used drugs known to result in vasculitis include these:

- Hydralazine
- Minocycline
- PTU (propylthiouracil)
- Allopurinol
- Phenytoin
- Penicillins/cephalosporins/quinolones
- Vaccines (hepatitis B, influenza)

CRYOGLOBULINEMIC VASCULITIS

Cryoglobulins are immunoglobulins that precipitate below 37°C. Type I is associated with myeloproliferative disorders; types II (mixed essential) and III (mixed polyclonal) are most often associated with hepatitis C. Cryoglobulinemic vasculitis can lead to immune complex deposition in vessel walls, resulting in cutaneous vasculitis, arthritis, and neuropathy, although on occasion life-threatening renal, GI, and pulmonary disease can also occur. Laboratory features include low-level C4, high RF, and elevated liver enzymes that may be indicative of hepatitis C infection. Therapy in severe cases consists of CS and sometimes other immunosuppressives such as cyclophosphamide (with concern for increased replication of hepatitis C), plasmapheresis, and consideration of treatment with antiviral therapy such as ribavirin and interferon-α if hepatitis C is present.

Other vasculitic syndromes in which immune complex deposition plays a significant role in pathogenesis include vasculitis related to rheumatic disorder such as SLE or RA, infection-associated vasculitis, malignancy-associated vasculitis, and Henoch-Schönlein purpura.

GIANT-CELL ARTERITIS AND TAKAYASU ARTERITIS

GCA and TA are both large-vessel vasculitides that are pathologically indistinguishable, often with evidence of granulomatous disease. Available evidence suggests that the etiologies of GCA and TA are related to cell-mediated processes and expression of various cytokines and chemokines such as IL-6, CCL-2, and interleukin-1B.

GCA is a large-vessel vasculitis with characteristic granulomatous and lymphocytic infiltration of arterial walls that presents in patents over the age of 50, but more often over the age of 60. Symptoms of GCA include:

- Headache, scalp tenderness
- Visual blurriness and visual loss including blindness
- Jaw claudication due to involvement of the facial artery
- Claudication of the upper and lower extremities
- Polymyalgia rheumatica
- Weight loss, fatigue, and fever

Laboratory evaluation frequently reveals elevated markers of inflammation such as CRP, ESR, and alkaline phosphatase, although in about 15% of patients the ESR may be normal. Regardless of the laboratory findings, if there is significant suspicion for the diagnosis, then a temporal artery biopsy should be performed. If the patient is experiencing visual symptoms at the time of consideration of the diagnosis, high-dose corticosteroid therapy should be instituted immediately to prevent permanent visual loss; then a temporal artery biopsy should be obtained as soon as possible. Biopsy findings may persist in patients with GCA for up to several weeks on corticosteroid therapy. If the initial biopsy is negative, the contralateral temporal artery may offer a small additional yield diagnostically, although in some patients in whom both biopsies are negative, it may be necessary to treat because the index of suspicion is high. In general, a negative biopsy evaluation (where both are done when the first is negative) has a negative predictive value of >91%. Ultrasound and magnetic resonance angiography (MRA) of the temporal arteries are under investigation as diagnostic tools.

Therapy with steroids involves prednisone at 1 mg/kg for at least 1 month and then a slow taper to about 20 mg per day at month 3 and then a continued taper to prevent relapse of symptoms. Therapy may last at least 2 years and many more years in other cases. Use of other steroid agents such as tumor necrosis factor (TNF) inhibitors has been disappointing in clinical studies, and other drugs such as methotrexate (MTX) or azathioprine may be useful, although studies supporting their use have shown mixed results.

TA is a large-vessel vasculitis that involves the aorta and branches of the aorta and affects predominately females up to the age of 50. Patients will typically present with claudication of the upper or lower extremities, especially involving the subclavian arteries, although the diagnosis should be considered in any young patient with diminished pulse and constitutional symptoms. The aorta on imaging can develop aneurysms; stenosis of the large vessels and aortic valve regurgitation may occur. Constitutional symptoms such as fatigue, headache, and weight loss are often noted prior to claudication, and hypertension can occur as well. CNS events secondary to carotid and vertebral artery involvement and intestinal ischemia have been noted.

Diagnosis should be suspected in a young patient, particularly female, with constitutional symptoms and absent or diminished pulses or bruits on examination. Although the ESR may be elevated, it may be only modestly elevated or normal in some cases and is not always indicative of disease activity. Areas of stenosis or aneurysm can be noted with MRA, computed tomography angiography (CTA), or conventional angiography. Treatment is high doses of corticosteroids, although some patients will not respond without addition of cytotoxic therapy. Emerging evidence suggests a role for TNF inhibitors and interventional vascular techniques such as stenting and angioplasty.

BEHÇET DISEASE

Behçet disease is characterized by the presence of recurrent aphthous or genital stomatitis that can, in a subset of patients, also exhibit vasculitis of various size vessels resulting in ocular involvement, intracranial hemorrhage, meningoencephalitis, and stroke. It is primarily a clinical diagnosis, and treatment can vary from colchicine for aphthous ulcers to corticosteroids and cytotoxic therapy in severe cases. TNF inhibition may be beneficial in some patients.

PRIMARY CNS VASCULITIS

Primary CNS vasculitis (PACNS) is a rare entity with protean manifestations including seizure, stroke, meningoencephalitis, and cranial nerve deficits. It is important to exclude secondary causes of CNS involvement of many of the above-mentioned vasculitides, other rheumatic diseases including SLE, APS, Sjögren disease, sarcoidosis, infections such as tuberculosis, HIV, and Lyme, and a variety of drugs including cocaine, methamphetamines, and heroin. Diagnosis is suggested by cerebrospinal fluid (CSF) abnormalities including elevated protein and cell counts and abnormalities on magnetic resonance imaging (MRI). Although angiography may in some cases show classic findings of vasculitis, a biopsy of suspected areas is frequently necessary to make the diagnosis. Treatment includes high doses of corticosteroids and sometimes cytotoxic agents, although there is a paucity of clinical trials to make definitive treatment recommendation with this rare disorder.

TREATMENT STRATEGIES IN VASCULITIS

It is important to note that morbidity in vasculitides can be tied not only to end-organ effects of disease but to the treatment used to control the underlying disease. Morbidity associated with corticosteroids is well documented, including diabetes, osteoporosis, infection, poor wound healing, cataracts, hypertension, and obesity, among many other side effects. Cytotoxic agents such as cyclophosphamide also have many side effects including heightening risk of opportunistic infection such as PCP, fungal infections, and the risk of cancer and sterility. As a consequence, four important points regarding vasculitis treatment need to be emphasized:

1. In a patient with known vasculitis who presents with clinical deterioration, a source of infection should be pursued aggressively prior to escalating immunosuppressive therapy.

2. In severe cases of vasculitis, aggressive immunosuppressive therapy such as cyclophosphamide is utilized, and then, after remission has been achieved, less toxic agents such as MTX, azathioprine, or mycophenolate mofetil are used in a step-down approach. Dose adjustments in renal failure are important to consider with both cyclophosphamide and methotrexate.

3. When patients are started on immunosuppressive therapy, prophylaxis for PCP should be used, immunizations against influenza and pneumococcal pneumonia should be given, and osteoporosis prophylaxis should be offered in appropriate circumstances.

4. The role of plasmapheresis and intravenous immunoglobulin is unclear in the vasculitides, but these may be considered in life-threatening cases where response to standard cytotoxic therapy with steroids is insufficient, especially in the pulmonary renal syndrome.

ADDITIONAL READING

Falk RJ, Jennette JC. ANCA disease: Where is this field heading? *J Am Soc Nephrol.* 2010;21(5):745–52.

Gómez-Puerta JA, Bosch X. Anti-neutrophil cytoplasmic antibody pathogenesis in small-vessel vasculitis: An update. *Am J Pathol.* 2009;175(5):1790–8.

Harper L. Recent advances to achieve remission induction in anti-neutrophil cytoplasmic antibody-associated vasculitis. *Curr Opin Rheumatol.* 2010;22(1):37–42.

Hellmich B. Update on the management of systemic vasculitis: What did we learn in 2009? *Clin Exp Rheumatol.* 2010;28(1 Suppl 57):98–103.

Jennett JC, Falk RJ. New insights in the pathogenesis of vasculitis associated with antineutrophil cytoplasmic autoantibodies. *Curr Opin Rheumatol.* 2008;20:55–60.

Krause I, Weinberger A. Behcet's disease. *Curr Opin Rheumatol.* 2007;20(1):82–7.

Maksimowicz-McKinnon K, Hoffman GS. Takayasu's arteritis: What is the long term prognosis. *Rheum Dis Clin North Am.* 2007;33(4):777–86.

Miller A, Chan M, Wiik A, Misbah SA, Luqmani RA. An approach to the diagnosis and management of systemic vasculitis. *Clin Exp Immunol.* 2010;160(2):143–60.

Stone JH, Calabrese LH, Hoffman GS, et al. Vasculitis: A collection of pearls and myths. *Rheum Dis Clin North Am.* 2001;27(4):677–728.

QUESTIONS

QUESTION 1. A 74-year-old male is hospitalized with hemoptysis over a period of a few days. He had a prodrome of malaise and arthralgia for several weeks. In the ICU his serum creatinine is 7.4 mg/dL, urinalysis shows 3+ protein, many

RBCs, and scattered red cell casts. He is intubated with copious bloody secretions evident from the endotracheal tube.

Which tests should be considered as part of the diagnostic evaluation in this patient?

A. Anti-Sm antibodies
B. Anti-GBM antibodies
C. pANCA MPO (myeloperoxidase)
D. cANCA PR3 (proteinase 3)
E. All of the above

QUESTION 2. A 45-year-old male with long-standing asthma is evaluated for new-onset fever, fatigue, skin rash, and worsening dyspnea. He had been using his albuterol inhaler more frequently and requiring more oral steroids and was recently started on a leukotriene antagonist. He complains of diffuse abdominal pain, and his CXR shows bilateral patchy infiltrates; his WBC count is 15,000/μL with 25% eos. His exam is notable for palpable purpura and weakness in the wrist flexors on his left.

Which of the following is the correct next step?

A. Increase inhaled steroids
B. Begin plasmapheresis
C. Increase his prednisone from 10 mg to 20 mg orally per day

D. Begin intravenous corticosteroids
E. Perform an open lung biopsy

QUESTION 3. A 70-year-old female with a history of hypertension presents with fatigue and pain in her shoulders and hips for 1 month. She notes pain in her jaw with chewing but no headaches or visual complaints. Her ESR was 18, CRP 2.0, and remaining labs normal. The exam is notable for a BP 140/80, HR 80, RR 12, weight 60 kg. Vision is normal, no scalp tenderness, but there is tenderness over the facial artery on the left.

What would be the next best step in the care of this patient?

A. Begin prednisone, 20 mg per day
B. Order a temporal artery biopsy
C. Repeat ESR and follow the patient carefully
D. Order a temporal artery ultrasound
E. Begin prednisone, 60 mg per day

ANSWERS

1. E
2. D
3. E

27.

COMMON SOFT TISSUE PAIN SYNDROMES

Simon M. Helfgott

The soft tissue pain syndromes are among the most common conditions that a primary care physician encounters in daily practice. They are characterized by local or regional pain and discomfort, often made worse by palpation of the adjacent soft tissue or movement of the nearby joint. When they involve the soft tissues near a joint, they can be associated with decreased range of motion of the joint, and the resultant loss of function can be significant. The diagnosis is clinical and based on the history and physical examination of the patient. Imaging and lab testing, when indicated, may help eliminate other diagnoses such as fracture or significant arthritis damage but rarely confirm a soft tissue pain syndrome. Thus, it may not be surprising that many patients are either undiagnosed or misdiagnosed, leading to costly evaluations including unnecessary imaging and costly therapeutics. This chapter reviews some of the more common forms of soft tissue pain syndromes, their clinical presentations, the physical examination findings, and the appropriate management of these conditions.

CLASSIFICATION OF DISORDERS

Soft tissue pain can be categorized into a few major categories. Some patients may have overlap features or more than one condition simultaneously. These are:

- Tendinitis (common shoulder problems such as supraspinatus or bicipital tendinitis)
- Bursitis (anserine, trochanteric, subacromial, olecranon)
- Epicondylitis (medial and lateral)
- Nerve entrapment syndromes (carpal or tarsal tunnel syndrome)
- Regional pain syndromes, characterized by widespread pain in a region of the body, such as the upper back, chest wall, or an entire extremity
- Generalized pain syndromes such as chronic widespread pain syndrome, fibromyalgia, whiplash injuries

PATHOPHYSIOLOGY

The pathophysiology of these conditions is poorly understood. Because tissue biopsy is rarely if ever indicated in any of these conditions, there are no good clinical-pathological correlations for most of these conditions with the exception of carpal tunnel syndrome. In this disorder, the histopathology of excised soft tissue demonstrates scarring and fibrosis sometimes associated with an inflammatory infiltrate surrounding the entrapped median nerve. However, in most other disorders the findings may be minimal: for example, in some patients with recurrent shoulder pain, there may be some thinning of the tendon sheaths with sparse inflammatory cell infiltrates and occasional fibrosis. Bursae are synovial lined sacs that help to facilitate tissue gliding. Generally there are two types of bursae, the subcutaneous and the deep forms. Subcutaneous bursae overlie prominences and permit the movement of skin overlying the bursae, thus provoking stretching or tearing. The deep bursae separate different tendon compartments or are present between tendons and bone. Generally, bursae contain trace amounts of synovial fluid, which contains a high content of hyaluronic acid with few leukocytes and a predominance of mononuclear cells.

The causes of chronic widespread pain syndrome, fibromyalgia, and regional pain syndromes remain unknown. The common feature to all these conditions is that the musculoskeletal areas that are symptomatic are not the actual pain-generating sites. There is mounting evidence to suggest that these disorders are caused by alterations in processing pain signals at the level of either the brain or the spinal cord.

PRESENTATION

The onset of soft tissue pain disorders can be acute or insidious. There may be an antecedent history of excessive physical activity that may have predisposed the patient to injury. Generally patients will complain of the onset of a localized discomfort, and they can usually point to an area of maximal pain. Descriptions of the pain include it being throbbing, dull, and aching. Pain symptoms are usually described as feeling worse during periods of inactivity and rest. For example, patients will often note the pain at night, and it may awaken them from sleep or prevent them from getting to sleep. A patient with trochanteric or subacromial bursitis may notice the pain mostly when lying on the affected side. Similarly, nerve entrapment pain such as carpal tunnel syndrome is often felt worse at night. Presumably, with sleep, the patient is unable to maintain a proper wrist position that would prevent irritation to the nerve. These nocturnal exacerbations are in contrast to the situation in patients with an inflammatory arthritis such as rheumatoid arthritis (RA). In those patients, nighttime pain is uncommon and, when present, suggests the development of a soft tissue pain disorder superimposed on the RA, a nerve entrapment syndrome, or severe destructive changes in a joint suggesting end-stage arthritis in that particular joint.

PATIENT DEMOGRAPHICS AND COMMON PRESENTATIONS

Soft tissue pain syndromes can affect patients of either sex with about equal frequency and at any age (table 27.1). The exception would be fibromyalgia, which is far more frequently seen in females. There are some specific types of soft tissue pain syndromes that can be seen in certain populations:

- Patients with shoulder pain due to supraspinatus tendinitis, subacromial bursitis, or bicipital tendinitis often present with an antecedent history of excessive use. In younger patients this might relate to athletic activities that require repeated external rotation and abduction at the shoulder. Sports such as baseball and tennis can precipitate these episodes. In older patients these shoulder problems can often be associated with some structural changes that have already occurred at the shoulder with aging. For example, the presence of an osteophyte near the rotator cuff mechanism (supraspinatus, infraspinatus,

and teres minor tendons) may result in a partial tear or fraying of the tendon mechanism. These patients often present with a marked limitation of mobility along with their pain. This may be in contrast to patients with a bursitis or tendinitis of the shoulder where pain limits motion but passive range of motion can easily be achieved.

- Medial and lateral epicondylitis are the most common causes of elbow pain. In long-standing cases, the pain can radiate distally toward the wrist and hand, mimicking other conditions such as carpal tunnel syndrome. It is often precipitated by repetitive hand squeezing and gripping maneuvers. The most common causes include excessive computer mouse use or work tools such as hammers or screwdrivers and sports that require a firm grip on the equipment such as tennis or golf.

- Carpal tunnel syndrome may be associated with repetitive overuse of the hands, although the data are conflicting. Other causes include marked obesity, pregnancy, inflammatory arthritis such as RA, hypothyroidism, diabetes mellitus, and rarely amyloidosis. These systemic disorders should he considered when patients present with bilateral symptoms.

- Trochanteric bursitis is usually seen in two groups of patients. The first includes moderately to extremely obese patients whose weight continually stresses the soft tissues surrounding the hip joint. The second group includes those patients who have rapidly increased their level of physical and athletic activities, resulting in excessive stresses around the hip and thigh.

- The most common soft tissue pains around the knee include pain due to anserine bursitis and patellofemoral dysfunction. The anserine bursa sits inferior and medial to the knee, and anserine bursitis can be distinguished from pain due to osteoarthritis by the presence of exquisite tenderness reproduced by the palpation over the bursa. These patients are older and usually have some degree of underlying medial knee joint cartilage loss consistent with osteoarthritis. Patellofemoral dysfunction results in pain being felt over the knee when attempting to initiate activities that require knee flexion and extension.

- Pain around the ankle and foot may include Achilles tendinitis as well as tendinitis affecting the extensor tendons (more often than the flexor tendons) of the foot. Tendinitis around the ankle and foot is often related to increased levels of physical activity or may be related to underlying altered foot biomechanics such as flat foot. Achilles tendinitis tends to occur in younger athletic individuals; a change in footwear may predispose certain patients to its development. A history of recent quinolone antibiotic use may predispose some patients to tendon rupture, especially the Achilles tendons.

Table 27.1 CLINICAL FEATURES OF SOFT TISSUE PAIN DISORDERS

Presentation	Acute or subacute
Location	Focal usually asymmetrical pain though it may radiate to a wider area
Pain description	Deep aching (tendonitis, bursitis) Paresthesias (nerve entrapment)
Time of discomfort	Often worst at night and with activities causing pressure over the area

SPECIFIC SOFT TISSUE PAIN DISORDERS

SHOULDER PAIN

Shoulder pain is a common disorder that may be caused by problems within the shoulder joints, that is, the glenohumeral, acromioclavicular, or sternoclavicular joints, or at one of the periarticular structures such as the rotator cuff or bicipital tendons, the shoulder joint capsule, or the subacromial bursa (table 27.2). Less commonly the pain is referred to the shoulder from a nerve impingement in the cervical spine, brachial plexus, or at the thoracic outlet. In some cases, the pain may originate from a lesion in the diaphragm or the right upper quadrant of the abdomen such as acute cholecystitis. Pain originating from the glenohumeral joint or the rotator cuff is generally felt just a few centimeters distal to the shoulder joint margin over the deltoid muscle area. Pain that is felt above the shoulder may not be emanating from the shoulder and suggests either a cervical radiculopathy or a soft tissue injury above the shoulder with radiation of the pain toward the shoulder. Pain that is felt behind the shoulder joint is most likely due to subscapularis tendon injuries or referred pain from cervical spine disease.

Bilateral shoulder pain may be a feature of a systemic disorder such as polymyalgia rheumatica or RA. On the other hand, osteoarthritis of the glenohumeral joint is very uncommon except in cases where there was antecedent shoulder joint injury or prior metabolic damage to the cartilage as seen in chondrocalcinosis.

Patients may describe a history of insidious onset of pain. Those who have an abrupt onset of pain during activity may be describing a partial tear of an affected tendon (e.g., rotator cuff tear). In those cases patients will often present with marked inability to raise the arm. Why does tendinitis occur so commonly in the shoulder region? This is because during shoulder abduction, the rotator cuff and long biceps tendons are subjected to impingement at the greater tuberosity of the humerus and the coracoacromial arch. With excessive or frequent repetitive overhead activities, there is tissue injury resulting in tears of the rotator cuff as well as tendinitis within the cuff mechanism. A viable rotator cuff is required for abduction and external rotation of the shoulder as well as stabilizing the glenohumeral joint and preventing the superior migration of the humeral head. Thus, an injured or damaged rotator cuff may be unable to prevent some degree of superior migration of the humeral head, which results in further damage to the rotator cuff and to the long biceps tendon (which sits on the humeral head), which are now being squeezed by the changing architecture of the joint. With time and recurrent injury, there may be osteophyte formation over the inferior surface of the acromioclavicular joint, and this will intensify the degree of impingement of the rotator cuff and the biceps tendon. Thus, the spectrum of these chronic impingement syndromes can range from episodes of mild tendinitis of the rotator cuff to the development of tears of the rotator cuff or the long head of the biceps tendon. Because the subacromial bursa is adjacent to the rotator cuff, many of these cases are also associated with a subacromial bursitis.

In some patients there may be the onset of an explosive exquisitely painful shoulder pain with marked difficulty with any range of motion. Patients are extremely uncomfortable and are very reluctant to comply with a physical exam of the shoulder. Radiographs of the affected shoulder demonstrate calcification within the rotator cuff tendon or subacromial bursa. These calcific deposits often disappear following resolution of the episode.

Physical Examination

The physical examination of the shoulder should begin with inspection for evidence of muscle wasting or bony hypertrophy over the acromioclavicular joint. These findings suggest a long-standing problem. Shoulder fullness (suggesting effusion) is unusual and not easily visualized because a shoulder joint effusion would be deep within the tissues and must be diagnosed through imaging such as magnetic resonance imaging (MRI) or shoulder ultrasound. Shoulder range of motion and function is assessed by having the patient place his or her arm by his or her side and slowly raise it laterally to assess the range of shoulder abduction. The first 30–40° of abduction is controlled by the deltoid muscle. Beyond 40°, abduction is performed using the rotator cuff mechanism. In patients with rotator cuff–related tendinitis or impingement syndromes, there will be a definite loss of motion and a description of pain with abduction beyond 40°. The patient

Table 27.2 **COMMON SOFT TISSUE DISORDERS BY SITE**

Shoulder	Rotator cuff tendonitis
	Bicipital tendonitis
	Subacromial bursitis
Elbow	Medial or lateral epicondylitis
	Olecranon bursitis
Wrist	De Quervain tenosynovitis
	Flexor tenosynovitis
	Dupuytren contracture
	Carpal tunnel syndrome
Hip/pelvis	Trochanteric bursitis
	Ischial bursitis
	Iliopsoas bursitis
Knee	Medial (no name) bursitis
	Anserine bursitis
	Pre- and infrapatellar bursitis
	Patellofemoral dysfunction
Ankle and foot	Achilles tendinitis
	Retrocalcaneal bursitis
	Plantar fasciitis
	Morton neuroma

continues this motion against the resistance of the examiner's hand, which is placed on the patient's elbow while applying downward pressure. The patient's ability to continue abduction against resistance is noted: if he or she complains of pain, the diagnosis of a rotator cuff–related injury (either tendinitis or tear or both) is made. A rotator cuff tear can be distinguished from tendinitis if the patient is unable to actively abduct the arm beyond 40° but can passively move the arm through this arc of motion without pain.

Patients who have a subacromial bursitis may note local tenderness on palpation of the subacromial bursa that sits at the top of the humerus just below the glenoid arch. Patients with a bicipital tendinitis often describe pain that is felt more anteriorly over the top part of the humerus corresponding to the biceps tendon insertion area. However, it should be noted that many patients may have features of each of these conditions because the affected areas lie in close proximity to one another.

ELBOW PAIN

The most common causes of elbow pain include medial and lateral epicondylitis. Although initially described as tennis elbow, lateral epicondylitis is more commonly seen with other activities such as excessive computer mouse use or repeated gripping of work tools such as screwdrivers and hammers. These activities all require repeated, frequent use of the hand flexor tendons. Although it was initially considered to be a form of tendinitis with suspected inflammation at the tendon bone insertion interface, it is now considered by some to be due to a cumulative trauma overuse disorder with repetitive mechanical overloading of the common extensor tendon particularly involving the portion derived from the extensor carpi radialis brevis tendon. In some histopathologic specimens of excised epicondylar tissue, there is evidence for fibroblastic hyperplasia and disorganized collagen bundles.

The pain is often insidious and sometime bilateral although usually involving the dominant arm. The pain is generally localized to the lateral epicondyle but over time may extend both distally toward the wrist and proximally upward toward the shoulder. It is exacerbated by any squeezing activities of the hands such as holding a pen, gripping, or lifting objects. This can be confirmed by having the patient try to squeeze an object such as a cup; this will often elicit the pain. Palpation over the lateral epicondylar area usually provokes intense pain and discomfort. However, the elbow range of motions such as flexion and extension as well as pronation and supination are maintained. One way to distinguish epicondylitis from a true elbow joint arthritis is to assess pronation and supination range of motion. In patients with elbow joint synovitis, there is a reduction in these motions, whereas there is no effect on these motions with either type of epicondylitis.

Medial epicondylitis is less commonly seen than the lateral form. Although it is known as "golfer's elbow," this condition is more commonly seen in patients who are at risk for lateral epicondylitis as well. Typically, there is an antecedent history of cumulative repetitive strain of the common flexor muscle of the forearm provoking pain and tenderness at the medial epicondylar region. The pain may radiate proximally and distally as well. The diagnosis is confirmed by noting pain over the medial epicondyle with either palpation or by the simultaneous forced full extension of the elbow and the wrist.

OLECRANON BURSITIS

The olecranon bursa sits below the tip of the elbow and can become swollen and sometimes painful from a number of conditions. These include trauma, inflammation (e.g., RA or gout), or sepsis. Because gouty bursitis and sepsis can both be associated with similar findings, such as increased warmth, swelling, and redness along with pain, it is generally necessary to aspirate the bursa for synovial fluid analysis including cell count, Gram stain, and culture of the joint fluid. Septic olecranon bursitis is usually the result of direct inoculation of bacteria via a skin abrasion and can occur in otherwise healthy individuals engaged in physical work that results in frequent trauma to the elbows. The most common pathogen is *Staphylococcus aureus*. Traumatic bursitis can occur with recurrent or incidental trauma to the elbow. Patients often present because of swelling that may be only minimally painful. The diagnosis is confirmed by joint aspiration demonstrating hemorrhagic joint fluid with few white blood cells, and no bacteria or crystals being present.

WRIST AND HAND DISORDERS
Carpal Tunnel Syndrome

Perhaps the most common soft tissue disorder involving the wrist and hand is the carpal tunnel syndrome. This is caused by entrapment of the median nerve within the carpal tunnel. It is characterized by painful paresthesias and sensory loss in a median nerve distribution (generally this involves the thumb, second digit, and half of the third digit). In more advanced cases there may be loss of motor power in the median distribution in the hands as well as atrophy of the thenar muscles. There is generally a history of nocturnal pain in the median nerve distribution. Percussion of the median nerve at the flexor retinaculum just radial to the palmaris longus tendon at the distal wrist crease (Tinel sign) will produce paresthesias in the median nerve distribution. Phalen sign is the development of paresthesias following sustained palmar flexion of the wrist for 20–30 seconds. The severity of the entrapment and the need for surgical decompression can be assessed by electromyography.

Flexor tendon entrapment syndromes of the digits can occur in patients without a history of an inflammatory arthritis or diabetes. Most cases are idiopathic although patients with diabetes and RA may be at increased risk for this condition. Patients present with triggering symptoms involving a digit especially following periods of inactivity such as arising in the morning. They often must use their other hand to help "unlock" the affected digit. A nodular thickening of the tendon is often present at the site of maximum tenderness that is generally in a part of the flexor tendon just proximal to the metacarpophalangeal (MCP) joint of the affected digit. The histopathology of the lesion consists of hypertrophy and fibrocartilaginous metaplasia of the ligamentous layer of the tendon sheath that results in stenosis of the tendon sheath canal and mechanical entrapment of the tendon.

De Quervain Tenosynovitis

De Quervain tenosynovitis is a disorder affecting the common tendon sheath of the abductor pollicis longus and extensor pollicis brevis tendons. It is characterized by pain over the radial aspect of the wrist that is aggravated by movements of the thumb during pinching, grasping, and lifting activities. It is actually a tendon entrapment syndrome resulting in thickening of the extensor retinaculum that covers the first compartment of the wrist and leads to a tendon entrapment. Palpation of the affected tendon sheath recreates pain and exquisite tenderness. In the Finkelstein test, the patient makes a fist with the fingers wrapped around the thumb and then is instructed to flex the thumb in the ulnar direction. This reproduces the pain and confirms the diagnosis.

Dupuytren Contracture

Dupuytren contracture is caused by a nodular thickening and contracture of the palmar fascia leading to marked flexion deformities of the fingers. Most often the ring finger is affected, but it can also involve any of the others. It can involve one or both hands. It may start in the ring finger flexor tendons and then continue to involve all the others. With the tendon scarring that develops, there is a gradual development of a flexion deformity of the fingers at the level of the MCP joints and an inability to fully extend the digits. The histopathology demonstrates fibrous nodules proliferating fibrosis and myofibrosis in the palmar fascia.

PELVIS AND HIP

There are three major bursae around the pelvis and hip region. These include the ischiogluteal, iliopsoas, and trochanteric bursae, with the latter being the most commonly affected. The trochanteric bursae are composed of three bursae with the largest and most important one clinically separating the fibers of the gluteus maximus muscle from the greater trochanter. The other two bursae lie between the greater trochanter and the gluteus medius and greater

trochanter, respectively. Trochanteric bursitis presents with a deep aching pain over the lateral aspect of the upper thigh made worse by walking but also noted to be painful at night when the patient is lying on the affected side. The diagnosis is confirmed by obtaining a history of pain both at rest and with activity but in the presence of a normal range of motion of the affected hip joint. Additionally, there is pain with palpation over the trochanteric bursae. The pain may radiate distally but rarely beyond the knee. Risk factors include overuse activities such as excessive walking or running and improper foot wear. The differential diagnosis of trochanteric bursitis includes lumbar radiculopathy involving the L1 and L2 nerve roots and the uncommon meralgia paresthetica, a syndrome characterized by entrapment of the lateral cutaneous nerve of the thigh resulting in discomfort in the same region. Unlike bursitis, these patients tend to have more dysesthesia symptoms than pain.

Ischiogluteal bursitis presents with pain felt over the ischial tuberosity. Previously known as "weavers bottom," it is caused by repeated leg flexion and extension in the sitting position or prolonged sitting on hard surfaces. Diagnosis is confirmed by eliciting tenderness on palpation over the ischial tuberosity with the patient lying supine and the hip and knee flexed.

The iliopsoas bursa lies over the anterior surface of the hip joint. In most cases of iliopsoas bursitis there appears to be communication between the hip joint and the bursa, and this may allow for a transfer of excess synovial fluid from one region to the other. The predisposing factors for excess synovial fluid include osteoarthritis, RA, and septic arthritis. The typical presentation consists of the onset of painful swelling in the inguinal area. When there is adjacent femoral vein or nerve compression, the resulting pain and or swelling may involve the entire leg.

SOFT TISSUE DISORDERS AROUND THE KNEE

There are three major bursae around the knee that can become inflamed or rarely infected, resulting in pain. These include the prepatellar, infrapatellar, and anserine bursae.

- The prepatellar bursa lies anterior to the patella and can become infected in patients who frequently kneel. Presumably there is skin breakdown resulting in bacterial infection, most commonly *Staphylococcus aureus*. There is superficial swelling over the dorsum of the patella with surrounding redness and erythema. Rarely there may be systemic complaints such as fever and chills. The infrapatellar bursa lies between the upper portion of the tibial tuberosity and the prepatellar ligament. It is separated from the knee joint synovium by a fat pad. Similar to prepatellar bursitis, excessive kneeling may predispose to skin breakdown in the region and infection. In other patients there may be a noninfectious inflammatory swelling of the bursa.

• The anserine bursa lies under and adjacent to the pes anserinus, which is the insertion of the thigh adductor complex consisting of the sartorius, gracilis, and semitendinosus muscles. This region is about 5 cm below the medial aspect of the knee joint space. Pain in this area is often referred to anserine bursitis. Predisposing factors include underlying osteoarthritis of the medial knee compartment and excessive physical stress to the knee. Patients will often describe nocturnal pain awakening them, and this can help them to distinguish this condition from osteoarthritis, which is rarely painful at night except if there is end-stage osteoarthritis in the knee that would require total knee replacement. Women more commonly develop anserine bursitis perhaps in part because they have a broader pelvic area leading to greater tension caused by greater angulation of the knee adductors. Obesity is another risk factor. There is a "no name bursa" that is found over the medial joint margin of the knee. Some clinicians believe that this bursa, when inflamed, can lead to intense medial knee pain. However medial knee pain can also be due to osteoarthritis, trauma, and ligamentous injury.

• The iliotibial band, which connects the ilium with the lateral tibia, can become painful from repetitive flexion and extension with running. This results in the *iliotibial band syndrome*. On examination, there is tenderness over the lateral femoral condyle approximately 2 cm above the joint line, with pain on weight bearing when the knee is flexed at about 40°. Correction of the problem with foot orthotics can be helpful.

• *Patellofemoral pain syndrome*, formerly known as chondromalacia patella, refers to poorly localized anterior knee pain often made worse when the patient initiates activities such as getting up from a seated position. There is pain felt over the entire knee and it is often made worse by forced flexion or extension of the affected knee. It is thought to result from anatomical abnormalities resulting in abnormal angulation of the patellar surface misaligning with the rest of the knee. Other theories include repetitive microtrauma to the patellar surface. This condition is more commonly seen in women but can occur in patients of either sex and at all ages. Radiographs of the knee are often unremarkable. Intensive physical therapy to enhance the strength of the medial aspect of the quadriceps mechanism is often helpful in alleviating symptoms.

FOOT PAIN

The most common soft tissue disorders around the ankle and feet include Achilles tendinitis, retrocalcaneal bursitis, and plantar fasciitis. They share a common causation in that these conditions are typically seen in patients who have a pes planus deformity resulting in altered foot biomechanics and excessive stress over other parts of the bone and soft tissue. The Achilles tendon can become inflamed and in rare cases can tear. Risk factors for tear also include recent use of quinolone antibiotics. Achilles tendinitis can also be the presenting manifestation of a spondyloarthropathy. Retrocalcaneal bursitis may be confused with Achilles tendinitis because the bursa lies between the tendon and a fat pad adjacent to the talus. Causes of bursitis include repetitive trauma, poor footwear, RA, and spondyloarthropathy. Plantar fasciitis is a common condition thought to be due to repetitive microtrauma at the attachment site of the plantar fascia to the calcaneus, resulting in injury and inflammation. There is localized pain over the heel with weight-bearing activities that is worst with the initiation of walking activities. Although the vast majority of patients with this condition do not have an underlying arthropathy, in younger individuals this might be the initial presentation of a spondyloarthropathy. A careful history and musculoskeletal exam can help identify these patients.

The tarsal tunnel syndrome refers to the compression of the posterior tibial nerve as it courses through the canal adjacent to the tarsal bone. It is similar to carpal tunnel syndrome with patients presenting with sensory dysesthesias involving the plantar aspect of the foot. Nocturnal symptoms are worse and often awaken the patient. Percussion of the flexor retinaculum reproduces the symptoms. There may be reduced vibratory sensation and decreased two-point discrimination over the plantar aspect of the foot and toes. Diagnosis can be confirmed by nerve conduction studies documenting a delay in the nerve conduction of the posterior tibial nerve across the ankle.

Morton's neuroma is a condition that presents with paresthesias or dysesthesias in the interdigital web spaces, particularly between the third and fourth interspaces. The pain is increased by weight bearing or by tight-fitting footwear. There is tenderness and a clicking sensation noted on simultaneous palpation of the webspace while squeezing the patient's metatarsal bones with the other hand (Mulder sign). The diagnosis can be confirmed by injection of a local anesthetic into the interspace, which should immediately, though temporarily, relieve symptoms.

FIBROMYALGIA

Fibromyalgia is a disorder characterized by widespread areas of achiness and pain with an otherwise unremarkable musculoskeletal exam (table 27.3). Laboratory tests are normal. To fulfill the clinical criteria for fibromyalgia patients generally must demonstrate tenderness over 11 of the 19 trigger points found in patients with fibromyalgia. Many of these trigger points actually correspond to the sensitive

Table 27.3 GENERALIZED SOFT TISSUE PAIN SYNDROMES

Fibromyalgia
Whiplash injuries (post–motor vehicle accident)
Chronic regional pain syndrome (CRPS)
Myofascial pain

periarticular areas (medial and lateral epicondyles, medial knee pain, chest wall, base of cervical and lumbar spines) that are discussed earlier in this chapter. The etiology of fibromyalgia remains unclear, and there is great debate as to whether the underlying causation relates to a pain perception disorder in the spinal cord or the higher structures of the central nervous system. There is a female preponderance, and the age of onset peaks between 30 and 50. Other chronic pain disorders such as migraine headaches, irritable bowel syndrome, temporomandibular joint pain syndrome, and bladder dysfunctions secondary to interstitial cystitis may all be seen more frequently in patients with fibromyalgia. The hallmark features include characterizations of widespread body pain and achiness along with some component of fatigue and malaise. The physical exam should confirm the absence of objective evidence for musculoskeletal inflammation such as no evidence for synovitis or myositis. Laboratory testing including complete blood count (CBC), hepatic, renal, and thyroid function, C-reactive protein (C-RP), erythrocyte sedimentation rate (ESR), and autoantibody production are all typically within normal limits.

ESTABLISHING THE DIAGNOSIS OF A SOFT TISSUE PAIN DISORDER

It is essential to take an accurate history and perform a thorough physical examination to rule out other causes that may mimic soft tissue pain syndromes. For example, radicular pain from cervical or lumbar spine nerve entrapment can mimic some of the conditions described earlier. These patients usually describe a wider area of pain and generally lack specific focal areas of tenderness on palpation. Another area of potential confusion, especially in the older patient, is the radiographic finding of osteoarthritis in adjacent joints. Sometimes these arthritic changes are ascribed as the underlying cause for the patient's pain syndrome. However, it is important to recall that soft tissue pain has some unique characteristics that help to distinguish it from pain due to osteoarthritis. These include the finding of intense pain on palpation of the affected area along with the history of pain that is worst with rest and at night. Generally, osteoarthritis pain follows a reverse pattern with pain improved with rest and sleep and made

worse with activity. Palpation of an osteoarthritic joint does not generally exacerbate the pain to the same degree as is seen in soft tissue pain disorders.

Systemic diseases that sometimes need to be considered include polymyalgia rheumatica (in patients over age 50 with persistent shoulder and hip girdle region discomfort), occult hypothyroidism, and, very rarely, vitamin D deficiency.

ANCILLARY STUDIES

For most soft tissue pain disorders laboratory investigation should be minimal. When appropriate, a CBC, ESR, and C-RP might be useful. If there is a question of an underlying infectious process, an aspiration procedure should be seriously considered. Imaging of the affected area can be helpful in some situations. For example in patients with an acute severe pain, fracture should be ruled out, especially if there is an antecedent history of trauma. If a calcific tendinitis is being considered, plain radiographs can confirm the diagnosis. In the case of periarticular knee pain thought to be due to bursitis, radiographs can assess the underlying cartilage loss already present and rule out other mimics such as avascular necrosis or a nondisplaced stress fracture.

THERAPY

Treatment for most soft tissue disorders (table 27.4) begins with the education of the patient. For example, in overuse syndromes it is necessary for the patient to understand the underlying mechanism that predisposes to the development of the pain syndrome and to be familiar with the measures that must be taken to avoid these repetitive stresses in the future. Second, referral to physical therapy for stretching

Table 27.4 THERAPEUTIC OPTIONS

Physical therapy	Stretching
	Massage
	Electrical stimulation
	Ultrasound
	Heat/ice
Occupational therapy	Splinting
	Joint immobilization
Medications	NSAIDs
	Acetaminophen
	Tramadol
	Mild narcotic analgesics
	Topical lidocaine
	Capsaicin creams
	Intralesional corticosteroids

and exercise programs can be useful. Therapeutic modalities such as ultrasound provide a heat energy that can penetrate into the deep soft tissues. For carpal tunnel syndrome, proper wrist splinting, especially at nighttime, can provide some symptom relief.

As mentioned earlier, if infection is a diagnostic concern, then an aspiration procedure should be seriously considered. Before injecting soft tissues one must be certain that an underlying infection is not the cause of the problem. Injection of a corticosteroid preparation combined with lidocaine can provide symptomatic relief. For example, the combination of 20–40 mg of methylprednisolone along with 1–2 mL of 2% lidocaine can he injected into a bursa or near painful tendon structures to provide symptomatic relief. Generally these injections can be performed at the bedside or in the office without assistive radiology guidance. There are data to suggest that patient injections are equal to those administered with radiographic assistance.

Nonsteroidal anti-inflammatory drugs (NSAIDs) can provide some modest pain relief. Other analgesics such as acetaminophen or tramadol can be useful. Narcotic analgesics should be avoided except for those circumstances requiring short-term management of severe pain. Systemic corticosteroids are not indicated for any of the soft tissue pain disorders.

For patients whose symptoms persist despite the therapeutic approaches listed above, one should consider the possibility that there is an underlying structural cause for the pain. At this point, if imaging has not yet been performed, it may be useful to assess the area radiographically. Patients who have more widespread and persistent achiness may have an underlying disorder such as fibromyalgia causing the persistence of symptoms.

ADDITIONAL READING

Andres BM, Murrell GA. Treatment of tendinopathy: What works, what does not, and what is on the horizon. *Clin Orthop Relat Res.* 2008;466:1539–54.

Barr KP. Review of upper and lower extremity musculoskeletal pain problems. *Phys Med Rehabil Clin N Am.* 2007;18(4):747–60.

Bennett R. Myofascial pain syndromes and their evaluation. *Best Practice Res Clin Rheumatol.* 2007;21:427–45.

Burbank KM. Stevenson JH, Czarnecki GR, Dorfman J. Chronic shoulder pain: Part 1. Evaluation and diagnosis. *Am Fam Physician.* 2008;77(4):453–60.

Matsen FA 3rd. Clinical practice. Rotator-cuff failure. *N Engl J Med.* 2008;358(20):2138–47.

Riley G. Tendinopathy—from basic science to treatment. *Nature Clin Pract Rheumatol.* 2008;4:82–9.

Sharmal P, Maffulli N. Biology of tendon injury: Healing, modeling and remodeling. *J Musculoskel Neuronal Interact.* 2006;6(2):181–90.

QUESTIONS

QUESTION 1. A 72-year-old female presents with a 6-week history of abrupt onset of stiffness around her neck and shoulders. She notes pain when trying to dress herself in the morning. She also notes difficulty at night and rolls from side to side seeking a comfortable position. She describes feeling better as the day progresses and then notes pains once again developing in the early evening. Past medical history notable for hypertension—on HCTZ. Rheumatologic examination shows a full range of motion in all joints tested except for some mildly decreased range of motion with external rotation in either shoulder. Motor strength appropriate in upper and lower extremities. Laboratory data: HCT 40.1, WBC 7.4, PLT 257k, TSH 1.3, ESR 12. What is the most likely diagnosis?

A. Polymyositis
B. Bilateral rotator cuff tendinitis
C. Fibromyalgia
D. Polymyalgia rheumatica
E. Metabolic myopathy

QUESTION 2. A 34-year-old colleague sees you for her left shoulder pain. She is a competitive tennis player and noticed some pain in her left deltoid area for the past 3 weeks. The pain is made worse by movements such as shoulder abduction or rotation. Rheumatological examination shows that there is full range of motion on abduction. Forced abduction is painful, but she can resist. Forward flexion and extension are maintained.

Which of the following is the most likely diagnosis?

A. Supraspinatus tendonitis
B. Full-thickness rotator cuff tear
C. Bicipital tendinitis
D. Calcific tendinitis
E. Deltoid myositis

QUESTION 3. A 55-year-old attorney is seeing you for left elbow pain. She developed this discomfort 2 months ago. She has trouble using her left arm for most activities and says she is beginning to drop items that she is holding. She denies trauma; she plays golf occasionally. Her only medication is simvastatin 40 mg qd. She is extremely concerned because of the worsening symptoms at night. The pain awakens her from sleep and radiates along the entire forearm. An x-ray of the elbow is normal.

Which of the following statements is correct?

A. She should stop the simvastatin
B. Check serum PTH and Fe
C. Arrange for elbow MRI
D. Arrange for EMG
E. Reassure patient and refer to physical therapy

QUESTION 4. When evaluating a patient for suspected trochanteric bursitis, which of the following statements is correct?

A. The pain is maximally felt over the lateral aspect of the affected thigh.
B. It is generally a bilateral condition.

C. The most common cause is an underlying arthritis of the ipsilateral hip.

D. Pain is worse with activity but improves at night.

QUESTION 5. A 28-year-old patient with RA is seen by you for acute foot pain and difficulty walking. She had been in her usual state of health until a few hours earlier when she felt a searing, sharp pain in her right Achilles tendon as she was walking out of her office. She fell and had to be assisted back on her feet. She realized that she could not bear weight on her right leg. She works out regularly but denies any recent injuries. She has had RA for 7 years and currently takes the following medications: methotrexate, 20 mg q week × 6 years; folate, 1 mg qd; ibuprofen, 400 mg bid prn; etanercept, 50 mg weekly 3 months, ciprofloxacin, 500 mg qd × 5 days, recently completed for a urinary tract infection, oral contraceptive × 4 years.

Which of the following statements is correct?

A. Stop the ibuprofen

B. Stop the oral contraceptive

C. Keep all meds; avoid ciprofloxacin in the future

D. Stop the methotrexate

E. Stop the etanercept

ANSWERS

1. D
2. A
3. E
4. A
5. C

28.

LABORATORY TESTS IN RHEUMATIC DISORDERS

Peter H. Schur

ACUTE-PHASE PROTEINS

The acute-phase response is a major pathophysiological phenomenon that accompanies inflammation. The acute-phase response accompanies both acute and chronic inflammatory states. It can occur in association with a wide variety of disorders, including infection, trauma, infarction, inflammatory arthritides, and various neoplasms.

Acute-phase proteins are defined as those proteins whose plasma concentrations change by at least 25% during inflammatory states. These changes largely reflect their production by hepatocytes.

Acute-phase proteins that increase include ceruloplasmin, several complement components, C-reactive protein (CRP), fibrinogen, alpha-1-antitrypsin, haptoglobin, and ferritin, while negative reactants include albumin, transferrin, and transthyretin.

Despite the lack of diagnostic specificity, the measurement of serum levels of acute-phase proteins is useful because it may reflect the presence and intensity of an inflammatory process. The most widely used indicators of the acute-phase protein response are the erythrocyte sedimentation rate (ESR) and CRP. The ESR depends largely on the plasma concentration of fibrinogen.

These tests may be useful both diagnostically, in helping to differentiate inflammatory from noninflammatory conditions, and prognostically. In addition, they may aid in monitoring activity of disease because they may reflect the response to therapeutic intervention and a need for closer monitoring. Serial measurements of CRP concentrations may provide prognostic information in rheumatoid arthritis.

COMPARISON OF ESR AND CRP

The ESR has a number of disadvantages compared to the CRP determination:

- The ESR is only an indirect measurement of plasma acute-phase protein concentrations; it can be greatly influenced by the size, shape, and number of red cells, as well as by other plasma constituents. Thus, results may be imprecise and sometimes misleading.

- As a patient's condition worsens or improves, the ESR changes relatively slowly; the CRP concentrations change rapidly.

- ESR values steadily increase with age (to approximately age in years divided by 2); plasma CRP concentrations also increase with age. One can roughly correct the CRP for age by using the following formula: the upper limit of the normal range (in mg/dL) equals age in years/50 for men and age/50 + 0.6 for women.

- Normal values for the ESR are slightly higher among women than men.

- Slight elevations of CRP may also reflect obesity, cigarette smoking, diabetes mellitus, or other noninflammatory causes.

RATIONALE FOR EMPLOYING MULTIPLE TESTS

Although elevations in multiple components of the acute-phase response commonly occur together, not all happen uniformly in all patients. Discordance between concentrations of different acute-phase proteins is common, perhaps because of differences in the production of specific cytokines or their modulators in different diseases. Knowing which acute-phase reactant has best correlated with an individual's disease in the past is helpful in choosing the test to follow over time.

The measurement of acute-phase reactants may be most helpful in assessing clinical activity in patients with rheumatoid arthritis (RA), polymyalgia rheumatica, and giant-cell arteritis, and perhaps to assess the prognosis of patients with malignancy, or to ascertain whether an infectious process (such as abscess, osteomyelitis, or endocarditis) has been eradicated.

Acute-phase reactants are usually of little use in distinguishing among early RA, osteoarthritis, and SLE.

Elevations in both CRP and ESR are associated with radiographic progression in RA.

Although polymyalgia rheumatica (PMR) and giant-cell arteritis (GCA) are frequently accompanied by markedly elevated levels of the ESR (often higher than 100 mm/hr), these elevated levels should not be regarded as a sine qua non for these disorders. In addition, a few patients with PMR have normal ESRs.

In patients with these diseases, CRP and ESR have been regarded as having nearly equal value in assessing disease activity. More recently, however, reports suggest that CRP levels may be more sensitive for the detection of active disease.

SYSTEMIC LUPUS ERYTHEMATOSUS

Systemic lupus erythematosus (SLE) represents an exception to the generalization that CRP concentrations correlate with the extent and severity of inflammation in patients with rheumatic disorders. Many patients with active SLE do not have elevated CRP concentrations, although they may have marked increases in CRP concentrations during bacterial infection. This finding can be applied to the differential diagnosis of fever in patients with SLE, but one must remember that CRP concentrations may be high in some patients with active lupus scrositis or chronic synovitis.

SYSTEMIC AUTOIMMUNE DISEASE

The sensitivity of the antinuclear antibody (ANA) for a particular autoimmune disease can widely vary (table 28.1). Other well-recognized disorders associated with a positive ANA titer include chronic infectious diseases such as mononucleosis, subacute bacterial endocarditis, tuberculosis, and some lymphoproliferative diseases in up to 90% of patients taking certain drugs, especially procainamide and

Table 28.1 SENSITIVITY OF THE ANA IN AUTOIMMUNE AND NONRHEUMATIC DISEASE

SENSITIVITY OF ANA

Autoimmune disease	
SLE	95–100%
Scleroderma	60–80%
Mixed connective tissue disease	100%
Polymyositis/dermatomyositis	61%
Rheumatoid arthritis	52%
Rheumatoid vasculitis	30–50%
Sjögren syndrome	40–70%
Drug-induced lupus	100%
Discoid lupus	15%
Pauciarticular juvenile chronic arthritis	71%
Nonrheumatic disease	
Hashimoto's thyroiditis	46%
Graves' disease	50%
Autoimmune hepatitis	100%
Primary autoimmune cholangitis	100%
Primary pulmonary hypertension	40%

hydralazine; however, most of these patients do not develop drug-induced lupus.

False-positive ANAs (i.e., ANAs in the absence of autoimmune disease) are more commonly found in normal women and in elderly patients (usually in low titer) but may also be detected in persons with infections or other nonrheumatic inflammatory disease. The presence of high concentrations of ANA (titer >1:640) should increase the suspicion that an autoimmune disorder is present. However, its presence alone is not diagnostic of disease. Therefore, it is routine practice to test for specific ANAs such anti-dsDNA, Sm, RNP, Ro, La, and Scl-70; their presence is more likely to facilitate making the diagnosis of a specific rheumatic disease (see below). If no initial diagnosis can be made, it is our practice to watch the patient carefully over time for the development of any ANA-associated diseases. The combination of low titers of antibody (<1:80) and no or few signs or symptoms of disease portend a much smaller likelihood of an autoimmune disease. As a result, these patients need to be reevaluated less frequently. Positive ANAs may also be found in the normal population including first-degree relatives of persons with ANA-associated rheumatic disease. A patient with a negative ANA and strong clinical evidence of a systemic autoimmune disorder may require specific antibody assays to accurately diagnosis a rheumatic disease. ANAs produce a wide range of different staining patterns (homogeneous, diffuse, peripheral, rim, speckled, nucleolar, anticentromere, etc.). The nuclear staining pattern has been recognized to have a relatively low sensitivity and specificity for different autoimmune disorders. The presence of antibodies directed at specific nuclear antigens is usually more useful; these include double-stranded DNA and the RNA-protein complexes Sm, RNP, Ro (SSA), and La (SSB).

ANTIBODIES TO DNA

Antibodies to DNA can be primarily divided into those that react with single-stranded DNA (ssDNA) and those recognizing double-stranded DNA (dsDNA).

ANTI-ssDNA ANTIBODIES

Anti-ssDNA antibodies have been reported in SLE, rheumatoid arthritis, drug-related lupus, healthy relatives of patients with SLE, and less commonly, in other rheumatic diseases (tables 28.2 and 28.3). However, they have limited usefulness for the diagnosis of SLE or other rheumatic diseases, and because they do not correlate well with disease activity, they are not useful for disease management.

ANTI-dsDNA ANTIBODIES

Anti-dsDNA antibodies are specific (95%) although not highly sensitive (70%) for SLE, making them very useful for

Table 28.2 ANA DISEASE ASSOCIATIONS

SENSITIVITY AND SPECIFICITY (%) OF DIFFERENT ANTINUCLEAR ANTIBODIES

	ANTIBODY							
	dsDNA	ssDNA	HISTONE	NUCLEOPROTEIN	Sm	RNP	Ro	La
SLE								
Sensitivity	70	80	30–80	58	25–30	45	40	15
Specificity	95		50	mod	mod	99	87–94	99
Drug LE								
Sensitivity		80	95	50	1%		low	low
Specificity	1–5%	50	high	mod				
RA								
Sensitivity		mod	low	25	1%	47	low	low
Specificity	1%	mod		low				
Scleroderma								
Sensitivity			<1	<1	<1	20		
Specificity	<1	low						
PM/DM								
Sensitivity			<1	<1	<1		low	
Specificity	<1	low						
Sjögren								
Sensitivity		mod	low	mod	1–5	5–60	8–70	14–60
Specificity	1–5	mod	low	mod			87	94

NOTE: Other associations: RNP: MCTD; Ro: SCLE, billary cirrhosis, vasculitis, CHB.

diagnosis when positive (table 28.2). They are occasionally found in other conditions, including rheumatoid arthritis, juvenile arthritis, drug-induced lupus, autoimmune hepatitis, and even in normal persons. Titers of anti-dsDNA antibodies often fluctuate with disease activity, especially in lupus nephritis, and are therefore useful in many patients for following the course of SLE (table 28.3).

The association between anti-DNA antibodies and other disease manifestations of SLE is far less clear. For example, there is no relationship between anti-dsDNA titer and disease activity of neuropsychiatric SLE.

Distinguishing active lupus manifestations from infectious complications or toxic effects of drugs and from unrelated disease is always a challenge. Anti-DNA antibodies may be helpful in some patients in making this distinction.

ANTI-SMITH (ANTI-Sм) ANTIBODIES AND ANTI-RIBONUCLEOPROTEIN (ANTI-RNP) ANTIBODIES

Anti-Sm antibodies are found in only 10% to 40% of patients with SLE, but infrequently in patients with other conditions, i.e., they are not sensitive but are highly specific (tables 28.2 and 28.3). Measurement of anti-Sm titers may be useful diagnostically, particularly at a time when anti-DNA antibodies are undetectable. Given their relatively low sensitivity, however, a negative value in no way excludes the diagnosis.

Anti-RNP antibodies are found in about 40–60% of patients with SLE but are not specific for SLE, being a defining feature of mixed connective tissue disease (MCTD) and in low titers and low frequencies in other rheumatic diseases including RA and scleroderma (tables 28.2 and 28.3).

The titers (levels) of anti-Sm or anti-RNP antibodies do not correlate with any clinical activity.

ANTI-Ro/SSA AND ANTI-La/SSB ANTIBODIES

Anti-Ro/SSA antibodies are found in approximately 50% of patients with SLE (table 28.2). They have been associated with photosensitivity, subacute cutaneous lupus, cutaneous vasculitis (palpable purpura), interstitial lung disease, neonatal lupus, and congenital heart block (table 28.3).

Anti-Ro/SSA antibodies are found in approximately 75% of patients with primary Sjögren syndrome (table 28.2), and high titers of these antibodies are

Table 28.3 CLINICAL ASSOCIATIONS OF SPECIFIC LUPUS AUTOANTIBODIES

ANTIGEN SPECIFICITY	SLE CLINICAL ASSOCIATIONS
dsDNA	Marker for active disease, titers fluctuates with disease activity, correlates best with renal disease
ssDNA	Nonspecific, no clinical utility
Ro/SSA	Subacute cutaneous lupus (75%), photosensitivity, neonatal lupus, complement deficiencies
La/SSB	Associated with Ro; low prevalence of renal disease; neonatal lupus (75%)
RNP (U1-RNP)	SLE generally in conjunction with Sm; in MCTD, required for diagnosis
Sm	Highly specific for SLE; not generally useful in management;
Phospholipids	Thromboembolic events in some patients;; thrombocytopenia, late trimester abortions; no clinical significance in others
Histones	>95% in many drug-related lupus; also present in RA, SLE, reported in systemic sclerosis with pulmonary fibrosis
Ribosomal P	Low sensitivity and high specificity for SLE; possible clinical associations

associated with a greater incidence of extraglandular features, especially purpura and vasculitis. By contrast, Ro/SSA antibodies are present in only 10% to 15% of patients with secondary Sjögren syndrome associated with rheumatoid arthritis. Therefore, the presence of anti-Ro/SSA or anti-La/SSB antibodies in patients with suspected primary Sjögren syndrome strongly supports the diagnosis.

Approximately 50% of patients with SLE who have anti-Ro antibody also have anti-La antibody, a closely related RNA-protein antigen. Similarly, most patients with Sjögren syndrome also have anti-La (SSB) antibodies. It is exceedingly rare to find patients with anti-La antibodies without anti-Ro antibodies.

Anti-Ro/SSA and anti-La/SSB have also been detected in patients with photosensitive dermatitis, and in 0.1% to 0.5% of healthy adults.

However, they have limited usefulness for the diagnosis of SLE or other rheumatic diseases, and because they do not correlate well with disease activity, they are not useful for disease management.

In our opinion, the indications for ordering anti-Ro/SSA and anti-La/SSB antibody tests are as follows:

- Women with SLE who are pregnant or may become pregnant in the future

- Women who have a history of giving birth to a child with heart block or myocarditis

- Patients with a history of unexplained photosensitive skin eruptions

- Patients strongly suspected of having SLE but who have a negative ANA test

ANTICENTROMERE ANTIBODIES

Anticentromere antibodies (ACA) are found almost exclusively in patients with limited cutaneous systemic sclerosis (lcSSc), especially in those with CREST. ACA has been observed in 57% of patients with CREST but has also been seen in patients with other conditions, including in some patients with Raynaud's phenomenon alone. ACA are typically detected by the characteristic immunofluorescent pattern on Hep-2 cells.

ANTI-SCL-70 (TOPOISOMERASE-1) ANTIBODIES

Approximately 15% to 20% of patients with scleroderma have antibodies to a 70-kDa protein (topoisomerase-1), subsequently named Scl-70. The usual method for detection is by ELISA. The presence of these antibodies appears to increase the risk for pulmonary fibrosis among patients with scleroderma and is quite specific for the disease.

ANTIRIBOSOMAL P PROTEIN ANTIBODIES

Antiribosomal P protein antibodies have been detected in 10% to 20% of U.S. patients with SLE, 40% to 50% of Asian SLE patients, but rarely in other rheumatic diseases. Testing for these antibodies may be useful when the diagnosis of SLE is uncertain because of the high specificity of this antibody for SLE, albeit with low sensitivity (table 28.3).

Antiribosomal P protein antibodies has limited diagnostic value for central nervous system (CNS) SLE, and is not helpful in differentiating clinical subtypes of SLE (table 28.3).

ANTIHISTONE ANTIBODIES

Antihistone antibodies are present in more than 95% of cases of drug-induced lupus (tables 28.2 and 28.3), particularly those taking procainamide, hydralazine, chlorpromazine, and quinidine; other autoantibodies are uncommon in this disorder. Antihistone antibodies are also seen in up to 80% of patients with idiopathic lupus (table 28.3); however, patients with SLE also form a variety of other autoantibodies, including those directed against DNA and small ribonucleoproteins.

It is important to note that although up to 80% of patients taking procainamide for 1–2 years will develop a positive ANA, most do not develop drug-induced lupus. Thus, screening for these antibodies in the absence of symptoms and stopping the drug if antibodies develop are not recommended.

RHEUMATOID FACTORS

Rheumatoid factors are antibodies directed against the Fc portion of IgG. The rheumatoid factor (RF) as currently measured in clinical practice is an IgM RF, although other immunoglobulin types, including IgG and IgA, have been described.

The presence of RF is generally detected by ELISA or nephelometry. Testing for RF is primarily used for the diagnosis of rheumatoid arthritis; however, RF may also be present in other rheumatic diseases and chronic infections.

CLINICAL DISORDERS ASSOCIATED WITH RF POSITIVITY

Patients with a variety of rheumatic disorders, many of which share similar features, such as symmetric polyarthritis and constitutional symptoms, may have detectable serum RF. These are shown in table 28.4.

Nonrheumatic disorders characterized by chronic antigenic stimulation (especially with circulating immune complexes or polyclonal B-lymphocyte activation) commonly induce RF production (table 28.4). Patients with indolent or chronic infection or chronic inflammation may also demonstrate RF positivity; examples include subacute bacterial endocarditis (SBE) or hepatitis B or C virus infection, inflammatory or fibrosing pulmonary disorders including sarcoidosis, malignancy, and primary biliary cirrhosis.

Rheumatoid factor positivity has also been detected in up to 5% of young, otherwise healthy individuals.

Table 28.4 RF AND ANTI-CCP IN RHEUMATIC AND OTHER DISEASES

	ANTI-CCP		RF	
	SENSITIVITY	SPECIFICITY	SENSITIVITY	SPECIFICITY
Normals	0.79			
RA	64	94	26–90	79
Juvenile arthritis	7.8		13.4	
Osteoarthritis	0			
Palindromic rheumatism	55		42	
Polymyalgia rheumatica	0			
Psoriatic arthritis	11.6		2–10	
Sjögren syndrome	5.4		75–95	
SLE	2.8		15–35	
MCTD			50–60	
Polymyositis/dermatomyositis			5–10	
Hepatitis C	0.5		30	
Mixed cryoglobulinemia			40–100	
Bacterial endocarditis			25–50	
Interstitial pulmonary fibrosis			10–50	
Primary biliary cirrhosis			45–70	

RF Titer

The higher the titer, the greater the likelihood that the patient has rheumatic disease. There are, however, frequent exceptions to this rule, particularly among patients with one of the chronic inflammatory disorders noted above. Furthermore, the use of a higher titer for diagnosis decreases the sensitivity of the test at the same time as it increases the specificity.

Prognostic Value

RF-positive patients with RA may experience more aggressive and erosive joint disease and extra-articular manifestations than those who are RF-negative. Similar findings have been observed in juvenile rheumatoid arthritis. These general observations, however, are of limited utility in an individual patient because of wide interpatient variability. In this setting, accurate prediction of the disease course is not possible from the RF alone.

ANTIBODIES TO CITRULLINATED PROTEINS (CCP)

There has been considerable interest in developing a better test for the diagnosis of RA that has greater sensitivity and specificity than the tests that detect RFs. Within the last decade, as an outgrowth of determining the molecular specificity of antifilaggrin, antikeratin, and antiperinuclear antibodies, it was recognized that many patients with RA have antibodies to citrullinated proteins. Proteins that are citrullinated have had an arginine replaced by citrulline, a minor amino acid. A number of peptides containing citrulline were created, and a cyclic peptide was used to develop an assay to detect antibodies thereto. This test (anti-CCP) has now been studied extensively, and it has better sensitivity and specificity than tests that detect RF for the diagnosis of RA. This is summarized in table 28.4.

In addition, antibodies to CCP were rarely found in patients with other rheumatic conditions and infectious diseases where RF is more frequently found. Anti-CCP is even found frequently before the diagnosis of RA. These observations suggest that the anti-CCP test may be more useful for the diagnosis of RA than are RF tests or at least should be part of the diagnostic algorithm.

ANTINEUTROPHIL CYTOPLASMIC ANTIBODIES (ANCA)

Two different immunofluorescence patterns can be seen when the patient's serum is incubated with ethanol-fixed normal human neutrophils:

- Cytoplasmic ANCA (cANCA) stain the cytoplasm diffusely; these antibodies are almost always directed against proteinase 3 (PR3). cANCA with anti-PR3 specificity is found primarily in patients with Polyangiitis (Wegener granulomatosis) (abbreviated currently as GPA) and microscopic polyarteritis, and occasionally in other diseases (table 28.5).

- Perinuclear ANCAs (pANCA) are usually directed against myeloperoxidase (MPO). The pANCA fluorescence pattern represents an artifact of ethanol fixation, with ethanol and positively charged granule constituents rearranging around and on the negatively charged nuclear membrane. pANCA directed primarily against MPO has been described in patients with a variety of rheumatic autoimmune diseases (table 28.6), whereas non-MPO pANCAs have been associated with several rheumatic and nonrheumatic diseases (table 28.6).

Although patients with rheumatic diseases have an increased frequency of vasculitis, data suggesting that ANCA positivity enhances the risk of vasculitis are contradictory. Nonvasculitic aspects of rheumatic disease activity, severity, and chronicity also fail to correlate consistently with ANCA status. As a result, there is little clinical utility for ANCA testing for patients in whom the presence of an ANCA-associated systemic vasculitis is not suspected on clinical grounds.

DRUG-ASSOCIATED ANCA

The administration of certain drugs has been reported to induce ANCA reactivity in association with varying symptoms. These include the following:

- Hydralazine-induced lupus with anti-MPO and anti-elastase antibodies

Table 28.5 SIGNIFICANCE OF CANCA DIRECTED AGAINST PROTEINASE 3

	FREQUENCY
Wegener's granulomatosis	90%
Microscopic polyarteritis	50%
PAN	5–10%
Churg Strauss angiitis	10%
Hypersensitivity vasculitis	Rare
Henoch-Schonlein purpura	Rare
IgA nephropathy	Rare
Postinfectious glomerulonephritis	Rare
Systemic lupus erythematosus	Rare
Controls	Very rare

Table 28.6 SIGNIFICANCE OF PANCA DIRECTED AGAINST MYELOPEROXIDASE

DISEASE	FREQUENCY (%)
Microscopic polyarteritis	50–70
Idiopathic necrotizing glomerulonephritis	50–85
Churg Strauss syndrome	70–85
Goodpasture (anti-GBM)	10–30
Wegener granulomatosis	5–10
Polyarteritisnodosa	+
Polyangiitis overlap	+
Systemic lupus erythematosus	+
Hydralazine-induced crescenteric glomerulonephritis	+

NOTE: +, reported to be present.

- Hydralazine- associated vasculitis and anti-MPO and antilactoferrin antibodies

- Minocycline-induced arthritis, fever, and livedoreticularis with anti-MPO antibodies

- Propylthiouracil-induced vasculitis and positive ANCA specificities to several different target antigens including PR3, MPO, and elastase

The role of sequential ANCA studies in patient care, after the diagnosis is established, is still unclear. If titers are sequentially followed and an increase is noted in an asymptomatic patient, surveillance should be increased to help detect a possible relapse. It is presently unknown whether it is cost-effective or prudent to sequentially follow ANCA titers.

ANTI-GBM ANTIBODY DISEASE

Antiglomerular basement membrane (GBM) antibody disease, which has similar renal and pulmonary manifestations to Wegener granulomatosis, may be associated with ANCA in 10% to 38% of cases.

The clinical significance of combined ANCA and anti-GBM antibodies is uncertain. Some patients have findings that are uncommon in anti-GBM antibody disease alone, suggesting that there is a concurrent systemic vasculitis. These include purpuric rash, arthralgias, granulomas in the kidney, and a more favorable renal prognosis.

ANTIPHOSPHOLIPID ANTIBODIES

Antiphospholipid antibodies (APL) are antibodies directed against either phospholipids or plasma proteins bound to

Table 28.7 SIGNIFICANCE OF PANCA DIRECTED AGAINST LACTOFERRIN, CATHEPSIN G, ELASTASE, AND LYSOZYME

DISEASE	FREQUENCY (%)
Giant cell arteritis	+
Rheumatoid arthritis	+
Systemic lupus erythematosus	25
Sjögren syndrome	+
Inflammatory bowel disease	+
Ulcerative colitis	+
Crohn disease	10–27
Primary sclerosing cholangitis	+
Unaffected relatives of patients with ulcerative colitis or primary sclerosing cholangitis	25–30
Chronic active hepatitis	+
Primary biliary cirrhosis	+

NOTE: +, reported to be present.

anionic phospholipids. Patients with these antibodies may have a variety of clinical manifestations including venous and arterial thrombosis, recurrent fetal losses, and thrombocytopenia (table 28.3). Patients with these antibodies have either the "primary antiphospholipid antibody syndrome (APS)" when it occurs alone or the secondary APS when it is seen in association with SLE or other rheumatic or autoimmune disorders.

Three major types of antiphospholipid antibodies have been characterized:

- Lupus anticoagulants

- Anticardiolipin antibodies

- Anti-beta-2-glycoprotein-I antibodies

LUPUS ANTICOAGULANTS

Lupus anticoagulants (LA) are antibodies directed against plasma proteins bound to anionic phospholipids. The LA blocks the in vitro assembly of the prothrombinase complex, resulting in a prolongation of in vitro clotting assays such as the activated partial thromboplastin time (aPTT), the dilute Russell viper venom time (RVTT), the kaolin clotting time, and rarely the prothrombin time. These abnormalities are not reversed when the patient's plasma is diluted 1:1 with normal platelet-free plasma, a procedure that will correct clotting disorders due to deficient clotting factors. The abnormal clotting test results can be largely reversed by incubation with a hexagonal-phase phospholipid, which neutralizes the inhibitor. Although these changes suggest impaired coagulation, patients with LA have a paradoxical increase in frequency of arterial and venous thrombotic events.

ANTICARDIOLIPIN ANTIBODIES

Anticardiolipin antibodies (aCL) react with phospholipids such as cardiolipin and phosphatidylserine. There is an approximately 85% concordance between the presence of a LA and aCL. In many cases, however, the LA is a separate population of antibodies from aCL. Thus, testing should be performed for both LA and aCL if APS is clinically suspected. LA positivity is probably associated with a somewhat greater risk for thrombosis than aCL.

Different immunoglobulin isotypes are associated with aCL, including IgG, IgA, and IgM. Elevated levels of IgGaCL incur a greater risk of thrombosis than do other immunoglobulin isotypes.

ANTI-BETA-2-GLYCOPROTEIN I ANTIBODIES

Antibodies to beta-2-glycoprotein I, a phospholipid-binding inhibitor of coagulation, are found in a large percentage of patients with primary or secondary APS. Although antibodies to beta-2-glycoprotein I are commonly found in those with other antiphospholipid antibodies, they are found without anticardiolipin antibodies in approximately 11% of patients with APS. Antibodies to beta-2-glycoprotein I correlate better with symptoms of APS than do antibodies to cardiolipin alone.

Although antiphospholipid antibodies are associated with a propensity for thromboembolic phenomena and (recurrent) miscarriages, especially after 10 weeks of gestation, and with various autoimmune disorders, they are found in up to 2–5% of normal individuals.

FALSE-POSITIVE SEROLOGIC TEST FOR SYPHILIS

Some patients, especially those with SLE, have a false-positive serologic test for syphilis (e.g., VDRL, RPR). Such patients have been noted to have fewer successful pregnancies, an increased number of thrombotic events, livedoreticularis, and migraine headaches, although this may be related to the presence of other antiphospholipid antibodies.

The false-positive STS should not be used to screen for APL because it has a low sensitivity and specificity.

ASSOCIATED DISORDERS

Antiphospholipid antibodies have been noted in increased frequency in patients with SLE: approximately 31% of patients have a LA and 40 to 47% have an aCL. On the other hand, only 50% of patients with a LA have SLE. Antiphospholipid antibodies also occur with increased frequency (5–10%) in women with more than three spontaneous recurrent miscarriages.

Both LA and aCL have also been found occasionally in patients with a variety of other autoimmune and rheumatic diseases; the clinical significance of these observations is not clear.

Antiphospholipid antibodies have also been noted in patients with infections and after the administration of certain drugs. These are usually IgMaCL antibodies, which are less commonly associated with thrombotic events. The infections that have been associated with these antibodies include hepatitis A, mumps, bacterial septicemia, HIV infection, syphilis, HTLV-I, malaria, *Pneumocystis carinii*, infectious mononucleosis, and rubella. Among the drugs that have been implicated are phenothiazines (chlorpromazine), phenytoin, hydralazine, procainamide, quinidine, quinine, valproate, amoxicillin, propranolol, cocaine, sulfadoxine, pyrimethamine, and streptomycin.

TESTING FOR LYME DISEASE

ENZYME-LINKED IMMUNOSORBENT ASSAY

The ELISA is currently the most common initial test to serologically confirm exposure to *B. burgdorferi*.

There are, however, false-positive results with this assay (see below); results that are positive or equivocal by ELISA should be confirmed by Western (immuno) blot analysis. "False seropositivity" is defined as a positive ELISA with a negative Western blot, analogous to the false-positive test for syphilis.

WESTERN BLOT

Western blot allows detection of antibodies to individual components of the organism and is therefore much more specific than the ELISA. Antibodies have been detected against a 41-kDa flagellin; multiple outer surface proteins of which ospA (31 kDa), ospB (34 kDa), and ospC (23 kDa) are best studied; heat shock proteins (60 and 66 kDa); and other prominent proteins, including those at 39, 75, and 83 kDa.

CAUTIONS TO BE USED IN INTERPRETATION

There are a number of issues that must be taken into account when evaluating the significance of a positive or negative serologic test for the presence of antibodies to *B. burgdorferi*.

False Positives with ELISA

Cross-reacting antibodies by ELISA can occur in patients with other Borrelial diseases (relapsing fever), spirochetal diseases (syphilis, leptospirosis, pinta, yaws), viral illnesses, autoimmune diseases (lupus, rheumatoid arthritis), and infectious diseases (including Epstein-Barr virus, malaria, and endocarditis). Finally, it is estimated that 5% or more of the normal population may test positive for Lyme disease by the ELISA due to cross-reacting antibodies elicited by other infections or by the immune response to normal flora.

Lack of Sensitivity in Early Disease

IgM antibodies directed against Borrelial antigens typically appear 2–4 weeks after EM, peak at 6–8 weeks, and decline to low levels after 4–6 months. IgG appears after 6–8 weeks, peaks at 4–6 months, and often remains elevated indefinitely despite therapy and resolution of symptoms.

Because most patients with early Lyme disease will not yet have produced detectable antibodies, those with clinically definite erythema migrans need not be serologically tested. If the true nature of the skin lesion is in doubt, serologic testing may be helpful, but a negative result does not rule out disease and should not necessarily discourage treatment in settings of high clinical suspicion. Serologic testing is clearly not cost-effective if treatment is to be administered independent of testing results.

In comparison to the findings in early disease, almost all untreated patients are antibody-positive in the later stages.

Effects of Antibiotic Therapy

The administration of antibiotics in early disease may abort seroconversion, even if inadequate therapy is given. This concern does not apply in patients with long-standing Lyme disease who have recently received antibiotics; these patients should have been seropositive on the basis of their chronic infection. The test will remain positive for some time after treatment is begun even though antibody production has ceased. However, some patients continue to make antibodies and therefore remain seropositive for long periods of time (see below).

Interlaboratory Variation

Results of ELISA tests from different laboratories may vary because of technique; therefore, it is best to compare results from the same laboratory.

Persistence of Positivity

As mentioned above, high levels of IgG are commonly sustained despite adequate therapy and resolution of symptoms. For this reason, follow-up serologic testing is of no value in assessing the patient who is cured or slowly improving.

The one setting in which follow-up testing may be helpful is the patient in whom there is either worsening of Lyme disease or the appearance of new features of possible Lyme disease (as with a patient with EM who is treated and months later develops monoarthritis). In this clinical setting, if sequential immunoblots performed in the same laboratory demonstrate the appearance of new "bands" (i.e., reactivity with proteins not previously recognized), the clinician should consider the possibility of ongoing infection. However, the immune response does not immediately cease simply because antibiotic therapy is begun, and new reactivity on immunoblot may appear despite effective antibiotic therapy. Thus, an expanding repertoire cannot be interpreted as reflecting ongoing infection unless worsening and/or evolution of the clinical signs is present.

USEFULNESS OF SEROLOGIC TESTS

If the test is utilized in a clinical setting in which Lyme disease is likely, such as isolated monoarthritis or bilateral facial nerve palsy in an endemic area, a positive test is likely to confirm the clinical suspicion of Lyme disease.

In disease of long duration, such as tertiary neuroborreliosis or Lyme arthritis, seroreactivity by ELISA and immunoblot is virtually universal. Absence of seroreactivity in such a patient, unless there is a plausible explanation, should raise significant doubts about the diagnosis of Lyme disease. In other words, the negative predictive power of a test in such a patient is high.

COMPLEMENT

Complement levels can be evaluated either by functional or antigenic assays. The most frequently used are immunoassays (antigenic assays) for C3 and C4 and the total hemolytic complement (CH50), which measures activation of the entire classical pathway.

CH50

The CH50 assesses the ability of the test serum to lyse sensitized sheep erythrocytes. All nine components of the classical pathway (C1 through C9) are required to give a normal CH50.

CH50 is a useful screening tool for detecting a deficiency of the classical pathway, either of a single component or of several components (as may be seen in SLE). The CH50 can also detect a homozygous deficiency of classical pathway components as indicated by a value of close to 0 units/mL. In contrast, with activation-induced reduction, several components, such as C4 and C3, will be decreased. In this setting, the CH50 is rarely <10 units/mL.

The CH50 assay requires appropriate collection, processing, and storage of specimens because several of the complement proteins are thermolabile. As a result, a common cause of a depressed CH50 is improper specimen handling. Serum samples should be assayed the day of collection or stored frozen at –70°C.

PLASMA C3 AND C4 LEVELS

Plasma C3 and C4 levels are usually measured in nephelometric immunoassays.

CLINICAL SIGNIFICANCE

Hypocomplementemia of CH50, C3, and C4 may be present in disorders associated with excessive levels of immune complexes, such as SLE, mixed cryoglobulinemia, certain glomerulonephritides, and certain vasculitides.

Assays of CH50, C1q, C4, and C3 may be valuable in following the course of these diseases.

- Classical pathway activation is indicated by low levels of C4 and C3 and normal levels of factor B

- Alternative pathway activation is indicated by decreased factor B and C3, and normal levels of C4, as in septicemia.

- Activation of the classical and alternative pathways is indicated by decreased levels of C1q, C4, C3, and factor B.

- Elevated levels of CH50, C3, C4, and factor B are common in many diseases associated with inflammation and represent an increase in hepatic synthesis as part of the acute-phase response.

INHERITED COMPLEMENT DEFICIENCY

A genetic deficiency of a single component is indicated by a virtually absent CH50, the fixed absence of a single component combined with normal levels of other complement components.

C1 INHIBITOR DEFICIENCY

A functional deficiency of C1 inhibitor (C1-Inh) produces the clinical syndrome of hereditary angioedema. In contrast to "allergic" angioedema, the edematous lesion lasts several days, is nonpruritic and nonerythematous, and is not associated with hives.

C1 inhibitor deficiency can be acquired or inherited in an autosomal dominant fashion. The acquired form is caused either by an autoantibody to C1-Inh or by excessive utilization (usually in the setting of malignancy).

A deficiency of functional C1 inhibitor prevents the proper regulation of activated C1. As a result, plasma levels of C4 and C2, the substrates of C1, are chronically reduced in most patients even between attacks and uniformly reduced during an attack.

URIC ACID

Uric acid determination may be helpful in certain clinical settings, particularly in suspected gout or in monitoring urate-lowering therapy. Because most patients with asymptomatic hyperuricemia will never develop gout or related problems, screening patients for hyperuricemia is not recommended. Whereas finding of an elevated or high-normal uric acid has little predictive value with respect to gout, patients with "low-normal" uric acid levels (e.g., 5.5 mg/dL or less) rarely develop gout.

If hyperuricemia is persistent, a thorough history, physical examination, and laboratory work should be performed and directed at discovering potential causes of hyperuricemia that may mandate treatment. As an example, lympho- and myeloproliferative disorders, polycythemia vera, vitamin B-12 deficiency, preeclampsia, and lead nephropathy (or lead exposure) may all lead to hyperuricemia and warrant treatment of the underlying disease. Treatment with many diuretics also causes elevations of serum uric acid levels.

Urinary collections for uric acid over a 24-hour period may be useful in the evaluation of nephrolithiasis, to classify a patient with gout as an overproducer or underexcreter, or if uricosuric therapy is under consideration.

SYNOVIAL FLUID

Synovial fluid analysis is inexpensive and may be diagnostic in patients with bacterial infections or crystal-induced synovitis. This analysis should be performed in the febrile patient with an acute flare of established arthritis to rule out superimposed septic arthritis as well as in any patient with an undiagnosed acute, inflammatory monoarthritis. In other situations, its main value is to permit classification into an inflammatory, noninflammatory, or hemorrhagic category and to monitor a condition (e.g., to determine whether an infection is clearing).

EXAMINATION OF SYNOVIAL FLUID

Normal joints contain a small amount of synovial fluid with the following characteristics:

- Highly viscous

- Clear

- Essentially acellular

- Protein concentration approximately one-third that of plasma

- Glucose concentration similar to that in plasma

If a synovial effusion is present and arthrocentesis is indicated, joint fluid should be routinely analyzed for volume,

Table 28.8 CATEGORIES OF SYNOVIAL FLUID

MEASURE	NORMAL	NONINFLAMMATORY	INFLAMMATORY	SEPTIC	HEMORRHAGIC
Volume, mL (knee)	<3.5	Often >3.5	Often >3.5	Often >3.5	Usually >3.5
Clarity	Transparent	Transparent	Translucent-opaque	Opaque	*Bloody*
Color	Clear	Yellow	Yellow to opalescent	Yellow	Red
Viscosity	High	High	Low	*Variable*	Variable
WBC per mm^3	<200	200–2000	2,000–50,000	>50,000*	200–2000
PMNs,%	<25	<25	>50	>75	50–75
Culture	Negative	Negative	Negative	Often positive	Negative
Total protein, g/dL	1–2	1–3	3–5	3–5	4–6
LDH (compared to levels in blood	Very low	Very low	High	Variable	Similar
Glucose, mg/dL	Nearly equal to blood	Nearly equal to blood	>25, lower than blood	<25, much lower than blood	Nearly equal to blood

NOTE: *Lower with infections caused by partially treated or low-virulence organisms.

clarity, color, viscosity, cell count with differential, Gram stain, culture, and crystals. In certain clinical settings, such as partially treated septic arthritis, synovial fluid glucose and protein may have utility as well.

Noninflammatory fluids generally have fewer than 2000 white blood cells/mm^3, with fewer than 75% polymorphonuclear leukocytes (table 28.8). An unexplained inflammatory fluid, particularly in a febrile patient, should be assumed to be infected until proven otherwise.

Synovial fluid is subsequently categorized as normal, noninflammatory, inflammatory, septic, or hemorrhagic based on the clinical and laboratory analysis (see table 28.8). The differential diagnosis of each of these specific categories is broad and not necessarily exclusive:

- *Noninflammatory*—The most common causes of a non-inflammatory joint effusion include degenerative joint disease (osteoarthritis), trauma, mechanical derangement (ligament or cartilage injury), neuropathic arthropathy, subsiding or early inflammation, hypertrophic osteoarthropathy, and aseptic necrosis.

- *Inflammatory*—The most common causes of inflammatory effusions include rheumatoid arthritis, acute crystal-induced synovitis, and spondyloarthropathy. SLE may be associated with an inflammatory or noninflammatory effusion.

- *Septic*—Septic effusions may be due to bacteria, mycobacteria, or fungus.

- *Hemorrhagic*—Hemorrhagic effusions may be caused by hemophilia or other hemorrhagic diathesis, calcium pyrophosphate deposition disease (pseudogout),

trauma with or without fracture, mechanical derangement,

- Neuropathic arthropathy, excessive anticoagulation, pigmented villonodular synovitis, or other neoplasm.

Infected fluid is usually purulent with a leukocyte count (most of which are neutrophils) of over 50,000 cells/mm^3. However, lower cell counts may be observed among immunocompromised patients and in infections due to mycobacterial, some Neisserial, and several Gram-positive organisms. Chemistry studies such as the concentrations of glucose, lactate dehydrogenase, or protein have only limited value: a reduction in glucose concentration and elevation in LDH concentration are consistent with bacterial infection but are not sufficiently sensitive or specific.

ROUTINE CULTURE

The synovial fluid samples are routinely sent for culture of the common nongonococcal causes of bacterial arthritis: staphylococci followed by streptococci and Gram-negative bacteria. These organisms are easily grown on routine culture media in the absence of concomitant antibiotic therapy. The diagnostic yield may be improved by inoculation of blood culture bottles, although the efficacy of this approach is controversial.

Gonococcal Arthritis

Gonococcal arthritis is a common cause of septic arthritis in which the organism cannot be cultured on routine culture media.

The joint aspirate should be cultured for *N. gonorrhoeae* when the history is suggestive. The yield can be increased if plates of chocolate agar or Thayer-Martin medium are inoculated with synovial fluid at the bedside along with cultures from the pharynx, urethra, cervix, rectum, and skin lesions (if present). Blood cultures are often positive in patients presenting with tenosynovitis and skin lesions alone but are frequently negative if a joint effusion is present.

Cultures of synovial fluid tend to be positive in less than 50% of cases of gonococcal arthritis. Use of polymerase chain reaction (PCR) techniques to detect gonococcal DNA in synovial fluid can increase the yield in culture-negative cases and permits monitoring of the response to therapy. However, this technique is not yet widely available, and its cost-effectiveness remains unproven.

When Should Cultures Be Sent for Unusual Organisms?

The history may reveal clues suggesting the possibility of an unusual cause of septic arthritis:

- A history of tuberculosis exposure
- A history of trauma or an animal bite
- Travel to or living in an area endemic with fungal infections or Lyme disease
- The presence of immune suppression
- A monoarthritis that is refractory to conventional therapy

SYNOVIAL FLUID CRYSTAL ANALYSIS

Aspiration of synovial fluid from the affected joint and analysis of the fluid by polarized light microscopy permits identification of sodium urate crystals in the great majority of instances of acute gouty arthritis. Joint aspiration is also helpful in distinguishing acute gout from pseudogout (calcium pyrophosphate crystal deposition, or CPPD, disease), although occasionally both crystals may be identifiable in the synovial fluid of patients in whom these disorders coexist.

Gout crystals are needle-shaped and display strongly negative birefrigence (i.e., they are yellow when parallel to the axis of the polarizer). CPPD crystals are pleomorphic, often in the shape of rhomboids with blunt ends, and are weakly positively birefringent (they appear blue when parallel to the axis of the polarizer). The clinical significance of intracellular crystals is often said to be greater than when they are extracellular, although no convincing evidence supports this suggestion.

The sensitivity of polarized microscopy in demonstrating negatively birefringent crystals in patients with acute gouty arthritis is at least 85%, and the specificity for gout is 100% if the results are unequivocal. However, gouty arthritis may occasionally coexist with another type of joint disease, such as septic arthritis or pseudogout. In some cases, needle-shaped crystals may be evident on a slide without polarized microscopy, especially when the crystals are abundant.

- Even during the asymptomatic intercritical period, extracellular urate crystals are identifiable in synovial fluid from previously affected joints in virtually all untreated gouty patients and approximately 70% of those administered uric acid-lowering therapy. This allows late establishment of the diagnosis in the majority of patients in whom the diagnosis was not made in the acute setting.

- Demonstration of urate crystals in aspirates of tophaceous deposits provides a convenient and specific means to corroborate the diagnosis in the small proportion of gouty individuals with tophi. Because these patients are typically treated with lifelong urate-lowering therapy, identification of tophaceous gout has significant therapeutic impact.

ACKNOWLEDGMENT

We are indebted to the work of many authors of *UpToDate in Medicine*, whose work provided a useful framework for the development of this chapter, as well as to Dr. Robert Shmerling, with whom I have written chapters on this same subject.

ADDITIONAL READING

American College of Physicians. Guidelines for laboratory evaluation in the diagnosis of Lyme disease. *Ann Intern Med.* 1997;127:1106.

American College of Rheumatology Ad Hoc Committee on Clinical Guidelines. Guidelines for the initial evaluation of the adult patient with acute musculoskeletal symptoms. *Arthritis Rheum.* 1996;39:1.

Breda L, Nozzi M, De Sanctis S, Chiarelli F. Laboratory tests in the diagnosis and follow-up of pediatric rheumatic diseases: An update. *Semin Arthritis Rheum.* 2010;40(1):53–72.

Joseph A, Brasington R, Kahl L, Ranganathan P, Cheng TP, Atkinson J. Immunologic rheumatic disorders. *J Allergy ClinImmunol.* 2010;125(2 Suppl 2):S204–15.

Miller A, Green M, Robinson D. Simple rule for calculating normal erythrocyte sedimentation rate. Brit Med J (Clin Res Ed). 1983;286:266.

Pincus T, Sokka T. Laboratory tests to assess patients with rheumatoid arthritis: Advantages and limitations. *Rheum Dis Clin North Am.* 2009;35(4):731–4, vi-vii.

Shmerling RH, Delbanco TL, Tosteson AN, Trentham DE. Synovial fluid tests. What should be ordered? *JAMA.* 1990; 264:1009.

Ton E, Kruize AA. How to perform and analyse biopsies in relation to connective tissue diseases. *Best Pract Res ClinRheumatol.* 2009;23(2):233–55.

Wener MH, Daum PR, McQuillam GM. The influence of age, sex, and race on the upper refrence limit of C-reactive protein concentration. 2000;27:2351.

QUESTIONS

QUESTION 1. A 48-year-old woman presents with a 4-week history of severe fatigue, painful joints, and a rash over her face. Examination shows normal vital signs, a malar maculopapular rash, and mildy erythematous proximal interphalangeal and metacarpal joints of both hands. Initial laboratory testing reveals an erythrocyte sedimentation rate of 68 mm/hr, normal electrolytes, and normal BUN and creatinine, liver function tests, and CBC. Serologies are requested. All of the following are correct statements EXCEPT:

A. An elevated ANA and anti-dsDNA titer would strongly support a diagnosis of SLE.

B. Anti-Sm (Smith) are specific antibodies for SLE, but Anti-Ro and anti-La antibodies are not specific for SLE.

C. Detection of antiribonucleoprotein (anti-RNP) antibodies is more likely to suggest a diagnosis of "mixed connective tissue disease."

D. The presence of antihistone antibodies should raise the possibility of drug-induced lupus.

E. Anti Scl-70 antibodies are likely to be elevated in this patient.

QUESTION 2. A 49-year-old patient suspected of acute gout of his right big toe undergoes synovial fluid aspiration. Which one of the following statements is correct?

A. Short, rhomboidal crystals would be typical of monosodium urate monohydrate (MSU).

B. Monosodium urate monohydrate (MSU) crystals show strong negative birefringence.

C. The synovial fluid WBC count is usually <200/mm^3.

D. Viscosity of the synovial fluid is high.

E. The synovial fluid usually has a reddish discoloration.

ANSWERS

1. E
2. B
3. B

29.

BOARD SIMULATION: RHEUMATIC AND IMMUNOLOGIC DISEASE

Elinor A. Mody

QUESTION 1. A 45-year-old woman with a 9-month history of joint pain, swelling, fatigue, and morning stiffness presents to her rheumatologist. On exam, she has swollen metacarpophalangeals (MCPs), proximal interphalangeals (PIPs) wrists, knees, and ankles. She also has metatarsophalangeal (MTP) squeeze tenderness. Her rheumatoid factor and anti-CCP antibody tests are positive. Her rheumatologist starts methotrexate at escalating doses starting at 10 mg a week, up to 20 mg a week. The patient improves, with her sedimentation rate dropping from 50 to 30, her morning stiffness improving to 30 minutes, and her joints are less swollen and tender. At this point, the most appropriate action is:

A. Continue methotrexate at 20 mg a week
B. Decrease methotrexate to 15 mg a week
C. Add a second agent

QUESTION 2. A 30-year-old man presents to his rheumatologist with a 4-month history of back pain and stiffness. He reports being stiff in the morning for up to 4 hours. Two years ago, he suffered anterior uveitis, treated with topical steroids. Sacroiliac radiographs show unilateral sacroiliitis. Indomethacin has helped with his back symptoms to a slight degree but has given him epigastric pain. At this point, the most appropriate action is:

A. Check for HLA-B27
B. Switch his anti-inflammatory to ibuprofen
C. Stop his indomethacin and add sulfasalazine at 2 g a day
D. Stop his indomethacin and add an anti-tumor necrosis factor (TNF) agent

QUESTION 3. A 22-year-old woman presents to a rheumatologist with a 3-month history of a scaling, erythematous eruption across her scalp and neck; there is some evidence of scarring. Apart from mild Raynaud's phenomenon, she has an otherwise negative review of systems. Her laboratories show normal complete blood count (CBC), chemistry profile, sedimentation rate, and urinalysis, but her antinuclear antibody (ANA) is positive at 1:640, with a positive Smith antibody and a minimally elevated anti-dsDNA antibody level. Biopsy of the rash reveals an interface dermatitis consistent with subcutaneous lupus erythematosus. At this point, the most appropriate action would be:

A. Start hydroxychloroquine
B. Counsel patient on sun protection
C. Consult nephrology for a renal biopsy
D. A and B
E. All of the above

QUESTION 4. An 80-year-old man with chronic renal insufficiency and coronary artery disease presents with a painful, swollen, warm right ankle for 2 days. He does not recall any trauma and denies recent sexual activity. He has no significant past medical history, other than stated above. At this point, the most appropriate initial action would be:

A. Aspiration of the ankle, with synovial fluid culture and crystal examination
B. Obtain a radiograph of the ankle
C. Obtain blood cultures
D. Bloodwork including CBC, uric acid level, creatinine level
E. Start allopurinol therapy

QUESTION 5. A 45-year-old woman with rheumatoid arthritis has been on methotrexate for 2 years, and for the past month has been on etanercept. Over the past week, she complains of a facial rash and chest pain. On exam, she has a malar rash. Her lungs are clear; however, her chest radiograph reveals a small pleural effusion. Her D-dimer level is not elevated. She has no dyspnea, just pain with a deep breath. At this point, the most appropriate action is:

A. Check her ANA titers, including an anti-dsDNA level
B. Start IV antibiotics for presumptive pneumonia
C. Increase the methotrexate dose
D. Stop the etanercept

QUESTION 6. A 20-year-old man is referred to you by his internist for treatment of rheumatoid arthritis. On exam, he has no evidence of synovitis, just tenderness of most of his joints. His rheumatoid factor is positive, but his anti-CCP antibody titer is negative. His erythrocyte sedimentation rate (ESR) and C-reactive protein (CRP) are also within normal limits. At this point, the most appropriate action is:

A. Start methotrexate and folic acid
B. Start an anti-TNF agent
C. Suggest to the patient that he try over-the-counter anti-inflammatory agents
D. Obtain hepatitis serologies.

QUESTION 7. A 30-year-old woman with a 10-year history of Raynaud's phenomenon, on exam, has telangiectasias, sclerodactyly distal to the wrists, and by history has significant acid reflux symptomatology. She is a smoker but quit recently. Her most likely diagnosis is:

A. Buerger disease
B. Scleroderma
C. CREST syndrome
D. Systemic lupus erythematosus

QUESTION 8. The woman described in the previous question reports recent-onset shortness of breath. She denies any recent infections. At this point, the most appropriate action is:

A. Prescribe an albuterol inhaler
B. Obtain a high-resolution chest computed tomography (CT) scan
C. Start nifedipine therapy
D. Obtain an echocardiogram

QUESTION 9. A 30-year-old man from Greece presents with painful, scarring oral ulcers, synovitis of his MCPs, wrists, and ankles. His rheumatoid factor is negative, and he has no history of colitis. The most likely diagnosis at this point is:

A. Crohn disease
B. Ulcerative colitis
C. Behçet disease
D. Ankylosing spondylitis

QUESTION 10. At this point in the case of question 9, the most appropriate action is:

A. Obtain an ophthalmology consult
B. Start colchicine therapy
C. Start IV cyclophosphamide therapy
D. Refer patient for a colonoscopy

QUESTION 11. A 69-year-old woman has a 1-month history of scalp pain, low-grade fevers, arthralgias, fatigue, and malaise. On exam, she has good temporal artery pulses and no evidence of scalp necrosis or tenderness. Her labs reveal an ESR of 99. At this point, the most appropriate action is:

A. Temporal artery biopsy
B. Start nonsteroidal anti-inflammatory drug (NSAID) therapy
C. Start methotrexate therapy
D. Obtain blood cultures

QUESTION 12. A 60-year-old man with a 20-year history of seropositive rheumatoid arthritis on methotrexate monotherapy presents with an open "sore" on his leg. He reports that he initially had a minor scrape in that area, which then became much larger and would not heal. On exam, he has a 5 cm in diameter open, draining, very tender lesion. Cultures are negative, including wound cultures. The most likely diagnosis is:

A. Cellulitis
B. Squamous cell carcinoma
C. Mycosis fungoides
D. Pyoderma gangrenosum

QUESTION 13. The most appropriate therapy for this patient is:

A. Excision
B. IV antibiotics
C. prednisone

QUESTION 14. A 55-year-old man with a 10-year history of plaque psoriasis and a diagnosis of osteoarthritis of his hands presents with a 2-week history of right ankle pain. On exam the ankle is swollen, with decreased range of motion and some tenderness. Of note, he has nail pitting and onycholysis. There is no history of trauma. His past medical history is only positive for bilateral Achilles tendinitis. The most likely diagnosis is:

A. Psoriatic arthritis
B. Gout
C. Rheumatoid arthritis
D. Osteoarthritis

QUESTION 15. A 55-year-old woman presents with a chief complaint of bilateral hand pain for several years. She denies wrist pain, significant arm stiffness, or other joint pain. Her past medical history is significant only for mild hyperglycemia. On exam, she has no obvious synovitis but significant bilateral MCP tenderness. Radiographs of her hands reveal joint space narrowing, sclerosis, and osteophyte formation at her third MCP joints bilaterally. At this point, the most appropriate action is:

A. Start methotrexate therapy
B. Inject both affected joints with hydrocortisone
C. Draw serum chemistries, including ferritin level
D. Start NSAID therapy

QUESTION 16. A 68-year-old woman presents with myalgias of a few weeks' duration. Her current medications include atorvastatin, alendronate, hydrochlorothiazide, and Premarin vaginal cream. On exam, she has no motor weakness, no synovitis, and her laboratories are normal, including a creatine phosphokinase level. The most likely cause of this patient's myalgias is:

A. Polymyositis
B. Inclusion body myopathy
C. Atorvastatin
D. Alendronate

QUESTION 17. A 30-year-old man felt a "pop" at the back of his left heel while running 1 day prior. He has pain and swelling in the area and has trouble standing on his toes on that foot. The most appropriate maneuver at this point is:

A. Thompson's
B. McMurray's
C. McBurney's
D. Schober's

QUESTION 18. A 50-year-old woman with rheumatoid arthritis on methotrexate is about to start infliximab therapy. A PPD is performed and is positive. The patient reports that she is an immigrant and had the bacille Calmette-Guérin (BCG) vaccination in her youth. A chest x-ray is negative. The most appropriate action at this point is:

A. Start isoniazid (INH) therapy
B. Start infliximab therapy
C. Perform three sputum cultures for acid-fast bacillus (AFB)
D. Increase methotrexate dose

QUESTION 19. A 26-year-old woman presents with a 2-week history of pain and swelling of her wrists, MCPs, and MTPs bilaterally, significant arm stiffness, and malaise. Her rheumatoid factor and CCP are negative. Of note, her two small children have had a recent viral infection, with fever and a rash. At this point, the most appropriate blood work to obtain is:

A. ANA titer
B. Hepatitis serologies
C. Parvovirus titers
D. Epstein-Barr virus (EBV) titers

ANSWERS

1. C. There is a significant amount of data to support the use of two agents in the treatment of rheumatoid arthritis for patients who do not fully remit on methotrexate alone.

2. D. This patient has a spondyloarthropathy with ongoing inflammatory back disease resistant to NSAIDs. The only other class of medications that has been shown to work in this disease with axial skeletal involvement is the anti-TNF class.

3. E. This patient has subcutaneous lupus erythematosus, and the treatment of choice is hydroxychloroquine, assuming there are no contraindications. Sun protection is extremely important, however, as sun exposure can greatly worsen SCLE and can cause other photosensitive rashes in these patients.

4. A. Although everything in this case points to an acute gouty flare, including the sudden-onset inflammatory process in a joint of the lower extremity, in the setting of renal insufficiency, the only way to prove it is to see intracellular crystals in the synovial fluid.

5. D. This patient's symptoms are temporally associated with starting etanercept. The anti-TNF drugs have all been associated with drug-induced lupus, which is the diagnosis most consistent with this patient's symptoms. Many patients on anti-TNF therapy will have a positive anti-dsDNA antibody level, which may or may not correlate with any clinical manifestations.

6. D. Hepatitis C can cause a false-positive rheumatoid factor. In this patient without synovitis and a negative anti-CCP antibody titer, which is a more specific test for rheumatoid arthritis, hepatitis C is a real possibility.

7. C. This patient has Raynaud's phenomenon (R), esophageal dysmotility (E), sclerodactyly (S), and telangiectasias (T). Evidence of calcinosis (C) is not given. However, Buerger disease does not cause telangiectasias and sclerodactyly, and these symptoms do not invoke SLE.

8. D. As this patient appears to have (calcinosis cutis, Raynaud's, esophageal dysmotility, sclerodactyly, and telangiectasia) the most likely reason for shortness of breath would be pulmonary artery hypertension, evidence of which can be found on echocardiogram.

9. C. Although inflammatory bowel disease cannot be completely ruled out, the absence of diarrhea in addition to the country of origin suggest that Behçet is the most likely diagnosis.

10. B. Colchicine therapy has been shown to work in mild Behçet disease.

11. A. This patient has a history suggestive of giant-cell arteritis. Of the choices available, temporal artery biopsy is the most appropriate. It would not be inappropriate to start corticosteroid therapy until temporal artery biopsy can be performed; this was not given as a choice, however. Any other therapy would not be appropriate initially in the setting of this potentially sight-threatening disease.

12. D. Pyoderma gangrenosum is seen in the setting of rheumatoid arthritis and is commonly a Koebner-like phenomenon. Given the open nature of the lesion and the negative cultures, infection is unlikely. Because of the short time period during which this has formed, cutaneous malignancy is unlikely.

13. C. Excision is contraindicated for a pyoderma lesion, as it can Koebnerize and become much worse. IV antibiotics are not helpful unless infection coexists, which is not common. Immunosuppression is the treatment of choice.

14. A. This patient has a history very suggestive of psoriatic arthritis, given his history of Achilles tendonitis, which is a common enthesitis in this disorder, nail changes, and

a 10-year history of plaque psoriasis. Gout is also possible, but a first flare would be unlikely to last for 2 weeks. Osteoarthritis does not cause an acute flare, and although rheumatoid arthritis is possible, it most commonly is a symmetric polyarthritis involving the hands and wrists.

15. C. Osteoarthritis of the MCPs is secondary osteoarthritis; and osteoarthritis of the third MCP is a classic presentation of hemochromatosis.

16. D. This is not a history consistent with polymyositis, as there is no motor weakness, nor is it consistent with myositis from HMG-CoA reductase inhibitors, as the CPK is normal. Although inclusion-body myositis is possible, the most likely scenario is myalgias caused by alendronate.

17. A. This history and exam are consistent with an acute Achilles tendon rupture; the appropriate maneuver to diagnose this is the Thompson's maneuver. The McMurray's maneuver is used to diagnose meniscal tears in the knee, McBurney's refers to a tender right upper quadrant due to acute cholecystitis, and the Schober's test is one of excursion of the lumbar spine.

18. A. According to CDC recommendations, BCG history should be ignored when interpreting a positive PPD. Therefore, as the PPD is positive, and infliximab therapy is to be started, of the choices available, starting INH therapy is the correct choice. Another appropriate choice is to obtain a chest radiograph to rule out active tuberculosis.

19. C. Parvovirus infection in adults often is not manifest as a rash and can cause a self-limited inflammatory arthritis, which can mimic rheumatoid arthritis.

30.

RHEUMATOLOGY SUMMARY

Derrick J. Todd and Jonathan S. Coblyn

Rheumatology is the study and treatment of diseases that affect the musculoskeletal system and connective tissues. This chapter provides an overview of the many different rheumatic disorders, reviews common tests used in the diagnosis or monitoring of rheumatic diseases, and highlights the various pharmacologic agents used in the treatment of these conditions.

Most rheumatic diseases can be conceptualized as either inflammatory or noninflammatory disorders. Idiopathic autoimmune diseases comprise the majority of inflammatory rheumatic disorders. Some inflammatory disorders have fibrosis as their principal manifestation. Inflammatory disorders with a better-defined origin include the microcrystalline diseases (e.g., gout and pseudogout) and the many infectious arthritides. Laboratory tests and imaging studies in rheumatology generally fall into two categories: those used to aid diagnosis and those used to monitor therapy. Most pharmacotherapy in rheumatic diseases is targeted against inflammation, pain, or both. In this chapter, laboratory testing, radiologic imaging, and treatment modalities are discussed within their respective disease contexts.

IDIOPATHIC AUTOIMMUNE DISORDERS

RHEUMATOID ARTHRITIS

Rheumatoid arthritis (RA) is a systemic autoimmune condition that primarily causes inflammation of synovial tissue (synovitis) with resultant inflammatory arthritis and tenosynovitis. RA classically presents as a symmetric polyarthritis of the small joints of the upper and lower extremities, although almost any joint can be involved. RA most commonly presents in patients with peak onset at ages 25–55 and ratio of 3:1 women to men. All ages, genders, and races may be affected, however. The hallmark pathologic process is proliferative synovitis, which can lead to cartilage destruction, bone erosion, and deforming arthritis. Patients with RA may experience extra-articular symptoms as well, most commonly constitutional and sicca symptoms, skin nodules, interstitial lung disease (ILD), serositis (pleural and pericardial effusions), anemia, and thrombocytosis. Less common complications include vasculitis, secondary amyloidosis, ocular disease, Felty syndrome, large granular lymphocyte syndrome, and lymphomas. Please see table 23.5 for a complete listing of extra-articular complications of RA.

The diagnosis of RA is aided by testing for serum rheumatoid factor (RF) and anti–cyclic citrullinated peptide (CCP) antibodies. These are present in approximately 80% of RA patients, with anti-CCP antibody testing being much more specific for RA than the serum RF. Importantly, about 20% of patients with RA never demonstrate abnormal RF or anti-CCP values. Laboratory markers of inflammation (table 30.1) are nonspecific but often correlate with disease activity. Analysis of synovial fluid in a patient with RA demonstrates >1500 WBC/mm³, but this finding is nonspecific and not diagnostic for RA. Arthrocentesis in this setting is used primarily to establish whether the effusion is inflammatory or not and to exclude other diagnoses (e.g., septic or microcrystalline arthritis). Plain film radiology may show soft tissue swelling, periarticular osteopenia, joint space narrowing, and marginal erosions. Magnetic resonance imaging (MRI) and musculoskeletal ultrasound are playing emerging roles in the diagnosis of RA.

Historically, nonsteroidal anti-inflammatory agents (NSAIDs) and analgesics were mainstays of RA therapy. More recently, however, great strides have been made in the treatment of RA. These treatments focus on interrupting the inflammatory proliferative synovitis. Corticosteroids have been able to accomplish this, but with many potential side effects (table 30.2). More recent treatment strategies aim to limit corticosteroid usage and impair disease progression through the use of disease-modifying antirheumatic drugs (DMARDs). For a list of DMARDs, their mechanisms of action, and side effect profiles, please see table 23.6. Examples of traditional DMARDs include methotrexate, leflunomide, hydroxychloroquine, sulfasalazine, gold, and

Table 30.1 COMMON LABORATORY ABNORMALITIES ASSOCIATED WITH INFLAMMATION

Elevated erythrocyte sedimentation rate

Elevated C-reactive protein

Thrombocytosis

Leukocytosis

Elevated complements

Elevated haptoglobin

Elevated ferritin

Table 30.3 DIFFERENTIAL DIAGNOSIS OF DISEASES ASSOCIATED WITH AN ERYTHROCYTE SEDIMENTATION RATE >100 MM/HR

Rheumatic diseases
  Polymyalgia rheumatica
  Systemic vasculitis, including giant cell arteritis
  Adult onset Still disease
  Unusually active rheumatic disorder (e.g., polyarticular gout, highly active RA)

Infectious diseases
  Endocarditis
  Osteomyelitis
  Septic arthritis

Malignant diseases
  Multiple myeloma
  Extensively metastatic disease

many others. The last decade has witnessed the advent of biological DMARD therapy, with drugs that antagonize the tumor necrosis factor-α (TNF-α) (etanercept, infliximab, and adalimumab), block T-cell costimulation (abatacept), or cause B-cell depletion (rituximab). These drugs, although potent immunosuppressive agents, have revolutionized the treatment of RA, creating a paradigm shift in treatment goals away from palliation and toward remission.

POLYMYALGIA RHEUMATICA

Polymyalgia rheumatica (PMR) is a systemic inflammatory disorder of individuals older than age 50. It typically presents as limb-girdle achiness of the shoulders and hips out of proportion to examination findings. Presentation is usually sudden in onset and is rarely associated with synovitis of the small joints. Laboratory tests show evidence of systemic inflammation (table 30.1). Erythrocyte sedimentation rate (ESR) may be >100 mm/hr, an uncommon finding (table 30.3). Up to 5–10% of patients with PMR will evolve

into an illness that resembles RA. Up to 15–20% of patients with PMR will develop symptoms of giant-cell arteritis (discussed below). Low-dose corticosteroids (<15 mg daily) are the primary treatment for PMR. Steroids are tapered as symptoms allow, sometimes over 1–2 years.

SPONDYLOARTHROPATHIES

The spondyloarthropathies are a collection of disorders that include ankylosing spondylitis, psoriatic arthritis, arthropathy associated with inflammatory bowel disease (IBD arthropathy), postinfectious (reactive) arthritis, and undifferentiated spondyloarthropathy. Unlike RA, peripheral arthritis is typically oligoarticular, asymmetric, and most pronounced in the lower extremities. Further distinguishing features of spondyloarthropathies include lumbosacral inflammation (spondylitis or sacroiliitis), enthesitis, and bone-forming lesions by radiography. Morning back stiffness in a young person should alert the clinician to the possibility of inflammatory back disease.

Ankylosing spondylitis (AS) has a >3:1 male-to-female predominance. AS primarily affects the spine and can lead to fusion (ankylosis) of the vertebrae. Women may develop AS in an atypical fashion with neck involvement before spine and sacroiliac (SI) joint involvement. Psoriatic arthritis and IBD arthropathy are associated with their respective disease entities, but spine involvement can cause "skip areas" rather than a uniform progression as one sees in AS. Arthritis may precede the skin or bowel disease in these disorders. Reactive arthritis is associated with antecedent infection by chlamydia or enteroinvasive bowel pathogens (*Shigella*, *Salmonella*, or *Yersinia*). Additional extra-articular manifestations of all the spondyloarthropathies may include dactylitis ("sausage digit"), uveitis, circinate balanitis, and scaly plantar lesions (keratoderma blennorrhagica). Rarely, these conditions are associated with proximal aortic aneurisms and pulmonary fibrosis.

Table 30.2 SIDE EFFECTS OF SYSTEMIC CORTICOSTEROIDS

Immunosuppression

Insulin resistance

Hypertension

Weight gain (cushingoid appearance)

Bone demineralization

Avascular necrosis

Cataracts

Adrenal suppression

Steroid myopathy

Increased cardiovascular risk

Laboratory workup of the spondyloarthropathies fails to reveal antinuclear antibodies (ANA), RF, or anti-CCP antibodies. Although nonspecific, laboratory tests may show systemic inflammation (table 30.1), and synovial fluid white blood cell (WBC) may be extremely elevated. Spinal involvement is closely associated with HLA-B27, but the diagnostic utility of testing HLA status is debatable. Enthesitis, ankylosis, and sacroiliitis are hallmark radiographic findings. The treatment of the spondyloarthropathies closely mirrors that of RA. Most DMARD therapies, including methotrexate and sulfasalazine, may help control peripheral arthritis, whereas the anti-TNF-α drugs have been remarkably effective for spinal disease.

SYSTEMIC LUPUS ERYTHEMATOSUS

Systemic lupus erythematosus (SLE) is a multisystem autoimmune disease characterized primarily by constitutional symptoms, hematologic abnormalities, and immune complex deposition in target organs. It tends to afflict women of childbearing age. Some patients with an inherited deficiency of complement are at increased risk to develop SLE. The potential manifestations of SLE are myriad (table 30.4), and the diagnosis of SLE requires a strong clinical suspicion, laboratory or pathologic evidence of disease, and exclusion of other possible infectious, rheumatic, and neoplastic conditions. Even in patients with established SLE, new clinical symptoms should not be attributed solely to SLE. Medication reactions and opportunistic infections occur commonly, and noninflammatory joint pain may indicate fibromyalgia or avascular necrosis (AVN) (table 30.5).

Lupus nephritis is the principal renal manifestation of SLE and is characterized by proteinuria and hematuria with red blood cell casts. Disease severity is classified based on histologic assessment of renal biopsy. Please see table 25.2, for the World Health Organization (WHO) classification of SLE nephritis. The degree of pathologic renal involvement cannot be predicted adequately by clinical criteria alone. Despite treatment, some patients still progress to end-stage renal disease (ESRD) and require dialysis therapy or renal transplantation. Renal vein thrombosis, interstitial nephritis, and antiphospholipid syndrome (APLS) may also lead to renal dysfunction in patients with SLE.

Autoantibody formation is the hallmark immunologic signature of SLE. ANA is detectable in essentially 100% of patients with SLE, but this test lacks specificity. Many other inflammatory conditions and upward of 20% of healthy patients may have a "positive ANA." Anti-double-stranded DNA (dsDNA) and anti-Smith antibody testing are much more specific but less sensitive assays. Anti-Ro (anti-SSA), anti-La (anti-SSB), and anti-ribonuclear protein (anti-RNP) antibodies may also be detectable in patients with SLE. A prevailing opinion is that these antibodies form circulating immune complexes that deposit in target tissues,

Table 30.4 MANIFESTATIONS OF SYSTEMIC LUPUS ERYTHEMATOSUS

CATEGORY	MANIFESTATIONS
Constitutional	Fever, weight loss, fatigue, malaise
Mucocutaneous	Mucosal ulcerations,[1] photosensitivity,[2] malar rash,[3] discoid lupus,[4] SCLE, alopecia, lupus profundus, lupus panniculitis, erythema nodosum, vasculitic purpura, urticarial vasculitis, angioedema
Kidney	Lupus nephritis,[5] interstitial nephritis, renal vein thrombosis
Musculoskeletal	Nonerosive inflammatory arthritis,[6] arthralgias, AVN, inflammatory myopathy
Lungs	Pleural effusion,[7] pulmonary hemorrhage, ILD, BOOP, pneumonitis, pulmonary embolism, pulmonary hypertension, "shrinking lung syndrome"
Cardiovascular	Pericardial effusion,[7] myocarditis, Libman-Sacks endocarditis, Raynaud's phenomenon, increased risk of cardiovascular disease
Nervous system	Seizures,[8] psychosis,[8] headache, cognitive or personality changes, mood disorders, meningoencephalitis, CNS vasculitis, transverse myelitis, chorea, mononeuritis multiplex
GI system	NSAID-related peptic ulcer disease, mesenteric ischemia, pancreatitis, and sterile peritonitis
CTD overlap	Erosive inflammatory arthritis, secondary Sjögren, CREST symptoms
Hematology	Leukopenia,[9] lymphopenia,[9] autoimmune hemolytic anemia,[9] anemia of chronic disease, thrombocytopenia,[9] ITP, TTP
Lab values	Presence of ANA,[10] anti-dsDNA,[11] anti-Smith.[11], anti-Ro, anti-La, anti-RNP, hypocomplementemia
APLS[11]	Livedo reticularis, stroke, pulmonary embolism, myocardial infarction, thrombotic microangiopathy of kidney and CNS, fetal loss
Pregnancy	Fetal loss, neonatal lupus (congenital heart block and photosensitive rash)

NOTES: Superscript numbers indicate manifestations that comprise the classification criteria, with 4 of 11 indicating SLE. ANA, antinuclear antibodies; APLS, antiphospholipid antibody syndrome; AVN, avascular necrosis; BOOP, bronchiolitis obliterans organizing pneumonia; CREST, calcinosis, Raynaud's, esophageal dysmotility, sclerodactyly, telangiectasia; CTD, connective tissue disease; GI, gastrointestinal; ILD, interstitial lung disease; ITP, idiopathic thrombocytopenia purpura; NSAID, nonsteroidal anti-inflammatory drug; SCLE, subacute cutaneous lupus erythematosus; TTP, thrombotic thrombocytopenia purpura.

recruit complement and other immunologic mediators, and cause end-organ disease.

Table 30.5 RISK FACTORS FOR AVASCULAR NECROSIS (AVN) IN ADULTS

Medications and toxins
 Corticosteroids (high dose or long duration)
 Bisphosphonates (AVN of the jaw)
 Alcohol

Permissive disease states
 Antiphospholipid syndrome
 Systemic lupus erythematosus
 Sickle cell anemia
 Gaucher disease
 Human immunodeficiency virus infection

Injury
 Trauma
 Radiation therapy
 Decompression illness (Caisson disease)

Corticosteroids remain the mainstay of treatment in SLE. High doses (1 mg/kg prednisone or equivalent) are often used for severe hematologic abnormalities or organ-threatening disease. Lower doses of corticosteroids or NSAIDs are often sufficient for cutaneous and serositis manifestations. Steroid-sparing agents are used to minimize steroid-related complications. These drugs include hydroxychloroquine, azathioprine, mycophenolate mofetil, methotrexate, cyclosporine, and possibly rituximab. Antimalarial agents (e.g., hydroxychloroquine) are well-tolerated drugs that play an important role in the treatment of SLE through poorly understood mechanisms. Cyclophosphamide is a cytotoxic agent reserved for the most severe manifestations of SLE (e.g., severe nephritis, pulmonary hemorrhage, severe central nervous system (CNS) disease, vasculitis). Acute complications of cyclophosphamide include hemorrhagic cystitis, bone marrow suppression, and profound immunosuppression. Lymphoma and urinary tract cancers are potential long-term adverse events. Plasmapheresis and intravenous immunoglobulin (IVIG) may be added to immunosuppressive therapy for life-threatening SLE. Anticoagulation is used in patients with thrombotic complications.

APLS is a hypercoagulable state in which a patient suffers a clot or fetal loss in the setting of having detectable serum antiphospholipid antibodies measured on two separate tests at least 12 weeks apart. Clots may be either venous, arterial, or even microvascular in nature. Fetal loss includes any three or more first-trimester miscarriages or any fetal loss after the first trimester. Antiphospholipid antibodies include anticardiolipin antibodies (IgG or IgM), antiprothrombin antibodies, anti-beta-2-glycoprotein I antibodies, or the lupus anticoagulant, which elevates the partial thromboplastin time (PTT) and is not corrected on mixing with normal serum. The term "secondary APLS" describes disease that occurs in the presence of an underlying autoimmune disease, most commonly SLE, whereas no such disorder is detected in "primary APLS." Catastrophic APLS is the syndrome of APLS with multiple clots, microvas-

cular thrombosis, and organ failure. It has a mortality rate reported at above 50%. All forms of APLS are treated with anticoagulation. Immunosuppression may also be used, and plasmapheresis may be added in cases of refractory APLS or catastrophic APLS.

Finally, drug-induced lupus (DIL) may occur with use of hydralazine, procainamide, isoniazid, methyldopa, quinidine, minocycline, or even anti-TNF-α agents. It is characterized primarily by constitutional symptoms, mucocutaneous findings, serositis, and elevated ANA. Organ-threatening disease should prompt consideration of an alternative diagnosis. Antihistone antibodies are a sensitive but not specific marker for DIL. Symptoms generally resolve with elimination of the offending drug.

SCLERODERMA

Scleroderma describes a family of rare but related disorders that share in common idiopathic dermal fibrosis. Scleroderma is categorized into localized disease (morphea and linear scleroderma) and systemic sclerosis (SSC). SSC is a disease characterized by both fibrosis and vasculopathy. SSC is subdivided into limited or diffuse disease based on the extent of fibrosis. In limited SSC, dermal fibrosis is restricted to the hands, feet, and face. Involvement of the proximal extremities, usually proximal to the MCPs, or trunk indicates diffuse SSC. Organ fibrosis represents a major source of mortality. It occurs principally in the lungs, heart, and GI tract. Vasculopathy accounts for pulmonary hypertension, scleroderma renal crisis, and the nearly universal Raynaud's phenomenon. Patients with SSC may manifest with the CREST symptoms (calcinosis cutis, Raynaud's, esophageal dysmotility, sclerodactyly, and telangiectasia), which have a high risk of developing pulmonary hypertension and can also occur independently of SSC. Serologic analysis of patients with SSC may demonstrate anticentromere antibodies or anti-SCL70 antibodies. The former are more often associated with limited disease such as CREST and pulmonary hypertension. The latter are associated with diffuse disease and cardiopulmonary fibrosis.

Treatment options exist for the vascular complications of SSC. Scleroderma renal crisis presents as hypertension, hematuria, and renal failure. Despite renal failure, renal crisis is treated with angiotensin-converting enzyme (ACE) inhibitors, angiotensin receptor blockers, or both. Aggressive use of these drugs to lower blood pressure has changed the natural history of scleroderma renal crisis such that patients may recover from or even avoid dialysis therapy. Pulmonary hypertension and digit-threatening Raynaud's disease are treated with vasodilator therapies. Dihydropyridine calcium channel blockers may be effective, but endothelin receptor antagonists (bosentan), phosphodiesterase inhibitors (e.g., sildenafil), and prostacyclins have markedly reduced mortality from pulmonary hypertension.

Pharmacologic treatment of fibrotic complications is sorely lacking. Immunosuppressive agents, including cyclophosphamide, have been used for pulmonary fibrosis, with only modest improvement in outcome. Additional therapy is symptom-directed. High-dose proton pump inhibitors are used for gastroesophageal reflux disease and should be administered to all patients with SSC to decrease the risk of esophageal strictures. Promotility agents (e.g., metoclopramide, erythromycin) are used for GI dysmotility, and oral antibiotics are used for bowel overgrowth syndrome.

Several other syndromes may cause cutaneous or systemic fibrosis and should be considered in the differential diagnosis of SSC. Eosinophilic fasciitis causes cutaneous fibrosis and results from infiltration of eosinophils into subcutaneous fascia. Graft-versus-host disease causes cutaneous and bowel fibrosis. Nephrogenic systemic fibrosis occurs in patients with severe renal insufficiency exposed to gadolinium-containing contrast agents often used in MRI procedures.

OTHER CONNECTIVE TISSUE DISEASES

Sjögren Syndrome

Sjögren syndrome (SS) may be a primary entity or may exist secondary to other CTDs such as SLE, RA, and SSC. Sicca describes the most predominant features of SS: dry mouth and dry eyes result from autoimmune destruction of salivary and lacrimal glands. Patients with SS often have positive ANA, anti-Ro, and anti-La antibodies, an elevated RF, and hypergammaglobulinemia. More serious complications include small-vessel vasculitis, interstitial lung disease, and lymphoma. Lymphomas typically occur in mucosal-associated lymphoid tissue and are heralded by a monoclonal gammopathy and drop in RF titer. Treatment for SS is typically directed at symptoms with artificial saliva and tears. Vasculitis or ILD requires high-dose corticosteroids or other intensive immunosuppressive therapy.

Idiopathic Inflammatory Myopathies

The idiopathic inflammatory myopathies (IIMs) include a collection of autoimmune diseases: dermatomyositis (DM), polymyositis (PM), malignancy-associated myositis, juvenile DM, and inclusion-body myositis (IBM). With the exclusion of IBM, these conditions present as proximal muscle weakness. Creatine kinase (CK) is typically elevated at least 5–10 times the upper limit of normal, and aldolase may also be elevated. DM, malignancy-associated myositis, and juvenile DM may have cutaneous manifestations. These include a malar rash that, unlike SLE, involves the nasolabial folds, a periorbital violaceous heliotrope rash, a photosensitive shawl sign over the precordium, Gottron papules over the dorsal knuckles, and

hyperkeratotic mechanic's hands. Interstitial lung disease may occur, usually in patients with anti-Jo-1 antibody. Oropharyngeal involvement may be life-threatening because of aspiration risk. Diagnosis is aided by electromyography (EMG) and confirmed by a muscle biopsy that shows an inflammatory infiltrate. Treatment consists primarily of high-dose corticosteroids, with additional immunosuppressive agents such as methotrexate or azathioprine used in patients who are unable to taper corticosteroids. Unlike the other IIMs, IBM presents as distal muscle weakness and atrophy in elderly patients. Diagnosis is made by electron microscopy of a muscle biopsy. Treatment is generally ineffective.

Adult-onset Still's Disease

Adult-onset Still's disease (AOSD) is a systemic inflammatory disease characterized by high fever, antecedent sore throat, evanescent rash, lymphadenopathy, hepatosplenomegaly, inflammatory arthritis, elevated liver transaminases, and markedly abnormal laboratory markers of inflammation, especially ferritin (table 30.1). It is a diagnosis of exclusion after ruling out RA, SLE, infectious, and malignant diseases. Treatment is similar to that of RA but may require higher doses of steroids. Notably, AOSD may respond rather dramatically to anakinra.

Mixed Connective Tissue Disease

Mixed connective tissue disease (MCTD) is an example of an overlap syndrome that manifests with various elements of several autoimmune diseases. Features may include inflammatory arthritis, sclerodactyly, Raynaud's syndrome, inflammatory myositis, pulmonary hypertension, and secondary Sjögren syndrome. Serology is notable for a positive ANA and high-titer anti-RNP. Treatment is directed at the individual manifestations.

THE VASCULITIDES

Collectively, the vasculitides represent a collection of diseases characterized by inflammation of blood vessels. The vasculitides are often categorized based on their involvement of large, medium, or small vessels (table 30.6). Patient demographics and serologic analysis are additional distinguishing features. Most vasculitides are serious conditions that are organ- or life-threatening. Fevers, constitutional symptoms, and abnormal inflammatory markers (table 30.1) are common features of most vasculitides. A definitive diagnosis often requires biopsy evidence of vascular inflammation. Immunosuppression with corticosteroids is a mainstay of treatment. Steroid-sparing agents (azathioprine, methotrexate, mycophenolate mofetil) or cytotoxic agents (cyclophosphamide) are often added to limit steroid

Table 30.6 CATEGORIZATION OF THE SYSTEMIC VASCULITIDES

VASCULITIS	HALLMARK FEATURES
Large-vessel vasculitides	Age >60, PMR symptoms
Giant cell arteritis	Pulselessness
Takayasu arteritis	
Medium-vessel vasculitides	Renal artery aneurisms
Polyarteritis nodosa	Disease of childhood
Kawasaki disease	
ANCA-associated small-vessel vasculitides	Normal/elevated complement
Wegener granulomatosis	cANCA, anti-PR3
Microscopic polyangiitis	pANCA, anti-MPO
Churg Strauss syndrome	Eosinophils
Immune-complex–mediated small-vessel	Low complement
vasculitides	IgA deposition
Henoch-Schönlein purpura	HCV infection
Cryoglobulin vasculitis	Offending drug
Hypersensitivity vasculitis	Associated CTD
CTD vasculitis	

NOTES: ANCA, antineutrophil cytoplasmic antibody; CTD, connective tissue disease; HCV, hepatitis C virus; MPO, myeloperoxidase; PMR, polymyalgia rheumatica; PR3, proteinase-3

toxicity and provide additional immunosuppression. For the most part, TNFα blockers are ineffective in systemic vasculitis.

LARGE-VESSEL VASCULITIDES

Giant-Cell Arteritis

Giant-cell arteritis (GCA) is the most common systemic vasculitis. Afflicted patients are exclusively >50 years old and usually of northern European ancestry. Patients typically fall into one of three types of presentation: cranial arteritis, aortitis, or fever of unknown origin (FUO). Approximately 30% of patients with GCA will have concurrent or pre-existing PMR, and 15–20% of patients with PMR will develop GCA. Patients with PMR should therefore be questioned routinely about symptoms of cranial arteritis. Cranial symptoms or visual changes in a patient with PMR are considered a rheumatologic emergency. Symptoms of cranial arteritis include scalp tenderness, new-onset head-ache, jaw claudication, persistent cough, and visual changes. A dreaded complication is ophthalmic artery involvement, which can lead to irreversible blindness. GCA may present as arm claudication or cough, but aortitis itself may be asymptomatic and found on postsurgical pathology. In patients >65 years old, GCA comprises 15–20% of FUO cases. Inflammatory markers are typically quite elevated in GCA (table 30.4). Regardless of presentation, a diagnosis of GCA is confirmed by histologic assessment of involved vasculature. Unilateral or sometimes bilateral temporal artery biopsy will often confirm the diagnosis in patients with cranial symptoms or FUO. The primary modality of treatment is corticosteroids (prednisone, 1 mg/kg) tapered over several months. Recent studies suggest that steroid-sparing agents

(e.g., methotrexate or azathioprine) may be considered for patients unable to taper steroids in a reasonable fashion.

Takayasu Arteritis

Takayasu arteritis is a large-vessel vasculitis that typically afflicts young women, which distinguishes it from GCA. The classic presentation is that of extremity claudication in a patient with asymmetric blood pressures, vascular bruits, or pulselessness. Proximal mesenteric or renal arteries may also be involved. Chronic arterial inflammation leads to fibrotic strictures, which account for symptoms. Tissue may be difficult to obtain, and a diagnosis may rely on imaging studies (conventional angiography, CT angiography, MR angiography, and positron emission tomography [PET] CT). ESR and CRP may be elevated, but not as reliably as in GCA. Corticosteroids are also the main treatment modality, although steroid-sparing agents may also be necessary.

MEDIUM-VESSEL VASCULITIDES

Polyarteritis Nodosa

Polyarteritis nodosa (PAN) is the prototypical medium-vessel vasculitis. Patients typically present with constitutional symptoms, purpuric skin lesions, and renal insufficiency. Additional organ involvement may include the pulmonary vasculature, intestine, gallbladder, testes, or ovaries. There is a cutaneous-limited variant of PAN as well. Serologic vasculitis workup is unremarkable. Diagnosis may be supported by renal or mesenteric angiogram showing aneurysmal disease. Biopsy of involved tissue shows necrotizing vasculitis of medium-size vessels. Treatment consists of corticosteroids, with steroid-sparing or cytotoxic agents added for more serious or refractory cases.

Kawasaki Disease

Kawasaki disease is a vasculitis of childhood, although cases have been reported in teenagers and young adults. It is a medium-vessel vasculitis that presents as fever >5 days, conjunctivitis, desquamative rash on the extremities, peripheral edema, and erythematous "strawberry" tongue in the setting of elevated ESR and CRP. Coronary artery involvement may cause life-threatening aneurisms or strictures. Although corticosteroids are helpful in controlling symptoms, the use of IVIG has changed the natural history of this disease by markedly reducing the incidence of coronary artery complications.

SMALL VESSEL VASCULITIDES

Vasculitides that affect the arterioles, capillaries, and venules are classified into two disease categories: those associated with antineutrophil cytoplasmic antibodies (ANCA) and those associated with immune-complex deposition. It is particularly important to exclude infectious endocarditis in the workup of a small-vessel vasculitis.

ANCA-Associated Vasculitides

ANCA-associated vasculitides (AAVs) include Wegener granulomatosis (WG), microscopic polyangiitis (MPA), and the Churg Strauss syndrome (CSS). AAVs cause necrotizing vasculitis of target tissues, which may include the sinuses, orbit, upper airway, alveoli, myocardium, glomeruli, CNS, peripheral nerves, GI tract, and skin. Renal involvement causes acute crescentic pauci-immune glomerulonephritis and may lead to ESRD. Life-threatening complications include pulmonary hemorrhage, myocarditis, mesenteric vasculitis, and CNS vasculitis. Lesions may be granulomatous in nature or, in the case of CSS, primarily eosinophilic. Patients may have associated arthralgias and laboratory evidence of systemic inflammation (table 30.1).

Serologic workup for AAV often reveals the presence of ANCA in a cytoplasmic ANCA (cANCA), perinuclear ANCA (pANCA), or nonspecific ANCA pattern. ANCA may be associated with antiproteinase-3 (anti-PR3) or antimyeloperoxidase (anti-MPO) antibodies by enzyme-linked immunosorbent assay (ELISA). A cANCA pattern with anti-PR3 ELISA is highly specific for WG, whereas the other AAVs tend to show a pANCA pattern with anti-MPO ELISA. Nonspecific ANCA or pANCA patterns in the absence of ELISA specificity may be observed in other inflammatory conditions, including ulcerative colitis, primary sclerosing cholangitis, and drug-induced vasculitis from such agents such as minocycline or propylthiouracil. Anti–glomerular basement membrane (anti-GBM) antibodies should also be tested in patients with AAV and pulmonary-renal symptoms. Complement levels are normal or elevated in AAVs.

Immunosuppressive therapy is central to the treatment of AAVs. High-dose corticosteroids (prednisone, 1 mg/kg) and cyclophosphamide or methotrexate are used to induce remission in any patient with organ- or life-threatening disease. Plasmapheresis may be added to those who are treatment refractory. Once remission is induced, methotrexate or azathioprine may be substituted for cyclophosphamide to minimize long-term toxicity of cyclophosphamide.

Immune Complex-Mediated Small Vessel Vasculitides

Immune-complex-mediated small-vessel vasculitides may be caused by several different disease processes. These include Henoch-Schönlein purpura (HSP), cryoglobulinemic vasculitis, hypersensitivity vasculitis, and vasculitis associated with connective tissue diseases (e.g., SLE, RA, Sjögren syndrome). These conditions have in common the deposition of immune complexes in target tissues. Serum complement levels are often depressed and correlate with disease activity. HSP is an IgA-mediated small-vessel vasculitis that primarily affects the skin, kidneys, and GI tract as purpura, glomerulonephritis, and bloody diarrhea. It is usually a self-limited disorder, but severe symptoms may necessitate corticosteroid therapy. Cryoglobulinemia may cause a vasculitis characterized by glomerulonephritis, peripheral neuritis, purpura, and, rarely, mesenteric vasculitis. Hepatitis C virus (HCV)-associated type II (mixed) cryoglobulins are the most likely to cause vasculitis. Treatment is directed at reducing the HCV viral load. Hypersensitivity vasculitis is typically drug-induced and limited to the skin as so-called leukocytoclastic vasculitis. Eliminating the offending agent is curative. CTD-associated vasculitides are discussed separately under each disease topic.

OTHER INFLAMMATORY ARTHRITIDES

MICROCRYSTALLINE ARTHRITIS

Gout and pseudogout typically present as an exuberant inflammatory monoarthritis, although patients may have polyarticular disease. Gouty arthritis occurs due to an inflammatory reaction against crystals of monosodium urate (MSU). Pseudogout has a similar presentation, but the pathogenic crystals are calcium pyrophosphate dihydrate (CPPD). In both cases, systemic inflammation from other causes (i.e., concurrent infection) may precipitate an attack of microcrystalline arthritis. Gouty arthritis tends to affect the lower extremities, whereas pseudogout prefers the knees and wrists. Although any joint may be affected by gout or pseudogout, the shoulders, hips, and spine tend to be spared.

Diagnosis of microcrystalline arthritis is confirmed by synovial fluid aspirate and observation of crystals by compensated polarized light microscopy. In the case of gout, crystals are long, needle-shaped, bright, and negatively birefringent. Customarily, this means that crystals are yellow when in the plane of the polarizing light and blue when perpendicular. On the other hand, the crystals of CPPD disease are short, rhomboid, dim, and positively birefringent (yellow when perpendicular with the polarizer). In both gout and pseudogout, joint fluid is inflammatory, often with $10–50 \times 10^3$ WBC/mm³ fluid. Concurrent septic arthritis should be excluded by Gram stain and culture of fluid, especially if the fluid WBC is $>100 \times 10^3$ WBC/mm³. Serum uric acid level has little role in the diagnosis of acute gouty arthritis because uric acid levels during an attack may not represent baseline levels. Chondrocalcinosis may be present on plain film of a patient with pseudogout but may be found in asymptomatic patients as well.

Acute gout or pseudogout arthritis may be managed with NSAIDs, corticosteroids, or oral colchicine. NSAIDs are effective and safe in patients without coagulopathy, renal insufficiency, or peptic ulcer disease. Corticosteroids may be administered systemically in low doses (prednisone 20 mg per day or less) or by intra-articular injection. Both are effective, although the former is more appropriate for polyarticular attacks. Oral colchicine is less effective than the others and plays a more important role in aborting an impending attack if taken at the first sign of symptoms. It should be dose-adjusted for renal insufficiency and may cause bone marrow suppression or liver toxicity if taken in excessive amounts. Intravenous colchicine should never be used because of its toxicity profile. Hyperuricemia is a risk factor for gout, and serum uric acid may be lowered by allopurinol or probenecid. These antihyperuricemic therapies are typically reserved for individuals with erosive gouty arthritis, uric acid nephropathy, uric acid nephrolithiasis, tophaceous gout, or frequent gouty attacks. They should not be initiated or adjusted in the midst of an episode of gouty arthritis. Rather, they are added several weeks after the attack, with appropriate prophylactic measures from colchicine, NSAIDs, or low-dose steroids. Allopurinol is excreted via the kidneys and can cause bone marrow suppression, hepatotoxicity, and, rarely, a distal-muscle myopathy. It potentiates the effect of azathioprine, so this combination should be used with great caution. Probenecid is generally ineffective in patients with any degree of moderate renal insufficiency (creatinine >2.0 mg/dL). When using antihyperuricemic agents, the goal serum uric acid is at least <6.0 mg/dL.

INFECTIOUS ARTHRITIS

Infectious arthritis should top the list of concerns in any patient with an acute monoarthritis. Bacterial septic arthritis is a rheumatologic emergency. Arthrocentesis is mandatory if septic arthritis is suspected. Risk factors are similar to those for endocarditis, including intravenous drug use, immunosuppression, breakdown of mucocutaneous barriers, and high-risk sexual activity. People with prosthetic joints and those affected by other inflammatory processes (e.g., RA) are also at risk. Although any joint may be involved, large joints are more commonly affected than small joints. Common bacterial pathogens include *Staphylococcus aureus*, *Streptococcus* species, and *Neisseria* species. In these cases, synovial fluid WBC is often very high ($>50 \times 10^3$ WBC/mm³) with $>95\%$ PMNs. Synovial fluid Gram stain may show organisms, and fluid culture is diagnostic. *Neisseria* species require chocolate agar for growth. Cultures may be negative in patients who have received antecedent antibiotics. It is prudent to seek a bacterial source because septic arthritis is most commonly the result of hematogenous seeding of a joint. Septic arthritis is treated with joint aspiration, intravenous antibiotics, and often surgical arthrotomy. Infection of a prosthetic joint is particularly problematic and typically warrants removal of hardware and prolonged antibiotics.

Spirochetes, mycobacteria, fungi, and parasites may cause a more chronic septic arthritis. For example, the typical presentation of Lyme arthritis (from *Borrelia burgdorferi*) is that of a chronic monoarthritis with swelling out or proportion to pain. Lyme arthritis tends to affect the knee or other large joint. It is a manifestation of chronic Lyme disease that occurs months after the offending tick bite. Diagnosis is based on clinical presentation and the presence of positive Lyme serology by ELISA and Western blot. One month of oral doxycycline is the first-line treatment for Lyme arthritis. Intravenous ceftriaxone may be used in treatment-refractory cases. A postinfectious Lyme arthritis may also develop and is treated with DMARDs such as hydroxychloroquine or methotrexate. In cases of undiagnosed chronic monoarthritis, synovial tissue biopsy is indicated to assess for mycobacteria, fungi, and parasites.

Polyarthritis is a less-common presentation of bacterial septic arthritis, although it is not unusual in the case of viral arthritis. Hepatitis B virus, hepatitis C virus, human immunodeficiency virus, parvovirus B19, and rubella virus are associated with a true inflammatory polyarthritis, whereas many other viruses may cause polyarthralgias without overt arthritis. Septic polyarthritis from bacterial sources may occur but is much less common. It is associated with a poor outcome because it reflects a high degree of bacteremia.

NONINFLAMMATORY RHEUMATIC DISORDERS

OSTEOARTHRITIS

Osteoarthritis (OA) is by far the most common cause of arthritis in the United States. It results from abnormal local mechanical forces that cause joint degeneration and cartilage injury over time. Risk factors for OA include age, obesity, family history, repetitive trauma, internal joint derangement, and prior inflammatory arthritis (e.g., RA, spondylarthritis, septic arthritis). OA is a chronic arthritis that typically affects the knees, hips, spine, /proximal interphalangeal (PIP) and distal interphalangeal (DIP) joints of older individuals. OA in younger individuals or OA affecting the wrists, elbows, shoulders, or ankles is uncommon. Such involvement may indicate secondary OA as a result of unrecognized internal joint derangement, inflammatory arthritis, congenital abnormality, avascular necrosis, chondrocalcinosis, hemochromatosis, or ochronosis from alkaptonuria.

Treatment options in OA are limited. Physical therapy, weight reduction, lifestyle changes, NSAIDs, and corticosteroid injections may be helpful interventions. Opiate analgesics should be used sparingly. Nutriceuticals such as glucosamine have no proven benefit. Prosthetic joint placement may be necessary in patients with debilitating pain that impacts function.

REGIONAL MUSCULOSKELETAL DISORDERS

Soft-tissue complaints account for a substantial percentage of doctor's office visits. Unlike inflammatory arthritis, morning stiffness is short-lived, and symptoms tend to be exacerbated by activity. Examination should include the involved region as well as proximal and distal structures. Processes such as tendinitis and bursitis tend to improve with ice, topical analgesics, NSAIDs, rest, or splinting. Physical or occupation therapy is an important adjunct. Corticosteroid injections usually provide only temporary relief even in refractory cases.

Common soft tissue syndromes of the proximal upper extremity include subacromial bursitis, impingement of the supraspinatus tendon, biceps tendinitis, rotator cuff tear, or cervical spine pathology. Injection of lidocaine into the shoulder should allow a patient to overcome any functional deficit if the symptoms are related to subacromial bursitis or supraspinatus tendon impingement but not rotator cuff tear. Patients with soft-tissue shoulder syndromes benefit greatly from physical therapy. It is crucial not to splint the shoulder or else risk adhesive capsulitis (frozen shoulder).

Common soft tissue syndromes of the distal upper extremity include lateral epicondylitis (tennis elbow), medial epicondylitis (golfer's elbow), and carpal tunnel syndrome (CTS). Despite their names, these conditions all represent overuse syndromes arising from the wrist. Epicondylitis is exacerbated by isometric resistance against the wrist. CTS presents as paresthesias in the distribution of the median nerve and is provoked by a Phalen or Tinel test. Wrist splints are an appropriate first-line treatment of these disorders. Bilateral CTS in a patient with no history of overuse may be the first sign of an inflammatory tenosynovitis as can occur in RA or other fluid-retentive disorders such as pregnancy or hypothyroidism.

Common soft tissue syndromes of the proximal lower extremity include trochanteric bursitis and iliotibial band syndrome. In trochanteric bursitis, patients complain of focal pain over the lateral trochanteric bursa that is worst when sleeping on that side or when directly palpated. It often reflects poor back mechanics and responds to back physical therapy. Iliotibial band syndrome is an overuse syndrome that affects the lateral thigh and knee in avid runners and cyclists. NSAIDs, ice, stretching, and modification of activities may provide relief.

Common soft tissue syndromes of the distal lower extremity include anserine bursitis, tarsal tunnel syndrome, and plantar fasciitis. Patients with anserine bursitis experience pain at the medial soft tissue just distal to the knee. It likely reflects poor foot mechanics and may respond favorably to orthotics. Tarsal tunnel syndrome is analogous to CTS and results from impingement of the posterior tibial nerve. Plantar fasciitis causes plantar pain on first awakening and with excessive activity. Stretching and supportive footwear are helpful.

FIBROMYALGIA

Fibromyalgia is a noninflammatory disorder in which patients experience musculoskeletal pain without an identifiable musculoskeletal source. Research advances support the notion that fibromyalgia represents one of many chronic pain disorders that may arise from a low pain threshold in the brain. Associated conditions include chronic lumbago, irritable bowel syndrome, seasonal affective disorder, chronic fatigue syndrome, interstitial cystitis, and noncardiac chest pain. Patients are often deconditioned, overweight, and have a coexisting mood disorder. Pain and fatigue are dominant symptoms of fibromyalgia. Physical examination may evoke exaggerated pain responses to minor pressure ("trigger points") along the soft tissue of the upper thorax, low back, and proximal extremities. Extensive workup with laboratory and imaging studies is unrevealing and often unwarranted. Immunosuppressive agents are of no benefit, and opiate analgesics should be avoided. Neurotransmitter-directed therapy is beneficial, and duloxetine and pregabalin have recently been approved for use in fibromyalgia.

SUMMARY

Musculoskeletal symptoms are a common cause for patients to seek medical attention. It is important for the treating physician to determine if a patient's complaints are related to an inflammatory or noninflammatory disorder. Medical history, physical examination, and some simple laboratory tests provide the best means to make this distinction. Inflammatory conditions are associated with acute or subacute symptoms, morning stiffness, and joints that are red, warm, and swollen. Inflammatory markers such as ESR and CRP are often elevated. Arthrocentesis is a safe and effective means to determine if a joint effusion is inflammatory, and it facilitates the diagnosis of microcrystalline or septic arthritis. Immunosuppressive therapy is often warranted for noninfectious, inflammatory rheumatic conditions such as connective tissue disease, vasculitis, and microcrystalline disease. Immunosuppression is generally ineffective for noninflammatory disorders, which are more responsive to NSAIDs, physical therapy, and lifestyle modifications.

ADDITIONAL READING

Arnold LM, Clauw DJ. Fibromyalgia syndrome: Practical strategies for improving diagnosis and patient outcomes. *Am J Med.* 2010;123(6):S2.

Becker MA, Ruoff GE. What do I need to know about gout? *J Fam Pract.* 2010;59(6 Suppl):S1–8.

Ea HK, Lioté F. Advances in understanding calcium-containing crystal disease. *Curr Opin Rheumatol.* 2009;21(2):150–7.

Rindfleisch JA, Muller D. Diagnosis and management of rheumatoid arthritis. *Am Fam Physician.* 2005;72(6):1037–47.

Schlesinger N. Diagnosing and treating gout: A review to aid primary care physicians. *Postgrad Med.* 2010;122(2):157–61.

So A, Thorens B. Uric acid transport and disease. *J Clin Invest.* 2010;120(6):1791–9.

Wilson JF. In the clinic. Gout. *Ann Intern Med.* 2010;152(3):ITC21. Erratum *Ann Intern Med.* 2010;152(7):479–80.

SECTION 4

PULMONARY AND CRITICAL CARE MEDICINE

31.

ASTHMA

Christopher H. Fanta

The 2007 National Asthma Education and Prevention Program Expert Panel defines asthma as "a common chronic disorder of the airways that is complex and characterized by variable and recurring symptoms, airflow obstruction, bronchial hyperresponsiveness, and an underlying inflammation. The interaction of these features of asthma determines the clinical manifestations and severity of asthma and the response to treatment."

EPIDEMIOLOGY

The prevalence of asthma has risen dramatically in recent decades. The estimated prevalence of active asthma in the United States increased from 3.1% in 1980 to 5.5% in 1996 to approximately 9% currently. At present, approximately 23 million persons in the United States have asthma, including 6.8 million children under age 18.

The potential cause(s) of this rise in the prevalence of asthma (and other allergic diseases) remains speculative. It has occurred most strikingly in industrialized and "Westernized" parts of the world. A seminal study that found the prevalence of asthma in the reunified Germany to be less in the former East Germany than the former West Germany weighs heavily against increasing levels of air pollution as the crucial factor. Other theories have invoked increased indoor allergen exposures, decreased exposure to endotoxin and other farm-based immunogenic stimulants, and decreasing levels of vitamin D in our increasingly indoor population.

Death due to asthma is uncommon and has decreased in the United States in recent years to approximately 4000 deaths/year. However, morbidity remains high, and the burden of disease in terms of both morbidity and mortality is inequitably distributed across ethnic and racial groups. African-American and Hispanic minorities have two to three times the frequency of urgent care visits, hospitalizations, and deaths compared to non-Hispanic whites. This discrepancy likely reflects both increased disease severity and poorer asthma care and tracks closely with lower socioeconomic status. For unknown reasons, asthma is more common in boys than girls prior to puberty and then more common in women than men in adulthood.

ASSESSMENT AND MANAGEMENT OF ASTHMA

Modern management of the asthmatic patient in the ambulatory setting has come to focus on the concept of asthma control. The goal of treatment is to achieve well-controlled asthma while minimizing medication side effects and preventing as much as possible severe asthmatic attacks. In this chapter we first define good asthma control and then outline a five-point plan describing how to achieve this goal.

DEFINING GOOD ASTHMA CONTROL

Well-controlled asthma, as defined by the Expert Panel 3 of the National Asthma Education and Prevention Program (Expert Panel Report 3, 2007), has two aspects or "domains." One aspect relates to ongoing asthmatic symptoms, which can be ascertained with a few simple questions.

- Do you have symptoms of your asthma requiring relief from your quick-relief bronchodilator more than twice per week?

- Do you wake with asthmatic symptoms more than twice per month?

- Does asthma interfere with your ability to exercise, limiting your usual physical activities?

- When we check your lung function with peak flow measurement or spirometry, is it less than normal (or less than your own best value)?

The other domain of asthma control relates to the risk of a serious asthmatic attack, based on the frequency of asthmatic attacks within the preceding year.

- Have you had more than one asthmatic attack requiring oral corticosteroids within the past year?

If the answer to any of these five questions is yes, then the patient's asthma is not well controlled, and asthma care should be intensified or "stepped up." If the answer to these questions is uniformly "no," then the goal of good asthma control has been achieved, and treatment can be continued unchanged or perhaps even reduced ("stepped down").

This approach to the assessment of asthma—based on the concept of control rather than severity—mirrors that used in other chronic diseases such as hypertension. Treatment is adjusted to achieve certain targets or goals of care. The previously recommended model, using categories of severity to make treatment recommendations (intermittent, mild persistent, moderate persistent, and severe persistent), can still be used in patients with newly diagnosed asthma or in patients being treated only with a quick-relief bronchodilator taken as needed. However, these categories of severity have proved inadequate when used to assess patients already taking regular controller medication for their asthma.

It is also good to remember that asthma control can change over time, necessitating reassessment of asthma control at each patient visit. For instance, a patient's treatment may need to be stepped up in the winter months, when his or her home is closed up and the forced hot-air heating is turned on (leading to increased exposure to dust mite antigen); or it may be possible to step down care when a new owner is found for the pet cat and the home is thoroughly cleaned of cat antigen.

ACHIEVING GOOD ASTHMA CONTROL

The five steps to achieving good asthma control as discussed in this chapter are to (1) make the correct diagnosis, (2) reduce environmental inciters of asthma, (3) treat with appropriate medications, (4) help patients prepare for asthmatic attacks, and (5) consult with a specialist when needed.

MAKING THE CORRECT DIAGNOSIS

For most adults with asthma, diagnosis simply involves review of a highly typical history dating back to childhood. Most patients with asthma are diagnosed before age 7 years (figure 31.1). However, occasional patients may be misdiagnosed in childhood, and asthma may have its onset in adulthood. Physicians are often confronted with adult patients whose symptoms raise the possibility of the new-onset asthma or who already have been given a quick-acting bronchodilator for symptoms that may or may not be due to asthma. Obviously, the approach to the patient whose cough, shortness of breath, and wheezing are due to

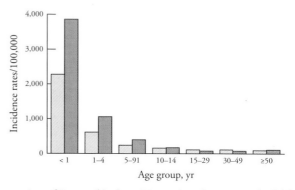

Figure 31.1. Age of Onset of Asthma. Most asthma begins in early childhood. This figure depicts the incidence of asthma among the general population in Rochester, Minnesota in the 1980s. Hatched bars = female; solid bars = male. Adapted from Yunginger JW, et al., *Am Rev Respir Dis.* 1992;146:888.

chronic obstructive pulmonary disease (COPD), recurrent infectious bronchitis, or diastolic dysfunction with intermittent congestive heart failure will be different from the stepped-care approach to asthma described below.

Historical features that point to a diagnosis of asthma include the intermittent nature of symptoms, characteristic triggers, and a favorable response to appropriate therapy. The following points bear emphasis. First, the exercise-induced bronchoconstriction of asthma characteristically occurs immediately *after* a short period (e.g., 5 min) of exercise and is characteristically worse if the air breathed during exercise is cold. Dyspnea on exertion, such as breathlessness climbing stairs or walking up an incline, should be distinguished from exercise-induced bronchoconstriction. Second, allergic triggers are unique to atopic asthma. For example, the patient who develops cough, wheezing, and chest tightness on exposure to cats almost surely has asthma. However, other triggers of asthmatic symptoms are nonspecific (e.g., exposure to smoke or strong fumes) and may be precipitants of symptoms in a variety of other respiratory diseases as well.

Third, for most patients with asthma, inhaled quick-acting bronchodilators bring rapid and effective relief of symptoms, if perhaps only temporarily; and typically a course of oral corticosteroids is dramatically successful in restoring normal breathing. Patients who report that they have tried these interventions in the past but found little benefit frequently will be found not to have asthma.

The characteristic diffuse, musical wheezing of asthma, prominent on exhalation, is familiar to most clinicians. It is worth remembering, however, that not all wheezing sounds are due to asthma. The single-toned, end-expiratory wheezing of COPD, repeated with little change at the end of each exhalation following deep breaths, can readily be distinguished from asthma. So, too, can a unilateral or focal wheeze raise the possibility of localized endobronchial obstruction (e.g., by a bronchial neoplasm or aspirated foreign body) and is atypical of asthma. Likewise, the low-pitched wheezing of persistent airway mucus, often associated with palpable vibration of the chest wall (tactile fremitus) and referred to as rhonchi, may indicate bronchiectasis or aspiration. This physical finding is less likely to suggest a diagnosis of asthma.

If after history and physical examination the diagnosis of asthma remains in doubt, confirmation (or exclusion) of the diagnosis is established by pulmonary function testing. Asthma is defined in terms of variable airflow obstruction, observed either on measurements made at multiple points over time or in response to bronchodilator administration. Although peak flow measurements are useful for screening purposes (e.g., in assessing for workplace-induced symptoms of occupational asthma) and for monitoring established asthma, the best test for identifying and quantifying expiratory airflow obstruction is spirometry. A 1-sec forced expiratory volume (FEV_1) that increases by more than 12% following bronchodilator is typical of asthma; the larger the increase (e.g., >15–20% increase following bronchodilator), the more likely the diagnosis of asthma and less likely the diagnosis of other obstructive lung diseases. A patient whose FEV_1 or peak expiratory flow (PEF) is consistently normal even when measurements are made during active respiratory symptoms probably does not have asthma.

In fully equipped pulmonary function testing laboratories, methacholine bronchoprovocation testing can be performed to evaluate for inducible bronchoconstriction in patients suspected of asthma whose lung function is repeatedly normal at the time of testing. Inhaled methacholine is administered in graded doses, and spirometry is repeated after each dose. A fall in FEV_1 in response to inhaled methacholine of at least 20% from baseline is found in nearly all patients with asthma; a fall in FEV_1 of ≥20% in response to a low provocative concentration of methacholine (PC_{20} ≤8 mg/mL) is relatively specific for asthma and uncommon in other obstructive lung diseases. Most helpful, failure to demonstrate bronchial hyperresponsiveness (FEV_1 does not fall to less the 80% of the baseline value even at the highest concentration of methacholine administered) excludes a diagnosis of asthma with at least 95% certainty (figure 31.2).

In the search for novel biological markers to diagnose asthma, to date measurement of the concentration of nitric oxide (NO) in the exhaled breath has proved to be the most useful biomarker of asthmatic airway inflammation. Commercially available devices can accurately record the concentration of exhaled NO in parts per billion (ppb) during a sustained exhalation at a steady expiratory flow. Among patients not taking anti-inflammatory medications (particularly inhaled steroids), values of >20 ppb argue against a diagnosis of asthma, whereas values <40 ppb are suggestive of asthma, even in the absence of airflow obstruction at the time of the measurement.

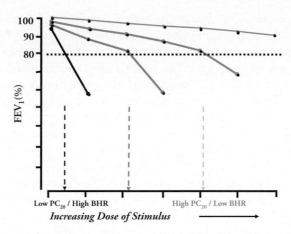

Figure 31.2. Bronchial Hyperresponsiveness in Asthma. Bronchoprovocative challenge illustrating the property of bronchial hyperresponsiveness in asthma. Lung function as the 1-sec forced expiratory volume (FEV_1) is expressed on the ordinate as the percentage of normal. Normal bronchial responsiveness is shown as the top line; the FEV_1 did not fall by >20% from baseline in response to the highest dose of the provocative agent (such as methacholine). Three examples of bronchial hyperresponsiveness are shown, consistent with three patients with asthma. They differ in the degree of their bronchial hyperresponsiveness. The patient whose FEV_1 falls to <20% below baseline in response to the smallest dose of provocative stimulus (line furthest to the left) has the most bronchial hyperresponsiveness, quantified by calculation of the provocative concentration of stimulus causing a 20% fall in FEV_1 (PC_{20}).

REDUCING ENVIRONMENTAL TRIGGERS OF ASTHMA

Some of the triggers of asthma, such as exercise, cause only transient bronchoconstriction. Others, however, cause both airway smooth muscle constriction and increased airway inflammation. Examples include allergen exposure (in the sensitized atopic asthmatic patient), viral respiratory tract infections, and noxious chemicals, such as ozone or cigarette smoke. The resulting increase in airway inflammation is associated with a heightened bronchial responsiveness that, even after a single exposure, may last for days. Therefore, in the atopic patient allergen exposure can precipitate not only an asthmatic attack but also worsened asthma in general.

In support of this hypothesis is the observation from the Cooperative Inner-City Asthma Study that among children living in poverty in inner-city communities, those with allergic sensitivities (demonstrated by positive allergy skin tests) and intense allergic exposures in the home environment (quantified by measuring antigen levels in dust vacuumed from the children's bedrooms) had more asthmatic symptoms and need for urgent asthma care than children without the combination of allergic sensitivity and high levels of allergen exposure. In this study, the most common offending allergen was cockroach antigen, but the principle confirmed by this study applies to all of the aeroallergens to which asthmatic patients may be sensitive.

Achieving good asthma control, therefore, begins with asking your patient about allergic (or noxious) exposures in the home or workplace, including cigarette smoking. The common allergens important in stimulating asthmatic inflammation are relatively few, leading to a short list of questions: Do you have a pet cat or dog or other furry animals (or birds)? Does your home have mold, particularly in a damp basement or bathroom? Do you have cockroaches, rats, or mice infesting your home? Does your asthma worsen when you dust or vacuum at home? Is there a large seasonal variation to your asthma, particularly with worsening in the spring (tree pollens), summer (grass pollens), or fall (weed pollens)?

With some patients you (or they) may suspect an allergic component but be uncertain based solely on their prior experiences. In this circumstance further testing is indicated and may include skin or blood testing for allergic sensitivities. The latter utilizes radioallergosorbent (RAST) testing to measure the amount of circulating immunoglobulin E (IgE) to specific allergens. For instance, you can order RAST testing for measurement of the circulating IgE to cat dander, dog dander, dust mite, cockroach, and common molds (e.g., *Aspergillus* and *Alternaria*). Positive test results combined with a consistent history point to a role for allergic exposure in worsening asthma control.

Although this is intuitively logical, until recently there has been little convincing evidence to demonstrate that reducing allergic exposures leads to improved asthma control in the allergic patient. However, in 2004 the Inner-City Asthma Study Group published the results of a randomized trial among impoverished households living in several inner-city communities. In one group, an intervention team helped families reduce allergen exposure in their homes; in the other group general encouragement to do so was offered, without equipment or educational reinforcement to help achieve those ends. Although symptoms lessened in both groups, presumably as the result of their participation in a formal research study, over the first year the intervention group had significantly greater improvement (fewer days with active asthma symptoms) than the control group. The interventions were conducted and reinforced over 1 year; of interest, the greater improvement in the intervention group was sustained for the entire 2 years of follow-up observations.

The interventions to reduce allergen exposures in these homes included the following: vacuum cleaners equipped with high-efficiency particulate air (HEPA) filters; stand-alone room HEPA filters for children with pets or dust mite allergy; cockroach and other pest extermination; and dust-impermeable covers for the children's mattress and pillows. Cigarette smokers were encouraged to quit smoking or not to smoke cigarettes indoors. A reasonable supposition is that if environmental control measures can help improve asthma control in these inner-city environments among families with low socioeconomic means and limited educational resources, they will likely be at least equally effective among patients with greater opportunities for their successful implementation.

TREATING WITH APPROPRIATE MEDICATIONS

The medications used to treat asthma are categorized as quick relievers or controllers. In the former category are the inhaled beta-agonist bronchodilators with a quick onset of action; in the latter category are inhaled corticosteroids, leukotriene-modifying drugs, long-acting inhaled beta-agonist bronchodilators, and, most recently, anti-IgE monoclonal antibody. Theophylline and inhaled chromones (e.g., cromolyn and nedocromil) have little role in modern asthma management and are not discussed in any detail in this review.

It has been an adage of asthma care for many years that the medications used to treat asthma should be individually tailored according to the severity of each patient's asthma. The *Guidelines for the Diagnosis and Management of Asthma* released by the Expert Panel 3 in 2007 confirms this recommendation but refocuses our thinking to consider the adequacy of asthma control in adjusting medications (that is, consider the activity of recent asthmatic symptoms, level of lung function, and the risk of a future asthmatic attack while minimizing medication side effects). These guidelines recommend that treatment be escalated along a six-step sequence until good asthma control is achieved (Expert Panel Report 3, 2007) (figure 31.3).

Step 1 is the recommended treatment for patients with intermittent asthma (symptoms necessitating quick-relief bronchodilator no more often than two days per week; nocturnal awakenings due to asthma no more often than two days per month; lung function within the normal range; and no more than one attack of asthma within the past year requiring a course of oral steroids). The term "mild intermittent asthma" has been modified to "intermittent asthma" to emphasize the point that even patients with intermittent asthma can suffer severe and life-endangering asthmatic attacks.

The treatment recommended at Step 1 of asthma care is an inhaled quick-acting beta-agonist bronchodilator used as needed for relief of symptoms. It is also helpful to remind (or inform) patients that they can take their quick-acting bronchodilator 10–15 min prior to physical exertion to prevent exercise-induced bronchoconstriction. The quick-acting beta agonists of short duration of action (4–6 hours) are albuterol, pirbuterol, and levalbuterol. All of these short-acting beta-agonist (SABA) bronchodilators have similar activity and side-effects profiles. Pirbuterol (Maxair) comes in a breath-actuated metered-dose inhaler called the Autohaler, where medication is released at the mouthpiece only in response to inspiratory flow detected at the beginning of an inhalation. Levalbuterol contains a single (dextrorotatory) stereoisomer from the racemic mixture that is albuterol; at half the dose (45 μg/puff), it has the same activity as albuterol.

Traditional albuterol metered-dose inhalers utilized chlorofluorocarbons (CFCs) as their propellant. Beginning in January 2009, all albuterol metered-dose inhalers are required to be CFC-free. The newer albuterol inhalers con-

Intermittent Asthma	Persistent Asthma: Daily Medication
	Consult with asthma specialist if step 4 care or higher is required.
	Consider consultation at step 3.

Step 1
Preferred:
SABA PRN

Step 2
Preferred:
Low-dose ICS
Alternative:
Cromolyn, LTRA
Nedocromil, or
Theophylline

Step 3
Preferred:
Low-dose
ICS + LABA
OR
Medium-dose ICS
Alternative:
Low-dose ICS+
either LTRA,,
Theophylline, or
Zileuton

Step 4
Preferred:
Medium-dose ICS
+ LABA
Alternative:
Medium-dose ICS
+ either LTRA,,
Theophylline, or
Zileuton

Step 5
Preferred:
High-dose
ICS + LABA

AND

Consider
Omalizumab for
patients who have
allergies

Step 6
Preferred:
High-dose
ICS + LABA + oral
corticosteroid

AND

Consider
Omalizumab for
patients who have
allergies

Step up if needed

(first, check adherence, environmental control, and comorbid conditions)

Assess control

Step down if possible

(and asthma is well controlled at least 3 months)

Each step: Patient education, environmental control, and management of comorbidities.
Steps 2–4: Consider subcutaneous allergen immunotherapy for patients who have allergic asthma (see notes).

Quick-Relief Medication for All Patients

- SABA as needed for Symptoms. Intensity of treatment depends on severity of symptoms: up to 3 treatments at 20-minute intervals as needed. Short course of oral systemic corticosteroids may be needed.
- Use of SABA >2 days a week for symptom relief (not prevention of EIB) generally indicates inadequate control and the need to step up treatment.

Figure 31.3. Step-Care Approach to Achieving Asthma Control. Step-care approach to achieving asthma control in children >12 years old and in adults. Source: Expert Panel 3 of the National Asthma Education and Prevention Program, www.nhlbi.nih.gov/guidelines/asthma

tain the propellant hydrofluoroalkane (HFA). No generic albuterol-HFA metered-dose inhalers are currently available; brand name albuterol-HFA inhalers are ProAir, Proventil, and Ventolin. The force of the medication plume as it exits the inhaler is slower with the HFA propellant compared to the traditional CFC-driven devices (figure 31.4). The medication consequently causes a different sensation in the pharynx; it feels lees forceful and less cold. Nonetheless, patients can be reassured that the medication effects are identical regardless of the propellant used for its delivery.

Step 2 involves a major transition in asthma care, from intermittent to daily medication use. Patients with mild persistent asthma have asthma that is not well controlled with intermittent use of an inhaled beta-agonist bronchodilator. Within the past month they have had daytime symptoms of their asthma more often than two days per week (but less often than daily, a feature of moderate persistent asthma); they have had nocturnal awakenings because of asthmatic symptoms more than twice per month (but fewer than five times per month); they have had a 1-sec forced expiratory volume (FEV_1) or peak expiratory flow (PEF) that is still within the normal range (≥80% of predicted); or within the past year they have had more than one attack of asthma requiring a course of oral steroids. It is recommended that these patients begin daily controller therapy for their asthma.

The preferred daily controller medication is an inhaled corticosteroid in low doses. Examples include beclomethasone (Qvar), 40 μg/puff, two puffs twice daily; budesonide (Pulmicort), 90 μg/inhalation, one inhalation twice daily; fluticasone (Flovent), 44 μg/puff, two puffs twice daily; ciclesonide (Alvesco) 80 μg/puff, two puffs twice daily; and mometasone (Asmanex), 220 μg/puff, one inhalation once daily. (Among the inhaled corticosteroids, budesonide has

the most favorable rating in pregnancy [category B]). Regular use of inhaled corticosteroids has been shown to improve lung function, reduce asthmatic symptoms and increase the number of symptom-free days, improve quality of life scores on asthma-related health questionnaires, and reduce the risk of asthmatic attacks.

Recent clinical trials have tested other options for the management of mild persistent asthma. One important study found that a strategy for periodic steroid use during the time of asthmatic symptoms (10 days of high-dose inhaled steroids or 5 days of oral steroids if symptoms worsened) led to no more frequent or severe asthmatic attacks in this select patient population than daily inhaled steroids. The latter strategy (daily inhaled steroids) was associated with a better asthma control score and more symptom-free days (estimated to be on average 26 more symptom-free days per year) than those using their inhaled steroids

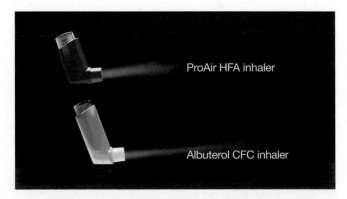

Figure 31.4. Albuterol Plumes with Different Propellants. Visual display of the difference in medication plume between albuterol delivered via a metered-dose inhaler with hydrofluoroalkane (HFA) propellant and one with traditional chlorofluorocarbon (CFC) propellant.

episodically. To date, the recommendations of national and international expert panels remain daily administration of controller medication for Step 2 of asthma care.

An alternative treatment option for those reluctant to begin an inhaled steroid is one of the leukotriene receptor antagonists, montelukast (Singulair) or zafirlukast (Accolate). The appeal of these medications includes the convenience of their oral administration as tablets once (montelukast) or twice (zafirlukast) daily and their freedom from side effects. For some patients they prove highly effective, but for others they are indistinguishable from placebo. At the present time a therapeutic trial of 2–4 weeks is necessary to determine their utility. Overall, they are less effective than inhaled steroids and so are considered a second-line option for mild persistent asthma.

Leukotriene-modifying drugs deserve special attention in patients with asthma and aspirin sensitivity. Such patients, if they ingest aspirin or any nonsteroidal anti-inflammatory drug (any inhibitor of cyclo-oxygenase-1), develop symptoms of asthma within 30–90 minutes, often provoking a severe asthmatic attack, frequently accompanied by nasal congestion and gastrointestinal upset. This subset of asthmatic patients, perhaps constituting 3–5% of adults with asthma, has a biochemical abnormality of arachidonic acid metabolism, leading to underproduction of certain prostaglandins and overproduction of leukotrienes. Inhibition of leukotrienes with a leukotriene receptor antagonist or with the lipoxygenase inhibitor, zileuton (Zyflo), makes particular sense in this group of patients and warrants a therapeutic trial. Zileuton is now available in an extended-release tablet formulation, making twice-daily dosing possible; a small incidence of drug-induced hepatic inflammation (2–4%) caused by zileuton necessitates initial monthly monitoring of liver function when beginning therapy with this drug.

Step 3 applies to the patient whose asthma is not well controlled despite regular use of a low-dose, inhaled corticosteroid. Review of the patient's technique using his inhaled medication is always appropriate to ensure adequate delivery of medication to the airways. Use of a valved holding chamber ("spacer") with metered-dose inhalers can increase deposition of medication onto the airways and minimize oropharyngeal deposition. Less oropharyngeal deposition reduces the risk of oral candidiasis ("thrush") and makes less steroid medication available to be swallowed and systemically absorbed.

There is controversy surrounding the choice of treatment for patients whose asthma is inadequately controlled despite Step 2 treatment, patients with moderate persistent asthma. Two options are given equal weight in the most recent set of expert guidelines: increase the dose of inhaled steroids to moderate doses (e.g., beclomethasone, 80 μg/puff, two puffs twice daily; fluticasone, 110 μg/puff, two puffs twice daily; budesonide, 180 μg/puff, two puffs twice daily; ciclesonide, 160 μg/puff, 2 puffs twice daily; or mometasone, 220 μg/puff, one puff twice daily) or continue low-dose inhaled steroid and add an inhaled long-acting beta-agonist (LABA) bronchodilator. The LABAs, formoterol (Foradil) and salmeterol (Serevent), are available in a single inhaler combined with an inhaled steroid: combination formoterol and budesonide (Symbicort), combination formoterol and mometasone (Dulera), and combination salmeterol and fluticasone (Advair). The first two are made available as a metered-dose inhaler in two different strengths (differing in the dose of inhaled steroid); the last is made available as a dry-powder inhaler or metered-dose inhaler in three different strengths (differing in the dose of fluticasone).

In terms of optimizing asthma control, the combination of low-dose inhaled steroid plus LABA proves to be the more effective strategy of these two options. The controversy enters because of questions raised about the safety of LABAs. In a large-scale 6-month-long trial of salmeterol combined with usual therapy versus placebo plus usual therapy, more deaths and near-deaths due to asthma occurred in the group of patients randomly assigned to receive salmeterol. The explanation for this startling finding is uncertain. The majority of patients in both treatment groups were not taking an inhaled steroid as part of their asthma therapy. It is possible that adding a LABA to other bronchodilator therapies provided temporary symptomatic relief while airway inflammation and mucus accumulation went unchecked, leading in some patients to respiratory failure and death due to asphyxia. It is unknown whether concomitant administration of an inhaled steroid with a LABA is protective.

Other explanations for the worse outcomes in the salmeterol-treated group are possible, including genetic differences in beta-agonist receptor response to chronic beta-agonist stimulation, inhibition of the activity of SABAs in a subset of patients treated with LABAs, and as yet unknown biochemical actions of LABAs. Because of this uncertainty, it is emphasized that LABAs should not constitute first-line treatment of asthma, and they should not be utilized without concomitant administration of an inhaled steroid. Combination low-dose inhaled steroid and LABA therapy is recommended for patients whose asthma is not well controlled on moderate-dose inhaled steroids. A leukotriene modifier added to low-dose inhaled steroids provides greater benefit than either agent alone, but this combination is not as effective as an inhaled steroid plus a LABA and so constitutes a second-line option for Step 3 care.

For patients whose asthma remains poorly controlled despite implementation of Step 3 medications, the recommended stepwise escalation of treatment is relatively straightforward. *Step 4* calls for moderate doses of an inhaled steroid plus a LABA. Examples of combination therapy are fluticasone/salmeterol by dry-powder inhaler (Advair Diskus) 250/50, one inhalation twice daily, and budesonide/formoterol by metered-dose inhaler (Symbicort) 160/4.5, two puffs twice daily. A less effective alternative is moderate doses of inhaled steroids plus a leukotriene modifier. *Step 5*, appropriate for patients with severe persistent asthma, recommends high-dose inhaled steroids plus a LABA (e.g., mometasone/formoterol by metered-dose inhaler (Dulera) 200/5, two puffs twice daily, or Advair Diskus 500/50, one inhalation twice daily), often combined with a leukotriene modifier. *Step 6* suggests the addition of systemic corticosteroids to high-dose combination therapy, using on a chronic basis the lowest possible dose of systemic steroids needed to achieve asthma control. Patients with allergic asthma requiring Step 5 or Step 6 treatment to gain good asthma control are potential candidates for the novel biological therapy, anti-IgE monoclonal antibody, which is discussed later when considering the subject of specialist referral.

Patients whose asthma remains well controlled for at least 3 months can be considered for "stepping down" their treatment. Stepping-down care is particularly appropriate when changes in the home or work environment might make one suspect a lessening of asthma severity, such as when your patient quits smoking, finds another home for the pet cat, or relocates to a mold-free apartment. Medication dose reduction can save time and money and decrease unnecessary risk of side effects. This latter is particularly relevant to patients taking high-dose inhaled steroids. At high doses (more than approximately 1000 μg/day of beclomethasone or the equivalent), systemic absorption of inhaled steroids can have consequences for the skin (ecchymoses and thinning), eyes (heightened risk of cataracts and elevated intraocular pressure), and bones (accelerated loss of bone mass). We need to be attentive to the bone health of our patients taking high-dose inhaled steroids, including ensuring adequate calcium and vitamin D intake and periodically monitoring bone density by bone densitometry.

HELPING PATIENTS PREPARE FOR ASTHMATIC ATTACKS

Once your patient has achieved good asthma control on the minimum amount of medication necessary, the proper use of the inhaler reviewed, and allergic and irritant exposures reduced as much as possible, your work as treating physician is not yet done. An important aspect of the care of the asthmatic patient remains: discussion of the steps the patient should take if his or her asthma were to worsen acutely. "What if," the discussion might begin, "your asthma were to get worse or you had a full-blown asthma attack? Do you have a plan as to what you can do at home to start getting better again?"

One of the first steps in developing such a plan, an "asthma action plan," is ensuring that patients are able to identify deterioration of their asthma. When they experience intense wheezing, cough, and dyspnea on light exertion following an obvious allergen exposure, most patients have no difficulty recognizing a severe asthmatic attack. However, at other times, the "diagnosis" may be more subtle. For instance, in the context of a respiratory tract infection, with low-grade fever, productive cough, chest congestion, and shortness of breath, it is easy to ascribe symptoms to a "bad chest cold." Patients and physician alike may wonder how much of this condition is due to a respiratory infection and how much to asthma.

In this instance (and other similar examples), a peak flow meter can provide useful information. In 1 minute or less, patients can check their expiratory flow and compare it with values recorded when they were feeling well. A peak flow reduced from the usual value by 20% or more indicates an asthmatic exacerbation, and treatment of the respiratory infection alone will be insufficient; the patient needs to have his or her asthmatic attack treated as well.

When tested in randomized clinical trials, asthma action plans based on peak flow measurements have not proven superior to action plans in which interventions are guided by the severity of symptoms alone. However, like having a thermometer at home to assess the degree of temperature elevation during an infection, the information provided by use of a peak flow meter—in the hands of a reliable patient—can't hurt, and it can be helpful to patient and physician alike. It is worth noting that on detailed investigation into the cause of asthmatic deaths, when asthmatic attacks progressed to the point of hypercapnic respiratory failure and asphyxiation, during the hours and days prior to death often neither patients nor their families (and sometimes, not their physicians as well) recognized the severity of the asthmatic attack. A peak flow measurement can help avoid this potentially fatal error.

A model widely used to help design an asthma action plan for your patient is based on three zones of severity—the "traffic-light model." When the patient feels well and has a peak flow ≥80% of their normal, they are said to be in their "green zone." When they experience increased asthmatic symptoms and have a peak flow between 50% and 80% of their normal, they are in their "yellow zone." The traffic-light analogy implies "slow down, take action, exhibit caution." If they have intractable coughing, repeated sleep disturbance due to asthma, and shortness of breath on light exertion, and if their peak flow is <50% of their normal, they are in their "red zone." The appropriate response is to "stop" one's usual activities and take action to get better; this represents a severe asthmatic attack.

The specific guidelines that you offer your particular patient as to how best to respond to a mild to moderate asthmatic attack (yellow zone) or severe asthmatic attack (red zone) will depend on the patient's usual medical regimen for asthma, other medications available to them at home, their experience managing prior asthmatic attacks, and your sense of their capabilities. The following is offered as very broad, general advice; specific asthma action plans need to be tailored to each individual patient.

Patients may need to be reminded that in the setting of an asthmatic attack, they can take their quick-acting inhaled bronchodilator more often than the usual "up to four times a day" recommendation for routine use. In the setting of a severe attack, they can safely repeat dosing every 20–30 min and can use four puffs with each dosing. If they are not improving after the first two or three doses, they should make medical contact for further advice. Some patients may substitute nebulized bronchodilator for metered-dose inhaler use in this circumstance. The two methods of delivery provide identical benefit when the metered-dose inhaler is properly used, preferably with an attached valved holding chamber, and with sufficient dosing. However, in the context of an asthmatic attack, some patients cannot properly coordinate their metered-dose inhaler and will derive additional benefit when drug administration can be achieved with the quiet, tidal breathing of nebulized medication.

During a mild to moderate asthmatic attack, patients may be advised to begin an inhaled steroid in high doses. Those already using an inhaled steroid in low doses can increase their dosing fourfold, with potential added benefit.

For patients already taking high-dose inhaled steroids or not improving despite increasing their usual dose of inhaled steroids or having a severe asthmatic attack (red zone), often oral steroids are needed. Practitioners tend to delay administration of oral steroids because of concern regarding potential serious side effects, but it is the oral steroids that most effectively reverse severe asthmatic attacks and have the greatest likelihood of preventing deterioration, hospitalization, and risk of death. Oral steroids are a routine part of the care of asthma attacks provided in hospital-based emergency rooms, and patients can be advised when to initiate therapy at home. Patients who have experienced previous severe asthmatic attacks may be given a supply of prednisone or methylprednisolone to have available at home and advised to begin 40–60 mg per day in the event of an asthmatic crisis and then call their physician.

Finally, as part of the discussion about asthma action plans, it is worth reminding your patient that self-initiation of care at home is not meant to substitute for treatment by healthcare professionals. The bottom line in all asthma action plans should be get help. If you as the patient are uncertain as to what to do, if your asthma is not improving with the measures that you have begun, if you are frightened and feel in danger, seek medical help—by phone, by medical visit, by emergency room care, or by 911, as necessary.

CONSULTING WITH A SPECIALIST

The Expert Panel 3 of the National Asthma Education and Prevention Program has offered the following indications for referral to an asthma specialist, typically either an allergist or a pulmonologist.

- Uncertainty as to the diagnosis

- Additional testing being needed for assessment of asthma or complicating medical conditions

- Patients not achieving and maintaining good asthma control and patients requiring Step 4 or higher care

- Patients who have had a life-threatening asthmatic attack, have required more than two courses of oral corticosteroids in the past year, or who have had an asthmatic attack necessitating hospitalization for their asthma

- Patients being considered for specialized treatments, such as allergen immunotherapy or anti-IgE monoclonal antibody

- Patients requiring extra time spent for education around issues of medication adherence and side effects or allergen avoidance strategies

Besides more time and expertise focused on this one medical problem, the consultant can offer a systematic approach to the patient with difficult-to-control asthma. Without going into depth about this approach, its elements are elucidated here. They include (1) evaluating in detail for inciters of asthma that are causing the patient's asthma to be severe; (2) exploring comorbid conditions (e.g., gastroesophageal reflux, rhinosinusitis, aspirin sensitivity, and allergic bronchopulmonary aspergillosis) that are aggravating the patient's asthma, (3) emphasizing the importance of medication understanding and adherence and exploring the barriers to compliance, and (4) ensuring that the diagnosis of asthma is correct and not being mimicked by other conditions (e.g., vocal cord dysfunction, tracheomalacia, COPD, bronchiolitis, or bronchiectasis).

One specialized therapy for patients with atopic asthma and sensitivity to a perennial allergen, approved by the Food and Drug Administration for use in severe asthma, is the anti-IgE monoclonal antibody omalizumab (Xolair). It is administered by subcutaneous injection every 2 or 4 weeks (depending on dose). The dose is adjusted according to body weight and level of total serum IgE. Treatment with omalizumab significantly reduces all circulating free IgE antibody, regardless of the allergen to which it has been formed. Because the routine assay for IgE measures both free IgE and IgE bound to omalizumab, it cannot be used to monitor IgE levels once therapy with omalizumab has been begun.

The most consistent beneficial effect of omalizumab has been a reduction in the number and severity of asthmatic attacks. Patients may also be able to reduce their steroid medications, use their quick-relief bronchodilator less frequently, and achieve stable to improved lung function. The circulating omalizumab-IgE complexes are small and not associated with immune-complex deposition diseases. Anaphylactic reactions to omalizumab have been observed with a frequency of approximately 1:1000, some delayed for hours after the injection, leading to the recommendations that patients be observed in the medical office for 2 hours after the first three injections and carry with them prefilled epinephrine-containing autoinjector syringes for a day or two after having received their injections. The cost of treatment is on the order of $20,000–$30,000 per year.

SUMMARY

In the vast majority of patients, good asthma control can be achieved—with a minimum of side effects—using currently available therapies in a stepped-care approach.

Achieving asthma control typically involves confirming the correct diagnosis, helping patients avoid allergic and irritant stimuli that exacerbate their asthma, periodically monitoring and readjusting therapy, and patient education in asthma comanagement skills. Patients should be equipped with an asthma action plan to help them initiate appropriate actions to counteract an asthmatic attack. Specialist consultation can help achieve these goals in difficult-to-manage patients. One approach to treatment of refractory allergic asthma is use of the novel biological therapy, anti-IgE monoclonal antibody, omalizumab.

ADDITIONAL READING

Expert Panel Report 3: *Guidelines for the Diagnosis and Management of Asthma* NIH Publication 07–4051. www.nhlbi.nih.gov/guidelines/asthma/asthgdln.pdf.

Fanta CH. Asthma. *N Engl J Med.* 2009;360(10):1002–14. Errata in *N Engl J Med.* 2009;361(11):1123 and *N Engl J Med.* 2009;360(16):1685.

Lazarus SC. Clinical practice. Emergency treatment of asthma. *N Engl J Med.* 2010;363(8):755–64.

Rust G. Drug therapy for asthma. *N Engl J Med.* 2009;360(24):2578.

Schatz M, Dombrowski MP. Clinical practice. Asthma in pregnancy. *N Engl J Med.* 2009;360(18):1862–9.

von Mutius E, Drazen JM. Choosing asthma step-up care. *N Engl J Med.* 2010;362(11):1042–3.

QUESTIONS

QUESTION 1. A 22-year-old woman without prior history of asthma complains of intermittent cough and chest tightness over the past 6 months. About 1 year ago she moved home to live with her parents, who own two cats. You suspect possible asthma. To evaluate her for asthma, you would order which of the following diagnostic tests:

A. Measurement of serum IgE
B. Allergy skin tests
C. Radioallergosorbent (RAST) tests for common aeroallergens
D. Spirometry pre- and postbronchodilator administration
E. Chest radiograph

QUESTION 2. Which of the following is NOT applicable to the assessment of a patient's asthma control?

A. Peak flow
B. FEV$_1$
C. Frequency of use of quick-acting bronchodilator for relief of symptoms
D. Frequency of nighttime awakenings due to asthma
E. Blood eosinophilia

QUESTION 3. Persons with atopic asthma are susceptible to making allergic reactions to a variety of allergens. If a patient with atopic asthma experiences worsening asthma control, common inciters of allergic inflammation that may be contributing to worsened symptoms include all of the following EXCEPT:

A. Dust mites
B. Cockroaches
C. Mice
D. Peanuts
E. Aspergillus

QUESTION 4. Over the last few weeks, a 30-year-old man with asthma reports needing to use his albuterol inhaler five or six times per week because of recurrent chest tightness and shortness of breath. He finds that he is no longer able to jog 2–3 miles comfortably and so has given up his daily exercise routine. He is taking the leukotriene receptor antagonist montelukast (Singulair) once daily and rarely misses a dose. His peak flow is 480 L/min, 80% of his usual. The recommended next step in his care would be:

A. Add combination inhaled corticosteroid and long-acting inhaled beta-agonist bronchodilator (e.g., fluticasone-salmeterol [Advair 250/50] by dry-powder inhaler, one inhalation twice daily)
B. Double the dose of montelukast (take 10 mg twice daily)
C. Change from the leukotriene receptor antagonist montelukast to the lipoxygenase inhibitor zileuton (Zyflo), 600 mg two tablets twice daily
D. Begin an inhaled steroid such as budesonide (Pulmicort Flexhaler 180), one inhalation twice daily
E. Review inhalational technique with his albuterol metered-dose inhaler, have him restrict his outdoor physical activity for 1 week, and continue montelukast at the present dose

QUESTION 5. Anti-IgE monoclonal antibody omalizumab (Xolair) is a novel therapy for the treatment of asthma. You would consider referral for this therapy in a patient who has which of the following characteristics:

A. Patients with features of both asthma and COPD
B. Patients with aspirin-sensitive asthma
C. Poorly controlled asthma despite Step 4 care
D. Asthma and nasal polyposis
E. Asthma with high peripheral blood eosinophil count

ANSWERS

1. D
2. E
3. D
4. D
5. C

32.

PLEURAL DISEASE

Ajay K. Singh

The pleural space is lined by the parietal and visceral pleurae. The parietal pleura covers the inner surface of the thoracic cavity, including the mediastinum, diaphragm, and ribs. The visceral pleura covers all lung surfaces, including the interlobar fissures. The right and left pleural spaces are separated by the mediastinum. The pleural space contains a relatively small amount of fluid, approximately 10 mL on each side (approximately 0.13 mL/kg of body weight). The pleural space plays an important role in respiration by coupling the movement of the chest wall with that of the lungs in two ways. First, a relative vacuum in the space keeps the visceral and parietal pleurae in close proximity. Second, the small volume of pleural fluid serves as a lubricant to facilitate movement of the pleural surfaces against each other in the course of respirations. The small volume of fluid is maintained through the balance of hydrostatic and oncotic pressure and lymphatic drainage, a disturbance of which may lead to pathology. A pleural effusion is defined as an abnormal amount of pleural fluid accumulation in the pleural space and is the result of an imbalance between excessive pleural fluid formation and pleural fluid absorption.

PLEURAL EFFUSION

A pleural effusion is a common clinical problem: the incidence of pleural effusions is estimated at 1 million per year in the United States. There are two types of pleural effusions: *transudative effusion*, which is caused by an increase in hydrostatic pressure within the pleural capillaries or a decrease in colloid osmotic pressure in the circulatory system, and *exudative effusion*, which is caused by an increase in capillary permeability resulting from an inflammatory or destructive process such as may be seen in infections and malignancies (table 32.1).

The common causes of transudative effusions are congestive heart failure and hypoalbuminemic states (e.g., cirrhosis), and those of exudative effusions are malignancy, infection (e.g., pneumonia), and pulmonary embolism.

Effusions may also be classified by systemic versus local causes (table 32.2).

CLINICAL FEATURES OF PLEURAL EFFUSIONS

The symptoms of a pleural effusion include dyspnea, pleural pain, and tachypnea. On examination, patients may have decreased movement of the chest wall, diminished tactile fremitus, dullness to percussion, diminished transmission of breath sounds (vocal resonance), and the presence of a friction rub. These features are usually evident when >500 mL of fluid has accumulated in the pleural cavity. Above the effusion, where the lung is compressed, there may be bronchial breathing and egophony ("E-to-A change"). With a large effusion (>1000 mL) there may be tracheal deviation and mediastinal shift away from the effusion.

Clinical features frequently provide clues to the diagnosis. Patients with a malignant pleural effusion usually present with dyspnea, a nonproductive cough, and evidence of anorexia and weight loss, whereas patients with an infectious etiology may present with fever, chest pain, and a productive cough. Systemic inflammatory causes of a pleural effusion are accompanied by joint pains, myalgia, rash, or evidence of abnormalities in other organ systems (for example, a pleural effusion from systemic lupus erythematosus [SLE] may be accompanied by a rash, arthralgias, mouth ulcers, and evidence of nephritis). Displacement of the trachea and mediastinum toward the side of the effusion is an important clue to obstruction of a lobar bronchus by an endobronchial lesion, which can be due to malignancy or, less commonly, a nonmalignant cause such as a foreign body.

COMMON TRANSUDATIVE AND EXUDATIVE PLEURAL EFFUSIONS

Transudative Effusions

Congestive Heart Failure
Congestive heart failure (CHF) is the most common cause for a transudative pleural effusion. Over 80% of

Table 32.1 CAUSES OF PLEURAL EFFUSION

	TRANSUDATE	EXUDATE
Common	Congestive heart failure Cirrhosis (hepatic hydrothorax) Atelectasis (which may be due to malignancy or pulmonary embolism) Hypoalbuminemia Nephrotic syndrome	Malignancy Parapneumonic effusions
Less common	Hypothyroidism Nephrotic syndrome Mitral stenosis Pulmonary embolism	Pulmonary infarction Autoimmune diseases (rheumatoid arthritis, lupus, sarcoidosis) Benign asbestos effusion Pancreatitis Post–myocardial infarction syndrome Tuberculosis Trauma Postcardiac injury syndrome Esophageal perforation Radiation pleuritis
Rare	Constrictive pericarditis Urinothorax Superior vena cava obstruction Ovarian hyperstimulation Meigs syndrome (ascites and pleural effusion due to a benign ovarian tumor)	Yellow nail syndrome Drugs (e.g., amiodarone, nitrofurantoin, phenytoin, methotrexate) Fungal infections

effusions from CHF are bilateral. Other causes of bilateral pleural effusions are shown in table 32.3. The most likely mechanism is pulmonary venous hypertension. Patients present with clinical features of CHF. The chest radiograph shows cardiomegaly and bilateral effusions of relatively equal size with evidence of vascular congestion. Treatment is directed at the underlying heart failure. Removal of a modest amount of fluid, 500–1000 mL, should be considered in patients who are refractory to medical therapy or are dyspneic because of large effusions. If therapeutic thoracentesis relieves the dyspnea but the effusion cannot be controlled with medical therapy, chemical pleurodesis with doxycycline or talc should be considered.

Hepatic Hydrothorax

Pleural effusions develop in approximately 6% of patients with hepatic cirrhosis. These effusions are usually unilateral

Table 32.2 SYSTEMIC AND LOCAL CAUSES OF PLEURAL EFFUSION

SYSTEMIC CAUSES OF PLEURAL EFFUSION	LOCAL CAUSES OF PLEURAL EFFUSION
Hydrothorax—Noninflammatory (e.g., related to heart failure, renal failure, liver failure) or inflammatory (e.g., related to malignancy or connective tissue disorders) collection of serous fluid in the pleural space	*Empyema*—Pus in pleural space resulting from infection *Hemothorax*—Blood in pleural space resulting from chest wall injuries, complications of surgery, etc. *Chylothorax*—Chyle accumulation in pleural space due to disruption of the thoracic duct

and right-sided but may occur on the left (16%) or be bilateral (16%). They may vary in size from small to massive. Large effusions may cause significant dyspnea. Therapy is directed at reducing the ascites with diuretics and sodium restriction. Therapeutic thoracentesis will bring only temporary relief because the ascitic fluid rapidly reaccumulates in the pleural cavity. Chemical pleurodesis may be attempted, but insertion of a chest tube involves risk. Tube thoracostomy may drain both the pleural fluid and the ascites, resulting in severe hypovolemia. If pleurodesis is not successful, thoracoscopy or thoracotomy to repair the diaphragmatic defects may be required to control the patient's symptoms.

Peritoneal Dialysis

Pleural effusions are observed in approximately 2% of continuous ambulatory peritoneal dialysis (CAPD) patients. Large, symptomatic effusions can develop within hours of initiating peritoneal dialysis. The dialysate moves from the peritoneal to the pleural cavity across the diaphragm in a manner analogous to the movement of ascitic fluid in the

Table 32.3 CAUSES OF BILATERAL EFFUSIONS

Generalized salt and water retention (CHF, nephrotic syndrome)
Ascites
Pulmonary infarction
Autoimmune disease (SLE, rheumatoid arthritis)
Tuberculosis
Malignancy

patient with cirrhosis. If this problem is going to occur, it usually develops in the first month after dialysis is initiated. However, it may be a year or more before the effusion develops in some patients. Most effusions are right-sided but left-sided or bilateral effusions do occur. Patients with dialysis-related effusions generally complain of dyspnea, but approximately 25% of the effusions cause no symptoms and are discovered on routine radiographs. Therapy comprises stopping the dialysis and draining the peritoneal fluid. The patient should be switched to hemodialysis. If this is not feasible, chemical pleurodesis should be performed prior to reinstituting CAPD. Small-volume peritoneal dialysis in the semierect position may be attempted while pleurodesis is being performed. The diaphragmatic defect may have to be repaired surgically if pleurodesis is unsuccessful.

Urinothorax

A urinothorax is a rare cause of a transudative effusion. The pleural effusion is due to the retroperitoneal leakage of urine that enters the pleural space via diaphragmatic lymphatics. It generally develops in association with obstructive uropathy but has been reported in patients with trauma, malignancy, kidney biopsy, and renal transplantation. Patients generally present with complaints related to the urinary tract obstruction. The pleural effusion is suspected because of dyspnea, or it may be asymptomatic and recognized on a routine chest radiograph. The pleural effusion is invariably ipsilateral to the urinary obstruction. Thoracentesis yields fluid that looks and smells like urine. The fluid has the characteristics of a transudate, but the pH may be high or low depending on the urine pH. The pleural fluid creatinine is always higher than the serum creatinine in a urinothorax. Relief of the urinary obstruction results in prompt resolution of the associated effusion.

Nephrotic Syndrome

Pleural effusions are frequently present in patients with the nephrotic syndrome. In one study radiographic evidence of effusions was found in 21% of 52 children with nephrosis. Hypoalbuminemia leads to a decrease in the plasma oncotic pressure, while salt retention produces hypervolemia and increased hydrostatic pressures, thereby favoring the development of transudative effusions. The effusions are bilateral and are frequently infrapulmonary. They are often associated with the presence of peripheral edema. Thoracentesis should be performed whenever an effusion is recognized in a patient with nephrotic syndrome, to confirm that the fluid is a transudate. If an exudate is found, thromboembolism is the most likely cause. These patients suffer from a hypercoagulable state, and venous thrombosis in the legs and at other sites is common. Treatment is directed at the underlying nephropathy. Therapeutic thoracentesis is indicated if there is severe dyspnea. Failure to medically control symptomatic effusions is an indication for chemical pleurodesis.

Exudative Effusions

Tuberculosis

Pleural effusions occur in approximately 30% of patients with tuberculosis (TB). Potential mechanisms for the exudative effusion are direct extension of tuberculous infection into the pleural space and rupture of a subpleural caseous focus into the pleural space, resulting in an immunological hypersensitivity reaction and subsequent accumulation of fluid. The clinical presentation is one of fever, chest pain, and weight loss. Workup should include a tuberculin skin test and diagnostic thoracentesis. The pleural fluid is rich in lymphocytes, but with <5% mesothelial cells. More definitive tests include culturing of *Mycobacterium tuberculosis* from pleural fluid and performing a parietal pleural biopsy looking for granulomas and acid-fast bacilli.

Chylothorax

A chylothorax occurs when there is damage to the thoracic duct (e.g., surgery, malignancy, or trauma) (table 32.4). The most common malignant cause is lymphoma. The pleural effusion is most commonly right-sided because the duct is in the right hemithorax, although a left-sided effusion may occur if the damage is at the level of the aorta. A true chylothorax has a milky gross appearance of the fluid (although this can be misleading because a tuberculous or rheumatoid pleural effusion can have a similar appearance, termed pseudochylothorax); it has a high fat content (>400 mg/dL of mostly triglyceride), and chylomicrons can be seen. A pleural fluid triglyceride level >110 mg/dL is highly suggestive of a chylothorax, whereas a pleural triglyceride level <50 mg/dL virtually excludes the diagnosis of chylothorax. Treatment strategies include treating the underlying cause (e.g., radiation of lymphomatous obstruction or surgical repair of a ruptured thoracic duct) and therapeutic thoracentesis for symptomatic effusions. In addition, because flow in the thoracic duct is also highly dependent on fat intake, manipulation of the diet can also be used to reduce flow. Consequently, switching to a low-fat diet with medium-chain triglycerides and parenteral nutrition has been used successfully. Concomitant medical therapy with somatostatin or octreotide can successfully decrease chylothorax formation in inoperable cases.

Table 32.4 CAUSES OF CHYLOTHORAX AND PSEUDOCHYLOTHORAX

CHYLOTHORAX	PSEUDOCHYLOTHORAX
Neoplasm: lymphoma, metastatic carcinoma	Tuberculosis
Trauma: operative, penetrating injuries	Rheumatoid arthritis
Miscellaneous: tuberculosis, sarcoidosis, lymphangioleiomyomatosis, cirrhosis, obstruction of central veins, amyloidosis	Inadequately treated empyema

Malignancy

A malignant pleural effusion is diagnosed when exfoliated malignant cells are found in pleural fluid or when malignant cells are seen in pleural tissue obtained by percutaneous pleural biopsy, thoracoscopy, or thoracotomy. Carcinoma of any organ can metastasize to the pleura. Carcinoma of the lung is the most common (table 32.5). Lung cancer can cause a pleural effusion either directly by metastasizing to the pleura, or indirectly by causing atelectasis, pneumonia, or lymphatic obstruction. Clinical features include the underlying tumor and the effects of the effusion (e.g., a large effusion may cause dyspnea). Workup should include a chest x-ray (carcinoma of the lung usually results in an effusion ipsilateral to the primary location of the tumor, and effusions are usually moderate to large). Notably, the presence of bilateral effusions in the absence of cardiomegaly is a clue suggesting a malignancy rather than CHF. Diagnostic thoracentesis may yield a serous, serosanguineous, or grossly bloody-appearing fluid that is an exudate rather than a transudate. Demonstrating the presence of malignant cells in pleural fluid or pleural tissue is key. Cytology is a more sensitive test for the diagnosis than percutaneous pleural biopsy because pleural metastases tend to be focal and may be missed on biopsy.

Autoimmune Diseases

Both SLE and rheumatoid arthritis (RA) are important causes of exudative pleural effusions. Effusions in SLE are small to moderate in size, whereas effusions with RA tend to be large. Effusions in SLE patients are usually accompanied by pleurisy, whereas RA effusions are frequently asymptomatic. Pleural analysis is key to diagnosis. For the diagnosis of an SLE effusion, measurement of pleural fluid antinuclear antibody levels (ANA) is recommended: an ANA titer >1:160 or a pleural to serum ANA ratio >1 indicates lupus pleuritis. With regard to RA effusions, measurement of rheumatoid factor in the pleural effusion is not helpful because an elevated RF level is nonspecific (also elevated in pneumonia, TB, malignancy, and SLE).

Asbestosis

Asbestos exposure may result in a benign asbestos effusion. Benign asbestos effusions are usually observed 10 to 15 years following asbestos exposure and commonly are associated with symptoms such as pleurisy, fever, and dyspnea. They usually resolve spontaneously after 3–4 months. On diagnostic thoracentesis, the pleural fluid is bloody in gross appearance and exudative. These effusions are usually not associated with the subsequent development of mesothelioma.

DIAGNOSTIC WORKUP OF A PLEURAL EFFUSION

Comprehensive clinical evaluation coupled with chest radiography is essential. In addition, diagnostic aspiration with analysis of pleural fluid is also frequently necessary in order to make a specific diagnosis.

Chest Radiography

Pleural effusion is confirmed by chest x-ray. Effusions greater than 175 mL in volume (usually in the >300 mL range) are apparent as blunting of the costophrenic angle on upright posteroanterior chest x-ray. A lateral decubitus chest x-ray (with the patient lying on his side) is more sensitive and can detect a 50-mL effusion. On supine chest x-ray (usually in the intensive care setting) moderate to large pleural effusions appear as a homogeneous increase in density spread over the lower lung fields. An elevation of the hemidiaphragm, lateral displacement of the dome of the diaphragm, or increased distance between the apparent left hemidiaphragm and the gastric air bubble suggests subpulmonic effusions.

Layering of an effusion on lateral decubitus films defines a freely flowing effusion and, if the layering fluid is ≥1 cm thick, indicates an effusion of >200 mL that is amenable to thoracentesis. Failure of an effusion to layer on lateral decubitus films indicates loculated pleural fluid or some other etiology causing the increased pleural density.

Pleural Aspiration/Thoracentesis

A pleural aspiration or diagnostic thoracentesis consists of placing a small needle through the chest wall using local anesthetic and aspirating from the fluid pocket to collect some fluid for analysis.

Relative contraindications to a diagnostic thoracentesis include a small volume of fluid (<1 cm thickness on a lateral decubitus film), bleeding diathesis or systemic anticoagulation, mechanical ventilation, and cutaneous disease over the proposed puncture site.

Mechanical ventilation with positive end-expiratory pressure does not increase the risk of pneumothorax after thoracentesis, but it increases the likelihood of severe complications (tension pneumothorax or persistent bronchopleural fistula) if the lung is punctured.

Complications of diagnostic thoracentesis include pain at the puncture site, cutaneous or internal bleeding, pneumothorax, empyema, and spleen/liver puncture.

Table 32.5 **TUMORS COMMONLY CAUSING MALIGNANT PLEURAL EFFUSIONS**

Lung
Breast
Lymphoma
Ovary
Stomach

Pneumothorax may complicate as many as 12–30% of thoracenteses in some series but requires treatment with a chest tube in less than 5% of cases.

The frequency of complications from thoracentesis is lower when a more experienced clinician performs the procedure and when ultrasound guidance is used. Postprocedure expiratory chest radiographs to exclude pneumothorax are not needed in asymptomatic patients after uncomplicated procedures (single needle pass without aspiration of air). However, postprocedure inspiratory chest radiographs are recommended to establish a new baseline for patients likely to have recurrent symptomatic effusions.

Pleural Fluid Analysis

The initial diagnostic consideration is distinguishing transudates from exudates. The gross appearance may provide a powerful clue. For example, frankly purulent-appearing pleural fluid indicates an empyema, whereas a milky, opalescent fluid suggests a chylothorax or pseudochylothorax. Grossly bloody fluid may result from trauma, malignancy, postpericardiotomy syndrome, and asbestos-related effusion, and this indicates the need for a hematocrit test of the sample. The presence of food indicates an esophageal rupture.

The simplest way to distinguish an exudate from a transudate is to measure the pleural fluid protein content. Exudates have a protein level of >3 g/dL, and transudates a protein level of <3 g/dL. However, if the patient's serum protein level is abnormal or the pleural protein level is close to the 3 g/dL cutoff point, using the criteria by Light is recommended. This requires measurement of serum and pleural fluid lactate dehydrogenase (LDH) and total protein levels.

Light's criteria are used for differentiating a transudate from an exudate. The fluid is considered an exudate if any of the following apply:

- Ratio of pleural fluid to serum protein >0.5

- Ratio of pleural fluid to serum LDH >0.6

- Pleural fluid LDH greater than two-thirds of the upper limits of normal serum value.

These criteria require concomitant measurement of pleural fluid and serum protein and LDH.

The criteria of Light et al. identify nearly all exudates correctly, but they misclassify approximately 20–25% of transudates as exudates, usually in patients on long-term diuretic therapy for CHF because of the concentration of protein and LDH within the pleural space. Using the criterion of serum minus pleural fluid albumin concentration of ≤1.2 g/dL rather than a serum/pleural fluid ratio of >0.5 more correctly identifies exudates in these patients.

The pleural fluid can be tested for other constituents, which may help in the differential diagnosis.

- *Differential cell counts on the pleural fluid:* Pleural lymphocytosis is common in malignancy and tuberculosis. An eosinophilic pleural effusion is defined as the presence of 10% or more eosinophils in the pleural fluid. The presence of pleural fluid eosinophilia is disappointingly not useful in the differential diagnosis of pleural effusions. It may be found in parapneumonic effusions, tuberculosis, drug-induced pleurisy, benign asbestos pleural effusions, Churg Strauss syndrome, pulmonary infarction, parasitic disease, and malignancy. Air or blood in the pleural space can elicit an eosinophilic response.

- *Cytology:* Consideration of a malignant etiology for pleural effusion should prompt cytologic evaluation. Cytology alone has an approximate sensitivity of 60%. If there is clinical suspicion of a malignancy, and if the first pleural fluid cytology specimen is negative, then it should be repeated a second time. Both cell blocks and fluid smears should be prepared for examination and, if the fluid has clotted, it needs to be fixed and sectioned as a histological section. Immunocytochemistry, as an adjunct to cell morphology, is becoming increasingly helpful in distinguishing benign from malignant mesothelial cells and mesothelioma from adenocarcinoma. Epithelial membrane antigen (EMA) is widely used to confirm a cytologic diagnosis of epithelial malignancy. When malignant cells are identified, the glandular markers for CEA, B72.3, and Leu-M1 together with calretinin and cytokeratin 5/6 will often help to distinguish adenocarcinoma from mesothelioma.

- *Pleural fluid amylase:* Amylase may be elevated in esophageal rupture (Boerhaave syndrome), pancreatitis, or pancreatic cancer. Amylase isoenzymes can be used to differentiate esophageal rupture (salivary isoenzymes) from a pancreatic source.

- *Pleural fluid glucose:* The glucose is characteristically decreased with malignancy, SLE, esophageal rupture, tuberculosis, empyema, and rheumatoid pleuritis. (The lowest glucose concentrations are found in rheumatoid effusions and empyema.)

- *Pleural fluid pH:* The pH of the normal pleural fluid is approximately 7.64 because of active transport of bicarbonate into the pleural space. Typically the pH is <7.2 with an empyema and indicates the need for drainage. Urinothorax is the only transudative effusion that can present with a low pleural fluid pH.

- *Pleural fluid Gram staining and culture:* The pleural space is normally sterile. The finding of bacteria on Gram stain or culture raises concern for empyema. The yield of mycobacteria on culture of pleural fluid in patients with tuberculous pleurisy is low (approximately 20–30%). If there is suspicion of tuberculosis, additional analysis can include measurement of pleural fluid adenosine deaminase and interferon-γ (markers for tuberculous pleurisy) and polymerase chain reaction (PCR) for tuberculous DNA.

If pleural fluid analysis does not provide an explanation as to the cause of pleural fluid formation, additional investigation may be required, including sampling of pleural tissue (thoracoscopic biopsy), as indicated in table 32.6.

TREATMENT OF PLEURAL EFFUSIONS

The treatment of a pleural effusion requires differentiating between a transudate and an exudate (table 32.7). Medical and surgical approaches then need to be considered.

Therapeutic Thoracentesis

Therapeutic thoracentesis to remove larger amounts of pleural fluid requires insertion of an intercostal drain (either pigtail catheter or thoracostomy tube). Indications include alleviation of dyspnea and to prevent ongoing inflammation and fibrosis in parapneumonic effusions. Two precautions are important to bear in mind: first, removal of 500 mL is usually sufficient to alleviate dyspnea; generally avoid removing >1000–1500 mL of fluid at one time to prevent development of reexpansion pulmonary edema. Second, monitor oxygenation closely during and after thoracentesis because arterial oxygen tension paradoxically might worsen after pleural fluid drainage as a result of shifts in perfusion and ventilation in the reexpanding lung. Consider use of empirical supplemental oxygen during the procedure. Larger amounts of pleural fluid can be removed if pleural pressure is monitored by pleural manometry. The onset of chest or shoulder pain during the removal of fluid typically indicates lung reinflation with apposition of inflamed pleural surfaces and is an indication to stop the procedure.

Tube Thoracostomy

Although small, freely flowing parapneumonic effusions can be drained by therapeutic thoracentesis, most larger effusions and complicated parapneumonic effusions or empyemas require drainage by tube thoracostomy. Traditionally, large-bore chest tubes (20–36F) have been used to drain thick pleural fluid and to break up loculations in empyemas. However, such tubes are not always well tolerated by patients and are difficult to direct correctly into the pleural space. More recently, small-bore tubes (7–14F) inserted at the bedside or under radiographic guidance have been shown to provide adequate drainage, even when empyema is present. These tubes cause less discomfort and are more likely to be placed successfully within a pocket of pleural fluid. In addition, long-term indwelling pleural catheters are being used with increasing frequency to treat malignant effusions in patients too frail to undergo pleural sclerosis, with good success over periods of weeks to months.

Pleural Sclerosis

Pleural sclerosis is considered for recurrent effusions, particularly symptomatic malignant effusions. Pleural sclerosis should be attempted only if the lung expands fully after fluid removal. The most commonly used sclerosing agents are doxycycline, talc slurry, bleomycin, and quinacrine. Doxycycline is the agent of first choice. Pleural sclerosis is usually well tolerated. Fever and self-limited chest pain occur in the minority of patients.

Surgical Management

Surgery is usually considered when sclerosis has failed, when lung expansion is prevented by a thickened pleura, or when organized tissue and clot will not drain via thoracostomy

Table 32.6 KEY FACTS ON ADDITIONAL IMAGING TESTS OR PROCEDURES

TYPE OF IMAGING/ PROCEDURE	KEY FACT
Ultrasound	Major indication is in differentiating solid lesions (e.g., tumor or thickened pleura) from fluid and in detecting abnormalities that are subpulmonic (under the lung) or subphrenic (below the diaphragm) Superior to CT scan for detection of fibrinous septations Guide thoracentesis in small or loculated pleural effusions to enhance safety
CT scan	Indications include distinguishing empyema from lung abscess, in detecting pleural masses (e.g., mesothelioma, plaques), in detecting lung parenchymal abnormalities "hidden" by an effusion, differentiating benign and malignant pleural thickening, and in outlining loculated fluid collections (loculated effusions on CT scans tend to have a lenticular shape with smooth margins and relatively homogeneous attenuation) Should routinely use contrast enhancement
Pleural biopsy	Indications for needle biopsy of the pleura include tuberculous pleuritis and malignancy of the pleura; for TB, consider pleural biopsy when tuberculous pleuritis is suspected and the pleural fluid adenosine deaminase or interferon-γ levels are not definitive; for malignancy, consider pleural biopsy when malignancy is suspected but cytologic study of the pleural fluid is negative and thoracoscopy is not readily available
Thoracoscopy	Indications include pleural effusions of unknown cause, particularly if mesothelioma, lung cancer, or tuberculosis is suspected; it can also be done to introduce sclerosing agents

Table 32.7 **TREATMENT STRATEGIES FOR TRANSUDATIVE AND EXUDATIVE PLEURAL EFFUSIONS**

Transudative pleural effusion	Treat the underlying medical disorder
	Large effusions, especially if refractory to treatment of the underlying etiology, require drainage
Exudative pleural effusion	Treat underlying etiology of the effusion
	Complicated parapneumonic effusions and empyemas should be drained to prevent development of fibrosing pleuritis
	Indications for urgent drainage of parapneumonic effusions
	Frankly purulent fluid
	Pleural fluid pH <7.2
	Loculated effusions
	Bacteria on Gram stain or culture
	Malignant effusions are usually drained to palliate symptoms and may require pleurodesis to prevent recurrence

tube. In this circumstance, pleural decortication becomes necessary, in which procedure the surgeon manually removes debris from the pleural space and strips fibrous tissue from the visceral pleural surface.

PLEURAL TUMORS

Most pleural neoplasms are metastatic in origin. Primary tumors of the pleura can be categorized as diffuse or localized. Diffuse malignant mesothelioma is more common, related to asbestos exposure, and associated with a poorer prognosis. Localized mesothelioma is also referred to as localized fibrous tumor of the pleura (LFTP) and solitary fibrous tumor of the pleura. It is a less common neoplasm of controversial histogenesis, unrelated to asbestos exposure.

LFTPs exist in benign and malignant forms. Only rarely is the localized fibrous tumor invasive or does it cause local recurrence after resection. The ratio of benign to malignant LFTPs is 7:1. The diagnosis of LFTP is important because the tumor is potentially resectable for cure despite its typically large size. In many cases, resection can repeatedly be used to treat recurrence, although usually with increasing difficulty.

ADDITIONAL READING

Kinasewitz GT. Transudative effusions. *Eur Respir J.* 1997;10:714–8.
Light RW. Diagnostic principles in pleural disease. *Eur Respir J.* 1997;10:476–81.

Light RW, Erozan YS, Ball WCJ. Cells in pleural fluid. Their value in differential diagnosis. *Arch Intern Med.* 1973;132:854–60.
Maskell NA, Butland RJA. BTS guidelines for the investigation of a unilateral pleural effusion in adults *Thorax.* 2003;58(Suppl II):ii8–ii17.
Rubins J. Pleural effusion: Treatment & management. http://emedicine.medscape.com/article/299959-treatment.

QUESTIONS

QUESTION 1. A 42-year-old man presents with gradually worsening dyspnea for the past 9 months. His past medical history is remarkable for long-standing rheumatoid arthritis. He also admits to sustaining a road traffic accident approximately 1 year previously. On examination, there is dullness to percussion of the right base. His chest x-ray shows a right-sided effusion. A diagnostic thoracentesis is performed and reveals cloudy fluid with a pleural protein level of 3.5 g/dL and pleural triglyceride level of 240 mg/dL.

The most likely diagnosis is which of the following:

A. Rheumatoid arthritis as the cause of his effusion
B. A chylothorax resulting from his road traffic accident
C. A malignant pleural effusion
D. Subclinical congestive heart failure
E. Langerhans cell granulomatosis (histiocytosis X)

QUESTIONS 2–5. Match the following pleural fluid results with the appropriate diagnoses:

PLEURAL/SERUM PROTEIN RATIO	PLEURAL/SERUM LDH RATIO	PH	GLUCOSE, MG/DL
2. 0.6	2.2	7.3	75
3. 0.2	0.4	6.9	94
4. 0.3	0.4	7.3	90
5. 0.7	5.0	7.2	25

A. Urinothorax
B. Uncomplicated parapneumonic effusion
C. CHF
D. Rheumatoid arthritis

ANSWERS

1. B
2. B
3. A
4. C
5. D

33.

CHRONIC OBSTRUCTIVE PULMONARY DISEASE

John J. Reilly

Virtually every health care practitioner who provides care to adults will encounter individuals with chronic obstructive pulmonary disease (COPD). Current estimates of the prevalence of the condition vary based on the method of ascertainment: most surveys show that approximately 6% of adults report a doctor's diagnosis of COPD but that approximately 25% have airflow obstruction when assessed by spirometry. COPD is common, morbid, mortal, and expensive: estimates are that >20 million U.S. adults have COPD and that it is responsible for >120,000 deaths annually with a cost to the U.S. economy of more than $38 billion. This chapter describes the definition of COPD, presenting clinical symptomatology and evaluation, natural history, differential diagnosis, current concepts of pathogenesis, therapeutic options, and the evaluation of a patient with known or suspected COPD considering surgery.

DEFINITION

The definition of COPD has undergone an evolution; originally presented as an umbrella term to encompass emphysema, chronic bronchitis, and chronic asthma, it has most recently been defined by the Global Initiative for Chronic Obstructive Lung Disease (2004) as

> a preventable and treatable disease with some significant extrapulmonary effects that may contribute to the severity in individual patients. Its pulmonary component is characterized by airflow limitation that is not fully reversible. The airflow limitation is usually progressive and associated with an abnormal inflammatory response of the lung to noxious particles or gases.

In contrast, the definition of emphysema is based on anatomic features: enlargement of the airspaces distal to the terminal bronchiole; and that of chronic bronchitis is based on symptoms: daily cough and phlegm for 3 months for two or more consecutive years; neither actually requires the presence of airflow obstruction.

PATHOGENESIS

There are compelling epidemiologic data relating inhalational exposure to tobacco smoke to the development of COPD. Exposure to tobacco smoke results in an inflammatory reaction in the lung in virtually everyone who smokes. As discussed below, however, the precise mechanisms by which tobacco smoke exposure results in COPD remain to be defined.

Observational human studies in the 1960s that identified the association of alpha-1-antiprotease deficiency with emphysema and work on animal models of disease led to the formulation of the *protease-antiprotease hypothesis,* which proposes that emphysema results from an imbalance of proteases and antiproteases in the lung. In the case of alpha-1-antiprotease, it is believed that the deficiency of this inhibitor allows unrestricted activity of neutrophil elastase, leading to alveolar destruction. It is not yet clear which proteases and antiproteases are involved in the pathogenesis of emphysema in smokers with normal alpha-1-antiprotease levels. There is experimental evidence supporting potential participation of elastases of several different classes, including macrophage metalloelastase, in the pathogenesis of emphysema. Inhibition of these enzymes or modulation of the protease–antiprotease balance by targeting relevant regulatory pathways are potential targets of new therapeutic agents.

In addition to the protease-antiprotease hypothesis, there is also evidence supporting the potential roles of oxidative stress, inflammatory cytokines, suppressed angiogenesis, and apoptosis in the pathogenesis of COPD. Also unanswered is the question of whether COPD is a disease of defective repair rather than excessive destruction.

There are also data to support the hypothesis that genetic factors may underlie the relative predisposition to or protection from the development of COPD as a result of exposure to cigarette smoke. Work to date has not convincingly identified a "COPD gene" other than alpha-1-antiprotease and current concepts of complex trait genetics suggest that there are likely a number of genes, each of which has a relatively small effect size.

CLASSIFICATION

A number of classification schemata have been proposed for COPD. They share the common property of characterizing severity by the degree of airflow obstruction present on spirometry. The presence of a reduction in the ratio of forced expiratory volume in 1 sec (FEV_1) to forced vital capacity (FVC) establishes the presence of obstruction; the degree of reduction in the FEV_1 is used to determine severity. The most recent, and currently most widely used, schema is the GOLD system, presented in table 33.1.

As the definition of COPD indicates, there are clinically significant manifestations of the disease in addition to airflow obstruction. The BODE Index, developed by Celli and colleagues, incorporates *b*ody mass index, airflow *o*bstruction, symptoms of *d*yspnea and *e*xercise tolerance in a scoring system that has been demonstrated to better predict mortality than using airflow obstruction alone. The BODE Index is presented in table 33.2.

The BODE Index more accurately correlates with prognosis than systems that use spirometry alone to classify patients.

CLINICAL PRESENTATION

The majority of persons diagnosed with COPD initially present for medical evaluation in one of two ways: with gradually progressive symptoms that include dyspnea on exertion or with an acute illness characterized by an abrupt increase in cough, sputum, and dyspnea (COPD exacerbation). In the latter scenario, questioning usually reveals antecedent gradual increase in exertional dyspnea and/or chronic cough.

Table 33.1 GOLD CLASSIFICATION SYSTEM OF COPD

Stage 1	Mild	FEV_1/FVC <0.70 FEV_1 ≥80% predicted
Stage 2	Moderate	FEV_1/FVC <0.70 50% pred ≤FEV_1 <80% pred
Stage 3	Severe	FEV_1/FVC <0.70 30% pred ≤ FEV_1 <50% pred
Stage 4	Very Severe	FEV_1/FVC <0.70 FEV_1 <30% pred

SOURCE: From the "Global Strategy for Diagnosis, Management, and Prevention of COPD, 2011" used with permission from the Global Initiative for Chronic Obstructive Lung Disease (GOLD), www.goldcopd.org.

DEMOGRAPHICS AND SYMPTOMS

The typical patient presents between the ages of 50 and 70 and frequently has a history of significant cigarette use. As mentioned above, the most frequently cited symptom is dyspnea on exertion, which has usually been gradually increasing for months to years. Given the age and demographic characteristics of patients with COPD, the increase in dyspnea is often attributed to aging, deconditioning, weight gain, or concomitant comorbid medical conditions. Cough, particularly morning cough with sputum production, is common and frequently accepted by patients as "a normal smoker's cough."

In addition to chronic symptoms, patients may also report episodic exacerbations in symptoms with a syndrome of increased cough, increase and/or change in characteristics of sputum production, and increased dyspnea. This may be accompanied by fever, myalgias, and other symptoms suggesting viral infection. Not infrequently, patients will report a repeated seasonal occurrence of such events, stating "every winter I get a cold and it settles in my chest" or similar descriptions.

PHYSICAL EXAM

In patients with mild or moderate disease, the history of symptoms in the appropriate exposure setting is the key to pursuing evaluation, as the physical exam is frequently normal. As airflow obstruction becomes more severe, the physical exam may reveal a prolonged expiratory phase of the respiratory cycle, inspiratory basilar rhonchi or crackles, and expiratory polyphonic wheezing. Supportive signs on the physical exam may include stigmata of cigarette smoking, including dental changes, skin thinning and wrinkling, and nicotine staining of fingers. Clubbing is *not* seen in COPD, and its presence should prompt evaluation for other causes, most frequently lung cancer.

In patients with severe or very severe COPD, there may be skeletal muscle wasting, and the use of accessory muscles of respiration at rest, with patients seeking positions that allow them to brace the shoulder girdle to provide mechanical advantage for these muscles. These positions include the classic "tripod" position while seated and using the handles on a shopping cart or wheelchair while ambulating. Examination of the chest reveals markedly prolonged expiratory phase, symmetrically diminished breath sounds, and medial and inferior displacement of the cardiac PMI to the subxiphoid position. It is unusual for patients to present with signs of overt right heart failure (cor pulmonale) or physical findings of severe pulmonary hypertension.

DIFFERENTIAL DIAGNOSIS

The differential diagnosis of a middle-aged person presenting with dyspnea on exertion is broad. It includes COPD, asthma, interstitial lung disease, anemia, congestive heart failure (CHF), coronary artery disease, and deconditioning.

Table 33.2 BODE INDEX (RANGE 0–10 POINTS)

BODE INDEX POINTS	FEV₁ (% PREDICTED)	6 MINUTE WALK DISTANCE (METERS)	MMRC DYSPNEA SCALE	BODY MASS INDEX
0	≥65	>350	0–1: Breathless only with strenuous exercise or when hurrying on the level or walking up a slight hill	>21
1	50–64	250–349	2: Walks slower than people of the same age on the level because of breathlessness or has to stop for breath when walking at own pace on the level	≤21
2	36–49	150–249	3: Stops for breath after walking about 100 yards or after a few minutes on the level	
3	≤35	≤150	4: Too breathless to leave the house or breathless when dressing or undressing	

SOURCE: Reprinted with permission from Celli R, Cote CG, Marin JM, et al. The body-mass index, airflow obstruction, dyspnea, and exercise capacity index in chronic obstructive pulmonary disease. *N Engl J Med.* 2004;350:1005–12. Copyright 2004 Massachusetts Medical Society. All rights reserved.

Given the nonspecificity of the presenting symptoms and physical exam, the ability to diagnose COPD depends on obtaining spirometry as part of the initial evaluation of the patient. The presence of airflow obstruction, as manifested by a reduction in the FEV₁/FVC that does not normalize after the administration of an inhaled bronchodilator, strongly supports the diagnosis (figure 33.1). The importance of ordering spirometry is underlined by the fact that NHANES 3 survey data suggest that at least 50% of patients with airflow obstruction have *not* been diagnosed with COPD and are not receiving any therapy (American Thoracic Society/European Respiratory Society, 2003).

PULMONARY FUNCTION TESTING

All patients with COPD have, by definition, incompletely reversible airflow obstruction on pulmonary function testing. Measurements of lung volumes will reveal increases in functional residual capacity (FRC), the ratio of residual volume to total lung capacity (RV/TLC), and total lung capacity (TLC), all indicative of hyperinflation, which is in proportion to the degree of airflow obstruction.

Measurement of the diffusing capacity for carbon monoxide (D1CO) may show a reduction. The magnitude of this reduction is in proportion to the amount of emphysematous destruction of the lungs in an individual patient.

ARTERIAL BLOOD GASES AND ASSESSMENT OF OXYGENATION

As discussed below, the data demonstrate that patients with COPD and *chronic resting hypoxemia,* defined as pO_2 <55 mm Hg or S_aO_2 <88%, benefit from supplemental oxygen therapy. It is appropriate to assess oxygenation with either an arterial blood gas (ABG) measurement or oximetry in patients with moderate or greater disease or those presenting with an increase in symptomatology. Measurement of ABGs provides information not only about oxygenation but also acid–base status and pCO_2. Knowledge of the latter two parameters is important in the assessment of acute respiratory failure.

THORACIC IMAGING

Imaging of the chest can be performed with conventional chest radiography, computed tomography (CT), and/or magnetic resonance imaging (MRI).

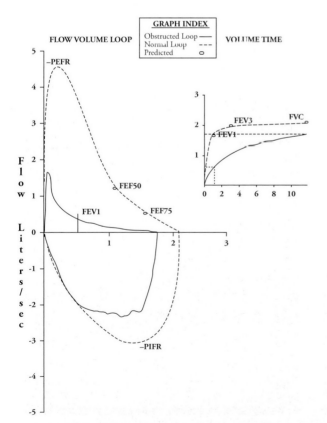

Figure 33.1. Spirogram and Flow-Volume Loops. Spirogram and flow-volume loop in airflow obstruction, compared to normal, showing reduced expiratory flow rates and "coving" of flow-volume loop.

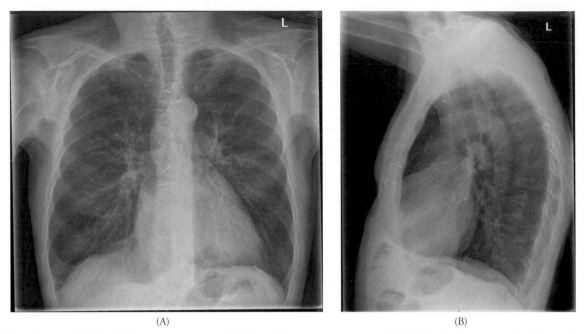

(A)   (B)

Figure 33.2. Chest X-rays in COPD. (A) Posterior-anterior and (B) lateral chest x-ray in patient with COPD showing increased A P dimension, flattened diaphragms, and increased retrosternal airspace.

Chest x-rays (CXRs) are frequently normal in patients with mild or moderate disease. Signs of hyperinflation with increase in anterior-posterior (AP) dimension and/or flattening of the diaphragms are nonspecific but are consistent with the presence of COPD (figure 33.2). Some smokers may manifest a nonspecific increase in interstitial markings ("dirty lungs"). In patients with more advanced disease, the images may demonstrate increased lucency of the lung fields, consistent with the tissue destruction of emphysema, a diminution in visualized vascularity, and medial and inferior displacement of the cardiac silhouette (figure 33.3). Focal areas of hyperlucency are suggestive of bullous disease. In patients presenting with acute respiratory decompensation, the x-ray should be carefully reviewed for evidence of CHF pneumonia, or pneumothorax. The latter can be difficult to distinguish from severe bullous changes in some individuals with marked underlying emphysema.

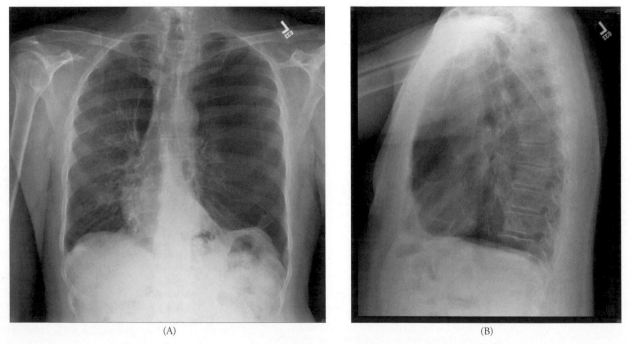

(A)   (B)

Figure 33.3. Chest X-rays in Severe COPD. (A) Posterior-anterior and (B) lateral chest x-ray in patient with severe COPD showing hyperlucency, flattened diaphragms, and inferomedial rotation of cardiac silhouette.

Chest CT scanning may be normal in mild disease. It is the current test of choice for assessing the presence of emphysema. It is much more sensitive than plain chest radiography for demonstrating emphysematous changes. Qualitatively, these changes can be described as consistent with centriacinar, panlobular, or paraseptal emphysema. In addition, the distribution of the changes can be described: upper-lobe predominant, lower-lobe predominant, or diffuse. The lower-lobe is suggestive of underlying alpha-1-antiprotease deficiency. More recently, tools are being developed to provide a more precise quantification of emphysema on CT scanning. Although still largely a research tool, these approaches have been used to evaluate patients considering surgical therapy for COPD. The CT scan is also the test of choice to evaluate for the presence of bronchiectasis. The presence of enlarged airways (greater in diameter than the associated blood vessel), nontapering airways, or airways visible within 1–2 cm of the pleural surface are findings of bronchiectasis; airway thickening may also be seen involving these structures.

Chest CT scanning with intravenous contrast is frequently used to evaluate patients with suspected pulmonary embolism and may be ordered in a patient with COPD presenting with chest pain or acute respiratory decompensation.

In addition to demonstrating emphysema, chest CTs performed in patients with significant smoking history and COPD frequently demonstrate pulmonary nodules (10–30%, depending on the definition used), a minority of which represent malignancy (figure 33.4). If such a nodule is detected, further evaluation is required. Published guidelines utilize the size of the nodule and the underlying risk factors of the patient to recommend evaluation and monitoring strategies (Foster et al., 2006).

The issue of whether to use chest CT scans to screen asymptomatic middle-aged smokers for the presence of lung cancer is controversial and currently the subject of a large government-funded multicenter trial in the United States (NLST). At the present time, guidelines do not recommend the routine use of CT scanning for this purpose. The current role of CT scanning in the assessment of a patient with known or suspected COPD is in evolution. Agreed-on indications include the evaluation of patients considering surgical therapy for COPD, such as bullectomy, lung volume reduction surgery, or lung transplantation; evaluation of large airways in patients in whom a focal anatomic abnormality is in the differential diagnosis; establishing the presence and extent of emphysema in individuals with alpha-1-antiprotease deficiency; and (with contrast) to evaluate possible pulmonary embolism in a patient with underlying COPD and acute decompensation.

MRI scanning of the chest has its greatest utility in visualizing the mediastinum, trachea, and proximal large airways. The nature of the lung parenchyma, with its large air content, limits the applicability of MRI in imaging the lung parenchyma. Although current research in the field includes the development of functional imaging techniques in COPD, there is currently little role for chest MRI scanning in the evaluation and management of patients with COPD.

BLOOD TESTS

There are no specific blood tests that establish the presence or absence of COPD. Traditionally, it has been recommended to obtain an alpha-1-antitrypsin (A1AT; also known as alpha-1-antiprotease) level in patients with a

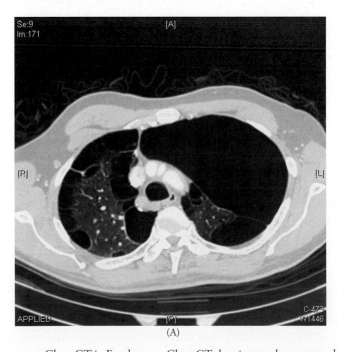
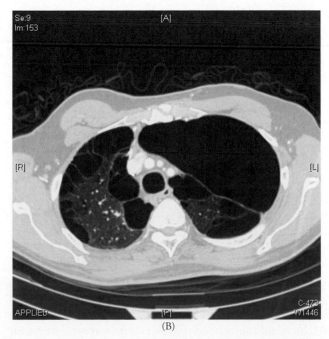

Figure 33.4. Chest CT in Emphysema. Chest CT showing emphysematous destruction of lung parenchyma and nodule in posterior aspect of left lung.

strong family history of COPD, patients presenting at a young age (<45–50), patients with basilar predominant emphysema, and patients with unexplained bronchiectasis and/or liver disease. More recent guidelines have recommended checking a level in every patient diagnosed with COPD. Those with a low A1AT level should be evaluated for replacement therapy and counseled concerning the genetics of A1AT deficiency. In patients with unexplained bronchiectasis, evaluation of IgG subclass deficiency (IgG2, IgG4), IgA deficiency, cystic fibrosis, and immotile cilia syndrome should be considered.

SUMMARY OF DIAGNOSIS OF COPD

Middle-aged or older patients complaining of unexplained or worsening dyspnea should be evaluated for COPD; this is particularly true of those individuals with a significant cigarette smoking history. For patients with mild to moderate disease, the physical exam may be relatively normal. Establishing the diagnosis requires consideration of COPD in the differential diagnosis and obtaining spirometry before and after bronchodilator. Spirometry alone is usually enough to establish the diagnosis; lung volumes and diffusing capacity provide additional information concerning degree of hyperinflation and emphysema and may be useful in situations where there is concern about the presence of an additional disease process (interstitial lung disease, weakness, neurologic disease), as a part of preoperative evaluation for chest surgery, or in patients being considered for therapy specific for emphysema.

CONTROVERSIES CONCERNING SCREENING FOR COPD

Given that COPD has a strong association with cigarette smoking and that over 20% of lifelong smokers will develop clinically significant COPD, there is a school of thought that advocates performing spirometry on all middle-aged smokers, regardless of the presence of symptoms. The logic is that identification of early airflow obstruction, prior to the onset of symptoms, will provide an opportunity for early intervention. The only intervention determined to influence the natural history of early COPD is smoking cessation. The available data are relatively limited, but those available do not establish that the knowledge of early signs of COPD results in a higher smoking cessation rate than smoking cessation interventions irrespective of spirometry results. The opposing school of thought reasons that (1) all smokers should be counseled to quit and provided appropriate cessation therapy regardless of the results of spirometry, and (2) the majority of smokers with normal lung function may be inappropriately reassured that they are not at risk for smoking-related disease(s). As a result, screening for COPD is not in widespread practice.

THERAPY FOR COPD

GOALS OF THERAPY

Treatment of any chronic disease has the goals of improving current symptoms, eliminating the disease or reducing the rate of progression, and reducing mortality. These combine to produce an improvement in health-related quality of life (HRQOL). In addition, the most desirable goal of therapy is to prevent the development of disease in the first place. COPD is somewhat unique in medicine, as the strategy to prevent development of disease in the majority of patients is very clear: prevent people from starting to smoke cigarettes.

Disease Prevention

As noted above, there is compelling evidence implicating cigarette smoking as the major risk factor for the development of COPD. There are data suggesting that there is (are) genetic predisposition(s) to develop COPD, and COPD is frequently cited as an example of gene × environment interactions. Although the majority of patients with COPD are cigarette smokers (80–90% or more in most series), the majority of smokers do not develop COPD.

Given that cigarette smoking is a risk factor for disease development, it is logical to assume that smoking cessation will have a favorable impact on disease course. This hypothesis is supported by data from the Lung Health Study, which demonstrate that individuals with early airflow obstruction who are able to cease smoking experience an improvement in the rate of decline of lung function back to normal rates for age and reduced mortality in 15-year follow-up (Sin et al., 2003).

Clearly, the most desirable approach is to prevent individuals from starting smoking. Public health campaigns have succeeded in reducing the proportion of U.S. adults who smoke, but the prevalence of smoking in the U.S. adult population is still approximately 20%. For such individuals who express a desire to quit, the current recommendations are to consider pharmacotherapy to aid in smoking cessation, based on reports that the chances of success are significantly improved with such therapy. Options for therapy are presented in table 33.3.

THERAPY OF CHRONIC STABLE DISEASE

A variety of pharmacologic and nonpharmacologic therapies are available for COPD. Pharmacologic therapy includes medications intended to produce bronchodilation, anti-inflammatory medications, mucolytics, antioxidants, and protease inhibitors. Although there is some controversy about their efficacy (discussed below), the majority of available data suggest that pharmacotherapy does not alter the rate of decline in lung function or mortality. Thus, they are best viewed as intended to improve current symptoms.

Other available therapies include supplemental oxygen, surgical therapy, and pulmonary rehabilitation. Of these,

Table 33.3 PHARMACOTHERAPY FOR SMOKING CESSATION

MEDICATION	TRADE NAME	FORM	SIDE EFFECTS
Nicotine		Lozenge Gum Nasal spray Transdermal patch	Nausea, insomnia (transdermal)
Bupropion	Zyban, Wellbutrin	Pill	May exacerbate seizures
Varenicline	Chantix	Pill	Nausea? Neuropsychiatric symptoms

supplemental oxygen and lung volume reduction surgery have been demonstrated to reduce mortality in appropriately selected patients.

The algorithm published by the Global Initiative on Chronic Obstructive Lung Disease recommends a stepwise escalation of therapy with worsening airflow obstruction. These recommendations are summarized in figure 33.5.

Vaccines

Influenza Vaccine

Available data support the use of the annual poly(tri)valent influenza vaccine in patients with COPD based on a reduction of serious exacerbations/hospitalizations related to influenza. It is recommended in the GOLD guidelines.

Pneumococcal Vaccine

The currently available polysaccharide vaccine is intended to stimulate antibody protection against the 23 most common serotypes of *Streptococcus pneumoniae* associated with human disease, including the six serotypes most commonly associated with invasive human infection. Despite the fact that pneumococcus is one of the three bacterial species associated with COPD exacerbations, there are very little available data addressing the efficacy of this vaccine in the COPD population. Nevertheless, many physicians recommend it to their patients with COPD on the premise that it has an excellent safety profile and it theoretically may reduce the risk of infection.

Pharmacotherapy

Short-Acting Beta Agonists

Examples of short-acting beta agonists include albuterol (also known as salbutamol), levalbuterol, pirbuterol, and fenoterol. As the name suggests, they have relatively rapid onset of action and last 4–6 hours. They are appropriate therapy for patients with intermittent symptoms or acute symptoms despite long-acting therapy. Side effects include tachycardia and tremor. The inhaled route of delivery is preferred, as side effects are more common with parenteral administration (usually oral, rarely subcutaneously).

Long-Acting Beta Agonists

Long-acting beta agonists (LABA) are available in inhaled form, via dry powder inhalers or nebulized solutions, and either alone or in combination with a corticosteroid. Examples include salmeterol and formoterol. The side-effect profile is similar to that of short-acting beta agonists, although less pronounced. The rate of onset of action is longer than that of short-acting medications, and the duration of action is 8–12 hours. They are indicated for patients with daily symptoms. Available data suggest that they provide modest improvements in FEV_1 and HRQOL. They have also been reported to reduce the risk of COPD exacerbation by 20–25%. The magnitude of benefit is similar to that seen with inhaled anticholinergic medications; combination of a LABA and an anticholinergic produces more bronchodilation than either medication alone. Currently, there are no available data to suggest that use of LABA is *disease-modifying* in terms of affecting the rate of decline in FEV_1 over time or in reducing mortality.

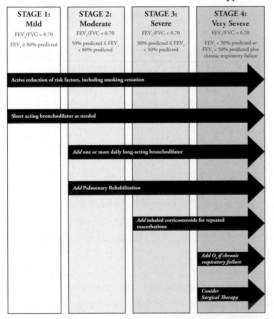

GOLD Recommendations for COPD Therapy

STAGE 1: Mild	STAGE 2: Moderate	STAGE 3: Severe	STAGE 4: Very Severe
$FEV_1/FVC < 0.70$ $FEV_1 \geq 80\%$ predicted	$FEV_1/FVC < 0.70$ 50% predicted $\leq FEV_1$ $< 80\%$ predicted	$FEV_1/FVC < 0.70$ 30% predicted $\leq FEV_1$ $< 50\%$ predicted	$FEV_1/FVC < 0.70$ $FEV_1 < 30\%$ predicted *or* $FEV_1 < 50\%$ predicted plus chronic respiratory failure

Active reduction of risk factors, including smoking cessation

Short acting bronchodilator as needed

Add one or more daily long-acting bronchodilator

Add Pulmonary Rehabilitation

Add inhaled corticosteroids for repeated exacerbations

Add O_2 *if chronic respiratory failure*

Consider Surgical Therapy

Figure 33.5. GOLD Recommendations for COPD Therapy. From the Global Strategy for Diagnosis, Management, and Prevention of COPD, 2010 used with permission from the Global Initiative for Chronic Obstructive Lung Disease (GOLD), www.goldcopd.org.

Short-acting inhaled anticholinergics, such as ipratropium bromide, can be used in the same manner as short-acting beta agonists: episodically for patients with intermittent symptoms. They may be used alone or in a combination with a short-acting beta agonist. The latter, inhaled albuterol/ipratropium, offers more bronchodilation than either agent alone. The choice of whether to use a short-acting beta agonist or anticholinergic therapy as initial intermittent therapy for patients with COPD is a matter of patient and physician preference; the magnitudes of benefit and costs are similar. Anticholinergics are less likely to produce tachycardia and tremor, although some patients do report dry mouth.

Long-Acting Anticholinergics

Tiotropium is an inhaled anticholinergic medication with a recommended dosing schedule of once daily. It produces improvement in maximal expiratory flow rates and HRQOL of a magnitude similar to LABA. It is available as a dry powder inhaler. As with ipratropium, the side-effect profile is related to anticholinergic properties, the most common being dry mouth. Tiotropium does not affect the rate of decline in FEV_1, nor has it been shown to affect mortality (Hancock and London, 2011). The choice between long-acting anticholinergic and LABA is one of patient and physician preference. Available data do suggest that combining these two classes of agents results in more improvement than either alone.

Inhaled Corticosteroids

The role of inhaled corticosteroids (ICS) in patients with COPD is incompletely defined. Examples include fluticasone, budesonide, and triamcinolone. There are good data demonstrating that inhalation of a combination of LABA and ICS produces more symptomatic benefit than an inhaled LABA alone, suggesting symptomatic benefit. There are also convincing data that ICS reduce exacerbation risk but also increase the risk of bacterial pneumonia. Studies to date involving different ICS preparations and somewhat different patient populations have consistently demonstrated that ICS do not affect the rate of decline in FEV_1 when used regularly for 3 years (Niewoehner, 2010; Gooneratne et al., 2010; Diaz-Guzman and Mannino, 2010). An unresolved controversy is the impact of ICS on COPD mortality; several retrospective analysis and observational studies suggest that ICS may reduce mortality in COPD, but in the recently published TORCH prospective study, the reduction in mortality in patients receiving LABA/ICS did not reach statistical significance.

Although ICS are commonly prescribed in patients with COPD, it should be noted that in the United States, the only ICS that has been approved for use is in combination with a LABA (salmeterol/fluticasone, Advair) on the basis of bronchodilator activity and exacerbation reduction. The GOLD guidelines recommend consideration of ICS in patients with recurrent exacerbations.

Parenteral Corticosteroids

Given the morbidity of long-term parenteral corticosteroid use and the absence of convincing evidence of benefit, they are not recommended for use in patients with stable COPD.

Aminophylline/Theophylline/Methylxanthines

Once a mainstay of COPD therapy, this class of medications has fallen into relative disfavor due to a high incidence of side effects, which include nausea, tremor, tachycardia and supraventricular arrhythmias, and seizures (rarely). They are available in either oral or intravenous preparations. They are mild bronchodilators and also may improve diaphragmatic contractility and respiratory drive. Their use as nocturnal therapy has largely been supplanted by LABAs.

More recently, it has been suggested that low-dose theophylline may restore glucocorticoid responsiveness in COPD patients due to their interaction with histone deacetylase. This clinical relevance of this observation awaits appropriately designed clinical trials.

Antioxidants/Mucolytics

Given the putative role of oxidative stress in the pathogenesis of COPD, as well as the incidence of mucous hypersecretion in some patients, multiple studies have investigated the utility of N-acetyl cysteine and other antioxidants. Although several smaller studies suggested benefit, the large BRONCUS trial failed to demonstrate any favorable impact on rate of decline in lung function or exacerbation rate. Thus, they are not recommended for use in COPD.

Alpha-1-Antiprotease Replacement Therapy

For patients with established alpha-1-antiprotease deficiency and evidence of lung disease (bronchiectasis, emphysema, and/or airflow obstruction), regular intravenous infusions of alpha-1-antiprotease protein are recommended. This recommendation is based on pathophysiologic principles and observational registry data suggesting a slower rate of decline in FEV_1 in patients on replacement therapy. Therapy is associated with inconvenience in the form of IV infusions every 1–4 weeks and with considerable expense. There is no role for replacement therapy in patients with COPD and normal alpha-1-antiprotease levels. Although there is controversy as to whether patients heterozygous for a deficient alpha-1-antiprotease allele are at increased risk for the development of COPD, there are no data to support the use of replacement therapy in such patients who do develop COPD.

Oxygen Therapy

The use of supplemental oxygen in appropriately selected patients is one of the few interventions that has been shown to improve mortality in patients with COPD. The Medical Research Council Trial and the Nocturnal Oxygen Therapy Trial demonstrated that supplemental oxygen dramatically reduces mortality in patients with *resting hypoxemia* (defined as P_aO_2 <55 mm Hg or 59 mm Hg with dependent edema, hematocrit >55%, or P pulmonale on electrocardiogram (EKG)) and that continuous therapy provided more benefit than nocturnal therapy. In current practice, resting oximetry is often substituted for measurement of ABGs a resting S_aO_2 of 88% or less is used as the threshold for therapy.

The role of supplemental oxygen in patients with COPD and nocturnal hypoxemia and/or exertional hypoxemia is less clear. For the latter, there is evidence that dyspnea may improve as well as exercise tolerance. In neither group has it been demonstrated that there is a mortality benefit from preventing episodic hypoxemia.

The role of oxygen therapy in patients with moderate resting hypoxemia is undefined and is currently the subject of a large multicenter trial.

Pulmonary Rehabilitation

The name is a misnomer, as it has been widely interpreted as suggesting an improvement in lung function as the result of an exercise program. It is more appropriately termed "rehabilitation of patients with lung disease." Most programs include two broad areas of intervention: education centered on strategies to minimize dynamic hyperinflation and to improve medication compliance and delivery, and physical conditioning primarily focused on improving cardiovascular conditioning. The latter emphasis is the result of studies demonstrating that deconditioning is a limiting factor for exertion in many patients with COPD, even accounting for their reduced ventilatory limit to exercise. In addition, some programs include strengthening specific target muscle groups, including the muscles of inspiration. Whether inspiratory muscle training results in clinically important patient improvement remains unclear.

It is clear, however, that pulmonary rehabilitation results in substantial improvements in symptoms and HRQOL. The magnitude of these improvements is as large as or larger than that reported for any available pharmacologic therapy. Although a mortality benefit has not been clearly demonstrated, short-term studies do demonstrate a reduction in health care resource utilization. The benefits of pulmonary rehabilitation wane with time if patients do not continue maintenance activities after completing the typical 6- to 8-week program.

In the GOLD guidelines, rehabilitation is recommended for patients with moderate or greater COPD. In common practice, it has often been reserved for patients with very severe disease and/or recurrent hospitalization. Of the available therapies for patients with symptomatic COPD, it is the most underutilized.

Surgical Therapy for COPD

There are three types of surgical intervention utilized in selected patients with COPD to improve symptoms. These are bullectomy, lung volume reduction surgery, and lung transplantation. In years past, a variety of other operative procedures for COPD have been tried and subsequently abandoned, including tracheotomy, glomectomy, and visceral denervation.

Bullectomy refers to the resection of a large dominant bulla(e) that prevents expansion of surrounding more functional lung tissue. Factors that have been identified that suggest bullectomy will achieve substantial physiologic benefit include size >60% of the hemithorax and the presence of adjacent "compressed normal" lung tissue. Patients with these characteristics are quite rare, but they do experience dramatic improvement in measured lung function and symptoms as a result of the procedure. Lung volume reduction surgery (LVRS) is based on a physiologic rationale similar to that used for bullectomy: resection of poorly functional lung tissue will improve elastic recoil, "reset" that resting volume of the respiratory system to a lower and more physiological level, and the result is improved symptoms and higher expiratory flow rates. First proposed in the early 1950s by Otto Brantigan, it was reintroduced in the 1990s. The National Emphysema Treatment Trial demonstrated that in patients with upper-lobe-predominant emphysema, as determined by review of chest CT scans, LVRS produced improvements in exercise performance and symptoms as compared to maximal medical therapy. In patients with upper-lobe-predominant emphysema and dramatically impaired exercise capacity, there was also a substantial mortality benefit of almost 50% during the observation period. The trial also demonstrated, however, that there is significant morbidity and mortality associated with LVRS, including a mortality rate of approximately 5% in the postoperative period. Current efforts in the area focus on the development of an endobronchial approach to lung volume reduction; several clinical trials are currently under way attempting to determine whether the same results may be achieved via a bronchoscopic approach, which would presumably eliminate some of the morbidity associated with the surgical procedure. Candidates for LVRS are patients with COPD that produces limiting symptoms despite appropriate pharmacotherapy and pulmonary rehabilitation, who have upper-lobe predominant emphysema on CT scan, and do not have pleural scarring, prior chest surgery, significant pulmonary hypertension, or other contraindications to the procedure. Such patients should be referred, if they so desire, to a center with expertise in providing the procedure.

Lung transplantation is the third surgical option for selected patients with COPD. COPD is the most common diagnosis for which patients receive a lung transplant. Common practice has been to do single lung transplantation in most patients with COPD despite theoretical concerns about hyperinflation of the contralateral lung and encroachment on the hemithorax containing the allograft. More recently, with publication of data suggesting better long-term outcomes in patients receiving bilateral lung transplantation, many centers are performing bilateral allografting procedures. Patients with COPD do well compared to other patients after lung transplant, with 1- and 5-year survival rates of 86% and 47%, respectively. Candidates for lung transplantation are patients with very severe airflow obstruction and disabling symptoms despite maximal medical therapy and pulmonary rehabilitation who are reasonably healthy other than having advanced COPD and have the capabilities and willingness to comply with a lifelong complex regimen of immunosuppressive and prophylactic medications. Most experts agree that in patients evaluated for transplant who have the characteristics suggesting a high likelihood of benefit from LVRS (as outlined above), LVRS should be offered first due to lower morbidity. Prior LVRS is not a contraindication to lung transplantation. Current concepts are that lung transplantation is a quality-of-life intervention for patients with COPD, as whether the intervention results in improvement in mortality remains controversial.

In summary, the approach to individuals with stable COPD should include the following:

- Spirometry should be obtained in individuals with exposure (smoke or occupational) with symptoms of dyspnea and considered in nonexposed individuals with unexplained cough or dyspnea.

- All smokers with COPD should be actively encouraged to quit smoking and, if willing to attempt to quit, offered pharmacotherapy.

- COPD patients should receive pneumococcal and influenza vaccines.

- In the absence of proof of disease modification, pharmacotherapy is indicated to improve symptoms. When possible, inhaled pharmacotherapy is preferred to parenteral therapy. Short-acting beta agonist and/or anticholinergics can be used in patients with intermittent symptoms; long-acting beta agonists and/or anticholinergics can be used in patients with frequent symptoms. Combining both classes of medications produces more benefit than either alone. The role of inhaled corticosteroids remains to be completely defined, but they may improve symptoms and reduce exacerbations and should be considered in those with persistent symptoms despite long-acting bronchodilators and/or with frequent exacerbations. The use of chronic parenteral corticosteroids for the treatment of COPD is not recommended.

- Patients reporting symptoms and/or limitation while on a long-acting agent should be considered for pulmonary rehabilitation.

- Patients with resting hypoxemia when clinically stable should be prescribed supplemental oxygen.

- Surgical therapy should be considered in patients with disabling symptoms and very severe airflow obstruction

despite use of maximal medical therapy and completion of a pulmonary rehabilitation program.

COPD Exacerbations

In addition to chronic symptoms in COPD, with associated exercise limitation and impact on HRQOL, many patients with COPD experience an episodic acute or subacute increase in symptomatology. These events, characterized by an increase in dyspnea and or cough, with a increase and/or change in character of phlegm, are often termed *acute exacerbations* and are often abbreviated as AECB (acute exacerbation of chronic bronchitis) or AECOPD (acute exacerbation of COPD).

Exacerbations are important for several reasons. Clinically, they are important as they are independent determinants of HRQOL and may be associated with an accelerated rate of decline. Hospitalized patients have a mortality of up to 11%. One-year mortality after hospitalization for AECOPD has been reported to range from 22% to 43%. Economically, they are important as they are responsible for 50–70% of COPD-associated health care expenditures in the United States (estimated at $21 billion/yr).

Definition
There is no universally agreed on definition, but the vast majority of those in current use incorporate major criteria of (1) increase in cough, (2) increase in dyspnea, (3) increase in volume of phlegm and/or increasing purulence of phlegm. Minor criteria include fever, myalgias, and fatigue. For clinical studies, the definition often requires that the constellation of symptoms results in a change in treatment for the patient.

Etiology
As one might expect from the presenting criteria, infectious etiologies are important and are responsible for the majority of exacerbations. There are strong data implicating viruses in the etiology of 30–50% of exacerbations, the most common being rhinovirus. Other viral etiologies include coronavirus, influenza A and B, parainfluenza, adenovirus, and respiratory syncytial virus (RSV). Bacterial infection plays a role in up to 50% of exacerbations, with *Haemophilus influenzae, Branhamella catarrhalis,* and *Streptococcus pneumoniae* being the three most commonly implicated species. Exposures to other irritants, such as ambient air pollution, are associated with increasing exacerbation rates. In 25–30% of cases, however, no etiology is identified.

Prevention
The inhaled agents prescribed for the treatment of chronic symptoms have all been reported to reduce the risk of having a COPD exacerbation. For any individual agent, the magnitude of this risk reduction is

approximately 20–25%. Combining more than one agent has been reported to reduce risk by up to 30%. It is important to note that there is a bimodal distribution of exacerbation frequency in patients with COPD: a significant proportion of patients with COPD have no or very infrequent exacerbations. At the present time, the best identifier for patients at risk of COPD exacerbation is a prior history of COPD exacerbations. For such patients, consideration can be given to providing pharmacotherapy to reduce the risk. It should be noted that regimens that contain inhaled corticosteroids, although clearly demonstrating a lower risk of exacerbation, have been reported to have an increased risk of pneumonia.

Current data and concepts are that the use of prophylactic antibiotics or parenteral corticosteroids *do not* reduce exacerbation risk and are not recommended. Clinical trials are currently under way to assess whether prophylactic or preemptive antibiotics have a role in management of patients at risk for exacerbation.

Assessment of the Patient with Exacerbation

The assessment of the patient presenting with symptoms of exacerbation has four goals: attempting to characterize the baseline severity of COPD and any comorbid conditions, ruling out other conditions that may produce similar symptoms, characterization of the severity of the exacerbation, and ascertainment of the etiology of the AECOPD.

Given these goals, the evaluation of the patient should include a history focused on determining baseline functional status and medication use, basis of the diagnosis of COPD and, if known, severity, comorbid condition, recent ill contacts, current symptoms, past history of exacerbations, smoking history (current, ex-, never), and risk factors for conditions producing similar symptoms (CHF pulmonary embolism, pneumothorax). The physical exam should include assessment of mental status, respiratory rate, presence or absence of paradoxical breathing pattern, use of accessory muscles of respiration, cyanosis, chest exam (breath sounds, prolonged expiration, focal findings or asymmetry). An objective assessment of oxygenation should be conducted. For patients with mild or moderate underlying COPD who are not tachypneic or in overt respiratory distress, this can be accomplished by use of pulse oximetry. For patients with abnormal mental status, severe underlying disease, tachypnea, or use of accessory muscles of respiration, an ABG should be performed. In addition to assessment of oxygenation, the ABG will provide pH and pCO_2; these parameters are important in the treatment algorithm for patients.

The CXR has been reported to be abnormal in up to 25% of patients being evaluated for an acute exacerbation, with the majority of findings being either pneumonia or CHF. The decision as to whether to obtain a CXR depends on the patient's baseline status and degree of distress at presentation. Many patients, for instance, will be treated with antibiotics (discussed below) regardless of the presence or absence of a focal opacity on CXR, suggesting that in patients who are not in respiratory distress and in whom the likelihood of CHF is small, the CXR can be omitted from the evaluation. In patients in whom CHF is more likely or in whom the history or exam suggests another etiology such as pneumothorax, the CXR may provide important information.

The decision concerning venue of treatment is complex, and no hard and fast guidelines exist. Patients with mild symptoms and mild to moderate underlying disease may be safely treated as outpatients. Patients with significant respiratory distress, hypercarbia and acute respiratory acidosis, multiple comorbid conditions, severe underlying disease, and/or poor social and family support structures are appropriate candidates for admission and inpatient therapy.

Treatment

The treatments for acute exacerbations include bronchodilators, antiinflammatory medications, antibiotics, and supportive therapies. The latter may include supplemental oxygen therapy and noninvasive or conventional mechanical ventilatory support.

Antibiotics: Most studies report that the use of antibiotics results in a faster clearing of symptoms than no antimicrobial therapy; this is particularly true in patients with two or more of the "major" exacerbation criteria. Antimicrobial therapy should be chosen with consideration of the most common pathogens—*Haemophilus influenzae, Moraxella catarrhalis*, and pneumococcus—and the local antibiotic resistance patterns within these species. Many recommend the use of fluoroquinolones, extended-spectrum macrolides, or amoxicillin/clavulanic acid, although studies using less expensive medications such as tetracyclines or trimethoprim/sulfamethoxazole have also shown benefit. The utility of sputum cultures in guiding decision-making concerning antibiotics is questionable, as many patients are chronically colonized with one or more of the species that are also associated with exacerbations.

Corticosteroids: Parenteral corticosteroids have been demonstrated to reduce returns to the emergency room in patients treated as outpatients in that setting and to shorten hospital length of stay in patients admitted for AECOPD. Although the optimal dose, route, and duration of therapy are unclear, a reasonable synthesis of the literature is that there is probably little difference between enteral and parenteral routes in patients able to take oral medications, the initial dose should be the equivalent of 40 mg or more of prednisone, and that 2 weeks of tapering therapy is as effective and less morbid than an 8-week taper.

Bronchodilators: Current guidelines recommend the use of beta agonists and anticholinergic inhaled agents during an exacerbation, with initial preference for short-acting agents delivered frequently, transitioning to longer-acting agents as patients improve. In patients capable of demonstrating good technique with metered-dose inhaler (MDI) devices, studies have shown use of MDIs is as effective, and less costly, than the use of nebulizer therapy. Many institutions have instituted pathways that transition patients from nebulizer therapy to MDI devices shortly after hospital admission.

The use of aminophylline or other xanthines has not been demonstrated to provide additional benefit over bronchodilators alone in the treatment of AECOPD.

Supportive Therapies: Many patients demonstrate hypoxemia when presenting with AECOPD. Supplemental oxygen should be provided and titrated to achieve a resting saturation of 90% or greater. This is true even in patients with hypercarbia. Although it is true that supplemental oxygen may alter ventilation/perfusion relationships and result in a modest rise in pCO_2, it does not alter minute ventilation and should not be withheld because of concerns about suppressing respiratory drive.

In addition to pharmacotherapy, patients with acute respiratory failure in the context of COPD exacerbation may benefit from mechanical ventilatory support. A series of recent studies have demonstrated that patients with AECOPD and respiratory decompensation manifested by tachypnea, signs of respiratory muscle fatigue, respiratory acidosis, and hypercarbia benefit from the institution of noninvasive positive-pressure ventilation (NIPPV). In such patients, institution of NIPPV has been demonstrated to reduce the need for endotracheal intubation and mechanical ventilation, ICU and hospital lengths of stay, and mortality. For patients unable to tolerate NIPPV or for whom NIPPV is ineffective at correcting acidosis/hypercarbia, endotracheal intubation and mechanical ventilation is indicated.

ACKNOWLEDGMENTS

Figures 33.2, 33.3, and 33.4 are courtesy of Dr. George Washko, Brigham and Women's Hospital. Figure 33.5 was prepared by Ms. Jimette Gilmartin.

ADDITIONAL READINGS

American Thoracic Society/European Respiratory Society. Standards for the diagnosis and management of individuals with alpha-1 antitrypsin deficiency. *Am J Respir Crit Care Med.* 2003;168:818–900.

Diaz-Guzman E, Mannino DM. Airway obstructive diseases in older adults: From detection to treatment. *J Allergy Clin Immunol.* 2010;126(4):702–9.

Foster TS, Miller JD, Marton JP, Caloyeras JP, Russell MW, Menzin J. Assessment of the economic burden of COPD in the U.S.: A review and synthesis of the literature. *COPD.* 2006;3:211–8.

Global Initiative for Chronic Obstructive Lung Disease. 2004. http://www.goldcopd.com/. Accessed August 4, 2005.

Gooneratne NS, Patel NP, Corcoran A. Chronic obstructive pulmonary disease diagnosis and management in older adults. *J Am Geriatr Soc.* 2010;58(6):1153–62.

Hancock DB, London SJ; CHARGE Pulmonary Function Working Group. Determinants of lung function, COPD, and asthma. *N Engl J Med.* 2011;364(1):86–7.

MacMahon H, Austin JH, Gamsu G, et al. Guidelines for management of small pulmonary nodules detected on CT scans: A statement from the Fleischner Society. *Radiology.* 2005;237:395–400.

Niewoehner DE. Clinical practice. Outpatient management of severe COPD. *N Engl J Med.* 2010;362(15):1407–16.

Sin DD, McAlister FA, Man SF, Anthonisen NR. Contemporary management of chronic obstructive pulmonary disease: Scientific review. *JAMA.* 2003;290:2301–12.

QUESTIONS

QUESTION 1. A 72-year-old white male presents to his physician's office with a 9-month history of wheezing, dyspnea on exertion, and daily sputum production. He is a 60-pack-year smoker. Examination shows markedly decreased breath sounds with mild wheezing at the end of expiration. Spirometry is consistent with a diagnosis of COPD. Which of the following interventions will be most effective for improving this patient's long-term survival?

A. Inhaled ipratropium
B. Long-term oral corticosteroids
C. Inhaled corticosteroids
D. Smoking cessation

QUESTION 2. A 66-year-old patient with COPD has repeated exacerbations (at least two episodes each year for the past 3 years) and has an FEV_1 45% predicted. She is currently being treated with salmeterol, two puffs twice per day, and albuterol, two puffs every 6 hours as needed. Which one of the following should be added to her treatment regimen?

A. Inhaled corticosteroid
B. Home oxygen therapy
C. Prophylactic antibiotic therapy
D. Long-term low-dose oral corticosteroid
E. Long-term theophylline therapy

QUESTION 3. A 68-year-old man with a 40-pack-year tobacco history presents with recent onset of pain in both knees and shins. Physical examination shows clubbing, gynecomastia, tenderness of both shins, and mild expiratory slowing of lung sounds.

The most likely diagnosis is:

A. RA with pulmonary involvement
B. IPF
C. Cryptogenic organizing pneumonia
D. Hypertrophic pulmonary osteoarthropathy
E. Acromegaly

ANSWERS

1. D
2. A
3. D

34.

VENOUS THROMBOEMBOLIC DISEASES

Gregory Piazza and Samuel Z. Goldhaber

Venous thromboembolism (VTE), including deep vein thrombosis (DVT) and pulmonary embolism (PE), is the third most common cardiovascular disorder in the United States after coronary artery disease and stroke. The incidence of VTE increases sharply after age 60 years in both men and women, with PE accounting for the majority of the increase. The mortality rate for acute PE exceeds 15% in the first 3 months and surpasses that of acute myocardial infarction. Sudden death may be the initial presentation of acute PE in nearly 25% of patients. Acute right ventricular (RV) failure accounts for the majority of deaths due to PE.

This chapter reviews the pathophysiology of VTE, including its risk factors and long-term consequences. Diagnostic algorithms that integrate clinical findings, laboratory testing, and imaging are described. The role of risk stratification for identification of high-risk PE patients is highlighted. Options for the management of VTE are reviewed. Finally, practical recommendations for the prevention of VTE are provided.

PATHOPHYSIOLOGY

CLINICAL RISK FACTORS

Most patients with VTE present with a combination of clinical risk factors (table 34.1). Advancing age, cancer, obesity, personal or family history of VTE, and recent surgery, trauma, or immobilization are well-recognized clinical risk factors. Prior recent hospitalization has been implicated in the development of VTE among outpatients. Common medical conditions, including acute infectious illness, chronic obstructive pulmonary disease, chronic kidney disease, and heart failure, increase the risk of VTE. Atherosclerotic cardiovascular disease and its associated risk factors, including obesity, smoking, diabetes, hypertension, and dyslipidemia, also increase the risk of VTE. Chronically indwelling central venous catheters or devices such as pacemaker or implantable cardiac defibrillator leads are associated with an increased incidence of upper extremity DVT.

VTE is an important women's health concern. Pregnancy is a well-recognized risk factor for VTE. In addition, oral contraceptive pills, especially those containing third-generation progestins, and estrogen plus progestin hormone replacement therapy have been associated with an elevated risk of VTE.

THROMBOPHILIA AND HYPERCOAGULABLE ASSESSMENT

A history of VTE at a young age, multiple family members with VTE, idiopathic or recurrent VTE, or recurrent spontaneous abortions should raise suspicion for thrombophilia. Laboratory evaluation for hypercoagulable states should focus on major thrombophilias such as factor V Leiden mutation resulting in activated protein C resistance, prothrombin gene mutation 20210, anticardiolipin antibodies, and lupus anticoagulant. The most serious of these is antiphospholipid antibody syndrome, probably best assessed by measuring quantitative levels of anticardiolipin antibodies. Deficiencies of antithrombin III, protein C, and protein S are less common, and testing for these disorders may be inaccurate in the setting of anticoagulation. Testing for hyperhomocysteinemia is unlikely to impact management because lowering homocysteine levels with folate, vitamin B-6, and vitamin B-12 has not been shown to reduce the risk of VTE.

PATHOPHYSIOLOGY OF DEEP VEIN THROMBOSIS

DVT most often results from a combination of pathophysiological states of stasis, hypercoagulability, and endothelial injury. Although the deep veins of the lower extremity are the most common location for DVT, thrombosis may also form in the veins of the upper extremity and pelvis. Damage from DVT may lead to dysfunction of the valves

Table 34.1. MAJOR RISK FACTORS FOR VENOUS THROMBOEMBOLISM

Clinical risk factors
- Advancing age
- Cancer
- Personal or family history of VTE
- Recent surgery, trauma, hospitalization, or immobilization
- Acute infectious illness
- Chronic obstructive pulmonary disease
- Chronic kidney disease including nephrotic syndrome
- Atherosclerotic cardiovascular disease and its associated risk factors (including obesity, smoking, diabetes, hypertension, dyslipidemia, diet)
- Heart failure
- Inflammatory bowel disease
- Pacemaker or implantable cardiac defibrillator leads and indwelling venous catheters
- Long-haul air travel
- Pregnancy, oral contraceptive pills, or hormone replacement therapy

Thrombophilias
- Factor V Leiden
- Prothrombin gene mutation 20210
- Anticardiolipin antibodies/lupus anticoagulant
- Antithrombin deficiency
- Protein C deficiency
- Protein S deficiency

of the deep venous system and, ultimately, the postthrombotic syndrome. Chronic lower extremity edema and calf discomfort characterize the postthrombotic syndrome and are associated with reduction in quality of life and impaired functional status. Postthrombotic syndrome is also associated with an increased risk of recurrent VTE.

PATHOPHYSIOLOGY OF PULMONARY EMBOLISM

The majority of pulmonary emboli originate from thrombus in the deep veins of the lower extremities. Thrombi embolize through the inferior vena cava and right heart and eventually lodge in the pulmonary arteries, where they result in hemodynamic and gas exchange abnormalities.

The size of the embolus, the patient's underlying cardiopulmonary reserve, and the extent of compensatory neurohumoral adaptations determine the hemodynamic impact of acute PE. Direct physical obstruction of the pulmonary arterial tree, hypoxemia, and release of potent pulmonary arterial vasoconstrictors as a result of PE cause an acute increase in pulmonary vascular resistance and RV afterload. Sudden RV pressure overload may lead to RV dilatation and hypokinesis, tricuspid regurgitation, and ultimately, acute RV failure. PE patients with acute RV failure may rapidly decompensate and manifest systemic arterial hypotension, cardiogenic shock, and cardiac arrest. In the setting of pericardial constraint, acute RV dilatation and an elevation in diastolic pressure result in flattening of the interventricular septum with deviation toward the left ventricle (LV) in diastole and impairment of LV filling. In addition, pressure overload may increase RV wall stress and result in ischemia or infarction by increasing myocardial oxygen demand while simultaneously limiting supply (figure 34.1).

Acute PE results in gas exchange abnormalities by a combination of ventilation-perfusion mismatch, increases in total dead space, and right-to-left shunt. Arterial hypoxemia and an increased alveolar-arterial (A-a) gradient are the most commonly observed abnormalities of gas exchange. Hypocapnia and respiratory alkalosis due to hyperventilation may also be encountered, especially in those with normal underlying pulmonary function.

Up to 4% of patients who survive acute PE may develop disabling chronic thromboembolic pulmonary hypertension.

DIAGNOSIS

DEEP VEIN THROMBOSIS

Clinical Findings

Patients with lower extremity DVT will often note a cramping or pulling sensation of the calf that may be exacerbated by ambulation. Patients with upper extremity DVT may report similar symptoms with activity. Physical findings of warmth, edema, tenderness, a palpable cord, or prominent venous collaterals may be present. Importantly, some patients may not demonstrate any abnormalities on physical examination.

Laboratory Evaluation

A nonspecific marker of endogenous fibrinolysis, D-dimer, is increased in VTE as well as in many other systemic illnesses. D-dimer is most useful in the evaluation of outpatients

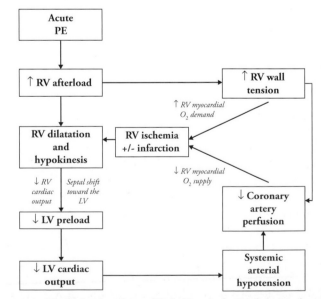

Figure 34.1. The Pathophysiology of Right Ventricular Dysfunction due to Acute Pulmonary Embolism. LV, left ventricular; O$_2$, oxygen; PE, pulmonary embolism; RV, right ventricular.

or emergency department patients with suspected VTE because a substantial proportion of inpatients will have elevated levels due to other conditions. These other conditions include acute myocardial infarction, pneumonia, cancer, the postoperative state, and second or third-trimester pregnancy. D-dimer offers the greatest accuracy in the evaluation of suspected DVT when used in conjunction with an assessment of clinical probability. However, D-dimer testing remains controversial for the evaluation of DVT and may produce false-negative results in the setting of a small thrombus burden such as isolated calf DVT.

Imaging

Duplex venous ultrasonography is the initial imaging test of choice in the evaluation of suspected lower and upper extremity DVT (figure 34.2). Noncompressibility of a vein is diagnostic of DVT. Alternative imaging modalities for assessment of patients with suspected DVT, including computed tomography (CT), magnetic resonance (MR), and contrast venography, may be warranted when ultrasonography is inadequate, such as when acute-on-chronic thrombosis is suspected. In addition, anatomical limitations may hinder ultrasonographic evaluation of the pelvic veins and upper extremity veins proximal to the clavicle.

PULMONARY EMBOLISM

Clinical Findings

Dyspnea is the most frequently reported symptom in patients with acute PE. Whereas pleuritic pain, cough, or hemoptysis may indicate a smaller peripherally located PE, severe dyspnea, cyanosis, or syncope suggest massive PE. Tachypnea is the most common physical finding. Patients without underlying cardiopulmonary disease may appear anxious but well compensated despite anatomically large PE. Systemic arterial hypotension, cardiogenic shock, or cardiac arrest suggests massive PE. Patients with submassive PE have preserved systolic blood pressure but may exhibit signs of RV failure, including tachycardia, jugular venous distension, tricuspid regurgitation, or an accentuated sound of pulmonic closure (P2).

Clinical Decision Rule

Simplified clinical decision rules assist clinicians in synthesizing important elements of the history and physical examination into an overall assessment of likelihood of PE. The combination of a simplified decision rule with laboratory testing and further imaging when indicated by clinical suspicion has been validated in major studies. In the Christopher study, the diagnosis of PE was excluded or established in three straightforward steps: (1) a dichotomized clinical decision rule (categorizing patients as high or nonhigh clinical probability for PE), (2) D-dimer testing, and (3) chest CT. Study investigators used a generally accepted clinical decision rule, known as the "Wells criteria," which assigns 3 points for symptoms and signs of DVT, 3 points for an alternative diagnosis less likely than PE, 1.5 points for heart rate >100 beats per minute, 1.5 points for recent surgery or immobilization, 1.5 points for previous VTE, 1 point for hemoptysis, and 1 point for malignancy undergoing therapy or palliation within 6 months of presentation (table 34.2). Patients are categorized as "PE unlikely" for scores ≤4 and "PE likely" for scores >4. Patients who were classified as "PE unlikely" underwent D-dimer testing and were referred to chest CT only if the result was positive, whereas patients in the "PE likely" category proceeded directly to chest CT.

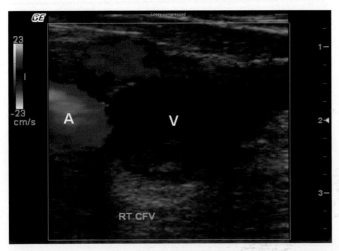

Figure 34.2. Venous Ultrasound Demonstrating a Dilated, Noncompressible Vein. Right common femoral vein (V) with absence of venous flow consistent with deep vein thrombosis in a 35-year-old woman with right leg swelling and discomfort at 38 weeks of pregnancy. The right common femoral artery (A) has normal arterial flow.

Table 34.2 A GENERALLY ACCEPTED CLINICAL DECISION RULE FOR THE EVALUATION OF PATIENTS WITH SUSPECTED PULMONARY EMBOLISM (THE WELLS CRITERIA)

VARIABLE	POINTS
Clinical symptoms and signs of DVT	3.0
Alternative diagnosis less likely than PE	3.0
Heart rate >100 beats per minute	1.5
Recent immobilization or surgery	1.5
Previous VTE	1.5
Hemoptysis	1.0
Malignancy undergoing treatment or palliation within 6 months	1.0

NOTES: DVT, deep vein thrombosis; PE, pulmonary embolism; VTE, venous thromboembolism; "PE unlikely" ≤ 4 points; "PE likely" > 4 points.

PE was excluded in patients categorized as "PE unlikely" with negative D-dimer results and in patients with negative chest CT scans. This simplified clinical algorithm permitted a management decision in 98% of patients and was associated with a low risk of VTE.

Laboratory Evaluation

D-dimer, as measured by enzyme-linked immunosorbent assay (ELISA), is particularly helpful in the evaluation of patients with suspected PE, especially in the emergency department setting. Because of its high negative predictive value, D-dimer can be used to exclude PE in outpatients with low clinical decision rule scores without the need for further costly testing. Inpatients should proceed directly to imaging as the initial test for PE because most will already have an increased D-dimer due to comorbid illness.

Electrocardiogram

The electrocardiogram plays an important role in the evaluation of patients with suspected PE because it may reveal the presence of RV strain while also suggesting alternative diagnoses such as myocardial infarction. Signs of RV strain due to PE include incomplete or complete right bundle branch block (RBBB), T-wave inversions across the anterior precordium, as well as an S wave in lead I and a Q wave and T-wave inversion in lead III (S1Q3T3). Some patients may demonstrate signs of increased adrenergic tone with resting sinus tachycardia, but others may not demonstrate any electrocardiographic abnormalities.

Imaging

The chest x-ray constitutes an important part of the evaluation of patients with suspected PE because it may suggest alternative diagnoses such as pneumonia. A normal or near-normal chest x-ray in a patient with dyspnea or hypoxemia suggests PE. However, the majority of patients with PE will have some radiographic abnormality such as cardiomegaly or pleural effusion.

Contrast-enhanced chest CT has emerged as the dominant diagnostic imaging modality for the evaluation of suspected acute PE (figure 34.3). The improved resolution of multidetector CT scanners has markedly reduced the frequency of nondiagnostic studies. In the Prospective Investigation of Pulmonary Embolism Diagnosis II (PIOPED II) trial, chest CT was found to be accurate for the exclusion of PE in patients with low and intermediate clinical probability. However, the results of PIOPED II also suggest that further testing to confirm or exclude the diagnosis of PE is warranted when clinical suspicion and chest CT results are discordant. The addition of venous phase imaging of the lower extremity veins to chest CT in

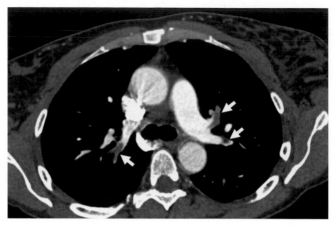

Figure 34.3. Contrast Enhanced Chest Computed Tomogram. CT demonstrating bilateral segmental pulmonary emboli (arrows) in a 48-year-old woman with acute dyspnea 2 days after left total knee replacement.

PIOPED II only modestly increased the negative predictive value when compared to chest CT alone. In general, CT venography as a routine "add-on" to chest CT is not recommended unless patients are at high risk of DVT due to active cancer or prior VTE.

Alternative imaging modalities utilized in the evaluation of patients with suspected PE include ventilation-perfusion lung scanning, MR angiography, and invasive contrast pulmonary angiography. Ventilation-perfusion lung scanning is most often used for patients with severe renal impairment, anaphylaxis to intravenous iodinated contrast, or pregnancy. Although it avoids the risks of iodinated contrast and ionizing radiation, MR angiography is not as sensitive as chest CT for detection of PE and has demonstrated more promise for the imaging of DVT. Invasive pulmonary angiography is reserved for the rare circumstance when other noninvasive imaging studies are inconclusive and a high clinical suspicion for PE persists.

Transthoracic echocardiography is insensitive for the diagnosis of PE, even though it plays a critical role in the risk stratification of patients with proven acute PE. Transthoracic echocardiography is superb for the detection of RV dysfunction due to RV pressure overload in the setting of acute PE. RV dilatation and hypokinesis, paradoxical interventricular septal motion toward the LV, tricuspid regurgitation, and pulmonary hypertension are characteristic echocardiographic findings (Piazza and Goldhaber, 2010a).

An Integrated Approach to Diagnosis

Both the Christopher study and PIOPED II highlight the importance of a diagnostic algorithm that integrates an assessment of clinical probability with laboratory testing and imaging with chest CT (figure 34.4). The use of an integrated algorithm permits management decisions to be made in the majority of patients with suspected PE and is associated with a low risk of VTE.

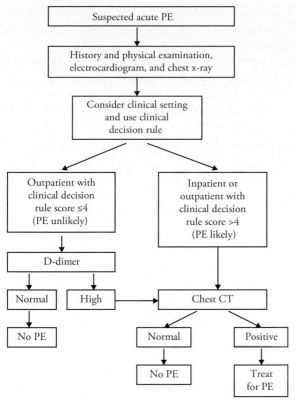

Figure 34.4. An Integrated Approach to Diagnosis of Acute Pulmonary Embolism. CT, computed tomography; PE, pulmonary embolism.

Risk Stratification for Pulmonary Embolism

A subset of normotensive patients with acute PE will abruptly deteriorate and suffer systemic arterial hypotension, cardiogenic shock, or cardiac arrest despite standard therapeutic anticoagulation. Risk stratification to identify these patients before they decompensate has become an essential step in the management of acute PE (figure 34.5).

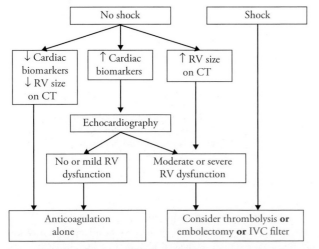

Figure 34.5. Risk Stratification of PE Patients. An algorithm for risk stratification of patients with acute pulmonary embolism. CT, computed tomography; IVC, inferior vena cava; RV, right ventricular.

The history and physical examination can provide important clinical clues for risk stratification of acute PE patients. Heart failure, chronic lung disease, cancer, systolic blood pressure <100 mm Hg, age >70 years, and heart rate >100 beats per minute have been demonstrated to be significant predictors of increased mortality.

Elevations in the cardiac troponins, heart-type fatty acid binding protein, and brain-type natriuretic peptide (BNP) correlate with the presence of RV dysfunction, an independent predictor of early mortality in acute PE patients. Normal levels of cardiac biomarkers accurately identify a low-risk subset of acute PE patients. Conversely, patients with acute PE and elevated cardiac biomarkers should undergo echocardiography to confirm the presence of RV dysfunction.

RV enlargement on chest CT, defined by a ratio of RV to LV diameter >0.9, is a predictor of increased 30-day mortality in patients with acute PE. Detection of RV enlargement by chest CT is a particularly convenient tool for risk stratification because it utilizes data acquired from the initial diagnostic scan.

Echocardiography remains the imaging study of choice for risk stratification of acute PE patients. Normotensive patients with acute PE and RV dysfunction on echocardiography demonstrate an increased risk of early mortality, whereas those without evidence of RV dysfunction generally have benign clinical courses. RV-to-LV end-diastolic dimension ratios >0.9 indicate RV enlargement and predict a more than doubling of hospital mortality for PE patients. Echocardiography is warranted in acute PE patients with clinical evidence of RV failure, elevated cardiac biomarkers, or unexpected clinical deterioration.

MANAGEMENT

SPECTRUM OF DISEASE

VTE describes a spectrum of diseases, including DVT and PE. Massive DVT describes thrombus that originates in the proximal veins of the lower extremity and extends into the pelvic veins. Proximal DVT involves the common femoral, superficial femoral, deep femoral, or popliteal veins. A common error is to assume that the "superficial" femoral vein is a "superficial" vein even though, in fact, it is a deep vein. Isolated calf DVT involves the venous system distal to the popliteal vein. Upper extremity DVT most often affects the subclavian, internal jugular, and axillary veins.

Massive PE describes a subset of acute PE patients presenting with syncope, systemic arterial hypotension, cardiogenic shock, or cardiac arrest. Normotensive patients with acute PE and evidence of RV dysfunction are classified as having submassive PE and have an increased risk of adverse events and early mortality. Acute PE patients with normal blood pressure and no evidence of RV dysfunction generally have a benign hospital course when treated with standard therapeutic anticoagulation alone.

ANTICOAGULATION

Immediate Anticoagulation

Immediate anticoagulation serves as the foundation of therapy for patients with VTE. Current agents for immediate anticoagulation in VTE include intravenous unfractionated heparin, low-molecular-weight heparin (LMWH), and fondaparinux (table 34.3). Three direct thrombin inhibitors, argatroban, bivalirudin, and lepirudin, are available for immediate anticoagulation in patients with documented or suspected heparin-induced thrombocytopenia (HIT).

Intravenous unfractionated heparin is administered as a bolus followed by a continuous infusion titrated to a target activated partial thromboplastin time (aPTT) of two to three times the upper limit of normal (approximately 60 to 80 sec). Weight-based protocols are widely utilized and may achieve therapeutic levels of anticoagulation more quickly. Because it can be discontinued and reversed rapidly, unfractionated heparin is preferred in patients undergoing fibrinolysis, catheter-assisted intervention, or surgery for VTE.

LMWHs and fondaparinux have longer half-lives, more consistent bioavailability, and more predictable dose responses than unfractionated heparin. LMWHs are administered subcutaneously according to weight and do not require dose adjustment or routine laboratory monitoring. Whereas unfractionated heparin is largely eliminated by the liver, LMWHs are cleared renally. Patients with impaired renal function, massive obesity, pregnancy, or unanticipated bleeding or thromboembolism will have altered pharmacodynamics. LMWH as monotherapy without transition to oral anticoagulation is a Food and Drug Administration–approved therapy in cancer patients with

VTE. This approach halved the rate of recurrent VTE when compared with warfarin in a randomized controlled trial (Lee, 2003).

Fondaparinux is administered subcutaneously in fixed once-daily doses of 5 mg for body weight <50 kg, 7.5 mg for 50–100 kg, and 10 mg for >100 kg. Fondaparinux does not require dose adjustment or routine laboratory monitoring. Because it is cleared by the kidneys, fondaparinux is contraindicated in severe renal impairment. Fondaparinux is not associated with HIT.

HEPARIN-INDUCED THROMBOCYTOPENIA

HIT is caused by heparin-dependent IgG antibodies directed against heparin–platelet factor 4 complexes and may result in limb-threatening and life-threatening arterial and, more commonly, venous thromboembolic complications. Although the risk is lower with LMWH, both unfractionated heparin and LMWH can result in HIT. A decline in platelet count of >50% from baseline or a new thromboembolic event while administering any heparin product, including heparin flushes, should raise concern for HIT and prompt the discontinuation of all heparin-containing products.

When HIT is confirmed or even suspected, a direct thrombin inhibitor such as argatroban, bivalirudin, or lepirudin should be administered to prevent arterial and venous thromboembolism. Argatroban is hepatically cleared and should be used cautiously in patients with impaired liver function, whereas bivalirudin and lepirudin require dose adjustment for renal impairment. Warfarin monotherapy, platelet transfusions, inferior vena cava (IVC) filter insertion, and LMWH should be avoided in HIT because all

Table 34.3. **OPTIONS FOR IMMEDIATE ANTICOAGULATION IN VENOUS THROMBOEMBOLISM**

AGENT	ADVANTAGES	DISADVANTAGES
Intravenous unfractionated heparin	Can be easily discontinued and rapidly reversed Preferred in patients undergoing fibrinolysis, surgery, or catheter-assisted embolectomy Can be used in severe renal insufficiency	Requires continuous infusion Associated with heparin-induced thrombocytopenia (HIT)
Low-molecular-weight heparin	Longer half-life Consistent bioavailability More predictable dose response Does not require dose adjustment or laboratory monitoring under usual circumstances Lower risk of HIT Preferred as monotherapy without warfarin in patients with active cancer	Renally cleared Patients with renal impairment, massive obesity, and pregnancy will have altered pharmacodynamics
Fondaparinux	Longer half-life Consistent bioavailability More predictable dose response Does not require dose adjustment or laboratory monitoring Does not cause HIT	Renally cleared Longer half-life is problematic if bleeding occurs No laboratory test to monitor level of anticoagulation

may perpetuate the tendency toward thromboembolism. Fondaparinux is often administered off-label to patients with HIT or suspected HIT who are at low risk of developing HIT with thrombosis.

CHRONIC ANTICOAGULATION

Warfarin remains the mainstay of outpatient anticoagulation for VTE. Oral anticoagulation for VTE is started concurrently with unfractionated heparin, LMWH, or fondaparinux and overlapped for a minimum of 5 days until full therapeutic efficacy has been achieved. The goal International Normalized Ratio (INR) is 2.0–3.0 for the majority of VTE patients. Dosing nomograms are available to assist clinicians with warfarin initiation (www. WarfarinDosing.org). Pharmacogenomics studies focusing on cytochrome P450 2C9 and the gene encoding vitamin K epoxide reductase complex 1 (VKORC1) have helped to explain the wide variation in warfarin dosing requirements and may provide a basis for individualized dosing nomograms.

Management of warfarin can be challenging due to many drug–food, drug–alcohol, and drug–drug interactions. Commonly implicated warfarin potentiators include acetaminophen, quinolone antibiotics, amiodarone, and antiplatelet agents such as clopidogrel. Home INR monitors can improve control of oral anticoagulation and lead to fewer bleeding and clotting complications. In March 2008, Medicare approved reimbursement of point-of-care self-testing INR devices for patients receiving >3 months of warfarin.

The optimal duration of warfarin therapy depends on the individual patient's risk for recurrent VTE. The risk of recurrence persists after completion of standard anticoagulation in patients with idiopathic or unprovoked VTE. Several studies have validated the safety and efficacy of indefinite duration anticoagulation for patients with idiopathic VTE.

Novel anticoagulants on the horizon, including dabigatran, rivaroxaban, and apixaban, show promise as oral anticoagulants that will not require routine laboratory monitoring.

PRIMARY THERAPY

FIBRINOLYSIS

Fibrinolysis for DVT should be catheter-directed and is most often used to treat upper extremity or iliofemoral DVT in young, otherwise healthy patients. This approach is usually combined with mechanical disruption of thrombus. Fibrinolytic therapy for PE is reserved for patients with either massive or submassive acute PE. Fibrinolysis is generally accepted as a life-saving intervention in patients with massive PE. Because there are a paucity of conclusive randomized, controlled trials, fibrinolysis for submassive PE remains controversial. The Management Strategies and Prognosis of Pulmonary Embolism-3 (MAPPET-3) trial evaluated tissue plasminogen activator (t-PA) in submassive PE patients. Although a mortality benefit was not shown, the MAPPET-3 trial demonstrated a reduction in the need for escalation of therapy among patients undergoing fibrinolysis with t-PA. The U.S. Food and Drug Administration has approved t-PA (alteplase), 100 mg, as a continuous peripheral infusion over 2 hours for massive PE. All patients being considered for fibrinolysis should be meticulously screened for contraindications (table 34.4). Bleeding, especially intracranial hemorrhage, is the most feared complication of fibrinolysis. The risk of intracranial hemorrhage may be as high as 3% among PE patients receiving fibrinolytics.

SURGICAL INTERVENTIONS

Surgical interventions are considered in patients with massive or severely symptomatic DVT and massive or submassive PE in whom fibrinolysis has failed or is contraindicated. At medical centers with experience in the management of such patients, surgical embolectomy is a safe and effective alternative for the treatment of massive and submassive PE.

CATHETER-ASSISTED TECHNIQUES

Catheter-assisted techniques may be utilized for treatment of DVT and PE when fibrinolysis and surgical intervention are contraindicated. Catheter-assisted embolectomy is an emerging technique for the treatment of massive and submassive PE patients.

INFERIOR VENA CAVA FILTERS

IVC filter insertion is considered for VTE patients in whom anticoagulation is contraindicated, those who experience recurrent PE despite adequate anticoagulation, massive or submassive PE patients with contraindications to fibrinolysis or embolectomy, and those undergoing surgical embolectomy. Although effective in the short-term prevention of PE, IVC filters have been shown to increase the long-term incidence of DVT. Retrievable IVC filters are safe and effective alternatives for patients with transient contraindications to anticoagulation.

Table 34.4 MAJOR CONTRAINDICATIONS TO FIBRINOLYTIC THERAPY FOR ACUTE PULMONARY EMBOLISM

Intracranial malignancy or tumor
History of intracranial hemorrhage
Recent cerebrovascular event or neurosurgical procedure
Recent surgery or trauma
Severe or uncontrolled hypertension
Recent prolonged cardiopulmonary resuscitation
Active or recent bleeding

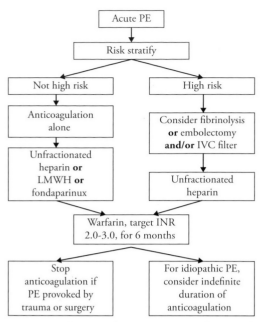

Figure 34.6 An Integrated Approach to Management of Acute Pulmonary Embolism. INR, International Normalized Ratio; IVC, inferior vena cava; LMWH, low-molecular-weight heparin; PE, pulmonary embolism.

AN INTEGRATED APPROACH TO MANAGEMENT

A therapeutic algorithm considers fibrinolysis or embolectomy for massive or submassive PE and incorporates the recommendation of indefinite anticoagulation for patients with idiopathic VTE (figure 34.6).

PREVENTION

Despite guidelines for the prevention of VTE, a large proportion of hospitalized patients at risk for VTE do not receive appropriate prophylaxis. Among hospitalized medical patients, including those in the intensive care setting, VTE prophylaxis is frequently omitted despite a high rate of comorbid conditions and VTE risk factors. Computerized provider order entry reminders alert healthcare providers to patients with an increased risk of VTE who are not receiving prophylaxis and represent one technique to improve implementation of VTE prophylaxis. Every hospital should adopt a formal VTE prophylaxis protocol and should audit compliance with its guidelines.

OPTIONS FOR PROPHYLAXIS

Pharmacological agents for the prevention of VTE include subcutaneously administered unfractionated heparin, LMWH, warfarin, and fondaparinux. Mechanical prophylaxis, including graduated compression stockings and pneumatic compression devices, is an alternative in patients who cannot receive prophylactic dose anticoagulation.

DURATION OF PROPHYLAXIS

When prescribed, VTE prophylaxis is usually administered while the patient is hospitalized and discontinued on discharge. However, the risk of VTE often persists in the

Table 34.5 REGIMENS FOR VENOUS THROMBOEMBOLISM PREVENTION

PATIENT POPULATION	PROPHYLAXIS
General surgery	Unfractionated heparin, 5000 units SC tid, *or* Enoxaparin, 40 mg SC qd, *or* Dalteparin, 2500 or 5000 units SC qd
Orthopedic surgery	Warfarin (target INR 2.0 to 3.0) *or* Enoxaparin, 30 mg SC bid, *or* Enoxaparin, 40 mg SC qd, *or* Dalteparin, 2500 or 5000 units SC qd, *or* Fondaparinux 2.5 mg SC qd
Oncologic surgery	Enoxaparin 40 mg SC qd
Medical patients	Unfractionated heparin, 5000 units SC tid *or* Enoxaparin, 40 mg SC qd, *or* Dalteparin 5,000 units SC qd, *or* Fondaparinux 2.5 mg SC qd (not FDA approved), *or* Graduated compression stockings/intermittent pneumatic compression for patients with contraindications to anticoagulation Consider combination pharmacological and mechanical prophylaxis for very high-risk patients such as intensive care unit patients Consider surveillance lower extremity ultrasonography for intensive care unit patients

NOTES: bid, twice daily; INR, International Normalized Ratio; qd, daily; SC, subcutaneous; tid, three times daily.

outpatient setting, as many patients continue to have limited mobility as well as other ongoing VTE risk factors. Many patients who suffer VTE in the outpatient setting have undergone recent surgery or hospitalization within the 3 months prior to diagnosis. Numerous studies have validated extended-duration prophylaxis for up to 4–6 weeks in high-risk patients, such as those who have undergone orthopedic or oncologic surgery.

RECOMMENDATIONS

Prophylactic regimens should consider the patient population as well as the individual patient's risk factors for VTE (table 34.5).

ADDITIONAL READING

Eikelboom JW, Weitz JI. New anticoagulants. *Circulation.* 2010; 121:1523–32.

Goldhaber SZ. Risk factors for venous thromboembolism. *J Am Coll Cardiol.* 2010;56:1–7.

Goldhaber SZ, Piazza G. Optimal duration of anticoagulation after venous thromboembolism. *Circulation.* 2011;123:664–7.

Kuo WT, van den Bosch MA, Hofman LV, Louie JD, Kothary N, Sze DY. Catheter-directed embolectomy, fragmentation, and thrombolysis for the treatment of massive pulmonary embolism after failure of systemic thrombolysis. *Chest.* 2008;134:250–4.

Lee AY, Levine MN, Baker RI, et al. Low-molecular-weight heparin versus a coumarin for the prevention of recurrent venous thromboembolism in patients with cancer. *N Engl J Med.* 2003;349:146–53.

Piazza G, Goldhaber SZ. Improving clinical effectiveness in thromboprophylaxis for hospitalized medical patients. *Am J Med.* 2009,122:230 2.

Piazza G, Goldhaber SZ. Management of submassive pulmonary embolism. *Circulation.* 2010a;122:1124–9.

Piazza G, Goldhaber SZ. Venous thromboembolism and atherothrombosis: An integrated approach. *Circulation.* 2010b;121:2146–50.

Piazza G, Goldhaber SZ. Fibrinolysis for acute pulmonary embolism. *Vasc Med.* 2010c;15:419–28.

Piazza G, Goldhaber SZ. Chronic thromboembolic pulmonary hypertension. *N Engl J Med.* 2011;364:351 60.

Spencer FA, Lessard D, Emery C, et al. Venous thromboembolism in the outpatient setting. *Arch Intern Med.* 2007;167:1471–5.

Stein PD, Fowler SE, Goodman LR, et al. Multidetector computed tomography for acute pulmonary embolism. *N Engl J Med.* 2006;354:2317–27.

Tapson VF. Acute pulmonary embolism. *N Engl J Med.* 2008; 358:1037–52.

van Belle A, Buller HR, Huisman MV, et al. Effectiveness of managing suspected pulmonary embolism using an algorithm combining clinical probability, D-dimer testing, and computed tomography. *JAMA.* 2006;295:172–9.

www.WarfarinDosing.org. Accessed January 3, 2011.

QUESTIONS

QUESTION 1. All of the following are risk factors for venous thromboembolism (VTE) except:

A. Chronic obstructive pulmonary disease (COPD)
B. Atherosclerotic cardiovascular disease
C. Shoveling heavy snow
D. Chronic kidney disease (CKD)
E. Heart failure

QUESTION 2. A 48-year-old woman with a history of hypertension and hyperlipidemia presents to the emergency department with sudden-onset right-sided pleuritic pain and dyspnea while gardening. She has no other medical conditions and takes a thiazide diuretic and statin daily. She does not smoke. On physical examination, she has a heart rate of 90 beats per minute, blood pressure of 160/90 mm Hg, respiratory rate of 20 breaths per minute, and oxygen saturation of 97% on room air. Cardiac examination reveals a regular rate and rhythm with no murmurs, rubs, or gallops. Her lungs are clear to auscultation. Her lower extremities are symmetric without edema. An electrocardiogram and chest x-ray are unremarkable. The most appropriate next step to evaluate for acute pulmonary embolism (PE) is:

A. Contrast-enhanced chest computed tomography (CT)
B. D-dimer testing
C. Lower extremity duplex ultrasonography
D. Ventilation-perfusion lung scanning

QUESTION 3. Which of the following does not identify acute pulmonary embolism (PE) patients at high risk for adverse outcomes?

A. Right ventricular (RV) dysfunction on echocardiography
B. RV enlargement on chest computed tomography (CT)
C. Elevated cardiac troponin levels
D. Age >70 years
E. Systolic blood pressure >170 mm Hg

QUESTION 4. All of the following statements regarding the management of venous thromboembolism (VTE) are true except:

A. Fibrinolysis may be considered for patients with massive or submassive pulmonary embolism (PE) and is associated with a negligible risk of bleeding.
B. Surgical embolectomy at tertiary medical centers skilled in this procedure is a safe and effective alternative for the treatment of acute PE patients with contraindications to fibrinolysis.
C. Inferior vena cava (IVC) filter insertion reduces the short-term risk of PE but may increase the long-term risk of deep vein thrombosis (DVT).
D. Appropriate agents for the immediate anticoagulation of VTE patients include intravenous unfractionated heparin, low-molecular-weight heparin (LMWH), and fondaparinux.
E. Indefinite-duration anticoagulation has been shown to reduce the risk of recurrence in patients with idiopathic VTE.

QUESTION 5. A 71-year-old man with a history of coronary artery disease, heart failure with a left ventricular ejection fraction of 30%, and diabetes mellitus is admitted to the telemetry floor with decompensated heart failure. Which of the following admission orders is not appropriate for venous thromboembolism (VTE) prophylaxis?

A. Unfractionated heparin, 5000 units subcutaneously 3 times a day
B. Enoxaparin, 40 mg subcutaneously daily
C. Dalteparin, 5000 units subcutaneously daily
D. Aspirin, 81 mg orally daily
E. Intermittent pneumatic compression devices

ANSWERS

1. C
2. B
3. E
4. A
5. D

35.

SLEEP APNEA

Douglas B. Kirsch and Lawrence J. Epstein

More has been learned about sleep in the last 60 years than in the preceding 6000 years, to paraphrase one sleep researcher, and sleep apnea is an area in which knowledge growth has been particularly exponential. In the last several decades, sleep specialists have learned how to study sleep, subdividing it into stages based on the sleep-related changes in the electroencephalogram (EEG), eye movements, and muscle tone. Additional measurements of airflow, respiratory effort, limb muscle movements, electrocardiogram (EKG), and oxygen saturation allow a full characterization of the changes and problems that occur during sleep. The process of studying physiological parameters during sleep, called polysomnography, has allowed sleep specialists to better understand the nocturnal rhythms of sleep and identify disruptors, one of the most common being obstructive sleep apnea (OSA). This chapter covers the epidemiology, pathophysiology, evaluation, and treatment of this common chronic disorder and its significant long-term effects on patient's well-being and health.

DEFINITION OF OBSTRUCTIVE SLEEP APNEA

The term apnea means no airflow. Apneas are subdivided into types, including *obstructive apneas*, meaning that there is ongoing respiratory effort in the muscles of respiration (thorax and abdomen) with no airflow; *central apneas*, in which there is neither effort nor airflow (the apnea is mediated by the central nervous system); and *mixed apneas*, during which the event begins as a central apnea and then becomes obstructive. OSA is caused by collapse of the upper airway, preventing or inhibiting airflow and causing disruption of sleep. Obstructive apneas are caused by total collapse of the airway and are defined as periods of complete stoppage of breathing for 10 seconds or more. Partial collapse of the airway results in hypopnea, which is a reduction in airflow lasting at least 10 seconds in association with a decrease in oxyhemoglobin saturation or an arousal from sleep.

Mild collapse can increase resistance in the airway, and the increased work necessary to overcome the resistance can cause arousals from sleep, called respiratory event-related arousals (RERA). The severity of OSA is often expressed as the apnea-hypopnea index (AHI): this index is determined by adding the number of apneas to the number of hypopneas and dividing by the hours of sleep during the study. Although the AHI is used quite frequently as a primary measure of apnea severity, the minimum oxygen saturation, arousal index (arousals per hour of sleep), and sleep architecture breakdown may also be useful in evaluating the severity of sleep apnea. The respiratory disturbance index (RDI), which is the numbers of apneas + hypopneas + RERAs per hour of sleep, is often used interchangeably with the AHI. Although polysomnography is the gold standard for evaluation, some variability still exists when attempting to compare different sleep laboratories, particularly depending on the criteria for hypopneas (which in some laboratories are scored with 3% desaturations versus 4% desaturations, 25% versus 50% airflow decreases, and thermistor versus nasal pressure transducers). The diagnostic criteria for OSA in an adult is an AHI ≥15 events/hr with or without symptoms or an AHI between 5 and 15 events/hr and patient complaints of unintended sleep episodes, daytime sleepiness, unrefreshing sleep or insomnia, waking up gasping or choking, or the bed partner reporting witnessed apneas. The criteria are different in children, where often a lower AHI is accepted as clinically significant.

EPIDEMIOLOGY

Several studies have been performed in order to estimate the prevalence of OSA in the U.S. and world population. Based on available population-based studies, the prevalence of OSA including sleepiness as a symptom is 3–7% for adult men and 2–5% for adult women in the general population. The prevalence of OSA is higher in the overweight population, older individuals, and possibly in some non-Caucasian racial groups (Asians, African Americans, and Hispanics). Other factors that increase the risk for OSA include craniofacial anatomy (small mandibular body length), family history of OSA, smoking and alcohol use, and some medical conditions (see table 35.1).

Little information is available from a standpoint of disease progression. Weight change can clearly play a role, subjects with a 10% increase in weight had a 32% increase in their AHI as compared to subjects with stable weight. However, in one study, even in the absence of weight change, 20% of men and 10% of women developed sleep apnea over a 5-year observational period.

PATHOPHYSIOLOGY

What happens during an apnea? As the patient falls asleep his or her airway collapses, with tongue and soft palate pressed against the back of the pharyngeal space. Worsening hypoxemia and hypercapnia stimulate repetitive efforts to breathe (thoracic and abdominal effort). Increasing effort causes marked reductions in intrathoracic pressure, which increases pulmonary artery pressure, venous return, and cardiac afterload. The hypoxemia stimulates peripheral artery chemoreceptors, triggering the response of peripheral vasoconstriction and increased arterial blood pressure. Increased respiratory efforts from hypoxemia and hypercarbia trigger a central nervous system arousal, awakening the person from sleep and causing the airway to open. The arousal causes a further increase in sympathetic stimulation that elevates blood pressure. With the airway open, a period of hyperpnea ensues to correct the blood gas derangements. The reoxygenation that then occurs may increase oxidative stress, leading to increasing inflammation and mitochondrial dysfunction. Once the blood gases return to normal values the person is able to fall asleep, allowing the airway to collapse and starting the cycle of events again. This sequence happens repetitively during the night, hundreds of times a night in severe cases.

Multiple factors contribute to the collapse of the airway and production of obstruction. These include upper airway anatomy, the functioning of upper airway musculature during sleep, stability of the respiratory control system, and the effect of lung volume on the previous factors.

UPPER AIRWAY ANATOMY

The airway, composed of muscles and soft tissue but without bony support, contains a collapsible portion from the hard palate to the larynx. It has three primary functions: speech, breathing, and swallowing. Patients with OSA have a smaller airway lumen than those without. This may be due to an increase in the lateral pharyngeal wall, increased tongue volume, adenotonsillar hypertrophy, or increase in the size of the parapharyngeal fat pads. The most common location of airway collapse is the retropalatal region; other areas of collapse may include the hypopharynx and retroglossal region.

UPPER AIRWAY MUSCLE CONTROL

During wakefulness, patients with OSA are able to maintain airway patency, even with a compromised airway, because of increased pharyngeal muscle tone. However, as they fall asleep, airway dilator muscle activity diminishes significantly compared to waking, allowing the airway to collapse.

COLLAPSIBILITY

The airway of OSA patients tends to be more collapsible, demonstrated by measurement of the closing pressure, P_{crit}. This value is the pharyngeal pressure at which the airway collapses, determined by the relationships among the soft tissue pressure, pharyngeal wall compliance, and upper airway muscle activity. P_{crit} is higher in those patients with OSA, meaning that the airway will collapse at a less negative pressure than a patient who does not have OSA. Conversely, a normal airway requires application of a more negative pressure to cause collapse than an airway of a patient with OSA.

FEEDBACK LOOPS

Ventilation is controlled by feedback loops. Increases in CO_2 and decreases in oxygen stimulate increased breathing, which reverses the blood gas changes, causing ventilation to decrease. Changes in the sensitivity or output of the system can promote unstable, irregular, or cyclical breathing patterns. Apneas tend to occur more frequently during unstable breathing and in a cyclical pattern.

LUNG VOLUME

Changes in lung volume modify upper airway mechanics; as lung volume decreases during sleep, upper airway resistance increases. Conversely, as end-expiratory lung volume

Table 35.1 **RISK FACTORS FOR OSA**

RISK FACTORS

Excess body weight
Advancing age
Male sex
Family/genetic predisposition
Tobacco use
Alcohol consumption
Medical conditions (polycystic ovarian syndrome, hypothyroidism, stroke)
Pregnancy
Menopause
Abnormal craniofacial anatomy

increases, airway collapsibility decreases, improving sleep disordered breathing in OSA. The underlying mechanisms of this action have not been well described.

CLINICAL EVALUATION OF OBSTRUCTIVE SLEEP APNEA

Although diagnosis of OSA is generally not based solely on a patient's symptoms and signs, the history and physical examination continue to a play a significant role in the evaluation of the patient. In many cases, particularly in patients with low AHIs, the symptom history may be the primary tool in determining the course of action.

Snoring, the most common reported symptom of OSA, occurs due to narrowing of the upper airway; the noise results from the vibration of the surrounding tissue by turbulent airflow through this constricted space. The rate of habitual snoring in the population is 25% in men and 15% in women; however, this rate increases with age. Given the epidemiological rates of OSA listed above, snoring does not have positive predictive value for OSA, but it is quite sensitive, as 95% of patients who have OSA also snore. Witnessed apneas, a common cause of referral to a sleep center, is more specific for OSA, though it may be observed in 6% of the normal population. Other nocturnal symptoms may include gasping arousals, choking, insomnia, frequent urination, and nocturnal sweating.

Daytime symptoms may also aid in the identification of patients with OSA. Excessive daytime sleepiness (EDS) is commonly reported by patients with OSA. Though OSA may be one of the most common medical causes of EDS, EDS by itself is not highly specific for OSA. In addition, many patients with OSA do not recognize their level of sleepiness or may report alternate symptoms such as fatigue or lack of energy. Other described daytime symptoms may include memory impairment, morning headaches, and depression.

Physical examination of the patient with OSA may be helpful in assessing pretest risk level for obstructive sleep apnea (see table 35.2). As body mass index rises, risk for OSA increases. Although high blood pressure is a common symptom in adults, it may be seen at a higher rate in patients with OSA. The majority of the assessment time should be spent on evaluation of the upper airway. The nasal examination should explore for reduced nasal airflow caused by either congestion or structural abnormalities. The oropharynx is inspected for evidence of airway narrowing. The Mallampati airway classification score, an assessment of airway crowding, has been shown to be predictive of OSA likelihood. Other features that may predispose to OSA include a high-arching soft palate, large tongue, soft palate redundancy, increased uvula size, abnormal molar occlusion, and retro- or micrognathia. Further evaluation of the upper airway may include use of cephalometry, fiberoptic laryngoscopy, and computed tomography (CT) or magnetic resonance imaging (MRI) of the upper airway. The complete examination should include palpation of the neck, a cardiorespiratory evaluation, and a neurological evaluation.

Subjective measures of daytime sleepiness have often been used to aid in the assessment of patients with sleep disorders. One of the most frequently used measures is the Epworth Sleepiness Scale (ESS), an eight-question scale with scores ranging from 0 (not sleepy) to 24 (very sleepy) (table 35.3). This scale assesses a patient's chronic level of sleepiness in different situations, from lying down to nap to driving a car. A score >10 suggests excessive sleepiness, and higher values on this scale (particularly >15) may be suggestive of a sleep disorder. The ESS is neither specific for OSA nor a replacement for objective testing.

The polysomnogram is the gold standard for objective testing for OSA, evaluating electroencephalography, electrooculography, respiratory parameters, oxyhemoglobin saturation, cardiac rhythms, and muscle activity during sleep (figure 35.1). Generally, the diagnostic test will last at least 6 hours, though some sleep centers have opted to perform "split-night" studies to minimize health care cost, in which the first half of the study is devoted to diagnosis and the second half is a positive-pressure treatment trial (figure 35.2). A technologist places all of the appropriate probes and wires on the patient at the beginning of the night and also observes that patient throughout the night, ensuring that the patient is medically stable and that the recorded data are accurate. The advantages of the polysomnogram are the assessment of sleep

Table 35.2 **PHYSICAL RISK FACTORS**

Obesity
Neck circumference (>17 inches in men, >16 inches in women)
Small, hypoplastic, and/or retroposed maxilla and mandible
Narrow posterior airway space
Inferiorly positioned hyoid bone
High and narrow hard palate
Abnormal dental overjet
Macroglossia
Tonsillar enlargement
Nasal obstruction

Table 35.3 **EPWORTH SLEEPINESS SCALE**

S.NO.	EACH QUESTION IS SCORED FROM 0 (NEVER DOZING OR SLEEPING) TO 3 (HIGH CHANCE OF DOZING OR SLEEPING); RANGE IS 0–24	RANGE
1	Sitting and reading	
2	Watching TV	
3	Sitting inactive in a public place	
4	Being a passenger in a motor vehicle for an hour or more	
5	Lying down in the afternoon	
6	Sitting and talking to someone	
7	Sitting quietly after lunch (no alcohol)	
8	Stopped for a few minutes in traffic while driving	

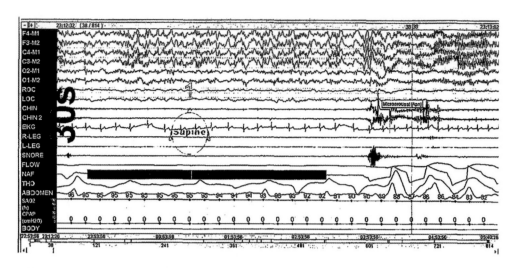

Figure 35.1. Monitoring Obstructive Apnea. This is a slide of a 37-year-old man demonstrating an obstructive apnea (30-sec epoch). Note the continuous thorax and abdominal effort with absent nasal airflow, increasing respiratory effort, the dropping oxygen saturation with a slight delay, and the EEG arousal (identified). The top 6 leads are EEG (right and left frontal, central, and occipital), followed by 2 eye leads (right and left), 2 chin leads, EKG, 2 leg leads (right and left), snore channel, oronasal thermistor, nasal pressure transducer, effort bands (thorax and abdomen), oxygen saturation, CPAP pressure, and body position.

stage and the effect of stage on sleep-disordered breathing, observer report and video for evaluation of patient behavior, scoring of EEG-based arousals from sleep, and ability to intervene to assure high-quality data and provide patient assistance.

In-home monitors have been developed for the diagnosis of OSA. These portable monitors measure only a subset of the parameters of a typical polysomnogram (e.g., airflow, respiratory effort, heart rate, and snoring). In-home testing is most likely to be successful for patients who have a high likelihood of moderate-to-severe OSA in the absence of comorbid medical conditions, such as lung disease, congestive heart failure, neuromuscular conditions, or other suspected sleep disorders. One limitation for most portable monitors is the lack of EEG leads; absence of brain wave measurement generally limits accurate sleep staging and identification of cortical arousals. Single-channel monitors, such as oximeters, may assess the efficacy of treatment of OSA; however, oximetry may poorly identify cases of OSA, especially mild apnea.

The diagnostic criteria for OSA are given in table 35.4. The primary value used by clinicians to assess severity of OSA is the AHI. OSA severity is defined as mild for AHI ≥5 and <15, moderate for AHI ≥15 and <30, and severe for AHI ≥30. However, sleep laboratories may use different criteria for scoring events and for defining apnea severity.

CONSEQUENCES OF OBSTRUCTIVE SLEEP APNEA

The long-term medical effects of OSA are the result of the physiological derangements that accompany the repetitive obstructive respiratory events (table 35.5). These are discussed in the following paragraphs.

HYPERTENSION

Hypertension is one of the most common medical conditions associated with OSA. Obstructive sleep-disordered breathing causes acute peripheral vasoconstriction and increased blood pressure during sleep. Typically, sleep is associated with decreased blood pressure compared to wakefulness (reduced 10–15%). This "dip" in blood pressure occurs to a lesser degree, or not at all, in many patients with OSA. The Wisconsin Sleep Cohort, looking at 709 subjects, demonstrated prospectively that the severity of OSA at baseline is associated with hypertension 4 years later. Compared to a reference AHI of 0, the odds ratios (95% confidence interval in parentheses) was 2.03 (1.29–3.17) for an AHI between 5 and 14.9 events/hr and was 2.89 (1.46–5.64) for an AHI ≥15 events/hr. In a large study of nurses aged 40–65, there was a higher incidence of hypertension in those women who reported snoring. Multiple studies have also demonstrated that treatment of OSA with continuous positive airway pressure (CPAP) therapy, will lower blood pressure in hypertensive patients, even in those patients who are considered refractory (poor control of blood pressure with use of three or more medications).

CARDIOVASCULAR MORBIDITY AND MORTALITY

The large multicenter Sleep Heart Health Study found that as OSA worsened, so did the prevalence of coronary heart disease. Another large prospective study demonstrated that over a mean observation period of 10 years, patients with severe OSA had a threefold higher risk of cardiovascular events than healthy controls. Prospective studies of patients from a sleep clinic evaluated 60 men with OSA and 122 men without sleep-disordered breathing and found that the

Table 35.4 DIAGNOSTIC CRITERIA FROM THE INTERNATIONAL CLASSIFICATION OF SLEEP DISORDER, 2ND EDITION

A. At least one of the following applies:
   a. The patient complains of unintentional sleep episodes during wakefulness, daytime sleepiness, unrefreshing sleep, fatigue, or insomnia
   b. The patient wakes with breath holding, gasping, or choking
   c. The bed partner reports loud snoring, breathing interruptions, or both during the patient's sleep

B. Polysomnographic recording shows the following
   a. Five or more scorable respiratory events (i.e., apneas, hypopneas, or RERAs per hour of sleep)
   b. Evidence of respiratory effort during all or a portion of each respiratory event

C. Polysomnographic recording shows the following
   a. Fifteen or more scorable respiratory events (i.e., apneas, hypopneas, or RERAs per hour of sleep)
   b. Evidence of respiratory effort during all or a portion of each respiratory event

D. The disorder is not better explained by another current sleep disorder, medical or neurological disorder, medication use, or substance use disorder

NOTE: A, B and D, or C and D satisfy the criteria.
SOURCE: Reprinted with permission from the American Academy of Sleep Medicine. Diagnostic Criteria from the International Classification of Sleep Disorder, 2nd edition. 2005.

OSA population had a higher incidence of cardiovascular disease (37%) than the controls (7%). Even snoring appears to be potentially associated with an increased risk of cardiovascular disease. The Nurses' Health Study discovered that occasional snorers had a 1.46 times age-adjusted relative risk of cardiovascular disease when compared to nonsnorers; frequent snorers have a 2.02 times increased risk.

OSA has been linked to arrhythmias in several studies. The Sleep Heart Health Study demonstrated that patients with a RDI >39 events/hr had a higher rate of atrial fibrillation, nonsustained ventricular tachycardia, and ectopic ventricular beats than those subjects with a RDI <5 events/hr. Among patients who had been electrically cardioverted for atrial fibrillation, the patients with untreated OSA had a recurrence rate two times that of patients treated with CPAP. Nocturnal hypoxemia from OSA has also been associated with the incidence of atrial fibrillation.

Table 35.5 POTENTIAL MEDICAL CONSEQUENCES OF OSA

Insulin resistance

Coronary artery disease

Hypertension

Stroke

Heart failure

Arrhythmias

Pulmonary hypertension

Depression

Gastroesophageal reflux

Motor vehicle accidents

A few studies suggest that treatment of OSA may improve cardiovascular disease, although the data are quite limited. One study compared patients who did not tolerate CPAP with those who were treated over a mean follow-up time of 7.5 years. Deaths from cardiovascular disease were more common in the untreated group compared to the treatment group (14.8% vs. 1.9%).

CEREBROVASCULAR DISEASE

Similarly to cardiovascular disease, an association of OSA and stroke has been observed in multiple studies. Subjects studied after a first stroke or transient ischemic attack (TIA) have a reported prevalence of sleep-disordered breathing of 63–70%. One longitudinal study found that an AHI >20 events/hr was a risk factor for stroke. In another >3-year study of more than 1000 subjects with OSA, severity of OSA correlated with risk of mortality from stroke and other causes. In addition, self-reported snoring has been found to be an independent risk factor for stroke in women. AHI also appears to predict mortality in patients with a first-time stroke or TIA within 2 years.

The cause and effect of cerebrovascular disease and sleep-disordered breathing is controversial; as above, some studies demonstrate that OSA is a risk factor for stroke. However, some researchers suggest that some forms of sleep-disordered breathing, particularly central sleep apnea, may be due to injury of brain respiratory centers or centrally mediated upper airway reflexes.

HEART FAILURE

OSA is associated with an increased frequency of congestive heart failure. Likely contributors include OSA-induced hypertension, large negative swings in intrathoracic pressure, hypoxemia, and increased sympathetic activity. The prevalence of patients with heart failure referred to a clinical sleep laboratory is nearly 40%. The effects of CPAP treatment on heart failure patients with OSA are currently controversial, with two interventional studies demonstrating improvement in left ventricular ejection fraction and one study that demonstrated no clear changes in cardiovascular function.

DIABETES MELLITUS TYPE 2

OSA is an often-observed comorbidity with diabetes type 2, possibly because of the common relationship to obesity. The Sleep Heart Health Study found that patients with AHI ≥5 events/hr had a two times greater risk of having impaired glucose tolerance, even after adjusting for confounding variables. The glucose tolerance impairment in these subjects was correlated with the severity of oxygen desaturation. The Wisconsin Sleep Cohort found similar information, demonstrating that 15% of subjects with AHI >15 events/hr had type 2 diabetes. Though the exact cause-and-effect relationship is not completely clear, some suggestions have included OSA causing stimulation of the sympathetic nervous system, stimulation of the hypothalamic-pituitary-adrenal axis, and increase in cytokine release. A role for intermittent hypoxia in the interaction between diabetes type 2 and OSA has also been raised.

MOTOR VEHICLE CRASHES

Though less of a "medical" risk factor, automobile crashes may be the most immediate source of danger from OSA. Patients with OSA may suffer from a twofold to a sevenfold increased risk of a motor vehicle accident when compared to the general population. One meta-analysis demonstrated that 800,000 drivers were involved with OSA-related motor vehicle accidents in 2000 with a cost of nearly $16 billion and 1400 lives. Although it is unclear whether the severity of OSA is directly correlated with the risk of crashes, it is clear that treatment of OSA with positive air pressure (PAP) therapy reduces that risk.

TREATMENT OF OSA

MEDICAL THERAPY

Not all patients demonstrate interest in or a preference for more aggressive therapies for obstructive sleep apnea, particularly depending on severity of the patient's symptoms. Obesity clearly is related to smaller airway size, promoting nocturnal airway collapse. Therefore, with patients who are obese, weight loss may play a major role in treatment of OSA. In some cases, self-motivating patients may be able to lose weight without much support; however, many patients have success in group programs or via a multidisciplinary team approach. In some cases, surgical approaches to weight

loss, such as gastric bypass surgery, are appropriate options for those who fail more conservative therapies. Gastric bypass surgery has been shown in several studies to cause a significant decrease in AHI as weight loss occurs.

Another common conservative treatment of OSA is positional therapy, as for many patients, sleep-disordered breathing may be significantly worse in the supine sleeping position. The cause of this positional predisposition is likely the effect of gravity on the tongue, causing closure against the posterior pharyngeal wall. One method of treatment would be to sleep with the head and trunk elevated (30°–60° to the horizontal), which has been shown to lessen airway opening pressure. Alternatively, the patient should avoid the supine position while lying horizontal. Methods to minimize sleeping on the back may include the use of a small backpack, sewing a pocket in the back of a t-shirt, which then would contain a tennis ball, or using a wedge pillow. It is necessary to demonstrate a person has positional OSA before implementing positional therapy.

Other areas to consider include avoidance of the use of tobacco, abstinence from alcohol or sedative-hypnotic medications prior to bedtime, and minimization of sleep deprivation. Cigarette smokers have a four to five times higher risk of at least moderate OSA compared to those who do not smoke, perhaps via upper airway edema. Alcohol may induce apneas in snorers and may increase the frequency of apneas in pre-existing apneics. There is some evidence, though limited and inconclusive, suggesting that benzodiazepines may have similar effects to alcohol. In addition, alcohol may worsen daytime sleepiness in patients with OSA. Acute sleep deprivation may increase the severity of sleep-disordered breathing. Medications such as rapid eye movement (REM)-suppressing tricyclic antidepressants and respiratory stimulants have not been effective in treating obstructive sleep apnea. Improvement in nasal airflow with saline rinses, medications, or nostril-opening adhesive strips may also provide mild reduction in snoring and apnea severity. Supplemental oxygen reduces the degree of hypoxemia but does not reverse the obstructive events; therefore, it should only be used as an adjunct to other therapies.

POSITIVE-PRESSURE THERAPY

The use of air pressure to maintain airway patency was introduced in Australia in 1981 by Colin Sullivan. Now, after the evolution of masks and breathing circuits over the last 25 years, continuous positive airway pressure (CPAP) is the first line treatment for OSA. CPAP acts as a pneumatic splint to maintain pharyngeal airway patency. The selection of the appropriate CPAP pressure has been classically done via an in-laboratory polysomnogram during which CPAP is titrated to the lowest possible pressure that eliminates snoring, respiratory-related arousals, and obstructive hypopneas and apneas. As this occurs, the patient's sleep architecture often improves, no longer fragmented by the repetitive airway collapse. Pressures set in the laboratory rarely need to be changed over time; some factors that may suggest the need for a pressure change include significant weight gain or loss, the return of snoring, or return of notable daytime symptoms that had been previously suppressed.

CPAP has been shown to improve daytime sleepiness, performance, and quality of life and to reduce automobile accidents. Studies often refer to CPAP use of more than 4 hours per night as being compliant; however, recent study has shown a dose-response relationship between improvement in symptoms and performance and time used. Patients should be encouraged to wear CPAP whenever sleeping. Compliance with PAP is often difficult for patients. The three primary factors that impact tolerance to CPAP are mask fit, PAP pressure, and nasal congestion. Different mask styles may include nasal masks, oral/nasal masks, and nasal prong style masks. Different patients will require different mask types; there is no "one-type-fits-all" mask. Though trial and error is often the method used to select mask style, some useful guidance may be offered by a patient's report of mouth-breathing (need for a chin-strap), nasal congestion (consider an oral/nasal mask), or claustrophobia (use less bulky nasal prong mask). If higher pressures lead to difficulty with tolerance or aerophagia, some consideration may be given to lowering the CPAP pressure for comfort, use of expiratory pressure adjustment (available on some CPAP machines), or switching to bilevel PAP therapy.

Humidification of PAP therapy can decrease nasal congestion and increase compliance.

Unlike the constant single pressure of CPAP, bilevel PAP therapy provides two different positive pressures, a higher one on inspiration and a lower one on expiration. Overall, compliance is not better with bilevel PAP than CPAP; however, some patients who will not tolerate CPAP can tolerate bilevel PAP. A separate titration study night is often recommended when trying to initiate bilevel PAP therapy, as the pressures required for treatment may be similar to, but not exactly the same as, those for CPAP.

AutoPAP, an autotitrating CPAP device, has been increasingly available and adjusts the PAP pressure via an internal algorithm to continuously eliminate respiratory events as the night goes on (during positional changes or sleep stage changes). The advantage of this device is that the pressure is only as high as necessary at any given time frame, potentially improving patient compliance and avoiding the need for an in-laboratory titration study.

ORAL APPLIANCES

When patients are unable to tolerate PAP therapy, one alternate option for treatment is using a custom-fit oral appliance. There are several types of appliances, though the two primary styles of devices are mandibular-advancing (more common) and tongue-retaining. The mandibular-advancing appliances are created to move the bottom jaw forward compared to the upper jaw, moving the tongue forward, in order

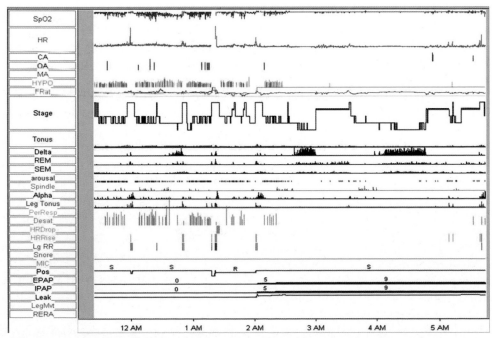

Figure 35.2. A Split-Night Study. This is an overnight hypnogram for a split-night study; first half of the night is diagnostic, the second half is a CPAP titration study. From the top down the horizontal images are oxygen saturation, heart rate, respiratory events (central apneas, obstructive apneas, mixed apneas, and hypopneas), sleep architecture (wake to deep sleep moving downward), PAP pressure, snoring, arousals, leg movements, and sleep position. Obstructive events (red, black, and pink) are eliminated as the PAP pressure is increased. Notice the improvement in the sleep architecture (fragmented in the first half, significantly improved in the second half).

to increase the size of the retropalatal airway. Preferably, specially trained dentists will make the appliances by taking an impression of the upper and lower teeth and building the appliance based on the molds. The mandibular-advancing devices may be either adjustable or nonadjustable. There are several advantages to the use of an oral appliance, though the most notable is the size. Easy for travel and without need for electricity, the appliance is a good choice for a rustic camper or frequent business traveler. Patients who were claustrophobic with CPAP may be more open to this style of treatment. However, the oral appliances as a group tend to be most successful for patients who have mild or moderate obstructive sleep apnea; in more severe cases of OSA, the reduction in severity from the use of the appliance may not improve the patient's symptoms or reduce cardiovascular risk. The appliances will work best in patients with a full set of teeth and with good jaw mobility; patients with poor dentition and with temporomandibular joint pain may not be good candidates. Tongue-retaining devices pull the tongue anteriorly in an attempt to reduce airway closure during the night but are less commonly used. Because the success rate for treating mild to moderate OSA with an oral appliance is 50–60%, patients should have a sleep study with the appliance in place to demonstrate effectiveness of the device.

SURGERY

Surgery is infrequently a cure for OSA, though often significant reductions in apnea severity can be observed. In order to increase the rate of a positive result, the presurgical evaluation should be oriented toward identifying the site of airway collapse (palate, base of tongue, or both). Although an external oronasal exam is helpful, often the use of fiberoptic nasopharyngolaryngoscopy and cephalometric radiography/CT scans may allow for more specific localization.

Tracheostomy was the first described surgical treatment for OSA and is nearly universally successful in the rare occasions that it is still performed. Its rarity is primarily related to patient disinterest combined with the knowledge that CPAP is an equally effective alternative. Tracheostomy may also be a temporary measure to maintain airway patency when performing other upper airway surgery.

Nasal reconstruction is rarely a sole intervention for OSA, though good nasal airflow may improve nocturnal respiration and increase the likelihood of CPAP tolerance. More frequently, this surgery may occur in combination with other upper airway surgeries.

Uvulopalatopharyngoplasty (UPPP) was first proposed in 1964 as a treatment for snoring. Overtime, this procedure has become quite popular, though the data supporting its use in all patients are variable. If the obstructive process is solely related to the retropalatal area, this surgery may be quite effective. UPPP involves removal of a portion of the soft palate, the uvula, and residual tonsillar tissue. Although the procedure is described by some surgeons as simple, there is significant throat pain described by patients postoperatively. Studies have demonstrated a 20–50% reduction in respiratory events with this procedure.

Laser-assisted uvulopalatoplasty is an ambulatory procedure that also focuses on oropharyngeal obstructive processes; through use of a carbon dioxide laser, the surgeon may shorten or amputate the uvula and tighten the palate. Less successful than the UPPP, this procedure rarely brings the AHI to a normal range and should be used primarily for treating primary snoring without OSA.

Mandibular osteotomy with genioglossus advancement attempts to prevent collapse of the hypopharyngeal space during sleep. A hole is created in the mandible, and part of the tongue muscle is pulled forward; however, no additional space is anatomically created.

Maxillomandibular advancement osteotomy is a more advanced surgery to improve refractory base-of-tongue obstruction, often after other surgeries fail (some surgeons consider this a second-phase surgery, to be performed after failure of a palatal surgery). In some patients with craniofacial disorders, such as mandibular deficiency, this surgery may be a first-line treatment. Movement of both the maxillary and mandibular complex forward by at least 10 mm via fracture creates physical room for the tongue. An orthodontist is also frequently involved in the procedure to manage dental occlusion.

RECENT INTERVENTIONS

Radiofrequency ablation delivers low heat energy to an area of tissue, which can reduce volume and create scar tissue, particularly directed to the soft palate. This intervention has improved snoring via repeated treatment sessions, but the data demonstrating improvement in OSA have been limited.

Placement of palatal implants is one of the most recently approved operations for snoring and OSA; by placing three polyester pieces into the soft palate and stiffening it, the frequency and volume of snoring has been reduced. The advantages to this system are low cost and low morbidity. However, although the data have demonstrated a small, but statistically significant improvement in mild OSA, this intervention has not been shown to be curative for OSA of any severity.

A BRIEF COMMENT ON CENTRAL SLEEP APNEA

Though both are associated with stoppage of breathing, obstructive sleep apnea should not be confused with central sleep apnea. Unlike the collapse of the airway, which prevents air movement in OSA, temporary loss of ventilatory effort is the cause of a central apnea. This disorder is rarer than obstructive sleep apnea, comprising 4–10% of the sleep laboratory population. Central sleep apnea has several different causes, most commonly related to congestive heart failure, though neurological disorders, medications, and high altitude are alternative options. Unlike OSA, central sleep apnea does not appear to confer the same medical risks, though sleep disruption and occasionally daytime sleepiness may occur.

SUMMARY

Obstructive sleep apnea is a common, though underrecognized, disorder caused by repetitive airway closure during sleep. Though not directly implicated in mortality, this disorder appears to significantly increase the likelihood of hypertension, coronary artery disease, and cerebrovascular disease. As well, there is a large impact on quality of life as a result of disrupted nocturnal sleep and production of excessive daytime sleepiness, including an increased risk of motor vehicle accidents. The primary treatments include weight loss, positional therapy, positive-pressure therapy, oral appliances, and surgical intervention.

ADDITIONAL READINGS

American Academy of Sleep Medicine. *The International Classification of Sleep Disorders: Diagnostic & Coding Manual* (2nd ed.). Westchester, IL: American Academy of Sleep Medicine, 2005.

Eckert D, Malhotra A. Pathophysiology of adult obstructive sleep apnea. *Proc Am Thorac Soc.* 2008;5:144–53.

Freedman N. Treatment of obstructive sleep apnea syndrome. *Clin Chest Med.* 2010;31(2):187–201.

Johns MW. A new method for measuring daytime sleepiness: The Epworth sleepiness scale. *Sleep.* 1991;14(6):540–54.

Kapur VK. Obstructive sleep apnea: Diagnosis, epidemiology, and economics. *Respir Care.* 2010;55(9):1155–67.

Kushida CA, Littner MR, Hirshkowitz M, et al.; American Academy of Sleep Medicine. Practice parameters for the use of continuous and bilevel positive airway pressure devices to treat adult patients with sleep-related breathing disorders. *Sleep.* 2006;29(3):375–80.

Kushida CA, Morgenthaler TI, Littner MR., et al. Practice parameters for the treatment of snoring and obstructive sleep apnea with oral appliances: An update for 2005. *Sleep.* 2006;29:240–3.

Malhotra A, Owens RL. What is central sleep apnea? *Respir Care.* 2010;55(9):1168–78.

McNicholas W. Diagnosis of obstructive sleep apnea in adults. *Proc Am Thorac Soc.* 2008;5:154–60.

Ramar K, Guilleminault C. Risk factors. In Kushida C, ed. *Obstructive Sleep Apnea: Pathophysiology, Comorbidity, and Consequences.* New York: Informa Healthcare; 2007: 197–222.

Riley R, Powell N, Li K, Guilleminault C. Surgical therapy for obstructive sleep apnea-hypopnea syndrome. In Kryger M, Roth T, Dement W, eds. *The Principles and Practice of Sleep Medicine* (2nd ed.). Philadelphia: W. B. Saunders; 2000: 913–28.

Sleep-related breathing disorders in adults: Recommendations for syndrome definition and measurement techniques in clinical research. The Report of an American Academy of Sleep Medicine Task Force. *Sleep.* 1999;22:667–89.

Ulualp SO. Snoring and obstructive sleep apnea. *Med Clin North Am.* 2010;94(5):1047–55.

Wickwire EM, Collop NA. Insomnia and sleep-related breathing disorders. *Chest.* 2010;137(6):1449–63.

Won C, Robert D. Morbidity and Mortality. In Kushida C, ed. *Obstructive Sleep Apnea: Pathophysiology, Comorbidity, and Consequences.* New York: Informa Healthcare; 2007: 259–74.

QUESTIONS

QUESTION 1. A 54-year-old man comes into your office with complaints of snoring and daytime sleepiness, to the point where he falls asleep while stopped at a red light commuting home in his car. He is 67 inches tall and 273 lb. The polysomnogram shows obstructive sleep apnea with an AHI of 55 events/hr and a minimal oxygen saturation of 83%. The patient's risk is most elevated for which of the following diseases:

A. Alzheimer dementia
B. Epilepsy
C. Stroke
D. Narcolepsy

QUESTION 2. According to International Classification of Sleep Disorders, second edition, guidelines, which of the following patients best fits criteria for diagnosis of obstructive sleep apnea?

A. A 57-year-old man with an AHI of 4 events per hour, a minimum oxygen saturation of 88%, and nocturnal shortness of breath
B. A 65-year-old woman with an AHI of 12 events/hr, a minimum oxygen saturation of 90%, and symptoms of daytime sleepiness
C. A 44-year-old man with an AHI of 8 events/hr, a minimum oxygen saturation of 89%, and symptoms only of restless legs
D. An 81-year-old woman with an AHI of 14 events/hr, a minimum oxygen saturation of 91%, and no other symptoms

QUESTION 3. A 68-year-old obese man has severe obstructive sleep apnea with an AHI of 111 events/hr and a minimal oxygen saturation of 68%. He is having difficulty with CPAP use on a nightly basis, including nasal congestion and morning mouth dryness. Which of the following interventions may help improve his tolerance to CPAP?

A. Use of a nasal steroid to treat nasal congestion
B. Use of a full-face CPAP mask
C. Use of a heated humidifier in line with CPAP
D. All of the above

QUESTION 4. The patient in question 3 decides that he will no longer use CPAP. Which of the following surgical options has the highest chance of complete elimination of OSA?

A. Uvulopalatopharyngoplasty
B. Tracheostomy

C. Laser-assisted uvulopalatoplasty
D. Genioglossus advancement

C. Supine sleep
D. Wedge pillow

QUESTION 5. A 23-year-old man with a height of 65 inches and a weight of 230 lb has a history of snoring and comes in for a sleep study. His sleep study demonstrates a RDI of 14 events/hr and a minimal oxygen saturation of 91%. What treatment would be LEAST likely to treat his OSA?

A. Weight loss
B. Alcohol reduction

ANSWERS

1. C
2. B
3. D
4. B
5. C

36.

PULMONARY FUNCTION TESTS

Jeremy B. Richards and David H. Roberts

OVERVIEW: CLINICAL INDICATIONS AND UTILITY

Pulmonary function tests (PFTs) include the measurement of velocity and volume of expiratory flow (spirometry), static volumes (lung volumes), diffusion of gases across the alveolar-capillary membrane (diffusion capacity), and respiratory muscle strength. PFTs can both identify patterns and quantify the severity of a variety of respiratory system diseases. The indications for performing PFTs in a given individual vary and may include diagnostic evaluation of symptoms, monitoring of disease stability or progression, assessing acute or long-term response to treatment, or providing preoperative pulmonary assessment.

TECHNICAL CONSIDERATIONS

SPIROMETRY: MEASUREMENT, VALUES, AND FLOW-VOLUME LOOPS

Spirometry is the determination of volume and flow rates of expiratory flow. The primary values of interest when obtaining spirometry include the forced expiratory volume in 1 second (FEV_1—the quantity of air in liters exhaled in 1 sec), forced vital capacity (FVC—the total quantity of air exhaled in a maximum voluntary exhalation), and peak expiratory flow rate (PEFR—the maximum velocity of air during a forced exhalation in liters/second). The ratio of FEV_1/FVC is useful in differentiating between obstructive (reduced ratio) and restrictive ventilatory (preserved or elevated ratio) deficits.

Results from spirometric measurements are effort dependent. To determine FEV_1 and FVC, a subject is instructed to inhale maximally to total lung capacity (TLC) followed by a vigorous, maximal forced expiratory effort to residual volume (RV). The subject exhales into a mouthpiece attached to a flow meter through which expiratory flow rates are measured and volume is integrated from the flow signal. Alternatively, expiratory volume may be measured by a volume-displacement spirometer, and flow is derived from the volume signal. Regardless of the method of assessing expiratory flow and

volume, standard practice is to perform at least three acceptable expiratory efforts. To account for differences in effort, the accepted consensus standard for spirometry requires performance of at least two expiratory efforts of similar flow and volume characteristics. Specifically, the largest FEV_1 and FVC should not vary from the second largest FEV_1 and FVC by >0.15 L (or by >0.1 L for a patient with a FVC of ≤1.0 L). More than three expiratory efforts may be performed if there is significant variation between efforts. There is no consensus on the maximum number of efforts that may be attempted; however, after 8–10 attempts the yield of further attempts is likely to be minimal. If two expiratory efforts in which the FEV_1 and FVC vary by less than 0.2 L cannot be achieved, the spirometry is termed to "lack reproducibility." In addition to assessing reproducibility, spirometry should be assessed for acceptability. Consensus guidelines define an "acceptable" expiratory effort as an expiratory effort that lasts ≥6 seconds. Particularly in younger individuals, the FVC may be achieved in less than 6 seconds, and a plateau in flow velocity of the expiratory effort of ≥2 seconds is considered by some as an alternative marker of acceptability.

Spirometry results are reported as both absolute values (i.e., FEV_1 = 2.5 L) as well as a percentage of what values would be predicted given certain individual characteristics (i.e., FEV_1 = 90% predicted). The specific characteristics used to generate predicted values for a given individual include height, race/ethnicity, age, and gender. Predictive equations have been derived from cross-sectional population studies; a number of equations are available in the literature. An American Thoracic Society (ATS) and European Respiratory Society (ERS) joint task force recommends using predictive equations derived from the National Health and Nutrition Examination Survey (NHANES) III cross-sectional study for individuals aged 8–80 years (Pelligrino et al., 2005; In patients whose true height cannot be accurately measured (i.e., due to kyphoscoliosis or an inability to stand due to neuromuscular disease), arm-span can be used as a surrogate metric (see table 36.1)). An individual's measured spirometric values can be compared to his or her predicted values to generate the "percentage predicted" value.

Table 36.1 USING ARM SPAN TO PREDICT A PATIENT'S STANDING HEIGHT

Arm span: height ratio	
White males	1.019
White females	0.999
Black males	1.044
Black females	1.035

Predictive equation:
Height (cm) = 67.904868 + (Arm span)(0.664182) – (Sex*)(2.816175) – (Race*)(4.05492) – (Age in years)(0.070892)

NOTE: *For sex, male = 1 and female = 2; for race, white = 1 and black = 2.
SOURCE: Reprinted with permission of the American Thoracic Society. Copyright © American Thoracic Society. From Parker JM, Dillard TA, Phillips YY. Arm span-height relationships in patients referred for spirometry. *Am J Respir Crit Care Med.* 1996;154:533–6.

These percentage predicted values for FEV_1 and FVC can also be used to grade the severity of disease. Deficits are typically described as mild, moderate, moderately severe, severe, or very severe depending on the degree of deviation from the predicted values (see table 36.2).

In addition to being characterized numerically, the measurements obtained while testing spirometry (FVC, PEFR) are typically displayed as a flow-volume loop. The flow-volume loop displays the expiratory effort with volume (in liters) on the x axis and flow (in liters per second) on the y axis. The expiratory effort starts at the intersection of the axes and terminates when the loop again intersects the x axis (i.e., when flow again equals zero.) The flow-volume loop typically displays the immediate posttest inspiration (below the x axis, when flow is negative). The shape of the flow-volume loop can be helpful in assessing the expiratory effort and the presence of certain disease states.

Table 36.2 USING CONFIDENCE INTERVALS TO GRADE SEVERITY OF DEFICITS IN SPIROMETRY

For Both FEV₁ and FVC (Using Confidence Intervals)	
Normal	<1.0 confidence interval from predicted value
Mild deficit	≥1.0–1.75 confidence intervals from predicted value
Moderate deficit	≥1.75–2.50 confidence intervals from predicted value
Severe deficit	≥2.50 confidence intervals from predicted value

For FEV₁ (Using Percentage Predicted)	
Mild	>70% predicted
Moderate	60–69% predicted
Moderately severe	50–59% predicted
Severe	35–49% predicted
Very severe	<35% predicted

A less-than-maximal expiratory effort is present when the terminal aspect of the inspiratory portion of the flow-volume loop (the portion below the x axis, when flow is negative) intersects the x axis left of the y axis. This implies that the subject did not maximally inhale prior to the expiratory effort or there was an air leak during exhalation (see figure 36.1). Other examples of less-than-maximal effort include a blunted peak flow or an abrupt drop to zero flow.

A classic finding of obstructive ventilatory disease is a "coved" appearance of the flow-volume loop. As discussed below (see Obstructive Ventilatory Deficits), airway resistance is increased in obstructive ventilatory deficits because of any process that narrows the airway lumen (i.e., bronchospasm in asthma or airway collapse in emphysema). The coved appearance of the flow-volume loop reflects this increased airway resistance as velocity of flow decreases precipitously compared to predicted values (see figure 36.2). Airways resistance is decreased in patients with restrictive ventilatory deficits while lung volumes are overall reduced (see Restrictive Ventilatory Deficits below), and the flow-volume loop may reflect this. PEFR may be higher than expected even though the FEV_1 and FVC may be reduced, and the FEV_1/FVC ratio may be preserved or even elevated (see figure 36.3). Finally, a fixed upper or central airway obstruction may cause a limitation on the upper maximum of flow velocity; the flow-volume loop reveals a decrease in PEFR with a "plateau" appearance without reduction in overall FVC (see figure 36.4). FEV_1 and FVC are not usually decreased in upper or central airway obstruction.

LUNG VOLUMES: MEASUREMENT AND VALUES

The lung volumes of most clinical interest include the total lung capacity (TLC—the volume of air in the lungs after maximal inhalation), residual volume (RV—the volume

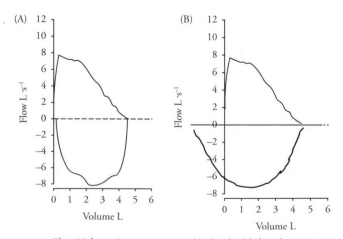

Figure 36.1. Flow-Volume Loop in a Normal Individual (A) and in an Individual Demonstrating Submaximal Expiratory Effort (B). Reprinted with permission from Miller MR, Hankinson J, Brusasco B, et al. Standardisation of spirometry. *Eur Respir J.* 2005;26:319–38. © 2005 European Respiratory Society.

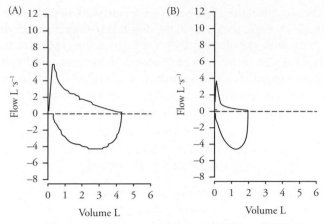

Figure 36.2. Flow-Volume Loop in Individuals with Obstructive Ventilatory Deficits: Asthma (A) and COPD (B). Reprinted with permission from Miller MR, Hankinson J, Brusasco B, et al. Standardisation of spirometry. *Eur Respir J.* 2005;26:319–38. © 2005 European Respiratory Society.

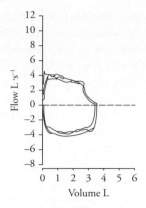

Figure 36.4. Flow-Volume Loop in Fixed Upper Airway Obstruction. Reprinted with permission from Miller MR, Hankinson J, Brusasco B, et al. Standardisation of spirometry. *Eur Respir J.* 2005;26:319–38. © 2005 European Respiratory Society.

of air remaining in the lungs after maximal exhalation), and functional residual capacity (FRC—the volume of air in the lung after a normal tidal volume breath is exhaled). The various lung volumes and lung capacities (a quantity of gas in the lungs calculated by addition or subtraction of two measured lung volumes) are depicted in figure 36.5. In brief, lung volumes are the RV, expiratory reserve volume (ERV), tidal volume (VT), and inspiratory reserve volume (IRV). Lung capacities are the sum of two or more lung volumes. The lung capacities are the inspiratory reserve capacity (IRC = VT + IRV), vital capacity (VC = ERV + IRC), functional residual capacity (FRC = RV + ERV), and TLC (RV + ERV + VT + IRV or VC + RV or FRC + IRC).

Lung volumes are typically measured by one of three techniques: helium dilution, nitrogen washout, or body plethysmography.

The *nitrogen washout method* allows for calculation of lung volumes using the initial concentration of nitrogen in the alveoli and the concentration after breathing 100% oxygen for up to 7 minutes (to "wash out" alveolar nitrogen). In addition, although truncated protocols have been proposed (i.e., breathing 100% oxygen for 5 as opposed to 7 minutes), the nitrogen washout method of measuring lung volumes is time consuming compared to plethysmography.

Plethysmography is based on Boyle's law: $P_1V_1 = k$, where k is a fixed constant. Technically, lung volumes are measured by plethysmography in a sealed chamber in which the volume of air is known and constant (referred to as a variable-pressure chamber). Because people enter into and are sealed within this chamber during testing, the chamber is colloquially referred to as a "body box." There is a mouthpiece within the chamber through which the individual breathes. When the respiratory cycle is at or near FRC, the mouthpiece is occluded by an automated shutter valve. The individual then pants (attempting to inhale and exhale against the closed mouthpiece.) The change in pressure at the mouthpiece, the change in pressure in the plethysmograph, and the known fixed volume of gas in the plethys-

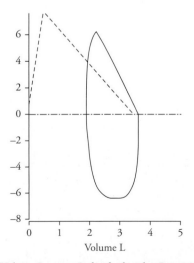

Figure 36.3. Flow-Volume Loop an Individual with a Restrictive Ventilatory Deficit. Reprinted with permission from Pellegrino R, Viegi G, Brusasco B, et al. Interpretative strategies for lung function tests. *Eur Respir J.* 2005;26:948–68. © 2005 European Respiratory Society.

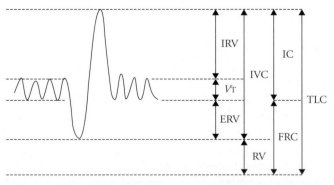

Figure 36.5. Lung Volumes and Capacities. Reprinted with permission from Wanger J, Clausen JL, Coates A, et al. Standardisation of the measurement of lung volumes. *Eur Respir J.* 2005;26:511–22. © 2005 European Respiratory Society.

mograph can be used to calculate the quantity of air in the lungs at FRC. After determining the volume of air in the lungs at FRC, exhalation to RV followed by inhalation to TLC is performed to determine their values of expiratory reserve volume (ERV) and inspiratory vital capacity (IVC), respectively. Plethysmography may overestimate lung volumes. The most important example of this overestimation of lung volumes occurs in patients with obstructive airways deficits and "air trapping" (see Obstructive Ventilatory Deficits, below, for formal definitions of air trapping and hyperinflation). When the shutter valve on the mouthpiece is closed and the patient pants, the assumption is that there is no flow of air (given the closed mouthpiece) and that changes in pressure reflect only changes in volume of the air in the lungs. However, particularly in patients with obstructive deficits, there may be flow between alveoli and extrathoracic airways. Air "trapped" in hyperinflated segments of lung may be liberated by the panting maneuver and flow to large airways; this airflow decreases measured pressure changes (as the pressure generated by panting leads to flow rather than compressed volume). Underestimating pressure changes leads to the volume of air in the lungs being overestimated.

Helium dilution is an alternative method of measuring lung volumes. The helium dilution method may be used when an individual is unable to perform plethysmography (due to dyspnea, claustrophobia, inability to perform the maneuvers, etc.) or when obstructive airways disease is present and there is concern for overestimating lung volumes.

Regardless of the method used to measure lung volumes, the values directly measured include FRC, ERV, and IVC. TLC and RV may be calculated in the following fashion:

$$RV = FRC - ERV$$
$$TLC = RV + IVC$$

As with spirometry (see above), lung volumes are reported as both measured values and as a percentage of a predicted value. Predicted values are generated from large cross-sectional studies. Determinants of predicted lung volumes include height, gender, race/ethnicity, and age. Due to continued lung growth and changes in body habitus and height, age is particularly important in determining predicted values in children and adolescents, and separate prediction equations are used for these populations. For individuals aged ≥18 years, a set of reference equations has been endorsed by the European Respiratory Society and appear to perform well in Caucasian, African-American, and Mexican-American populations. The American Thoracic Society has adopted predictive equations for subjects aged 8–80 years old.

At least two measurements of lung volumes should be performed regardless of the method used, and as noted above, performing three separate measures of ERV and IVC is appropriate to account for effort-dependent variation. Lung volume measurements are considered to be reproducible if the TLC values are within 0.2 L of each other, and in that case the mean of the measured values is reported.

As with spirometry, 95% confidence intervals may be used to grade the severity of abnormalities in measured compared to predicted lung volumes (see table 36.3). Deviations from the predicted values for lung volumes can be quantified as mild, moderate, or severe in nature.

D_LCO: MEASUREMENT AND CORRECTION FACTORS

The diffusing capacity for carbon monoxide (D_LCO) is a test that quantifies the diffusing properties of the alveolar-capillary membrane. The D_LCO provides information about the efficiency of gas exchange at the level of the alveolus and capillary.

The D_LCO is typically measured by a single-breath method. While breathing through a mouthpiece, the patient takes a breath to RV from TLC, inhaling a mixture of air that typically contains a known quantity of an insoluble gas (typically 10% of a gas such as helium, methane, argon, or neon) and 0.3% carbon monoxide (CO). The breath is then held for 10 seconds before exhaling. The first 0.75–1.0 L of the exhaled breath is discarded, as it represents dead space of the tubing and upper airways (if the FVC is <2.0 L, then the first 0.5 L is discarded.) The next 0.5 to 1 L of air is analyzed, and the quantity of the insoluble gas present in the exhaled air indicates the degree of dilution of the inhaled gas with the air already in the alveoli.

Exhaled CO is measured and corrected for dilution by gas already in the alveoli (using the known dilution of the insoluble gas). The difference between the amount of CO inhaled and the amount present in the exhaled gas (corrected for dilution) represents the uptake of CO across the alveolar-capillary membrane. By convention, D_LCO is reported in units of mL/[(min) (mm Hg)], where mL indicates the volume of CO taken up across the alveolar-capillary membrane and mm Hg indicates the partial pressure of CO

Table 36.3 USING CONFIDENCE INTERVALS TO GRADE SEVERITY OF DEFICITS IN TOTAL LUNG CAPACITY: DIFFERENCE OF PREDICTED MINUS MEASURED VALUE FOR MEN AND WOMEN

	MEN	WOMEN
Normal: <1 confidence interval from predicted value	<1.61 L	<1.08 L
Mild deficit: ≥1.0 to 1.5 CI from predicted value	1.61–2.41 L	1.08–1.61 L
Moderate deficit: ≥1.5 to 2.0 CI from predicted value	2.41–3.21 L	1.62–2.15 L
Severe deficit: ≥2.0 CI from predicted value	≥3.22 L	≥2.16 L

in the alveolus. Because the partial pressure of CO in the pulmonary capillaries is normally zero, the partial pressure of CO in the alveolus is essentially the driving pressure of CO across the alveolar-capillary membrane. To account for the length of time of the breath-hold maneuver to allow for transfer of CO across the alveolar-capillary membrane, units of time are present in the denominator. $D_L CO$ may be considered via the following equation:

$$D_L CO = \text{total CO uptake}/(\text{time} \times PA_{CO})$$

The European Respiratory Society prefers to report the amount of CO taken up across the alveolar membrane in millimoles and the partial pressure of CO in kilopascals (i.e., $D_L CO$ is reported as mmol/[(min) (kPa)]).

Correcting for a patient's hemoglobin is a more clinically relevant adjustment of $D_L CO$, as CO binding to hemoglobin is a requisite for CO uptake across the alveolar membrane. The calculation adjusting $D_L CO$ for hemoglobin (Hb) is expressed as follows:

For men: $D_L CO$ (Hb) = $D_L CO \times (1.7 Hb/(10.22 + Hb))$
For women: $D_L CO$ (Hb) = $D_L CO \times (1.7 Hb/(9.38 + Hb))$

The units of hemoglobin in this equation are g/dL. These equations are relevant for Hb concentrations of ≥ 7 g/dL.

OBSTRUCTIVE VENTILATORY DEFICITS

DEFINITION AND CHARACTERISTICS

Obstructive ventilatory deficits are defined by a reduction of expiratory flow as measured by FEV_1 or PEFR. Pathophysiologically, obstructive ventilatory deficits are characterized by increased airways resistance. Increased airways resistance results in impaired air flow. In the later stages of obstructive ventilatory diseases, incomplete exhalation due to increased airways resistance and impaired flow may result in hyperinflation and intrinsic positive end-expiratory pressure (PEEP).

There are a variety of pathologic processes that can cause obstructive ventilatory deficits, ranging from reversible air flow obstruction (i.e., asthma) to permanent changes in the lung parenchyma and airways (i.e., emphysema). Regardless of the underlying process, the primary manifestation of an obstructive ventilatory deficit is a decreased FEV_1 as measured by spirometry. Typically, FVC is *relatively* preserved in obstructive ventilatory diseases compared to the decrease in FEV_1. The relative preservation of FVC occurs as the volume of air in the lungs is not decreased, and given adequate time a patient can exhale a relatively larger quantity of air than possible in 1 second.

In the setting of a decreased FEV_1 and a relatively preserved FVC, the FEV_1/FVC ratio is decreased. This constellation of findings (decreased FEV_1 as compared to FVC and decreased FEV_1/FVC) is the hallmark of obstructive ventilatory deficits.

As described above (see Spirometry above and figure 36.2), the classic coved appearance of a flow-volume loop in a patient with an obstructive ventilatory deficit is due to decreased expiratory flow rates. As depicted on a flow-volume loop, the overall volume of air exhaled may not be significantly decreased compared to predicted values. As the underlying disease process progresses, FVC may decrease (for example, due to progressive air trapping in emphysema); however, the decrease in FEV_1 is by definition out of proportion to the decrease in FVC. However, reduced FEV_1 and reduced FVC with a normal FEV_1/FVC has been reported to occur in up to 10% of patients with a clinical diagnosis of COPD and normal TLC.

Lung volumes may be abnormal in certain obstructive ventilatory deficits. Particularly in emphysema, hyperinflation or air trapping may be present. Air trapping is defined by an increase in RV of >120% of predicted. Hyperinflation is defined as a TLC >120% of predicted and an RV >140% of predicted. Lung volumes can occasionally be elevated without spirometric evidence of an obstructive deficit in normal patients.

DIFFERENTIAL DIAGNOSIS

Any process that increases airways resistance and reduces airflow velocity in a clinically significant manner can result in an obstructive ventilatory deficit. Differentiating between reversible and irreversible processes may be a clinically useful way to approach obstructive ventilatory deficits. The presence of bronchodilator responsiveness (discussed below) is helpful in determining the presence (or absence) of reversibility in most cases. Of course, some pathologic processes may be "partially" reversible, thereby complicating determining the cause of obstruction.

An alternative approach to obstructive ventilatory deficits that may aid in understanding the causative pathophysiological process is to consider the structural deficit leading to airways obstruction. Specifically, abnormalities in the airway lumen, in the wall of the airway, or in the peribronchial structures may each result in an obstructive deficit.

Possible causes of an obstructive ventilatory deficit include chronic obstructive pulmonary disease (COPD) including emphysema and chronic bronchitis as well as asthma, congestive heart failure, bronchiectasis, pneumonia, foreign body aspiration, or bronchiolitis.

GOLD CRITERIA AND CONFIDENCE INTERVALS

COPD is one of the most important and common causes of an obstructive ventilatory deficit. There are various methods for classifying severity of COPD. One of the most disseminated and widely used classification schemes is the GOLD criteria (Global Initiative for Chronic Obstructive Lung Disease).

The GOLD criteria are widely accessible and easy to use for diagnosing and grading the severity of COPD and have raised awareness about COPD (www.goldcopd.com). Although not a perfect tool for classification of severity, the GOLD criteria are useful in considering treatment and prognosis for a symptomatic patient with COPD (see table 33.1 in chapter 33).

BRONCHODILATOR RESPONSIVENESS

Assessing for bronchodilator responsiveness is commonly done in the evaluation of obstructive ventilatory deficits. Bronchodilator response can be assessed in one testing session by administering a short-acting medicine or over the course of two (or more) testing sessions with interval longitudinal treatment with a bronchodilator(s).

Bronchodilator responsiveness is defined as an increase in the percentage predicted FEV_1 and/or FVC of at least 12% and 0.2 L above baseline. Changes of <8% or <0.15 L are thought to be due to test-to-test variability and not due to a medication effect. Although not commonly measured as a marker of bronchodilator responsiveness, improvement in distance walked in the 6-minute walk test is another very reproducible marker of the effectiveness of bronchodilator responsiveness.

The drug, dose, and method of delivery of the bronchodilator for responsiveness assessment are not standardized. Typically when testing bronchodilator responsiveness in one testing session, a short-acting inhaled medicine is appropriate. Inhaled albuterol (four puffs of a 90-µg metered dose inhaler) through a spacer is a typical regimen. An interval of 15–20 minutes between measuring baseline spirometry and postbronchodilator spirometry values allows time for any effect of the medicine to occur. If of particular clinical interest, a different short-acting medication (such as ipratropium) can be used at the request of the ordering physician. Of note, one large study reported >50% bronchodilator responsiveness in patients with moderate to severe COPD when a combination of an inhaled anticholinergic plus an inhaled beta agonist was administered in one testing session.

The clinical relevance of bronchodilator responsiveness (or the absence thereof) is nebulous. Although some individuals may have a correlation between bronchodilator responsiveness and symptom improvement, others may experience significant subjective improvement after treatment with an inhaled bronchodilator despite the lack of improvement in FEV_1 or FVC. A possible explanation for this apparent discordance is that bronchodilators affect airway resistance and airway flow most at tidal volumes. FRC has been shown to decrease after bronchodilator therapy, which may partially explain an improved sense of dyspnea. Therefore, assessing for changes in FEV_1 and FVC by forcibly exhaling from TLC (i.e., performing a FVC breath) may not adequately represent these changes at tidal volume breathing.

HOW PFTs GUIDE TREATMENT

Primarily with regard to COPD, the degree of decrease of the FEV_1 can guide treatment. Treatment for other obstructive ventilatory deficits may be driven by the measured FEV_1; however, for COPD, a structured treatment approach is based primarily on FEV_1 decrement.

For all patients with COPD, risk reduction is appropriate. Specifically, when applicable, encouragement of and assistance with smoking cessation is of the utmost importance. Appropriate vaccinations (influenza and pneumococcal vaccines) are appropriate for all patients with COPD. For patients with mild disease (GOLD stage 1), short-acting bronchodilators on an as-needed basis are usually considered to be sufficient. Patients with moderate (GOLD stage 2) disease should receive long-acting bronchodilators (typically long-acting beta agonists) in addition to short-acting as-needed inhalers. Inhaled corticosteroids are added to the regimen of patients with severe disease (GOLD stage 3). Finally, very severe disease (GOLD stage 4) may necessitate oxygen treatment depending on the patient's oxygenation. Lung volume reduction surgery may be offered to a very select group of patients with primarily apical bullous disease.

The value of continued patient education is important in improving patients' understanding of their disease. Pulmonary rehabilitation has been demonstrated to improve patients' quality of life, although there has not been a demonstrable effect on mortality. When to consider referral to pulmonary rehabilitation is unclear, but the GOLD criteria advocate early (i.e., GOLD stage 1) referral.

The BODE score is a multifactorial index used to grade the severity of disease in patients with COPD. BODE is an acronym for *b*ody mass index, airflow *o*bstruction (as measured by FEV_1), symptoms of *d*yspnea, and *e*xercise capacity (as measured by a 6-minute walk). The BODE score has been shown to be better than FEV_1 alone for predicting mortality in patients with COPD and can be a guide to treatment.

RESTRICTIVE VENTILATORY DEFICITS

DEFINITION AND CHARACTERISTICS

Restrictive ventilatory deficits are defined by abnormally reduced lung volumes. Typically, confidence intervals around the percentage predicted values of lung volumes are used to determine the degree of restriction. In restrictive diseases, lung volumes are decreased below their expected values

Spirometry has been shown to be sensitive in ruling out restrictive ventilatory deficits; in one large retrospective study, a normal FVC was associated with restrictive disease in less than 3% of cases. An abnormal FVC with a normal FEV_1/FVC ratio, however, was present in patients with normal lung volumes in >40% of cases. Therefore, spirometric measurements of FVC can be considered relatively sensitive but not specific. Measuring lung volumes is necessary to confirm a restrictive ventilatory deficit when the FVC is abnormally low with a normal FEV_1/FVC.

It is important to emphasize that in restrictive ventilatory deficits caused by parenchymal diseases (such as fibrosis), airways resistance is not increased. In fact, PEFR may be increased compared to predicted values. This may be due to the airways being in effect "tethered" open by fibrotic changes of the lung parenchyma. Not all restrictive disease is due to pulmonary fibrotic changes, however, so an increase in PEFR, although suggestive, is not diagnostic of a restrictive ventilatory deficit.

DIFFERENTIAL DIAGNOSIS

Restrictive ventilatory deficits can be due to any process that results in decreased lung volumes. Fibrotic changes in the lung parenchyma itself can manifest as a restrictive deficit as the lung tissue becomes less compliant. The loss of compliance leads to lower lung volumes as a given inspiratory effort results in less inhaled volume.

Restrictive deficits can also occur from extrapulmonary processes. Pleural diseases, from pleural effusions to pleural scarring and fibrosis, can limit lung expansion and manifest as low lung volumes and a restrictive ventilatory pattern. The lungs themselves may have normal elastic properties, but the extrinsic compression from diseased pleura may limit the volume that can be inhaled.

Chest wall pathology can similarly result in a restrictive deficit. Kyphosis and/or scoliosis may result in restrictive physiology because the muscles of respiration are placed at a mechanical disadvantage. With severe curvature of the vertebral column, the diaphragm and accessory muscles may not be able to generate maximal inspiratory forces leading to decreased lung volumes. Chest wall trauma, including broken ribs or scarring (i.e., secondary to burns), may result in decreased mobility of the chest wall, extrinsic compression of the lungs, and a restrictive ventilatory deficit. Similarly, extreme obesity can cause a restrictive ventilatory deficit by a similar mechanism: extrinsic compression by excess adipose tissue can limit maximal expansion of the respiratory system.

Finally, neuromuscular diseases may cause a restrictive ventilatory deficit. Weakened or poorly functioning respiratory muscles (whether due to a myopathy or neuropathy) can limit a patient's ability to ventilate, resulting in low lung volumes. One way of distinguishing the neuromuscular disorders from other types of restrictive disease is through the use of respiratory muscle forces (often reduced) as described below. Additionally, because the ability to exhale completely to RV is an effort-dependent process, the RV may actually be elevated in neuromuscular weakness.

From the above considerations, specific pathologic processes that may result in a restrictive ventilatory deficit include pulmonary fibrosis, sarcoidosis, hypersensitivity pneumonitis, medication/toxic pneumonitis, collagen-vascular diseases (i.e., scleroderma, systemic lupus erythematosus, rheumatoid arthritis), pneumothorax, pleural effusion, pleural fibrosis, severe morbid obesity, scoliosis, kyphosis, chest wall trauma or scarring, and ankylosing spondylitis. Possible neuromuscular causes of restrictive ventilatory deficits include Guillain-Barré, amyotrophic lateral sclerosis, myasthenia gravis, and muscular dystrophies.

GRADING SEVERITY

As mentioned above, confidence intervals below the predicted values of lung volumes can serve to grade the severity of the restrictive deficit. As detailed in table 36.3, the quantitative decrease of the measured TLC below the predicted value is used to grade the severity of the restrictive deficit.

Unlike obstructive deficits (COPD in particular), the severity of restrictive ventilatory deficits does not necessarily guide treatment. Treating the underlying pathologic process causing the restrictive ventilatory deficit is appropriate.

REDUCED $D_L CO$

DEFINITION, CHARACTERISTICS, AND PHYSIOLOGY OF DECREASED $D_L CO$

Decreased diffusing capacity for carbon monoxide ($D_L CO$) indicates impaired diffusion of carbon monoxide (CO) across the alveolar-capillary membrane into the bloodstream and is thought to correlate with impaired diffusion of oxygen across the alveolar-capillary membrane. However, CO uptake is dependent not only on diffusion across the alveolar-capillary membrane but also on binding to hemoglobin. Therefore, the term "diffusing capacity" is inaccurate in that it implies that the transfer of CO from the alveolus to the bloodstream is dependent on diffusion alone. As such, the term *transfer factor* (TLCO), rather than $D_L CO$, is used outside of the United States.

The $D_L CO$ may be conceptualized through the following equations:

$$D_L CO = \text{total CO uptake}/(\text{time} \times PA_{CO})$$
$$\text{or}$$
$$D_L CO = VCO/(PA_{CO} - Pc_{CO})$$

where VCO is the uptake of CO (mL CO/min), PA_{CO} is the alveolar pressure of CO, and Pc_{CO} is the average pulmonary capillary pressure of CO. The Pc_{CO} is usually zero.

As with measurements of spirometry and lung volume, confidence intervals are used to grade the severity of reductions in $D_L CO$. Reductions in percentage predicted of $D_L CO$ can also be used to grade severity. Table 36.4 delineates a schema for grading the severity of reductions in $D_L CO$.

Table 36.4 USING CONFIDENCE INTERVALS TO GRADE SEVERITY OF DECREASES IN D$_L$CO: DIFFERENCE OF PREDICTED MINUS MEASURED VALUE FOR MEN AND WOMEN

	MEN	WOMEN
Normal: <1 confidence interval from predicted value	<7.99	<6.50
Mild deficit: ≥1.0–1.75 CI from predicted value	≥7.99–13.98	≥6.5–11.37
Moderate deficit: ≥1.75–2.5 CI from predicted value	13.99–19.97	11.38–16.24
Severe deficit: ≥2.5 CI from predicted value	≥19.98	≥16.25

NOTE: Units are in mL/[(mm Hg)(min)].

As described above, the D$_L$CO may be "corrected" for hemoglobin level. This is a physiologically meaningful correction as CO uptake is directly dependent on hemoglobin concentration. Decreases in D$_L$CO corrected for hemoglobin concentration [D$_L$CO(Hb)] may be graded with confidence intervals.

CLINICAL UTILITY AND MEANING OF D$_L$CO

The D$_L$CO can provide useful information about the functional relationship of the alveoli and the pulmonary capillaries. By extension, the D$_L$CO may provide some information about gas exchange in general. Given similarities of the mechanism of CO uptake (diffusing across the alveolar membrane and being taken up by hemoglobin) to oxygen uptake, clinicians extrapolate the results of D$_L$CO measurements to oxygen uptake. When D$_L$CO is extrapolated in this fashion, it at best provides a rough guide of actual oxygen diffusion and uptake.

DIFFERENTIAL DIAGNOSIS

D$_L$CO may be decreased or increased as compared to the predicted value. As with spirometry and lung volumes, the predicted value of D$_L$CO is determined by predictive equations that take into account age, height, gender, and ethnicity/race. The grade of severity of the difference in the measured D$_L$CO from the predicted D$_L$CO is determined by confidence intervals (see table 36.4).

D$_L$CO may be increased by a number of processes. Increased CO uptake is primarily dependent on the increased availability of hemoglobin for binding CO, as the pressure gradient across the alveolar membrane is constant from test to test, and changes in the alveolar-capillary membrane only serve to decrease CO diffusion and subsequent uptake. Conditions that result in increased cardiac output through the pulmonary circulation can result in increased measured D$_L$CO compared to the predicted value. Specifically, exercise is a condition in which cardiac output is increased, pulmonary vascular resistance (PVR) decreases, and minute ventilation increases. These physiological changes result in increased pulmonary capillary blood volume; therefore, when measured immediately after exercise, D$_L$CO is increased compared to predicted values. Obesity is associated with an increased D$_L$CO; the mechanism of this is unclear but is thought to be related to increased cardiac output and increased blood volume in the pulmonary circulation. When measured in the supine position, the D$_L$CO may be modestly, but not clinically significantly, increased. This is thought to be to due to increasing the proportion of the lung that is well perfused (West zone 3). Polycythemic states may result in an increased D$_L$CO as more hemoglobin is available for CO binding. Similarly, intra-alveolar hemorrhage may result in an increased D$_L$CO, even in cases where the alveolar-capillary membrane is abnormal, as CO may bind to hemoglobin without having to pass through the alveolar-capillary membrane. Finally, left-to-right intracardiac shunts may increase D$_L$CO due to increased cardiac output and blood volume through the pulmonary circulation.

Decreased D$_L$CO is typically due to conditions in which the alveolar membrane is abnormal, the cardiac output through the pulmonary circulation is decreased, or conditions in which there is a decrease in hemoglobin available for binding CO. D$_L$CO may occur with restrictive lung deficits (i.e., pulmonary fibrosis) or obstructive ventilatory deficits (i.e., COPD.) In these conditions, lung parenchymal changes lead to perturbations in pulmonary capillary perfusion, which in turn result in a decrease in the hemoglobin available to bind CO and thereby decrease uptake.

When a decreased D$_L$CO is encountered in a patient with other PFT abnormalities (such as decreased lung volumes and/or decreased FEV$_1$), a unifying diagnosis to explain all the abnormalities should be sought. For example, a patient with reduced lung volumes and a reduced D$_L$CO may have idiopathic pulmonary fibrosis causing a restrictive ventilatory deficit (due to parenchymal fibrosis and decreased lung compliance) and a decreased D$_L$CO (due to fibrotic changes of the alveolar membrane and loss of alveolar surface area, leading to impaired diffusion of CO).

When the D$_L$CO is decreased and other PFTs are normal, there is a limited differential diagnosis. Conditions that affect the pulmonary circulation and thereby reduce functional pulmonary capillary circulation may cause a decreased D$_L$CO. Specifically, pulmonary vascular disease (including both pulmonary arterial hypertension and thromboembolic disease) is a possible explanation for a reduced D$_L$CO and otherwise normal PFTs. Pulmonary hypertension results in elevated PVR and decreased blood volume in the pulmonary circulation with decreased hemoglobin available for CO binding. Methemoglobinemia or carboxyhemoglobinemia can result in a decreased D$_L$CO with otherwise normal PFTs, as even though there may be a normal quantity of hemoglobin passing through the pulmonary circulation, the binding sites are already occupied. In carboxyhemoglobinemia, there is increased partial pressure of CO in pulmonary blood, which decreases the diffusion gradient for CO across the alveolar membrane. In methemoglobinemia, the binding sites for CO have undergone a conformational change and cannot bind CO. Anemia can also result in a reduced D_LCO.

ASSOCIATION OF D_LCO WITH FUNCTIONAL CAPACITY

With worsening measured D_LCO, functional capacity decreases. As described above, although CO and oxygen have similar properties of diffusion and hemoglobin binding, there are important differences that make direct comparisons difficult; for this reason, the relationship between D_LCO and function capacity is not linear.

One manner in which D_LCO represents functional capacity is in its role as a marker of a patient's ability to tolerate surgery. Specifically, D_LCO has been observed to predict postoperative complications in lung resection surgeries. A predicted postoperative D_LCO of <40% predicted is associated with increased mortality in several studies, and a preoperative D_LCO of <60% predicted has been associated with increased mortality in some studies.

MIXED DISORDERS: INTERPRETING MIXED OBSTRUCTIVE AND RESTRICTIVE DEFICITS

Obstructive and restrictive ventilatory deficits may both occur simultaneously. As previously described, the FEV_1/FVC ratio is helpful in determining the presence of an obstructive versus restrictive deficit. A decreased FEV_1 and a decreased measured FEV_1/FVC ratio compared to the predicted value indicate an obstructive ventilatory deficit. A decreased FEV_1 with a normal measured FEV_1/FVC ratio is consistent with a restrictive deficit (although this should be confirmed by measuring lung volumes).

It is not possible by spirometry alone to diagnose a mixed obstructive and restrictive ventilatory disorder. However, a decreased FEV_1/FVC ratio in the setting of *both* a low FEV_1 *and* FVC is suggestive of a mixed obstructive and restrictive ventilatory deficit. If this pattern is observed, then lung volumes can be measured to confirm a diagnosis of a restrictive deficit (in addition to an obstructive deficit diagnosed by spirometry). Mixed deficits are commonly characterized by a normal FRC, decreased TLC and increased RV. An increased RV is indicative of air trapping in the setting of an obstructive deficit, whereas a decreased TLC reflects the restrictive process.

The differential diagnosis of a mixed restrictive and obstructive ventilatory deficit is broad and can include any combination of restrictive and obstructive processes. Most commonly seen is the combination of a restrictive process (such as interstitial lung disease) and COPD. Less commonly, processes that are classically restrictive may have an obstructive component; examples include lymphangioleiomyomatosis, tuberous sclerosis, chronic hypersensitivity pneumonitis, sarcoidosis, and eosinophilic granulomatosis.

RESPIRATORY MUSCLE FORCES: MIP AND MEP

DEFINITION

Maximal inspiratory pressure (MIP) and maximal expiratory pressure (MEP) are the primary measurements of pressures generated by respiratory muscles. By extension, the MIP and MEP provide information about respiratory muscle strength and function.

MIP and MEP are particularly useful measurements in assessing patients with and for neuromuscular disease, whether they are inherent (Duchenne, amyotrophic lateral sclerosis) or acquired (myasthenia gravis, Guillain-Barré, critical illness neuropathy, steroid-induced polymyoneuropathy).

MIP is used as a marker of readiness for extubation in mechanically ventilated patients. An adequate, coordinated maximal inspiratory effort is considered one predictor of successful extubation. In this setting, the term NIF or negative inspiratory force is often used in place of MIP.

Normal measured values for MIP are approximately -70 to -100 cm H_2O, and a normal measured MEP is approximately 100 to 150 cm H_2O. As with other parameters of pulmonary function, predicted values for MIP and MEP may be generated by using reference equations. There is no consensus as to which reference equation is the standard for determining predicted MIP or MEP. Regardless of the equation used, the measured MIP and MEP are displayed as both a measured value (in centimeters of H_2O) and as the percentage predicted.

Low values for MIP in particular may be related to submaximal subject effort. Performing a MIP test can be uncomfortable for a subject, and early termination of inspiratory effort before generating a true maximal inspiratory effort is common.

DIFFERENTIAL DIAGNOSIS

Respiratory muscle weakness as diagnosed by abnormal MIP and/or MEP can by due to a variety of processes. Neuromuscular pathologies are the most common causes of decreased MIP and MEP. Inherent or congenital neuromuscular processes that can lead to respiratory muscle weakness include muscular dystrophies (such as Duchenne), spinal cord processes (amyotrophic lateral sclerosis), or other primary neuromuscular pathologies.

Acquired neuromuscular diseases include Guillain-Barré, myasthenia gravis, critical illness neuropathy, and steroid-induced polymyoneuropathy. Vasculitis, dermatomyositis, polymyositis, and Eaton-Lambert syndrome may all cause compromised neuromuscular function.

Diaphragmatic dysfunction or paralysis may occur from a variety of causes; unilateral diaphragmatic paralysis is usually well tolerated clinically but may result in decreased MIP and MEP and occasionally to symptoms of dyspnea. Bilateral diaphragmatic paralysis typically causes symptoms of dyspnea, particularly worse in the supine position, and results in decreased MIP and MEP.

Central nervous system pathology can lead to decreased respiratory muscle function as well. Infections such as viral encephalopathies (poliomyelitis, West Nile virus, etc.) may lead to depressed respiratory muscle function and decreased MIP and MEP. Spinal cord compression, particularly in the high cervical cord, can lead to decreased MIP and MEP by causing compromised phrenic nerve activity and diaphragmatic dysfunction

Finally, toxic exposures or metabolic abnormalities may cause decreased MIP and MEP. Specifically, hypokalemia, hypophosphatemia, botulism, organophosphate poisoning, and heavy metal toxicities are all possible causes of respiratory muscle compromise and decreased MIP and MEP.

CLINICAL UTILITY: WHEN TO ORDER, HOW TO INTERPRET, FURTHER TESTING

Measuring MIP and MEP in patients with unexplained dyspnea may be useful in identifying an underlying diagnosis, particularly when a neuromuscular process is suspected. When orthopnea is a component of shortness of breath and diaphragmatic dysfunction is suspected, measuring respiratory muscle forces may be diagnostically helpful.

When the MIP and MEP are low, further workup can include an electroneurogram (ENG) and/or electromyogram (EMG). These tests are useful in determining a neuronal versus muscular contribution to respiratory muscle weakness. Phrenic nerve ENG may be performed to identify diaphragmatic dysfunction. The "sniff test" is a less sensitive test of diaphragmatic dysfunction; the patient is asked to rapidly inhale (i.e., "sniff") while diaphragmatic movement (or the lack thereof) is monitored fluoroscopically.

Muscle biopsy in selected patients can be diagnostic for polymyositis, mitochondrial diseases, and myopathies.

ADVANCED PFTs

RESISTANCE AND COMPLIANCE

The resistance of the airways to airflow may be estimated when performing PFTs. A number of assumptions are made in estimating airways resistance, and the clinical utility of this measured value in isolation is uncertain. However, measured airways resistance, when correlated with the patient's symptoms and other measures of pulmonary function (such as spirometry), can serve to further characterize a patient's pulmonary physiology.

The resistance to airflow is determined by both the airways (determined by endobronchial obstruction, bronchospasm, and/or flow limitation) and the pulmonary parenchyma (specifically in the setting of noncompliant lungs). Typically, the majority of resistance to flow is from the airways rather than the pulmonary parenchyma. It is estimated that the airways account for approximately 80% of the resistance to airflow. The measured resistance reported with PFTs is assumed to reflect the resistance of the airways, although in the setting of decreased lung compliance this may be an inaccurate assumption.

Resistance is defined as the change in pressure divided by flow:

$$\text{Resistance} = \text{Pressure difference (cm } H_2O)/\text{Airflow (L/sec)}$$

The pressure gradient between the mouth and the alveoli is the gradient of interest when estimating resistance. Changes in pressure are measured via plethysmography as described above. Airflow at the mouth can be measured at the same time, and resistance can be calculated. Resistance may be measured while the patient is panting or during tidal breathing.

In considering airways resistance, it is worthwhile to recall that as described by Poiseuille's law, the resistance of a tube is dependent on viscosity of air flowing, the length of the tube, and the fourth power of the radius of the tube.

$$R = (8 \times \text{viscosity} \times \text{length})/(\pi \times \text{radius}^4)$$

This measured resistance may be quite variable between measurements, and the normal range for airways resistance is poorly characterized. The resistance to airflow is of uncertain clinical utility.

Lung *compliance* is the ability of the lungs to stretch to accommodate volume. Compliance is defined as the change in volume divided by the change in pressure:

$$\text{Compliance} = \text{Volume difference}/\text{Pressure difference}$$

Compliance is affected by numerous pathologies. COPD results in parenchymal destruction, loss of the innate elastic recoil of the lungs, and increased compliance. Pulmonary fibrosis results in decreased distensibility and decreased compliance. As with airways resistance, the clinical utility of measured compliance in isolation is questionable. However, when correlated with the clinical scenario and other pulmonary function tests, the measured compliance may provide useful or corroborating information.

BRONCHOPROVOCATION

Methacholine challenge is the most common method of performing bronchoprovocation in an effort to diagnose hyperreactivity of the airways and the clinical disorder of asthma. Methacholine challenge is reserved for patients in whom the diagnosis of asthma is elusive despite prior investigations, such as spirometry performed pre- and post–bronchodilator administration. Methacholine challenge is very sensitive but not specific. Patients with COPD, CHF, bronchitis, cystic fibrosis, and other conditions may have airways hyperreactivity and therefore a positive methacholine challenge test.

Contraindications to methacholine challenge include a FEV_1 <1.0 L (or <50% predicted), a heart attack or stroke within 3 months, uncontrolled hypertension (>200/100 mm Hg), and aortic aneurysm (ATS, 2000).

There are different protocols for the administration of methacholine during testing. In all protocols, increasing concentrations of aerosolized methacholine are administered, and subsequently spirometry is performed. One method of administering methacholine uses increasing concentrations of methacholine, with diluents at 0.0625, 0.25, 1.0, 4.0, and 16 mg/mL of methacholine (ATS, 2000). Five doses of each concentration of methacholine are administered prior to measuring spirometry. Two acceptable efforts should be performed after each concentration of methacholine.

If FEV_1 *decreases* by ≥20% from the baseline (diluent) level after a given concentration of methacholine, then no further doses should be given. Similarly, if the FEV_1 does not decrease by ≥20% after the highest concentration of methacholine (16 mg/mL), no further doses of methacholine should be given.

The PC20 is the concentration of methacholine that causes significant bronchoconstriction as defined by a decrease in FEV_1 of ≥20%. If a decrease in FEV_1 of ≥20% is not reached by 16 mg/mL of methacholine, then the PC20 is reported as >16 mg/mL. A PC20 of >8 mg/mL represents normal bronchial responsiveness. A PC20 of 4–8 is a borderline test, a PC20 of 1–4 indicates mild bronchial hyperresponsiveness, and a PC20 of <1.0 indicates moderate to severe bronchial hyperresponsiveness.

The results of the methacholine test alone do not determine whether the patient has asthma. Rather, the PC20 must be correlated with the likelihood that a patient has asthma based on his or her clinical symptoms. Patients who smoke or who have allergic rhinitis are prone to have reactive airways and thereby a low PC20. Correlating clinical symptoms with PC20 reduces false-positive methacholine challenges.

False-negative results are uncommon; as noted above, the methacholine challenge is sensitive for bronchial hyperreactivity. When the pretest probability of asthma is 30–70%, the negative predictive value of the methacholine challenge is 90% (Gilbert, 1990).

False-positive results are more likely to occur in patients with allergic rhinitis and in smokers with COPD. In addition, methacholine challenge may result in acute inspiratory vocal cord adduction without reactive airways disease, resulting in a false-positive result.

Methacholine is not the only manner in which to perform bronchoprovocation. Exercise can be used as a challenge in an effort to induce bronchial hyperreactivity. There are various protocols for performing bronchoprovocatory exercise. Typically, 4–6 minutes of near-maximum exercise is performed on a treadmill or a cycle ergometer. The cool, dry air the patient breathes during the test is also thought to contribute to bronchial hyperreactivity.

ADDITIONAL READING

Aaron SD, Dales RE, Cardinal P. How accurate is spirometry at predicting restrictive pulmonary impairment? *Chest.* 1999;115:869–73.

American Thoracic Society. ATS statement: Guidelines for Methacholine and Exercise Challenge Testing 1999. *Am J Respir Crit Care Med.* 2000;161:309–29.

American Thoracic Society. ATS statement: Guidelines for the Six-Minute Walk Test. *Am J Respir Crit Care Med.* 2002;166:111–7.)

Brand PL, Quanjer PH, Postma DS, et al. Interpretation of bronchodilator response in patients with obstructive airways disease. The Dutch Chronic Non-Specific Lung Disease (CNSLD) Study Group. *Thorax.* 1992;47:429–36.

Brusasco V, Crapo R, Viegi G; American Thoracic Society; European Respiratory Society. Coming together: The ATS/ERS consensus on clinical pulmonary function testing. *Eur Respir J.* 2005;26(1): 1–2.

Crapo RO. Pulmonary-function testing. *N Engl J Med.* 1994; 331(1):25–30.

Gilbert R, Auchincloss JH Jr. Post-test probability of asthma following methacholine challenge. *Chest.* 1990;97(3):562–5.

MacIntyre N, Crapo RO, Viegi G, et al. Standardisation of the single-breath determination of carbon monoxide uptake in the lung. *Eur Respir J.* 2005;26:720–35.

Miller MR, Crapo R, Hankinson J, et al; ATS/ERS Task Force. General considerations for lung function testing. *Eur Respir J.* 2005; 26(1):153–61.

Miller MR, Hankinson J, Bruasasco V, et al. Standardisation of spirometry. *Eur Respir J.* 2005;26:319–38.

Newth CJ, Enright P, Johnson RL. Multiple-breath nitrogen washout techniques: Including measurements with patients on ventilators. *Eur Respir J.* 1997;10:2174–85.

Pellegrino R, Viegi G, Bruasasco V, et al. Interpretative strategies for lung function tests. *Eur Respir J.* 2005;26:948–68.

Swanney MP, Jensen RL, Crichton DA, Beckert LE, Cardno LA, Crapo RO. FEV_6 is an acceptable surrogate for FVC in the spirometric diagnosis of airway obstruction and restriction. *Am J Respir Crit Care Med.* 2000;162:917–9.

Tashkin DP, Celli B, Decramer M, et al. Bronchodilator responsiveness in patients with COPD. *Eur Respir J.* 2008;31:742–50.

QUESTIONS

QUESTION 1. A 63-year-old man presents to clinic with a chief complaint of intermittent wheezing, chest tightness, and dyspnea that primarily occurs with exertion. He has smoked a pack of cigarettes daily for almost 40 years. The wheezing, chest tightness, and dyspnea with exertion have occurred intermittently over the years but became progressively more frequent approximately 2 years ago. He has no other associated symptoms or known past medical history. As part of his evaluation, he undergoes PFTs.

The most likely finding would be:

A. $FEV_1/FVC < 0.7$ due to obstructive airways disease
B. TLC decreased due to accumulation of mucus in his airways
C. Normal FEV_1 and decreased FVC due to goblet cell proliferation
D. Increased D_LCO due to increased cardiac output
E. Low FEV_1 and FVC with a normal FEV_1/FVC

QUESTION 2. A 65-year-old man presents to clinic with dyspnea and dry cough. He has been feeling more and more short of breath over the last 8 months, particularly with exertion. He doesn't recall any new exposures or recent illnesses. He has no other complaints. His exam reveals a heart rate of 115 beats per minute, a blood pressure of 110/60 mm Hg, a respiratory rate of 16, and a resting oxygen saturation of 89% on room air at rest. His pulmonary exam is notable for bilateral diffuse dry crackles on inhalation. He undergoes PFTs.

The most likely finding would be:

A. Low FEV_1, FVC, and FEV_1/FVC
B. Low FEV_1 with a normal FVC
C. Increased D_LCO due to increased cardiac output
D. Decreased TLC but normal RV
E. Low FEV_1 and FVC with a normal or elevated FEV_1/FVC

QUESTION 3. A 23-year-old woman with a history of asthma presents to the emergency department with 2 days of worsening cough, wheezing, chest tightness, and dyspnea. She ran out of her inhalers a week ago and has been taking no medicine for her asthma during that time. Her peak flow rate on presentation is 150 L/min; her normal, baseline peak flow rate is 400 L/min. On exam, her heart rate is 140 beats per minute, her blood pressure is 150/90 mm Hg, her respiratory rate is 24 breaths per minute, and her oxygen saturation is 94% on room air at rest. She is uncomfortable appearing, in severe respiratory distress. She has poor air movement with inspiratory and expiratory wheezing on pulmonary auscultation. She does not respond to nebulizer treatments and steroids and is ultimately intubated.

Which of the following ventilatory parameters would you expect to find?

A. Low compliance
B. Low peak inspiratory pressure with elevated plateau pressure

C. Elevated peak inspiratory pressure with normal airways resistance
D. Elevated peak inspiratory pressure with elevated airways resistance
E. A Pao_2/Fio_2 of <100

QUESTION 4. A 45-year-old man is admitted after a motor vehicle accident. He has suffered multiple fractures and has a pulmonary contusion. He is hypoxemic on room air with diffuse pulmonary infiltrates. An arterial blood gas on room air prior to intubation demonstrates pH 7.48, $Paco_2$ 32, Pao_2 45. He is intubated and placed on mechanical ventilation. A chest x-ray demonstrates bilateral fluffy infiltrates. He has no history of heart disease and has no clinical signs of congestive heart failure. The respiratory therapist checks the patient's mechanics on the ventilator.

You would predict that she will find:

A. Increased resistance and normal compliance
B. Increased resistance and increased compliance
C. Normal resistance and increased compliance
D. Normal resistance and decreased compliance
E. Normal resistance and normal compliance

QUESTION 5. A 48-year-old man with a known history of advancing amyotrophic lateral sclerosis presents to clinic for follow-up. His wife has noticed that he has been breathing more rapidly over the past few weeks, and the patient feels that he is subjectively working harder to breathe. He feels particularly short of breath when he lies down at night, and he awakens several times a night gasping for breath. These episodes are relieved when his wife helps him sit up.

Which of these findings would support his restrictive physiology being a result of neuromuscular weakness and *not* decreased lung compliance or chest wall stiffness?

A. Decreased TLC and decreased RV
B. Decreased TLC and normal RV
C. Decreased TLC and normal FRC
D. Normal TLC and decreased RV
E. Normal TLC and normal FRC

ANSWERS

1. A
2. E
3. D
4. D
5. C

37.

CHEST X-RAY REFRESHER

Christopher H. Fanta

This exercise provides an opportunity to consider common radiographic patterns in pulmonary diseases, identify specific images helpful in the diagnosis of pulmonary diseases, and review certain topics discussed elsewhere in the Pulmonary Medicine section of the *Intensive Review of Internal Medicine* course. Discussing the findings on your patient's chest radiograph with your local radiologist—you providing clinical data and a grounding in internal medicine and the radiologist offering insights into the radiographic findings and potential causes for those findings—is one of the more enjoyable clinical interactions in medicine. I encourage you at any opportunity to review the actual chest images obtained on your patients rather than relying exclusively on the written reports, just as you might want to inspect your patient's actual electrocardiogram tracing when considering his or her cardiac status. Pattern recognition remains an important part of how we process medical information, and like any skill it improves with practice.

This *Chest X-Ray Refresher* is organized as a game. For each of the three topics to be discussed, we offer four chest x-rays and four clinical histories. The order of each set is random. The exercise asks that you consider the clues in the history and the findings on chest x-ray to match the history with the x-ray. In many instances, the combination will suggest a diagnosis or a limited differential of diagnostic possibilities. The three topics to be discussed are hemoptysis, chronic interstitial lung diseases, and obstructive lung diseases.

HEMOPTYSIS

After obtaining a history and performing a physical examination, the next step in the evaluation of the patient with hemoptysis is usually a chest x-ray. Even episodes of minor hemoptysis warrant an initial chest x-ray because serious illnesses (such as lung cancer, pneumonia, tuberculosis, and pulmonary embolism) can present with small amounts of expectorated blood. An abnormal chest x-ray may point to the source of bleeding and to its cause. Further workup is often then directed at determining the cause of the radiographic abnormality. Diagnostic evaluation and treatment may vary widely depending on chest x-ray findings, as illustrated by our four examples (figures 37.1–4).

- Case 1. Expectoration of blood-streaked sputum preceded by chronic early morning cough in a 2-pack-per-day cigarette smoker. Physical exam notable for clubbing and obvious weight loss.

- Case 2. Several days of hemoptysis with progressive shortness of breath; dark-colored urine and serum creatinine of 2.5 mg/dL.

- Case 3. Four weeks of cough with discolored sputum intermittently mixed with blood; fevers, night sweats, and significant weight loss.

- Case 4. Hemoptysis and pleuritic chest pain on the third postoperative day.

The first chest film (figure 37.1) has several areas of abnormality within the lung parenchyma. Abnormal opacities can be seen within the right upper lobe, right middle lobe (obscuring the normal sharp silhouette made by juxtaposition of the right heart border and aerated lung tissue in the right middle lobe), and the left mid-lung zone. Most striking is the abnormality in the right upper lobe. On close inspection, there are two distinct features to this area of opacities. First, in the right apex one can make out a ring of opacity surrounding aerated lung—a thick-walled lung cavity. The rim of this cavity is several millimeters thick (4–5 mm) and irregular along its inner margin. Second, the base of the opacities in the right upper lobe is curvilinear, making an upward bowing arc from hilum to lateral pleural surface. This linear opacity bears the characteristic shape of the minor fissure pulled cephalad by right upper lobe volume loss.

The differential diagnosis of a pulmonary cavity includes tuberculosis, cavitary bacterial lung abscess, cavitary lung

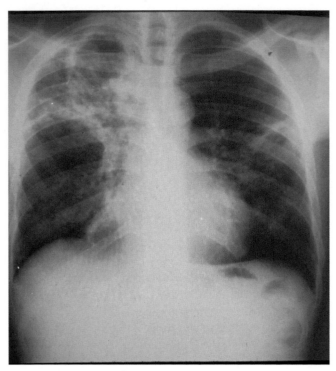

Figure 37.1. Hemoptysis: Chest X-ray 1.

cancer, and pulmonary vasculitis (e.g., Wegener granulomatosis). The upper lobe location and associated volume loss are suggestive of mycobacterial disease such as tuberculosis. Which of the four clinical histories might fit with this x-ray appearance? Our choice is case history 3, the patient with subacute to chronic purulent sputum production with blood admixed plus night sweats, fever, and weight loss. The chest x-ray together with this brief history raise high the suspicion of cavitary tuberculosis, with multifocal spread of infection in both lungs. Consider the initial evaluation and treatment in this patient: have the patient wear a face mask; if hospitalized, request a negative-pressure isolation room; sputum is to be sent on at least three occasions for mycobacterial (acid-fast bacilli or AFB) culture and smear; and antituberculous therapy with three or four drugs is likely soon to be initiated.

The second chest x-ray in this series (figure 37.2) has two major left-sided abnormalities notable as one inspects the normal contours of the hilar and mediastinal structures and of the diaphragms and pleural surfaces. There is a large, rounded opacity that at its top begins at the level of the arch of the aorta and then obliterates both the aortopulmonary recess and the left hilar shadows. It looks like a large mass. In addition, the left hemidiaphragm is raised cephalad several centimeters above its usual position. A third finding of note on this chest x-ray is the hazy fanlike opacity with sharp medial border that extends "northeast" from the hilar area into the region of the left upper lobe. It is this appearance that is particularly worth remembering: the image of left upper lobe collapse. Unlike the right upper lobe, which collapses as an opacity that fills the right apex, the left upper

lobe collapses anteriorly (its apex still tethered at the hilum), allowing aerated left lower lobe tissue to fill the left apex.

As in any lobar atelectasis, there must be adjustment of other structures to compensate for the volume loss—cephalad movement of the ipsilateral diaphragm, shifting of mediastinal structures (sometimes including the heart) toward the side of collapse, and overexpansion of the remaining ipsilateral lobe(s) of the lung. In this example the left hemidiaphragm has shifted dramatically upward, perhaps in compensation for left upper lobe collapse, perhaps also due to phrenic nerve injury with hemidiaphragmatic paralysis.

What is the cause of left upper lobe collapse in this case? It is likely the result of proximal obstruction of the left upper lobe bronchus by the large medial mass. In a patient with hemoptysis, we would strongly suspect a neoplasm, probably a lung cancer. Case history 1 seems the best fit: a cigarette smoker with symptoms of chronic bronchitis (daily early morning cough) and weight loss whose physical examination indicates (among other likely findings) clubbing of the digits. Evaluation of this patient with hemoptysis might include further imaging (chest computed tomography [CT]), sputum for cytology, and probable bronchoscopy for visualization of the airway obstruction and tissue sampling. Treatment will depend on the type of neoplasm and the anatomic extent of tumor involvement (both within and outside the thorax) but might include external beam radiation, chemotherapy, and possibly endobronchial approaches to opening the left upper lobe bronchus.

The third chest x-ray to consider (figure 37.3) has diffuse parenchymal opacities bilaterally, left more than right.

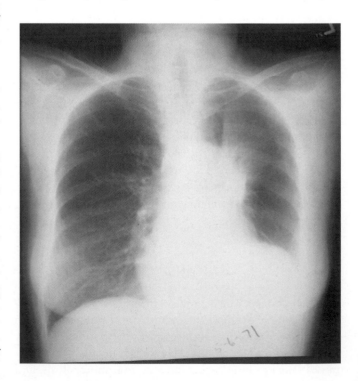

Figure 37.2. Hemoptysis: Chest X-ray 2.

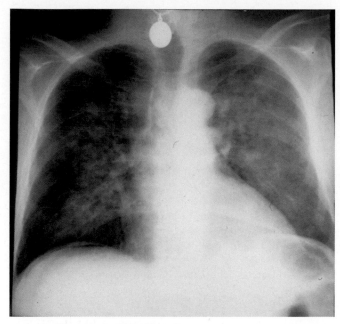

Figure 37.3. Hemoptysis: Chest X-ray 3.

(for Wegener's granulomatosis) or plasmapheresis (for Goodpasture syndrome).

By process of elimination we can match the fourth chest x-ray in this series with case history 4, a patient with hemoptysis and pleuritic chest pain 3 days after a surgical procedure. Based on the history alone, the possibility of pulmonary embolism jumps to mind. Other potential causes might include pneumonia, perhaps upper airway bleeding following intubation, or postsurgical bleeding following thoracic surgery, but pulmonary embolism is the potentially fatal etiology that we will not want to miss. The chest x-ray that we obtain (figure 37.4) has opacity at the left base. There is "blunting" of the left costophrenic angle consistent with a small pleural effusion (a lateral chest film would be helpful here for confirmation) and loss of the normal silhouette along the medial portion of the left hemidiaphragm, perhaps due to pleural effusion and perhaps due to a component of subsegmental atelectasis, causing the left hemidiaphragm to be raised up slightly and higher than the right hemidiaphragm (the reverse of normal).

A small pleural effusion and minor subsegmental atelectasis are common findings following cardiothoracic and upper abdominal surgery and are nonspecific. And that's the point, here. The findings of pulmonary embolism on plain chest radiography are typically none (a normal chest film) or nonspecific (with pleural effusion and minor atelectasis being the most common abnormalities). Only very rarely in pulmonary embolism will one find the dramatic pleural-based, wedge-shaped consolidation with rounded apex (so-called Hampton's

Especially on the left side, the appearance is that of diffuse "ground-glass" opacities. This ground-glass appearance is uniform in its "texture," not so dense (like consolidation) that one cannot see aerated lung throughout, and not linear and nodular (like an interstitial process). It reminds one of the glass door of a shower stall made opaque by grinding the surface of the glass. The pathologic correlate of this radiographic pattern is partial or incomplete airspace filling, sometimes with edema fluid (e.g., congestive heart failure), sometimes with inflammatory material (e.g., *Pneumocystis* pneumonia), and sometimes with blood (e.g., diffuse alveolar hemorrhage).

In our patient with hemoptysis, this radiograph raises a relatively limited differential diagnosis. Diffuse alveolar hemorrhage (in the absence of severe coagulopathy and/or platelet disorder) makes one think of a pulmonary vasculitis, and if we add in the "dark-colored urine and serum creatinine of 2.5 mg%" of case history 2, it specifically focuses us on pulmonary-renal hemorrhage syndromes. Diagnostic considerations include Goodpasture syndrome, Wegener's granulomatosis, and collagen-vascular disorders, especially systemic lupus erythematosus. To establish a specific diagnosis, we may rely on serologic information, such as anti–glomerular basement membrane (anti-GBM) antibody, antinuclear cytoplasmic antibody (ANCA), and antinuclear antibody (ANA), or we may obtain tissue for histologic analysis via lung or kidney biopsy. In fact, in this patient the finding on chest x-ray of free air under the right diaphragm (extra credit for all who noticed this finding!) suggests that a renal biopsy may have recently been performed. Treatment of hemoptysis in this patient is likely to involve high-dose systemic corticosteroids with potential addition of other modalities such as cyclophosphamide

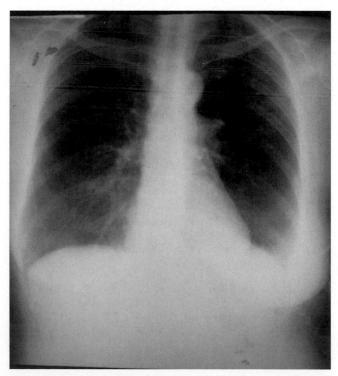

Figure 37.4. Hemoptysis: Chest X-ray 4.

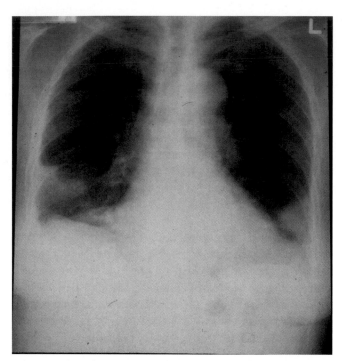

Figure 37.5. Bilateral Hampton's Humps Suggestive of Pulmonary Infarcts.

hump) (figure 37.5) that is characteristic of pulmonary infarction. Were one to wait to see this plain film manifestation of pulmonary embolism, one would miss a lot of pulmonary emboli!

For our last patient with hemoptysis, then, evaluation will likely involve either a ventilation-perfusion lung scan or chest CT angiogram. If a diagnosis of pulmonary embolism is confirmed, then treatment of this patient with hemoptysis will be, paradoxically, anticoagulation.

CHRONIC INTERSTITIAL LUNG DISEASES

Alveolar walls and their constituents (epithelial lining cells, macrophages, collagen and elastin, and pulmonary capillaries) make up the pulmonary interstitium. As discussed elsewhere in this volume, a broad collection of chronic inflammatory lung diseases affect primarily the pulmonary interstitium. Common categories include idiopathic pulmonary fibrosis, sarcoidosis, hypersensitivity pneumonitis, pneumoconiosis, and "other." The plain film radiographic hallmarks of these interstitial pulmonary processes are linear and nodular opacities. As shown in the accompanying cartoon (figure 37.6), this pattern is made up of some combination of opaque lines of varying length and thickness and dots (nodules) of varying size. The combination of linear shadows and dots gives a lacelike pattern generally readily distinguishable from consolidation (dense white opacity) or ground-glass appearance (as discussed above). High-resolution chest CT imaging (HRCT) has proved very useful in distinguishing distinctive patterns of

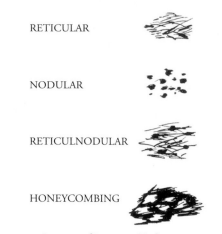

RETICULAR

NODULAR

RETICULNODULAR

HONEYCOMBING

Figure 37.6. Patterns of Interstitial Inflammation on Chest X-Ray.

interstitial inflammation, helping further to identify specific diseases or disease patterns within this broad category. Obtaining an HRCT is the appropriate next step in the radiographic evaluation of most instances of chronic interstitial lung disease.

Often the finding of diffuse linear and nodular opacities on chest film is nonspecific. A specific etiologic diagnosis will require additional history, further chest imaging (HRCT), and perhaps lung biopsy (either bronchoscopic or thoracoscopic). However, on occasion the history and characteristic chest x-ray appearance will point to a specific diagnosis or limited group of diagnoses, as illustrated by

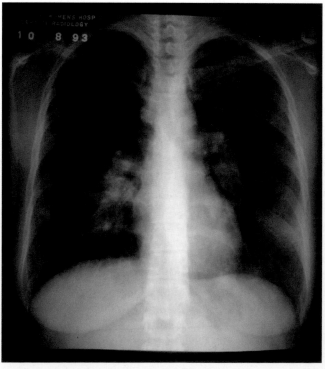

Figure 37.7. Chronic Interstitial Lung Disease: Chest X-Ray 1.

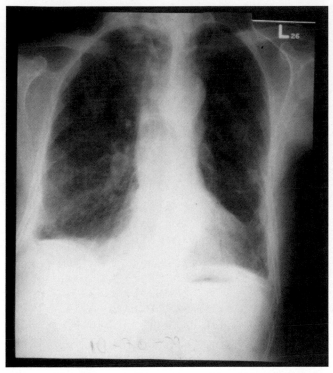

Figure 37.8. Chronic Interstitial Lung Disease: Chest X-Ray 2.

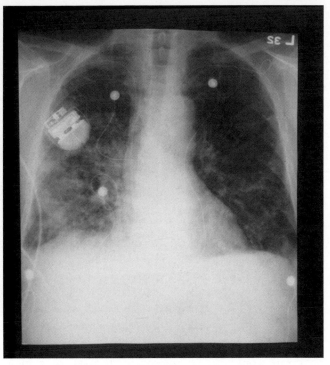

Figure 37.10. Chronic Interstitial Lung Disease: Chest X-Ray 4.

the following examples (figures 37.7–10). Four brief case histories follow (to be matched to the four accompanying chest x-rays). Each of these four patients presented with nonproductive cough and progressive dyspnea on exertion of several months' duration.

- Case 1. Inoperable gastric cancer
- Case 2. Work as a stonecutter in a quarry for 20 years, now retired for 10 years
- Case 3. Prior episodes of erythema nodosum and uveitis
- Case 4. Work cleaning and insulating boilers for 30 years

The first chest x-ray in this series (figure 37.7) has fairly subtle parenchymal opacities, left lower lung zone more than right, with what appear to be fine nodular opacities. Most striking is an ancillary finding: large hilar shadows bilaterally. The lobulated appearance suggests enlarged hilar lymph nodes. Bilateral hilar adenopathy can often be confirmed on lateral chest x-ray with the so-called "doughnut" or "bagel" sign: a ring of opacification surrounding the major bronchi at the distal end of the tracheal air column (figure 37.11). On the posteroanterior chest film one can probably make out bilateral mediastinal adenopathy as well: an enlarged azygous node along right margin of the inferior portion of the trachea and aortopulmonary adenopathy suggested by blunting of the normal recess between the aortic arch and the upper margin of the left main pulmonary artery.

The differential diagnosis for interstitial lung disease with bilateral hilar lymphadenopathy includes sarcoidosis, berylliosis, granulomatous (mycobacterial) infection, and lymphoma. A clinical history that would fit with this image is case history 3, a patient with persistent nonproductive cough, dyspnea on exertion, and a prior history of erythema nodosum and uveitis. These latter findings are among the more common extrapulmonic manifestations of sarcoidosis. In fact, given this history and chest x-ray, many pulmonary

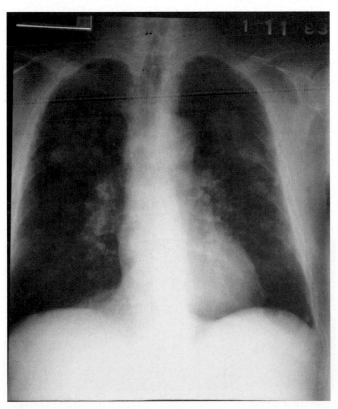

Figure 37.9. Chronic Interstitial Lung Disease: Chest X-Ray 3.

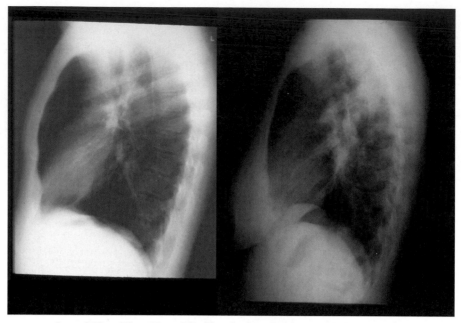

Figure 37.11. Lateral Chest Films: Normal (Left) and Bilateral Hilar Lymphadenopathy (Right).

physicians would make a presumptive diagnosis of sarcoidosis and not feel it necessary to obtain histologic confirmation (either by bronchoscopic transbronchial lung biopsy or mediastinoscopy).

Our next chest image (figure 37.8) is full of abnormalities. One can see bilateral linear and nodular opacities, especially prominent at the right base. This finding alone is nonspecific and can be seen in more than 100 chronic interstitial lung diseases. However, as we look further, there are additional clues. The costophrenic recesses are blunted, and pleural opacification extends up the lateral pleural borders bilaterally, indicative of loculated pleural effusion or pleural thickening. Perhaps you can make out (on this underpenetrated reproduction) dense white arcs paralleling each of the diaphragmatic shadows. The intensity of these white lines implies calcification, most likely calcification along the diaphragmatic pleura. A close-up of the diaphragms on this patient's lateral chest film brings out this finding more clearly (figure 37.12). Finally, there are nodular densities to be accounted for, in the left mid-lung zone laterally and in the right upper lobe. We will come back to these nodular opacities in a moment.

Chronic interstitial lung disease with pleural thickening and extensive pleural calcifications suggests a diagnosis of asbestosis. Asbestosis refers the interstitial inflammation and fibrosis secondary to chronic inhalation of asbestos fibers. It typically develops only after many years of intense asbestos exposure and with a latency period of decades, appearing 20–30 years after exposure began. The exposure may have been work cleaning and insulating asbestos-lined boilers, as in case history 4. Pleural fibrosis and plaques, with or without calcification, are indicators of asbestos exposure. They are often asymptomatic and may or may not be accompanied by diffuse interstitial inflammation and fibrosis.

Now, what about the nodular opacities? On the left, I suspect a pleural plaque. When the plaque occurs along the anterior or posterior aspect of the pleura, surrounded by aerated lung and imaged "*en face*," it can mimic an intra-parenchymal nodule. On the other hand, the right upper lobe nodule proved to be a lung cancer. It reminds us that the most common cancer associated with asbestos exposure, especially common among cigarette smokers, is lung cancer. The pleural malignancy, mesothelioma, is more specifically associated with asbestos exposure, but it is far less common.

The next image (figure 37.9) is classic, virtually pathognomonic, and now rare. It belongs in the category of "interstitial" diseases because of the presence of many small lung nodules throughout the lung parenchyma, but the major findings are elsewhere. There are large consolidated opacities in the upper lobes, bilaterally symmetric, and suspicious for malignancy. However, their size and shape have not changed over many months. And the appearance of the hila is distinctive; they are full and very radiopaque (whiter than usual). Perhaps on the left you can make out discrete, enlarged hilar lymph nodes as part of the hilar shadows.

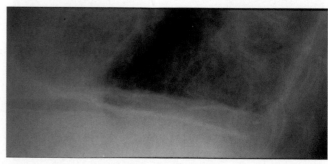

Figure 37.12. Pleural Calcifications Along Diaphragmatic Pleura (Close-Up of Lateral Chest Film).

They are so radiopaque and distinct because they are calcified. Calcified hilar lymph nodes make one think of granulomatous lung infections (e.g., tuberculosis, histoplasmosis, and coccidioidomycosis), chronic sarcoidosis, and silicosis. In a patient with many years of silica dust exposure (as a stonecutter in a quarry for 20 years, as in case history 2), one can make a diagnosis of silicosis based on this chest image. Sometimes calcification of the hilar nodes occurs only along their rim, giving a distinctive appearance referred to as "eggshell calcification," seen in silicosis and occasionally sarcoidosis. Figure 37.13 offers a close-up view of a patient with "eggshell calcification" of right hilar and mediastinal lymph nodes due to silicosis.

Multiple small silicotic nodules throughout the lungs can be asymptomatic, referred to as simple silicosis. This patient has more advanced disease, however. In the upper lobes, a dense conglomeration of silicotic nodules and inflammatory reaction has formed masslike lesions, called "progressive massive fibrosis." The symmetric involvement and upper lobe location have led to the description of an "angel's wings" distribution of these opacities. Characteristically, in progressive massive fibrosis there may be progressive upper lobe scarring years after silica dust exposure has ceased.

The last of the four chest images in this series (figure 37.10) must belong, then, with the patient with inoperable gastric cancer (case 1). Even knowing this history, one is strongly tempted to make a diagnosis of congestive heart failure. Besides linear and nodular opacities in the left lower lobe and a mixture of linear and nodular opacities combined with more confluent (airspace) opacities in the right lower lobe, there are probably small bilateral pleural effusions (although on both sides the film fails to include the lateral margins of the chest). In addition, if one had the opportunity to look at the x-ray close-up, one might be able to pick out Kerley B lines (thin, horizontal lines extending approximately 1 cm in length and ending laterally at the pleural margin) and a Kerley A line (thin, longer line, not oriented horizontally, that also indicates fluid in the interlobular septa). And then there is the circumstantial evidence of a cardiac pacemaker (with old, disconnected pacer wires still in place on the left).

However, this patient does not have congestive heart failure. Of interest, the cardiac silhouette is normal in size. Additional history is that diuresis to the point of prerenal azotemia brought no improvement. As we expand our differential diagnosis of interstitial infiltrates with Kerley lines and pleural effusions, the history of inoperable gastric cancer becomes relevant. What is filling the interstitial spaces and especially the interlobular septa in this case is not edema fluid but malignant cells and associated desmoplastic reaction. This patient has lymphangitic carcinomatosis, the spread of malignancy (almost always adenocarcinoma) through lymphatic channels. Common primary cancers are lung and breast and also stomach, pancreas, and thyroid. A close-up image (figure 37.14) highlights the nodular component of the interstitial pattern in this case along with the Kerley A and B lines.

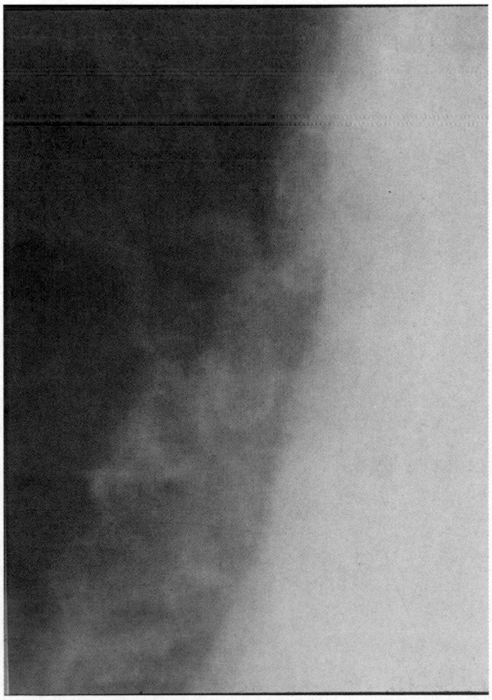

OBSTRUCTIVE LUNG DISEASES

Obstructive lung diseases are grouped together based to their shared physiological (rather than radiographic) pattern: airflow obstruction on the forced expiratory maneuver of spirometry. Common among the obstructive lung diseases

Figure 37.13. Pattern of "Eggshell Calcification" of Hilar and Mediastinal Lymph Nodes (Close-Up of Right Lung, Medially, on Posteroanterior Chest Film).

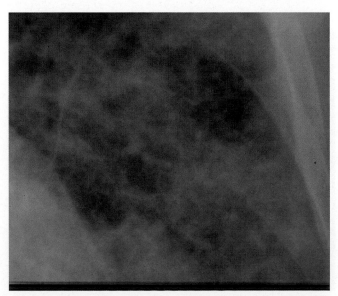

Figure 37.14. Linear and Nodular Opacities, Including Kerley A and B Lines (Close-Up of Left Paracardiac Area on Posteroanterior Chest Film).

are asthma, chronic bronchitis, and emphysema (referred to collectively as chronic obstructive pulmonary disease [COPD]), bronchiolitis, diffuse bronchiectasis, and upper airway obstruction. In addition, other lung diseases may frequently manifest with airflow obstruction even though they are not primarily thought of in this category. Examples include congestive heart failure (remember wheezing due to heart failure, referred to as "cardiac asthma"), sarcoidosis (as many as one-quarter of patients with sarcoidosis will have primarily obstructive rather than restrictive physiology), and the rare entity, discussed in this course under the heading of "interstitial lung diseases," called lymphangioleiomyomatosis (LAM).

When the primary abnormality is airway narrowing, the chest radiograph may be normal or reveal only hyperinflation. Consider this example, for instance, of a patient with severe COPD due primarily to chronic bronchitis (figure 37.15). The chest film has only a minor, nonspecific increase of lung markings at the bases bilaterally. On close inspection one can see a ring shadow in the left hilar region, representing a thickened bronchial wall cut in cross section. Despite the severity of airflow obstruction, the chest x-ray has only few abnormalities.

Still, the chest x-ray may provide valuable diagnostic clues in patients with chronic airflow obstruction, as illustrated by the next series of four chest x-rays (figures 37.16–19). Each of these patients has cough, shortness of breath, and intermittent wheezing. In addition, the following histories were obtained:

- Case 1. The patient's father and older brother died in their 40s of emphysema.

- Case 2. The patient has had a chronic productive cough and recurrent sinusitis since childhood and now presents for evaluation of infertility.

- Case 3. The patient, a nonsmoker, had recurrent pneumothoraces in the past and a pleural effusion that was said to look "milky" when drained.

- Case 4. The patient complains of weight loss, chronic diarrhea, and sinusitis. Mucoid pseudomonas has been grown from the sputum.

This first image (figure 37.16) is quite striking: the lungs are large and very black ("hyperlucent"); and the diaphragms are flattened, lacking the normal rounded arc of their silhouettes. The film is cut off at the lung apices, making it difficult to count rib numbers accurately, but it is clear that the diaphragms are positioned very low in the chest, probably at the level of the 11th or 12th ribs posteriorly (normal is at 9th to 10th ribs). The pulmonary arteries centrally are brought into stark relief by the surrounding overinflated lung tissue. (An incidental note is made of an accessory [azygos] fissure in the right upper lung zone and a callus formed along the rib in the right lower lung zone.)

This pattern of hyperinflated and hyperlucent lungs is readily identified as that of emphysema, with destruction of alveolar tissue and consequent excessive lung compliance. However, this chest film holds additional clues as to etiology. The distribution of lucency is not uniform, apex to base. The blackest areas are at the lung bases. The cause is clear if we look for vascular markings: the blood vessels can be traced in the upper lung zones with almost none coursing inferiorly. These areas of hyperlucent lung tissue with absence of vascularity suggest bullae.

The location of these bullae at the lung bases is atypical. In most cigarette smokers with bullous emphysema, the

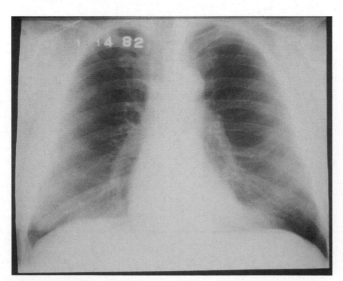

Figure 37.15. Patient with Severe Obstructive Lung Disease Caused by Chronic Bronchitis.

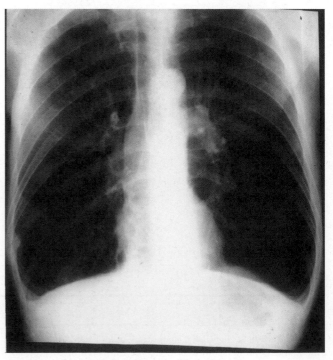

Figure 37.16. Obstructive Lung Disease: Chest X-Ray 1.

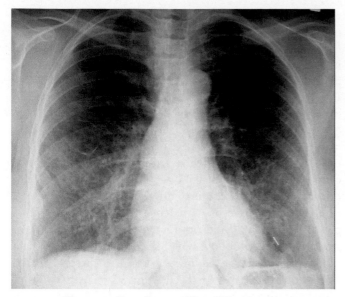

Figure 37.17. Obstructive Lung Disease: Chest X-Ray 2.

bullae are located at the apices. The bibasilar location of the bullae in this example of emphysema suggests a specific etiology: alpha-1-antitrypsin deficiency. Consequently, we have no difficulty matching this chest x-ray with a clinical history. It belongs to the patient with a strong family history of emphysema that develops at a relatively young age (case 1).

Confirmation of a suspicion of alpha-1-antitrypsin deficiency is easy: on a routine blood requisition form, request measurement of the alpha-1-antitrypsin level.

Patients homozygous for the abnormal alpha-1-antitrypsin gene will have blood levels on the order of 10–15% of normal. Further specialized genetic or phenotypic testing can then be requested to identify the specific genetic abnormality, but the initial screening test simply involves a routine blood test.

The second chest x-ray in this series (figure 37.17) has evidence for hyperinflation (the diaphragms are flattened and at the level of the 11th ribs posteriorly), but it is not hyperlucent—just the opposite. It is hard to make out many details on this film, other than to say that it is not what we would expect in obstructive lung disease due to asthma or COPD. Close-up inspection helps somewhat (figure 37.20): it appears that the increased markings are due to thickened walls of cystic spaces (and a very opaque linear shadow suggests a surgical clip, as at the left lung base). Potential etiologies of diffuse cystic lung disease that come to mind include emphysema, Langerhans cell granulomatosis, and LAM. Further evaluation is likely to include a chest CT scan, as shown in figure 37.21.

On the CT scan loculated pneumothoraces are visible on the right, and the myriad bilateral cystic spaces are dramatically demonstrated. The cyst walls are very thin, barely detectable in some instances, as is typical in emphysema and LAM. In this young nonsmoker with a history of recurrent pneumothoraces and chylous pleural effusion (case history 3), the likely diagnosis is LAM.

LAM is a distinctive disorder characterized by neoplastic-like proliferation of abnormal smooth muscle–like cells

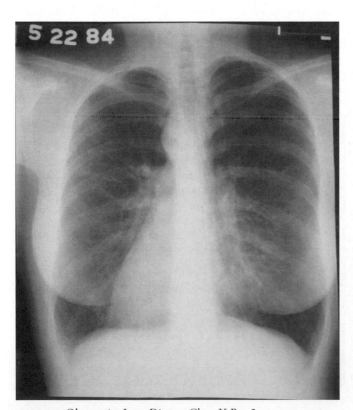

Figure 37.18. Obstructive Lung Disease: Chest X-Ray 3.

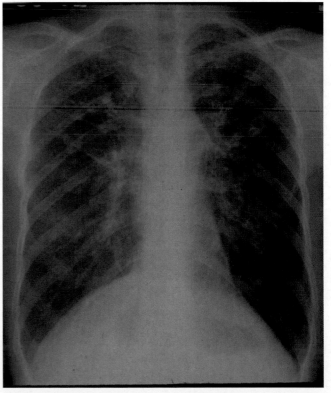

Figure 37.19. Obstructive Lung Disease: Chest X-Ray 4.

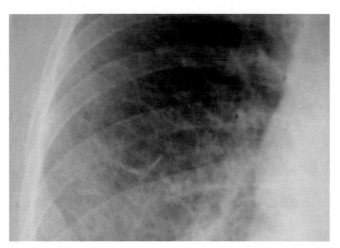

Figure 37.20. Obstructive Lung Disease, Chest X-Ray 2: Close-Up View of Right Mid-Lung Zone.

along small airways and alveolar walls. It is part of a broader syndrome of abnormalities, tuberous sclerosis complex, for which genetic defects have been identified. It occurs exclusively in women of childbearing age, suggesting a strong hormonal influence, and it commonly progresses to severe airflow obstruction and respiratory failure. Traditional therapies (oophorectomy and antiestrogen medications) have proved of limited benefit. In an exciting development, a recent randomized trial found that sirolimus halts the progression of airflow obstruction in LAM.

There is something very wrong with the next chest x-ray (figure 37.18)! It is either displayed in reverse (left side inverted to the right), or the patient has dextrocardia. If there were gas in the stomach, the location of gastric lucency under one of the diaphragms ("stomach bubble") would indicate whether or not the dextrocardia were part of more generalized situs inversus.

Looking beyond this most striking finding, one can also note an abnormality of the lung parenchyma. The normal silhouette made by aerated lung tissue abutting the right ventricle (now on the right side of the film) has been lost. The heart margin is indistinct, and there are increased non-homogeneous opacities in the region of the adjacent lung tissue. The appearance suggests a possible pneumonia, but with additional information we find that the abnormality is unchanging, identical on prior chest films over a period of years. In a patient with symptoms of airway disease—chronic productive cough and intermittent wheezing—the possibility of bronchiectasis comes to mind. The radiographic opacities in bronchiectasis are due to thickened airway walls and inflammation/infection in surrounding (peribronchial) lung tissue, often with associated atelectasis.

This combination of dextrocardia and bronchiectasis triggers a synapse: Kartagener's syndrome. Manes Kartagener described patients with situs inversus, bronchiectasis, and chronic sinusitis; men with this syndrome have immotile or dysmotile sperm and consequent infertility. The pathogenesis of Kartagener's syndrome has been

explicated: abnormal ciliary function underlies all of its manifestations. As a result, alternative names for this syndrome are utilized, including immotile cilia syndrome and, more precisely, primary ciliary dyskinesia. Primary ciliary dyskinesia is inherited as an autosomal recessive disorder. In some examples of this molecularly heterogeneous syndrome, an ultrastructural abnormality can be identified on electron microscopy of ciliated epithelial cells (obtained on nasal biopsy or bronchoscopic bronchial biopsy) or of the tails of sperm. Absence of the dynein arm connecting adjacent microtubule doublets in the "spoke and wheel" architecture of cilia is the classic finding.

The history that best matches this x-ray is case 2, a patient with a chronic productive cough and recurrent sinusitis since childhood, now presenting for evaluation of infertility. The breast shadows seen on this chest x-ray suggest that the patient is a woman. Some women with immotile cilia syndrome have infertility, presumably due to ciliary dysfunction in the fallopian tubes.

By way of "full disclosure," although this patient has airway disease and we have included bronchiectasis in our discussion of obstructive lung diseases, it is possible that this patient will not have significant airflow obstruction on pulmonary function testing. Localized bronchiectasis may have little impact on lung function, or it may manifest as restriction due to lung destruction, consolidation, and/or atelectasis.

The final chest x-ray (figure 37.19) is one of our most striking. Like the second film in this series (figure 37.17), it has the unusual combination of hyperinflation and widespread parenchymal opacities. On closer inspection, these opacities have some distinctive features. First, they are distributed more in the upper lobes than in the lower lobes. Second, they appear generally aligned in the same orientation as the bronchovascular bundles, radiating out from the hila in "northwesterly" (in the right upper lobe)

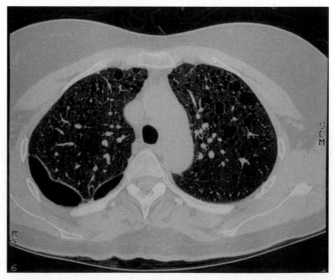

Figure 37.21. Chest CT Scan with Multiple Thin-Walled Cysts and Loculated Right Pneumothoraces.

and "northeasterly" (in the left upper lobe) directions. Third, on close inspection one can make out cysts within these opacities, some of which are oval and share the same general orientation described above. In fact, these are bronchi with cystic dilatation—cystic bronchiectasis. You have likely made a diagnosis already, based on the history (case 4) of weight loss, chronic diarrhea, and sinusitis, with mucoid *Pseudomonas* grown on sputum culture. This is an example of cystic fibrosis, Its upper lobe predominance puts it in a relatively small group of chronic lung diseases manifesting bilateral upper more than lower lobe opacities, including sarcoidosis, ankylosing spondylitis, and tuberculosis (and other chronic granulomatous infections).

Cystic fibrosis is recognized with increasing frequency among adults, not only because children with the disease are living longer (average age of survival is now projected into the mid-30s) but because variant forms of cystic fibrosis exist that can first manifest in adulthood. Often, chest disease (bronchiectasis) is the dominant manifestation of adult-onset cystic fibrosis. Diagnosis can be established by specialized genetic testing (with more than 100 abnormal alleles now identified in the cystic fibrosis transmembrane conductance regulator gene) or by the traditional sweat chloride test (sweat chloride level >60 meq/L).

ADDITIONAL READING

Fraser RS, Muller NL, Colman NC, Pare PD. *Fraser and Pare's Diagnosis of Diseases of the Chest*, 4th ed. Philadelphia: W. B. Saunders; 1999.

Kang J, Litmanovich D, Bankier AA, Boiselle PM, Eisenberg RL. Manifestations of systemic diseases on thoracic imaging. *Curr Probl Diagn Radiol.* 2010 Nov-Dec;39(6):247–261.

Novelline RA, *Squire's Fundamentals of Radiology*, 6th edition, (Cambridge: Harvard University Press; 2004).

Washko GR. Diagnostic imaging in COPD. *Semin Respir Crit Care Med.* 2010 Jun;31(3):276–285. Epub 2010 May 21.

38.

MECHANICAL VENTILATION

Patricia A. Kritek

Patients receive mechanical ventilation for a variety of reasons. The general practitioner should understand the broad categories for initiation of mechanical ventilation as well as be able to determine when a patient can be liberated from a ventilator. The majority of this chapter focuses on the common modes of ventilation, the difference between pressure- and volume-cycled breath delivery and how these different modes are monitored.

REASONS FOR INITIATION

Patients may require mechanical ventilatory support for a variety of reasons (table 38.1). These can be broadly categorized as impaired oxygenation (low Pao_2) or impaired alveolar ventilation (increased $Paco_2$). In addition, some patients with insufficient protective reflexes require intubation for airway protection even if both oxygenation and ventilation are currently adequate.

Although there is no absolute threshold of supplemental oxygen to determine when mechanical ventilation is indicated, if a patient can not maintain a Pao_2 >60 mm Hg or an oxygen saturation >90% despite high levels of supplemental oxygen (e.g., 60% or higher), it is appropriate to consider initiating mechanical ventilation regardless of the $Paco_2$. Pathophysiological causes of hypoxemia include increased shunting, ventilation-perfusion $(\dot{V}/\dot{Q})$ mismatch, hypoventilation, and low inspired fraction of oxygen. Only shunt and $\dot{V}/\dot{Q}$ mismatch result in a widened alveolar-arterial (Aa) difference. Common clinical causes of hypoxemic respiratory failure are the acute respiratory distress syndrome (ARDS), cardiogenic pulmonary edema, and pneumonia.

Inadequate alveolar ventilation causes progressive hypercarbia and elevated $Paco_2$. In this situation, hypoxemia is caused by a decrease in the alveolar oxygen concentration and not an increased Aa difference. Ventilatory failure can result from inadequate respiratory drive, mechanical impairment of the chest wall, neuromuscular system disease, or increased airways resistance. Hypoventilation and respiratory failure may result from an overdose of drugs (e.g., benzodiazepines, narcotics) that impair central nervous system respiratory centers. Mechanical restriction of the chest wall can be the result of severe kyphoscoliosis or morbid obesity although this is usually a more chronic process. Patients with neuromuscular weakness (e.g., Guillain-Barré syndrome, amyotrophic lateral sclerosis) may not be able to maintain adequate alveolar ventilation. Perhaps most commonly, patients with exacerbations of underlying obstructive lung disease present with ventilatory failure requiring mechanical ventilation. Patients with severe asthma can present with acute respiratory failure due to a sudden, marked increase in airways resistance. More commonly, those with COPD can develop acute on chronic respiratory failure with intercurrent illnesses such as a viral upper respiratory tract infection or bacterial bronchitis.

As previously noted, some patients are intubated for support of neither oxygenation nor ventilation but because of a need to "protect the airway." The loss of protective airway reflexes is an indication for intubation. A patient with pooling secretions is at risk for aspiration and may require placement of an endotracheal tube to protect against this. Although this is not truly an indication for mechanical ventilatory support, this is a common reason for emergent intubation, especially in unstable patients requiring imaging or other diagnostic procedures.

Not all patients require tracheal intubation in order to receive mechanical ventilatory support. Noninvasive positive-pressure ventilation (NIPPV) consists of the provision of positive-pressure ventilation without the need for intubation and can be beneficial both for hypoxemia and hypercarbia in specific clinical situations.

Table 38.1 POTENTIAL INDICATIONS FOR INVASIVE MECHANICAL VENTILATION

Failure of noninvasive positive-pressure ventilation (NIPPV)

Severe hypoxemia (PaO_2 <60 mm Hg or O_2 saturation <90%) despite high concentrations of supplemental oxygen that can be delivered without intubation (e.g., ~60% FiO_2)

Respiratory acidosis producing a pH less than approximately 7.25 (or progressive respiratory acidosis without likelihood of short-term improvement)

Insufficient reserve to maintain ventilation in the setting of increased work of breathing (e.g., evidenced by use of accessory muscles and/or paradoxical abdominal motion)

Respiratory arrest

Inability to protect airway

Cardiovascular complications: shock, severe heart failure, hypotension, arrhythmia

ROLE OF PULMONARY MECHANICS

Patients are supported with mechanical ventilation for a variety of reasons, often in complex clinical scenarios with multiple possible etiologies for respiratory failure. Measuring a patient's airways *resistance* and respiratory system *compliance* can be a helpful way to tease out the underlying pathophysiological process (or processes). Similarly, pulmonary mechanics can be used to assess responses to therapy or to help understand sudden changes in a patient's respiratory status while being supported by the ventilator.

Compliance is a measure of distensibility, the change in volume that occurs in response to a change in pressure ($\Delta V/\Delta P$). In the lung, compliance is the volume achieved when a distending pressure is applied (e.g., the positive pressure from a mechanical ventilator). While we refer to compliance of the lung, this value actually reflects the distensibility of the respiratory system as a whole, including the lung and the chest wall. Airway resistance opposes the flow of gas; the more resistance, the greater the driving force required to move air. Airway resistance is predominantly dependent on the caliber (radius) of the airway. Once again, for patients on a ventilator, "airway" resistance not only encompasses the trachea, main stem bronchi, smaller bronchi, and bronchioles but also the endotracheal tube and the ventilator tubing connecting the patient to the ventilator.

To move air into the chest, the ventilator must overcome both the compliance of the respiratory system and airway resistance. The peak inspiratory pressure (PIP) reflects the force required to overcome both of these (respiratory system compliance and airway resistance). If airflow is eliminated, there is no airway resistance and the remaining pressure (the "plateau pressure") is a reflection of what is needed to overcome compliance. The plateau pressure is measured by performing an "inspiratory pause" during which all airflow is stopped and the lung volume held steady (see figure 38.1).

Knowing the pressure applied by the ventilator (ΔP) and the resultant tidal volume (ΔV) enables a calculation of respiratory system compliance ($\Delta V/\Delta P$). The ΔV is measured as the exhaled tidal volume (in milliliters) and the ΔP by the plateau pressure (in cm H_2O) minus any positive end expiratory pressure (PEEP) in use. Based on Ohm's law ($V = IR$), the equation for airways resistance is R = ΔP/flow. In this case, the change in pressure is the difference between the inspiratory pressure measured when there is flow in the system (peak inspiratory pressure) and when flow is halted with an inspiratory pause (plateau pressure). The flow (measured in liters per second) is a value that is set on the ventilator. It is usually reported in liters per minute and thus needs to be converted to liters per second prior to any calculations.

$$\text{Compliance} = \Delta V/\Delta P = V_t/(\text{Plateau} - \text{PEEP})$$
$$\text{Resistance} = \Delta P/\text{flow} = (\text{PIP} - \text{Plateau})/\text{flow}$$

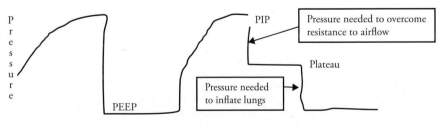

Figure 38.1. Pressure–Time Curve from a Volume-Targeted Breath. The peak inspiratory pressure (PIP) is determined from the resistance of the airways, the compliance of the respiratory system, and the inspiratory flow rate. In contrast, the plateau pressure, which is determined by pausing at the end of inspiration, thus eliminating airflow, reflects solely the compliance of the respiratory system. The baseline pressure is the set positive end expiratory pressure (PEEP).

Table 38.2 CAUSES OF INCREASED PEAK INSPIRATORY PRESSURES

Increased resistance	Bronchospasm
	Kinked ventilator tubing
	Secretions in airways, endotracheal tube, or ventilator tubing
	Patient biting on the endotracheal tube
	Pulmonary edema
Decreased compliance	Right mainstem intubation
	Large mucus plug → lobar collapse
	Pneumothorax
	Worsening airspace disease: ARDS, pneumonia
	Pulmonary edema
Agitation	Dyssynchrony with the ventilator

Normal airways resistance, while on a ventilator, is usually <5 cm H_2O/(L/sec). Normal respiratory system compliance is >50 mL/cm H_2O.

Determination of airways resistance and respiratory system compliance is useful in making an initial diagnosis but perhaps even more helpful as a way of assessing an acute change in a patient. If a patient suddenly has an increase in measured PIP, it is important to determine if this is because of a fall in compliance, an increase in resistance, or both. A sudden fall in compliance may be due to a pneumothorax as a result of barotrauma while on the ventilator or because of migration of the endotracheal tube into the right mainstem, resulting in delivery of the same tidal volume to only one lung instead of two. Increased airways resistance may have a variety of causes including acute bronchospasm, kinking of ventilator tubing, or secretions in the endotracheal tube. Another common reason for a sudden increase in PIP is patient agitation resulting in dyssynchrony with the ventilator and patient exhalation while the ventilator delivers a breath. A more complete list of common causes of increased resistance and decreased compliance is included in table 38.2.

MODES OF VENTILATION

There are several different modes of ventilation that determine the way that breaths are initiated and the pattern of breath delivery over time (table 38.3). The most commonly used modes include assist control (AC), pressure support (PSV), and synchronized intermittent mandatory ventilation (SIMV). For all of these modes, both positive end-expiratory pressure (PEEP) and the fraction of inspired oxygen (FiO_2) must also be specified; the major differences are in how each breath is initiated and the pattern of breathing over time.

In AC ventilation, the patient's initiation of a breath triggers the ventilator to deliver a fully supported inspiration (either volume-targeted or pressure-targeted). When clinicians refer to AC, they are usually referring to volume-targeted AC. However, AC can also be used for delivery of pressure-targeted breaths, in which case the term pressure-controlled ventilation (PCV) is used. In either case, the respiratory rate set by the clinician is the minimum number of breaths that the patient will receive; when the patient breathes at a rate above that level, each additional breath is fully supported to the specified volume or pressure target. Therefore, the respiratory rate setting on the ventilator becomes relevant only when the patient is not spontaneously initiating at least that number of breaths. With a volume-targeted AC mode, the

Table 38.3 MODES OF VENTILATION

MODE	CLINICAL USE	INDEPENDENT VARIABLES (SET BY THE CLINICIAN)	DEPENDENT VARIABLES (DETERMINED BY INTRINSIC PROPERTIES OF THE LUNG)
Volume assist control (AC)	Full ventilatory support	Minimum respiratory rate, tidal volume	Peak inspiratory pressure, plateau pressure
Pressure control ventilation (PCV)	Full ventilatory support	Minimum respiratory rate, inspiratory time, inspiratory to expiratory (I:E) ratio, peak inspiratory pressure	Tidal volume, minute ventilation
Pressure support ventilation (PSV)	Weaning or partial ventilatory support	Peak inspiratory pressure	Respiratory rate, tidal volume, minute ventilation
Synchronized intermittent mandatory ventilation (SIMV)	Full or partial ventilatory support	Respiratory rate, tidal volume (for fully supported breaths), peak inspiratory pressure (for patient-triggered breaths in patients also receiving PSV)	Minute ventilation, peak inspiratory pressure, plateau pressure

patient is assured of receiving a minimum minute ventilation, which is the product of the tidal volume and the respiratory rate setting ($V_t \times f$). With a pressure-targeted AC mode (PCV), the volume delivered with each breath (and therefore the total minute ventilation) is not assured, as it will depend on the lung compliance and the airway resistance.

In SIMV, the ventilator is set to deliver a specified number of breaths at a particular tidal volume. There is some flexibility in the timing of a breath so that it is ideally synchronized with the patient's own inspiratory effort. If the patient spontaneously initiates a breath outside of the time window when the ventilator should deliver a breath, the ventilator does not assist the spontaneous breath, and the volume of the breath is determined solely by the patient's inspiratory effort. It is also possible to combine SIMV with pressure support ventilation (PSV). In this situation, the patient's spontaneous breaths that are not fully supported by the ventilator can be given partial support through use of PSV.

Pressure support ventilation (PSV) is used only when a patient is awake enough to initiate breaths on his or her own. In this mode, the preset independent parameter is the inspiratory pressure, which is triggered by and delivered with each patient-initiated breath. Each breath is terminated when the flow diminishes to a preset percentage of the peak inspiratory flow rate, usually 25%. While the positive pressure decreases the patient's work of breathing, the patient determines the flow rate, inspiratory time, tidal volume, and respiratory rate. Many clinicians feel this mode is more comfortable for the alert patient, and it is commonly used when a patient is clinically improving and moving toward extubation. The disadvantage of this mode is that there is no guaranteed minimum minute ventilation, and it is not suited for a patient with waxing and waning respiratory drive (e.g., some patients who are deeply sedated or who have suffered CNS injury). PSV may also be inappropriate when, despite an intact CNS drive to breathe, the patient lacks sufficient muscular strength to reliably generate adequate tidal volumes (e.g., with neuromuscular disorders).

There are several other, less commonly used ventilator modes including airway pressure release ventilation (APRV), bilevel ventilation, and volume-targeted pressure-cycled ventilation. These advanced modes are beyond the scope of this chapter.

PRESSURE VERSUS VOLUME BREATH DELIVERY

The physician ordering mechanical ventilation for a patient must decide the overall pattern of ventilatory support (the "mode") and whether for each supported breath the ventilator will deliver a preset tidal volume or preset inspiratory pressure (the form of "breath delivery").

The ventilator can be set to deliver either a specified tidal volume (V_t) or a specified PIP for each breath. When volume-targeted breaths are chosen, a tidal volume is set by the clinician. Additional parameters, usually set by the respiratory therapist, include the peak flow rate and the pattern in which the ventilator will deliver this volume. In contrast, when pressure-targeted breaths are chosen, a PIP is specified by the clinician. This is often called the inspiratory pressure or the driving pressure. In either form of breath delivery, the resultant volumes and pressures are determined by the intrinsic properties of the patient's lungs.

In volume-targeted ventilation, the V_t and flow rate are independent (determined by the clinician or respiratory therapist), whereas the resultant PIP and plateau pressure are dependent on the volume and airflow settings, how stiff the lungs are, and the airway (including the endotracheal tube and ventilator tubing) resistance. The PIP and the plateau pressure that result from delivering a set V_t will be higher in a patient whose lungs have become stiffened (e.g., in acute respiratory distress syndrome, ARDS) than in a patient whose lungs have lost much of their elastic recoil properties (e.g., in emphysema).

In contrast, when a pressure-targeted breath is delivered, the peak airway pressure is the independent variable (determined by the clinician or respiratory therapist) and the resultant tidal volume is determined by the intrinsic properties of the lung. The same amount of pressure will result in small V_t in patients with stiff lungs (e.g., pulmonary fibrosis) and in larger volumes in patients with more compliant lungs (e.g., emphysema).

There are no data demonstrating a superiority of either pressure-targeted or volume-targeted breath delivery with respect to mortality or liberation from the ventilator. They both can achieve adequate oxygenation and ventilation in most scenarios. The main advantage of volume-targeted ventilation modes is that a minimum minute ventilation can be guaranteed as both a tidal volume and a minimum respiratory rate are predetermined and set. Volume-targeted breath delivery also makes it easier to assure low tidal volumes are maintained in conditions where this is warranted such as in ARDS. Pressure-targeted ventilation, on the other hand, has the advantage of being able to limit airway pressures, but tidal volume can vary with changes in the mechanical properties of the lungs and airways. Pressure-targeted ventilation may be useful in situations in which high airway pressures are encountered and there is concern for development of barotrauma. It also allows variability in flow rates and patterns that may result in greater patient comfort. It is difficult, however, to predict which ventilator settings will be most comfortable for an individual patient as significant variability occurs.

DISCONTINUATION OF MECHANICAL VENTILATION

The longer a patient is intubated, the greater the risk of complications associated with mechanical ventilation, most significantly ventilator-associated pneumonia. Because of this risk, patients should be assessed on a regular basis for extubation readiness. When a patient can maintain adequate oxygenation (Sao_2 >90% on Fio_2 ≤40%) and ventilation (pH >7.30), it is reasonable to consider extubation. In most situations, a patient should also be hemodynamically stable and alert enough to follow commands, though there are exceptions to this rule. Additionally, a patient being assessed for extubation should have an adequate cough and the ability to safely clear his or her secretions. Patients who meet these criteria should undergo a spontaneous breathing trial in which they breathe with minimal continuous positive airway pressure (CPAP) support or on a T-piece for 30–120 minutes. If patients tolerate this trial without deterioration of gas exchange or hemodynamic instability, extubation can be attempted.

Some clinicians include the rapid shallow breathing index (RSBI) as part of the assessment for extubation. The RSBI is the respiratory rate divided by the tidal volume in liters (RSBI = f/V_t). If elevated (>105), the RSBI identifies patients at high risk for extubation failure. In general, a patient who is achieving adequate minute ventilation by taking fewer and larger breaths is more likely to do well than a patient who is achieving the same minute ventilation by taking more shallow breaths. While not a particularly specific test, in one meta-analysis the RSBI was a sensitive test for extubation readiness. As with all weaning tests, the RSBI is not a single predictor of extubation success but can be used in conjunction with other parameters to decide on timing of extubation.

Practices that promote regular assessments of a patient's readiness to breathe independently have been shown to decrease the mechanical ventilator time. Most often, these have involved the use of "protocols" that allow respiratory therapists and nurses to evaluate a patient's ability to breathe spontaneously at least daily, without the need for a physician order with each assessment (provided specified safety parameters are met). The most commonly employed protocol involves a daily spontaneous breathing trial as described above. In a randomized controlled trial of 300 mechanically ventilated patients, a daily spontaneous breathing trial resulted in fewer days on the mechanical ventilator, fewer complications, and lower cost. The daily interruption of sedative drugs is also suggested as a means of hastening a patient's readiness to breathe spontaneously, and in a randomized controlled trial of 128 patients at a single center, this practice reduced both mechanical ventilator and ICU time.

SUMMARY

Mechanical ventilation is used when a patient develops hypoxemia, hypercarbia, or both. Ventilator settings are chosen to improve oxygenation (Fio_2 and PEEP) as well as to maintain ventilation. The different modes of ventilation and the different types of breath delivery (pressure-cycled vs. volume-cycled) are simply different ways to achieve ventilation. When a pressure-cycled mode is used, the clinician needs to monitor volumes, as they are a reflection of the patient's airways resistance and respiratory system compliance. Conversely, when ventilation is maintained with a volume-cycled mode, the pressures (PIP and plateau) will be a reflection of the patient's respiratory system mechanics.

ADDITIONAL READING

Ely EW, Baker AM, Dunagan DP, et al. Effect on the duration of mechanical ventilation of identifying patients capable of breathing spontaneously. *N Engl J Med.* 1996;335:1864–9.

Esteban A, Frutos F, Tobin MJ, et al. A comparison of four methods of weaning patients from mechanical ventilation. Spanish Lung Failure Collaborative Group. *N Engl J Med.* 1995;332:345–50.

Kress JP, Pohlman AS, O'Connor MF, Hall JB. Daily interruption of sedative infusions in critically ill patients undergoing mechanical ventilation. *N Engl J Med.* 2000;342:1471–7.

Soo Hoo GW. Noninvasive ventilation in adults with acute respiratory distress: A primer for the clinician. *Hosp Pract (Minneap).* 2010;38(1):16–25.

QUESTIONS

QUESTION 1. A 22-year-old college student with asthma presents to the ED with a severe flare. She had a recent URI and then progressive shortness of breath/wheezing. She has been using her albuterol MDI 12–16 times a day. She is intubated in the ED because of extreme work of breathing. On exam, she is intubated and appears agitated with heart rate 135, blood pressure 95/47. There are no audible wheezes, but she is tachycardic with cool extremities. The patient's initial ventilator settings are Assist Control Ventilation, V_t 450, rate 16, Fio_2 40, PEEP 10 cm H_2O. She is over-breathing at 19 and her PIP are 48–54 cm H_2O.

The patient is given intravenous Solu-Medrol and continuous albuterol via MDI. She is fully sedated with fentanyl and midazolam although she still seems to be interacting with the ventilator and continues to have high peak airways pressures (PIP). In addition to dyssynchrony, what do think is contributing to the patient's high PIPs?

A. Increased autoPEEP, high airways resistance, and high lung compliance

B. Increased autoPEEP alone

C. Low airways resistance and low lung compliance
D. Increased autoPEEP, high airways resistance, and low lung compliance
E. Low airways resistance alone

QUESTION 2. In order to adequately ventilate the patient, the next step with the patient's ventilator settings would include:

A. $\downarrow V_t$ and $\downarrow$ inspiratory flow rate
B. $\uparrow V_t$ and $\uparrow$ respiratory rate
C. $\downarrow V_t$ and $\uparrow$ inspiratory flow rate
D. $\downarrow V_t$ and $\uparrow$ expiratory flow rate
E. $\uparrow$ respiratory rate and $\uparrow$ inspiratory flow rate

ANSWERS

1. D
2. C

39.

SEPSIS SYNDROME

Joshua A. Englert and Rebecca Marlene Baron

epsis is a clinical syndrome characterized by systemic inflammation leading to tissue injury that arises as a complication of an infection. According to current paradigms, sepsis arises as a result of the infection of a normally sterile body compartment. Infection leads to activation of the innate immune system to produce a systemic inflammatory response. This response is a necessary component of the body's defense against infection under normal conditions, but it is the lack of regulation of this response that is central to the pathogenesis of sepsis. As discussed in more detail below, this dysregulated inflammatory state can lead to tissue injury and dysfunction in organs not involved in the original infectious insult. Although sepsis remains a condition with exceedingly high morbidity and mortality, recent early management and treatment strategies have demonstrated exciting improvements in overall outcomes.

DEFINITIONS

Our current characterizations of patients along the critical illness spectrum (ranging from the systemic inflammatory response syndrome to sepsis to severe sepsis to septic shock) are based upon Consensus Conference definitions. The response to inflammation manifests itself clinically as the systemic inflammatory response syndrome (SIRS) (see table 39.1). SIRS is defined as two or more of the following: (1) fever or hypothermia, (2) tachypnea, (3) tachycardia, (4) leukocytosis or leukopenia; it can be caused by both infectious etiologies and noninfectious causes. Sepsis is defined as evidence of SIRS in the presence of an infection. When sepsis is accompanied by organ hypoperfusion or dysfunction (see table 39.2), it is designated as "severe sepsis." Septic shock occurs when sepsis is accompanied by hypotension (defined as an absolute systolic blood pressure of <90 mm Hg or of 40 mm Hg less than the patient's baseline despite adequate fluid resuscitation).

EPIDEMIOLOGY

Sepsis affects approximately 750,000 people in the United States annually and is associated with a mortality rate of 40%–70% in its most severe form. The incidence continues to increase as the American population ages and as increasingly complex treatments are applied for conditions such as cancer and organ transplantation that require significant immunosuppression of the host. A majority of cases occur in patients with significant comorbidities. Significant risk factors include increasing age, immunosuppression, and chronic illnesses (such as chronic obstructive pulmonary disease or diabetes mellitus). Various risk stratification tools, including the Acute Physiology and Chronic Health Evaluation (APACHE) II score, can be used to quantify the severity of illness and estimate the risk of death from sepsis.

CLINICAL PRESENTATION AND DIAGNOSIS

The clinical manifestations of sepsis can vary greatly from one patient to another. Not infrequently, this variability in presentation contributes to diagnostic uncertainty in cases of sepsis, especially early in the course of illness. Difficulty in early recognition of the septic response has hampered the identification of patients who might benefit from early aggressive management of sepsis, as described below. All too often, patients are identified further into the course of the inflammatory "storm," by which time rescue strategies to restore adequate tissue perfusion and oxygen delivery are likely not as effective. There is no single specific diagnostic test for sepsis; rather, the diagnosis hinges on physical findings and laboratory values consistent with SIRS in the presence of suspected or identified underlying infection. Moreover, early localization of the primary source of infection is critical for optimal therapy. Thus, the clinician must be on the lookout for signs and symptoms attributable to the primary infection as well as to those that might reflect the inflammatory

Table 39.1 THE SYSTEMIC INFLAMMATORY RESPONSE SYNDROME (SIRS)

DEFINED AS TWO OR MORE OF THE FOLLOWING CRITERIA

1. Temperature: >38°C or <36°C
2. Heart rate >90 beats per minute
3. White blood cell count: >12,000 cells/mm³ or <4000 cells/mm³ or >10% bands
4. Respiratory rate >20 breaths per minute or $PaCO_2$ <32 mm Hg

response to infection. It is equally important to keep an open mind in the diagnostic process, as many patients who present with signs or symptoms consistent with SIRS and shock may have alternative or concomitant diagnoses (e.g., cardiogenic or hemorrhagic shock) that explain their presentation.

As noted above, the four signs that comprise SIRS (table 39.1) are common but not requisite in sepsis. One example of the variability in the clinical presentation is that elderly patients with sepsis often present without fever. Other common findings on physical exam include delirium, confusion, and tachypnea that might represent nonspecific effects of a variety of different possible sources of infection. Thus, it is important to search for manifestations of the primary infectious insult that are specific to the initial site of infection. For example, patients with sepsis due to pneumonia may present with fever, a productive cough, evidence of lung consolidation on percussion and auscultation of the chest, and presence of an infiltrate on chest radiography. Sepsis originating from an infection of the urinary tract can present with dysuria, urinary frequency or incontinence, suprapubic tenderness on physical examination, and the presence of pyuria on examination of a urine specimen. An abdominal source of infection might manifest itself with nausea, vomiting, diarrhea, and/or the presence of rebound or guarding on physical examination. The wide variability in clinical presentation requires vigilance on the part of the providers caring for patients with sepsis.

Laboratory abnormalities in septic patients can some times help point toward a source of sepsis (e.g., elevated

Table 39.2 DEFINITION OF SEVERE SEPSIS

Severe sepsis: Sepsis with evidence of organ hypoperfusion or organ dysfunction as defined by the following criteria:

Organ Hypoperfusion
Oliguria
Signs of abnormal peripheral circulation (*e.g.* mottled skin)
Altered mental status
Increased serum lactate levels

Organ Dysfunction
Pulmonary: PaO_2/FiO_2 <250
Cardiovascular: systolic blood pressure <90 mm Hg or mean arterial pressure (MAP) <70 mm Hg
Renal: urine output <0.5 cc/kg per hour despite adequate volume resuscitation
Gastrointestinal: hyperbilirubinemia
Hematologic: platelet count <80,000 mm³ or a 50% decrease in the platelet count from the highest value during the 3 preceding days

bilirubin and alkaline phosphatase levels in cholecystitis) but more often reveal nonspecific indices of infection and inflammation, including a leukocytosis with a left shift and thrombocytopenia. Arterial blood gas analysis early in the course of this syndrome often reveals a respiratory alkalosis. If untreated, patients can develop an anion gap acidosis due to the accumulation of lactic acid in the setting of organ hypoperfusion. In fact, an elevated lactate level has been proposed by some as a possible marker that should heighten suspicion for the presence of sepsis, even though the lactate level can be elevated from other causes of tissue hypoperfusion (e.g., ischemic bowel). Unfortunately, once the lactate level is elevated in sepsis, end-organ hypoperfusion and damage may already have occurred. This end-organ effect has been referred to as the multiple organ dysfunction syndrome (MODS), and laboratory evidence of renal and hepatic insufficiency are often hallmarks of this syndrome. Additionally, coagulopathy can occur due to the development of disseminated intravascular coagulation. Hyperglycemia is a common finding among patients with underlying diabetes, and even in patients without previously diagnosed underlying diabetes, elevated glucose levels are often seen during critical illness, likely as a result of a stress response.

In patients with suspected infection who do not manifest focal signs, symptoms, physical findings, or laboratory data pointing at source of sepsis, a continued search must be pursued while the patient is treated with broad-spectrum antibiotics and stabilized. Cultures of blood, urine, and sputum should be obtained on presentation. Samples of fluid from other potential sources of infection should also be sent for culture as the clinical scenario dictates (e.g., spinal fluid if meningitis is suspected, or ascitic fluid if spontaneous bacterial peritonitis might be a concern). If the patient's condition deteriorates on empirical antibiotic therapy with an unknown source of infection and/or the initial microbiological workup is negative, a more aggressive workup may be indicated, including early consideration of additional imaging by computed tomography. More invasive testing is often necessary in critically ill patients to identify (or exclude) possible sources of infection. For example, if a patient with suspected bacterial pneumonia worsens on broad-spectrum antibacterial agents, bronchoscopy with bronchoalveolar lavage in order to culture the pathogenic organism may be helpful.

PATHOPHYSIOLOGY

As described above sepsis can develop following microbial infection of a normally sterile cavity. One useful framework for thinking about the pathogenesis of sepsis is the "PIRO" concept that was described by an international panel of experts at the 2001 Symposium on Intensive Care and Emergency Medicine. PIRO is an acronym that stands for *p*redisposition, *i*nfection, *r*esponse, and *o*rgan dysfunction.

With regard to predisposition, the response to a particular infection varies greatly from one individual to another. For example, it is not uncommon for an elderly patient to present with a urinary tract infection and subsequent bacteremia as a result of translocation of the organisms into the bloodstream. Some of these patients will have a fulminant course complicated by septic shock and organ dysfunction. In contrast, other patients will remain normotensive and asymptomatic despite the circulating microbes. The predisposition of some patients to developing sepsis is likely related to a combination of genetic and environmental factors. Immune suppression, either drug induced or due to comorbid conditions such as malignancy or cirrhosis, weakens the host response to infection and predisposes patients toward the development of sepsis. It is likely that genetic variation also plays an important role in the response to infection, as demonstrated by studies that have shown possible differences in the risk of sepsis among individuals with polymorphisms in various inflammatory genes.

The site and microbiology of the antecedent infection plays a key role in the pathogenesis of this syndrome. The microbiology of sepsis has changed somewhat over time. Prior to 1990, intra-abdominal infections were the most common. Recently, studies have shown that pulmonary infection (i.e., pneumonia) is the most frequent source, accounting for approximately 40% of sepsis cases. Moreover, although a large percentage of sepsis cases had traditionally been attributed to infection with Gram-negative bacterial organisms, recent years have seen an increase in numbers of infections attributed to Gram-positive bacteria and infections with nonbacterial organisms such as fungi or viruses. Increasing prevalence of infections with fungi and viruses has been associated with an increase in numbers of immunocompromised hosts as a result of chemotherapy treatments for cancer or immune suppression for organ transplantation.

The host response to infection is one of the key determinants in the pathophysiology of sepsis. Recognition of microbes by cells of the innate immune system results in the release of numerous proinflammatory cytokines. Downstream effects of this inflammatory response include recruitment of neutrophils to the tissues and development of hypotension as a result of vasodilation. Cytokines that are thought to be important to the inflammatory response include, but are not limited to, tumor necrosis factor (TNF)-α, interferon (IFN)-γ, and interleukin (IL)-1β. Many of these cytokines are known to be important early in the course of sepsis (i.e., within the first 6–24 hours), and there is increasing evidence that the inflammatory response is mediated by other proteins later in the course of sepsis. Recently, extracellular high-mobility group B-1 (HMGB1) was identified as a late-acting mediator in the course of sepsis. This cytokine-like protein is not released until nearly 24 hours into the course of sepsis and may play a key role in the development of organ dysfunction later in the course of this syndrome. Following the production of proinflammatory cytokines, it has been proposed that the host can develop a compensatory response through production of anti-inflammatory cytokines, such that a period of relative "immune compromise" for the host can develop later in the septic response.

Other key components of the host's response to sepsis include activation of the coagulation and neuroendocrine systems. Endothelial damage leads to expression of tissue factor and subsequent activation of the clotting cascade followed by the formation of thrombin. Some experts hypothesize that this process may play a role in containing invading pathogens. Deficiency of several fibrinolytic proteins, including protein C, further enhances the procoagulant milieu. The stress response also results in the development of peripheral insulin resistance and hyperglycemia, as well as in activation of the hypothalamic-pituitary axis and secretion of a number of key hormones, including adrenocorticotropic hormone (ACTH) and vasopressin. Insufficient production of these hormones during sepsis have led to the concepts that critical illness might result in states of relative adrenal insufficiency and vasopressin deficiency, respectively. Management strategies that have arisen in response to the appreciation of these pathophysiological processes are discussed in more detail below.

Although the exact mechanism of organ dysfunction in patients with severe sepsis is unknown, tissue hypoperfusion as a result of hypotension and vasodilatation likely plays an important role. Moreover, significant interest has arisen in the concept of microcirculatory dysfunction as an important contributor to this process. Inflammation and a local activation of clotting mechanisms are needed to combat infection as described above, but if left unchecked, these processes can lead to progressive organ dysfunction. Thrombosis of the microvasculature can lead to shunting of blood flow away from vital organs and result in impaired local oxygen delivery to the tissues. As an alternative or perhaps coexisting phenomenon, inability of the tissues to use delivered oxygen as a result of the development of mitochondrial dysfunction has been proposed as a possible mechanism of organ dysfunction.

MANAGEMENT

The prompt recognition and treatment of severe sepsis is necessary in order to correct metabolic derangements, optimize oxygen delivery, and prevent the development of organ dysfunction. The initial approach to the patient involves stabilization of hemodynamics and respiratory status. Intubation of the airway with an endotracheal tube and support of breathing with mechanical ventilation is necessary for those patients who are unable to protect their airway or for those who present with inability to sustain adequate oxygenation or ventilation. Assessment of the blood pressure, pulse, and signs/symptoms of perfusion as described above are important to ensure presence of adequate circulation. Obtaining early intravenous access with large-bore peripheral catheters and/or central venous catheters is critical for the facilitation of aggressive volume resuscitation and administration of medications.

A key component in the management of patients with sepsis is controlling the source of the infection. This requires the early administration of broad-spectrum antibiotics as well as drainage or removal of any indwelling sources of infection. Examples of infectious sources that require removal include infected venous catheters, soft tissue abscesses, and empyema (table 39.3). It is recommended that broad-spectrum antibiotics be administered within the first hour of presentation, and each hour of delay in antibiotic treatment has been associated with an increased mortality rate. If cultures reveal a specific organism, the antibiotic regimen can be tailored accordingly. Recommended duration of antibiotic therapy varies greatly depending on the initial source and severity of infection.

Early optimization of tissue perfusion and oxygen delivery is most important step in the management strategy of septic patients. In a landmark randomized, controlled clinical trial, Rivers et al. (2001) demonstrated an absolute 16% reduction in in-hospital mortality using a protocolized resuscitative strategy targeted to achieve specific goals in a number of parameters (e.g., central venous pressure, mean arterial pressure, urine output, central venous saturation). One important way in which this trial was unique compared with previous studies is that the resuscitative strategy was applied within the emergency department during the first 6 hours of the patient's hospitalization. Patients were randomized to the protocolized approach (i.e., "early goal-directed therapy" [EGDT] group), versus a group of patients who received standard management. Subsequent analysis of the study revealed that early administration of large volumes of intravenous fluid was an important contributor to the beneficial outcome. Although the total volume of administered fluid for the duration of the hospitalization was similar for all patients, the EGDT group received substantially more fluids within the first 6 hours.

This protocolized approach, referred to as EGDT (figure 39.1), has been widely adopted and incorporated into consensus guidelines for the initial management of severe sepsis and septic shock. We therefore review the details of the protocol. All patients had arterial and central venous catheters placed for hemodynamic monitoring. The protocol targeted specific hemodynamic goals, including maintaining a central venous pressure (CVP) of 8–12 mm Hg with 500 cc of IV fluids every 30 minutes. Once the CVP goal was attained, a goal mean arterial pressure (MAP) between 65–90 mm Hg was targeted, using vasopressors as needed (usually norepinephrine). Once the MAP goal was obtained, a central venous saturation was measured as a marker of adequate oxygen delivery to the tissues. If the central venous saturation was <70% and the hematocrit was <30%, packed red blood cells were transfused to a goal hematocrit ≥30%. If the central venous saturation was <70% and the hematocrit was >30%, inotropic agents were used in order to improve oxygen delivery to the periphery and obtain the central venous saturation goal. Finally, once all these goals were obtained, the patients were admitted to the hospital for further evaluation and treatment.

As noted previously, a relatively thrombophilic state occurs in septic patients. This procoagulant milieu can lead to progressive microcirculatory tissue thrombosis and tissue hypoxia. Although approaches such as EGDT are critical for restoring the macrocirculation, it is likely that microcirculatory dysfunction and tissue injury had already ensued by the time patients presented for treatment. One possible contributing factor to this procoagulant state is a relative deficiency of protein C in patients with sepsis. A placebo-controlled trial of recombinant human activated protein C (rhAPC) in patients with severe sepsis and a high risk of death showed a statistically significant decrease (6.1%) in 28-day mortality in patients who received rhAPC when compared to controls (PROWESS trial). Subsequent subgroup analysis revealed a more pronounced benefit of rhAPC in the sickest patients (i.e., patients with an APACHE II score ≥25). Moreover, in a separate trial, rhAPC did not reduce mortality in septic patients at lower risk for death (ADDRESS trial). These trials and others have raised concern for increased risk of serious bleeding (i.e., intracranial hemorrhage) in patients receiving rhAPC. While there was initial enthusiasm for use of Activated Protein C in the sickest patients with sepsis, in

Table 39.3 EXAMPLES OF SOURCES OF INFECTION THAT REQUIRE INTERVENTION IN ADDITION TO ANTIBIOTIC THERAPY

SOURCE OF INFECTION	PROCEDURE
Soft tissue abscess	Surgical or radiographically guided drainage
Empyema	Chest tube placement or surgical evacuation
Cholangitis	ERCP with biliary decompression
Catheter- or device-related bacteremia	Remove the infected catheter/device
Septic arthritis	Arthrocentesis +/– debridement
Endocarditis/valvular abscess	Consider valvular replacement

NOTE: ERCP, endoscopic retrograde cholangiopancreatography.

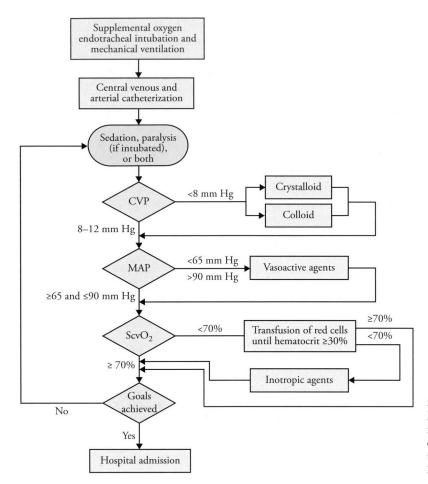

Figure 39.1. Schematic Representation of the Protocol for Early Goal-Directed Therapy. Reprinted with permission from Rivers E, Nguyen B, Havstad S, et al. Early goal-directed therapy in the treatment of severe sepsis and septic shock. *N Engl J Med.* 2001;345(19):1368. Copyright 2001 Massachusetts Medical Society. All rights reserved.

October 2011, Eli Lilly and Company withdrew Activated Protein C from the market. The company stated that newer data from the PROWESS-SHOCK study demonstrated a lack of efficacy, thus calling into question the risk-benefit profile of Activated Protein C. The company also stated that improvement in management of sepsis over the last 10 years might have played a role in the different outcomes of this more recent trial.

One recurring controversy in the management of septic patients is the use of corticosteroids. Given that the activation of inflammatory pathways plays a key role in the pathophysiology of sepsis, it seems logical that inhibiting these pathways could prevent the development of end-organ damage. However, several trials of high-dose steroids in septic patients have demonstrated that this strategy did *not* improve outcomes. Although high-dose steroids are not effective for treating sepsis, there are data to suggest that low-dose steroids (e.g., hydrocortisone, 50 mg IV q6h) may be beneficial in a subset of patients with relative adrenal insufficiency (Annane et al., 2002). In a randomized, placebo-controlled trial of hydrocortisone and fludrocortisone in 300 patients with hypotension despite use of fluids and vasopressors, 28-day mortality was significantly lower in a subgroup of patients who did not respond to an ACTH stimulation test with an increase in cortisol of at least 9 μg/dL

(termed "nonresponders"). Of note, there was no significant difference in the primary endpoint (i.e., 28-day mortality) when all patients (responders and nonresponders) were included in the analysis. This study led to increased use of corticosteroid treatment for septic patients with no response to a 250 μg ACTH stimulation test. More recently, a larger trial of corticosteroids (hydrocortisone alone without addition of fludrocortisone) in patients with septic shock demonstrated no significant difference in 28-day mortality in the entire study population, nor in the nonresponder subgroup of patients who did not have an appropriate increase in serum cortisol following stimulation with ACTH (CORTICUS trial). Notably this population of patients was less sick overall than the group included in the trial by Annane et al. in that the CORTICUS trial included patients who had restored adequate perfusion parameters with fluids and vasopressors. Hydrocortisone treatment led to faster reversal of shock in patients in whom shock was ultimately reversed, but there was also a suggestion of increased rates of infection with steroid administration. Thus, although significant debate still exists with regard to the role of low-dose steroids in septic shock, the most recent consensus guidelines have suggested that low-dose hydrocortisone be considered only for patients who remain hypotensive after fluid and vasopressor administration.

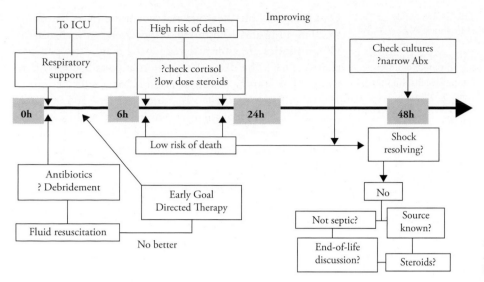

Figure 39.2. Schematic Overview of an Approach to Management of Sepsis Syndrome.

Given the high frequency of hyperglycemia in critically ill patients, there have been many studies examining whether restoration of euglycemia improves outcomes from sepsis. One notable study of patients in a surgical ICU showed improved mortality when "intensive" insulin therapy was used to lower glucose levels to the range of 80–110 mg/dL (Van den Berghe et al., 2001). A subsequent study of all patients in a medical ICU (i.e., patients with sepsis as well as other diagnoses and who were assumed to require at least 3 days of ICU-level care) showed no improvement in overall mortality with intensive insulin therapy (Van den Berghe et al., 2006). Although subgroup analysis revealed a benefit of intensive insulin therapy for patients who required a medical ICU stay of longer than 3 days, the subgroup of patients in the ICU for less than 3 days exhibited an increased mortality rate. More recently, a large, international, randomized trial (NICE-SUGAR study) demonstrated increased mortality in ICU patients who received intensive glucose control. Thus, more recent consensus guidelines have favored less intensive glucose control, perhaps more liberally targeting glucose levels to <150 mg/dL in critically ill patients.

Thus, although morbidity and mortality remain high in critically ill patients with sepsis and septic shock, recent studies have taught us that early and aggressive resuscitative care for septic patients improves outcomes (figure 39.2). From the time concern for sepsis is raised, early goal-directed therapy should be instituted, while broad-spectrum antibiotics are administered, and a search for a possible source of infection should be undertaken. In patients who remain at a high risk for death after the early resuscitative phase, adjunctive supportive therapies can be considered, including low-dose steroids, and insulin therapy to avoid significant hyperglycemia, while also maintaining care to avoid episodes of hypoglycemia. This is an exciting time in development of treatment strategies for sepsis, as ongoing and future trials will continue to optimize our care of these critically ill patients.

ADDITIONAL READING

Abraham E, Laterre P-F, Garg R, et al.; ADDRESS trial. Drotrecogin alpha (activated) for adults with severe sepsis and a low risk of death. *N Engl J Med.* 2005;353:1332–41.

American College of Chest Physicians/Society of Critical Care Medicine Consensus Conference. Definitions for sepsis and organ failure and guidelines for use of innovative therapies in sepsis. *Crit Care Med.* 1992;20:864–74.

Angus DC, Linde-Zwirble WT, Lidicker J, Clermont G, Carcillo J, Pinsky MR. Epidemiology of severe sepsis in the United States: Analysis of incidence, outcome, and associated costs of care. *Crit Care Med.* 2001;29:1303–10.

Annane D, Sebille V, Charpentier C, et al. Effect of treatment with low doses of hydrocortisone and fludrocortisone on mortality in patients with septic shock. *JAMA.* 2002;288:862–71.

Baron RM, Baron MJ, Perrella MA. Pathobiology of sepsis: Are we still asking the same questions? *Am J Respir Cell Mol Biol.* 2006;34:129–34.

Bernard GR, Vincent JL, Laterre PF, et al.; PROWESS trial. Efficacy and safety of recombinant human activated protein C for severe sepsis. *N Engl J Med.* 2001;344:699–709.

de Oliveira JM, Lisboa L de B. Hospital-acquired infections due to gram-negative bacteria. *N Engl J Med.* 2010;363(15):1483–4.

Hotchkiss RS, Karl IE. The pathophysiology and treatment of sepsis. *N Engl J Med.* 2003;348:138–50.

Hotchkiss RS, Opal S. Immunotherapy for sepsis—a new approach against an ancient foe. *N Engl J Med.* 2010;363(1):87–9.

Lee WL, Slutsky AS. Sepsis and endothelial permeability. *N Engl J Med.* 2010;363(7):689–691.

Levy MM, Fink MP, Marshall JC, et al. International Sepsis Definitions Conference. *Crit Care Med.* 2003;31:1250–6.

NICE-SUGAR Investigators. Intensive versus conventional glucose control in critically ill patients. *N Engl J Med.* 2009;360:1283–97.

Rivers E, Nguyen B, Havstad S, et al. Early goal-directed therapy in the treatment of severe sepsis and septic shock. *N Engl J Med.* 2001;345:1368–77.

Sprung CL, Annane D, Keh D, et al.; CORTICUS study group. Hydrocortisone therapy for patients with septic shock. *N Engl J Med.* 2008;358:111–24.

Surviving Sepsis Campaign. International guidelines for management of severe sepsis and septic shock. *Crit Care Med.* 2008;36:296–327.

Van den Berghe G, Wouters P, Weekers F, et al. Intensive insulin therapy in critically ill patients. *N Engl J Med.* 2001;345:1359–67.

Van den Berghe G, Wilmer A, Hermans G, et al. Intensive insulin therapy in the medical ICU. *N Engl J Med.* 2006;354:449.

QUESTIONS

QUESTION 1. A 67-year-old man with a history of hypertension and prostate cancer presents to the ED with fevers and confusion. Physical examination is notable for a systolic blood pressure of 50 mm Hg, heart rate 150 beats per minute, respiratory rate 40 breaths/min, and an O_2 saturation of 94% on room air. Microscopic examination of the urinary sediment reveals >200 white blood cells/hpf and innumerable bacteria. What is the next most appropriate step in the management of his hemodynamic status:

A. Vasopressin
B. Norepinephrine
C. Neo-Synephrine
D. Central line insertion
E. Dopamine

QUESTION 2. A 47-year-old man with a history of alcohol-induced cirrhosis is brought to the emergency room with fevers, confusion, and worsening ascites. Blood pressure on presentation is 60/30 mm Hg. Sepsis due to spontaneous bacterial peritonitis is suspected, and central venous and arterial catheters are placed. He receives 8 L of normal saline, and his blood pressure improves to 70/40 mm Hg with a central venous pressure of 2 mm Hg. What is the most appropriate next step?

A. Initiate treatment with IV vasopressin
B. Bolus with normal saline
C. Start dobutamine
D. Start stress-dose steroids (i.e., hydrocortisone, 50 mg IV q6h)

QUESTION 3. His mean arterial pressure and CVP improve to 70 mm Hg and 10 mm Hg, respectively, with treatment. IV antibiotics are administered, and a diagnostic paracentesis confirms the diagnosis of spontaneous bacterial peritonitis. Laboratory testing is notable for a white count of 17,000/mL, hematocrit 19%, and platelets 105,000/mL. Electrolytes and coagulation studies are within normal limits. Venous blood gas testing reveals a normal pH and a central venous saturation of 60%. What is the next most appropriate step?

A. Airway intubation in order to initiate mechanical ventilation
B. Start intravenous dobutamine
C. Bolus with normal saline
D. Transfuse 1 unit of packed red blood cells

QUESTION 4. An 82-year-old woman with a history of diabetes and recurrent lower extremity ulcers due to infections with multi-drug-resistant organisms is admitted from the skilled nursing facility where she resides, with hypoxia and altered mental status. Per report of the nursing home staff she developed a cough productive of purulent sputum 3 days prior to admission. Physical exam reveals a temperature of 102.5°F, heart rate 120 beats per minute, blood pressure 70/40, and an oxygen saturation of 88% on 4 L via nasal cannula. Chest imaging shows bilateral airspace opacities consistent with pneumonia. After initial stabilization of the patient, what is the most appropriate initial antibiotic regimen?

A. Azithromycin
B. Vancomycin
C. Piperacillin/tazobactam
D. Cefepime and vancomycin

ANSWERS

1. D
2. B
3. D
4. D

40.

HEMODYNAMIC MONITORING IN THE ICU

Patricia A. Kritek

Hemodynamic monitoring is a central part of the care of many patients in the intensive care unit (ICU). The most invasive form of hemodynamic monitoring is a pulmonary artery catheter (PA catheter), often referred to as a Swan-Ganz catheter after its coinventors Jeremy Swan and William Ganz. More commonly, a patient's central venous pressure and arterial pressure will be monitored via a central venous catheter and an arterial line, respectively. There are limited data that use of hemodynamic monitoring impacts mortality of critical patients. In fact, the use of PA catheters has been a subject of great debate for nearly four decades. That being said, many intensivists believe the data from these devices contribute to better management of patients in the ICU and can have a role in diagnosing certain life-threatening conditions. The majority of this chapter focuses on the use of pulmonary artery catheters including their potential roles in the ICU, the placement of these devices, the measurements they provide, and the subsequent interpretation of these data.

ROLE OF HEMODYNAMIC MONITORING

Right heart catheterization is the gold standard for diagnosis of pulmonary artery hypertension (PAH). Although this is often performed in a catheterization laboratory, it is not uncommon to diagnosis pulmonary hypertension in patients in the ICU. Pulmonary artery catheters can also be used to determine the presence of a left-to-right cardiac shunt, cardiac tamponade, and valvular disease. Data available from a PA catheter, including cardiac output, filling pressures, and systemic venous resistance, can help in determining the etiology of shock.

With respect to the ongoing management of critically ill patients, protocolized care of patients guided by central venous pressure monitoring and central venous oxygenation has been shown to decrease mortality when employed early in the treatment of septic patients. There are no convincing data

that the use of a PA catheter impacts outcome in septic patients similarly. There are small studies that support the use of arterial monitoring and measurement of pulse pressure variability to assess volume responsiveness in mechanically ventilated critically ill patients. In the largest trial designed to assess the role for PA catheter-directed volume management of patients with the acute respiratory distress syndrome (ARDS), there was no benefit guiding therapy by PA-catheter–measured pressures (pulmonary artery occlusion pressure, PAOP) as compared to central venous catheter pressures (central venous pressure, CVP). Although earlier research supported the use of PA-catheter data to guide medication adjustment in patients with severe cardiomyopathy and heart failure, the largest study of these patients did not show a mortality benefit to PA-catheter guidance over clinical assessment alone. PA-catheter guidance is still often recommended in the care of patients with severe, refractory heart failure, although convincing data for this practice do not exist.

The potential value of a PA catheter over central venous monitoring is that is allows an estimation of left atrial pressure (LAP) as well as right atrial pressure (RAP). The catheter, when appropriately positioned, can occlude a branch pulmonary artery, resulting in the cessation of flow between that branch of the pulmonary artery and the left atrium. The pressure measured will be an approximation of the left atrial pressure (LAP). This pressure is referred to as the pulmonary artery occlusion pressure (PAOP), the pulmonary artery wedge pressure (PAWP), or the pulmonary capillary wedge pressure (PCWP). In order for this measurement to be accurate, the PA catheter must be placed in a location where both pulmonary arterial and venous pressures are greater than alveolar pressures. If this is not the case, the PAOP will reflect, at least partially, alveolar pressure. This ideal position is referred to as West lung zone 3 (figure 40.1).

If truly a reflection of LAP, this information gives the clinician an idea of the left ventricular end-diastolic pressure (LVEDP) and in turn the left ventricular end-diastolic volume (LVEDV). This information can be used to assess cardiac filling and cardiac function. It also allows the

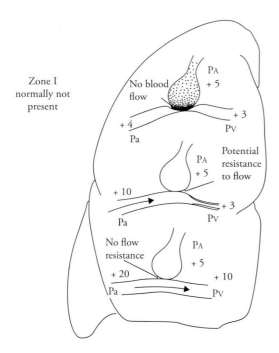

Potential Zones in the Lung

Zone I
normally not
present

No blood
flow

PA
+ 5

+ 4
Pa

+ 3
PV

Zone I   Pa<PA>PV

PA
+ 5

Potential
resistance
to flow

+ 10
Pa

+ 3
PV

Zone II   Pa>PA>PV

No flow
resistance

PA
+ 5

+ 20
Pa

+ 10
PV

Zone III   Pa>PA<PV

Figure 40.1. West Lung Zones.

calculation of pulmonary vascular resistance. Additionally, a PA catheter can be used to calculate cardiac output and systemic vascular resistance.

PULMONARY ARTERY CATHETER PLACEMENT

A pulmonary artery catheter, when placed in the ICU, is inserted through a cordis in one of the large veins of the neck or chest. Internal jugular and subclavian veins on either the left or right are acceptable locations for access, but the PA catheter is more easily positioned when the right internal jugular or the left subclavian vein is used. These vessels provide a straighter path to the right atrium and afford a higher likelihood of the catheter successfully passing through the central vein to the right atrium and beyond.

After a cordis is placed under sterile conditions, the patient is generally redraped for placement of the PA catheter. At times, clinicians will reglove for the procedure, as sterility is essential. The catheter is inserted and advanced 20 cm so that it is clear of the cordis. At this time, the balloon at the tip of the catheter (see figure 40.2) is inflated with 1–1.5 cc of air, which allows the catheter to "float" in the bloodstream. The catheter is then advanced, being guided by the appearance of varying waveforms, through the central vein to the right atrium, through the tricuspid valve, into the right ventricle (RA), and eventually into the right pulmonary artery. At this point, the clinician slowly advances the catheter until it "wedges" in a more distal pulmonary artery, resulting in occlusion of flow. This position is determined by distance advanced and waveform appearance. These waveforms are the focus of the following section.

At times, it can be difficult to place a PA catheter. As already mentioned, placement via the left internal jugular or right subclavian approach can be challenging because of the more acute turns the catheter must take. If a patient has significant tricuspid regurgitation, it can be difficult to advance from the right atrium to the right ventricle. Similarly, if a patient has a dilated right ventricle, it is sometimes difficult to navigate out of the ventricle and advance into the pulmonary artery. In these circumstances, PA catheter placement can be aided by fluoroscopic guidance.

In addition to the risks associated with placement and use of a central venous catheter (e.g., bleeding, infection, pneumothorax), PA catheter placement and maintenance have multiple potential complications. While floating a PA line, particularly while traversing the right ventricle,

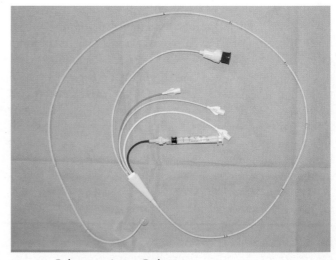

Figure 40.2. Pulmonary Artery Catheter.

there is a risk of inducing ventricular tachycardia from contact with the conduction system of the heart. Similarly, it is possible to induce a right bundle branch block during placement, a life-threatening complication in a patient with an underlying left bundle branch block at baseline. During pulmonary artery occlusion, there is a small risk of pulmonary infarction and less commonly pulmonary artery rupture. Finally, over time, a pulmonary artery catheter can become knotted in the right ventricle. This complication generally requires surgical intervention. Because of rare but potentially life-threatening complications, PA catheter placement should be done with care and after thoughtful decision-making about the value of the data provided.

WAVEFORM ANALYSIS

RIGHT ATRIAL PRESSURE

The initial pressure that is seen when a PA catheter is placed is that of the central vein (CVP). This is usually apparent after the catheter is advanced 20 cm and is clear of the cordis. The CVP is an approximation of the right atrial pressure (RAP), and the waveform in the central vein and the right atrium will look the same.

The RAP waveform can demonstrate three distinct deflections, although the fidelity of a PA catheter tracing in the ICU is often not good enough to distinguish each. The first upward deflection is the "a-wave" and is a reflection of atrial contraction. This is followed by the "x descent" as pressures fall with atrial relaxation. The second upward deflection, termed the "c-wave," which is often not discernible, is a small rise associated with closure of the tricuspid valve. The final upward deflection, the "v-wave," is associated with passive filling of the atrium and occurs at the time of ventricular contraction. This is followed by the "y descent" as the tricuspid valve opens and blood flows into the ventricle.

In order to interpret the CVP or RAP tracing, a synchronous electrocardiogram (EKG) is used. As mechanical activity in the heart follows slightly on electrical activity, the EKG changes will precede the pressure tracing changes. Accordingly, the CVP a-wave will follow the P wave on the EKG, and the v-wave will follow the T wave, as shown in figure 40.3. The measurement of the CVP or RAP is by convention taken as the mean of the a-wave. As valvular pathology can result in large v-waves, the maximal deflection of the tracing is not used. Normal values for CVP range from 2 to 8 mm Hg, although there is considerable variability.

RIGHT VENTRICULAR PRESSURE

There is a dramatic change in the waveform as the catheter moves from the right atrium to the right ventricle, as demonstrated in figure 40.4. This will happen when the catheter is advanced 25–30 cm, varying based on site of vascular access and patient anatomy. As shown, there is a rapid rise in pressure as the right ventricle contracts and then a rapid fall as the right ventricle relaxes. Right ventricular pressures are reported with a systolic, diastolic, and mean value. Normal values are in the range of 15–25 mm Hg systolic and 4–10 mm Hg diastolic. This tracing should only be seen during the floating of the PA line, as the catheter tip should not remain in the right ventricle, where there is a greater risk of inducing arrhythmias and none of the catheter measurement ports will remain in the RV if the catheter is appropriately positioned.

PULMONARY ARTERY PRESSURE

Close attention must be paid as the PA catheter is advanced from the right ventricle into the pulmonary artery, usually 5–10 cm after the RV tracing is seen. The waveform will have three distinct changes in appearance after this transition. While the systolic pressure will remain essentially constant (15–25 mm Hg), the diastolic pressure will rise in the

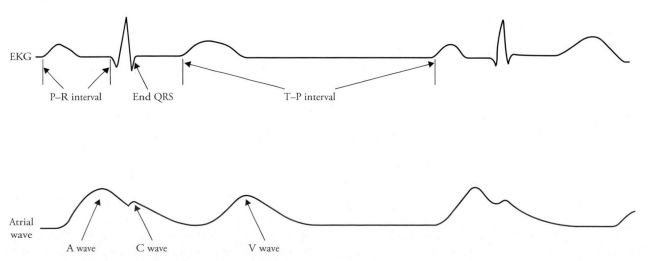

Figure 40.3. Central venous pressure tracing with electrocardiogram.

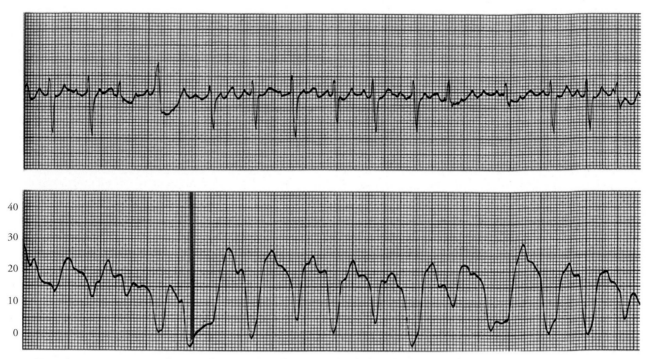

Figure 40.4. Central venous pressure to right ventricle tracing. This figure was published in Aherns TS, Taylor LA. Hemodynamic Waveforms Analysis. 1992, p.109. Copyright Elsevier.

pulmonary artery (normal range 8–15 mm Hg). The waveform will have a dicrotic notch (see figure 40.5), which is a reflection of pulmonic valve closure. Finally, the diastolic portion of the curve will now be downsloping, as pressures fall during diastole with run off into the pulmonary vascular bed between cardiac contractions.

PULMONARY ARTERY OCCLUSION PRESSURE

Once the catheter is in the pulmonary artery, the clinician will slowly advance it until a waveform similar to the CVP is attained, usually at approximately 45 cm. This new tracing is the pulmonary artery occlusion pressure (PAOP) or "wedge" pressure. It is, as previously discussed, an approximation of left atrial pressure. It has similar deflections and descents as the RAP, although there is a greater lag between the electrical events on the EKG and the mechanical events reflected on the tracing, and the PAOP will be higher than the RAP. Once again, an incompetent mitral valve can result in large v-waves, which should not be incorporated in the measurement of the PAOP. Normal values range from 8 to 12 mm Hg.

8283 04 MAR 90 1735 P1 WAVE:0-100 HR:93 P1:60/26 (39) P2:279/278 (278)

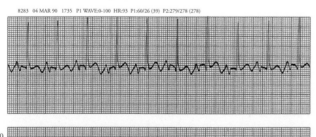

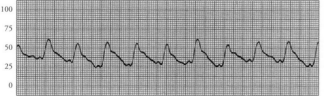

Figure 40.5. Pulmonary Artery Tracing with Notation of Dicrotic Notch. This figure was published in Aherns TS, Taylor LA. Hemodynamic Waveforms Analysis. 1992, p.115. Copyright Elsevier.

READING PRESSURES

Prior to any measurements being made, the PA catheter transduction apparatus must be "zeroed" or opened to air so as to establish atmospheric pressure as zero. The transduction system must also be set at a mid-chest level on the patient, usually at the fourth intercostal space. This position, in most patients, will most closely approximate the level of the heart and improve accuracy of pressure measurements. Perhaps most importantly, this position must be consistent from measurement to measurement in an individual patient.

Respiratory pressure changes can affect PA catheter readings, although ideally the catheter is placed in lung zone 3 (figure 40.1) where alveolar pressure is less than both pulmonary artery and venous pressures. This position can be hard to achieve when patients are on mechanical ventilation and have abnormally high alveolar pressures due to the delivery of high positive end-expiratory pressures (PEEP). By convention, PA catheter pressure tracings are read at end-expiration, when alveolar pressures should have the least impact on arterial pressure readings.

INTERPRETATION OF DATA

ELEVATED PRESSURES

An elevated CVP is generally consistent with increased filling of the right cardiac chambers, although there are exceptions to this rule. Similarly, high PAOP generally indicates volume overload and increased left ventricular end-diastolic volume. These pressures can also be elevated due to pericardial disease or be artificially "increased" by the transmission of alveolar pressures to the PA catheter. Because of this potential for artifact in measurement, care must always be taken in interpretation of data from a PA line. Similarly, for each individual, the ideal filling pressures to maximize cardiac output will vary; thus, there is no one "normal" value to which a patient's therapy should be tailored.

As mentioned previously, regurgitant flow through either the tricuspid valve or the mitral valve can result in very large v-waves in the CVP or the PAOP, respectively. This finding should alert the clinician to valvular pathology, and these large v-waves should not be taken into account when estimating pressures. In the setting of atrial fibrillation, when there is no regular contraction of the atrium, there will not be true a-waves, and a mean of the entire waveform should be used for pressure measurement (assuming minimal mitral or tricuspid regurgitation). If there is loss of atrial–ventricular synchrony, there can be atrial contraction against a closed tricuspid valve. This will results in a much larger deflection called a "cannon a-wave." This also should not be included in estimation of filling pressures, as it is an artifact of the dyssynchrony between the atria and ventricles.

HEMODYNAMIC CALCULATIONS

A pulmonary artery catheter allows the calculation of cardiac output in two ways: thermodilution and the Fick equation. Data provided can also be used to calculate systemic vascular resistance (SVR) and pulmonary vascular resistance (PVR).

Thermodilution

The thermodilution technique works on the principle that flow (or cardiac output) is inversely proportional to the mean concentration of an indicator, in most cases cold water, as measured over time at a static point. Simplistically, a 5 cc bolus of cold water is injected out of a proximal port in the right ventricle and the temperature of the blood is measured,

over time, at a distal port in the pulmonary artery. The area under the curve of the temperature–time plot is inversely proportional to the cardiac output. This technique is limited by pathology that will interfere with consistent forward flow such as significant tricuspid regurgitation. In this setting, some of the cold water bolus can move backward toward the right atrium, and cardiac output can be underestimated.

Fick Calculation

The Fick equation allows calculation of the cardiac output based on the difference in oxygen saturation between the arterial and venous blood as well as the systemic oxygen consumption. The arterial oxygen saturation (SaO_2) is obtained from an arterial blood gas, and the venous saturation is obtained from a blood sample from the tip of the PA catheter when it is not in wedge position (called a mixed venous saturation or SvO_2). In most cases, the oxygen consumption used in the calculation of cardiac output is an assumed value based on a patient's size, although it is possible to measure this directly. The Fick equation is:

$$CO = \frac{\text{oxygen consumption}}{\text{arterial oxygen content} - \text{venous oxygen content}}$$

Error in measurement of cardiac output via the Fick equation usually results from the assumption of a value for oxygen consumption, as many critically ill patients will have a markedly increased oxygen consumption due to infection or other inflammatory processes. Normal values of cardiac output range from 4 to 7 L/min. Some clinicians prefer to use cardiac index (CI), which is cardiac output normalized by body surface area (BSA) and can be easily calculated from cardiac output (CI = CO/BSA). The range of normal for CI is 2.5–4 L/min/m².

Vascular Resistance

Both systemic vascular resistance (SVR) and pulmonary vascular resistance (PVR) can be calculated from the data provided by a PA catheter. The equations are:

$$SVR = [(MAP - RAP)/CO] \times 80$$
$$PVR = [(mPAP - PAOP)/CO] \times 80$$

where MAP = mean arterial pressure, RAP = right atrial pressure, mPAP = mean pulmonary artery pressure, and PAOP = pulmonary artery occlusion pressure.

Normal values for SVR range from 900 to 1300 dynes/sec/cm⁵. Because the pulmonary circulation is a much lower resistance system, normal values are much lower, in the range of 40–150 dynes/sec/cm⁵. It is important to note that these values will be calculated from a calculated cardiac output as well as from pressures measured from the PA catheter, allowing for multiple potential points for error.

Table 40.1 DIFFERENTIATION OF THE TYPES OF SHOCK

CAUSE OF SHOCK	CO/CI	RAP	PAOP	SVR
Hypovolemic	↓	↓	↓	↑
Distributive	↑ (or ↓)	↓	↓	↓
Cardiogenic	↓	↑	↑	↑

NOTES: CO = cardiac output, CI = cardiac index (CO/body surface area), PAOP = pulmonary artery occlusion pressure, RAP = right atrial pressure, SVR = systemic vascular resistance.

Distinguishing Types of Shock

Often the calculated cardiac output and systemic vascular resistance as well as filling pressures are used to distinguish among different types of shock: hypovolemic, distributive, and cardiogenic. An extensive discussion of this topic is beyond the scope of this chapter, but table 40.1 is a simplification of the distinctions among these different clinical pictures, and table 40.2 give some clinical examples of these types of shock.

SUMMARY

Hemodynamic monitoring can help in the diagnosis and management of critically ill patients. The PA catheter allows assessment of cardiac filling pressures as well as calculation of cardiac output and vascular resistance. As with all invasive procedures, there are known complications of PA catheters, as well as challenges in the interpretation of the data provided. For these reasons, clinicians should carefully weigh the risks and benefits of placement before deciding on the use of this invasive device.

Table 40.2 EXAMPLES OF TYPES OF SHOCK

TYPE OF SHOCK	CLINICAL EXAMPLE
Hypovolemic	Gastrointestinal bleeding Bleeding from trauma Massive diarrhea or vomiting Third-spacing from pancreatitis Large surface area burns
Distributive	Sepsis SIRS Spinal cord injury Anaphylaxis Adrenal insufficiency Pancreatitis
Cardiogenic	Ischemic cardiomyopathy Acute mitral regurgitation Pulmonary embolism Cardiac tamponade Ventricular tachycardia

ADDITIONAL READING

Bernard GR, Sopko G, Cerra F, et al. Pulmonary artery catheterization and clinical outcomes: National Heart, Lung, and Blood Institute and Food and Drug Administration Workshop Report. Consensus Statement. *JAMA.* 2000;283(19):2568–72.

Binanay C, Califf RM, Hasselblad V, et al. *Evaluation study of congestive heart failure and pulmonary artery catheterization effectiveness: The ESCAPE trial. JAMA.* 2005;294(13):1625–33.

Kahwash R, Leier CV, Miller L. Role of the pulmonary artery catheter in diagnosis and management of heart failure. *Heart Fail Clin.* 2009;5(2):241–8.

Kramer A, Zygun D, Hawes H, Easton, P, Ferland A. Pulse pressure variation predicts fluid responsiveness following coronary artery bypass surgery. *Chest.* 2004;126(5):1563–8.

Rivers E, Nguyen B, Havstad S, et al. Early goal-directed therapy in the treatment of severe sepsis and septic shock. *N Engl J Med.* 2001;345(19):1368–77.

Sandham JD, Hull RD, Brant RF, et al. A randomized, controlled trial of the use of pulmonary-artery catheters in high-risk surgical patients. *N Engl J Med.* 2003;348(1):5–14.

Shah MR, Hasselblad V, Stevenson LW, et al. Impact of the pulmonary artery catheter in critically ill patients: meta-analysis of randomized clinical trials. *JAMA.* 2005;294(13):1664–70.

Shah MR, Miller L. Use of pulmonary artery catheters in advanced heart failure. *Curr Opin Cardiol.* 2007;22(3):220–4.

Vieillard-Baron A, Chergui K, Augarde R, Prin S, Page B, Beauchet A, Jardin F. Cyclic changes in arterial pulse during respiratory support revisited by Doppler echocardiography. *Am J Respir Crit Care Med.* 2003;168(6):671–6.

Wheeler AP, Bernard GR, Thompson BT, et al. Pulmonary-artery versus central venous catheter to guide treatment of acute lung injury. *N Engl J Med.* 2006;354(21):2213–24.

QUESTIONS

QUESTION 1. A 67-year-old woman presents with lethargy, fever, and dysuria. She has a history of hypertension and medically treated CAD. Her medications include atenolol, lisinopril, aspirin, and simvastatin. Her husband reports that today "she has not been herself." On exam, she is lethargic but arousable. Vital signs: heart rate 126, BP 70/46, RR 24. Her lungs are clear. She is tachycardic

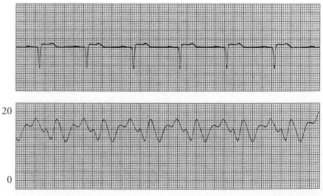

Figure 40.6. Central venous pressure tracing for patient in Question #1. This figure was published in Aherns TS, Taylor LA. Hemodynamic Waveforms Analysis. 1992, p.51. Copyright Elsevier.

without murmurs. Jugular venous pressure (JVP) is flat, and her abdomen is soft and nontender. She has no CVA tenderness. WBC 13,000 with a left shift, hematocrit 42. Urinalysis with a large number of white blood cells, many bacteria, positive nitrites, positive leukocyte esterase. CXR and EKG are unremarkable. The patient receives 2 L normal saline in 500-cc boluses. A central line is placed. A CVP is measured. The tracing is shown in figure 40.6.

The patient's CVP is

A. 12 mm Hg
B. 15 mm Hg
C. 12/17 mm Hg
D. 12/15 mm Hg
E. Unable to determine due to respiratory variation

QUESTION 2. A patient is admitted to the ICU with endocarditis and hypotension. Because it is difficult to determine whether the hypotension is caused by sepsis or cardiogenic shock from acute mitral regurgitation, a PA catheter is placed. What data would be needed to calculate SVR?

A. RAP, PAOP, and CO
B. CI and PAOP
C. RAP, MAP, and SaO$_2$
D. RAP, MAP, and CO
E. CI, MAP, and PAOP

QUESTION 3. Which of the following sets of data would suggest that the etiology of the shock is due to sepsis?

A. SVR 550, CI 6.0, RAP 3
B. SVR 900, CI 6.0, RAP 5
C. SVR 800, CI 3.2, RAP 10
D. SVR 1200, CI 1.5, RAP 15
E. SVR 1500, CI 2.4, RAP 4

ANSWERS

1. B
2. D
3. E

41.

ARTERIAL BLOOD GASES

Jeremy B. Richards and David H. Roberts

OVERVIEW: CLINICAL INDICATIONS AND UTILITY

An arterial blood gas (ABG) provides clinically useful information about an individual's acid–base status, the partial pressure of arterial carbon dioxide, the partial pressure of arterial oxygen, and the arterial oxygen saturation. Hypoxia, dyspnea, or suspected acid–base disturbance are clear indications to check an ABG. Altered mental status, critical illness, and acute respiratory distress syndrome (ARDS) are specific clinical syndromes or presentations that warrant checking an ABG.

An ABG is helpful in evaluating pulmonary pathophysiology as the presence and severity of hypoxia and/or hypercapnia can be quantified. Because an ABG can rapidly provide information about oxygenation, ventilation, and acid–base status, ABGs are particularly useful and common in the critical care setting.

TECHNICAL CONSIDERATIONS: HOW TO OBTAIN AN ABG

An ABG may be obtained from any artery. Relative contraindications to performing an ABG include uncontrolled coagulopathy, superficial infection over the artery, the absence of a detectable pulse, or an AV fistula.

Because arterial puncture carries the potential complication of arterial laceration and/or hematoma with compromise of blood flow to distal tissues, ideally easily accessible arteries perfusing tissue with adequate collateral circulation should be used. Large arteries that are accessible may be accessed in the absence of collateral circulation, as it is unlikely that a hematoma would cause occlusion or a laceration would compromise distal flow.

The radial artery is easily accessible in that it is superficial and has adequate collateral circulation (the ulnar artery coursing along the medial arm). The femoral, dorsalis pedis, brachial, and axillary arteries are potential alternative sites

for obtaining an ABG when the radial arteries cannot be accessed.

Prior to obtaining an ABG from the radial artery, an Allan's test should be performed. The hand is held above the level of the heart and a fist is made while the radial and ulnar arteries are compressed. The hand is then lowered below the level of the heart and the fist is opened. Compression of the ulnar artery is released while maintaining compression of the radial artery; the hand should reperfuse within 6 seconds if the ulnar artery is adequately perfusing the hand. If the Allan's test is negative (i.e., color does not return to the hand within 6 seconds, indicating inadequate perfusion), the contralateral radial and ulnar arteries should be assessed. If both hands demonstrate inadequate ulnar circulation, alternative sites for obtaining an ABG should be considered to avoid causing decreased tissue perfusion and possible damage to the hands.

If the individual is awake and alert, a small amount of subcutaneous lidocaine may be administered prior to obtaining the ABG. The lidocaine should not be injected directly over the artery, rather slightly lateral or medial to avoid creating a weal directly over the vessel. Superficial anesthetic is typically sufficient, administering deeper dermal lidocaine is usually not necessary to ensure comfort.

To perform an ABG, prepackaged kits of the requisite supplies are typically available. The kits contain a syringe preloaded with heparin powder (to minimize clotting), a needle (typically 22 gauge for the radial artery), and a filter cap to place on the syringe for transport.

The clinician may palpate the pulse while attempting to access the artery; however, care should be taken not to apply too much pressure to the artery proximally so as to occlude the artery and obstruct flow to the access site. Palpating the artery distal to the access site may prevent this complication. Alternatively, light palpation proximal to the puncture site is acceptable. The needle should be oriented with the bevel up. When the needle enters the artery a flash of blood will appear in the syringe. If the aperture of the needle is within the artery, blood will spontaneously fill the syringe without one needing to apply suction to the syringe. After an acceptable quantity of blood has been collected, the needle is withdrawn and protected, and pressure is applied over the access site. The protected needle is removed and safely discarded and the filter cap is placed on the syringe. Bubbles should be removed by expelling them through the filter cap.

The capped syringe should be rapidly transported to the lab for processing. Some recommend placing the syringe on ice prior to transport to minimize cell degradation, clotting, and changes in the partial pressure of the gases of interest.

When multiple serial ABGs are needed, an arterial catheter may be placed to facilitate frequent measurements and minimize repeated needle sticks.

HYPOXEMIA

PaO_2 VERSUS SaO_2 VERSUS CaO_2

Oxygen is present in arterial blood in two forms—bound to hemoglobin and dissolved in the plasma. The oxygen saturation (SaO_2) represents oxygen bound to hemoglobin, while the partial pressure of oxygen (PaO_2) represents oxygen dissolved in plasma.

PaO_2 reflects only molecules dissolved in the plasma, as oxygen bound to hemoglobin does not influence the measured partial pressure in the plasma. PaO_2 is measured directly by an electrode that senses oxygen molecules not bound to hemoglobin.

SaO_2 reflects the percentage of available hemoglobin binding sites to which oxygen is bound. For example, a SaO_2 of 90% means that out of 100 available hemoglobin binding sites, 90 are bound by oxygen. SaO_2 should be directly measured by co-oximetry rather than extrapolated from the measured PaO_2.

There is a well-defined relationship between PaO_2 and SaO_2. When a molecule of oxygen passes from the alveolus to the pulmonary capillary it is initially dissolved in the plasma. The oxygen molecule then rapidly binds to an available hemoglobin binding site. When bound to hemoglobin, the molecule of oxygen does not contribute to the pressure gradient of oxygen between the alveolus and pulmonary capillary, thereby allowing for more oxygen to diffuse from the alveolus into the bloodstream. In general, the more dissolved oxygen molecules there are (i.e., the higher the PaO_2), the more oxygen will bind to hemoglobin (i.e., the higher the SaO_2).

Therefore, the PaO_2 may be considered a "driver" of SaO_2. The relationship of SaO_2 and PaO_2 is graphically described by the oxygen dissociation curve (see figure 41.1).

Although they are clinically valuable parameters, neither PaO_2 nor SaO_2 provides quantitative information about the amount of oxygen in arterial blood. The total quantity of oxygen in arterial blood is referred to as the arterial oxygen content (CaO_2) and is described by the equation:

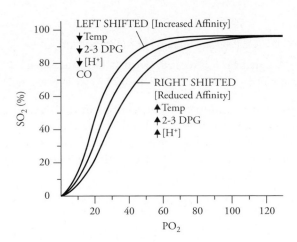

Figure 41.1. Oxygen Dissociation Curve. This figure was published in Walker HK, Hall WD, Hurst HW. *Clinical Methods*, 3rd ed. 1990: 256. Boston: Butterworths. Copyright Elsevier.

$$CaO_2 = (1.34)(Hb)(SaO_2) + (PaO_2)(0.003)$$

Where Hb is hemoglobin (in g/dL), 1.34 is the volume of oxygen (mL) that can be bound by a gram of hemoglobin, and 0.003 is the solubility coefficient of oxygen in plasma. CaO_2 is expressed in milliliters of oxygen per deciliter.

The arterial oxygen content, therefore, is essentially the sum of the SaO_2 and PaO_2 (corrected for hemoglobin content and solubility, respectively). CaO_2 is the most physiologically relevant estimation of the quantity of oxygen delivered to peripheral tissues.

A-a GRADIENT AND THE ALVEOLAR GAS EQUATION

The transfer of oxygen from the alveolus to the blood in the pulmonary capillaries is described by the alveolar (A) to arterial (a) gradient. The A-a gradient provides a rough estimation of the relative ease by which oxygen transfers across the alveolar-capillary membrane. The partial pressures of oxygen in the alveolar and arterial compartments are used to determine the A-a gradient.

The partial pressure of oxygen in arterial blood (the PaO_2) is directly measured by obtaining an ABG. The partial pressure of oxygen in the alveoli (PAO_2) must be calculated by the alveolar gas equation:

$$PAO_2 = PIO_2 - (PaCO_2/R)$$

where $PIO_2 = (P_{bar} - PH_2O) \times FiO_2$, P_{bar} is barometric pressure (760 mm Hg at sea level), PH_2O is the partial pressure of water vapor (47 mm Hg), and FiO_2 is the fraction of inhaled oxygen. $PaCO_2$ is the partial pressure of carbondioxide in arterial blood and R is the respiratory quotient (estimated to be 0.8).

If the patient is breathing room air $(FiO_2 = 0.21)$ at sea level, the equation can be simplified:

$$PAo_2 = (Fio_2 \times 713) - (5/4) Paco_2$$
$$\text{Or } PAo_2 = 150 \text{ mm Hg} - (1.25 \times Paco_2)$$
$$\text{A-a gradient} = PAo_2 \text{ (calculated)} - Pao_2 \text{ (measured)}$$
Normal range = 0–10 mm Hg or 2.5 + 0.21 × (age in years) mm Hg

There are a number of assumptions in the alveolar gas equation that need to be considered when using the A-a gradient clinically. The respiratory quotient is the amount of carbon dioxide produced divided by the amount of oxygen consumed, described as:

$$R = \dot{V}co_2/\dot{V}o_2$$

where $\dot{V}co_2$ is the carbon dioxide production and $\dot{V}o_2$ is oxygen consumption.

The amount of carbon dioxide produced may vary markedly depending on the patient's metabolic state. Patients with sepsis and systemic inflammation may initially have very high CO_2 production. Sepsis is also characterized by decreased oxygen uptake, further skewing the respiratory quotient from its assumed value of 0.8.

Fio_2 may influence the A-a gradient, as higher Fio_2 is associated with a higher A-a gradient. Increasing age is also associated with a higher A-a gradient. These factors need to be considered to determine whether the calculated A-a gradient actually represents abnormal oxygen transfer and uptake.

Hypoxemia can be caused by a variety of pathophysiological processes including ventilation/perfusion (V/Q) mismatch, shunt, alveolar hypoventilation, reduced partial pressure of oxygen in the inhaled air, or a diffusion abnormality (typically does not cause hypoxemia at rest at sea level). A truly elevated A-a gradient is consistent with V/Q mismatch, shunt, or a diffusion abnormality. In cases of hypoxemia due to alveolar hypoventilation or reduced partial pressure of oxygen, the A-a gradient is normal.

The Pao_2/Fio_2 ratio is another metric that is frequently used in the critical care setting. The normal Pao_2/Fio_2 is 300–500. A Pao_2/Fio_2 ratio of <250 indicates a clinically significant gas exchange derangement.

EFFECTS OF SUPPLEMENTAL OXYGEN

Supplemental oxygen increases the PAo_2 in patients who are ventilating normally by increasing the Fio_2. Increased PAo_2 leads to an increased driving pressure of oxygen across the alveolar membrane. In a patient with V/Q mismatch, increased PAo_2 leads to an increased Pao_2. In the setting of shunt, in which blood passes through the lungs without making contact with the alveolus for gas exchange to occur, supplemental oxygen does not improve hypoxemia.

In the absence of a complete shunt, the amount of increase of Pao_2 for a given amount of supplemental oxygen can be estimated. It should be emphasized that measurements of Pao_2 do vary over time without any significant change in clinical status, so the fidelity of equations predicting changes in Pao_2 for a given increase in Fio_2 is limited. Additionally, methods of administering oxygen make estimating the precise percentage of oxygen inhaled difficult. Specifically, an awake patient receiving oxygen by nasal cannulae, may inhale through his or her mouth, decreasing the relative contribution of the nasally delivered oxygen. Figure 41.2 demonstrates the approximate relationship between increased Fio_2 and Pao_2 in hypothetical patients with varying degrees of V/Q mismatch.

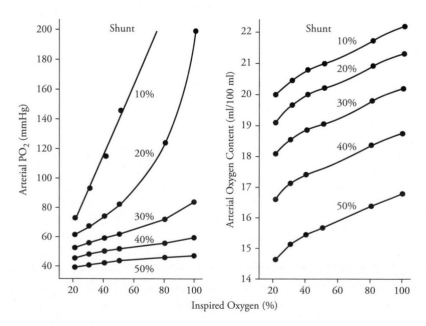

Figure 41.2. Changes in Pao_2 with Increasing Fio_2 with Varying Degrees of V/Q Mismatch. Reprinted with permission from Tobin MJ. *Principles and Practice of Mechanical Ventilation*. New York: McGraw-Hill; 2006: 760.

Plane travel is an interesting circumstance in which supplemental oxygen may be necessary for patients who normally do not require it. The alveolar gas equation reminds us that barometric pressure is the primary driving force of gas into the alveoli. By law, the cabin pressure of planes is set at the equivalent of no higher than 8000 feet (~560 mm Hg); usually cabin pressure is the equivalent of 6000–8000 feet. For people without lung disease or shunt, this decrease in barometric pressure is well tolerated. However, for patients with pulmonary disease, depressurization to approximately 8000 feet may be dangerous. Prior to flying, the predicted PaO_2 at 8000 feet should be calculated for such patients using the following equation:

$$\text{Predicted PaO}_2 \text{ at 8000 feet} = 0.294 \,(\text{PaO}_2 \text{ on RA at sea level}) + 0.086 \,(\text{percentage predicted FEV}_1) + 23.211$$

If the patient's predicted PaO_2 is unacceptably low (i.e., <60 mm Hg), providing supplemental oxygen to increase the patient's FiO_2 can counterbalance the effects of decreased barometric pressure while flying. Alternative methods for assessing whether a patient would tolerate plane travel include having the patient breathe hypoxic gas (15.1% oxygen, called the hypoxia altitude simulation test) or measuring PaO_2 in a hypobaric chamber. These methods may be more accurate but may also require additional equipment compared with the aforementioned equation.

CARBOXYHEMOGLOBINEMIA AND METHEMOGLOBINEMIA

Hemoglobin molecules can lose affinity for oxygen by binding to carbon monoxide or by transforming into methemoglobin. Carbon monoxide avidly and irreversibly binds to hemoglobin, thereby decreasing the binding sites available for oxygen to bind hemoglobin. Hemoglobin bound to carbon monoxide is referred to as carboxyhemoglobin.

Methemoglobin is formed when ferrous ion (Fe^{2+}) is oxidized to the ferric state (Fe^{3+}); this oxidative change prevents oxygen from binding methemoglobin. Methemoglobinemia can be congenital or acquired. Congenital forms of methemoglobinemia may be due to enzyme deficiencies (such as diaphorase I deficiency). More commonly, methemoglobin is acquired as a result of oxidizing medications causing ferrous ion to convert to the ferric state. Dapsone, nitrates, local anesthetics (such as benzocaine), trimethoprim, and sulfonamides are potential causes of methemoglobinemia.

In these conditions, ABG analysis may reveal a normal PaO_2. The measured SaO_2, however, is abnormal as the amount of oxygen bound to hemoglobin is decreased. It is important to recognize that peripherally measured oxygen saturation levels with pulse oximetry will be normal—an ABG is necessary to determine the true degree of hypoxia in these conditions. Pulse oximetry is normal (or near normal) in these conditions, as light emitted by the pulse oximeter is increased by carboxy- and methemoglobin, which the oximeter reports as oxygen (rather than carbon monoxide saturation or methemoglobin levels).

Both carboxyhemoglobinemia and methemoglobinemia are treated with supplemental oxygen (including intubation and mechanical ventilation if necessary). Methemoglobinemia may be treated with methylene blue (1–2 mg/kg over 5 min), as it reduces the iron ion in hemoglobin to its ferrous (Fe^{2+}) state, thereby allowing the Hb to bind and carry oxygen. Carboxyhemoglobinemia may require treatment in a hyperbaric oxygen chamber. Increasing the PAO_2 (by increasing the barometric pressure) may make the pressure gradient for oxygen across the alveolar membrane high enough for oxygen to displace avidly bound carbon monoxide from hemoglobin.

ACID–BASE DISORDERS

HYPERCAPNIA AND ACUTE RESPIRATORY ACIDOSIS

Increased carbon dioxide levels (referred to as hypercapnia) occur in the setting of hypoventilation. Carbon dioxide readily diffuses from the bloodstream across the alveolar-capillary membrane; it is removed from alveoli by the process of ventilation. The limiting step in the elimination of carbon dioxide is not diffusion from the pulmonary circulation to the alveoli, rather it is the efficiency and efficacy of ventilation. This relationship is described via the following equation:

$$\dot{V}A = (\dot{V}CO_2 \times k)/PaCO_2$$

where $\dot{V}A$ is alveolar ventilation, $\dot{V}CO_2$ is the metabolic production of CO_2, k is a proportionality constant, and $PaCO_2$ is the partial pressure of carbon dioxide in arterial blood (in mm Hg).

When alveolar ventilation ($\dot{V}A$) decreases, $PaCO_2$ must increase proportionally, assuming that $\dot{V}CO_2$ does not change. Understanding that hypoventilation is the primary cause of elevated blood levels of carbon dioxide is important in diagnosing and treating hypercapnia.

Alveolar ventilation cannot be readily measured in the clinical setting. However, minute ventilation ($\dot{V}E$) is easily determined:

$$\dot{V}E = \text{Respiratory rate} \times \text{Tidal volume}$$

$\dot{V}A$ is the portion of the $\dot{V}E$ that does not include deadspace ventilation:

$$\dot{V}A = \dot{V}E \,(1 - v_d/v_t)$$

where v_d/v_t is deadspace fraction.

The v_d/v_t may be measured by the ventilator in mechanically ventilated patients. Specifically, expired carbon dioxide is collected and measured over a certain period of time; v_d/v_t can be calculated via the following relationship:

$$v_d/v_t = (Paco_2 - PEco_2)/Paco_2$$

where $PEco_2$ is the expired CO_2.

Clinically, therefore, the relationship between $\dot{V}A$ and $Paco_2$ can be represented by the following equation:

$$\dot{V}E(1 - v_d/v_t) = (\dot{V}co_2 \times k)/Paco_2$$

$\dot{V}E$, v_d/v_t, and $Paco_2$ are all easily measured parameters and $\dot{V}co_2 \times k$ is thought to be relatively constant. When $\dot{V}E$ decreases, $Paco_2$ must increase. When v_d/v_t increases, $Paco_2$ must increase. Both of these situations (increased v_d/v_t and decreased $\dot{V}E$) result in alveolar hypoventilation (decreased $\dot{V}A$).

Acute respiratory acidosis occurs when $\dot{V}A$ decreases suddenly. As the continued, efficient elimination of carbon dioxide is important for preservation of a neutral acid–base status, a sudden decrease in $\dot{V}A$ and a sudden increase in $Paco_2$ causes a rapid decrease in pH.

Causes of decreased $\dot{V}A$ are classically divided into central and peripheral processes. Central hypoventilation may occur for a variety of reasons. Intoxication, particularly with opiates or other central nervous system (CNS) depressants, may result in a blunted central respiratory drive and decreased $\dot{V}A$.

Peripheral causes of decreased $\dot{V}A$ include neuromuscular disorders or neuromuscular blocking medications that cause weakened or inefficient muscles of respiration. When tidal volume and/or respiratory rate decreases, $\dot{V}E$ decreases, and $Paco_2$ rises. Severe airways obstruction, such as a chronic obstructive pulmonary disease (COPD) exacerbation, may also result in acute hypoventilation and hypercapnia.

It is rare that small increases in v_d/v_t alone result in hypercapnia. Carbon dioxide so readily diffuses across the alveolar membrane that minimal increases in $\dot{V}E$ can compensate for small increases in v_d/v_t and maintain a normal or near-normal CO_2.

Treatment of hypercapnia is centered on treatment of the underlying process. In certain circumstances, mechanical ventilation may be necessary to provide adequate $\dot{V}E$ and $\dot{V}A$ to correct hypercapnia.

COMPENSATORY MECHANISMS CHRONIC RESPIRATORY ACIDOSIS

Chronic respiratory acidosis is an interesting condition in which a patient experiences persistent alveolar hypoventilation. Persistent alveolar hypoventilation and persistently elevated $Paco_2$ result in changes in kidney function in an effort to restore acid–base neutrality. Specifically, normally functioning kidneys respond to persistent acidemia by increasing retention of bicarbonate while increasing excretion of hydrogen ion. Over several days, the kidneys' response results in elevated serum bicarbonate levels and the return of serum pH toward normal.

Reasons for chronic alveolar hypoventilation, and thereby chronic respiratory acidosis, include central and peripheral processes (table 41.1). Central processes include pathologies such as obesity hypoventilation syndrome (aka OHS, or the Pickwickian syndrome.) In patients with OHS, chronic hypoventilation leads to a "reset" of the carotid bodies and the central medullary respiratory centers. The physiologically acceptable $Paco_2$ is liberalized, and the centrally mediated respiratory drive is relatively decreased due to increased tolerance for elevated $Paco_2$ by the central respiratory centers. Similarly, rarely, a stroke in the medullary respiratory center can result in central hypoventilation.

As with acute respiratory acidosis, neuromuscular diseases or advanced obstructive diseases such as COPD can result in chronic respiratory acidosis. If untreated, a neuromuscular process such as amyotrophic lateral sclerosis (ALS) can lead to chronically decreased minute ventilation and/or respiratory rate. Over time, a persistently elevated $Paco_2$ will lead to changes in renal function and a compensatory metabolic alkalosis. The central respiratory drive will still respond to the elevated $Paco_2$, but the muscles of respiration will not be able to adequately increase $\dot{V}A$.

Similarly, patients with advanced COPD may be unable to perform efficient ventilation due to airways obstruction and hyperinflation. Over time, elevated $Paco_2$ leads to a chronic respiratory acidosis and a compensatory metabolic alkalosis.

As in acute respiratory acidosis, treatment of a chronic respiratory acidosis must be focused on the underlying cause. Supportive care is typically appropriate, given that many

Table 41.1 CAUSES OF RESPIRATORY ACIDOSIS

Chronic obstructive pulmonary disease: Emphysema, severe asthma, chronic bronchitis

Neuromuscular diseases: Amyotrophic lateral sclerosis, diaphragm dysfunction and paralysis, Guillain-Barré syndrome, myasthenia gravis, muscular dystrophy

Chest wall disorders: Severe kyphoscoliosis; status post-thoracoplasty; flail chest; less commonly, ankylosing spondylitis, pectus excavatum, or pectus carinatum

Obstructive sleep apnea

Obesity-hypoventilation syndrome

CNS depression: Drugs (e.g., narcotics, barbiturates, benzodiazepines, other CNS depressants), neurologic disorders (e.g., encephalitis, brainstem disease, trauma), primary alveolar hypoventilation

Other lung and airway diseases: Laryngeal and tracheal stenosis

Lung-protective ventilation in ARDS

causes of chronic respiratory acidoses are not reversible or easily treatable. Mechanical ventilation, particularly noninvasive positive-pressure ventilation (NIPPV), is appropriate treatment for many causes of chronic respiratory acidosis. Particularly for patients with OHS or other central causes of chronic respiratory acidosis, nocturnal NIPPV can delay the progression of disease and the worsening of chronic respiratory acidosis.

For patients with advanced COPD, treatment of the underlying disease with appropriate medical therapy and judicious use of NIPPV is appropriate.

RESPIRATORY ALKALOSIS

Respiratory alkalosis is defined as an increased pH due to a decreased $PaCO_2$. Just as respiratory acidosis may be considered a consequence of decreased alveolar ventilation, increased alveolar ventilation is considered the primary cause of respiratory alkalosis. Any process that leads to an increase in minute ventilation without a substantive increase in deadspace ventilation will result in a respiratory alkalosis.

Most commonly, respiratory alkaloses are acute (table 41.2). Increases in respiratory rate and/or tidal volume due to pain, anxiety, stress, fever (which may stimulate the medullary respiratory centers), drugs (methamphetamines, caffeine, or other stimulant use), or hypoxia can lead to increased elimination of carbon dioxide and a respiratory alkalosis. It should be emphasized that in an awake and alert patient with hypoxemia, it is not uncommon for a mild respiratory alkalosis to be present. Aspirin is a unique example, as it classically causes a centrally mediated respiratory alkalosis and a metabolic acidosis.

Chronic respiratory alkalosis is a relatively rare phenomenon; chronic causes of persistently increased alveolar ventilation are almost exclusively related to central nervous system pathologies. Stroke, infection (such as meningitis), and subarachnoid hemorrhage are all potential causes of chronic respiratory alkalosis due to direct brainstem stimulation. Additional etiologies of chronic respiratory alkaloses are high-progesterone states, including pregnancy, and advanced liver disease and cirrhosis.

Table 41.2 **CAUSES OF RESPIRATORY ALKALOSIS**

Iatrogenic

Psychiatric: Anxiety, hysteria, stress

Medications: Doxapram, aspirin, caffeine

CNS: Stroke, subarachnoid hemorrhage, meningitis

Pulmonary disease: Pneumonia

General: Fever, pregnancy, sexual activity, hepatic failure (high ammonia levels), high altitude

The treatment of an acute respiratory alkalosis is primarily centered on treatment of the underlying process. In an anxious patient, redirection and judicious use of anxiolytics is appropriate. In a patient with pain, analgesia is appropriate. In a hypoxic patient, treatment of the underlying process and providing supplemental oxygen are appropriate interventions.

Chronic respiratory alkaloses are more difficult to treat as they are typically centrally mediated. Therapeutic efforts are focused on supporting and reversing (if possible) the underlying central process.

METABOLIC ACIDOSIS

Acute metabolic acidosis is defined as a decrease in serum bicarbonate levels with a concomitant decrease in pH. Bicarbonate (HCO_3^-) is an important physiological buffer; when hydrogen ion is increased, bicarbonate is consumed via the following relationship:

$$HCO_3^- + H^+ \rightarrow H_2CO_3 \rightarrow H_2O + CO_2$$

where H_2CO_3 is a transient, unstable state.

The relationship between carbon dioxide and bicarbonate can also be described by the Henderson-Hasselbalch equation:

$$pH = pK + \log[(HCO_3^-)/(0.03 \times PaCO_2)]$$

The Henderson-Hasselbalch equation demonstrates the important point that pH is dependent on the ratio of bicarbonate to carbon dioxide. This concept explains the importance of so-called "compensatory" mechanisms. In an effort to preserve pH near normal, changes in bicarbonate level lead to changes in respiration and minute ventilation in an effort to adjust the carbon dioxide levels.

Most metabolic acidoses are acute in nature, as a sudden increase in hydrogen ion production is usually due to an acute event. Chronic metabolic acidoses are simply processes in which acids are produced (and buffered) over time. The primary differentiation between an acute metabolic acidosis is that alternative buffers such as bone and hemoglobin may be used as bicarbonate is depleted.

Metabolic acidoses may be divided into anion-gap and non-anion-gap metabolic acidoses. Anion-gap metabolic acidoses are processes in which an unmeasured anion is produced, leading to an increase in the anion gap. The anion gap represents the presence of anions that are not measured in the basic chemistry panel. Negatively charged proteins (particularly albumin) form the majority of unmeasured anions. The anion gap is calculated in the following manner:

$$Na^+ - (Cl^- + HCO_3^-) = \text{anion gap}$$

A normal anion gap is approximately 10–12. When albumin is lower than normal, the upper limit of the anion gap is reduced. This reduction can be approximated by lowering the upper limit of the anion gap by 2 for every 1 g/dL decrease in serum albumin. For example, an anion gap of 10 would be normal in a patient with a normal serum albumin; however, in a patient with a serum albumin of 2 g/dL an anion gap of 10 would be considered elevated (as the upper limit of normal of the anion gap in this patient would be ~6–8).

Processes that produce unmeasured anions cause an anion-gap metabolic acidosis. Methanol ingestion, uremia, diabetic ketoacidosis, paraldehyde, iron toxicity, lactic acidosis, ethylene glycol ingestion, and salicylate toxicity are all potential causes of an anion-gap metabolic acidosis (the acronym MUDPILES can be helpful in recalling these conditions).

Non-anion-gap metabolic acidoses result from depletion of bicarbonate without an increase in unmeasured anions. Bicarbonate may be lost from the GI tract (diarrhea), the kidneys (renal tubular acidoses), or in the setting of rapid volume resuscitation with normal saline (hyperchloremic metabolic acidosis).

The urine anion gap (UAG) is helpful in the workup of a normal anion-gap metabolic acidosis. The three main causes of normal anion gap acidosis are (1) loss of HCO_3^- from the gastrointestinal tract (e.g., diarrhea), (2) loss of HCO_3^- from the kidneys (e.g., renal tubular acidosis, RTA), and (3) administration of acid. The urine anion gap = unmeasured anions – unmeasured cations, or: $[Na^+] + [K^+] – [Cl^-]$.

Distinguishing among the above three groups of causes is usually clinically obvious, but occasionally it may be useful to have an extra aid to help in deciding between a loss of base via the kidneys or the bowel. Calculation of the urine anion gap may be helpful diagnostically in these cases.

In normal subjects, the urine anion gap is usually near zero or is positive. In metabolic acidosis, the excretion of NH_4^+ (which is excreted with Cl^-) should increase markedly if renal acidification is intact. Because of the rise in urinary Cl^-, the urine anion gap, which is also called the urinary net charge, becomes negative, ranging from –20 to more than –50 meq/L. The negative value occurs because the Cl^- concentration now exceeds the sum total of Na^+ and K^+.

In contrast, if there is an impairment in kidney function resulting in an inability to increase ammonium excretion (e.g., renal tubular acidosis), then Cl^- ions will not be increased in the urine, and the urine anion gap will not be affected and will be positive or zero. In a patient with a hyperchloremic metabolic acidosis, a negative UAG suggests GI loss of bicarbonate (e.g., diarrhea), whereas a positive UAG suggests impaired renal acidification (i.e., renal tubular acidosis).

When serum bicarbonate decreases, alveolar ventilation increases to decrease $PaCO_2$ in an effort to maintain the pH near normal. Normally, the $PaCO_2$ decreases by 1 mm Hg for each 1 millimolar decrease in serum bicarbonate.

In most cases, treatment of metabolic acidoses centers on treating the underlying disorder. In specific instances, such as in a type 1 renal tubular acidosis, replacement of bicarbonate is appropriate. However, in most cases of metabolic acidosis (particularly anion-gap metabolic acidosis) bicarbonate replacement is not necessary. In cases of extreme acidosis such as a pH <7.15, bicarbonate replacement may be considered while the underlying process is addressed.

METABOLIC ALKALOSIS

Metabolic alkalosis is defined as an increase in serum bicarbonate levels with a concomitant increase in pH. Conceptually, the causes of metabolic alkaloses are an overall loss of hydrogen ion or retention of bicarbonate.

Loss of hydrogen ion may occur due to vomiting or nasogastric suctioning. Normally, when acidic gastric secretions pass into the duodenum they result in the release of relatively basic pancreatic secretions. However, in the setting of vomiting or gastric suctioning, the release of bicarbonate-rich pancreatic secretions does not occur, and a metabolic alkalosis ensues.

Diuretics such as thiazides or loop diuretics (such as furosemide) cause increased hydrogen ion secretion in the urine and thereby cause a metabolic alkalosis. Hyperaldosteronism may cause a metabolic alkalosis as well. A variety of relatively rare syndromes may result in metabolic alkalosis.

An increase in serum bicarbonate level results in alveolar hypoventilation with an increase in $PaCO_2$ in an effort to maintain a near-neutral pH. Typically, $PaCO_2$ will increase by 0.7 mm Hg for every 1 millimolar increase in the serum bicarbonate.

Treatment of metabolic alkalosis is focused on treatment of the underlying process. Patients with excessive vomiting should receive antiemetics, and the cause of the vomiting should be addressed. Diuretics should be stopped or adjusted when appropriate. Spironolactone (an aldosterone receptor antagonist) may be considered in patients with hyperaldosteronism.

MIXED DISORDERS

Expected Compensation

As described in the previous sections, carbon dioxide and bicarbonate levels will vary in a predictable fashion in response to an acid–base abnormality. The Henderson-Hasselbalch equation describes the relationship between carbon dioxide and bicarbonate:

$$pH = pK + \log\left[(HCO_3^-)/(0.03 \times PaCO_2)\right]$$

Specifically, in the setting of a metabolic acidosis, the central respiratory centers are stimulated to increase minute ventilation and thereby increase elimination of carbon dioxide. Predictably, carbon dioxide should decrease 1mm Hg for every 1 millimolar decrease in bicarbonate.

This anticipated change in carbon dioxide may be estimated by using Winters' formula:

$$\text{Estimated Paco}_2 = [1.5 \times \text{bicarbonate}] + 8 \pm 2$$

If the measured carbon dioxide varies from the estimated Paco_2, then a secondary independent acid–base process is likely occurring.

A metabolic alkalosis causes increased pH which decreases the respiratory drive and leads to relative hypoventilation. This results in an increase in Paco_2. The carbon dioxide should increase by 0.7 mm Hg for each 1 millimolar increase in bicarbonate.

Compensation for respiratory disorders may be either acute or chronic. Acute compensation is primarily performed by intracellular buffers and is relatively modest.

Chronic compensation is accomplished by alterations in kidney function by either increased excretion of bicarbonate (in respiratory alkalosis) or increased reabsorption of bicarbonate (in respiratory acidosis).

In acute respiratory alkalosis, alveolar hyperventilation leads to increased elimination of carbon dioxide and a decrease in pH. Acutely, serum bicarbonate decreases by 0.1 millimolar for each 1 mm Hg decrease in Paco_2. By extension, serum bicarbonate decreases by 2 millimoles for each 10 mm Hg decrease in Paco_2.

Chronic respiratory alkalosis allows for changes in kidney function and increased bicarbonate excretion. In the chronic setting, serum bicarbonate is expected to decrease

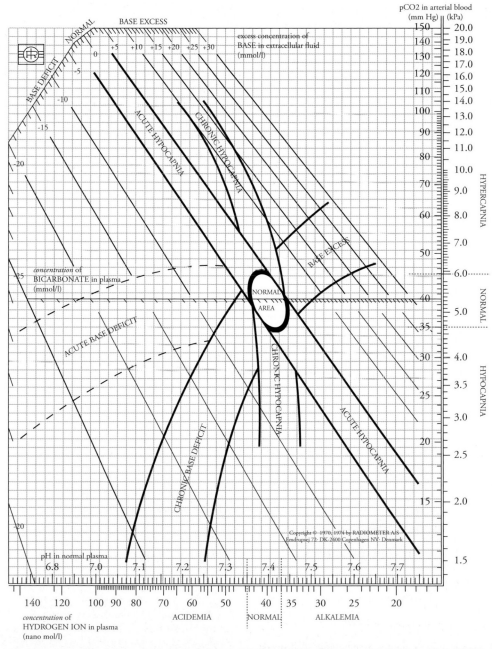

Figure 41.3. Acid–Base Compensation Chart. From Siggaard-Andersen O. The Siggaard-Andersen curve nomogram. *Scand J Clin Lab Invest.* 1962;14:598–604.

Table 41.3 RED FLAGS SUGGESTING A MIXED ACID–BASE DISORDER

The expected compensatory response does not occur.

Compensatory response occurs, but level of compensation is inadequate or too extreme.

Whenever the P_{CO_2} and $[HCO_3^-]$ become abnormal in the opposite direction (i.e., one is elevated while the other is reduced). In simple acid–base disorders, the direction of the compensatory response is always the same as the direction of the initial abnormal change.

pH is normal but P_{CO_2} or HCO_3^- is abnormal.

In anion-gap metabolic acidosis, if the change in bicarbonate level is not proportional to the change of the anion gap. More specifically, if the Δ ratio is greater than 2 or less than 1.

In simple acid–base disorders, the compensatory response should never return the pH to normal. If that happens, suspect a mixed disorder.

---

by 0.5 millimoles for each 1 mm Hg decrease in Pa_{CO_2} (or a decrease of 5 millimoles for each decrease of 10 mm Hg).

Acute respiratory acidosis is defined by alveolar hypoventilation and an increase in carbon dioxide. In the acute setting, bicarbonate increases by 0.05 millimoles for each 1 mm Hg increase in carbon dioxide (or a 1 millimole increase for every increase of 10 mm Hg of carbon dioxide).

The serum bicarbonate is expected to rise by 0.4 millimoles for every 1 mm Hg increase in carbon dioxide (or a rise of 4 millimoles for every increase of 10 mm Hg of carbon dioxide).

There are more complicated equations for predicting the appropriate compensatory response for a given acid–base situation; however, for practical purposes the simple relationships described are more than adequate.

In addition, graphic representations of the relationship between carbon dioxide and bicarbonate are available as aids to determine expected compensatory responses (see figure 41.3).

TRUE MIXED ACID–BASE DISORDERS

True mixed acid–base disorders occur when two or more independent processes are occurring, both of which affect either the bicarbonate or carbon dioxide levels and thereby affect pH (table 41.3). The simplest manner by which to identify multiple acid–base processes is to recognize when the expected compensatory response is not present. In this instance, a second, independent process is likely the cause of the lack of expected compensation. The Δ-Δ is also helpful in sorting out mixed acid-base disorders (table 41.4).

The delta ratio is calculated as follows:

$$\text{Delta ratio} = \Delta \text{ anion gap}/\Delta [HCO_3^-] \text{ or } \uparrow\text{anion gap}/\downarrow [HCO_3^-]$$

$$\Delta\text{-}\Delta = (\text{measured anion gap} - \text{normal anion gap})/$$
$$(\text{normal } [HCO_3^-] - \text{measured } [HCO_3^-])$$

$$= \Delta\text{-}\Delta = (AG - 12)/(24 - [HCO_3^-])$$

A Δ-Δ value below 1:1 indicates a greater fall in $[HCO_3^-]$ than one would expect given the increase in the anion gap. This can be explained by a mixed metabolic acidosis, that is, a combined elevated anion gap acidosis and a normal anion-gap acidosis, as might occur when lactic acidosis is superimposed on severe diarrhea. In this situation the additional fall in HCO_3^- is due to further buffering of an acid that does not contribute to the anion gap. (i.e., addition of HCl to the body as a result of diarrhea).

A Δ-Δ value of 1:2 is usual for an uncomplicated high-AG acidosis. In patients with a lactic acidosis the average value is 1.6, whereas in patients with a diabetic ketoacidosis (DKA), the Δ-Δ ratio is more likely to be closer to 1 due to urine ketone loss. A further complication is that DKA patients are often fluid resuscitated with "normal saline" solution, which results in an increase in plasma chloride and a decrease in anion gap and development of a hyperchloremic normal-anion-gap acidosis superimposed on the ketoacidosis. The result is a further drop in the Δ ratio.

A value above 2:1 indicates a lesser fall in $[HCO_3^-]$ than one would expect given the change in the anion gap. This can be explained by another process that increases the $[HCO_3^-]$—a concurrent metabolic alkalosis. Another situation to consider is a pre-existing high HCO_3^- level as would be seen in chronic respiratory acidosis.

ACKNOWLEDGMENTS

The authors would like to thank Mr. Richard Johnston for his thoughtful review of this chapter.

ADDITIONAL READING

Adrogué HJ, Madias NE. Management of life-threatening acid-base disorders. First of two parts. *N Engl J Med*. 1998;338(1):26–34. Erratum *N Engl J Med*. 1999;340(3):247.
Adrogué HJ, Madias NE. Management of life-threatening acid-base disorders. Second of two parts. *N Engl J Med*. 1998;338(2):107–11.
Ayers P, Warrington L. Diagnosis and treatment of simple acid-base disorders. *Nutr Clin Pract*. 2008;23(2):122–7.

Table 41.4 DIFFERENTIAL DIAGNOSIS OF A Δ-Δ

Δ	DIFFERENTIAL DIAGNOSIS
<0.4	Hyperchloremic normal-anion-gap acidosis
<1	High-AG and normal-AG acidosis
1 to 2	Pure anion-gap acidosis (lactic acidosis)
>2	High-AG acidosis and a concurrent metabolic alkalosis or a pre-existing compensated respiratory acidosis

Budweiser S, Jörres RA, Pfeifer M. Treatment of respiratory failure in COPD. *Int J Chron Obstruct Pulmon Dis.* 2008;3(4):605–18.

Gunnerson KJ, Kellum JA. Acid-base and electrolyte analysis in critically ill patients: Are we ready for the new millennium? *Curr Opin Crit Care.* 2003;9(6):468–73.

Laffey JG, Kavanagh BP. Hypocapnia. *N Engl J Med.* 2002;347 (1):43–53.

Moe OW, Fuster D. Clinical acid-base pathophysiology: Disorders of plasma anion gap. *Best Pract Res Clin Endocrinol Metab.* 2003;17(4):559–74.

Morris CG, Low J. Metabolic acidosis in the critically ill: Part 1. Classification and pathophysiology. *Anaesthesia.* 2008;63(3):294–301.

QUESTIONS

QUESTION 1. A 72-year-old man with severe COPD presents to the ED with increased cough, phlegm, and shortness of breath. He has increased his MDI use without change in his symptoms. On exam, he is "tripoding" and in moderate distress. Vital signs: heart rate 126, blood pressure 110/62, respiratory rate 22, O_2 sat 85% on room air. He has very little air movement and is tachycardic and mildly cyanotic.

ABG reveals pH 7.22, $PaCO_2$ 71, PaO_2 55.

CXR shows hyperinflation but no new opacities.

Your interpretation of his arterial blood gas would be:

A. Acute respiratory acidosis

B. Acute metabolic acidosis

C. Metabolic acidosis with superimposed respiratory alkalosis

D. Chronic respiratory acidosis with superimposed acute respiratory acidosis

E. Metabolic acidosis and respiratory acidosis

QUESTION 2. A 47-year-old female with known peptic ulcer disease presents with a 3-day history of epigastric pain, profuse vomiting, and inability to tolerate oral fluids. On examination, she is in moderate pain. Blood pressure is 88/42, pulse rate 97, and mucous membranes are dry.

Laboratory studies yield serum sodium 124 meq/L, serum potassium 3.0 meq/L, serum chloride 65 meq/L, serum bicarbonate 40 meq/L, blood urea nitrogen 56 mg/dL, serum creatinine 2.1 mg/dL.

Arterial blood studies on room air reveals pH 7.65 and PCO_2 38 mm Hg.

Which of the following best describes the acid-base disorder in this patient?

A. Metabolic alkalosis and respiratory acidosis

B. Metabolic alkalosis and respiratory alkalosis

C. Metabolic alkalosis, respiratory acidosis, and respiratory alkalosis

D. Metabolic acidosis, metabolic alkalosis, and respiratory alkalosis

E. None of the above

QUESTION 3. A 22-year-old female presents with fatigue and generalized muscle weakness. Blood pressure is 92/65, pulse rate 62, weight 60 kg, height 5 ft 9 in.

Laboratory studies yield serum sodium 136 meq/L, serum potassium 3.3 meq/L, serum chloride 98 meq/L, serum bicarbonate 32 meq/L, blood urea nitrogen 12 mg/dL, serum creatinine 0.6 mg/dL.

Arterial blood studies on room air reveals pH 7.46 and PCO_2 47 mm Hg.

What is the likely cause of this patient's acid–base disturbance?

A. Surreptitious vomiting

B. Laxative abuse

C. Thiazide diuretic abuse

D. Gitelman syndrome

E. Hepatic encephalopathy

ANSWERS

1. D
2. D
3. A

CRITICAL CARE BOARD REVIEW

Rebecca Marlene Baron

QUESTIONS

QUESTION 1. A 65-year-old man with a history of insulin-dependent diabetes, hypertension, and end-stage renal disease (on home hemodialysis) is admitted to the hospital for treatment of lower extremity cellulitis. At the registration area of the emergency room he collapses. The code team is activated, and on arrival he is unresponsive without detectable respirations or blood pressure. A monitor/defibrillator is attached, and the rhythm is shown in figure 42.1. Patient has been given effective bag mask ventilation and five cycles of appropriate chest compressions. He remains without detectable blood pressure.

Treatment at this point should be:

A. Biphasic shock at 200 J
B. Monophasic shock at 100 J
C. Epinephrine, 1 mg IV
D. Lidocaine, 1 mg/kg IV

QUESTION 2. A 50-year-old woman with a history of hypertension is brought to the emergency room after an extensive house fire. On presentation she is afebrile, her heart rate is 120, blood pressure is 105/45, respiratory rate is 23 and unlabored. Her Sao_2 is 98% (pulse oximetry). The best next step in her evaluation would be:

A. Bronchoscopy to exclude lower airways thermal injury
B. Arterial blood gas for Pao_2 determination
C. Administration of methylene blue and check cyanomethemoglobin level
D. Arterial blood gas with co-oximetry

QUESTION 3. Which of the following statements is true regarding central venous catheters?

A. The frequency of mechanical complications of central line placement (arterial puncture, hematoma, and pneumothorax) is twice as high for internal jugular catheterizations as for subclavian vein catheterizations.

B. Femoral vein cannulation carries a higher risk of arterial puncture than internal jugular or subclavian site.
C. Subclavian vein catheterization is associated with a higher infection rate than internal jugular vein catheterization.
D. Routine exchanges of catheters every 7 days is associated with a decreased rate of catheter infection.

QUESTION 4. A 35-year-old woman is admitted to the intensive care unit with crush injury after a motor vehicle accident. After 48 hours of admission, she develops an increased oxygen requirement. She is intubated, and mechanical ventilation is initiated. Which of the following interventions is *not* recommended to reduce incidence of ventilator-associated pneumonia?

A. Continuous aspiration of subglottic secretions
B. Selective decontamination of the digestive tract
C. Elevation of the head of the bed to >30°
D. Changes of ventilator circuit only when visibly soiled

QUESTION 5. A 23-year-old college student is brought to the emergency room after ingestion of 60 mL of wintergreen oil in a suicidal gesture. She is lethargic and unable to answer questions. On presentation she has a RR = 28 with deep respirations. Oral T = 100.5°F, HR = 128 bpm, BP = 124/60 mm Hg. Skin has no rashes. There is no evidence of external trauma. Lungs are clear. CV shows a regular rate and rhythm with a normal S1 and S2. Abdomen is soft with mild diffuse tenderness. Neuro exam is nonfocal. Her labs reveal a Na^+ = 136, K^+ = 3.8, Cl^- = 100, HCO_3^-= 18, Creat = 0.6, Glucose = 90, WBC = 12,000, Hct = 42, Plt = 300K. ABG on 2 L via NC reveals pH = 7.44, Pco_2 = 22, Po_2 = 100. Chest x-ray (CXR) is normal. Electrocardiogram (EKG) reveals NSR without ischemia. The remainder of her laboratory studies are pending. In the emergency room she was begun on IV normal saline. Activated charcoal was given. Your next step should be to:

A. Administer acetazolamide
B. Begin mechanical ventilation
C. Change IVF to bicarbonate-containing solution

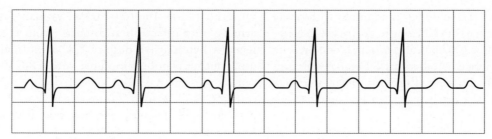

Figure 42.1. Rhythm Strip of Patient in Question 1.

D. Begin beta blocker

E. Administer N-acetylcysteine (NAC)

QUESTION 6. A decision is made to intubate an asthmatic patient for impending respiratory failure. During intubation patient receives sedation and a short-acting paralytic agent. Initial ventilator settings are assist control, respiratory rate = 16/min, tidal volume = 500 mL, positive end-expiratory pressure (PEEP) = 5 cm H_2O, Inspiratory flow rate = 60 L/min, FiO_2 = 1.0. An end-inspiratory pause is administered, and the peak inspiratory pressure (PIP) and plateau pressure (P_{plat}) are measured. Compliance (C_{stat}) and airway resistance (R_{aw}) are calculated. In this patient with status asthmaticus the most likely findings would be:

A. PIP = 35 cm H_2O, P_{plat} =15 cm H_2O, C_{stat} = 50 mL/cm H_2O, R_{aw} = 20 cm H_2O/L/sec

B. PIP = 17 cm H_2O, P_{plat} = 15 cm H_2O, C_{stat} = 50 mL/cm H_2O, R_{aw} = 2 cm H_2O/L/sec

C. PIP = 32 cm H_2O, P_{plat} = 30 cm H_2O, C_{stat} = 20 mL/cm H_2O, R_{aw} = 2 cm H_2O/L/sec

D. PIP = 35 cm H_2O, P_{plat} = 15 cm H_2O, C_{stat} = 40 mL/cm H_2O, R_{aw} = 2 cm H_2O/L/sec

QUESTION 7. After 4 hours on these ventilator settings PIP is noted to now be 50 cm H_2O. Review of the ventilator waveforms indicates the flow-time curve graphic shown in figure 42.2.

Which ventilator change should be considered next?

A. Increase the set respiratory rate

B. Decrease the FiO_2

C. Decrease the set inspiratory time

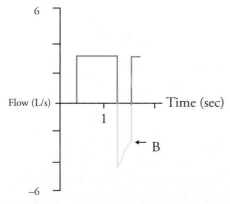

Figure 42.2 Ventilator Waveform (flow-time curve) for Patient in Question 7.

D. Increase the inspiratory flow rate

E. Decrease the tidal volume

QUESTION 8. Which of the following statements is false regarding the fat embolism syndrome (FES)?

A. FES refers to the triad of respiratory dysfunction, neurological changes, and renal failure caused by entry of fat particles into the microcirculation.

B. FES occurs in 5–10% of patients with multiple long bone fractures or concomitant pelvic fractures.

C. There is commonly a latent period after the injury before clinical manifestation is noted.

D. FES without pulmonary involvement is uncommon.

QUESTION 9. A 50-year-old male smoker with chronic obstructive pulmonary disease (COPD) and diabetes mellitus (DM) type 2 is admitted to the ICU with pneumonia and respiratory failure. He is intubated, and mechanical ventilation is initiated. Labs on presentation reveal Sodium = 140, WBC =19,000 (89% polys, 4% bands), Potassium = 4.6, Hct = 38%, Chloride = 110, Plt = 190,000, Bicarbonate = 26, Glucose = 230.

IV vancomycin, levofloxacin, Solu-Medrol, and bronchodilator therapy are ordered. A ventilator bundle is implemented including elevation of head of bed, daily assessment of readiness to extubate, daily sedation holiday, GI prophylaxis with IV Pepcid, and deep vein thrombosis (DVT) prophylaxis with heparin SC. IV insulin is begun with goal glucose of 150 mg/dL.

On hospital day 7 patient remains intubated. He has new right lower extremity pain. Right dorsalis pedis and posterior tibialis pulses are newly absent.

Labs reveal Sodium = 136, WBC = 12,000 (93% polys, 0% bands), Potassium = 3.6, Hct = 36%, Chloride = 106, Plt = 40,000, Bicarbonate = 22, Glucose = 114.

PF4 antibodies and vascular imaging studies are ordered. In addition to surgical consultation, appropriate treatment includes:

A. Stop unfractionated heparin and begin platelet infusion

B. Stop unfractionated heparin and monitor platelets daily

C. Stop unfractionated heparin and begin low-molecular-weight heparin

D. Stop unfractionated heparin and begin argatroban

E. Stop unfractionated heparin and begin warfarin

QUESTION 10. A 60-year-old man is admitted with severe midepigastric abdominal pain radiating to the back. Oral temperature is 103°F. HR is 100 bpm, and current blood pressure is 110/60. Lipase is elevated. Abdominal CT scan reveals pancreatic inflammation with areas of necrosis. Biliary ducts are not dilated. The best next step in management would be:

A. Begin enteral nasojejunal feeds
B. Normal saline
C. Empirical antibiotic treatment with aminoglycoside
D. Empirical antifungal therapy

QUESTION 11 Decisions regarding end-of-life care are guided by all the ethical principles outlined below except one.

A. Autonomy
B. Nonmaleficence
C. Beneficence
D. Social Justice

QUESTION 12. A 75-year-old man is admitted to the intensive care unit with increased respiratory distress. He is a current smoker (75-pack-year history). Most recent outpatient spirometry revealed an FEV_1 of 50% of predicted. At home he is on inhaled tiotropium and an albuterol inhaler prn. Treatment was initiated with supplemental oxygen, 4 L/min via nasal cannula, intravenous steroids, inhaled bronchodilators, and broad-spectrum antibiotics. He notes progressive dyspnea. On evaluation he appears fatigued but follows all commands. He is currently afebrile, heart rate is 96 bpm, blood pressure is 104/62 mm Hg, and his respiratory rate is 32/min with use of accessory muscles. Oxygen saturation is 92%. Auscultation of lungs reveals bilateral expiratory wheezes. Arterial blood gas reveals pH = 7.30, Pco_2 = 49 and Po_2 = 66.

What would be the best next treatment?

A. Increase Fio_2 to 6 L via nasal cannula
B. Diuresis
C. Initiation of noninvasive ventilation
D. Intubation and initiation of mechanical ventilation

QUESTION 13. A 67-year-old woman with a history of hypertension and coronary artery disease presents with 72 hours of progressive lethargy, fever, and dysuria. On evaluation in the emergency department, she is lethargic but arousable. Her heart rate is 126 bpm and regular, BP = 70/46 mm Hg, RR = 24/min unlabored. Jugular venous pressures do not appear to be elevated. Lungs are clear to percussion and auscultation. Cardiac exam reveals a tachycardia but regular rate and rhythm. There are no murmurs noted. Abdomen is soft and nontender. WBC = 13,000 with a left shift. Hematocrit is 42. Urinalysis reveals too numerous to count WBCs. EKG is unremarkable. Urine and blood cultures are obtained. Antibiotics are initiated. What is the most appropriate next step in treatment?

A. Initiation of vasopressin drip
B. Administration of IV normal saline
C. Empirical stress-dose steroids
D. Initiation of norepinephrine drip

QUESTION 14. The 67-year-old woman with presumed urinary tract infection and sepsis (from the case above) remains hypotensive despite 8 L of normal saline. Her urine output is poor. Blood pressure is 80/50, and central venous pressure has been measured at 12 mm Hg. Blood cultures have grown Gram-negative rods (speciation pending). What would the best treatment for hypotension be now?

A. Intubation and mechanical ventilation
B. Additional fluid resuscitation with normal saline
C. Placement of a Swan-Ganz catheter
D. Initiation of vasopressors

QUESTION 15. Which of the following medications has the least amount of alpha activity?

A. Dopamine
B. Dobutamine
C. Epinephrine
D. Norepinephrine
E. Phenylephrine

QUESTION 16. A 64-year-old man is admitted to the intensive care unit with nausea, hematemesis, and melena. Upon arrival he is alert. He is afebrile, heart rate is 126 bpm, and blood pressure is 92/58 mm Hg.

Which treatment has been shown to reduce the need for endoscopic therapy?

A. Continuous intravenous H_2 blocker
B. Intermittent bolus dose H_2 blocker
C. Continuous intravenous proton pump inhibitor
D. Continuous intravenous octreotide

QUESTION 17. Which of the following represents a significant risk of administration of activated protein C?

A. Anaphylaxis with repeated use
B. Intracranial hemorrhage
C. Congestive heart failure
D. Pneumonia

QUESTION 18. You are asked to evaluate a 50-year-old man (70 kg) admitted to the ICU with alcoholic pancreatitis 72 hours earlier. He has now developed bilateral pulmonary infiltrates requiring mechanical ventilation. His Fio_2 is 0.8. Vent settings: Volume cycle CMV rate = 12, V_t =1000 mL, PEEP = 10. ABG reveals pH = 7.32, $Paco_2$ = 56, and Pao_2 = 68. CVP = 12 mm Hg. Echocardiogram reveals normal LV function. The next step in management should be:

A. Initiation of prone-positioning ventilation
B. Increase PEEP to 15 cm H_2O
C. Reduce tidal volumes to 500 mL
D. Convert to pressure-cycle CMV (pressure control) ventilation
E. Trial of diuresis

QUESTION 19. Therapeutic hypothermia has been shown to be effective in which of the following clinical situations?

A. 60-year-old male now unresponsive 30 minutes/pVT arrest on postoperative day 2 after colon resection for newly diagnosed colon carcinoma
B. 19-year-old female intubated, unresponsive s/p lorazepam overdose 2 hours earlier
C. 82-year-old female with history of DM type 2 now comatose s/p VF arrest 4 hours earlier
D. 50-year-old male transferred from an outside hospital unresponsive s/p pulseless electrical activity (PEA) arrest at home 24 hours earlier

QUESTION 20. A 50-year-old woman with insulin-dependent diabetes presents to the emergency room with 24 hours of rhinorrhea, cough, and crampy abdominal pain. On physical exam, she appears ill with T 38°C, HR 130 bpm, BP 100/64 mm Hg, SaO_2 = 96% on RA. There is mild abdominal tenderness without rebound or guarding. Labs reveal Sodium = 134, Potassium = 4.9, Chloride = 86, Bicarbonate = 14, Glucose = 660; ABG pH = 7.20, $PaCO_2$ = 25, PaO_2 = 80. Treatment is initiated with NS, 250 mL/hr. Insulin is begun at 4 units per hour. Six hours later, labs reveal Sodium = 138, Potassium = 3.6, Chloride = 100, Bicarbonate = 18, Glucose = 160. What should you do next?

A. Decrease insulin infusion rate to 1 U/hr
B. Administer NPH insulin (patient's home dose)
C. Change NS to D5NS
D. Change NS to ½NS with bicarbonate
E. Continue the current therapy

ANSWERS

1. C. The patient has suffered loss of a detectable pulse in the setting of continued electrical activity and therefore has PEA. PEA accounts for about 20% of out-of-hospital cardiac arrests and about 60% of in-hospital cardiac arrests. The differential diagnosis for underlying contributing conditions to a PEA arrest include the "H's and the T's," i.e., hypoxemia, hyper- or hypokalemia, hypovolemia, hypoglycemia, hydrogen ions (acidosis), hypothermia, hypocalcemia, tension pneumothorax, tamponade, thrombosis (cardiac or pulmonary), toxins (e.g., tablets), and trauma. There is no indication for administration of shocks or for administration of lidocaine.

In summary, pulseless electrical activity (PEA) can be caused by a number of underlying conditions (e.g., the "H's and the T's," see above), and primary treatment should be directed toward alleviating the underlying problem. Adjunctive support during a PEA arrest, in addition to effective CPR, can include administration of epinephrine and other ACLS code algorithm medications.

2. D. Smoke inhalation injury can arise from a variety of mechanisms, including thermal damage (oropharyngeal injury or lower airways injury from steam or explosive gases), asphyxiation (hypoxemia as a result of reduced oxygen tensions from combustion, carbon monoxide [CO] toxicity resulting in decreased oxygen-carrying capacity of hemoglobin, cyanide toxicity as a result of interfering with cellular respiration, particularly as a result of burning of polyurethane or wool, methemoglobinemia), and pulmonary parenchymal inflammation. The most common toxic inhalation as a result of house fires is carbon monoxide toxicity. Standard pulse oximetry will not distinguish between oxygenated hemoglobin and CO-bound hemoglobin, so co-oximetry is required for detection of CO-intoxication.

In summary, a variety of injuries can occur as a result of smoke inhalation, including direct thermal injury and toxic inhalations. Detection of carbon monoxide toxicity requires an arterial blood gas with co-oximetry.

3. B. A variety of complications can arise from central line placement, including bleeding (hematoma, arterial puncture), pneumothorax, air embolization (0.5%), loss/migration of catheter or wire, arrhythmia (68% ectopy, 6–12% right bundle branch block), cardiac tamponade, injury to nonvascular structures (e.g., nerves, thoracic duct), line misplacement, thrombosis (21% femoral, 1.9% subclavian), infection. Risks of central line insertion vary by site, with infection risk highest at the femoral site (femoral > internal jugular > subclavian), arterial puncture risk highest at femoral site (femoral > internal jugular > subclavian), and pneumothorax risk higher at subclavian than at internal jugular vein site. Catheter-associated bloodstream infections can cause significant morbidity in the ICU, and mechanisms of line-site infection can include subcutaneous skin tract colonization (85%), contamination of the catheter hub or stopcock, infusate contamination, or seeding of the blood from a remote site. Adoption of standardized techniques in line insertion has been shown to reduce rates of line-associated infections, and these protocols include hand hygiene, use of chlorhexidine skin prep, full barrier precautions and full body draping, avoidance of the femoral site, strict maintenance of sterile field during insertion, and removal of catheters when no longer necessary.

In summary, risks of arterial puncture and line-associated infection are highest at the femoral site for line insertion. The use of protocolized checklists for line insertion can reduce development of line-associated infections.

4. B. Ventilator-associated pneumonia (VAP) has a reported incidence of 7–40% and results in prolonged time on the ventilator, longer ICU stays, and higher morbidity. A number of strategies have been proven to decrease development of VAP, presumably through decreasing entrance of oral and GI microbes into the lower respiratory tract. These include elevation of the head of the bed >30° (at least 3× risk reduction in VAP), use of enteral feeds rather than

parenteral feeds, and continuous suctioning of subglottic secretions. While selective digestive tract decontamination (SDD) using topical and IV antibiotics has been shown to reduce mortality, significant concern has been raised for this technique resulting in development of increased drug resistance. No benefit has been demonstrated for prophylactic changes of the ventilator circuit tubing.

In summary, VAP results in significant morbidity in the ICU, and extubation as soon as is feasible should be a primary goal of ICU care. Strategies such as elevation of the head of the bed >30° and continuous subglottic suctioning should be employed to minimize the risk of VAP development.

5. C. Oil of wintergreen (methyl salicylate) is a plant product that has been used in topical pain relief products and as a flavoring in small doses. Salicylate is the major metabolite of methyl salicylate, and one teaspoon of this substance contains 7 g of salicylate, which is approximately equivalent to 23 tablets of 325 mg aspirin. Thus, ingestion of 60 mL of oil of wintergreen likely has resulted in salicylate toxicity in this patient. Consistent with salicylate toxicity is the presence of an anion-gap acidosis and a respiratory alkalosis. Other features of salicylate intoxication can include lethargy, depressed mental status, tinnitus, noncardiogenic pulmonary edema, hepatic failure, and coma. In addition to supportive care, treatment for salicylate toxicity includes alkalinization of the urine to increase renal clearance of the drug and hemodialysis in severe cases of toxicity.

In summary, salicylate intoxication classically presents with a combined anion-gap metabolic acidosis and respiratory alkalosis. The treatment for salicylate toxicity includes standard supportive care and urine alkalinization to enhance clearance of the drug.

6. A. Patients with severe asthma usually exhibit elevated airways resistance with reasonably conserved lung compliance, and option A is the only choice with this combination. Resistance and compliance are calculated using a plateau pressure measured at end-inspiration (in a sedated patient). Resistance is equal to the difference between the peak inspiratory pressure and plateau pressure, divided by the flow, with a normal resistance being in the range of 5–12 cm H_2O/L/sec. Compliance is equal to the tidal volume divided by the difference between the plateau pressure and PEEP (positive end expiratory pressure), with a normal compliance being in the range of 40–70 mL/cm H_2O.

In summary, patients with diseases involving airflow limitation exhibit an increased resistance, whereas patients with diseases involving the alveolar space exhibit a reduced compliance. Resistance and compliance can be calculated from the ventilator with use of an end-inspiratory pause to measure the plateau pressure (see equations above).

7. E. The waveform demonstrates inadequate time for exhalation (as seen by the yellow waveform not reaching baseline before the next breath, labeled "B"). This pattern of breathing is likely to result in increased development of intrinsic PEEP (i.e., auto-PEEP) and risk of barotrauma if not treated. Increasing the respiratory rate will likely worsen gas trapping with a further reduction in exhalation time. Although increasing the inspiratory flow rate and decreasing inspiratory time might also lead to increased time for exhalation, it is generally felt that these maneuvers are likely not as effective as decreasing the respiratory rate and/or tidal volume in minimizing gas trapping.

In summary, patients with severe airflow obstruction are at risk for development of auto-PEEP as a result of gas trapping. In addition to treatment of the underlying cause (e.g., bronchodilators, steroids, etc., for asthma) and adequate sedation on the ventilator, maneuvers to minimize auto-PEEP include decreasing the respiratory rate and the tidal volume with careful monitoring of acid–base status and the overall clinical condition.

8. A. The classic triad of fat embolism syndrome is respiratory failure, mental status changes, and a petechial rash that results most often from long-bone and pelvic fractures (more often with closed than open fractures) and usually develops 24–72 hours after the insult. Neurological symptoms often develop after respiratory symptoms and can include confusion, lethargy, seizures, and focal deficits. Mortality has been reported to range from 5% to 15%.

In summary, consider fat embolism syndrome in patients who develop respiratory failure, mental status changes, and a petechial rash in the 24- to 72-hour window after long-bone fracture.

9. D. The patient has developed >50% reduction in his platelet count over a 7-day period, during which time he was treated with subcutaneous unfractionated heparin and thus most likely had developed heparin-induced thrombocytopenia with thrombosis (HITT). Treatment includes discontinuation of unfractionated heparin and initiation of a direct thrombin inhibitor such as argatroban. Solely stopping unfractionated heparin will not be sufficient to treat the thrombosis. Although low-molecular-weight heparin (LMWH) is associated with a lower risk of developing HIT, once HITT has developed, LMWH has sufficient cross-reactivity with unfractionated heparin that it cannot be used. Transfusing platelets is not advised, given theoretical risk of worsening thrombosis risk. Transition to longer-term warfarin (with at least 5 days of overlap with a direct thrombin inhibitor) should be considered only once the platelet count has recovered and once the patient has been stably anticoagulated on a direct thrombin inhibitor.

In summary, suspect heparin-induced thrombocytopenia in patients who develop a >50% drop in their platelet count in the setting of receiving heparin products. The treatment for HITT includes discontinuation of heparin and initiation of anticoagulation with an alternative agent such as a direct thrombin inhibitor.

10. B. The patient likely has necrotizing pancreatitis, and the primary initial approach involves aggressive fluid resuscitation, given the intravascular volume depletion that arises from third-spaced fluid. Inadequate fluid resuscitation can result in the development of acute tubular necrosis, and there is concern that volume depletion can worsen the pancreatic microcirculation and further aggravate pancreatic necrosis. The other answer choices might be treatment considerations during the course of therapy, but the primary initial goal of management involves adequate rehydration.

In summary, patients with necrotizing pancreatitis require aggressive fluid resuscitation and close monitoring, given third-spaced fluid and intravascular volume depletion.

11. D. *Autonomy:* The patient has the right to choose among offered therapies and the right to refuse any treatment even though this decision could result in the patient's death. *Nonmaleficence* is a companion of beneficence—not inflicting evil or harm. Physicians must refrain from providing interventions that are more likely to be of harm than benefit. *Beneficence* means that the physician ought to do and promote good and must remove evil or harm. *Social Justice*—the resources of a particular group can be allocated based on various material principles (need, merit, effort).

12. C. The patient likely has underlying COPD and is experiencing an exacerbation, with increased respiratory distress and increased work of breathing. Noninvasive positive-pressure ventilation refers to delivery of positive-pressure ventilation via face mask, and appropriate patients with COPD exacerbations have been shown to respond well to this support, with the goal of avoiding mechanical ventilation if at all feasible. Contraindications to noninvasive ventilation use include cardiac/respiratory arrest, inability to protect the airway, copious secretions, altered mental status, facial trauma/deformity, and high risk of aspiration. Patients receiving noninvasive ventilation require close monitoring.

In summary, noninvasive ventilation can improve outcomes in patients with COPD exacerbations who are appropriate candidates for this type of support. Altered mental status, copious secretions, and significant aspiration risk are contraindications to use of noninvasive ventilation.

13. B. This patient has presented in septic shock, likely from urosepsis. In addition to source control and administration of early appropriate antibiotics, initiation of early goal-directed therapy (EGDT *NEJM* 2001;345:1368) has been shown to improve mortality from severe sepsis and septic shock. The first step in the algorithm involves catheter-guided fluid resuscitation, using colloid or crystalloid to target a CVP >8 mm Hg. Once the CVP goal has been met, use of vasoactive agents (norepinephrine was used in the study) is advised to target the mean arterial pressure in the 65–90 mm Hg range. The protocol next uses a central venous saturation (Svo_2) target of 70% to guide use of packed red blood cells and inotropic agents.

In summary, in patients with sepsis, early source control and appropriate antibiotics are key management strategies. The use of EGDT to guide resuscitative and management strategies in severe sepsis and septic shock has been shown to reduce mortality.

14. D. As described above, the patient has been fluid resuscitated to a goal CVP in the 8–12 mm Hg range, and she remains with a MAP<65 mm Hg. Thus the next step would be addition of vasoactive agents.

15. B. Vasopressors (such as dopamine, norepinephrine, and epinephrine) increase MAP through vasoconstriction and have actions to varying degrees via alpha-adrenergic receptors and beta-adrenergic receptors (with dopamine at low doses acting as well through dopamine receptors). Phenylephrine has sole alpha-adrenergic activity. Inotropes (such as dobutamine) act to increase cardiac contractility predominantly through beta-1 adrenergic receptors.

16. C. A 2007 *N Engl J Med* article (356:1631) evaluated the effect of IV omeprazole (bolus followed by infusion) versus placebo prior to endoscopy in decreasing the need for endoscopic intervention. Omeprazole significantly reduced the need for endoscopic therapy at the first endoscopy (primary endpoint), as well as length of hospital stay and the number of actively bleeding ulcers (secondary endpoints).

In summary, high-dose omeprazole infusion before endoscopy reduced the need for endoscopic intervention and accelerated resolution of signs of bleeding.

17. B. While there was initial enthusiasm for use of activated protein C in the sickest subgroup of sepsis patients after analyses of trials in 2001 and 2005, a more recent trial has not supported efficacy of activated protein C. Thus, given risks of life-threatening hemorrhage with activated protein C, Eli Lilly and Company withdrew activated protein C from the market in October 2011, further calling into question the risk-benefit profile of the drug.

18. C. This patient has developed ARDS (consensus conference criteria for ARDS definition include acute onset of bilateral infiltrates, Pao_2/Fio_2 ratio <200, absence of heart failure or LV dysfunction as a contributor) likely as a result of pancreatitis. The ARDSnet trial (*NEJM* 2000;342:1301) demonstrated a mortality benefit in ARDS patients ventilated with 6 cc/kg tidal volumes, as compared with 12 cc/kg tidal volumes. They targeted a maximal plateau pressure of <30 cm H_2O and adjusted Fio_2 and PEEP per protocol to target Pao_2 values of 55–80 mm Hg. Despite multiple trials, optimal PEEP in ARDS is not clear, and thus, many practitioners target PEEP for adequate oxygenation.

In summary, low-tidal-volume ventilation in ARDS (6 cc/kg) reduced mortality compared with higher tidal volume (12 cc/kg).

19. C. Two randomized controlled trials (*NEJM* 2002;346:549 and *NEJM* 2002; 346:557) demonstrated improved neurological outcomes for patients resuscitated

after VF arrests who were subjected to mild to moderate hypothermia for a period of 12–24 hours after arrest. Although there may be similar benefits for patients who have suffered from other precipitants resulting in cardiac arrest (and many centers treat these patients similarly), rigorous data are not available for these other groups of patients.

In summary, therapeutic hypothermia has been shown to improve neurological outcomes in patients who have been successfully resuscitated after a VF arrest.

20. C. This patient has diabetic ketoacidosis (DKA), perhaps triggered by a viral syndrome. Key aspects of DKA management include fluid resuscitation (usually with 0.9% normal saline) to replete intravascular volume and insulin administration with close glucose monitoring. Once the glucose level falls below 200 mg/dL, it is advised to add D5 to the administered fluids, both so that glucose levels do not fall precipitously (with risk of cerebral edema) and to facilitate continuation of the IV insulin drip (even at a low level) so that DKA is not reprecipitated by discontinuation of insulin.

In summary, fluid resuscitation and insulin administration with glucose monitoring are key aspects of DKA management. Careful attention also needs to be paid to potassium levels in patients with DKA, as these patients usually have marked potassium depletion.

43.

BOARD SIMULATION: PULMONARY MEDICINE

Christopher H. Fanta

QUESTIONS

QUESTION 1. An elderly woman is admitted to a nursing home. She feels well; hypertension is the only medical problem identified in her history. As part of her initial evaluation, a purified protein derivative (PPD) skin test is performed. It demonstrates 12 mm of induration. Her physical examination is normal, and routine laboratory studies (complete blood count and chemistry profile) are likewise normal. A chest x-ray is obtained and reveals minor apical scarring on the right and a localized, poorly defined area of opacity in the right upper lobe posteriorly. Prior chest films are not available for comparison.

As the patient's physician, which of the following do you recommend?

A. Follow-up evaluation with repeat chest x-ray in 3 months to assess for change
B. Administer isoniazid (INH), 300 mg/day, for 9 months to treat for latent tuberculous infection
C. Obtain three induced sputum samples and await the results of mycobacterial culture and smear
D. Obtain three induced sputum samples and immediately begin antituberculous therapy with INH, rifampin, and ethambutol
E. Empirically begin treatment for tuberculosis with INH and ethambutol

QUESTION 2. All of the following conditions may be found in a patient with cystic fibrosis *except* which?

A. Bronchiectasis
B. Nasal polyps
C. Mixed obstructive and restrictive lung disease
D. Azoospermia
E. Systemic pseudomonas infection

QUESTION 3. Which of the following radiographic findings of thoracic diseases is *not* associated with chronic asbestos exposure?

A. Fibrocalcific parenchymal disease, predominantly involving the upper zones of the lung

B. Pleural plaques
C. Malignant mesothelioma
D. Benign pleural effusions
E. Bronchogenic carcinoma

QUESTION 4. A 65-year-old woman with a 60-pack-year history of cigarette smoking presents with cough and shortness of breath. She reports an increase in her usual amount of sputum production with yellow discoloration of the sputum. She has a low-grade fever (99.6°F). Chest examination reveals scattered expiratory rhonchi, and a chest x-ray is normal. A sample of sputum is sent for routine culture. The sputum Gram stain describes 4+ polys and many Gram-negative cocci in pairs.

Based on the history and Gram stain, an appropriate choice of antibiotics would be which of the following?

A. Ampicillin, orally
B. Amoxicillin-clavulanic acid, orally
C. Procaine penicillin G, intramuscularly twice a day
D. Cefotaxime, intravenously
E. Cephalexin, orally

QUESTION 5. Which of the following outcomes can one expect from an outpatient pulmonary rehabilitation program in a patient with severe chronic obstructive pulmonary disease?

A. Increased survival
B. Improved cardiovascular function
C. Increased exercise tolerance
D. Increased expiratory airflow (FEV_1)
E. Decreased use of inhaled bronchodilators and/or corticosteroids

QUESTION 6. A 23-year-old man presents with nosebleeds and a petechial rash. A complete blood count reveals pancytopenia with a white blood cell count of 400 cells/μL, hematocrit of 24%, and platelet count of 12,000/μL. A diagnosis of acute myelogenous leukemia is made, and chemotherapy is begun. Ten days into his course of induction chemotherapy he develops a fever (101°F) and cough. He expectorates minimal mucoid sputum. A chest x-ray reveals new localized nonhomogeneous opacities in the left lower lobe. A sample of induced sputum is obtained; Gram stain shows no polys or microorganisms.

The pathogen most likely to cause this illness is which of the following?

A. Aspergillus
B. Cytomegalovirus
C. Nocardia
D. Gram-negative bacteria
E. Candida

QUESTION 7. Five potential diagnoses are provided below. Which diagnosis fits best with the following set of arterial blood gases obtained with the patient breathing air: Po_2 40 mm Hg, Pco_2 80 mm Hg, and pH 7.10?

A. Adult respiratory distress syndrome
B. Severe attack of asthma
C. Severe bilateral bacterial pneumonia
D. Acute exacerbation of severe chronic obstructive pulmonary disease
E. Sedative drug overdose

QUESTION 8. A 60-year-old man was recently seen in the emergency department following a fall from a ladder. No rib fracture or lung contusion was sustained, but chest x-ray revealed a 1.8 by 1.4 cm nodule in the left lower lobe. A chest computed tomography (CT) scan was obtained, which confirmed the presence of the nodule within the lung parenchyma. No other nodules were seen, and no abnormal hilar or mediastinal lymph node enlargement was found. The nodule has sharp margins without calcification.

The patient smoked cigarettes only briefly in college. He grew up in Arkansas until age 15, then moved to New England. He works as a college administrator.

Which of the following would you recommend as the next step in his workup?

A. Obtain a chest positron emission tomography (PET)-CT scan
B. Order a transthoracic needle aspirate
C. Ask a pulmonologist to perform bronchoscopy
D. Review prior chest x-rays for comparison
E. Order chest magnetic resonance imaging (MRI)

QUESTION 9. A 56-year-old man presents with a 6-week history of nonproductive cough, moderate exertional dyspnea, and intermittent low-grade fevers (to 100.4°F). He had been in good health but smoked a pack of cigarettes each day for the last 35 years. The patient has received two courses of clarithromycin (500 mg orally twice daily for 10 days) without improvement in symptoms. He denies any history of ocular inflammation, skin rash, or arthritis.

The physical examination shows no clubbing or cyanosis. There is no peripheral lymphadenopathy or jugular venous distension. Chest examination reveals inspiratory crackles in the lower posterior lung zones bilaterally; no wheezing.

Laboratory studies include the following: hematocrit 34%; white blood cell count, 11,100/μL with 18% lymphocytes, 64% polys, 7% bands; 6% monocytes, and 5% eosinophils; platelets 250,000/μL.

Serum blood urea nitrogen is 22 mg/dL, and creatinine 0.8 mg/dL.

Urinalysis is normal.

The chest x-ray shows airspace disease at both lung bases (see figure 43.1).

The most likely diagnosis is:

A. Pneumococcal pneumonia
B. Legionnaires' disease
C. Wegener granulomatosis
D. Idiopathic pulmonary fibrosis
E. Bronchiolitis obliterans organizing pneumonia (cryptogenic organizing pneumonia)

QUESTIONS 10–14. For each of the five following phrases or statements (10–14), indicate whether it pertains to patients with asthma, chronic obstructive pulmonary disease (COPD), neither, or both.

A. Asthma
B. COPD
C. Neither
D. Both

10. Disease severity correlates directly with the reduction in the forced expired volume in 1 sec (FEV_1).

11. Leukotriene receptor antagonists such as montelukast (Singulair) are indicated in patients with mild or moderate disease.

12. The short-acting inhaled anticholinergic bronchodilator, ipratropium, is equally effective with potentially fewer side effects compared to inhaled beta-adrenergic agonists.

13. Alpha-1-antitrypsin augmentation therapy may improve lung function (increase FEV_1) in some patients.

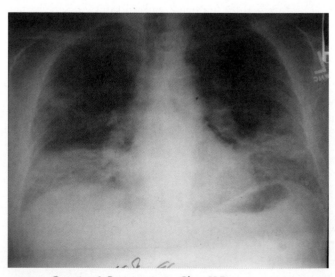

Figure 43.1. Question 9, Posteroanterior Chest X-Ray.

14. Antibiotics are generally indicated for exacerbations of the disease when the patient reports cough and discolored sputum.

QUESTIONS 15–19. For each of the five following phrases or statements (15–19), indicate whether it pertains to patients with sarcoidosis, idiopathic pulmonary fibrosis, neither, or both.

    A. Sarcoidosis
    B. Idiopathic pulmonary fibrosis
    C. Neither
    D. Both

15. Rarely seen in children

16. May be a cause of chronic airflow obstruction on pulmonary function testing

17. Associated with an increased risk of lung cancer

18. Predominantly involves the lower lung zones

19. A definitive infectious pathogen has been identified as the cause

QUESTIONS 20–24. INH treatment for latent tuberculous infection (INH 300 mg daily for 9 months) should be given to which of the following patients?

20. A 21-year-old healthcare worker with a PPD skin test reaction of 12 mm of induration. His chest x-ray is normal. His skin test reaction last year had 10 mm of induration.

    A. Yes
    B. No

21. A 45-year-old former intravenous drug abuser known to be human immunodeficiency virus (HIV) positive has a clear chest x-ray, and the PPD skin test shows 5 mm of induration. Prior skin tests are reported as "equivocal."

    A. Yes
    B. No

22. A 74-year-old man with no known tuberculosis exposure and a clear chest x-ray has a PPD skin test showing 5 mm of induration. The patient does not recall any previous tuberculin skin tests. Repeat testing 1 week later now shows 15 mm of induration.

    A. Yes
    B. No

23. A 53-year-old woman with no known medical illnesses and a clear chest x-ray has a PPD skin test reaction with 8 mm of induration. She has never before had skin testing but has been tested now because her husband has just had active tuberculosis diagnosed after a 6-month illness.

    A. Yes
    B. No

24. A 26-year-old homeless man has a PPD skin test demonstrating 15 mm of induration. He has no symptoms, but his chest x-ray shows nonhomogeneous opacities with some nodularity in the left upper lobe.

    A. Yes
    B. No

ANSWERS

1. D. The correct answer is D. An elderly woman admitted to a nursing home has a positive PPD skin test and an abnormal chest x-ray with evidence of "a localized, poorly defined area of opacity in the right upper lobe posteriorly." This description is suspicious for reactivation tuberculosis with a tuberculous pneumonia in the right upper lobe. The anatomic location is typical for reactivation tuberculosis, which most often begins in the posterior and apical segments of the upper lobes or in the superior segment of the lower lobes. A pneumonia localized to the anterior segment of the upper lobe is unlikely to be tuberculosis.

What is surprising in the brief description of her condition—and what may cause some doubt about the correct answer—is that she is asymptomatic, free of cough, sputum production, fever, or weight loss. Do not let this observation dissuade you from the possibility that she has active pulmonary tuberculosis. In its early stages, active tuberculosis may be asymptomatic. Nor should it be reassuring to those around her that she has no cough. She may develop a cough any day, and the risk of contagion is real, especially in a nursing home residence where she will likely be in contact with a vulnerable population of people, many with chronic illness.

With active tuberculosis as a possibility, your proper management plan is to attempt diagnosis (such as with analysis of sputum induced by inhalation of nebulized hypertonic saline or with bronchoscopy with bronchoalveolar lavage) and, while awaiting the results of sputum acid-fast stain and culture, initiate therapy for presumed active tuberculosis (answer D). The patient will also need to be kept in respiratory isolation until either three sputum samples have returned negative for acid-fast bacilli on smear or until she has completed 2 weeks of antimycobacterial therapy. A three-drug regimen of antituberculous medications, such as offered in answer D, is appropriate for a patient at low risk for primary drug-resistant tuberculosis.

The other proposed options for her management are not appropriate. "Watchful waiting," as in answer A, puts both the patient and those around her at risk. It might be an appropriate course if an old chest x-ray from a year or two previously had been identical, indicating that the right upper lobe abnormality was a chronic radiographic finding, but not in the absence of such information.

Until you are certain that this patient does not have active pulmonary tuberculosis, it would be inappropriate to treat with a single antituberculous medication for latent tuberculous infection (answer B). Doing so might induce an INH-resistant strain of *Mycobacterium tuberculosis*. Besides, the indication for chemoprophylaxis in this elderly woman with a positive PPD skin test is unclear. We will discuss these indications further is a subsequent portion of the Board Simulation exercise (Questions 20–24).

Identification of *M. tuberculosis* by traditional culture techniques can take up to 6–8 weeks. Waiting several weeks without initiating antituberculous therapy (answer C) again places the patient at risk for worsening disease and those around her at risk for acquiring tuberculous infection. Finally, immediate treatment with a two-drug regimen (answer E) is wrong because (1) it fails to obtain a diagnostic sample for culture and sensitivity testing, (2) it employs an old-fashioned treatment regimen that requires 18 months of therapy, and (3) it does not address the possibility of infection with a primary INH-resistant strain of tuberculosis.

2. E. You may have difficulty choosing the correct answer to this question because all of the options strike you as correct. You know that the pulmonary disease of cystic fibrosis is bronchiectasis (answer A) and that chronic sinusitis and nasal polyps are common in cystic fibrosis (answer B). (As a general rule, if you identify a *child* with nasal polyps, think cystic fibrosis rather than asthma and allergies, because nasal polyps rarely complicate allergies and asthma until later in life.) You are aware that diffuse bronchiectasis can cause both airflow obstruction (due to airway narrowing and intraluminal secretions) and restriction (due to destruction of lung tissue, consolidation due to infection and inflammation, and atelectasis) as in answer C. You recall that men with cystic fibrosis generally have azoospermia due to bilateral absence of the vas deferens (answer D). And of course, *Pseudomonas* commonly infects the bronchiectatic airways in cystic fibrosis (as well as in bronchiectasis of other causes). But wait—answer E specifically refers to *systemic Pseudomonas* infections, and in fact, *Pseudomonas* bacteremia or disseminated *Pseudomonas* infection involving skin, kidneys, liver, and so forth, is unheard of in cystic fibrosis. You know this fact; the challenge in this question is simply careful reading of the potential choices offered!

3. A. The term asbestosis is sometimes loosely and inappropriately used to describe any thoracic manifestation that results from extensive asbestos fiber inhalation. In fact, the term should be reserved to describe specifically the diffuse interstitial inflammation and fibrosis that results from many years (decades) of intense asbestos exposure. The radiographic appearance typically involves a pattern of interstitial opacities (linear and nodular shadows) predominantly in the lower lung zones bilaterally. Calcification, if present, involves pleural surfaces. The description offered as answer A, "fibrocalcific parenchymal disease, predominantly involving the upper zones of the lung," does not evoke asbestosis. It is rather a description of chronic granulomatous lung disease, such as tuberculosis. A sample chest x-ray with this pattern is seen in figure 43.2. It shows bilateral upper lobe scarring, calcified nodules in the right upper lobe, and cephalad retraction of the hila in a patient with treated reactivation tuberculosis.

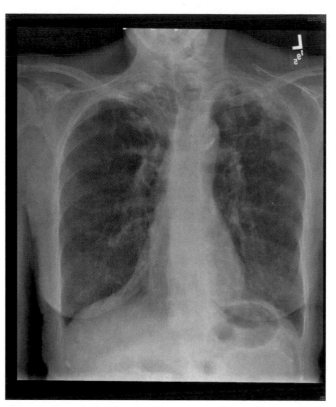

Figure 43.2. Fibrocalcific Parenchymal Disease Predominantly Involving the Upper Zones of the Lung.

The other choices, pleural plaques, mesothelioma, benign pleural effusions, and bronchogenic carcinoma, are indeed all potential consequences of chronic asbestos fiber inhalation. Perhaps least well known is answer D, benign pleural effusions. Benign exudative effusions, often bloody and often bilateral, may develop with a latency period of ≥10 years after asbestos inhalation, a relatively short latency period compared to other asbestos-related diseases. Because mesothelioma often manifests as a unilateral pleural effusion, the challenge for the clinician in a patient with unilateral pleural effusion and a history of asbestos exposure is to exclude malignancy as the cause.

The radiographic images of asbestos-related pleural plaques and of mesothelioma can be distinctive. Figure 43.3 is the posteroanterior chest x-ray of a patient with asbestos-related pleural plaques. It shows multiple bilateral nodular opacities, and one's immediate response to the image may well be to think of metastatic lung nodules. However, many of the opacities are pleural-based, and at least one (on the left lateral margin) is not spherical but rather is shaped like a bluff or plateau with its long diameter paralleling the pleural surface, a clue to its pleural origin. Adjacent and more medial to this plaque is a round-appearing nodule. It too is a pleural plaque, not located in the substance of the lung but along the pleural surface. It is located along an anterior or posterior portion of the pleura and when seen *en face* gives a rounded appearance. The pleural location of these asbestos-related plaques is best visualized on the transverse

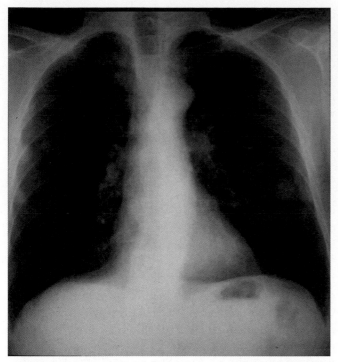

Figure 43.3. Asbestos-Related Pleural Plaques on Posteroanterior Chest X-Ray.

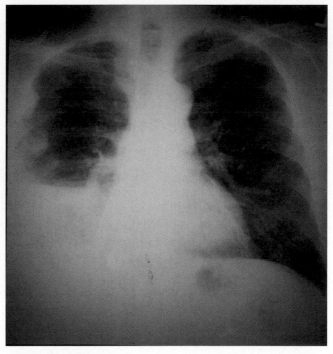

Figure 43.5. Mesothelioma.

image of a chest CT scan, as seen in figure 43.4 (in a chest CT image from a different patient). Although not illustrated by these images, pleural plaques may become calcified. They are not pre-cancerous lesions and do not evolve into mesothelioma.

Figure 43.5 is the posteroanterior chest x-ray of a patient with mesothelioma. There is a large right pleural effusion. In addition, one sees distinctive lobulated opacities along the upper portion of the lateral pleural surface on the right. These opacities may represent loculated pleural fluid, but their nodularity suggests more mass-like tissue invasion along the chest wall. We are likely visualizing both tumor mass growing along the pleural surface as well as associated malignant pleural effusion. Mesothelioma is the disease manifestation related to asbestos fiber inhalation that may

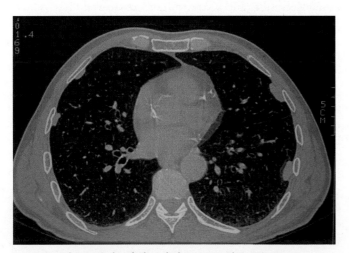

Figure 43.4. Asbestos-Related Pleural Plaques on Chest CT Image.

develop with relatively minor exposure, such as a summer or two spent working closely with asbestos in a shipyard 20 years earlier.

4. The correct answer is B. This 65-year-old cigarette-smoking woman with a chronic productive cough most likely has chronic bronchitis (chronic productive cough related to cigarette smoking) and possibly also has chronic airflow obstruction related to cigarette smoking (COPD). She has developed shortness of breath, increased cough, discolored sputum production, and a low-grade fever. You readily diagnose a respiratory tract infection and attribute her symptoms to an acute exacerbation of her COPD. Her chest examination is confirmatory (expiratory low-pitched wheezes or "rhonchi" indicative of accumulated central airway secretions), and her chest x-ray helps to exclude pneumonia.

In most instances you will treat this condition with empirical antibiotics chosen to cover the common pathogens that cause acute infectious exacerbations of COPD, such as streptococcus, *Haemophilus influenzae*, *Moraxella catarrhalis*, and Gram-negative rods. In this instance a sputum sample was sent for culture, and you are asked to interpret the significance of the many "Gram-negative cocci in pairs" seen on Gram stain. Although perhaps tempted to dismiss this finding as typical of the *Neisseria* species that are "normal flora" of the oropharynx, in fact Gram-negative cocci can be pathogenic. This is the Gram-stain appearance of *M. catarrhalis* (formerly *Branhamella catarrhalis*), a potential cause of bronchitis and pneumonia, particularly in patients with COPD.

Not satisfied with your knowledge of the microscopic appearance of *Moraxella*, the question further asks about this pathogen's usual pattern of antibiotic sensitivities. In particular, you are asked to remember that almost universally these are beta-lactamase-producing bacteria. Consequently, they will be resistant to ampicillin and penicillin (answers A and C) but sensitive to ampicillin combined with clavulanic acid (Augmentin), answer B. They are likely also to be sensitive to cephalosporin antibiotics, but intravenous antibiotics such as cefotaxime (answer D) are not indicated, and the orally administered cephalexin (Keflex) has poor lung penetration and would be a "second-best" option (answer E).

5. C. Outpatient pulmonary rehabilitation is recommended for patients with disabling exertional dyspnea due to their COPD. It is designed to interrupt the vicious cycle by which shortness of breath on exercise (due to severe airflow obstruction) leads to physical inactivity, which promotes decreased physical conditioning and consequent worsened exertional dyspnea. Most pulmonary rehabilitation programs include supervised upper and lower body exercising, typically two to three times per week for a period of 6–12 weeks. Additional components of most programs include education about lung diseases and psychosocial support, not the least of which comes from sharing experiences with other people in a group with similar medical problems.

The most consistent benefit at the end of such training programs is an improved exercise capacity (answer A) with associated reduced sense of dyspnea, the result of improved oxygen uptake and utilization by exercising muscles. Some studies have also found a reduction in the number of hospitalizations and urgent care visits following outpatient pulmonary rehabilitation. Patients with severe COPD cannot achieve maximal heart rate targets for exercise and do not stimulate improved cardiac output (answer B). No study has been able to demonstrate improved long-term survival in COPD as the result of outpatient pulmonary rehabilitation (answer C). Expiratory airflow in COPD is not limited by muscle strength and does not improve with improved conditioning (answer D). Although a reduced sense of dyspnea may conceivably lead patients to rely less on their bronchodilator inhalers, decreased medication use has not been a well-documented benefit of pulmonary rehabilitation (answer E).

6. D. A young man with newly diagnosed acute myelogenous leukemia, 10 days into his course of induction chemotherapy, develops a fever and localized pulmonary opacities consistent with a diagnosis of pneumonia. In this question, we are asked to consider the most likely pathogens causing pneumonia in this context. We can readily invoke the rubric of "pneumonia in an immunocompromised host," but we must also acknowledge that not all immunocompromising conditions are the same. The patient with compromised immunity due to splenectomy will be prone to one set of pathogens (such as *Streptococcus, Klebsiella,* and *Haemophilus*); another patient with immunocompromise following solid organ transplant will be vulnerable to other pathogens (including certain viruses such as cytomegalovirus and fungi such as *Pneumocystis, Nocardia,* or *Cryptococcus*).

The patient in this question is susceptible to a broad array of pathogens primarily due to his neutropenia, plus whatever other direct suppressive effects his chemotherapeutic medications may have. Neutropenic patients are especially vulnerable to bacterial infections, especially *Staphylococcus* and Gram-negative bacilli, and fungal infections, including *Aspergillus* and mucormycosis. The fact that his sputum is scant and mucoid should not dissuade us from an infectious cause of his pulmonary disease. Due to his severe neutropenia he lacks sufficient numbers of polymorphonuclear leukocytes to generate sputum purulence; and often microorganisms do not appear in expectorated (or induced) sputum despite true lower respiratory tract infection.

The timing of the onset of this infection provides helpful information. Among neutropenic patients, fungal infections typically do not develop within the first 30 days of illness. Gram-negative bacilli are the most common cause of pneumonia in this timeframe (answer D). Thereafter, *Aspergillus* pneumonia (answer A) would be plausible, especially in a patient who might have recently received broad-spectrum antibiotics. On the other hand, *Candida* pneumonias (answer E) are rare, except perhaps preterminally, typically following aspiration in a patient with oropharyngeal candidiasis or as a complication of candidemia. Pneumonia due to cytomegalovirus (answer B) or nocardia (answer C) is statistically far less common in this setting than Gram-negative bacterial pneumonia. They are found more commonly in disorders with profound lymphopenia (such as certain lymphomas/leukemias, acquired immunodeficiency syndrome, and following solid organ transplantation secondary to antirejection medications).

7. E. This question is strictly an exercise in arterial blood gas interpretation. It does not involve clinical decision-making because we are not provided with any other patient information, including symptoms, past medical history, physical examination, or other laboratory data. Some physicians may be able simply to look at these arterial blood gas results and intuit the correct answer. Here is how I come to this conclusion.

The patient with these arterial blood gases has profound hypoxemia, hypercapnia, and acidemia. The acidemia is respiratory in etiology, a consequence of the profound CO_2 retention. Although all five of the disease states offered as potential answers can cause profound hypoxemia, acute respiratory distress syndrome (ARDS) (answer A) and severe bilateral bacterial pneumonia (answer C) are far less likely than the others to cause hypercapnia. Alveolar hyperventilation with hypocapnia would be the norm in ARDS and severe pneumonia, except perhaps in patients with very advanced disease or with other underlying cardiorespiratory illness.

Of the remaining choices, an acute asthmatic attack (answer B) and sedative drug overdose (answer E) would be expected to cause an acute respiratory acidosis, whereas an acute exacerbation of severe COPD (answer D) would more likely be associated with chronic hypercapnia or perhaps acute worsening of chronic hypercapnia (acute-on-chronic respiratory acidosis). It is helpful, then, to determine whether this set of arterial blood gases suggests an acute or an acute-on-chronic respiratory acidosis. One method to calculate the distinction is as follows:

- Acute respiratory acidosis: Predicted fall in pH below 7.40 = rise in P_{CO_2} above 40 mm Hg × 0.008
- Chronic respiratory acidosis: Predicted fall in pH below 7.40 = rise in P_{CO_2} above 40 mm Hg × 0.003
- Acute-on-chronic respiratory acidosis: Predicted fall in pH below 7.40 = rise in P_{CO_2} above 40 mm Hg × 0.005

In our example, the patient's P_{CO_2} of 80 mm Hg represents a rise in P_{CO_2} above 40 mm Hg of 40. The pH of 7.10 is 0.3 units below 7.40. The best approximation for this value is 40 × 0.008 (= 0.32), consistent with an acute respiratory acidosis. A patient with a P_{CO_2} of 80 mm Hg due to chronic CO_2 retention with appropriate renal compensation would be expected by these calculations to have a pH of approximately 7.28 (40 × 0.003 = 0.12 units below 7.40); and a patient with a P_{CO_2} of 80 mm Hg due to acute-on-chronic hypercapnia would be expected to have a pH of approximately 7.20 (40 × 0.005 = 0.2 units below 7.40). Our patient's profound acidemia reflects the acuteness of this pulmonary process, without time for compensatory renal retention of bicarbonate.

We still need to choose between answers B (acute asthmatic attack) and E (sedative drug overdose). The former is associated with airway disease and hypoxemia that is at least in part due to mismatching of the distribution of ventilation and perfusion. Besides hypoventilation, lung zones with low ventilation for the amount of perfusion that they are receiving contribute to hypoxemia. The latter (sedative drug overdose) may have no intrinsic lung disease; the hypoxemia may be entirely due to depressed respiratory drive with central hypoventilation. We can utilize the alveolar gas equation to distinguish between these two possibilities. The alveolar gas equation allows us to calculate a predicted alveolar partial pressure of oxygen (PA_{O_2}). We can then compare our predicted PA_{O_2} with the measured arterial blood oxygen (Pa_{O_2}) to derive an alveolar-to-arterial difference (or gradient) for oxygen (A-aD_{O_2}). In the absence of intrinsic lung disease with ventilation/perfusion (V/Q) mismatching, the A-aD_{O_2} will be normal (≤25 mm Hg); in the presence of V/Q mismatching or shunt, the A-aD_{O_2} will be increased.

An abbreviated version of the alveolar gas equation is the following:

$$PA_{O_2} (mm\ Hg) = [(P_B - 47) \times FI_{O_2}] - P_{CO_2}/R),$$

where P_B is ambient barometric pressure, FI_{O_2} is the fraction of oxygen in the inspired gas, and R is the respiratory exchange ratio, in most instances presumed to be 0.8. For patients breathing air at sea level, this equation simplifies to:
$$PA_{O_2} (mm\ Hg) = [(760 - 47) \times 0.21] - P_{CO_2}/0.8$$
$$= 150 - P_{CO_2}/0.8$$
For our patient, the calculated alveolar P_{O_2} is as follows:
$$PA_{O_2} = 150 - 80/0.8$$
$$= 50\ mm\ Hg$$

The measured arterial P_{O_2} in this example is 40 mm Hg, giving an A-aD_{O_2} (that is, $PA_{O_2} - Pa_{O_2}$) of 10 mm Hg, a normal value. The absence of a widened A-a gradient for oxygen fits best with answer E, a sedative drug overdose with pure alveolar hypoventilation as the cause of hypoxemia.

8. D. This 60-year-old man is discovered by serendipity to have an asymptomatic solitary pulmonary nodule on chest x-ray. Our task is to determine whether the nodule is benign or malignant. Features favoring benignity are its sharp margins and the patient's lack of a significant cigarette smoking history. His prior residence in Arkansas raises the possibility of a lung nodule related to endemic fungal infection, specifically a histoplasmoma. Features that raise the possibility of malignancy are his age (lung cancer is uncommon below the age of 40, but increases in incidence with increasing age) and the relatively large size (greatest diameter >1 cm) of the nodule. A completely calcified lung nodule or a nodule with a characteristic pattern of calcification (e.g., "bull's eye" lesion with dense central calcification, as in granulomas, or "popcorn ball" calcifications, as in hamartomas) would clinch a benign diagnosis, but his nodule is noncalcified.

The decision regarding further workup should be easy. If available, obtain prior chest images for comparison. This search for old films may be labor-intensive or time-consuming, but it is cost-effective and safe. A nodule such as this one that can be shown not to have grown in size over a period of 2 years or more is benign; no further evaluation will be necessary. Rare exceptions to this rule may be very slow-growing adenocarcinomas of the bronchoalveolar cell type, but their radiographic appearance is not that described here. They tend to be less uniformly dense and less well circumscribed; they may have a ground-glass texture, air bronchograms within their margins, or focal, persistent consolidation.

If old chest images are not available for comparison, a positron emission tomography (PET) scan combined with chest CT imaging (PET-CT scan) (answer A) would be an appropriate next step. A negative PET-CT scan in this patient (uptake of glucose in the nodule no greater than in surrounding normal lung tissue) would indicate with 95% certainty that the nodule is benign. (Again, the exceptions to this rule, giving the test a false-negative rate of approximately 5%, are bronchoalveolar-type adenocarcinomas).

A transthoracic needle aspirate (answer B) is tempting in an effort to establish a definitive diagnosis without surgery; and in some centers with special expertise this procedure would be routinely attempted. However, at most institutions the false-negative rate for needle aspirates reported as "nondiagnostic, with no malignant cells seen" is unacceptably high, on the order of 20%. The procedure carries with it a risk of iatrogenic pneumothorax of 7–10%. The accuracy of fiberoptic bronchoscopy (answer C) in the evaluation of peripheral lung nodules is even lower than that of transthoracic needle aspirates. Specific benign etiologies (such as histoplasmoma) are rarely established (<5%), and the risk of false-negative results (no malignant cells identified in a patient with a malignant lung nodule) is high (well above 20%). Thoracic magnetic resonance imaging (MRI) (answer E) has no role in the evaluation of lung nodules or parenchymal lung abnormalities in general.

9. E. For this question we are asked to make a diagnosis. The patient, a middle-aged cigarette smoker, has had a nonproductive cough, dyspnea on exertion, and intermittent fevers for the last 6 weeks, persistent despite two courses of macrolide antibiotics (clarithromycin). His chest examination reveals bilateral inspiratory crackles in the lower lung zones, and his chest x-ray has extensive bilateral lower-lobe airspace opacities. On the image shown (figure 43.1) one can make out air bronchograms, evidence of lung consolidation with an alveolar filling process.

We would expect that after two courses of antibiotics, pneumococcal pneumonia (answer A) would have resolved; or were this a macrolide-resistant strain of *Streptococcus pneumoniae*, it would have worsened considerably over this time period. Similarly, pneumonia due to *Legionella pneumophila* (answer B) should have been adequately treated with clarithromycin; we would expect the patient to be on the mend after two rounds of antibiotics. The clinical features (and remaining three answers from which to choose) encourage us to think about noninfectious causes for his illness.

History and physical examination offer no additional clues: he denies ocular, cutaneous, or joint manifestations that might point to a diagnosis of sarcoidosis, vasculitis, or lung disease associated with collagen-vascular disease. He has no clubbing, as may be seen in chronic inflammatory lung diseases, especially idiopathic pulmonary fibrosis (IPF) (answer D). In fact, the subacute duration of his illness (6 weeks) does not invoke *chronic* inflammatory diseases such as IPF, which tend to have a time course of many months to years. The radiographic pattern of IPF is likewise very different from that of our patient, with linear and nodular opacities and sometimes honeycombing, rather than consolidation with alveolar filling.

Wegener's granulomatosis (answer C) can present with diffuse alveolar hemorrhage, giving airspace opacities as seen in this patient. More often, however, it presents with lung nodules, with or without cavitation; and in this patient the absence of renal abnormalities on blood studies and urinalysis further dissuade us from a systemic vasculitis with pulmonary and renal involvement, such as Wegener's.

By process of elimination, we are drawn to the diagnosis of bronchiolitis obliterans organizing pneumonia (BOOP), also known as cryptogenic organizing pneumonia (COP). In fact, we may recognize that this diagnosis is compelling: a pulmonary process with (1) bilateral airspace pulmonary opacities, (2) mimicking an infectious pneumonia, (3) unresponsive to antibiotics, (4) with a time course of several weeks. A bronchoscopy might be useful to rule out infection, hemorrhage, and malignancy. A transbronchial lung biopsy occasionally provides sufficient lung tissue to see the characteristic pathologic features of BOOP: organizing pneumonia plus bronchiolar inflammation with endobronchial polypoid tissue. Some physicians might make a presumptive diagnosis of BOOP and begin systemic steroids, observing for a clinical response over the next few days. BOOP tends to be highly responsive to treatment with systemic steroids (with resolution of symptoms and clearing of pulmonary opacities), although in up to one-third of cases the disease may recur with steroid dose reduction and withdrawal.

It is important to emphasize the distinction between bronchiolitis obliterans (or constrictive bronchiolitis), an obstructive lung disease often refractory to treatment with systemic steroids, and bronchiolitis obliterans organizing pneumonia, a steroid-responsive inflammatory lung disease as described above. Some of the differences between the two entities are summarized in table 43.1. Part of the confusion between these two conditions is based on nomenclature, hence the preference of some physicians for the term, cryptogenic organizing pneumonia.

10. D. Questions 10–14 ask us to compare and contrast asthma with COPD.

Both asthma and COPD are characterized by airflow obstruction, intermittent in the former, chronic in the latter. The *presence* of airflow obstruction is identified on

Table 43.1 DIFFERENTIATION BETWEEN BRONCHIOLITIS OBLITERANS AND BRONCHIOLITIS OBLITERANS ORGANIZING PNEUMONIA

	CRYPTOGENIC ORGANIZING PNEUMONIA (BOOP)	CONSTRICTIVE BRONCHIOLITIS (BO)
Presentation	Pneumonia-like	Emphysema-like
Chest x-ray	Multifocal or diffuse pulmonary opacities	Hyperinflammation
Physiology	Restrictive	Obstructive
Response to steroid treatment	Good	Poor

spirometry by a reduction in the ratio of FEV_1 to FVC (FEV_1/FVC). On the other hand, the *severity* of airflow obstruction is characterized by the extent of the reduction in FEV_1. In both asthma and COPD, the frequency and severity of symptoms, need for medications, and frequency of urgent care visits and hospitalizations correlate directly with the degree to which FEV_1 is decreased.

11. A. Leukotriene receptor antagonists such as montelukast (Singulair) and zafirlukast (Accolate) have proven effective in the treatment of mild to moderate asthma. They have not been found to be effective in COPD. Our understanding of the pathobiology of these two diseases would lead us to predict that leukotrienes (released by mast cells, eosinophils, and to some extent epithelial lining cells) play an important role in some patients with asthma but have little pathogenetic role in COPD.

12. B. One might predict that inhibition of cholinergic neural traffic to the airways (via the vagus nerve) would be of great benefit in asthma. However, clinical studies in asthma have found that, compared to inhaled beta-adrenergic bronchodilators, short-acting anticholinergic bronchodilators are less effective (as well as slower in their onset of action). By contrast, in COPD the bronchodilator response to anticholinergics is comparable to that observed with beta agonists. The appeal of anticholinergic bronchodilators in the older-aged population in whom COPD tends to develop is their lack of cardiovascular stimulatory side effects.

13. C. It is estimated that approximately 1% of patients with COPD have a genetic deficiency of alpha-1-antitrypsin protein. Those who are homozygous for this abnormality may benefit from alpha-1-antitrypsin augmentation therapy, with concentrated alpha-1-antitrypsin protein given as an intravenous infusion once weekly. The benefit, however, is one of slowing or arresting the accelerated decline in lung function observed in patients with alpha-1-antitrypsin deficiency. One would not expect *improvement* in lung function.

14. B. Antibiotics are recommended for acute exacerbations of COPD. Many of these exacerbations are due to bacterial tracheobronchitis. Although there are other potential causes for increased cough and discolored sputum production in patients with COPD, both viral and noninfectious, withholding antibiotics in this setting puts the patient at risk for serious deterioration. On the other hand, most exacerbations of asthma are due to viral infections. Antibiotics are not recommended for treatment of exacerbations of asthma in the absence of comorbidities such as pneumonia or bacterial sinusitis.

15. D. Questions 15–19 ask us to compare and contrast sarcoidosis with IPF.

Both sarcoidosis and IPF are rare in childhood. The incidence of sarcoidosis is highest in young adults between ages 20 and 40 years; IPF most commonly begins after age 50 years.

16. A. Approximately 25–30% of patients with sarcoidosis will have a predominantly obstructive physiology. The mechanism is presumably airway narrowing due to endobronchial and peribronchial granuloma formation. By contrast, IPF is a quintessential restrictive lung disease, with low lung compliance and extensive interstitial inflammation and fibrosis.

17. B. Patients with IPF are at increased risk for the development of bronchogenic carcinoma, even the absence of prior cigarette smoking. Sarcoidosis is not associated with an increased risk of lung cancer.

18. B. Sarcoidosis is protean in its thoracic radiographic presentations, but it is more likely to present with bilateral upper lobe opacities than lower lobe opacities. IPF on the other hand, typically predominates in the lower lobes, although it frequently progresses to diffuse lung involvement.

19. C. No infectious pathogen has been found as the causative agent for either sarcoidosis or IPF both remain "idiopathic" in etiology. Much research has attempted to identify a microbiologic cause of sarcoidosis, with interest focusing on mycobacterial antigens and cell wall–deficient bacteria such as *Mycoplasma*. However, confirmation of a causative role for these organisms is lacking.

20. A. The patients in questions 20–24 have all undergone skin testing with PPD using the intermediate strength (5 tuberculin units). In follow-up, a chest x-ray was obtained. You are then asked to consider whether, based on the information given, you would recommend treating this patient for latent tuberculous infection with INH.

The following "rules" have been recommended to guide your decision making. First, what constitutes a positive PPD skin test reaction? These measurements, based on the longest diameter of induration recorded approximately 48 hours after intradermal administration, are designed to maximize true positive reactions to *M. tuberculosis* and minimize false-positive cross reactivity due to infection with other mycobacterial species—that is, to maximize the sensitivity and specificity of the test for latent tuberculous infection.

- ≥5 mm induration for *high-risk* populations: patients with HIV/AIDS or other immunosuppressing illness or treatment; patients who have recently been in close contact with a patient with active pulmonary tuberculosis; or patients with prior pulmonary tuberculosis and residual pulmonary scarring on chest imaging who have never received adequate antituberculous drug therapy.

- ≥10 mm induration for *moderate-risk* populations: patients who are at increased risk of having had exposure to tuberculosis (recent immigration from countries with a high prevalence of tuberculosis; intravenous drug abusers, persons living in shelters; nursing home residents, healthcare workers; and children exposed to high-risk adults); or patients who are at increased risk of activation of their tuberculous infection (diabetes, chronic renal failure, loss of weight of >10% of ideal body weight); postgastrectomy; underlying malignancies).

- ≥15 mm induration for *low-risk* populations: all other patients.

Second, which patients with evidence for latent tuberculous infection (based on a positive PPD skin test) should be treated with antituberculous medication ("chemoprophylaxis") to prevent activation of infection and development of disease? Here the decision-making tries to weigh the risks in an asymptomatic patient of activation of tuberculosis (over the course of a lifetime) versus drug-induced toxicity, particularly hepatotoxicity (over the duration of therapy). The usual recommended treatment is INH, 300 mg/day for 9 months. The following are considered indications for treatment of latent tuberculous infection, *regardless of the age of the patient*:

- Household contact of a patient with active pulmonary tuberculosis.

- Recent converter; that is, a person whose PPD skin test has gone from negative on prior testing to positive with an increase of at least 6 mm in diameter.

- Patient with prior pulmonary tuberculosis and residual pulmonary scarring on chest imaging who has never received adequate antituberculous drug therapy.

- Patient with "special circumstances" increasing the risk of activation of infection, such as diabetes, HIV infection, dialysis, receiving immunosuppressing drugs, major weight loss, silicosis, or recent immigration from an endemic area.

A more controversial indication, previously recommended by panels of experts and now left to the discretion of the treating physician, is treatment of any patient under age 35 years (regardless of special risk factors). The motivation to treat this population of patients with latent tuberculous infection is that their lifetime risk of activation of tuberculosis spans many decades, whereas their risk of INH hepatotoxicity (which increases with increasing age) is less than 0.1%.

Based on these recommendations, I would choose to treat the 21-year-old healthcare worker with 12 mm of induration on his PPD skin test (Question 20). Because of his increased risk of exposure to active tuberculosis in his work, 12 mm of induration is considered a positive result. His chest x-ray shows no evidence for active pulmonary tuberculosis. He is not a "recent converter"; the 2-mm difference between the diameter of his previous skin test response and the current one is inconsequential. However, he is under age

35 years of age, with very low risk of INH hepatotoxicity during treatment. One can make the argument that protecting this young man from activation of tuberculosis may benefit not only him but others to whom he might spread infection, should he remain in the healthcare profession and ever develop active pulmonary tuberculosis.

21. A. In a patient with HIV infection, a skin test reaction of only 5 mm induration is considered positive, sufficient in size to suggest latent tuberculous infection. Because of his or her HIV-related immunodeficiency, treatment of latent tuberculous infection is indicated, regardless of age.

22. B. This 74-year-old man without known risk factors for tuberculosis exposure or activation has an initial negative skin test (5 mm of induration) that on repeat testing 1 week later is positive (15 mm of induration). This is *not* a recent converter; he did not develop cellular immunity to tuberculosis in the week between the two skin tests. Rather, he has a latent tuberculous infection that was not detected on the first skin test (false-negative result) but became apparent on the repeat test (true-positive result). Skin testing was repeated after just 1 week because of the well-known tendency of cellular immunity to mycobacterial infection (as judged by cutaneous reactions) to wane with advancing age. The initial skin test with its intradermal administration of a small amount of tuberculin protein is sufficient to revive an amnestic immune response, with an appropriate cutaneous response (positive skin test) on repeat intradermal exposure to tuberculin protein. This two-step testing is widely practiced in older-aged persons (in some institutions, in any person over age 50 years of age), and the eliciting of a true-positive result after an initial false-negative response is referred to as the "booster phenomenon." Note that in a patient without latent tuberculous infection, repeat PPD skin testing, even if done multiple times in a relatively short period, will not provoke a positive result.

Now that it has been established that this 74-year-old man without known tuberculosis exposure has latent tuberculous infection and a normal chest x-ray, should he receive treatment with INH for chemoprophylaxis? No. He has no known indications for treatment, as listed above. We do not know the duration of his latent tuberculous infection. The risk of activation of infection is greatest in the 2–3 years after initial exposure. If he has had latent tuberculous infection for many decades, his risk of reactivation at this age is very low, whereas the risk of INH toxicity is not negligible. Risk–benefit analysis suggests that he not receive treatment.

23. A. This patient is at high risk for latent tuberculous infection: she has been intensely exposed to someone with active pulmonary tuberculosis (as a "household contact") over a period of several months. Based on her high risk for exposure, a PPD skin test with 8 mm of induration should be considered a positive test result. Given her likely recent acquisition of tuberculous infection, she is currently at greatest risk for progressing to active disease. She meets

the criteria for treatment of latent tuberculous infection (regardless of age).

24. B. This patient, at increased risk for tuberculous infection because of his homelessness, has a positive skin test (≥10 mm of induration, given his moderate-risk status). However, the next step in evaluating a patient with a positive PPD skin test reaction is to obtain a chest x-ray. This patient's chest x-ray reveals "nonhomogeneous opacities with some nodularity in the left upper lobe." We are left wondering if his positive PPD skin test is evidence for latent tuberculous infection or active tuberculous pneumonia (reactivation tuberculosis in the upper lobe). If it is possible that he has active pulmonary tuberculosis, treatment with INH alone would be anathema. It would be inadequate treatment for active tuberculosis and might induce INH-resistant *M. tuberculosis*. Before initiating treatment for latent tuberculous infection, it is imperative to exclude active disease.

44.

PULMONARY AND CRITICAL CARE MEDICINE SUMMARY

Patricia A. Kritek

Patients commonly present to their primary care doctors or to the emergency room complaining of dyspnea and cough. These cardinal symptoms of lung disease are features of a myriad of respiratory illnesses. Acute dyspnea and cough are often associated with infections such as bronchitis or pneumonia, whereas more chronic symptoms are commonly suggestive of asthma or chronic obstructive pulmonary disease (COPD). Although these are often the first diagnoses considered, there is a much wider differential of causes of these symptoms including the diffuse parenchymal lung diseases (DPLD), malignancies affecting the lung, pleural disease, and pulmonary vascular disease. For many patients, a diagnostic evaluation including history and physical exam as well as a combination of chest radiography, pulmonary function testing, and arterial blood gas sampling are required to reveal the underlying cause of dyspnea or cough.

DIAGNOSTIC EVALUATION OF LUNG DISEASE

Initial evaluation of a patient with respiratory symptoms begins with a comprehensive history and physical exam. Particular emphasis is placed on history of cigarette smoking or other inhalational exposures, as these are linked to a variety of lung diseases. On exam, focus is placed on signs of small airway obstruction (wheezes) and evidence of alveolar filling or interstitial fibrosis (crackles) or secretions in the larger airways (rhonchi) in addition to looking for signs of pleural disease or right heart failure. Even with a thorough initial evaluation, many patients will require a chest radiograph as well as pulmonary function testing.

CHEST RADIOGRAPHY

One of the most commonly obtained radiologic images is a chest x-ray. A systematic, stepwise approach to the interpretation of a chest radiograph is important, as subtle abnormalities are missed when one jumps to the most obvious finding immediately.

Evaluation of a film begins with ascertainment of the correct patient name and the date of the study. Additionally, the technique of the film should be reviewed. The gold standard film is a posteroanterior (PA) film with accompanying lateral film. When a patient is too ill to stand, a portable anteroposterior film (AP) is often obtained. As this projection results in slightly different dimensions, the clinician is cautioned about making assessments of cardiac size with this technique. Finally, before true interpretation begins, one should assess the quality of penetration with an ideal film just barely revealing the thoracic vertebrae in the lower chest.

One approach to the chest radiograph proceeds from "outside in," beginning with the soft tissues and bones. This is followed by examining the pleural reflections, assessing for pleural effusions or pneumothoraces. Significant attention should be paid to the lung parenchyma, comparing right to left, upper lung zones to lower long zones, and the periphery to more central areas of lung. Opacities are described as reticular, reticulonodular, fluffy, or confluent. Rounded abnormalities are termed nodules or masses based on size, usually the former being <3 cm in diameter. The mediastinum should be reviewed focusing on the tracheal position and contour, any enlargements in the paratracheal stripe, the hila, and the aortic shadow. Finally, the heart size with attention to all four chambers should be assessed.

Although pattern recognition is important when examining chest radiographs, a systematic approach will result in the most comprehensive assessment of a film and yield the greatest diagnostic value. As with all studies, a collaborative approach between the radiologist and the internal medicine physician often results in the most clinically helpful interpretation.

PULMONARY FUNCTION TESTING

Pulmonary function tests (PFTs) are commonly among the first steps in the evaluation of patients with dyspnea and other respiratory complaints. PFTs are used to establish obstructive or restrictive pathophysiology as well as gas-exchange abnormalities. They can assist with diagnosis of some respiratory disorders (e.g., asthma) as well as track progression of many pulmonary diseases, assess for side effects of medications, or evaluate for disability.

The initial study most often obtained is spirometry. This test, in which a patient forcefully exhales from total lung capacity (TLC) down to residual volume (RV), provides information on both volumes and flows. The parameters of greatest utility are the forced vital capacity (FVC) and the forced expiratory volume in 1 sec (FEV_1). A decreased ratio of these two values (FEV_1/FVC) defines obstructive pathophysiology and focuses the clinician on diseases such as asthma or COPD. The cutoff often used is FEV_1/FVC <70%. Asthma is more likely if the FEV_1 or FVC improves after the administration of a quick-acting bronchodilator (e.g., albuterol), although this can also be seen in COPD. If the FEV_1 and FVC are decreased symmetrically, this suggests restrictive pathophysiology, and further testing is required.

Decreased TLC defines restrictive pathophysiology. This measurement is determined by the assessment of lung volumes either through helium dilution or plethysmography. In addition to TLC, lung volume measurement also provides the RV and the functional residual capacity (FRC). When assessing for restrictive pathophysiology, the diffusion capacity for carbon monoxide (D_LCO) is also often obtained, as if this is impaired it suggests parenchymal lung disease (see DPLD below). There are a variety of other studies available in the PFT laboratory, including measurement of maximal inspiratory and expiratory pressures (MIP and MEP, respectively), bronchoprovocation testing with either exercise or methacholine, arterial blood gas sampling, and cardiopulmonary exercise testing. These tests are used alone or in combination to further evaluate dyspnea and gas exchange abnormalities.

RESPIRATORY DISORDERS

ASTHMA

Asthma is characterized by reversible airflow obstruction as a result of airway inflammation and smooth muscle constriction. These events usually occur as a response to one of many triggers including exercise, allergens (e.g., cat dander or pollen), and irritants such as tobacco smoke or perfumes. In addition to a history of intermittent dyspnea related to specific triggers, physical exam will often reveal diffuse, polyphonic wheezes. It should be noted that "all that wheezes is not asthma," and a diagnosis of asthma should be confirmed by demonstration of airflow obstruction on spirometry. Additionally, if the FEV_1 increases by more than 12% following bronchodilator administration, the diagnosis of asthma becomes much more likely.

The main focus of the treatment of asthma is on the control of symptoms. The first step in this process is to eliminate triggers as much as feasible. This may include avoidance of allergens, for which radioallergosorbent (RAST) testing may help identify particularly potent stimuli. Use of high-efficiency particulate air (HEPA) filters, smoking cessation, and avoidance of secondary tobacco smoke may all help. If symptoms persist despite efforts to decrease triggers of asthma, patients need to be treated with a combination of a controller medication (perhaps used intermittently) and a quick-relief medication, usually an inhaled beta agonist.

The *Guidelines for the Diagnosis and Management of Asthma* released by the Expert Panel of the National Asthma Education and Prevention Program in 2007 focuses on assessment of the control of symptoms, lung function, and risk of future asthmatic attack in adjusting medications. These guidelines recommend that treatment be escalated along a six-step sequence until good asthma control is achieved (see figure 44.1). Briefly, the six steps include:

1. *Intermittent asthma*—which is defined as symptoms necessitating a quick-relief bronchodilator no more often than two days per week; nocturnal awakenings due to asthma no more often than two days per month; lung function within the normal range; and no more than one attack of asthma within the past year requiring a course of oral steroids—should be treated with an "as needed" short-acting bronchodilator, usually a beta agonist.

2. *Mild persistent asthma* that is not controlled with just a quick-relief medication requires the addition of a controller medication, which could either be a low-dose inhaled steroid or a leukotriene modifier.

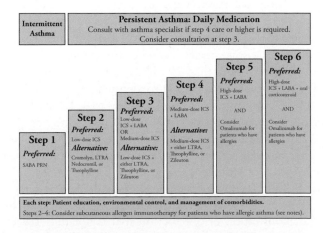

Figure 44.1. NAEPP Stepwise Approach to Asthma Therapy. Source: National Asthma Education and Prevention Program: Expert Panel Report 3: Guidelines for the diagnosis and management of asthma: National Institutes of Health Publication No. 08-4051. Bethesda, MD, 2007.

3. Recommendations for patients with *moderate persistent asthma* are in evolution, but clinicians generally increase the dose of inhaled steroid, add a long-acting beta agonist (LABA) to a low-dose inhaled steroid, or supplement with a leukotriene modifier. Recent studies have revealed an increased risk of death in patients treated with LABAs alone. Although many clinicians feel comfortable adding LABA to an inhaled steroid, it is unknown whether concomitant administration of an inhaled steroid with a LABA is protective.

4. If symptoms persist despite an additional agent or an increased dose of steroid, the recommendations are for use of a moderate-dose inhaled steroid plus LABA.

5. *Severe persistent asthma* is treated with a high-dose inhaled steroid combined with LABA, often in conjunction with a leukotriene modifier. Monoclonal antibodies to IgE are also considered in this step.

6. Refractory asthma is treated with biologic agents (as above) and/or oral glucocorticoids.

As control of symptoms is achieved, patients are "stepped down" in therapy as appropriate with the goal of minimizing symptoms and maintaining lung function with the least medication necessary. Once control has been achieved, clinicians should work with patients to develop an "action plan" based on symptoms and peak flow measurement. Each plan is individually tailored and can allow a reliable patient to treat an exacerbation early before severe symptoms and a true asthmatic attack ensue.

COPD

The Global Initiative for Chronic Obstructive Lung Disease characterizes COPD as a disease of "airflow limitation that is not fully reversible. The airflow limitation is usually progressive and associated with an abnormal inflammatory response of the lung to noxious particles or gases." Most commonly, the noxious particles and gases are from cigarette smoke. This disease, in its myriad of presentations, conservatively affects more than 20 million Americans and is the third leading cause of death in the United States. With this in mind, it is important for all clinicians to be familiar with the diagnosis and treatment of COPD.

Patients with intermittent dyspnea and cough who have long-term exposure to cigarette smoke should be assessed for evidence of airflow obstruction by spirometry. As is the case in asthma, obstruction is generally defined as a ratio of FEV_1/FVC <70%. The diagnosis of COPD is made by the demonstration of obstruction that is not fully reversible with a short-acting bronchodilator in the setting of the appropriate exposure history. Spirometry is particularly helpful as the severity of COPD is based on the measured FEV_1 (see table 44.1). Additional testing including lung

Table 44.1 GOLD CLASSIFICATION SYSTEM OF COPD

Stage 1	Mild	FEV_1/FVC <0.70
		FEV_1 ≥80% predicted
Stage 2	Moderate	FEV_1/FVC <0.70
		50% pred ≤FEV_1 <80% pred
Stage 3	Severe	FEV_1/FVC <0.70
		30% pred ≤FEV_1 <50% pred
Stage 4	Very severe	FEV_1/FVC <0.70
		FEV_1 <30% pred or
		FEV_1 <50% pred plus chronic respiratory failure

SOURCE: From the "Global Strategy for Diagnosis, Management, and Prevention of COPD, 2010" used with permission from the Global Initiative for Chronic Obstructive Lung Disease (GOLD), www.goldcopd.org

volumes, D_LCO, blood gas sampling, and chest tomography do not need to be routinely obtained but should be considered on an individual basis, particularly in those patients who have severe symptoms, resting hypoxemia, or severely impaired lung function.

The most important step in the treatment of COPD is to prevent its development through smoking cessation. Similarly, patients with established COPD will slow the rate of decline in lung function when they quit smoking. Therapies for smoking cessation include both nonpharmacologic approaches (e.g., support groups) and medications (see table 44.2). Physicians should inquire about smoking cessation on each patient visit.

Pharmacologic therapy for stable, chronic COPD includes both short- and long-acting inhaled bronchodilators including beta agonists and anticholinergics as well as inhaled steroids. In contrast to asthma treatment, multiple studies support the use of LABAs alone in the treatment of COPD without the evidence of increased mortality. Most patients are initially treated with either a long-acting anticholinergic or LABA. Inhaled steroids are reserved for patients with moderate to severe COPD (based on FEV_1) and recurrent exacerbations of disease. All patients should also receive pneumococcal and influenza vaccines.

Patients with more severe disease may develop resting hypoxemia. When oxygen saturation is <88% at rest, supplemental oxygen should be initiated, as there is a clear mortality benefit to this therapy. Patients with more severe disease also benefit from pulmonary rehabilitation. The clinician should consider referral of such patients to a specialist because certain subsets of COPD patients may benefit from lung volume reduction surgery, lung transplantation, or other novel therapies.

DIFFUSE PARENCHYMAL LUNG DISEASES

There are a variety of less common diseases that diffusely affect the lung parenchyma. In the past, these conditions were referred to as the interstitial lung diseases (ILD).

Table 44.2 PHARMACOTHERAPY FOR SMOKING CESSATION

MEDICATION	TRADE NAME	FORM	SIDE EFFECTS
Nicotine		Lozenge Gum Nasal spray Transdermal patch	Nausea, insomnia (transdermal)
Bupropion	Zyban Wellbutrin	Pill	May exacerbate seizures
Varenicline	Chantix	Pill	Nausea Neuropsychiatric symptoms

Because these processes often affect more than the interstitium, the grouping is now commonly called DPLDs. The classic DPLD is idiopathic pulmonary fibrosis (IPF), but there are a myriad of other poorly understood diseases including sarcoidosis, cryptogenic organizing pneumonia (COP), and hypersensitivity pneumonitis included in the DPLDs.

IPF is an insidious disease of presumed abnormal wound healing that results in progressive scarring of the lungs with impaired gas exchange and restrictive pathophysiology. The cause of IPF, as the name implies, is unknown. Patients present with progressive dyspnea on exertion and nonproductive cough, often initially misdiagnosed as asthma or pneumonia. On exam, basilar crackles and clubbing are common, and most patients progress to resting hypoxemia. Diagnosis is occasionally made by classic computed tomography (CT) scan appearance with basilar, subpleural honeycombing with a lack of ground glass infiltrates, however most patients require a lung biopsy for definitive diagnosis. On biopsy, subpleural changes including "fibroblastic foci" within heterogeneous areas of injury and fibrosis are pathognomonic for IPF. Unfortunately, at this time there are no effective therapies for IPF. Patients should be referred early in their course for evaluation for possible lung transplantation.

Other DPLDs can be grouped into those with known causes and those of unknown etiology, with, unfortunately, many more diseases in the latter category. Changes in the lung related to inorganic inhalational exposures are termed pneumonconioses. The best-described pneumoconiosis is asbestosis. This disease is quite similar pathologically to IPF but is secondary to chronic asbestos exposure. As with IPF, there is no known therapy for asbestosis, although it is rarely as aggressively progressive as IPF. In contrast, inhalation of *organic* substances can lead to a granulomatous inflammation along the bronchovascular bundles called hypersensitivity pneumonitis (HP). A variety of materials can result in HP, and well-described exposures include actinomycetes, pigeon droppings, atypical mycobacteria (commonly from hot tubs), and *Aspergillus*. The initial therapy is removal of the offending agent. In the acute phase, these reactions are generally responsive to glucocorticoids; however, with chronic exposure the parenchymal changes can become irreversible.

There are a series of poorly understood DPLDs related to cigarette smoking. These include desquamative interstitial pneumonitis (DIP), respiratory bronchiolitis interstitial lung disease (RBILD), and pulmonary Langerhans-cell histiocytosis (PLCH). All of these are much less common than COPD, which should be suspected first in patients with a history of tobacco exposure and new dyspnea or cough.

Sarcoidosis is a multiorgan disease of unknown etiology. The pathology is caused by diffuse noncaseating granulomatous inflammation. The lung disease of sarcoid ranges from benign and asymptomatic hilar lymphadenopathy to end-stage fibrosis. Most lung disease is at least initially responsive to glucocorticoids, although many patients will require no therapy. Other organs commonly affected by sarcoid include the skin (e.g., erythema nodosum, lupus pernio), heart, liver, central nervous system, and eyes.

VENOUS THROMBOEMBOLIC DISEASE

Although the incidence markedly increases after the age of 60, patients of all ages, with a variety of risk factors and underlying diseases, may develop venous thrombolic disease (VTE), which encompasses both deep venous thrombosis (DVT) and pulmonary embolism (PE). The majority of patients who develop VTE have one or more clinical risk factors including underlying malignancy, cigarette smoking, oral contraceptive use, recent surgery, trauma, or immobilization. In addition, those patients with a personal or family history are at increased risk, suggesting a genetic risk factor such as factor V Leiden or prothrombin gene mutation.

Patients with DVT usually present with symptoms related to lower extremity swelling and discomfort. Patients with PE classically present with dyspnea, pleuritic chest discomfort and mild hypoxemia; however, PE can be clinically silent or result in hemodynamic collapse, refractory hypoxemia, and death. For this reason, clinicians need to always be alert to the possibility of PE, particularly in patients with multiple risk factors for VTE.

Diagnosis of VTE can be quite challenging. The gold standard for confirmation of DVT is a duplex venous ultrasound, but CT, magnetic resonance (MR) angiography, and contrast venography are also used in certain clinical situations. In the recent 5–10 years, contrast CT scan has become the modality by which most pulmonary emboli are diagnosed, whereas in the past ventilation-perfusion scans were more common. MR and pulmonary angiography remain other options; however, timeliness and invasiveness (respectively) are issues with these studies. In many clinical situations, it is more important to "rule out" pulmonary embolism, particularly when there is a low clinical probability. In these settings, the measurement of a D-dimer may be helpful, as it has a strong negative predictive value in outpatient populations with low clinical likelihood of PE.

The mainstay of treatment of VTE is anticoagulation either with heparin products, warfarin, or fondaparinux. For patients who can not be anticoagulated, placement of an inferior vena cava filter can acutely protect against a DVT resulting in a PE but may have significant long term morbidity. The use of thrombolytic agents, catheter, or surgical intervention in the setting of massive pulmonary emboli remains an area of ongoing debate. As all of these interventions have limitations, it is encouraging that new therapies are on the horizon for all aspects of VTE.

OBSTRUCTIVE SLEEP APNEA

Obstructive sleep apnea (OSA) is an underdiagnosed disease that is estimated to affect approximately 5% of the adult population. Because there are many long-term health consequences of OSA, it is important for all clinicians to consider the possibility of this diagnosis in their patients. Patients with OSA have increased rates of hypertension, coronary artery disease, heart failure, diabetes, and stroke, as well as significantly increased risk of motor vehicle accidents.

The hallmark of OSA is the obstructive apnea where there is full collapse of the airway resulting in complete cessation of breathing for at least 10 seconds. The diagnosis of OSA, however, relies on the number of apneas and hypopneas (i.e., reduced airflow for at least 10 seconds due to partial collapse) per hour of sleep often referred to as the apnea-hypopnea index (AHI). Most clinicians use a threshold of at least 15 episodes per hour to diagnose OSA in asymptomatic patients and between 5 and 15 events per hour in symptomatic patients. In some settings, the number of respiratory event–related arousals (RERA) per hour is also tabulated, as these events related to increased work of breathing due to partial airway collapse are also disruptive to sleep.

Risk for OSA correlates with obesity and advanced age. There are a variety of other risk factors, some of which are modifiable, which should be assessed in any patient suspected of having OSA (see table 44.3). In addition, an individual patient's upper airway anatomy impacts the risk of OSA, as smaller upper airway lumens are more likely to collapse. This can be affected by large tonsils, large tongue, and increased adipose tissue.

Several symptoms should suggest a diagnosis of OSA. These include snoring (the most commonly reported

Table 44.3 RISK FACTORS FOR OSA

Excess body weight

Advancing age

Male sex

Family/genetic predisposition

Tobacco use

Alcohol consumption

Medical conditions (polycystic ovarian syndrome, hypothyroidism, stroke)

Pregnancy

Menopause

Abnormal craniofacial anatomy

Neck circumference (>17 inches in men, >16 inches in women)

Small, hypoplastic, and/or retroposed maxilla and mandible

Narrow posterior airway space

Inferiorly positioned hyoid bone

High and narrow hard palate

Abnormal dental overjet

Macroglossia

Tonsillar enlargement

Nasal obstruction

symptom), daytime sleepiness, morning headaches, memory impairment, and depression. Patients are often formally evaluated with the Epworth Sleepiness Scale, which is a validated tool to assess for excessive daytime sleepiness. On exam, obesity and hypertension should raise a clinician's suspicion; however, the airway exam is most helpful. Mallampati airway scores have been shown to predict risk for OSA.

Although the history and physical exam may raise the possibility of OSA, a polysomnogram is required for definitive diagnosis. This study records electrocardiogram (EKG), electroencephalogram (EEG), eye movements, chest wall movements, oxygen saturation, and muscle activity during sleep, which allow the calculation of an AHI as well as measurement of a variety of other parameters. Many centers offer a split-night sleep study, which allows a patient to be diagnosed in the first half of the night and then to begin therapy with continuous positive airway pressure (CPAP) in the latter half of the night's sleep.

There are a variety of therapies for OSA. Weight loss may help many patients, but it is often very difficult to achieve. Other modifiable risk factors, such as cigarette smoking and excessive alcohol intake, should also be addressed. Patients may have relief of symptoms by positional therapy, as OSA is worse in most patients in the supine position. Many patients, however, will require CPAP to maintain an open airway. CPAP has been shown to decrease the majority of symptoms associated with OSA. For patients who do not tolerate CPAP, there are dental appliances and surgery as additional options for therapy. Most importantly, all of these therapies require the clinician to first look for and diagnose OSA, a generally underdiagnosed disease.

CRITICAL CARE

As the population of the United States ages, more and more patients will spend time in an intensive care unit (ICU). Although many clinicians will not directly deliver care to patients in an ICU, a familiarity with ventilator management and therapies for shock and sepsis are important for understanding the severity of illness of one's patient.

SHOCK AND SEPSIS

One of the most common causes of admission to an ICU is a fall in blood pressure (i.e., hypotension) despite adequate volume resuscitation, resulting in poor end-organ perfusion. This state, termed "shock," results in significant morbidity and mortality. Shock can be categorized broadly into hypovolemic, cardiogenic, obstructive, or distributive.

Hypovolemic shock is usually the result of profound dehydration or severe bleeding as associated with gastrointestinal disease or major trauma. The cornerstone of therapy for hypovolemic shock is rapid volume replacement with either crystalloid or colloid (e.g., packed red blood cells) and resolution of the underlying disorder. Cardiogenic shock results from impairment of cardiac output from a variety of causes including cardiomyopathy, ischemia, valvular dysfunction, or arrhythmia. Obstructive shock can be considered a subset of cardiogenic shock as it results from blockage of forward flow from the heart. The most common cause of obstructive shock is massive pulmonary embolism, but cardiac tamponade and tension pneumothorax can result in the same pathophysiology.

Distributive shock is the result of severe vasodilation. Although anaphylaxis and spinal cord injury can result in distributive shock, the most common cause is sepsis. Sepsis is defined as the systemic inflammatory response (SIRS) with a probable source of infection. SIRS is manifest by a combination of tachycardia, tachypnea, fever, and elevated white blood cell count. Common causes of sepsis include pneumonia, pyelonephritis, and biliary tract obstruction. Prompt administration of antibiotics and source control are the keys to treatment of sepsis, but patients will often require vasopressor agents as well to support their blood pressure before the infection has resolved.

After rapid and aggressive volume resuscitation, vasoactive agents are initiated to maintain an adequate mean arterial pressure (MAP). Guidelines recommend the use of norepinephrine (an alpha and beta agonist) or dopamine (a dopaminergic as well as alpha and beta agonist) as an initial agent. Some intensivists augment one of these agents with intravenous vasopressin, although there is no evidence that this provides a mortality benefit. These medications are titrated to a MAP that results in adequate tissue perfusion as demonstrated by clinical features such as improved mental status and urine output.

MECHANICAL VENTILATION

Patients receive mechanical ventilation because of problems with oxygenation, ventilation, or excessive work of breathing. Sometimes a patient has an endotracheal tube placed not because of a respiratory problem but instead for "airway protection" in the setting of altered mental status. Although these patients will also receive mechanical ventilation while intubated, they do not truly require this support.

Although this is somewhat of an oversimplification, the degree of oxygenation is determined by the fraction of inspired oxygen (FiO_2) and the positive end-expiratory pressure (PEEP). Mechanistically, one can think of PEEP as holding alveoli open in order to increase surface area for gas exchange and thus improving oxygenation. The clinician needs to set the FiO_2 and the PEEP for all patients receiving mechanical ventilation.

In contrast, ventilation (or clearance of CO_2) is determined by a patient's minute ventilation (VE). Minute ventilation is calculated as the product of the respiratory rate and the tidal volume ($VE = RR \times V_t$). The different ventilator modes are used to provide a patient's minute ventilation. Some modes fully support a patient's breathing (e.g., assist control), whereas others allow a patient to initiate breaths and interact more with the ventilator (e.g., pressure support). In general, a ventilator is set to deliver either a given volume or a given pressure with each breath. If the mode is set to deliver a specific volume each breath, the resulting pressures will reflect the patient's respiratory system compliance and airways resistance. The converse is also true, as the pressure-delivered breaths will vary in size based on the patient's physiology. Clinicians monitor these measurements as well as gas exchange (usually via pulse oximetry and arterial blood gas sampling) to assess a patient's condition while receiving mechanical ventilation.

ARTERIAL BLOOD GAS INTERPRETATION

An arterial blood gas (ABG) provides information about both a patient's oxygenation and acid–base status. Both aspects should be interpreted on any ABG obtained.

The PaO_2 reflects the amount of dissolved oxygen in plasma, and the SaO_2 is a measure of the amount of oxygen bound to hemoglobin. Although oxygen saturation (SaO_2) can be obtained noninvasively with a pulse oximeter, an ABG is required for the measurement of PaO_2. In many ways the SaO_2 is more useful to the clinician, as it is the major determinant of blood oxygen content. The following equation reflects this relationship:

$$CaO_2 = (SaO_2 \times Hb \times 1.34) + (PaO_2 \times 0.003)$$

The particular value of the PaO_2 is that is allows calculation of the alveolar-arterial oxygen difference ($AaDO_2$).

$$AaDO_2 = PAO_2 - PaO_2$$
$$PAO_2 = (FiO_2 \times 713) - (PaCO_2/0.8).$$

The $AaDO_2$ is used to determine the pathophysiological cause of hypoxemia. Although hypoventilation and low FiO_2 result in a normal $AaDO_2$, shunt and ventilation-perfusion mismatch cause a widened $AaDO_2$. Normal values for $AaDO_2$ vary with age, but in general $AaDO_2$ in the range of 8–14 is considered normal.

Acid–base status, including pH, $PaCO_2$, and calculated HCO_3 can also be assessed with an ABG. Normal pH is generally thought to range from 7.38 to 7.42. When a patient's blood pH falls lower than 7.38, this is called acidemia, and an elevated pH is termed alkalemia. The processes that result in these changes in pH are respectively acidoses and alkaloses. An acidosis or an alkalosis can either be respiratory or metabolic in origin.

A respiratory acidosis, as indicated by an elevated $PaCO_2$, is a result of inadequate minute ventilation for the amount of CO_2 produced. This can be because of low tidal volumes, low respiratory rate, or overwhelming work of breathing. Common causes of a respiratory acidosis include severe airways obstruction (e.g., COPD exacerbation), neuromuscular weakness, or depressed mental status. In contrast, a respiratory alkalosis results from an increased minute ventilation, most commonly due to pain or anxiety.

Metabolic acidosis is a result of the production of increased acids causing a subsequent fall in the measured bicarbonate level. Metabolic acidoses are categorized as anion-gap (AG) or non-AG processes. The anion gap is calculated as the difference between the serum Na and the serum Cl + HCO_3. This difference is usually 8–12. If there is an increased AG it is an indication of unmeasured anions (acids). Common AG acidoses include diabetic ketoacidosis (DKA) and lactic acidosis associated with poor tissue perfusion. Falls in bicarbonate not associated with an increased AG fit into the category of non-AG metabolic acidoses, examples of which are renal tubular acidosis (RTA) and severe diarrhea. Finally, loss of acid can result in a metabolic alkalosis. Most commonly this is due to dehydration or profound vomiting.

A comprehensive evaluation of an ABG can reveal multiple respiratory and metabolic processes. Each ABG should be systematically reviewed for all acid–base disorders as well as hypoxemia and its potential etiologies.

ADDITIONAL READING

Agnelli G, Becattini C. Acute pulmonary embolism. *N Engl J Med.* 2010;363(3):266–74.

Dempsey OJ, Kerr KM, Remmen H, Denison AR. How to investigate a patient with suspected interstitial lung disease. *BMJ.* 2010;340: c2843.

Dixon S, Benamore R. The idiopathic interstitial pneumonias: Understanding key radiological features. *Clin Radiol.* 2010;65(10): 823–31.

Eickelberg O, Selman M. Update in diffuse parenchymal lung disease 2009. *Am J Respir Crit Care Med.* 2010;181(9):883–8.

Fanta CH. Asthma. *N Engl J Med.* 2009;360(10):1002–14. Errata *N Engl J Med.* 2009;361(11):1123; and *N Engl J Med.* 2009;360(16):1685.

Lazarus SC. Clinical practice. Emergency treatment of asthma. *N Engl J Med.* 2010;363(8):755–64.

Niewoehner DE. Clinical practice. Outpatient management of severe COPD. *N Engl J Med.* 2010;362(15):1407–16.

Papanikolaou IC, Drakopanagiotakis F, Polychronopoulos VS. Acute exacerbations of interstitial lung diseases. *Curr Opin Pulm Med.* 2010;16(5):480–6.

SECTION 5

ENDOCRINOLOGY

45.

PITUITARY DISORDERS

Florencia Halperin and Ursula B. Kaiser

PITUITARY ANATOMY AND PHYSIOLOGY

The pituitary gland sits in a depression in the base of the skull, the sella turcica, directly below the optic chiasm and is connected to the hypothalamus by the pituitary stalk. On each side, the pituitary is bordered by the cavernous sinus, through which run cranial nerves III, IV, VI, and the first and second branches of cranial nerve V (figure 45.1).

The pituitary gland is divided into an anterior and a posterior portion. The anterior pituitary, also known as the adenohypophysis, is composed of five distinct cell types, each of which secretes a distinct hormone. The anterior pituitary forms part of a tightly coordinated system of hypothalamic-pituitary-target organ axes, in which hormonal signals from the hypothalamus stimulate or inhibit secretion of anterior pituitary hormones, which in turn act on specific organs, as follows. Hypothalamic neurons produce gonadotropin-releasing hormone (GnRH), which stimulates pituitary production of luteinizing hormone (LH) and follicle-stimulating hormone (FSH), and these signal the ovaries to secrete estrogen and progesterone or the testes to secrete testosterone. Hypothalamic corticotropin-releasing hormone (CRH) induces pituitary adrenocorticotropic hormone (ACTH) production, which regulates adrenal cortisol synthesis. Thyrotropin-releasing hormone (TRH) stimulates thyroid-stimulating hormone (TSH), which in turn regulates thyroid hormone production. Hypothalamic growth hormone releasing hormone (GHRH) is responsible for pituitary growth hormone (GH) production, which leads to insulin-like growth factor-1 (IGF-1) production in the liver. While most hypothalamic hormones have a stimulatory effect on the anterior pituitary, somatostatin plays an inhibitory role; it inhibits the secretion of GH and TSH. Finally, prolactin secretion is tonically inhibited by hypothalamic dopamine (figure 45.2).

The hypothalamic-pituitary-target gland axes tend to function as negative-feedback systems in which hormones secreted by target organs suppress hypothalamic and/or

pituitary activity. A hormone deficiency can be primary, caused by target gland failure, or secondary or tertiary, caused by failure of the pituitary or hypothalamus, respectively, to stimulate the target gland.

The posterior pituitary, also known as the neurohypophysis, is the site of storage and secretion of vasopressin (AVP) and oxytocin, which are both synthesized in neurons in the hypothalamus.

PITUITARY LESIONS

Pituitary lesions can be of multiple etiologies and thus have a broad differential diagnosis. Tumors of several types can involve the pituitary gland. Benign tumors of anterior pituitary cell origin are known as adenomas. Very rarely, these can become carcinomas. Other tumors that can affect the pituitary gland include craniopharyngiomas, Rathke's cleft cysts, and germinomas. Malignancies from multiple primary sites, including hematologic malignancies, can metastasize to the pituitary. Last, granulomatous, infectious, infiltrative, and inflammatory processes such as sarcoidosis, eosinophilic granulomatosis, tuberculosis, mycosis, abscesses, hemochromatosis, and lymphocytic hypophysitis can all cause pituitary lesions (table 45.1).

PITUITARY ADENOMAS

By far the most common pituitary lesion is the pituitary adenoma, with a prevalence of approximately 1 in 1000 to 1 in 10,000 individuals. In formulating a clinical approach to the diagnosis and management of a patient with a pituitary adenoma, two major factors need to be considered: *mass effects* and *effects on pituitary function*.

Mass effects are neurological and hormonal abnormalities that develop secondary to the intracranial space occupied by the lesion or to its proximity to important anatomical structures. Patients who develop *mass effects* from a pituitary lesion may complain of headaches. Temporal visual field deficits may develop as a result of compression of the optic chiasm.

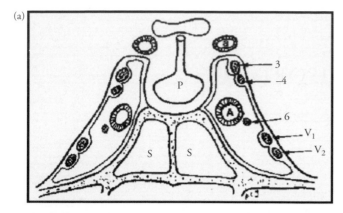

(a)

(b)

Figure 45.1. Pituitary Anatomy. (A) P, pituitary gland; S, sphenoid sinus; A, carotid artery; 3,4,6, cranial nerves III, IV, and VI; V1,V2, branches 1 and 2 of cranial nerve V. *Source*: Reprinted from Naidich MJ and Russell EJ. Current Approaches to Imaging of the Sellar Region and Pituitary. *Endocrinol Metab Clin North Am.* 1999; 28(1):45–79, with permission from Elsevier. (B) MRI of normal pituitary gland. *Source*: Reprinted with permission from Vance ML. Hypopituitarism. *N Engl J Med.* 1994; 330(23):1651–62. Copyright 1994 Massachusetts Medical Society. All rights reserved.

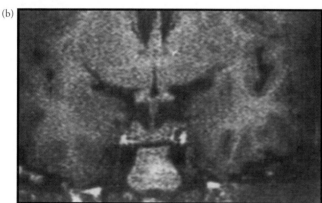

Figure 45.2. Schematic of Hypothalamic-Pituitary-Target Organ Regulation. GnRH, gonadotropin-releasing hormone; CRH, corticotropin-releasing hormone; TRH, thyrotropin-releasing hormone; DA, dopamine; GHRH, growth hormone-releasing hormone; LH, leuteinizing hormone; FSH, follicle-stimulating hormone; ACTH, corticotropin; TSH, thyroid-stimulating hormone; PRL, prolactin; GH, growth hormone; IGF-1, insulin-like growth factor-1.

Table 45.1 DIFFERENTIAL DIAGNOSIS OF SELLAR/ PARASELLAR LESIONS

Tumors
Pituitary adenoma
Pituitary carcinoma
Meningioma
Craniopharyngioma
Rathke's cleft cyst
Germinoma
Dermoid
Teratoma
Oligodendroglioma
Ependymoma
Astrocytoma
Tumor metastasis
Hematologic malignancy

Infections
Abscess
Tuberculosis
Mycoses

Granulomatous diseases
Sarcoidosis

Inflammatory diseases
Eosinophilic granulomatosis
Lymphocytic hypophysitis

Vascular lesions
Miscellaneous
Empty sella syndrome

Ocular nerve palsies and diplopia can occur if cranial nerves III, IV, or VI, which travel in the cavernous sinus, are compressed; facial numbness and pain can result if cranial nerve V is affected (figure 45.1). Additionally, the presence of a pituitary mass can distort regional anatomy sufficiently to decrease hormone production by adjacent cells. This can lead to various degrees of hypopituitarism. Hyperprolactinemia can result from compression of the pituitary stalk, as this interrupts inhibitory dopamine signaling.

The second important consideration when evaluating a patient with a pituitary lesion is its *effect on pituitary hormone production*. Adenomas can be nonfunctioning (15% of all adenomas), or they can secrete one or more pituitary hormones in excess. The most common type of hyperfunctioning lesions (60%) are lactotroph adenomas, which produce prolactin. GH-secreting adenomas (15%) result in the disease known as acromegaly, and 6% of adenomas secrete ACTH, resulting in Cushing disease. Adenomas that secrete bioactive LH, FSH, or TSH are very rare.

At the same time, as mentioned above, whether an adenoma is hyperfunctioning or nonfunctioning, it can cause pituitary hypofunction by compression of nearby normal anterior pituitary cells. Indeed, a pituitary tumor could cause impaired secretion of all hormones except for the one that it secretes in excess. The clinical manifestations and differential diagnosis of hypopituitarism are addressed in detail below.

Prolactinomas

Clinical Presentation

The most common symptoms of high prolactin levels, or hyperprolactinemia, in premenopausal women are menstrual abnormalities (oligomenorrhea or amenorrhea) and anovulation. Galactorrhea occurs in about 50–80% of women. In men, hyperprolactinemia can cause decreased libido, impotence, and infertility; galactorrhea is less common. The reproductive abnormalities seen in both sexes are thought to be secondary to a direct suppressive effect of prolactin on hypothalamic gonadotropin-releasing hormone (GnRH) production; this inhibits gonadotropin (LH and FSH) release, and consequently impairs gametogenesis and gonadal steroidogenesis. Prolonged estrogen and androgen deficiency also leads to decreased bone density. The clinical presentation of a prolactinoma may also include symptoms from mass effect, including headache and visual field cuts, especially in men, who generally present with larger tumors.

Differential Diagnosis of Hyperprolactinemia

Prolactinomas are not the only cause of hyperprolactinemia (table 45.2). As previously stated, prolactin secretion is under tonic inhibitory control by dopamine, and any process that interferes with hypothalamic dopamine secretion or its delivery to the pituitary gland can result in hyperprolactinemia. There are also factors that stimulate prolactin release, including stress, exercise, sleep, chest wall stimulation (via afferent neural pathways), thyrotropin-releasing hormone (TRH), serotonin, estrogen, and others.

There are *physiological* states of hyperprolactinemia, such as pregnancy and lactation. During pregnancy, rising estrogen levels stimulate prolactin, which can increase 10- to 20-fold. The stimulus of suckling maintains high prolactin levels during lactation. There are also multiple *pharmacologic* agents that elevate prolactin. The majority of these are dopamine antagonists, such as the antipsychotic agents (risperidone, haloperidol) and metoclopramide. Last, there are *pathophysiological* states that result in hyperprolactinemia. Pituitary stalk compression secondary to tumors or infiltrative diseases interferes with dopamine inhibition of prolactin. Primary hypothyroidism results in elevation of TRH, which stimulates both TSH and prolactin (and in such cases, treatment of hypothyroidism should normalize prolactin). Chronic renal failure causes hyperprolactinemia secondary to decreased clearance of the hormone. Finally, prolactinomas are a major cause of prolactin elevation; occasionally, adenomas cosecrete prolactin with other anterior pituitary hormones.

Diagnosis

A patient who presents with symptoms of hyperprolactinemia can be evaluated with a random measurement

Table 45.2 **CAUSES OF HYPERPROLACTINEMIA**

Physiological
Pregnancy
Lactation
Nipple or chest wall stimulation
Stress

Pharmacologic
Dopamine antagonists
Phenothiazines
Haloperidol
Risperidone
Metoclopramide
Domperidone
Amitriptyline
Selective serotonin reuptake inhibitors
Antihypertensives
Methyldopa
Reserpine
Verapamil
Cimetidine
Estrogens

Pathophysiological
Primary hypothyroidism
Chronic renal failure
Chest wall lesions
Hypothalamic or pituitary lesions that cause pituitary stalk compression
Prolactinoma
Cosecretion of prolactin and other hormones from a pituitary adenoma
Idiopathic

of serum prolactin. If the prolactin level is mildly elevated, the measurement should be repeated, given the various physiological factors (listed above) that can transiently elevate prolactin. If the level remains high, further evaluation should include a detailed history of recent medication use, a pregnancy test (if the patient is female), and thyroid and renal function tests. If no secondary cause of hyperprolactinemia is identified, the patient should be evaluated for the presence of a pituitary mass by gadolinium-enhanced magnetic resonance imaging (MRI).

Pituitary adenomas are classified as a microadenoma if they are <10 mm in size and as macroadenomas if they ≥10 mm in size. In general, in the case of prolactinomas, the magnitude of prolactin elevation correlates well with radiographic estimates of tumor size. Macroadenomas are generally associated with prolactin levels greater than 200–250 μg/L. Therefore, a mild prolactin elevation in the presence of a macroadenoma should raise suspicion that the tumor is not in fact prolactin-secreting, but is causing hyperprolactinemia secondary to compression of the pituitary stalk. In such cases, treatment with dopamine agonists will lower prolactin levels, but will not cause a decrease in tumor size (see below).

Management

The indications for treatment of a prolactin-secreting adenoma depend on the size of the tumor, the presence of hypogonadism, menstrual irregularities, bothersome symptoms such as galactorrhea, and the patient's desire for fertility.

The presence of a macroadenoma is an absolute indication for therapy, as there is significant potential for tumor expansion (figure 45.3). Patients with macroadenomas that extend beyond the sella turcica should undergo visual field testing and evaluation of anterior pituitary function. The goals of treatment are to normalize prolactin levels and achieve remission of symptoms, reduce tumor size, and prevent disease progression.

On the other hand, most microadenomas do not increase in size over time. As a result, these patients require treatment only if they desire fertility, have amenorrhea, hypogonadism, or troublesome galactorrhea, or if the adenoma enlarges. Patients with microadenomas without these indications for treatment can be followed with periodic prolactin measurements and MRI if their clinical symptoms progress (figure 45.3). Women can also safely be treated with oral contraceptives or estrogen/progesterone replacement to prevent bone loss.

The first line of treatment for prolactin-secreting tumors is a dopamine agonist, of which two are approved for this indication in the United States: bromocriptine and cabergoline. Both medications effectively lower serum prolactin levels, restore gonadal function, and reduce tumor size. Cabergoline may be more effective than bromocriptine, is usually better tolerated, and can be administered once or twice weekly rather than daily. Both bromocriptine and cabergoline are usually started at low doses and titrated until prolactin levels normalize. Side effects include nausea, headache, and dizziness. In women attempting to conceive, because of more extensive safety data, bromocriptine is generally preferred. The medication should be discontinued when pregnancy is achieved.

Dopamine agonists may not be necessary indefinitely; when dopamine agonist therapy is discontinued, 20–25% of patients remain normoprolactinemic. Therefore, after 1–2 years of therapy, it is reasonable to taper the dopamine agonist therapy while monitoring prolactin levels, to determine if permanent remission of hyperprolactinemia has occurred.

It is worth noting that the ergot-derived dopamine agonists, pergolide and cabergoline, have recently been associated with increased risk of cardiac valve regurgitation in patients treated with these medications for Parkinson disease. However, the doses used for the treatment of Parkinson disease are much higher than those used for hyperprolactinemia, and there is no evidence that valvulopathy occurs at the lower cumulative doses used for this indication. A possible mechanism for the valvular disease associated with these drugs is the activation of cardiac serotonin receptor subtype 5-HT_{2B}; valvulopathies associated with carcinoid syndrome and fenfluramine also occur through this mechanism.

In addition to dopamine agonists, treatment options for prolactinomas include surgery and external radiation. Transsphenoidal removal of a prolactinoma is indicated when a macroadenoma does not respond to medical therapy or when there is tumor growth despite medical treatment. If a substantial amount of tumor remains after surgical excision, external radiation may occasionally be necessary.

Acromegaly

Clinical Presentation

Acromegaly is rare, with an incidence of approximately three cases per 1 million persons per year. The vast majority of cases are caused by pituitary GH-secreting adenomas. The clinical manifestations of acromegaly are varied. Accelerated growth and gigantism occur only if the disease develops in adolescence before epiphyseal plates are closed. In adults, the most common clinical features are coarsening

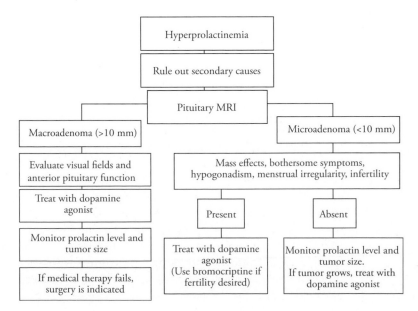

Figure 45.3. Treatment Algorithm for Hyperprolactinemia.

Table 45.3 CLINICAL FEATURES OF ACROMEGALY IN ADULTS

Coarsening of facial features (frontal bone bossing; jaw prognathism)

Soft-tissue swelling (acral enlargement: increased ring, shoe, hat size)

Arthralgias

Osteoarthritis

Excessive sweating

Menstrual irregularities

Hyperglycemia

Hyperlipidemia

Cardiac abnormalities (hypertension, heart failure, arrhythmias, valvular disease)

Sleep apnea

---

of facial features, such as frontal bone bossing and jaw prognathism, and soft-tissue swelling that can lead to increases in ring, shoe, or hat size. Patients also frequently complain of increased sweating, and premenopausal women may note menstrual irregularities. Arthralgias and osteoarthritis are a source of significant functional disability. Metabolic complications include hyperglycemia and hyperlipidemia. Cardiac abnormalities such as arrhythmias, hypertension, valvular disease, and heart failure, as well sleep apnea secondary to airway soft-tissue swelling, may develop (table 45.3). Additionally, acromegaly is associated with an increased risk of certain tumors, such as colonic polyps.

More than 75% of patients with acromegaly have a macroadenoma at diagnosis, and if that is the case they may additionally present with symptoms of mass effect, such as headaches, visual field defects, and pituitary hormone deficiencies. About 25% of GH adenomas cosecrete prolactin, and in these instances galactorrhea may be present.

Diagnosis

Under normal physiological conditions, GH is released in a pulsatile fashion, which results in considerable variation in circulating levels. A random serum GH level is therefore not an accurate indicator of GH excess. GH induces the synthesis of IGF-1 from tissues such as the liver. Circulating IGF-1 concentrations reflect peripheral GH levels, but unlike GH, IGF-1 has a long half-life and can be reliably measured at any time of day. As a result, measurement of serum IGF-1 is the best screening test for acromegaly. IGF-1 levels should be compared against age- and gender-matched normative data.

If IGF-1 levels are elevated, the diagnosis of acromegaly can then be confirmed by documenting failure of suppression of GH secretion. This is best accomplished by performing a 75-g oral glucose tolerance test, during which GH levels are obtained. The most widely used diagnostic criterion is a GH level 2 hours after glucose ingestion of >1 µg/L Conventionally, both an elevated IGF-1 level and failure of GH suppression are required for a diagnosis of acromegaly (table 45.5). In clinical practice, however, GH suppression testing is not always necessary if the clinical picture is highly suggestive, IGF-1 levels are elevated, and a pituitary mass is present.

Indeed, the evaluation of a patient with suspected acromegaly should also include a gadolinium-enhanced pituitary MRI to establish the presence and dimensions of a pituitary tumor, as well as its proximity to the optic chiasm. In addition, given the significant number of patients who present with macroadenomas, these patients should undergo evaluation of other pituitary hormones to rule out hypopituitarism. This should include measurement of morning serum cortisol, TSH and free T_4, testosterone levels in men, and a menstrual history in premenopausal women. Because many adenomas cosecrete growth hormone and prolactin, the latter should also be measured.

Management

The goals of treatment for acromegaly are to control GH and IGF-1 levels (GH <1 µg/L after oral glucose tolerance, and IGF-1 levels in the normal range for age and gender) as well as to reduce tumor size and mass effects and improve comorbid conditions, including restoration or preservation of pituitary function. Patients with acromegaly have increased risk of premature mortality, and epidemiologic studies suggest that normalizing GH and IGF-1 levels helps to reduce complications and normalize mortality rates. During treatment for acromegaly, it is important to continue monitoring for associated morbidities including pituitary insufficiency, cardiovascular dysfunction, sleep apnea, hyperglycemia, musculoskeletal diseases, and colonic polyps.

Transsphenoidal surgery is the treatment of choice for acromegaly in most patients. This is the only treatment with potential for definitive cure. Surgery reduces tumor size and relieves complications from mass effect. Surgical outcomes depend on several factors. Certain tumor characteristics, such as size, presence of extrasellar growth, and dural invasion, are associated with lower rates of cure. Individual surgical expertise is another major determinant of outcome. Postoperatively, IGF-1 and nadir glucose-suppressed GH levels should be measured to determine the success of the procedure. In one series, after 12 months of postoperative follow-up, about 70% of patients had normal IGF-1 levels, and about 60% had nadir glucose-suppressed GH levels <1 µg/L.

When surgery fails to normalize the biochemical parameters, or when patients refuse or have a contraindication to surgery, medical therapy should be initiated. The first line of treatment in such cases is a somatostatin analogue (octreotide or lanreotide). These drugs suppress pituitary GH secretion and block the synthesis of IGF-1 in the liver. They are administered subcutaneously or intramuscularly, have long-acting forms that can be injected monthly, and are generally well tolerated, although gastrointestinal side effects such as nausea, vomiting, and diarrhea are common, and risk of gallstone formation and hyperglycemia is increased. When used as adjunctive therapy postoperatively, somatostatin analogues normalize IGF-1 levels in about 60% of patients and result in symptomatic improvement and decreased soft-tissue swelling in about 80%, but tumor size is reduced in only about 30% of cases. GH and IGF-1 assessment should be performed a few months after initiation of treatment to establish dose adequacy.

When surgery and somatostatin analogues both fail to normalize biochemical parameters, another available drug is pegvisomant, a GH receptor antagonist. Importantly, because the drug acts peripherally but does not affect the pituitary secretion of GH, it does not lower GH or reduce tumor size, and therefore, patients on pegvisomant should be monitored biochemically with IGF-1 levels and radiographically for tumor growth. Pegvisomant is administered subcutaneously on a daily basis and normalizes IGF-1 levels in over 85% of cases.

Somatotroph adenomas express dopamine receptors, and dopamine agonists have been used in the management of acromegaly, but they are not as effective as other agents. Radiation therapy is generally reserved as a last resort for patients who have undergone surgery and subsequently were resistant to or intolerant of medical treatment. Radiotherapy slows tumor growth and can effectively normalize biochemical parameters, but its effects are delayed, and hypopituitarism is a common adverse effect.

Cushing Disease

Pituitary adenomas of corticotroph origin secrete ACTH, which in turn causes excess adrenal production of cortisol and results in Cushing disease. Note that Cushing disease refers specifically to an ACTH-producing pituitary adenoma, whereas Cushing syndrome refers to the clinical manifestations of cortisol excess of any etiology. Clinical features of Cushing syndrome include fatigue, weight gain, hirsutism, proximal muscle weakness, hypertension, hyperglycemia, and hypokalemia, as well as loss of bone mineral density. Patients with Cushing syndrome have a characteristic physical appearance, with facial plethora, moon-shaped facies, and supraclavicular and dorsocervical fat pads, and they may have wide purple striae or ecchymoses. The etiologies of endogenous Cushing syndrome include adrenal cortisol-secreting tumors and ectopic ACTH production, for example from small cell lung cancer, in addition to ACTH-producing pituitary adenomas, which are the most common cause.

Screening for Cushing syndrome can be done by 24-hour urinary free cortisol measurement, dexamethasone suppression testing (1 mg given overnight or 2 mg given over 48 hours, followed by morning serum cortisol measurement), or late-night salivary cortisol (two independent measurements). If the result of one of these tests is abnormal, it should be confirmed by performing another test. If values are elevated on both tests, further evaluation is required to determine the etiology of the disease. ACTH levels can be used to establish if the cause of excess cortisol is ACTH-dependent, in which ACTH levels are elevated or inappropriately normal, as is seen in pituitary or ectopic ACTH production, versus ACTH-independent, in which ACTH levels are low, as seen in adrenal cortical tumors. If ACTH levels are elevated or normal, follow-up testing with high-dose (8 mg) dexamethasone suppression can be used to distinguish between a pituitary source, in which case cortisol should suppress, or an ectopic source, which will not respond to dexamethasone. If the results suggest a pituitary source, the pituitary gland should be imaged. Most clinicians favor proceeding at this point with catheterization and sampling of the inferior petrosal sinus veins to establish a central-to-peripheral gradient, as well as try to lateralize the source of ACTH hypersecretion. If sampling results are consistent with Cushing disease, transsphenoidal surgery is the treatment of choice. For a complete review of the diagnosis and management of Cushing syndrome, please see chapter 48 on adrenal gland disorders.

TSH- AND GONADOTROPIN-PRODUCING PITUITARY ADENOMAS

Pituitary tumors that secrete biologically active LH or FSH are rare. Tumors of gonadotropic origin may also secrete gonadotropin subunits or proteins without functional activity. In fact, many adenomas considered nonfunctional are actually gonadotropic in origin. The diagnosis of gonadotroph adenoma can be difficult to make because tumors that secrete gonadotropins or gonadotropin subunits usually do not result in a specific clinical syndrome. When they become sufficiently large, like all other pituitary tumors, gonadotroph adenomas can cause mass effects. Patients suspected of having gonadotropin-secreting adenomas should undergo pituitary MRI as well as testing of pituitary function. Transsphenoidal surgery is the treatment of choice.

Adenomas that secrete TSH are exceedingly rare. Clinically, these tumors present with hyperthyroidism. They are usually large at the time of diagnosis, and as a result are usually also associated with mass effects. This diagnosis should be suspected in patients with elevated serum T_4 and T_3 levels, but with an inappropriately normal or elevated TSH concentration (rather than suppressed TSH values, as would be expected in primary hyperthyroidism). The primary treatment for TSH-producing adenomas is trans sphenoidal excision. In cases of residual tumor or contraindications to surgery, somatostatin analogues are an alternative therapeutic option.

GENETIC SYNDROMES ASSOCIATED WITH PITUITARY TUMORS

Some genetic syndromes are associated with the formation of pituitary tumors or hypopituitarism. Genetic syndromes associated with pituitary defects exclusively include the familial isolated pituitary adenomas (FIPA) syndrome, and mutations in the transcription factors PROP-1 and PIT-1, which cause combined pituitary hormone deficiencies. On the other hand, multiple endocrine neoplasia type 1 (MEN-1) is characterized by tumors in multiple endocrine glands, including pituitary adenomas but also parathyroid adenomas, pancreatic and gastrointestinal neuroendocrine tumors, and, less frequently, other endocrine tumors. MEN-1 is an autosomal dominant disorder that results from a mutation in the gene that encodes menin, a tumor suppressor protein. Anterior pituitary tumors develop in approximately 65% of patients with MEN-1.

The MEN-2 syndromes (MEN-2A, MEN-2B, and familial medullary thyroid cancer) are autosomal dominant and caused by germ-line mutations in the RET proto-oncogene. In contrast to the MEN-1 syndrome, the MEN-2 syndromes do not involve the pituitary gland. The MEN-2 syndromes are all characterized by medullary thyroid cancer (MTC), which is fully penetrant in all affected individuals. MEN-2B is also associated with pheochromocytoma, mucosal and intestinal neuromas, and marfanoid habitus; MEN-2A is associated with MTC, pheochromocytoma, and parathyroid tumors.

Hypopituitarism

Hypopituitarism is characterized by decreased secretion of one or more anterior pituitary hormones, which include GH, ACTH, TSH, FSH, LH, and prolactin. Deficiencies may be partial or complete. Panhypopituitarism refers to a deficiency of all pituitary hormones.

Differential Diagnosis

A pituitary hormone deficiency may result from intrinsic pituitary disease or from a derangement in the pituitary stalk or hypothalamus that results in a deficiency in the hypothalamic hormones that stimulate pituitary function. The causes of acquired hypopituitarism are myriad (table 45.4), and the most common are described below.

Mass lesions in or near the hypothalamus or pituitary gland can cause partial or complete hypopituitarism. By far the most common such lesions are *pituitary adenomas*, which may be functioning or nonfunctioning. As has been previously reviewed, a mass lesion causes hormone insufficiencies either by mechanical compression or by impairment of blood flow to adjacent pituitary tissue or by interference with the delivery of hypothalamic regulating factors through the hypothalamic-hypophyseal portal system (figure 45.4). Excision or shrinkage of the tumor may result in restoration of pituitary function, although if pituitary tissue has been destroyed, this is unlikely, and lifelong hormone-replacement therapy will be required.

In addition to benign tumors that affect the pituitary gland, many types of cancer, most commonly breast and

Table 45.4 **CAUSES OF ACQUIRED HYPOPITUITARISM**

Pituitary causes
Mass lesions
Pituitary tumors
Metastatic tumors
Iatrogenic
Surgical destruction
Radiation
Infarction or ischemia
Pituitary apoplexy
Sheehan syndrome (postpartum)
Empty sella syndrome
Traumatic brain injury
Granulomatous disease
Sarcoidosis
Giant cell granuloma
Eosinophilic granuloma
Wegener granulomatosis
Infiltrative disorders
Hemochromatosis
Lymphocytic hypophysitis
Infections
Meningitis
Abscess
Genetic
Prop-1 and Pit-1 mutations
Idiopathic

Destruction of the pituitary stalk
Trauma
Compression by masses
Surgical damage

Hypothalamic causes
Trauma
Masses
Craniopharyngioma
Meningioma
Other tumors
Tumor metastases
Radiation
Functional
Starvation/anorexia nervosa
Stress/critical illness

lung, can metastasize to the hypothalamus or the pituitary and cause hypopituitarism. Metastases tend to occur in the posterior pituitary initially, causing diabetes insipidus.

Iatrogenic causes of pituitary deficiency may ensue after *pituitary surgery* or after *radiation therapy*. Postoperative patients should undergo biochemical evaluation to detect changes in pituitary function. Patients who undergo pituitary radiation, either for functioning adenomas after incomplete resections or for brain tumors, should be screened at regular intervals, as most will eventually develop some degree of hypopituitarism.

Pituitary apoplexy is the infarction of or hemorrhage into the pituitary gland, causing abrupt damage to the tissue. This usually occurs in the setting of an undiagnosed

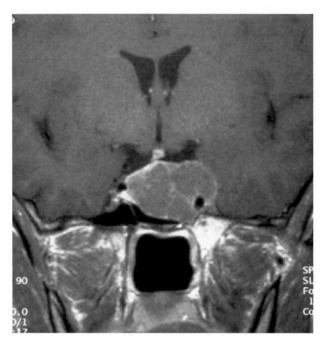

Figure 45.4. Pituitary Mass. Note compression of nearby structures.

pituitary adenoma. It presents clinically with the sudden onset of severe headache, visual field loss, and sometimes cranial nerve palsies (III, IV, or VI). Evaluation should include an MRI scan and neurological assessment with formal visual field testing. *Sheehan syndrome*, which is pituitary necrosis after postpartum hemorrhage, is characterized by hypopituitarism and inability to breast-feed and can present immediately or several years after childbirth.

Less common causes of hypopituitarism include *empty sella syndrome*, which results from either a congenital or an acquired sellar diaphragmatic defect, through which arachnoid herniates and enlarges the pituitary fossa. Most patients with a congenital empty sella have normal pituitary function; approximately 15% have mild hyperprolactinemia. *Traumatic brain injuries* can lead to hypothalamic or pituitary damage, either immediately or years afterward, and patients should be monitored for hypopituitarism.

Granulomatous diseases, including sarcoidosis, giant-cell granuloma, eosinophilic granuloma, and Wegener granulomatosis can affect the hypothalamus or pituitary and thus lead to hypopituitarism. *Lymphocytic hypophysitis*, a diffuse infiltration of the anterior pituitary, occurs predominantly in women and is often first evident during pregnancy or after delivery. In *hemochromatosis*, iron infiltrates the pituitary and results in one or more hormonal deficiencies. In addition, several types of *infections*, such as meningitis or an abscess, can involve the hypothalamus or pituitary and cause pituitary insufficiency. Certain genetic mutations, for example in PROP-1 and PIT-1, cause combined pituitary hormone deficiencies. Finally, there can be functional hypopituitarism: reversible suppression of hypothalamic function from severe stress such as starvation or critical illness.

Clinical Presentation, Diagnosis, and Management of Pituitary Hormone Deficiencies

The clinical presentation of hypopituitarism depends on the rapidity of its onset as well as on which pituitary hormones are deficient and the degree of deficiency. The clinical manifestations of the endocrine abnormalities result from dysfunction of the target organs regulated by the deficient pituitary hormones, and the symptoms are similar to those of primary target organ failure—for example, in the case of TSH deficiency, the clinical presentation is similar to that of primary hypothyroidism caused by intrinsic thyroid disease. Depending on the etiology of the hypopituitarism, patients may additionally present with symptoms of mass effects, including headaches and visual field deficits or other neurological abnormalities.

Pituitary adenomas and other tumors that affect this region are typically slow-growing, so endocrine deficiencies and mass effects tend to develop slowly. However, when symptoms are acute in onset or abruptly exacerbated, an event such as pituitary apoplexy associated with rapid expansion in size and infarction of the gland should be considered.

In general, the diagnosis of hypopituitarism cannot be made by measurement of pituitary hormone levels in serum because there are substantial overlaps between normal and deficient ranges. Instead, in most cases, serum levels of the hormones made by target organs (in response to stimulation from the pituitary) are used to assess the status of pituitary function. For example, T_4 is measured to assess adequacy of TSH production. If the concentrations of target organ hormones are equivocal, subsequent stimulation tests can be performed to determine pituitary function. The dynamic studies that are appropriate for testing each hypothalamic-pituitary-target organ axis are described below.

After the clinical and biochemical diagnosis of hypopituitarism has been established, a radiographic study is indicated to determine whether a mass, or other abnormality, is present. The most informative imaging study of the pituitary gland is a gadolinium-enhanced MRI.

Patients with panhypopituitarism on standard replacement therapies have increased prevalence of obesity as well as osteopenia and fractures. They report decreased quality of life on neuropsychiatric evaluation. In addition, for reasons that remain poorly understood, cardiovascular mortality is increased in these patients. Deficiency of each pituitary hormone has a unique presentation, diagnostic strategy, and management, and these are addressed below.

ACTH (CORTICOTROPIN) DEFICIENCY

The symptoms of ACTH deficiency include fatigue, weakness, headache, anorexia, weight loss, nausea, vomiting, and abdominal pain; hypoglycemia can also occur. If left untreated, particularly in the context of physiological stressors such as illness, secondary adrenal insufficiency can lead to vascular collapse and death. On physical examination, orthostatic hypotension may be present and should be assessed. Cortisol deficiency leads to inadequate vascular tone, increased vasopressin, and water retention and hyponatremia may ensue.

There are two important clinical distinctions between primary and secondary adrenal insufficiency. In patients with secondary adrenal insufficiency, ACTH is not elevated, and therefore hyperpigmentation is not present. In addition, in secondary adrenal insufficiency, adrenal aldosterone production is preserved, so serum potassium concentration should be normal; in primary disease, aldosterone deficiency may result in both hyponatremia and hyperkalemia.

A serum cortisol level is the best screening test for ACTH deficiency (table 45.5); because of diurnal variation, cortisol should be measured in the early morning. Measurement of ACTH is not useful for the diagnosis of secondary adrenal insufficiency. However, ACTH measurement is helpful to distinguish between etiologies of adrenal insufficiency: in primary (adrenal) disease, the ACTH level will be high, whereas in secondary (pituitary) disease, the ACTH level will be low or inappropriately normal in the context of a low serum cortisol.

In general, a morning serum cortisol value of <3 μg/dL indicates adrenal insufficiency. The level of morning serum cortisol that accurately predicts normal hypothalamic-pituitary-adrenal (HPA) function remains less clear: some studies suggest that levels above 11–14 μg/dL accurately predict normal adrenal function on dynamic testing. However, it is well accepted that patients with morning cortisol levels above 18 μg/dL can be considered to have normal HPA function and do not need further testing. Therefore, conventionally, if the morning serum cortisol concentration is between 3 and 18 μg/dL, dynamic testing of hypothalamic-pituitary-adrenal function is indicated (table 45.5). The easiest and most widely used dynamic test is the corticotropin stimulation test, which consists of measuring serum cortisol concentrations before and 30 and 60 minutes after an intravenous injection of 250 μg of corticotropin. An increase in the serum cortisol concentration to 18–20 μg/dL or more is considered a normal response. In patients with severe corticotropin deficiency the adrenal glands atrophy, and therefore, the serum cortisol response to stimulation will be diminished (abnormal). Of note, this test is not useful in the acute setting: test results will be normal before adrenal atrophy has occurred, and this can take weeks to months to develop.

Other dynamic tests are available, including the insulin tolerance test, in which insulin-induced hypoglycemia leads to an increase in corticotropin-releasing hormone (CRH), corticotropin (ACTH), and subsequently cortisol. Although this test is considered the gold standard for diagnosis of secondary adrenal insufficiency, it is rarely conducted because of the safety concerns of inducing hypoglycemia.

When the diagnosis of adrenal insufficiency is made, or when clinical suspicion is high, glucocorticoid therapy

Table 45.5 SUMMARY OF SELECTED ENDOCRINE DERANGEMENTS AND DIAGNOSTIC STRATEGIES

ENDOCRINE DERANGEMENT	SCREENING TEST	CONFIRMATORY TEST	CONFIRMATORY RESULT
Acromegaly (GH overproduction)	IGF-1	Oral glucose tolerance with measurement of GH	Elevated IGF-1 and glucose suppressed GH >1 μg/L
ACTH deficiency	Morning cortisol (μg/dL) <3: deficient >18: normal 3–18: confirmatory test	Corticotropin stimulation	Stimulated cortisol <18 μg/dL
TSH deficiency	TSH and free T$_4$		Low free T$_4$ and low or normal TSH
LH and FSH deficiency	Men: Testosterone	LH and FSH	Low testosterone, low or normal LH and FSH
	Women: Premenopausal: menstrual history		
	Postmenopausal:	LH and FSH	Low or premenopausal range LH and FSH
GH deficiency	IGF-1	Growth hormone-releasing hormone and arginine stimulation test	Failure to stimulate GH
Diabetes insipidus		Water deprivation test	Urine osmolality <600 when plasma osmolality >300 mosm/kg H$_2$O

NOTE: ACTH, corticotrophin; FSH, follicle-stimulating hormone; IGF-1, insulin-like growth Factor-1; GH, growth hormone; LH, luteinizing hormone; TSH, thyroid-stimulating hormone; T$_4$, thyroxine.

should be initiated immediately. Patients can be treated with hydrocortisone, 20–30 mg daily, administered in divided doses in the morning and afternoon. Overtreatment should be avoided to decrease risks of iatrogenic hypercortisolism, such as bone loss. Patients should be instructed to double or triple their steroid doses for periods of stress such as febrile illnesses. Mineralocorticoid replacement is not necessary in patients with secondary adrenal insufficiency, as aldosterone production is intact. All patients with adrenal insufficiency should wear medical alert bracelets.

TSH (THYROTROPIN) DEFICIENCY

Symptoms and signs of TSH deficiency are similar to those of primary hypothyroidism, and include fatigue, weight gain, constipation, cold intolerance, bradycardia, periorbital puffiness, and delayed relaxation of tendon reflexes. Laboratory findings may include mild hyponatremia and anemia.

In order to make a diagnosis of TSH deficiency, serum TSH and free thyroxine (T_4) concentrations should be measured simultaneously (table 45.5). Patients with secondary hypothyroidism most commonly have low free T_4, with normal or low serum TSH concentrations, and therefore, TSH should never be used alone as a screening test for central hypothyroidism. A normal or low TSH value is inappropriate in the context of a low serum thyroxine concentration, and indicates TSH insufficiency. Occasionally, patients with central hypothyroidism may have an elevated serum TSH due to the formation of an abnormal TSH molecule that has reduced biological activity but is recognized by the immunoassay.

The treatment for secondary hypothyroidism is thyroid hormone replacement with levothyroxine. In patients with multiple pituitary hormone deficiencies, it is important to treat adrenal insufficiency before starting thyroid hormone replacement. This is because levothyroxine will increase the metabolism of cortisol, and an adrenal crisis can be precipitated. Laboratory studies should be repeated 4–6 weeks after initiation of therapy to evaluate appropriateness of dose. In patients with secondary hypothyroidism, free T_4 (not TSH) should be used to monitor treatment, and the goal of therapy is a free T_4 concentration in the normal range.

LH AND FSH (GONADOTROPIN) DEFICIENCY

In general, LH and FSH deficiencies result in decreased production of gonadal steroids and present differently in men and in women. Gonadotropin deficiency before puberty results in failure to progress through sexual maturation. In adult premenopausal women, estrogen deficiency manifests as infertility, anovulatory cycles, and oligomenorrhea or amenorrhea. Other symptoms include hot flashes, decreased libido, and vaginal dryness. Because estrogen levels are low at baseline in postmenopausal women, if they develop hypopituitarism they usually present with symptoms of other hormonal deficiencies or of mass effects. Men with hypogonadism experience decreased libido and erectile dysfunction. Long-standing testosterone deficiency results in sparse facial and body hair and testicular atrophy. Both men and women can develop bone loss from chronic gonadal steroid deficiency.

Gonadotropin deficiency can occur secondary to all of the causes of hypopituitarism listed in table 45.4, and in addition, there are various syndromes of isolated gonadotropin deficiency. A congenital condition known as idiopathic hypogonadotrophic hypogonadism (IHH) presents with failure to undergo puberty and persistently low gonadotropin levels. Kallmann syndrome is characterized by IHH plus anosmia. An acquired form of IHH has been described in men who develop hypogonadism in adulthood without any identifiable cause. Physiological stress can also cause acquired derangements in the hypothalamic-pituitary-gonadal axis. Women who suffer from anorexia nervosa or who exercise excessively can develop what has been termed hypothalamic amenorrhea: abnormal secretion of GnRH and gonadotropins resulting in menstrual dysfunction and other complications such as bone loss.

Appropriate evaluation for gonadotropin deficiency depends on age and gender. In women, serum LH, FSH, and estradiol concentrations may be low or normal. In premenopausal women, the best assessment of gonadotropin status is the menstrual history; regular menses indicate at least some gonadotroph function, and measurement of gonadotropins or estradiol provides little additional information. In contrast, in postmenopausal women, measurement of LH and FSH concentrations is useful (table 45.5). In these patients, gonadotropin levels are normally high, so low or normal levels are inappropriate and confirm gonadotropin deficiency and anterior pituitary dysfunction. In men, central hypogonadism results in low serum testosterone and low or normal LH and FSH levels; in the setting of low testosterone, even normal values of gonadotropins are inappropriate and indicate deficiency. A serum testosterone concentration should always be measured as part of the diagnostic workup (table 45.5). Measurement of gonadotropins is helpful only if the etiology is uncertain, to distinguish between primary (testicular disease, high LH and FSH) and secondary hypogonadism (hypothalamic or pituitary disease, low or normal LH and FSH).

Treatment for hypogonadism consists of gonadal steroid replacement unless fertility is desired. In women of reproductive age, estrogen and progesterone therapy is recommended to restore the normal hormonal milieu and prevent bone loss. If fertility is desired, it can be achieved with exogenous gonadotropin therapy. For men with hypogonadism, testosterone replacement can be provided by intramuscular injection or in patches and gels. Serum testosterone levels should be monitored during treatment, and supraphysiological doses should be avoided because of risks of prostate stimulation and elevated hematocrit.

GROWTH HORMONE (SOMATOTROPIN) DEFICIENCY

Symptoms and signs attributed to GH deficiency in adults include a diminished sense of well-being, decreased muscle strength and exercise tolerance, and changes in body composition including decreased lean body mass, increased central adiposity, and decreased bone density. GH deficiency also leads to increased total and low-density lipoprotein (LDL) cholesterol and increased risk of cardiovascular disease. In children, prior to epiphyseal plate closing, GH deficiency results in short stature.

For the diagnosis of GH deficiency, a single random measurement is not useful because even under physiological conditions GH is secreted in pulses and remains low during most of the day. A low serum IGF-1 level is suggestive of GH deficiency, but normal levels do not exclude it. Therefore, to formally establish the diagnosis, provocative testing is required, and multiple options exist. One widely used option is the growth hormone-releasing hormone and arginine test, in which these stimulants of GH secretion are infused, and GH is subsequently measured (table 45.5). Another option is the insulin tolerance test, in which insulin-induced hypoglycemia is the stimulus for GH secretion, though because of the risks associated with inducing hypoglycemia, this test is used less frequently. Arginine alone and glucagon are other stimulants of GH secretion used for diagnostic testing. A diminished response to these stimuli is considered diagnostic of GH deficiency.

Treatment for GH deficiency is available with injectable recombinant human GH. Therapy is indicated in GH-deficient children and should be given before epiphyses are closed, to promote growth. In GH-deficient adults, there is evidence that GH therapy increases lean body mass and bone density, improves certain cardiac indices and LDL cholesterol, and improves quality of life.

PROLACTIN DEFICIENCY

The serum prolactin concentration is rarely low in hypopituitarism. If prolactin deficiency exists, it manifests as an inability to lactate and typically reflects complete or near complete destruction of the anterior pituitary. As previously described, prolactin may in fact be elevated in patients with hypothalamic-pituitary disease of any cause if there is interference with the transport of dopamine to the pituitary. Serum prolactin should always be measured as part of the evaluation of hypopituitarism because it may provide valuable information about the cause of hypogonadism and the location of a mass.

POSTERIOR PITUITARY DEFICIENCY

Deficiency AVP, which is secreted from the posterior pituitary, is known as central diabetes insipidus (DI); it can be partial or complete.

Etiology

In 30–50% of cases, DI is idiopathic and may be autoimmune in nature. Trauma, commonly pituitary surgery, as well as tumors, tumor metastases, and infiltrative disorders of the hypothalamus or pituitary can all cause central DI. The differential diagnosis of DI includes nephrogenic DI, which is due to resistance to the effects of AVP at the level of the kidneys, primary polydipsia, or osmoreceptor dysfunction.

Clinical Presentation

DI presents with polyuria, which is defined as urine output ≥50 mL/kg per 24 hours, usually including nocturia, as well as polydipsia. If there are alterations in serum sodium concentration and serum osmolality, patients may also have neurological symptoms such as confusion and lethargy.

Diagnosis

Evaluation of a patient with polyuria and polydipsia should include serum osmolality, sodium, potassium, glucose, calcium, blood urea nitrogen (BUN) and creatinine, and urinalysis, including measurement of urine osmolality and glucose. The diagnosis is unlikely if the urine osmolality is >600 mosm/kg H_2O, and a serum osmolality >300 mosm/kg H_2O with a urine osmolality <300 mosm/kg H_2O, is suggestive of the diagnosis. But the diagnosis is best confirmed by a water deprivation test (table 45.5). This consists of depriving the patient of oral intake while monitoring his or her weight, vital signs, serum sodium, osmolality, and serum AVP as well as urine sodium, osmolality, and volume on an hourly basis. If at any time during the test the urine osmolality exceeds 600 mosm/kg H_2O, this indicates normal ability to concentrate urine, and the patient does not have DI. If the serum osmolality rises above 300 mosm/kg H_2O and the urine osmolality remains below 600 mosm/kg H_2O, the test is diagnostic of DI. If a diagnosis of DI is made, DDAVP is given to differentiate between central and nephrogenic DI (in the latter there will be little response to DDAVP).

Management

Water is the mainstay of therapy for DI. Thirst is an excellent defense mechanism against hypertonicity, and if free water losses can be adequately replaced, patients with DI will not develop hypernatremia. DDAVP, a synthetic vasopressin receptor agonist, is also available for symptomatic management. Because of significant variations in the duration of action of the drug, it is recommended that dose and dosing intervals be individualized; patients are advised to wait for symptoms of polyuria and polydipsia to restart before administering the next dose of medication. Typically the drug is taken once or twice daily, and can be taken intranasally or orally.

ADDITIONAL READING

Arafah BM. Medical management of hypopituitarism in patients with pituitary adenomas. *Pituitary.* 2002;5:109–17.

Chamarthi B, Morris CA, Kaiser UB, Katz JT, Loscalzo J. Clinical problem-solving. Stalking the diagnosis. *N Engl J Med.* 2010; 362(9):834–9.

Grossman AB. Clinical review: The diagnosis and management of central hypoadrenalism. *J Clin Endocrinol Metab.* 2010;95:4855–63.

Ho KK; GH Deficiency Consensus Workshop Participants. Consensus guidelines for the diagnosis and treatment of adults with GH deficiency II: A statement of the GH Research Society in association with the European Society for Pediatric Endocrinology, Lawson Wilkins Society, European Society of Endocrinology, Japan Endocrine Society, and Endocrine Society of Australia. *Eur J Endocrinol.* 2007;157:695–700.

Klibanski A. Clinical practice. Prolactinomas. *N Engl J Med.* 2010; 362:1219–26.

Kreutzer J, Vance ML, Lopes MB, Laws ER Jr. Surgical management of GH-secreting pituitary adenomas: An outcome study using modern remission criteria. *J Clin Endocrinol Metab.* 2001;86:4072–7.

Melmed S. Medical progress: Acromegaly. *N Engl J Med* 2006;355: 2558–73.

Melmed S, Colao A, Barkan A, et al.; Acromegaly Consensus Group. Guidelines for acromegaly management: An update. *J Clin Endocrinol Metab.* 2009;94:1509–17.

Nieman LK, Biller BM, Findling JW, et al. The diagnosis of Cushing's syndrome: An Endocrine Society Clinical Practice Guideline. *J Clin Endocrinol Metab.* 2008;93:1526–40.

Schlechte JA. Long-term management of prolactinomas. *J Clin Endocrinol Metab.* 2007;92:2861–5.

Vance ML. Hypopituitarism. *N Engl J Med.* 1994;330:1651–62.

QUESTIONS

QUESTION 1. A 35-year-old woman presents for initial evaluation and complains of amenorrhea. Previously, her menstrual periods had been regular until about 2 years ago, when they became less frequent, and they stopped altogether 1 year ago. She also mentions that she occasionally has milky discharge from her breasts, although she is nulliparous. She is taking no medications. A prolactin level is found to be 55 ng/mL on two separate occasions. All other blood tests are normal.

What should be the next step in her evaluation?

A. She should be started on cabergoline, a dopamine agonist.

B. She should be started on cabergoline, a dopamine antagonist.

C. A gadolinium-enhanced pituitary MRI should be obtained.

D. She should be started on oral contraceptive pills.

QUESTION 2. A 27-year-old woman presents with fatigue, constipation, and weight gain. Her menstrual periods have been irregular over the last year but previously had been normal. On physical examination, her thyroid is mildly enlarged. She has mild expressible galactorrhea. Her deep tendon reflexes exhibit delayed relaxation phase. She is taking no medications. Laboratory studies reveal a prolactin level of 35 ng/mL and a TSH level of 24 mIU/L.

What should be the next step in the management of this patient?

A. She should be started on bromocriptine for treatment of hyperprolactinemia.

B. A gadolinium-enhanced pituitary MRI should be obtained.

C. She should be started on levothyroxine for treatment of hypothyroidism.

D. She should be referred to a neurologist for full neurological evaluation.

QUESTION 3. A 60-year-old woman with a long-term history of smoking presents for evaluation of an unsteady gait. She describes loss of balance and frequent falls at home. On review of systems, she has a chronic cough, which has been worsening, and has lost 15 lb. Furthermore, she has been feeling extremely thirsty for many weeks and gets up several times per night to drink and urinate, which is when many of her falls occur. Laboratory studies show a serum sodium of 142 meq/L. A chest x-ray shows a mass in the right hilum, and a head CT scan shows several masses in her brain. The patient is referred to oncology. Diabetes insipidus is suspected. All of the following results could be consistent with that diagnosis EXCEPT:

A. A plasma osmolality of 290 mosm/kg H_2O and a urine osmolality of 700 mosm/kg H_2O

B. A plasma osmolality of 305 mosm/kg H_2O and a urine osmolality of 200 mosm/kg H_2O

C. A urine specific gravity of 1.005

D. A serum sodium of 146 mEq/L and a urine osmolality of 180 mosm/kg H_2O

QUESTION 4. A 37-year-old construction worker falls from a roof and sustains a basilar skull fracture. One year later, he is found to have testosterone deficiency, adrenal insufficiency, and hypothyroidism. Replacement therapy with testosterone injection, hydrocortisone, and levothyroxine is initiated. A few months later, he returns for evaluation to a new primary care physician and complains of profound fatigue, constipation, and weight gain. His doctor suspects inadequate thyroid hormone replacement and checks a TSH level, which is 1.0 mIU/L.

What is the best next step in this man's management?

A. Reassure the patient that his symptoms will take some time to resolve.
B. Decrease his hydrocortisone dose to help him lose weight.
C. Check a morning cortisol level.
D. Check a serum free T$_4$ level.

QUESTION 5. A 44-year-old woman presents to the emergency room with a severe headache, which has been present constantly for 2 days and is not alleviated by analgesics at home. She has had dizziness and nausea but no vomiting. She takes oral contraceptive pills. Her blood pressure is 80/60 mm Hg, and heart rate is 95. A contrast-enhanced MRI is ordered and reveals a 3-cm sellar mass with suprasellar extension and a large area of hemorrhage within the mass. Laboratory testing and a neurosurgical consult are ordered. Of the following physical exam findings, which is the *least* likely to be present?

A. Bitemporal hemianopsia
B. Diplopia
C. Tall stature
D. Galactorrhea

ANSWERS

1. C
2. C
3. A
4. D
5. C

46.

THYROID DISEASE

Erik K. Alexander

The thyroid is an organ preserved throughout vertebrate evolution. Its primary function is to assist with the regulation of whole-body metabolism through the production and release of thyroid hormone. The thyroid gland releases two forms of thyroid hormone: thyroxine (T_4) and triiodothyronine (T_3). All T_4 in the human body is made within the thyroid gland, whereas 80% of T_3 is derived in the peripheral tissues. T_3 affects the physiological function of almost all bodily tissues through binding with a specific nuclear receptor and thereby regulates the transcription of thyroid-dependent genes. The peripheral conversion of T_4 to T_3 is decreased by various medications, including propranolol, glucocorticoids, propylthiouracil, and amiodarone, and is down-regulated during the course of acute illness such as sepsis or surgery.

The synthesis and release of thyroid hormone are controlled by the pituitary-derived thyroid-stimulating hormone (TSH) under the influence of thyrotropin-releasing hormone from the hypothalamus. TSH stimulates basic thyrocyte functions such as iodine uptake and organification and the synthesis and release of thyroid hormone. Both T_3 and T_4 are bound to protein in the circulation, which serves the dual purpose of preventing excessive tissue uptake and maintaining a readily accessible reserve of hormone. Several common medications (e.g., estrogen) affect levels of thyroxine-binding globulin without generally affecting the free thyroid hormone levels. Free thyroxine measurements (or estimates) are therefore most reflective of the active hormone in the serum.

Although the thyroid is a relatively small organ in the body, thyroid illnesses such as hyperthyroidism and hypothyroidism can cause profound systemic effects given the endocrine properties of thyroid hormone. Hyperthyroidism can be either transient or permanent depending on the etiology, although its incidence in adults appears independent of patient age. In contrast, the epidemiology of hypothyroidism is notable for an increasing incidence with greater patient age. Nearly all thyroid illnesses (with only a few exceptions) show a substantial female predominance,

although the underlying mechanism for this is unclear. Separate from thyroid hormonal illnesses such as hyperthyroidism and hypothyroidism, thyroid nodular disease is also very common and often unrelated to gland function. Although most thyroid nodules are benign and inconsequential, some prove cancerous and can be dangerous to a patient's overall health. Thyroid cancer remains one of the few malignancies increasing in incidence over the last two decades, even though disease-related mortality remains very low and unchanged.

Below a broader discussion ensues regarding screening for thyroid disease, followed by a more in-depth discussion of the evaluation, treatment, and follow-up options for hyperthyroidism, hypothyroidism, and thyroid nodular disease and cancer.

SCREENING FOR THYROID DISEASE

Screening for hypothyroidism and hyperthyroidism is not recommended for the general population, but it is considered for certain higher-risk populations. It is reasonable to screen women aged >50 years using a sensitive TSH test given the increased prevalence of hypothyroidism in this population. Screening other high-risk populations is also appropriate (see table 46.1). In particular, measuring TSH is appropriate in the following patients: those patients with evidence of Hashimoto disease or Graves disease in a first-degree relative; patients with other autoimmune diseases such as type 1 diabetes; those with a history of any prior thyroid dysfunction, even if self-limited; patients living in an iodine-deficient region of the world; patients anticipating a pregnancy or currently pregnant; and patients with conditions that may be explained or aggravated by hyperthyroidism such as cardiac arrhythmias, weight loss, osteoporosis, and anxiety.

Of particular note is the population of young women with hypothyroidism receiving adequate levothyroxine replacement therapy who desire to be (or are currently)

Table 46.1 SCREENING FOR THYROID DYSFUNCTION

- Examination of the thyroid is encouraged as part of an annual evaluation. Enlargement, asymmetry, or the presence of a nodule should prompt further investigation.

- Population-wide screening for abnormal thyroid function (TSH) is *NOT* recommended.

- However, screening selective populations *IS* recommended given high rates of thyroid illness as well as greater potential for harmful effects. These populations include:

  - Women aged >50 years.

  - Patients whose first-degree relatives are diagnosed with Hashimoto disease or Graves disease.

  - Patients with autoimmune illnesses such as type 1 diabetes mellitus or multiple sclerosis.

  - Patients with a history of prior thyroid dysfunction or currently living in an iodine-deficient part of the world.

  - Women anticipating a pregnancy or currently pregnant.

  - Patients in whom thyroid illness may substantially aggravate or explain concurrent illness (such as atrial fibrillation, unexplained osteoporosis).

pregnant. During pregnancy the daily thyroid hormone requirement increases by approximately 30–40% above baseline beginning very early in gestation. In patients with hypothyroidism, the dose of levothyroxine must be increased. Failure to do so results in maternal (and possibly fetal) hypothyroidism, which can be associated with substantial morbidity to both the mother and the fetus. For this reason prepregnancy or pregnancy screening of women for hypothyroidism is important. Patients on thyroid replacement should be counseled to contact their physician as soon as pregnancy is confirmed so that levothyroxine dose adjustment can be made early to maintain a euthyroid state throughout gestation. Finally, an annual evaluation of serum TSH is recommended in patients receiving levothyroxine therapy, as studies have demonstrated that up to 30% of such patients may be unintentionally under- or overreplaced.

Screening for thyroid nodules and thyroid cancer is not recommended. However, as most thyroid nodules are asymptomatic and unlikely to be noted by patients until very large, routine examination of the anterior neck is recommended during annual patient physicals. The neck should be palpated just below the cricoid cartilage. The patient should be asked to swallow, which raises the thyroid and improves the sensitivity of examination. In general, the left lobe, the right lobe, and isthmus should all be examined separately for symmetry, overall size, and the presence of nodules via this mechanism.

HYPERTHYROIDISM

The diagnosis of hyperthyroidism should be considered in patients with signs or symptoms of thyrotoxicosis (table 46.2) or in those with diseases known to be caused or aggravated by thyrotoxicosis (such as atrial fibrillation). In hyperthyroidism, the TSH is low or undetectable, and the free T_4 concentration is elevated. If the TSH is suppressed

and the free T_4 is normal, measure the serum T_3 concentration. T_3 thyrotoxicosis (suppressed TSH, normal T_4, elevated T_3) is seen with increased frequency in patients with toxic multinodular goiter and autonomously functioning thyroid nodules. Physicians should look for "apathetic thyrotoxicosis" in elderly patients characterized by a lower frequency of goiter (found in 50%), fewer hyperadrenergic symptoms, and a predominance of cardiac findings including heart failure and atrial fibrillation. Patients with a low or undetectable TSH and a normal free T_4 have subclinical hyperthyroidism. Typically, the TSH is only mildly suppressed in this situation, with a value between 0.1 and 0.5 mIU/L. This distinction is important, however, because subclinical hyperthyroidism can be followed with periodic thyroid function tests in otherwise healthy patients <60 years old.

Most thyrotoxicosis is due to Graves disease or thyroiditis. Rarely, a toxic ("hot") adenoma, toxic multinodular goiter, factitious hyperthyroidism due to thyroid hormone consumption, or a struma ovarii may be causative. Pregnant women are often found to have mild to moderately suppressed TSH values during the first trimester, in relation to physiological stimulation of the thyroid gland from the hormone human chorionic gonadotropin (hCG). This is self-limited and not pathologic. Occasionally, however, differentiation between physiological TSH suppression during pregnancy (due to hCG stimulation) and true hyperthyroidism can be difficult. In such cases, endocrine consultation should be obtained. An important albeit rare etiology of hyperthyroidism is amiodarone administration. Thyrotoxicosis in this setting can be caused by multiple mechanisms, and endocrine consultation is required.

In almost all cases, a radioactive iodine uptake (RAIU) is the optimal test to differentiate between thyrotoxicosis from excess thyroid hormone *production* (Graves disease or a toxic adenoma) and increased hormone *release* from a damaged thyroid (thyroiditis). An elevated RAIU is consistent with excess thyroid hormone production (figure 46.1),

Table 46.2 COMMON SIGNS AND SYMPTOMS OF HYPERTHYROIDISM AND HYPOTHYROIDISM

HYPERTHYROIDISM	HYPOTHYROIDISM
Common symptoms • nervousness or emotional lability • insomnia • increased sweating • heat intolerance • palpitations • fatigue • weight loss • hyperdefecation • menstrual irregularity	Common symptoms • fatigue and excessive sleep • weight gain • alopecia • cold intolerance • sluggish affect or depression • bradycardia and fluid retention • delayed deep tendon reflexes • poor concentration • constipation
Common signs • tremors • tachycardia or evidence of atrial fibrillation • proptosis of the eyes or extraocular muscle palsy • stare, lid lag, or signs of Graves orbitopathy • goiter • pretibial myxedema	Common signs • dry, course skin and hair • periorbital puffiness • bradycardia • slow movements and speech • hoarseness • goiter • dementia or confusion

whereas a suppressed RAIU (usually <5%) is consistent with hormone release from an inflamed thyroid gland. An RAIU should not be performed if a patient is suspected or confirmed to be pregnant. Patients with acute nonthyroidal illness may have TSH suppression that is part of the *euthyroid sick syndrome* and not due to underlying thyrotoxicosis. The free T_4 is most often normal or low. Additional testing over a period of days or weeks is sometimes required to conclusively make the diagnosis of euthyroid sick syndrome.

Thyroid storm is defined as a life-threatening condition manifested by an exaggeration of the clinical signs and symptoms of thyrotoxicosis accompanied by systemic decompensation. It is usually caused by rapid release of thyroid hormone (e.g., large iodine load, withdrawal of antithyroid drugs, or treatment with radioactive iodine) in the setting of other illness such as surgery, infection, or trauma. Most often the diagnosis of thyroid storm is made when hyperthyroidism also causes coexistent cardiovascular, neurological, or gastroenterologic compromise. Early recognition, prompt hospitalization, and consultation with endocrinology are the keys to a successful outcome. Thyroid storm is a clinical diagnosis, and there is no concentration of thyroid hormone elevation diagnostic of the illness.

The risks of hyperthyroidism are primarily related to cardiac function and arrhythmias, bone loss and osteoporosis, and a hypermetabolic state. Graves' ophthalmopathy (soft tissue inflammation, proptosis, extraocular muscle dysfunction, and optic neuropathy) is present in 10–25% of affected patients, although subclinical enlargement of extraocular muscles may be present in up to 50–70% of patients without overt eye disease. Pretibial myxedema (infiltrative dermopathy characterized by nonpitting scaly thickening and induration of the skin) is a rare complication of Graves disease. Once it has been treated effec-

(A)   (B)

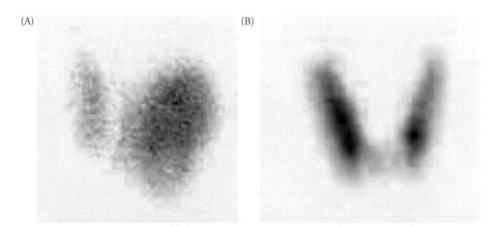

Figure 46.1. Radioactive Iodine Uptake Scans. Both images are of hyperthyroid patients with suppressed TSH concentrations. (A) Left toxic adenoma: a large left-sided toxic "hot" adenoma, with relative suppression of right-sided activity. (B) Graves disease: bilateral diffuse uptake consistent with Graves disease.

tively, the overall risk associated with hyperthyroidism can be substantially diminished. Early in the treatment of thyrotoxicosis, iodine avoidance (such as the contrast agent used in computed tomography (CT) scans) and exercise restriction are recommended.

If thyroiditis is suspected, a conservative follow-up and repeated measurements of thyroid function (monthly) are indicated over a 3- to 4-month period. Thyrotoxicosis due to thyroiditis is managed conservatively because it is often self-limited. Beta blockers can be used to treat sympathomimetic symptoms such as tachycardia, tremor, and anxiety. Nonsteroidal anti-inflammatory drugs and, rarely, glucocorticoids, can also be administered to reduce inflammation and discomfort. For patients with Graves disease and autonomously functioning thyroid nodules, antithyroid drugs or radioiodine should be considered (table 46.3), although patient preference, patient age, comorbidity, severity of thyrotoxicosis, and the presence of Graves' ophthalmopathy must be taken into account. Antithyroid drugs are used for primary therapy of thyrotoxicosis, to attain a euthyroid state in preparation for thyroidectomy, and for use in conjunction with radioiodine therapy in selected patients. Antithyroid drugs are also preferred to radioactive iodine in the presence of severe Graves' ophthalmopathy and thyroid storm. Most patients in the United States, however, ultimately select radioiodine (^{131}I) as therapy for thyrotoxicosis caused by Graves disease, toxic multinodular goiter, or autonomously functioning thyroid nodules. Radioiodine is also indicated in patients failing to achieve a remission after a course of antithyroid drugs. When administered, radioactive iodine is likely to cause permanent thyroid destruction requiring life-long levothyroxine therapy.

When antithyroid drugs are prescribed, methimazole is effective for most patients and usually initiated at an oral dose of 10 mg twice daily. Alternatively, propylthiouracil may be preferred in pregnant patients and in those with an allergy to methimazole, although recent data suggest propylthiouracil is associated with a higher side-effect profile.

Table 46.3 INITIAL TREATMENT REGIMENS FOR HYPERTHYROIDISM

Etiology: Unregulated Production of Excessive Thyroid Hormone

Possible diagnosis:

   Graves disease
   Functional ("hot") nodule or toxic adenoma
   Pregnancy (late first trimester)

Biochemical and laboratory findings:

   Suppressed thyroid-stimulating hormone (TSH)
   Elevated T_4 (or T_3)
   Detectable (or elevated) iodine uptake on thyroid scintigraphy (Note: radionuclide imaging is contraindicated in any pregnant individual)

Treatment:

If pregnant, involve endocrine and high-risk obstetrical services
All other cases, consider:

   (a) Methimazole (starting dose: 20 mg daily; 5–60 mg daily titrated to normalization of free T_4 concentration) *or*
       Propylthiouracil (starting dose: 50–150 mg tid; 100–900 mg total daily dose titrated to normalization of free T_4 concentration)
   (b) Beta blocker (titrated to avoid hypotension, yet reduce heart rate modestly)
   (c) SSKI: Inorganic iodine (rarely needed, only in severe cases), starting dose: 3 drops in 8 oz liquid bid × 7 days)

Etiology: Release of Preformed (Stored) Thyroid Hormone

Possible diagnosis:

   Silent thyroiditis
   Postpartum thyroiditis
   Painful (DeQuervain) thyroiditis

Biochemical and laboratory findings:

   Suppressed TSH
   Elevated T_4 (or T_3)
   Undetectable (or absent) iodine uptake on thyroid scintigraphy

Treatment:

Conservative therapy usually indicated unless patient severely symptomatic
As needed, consider:

   (a) Beta blocker (titrated to avoid hypotension, yet reduce heart rate modestly)
   (b) Glucocorticoid (rarely needed for severe pain and thyroid inflammation; starting dose prednisone 20 mg twice daily × 7 days)

When administered, propylthiouracil is frequently initiated at a dose of 50–150 mg three times daily, depending on the severity of the illness. With either drug, patients should be counseled for the risk of hepatitis and agranulocytosis, both rare but potentially severe side effects. Propylthiouracil has also been associated with vasculitis and concomitant renal dysfunction. If immediate control of severe thyrotoxicosis is required, inorganic iodine (saturated solution of potassium iodine [SSKI]) can be administered orally and is highly effective. This therapy, however, is self-limited in duration (usually ~3 weeks) and precludes further use of radioactive iodine for months thereafter. Thyroidectomy is rarely considered but is a reasonable choice in thyrotoxic patients with concomitant suspicious (malignant) nodules and also in patients who either cannot tolerate or who refuse radioactive iodine or antithyroid drugs described above.

Managing Graves' hyperthyroidism during pregnancy is highly complex given the differential effects of antithyroid drugs on the fetus in comparison to the mother. In general the developing fetus is much more sensitive to both methimazole and propylthiouracil. Therefore, a biochemical euthyroid state in the mother does not predict safety and normal development for the fetus. As a rule, endocrine consultation should be sought in these situations and the lowest dose of antithyroid medication administered whenever possible.

Graves' ophthalmopathy is often treated conservatively in patients with mild to moderate disease. In more severe cases, an intravenous or oral steroid course may be considered, although it should be administered by physicians with expertise and experience with this illness. Rarely, surgical decompression of the orbit is required to preserve vision.

HYPOTHYROIDISM

Hypothyroidism has a wide range of clinical symptoms and signs (table 46.2). The serum TSH is elevated ($>10\,\mu U/mL$) in primary hypothyroidism (thyroid gland failure) and is low or normal in conjunction with a low free T_4 in rare cases of hypothyroidism due to pituitary or hypothalamic disease (secondary hypothyroidism). Patients with a mildly elevated TSH (5–$10\,\mu U/mL$) and a normal free T_4 have subclinical hypothyroidism. This distinction is important because patients with subclinical hypothyroidism may not require treatment if asymptomatic and not desiring pregnancy (or not currently pregnant).

The most common causes of hypothyroidism are chronic lymphocytic thyroiditis (Hashimoto disease), previous thyroidectomy, or a history of radioactive iodine (^{131}I) administration. Hashimoto disease is an autoimmune disease that may present at any age but increases in prevalence as patients are older. Onset is usually insidious and is usually associated with a goiter. The presence of elevated concentrations of thyroid peroxidase antibody (TPO antibody) in the serum is highly correlated with the presence of Hashimoto

disease and can be useful in confirming the disease or assessing the risk of developing hypothyroidism in the future. Subacute and painful thyroiditis are other illnesses that can lead to hypothyroidism, although nearly all patients follow a triphasic thyroid hormone response once activated—mild hyperthyroidism initially, followed by mild hypothyroidism, and then followed by normalization of TSH values. This triphasic pattern occurs over a 2- to 4-month duration. If the final phase of TSH normalization is impaired, hypothyroidism will persist. This occurs most often in patients with TPO antibody positivity.

Levothyroxine (L-T_4) is the preferred treatment of hypothyroidism, and it safely, effectively, and reliably relieves symptoms and normalizes lab tests in hypothyroid patients. Levothyroxine is converted to T_3 (the active hormone) primarily in peripheral tissues at an appropriate rate for overall metabolic needs. Treatment with a combination of T_4 and T_3 is not recommended. Although all patients with overt hypothyroidism (TSH $>10\,\mu U/mL$) should be treated, there is limited evidence that treatment of subclinical hypothyroidism is beneficial in nonpregnant, asymptomatic patients. At present most patients with subclinical hypothyroidism can be safely monitored with TSH measurements every 4–6 months, evaluating for progression of disease. This recommendation excludes women seeking pregnancy or currently pregnant, who should be treated once TSH is outside the normal range because of greater maternal and fetal risk.

During initial management, the degree of hypothyroidism should be assessed in affected individuals. Biochemical and clinical parameters often correlate, although at times they may be discordant. For patients with severe hypothyroidism (TSH $>100\,\mu U/mL$), several important facts in their care must be considered when thyroid hormone replacement is instituted. Importantly, morbidity and mortality in such patients are most often related to simultaneous (though often silent) infection, hypoventilation, or medication overdose. For these reasons sedatives and narcotics should be avoided, or their doses significantly reduced, given reduced drug clearance caused by hypothyroidism. For patients with mild to moderate hypothyroidism, these considerations usually do not apply.

A full replacement dose of levothyroxine can be approximated by multiplying 1.7 μg/day × patient weight (kg). The severity of hypothyroidism should determine the urgency for replacement therapy. When possible, however, a modest dose of levothyroxine (50–75 μg daily) is preferred during the first week of therapy in those patients who are not in acute danger. An acute rise in thyroid hormone concentration can rarely induce increased cardiac demand and potential ischemia. For this reason caution should be exercised in those with known coronary artery disease or in patients over 80 years of age. Mild to moderate hypothyroidism can often be treated with 50–100 μg of levothyroxine daily. Once initiated, levothyroxine treatment is usually lifelong, and the goal TSH concentration is within the normal range. Long term, most patients can be safely monitored with TSH measurements every 6–12 months, evaluating for progression of disease.

Myxedema coma is a rare and extreme form of hypothyroidism manifested by features such as delayed reflexes, sparse hair, dry skin, and puffy or edematous facies. It is considered severe, life-threatening hypothyroidism. Frequently, hypothermia (core temperature <95°F) as well as impaired cardiovascular, neurological, and gastroenterologic functions are documented. Similar to thyroid storm, myxedema coma is a clinical diagnosis, and no specific thyroid hormone level defines this illness. Treatment is with thyroid hormone administration. Because this condition is life-threatening, however, both T_3 and T_4 preparations are often used initially following consultation with an endocrinologist. Intravenous preparations are often preferred, given hypothyroidism-associated bowel edema that can impair the absorption and action of oral hormone. Severely myxedematous patients should be considered for prophylactic antibiotic medication. Additionally, the possibility of adrenal insufficiency should be considered. In severe cases concomitant treatment of thyroid hormone and glucocorticoids may be considered.

THYROID NODULES

Thyroid nodules are common, occurring more frequently in women and with increasing age. Most nodules are asymptomatic and come to clinical attention following a routine physical examination or imaging procedure performed for another indication. Differentiating patients with malignant nodules from those with benign nodules is the most important consideration. A secondary consideration for evaluation is nodule size, as some large nodules (usually larger than 4 cm in diameter) can cause tracheal deviation or compressive symptoms prompting further intervention. However, most clinically relevant nodules measure between 1 and 3 cm in diameter, are nonmalignant, and cause no adverse symptoms. Such nodules are almost always followed conservatively without further intervention or surgery.

Approximately 10–15% of thyroid nodules >1 cm are cancerous, and this forms the rationale for investigating patients with nodular disease. Ironically, thyroid cancers smaller than 1 cm in diameter (often termed "microcarcinomas") are almost always indolent and pose little or no risk to the patient. Epidemiological evidence suggests that the properties of well-differentiated thyroid carcinomas appear to change once growth exceeds 1 cm in diameter, and tumors increasingly gain potential to spread, invade, and ultimately metastasize. There are few exceptions to this dogma, most of which are primary well-differentiated thyroid cancers measuring 8–9 mm in size. Given these findings, combined with known interobserver variability associated with both ultrasound and histopathologic measurement of tumors, consensus expert opinion has recommended that only thyroid nodules larger than 1 cm in diameter undergo further evaluation in the typical patient without cancer risk factors.

In patients with one or more thyroid nodules larger than 1 cm in diameter, initial evaluation is assessment of thyroid function. This is most accurately measured by obtaining a serum TSH measurement. Patients with suppressed TSH levels (~5–10%) may have an autonomously functioning nodule (figure 46.1A). This is important because such nodules pose virtually no risk of being cancerous and are often ablated with radioactive iodine (^{131}I). Patients with normal or elevated TSH values should be considered for fine-needle aspiration (FNA) for full diagnostic evaluation

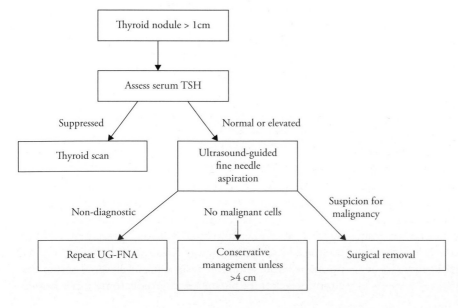

Figure 46.2. Evaluation of a Patient with a Thyroid Nodule Larger Than 1 cm in Diameter.

(figure 46.2). Most experts recommend FNA be performed with ultrasound guidance, as improved accuracy and decreased diagnostic error (false-negative results) have been demonstrated. FNA of a thyroid nodule is a safe and relatively painless procedure in most cases, especially when performed by an experienced clinician.

Findings on FNA cytology determine further evaluation or intervention. Approximately 66% of aspirates will reveal no evidence of malignancy. This is a highly accurate diagnosis when the aspirate is performed with ultrasound guidance. Such nodules are considered benign, and generally a 1- to 2-year follow-up is recommended. It is currently believed that benign thyroid nodules do not "transform" to malignant lesions. Rather, slow growth over time is often expected, often at the rate of 1 mm or less annually. Growth beyond this rate may prompt further repeat evaluation, although data are insufficient to provide clear recommendations. Approximately 10% of aspirates will be insufficient for evaluation (nondiagnostic) at initial FNA. In such cases repeat FNA is recommended, as a diagnostic sample is often obtained on the second procedure. The remaining aspirates (~25%) return positive or suspicious for malignancy. Often such cytology varies, however, in terms of final terminology used to describe abnormal cellular features. Unfortunately, such patients are advised that thyroid cancer cannot be excluded based on their cytology findings, and thus surgical hemithyroidectomy, or near-total thyroidectomy, is often advised.

Importantly, risk of cancer is similar in patients with solitary nodules >1 cm compared to those with multiple nodules each >1 cm. Because of this, patients with multinodular glands are usually recommended for aspiration of numerous nodules >1 cm when present. Thyroid hormone therapy with the goal of suppressing serum TSH concentrations should not be utilized in the evaluation and treatment of patients with nodular disease. Randomized controlled trials of this intervention demonstrate no effect on nodule size, and excessive thyroid hormone can cause adverse effects on the cardiovascular and skeletal systems.

SUMMARY

Thyroid disorders are common. Given the association of most thyroid illness with female sex and increasing patient age, it is likely that the extent of patients diagnosed with such illness in the United States will greatly increase in the 30–50 years ahead. Understanding the common presentations of hyperthyroidism, hypothyroidism, and thyroid nodular disease is critical for effective diagnosis and subsequent care of the patient. Although many types of thyroid illness can be effectively managed by primary care physicians, complex cases involving severe disease, unique situations, or thyroid illness during pregnancy should prompt consultation with an endocrinologist. Fortunately, most thyroid illnesses are readily treatable in experienced hands.

ADDITIONAL READING

Alexander EK, Marqusee E, Lawrence J, Jarolim P, Fischer GA, Larsen PR. Timing and magnitude of increases in levothyroxine requirements during pregnancy in women with hypothyroidism. *N Engl J Med.* 2004;351:241–9.

American Association of Clinical Endocrinologists Medical Guidelines for Clinical Practice for the Evaluation and Treatment of Hyperthyroidism and Hypothyroidism. *Endocr Pract.* 2002;8(6):457–69.

Cooper DS. Drug therapy: Antithyroid drugs. *N Engl J Med.* 2005;352:905–17.

Cooper DS, Doherty GM, Haugen BR, et al. Revised American Thyroid Association management guidelines for patients with thyroid nodules and differentiated thyroid cancer. *Thyroid.* 2009;19:1167–1214.

Fatourechi V, Aniszewski JP, Fatourechi GZ, Atkinson EJ, Jacobsen SJ. Clinical features and outcome of subacute thyroiditis in an incidence cohort: Olmsted County, Minnesota. *J Clin Endocrinol Metab.* 2003;88:2100–5.

Fish LH, Schwartz HL, Cavanaugh J, Steffes MW, Bantle JP, Oppenheimer JH. Replacement dose, metabolism, and bioavailability of levothyroxine in the treatment of hypothyroidism. Role of triiodothyronine in pituitary feedback in humans. *N Engl J Med.* 1987;316:764–70.

Ringel MD. Management of hypothyroidism and hyperthyroidism in the intensive care unit. *Crit Care Clinics.* 2001;17:59–74.

Surks MI, Ortiz E, Daniels GH, et al. Subclinical thyroid disease. Scientific review and guidelines for diagnosis and management. *JAMA.* 2004;291:228–38.

Toft AD. Thyroxine therapy. *N Engl J Med.* 1994;331:174.

Wartofsky L. Acute presentation of thyroid disease. In Wachter RM, Goldman L, Hollander H (Eds.), *Hospital Medicine.* Baltimore: Williams & Wilkins, 2005:1093–102.

Woeber K. Update on the management of hyperthyroidism and hypothyroidism. *Arch Fam Med.* 2000;9:743–7.

QUESTIONS

QUESTION 1. A 29-year-old woman who works as a jewelry maker presents with restlessness, difficulty concentrating at work, and complains of a tremor for the past 6 weeks. She also complains of feeling hot. Although noting increased intake of food, she reports losing 11 lb of weight in the past 2 months. She has had difficulty sleeping. On physical examination the patient's temperature is 37.5°C, pulse 101/min, respiratory rate 22/min, and blood pressure 145/85 mm Hg. Which of the following laboratory findings is most likely to be present in this woman?

A. Decreased catecholamines
B. Decreased iodine uptake
C. Decreased plasma insulin
D. Decreased TSH
E. Increased ACTH
F. Increased calcitonin

QUESTION 2. A 62-year-old woman has noted painless enlargement of her anterior neck region over the past 6 months. On physical examination she has diffuse, symmetrical thyroid enlargement without tenderness. FNA of the thyroid yields cells suspicious for malignancy. She has normal thyroid function tests, but an elevated serum calcitonin level of 42 pg/mL. A thyroidectomy is performed.

Pathology reveals malignant cells with positive staining for calcitonin. In the stroma green birefringence on Congo red staining is seen. The most likely diagnosis is:

A. Papillary thyroid carcinoma
B. Medullary carcinoma
C. Anaplastic carcinoma
D. Follicular carcinoma
E. Parathyroid carcinoma

QUESTION 3. A 49-year-old woman has had increasing cold intolerance, feeling of being tired and sluggish, and a weight gain of 8 lb over the past 18 months. Physical examination reveals dry, coarse skin and alopecia of the scalp. Her thyroid is not palpably enlarged. Her serum TSH is 18.7 mU/L with total thyroxine concentration of 3.1 μg/dL. On further workup, anti–thyroid peroxidase antibodies are detected at high titer. Which of the following thyroid diseases is she most likely to have?

A. DeQuervain disease
B. Papillary carcinoma
C. Hashimoto thyroiditis
D. Nodular goiter
E. Graves disease

QUESTION 4. What one of the following statements about propylthiouracil is correct:

A. The FDA has issued a notice of serious liver injury associated with propylthiouracil use.
B. Propylthiouracil is first-line therapy for Graves disease.
C. Methimazole should be used in place of propylthiouracil in the first trimester of pregnancy.

D. Propylthiouracil is recommended in pediatric patients unless the patient is allergic to it, in which case methimazole should be used.
E. Propylthiouracil administration is contraindicated in breast-feeding women.

QUESTION 5. What one of the statements regarding amiodarone's effect on the thyroid is incorrect?

A. In the United States amiodarone-associated thyrotoxicosis is much more commonly seen than amiodarone-associated hypothyroidism.
B. Each 200-mg tablet of amiodarone is estimated to contain about 75 mg of organic iodide.
C. Amiodarone and its metabolites may have a direct cytotoxic effect on the thyroid follicular cells, which causes a destructive thyroiditis.
D. Serum thyrotropin (TSH) levels usually rise after the start of amiodarone therapy but return to normal in 2–3 months.
E. Amiodarone-induced hypothyroidism does not necessitate discontinuation of amiodarone administration, as levothyroxine can be administered simultaneously.

ANSWERS

1. D
2. B
3. C
4. A
5. A

47.

ANDROGENIC AND REPRODUCTIVE DISORDERS

Maria A. Yialamas

FEMALE REPRODUCTIVE ENDOCRINOLOGY

Normal menstrual cycle function requires careful coordination between the hypothalamus, pituitary gland, and ovaries. The hypothalamus releases gonadotropin-releasing hormone (GnRH) in a pulsatile manner. The frequency of the GnRH pulses varies across the menstrual cycle in order to promote follicular development and ovulation. GnRH, in turn, stimulates the pituitary gland to release follicle-stimulating hormone (FSH) and luteinizing hormone (LH). FSH and LH stimulate the ovaries for follicular development with subsequent estrogen, progesterone, inhibin A, and inhibin B production.

A normal menstrual cycle length is 25–35 days. Menstrual cycles <25 days or >35 days are likely anovulatory. The follicular phase can vary in length from cycle to cycle; the luteal phase is typically constant at 12–14 days. Menstrual disorders can occur as a result of a defect in the hypothalamus, pituitary gland, or ovary.

This chapter reviews the evaluation and etiologies of amenorrhea with a special emphasis on hypothalamic amenorrhea (HA) and polycystic ovary syndrome (PCOS).

AMENORRHEA

Primary amenorrhea is defined as the absence of menses by age 16, and secondary amenorrhea is defined as the absence of menses for a period of 3 months. The pathophysiological considerations are the same for both primary and secondary amenorrhea, but uterine and outflow tract abnormalities are much more common in patients with primary amenorrhea.

The most common cause of amenorrhea is pregnancy, and this diagnosis must always be excluded. The other two main categories to consider are (1) ovulatory disorders and (2) structural disorders of the uterus or outflow tract. *Ovulatory disorders* are due to impaired hormone production at (1) the hypothalamus and/or pituitary gland or at (2) the ovary.

Hypothalamic and Pituitary Gland Disorders

In menstrual cycle disorders due to hypothalamic and/or pituitary gland defects, estradiol is low, and FSH and LH are low or normal (hypogonadotropic hypogonadism). There are many etiologies for hypogonadotropic hypogonadism, the most common of which is functional HA. HA occurs because of a stress to the system, whether physical or psychological, or from an energy imbalance when energy output exceeds energy input. This energy imbalance can be observed in those women with eating disorders, weight loss, or excessive exercise. Leptin appears to be the hormone that plays the important role of signaling to the brain that there are adequate fat stores and proper energy balance for reproduction. This important role of leptin was delineated in a recent study in which physiological doses of leptin were administered to women with HA, with follicle growth and ovulation in many of these women. Recovery of menstrual function in women with HA depends on the etiology, with stress and weight loss having the best prognoses.

Other common etiologies for hypogonadotropic hypogonadism include hyperprolactinemia and thyroid disease (hypothyroidism or hyperthyroidism). Other less common etiologies include Sheehan syndrome, lymphocytic hypophysitis, hypothalamic or pituitary tumors, infiltrative diseases (i.e., hemochromatosis, sarcoidosis, tuberculosis), and genetic disorders such as idiopathic hypogonadotropic hypogonadism/Kallmann syndrome.

Ovarian Dysfunction (Spontaneous Primary Ovarian Insufficiency (POI)/Premature Ovarian Failure)

In menstrual cycle disorders due to ovarian dysfunction (hypergonadotropic hypogonadism), estradiol is low, and FSH and LH are elevated. Primary Ovarian Insufficiency (POI) is defined as a woman <40 years with amenorrhea and an elevated FSH. The FSH should always be repeated in the follicular phase to confirm the diagnosis. Etiologies of POF include Turner syndrome, X chromosome deletions/

translocations, Fragile X premutations, autoimmune disease, chemotherapy, or radiation therapy to the pelvic area. In patients with POI diagnostic testing should include a karyotype, especially in women <35 years of age. Many women with Turner syndrome demonstrate mosaicism and may not have the full features of Turner syndrome on physical exam, and therefore, they can only be diagnosed on karyotype testing. Fragile X premutation carriers have increased risk of POI, and consequently, screening is important because women with POI may intermittently ovulate and conceive. Antiovarian antibodies have no utility because of their low specificity, and ovarian biopsy is not helpful in most cases.

Polycystic Ovary Syndrome

Polycystic ovary syndrome (PCOS) is a common cause of amenorrhea as well as irregular menses and is characterized by a normal estradiol level and elevated ratio of LH:FSH. It is a complicated disorder characterized by increased ovarian androgen production, disordered GnRH pulsatility, and insulin resistance. In 1990, a National Institutes of Health (NIH) Conference defined PCOS as a disorder characterized by oligomenorrhea and either biochemical or clinical evidence of hyperandrogenism in the absence of other known disorders, such as thyroid disease, hyperprolactinemia, and congenital adrenal hyperplasia. Using these criteria, studies have shown a prevalence of PCOS of 4–7% in reproductive-aged women. In fact, PCOS may be the most common endocrinopathy in young women and is the most common cause of female infertility. In 2003 the definition for PCOS was revisited by the American Society for Reproductive Medicine and European Society for Human Reproduction and Embryology (table 47.1). The new Rotterdam criteria stated that PCOS was present if two of the following three criteria were present in the absence of other known disorders: (1) oligo- or anovulation; (2) clinical and/or biochemical evidence of hyperandrogenism; and (3) polycystic ovary morphology (PCOM). PCOM was defined when at least one ovary is at least 10 cm^3 in volume or has 12 or more follicles, 2–9 mm in diameter.

The main clinical manifestations of PCOS are oligo-ovulation or anovulation, hyperandrogenism, infertility, and insulin resistance. The oligo- and anovulation can lead to infertility as well as endometrial hyperplasia and increased risk of endometrial cancer. Hyperandrogenism can present

as hirsutism, acne, and/or alopecia. One of the clinically most worrisome features of PCOS is the insulin resistance that can be present. The prevalence is not trivial, with as many as 31–35% with impaired glucose tolerance (IGT) and 7.5–10% with type 2 diabetes as defined by the oral glucose tolerance test (OGTT). The insulin resistance that is seen in PCOS can be present in both lean and obese women with the disorder and differs from that seen in obesity alone, a frequent component of this disorder. Because abnormalities have been shown in lean women as well as obese women with PCOS, there appears to be an intrinsic insulin resistance that is present in this disorder. Therapeutic studies in PCOS women have shown that reductions in insulin resistance with weight loss, metformin, and thiazolidinediones result in a decrease in serum androgen levels and/or serum luteinizing hormone (LH) levels. In fact, patients treated with metformin or thiazolidinediones have not only improved insulin sensitivity, androgen levels, and LH levels but also improved ovulatory rates. These data strongly suggest that the underlying insulin resistance of PCOS is responsible for the oligomenorrhea and hyperandrogenism seen in this disorder.

More recent studies have suggested that the insulin resistance observed in women with PCOS confers an increased risk of fatty liver disease, metabolic syndrome, and sleep apnea.

Uterus/Outflow Tract Disorders

Uterine/outflow tract disorders are characterized by normal estradiol, FSH, and LH levels. Many of these disorders present as primary amenorrhea in adolescence. Etiologies include absent cervix, imperforate hymen, and Mayer-Rokitansky-Kuster-Hauser syndrome (absent vagina and/or uterus). Androgen insensitivity syndrome can also present with amenorrhea; this is diagnosed with a karyotype. In adults, amenorrhea due to Asherman syndrome can occur after instrumentation or infections of the uterus.

Evaluation of the Patient with Amenorrhea

History

Because of the many possible etiologies described above, a detailed history must be obtained from patients who present with amenorrhea. Important historical points include unprotected sexual intercourse to assess for the possibility of pregnancy. A history of headaches or neurological symptoms, galactorrhea, or excessive exercising or dieting may point to a hypothalamic or pituitary etiology. Because thyroid disease is so common in women, a careful review of signs and symptoms of hypothyroidism and hyperthyroidism should be discussed with the patient. Hot flushes, night sweats, and insomnia may make POF a likely diagnosis. Classic symptoms for outflow tract obstruction or uterine abnormalities include cyclic menstrual pain or premenstrual symptoms without menses.

Table 47.1 **1990 NIH CRITERIA AND ROTTERDAM CRITERIA FOR THE DIAGNOSIS OF PCOS**

NIH CRITERIA	ROTTERDAM CRITERIA
Oligo/anovulation and hyperandrogenism	Two of the following: • Oligo/anovulation • Hyperandrogenism • PCOM*

NOTE: NIH, National Institutes of Health; PCOM, polycystic ovary morphology.

Physical Exam

Important physical exam findings begin with the general appearance of the patient, especially young women with primary amenorrhea. It is important to assess these patients for any evidence of Turner syndrome and note the amount of breast development. The skin examination is also extremely important. For example, hirsutism, acne, and male pattern balding may indicate that PCOS is the etiology of the menstrual abnormality. Vitiligo may indicate autoimmune disease and increase the probability of POI. Other aspects of the exam that should be carefully assessed include the thyroid exam, the presence of galactorrhea, the neurological exam with a special focus on the visual field exam, and the pelvic exam to assess the external genitalia as well as the uterus and ovaries.

Laboratory Evaluation and Diagnostic Tests

Every patient with amenorrhea should have hCG, prolactin, thyroid-stimulating hormone (TSH), and FSH tests to exclude pregnancy, hyperprolactinemia, thyroid disease, and POI, respectively. FSH is the single best marker of ovarian reserve; LH and estradiol are not needed in the initial evaluation (table 47.2). If any signs or symptoms of hyperandrogenism are present and PCOS is suspected, a total testosterone and dehydroepiandrosterone (DHEAS) should be drawn to exclude an ovarian or adrenal neoplasm. Levels that increase suspicion of a malignancy include a testosterone >200 ng/dL and a DHEAS >800 µg/dL.

Often, all of the laboratory test results return normal, and the underlying etiology of the amenorrhea is unclear. In these cases a Provera challenge test is helpful. If there is no withdrawal bleed, this indicates a low-estrogen state and possibly a hypothalamic or pituitary etiology for the amenorrhea. If there is a withdrawal bleed, this indicates adequate estrogen production and PCOS as the possible diagnosis.

The question of whether a women with HA needs pituitary magnetic resonance imaging (MRI) imaging often arises. Most women diagnosed with HA do not require brain imaging. Exceptions include patients with an elevated prolactin (even if it is a mild elevation), headaches or neurological symptoms, primary amenorrhea that is due to hypogonadotropic hypogonadism, or if an underlying etiology for the HA cannot be elicited.

Table 47.2 **THE INITIAL LABORATORY EVALUATION FOR AMENORRHEA ASSESSES FOR PREGNANCY, PREMATURE OVARIAN FAILURE, HYPERPROLACTINEMIA, AND THYROID DISEASE**

LABORATORY EVALUATION OF AMENORRHEA

- β-hCG (rule out pregnancy)
- Follicle-stimulating hormone (best test for ovarian function)
- Prolactin
- Thyroid-stimulating hormone
  If all labs normal: Provera challenge

For patients with amenorrhea due to a low-estrogen state (hypothalamic and pituitary sources as well as POF), bone mineral density testing to assess for bone loss due to estrogen deficiency may be considered if the amenorrhea has been present longer than 6 months.

Treatment

Hypothalamic Amenorrhea

Treatment includes changing the energy imbalance by increasing weight or decreasing exercise. Oral contraceptive pills (OCPs) and calcium and vitamin D supplements are also important to preserve bone health. If fertility is desired, gonadotropins are administered.

Premature Ovarian Failure

A major concern for women with POF is the preservation of bone health, and therefore, OCPs or hormone replacement therapy is prescribed.

Polycystic Ovary Syndrome

Treatment options for PCOS target which symptom is most problematic for the patient. If the most concerning symptom is the hyperandrogenism, the most commonly prescribed treatment is an OCP, sometimes with the antiandrogen spironolactone. OCPs are also useful for providing endometrial protection for women with anovulation. For those women with anovulation who do not wish to be on OCPs, treatment with cyclic progesterone is another option to promote endometrial protection. Other possible treatment options for the hyperandrogenism and oligomenorrhea include weight loss and metformin. For infertility, clomiphene is the most commonly prescribed treatment, often in conjunction with metformin and weight loss.

MALE REPRODUCTIVE ENDOCRINOLOGY

The hypothalamic-pituitary-testicular axis tightly regulates testosterone production in men. GnRH is released in a pulsatile fashion, approximately every 2 hours and stimulates the pituitary gland to produce LH and FSH, which in turn stimulate testosterone production and spermatogenesis in the testes. Testosterone plays a number of important physiological roles in men. It is necessary for virilization, normal sexual function, and normal bone and muscle mass.

The following section reviews the diagnosis and evaluation of male hypogonadism.

MALE HYPOGONADISM SYMPTOMS

Symptoms of hypogonadism include low libido, erectile dysfunction, infertility, fatigue, low mood, decreased strength, and gynecomastia. Many of these symptoms are nonspecific, and therefore, the diagnosis of hypogonadism is difficult to obtain on history alone in many cases.

Physical Exam

The physical exam is extremely important when evaluating a patient for hypogonadism. Important signs include the presence of eunuchoidal proportions, the distribution of body hair, the presence of gynecomastia, and, most importantly, the testicular size.

Laboratory Assessment

Because the symptoms of hypogonadism are nonspecific, testosterone measurements are extremely important in confirming the diagnosis. When assessing the reproductive axis in men, the single best test is the total testosterone level. With the exception of the free testosterone by equilibrium dialysis assay, most free testosterone assays are inaccurate. The timing of the blood draw is also important. Testosterone secretion is diurnal, with the highest levels in the morning and lowest in the afternoon. Therefore, early morning total testosterone levels are the most diagnostic in assessing whether a patient has hypogonadism. Testosterone measurements should always be checked on two separate occasions when assessing for hypogonadism because there can be variability from day to day.

If hypogonadism is confirmed, then LH and FSH should be obtained to determine whether primary or secondary hypogonadism is present (figure 47.1). Primary hypogonadism is defined as hypogonadism due to a testicular defect and is characterized by a low testosterone and elevated LH and FSH levels. Secondary hypogonadism is defined as hypogonadism due to a hypothalamic or pituitary defect and is characterized by a low testosterone and inappropriately low or normal LH and FSH.

In addition to assessing the etiology of the hypogonadism, it is also important to assess the end-organ effects of the patient's hypogonadism. These assessments may include a semen analysis to assess sperm counts, hematocrit to assess for anemia, and bone mass density (BMD) scan to assess for osteopenia/osteoporosis.

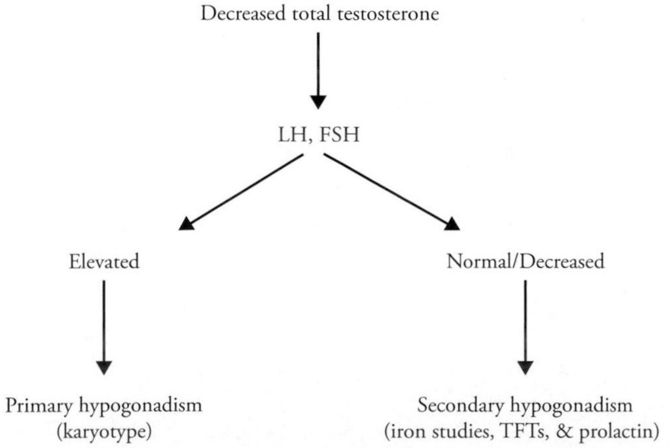

Primary Hypogonadism

Primary hypogonadism may be congenital or acquired (table 47.3). The most common congenital etiology is Klinefelter syndrome, which has been described to occur in 1 in 800 live births. In patients with Klinefelter mosaicism, the hypogonadism may not present until later in life. Therefore, all patients with primary hypogonadism should have a karyotype.

Acquired etiologies for primary hypogonadism include infectious etiologies such as mumps, chemotherapy, or radiation therapy to the pelvic area.

Secondary Hypogonadism

Secondary hypogonadism may also be congenital or acquired. Congenital etiologies include idiopathic hypogonadotropic hypogonadism, with or without anosmia. Acquired etiologies include hemochromatosis, hyperprolactinemia, opiate use, and pituitary or hypothalamic tumors.

All patients with secondary hypogonadism require a transferrin saturation to assess for hemochromatosis and a prolactin level to assess for hyperprolactinemia. All patients under the age of 60 with secondary hypogonadism require imaging of their pituitary gland to exclude a pituitary neoplasm.

Treatment

Treatment depends on the patient's goals. Testosterone replacement therapy is prescribed in men without immediate desire for fertility. Various formulations are available, including intramuscular injections, transdermal patches, transdermal gels, and buccal tablets. Older oral formulations are no longer available in the United States because of the significant hepatotoxicity associated with them.

If a patient desires fertility and has secondary hypogonadism, then testosterone is not recommended because it can impair spermatogenesis. Instead, these men are treated with gonadotropins.

Figure 47.1. Evaluation of Male Hypogonadism.

Decreased total testosterone → LH, FSH → Elevated → Primary hypogonadism (karyotype); Normal/Decreased → Secondary hypogonadism (iron studies, TFTs, & prolactin)

Table 47.3 **ETIOLOGIES OF PRIMARY AND SECONDARY HYPOGONADISM**

PRIMARY HYPOGONADISM	SECONDARY HYPOGONADISM
Klinefelter syndrome	Hyperprolactinemia
Orchitis (i.e., mumps)	Hemochromatosis
Trauma	Opiates
Chemotherapy	Chronic illness
Radiation therapy	Pituitary adenoma
Alcohol	Hypothalamic tumor
	Cushing syndrome
	Head trauma
	Head irradiation
	IHH/Kallmann syndrome
	Alcohol

Potential dangers of testosterone overreplacement include exacerbation of sleep apnea, increase in hematocrit exceeding the normal range, and possibly an increase in prostate cancer.

ADDITIONAL READING

Bhasin S, Cunningham GR, Hayes FJ, et al. Testosterone therapy in men with androgen deficiency syndromes: An Endocrine Society clinical practice guideline. *J Clin Endocrinol Metab.* 2010;95:2536–59.

Ehrmann DA. Polycystic ovary syndrome. *N Engl J Med.* 2005;352(12): 1223–36.

Gordon CM. Clinical practice. Functional hypothalamic amenorrhea. *N Engl J Med.* 2010;363(4):365–71.

Klibanski A. Clinical practice. Prolactinomas. *N Engl J Med.* 2010;362 (13):1219–26.

Lord JM, Flight IH, Norman RJ. Metformin in polycystic ovary syndrome: A systematic review and meta-analysis. *BMJ.* 2003;327:951.

Martin KA, et al. Evaluation and treatment of hirsutism in premenopausal women: An Endocrine Society clinical practice guideline. *J Clin Endocrinol Metab.* 2008;93(4):1105–20.

Rosenfield RL. Clinical practice. Hirsutism. *N Engl J Med.* 2005;353(24): 2578–88.

QUESTIONS

QUESTION 1. A 24-year-old woman with a 6-month history of amenorrhea comes in for evaluation. Her thyroid review of systems is negative. She does not have hot flushes, night sweats, or galactorrhea. She is on no medications. Physical exam is unremarkable. hCG is negative. FSH and TSH are normal. Prolactin is slightly elevated at 30 ng/mL (<18 ng/mL) and confirmed on repeat evaluation. What is the best next step?

A. Treat with bromocriptine/cabergoline.
B. Treat with an oral contraceptive pill.
C. Give a progesterone challenge.
D. Obtain a pituitary MRI.
E. Repeat the prolactin in 3 months. No treatment for now.

QUESTION 2. A 34-year-old woman with a 4-month history of amenorrhea comes to see you for evaluation. Her menses had occurred every 2 months before they stopped. Her exercise routine is unchanged; she runs about 25 miles per week. She has had no hot flushes or night sweats. Her thyroid review of systems is negative. Physical exam reveals some terminal hair growth of her face. TSH, FSH, prolactin, total testosterone, and DHEAS are normal; hCG is negative. What would you do next?

A. Provera challenge
B. Treat with OCPs
C. Treat with metformin

D. MRI of the pituitary gland
E. Pelvic ultrasound

QUESTION 3. An 18-year-old woman presents for evaluation of primary amenorrhea. Her review of systems is remarkable for normal breast development and increasing headaches over the last few months. Physical exam is unremarkable with normal visual field, thyroid, and pelvic exams and no galactorrhea. Her hCG, TSH, and prolactin are all normal. FSH is 50 IU/L (nL 3–12). Which of the following is *not* appropriate at this time?

A. Karyotype
B. Fragile X premutation carrier testing
C. Pituitary MRI
D. Bone mineral density scan
E. Antiadrenal antibody testing

QUESTION 4. A 22-year-old woman presents with a 6-month history of amenorrhea. She had normal menarche until 6 months ago. Over the last year she has had a 30-lb weight gain. During this time, she also noted worsening acne and some upper-lip terminal hair growth. Her hCG, prolactin, TSH, and FSH are all normal. What would be your next step?

A. Pelvic ultrasound
B. Total testosterone and DHEAS levels
C. LH and estradiol levels
D. Pituitary MRI
E. Adrenal CT scan

QUESTION 5. A 30-year-old man presents with symptoms of low libido and erectile dysfunction. He had normal pubertal development, and his symptoms started about 4 months prior. His total testosterone level is decreased at 150 ng/dL (300–1000). This is confirmed on a repeat early morning blood draw. His LH and FSH are in the normal range. Which of the following laboratory tests are appropriate in the next phase of your evaluation?

A. Iron studies
B. Prolactin level
C. Karyotype
D. A and B
E. A and C

ANSWERS

1. D
2. A
3. C
4. B
5. D

48.

ADRENAL DISORDERS

Subbulaxmi Trikudanathan and Robert G. Dluhy

The adrenal gland consists of the cortex and medulla. The adrenal cortex secretes three classes of steroid hormones: glucocorticoids, mineralocorticoids, and androgens. The outer zona glomerulosa secretes the mineralocorticoid aldosterone, which performs a key role in the maintenance of blood pressure, vascular volume, and potassium homeostasis. The central zona fasciculata produces cortisol, which is crucial in the stress response and controls intermediary metabolism and immune functions. The inner layer, the zona reticularis, produces androgens, which serve as precursors of testosterone and androstenedione; they play a role in the development of secondary sexual characteristics in females.

GLUCOCORTICOIDS

The adrenal cortex upon stimulation by adrenocorticotropic (ACTH) hormone through a steroidogenic acute regulatory protein (StAR) takes up cholesterol, the primary substrate for steroidogenesis. The specific hormones for the three zones of the adrenal cortex are then produced through a series of coordinated steps of cytochrome P450 enzymes. Cortisol circulates in the plasma as free and protein-bound cortisol and cortisol metabolites. Free or unbound cortisol, which is approximately 5% of the total cortisol, is the physiologically active hormone acting at tissue sites. The circulating half-life of cortisol is 70–120 minutes.

REGULATION OF THE HYPOTHALAMIC-PITUITARY-ADRENAL AXIS

ACTH secreted by the anterior pituitary gland regulates adrenal cortisol synthesis. ACTH is processed from a large precursor molecule, pro-opiomelanocortin (POMC), along with a number of other peptides including beta-lipotropin, endorphins, and melanocyte-stimulating hormone. Corticotropin-releasing hormone (CRH), produced in the hypothalamus, stimulates the release of ACTH and its related peptides (see figure 48.1).

Several factors influence ACTH release—CRH, arginine vasopressin (AVP), circadian rhythm, stress, and free cortisol levels. ACTH has a pulsatile secretion pattern and follows a circadian rhythm, with the peak levels prior to waking and nadir values in the late evening. The sleep–wake pattern, which is disturbed by long-distance travel across time zones or by night-shift working, takes about 2 weeks to reset. Stress such as fever, surgery, hypoglycemia, exercise, and acute emotions trigger the release of CRH, AVP, and subsequently ACTH; the sympathetic nervous system is also activated. Immune-endocrine interaction occurs when proinflammatory cytokines (particularly interleukin-1, interleukin-6, and tumor necrosis factor-α) augment the effects of CRH and AVP on ACTH secretion. Finally, negative feedback control of ACTH secretion is exerted by free plasma cortisol, whereby cortisol inhibits POMC gene transcription in the anterior pituitary gland and CRH and AVP secretion in the hypothalamus. Cortisol also stimulates the higher brain centers (such as the hippocampus and reticular system) and inhibits the locus coeruelus/sympathetic system. Chronic administration of corticosteroids suppresses the hypothalamic-pituitary-adrenal (HPA) axis, which persists for months after cessation of treatment.

PHYSIOLOGICAL ACTIONS OF GLUCOCORTICOIDS

Glucocorticoids play a pivotal role in the intermediary metabolism of carbohydrate, protein, and fat. Glucocorticoids increase the blood glucose concentration by increasing hepatic glycogen synthesis and stimulating gluconeogenesis. Glucocorticoids also exert an anti-insulin action in the peripheral tissues by reducing glucose uptake. Consequently, increased glucocorticoid actions result in insulin resistance and an increase in blood glucose concentrations in the setting of increased protein and lipid catabolism.

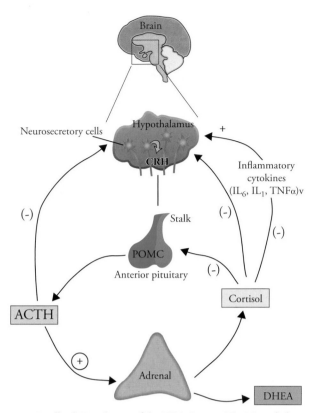

Figure 48.1. Feedback Regulation of the HPA System. The Hypothalamic–Pituitary–Adrenal Axis. The main sites for feedback control for plasma cortisol are the pituitary gland, hypothalamus, and higher centers of the brain. There is a short feedback loop involving the inhibition of CRH by ACTH. There is a negative feedback control of cortisol over the pituitary and hypothalamus. Inflammatory cytokines in response to stress lead to increased cortisol via the hypothalamus and the cortisol produced in turn suppress the proinflammatory cytokines. (–) suppression; (+) stimulation; ACTH, adrenocorticotropic hormone; CRH, corticotropin releasing hormone; DHEA, dehydroepiandrostenedione; POMC, proopiomelanocortin; IL, interleukin; TNF, tumor necrosis factor. Source: Reproduced from Adrenal Imaging, 2009, Adrenal Cortical Dysfunction, Trikudanathan S, Dluhy RG, Fig 2.2. With kind permission of Humana Press part of Springer Science and Business media.

Table 48.1 CAUSES OF CUSHING SYNDROME

ACTH-Dependent
Pituitary-hypothalamic dysfunction
ACTH-producing pituitary adenoma
Ectopic ACTH/CRH-producing nonendocrine tumors*

ACTH-Independent
Adrenocortical adenoma
Adrenocortical carcinoma
Primary pigmented nodular adrenocortical disease (PPNAD)**
Adrenal macronodular hyperplasia^
Exogenous use of glucocorticoids

NOTES: *Nonendocrine tumors: bronchogenic carcinoma, carcinoid tumors, pancreatic carcinoma.
**PPNAD: sporadic or part of familial Carney syndrome.
^Abnormal cortisol response to ectopic expression of gastric inhibitory peptide or luteinizing hormone in the adrenal cortex.
ACTH, adrenocorticotropic hormone; CRH, corticotropin-releasing hormone.

Excess cortisol leads to increased deposition of adipose tissue centrally in the viscera as opposed to the periphery. Excess glucocorticoids cause muscle atrophy by catabolic actions as well as by reducing the protein synthesis in muscle. In the skeleton, osteoblastic activity is inhibited leading to osteoporosis in glucocorticoid excess. Glucocorticoids suppresses the inflammatory cytokines and impairs cell-mediated immunity. Glucocorticoids increase neutrophil counts by demargination of neutrophils with depletion of the eosinophils. Changes in cortisol levels affect mood, implicating the brain as an important target of this hormone.

CUSHING SYNDROME

Cushing syndrome results from prolonged and inappropriate exposure to elevated levels of glucocorticoids. Endogenous hypercortisolism or Cushing syndrome is caused by excessive secretion of ACTH secretion from either the pituitary (Cushing disease—70%), or from ectopic nonpituitary source/tumors (15%), or from excessive cortisol secretion by adrenal tumors (15%). However, the most common cause of Cushing syndrome is iatrogenic from medical prescription of steroids. Table 48.1 enumerates the causes of Cushing syndrome.

Clinical Features of Cushing Syndrome

The prominent features of Cushing syndrome include central or truncal obesity with increased fat depots in distinctive sites such as the dorsocervical area (buffalo hump), supraclavicular fat pads, and the mesenteric bed. The extremities are depleted of fat and appear thin. Patients develop moon face, hirsutism, and facial plethora. Signs of protein wasting are characteristically seen with thin skin, easy bruisability, broad violaceous cutaneous striae, and proximal myopathy. Osteoporosis may occur with vertebral fractures. Glucose intolerance occurs owing to insulin resistance, with overt diabetes mellitus in about 20% of the patients. Imaging studies show hepatic steatosis and increased visceral fat. Cortisol excess predisposes to hypertension and thereby increases the cardiovascular risk. In women increased levels of adrenal androgens can lead to acne, hirsutism, and menstrual abnormalities such as oligomenorrhea and amenorrhea. Emotional dysfunction ranging from irritability to depression or even frank psychosis may occur. Wound infections are common and contribute to poor wound healing. The spectrum of clinical presentation is broad and overlaps with many common conditions such as simple obesity, and hence, the diagnosis can be challenging. The morbidity and mortality from Cushing syndrome occur mostly from cardiovascular complications followed by infectious causes.

Screening for Cushing Syndrome

Initial testing for Cushing syndrome should be done in patients with clinical features suggestive of Cushing syndrome or in patients with adrenal incidentaloma. It is reasonable to screen patients with unusual features for their age that could reflect hypercortisolism such as osteoporosis, hypertension, or easy bruising. Studies have shown that Cushing syndrome is prevalent in 2–5% of poorly controlled diabetic patients.

Initial screening for Cushing syndrome should demonstrate increased cortisol production and/or failure to suppress cortisol secretion when exogenous glucocorticoid (dexamethasone) is administered. Once the diagnosis of hypercortisolism is ascertained, the etiology should be sought. The following tests are useful and complementary as initial diagnostic studies for Cushing syndrome: measurement of urinary free cortisol levels, late-night salivary cortisol, overnight dexamethasone suppression test (DST), and low-dose DST.

Measurement of 24-hour urinary free cortisol (along with urinary creatinine to ascertain the completeness of collection) is useful to diagnose hypercortisolism. It measures the cortisol that is not bound to CBG, which is filtered by the kidney unchanged and not reabsorbed. Urinary free cortisol (UFC) should not be measured in patients with moderate to severe renal impairment. UFC can also be normal if a patient has cyclic disease or mild Cushing syndrome. False-positive results are seen in any physiological state that increases cortisol production; hence, two measurements done on separate occasions may be needed. Normal values are <220–330 nmol/24 hr depending on the assay. The normal circadian rhythm is lost in Cushing syndrome; values of plasma midnight cortisol >2 µg/dL are diagnostic. Although this is a sensitive test and specific, patients require hospitalization for this investigation to avoid any patient influence of stress on cortisol levels. As a result it is not a widely used screening test. Salivary cortisol also reflects the amount of free circulating cortisol; a midnight level or a late-night salivary sample collected between 2300 and 2400 hours can be a valuable test and obviates hospitalization. Alteration of sleep–wake cycles (e.g., shift work) can produce false-positive results.

A simple outpatient screening test is the overnight DST (1 mg of dexamethasone at bedtime). Currently to enhance the sensitivity of this test, a cortisol level >1.8 µg/dL (50 nmol/L) the next morning between 8 and 9 a.m. supports the diagnosis of Cushing syndrome. This may be followed by the low-dose DST (0.5 mg every 6 hours for 48 hours), which has greater specificity. Failure of urinary cortisol to fall <25 nmol/day or of plasma cortisol to fall <1.8 µg/dL (50 nmol/L) establishes the diagnosis of autonomous cortisol production.

Investigations to Identify the Cause of Cushing Syndrome

Once a diagnosis of hypercortisolism is confirmed, the next step is to confirm the etiology. Measurement of plasma ACTH level would help distinguish between the ACTH-dependent and ACTH-independent causes. A low or undetectable ACTH level (<2 pmol/L) diagnoses primary adrenal disorders. In pituitary ACTH-secreting microadenomas (Cushing disease) the ACTH levels are inappropriately normal or modestly elevated (6–30 pmol/L), whereas in pituitary macroadenomas and ectopic ACTH syndrome, ACTH values will be two- or threefold elevated (>110 pmol/L).

In cortisol-producing adrenal adenomas the ACTH level is suppressed or undetectable. There is also suppression in plasma dehydroepiandrosterone sulfate (DHEAS) as adrenal androgen production is reduced as a result of ACTH suppression. In adrenal carcinomas hypercortisolism is often accompanied by increased androgen secretion. The steroid production in adrenal carcinoma is usually resistant to ACTH stimulation and dexamethasone suppression. Patients with primary adrenal disorders should undergo high-resolution computed tomography (CT) scanning of the abdomen.

To distinguish the etiologies of ACTH-dependent Cushing syndrome, high-dose dexamethasone suppression testing (HDDST) (2 mg every 6 hours for 2 days) may be used. Pituitary macroadenoma and ectopic ACTH production show no suppression, whereas there is usually suppression of 50% or greater of plasma cortisol in ACTH-secreting pituitary microadenomas.

Imaging study of the pituitary (usually magnetic resonance imaging [MRI] with gadolinium) is the initial imaging study in ACTH-dependent Cushing syndrome; however, it may not always demonstrate a pituitary lesion in patients with Cushing disease. It is also important to keep in mind that 10–20% of normal patients have nonfunctioning pituitary "incidentalomas." In most circumstances inferior petrosal sinus sampling (IPSS) is needed to prove pituitary hypersecretion of ACTH. Blood from each half of the pituitary drains into the cavernous sinus and then into ipsilateral inferior petrosal sinus. Catheterization and venous sampling for measurement of ACTH from both the sinuses simultaneously compared to a peripheral sample would differentiate a pituitary source from an ectopic source. In pituitary ACTH-secreting tumor the ratio of ACTH concentrations from the inferior petrosal sinus to simultaneously drawn peripheral blood would be greater than twofold basally and greater than threefold after CRH injection. Thus, IPSS is a highly sensitive and specific test to distinguish between pituitary and nonpituitary sources of ACTH excess. However, IPSS is technically demanding, and complications such as thrombosis can occur. As a result this test should be performed in an experienced center.

To locate sources for ectopic ACTH production, it would be reasonable to start with a CT scan of the chest and abdomen searching for a mass. Positron emission tomography (PET) scanning would be a second test if CT scanning is negative. Octreotide scanning can also be useful to image ACTH-producing neuroendocrine tumors such as carcinoids. In spite of meticulous investigations, the ectopic ACTH cause for Cushing syndrome can remain occult in about 5–15% of patients; such patients need periodic radiographic reassessment.

DIFFERENTIAL DIAGNOSIS

Pseudo-Cushing Syndrome

Obesity, chronic alcoholism, and depression can mimic the biochemical abnormalities seen in Cushing syndrome. For example, chronic excessive alcohol intake and depression may cause mild elevation in urinary free cortisol, blunted circadian rhythmicity, and resistance to suppression with dexamethasone. However, these patients usually do not have the more reliable clinical features of Cushing syndrome such as proximal myopathy and easy bruisability. Following discontinuation of alcohol or with relief of depression, steroid testing returns to normal.

Management

Surgical resection of the pituitary adenoma using the transsphenoidal approach is the first line of therapy for Cushing disease. Remission in the hands of an experienced surgeon is in the range of 65–90% for microadenomas and 50% for macroadenomas. After removal of the ACTH-producing pituitary adenoma, the normal corticotropes are suppressed; hence, patients need glucocorticoid treatment postoperatively until the HPA axis recovers. A postoperative morning serum cortisol level of <2 μg/dL the day after surgery is suggestive of remission and possible surgical cure. In the past, bilateral adrenalectomy was performed for Cushing disease; that led to the subsequent development of Nelson syndrome in 10–20% of patients—an aggressive ACTH-secreting pituitary macroadenoma. Presumably the ACTH-secreting pituitary tumor escaped feedback inhibition of the hypercortisolism. Pituitary irradiation may be used for patients with postoperative recurrence and in Nelson syndrome. In other centers, gamma knife and stereotactic techniques have been used to treat pituitary adenomas.

In ectopic ACTH syndrome, tumor-directed therapy involving resection of the primary tumor (e.g., bronchial carcinoid) can lead to cure. However, the prognosis remains poor for small cell lung tumors, and medical therapy inhibiting steroidogenesis is indicated for symptoms of cortisol excess.

Laparoscopic adrenalectomy is preferred for adrenal adenomas. Adrenal carcinomas carry a poor prognosis with dismal 5-year survival rates. Adrenal carcinomas are neither radiosensitive nor chemosensitive, although mitotane has been shown to improve disease-free survival if administered adjunctively following surgical resection of the neoplasm. The best predictor of outcome is the ability to do a complete surgical resection.

Medical Therapies for Cushing Syndrome

Drugs can be used to treat hypercortisolism by inhibiting steroidogenesis: metyrapone, ketoconazole, and mitotane. Metyrapone inhibits 11β-hydroxylase while ketoconazole blocks cytochrome P450-dependent enzymes. These drugs can be used preoperatively or as adjunctive treatment following surgery or radiotherapy. Mitotane inhibits steroidogenesis but in some patients is also cytotoxic to the adrenal gland. Its use is primarily for adrenal carcinoma because of its potential cytotoxicity.

ADRENAL INSUFFICIENCY

Primary adrenal insufficiency (Addison disease) results from the destruction of the adrenal cortex and further results in a deficiency in aldosterone, cortisol, and adrenal androgen production. Secondary hypoadrenalism results from decreased ACTH production leading to reduced cortisol and adrenal androgen secretion; aldosterone production is normal, as the renin-angiotensin axis remains intact in such patients. Although Addison disease is uncommon, it carries significant morbidity and mortality if left untreated.

ETIOLOGY

In the Western world the most common cause of Addison disease is autoimmune adrenalitis with the majority of the patients having autoantibodies directed toward 21-hydroxylase and side-chain cleavage enzymes. Primary adrenal insufficiency can occur as a part of autoimmune polyendocrine syndromes (APS) I and II.

In the developing world primary adrenal insufficiency is mainly due to infections, especially tuberculosis. Other causes of adrenal insufficiency are listed in table 48.2.

CLINICAL FEATURES

Symptoms of chronic adrenal insufficiency are nonspecific and include fatigue, weakness, listlessness, anorexia, and weight loss. Gastrointestinal symptoms such as nausea, vomiting, diarrhea, and abdominal cramps can occasionally be the only presenting complaint. A specific sign of primary adrenal insufficiency is cutaneous and mucous hyperpigmentation, which occurs due to elevated ACTH from the absence of negative cortisol feedback. Darkening of the skin is typically seen in the sun-exposed areas, recent scars, palmar creases, and buccal mucosa. Orthostatic hypotension may be marked in primary adrenal insufficiency due to aldosterone deficiency; salt craving is a frequent complaint. Women may note loss of axillary and pubic hair, as a result of the adrenal androgen deficiency. Biochemical abnormalities include hyponatremia (frequent), hyperkalemia, hypoglycemia, elevation of blood urea, mild hypercalcemia, mild normocytic anemia, lymphocytosis, and eosinophilia. In primary adrenal insufficiency hyponatremia occurs due to aldosterone deficiency and sodium wasting, whereas in secondary hypoadrenalism it is dilutional due to cortisol deficiency, which is associated with increased antidiuretic hormone levels and ineffective free water clearance.

Table 48.2 **CAUSES OF ADRENAL INSUFFICIENCY**

Primary

Autoimmune–sporadic: APS I* and II**

Infections: tuberculosis, fungal infections, cytomegalovirus, HIV†

Hemorrhage: anticoagulant therapy, CAPS‡, Waterhouse-Friderichsen syndrome

Invasion: metastatic disease

Infiltrative disorders: amyloid, hemochromatosis

Drugs: enzyme inhibitors of steroidogenesis, cytotoxic agents

Miscellaneous: congenital adrenal hyperplasia, adrenoleukodystrophy

Secondary

Pituitary tumors

Pituitary surgery

Pituitary apoplexy

Sheehan syndrome

Lymphocytic hypophysitis

Granulomatous disease: sarcoid, eosinophilic granuloma

Exogenous glucocorticoid therapy

NOTES: *Autoimmune polyglandular syndrome type I: Addison disease, chronic mucocutaneous candidiasis, hypoparathyroidism, dental enamel hypoplasia, alopecia, primary gonadal failure. **Autoimmune polyglandular syndrome type II: Addison disease, primary hypothyroidism, primary hypogonadism, insulin-dependent diabetes, pernicious anemia, vitiligo.
‡CAPS, catastrophic antiphospholipid syndrome.
†HIV, human immunodeficiency virus.

Acute adrenal insufficiency, when caused by adrenal hemorrhage or precipitated by acute infection, presents as hypotension, acute circulatory failure, confusion, abdominal pain, and fever, and prompt recognition is extremely important. In secondary adrenal insufficiency, pallor, scanty axillary and pubic hair with headache and visual symptoms may point toward hypothalamic-pituitary disease. Hyperkalemia is not seen, as there is normal aldosterone secretion.

DIAGNOSIS

A morning plasma cortisol level of ≤3 μg/dL (83 nmol/L) is diagnostic of adrenal insufficiency and precludes the need for further testing; levels ≥19 μg/dL (525 nmol/L) rule out the disorder.

The most commonly used diagnostic test for adrenal insufficiency is the ACTH stimulation test wherein 250 μg of cosyntropin is given intramuscularly or intravenously, and the cortisol response is measured at 0, 30, and 60 minutes. The normal response is a basal or peak cortisol response >18 μg/dL (495 nmol/L). This test is useful in diagnosing primary destruction of tissue and long-standing secondary adrenal insufficiency. This test may be normal in patients with mild or recent-onset secondary adrenal insufficiency. In early morning plasma, ACTH level is useful to distinguish primary from secondary adrenal insufficiency if the cortisol levels are abnormal. The plasma ACTH values are usually elevated (above 100 pg/mL) in primary adrenal insufficiency as opposed to secondary hypoadrenalism, where the plasma ACTH values may be low or "inappropriately" normal. Other tests such as the insulin tolerance test, metyrapone test, and CRH test are uncommonly used to diagnose secondary adrenal insufficiency.

Adrenal autoantibodies (e.g., 21-hydroxylase) can be measured by radioimmunoassay to diagnose autoimmune adrenalitis. CT scan of the adrenal glands may show enlargement (e.g., hemorrhage) or calcification depending on the etiology of the adrenal failure. In secondary adrenal insufficiency there is normal aldosterone secretion, and hyperkalemia is not seen. Pituitary MRI scans and assessment of anterior pituitary functions are usually needed in these patients for concomitant deficiencies of other pituitary hormones.

Individuals receiving long-term high-dose steroid therapy will develop prolonged HPA suppression leading to adrenal atrophy. Recovery takes months to over 1 year after glucocorticoid withdrawal. Early morning cortisol levels and ACTH stimulation testing should be used to assess adrenal recovery.

DIFFERENTIAL DIAGNOSIS

Chronic nonspecific symptoms such as fatigue, weakness, and malaise should make the possibility of a diagnosis of adrenal insufficiency. When insidious in onset, adrenal insufficiency is frequently mistaken for chronic fatigue syndrome. Occasionally such patients have been misdiagnosed with anorexia nervosa or depression. However, hyperpigmentation, weight loss, and gastrointestinal symptoms should alert the clinician to consider adrenal insufficiency. It is also reasonable to look for other organ-specific autoimmune diseases in the context of polyglandular syndromes.

MANAGEMENT

In the setting of adrenal crisis, parenteral treatment with high doses of hydrocortisone should be immediately initiated along with fluid resuscitation with normal saline. In nonacute situations, replacement doses of oral hydrocortisone at a dosage of 8–10 mg/m²/day should be started in divided doses. To mimic the diurnal pattern of steroid secretion, two-thirds of the total dose is given in the morning and one-third is given in late afternoon with mealtime or snack. In secondary adrenal insufficiency, only glucocorticoid therapy is needed.

In primary adrenal insufficiency, mineralocorticoid insufficiency is replaced with fludrocortisone, administered at a daily dose of 0.05–0.1 mg orally. Plasma renin activity, blood pressure, and serum electrolytes are useful parameters to titrate the dose of fludrocortisone. In female patients some studies have suggested the benefit of androgen treatment with 25–50 mg per day of DHEA orally to improve sexual function and general well-being.

Patient education and daily replacement therapy form a cornerstone in the management of primary adrenal insufficiency. Patients are advised to double the dose of hydrocortisone during periods of intercurrent illness or surgery. All patients should wear a medical alert bracelet and should be instructed in self-injection of steroids if they cannot take their dosing orally.

REGULATION OF RENIN-ANGIOTENSIN-ALDOSTERONE AXIS

Renin is formed in the juxtaglomerular cells (JG), located in the renal afferent arteriole of the glomerulus. Renin acts on the substrate angiotensinogen (hepatic origin) to form the angiotensin I. Angiotensin I is converted to angiotensin II by angiotensin-converting enzyme (ACE). Angiotensin II is a potent vasoconstrictor and also stimulates the zona glomerulosa of the adrenal cortex to increase aldosterone secretion. The hexapeptide angiotensin III also acts as a potent secretagogue of aldosterone secretion (see figure 48.2). The control of adrenal aldosterone secretion includes the renin-angiotensin system, potassium, and ACTH. Aldosterone serves two important functions: regulation of extracellular fluid volume and potassium homeostasis. Chronic exposure to aldosterone over 3–5 days leads to an "escape" from mineralocorticoid action; after an initial period of sodium retention and a gain of several kilograms, sodium balance is reestablished. Therefore edema does not develop. An increase in atrial natriuretic peptide and interplay of renal hemodynamic factors play a role in the "escape" from the sodium-retaining action of aldosterone. However, it is important to realize that there is no "escape" from the potassium-losing effects of chronic mineralocorticoid exposure.

Nonepithelial toxic action of aldosterone includes inflammation, necrosis, and subsequent fibrosis in a variety of tissues including the heart, kidney, and vasculature. These pathophysiological situations occur when aldosterone levels are inappropriately elevated on a high-salt intake such as in primary aldosteronism.

PRIMARY ALDOSTERONISM

Primary aldosteronism (PA) is now recognized to be the most common form of secondary hypertension, prevalent in nearly 10% of all patients with hypertension. It is caused by autonomous secretion of aldosterone from a unilateral adrenal adenoma or from bilateral adrenal hyperplasia. Hypokalemic patients with PA present with nonspecific

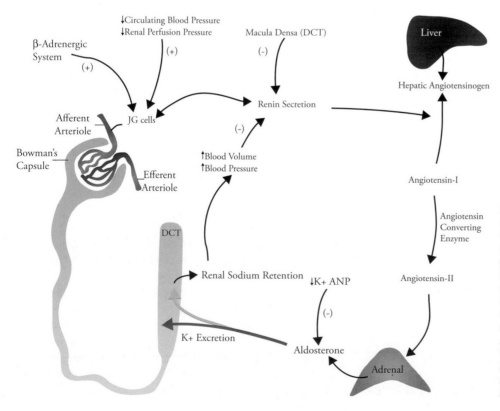

Figure 48.2. Renin-Angiotensin-Aldosterone System. This figure shows the interplay of various signals from the nephron in the kidney, liver, and adrenal gland that form the feedback loop to maintain circulating blood volume and aldosterone secretion. (−) suppression; (+) stimulation; DCT, distal convoluted tubule; K+, potassium; and ↑ shows an increase. *Source*: Reproduced from Adrenal Imaging, 2009, Adrenal Cortical Dysfunction, Trikudanathan S, Dluhy RG, Fig. 2.3. With kind permission of Humana Press part of Springer Science and Business media.

symptoms such as muscle cramping, weakness, headaches, palpitations, polyuria, and nocturia. However, recent studies have shown that hypokalemia occurs in 9–37% of patients with proven PA. Normokalemic hypertension remains the more common form of presentation of this disorder and likely reflects earlier detection. A diagnosis of PA should be considered in hypertensive patients with refractory hypertension, which is poorly controlled blood pressure on three antihypertensive agents (including a diuretic). Several studies have also shown that patients with PA have a higher cardiovascular morbidity and mortality when compared to age-matched patients with essential hypertension.

DIAGNOSIS

The recent clinical guidelines by the endocrine society have recommended case detection for PA in high-risk groups as enumerated in table 48.3. These guidelines also recommend the use of plasma aldosterone:renin ratio (ARR) to detect PA in these patient groups. Testing should be performed in the morning in a seated ambulatory patient who has been on unrestricted dietary salt intake. It is important to correct hypokalemia with supplements before measuring aldosterone levels. Certain medications can affect the ARR mainly by altering PA levels and should be withdrawn for at least 4 weeks before testing; these include spironolactone, eplerenone, amiloride, triamterene, and beta blockers. Beta blockers can reduce the renin and aldosterone levels, thereby falsely increasing the ratio, whereas ACE inhibitors and angiotensin receptor blockers (ARB) can increase the renin level and cause false negative results. If controlling hypertension becomes difficult when these medications are discontinued, drugs

Table 48.3 CASE DETECTION FOR PA IN HIGH-RISK GROUPS

Moderate/severe hypertension*

Drug-resistant hypertension**

Hypertension with spontaneous or diuretic-induced hypokalemia

Hypertension with adrenal incidentaloma

Hypertension and a family history of a early-onset hypertension or cerebrovascular accident at a young age (<40 years)

First-degree relatives of patients with PA

Onset of hypertension at a young age (< 20 years)

NOTES: *JNC stage 2 (>160–179/100–109 mm Hg), stage 3 (>180/110 mm Hg). **>140/90 mm Hg despite three antihypertensive medications.

that do not interfere with levels should be used such as verapamil slow release, hydralazine, or alpha blockers, as they have minimal effects on plasma aldosterone levels. The rationale for this test is that autonomous hyperaldosteronism results in sodium retention and suppression of plasma renin activity (PRA). The normal PA–PRA ratio in normal subjects and in patients with essential hypertension should be <30 (when PA is in ng/dL and PRA is in ng/mL/hr). Some studies suggest that an elevated plasma aldosterone level (aldosterone >15 ng/dL) is required in addition to the ARR (see figure 48.3).

Patients with an abnormal ARR usually need a confirmatory test to diagnose PA. Any of the four testing procedures can be used: oral sodium loading, saline infusion, fludrocortisone suppression, and captopril challenge. The endpoint for testing in these tests is to demonstrate autonomy

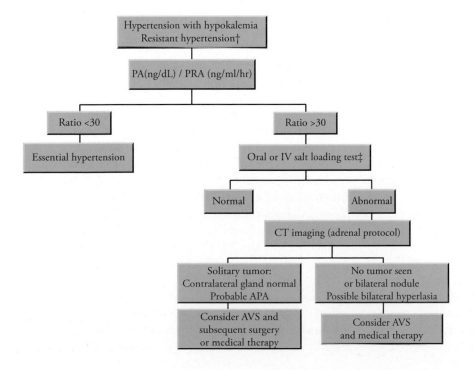

Figure 48.3 Algorithm for Diagnosis of Primary Aldosteronism. †Inadequate control of hypertension on three antihypertensives (including a diuretic). ‡Oral/IV salt loading: 2 gm of sodium chloride tablets for 3 days or 2 L of isotonic saline over 4 hrs intravenously. 24 hr urinary aldosterone collected on day 3. Dedicated adrenal protocol CT examination— see text in the chapter. AVS, adrenal venous sampling. Source: Reproduced from Adrenal Imaging, 2009, Adrenal Cortical Dysfunction, Trikudanathan S, Dluhy RG, Fig 2.8. With kind permission of Humana Press part of Springer Science and Business media.

of aldosterone secretion. There is inadequate evidence to recommend one test over the others, and the choice of testing is often center specific. For oral sodium-suppression testing, patients are instructed to take sodium chloride tablets (2 g) with each meal on a normal-salt diet for 4 days. On the fourth day a 24-hour urinary aldosterone excretion >12 µg/24 hr in the presence of urinary sodium excretion >250 mmol/day is diagnostic of autonomous aldosterone production. It should be noted that an oral sodium-loading test and intravenous saline infusion test should not be performed in patients with hypokalemia, severe uncontrolled hypertension, or congestive heart failure.

After biochemical diagnosis of PA, all patients should have an adrenal CT scan. Bilateral adrenal venous sampling (AVS) is then needed to guide treatment decisions in patients with PA. Because imaging cannot differentiate nonfunctioning incidentalomas (see below) from aldosterone-producing adenomas, it is essential to lateralize the source of aldosterone overproduction to the adenoma, especially in patients who are considering surgical intervention. AVS should be performed in a center with experienced radiologists to ensure a successful catheterization and to minimize the risk of adrenal hemorrhage and venous thrombosis.

TREATMENT

Patients diagnosed with unilateral aldosterone-producing adenoma (APA) should be offered unilateral laparoscopic adrenalectomy. This leads to improvement in both blood pressure and serum potassium concentrations in all patients. Hypertension is cured in about 50% of patients after unilateral adrenalectomy; persistent hypertension after adrenalectomy in APA patients is due to coexistent essential hypertension, older age, renal insufficiency, and longer duration of the hypertension.

In patients with bilateral adrenal disease or when APA patients are not surgical candidates for adrenalectomy, they should be treated with a mineralocorticoid antagonist (spironolactone or eplerenone). In male patients who develop predictable dose-related side effects from spironolactone such as gynecomastia, decreased libido, and impotence, eplerenone, a selective MR antagonist devoid of antiandrogen and progesterone actions, should be used. Other useful agents include the potassium-sparing diuretics amiloride and triamterene.

GLUCOCORTICOID-REMEDIABLE ALDOSTERONISM

Glucocorticoid-remediable aldosteronism (GRA), inherited as an autosomal dominant disorder, results from a chimeric gene duplication, which is the result of an unequal crossover between the homologous 11β-hydroxylase and aldosterone synthase genes. As a result there is ectopic expression of the aldosterone synthase enzyme in the cortisol-producing zona fasiculata, under the regulation of ACTH. GRA is characterized by early-onset hypertension, hemorrhagic stroke, and suppressed plasma renin levels. Genetic testing using Southern blot technique should be considered for PA patients with a family history of PA, or family history of hemorrhagic strokes at a young age (<30 years), or with early-onset hypertension. A 24-hour urine collection would reveal marked elevation in the levels of the "hybrid" steroids 18-oxocortisol and 18-OH-cortisol. Treatment with a long-acting glucocorticoid will suppress the ACTH-regulated aldosterone secretion. The smallest effective dose should be used to control blood pressure while minimizing the risk of Cushing syndrome. Alternative treatments include mineralocorticoid receptor and sodium-epithelial channel antagonists.

SECONDARY HYPERALDOSTERONISM

In secondary hyperaldosteronism there is an appropriate increase in aldosterone production due to elevated circulating levels of renin. The elevated renin production may occur in the setting of reduced effective circulating blood volume (e.g., cirrhosis, nephrotic syndrome, and congestive cardiac failure) or decreased renal perfusion. Atherosclerotic renal artery stenosis or fibromuscular hyperplasias are examples of renin overproduction due to decreased renal perfusion. These patients may have hypokalemic alkalosis as a result of hyperaldosteronism and moderate to marked increases in plasma renin activity.

OTHER CAUSES OF HYPERMINERALOCORTICOIDISM

HYPERALDOSTERONISM WITH SUPPRESSED PLASMA RENIN ACTIVITY

Apparent mineralocorticoid excess (AME) can occur in both heritable and acquired forms of impaired activity of the renal enzyme 11β-hydroxysteroid dehydrogenase (11β–HSD II). The enzyme deficiency results in the failure to degrade cortisol to the biologically inactive cortisone in renal tubules. As a result, cortisol binds to the MR exerting mineralocorticoid actions. The acquired form of this syndrome is caused by the ingestion of certain licorices or chewing tobacco, which contains glycyrrhizinic acid. These patients demonstrate hypertension and hypokalemia; PRA and aldosterone levels are suppressed. Cortisol levels are normal because the ACTH feedback loop is intact. Small doses of dexamethasone can be used to suppress the endogenous cortisol production.

Liddle syndrome is an autosomal dominant disorder caused by gain-of-function mutations in the subunits of the renal sodium epithelial channel that is normally regulated by aldosterone. Constitutive activation of the channel results in sodium retention, hypokalemia, and low renin/aldosterone levels.

HYPERALDOSTERONISM WITH ELEVATED PLASMA RENIN ACTIVITY

Bartter syndrome (BS) patients exhibit hypokalemic alkalosis, hypercalciuria, normal blood pressure, and absence of edema. In BS, loss-of-function mutation in the loop of Henle Na-K-2Cl cotransporter gene results in activation of the renin-angiotensin-aldosterone system and hence renal wasting of sodium. Patients with Gitelman syndrome (GS) have similar features to BS except that they are hypocalciuric. GS results from loss-of-function mutations in the thiazide-sensitive Na-Cl cotransporter in the distal convoluted tubule of the kidney.

HYPOALDOSTERONISM

Hyporeninemic hypoaldosteronism, usually occurring in diabetic adults with mild renal impairment, results in hyperkalemia and metabolic acidosis that are out of proportion to the level of renal failure. Isolated aldosterone deficiency with low renin levels also occurs postoperatively following removal of an aldosterone-producing adenoma and following long-standing heparin treatment.

THE SYMPATHOADRENAL SYSTEM

The sympathoadrenal system is derived from the neural crest and consists of the ganglia of the sympathetic nervous system and the adrenal medulla. Epinephrine, synthesized in the adrenal medulla, and norepinephrine at the peripheral nerve endings, are formed from the amino acid tyrosine. The rate-limiting enzyme in the biosynthetic pathway is tyrosine hydroxylase. Metabolism of epinephrine and norepinephrine to biologically inactive compounds by catecholamine-O-methyl transferase (COMT) results in metanephrine and norepinephrine, respectively. Further oxidation results in vanillylmandelic acid (VMA).

PHEOCHROMOCYTOMA

Pheochromocytomas are neuroectodermal tumors arising from the chromaffin cells. These catecholamine-secreting tumors mostly arise from the adrenal medulla; if these chromaffin tumors arise in the parasympathetic or sympathetic ganglia, they are referred to as paraganglionomas. Taken together pheochromocytoma and paragangliomas occur in 0.1–0.2% of hypertensive patients with a mean age of diagnosis at around 40 years.

The rule of 10 has been used to describe pheochromocytoma whereby 10% are extra-adrenal and, of those, 10% are extra-abdominal; 10% are bilateral; 10% are malignant, and 10% do not have hypertension. These tumors occur sporadically or as part of a genetic syndrome such as multiple endocrine neoplasia (MEN) type 2. Most of the tumors occur sporadically, but recent studies suggest that 20–30% of pheochromocytomas are associated with germline mutations. The clinical presentation varies from essential hypertension to the classic paroxysmal hypertensive crises. Failure to diagnose and treat pheochromocytoma can lead to hypertensive crises and fatality.

CLINICAL FEATURES

Classically, patients present with paroxysms of severe hypertension and palpitations; however, sustained hypertension occurs in approximately 50% of the patients. Generalized sweating and headache are other frequent symptoms. Weakness, weight loss, pallor, nausea, and abdominal pain have also been associated with pheochromocytoma. Patients with predominantly epinephrine-secreting tumor usually present with periodic attacks of anxiety and hypotension. Occasionally patients with adrenal incidentaloma or those undergoing periodic screening for a familial syndrome can be asymptomatic. Table 48.4 summarizes indications for screening for pheochromocytoma.

DIAGNOSIS

Because catecholamines (norepinephrine and epinephrine) are typically secreted in an episodic fashion and have short half-lives, random levels may miss the diagnosis unless they are checked during a paroxysmal attack. Since the metabolism of catecholamines produced by pheochromocytoma are largely intratumoral, there is a continuous release of O-methylated metabolites, that is, metanephrine and normetanephrines. As a result, measurement of metanephrines in blood or urine has become the preferred diagnostic test.

Table 48.4 **SCREENING FOR PHEOCHROMOCYTOMA**

Hypertension with episodic features
Refractory hypertension
Prominent lability of blood pressure
Severe pressor response during anesthesia, surgery, or an angiography
Unexplained hypotension during anesthesia, surgery, or pregnancy
Family history of pheochromocytoma, MEN-2,* VHL** disease, neurofibromatosis
Adrenal incidentalomas
Idiopathic dilated cardiomyopathy

NOTES: *MEN-2, multiple endocrine neoplasia-2. **VHL, Von Hippel Lindau syndrome.

There is no consensus regarding the best diagnostic test. Plasma free metanephrines or a 24-hour urine collection for fractionated catecholamines and metanephrines can alternatively be used as reliable screening tests. Plasma free metanephrines have the advantage of a simple random blood test in the office. Plasma metanephrines have a high negative predictive value except in patients with early preclinical disease or dopamine-secreting tumors. On the other hand a 24-hour urine collection for fractionated catecholamines and metanephrines is also a reliable test to diagnose pheochromocytoma. Blood or urinary catecholamine levels that are two- or threefold elevated above the upper limit of normal are considered diagnostic of pheochromocytoma. Interfering medications, such as acetaminophen, tricyclic antidepressants, levodopa, and sympathomimetics, should be stopped for at least 2 weeks prior to testing. If the testing is equivocal and the clinical suspicion for pheochromocytoma is high, clonidine suppression testing can be considered.

After biochemical confirmation of catecholamine excess, CT or MRI scanning of the abdomen usually diagnoses adrenal pheochromocytoma because most tumors are ≥ 3 cm in size. Functional imaging, such as ^{123}I-metaiodobenzylguanidine (MIBG) scintigraphy, is done if adrenal imaging is negative. MIBG is taken up into adrenergic neurosecretory granules and hence images chromaffin tumors. Other imaging techniques to locate catecholamine-producing tumors include octreotide scan and ^{18}F-flurodeoxyglucose PET scanning.

TREATMENT

Surgical removal of the pheochromocytoma is the treatment of choice, but it is essential to preoperatively treat the patient with alpha-adrenergic blockade. Alpha-adrenergic blockers include phenoxybenzamine, a noncompetitive, nonselective drug, or selective alpha blockers such as doxazosin or prazosin. Beta blockers should not be initiated before adequate alpha blockade because unopposed alpha-receptor stimulation can further raise blood pressure. After alpha blockade has been established, beta blockers may be used to control tachycardia or arrhythmias. Metyrosine, an inhibitor of catecholamine synthesis, may be used preoperatively in some situations. Preoperatively increased volume expansion with high sodium intake should be prescribed routinely because pheochromocytoma patients are known to be plasma volume contracted. Following resection of a pheochromocytoma, catecholamine levels should be periodically measured to rule out malignant disease.

MALIGNANT PHEOCHROMOCYTOMA

About 10% of pheochromocytomas are malignant, which is detected by local invasion of the tumor or from distant metastasis to lungs, liver, and bone. Patients with succinate dehydrogenase (SDHB) mutation are at a particularly high risk of malignancy, and extra-adrenal location is an independent risk factor. Surgical removal for tumor debulking followed by MIBG radiotherapy or in combination with chemotherapy has been used with limited results. Alpha blockers are used for control of blood pressure. The 5-year survival for malignant pheochromocytoma in the presence of distant metastasis is approximately 50%.

PHEOCHROMOCYTOMA AND GENETIC SYNDROMES

Pheochromocytoma usually occurs sporadically; yet 10–20% are a part of familial syndromes that include Von Hippel-Lindau (VHL) syndrome, MEN 2A and 2B, and neurofibromatosis type 1, all of which are inherited in an autosomal dominant fashion. In VHL syndrome pheochromocytoma is frequently bilateral and is associated with retinal angiomas, cerebellar hemangioblastoma, renal and pancreatic cysts, and renal cell carcinoma. MEN syndrome conditions are associated with mutations in the RET proto-oncogene. The MEN 2A phenotype includes pheochromocytoma, medullary carcinoma (MCT) of the thyroid, and hyperparathyroidism. In MEN 2B, pheochromocytoma is seen with MTC with mucosal neuromas and marfanoid body habitus.

Familial paraganglioma is an autosomal dominant disorder that is caused by mutations in succinate dehydrogenase (SDH) subunit genes SDHB, SDHC, and SDHD. Paragangliomas are located in head and neck and also in thorax, abdomen, and pelvis. Table 48.5 illustrates the situations where genetic testing for mutations in VHL, RET oncogene, SDHD, and SDHB should be performed.

ADRENAL INCIDENTALOMA

An adrenal mass >1 cm serendipitously discovered on radiological imaging is termed an "adrenal incidentaloma." The prevalence of adrenal incidentaloma increases with age, and they are seen in up to 7% among persons older than 70 years of age. Conversely, incidentalomas are uncommon in patients younger than 30 years. Two important issues need to be addressed regarding incidentaloma: are they hypersecretory, and are they malignant?

The first step in evaluation should be a careful review of history and physical examination searching for clues of

Table 48.5 GENETIC SCREENING RECOMMENDATIONS FOR PHEOCHROMOCYTOMA

Paraganglioma
Bilateral adrenal pheochromocytoma
Unilateral adrenal pheochromocytoma and a family history of pheochromocytoma/paraganglioma
Unilateral adrenal pheochromocytoma onset at a young age (<20 years)

excessive hormonal secretion. The National Institutes of Health (NIH) consensus panel recommended hormonal evaluation for pheochromocytoma and Cushing syndrome in all patients with adrenal incidentaloma and screening for primary aldosteronism in hypertensive patients. If clinical features of androgen hypersecretion are observed in women, DHEAS levels should be measured.

The next concern is whether the mass is malignant. Radiological features that predict malignancy include tumor size and imaging phenotype. Masses >6 cm are more likely to be malignant and should be resected. Benign adrenal adenomas are typically <4 cm (usually 1–2 cm), homogeneous with smooth margins, and characteristically lipid-rich by CT or MRI criteria. Benign adrenal adenomas are lipid-rich, typically <10 Hounsfield units on unenhanced CT scan. Benign adenomas also have a rapid washout of contrast medium on contrast-enhanced CT scanning. Lesions between 4 and 6 cm lie in the gray area, and decision to surgically resect should be based on patient's age, imaging phenotype, and coexisting conditions. To diagnose metastatic disease, fine-needle aspiration biopsy can be used in a patient with a history of malignancy. This should be performed only after ruling out pheochromocytoma.

In summary, for lesions that are hypersecretory or >6 cm in diameter, surgical resection should be performed. For lesions likely to be benign, repeated imaging should be done at 6, 12, and 24 months. An increase in size >1 cm/year should raise concern for possible malignancy, and resection should be considered (see table 48.6).

CONGENITAL ADRENAL HYPERPLASIA

Congenital adrenal hyperplasia (CAH) is an autosomal recessive disorder resulting from loss-of-function mutations of enzymes involved in cortisol synthesis. The most frequent enzymatic deficiency is 21-hydroxylase deficiency. Patients with 21-hydroxylase deficiency have impaired synthesis of cortisol; as a result, compensatory ACTH secretion results in the shunting of precursors into the androgen pathway. The phenotype ranges from ambiguous genitalia in newborn girls to hirsutism in adulthood and to sexual precocity in males. Aldosterone synthesis is also impaired, resulting in salt wasting, failure to thrive, and hypotension.

In late-onset CAH there is a partial enzymatic 21-hydroxylase deficiency resulting in hirsutism and oligomenorrhea in adult women. This diagnosis is established by documenting elevated morning levels of 17-hydroxyprogesterone (17-OHP) or an abnormal increase in 17-OHP levels following ACTH stimulation. The therapeutic goal in adults with late-onset CAH is the minimal dose of long-acting steroids to suppress androgen production. Typically 5 mg of prednisone or 0.25–0.5 mg of dexamethasone is given at bedtime to suppress adrenocortical androgen production.

ADDITIONAL READING

Bertagna X, Guignat L, Groussin L, Bertherat J. Cushing's disease. *Best Pract Res Clin Endocrinol Metab.* 2009;23(5):607–23.

Gomez-Sanchez CE, Rossi GP, Fallo F, Mannelli M. Progress in primary aldosteronism: Present challenges and perspectives. *Horm Metab Res.* 2010;42(6):374–81.

Mulatero P, Monticone S, Bertello C, et al. Evaluation of primary aldosteronism. *Curr Opin Endocrinol Diabetes Obes.* 2010;17(3):188–93.

Neary N, Nieman L. Adrenal insufficiency: Etiology, diagnosis and treatment. *Curr Opin Endocrinol Diabetes Obes.* 2010;17(3):217–23.

Nieman LK. Approach to the patient with an adrenal incidentaloma. *J Clin Endocrinol Metab.* 2010;95(9):4106–13.

Pelosof LC, Gerber DE. Paraneoplastic syndromes: An approach to diagnosis and treatment. *Mayo Clin Proc.* 2010;85(9):838–54.

Willatt JM, Francis IR. Radiologic evaluation of incidentally discovered adrenal masses. *Am Fam Physician.* 2010;81(11):1361–6.

Table 48.6 EVALUATION OF ADRENAL INCIDENTALOMA

Clinical
± History of prior malignancy
Hypertension (± paroxysmal symptoms)
± Cushingoid features
± Hypokalemia

Hormonal
Overnight dexamethasone suppression test
Plasma free metanephrines
Plasma aldosterone and plasma renin activity (if hypertensive)
DHEAS* (female with signs of androgen excess)

Radiographic Evaluation of Tumor Phenotype
Size, regular/irregular margins and homo/heterogeneity
Attenuation coefficient (Hounsfield units) on unenhanced CT scan
Rapidity of washout of on contrast-enhanced CT scan

NOTE: *DHEAS, dehydroepiandrosterone sulfate.

QUESTIONS

QUESTION 1. A 42-year-old female comes to see her primary care physician for fatigue and weakness over the last few months. Her medical history is unremarkable. She is not on any medications. During her last physical examination 2 years ago, her blood pressure was within normal limits, but during this visit it was elevated, 180/100 mm Hg. The remainder of her physical examination was unremarkable. Laboratory studies so far reveal a low plasma renin activity and serum potassium level of 3.2 mEq/L. What would be the most appropriate next step in evaluating this patient?

A. Plasma free metanephrines
B. CT scan of adrenal gland
C. Salt suppression of aldosterone excretion
D. MR angiography of renal arteries
E. Plasma aldosterone/plasma renin activity ratio after potassium repletion

QUESTION 2. A 38-year-old female was admitted in the hospital for the management of acute myelogenous leukemia. During her hospitalization she complains of bilateral upper quadrant pain. Subsequently she develops fever to 102°F and hypotension (80/50 mm Hg). Physical examination reveals no cutaneous or buccal pigmentation; abdominal examination shows mild tenderness in both her upper quadrants with no rigidity or guarding. Her laboratory values indicate sodium 131 mEq/L, potassium 5.0 mEq/L, BUN 24 mg/dL, Cr 1.0 mg/dL. Her CBC also reveals Hct 31%, WBC 24.3 k/mm^3, and platelets 20,000 k/mm^3. What would be your next diagnostic approach?

A. 8 a.m. ACTH levels
B. 8 a.m. cortisol level
C. CT scan abdomen/pelvis
D. Administer dexamethasone followed by a cosyntropin test
E. Treat with intravenous fluids and recheck electrolytes

QUESTION 3. A 60-year-old male smoker has a CT scan of chest performed for cough. His past medical history is unremarkable, and he takes no medications. On physical examination blood pressure is 128/74 mm Hg. His CT scan/contrast-enhanced study that included the upper quadrants of the abdomen demonstrates a 1.3-cm mass in his left adrenal gland. What would be the next radiological study?

A. Unenhanced CT scan of the abdomen
B. I-MIBG scan
C. Unenhanced CT scan followed by contrast washout adrenal protocol
D. CT-guided fine-needle aspiration biopsy of the mass
E. PET scan

QUESTION 4. Which of the following biochemical evaluations should be performed on the patient of Question 3?

A. 24-hour urine for 17-ketosteroids
B. Plasma free metanephrine and overnight dexamethasone suppression test

C. Overnight dexamethasone suppression test and ARR
D. ACTH stimulation test
E. Salt suppression of aldosterone excretion

QUESTION 5. A 25-year-old female presents with symptoms of paroxysmal hypertension, sweating, and tachycardia. Her father had died of metastatic extra-adrenal paraganglioma. During episodes her pulse rate was 100 bpm, blood pressure 188/100 mm Hg. Which is the best diagnostic study?

A. 24-hour urine for VMA
B. Plasma norepinephrine/epinephrine
C. Plasma free metanephrines
D. MRI of the abdomen
E. MIBG scan

QUESTION 6. A 38-year-old female was seen in the hematology clinic for easy bruisability. Her physical examination showed mild facial plethora, acne on her back, increased facial hair, supraclavicular and dorsocervical fat pads. Examination of the abdomen showed truncal obesity but no cutaneous striae. She has been on oral contraceptive for several years. Which of the following would be your next step?

A. Low-dose 48-hour dexamethasone suppression test
B. MRI of pituitary gland
C. CT scan abdomen-adrenal protocol
D. 24-hour urinary cortisol or midnight salivary cortisol
E. Inferior petrosal sinus sampling for the measurement of ACTH

ANSWERS

1. E
2. D
3. C
4. B
5. C
6. D

49.

DISORDERS OF CALCIUM METABOLISM

Carolyn B. Becker

Calcium is vital for the regulation of a vast array of human physiological processes including cell division, cell adhesion, plasma membrane integrity, protein and hormone secretion, muscle contraction, neuronal excitability, glycogen metabolism, platelet aggregation, and blood coagulation. Given this list, it is not surprising that calcium levels are very tightly regulated.

The human body contains about 1000 g of calcium, of which more than 99% resides in the skeleton. This leaves less than 1% of total body calcium in the soluble phase, divided between intracellular and extracellular fluid compartments. The concentration of extracellular calcium is approximately 10,000-fold higher than the concentration of intracellular calcium, yet both are critical for the proper functioning of physiological processes. Of the extracellular calcium, 50% is bound (40% to albumin; 10% to citrate, phosphate, and other ions), while the other 50% is unbound or "ionized." It is only the ionized calcium that is biologically active and only this fraction that is regulated hormonally. To adjust the calcium level for elevations in plasma proteins, total serum calcium should be reduced by 0.8 mg/dL for every 1 g/dL of albumin above the normal range.

The exquisite regulation of ionized calcium is truly remarkable, given the ever-changing supply of calcium from the diet versus the constant demands for calcium by various tissues throughout the body. Given the complexity of the system, it is not surprising that four different organs and at least two different hormones are needed to maintain calcium homeostasis around a desired "set point." The four key organs are the parathyroids, intestine, kidneys, and skeleton, whereas the most critical regulatory hormones are parathyroid hormone (PTH) and vitamin D. Magnesium and phosphorus, as well as calcitonin and fibroblast growth factor 23 (FGF-23) contribute to mineral homeostasis as well (Bringhurst, Demay, and Kronenberg, 2008; Shoback, Sellmeyer, and Bikle, 2007).

When serum calcium rises 2–3% above the genetically determined set point, homeostatic mechanisms are quickly activated to return the level to normal. First, at the parathyroid glands excess calcium acts via innumerable calcium sensing receptors (CaSRs) to immediately shut down PTH secretion. The CaSRs are G-protein-coupled transmembrane receptors that are exquisitely sensitive to changes in ionized calcium concentration (figure 49.1). Reduction in PTH decreases calcium resorption from bone, increases renal excretion of calcium at the distal tubule, and reduces the renal synthesis of calcitriol (1,25-dihydroxyvitamin D), thus decreasing the intestinal absorption of calcium. Activation of the CaSR at the kidneys by excess ionized calcium also directly inhibits tubular reabsorption of calcium and inhibits urinary concentrating ability in the distal collecting duct. In most cases the reduced bone resorption, combined with reduced GI calcium absorption and enhanced renal excretion of calcium, restores serum calcium to normal. Note that because the kidneys filter 10,000 mg of calcium per day, anything that impairs renal function will greatly impact the body's ability to regulate calcium loads. In the converse situation, when serum calcium falls by 2–3% below the desired set point, the opposite cascade occurs (figure 49.2): a drop in ionized calcium stimulates PTH release from the parathyroids; higher PTH increases calcium flux from bone, decreases renal excretion of calcium at the distal tubule, and stimulates the synthesis and secretion of calcitriol, enhancing absorption of calcium from the gut. Homeostasis is restored.

THE PARATHYROID GLANDS AND PARATHYROID HORMONE

The four parathyroid glands derive from the third and fourth branchial pouches and reside adjacent to the thyroid gland in the neck. They are very small, each weighing only about 40 g. The predominant epithelial cell in the parathyroid glands is called the "chief cell," which has a clear cytoplasm and is distinct from the larger oxyphil cell, which has an eosinophilic granular cytoplasm. Both cell types contain PTH.

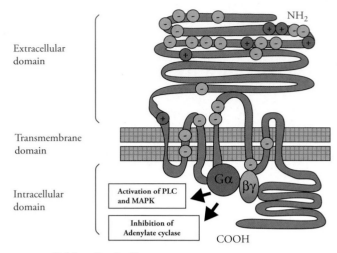

Extracellular domain

Transmembrane domain

Intracellular domain

Activation of PLC and MAPK

Inhibition of Adenylate cyclase

Figure 49.1. Calcium-Sensing Receptor.

The parathyroid cells "sense" the level of ionized calcium by way of the CaSRs that are expressed on the surface of the cells. The relationship between the extracellular ionized calcium concentration and PTH is a steep sigmoid curve in which small changes in ionized calcium produce marked changes in PTH (figure 49.3).

The initial effect of a decrease in extracellular ionized calcium is to stimulate the secretion of preformed PTH via exocytosis from storage granules in the parathyroid cells. Interestingly, most cells in the body *require calcium* to stimulate the process of exocytosis. How, then, can parathyroid cells release PTH via exocytosis in an environment of calcium deficiency? It appears that this critical role is played by intracellular *magnesium* in the parathyroid cells. This explains why severe prolonged magnesium deficiency essentially paralyzes PTH secretion, inducing reversible hypoparathyroidism. Interestingly, more moderate hypomagnesemia stimulates PTH secretion, whereas hypermagnesemia inhibits it, similar to the effects of hypo- and hypercalcemia (Shoback et al., 2007).

Changes in serum calcium regulate both the secretion of preformed PTH and the de novo synthesis of PTH at the level of gene transcription. Vitamin D also plays a role in PTH gene regulation in that high levels of calcitriol [1,25(OH)$_2$] inhibit PTH gene transcription. This allows calcitriol or vitamin D analogues to be used in the treatment of secondary hyperparathyroidism in patients with renal failure.

HYPERCALCEMIA

The differential diagnosis for hypercalcemia is shown in table 49.1. The first question to ask in any case of hypercalcemia is: what is the PTH level? If PTH is frankly high or even inappropriately "normal" in the setting of hypercalcemia, the diagnosis is primary hyperparathyroidism (PHPT). There are a few other diagnoses that should be considered. These include tertiary hyperparathyroidism (from chronic renal failure) and use of lithium or thiazides, possibilities that are easily eliminated. A fourth possibility is the very rare autosomal dominant condition known as familial benign hypercalcemia or familial hypocalciuric hypercalcemia (FHH). Individuals with FHH have inactivating mutations of the CaSR, rendering the receptor less sensitive or resistant to the ambient serum calcium concentration at both the parathyroids and kidneys. In other words, these individuals require *higher* serum calcium levels to maintain normal calcium homeostasis (Brown, 2007). The hallmark of FHH is an inappropriately low urinary calcium excretion that can be easily calculated using a simple formula:

$$CaCl/CrCl = (urinary\ calcium \times plasma\ creatinine)/(plasma\ calcium \times urinary\ creatinine)$$

Urine CaCl/CrCl <0.01 is consistent with FHH. These patients should not be sent for parathyroid surgery. Genetic

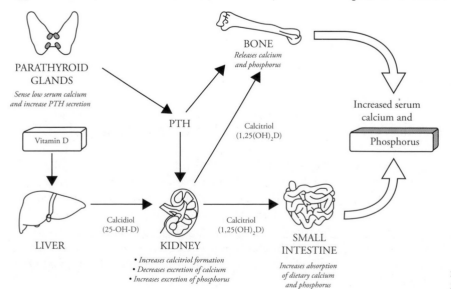

Figure 49.2. Calcium Homeostasis in Setting of Low Serum Calcium.

PARATHYROID GLANDS
Sense low serum calcium and increase PTH secretion

Vitamin D

PTH

Calcitriol (1,25(OH)$_2$D)

BONE
Releases calcium and phosphorus

Increased serum calcium and

Phosphorus

Calcidiol (25-OH-D)

Calcitriol (1,25(OH)$_2$D)

LIVER

KIDNEY
• *Increases calcitriol formation*
• *Decreases excretion of calcium*
• *Increases excretion of phosphorus*

SMALL INTESTINE
Increases absorption of dietary calcium and phosphorus

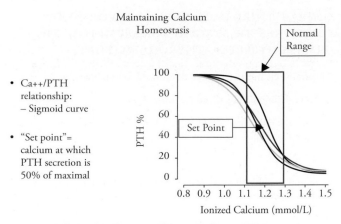

Maintaining Calcium Homeostasis

- Ca++/PTH relationship:
  - Sigmoid curve

- "Set point"= calcium at which PTH secretion is 50% of maximal

Figure 49.3. Relationship Between Changes in Serum Calcium and Intact PTH.

testing for mutations of the CaSR can be done if the diagnosis is uncertain.

PRIMARY HYPERPARATHYROIDISM

Primary hyperparathyroidism (HPT) accounts for 80–90% of hypercalcemia in asymptomatic individuals and is, by far, the most common cause of hypercalcemia in healthy outpatients. The vast majority (80%) of cases of PHPT are due to solitary adenomas. Around 15% of patients will have four-gland hyperplasia, and 2–4% will have multiple adenomas. Parathyroid hyperplasia is most commonly found in three autosomal-dominant inherited syndromes: multiple endocrine neoplasia (MEN) 1, MEN 2A, and isolated familial hyperparathyroidism. Parathyroid carcinoma represents less than 0.5% of cases.

The classic signs and symptoms of PHPT have been referred to as "stones, bones, abdominal groans, and psychic moans." These are listed in table 49.2. Prior to the introduction of multiphasic chemistry screening, most patients with PHPT presented with renal manifestations (stones, nephrocalcinosis, renal failure) and/or the classic bone disease, osteitis fibrosa cystica. Now, up to 85% of individuals with PHPT are asymptomatic. Kidney stones occur in fewer than 15% of patients with PHPT, whereas the most common bone disorder, osteoporosis, mainly affects skeletal sites rich in cortical bone (such as the distal one-third of the radius). Other manifestations of mild PHPT include dyspepsia, nausea, and constipation ("abdominal groans") as well as fatigue, lethargy, depression, and difficulty concentrating ("psychic moans"). Myalgias, muscle weakness, chondrocalcinosis, polyuria/polydipsia, and nocturia can also occur. Nonclassical manifestations of PHPT such as cardiovascular and neurological dysfunction are under active investigation at this time.

Laboratory findings in PHPT typically show elevated serum calcium (corrected for serum albumin) with a simultaneously elevated serum intact PTH. However, many patients with mild PHPT have serum calcium levels that

Table 49.1 **DIFFERENTIAL DIAGNOSIS OF HYPERCALCEMIA**

PTH-Mediated
Sporadic primary hyperparathyroidism
Familial syndromes
Associated with MEN 1 or 2A
Isolated familial hyperparathyroidism
Familial hypocalciuric hypercalcemia (FHH)
Parathyroid carcinoma
Tertiary hyperparathyroidism (in end-stage renal disease or post–renal transplant)
Drugs
Lithium
Thiazide diuretics

Non-PTH-Mediated
Absorptive
Milk-alkali syndrome
Resorptive (benign)
Hyperthyroidism
Immobilization
Vitamin A intoxication
Paget disease
Resorptive (malignant)
Humoral (PTHrP-mediated) hypercalcemia of malignancy
Solid tumors, especially squamous and renal cell carcinomas
Adult T-cell leukemias
Vitamin D [1,25(OH)$_2$D]-mediated
Lymphomas
Local osteolytic hypercalcemia
Multiple myeloma
Leukemia
Lymphoma
Metastatic breast cancer
Mixed (absorptive and resorptive)
Exogenous vitamin D intoxication
Endogenous vitamin D excess [1,25(OH)$_2$D-mediated]
Granulomatous diseases (sarcoidosis)
Lymphomas
Miscellaneous
Adrenal insufficiency
Pheochromocytoma
VIPoma

fluctuate in and out of the normal range. Similarly, serum PTH levels may be in the middle or upper level of normal range, although such levels are still "inappropriate" within the context of hypercalcemia. Even "low normal" PTH levels may be associated with PTH-secreting parathyroid adenomas (Lafferty, 2006). Serum phosphorus levels tend to be below 3.5 mg/dL due to the phosphaturic effect of PTH on the renal tubules. Note that concomitant vitamin D deficiency is very common in patients with PHPT and in some cases may "mask" the hypercalcemia. Recent guidelines recommend checking 25-hydroxyvitamin D levels in all patients with PHPT and correcting any deficiencies to maintain levels above 50 nmol/L (Eastell et al., 2009).

Parathyroidectomy remains the definitive treatment for PHPT. For individuals with mild, asymptomatic

Table 49.2 SIGNS AND SYMPTOMS OF PRIMARY HYPERPARATHYROIDISM

Stones
Renal stones
Nephrocalcinosis
Polyuria
Polydipsia
Uremia

Bones
Osteitis fibrosa cystica (subperiosteal resorption, osteoclastomas, bone cysts)
Osteoporosis and fractures
Osteomalacia or rickets
Arthritis

Abdominal Groans
Constipation
Indigestion, nausea, vomiting
Peptic ulcers
Pancreatitis

Psychic Moans
Lethargy, fatigue
Depression
Memory loss
Psychoses-paranoia
Personality change, neurosis
Confusion, stupor, coma

Other
Proximal muscle weakness
Keratitis, conjunctivitis
Itching
Hypertension?
Coronary artery disease?

SOURCE: Shoback et al. (2007).

Table 49.3 THIRD INTERNATIONAL WORKSHOP GUIDELINES FOR SURGERY FOR ASYMPTOMATIC PRIMARY HYPERPARATHYROIDISM (PHPT)

Creatinine clearance (calculated) reduced to <60 mL/min[a]

Serum calcium > 1 mg/dL above normal

Bone mineral density (BMD) T-score of −2.5 or lower at the spine, hip, or distal third of radius[b]

Age <50 years

Situations in which long-term medical surveillance is neither desired nor possible

NOTES:
[a] Some physicians still regard 24-hour urinary calcium excretion >400 mg as an indication for surgery.
[b] Consistent with the position established by the International Society for Clinical Densitometry, the use of Z-scores instead of T-scores is recommended in evaluating BMD in premenopausal women and men younger than 50 years.
SOURCE: Bilezikian et al. (2009).

of vitamin D deficiency, good hydration, and, in select cases, antiresorptive therapy with bisphosphonates or other anti-resorptive agents. The calcimimetic, cinacalcet, is FDA approved for secondary HPT and parathyroid cancer, but in recent trials, it has successfully controlled hypercalcemia in patients with PHPT for up to 3–5 years. Unfortunately, cinacalcet did not improve bone density in patients with PHPT even though serum calcium was normalized and PTH levels were reduced (Peacock, 2005; Peacock, 2010).

NON-PTH-MEDIATED HYPERCALCEMIA

Etiologies of non-PTH-mediated hypercalcemia can be divided into three broad categories: absorptive, resorptive, or mixed. Absorptive hypercalcemia, from excess calcium, is characterized by increased absorption of calcium from the gut. The best example of this is ingestion of excessive calcium carbonate leading to the milk-alkali syndrome. Mixed disorders with both absorptive and resorptive hypercalcemia include vitamin D–mediated hypercalcemia such as exogenous vitamin D intoxication or excess 1,25-dihydroxyvitamin

Table 49.4 GUIDELINES FOR FOLLOW-UP OF NONSURGICALLY TREATED PATIENTS WITH ASYMPTOMATIC PHPT

Serum calcium annually
24-hour urine calcium: not recommended
Creatinine clearance: not recommended
Serum creatinine: annually
Bone density: every 1–2 years (three sites)
Abdominal x-ray (ultrasound): not recommended

SOURCE: Bilezikian et al. (2009).

PHPT, a 2008 international workshop of experts developed guidelines for surgical intervention (Bilezikian, 2009) (table 49.3). Patients who do not meet any of these criteria (up to 50% in some series) may be monitored with annual serum calcium, serum creatinine, and bone mineral density (BMD) measurements every 1–2 years (see table 49.4). Longitudinal studies of patients with asymptomatic PHPT show remarkable biochemical stability over 10–15 years, although up to 25% ultimately require surgery. Following surgical cure of PHPT, there are dramatic improvements in BMD and 90–95% reduction in renal stone formation in those with previous nephrolithiasis (Silverberg et al., 1999; Bilezikian and Silverberg, 2004). Recent clinical trials randomizing subjects with PHPT to either parathyroidectomy or observation have found improvements in bone density in the surgical groups but variable effects on quality of life and symptoms (Bollerslev, 2007; Ambrogini, 2007).

For nonsurgical patients, medical management includes moderate calcium intake of 1000 mg/day (but lower in those with high calcitriol or high urinary calcium levels), correction

D production from activated macrophages in granulomatous diseases (e.g., sarcoidosis) or certain lymphomas.

Resorptive hypercalcemia occurs whenever excessive osteoclastic bone resorption is the primary mechanism underlying the hypercalcemia. Although a number of benign disorders may be associated with non-PTH-mediated resorptive hypercalcemia, (including hyperthyroidism, immobilization, Paget disease, vitamin A intoxication), the majority of cases are due to malignancies. Mechanisms of malignant hypercalcemia include local release of osteoclast-activating cytokines in bone (multiple myeloma), osteolytic destruction of bone from metastases (breast cancer), or PTHrP (parathyroid hormone–related peptide)-mediated skeletal resorption from distant tumors (squamous and renal cell carcinomas most commonly). Among inpatients with symptomatic hypercalcemia, 45% have malignancies, 25% have PHPT, and 10% have renal insufficiency. Remember that PHPT and malignancies may coexist in the same patient. In addition, there are a number of rare causes of hypercalcemia reported in the literature (Jacobs and Bilezikian, 2005).

Symptoms of hypercalcemia depend on the severity of the calcium elevation as well as the rapidity of the rise. In general, rapid rises in calcium cause more symptoms than slower, more gradual increases. Patients with non-PTH-mediated hypercalcemia tend to have more severe symptoms affecting the central nervous system (lethargy, psychosis, stupor, and coma), cardiovascular (bradycardia, asystole, and shortened QT intervals), and gastrointestinal (anorexia, nausea, vomiting, and constipation) systems.

Workup of the symptomatic patient with hypercalcemia requires a very careful history and physical examination, followed by judicious laboratory testing (table 49.5). Useful laboratory tests include routine CBC and chemistries, phosphorus, magnesium, intact-PTH, 25-hydroxy-vitamin D (the key test in vitamin D intoxication), 1,25-dihydroxyvitamin D (the key test in granulomatous diseases and some lymphomas), and SPEP and UPEP (multiple myeloma). Serum PTHrP is rarely needed to make the diagnosis of humoral hypercalcemia of malignancy but can be confirmative in cases where the primary tumor is elusive. Other useful tests can be chest x-ray, bone scan, mammography, computed tomography (CT) scans of chest/abdomen/pelvis, and lymph node or tissue biopsy.

Management of symptomatic, severe hypercalcemia, regardless of the cause, begins with vigorous hydration and restoration of the glomerular filtration rate to normal, if possible (table 49.6). This enhances renal clearance of calcium and reduces serum calcium substantially. Loop diuretics should be used to enhance renal calcium excretion only after euvolemia has been restored and are often unnecessary. In the milk-alkali syndrome, adequate hydration and cessation of the calcium source completely reverse the hypercalcemia. However, in most of the other conditions, antiresorptive therapy is needed to achieve and maintain normocalcemia. Intravenous bisphosphonates rapidly reduce resorptive and mixed hypercalcemia in the well-hydrated patient by causing apoptosis of activated osteoclasts. Either pamidronate or zoledronic acid may lower serum calcium to the normal range within a few days. Adverse side effects from IV bisphosphonates include acute-phase reactions, renal insufficiency, and hypocalcemia. Frequent, high-dose IV bisphosphonate therapy for malignant disease may result in osteonecrosis of the jaw. Finally, in patients with hypercalcemia from multiple myeloma, lymphoma, sarcoidosis, or vitamin A or D intoxication, glucocorticoids are extremely effective treatments. The success in treating non-PTH-mediated hypercalcemia ultimately depends on treatment of the underlying disorder (Stewart, 2005).

Table 49.6 MANAGEMENT OF ACUTE HYPERCALCEMIA

Fluids
0.9% NaCl IV
Loop diuretic in those with CHF or evidence of volume overload

Medications
Bisphosphonates
Pamidronate 60–90 mg IV
Zoledronic acid 4 mg IV
Calcitonin 4 IU/kg SC q 12 hours
Glucocorticoids 20–100 mg prednisone daily
Plicamycin 15–25 mg/kg IV
Gallium nitrate 200 mg/m²/day continuous infusion for 5 days
Cinacalcet 30–90 mg daily for PTH-mediated hypercalcemia

Other
Therapy directed at primary tumor
Surgery
Chemotherapy
Radiation
Decrease calcium and vitamin D intake
Maintain hydration
Mobilization

Table 49.5 WORKUP FOR NON-PTH-MEDIATED HYPERCALCEMIA

SPEP, UPEP	CXR
25(OH)-vitamin D	Bone scan
1,25(OH)$_2$-vitamin D	Mammography
Serum ACE (if indicated)	CT scan of chest, abdomen, pelvis
PTHrP (rarely necessary)	Lymph node or tissue biopsy
PSA (rarely; usually osteoblastic)	

HYPOCALCEMIA

Hypocalcemic disorders can result from a number of abnormalities of the calcium regulatory system: PTH deficiency, abnormal responsiveness to PTH, vitamin D disorders, or complexation or deposition of calcium (table 49.7). The rare inherited disorders of vitamin D resistance (vitamin D-dependent and vitamin D-resistant rickets) will not be discussed here. It is important to note that hypoalbuminemia results in low total serum calcium due to a reduction in the protein-bound fraction of calcium; however, ionized calcium remains normal.

Hypocalcemia may present dramatically with symptoms of perioral numbness, paresthesias, carpopedal spasm,

Table 49.7 DIFFERENTIAL DIAGNOSIS OF HYPOCALCEMIA

Hypoparathyroidism
Surgical
Idiopathic
Neonatal
Familial
Autoimmune
Metal deposition (iron, copper, aluminum)
Postradiation
Infiltrative
Functional (severe hypomagnesemia)
Abnormal regulation (CaSR mutations)

Resistance to PTH Action
Pseudohypoparathyroidism
Renal insufficiency

Medications that Prevent Osteoclastic Bone Resorption
Plicamycin
Calcitonin
Bisphosphonates

Vitamin D Disorders
Deficiency of 1,25-$(OH)_2$D
Renal failure
Severe substrate deficiency (malabsorption syndromes)
Hereditary vitamin D–dependent rickets, type 1 (deficiency of renal 1-alpha-hydroxylase)
Resistance to 1,25-$(OH)_2$D action
Hereditary vitamin D–dependent rickets, type 2 (defective vitamin D receptor)

Acute Complexation or Deposition of Calcium
Acute hyperphosphatemia
Crush injury with muscle necrosis
Rapid tumor lysis
Parenteral or enteral phosphate administration
Acute pancreatitis
Transfusions with citrated blood
Rapid, excessive skeletal mineralization
Hungry bones syndrome (postparathyroidectomy)
Osteoblastic metastases

SOURCE: Shoback et al. (2007).

seizures, or tetany or may be relatively asymptomatic. Most of the symptoms are due to increased neuromuscular excitability. The classic muscular manifestation of hypocalcemia is carpopedal spasm, a painful involuntary muscular contraction of the hands in which there is adduction of the thumb, flexion of the metacarpophalangeal joints, extension of the interphalangeal joints, and flexion of the wrists (figure 49.4). Tetany may also present as laryngospasm, which can be fatal. Latent tetany can be elicited by testing for Chvostek's sign (tapping on the facial nerve to produce contraction of the ipsilateral facial muscles) and Trousseau's sign (inflating a blood pressure cuff to 20 mm Hg above systolic pressure to elicit ipsilateral carpal spasm). Note that 25% of normal people can have a mild Chvostek's sign. In addition to tetany, other serious manifestations of hypocalcemia can include seizures and prolongation of the QT interval on electrocardiogram (EKG) testing (due to delay in repolarization), resulting in serious arrhythmias and congestive heart failure.

HYPOPARATHYROIDISM

Syndromes of hypocalcemia associated with low PTH levels include postsurgical hypoparathyroidism, "hungry-bone syndrome," following parathyroid surgery, hypomagnesemia, critical illness, autoimmune or infiltrative destruction of the parathyroid glands, as well as inherited disorders including autosomal dominant hypocalcemia (Marx, 2000). In this disorder, the "flip side" of FHH, *activating* mutations of the CaSR, result in increased sensitivity to calcium and a lower set point for Ca and PTH (Brown, 2007).

Surgical hypoparathyroidism is the most common cause of PTH deficiency. It results from removal or destruction of the parathyroid glands during surgery for cancer of the head or neck, total thyroidectomy, or parathyroidectomy. Laboratory studies show hypocalcemia, hyperphosphatemia, and undetectable PTH. Other causes of hypoparathyroidism such as autoimmune destruction of the parathyroid glands and inherited disorders (familial hypoparathyroidism, DiGeorge syndrome) are far less common. Infiltrative destruction of the parathyroids by iron (thalassemia), copper (Wilson disease), metastatic disease, or infections is also unusual.

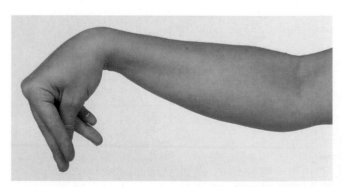

Figure 49.4. Carpal Spasm in Hypocalcemia.

An important and reversible cause of hypoparathyroidism is severe, chronic magnesium deficiency that paralyzes the secretion of PTH from vesicles in the parathyroid glands while blunting the peripheral actions of PTH. The hypocalcemia responds quickly to administration of magnesium.

PSEUDOHYPOPARATHYROIDISM

This category includes two inherited, rare disorders of target-organ resistance to PTH, referred to as PHP 1A and PHP 1B. Biochemically, the syndromes present exactly like hypoparathyroidism with hypocalcemia and hyperphosphatemia, but PTH is elevated rather than undetectable. PHP 1A is associated with a classic phenotype known as Albright hereditary osteodystrophy in which patients are short, have round faces, short necks, mental retardation, and shortening of the fourth and/or fifth metacarpals. Patients with PHP 1B have no somatic phenotype and otherwise appear normal. The genetic mutations and inheritance of both syndromes have now been fully elucidated.

VITAMIN D DEFICIENCY

Patients with hypocalcemia due to vitamin D deficiency have *elevated* PTH levels (so-called secondary hyperparathyroidism). The most common causes of vitamin D deficiency are shown in table 49.8. Note that hypocalcemia rarely occurs from depletion of 25-hydroxyvitamin D alone, even when levels are undetectable, due to the ability of high PTH levels to mobilize calcium from bone.

CHRONIC KIDNEY DISEASE

One of the most important causes of secondary hyperparathyroidism is chronic kidney disease (CKD). Patients on dialysis often have extremely elevated levels of PTH and PTH fragments (not all are bioactive) due to the decline in 1,25-dihydroxyvitamin D levels and increases in serum phosphate associated with progressive renal failure. The disordered mineral metabolism associated with CKD can result in renal osteodystrophy, soft tissue and vascular calcifications, cardiovascular disease, and high cardiovascular

Table 49.8 CAUSES OF VITAMIN D DEFICIENCY

Inadequate sun exposure
Inadequate dietary intake
Malabsorption syndromes
Anticonvulsants
Nephrotic syndrome
Chronic renal failure/end-stage renal disease
Inherited disorders (see table 49.7)

mortality. In the past the only treatments available for secondary hyperparathyroidism due to CKD were large doses of calcium to serve as phosphate binders as well as vitamin D sterols to lower PTH. These interventions often aggravated the abnormal mineral metabolism by increasing the calcium × phosphate product and worsening vascular and ectopic calcification. The calcimimetic, cinacalcet, has offered an attractive alternative to the traditional treatment of secondary hyperparathyroidism in CKD. By mimicking calcium at the CaSR, cinacalcet reduces PTH without raising serum calcium, phosphate, or the calcium × phosphate product. It has greatly improved calcium-phosphate homeostasis in patients on dialysis (Block, 2004).

MISCELLANEOUS

A number of other disorders can result in hypocalcemia including hyperphosphatemia from rhabdomyolysis or tumor lysis syndrome, calcium malabsorption from celiac disease or other malabsorption states, transfusions with citrated blood, widespread osteoblastic skeletal metastases, and acute pancreatitis, among others. Acute respiratory alkalosis from hyperventilation can cause symptomatic, reversible hypocalcemia due to a shift of ionized calcium onto albumin within the alkalotic environment.

TREATMENT

Treatment of hypocalcemia depends on the cause, the severity, and the degree of symptomatology but generally includes both calcium and vitamin D supplementation. Acute hypocalcemia associated with tetany or incipient tetany is a medical emergency and requires immediate intravenous calcium administration (table 49.9). Two to three ampules of calcium gluconate (90 mg elemental calcium per 10-mL ampule) can be given intravenously over several minutes followed by an infusion of 10 ampules in 1 L of IV fluids over 24 hours. Simultaneously, the patient should be started on calcitriol (activated vitamin D) and oral calcium. For chronic hypocalcemia due to hypoparathyroidism, the goal is to keep serum calcium in the 8.5–9.0 mg/dL range, high enough to prevent symptoms but low enough to avoid hypercalciuria. Periodic monitoring of 24-hour urinary calcium excretion is desirable to detect hypercalciuria. Treatment with thiazide diuretics can help reduce urinary calcium excretion. The goal is to maintain 24-hour urinary calcium levels below 4 mg/kg/day. At least 1.5–3.0 g of oral elemental calcium should be given daily in divided doses along with activated vitamin D (calcitriol). Large doses of ergocalciferol (vitamin D_2) or cholecalciferol (vitamin D_3) may be used in place of calcitriol but may accumulate and cause vitamin D intoxication. Clinical trials using teriparatide (PTH_{1-34}) in adults (Winer, 2003) and children (Winer, 2008) with hypoparathyroidism have shown promising results.

Table 49.9 MANAGEMENT OF HYPOCALCEMIA

Acute

2–3 ampules of calcium gluconate (90 mg elemental calcium per 10-mL ampule) IV, followed by

Infusion of 10 ampules calcium gluconate in 1 L of IV fluids over 24 hours

Calcitriol 0.25–1.0 μg PO daily

Calcium carbonate 1250 mg (500 mg elemental calcium per tab) 1–2 tabs tid with food

Correct Mg deficiency with parenteral magnesium

Chronic

Keep serum calcium in 8.5–9.0 mg/dL range

Monitor 24-hour urinary calcium excretion to detect hypercalciuria

Thiazide diuretics if significant hypercalciuria >4 mg/kg/day

1.5–3.0 g of oral elemental calcium daily in divided doses

Calcitriol 0.25–0.75 μg daily

ADDITIONAL READING

Ambrogini E, Cetani F, Cianferotti L, et al. Surgery or surveillance for mild asymptomatic primary hyperparathyroidism: a prospective, randomized clinical trial. *J Clin Endocrinol Metab.* 2007;92:3114–21.

Bilezikian JP, Khan AA, Potts JT, et al. Guidelines for the management of asymptomatic primary hyperparathyroidism: Summary statement from the third international workshop. *J Clin Endocrinol Metab.* 2009;94:335–9.

Bilezikian JP, Silverberg SJ. Asymptomatic primary hyperparathyroidism. *N Engl J Med.* 2004;350:1746–51.

Bilezikian JP, Potts JT Jr, Fuleihan Gel-H, et al. Summary statement from a workshop on asymptomatic primary hyperparathyroidism: A perspective for the 21st century. *J Clin Endocrinol Metab.* 2002;87:5353–61.

Block GA, Martin KJ, de Francisco AL, et al. Cinacalcet for secondary hyperparathyroidism in patients receiving hemodialysis. *N Engl J Med.* 2004;350:1516–25.

Bollerslev J, Jansson S, Mollerup CL, et a. Medical observation, compared with parathyroidectomy, for asymptomatic primary hyperparathyroidism: a prospective, randomized trial. *J Clin Endocrinol Metab.* 2007; 92:1687–92.

Bringhurst RF, Demay MB, Kronenberg HM. Hormones and disorders of mineral metabolism. In *Williams Textbook of Endocrinology* (pp. 1203–68). Philadelphia: Elsevier; 2008.

Brown EM. Clinical lessons from the calcium sensing receptor. *Nat Clin Pract Endocrinol Metab.* 2007;3(2):122–33.

Eastell R, Arnold A, Brandi L, et al. Diagnosis of asymptomatic primary hyperparathyroidism: Proceedings of the third international workshop. *J Clin Endocrinol Metab.* 2009;94:340–50.

Jacobs TP, Bilezikian JP. Rare causes of hypercalcemia. *J Clin Endocrinol Metab.* 2005;90:6316–22.

Lafferty FW, Hamlin CR, Corrado KR, Arnold A, Shuck JM. Primary hyperparathyroidism with a low-normal, atypical serum parathyroid hormone as shown by discordant immunoassay curves. *J Clin Endocrinol Metab.* 2006; 91:3826–9.

Peacock M, Bilezikian JP, Klassen PS, Guo MD, Turner SA, Shoback D. Cinacalcet hydrochloride maintains long-term normocalcemia in patients with primary hyperparathyroidism. *J Clin Endocrinol Metab.* 2005; 90:135–41.

Peacock M. Bilezikian JP, Bolognese MA, et al. Cinacalcet HCl reduces hypercalcemia in primary hyperparathyroidism across a wide specturm of disease severity. *J Clin Endocrinol Metab.* 2011; 96:E9–18.

Marx SJ. Hyperparathyroid and hypoparathyroid disorders. *N Engl J Med.* 2000;343:1863–75.

Shoback D, Sellmeyer D, Bikle DD. Metabolic bone disease. In *Greenspan's Basic and Clinical Endocrinology.* 8th ed. (pp. 281–345). New York: McGraw-Hill; 2007.

Silverberg SJ, Shane E, Jacobs TP, Siris E, Bilezikian JP. A 10-year prospective study of primary hyperparathyroidism with or without parathyroid surgery. *N Engl J Med.* 1999;341:1249–55.

Stewart AF. Clinical practice. Hypercalcemia associated with cancer. *N Engl J Med.* 2005;352:373–9.

Winer KK, Ko CW, Reynolds JC, et al. Long-term treatment of hypoparathyroidism: a randomized controlled study comparing parathyroid hormone (1-34) versus calcitriol and calcium. *J Clin Endocrinol Metab.* 2003;88:4214–20.

Winer KK, Sinaii N, Peterson D, Sainz B Jr, Cutler GB Jr. Effects of once versus twice-daily parathyroid hormone 1-34 therapy in children with hypoparathyroidism. *J Clin Endocrinol Metab.* 2008; 93:3389–95.

QUESTIONS

QUESTION 1. A 55-year-old woman has a routine physical. She entered menopause at age 52 and is doing well. She is not on any medications. She takes 500 mg calcium twice daily and has very little dairy in her diet. Review of systems reveals some fatigue.

Labs find calcium 10.8 mg/dL (normal 8.6–10.4) and albumin 4.0 g/L.

What is the next best step?

A. Check a 24-hour urine for calcium excretion.
B. Check PTH, SPEP, PTHrP, 1,25-D, and 25-OHD.
C. Repeat serum calcium and intact PTH.
D. Stop all calcium intake and repeat serum calcium in 2 months.

QUESTION 2. A 65-year-old woman is diagnosed with asymptomatic primary hyperparathyroidism. Her serum calcium is 11.0 mg/dL (normal 8.6–10.4) with intact PTH 85 pg/mL (normal 1–65 pg/mL). What should you order next?

A. Bone mineral density (including one-third distal radius)
B. 25-Hydroxyvitamin D
C. 1,25-Dihydroxyvitamin D
D. A and B
E. All of the above

QUESTION 3. A previously healthy 55-year-old man is brought to the hospital because of nausea, vomiting, lethargy, and severe back pain. Labs reveal serum calcium 15.8 mg/dL (8.6–10.4), PTH <10 pg/mL, creatinine 2.8 mg/dL, and Hct 35%.

In addition to checking vitamin D levels, what other key test should you order?

A. PTHrP
B. PSA
C. SPEP

D. Phosphate
E. 24-Hour urine calcium

QUESTION 4. A 43-year-old woman with ESRD on hemodialysis has serum calcium 11.4 mg/dL, intact PTH >1200 pg/mL, and evidence of osteitis fibrosa cystica on a skeletal survey. She is taken to surgery, where 3.5 parathyroid glands are removed. Postoperatively, her serum calcium plummets to 7.0 mg/dL with serum phosphate 2.0 mg/dL and magnesium 1.7 mEq/L. Despite treatment with high doses of oral calcium and calcitriol, she continues to require intravenous calcium infusions for over 5 days. What is the most likely cause of the persistent hypocalcemia?

A. Postoperative hypoparathyroidism
B. Hungry bone syndrome
C. Magnesium deficiency
D. 25-Hydroxyvitamin D deficiency
E. Adynamic bone disease

QUESTION 5. A 35-year-old man is admitted because of nausea, vomiting, and dizziness. He has had epigastric pain for several months and admits to excess alcohol intake. His only medication is Tums for "heartburn." On exam, he is alert and oriented × 3 with BP 120/60 mm Hg, P 110, epigastric tenderness, but is otherwise in no distress. Labs reveal serum calcium 16.8 mg/dL, HCO_3 38 mg/dL, intact PTH <10 pg/mL, and creatinine 3.0 mg/dL. The most likely cause of his hypercalcemia is

A. Milk alkali syndrome
B. Malignancy
C. Adrenal insufficiency
D. Renal failure

ANSWERS

1. C
2. D
3. C
4. B
5. A

50.

DIABETES MELLITUS

Rajesh K. Garg and Merri Pendergrass

Diabetes mellitus is one of the most challenging problems facing healthcare providers today. According to the Centers for Disease Control and Prevention (CDC), 24 million people or 8% of the U.S. population had diabetes in the year 2008. An additional 57 million Americans had prediabetes, a condition that substantially increases the risk for future type 2 diabetes.

The high prevalence of diabetes leads to a tremendous overall burden of disease because diabetes is associated with multiple complications including cardiovascular disease (CVD), blindness, renal failure, lower extremity amputations, adverse pregnancy outcomes, increase in fractures, and premature death. The financial cost is staggering, with one in five healthcare dollars spent on treating diabetes or its complications. The true burden of the disease actually exceeds cost estimates because they do not include the social cost of intangibles such as pain and suffering, care provided by nonpaid caregivers, excess medical costs associated with undiagnosed diabetes, and diabetes-attributed costs for healthcare expenditure categories not studied.

This chapter begins with a discussion of the diagnosis and classification of diabetes. Strategies to prevent diabetes and its complications are reviewed. The major focus of the presentation will be glucose management.

CLASSIFICATION

Diabetes mellitus is a group of metabolic abnormalities characterized by hyperglycemia that results from defects in insulin secretion, insulin action, or both (table 50.1). The vast majority of cases fall into two broad categories: type 1 diabetes (T1DM) and type 2 diabetes (T2DM). Some patients cannot be clearly classified into either category due to overlap between them (see table 50.2).

TYPE 1 DIABETES

Type 1 diabetes accounts for 5–10% of diabetes cases in the United States. The condition results from an absolute deficiency of insulin secretion, typically due to cellular-mediated auto-immune destruction of pancreatic beta-cells. Markers of the immune destruction include antibodies to biochemically characterized antigens such as insulin, glutamic acid decarboxylase (GAD), islet antigen 2 (IA-2), and zinc transporter 8 (ZnT8). One, and usually more, of these autoantibodies are present in the majority of patients at the time of diagnosis. A minority of patients with T1DM have no evidence of autoimmunity.

TYPE 2 DIABETES

Type 2 diabetes, which accounts for 90–95% of diabetes in the United States, is a heterogeneous disease resulting from multiple dysregulated metabolic pathways. The two major abnormalities are: (1) insulin resistance in skeletal muscle, liver, and adipocytes; and (2) a progressive decline in insulin secretion by beta-cells. Insulin resistance results from both environmental factors (e.g., obesity and physical inactivity) and genetic factors that have yet to be fully identified. Early in the natural history of T2DM, insulin-resistant prediabetic individuals compensate by secreting increased amounts of insulin. Insulin levels therefore tend to be high in prediabetes and early T2DM. As the capacity of the pancreas to secrete insulin deteriorates, endogenous insulin production is insufficient to overcome insulin resistance, and hyperglycemia ensues. In later stages of T2DM, insulin levels may be low or absent. Although T2DM is not thought of as an auto-immune disease, a small minority of patients with T2DM also have been shown to have diabetes-related autoantibodies, particularly to GAD. One explanation for this finding is that patients may have been misdiagnosed and actually have T1DM. These cases are increasingly referred to as *latent autoimmune diabetes of adults (LADA)*. Another possibility is that T1DM and T2DM represent two ends of a spectrum, with many patients having characteristics of both types.

GESTATIONAL DIABETES MELLITUS

Gestational diabetes mellitus (GDM) refers to glucose intolerance with onset or first recognition during pregnancy.

Table 50.1 CLASSIFICATION OF DIABETES MELLITUS

TYPE OF DIABETES	DESCRIPTION
Type 1 diabetes mellitus	Pancreatic beta-cell destruction (usually autoimmune) results in *absolute* insulin deficiency
Type 2 diabetes mellitus	Combination of (1) insulin resistance (which results in decreased peripheral glucose uptake and increased hepatic glucose production) and (2) *relative* insulin deficiency
Gestational diabetes mellitus	Any degree of glucose intolerance with onset or first recognition during pregnancy
Other specific types	Heterogeneous group of disorders including genetic disorders of beta-cell function or insulin action, exocrine pancreatic disorders, endocrinopathies, drug- or chemical-induced pancreatic processes, and infections

GDM complicates approximately 4% of pregnancies in the United States, with a prevalence ranging between 1% and 14%, depending on the population studied. Patients who develop GDM tend to have risk factors for T2DM, including older age, obesity, and nonwhite ethnicity. GDM is typically recognized during the third trimester and resolves following delivery. However, GDM is a strong risk factor for the future development of T2DM.

OTHER SPECIFIC TYPES

When diabetes occurs as the result of another medical condition, it is categorized as *secondary diabetes* or "another specific type." Examples include diseases of the exocrine pancreas (e.g., cystic fibrosis, chronic pancreatitis), endocrinopathies (e.g., Cushing syndrome), drug-induced (e.g., steroids, protease inhibitors, atypical antipsychotics, thiazides), genetic disorders of beta-cell function or insulin action, and uncommon immune-mediated forms (e.g., stiff-man syndrome).

DIAGNOSIS

DIABETES

Diabetes in nonpregnant patients may be diagnosed by one of the following ways: hemoglobin A1c (A1C), a fasting plasma glucose (FPG), oral glucose tolerance test (OGTT), or a random glucose value (table 50.3). Symptoms of hyperglycemia and random plasma glucose ≥200 mg/dL can be used to make the diagnosis without the need to repeat the test. For routine screening in asymptomatic people, A1C or FPG or OGTT may be used. The A1C, recently added to the diagnostic criteria of diabetes, is an attractive option because it can be obtained at any time of the day without fasting, is a measure of long-term glycemia, and can be used to make treatment decisions. In the absence of unequivocal hyperglycemia, a positive test for diabetes must be repeated and confirmed. The American Diabetes Association (ADA) recommends repeating the same test that was obtained in the first instance. For example, if A1C was obtained for screening and found to be abnormal, A1C should be repeated. If FPG was obtained for screening and found to be abnormal, then FPG should be repeated. However, if two abnormal results are already available from different tests (e.g., FPG and A1C), diagnosis may be made without repeating the tests.

There is no consensus about how to best screen and diagnose GDM. Various strategies are used, and all require an OGTT for the majority of patients. Screening is typically done at the beginning of the third trimester. Lower glucose cutoffs than the ones used for nonpregnant patients are used to make the diagnosis of GDM.

Table 50.2 CLINICAL CLUES TO TYPE 1 DIABETES VERSUS TYPE 2 DIABETES

	TYPE 1 DIABETES	TYPE 2 DIABETES
Age	~10% of newly diagnosed adults ~50% of newly diagnosed children	~90% of newly diagnosed adults ~50% of newly diagnosed children
Ethnicity	More common in non-Hispanic whites	More common in nonwhite groups
Weight	~20% overweight	~90% overweight
Family history	~10% with relative with diabetes	>50% with relative with diabetes
DKA	Frequently occurs	Sometimes occurs
Glucose levels	More variable	Less variable
Hypoglycemia	More frequent and severe	Less frequent and severe
Antibodies	Usually positive	Not usually positive
C-peptide	Usually low or undetectable	Usually detectable

Table 50.3 CATEGORIES OF GLUCOSE TOLERANCE

	FASTING PLASMA GLUCOSE (Mg/dL)	2-HOUR OGTT GLUCOSE (Mg/dL)	HBA1c (%)
Normal	≤100	≤140	<5.7
Categories of increased risk for diabetes	101–125	140–199	5.7–6.4
Diabetes	≥126	≥200	≥6.5

NOTE: OGTT, oral glucose tolerance test.

CATEGORIES OF RISK FOR DIABETES

The ADA recognizes an intermediate group of people whose glucose levels do not meet criteria for diabetes but still are too high to be considered normal (see table 50.3). These individuals were previous labeled as having "prediabetes" but are now simply called to be at risk for diabetes to avoid a distinct disease label. Other important risk factors for diabetes include advanced age, excess adiposity, sedentary lifestyle, family history of diabetes, high-risk ethnic group, history of gestational diabetes, hypertension, dyslipidemia, polycystic ovarian syndrome, and history of vascular disease (see table 50.4).

Stress Hyperglycemia

Although the ADA does not define stress hyperglycemia as a unique category, this term is frequently used to describe the transient elevation of the blood glucose that occurs in some individuals during a serious acute illness. Stress hyperglycemia is strongly associated with poor outcomes in hospitalized patients. Although stress hyperglycemia

Table 50.4 RISK FACTORS FOR TYPE 2 DIABETES

- Overweight or obese (BMI >25 kg/m²)
- Physical inactivity
- First-degree relative with diabetes
- Members of a high-risk ethnic population (e.g., African American, Latino, Native American, Asian American, and Pacific Islander)
- Women who delivered a baby weighing >9 lb or were diagnosed with GDM
- Hypertension (>140/90 mm Hg or on therapy for hypertension)
- HDL cholesterol level < 35 mg/dL (0.90 mmol/L) and/or a triglyceride level >250 mg/dL (2.82 mmol/L)
- Women with polycystic ovarian syndrome (PCOS)
- IGT or IFG on previous testing
- Other clinical conditions associated with insulin resistance (e.g., severe obesity and acanthosis nigricans)
- History of CVD

resolves with resolution of the acute illness, patients who experience hyperglycemia in the setting of stress appear to be at increased risk for the future development of T2DM. Regular screening for diabetes should be incorporated into their subsequent medical care.

SCREENING FOR DIABETES

Periodic screening for T2DM is recommended in asymptomatic adults who are overweight and have one or more of additional risk factors, as shown in table 50.4. In individuals without these risk factors, testing should begin at age 45. If tests are normal, repeat testing should be carried out at least every 3 years.

PREVENTION OF DIABETES AND ITS COMPLICATIONS

PREVENTION OF TYPE 1 DIABETES

Multiple strategies to prevent T1DM, for example, parenteral insulin, oral insulin, and oral nicotinamide, have been evaluated in large randomized controlled trials. Unfortunately, no strategy has been found to be effective. Nevertheless, this remains an area of intense investigation. Additional trials aimed to prevent T1DM or to delay the progressive loss of beta-cell function in newly diagnosed patients are currently in progress.

PREVENTION OF T2DM

The major T2DM prevention trials are summarized in table 50.5. Although lifestyle changes and pharmacologic treatment have been shown to reduce rates of progression to T2DM among high-risk patients, it remains unknown whether these interventions truly prevent diabetes or simply delay its inevitable diagnosis. Lifestyle modification, with a goal of achieving moderate weight loss (~5–10% body weight) and regular physical activity (~30 min per day of moderately increased physical activity), remains the preferred approach to diabetes prevention for most patients. However, because lifestyle modification is difficult

Table 50.5 MAJOR TYPE 2 DIABETES PREVENTION TRIALS

STUDY	NUMBER OF SUBJECTS	ENTRY CRITERIA	INTERVENTION(S)	RELATIVE RISK REDUCTION
Finnish Diabetes Prevention Study	522	IGT	Lifestyle modification	58%
Diabetes Prevention Program (DPP)	3234	IGT	Lifestyle modification Metformin	Lifestyle modification: 58% Metformin: 31%
Study to Prevent Non-Insulin-Dependent Diabetes Mellitus (STOP-NIDDM)	1429	IGT	Acarbose	25%
Troglitazone in Prevention of Diabetes (TRIPOD)	266	Hispanic women with previous GDM (70% with IGT)	Troglitazone	55%
Diabetes Reduction Assessment with Ramipril and Rosiglitazone Medication (DREAM)	5269	IFG or IGT	Rosiglitazone Ramipril	Rosiglitazone: 60% Ramipril: not significant
Nateglinide and Valsartan in the Prevention of Diabetes and Cardiovascular Outcomes (NAVIGATOR)	9306	IGT	Valsartan Nateglinide	Valsartan: 14% Nateglinide: not significant

NOTES: IGT, impaired glucose tolerance; GDM, gestational diabetes mellitus.

to achieve and maintain, metformin is recommended for certain very high-risk patients, as shown in table 50.6.

STRATEGIES FOR PREVENTION OF DIABETES COMPLICATIONS

Diabetes complications are generally categorized as resulting from microvascular disease (i.e., retinopathy, neuropathy, nephropathy) or macrovascular disease (i.e., CVD, peripheral vascular disease, cerebrovascular disease).

Glycemic Control

Improved glycemic control clearly reduces diabetes microvascular complications in both T1DM and T2DM. Potential benefits of glycemic control on macrovascular

Table 50.6 THERAPY FOR DIABETES PREVENTION

POPULATION	TREATMENT
IFG or IGT or A1C 5.7–6.0%	Lifestyle modification (i.e., 5–10% weight loss and ~30 min/day moderately intense physical activity)
IFG and IGT and any of the following: • Age < 60 years • BMI > 35 kg/m² • First-degree relative with diabetes • Triglycerides > 250 mg/dL • HDL < 35 mg/dL • A1C > 6%	Lifestyle modification and/or metformin (850 mg bid)

disease are not as well established and appear to be more modest.

In the Diabetes Control and Complications Trial (DCCT), intensive glycemic control in T1DM (A1C 7.2% versus 9.1%) reduced the risk of retinopathy by 76%, the risk of microalbuminuria by 34%, and the risk of neuropathy by 69%. Although CVD event rates were not reduced in the initial study, observational follow-up studies of DCCT participants 6–10 years after completion of the initial trial revealed significant reductions in CVD among the participants who had originally been assigned to intensive therapy.

In the United Kingdom Prospective Diabetes Study (UKPDS) of patients with newly diagnosed T2DM, a 1% reduction in A1C was associated with a 25% reduction in microvascular complications in the intensively treated group (median A1C = 7.0%) compared with the conventionally treated group (median A1C = 7.9%) after 10 years of follow-up. There was a nonsignificant ($p = 0.052$) trend for a 16% reduction in myocardial infarction in the intensively treated group, but the rate of myocardial infarction was significantly reduced in patients treated with metformin ($p = 0.01$). Further follow-up of UKPDS patients for 10 years after the end of the main study showed a significant reduction in myocardial infarction in patients treated with sulfonylureas and insulin as well ($p = 0.01$).

Glycemic Goals

Recommended glycemic goals for nonpregnant adults are shown in table 50.7. A1C, a measure of long-term glycemic

Table 50.7 SUMMARY OF TREATMENT GOALS

Glycemic control	
A1C	<7.0%*
Preprandial plasma glucose	70–130 mg/dL
Peak postprandial plasma glucose	<180 mg/dL
Blood Pressure	<130/80 mm Hg
Lipids	
LDL	<100 mg/dL
Triglycerides	<150 mg/dL
HDL	>40 mg/dL

NOTE: *Referenced to a DCCT-based assay.

control, is the primary predictor of diabetes complications and therefore the primary target of therapy. Some surrogate measures of CVD, such as endothelial dysfunction, may be associated with increased postprandial glucose, independent of fasting glucose levels. However, no interventional studies have proven that specifically targeting postprandial hyperglycemia will improve outcomes. It is therefore recommended that postprandial glucose should only be targeted for treatment with a goal of reducing the A1C.

The glycemic goals outlined in table 50.7 should be interpreted as general guidelines. Available data do not identify the optimal level of control for individual patients. Epidemiologic studies suggest a continuous association between A1C and diabetic complications without any threshold. Thus, there may be incremental (albeit, small) benefit to lowering A1C from 7% into the normal range in selected patients if achieved without significant hypoglycemia or lifestyle burden. On the other hand, some patients may have greater risks associated with hypoglycemia, weight gain, and other adverse effects of antihyperglycemic therapies. Recently, three large clinical trials (Action to Control Cardiovascular Risk in Diabetes [ACCORD], Action in Diabetes and Vascular Disease: Preterax and Diamicron Modified Release Controlled Evaluation [ADVANCE], and Veterans Affairs Diabetes Trial [VADT]) failed to show benefits of targeting A1C into the normal range (<6–6.5%) in type 2 diabetic patients with CVD or at high risk of CVD. In fact, the ACCORD trial was stopped prematurely due to increased mortality in the intensive treatment group. Patients enrolled in these trials were older, had been diagnosed with diabetes for about 10 years, and had multiple comorbidities. Less stringent treatment goals therefore may be appropriate for patients with limited life expectancies or serious comorbid conditions.

TREATMENT OF CARDIOVASCULAR RISK FACTORS

Aggressive treatment of established CVD risk factors remains an essential component of diabetes management (see table 50.7). Diabetes is widely considered a coronary heart disease risk equivalent, and patients with diabetes should be treated with the same aggressive therapy that is recommended for nondiabetic patients with known CVD. Adequate treatment of hypertension and dyslipidemia is as important as the treatment of hyperglycemia. Aspirin therapy for primary prevention is generally recommended only in diabetic men >50 years of age and women >60 years of age with another cardiovascular risk factor (i.e., hypertension, family history, dyslipidemia, microalbuminuria, cardiac autonomic neuropathy, or smoking). Treatment of CVD risk factors is presented in detail in other chapters and not discussed further here.

PREVENTIVE CARE PRACTICES

In addition to optimizing glycemic control and CVD risk factors, other diabetes preventive care practices should be performed. Annual eye, foot, dental, microalbumin, and creatinine clearance examinations are recommended. Annual influenza vaccine is recommended for all patients >6 months of age. At least one lifetime pneumococcal vaccine is recommended for adults ≥2 years of age, with a one-time revaccination for individuals >64 years of age if the last vaccine was administered when they were <65 years and it is >5 years since the administration.

TREATMENT OF HYPERGLYCEMIA

Treatment of hyperglycemia in nonpregnant adults is reviewed in this section.

Treatment for secondary forms of diabetes should be targeted at the underlying cause. If this is not possible, treatment strategies are similar to those outlined here for T1DM and T2DM.

Type 1 Diabetes

Insulin

Because patients with T1DM make little or no insulin, treatment is initiated with a goal of mimicking physiological insulin patterns as closely as possible. This is achieved by using multiple daily injections (MDI) of insulins with different times of onset and durations of action (table 50.8) or insulin-pump therapy. Although it has been proposed that pharmacokinetic properties of insulin analogues may translate into improved clinical efficacy, this has not been convincingly demonstrated in clinical trials. Recent meta-analyses of published clinical trials suggest that, compared with human regular insulin, the rapid-acting analogues (lispro, aspart, glulisine) provide only a small advantage in terms of A1C reductions and no advantage for hypoglycemia. Compared with human NPH insulin, basal analogues (glargine and detemir) have no advantage for A1C and only minor reductions in nocturnal hypoglycemia.

Table 50.8 APPROXIMATE DURATION OF ACTION OF INSULIN PREPARATIONS

	INSULIN	ONSET OF ACTION	PEAK ACTION	DURATION OF ACTION
Bolus	Rapid-acting			
	Insulin aspart (Novolog®)	5–15 min	30–90 min	<5 hours
	Insulin lispro (Humalog®)	5–15 min	30–90 min	<5 hours
	Insulin glulisine (Apidra®)	5–15 min	30–90 min	<5 hours
	Short-acting			
	Human regular insulin	30–60 min	2–3 hours	5–8 hours
Basal	Intermediate-acting			
	Human NPH insulin	2–4 hours	4–10 hours	10–16 hours
	Long-acting			
	Insulin glargine (Lantus®)	2–4 hours	None	20–24 hours
	Insulin detemir (Levemir®)	2–4 hours	None	14–20 hours

Effective regimens in T1DM usually consist of at least one daily injection of basal insulin in addition to injections of rapid-acting insulin given before each meal. There are three components of effective insulin regimens for patients with T1DM: (1) *basal insulin,* which is used to suppress hepatic glucose production and control glucose levels in the fasting state and between meals; (2) *nutritional insulin,* which is used to control the hyperglycemia that results from nutritional sources; and (3) *supplemental insulin* boluses, which are used to correct hyperglycemia that occurs despite basal and nutritional insulin treatment. Basal insulin is typically provided by an intermediate- to long-acting preparation (i.e., NPH, glargine, or detemir), which is usually administered once or twice daily. Nutritional and supplemental insulin is typically provided by a short- (i.e., regular) or rapid-acting (i.e., lispro, aspart, or glulisine) insulin preparation administered before meals. Continuously infused short- or rapid-acting insulin delivered subcutaneously via an insulin pump also can be used to provide basal insulin coverage. Nutritional and supplemental insulin boluses are administered via the pump as well. The choice between MDI and insulin pump therapy depends on multiple considerations including cost, patient preference, and an individual's personal glycemic profile. Neither strategy can be considered superior for all patients.

A person with T1DM requires approximately 0.5–0.7 units/kg/day of insulin. However, the total daily dose (TDD) of insulin required for treatment of T1DM is highly variable. The TDD should be divided into its two main components: approximately half of the TDD should be given as basal insulin and approximately half of the TDD should be given as nutritional insulin (with the nutritional insulin divided among the different meals) (figure 50.1). Frequent insulin adjustments based on fasting, premeal, and post-meal blood glucose values must be made in order to achieve and maintain euglycemia. Continuous glucose monitoring devices may be helpful in selective type 1 diabetic patients.

Amylin Analogues

Pramlintide, a synthetic analogue of amylin, is an injectable agent approved for use in both T1DM and T2DM. Amylin is a hormone that is synthesized by pancreatic beta-cells and cosecreted with insulin in response to a meal. It slows gastric emptying, suppresses postprandial glucagon secretion, and increases satiety. Fixed-dose injections of pramlintide added to premeal insulin lead to mild reductions in A1C (~0.3%) and weight loss. Pramlintide does not cause hypoglycemia by itself, but it can increase the risk imparted by coadministered insulin. The main adverse effect is dose-dependent nausea.

Type 2 Diabetes

Lifestyle Measures

Diet and exercise are central components of any therapeutic regimen. Healthy eating and a physically active lifestyle improve insulin sensitivity and allow endogenous or exogenous insulin to exert a greater glucose-lowering effect.

Initial Insulin Regimen for T1DM

Estimate* Total Daily Dose (TDD)

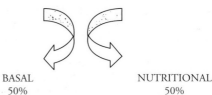

BASAL	NUTRITIONAL
50%	50%

*0.5–0.7 units/kg/day

Figure 50.1. Initial Insulin Regimen for T1DM.

Diet. It is recommended that the term "ADA diet" no longer be used because the ADA no longer endorses a single nutrition plan. Meal plans should be individualized to accommodate personal preferences, medication regimens, provide flexibility, and accommodate lifestyle, age, and overall health status.

Because most patients with T2DM are overweight, the primary dietary strategy to optimize glycemic control is decreased calorie intake to promote weight reduction. ADA nutritional guidelines do not give specific targets for the amounts of dietary carbohydrate, protein, and fat. They encourage patients to make healthy choices from a wide variety of foods. Monitoring carbohydrate, whether by carbohydrate counting, exchanges, or experience-based estimation, remains a key strategy in achieving glycemic control. However, carbohydrate restriction should not routinely be recommended for all patients. A diet that includes carbohydrates from fruits, vegetables, whole grains, legumes, and low-fat milk is encouraged because excessive elimination of carbohydrates reduces important nutrient intake and diet palatability.

Exercise. Exercise in diabetes is associated with potential risks as well as benefits. Patients should be counseled about what types of exercises can be performed and how much exercise is recommended. A pre-exercise evaluation should be conducted to determine whether the patient has any long-term diabetes complications that may constitute a contraindication for certain exercises. For example, patients with severe diabetic retinopathy should exercise caution with exercises that involve Valsalva (e.g., lifting heavy weights), pounding (e.g., tennis), or contact sports (e.g., boxing). Patients with severe peripheral neuropathy should avoid repetitive stepping exercise (e.g., jogging), which may increase the risk of a foot ulcer. Because of the high prevalence of CVD in patients with diabetes, all patients should be assessed to determine whether formal cardiac testing is indicated. Those with typical or atypical cardiac symptoms or an abnormal resting ECG should undergo further cardiac testing. There is no clinical utility of screening asymptomatic diabetic patients for CAD.

In the absence of contraindications, the exercise program should include both aerobic and resistance exercises (table 50.9). Patients also should be counseled about how to coordinate timing of exercise, meals, medications, and glucose monitoring. Fortunately, low- to moderate-intensity exercise, such as walking, has been shown to have significant benefits and minimal associated risks. As long as there are no contraindications, the benefits of walking almost certainly outweigh the risks in the majority of people with diabetes. Nevertheless, high-risk patients should be encouraged to start with short periods of low-intensity exercise and increase the intensity and duration slowly.

Noninsulin Therapies

Nine different classes of medication, in addition to insulin and pramlintide, are currently approved specifically for treatment of hyperglycemia in T2DM (table 50.10). Beneficial effects of antihyperglycemic agents appear to be mediated predominantly through their ability to lower blood glucose. There is no conclusive evidence that any particular agent (or treatment strategy) has any advantages, beyond glucose lowering, in terms of reducing cardiovascular endpoints.

Unfortunately, there are few high-quality, head-to-head comparison trials evaluating the ability of available agents to achieve recommended glycemic targets. This is important because the glucose-lowering effectiveness of individual medications is strongly influenced by patient baseline characteristics such as A1C, duration of diabetes, and previous therapy. With these limitations in mind, the relative glucose-lowering effectiveness of available agents is shown in table 50.11.

Biguanides. Metformin, the only biguanide available in the United States, works primarily by decreasing hepatic glucose production. The ADA recommends that metformin be prescribed at the time of diabetes diagnosis, concurrent with lifestyle modification. This is based on the fact that (1) lifestyle interventions typically fail to achieve or maintain goals, and (2) metformin is a potent glucose-lowering agent that has a low cost and few side effects. Metformin has the advantages of not causing hypoglycemia and being associated with weight loss. The most common adverse effects are gastrointestinal. Lactic acidosis, a potentially fatal adverse effect, is extremely rare and is associated almost exclusively with other risk factors such as renal or hepatic disease.

Sulfonylureas. Sulfonylureas (SUs) reduce blood glucose levels by stimulating insulin secretion by the pancreatic beta-cells. The combination of their proven efficacy, low incidence of adverse events, and low cost has contributed

Table 50.9 SUMMARY OF ADA EXERCISE RECOMMENDATIONS

TYPE	FREQUENCY	AMOUNT
Aerobic	3 days/week No more than 2 consecutive days without exercise	150 min/week moderate-intensity (50–70% of HR_{max}) OR 90 min/week vigorous-intensity (>70% of HR_{max})
Resistance	3 days/week for all muscle groups (i.e., hip and legs, chest, shoulders, back, arms, abdominal muscle groups)	Progress to 3 sets of 8–10 repetitions at a weight that cannot be lifted >8–10 times

Table 50.10 MECHANISMS OF ACTION

CLASS	MECHANISM OF ACTION
Biguanides	Decrease glucose production (liver)
Sulfonylureas	Increase insulin secretion (pancreas)
Glinides	Increase insulin secretion (pancreas)
Thiazolidinediones	Increase glucose uptake (muscle, fat)
α-Glucosidase inhibitors	Delay carbohydrate absorption (gut)
Gliptins	Prolongs effect of GLP-1 ($\uparrow$ insulin, $\downarrow$ glucagon, $\uparrow$ satiety)
Incretin mimetics	Similar effects as GLP-1 ($\uparrow$ insulin, $\downarrow$ glucagon, $\uparrow$ satiety, delays gastric emptying)
Amylin analogues	Similar effects as amylin ($\downarrow$ glucagon, $\uparrow$ satiety, delays gastric emptying)
Bile acid sequestrants	Not known
Bromocriptine	Not known

to their success and continued use. First-generation SUs (acetohexamide, chlorpropamide, tolbutamide) should not be used because of increased risk of hypoglycemia and drug interactions. Second-generation SUs (glipizide, glyburide, and glimepiride) are the most common agents added to initial treatment with metformin. The major adverse effect of SU treatment is hypoglycemia, which appears to occur most frequently in the elderly. A weight gain of approximately 2 kg is commonly associated with SU therapy, and this potentially could have an adverse impact on CVD risk. However, increased CVD risk with SUs has not been established.

Glinides. Two agents, repaglinide and nateglinide, are available in this class. Like SUs, they stimulate insulin secretion by binding to the SU receptor. They have a more rapid onset and shorter duration of action than the SUs and are designed to target postprandial hyperglycemia. They should be taken just prior to meals. Compared to SUs, the risk for hypoglycemia is similar with repaglinide but less frequent with nateglinide. Glinides are not commonly used in the United States because of their higher cost, more frequent dosing, and reduced efficacy (nateglinide) compared to SUs.

Thiazolidinediones. Two thiazolidinediones (glitazones or TZDs), rosiglitazone and pioglitazone, are currently available. They improve glycemia primarily by increasing insulin-mediated glucose uptake in muscle and adipocytes. To a lesser extent they decrease hepatic glucose production. Like metformin, TZDs do not cause hypoglycemia when used as monotherapy. The major side effects of TZDs are weight gain and fluid retention. The fluid retention typically manifests as peripheral edema, although new or worsened congestive heart failure can occur. There has been considerable interest regarding the effect of TZDs on cardiovascular risk. A meta-analysis suggested an increased risk of CVD with rosiglitazone. Another recent meta-analysis showed increased risk of myocardial infarction in association with rosiglitazone use and led the FDA to restrict its sales to patients either currently benefiting from its use or unable to achieve adequate diabetes control with other antidiabetic agents and unwilling or unable to take pioglitazone. Prescribers and patients must enroll into the rosiglitazone medicine access program as part of the FDA's risk evaluation and mitigation strategy. The drug is then delivered to patients by a restricted number of pharmacies. However, a large clinical trial suggested against this possibility. Clinical trial data suggest some cardioprotective effects of pioglitazone. Both agents may increase the risk of fracture, which is greater in diabetic than nondiabetic patients.

Alpha-glucosidase inhibitors. Acarbose and miglitol are the two agents in the alpha-glucosidase inhibitor (AGI) class of antihyperglycemic compounds. Alpha-glucosidase inhibitors reduce the rate of digestion of polysaccharides in the proximal small intestine. When used before meals, they delay the absorption of complex carbohydrates and blunt postprandial hyperglycemia, resulting in modest reductions in A1C. They are not associated with weight changes or hypoglycemia. AGIs are infrequently used in the United States. The main limitations to their widespread use are the need for frequent dosing, poor tolerability due to frequent gastrointestinal side effects, and only modest antihyperglycemic effects.

Incretin (GLP-1) agonists. Exenatide and liraglutide are members of this class of agents that work through the incretin system. Both these drugs are resistant to degradation by dipeptidyl peptidase IV (DPP-IV), the enzyme that normally inactivates GLP-1. Both agents enhance glucose-dependent insulin secretion, suppress glucagon secretion, slow gastric emptying, and reduce food intake. These drugs do not cause hypoglycemia by themselves and are associated with weight loss. The major limitations are the relatively high frequency of gastrointestinal side effects and the requirement for injections once (liraglutide) or twice (exenatide) daily. Intriguing results in animal studies suggest that GLP-1 agonists may preserve beta-cell function. There are some concerns about

Table 50.11 PRESCRIBING CONSIDERATIONS

CLASS AGENT (TRADE NAME)	A1C LOWERING* (%)	DOSING CHARACTERISTICS		PRIMARY PRECAUTIONS/ CONTRAINDICATIONS	HYPO GLYCEMIA	PRIMARY ADVERSE EFFECTS	BODY WEIGHT
		ROUTE	FREQUENCY				
Biguanides Metformin (Glucophage®)	1–2	Oral	qd-bid	Creatinine >1.5 man, >1.4 woman Acute, unstable illness	No	Diarrhea	Decreases
Sulfonylureas Glipizide, Glyburide, Glimepiride, Others	1–2	Oral	qd-bid	Predisposition to hypoglycemia	Yes	Hypoglycemia	Increases
Glinides Repaglinide (Prandin®) Nateglinide (Starlix®)	1.0–1.5	Oral	tid ac	Predisposition to hypoglycemia	Yes	Hypoglycemia	Increases
Thiazolidinediones Pioglitazone (Actos®) Rosiglitazone (Avandia®)	0.5–1.4	Oral	qd-bid	ALT >25 times ULN CHF	No	Edema/CHF Fractures Potential ↑ or ↓ MI (see text)	Increases
Alpha-glucosidase inhibitors Acarbose (Precose) Miglitol (Glycet)	0.5–0.8	Oral	tid ac	Chronic intestinal disorders Cirrhosis Creatinine >2.0	No	Flatulence	Neutral
Gliptins Sitagliptin (Januvia) Saxagliptin (Onglyza) Linagliptin (Tadjenta)	0.5–0.8	Oral	qd	None	No	Rare	Neutral
Incretin agonists Exenatide (Byetta) Liraglutide (Victoza)	0.5–1.0	Parenteral	qd-bid	Severe renal insufficiency (CrCl <30) Pancreatitis Personal or family history of medullary thyroid carcinoma (liraglutide only)	No	Nausea	Decreases
Amylin analogues Pramlintide (Symlin)	0.5–1.0	Parenteral	tid	None	No	Nausea	Decreases
Bile acid sequestrants Colesevelam (Welchol)	0.5	Oral	qd-bid	Very high triglyceride levels	No	Rare	Neutral
Bromocriptine Cycloset	0.3–0.4	Oral	qd	None	No	Nausea	Neutral

NOTE: *Values shown are approximations. Greater A1C reductions are expected with higher baseline A1C values and in drug-naïve patients.

the association of GLP-1 agonists with acute pancreatitis and acute renal failure and also the association of liraglutide with medullary thyroid carcinoma.

Dipeptidyl peptidase IV inhibitors. Sitagliptin, linagliptin, and saxagliptin are currently approved in the United States. By inhibiting DPP-IV these agents prolong the glucoregulatory actions of GLP-1. DPP-IV inhibitors modestly reduce A1C levels, are generally very well tolerated, are not associated with hypoglycemia, and are weight neutral. Despite these attractive properties, which have been demonstrated in short-term studies, the long-term effects of these agents remain unknown. DPP-IV is present in multiple other biological systems, including ones involved in immunity and other hormones. This raises the theoretical risk that inhibition of DPP-IV may adversely affect functioning of other systems.

Bile acid sequestrants. Colesevelam, a bile acid sequestrant that has been used for some time as a lipid-lowering agent, received FDA approval for the indication of improvement of glycemic control in patients with T2DM. The exact mechanism by which colesevelam improves glycemic control is unknown. It has been shown to reduce A1C levels by approximately 0.3%, relative to baseline.

Bromocriptine. Bromocriptine was recently approved for treatment of T2DM. Its mechanism of action for the glucose-lowering effect is not clear but involves dopaminergic effects in the hypothalamus. It has been shown to reduce A1C levels by 0.4%, compared to placebo.

Insulin. In contrast to patients with T1DM, most patients with T2DM secrete some endogenous insulin. Because of this, they frequently can be controlled with only a single daily injection of insulin. Their endogenous insulin secretion helps fine-tune their glycemic control. In later stages of T2DM, patients may make very little insulin. Thus, they may require multiple daily injections of insulin, similar to the regimens used for T1DM.

The most widely recommended strategy for initiating insulin in T2DM is to add a single bedtime injection of basal insulin (i.e., NPH, glargine, detemir) to the patient's oral medications (table 50.12). This regimen has been found to be effective in numerous studies and controls hyperglycemia in up to 60% of patients. Despite a prevailing misconception that NPH must be given twice a day, it has long been recognized that, in T2DM, a single daily injection of NPH yields similar improvements in control as two daily injections. Other possibilities for initial insulin therapy include adding a single injection of glargine or detemir in the morning, or premix insulin at suppertime. Although initial treatment with multiple daily injections of insulin also may be effective, this strategy has not been shown to be superior to a single injection and may be less acceptable to patients. If the patient is treated with a single bedtime injection of insulin and the fasting glucose level is within the target range, but the A1C level remains above goal, additional insulin injections are likely to be beneficial. Additional injections

Table 50.12 EXAMPLE STRATEGY FOR INSULIN INITIATION AND ADVANCEMENT IN TYPE 2 DIABETES

1. Start basal insulin (e.g., 10 units NPH or glargine or detemir) at bedtime

2. Continue metformin. Stop all other antihyperglycemic medications.

3. Have patient check daily FBG

4. Increase insulin frequently (e.g., every few days) until the FBG averages <100 mg/dL

5. If A1C remains above goal, and FBG has been ~70–130 mg/dL for 2–3 months,
   - Add premeal rapid-acting insulin before the largest meal of the day
   - Increase premeal insulin frequently until BG 1–2 hours after meal is below 180 mg/dL

6. If A1C remains high, consider adding rapid-acting insulin before additional meals

NOTE: FBG, fasting blood glucose.

typically are given as premeal boluses of rapid-acting insulin (i.e., lispro, aspart, glulisine).

The key factor contributing to the success of the regimen is not what type of insulin is given or the number of injections that are initially used. Rather, the key factor to success is whether enough insulin is given. For a regimen to be effective, the insulin dose must be increased frequently until targets are achieved. Multiple protocols for initiating and increasing insulin have been found to be effective. Furthermore, having patients self-titrate their own doses, according to protocol, appears to be similarly effective as having the insulin adjusted by a healthcare provider.

Selection of the Agents

Choice of therapy is complex and depends on multiple factors including the patient's initial A1C, the agent's effect on glucose lowering, cost, side effects, contraindications, dosing frequency, and acceptability to patients.

There is an emerging consensus that, as long as there are no contraindications, metformin should be initiated, concurrent with lifestyle intervention, at the time of diabetes diagnosis. The recommendation is based on the fact that patient adherence with diet, weight reduction, and regular exercise is not sustained in most patients, and most patients ultimately will require treatment. Since metformin is usually well-tolerated, does not cause hypoglycemia, has favorable effects on body weight, and is relatively inexpensive, potential benefits of early initiation of medication appear to outweigh potential risks.

Combination Therapy

Even if oral agent monotherapy is initially effective, glycemic control is likely to deteriorate over time due to progressive loss of beta-cell function in T2DM. Although metformin is generally recommended as first-line therapy,

Table 50.13 POTENTIAL STRATEGY FOR TREATMENT OF HYPERGLYCEMIA IN TYPE 2 DIABETES

	USUAL APPROACH	ALTERNATIVE APPROACH
First line	Lifestyle modification plus metformin*	Insulin#
Second line	Add a second noninsulin agent (Table 50.11), based on expected A1C lowering, contraindications, side effects, costs, and patient preferences	Insulin#
Third line	Add insulin	

NOTES: *If no contraindications. #Choose if very hyperglycemic, ketotic, thin and/or losing weight.

there is no consensus as to what the second-line agent should be. Numerous two-drug combinations have been studied and have been found to be effective. Selection of a second agent should be made based on potential advantages and disadvantages of each agent for any given patient. Sulfonylureas are the most commonly used second-line agents, although thiazolidinediones, incretin mimetics, and DPP-IV inhibitors are increasingly being used. Insulin may be preferred if the patient has very high initial blood glucose levels, is underweight, losing weight, or is ketotic. From a practical standpoint, glinides, alpha-glucosidase inhibitors, and pramlintide, are seldom used due to low glucose-lowering potential, poor patient tolerability, and/or the need for injection.

If patients progress to the point where dual therapy does not provide adequate control, either a third noninsulin agent or insulin can be added. In patients with modestly elevated A1C level (below ~8), addition of a third noninsulin agent may be equally effective as (but more expensive than) addition of insulin. Patients with significantly elevated A1C levels on two noninsulin agents usually should have insulin added to their regimens. A potential treatment algorithm is outlined in table 50.13.

SPECIAL POPULATIONS

Pregnancy

Patients with diabetes in pregnancy typically are considered as having either (1) pregestational diabetes or (2) GDM. Hyperglycemia during the first trimester, which may occur with pregestational diabetes, increases the risk for congenital malformations in the fetus. Diabetic patients therefore should be counseled to use effective contraception until A1C is controlled. Hyperglycemia that occurs during the third trimester, when GDM is typically diagnosed, increases the risk for fetal macrosomia and associated complications. Strict glucose control during pregnancy reduces this risk. Although expert opinion varies about the specific target glucose levels, glucose goals during pregnancy are considerably lower than for nonpregnant adults. Recommendations for fasting and premeal values are generally below 90 mg/

dL and recommendations for postprandial values are generally below 120 mg/dL. Insulin is the preferred agent for diabetes treatment during pregnancy. Regular, NPH, aspart, and lispro are commonly used. There are fewer safety data for glargine, detemir, and glulisine, so these are not recommended. Emerging evidence indicates metformin and glyburide also may be safe and effective, and both of these agents are increasingly used to treat patients with GDM.

Hospitalized Patients

Diabetes mellitus and/or inpatient hyperglycemia are common comorbid conditions in hospitalized patients. Observational studies have shown that hyperglycemia in hospitalized patients is associated with adverse outcomes including infections, increased length of stay, and increased mortality. Randomized controlled trials have been conducted only in the intensive care unit (ICU) setting, and their results are contradictory. Based on the available data, the ADA recommends moderate metabolic control, as shown in table 50.14. Insulin is the preferred agent in view of the rapidly changing requirements. Insulin drips are recommended for patients in the ICU. In non-ICU patients, subcutaneous insulin regimens should include each of three components: (1) basal insulin, which controls fasting and between-meal glucose levels; (2) nutritional insulin, which controls glucose from nutritional sources, such as discrete meals or tube feeds; and (3) supplemental insulin (aka "sliding scale"), which controls unexpected hyperglycemia that occurs despite scheduled basal and nutritional insulin. Regimens that use sliding scale insulin alone are not effective and should not be used.

Table 50.14 GLUCOSE GOALS IN INPATIENTS

	GOAL (Mg/dL)
Critically ill patients	140–180
Non–critically ill patients	
Premeal	<140
Random	<180

ADDITIONAL READING

American Diabetes Association. Clinical Practice Recommendations. *Diabetes Care.* 2010;33:Suppl 1.

Gough SC. A review of human and analogue insulin trials. *Diabetes Res Clin Pract.* 2007;770:1–15.

Kahm RP, Buse IF, Ferrannini E, Stem M. The metabolic syndrome: Time for a critical appraisal. Joint statement from the American Diabetes Association and the European Association for the Study of Diabetes. *Diabetes Care.* 2005;28:2289–2304.

Moghissi ES, Korytkowski MT, DiNardo M, et al.; American Association of Clinical Endocrinologists, American Diabetes Association. American Association of Clinical Endocrinologists and American Diabetes Association consensus statement on inpatient glycemic control. *Diabetes Care.* 2009;32:1119–31.

Nathan DM, Davidson MB, DeFronzo BA, et al. Impaired fasting glucose and impaired glucose tolerance: Implications for care. *Diabetes Care.* 2007;30:753–9.

Nathan DM, Buse TB, Davidson MB, et al. Medical management of hyperglycemia in type 2 diabetes: A consensus algorithm for the initiation and adjustment of therapy. A consensus statement from the American Diabetes Association and the European Association for the Study of Diabetes. *Diabetes Care.* 2009;32:193–203.

Rodbard HW, Jellinger PS, Davidson JA, et al. Statement by an American Association of Clinical Endocrinologists/American College of Endocrinology consensus panel on type 2 diabetes mellitus: An algorithm for glycemic control. *Endocrinol Pract.* 2009;15:768–70.

Sigal RJ, Kenny JP, Wasserman DH, Castaneda-Sceppa C. Physical activity/exercise and type 2 diabetes. *Diabetes Care.* 2004;27:2518–39.

QUESTIONS

QUESTION 1. A patient has been taking the maximal dose of a sulfonylurea and metformin for the past 6 months. The A1C is now 9.5%. Which of the following should be added?

A. Pioglitazone (Actos)
B. Exenatide (Byetta)
C. Sitagliptin (Januvia)
D. Insulin

QUESTION 2. A patient with T2DM is taking metformin and bedtime NPH. The fasting blood glucose ranges from 80 to 100 mg/dL, and the A1C is 7.5%. What would you do now?

A. Add morning NPH
B. Stop NPH and start bedtime glargine (Lantus)

C. Add aspart (Novolog) before the largest meal of the day
D. Change to an insulin pump

QUESTION 3. A nondiabetic patient is 5 feet 3 inches tall and weighs 200 lb (body mass index [BMI] 34.4 kg/m^2). The patient should be advised he will reduce his risk of diabetes if he

A. Loses at least 30 lb
B. Loses 5–10% of his body weight
C. Loses enough weight to reduce his BMI to <30 kg/m^2
D. Loses enough weight to reduce his BMI to <27 kg/m^2

QUESTION 4. Which of the following diets will be most likely to improve glycemic control in an obese patient with type 2 diabetes?

A. Reduced calorie intake
B. Low carbohydrate
C. Low glycemic index
D. ADA diet

QUESTION 5. A patient with type 2 diabetes is admitted to the hospital (non-ICU) with sepsis. He has been treated at home with glyburide. A recent A1C was 7.5%. Admission glucose (nonfasting) is 250 mg/dL. His appetite is poor. What medication regimen should be prescribed?

A. Continue glyburide and start sliding scale regular insulin before meals and bedtime.
B. Stop glyburide and start sliding scale regular insulin before meals and bedtime.
C. Stop glyburide and start NPH, premeal aspart, and premeal sliding scale aspart before meals and bedtime.
D. Stop glyburide and start an insulin drip.

ANSWERS

1. D
2. C
3. B
4. A
5. C

51.

DIABETES MELLITUS
CONTROL AND COMPLICATIONS

Deborah J. Wexler and David M. Nathan

Acutely uncontrolled diabetes, characterized by hyperglycemia and tissue catabolism, can cause fatigue, polyuria, polydipsia, weight loss, visual changes, coma, and death. Although the risk for ketoacidosis is markedly higher in type 1 diabetes, characterized by absolute insulin deficiency, it can also occur in type 2 diabetes (usually in the setting of major stress). With the development of effective therapies to control symptomatic hyperglycemia, the chief concern of chronic diabetes management has moved on to the prevention of long-term complications associated with hyperglycemia, including the microvascular complications of retinopathy, nephropathy, and neuropathy, and macrovascular (cardiovascular) disease. Maintaining glycemia as close to normal as possible without unacceptable hypoglycemia and controlling blood pressure and cholesterol have been demonstrated to prevent or delay progression of complications of diabetes.

Diabetes affects an estimated 8% of the U.S. population, or about 24 million people, with the vast majority having type 2 diabetes. Approximately 6 million of the more than 24 million with type 2 diabetes, based on National Health and Examination Survey (NHANES) fasting glucose levels, are undiagnosed. The epidemic of type 2 diabetes disproportionately affects older and minority populations.

Type 1 diabetes, formerly known as juvenile-onset or insulin-dependent diabetes, affects about 1 million Americans. Type 1 diabetes is caused by autoimmune destruction of pancreatic beta-cells leading, ultimately, to complete insulin deficiency and an absolute requirement for exogenous insulin for survival. Type 1 diabetes is one of the most common chronic diseases with onset during childhood and adolescence, but adults may also develop type 1 diabetes. It should be suspected in lean patients with a prominent family history of type 1 diabetes or other autoimmune diseases, such as Graves disease or hypothyroidism, pernicious anemia, or celiac disease, who have positive anti-islet cell antibodies and fail oral antidiabetic medications. The presence of ketonuria also suggests type 1 diabetes.

Although the incidence of type 1 diabetes is increasing, the diabetes epidemic is largely due to the fivefold increase in type 2 diabetes during the past 20 years. What is commonly called type 2 diabetes likely represents a group of pathophysiologically distinct subcategories of hyperglycemic disorders in which some degree of beta-cell function is maintained. Nonetheless, all patients with type 2 diabetes have a relative deficit in insulin secretion with varying degrees of insulin resistance. Type 2 diabetes, which has a polygenic basis, is frequently unmasked by the increasing insulin resistance associated with advancing age, weight gain, intercurrent illness, or, in the case of gestational diabetes, pregnancy. There are many other, relatively rare causes of diabetes including monogenic defects in beta-cell function (the maturity-onset diabetes of the young, or MODY, disorders), pancreatic diseases such as chronic pancreatitis and cystic fibrosis, and other endocrinopathies (i.e., Cushing disease/syndrome, acromegaly).

MONITORING GLYCEMIC CONTROL

Patients self-monitor short-term glycemic control using glucose meters to check fasting, preprandial, and/or postprandial glucose levels. In type 1 diabetes, self-monitoring is necessary to guide selection of doses of rapid-acting insulins before meals and to prevent and detect hypoglycemia. In type 2 diabetes, self-monitoring is necessary for safety and to adjust doses in patients taking insulin or oral agents that can cause hypoglycemia (i.e., sulfonylureas). Although the role of self-monitoring is less clear for type 2 diabetic patients treated with diet alone or other medications that do not cause hypoglycemia, self-monitoring can also be used for behavioral feedback. Long-term glycemia is monitored by hemoglobin A1c levels, which reflect mean glucose levels over the preceding 2 to 3 months. The development of the HbA1c assay facilitated the testing and proof of the "glucose hypothesis" (that reducing mean levels of chronic glycemia would prevent or delay the progression of complications

Table 51.1 SUMMARY OF SCREENING AND TREATMENT GOALS IMPLEMENTED BY INTERNISTS FOR ADULTS WITH DIABETES

TEST/THERAPY	TARGET	FREQUENCY
Hemoglobin A1c	<7%, individualized to patient comorbidities	Every 3 months
Blood pressure	<140/90, and possibly <130/80 mm Hg, depending on comorbidities, with regimen including ACEi or ARB if microalbuminuria is present	Every visit
Urine microalbuminuria	<30 mg/g creatinine	Annually, confirm two or three times if positive on screen
Lipids	Total cholesterol <200 mg/dl, LDL cholesterol <100 mg/dL, HDL cholesterol >40 mg/dL in men, >50 mg/dl in women, and triglycerides <150 mg/dL	Annual screen, then every 3–6 months on treatment
Aspirin	81–325 mg	For patients older than 40 years, CAD, or CVD risk factors
Smoking	Cessation	Every visit
Depression		Screen patients with difficulty with adherence

of diabetes). The hemoglobin A1c assay is unreliable when red cell turnover is altered as in, for example, hemolysis. In addition certain assays may be affected by hemoglobinopathies, for example, with hemoglobin S causing a spuriously low and hemoglobin F a spuriously high HbA1c result with some high-performance liquid chromatography methods. In these circumstances, an affinity method or immunoassay methods can accurately measure HbA1c independent of any hemoglobinopathies.

As outlined below several trials have shown that every 1% drop in hemoglobin A1c levels reduces the risk of microvascular complications by approximately 40%.

THE GLUCOSE HYPOTHESIS

Several landmark clinical trials published in the 1990s demonstrated the beneficial effect of intensive glycemic control on long-term complications of diabetes. The Diabetes Control and Complications Trial (DCCT) has provided the longest follow-up, now with almost 25 years since recruitment of the study cohort between 1983 and 1989. The DCCT randomly assigned 1441 patients with type 1 diabetes to intensive treatment in which multiple daily insulin injections or continuous insulin infusion with external pumps were used to achieve glycemic levels as close to the nondiabetic range as possible or to conventional treatment, in which twice-daily insulin injections were given with a goal of avoiding symptomatic hyper- and hypoglycemia. Patients were 13–39 years old at study entry. Those with fewer than 5 years of diabetes and no signs of complications were enrolled in a primary prevention cohort, whereas those in the secondary prevention cohort had had diabetes for 1–15 years, at least one microaneurysm but no more

than moderate nonproliferative diabetic retinopathy, and <200 mg of albuminuria per 24 hours. Over the 6.5-year average duration of DCCT follow-up, the intensive group achieved a mean hemoglobin A1c of 7%, while the conventional group maintained a mean hemoglobin A1c of 9%. As discussed in detail below, the DCCT demonstrated a large reduction in retinopathy, microalbuminuria, and neuropathy at the cost of a two- to threefold increased risk of severe hypoglycemia. This cohort has continued to be followed in the Epidemiology of Diabetes and Complications (EDIC study), in which hemoglobin A1c levels in both groups have been about 8%.

The United Kingdom Prospective Diabetes Study (UKPDS) studied patients with newly diagnosed type 2 diabetes to determine whether intensive therapy was superior to conventional (dietary) intervention. The UKPDS had two substudies. In the first, 3876 subjects, mean age 54, were randomly assigned to intensive control with

Table 51.2 SUMMARY OF REFERRALS FOR ADULTS WITH DIABETES

Dilated fundoscopic exam	
Type 1 diabetes	5 years after diagnosis, then annually
Type 2 diabetes	Annually
Podiatry	When neuropathy is present
Dentistry	Annually
Certified diabetes educator for diabetes self-management education	At diagnosis and as indicated
Registered dietician for medical nutrition therapy	At diagnosis and as indicated
Mental health professional	As indicated

sulfonylurea or insulin versus conventional control. In the second, 753 obese patients, mean age 53, were randomly assigned to metformin versus conventional control. The intensive strategy aimed for a goal fasting glucose of <108 mg/dL. Conventional control was pursued with diet, and medications were added for symptoms of hyperglycemia or fasting plasma glucose >270 mg/dL. The majority of the conventional group crossed over to the treatments given in the intensive groups, and more than 20% of the intensive groups had additional medications added, complicating interpretation of the results. Nonetheless, the intensive group maintained a mean hemoglobin A1c of 7% compared to 7.9% in the conventional group. Intention-to-treat analyses showed a 12% reduction in aggregate diabetes outcomes, which was largely due to a 25% reduction in severe treatment for retinopathy. The intensive group gained 2.9 kg more, on average, and had more hypoglycemia. In the metformin cohort, the intensive group maintained a mean hemoglobin A1c of 7.4% compared to 8% in the control group. Intention-to-treat analysis showed that patients assigned to the metformin group had a significant 32% risk reduction for any diabetes-related endpoint and a 36% reduction in all-cause mortality. Ten-year follow-up of this cohort showed persistent benefits in any diabetes-related endpoint as well as lower rates of myocardial infarction and death in both intensively treated groups. Subsequent analyses of these studies have yielded further information on the role of blood pressure control in contributing to reduction in complications, as outlined below.

The Kumamoto trial in Japanese patients with type 2 diabetes, modeled after the DCCT, randomly assigned 110 patients to intensive control with multiple insulin injections, achieving a mean hemoglobin A1c of 7.1%, or to conventional insulin treatment, associated with a mean HbA1c of 9.4%, over the 6 years of the study. Intensive treatment was associated with significant reductions in retinopathy, neuropathy, and nephropathy, similar in magnitude to the results in the DCCT.

PRESERVING PANCREATIC FUNCTION

In addition to reducing the long-term complications of diabetes, better glycemic control may improve, and potentially preserve, beta-cell function, which, in turn, sustains glycemic control and reduces complications. Acutely, glucose and free fatty acids stimulate insulin secretion; however, chronically elevated levels of glucose and free fatty acids desensitize and may poison the beta-cell. Early in the course of type 1 diabetes and in type 2 diabetes, residual beta-cell function can be improved by reducing high ambient glucose and free fatty acid levels, which adversely affect beta-cell function through glucotoxicity and lipotoxicity, respectively. The reduction of glucotoxicity and lipotoxicity with resultant improvement in beta-cell function has been achieved with intensive insulin treatment in type 1

and type 2 diabetes. In type 2 diabetes, reduction of glucotoxicity may also be accomplished by other pharmacologic or nonpharmacologic means. In addition to contributing to improved glycemia and reduced long-term complications, preserved beta-cell function promotes hypoglycemia awareness, allowing the safe application of intensive therapy.

RETINOPATHY

In the United States, diabetic retinopathy is the leading cause of vision loss among adults, with 12,000–24,000 new cases of blindness annually and with 21% of all adults with diabetes reporting some visual impairment. Diabetic retinopathy is related to the duration of diabetes, the degree of glycemic control, hypertension, and dyslipidemia. Glaucoma and cataracts are more common in diabetes and also contribute to loss of vision.

SCREENING

Because retinopathy is estimated to develop only after 5 years of hyperglycemia, and the onset of hyperglycemia is usually easily recognized in type 1 diabetes, patients with type 1 diabetes should be screened with a dilated funduscopic examination 5 years after diagnosis. Patients with type 2 diabetes, who frequently have an indolent onset of diabetes and may therefore have unrecognized prior diabetes and complications at the time of diagnosis, should be screened for retinopathy at the time of diabetes diagnosis. In general, screening should be repeated annually.

PREVENTION

Glycemic control has been shown to reduce the risk of development and progression of retinopathy; every 1% reduction in hemoglobin A1c is associated with an approximately 40% reduction in retinopathy in both type 1 (DCCT; see figure 51.1) and type 2 diabetes (UKPDS; see figure 51.2). Blood pressure control reduces the risk of progression of retinopathy in type 2 diabetes. Lowering triglyceride levels reduces the risk of retinopathy in type 2 diabetes. Notably, intensification of glycemic control in patients with previously poorly controlled diabetes and pre-existing retinopathy can precipitate worsening retinopathy, at least transiently; close monitoring by an ophthalmologist is warranted in such patients. Efforts at screening and more intensive interventions correspond to a decrease in the prevalence of visual impairment from diabetes from 26% in 1997 to 21–22% in 2005.

PATHOPHYSIOLOGY AND TREATMENT

Diabetic retinopathy occurs in two forms: nonproliferative retinopathy, characterized by abnormal microvasculature resulting in leakage of serum proteins and manifested

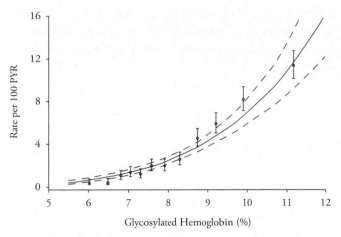

Figure 51.1 Rate of complications per 100 person-years of observation by mean HbA1c. Reprinted with permission from The absence of a glycemic threshold for the development of long-term complications: the perspective of the Diabetes Control and Complications Trial. *Diabetes* 1996; 45:1289–1298.

as microaneurysms and hard exudates, and the more advanced preproliferative and proliferative retinopathy. Preproliferative retinopathy is caused by occlusion of the small vessels leading to retinal ischemia with retinal infarcts, manifested as soft "cotton wool" exudates. Retinal ischemia promotes the secretion of growth factors such as vascular endothelial growth factor (VEGF), which, in turn, trigger *neovascularization*, proliferation of friable vessels in the fundus and into the vitreous.

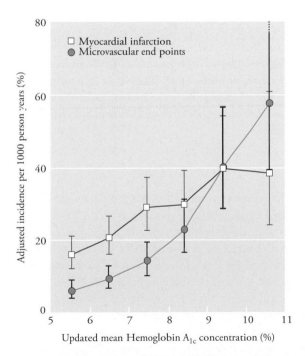

Figure 51.2 Incidence rates and 95% confidence intervals for myocardial infarction and microvascular complications by category of updated mean hemoglobin A1c concentration, adjusted for age, sex, and ethnic group, expressed for white men aged 50–54 years at diagnosis and with mean duration of diabetes of 10 years.

Loss of vision in diabetic retinopathy is due to one or a combination of the following: macular edema resulting from leaking capillaries near the maculae, macular ischemia from obstructed vessels supplying the maculae, retinal detachment related to traction from proliferative retinopathy vessels and fibroproliferative scarring, vitreous hemorrhage, and neovascular glaucoma. Because patients may be asymptomatic even in the presence of severe disease, and treatment prevents development and progression rather than reversing loss of vision, primary prevention by control of glycemia, blood pressure, and lipids, coupled with regular screening, is of paramount importance.

Laser photocoagulation therapy is used to treat macular edema and proliferative retinopathy, according to indications established by the Diabetic Retinopathy Study and Early Treatment Diabetic Retinopathy Study. Macular edema, which is difficult to appreciate on direct ophthalmoscopy, is treated with focal photocoagulation, which reduces the risk of progression of visual loss in macular edema from 20% to 8%. Severe nonproliferative diabetic retinopathy (with intraretinal hemorrhages in all four quadrants of the eye) and proliferative diabetic retinopathy (with neovascularization of the optic disk or neovascularization of a significant portion of the retina elsewhere) are treated with panretinal photocoagulation, which reduces the risk of severe vision loss from 15.9% to 6.4% (>50% reduction). This treatment sacrifices the damaged portion of the retina outside of the macula to decrease the ischemic stimulus to neovascularization. Aspirin (for prophylaxis of cardiovascular disease) is not contraindicated in the presence of retinopathy but does not appear to reduce retinopathy.

NEPHROPATHY

Diabetic nephropathy is the leading cause of end-stage renal disease (ESRD) in the United States, with about 43,600 people beginning treatment for ESRD due to diabetes in 2002. Twenty to thirty percent of patients with diabetes develop diabetic nephropathy, with nonwhite groups having a higher rate of progression. The rate of increase in new cases and the frequency of progression to ESRD have declined since 1997, probably owing to intensive treatment of hyperglycemia and hypertension.

The earliest sign of diabetic nephropathy is an elevated level of urinary albumin excretion, called microalbuminuria, which can be detected on a spot urine collection. Conventional urine dipstick testing only detects levels >300 mg/day, usually called clinical proteinuria. Presence of microalbuminuria is correlated not only with risk for progression to more severe kidney dysfunction but also with high cardiovascular disease risk in patients with and without diabetes. Thirty percent of patients with type 1 diabetes have microalbuminuria after 15 years of diabetes. Half of this population progresses to overt nephropathy, characterized by albuminuria (>300 mg/24 hours). The development of microalbuminuria late in the course of diabetes corresponds to a lower risk of progression to nephropathy. Twenty-five to forty percent of patients with type 2 diabetes have microalbuminuria after 10–15 years of diabetes, and approximately one-half of these will progress to overt nephropathy. Risk of progression is increased in African Americans and with hyperglycemia, hypertension, and smoking. Overt nephropathy almost always progresses to decreasing glomerular filtration rate and, given enough time, kidney failure.

SCREENING

Screening for diabetic nephropathy includes an annual test for urine microalbumin excretion in a spot urine sample in which albumin in milligrams is standardized to grams of urine creatinine. This ratio roughly approximates the daily albumin excretion in milligrams per day. Less than 30 mg albumin per gram of creatinine is considered normal (although normal levels of albuminuria are probably closer to 10 mg per gram creatinine); values between 30 and 300 represent microalbuminuria and early nephropathy, and values >300 are consistent with overt nephropathy (sometimes called clinical proteinuria). Vigorous exercise, acute hyperglycemia, fever, infection, congestive heart failure (CHF), severe hypertension, and low muscle mass can falsely elevate the degree of microalbuminuria, so a positive screen should be confirmed with two of three midmorning samples. In addition, serum creatinine should be measured yearly to estimate glomerular filtration rate and stage the degree of chronic kidney disease (CKD). Referral to a nephrologist is recommended as stage 3 CKD develops (eGFR <60 mL/min).

PREVENTION

Optimizing glycemia has been shown to prevent development and slow the rate of progression of nephropathy in both type 1 and type 2 diabetes. Maintaining blood pressure at <130/80 mm Hg also prevents development and progression of proteinuric kidney disease, has been shown to have additive benefit to glycemic control in patients with type 2 diabetes, and likely has the same effect in type 1 diabetes.

TREATMENT

When microalbuminuria develops, angiotensin-converting enzyme inhibitors (ACEi) have been shown to prevent progression of nephropathy in patients with type 1 diabetes, and both ACEi and angiotensin receptor blockers (ARB) have been shown by UKPDS to prevent progression in patients with type 2 diabetes. The dose of the ACEi or ARB should be maximized in patients with microalbuminuria or nephropathy, with monitoring for hyperkalemia and other side effects. ACEi should be initiated first based on their lower cost; if ACEi are not tolerated, an ARB can be substituted. The addition of an ARB to an ACEi, in general, results in higher cost and more side effects without reduction of cardiovascular disease (CVD) events; however, it may lower blood pressure, benefit patients with CHF, and further reduce microalbuminuria. Whether the rate of loss of glomerular filtration rate (GFR) is attenuated by adding an ARB to an ACEi is not known.

There are currently no randomized controlled trial data to support the use of an ACEi or ARB in place of other antihypertensive agents prior to the development of microalbuminuria or hypertension. If hypertension develops in a patient with diabetes, the choice of initial antihypertensive agent should be based on patient comorbidities and medication side-effect profile.

NEUROPATHY AND LOWER EXTREMITY DISEASE

Diabetic neuropathy (DN) affects both the peripheral and autonomic nervous systems. The diabetic neuropathies can result in lower extremity ulcers and amputations, especially when compounded by peripheral vascular disease. Some form of neuropathy affects up to 70% of people with diabetes; the lifetime risk of a foot ulcer is 15%. Once an ulcer has developed, treatment costs an average of $28,000 over the subsequent 2 years. Duration and severity of hyperglycemia are the major risk factors for development of neuropathy, but elevated triglycerides, body mass index (BMI), smoking, and hypertension increase risk as well. Patients with type 1 diabetes usually do not develop neuropathy until several years after diagnosis, but 10–18% of patients with type 2 diabetes have peripheral neuropathy at the time of diabetes diagnosis, reflecting the role of even a mild degree of hyperglycemia, combined with other risk factors, in contributing to nerve damage. The most common form of DN is distal symmetric polyneuropathy.

SCREENING

Screening for distal symmetric polyneuropathy (DPN) is recommended at diagnosis for patients with type 2 diabetes and 5 years after diagnosis for patients with type 1 diabetes. The most sensitive indicator of DPN is loss of vibratory sense, determined by loss of perception of a vibrating 128 Hz tuning fork on the interphalangeal joint of the hallux, compared to a more proximal point on the body or to the examiner's perception, or by ability to sense cessation of vibration. Loss of perception of pressure applied with a 10-g Semmes-Weinstein monofilament at any of 12 spots on the plantar surfaces of the feet predicts ulcer risk. Assessment of ankle reflexes, integrity of the skin and nails, loss of hair, pedal pulses, and any bony deformities complete the lower extremity evaluation.

PREVENTION

In both type 1 and type 2 diabetes, optimizing glycemic control prevents the development of neuropathy. Patients should be instructed to trim toenails carefully, following the natural nail bed and filing sharp edges, and to examine their feet for any lesions, as most ulcers can be traced to a minor injury that might have healed properly with evaluation and treatment. Routine nail care should be carried out by a podiatrist in frail patients, those with limited vision, and in those with severe neuropathy (loss of light touch) or a prior history of a foot ulcer.

SYNDROMES AND TREATMENT

Distal Symmetric Polyneuropathy

DPN is usually asymptomatic or characterized by minimal paresthesias (numbness or pins-and-needles sensation), most often in the toes or feet. It can progress to involve the lower leg and fingers and distal arm. DPN can rarely be painful. The pain is often greater at night, interfering with sleep, and can include hypersensitivity to light touch, so even the weight of a sheet is uncomfortable (dysesthesias). In contrast to intermittent claudication associated with peripheral vascular disease, neuropathic pain often decreases—or is less noticeable—with walking. Pain medication should be initiated for pain that affects sleep or quality of life. The choice of medications to treat painful neuropathy should be based on effectiveness, side-effect profile, and patient comorbidities. Options include low-dose tricyclic antidepressants, anticonvulsants, and serotonin- and norepinephrine-reuptake inhibitors. Narcotic analgesics should be avoided.

Mononeuropathies

Mononeuropathies are much less common than the distal symmetric polyneuropathies. They are thought to be secondary to an ischemic infarct, perhaps from microvascular disease of a vasa nervorum. Depending on the specific nerve affected, a mononeuropathy may cause, for example, a foot drop (peroneal nerve) or an ocular or facial palsy (cranial nerves III, IV, VI, or VII). These predominant motor neuropathies must be evaluated to distinguish them from other causes of mononeuropathy, as diabetic mononeuropathy is established as a diagnosis of exclusion. No specific therapy is usually necessary, and they typically recover spontaneously, usually in 6 weeks to 3 months.

Autonomic Neuropathy

Autonomic neuropathies include cardiovascular (resting tachycardia, orthostatic hypotension), gastrointestinal (gastroparesis, constipation, diarrhea, fecal incontinence), genitourinary (erectile dysfunction, bladder atony with urinary retention), and sudomotor dysfunction (impaired sweating leading to skin breakdown, and gustatory sweating) and hypoglycemia unawareness.

Normalizing glucose control can improve gastroparesis and hypoglycemia unawareness even after these have developed. Otherwise, treatment is symptom-targeted and supportive. In all cases, medication side effects and other disorders must be ruled out as causes.

Diabetic Foot Pathology

Diabetic foot disease is multifactorial. Impaired sensation prevents recognition of barotrauma and leads to delayed detection of even minor injury. Motor neuropathy of the small fibers of the feet leads to characteristic deformities (claw toes) and altered foot architecture that can predispose to mal perforans ulcers. In severe cases Charcot joints can develop. Dry, cracked skin due to sudomotor dysfunction diminishes barriers to infection. Vascular insufficiency and diseased capillaries impair wound healing. Treatment is directed at the contributing causes and may involve podiatrists, vascular surgeons, and infectious disease specialists in addition to internists and endocrinologists.

CARDIOVASCULAR DISEASE

CVD is the leading cause of death among people with diabetes, with heart attack and stroke accounting for at least 65% of deaths in this population. Diabetes is associated with a cardiovascular risk profile similar to that of having had a prior heart attack in the absence of diabetes and is associated with a two- to fourfold increased risk of cardiovascular death and stroke compared to nondiabetics. Although hyperglycemia is clearly associated with increased rates of CVD in patients with type 1 and type 2 diabetes, traditional cardiovascular risk factors such as age, hypertension, hypercholesterolemia, smoking, and kidney failure are the main drivers of CVD risk; thus they are the main focus of interventions to prevent CVD in people with diabetes.

GLYCEMIA AND CARDIOVASCULAR DISEASE

Although insufficient cardiac events accrued among the young participants during the DCCT to assess the effect of intensive glycemic control on cardiovascular outcomes, continuing follow-up of DCCT participants in the EDIC trial demonstrated a long-term protective effect of intensive treatment on macrovascular outcomes. Intensive treatment during the DCCT was associated with a 57% lower risk of nonfatal myocardial infarction (MI), stroke, and cardiovascular death over 18 years of follow-up in EDIC. In type 2 diabetics in the UKPDS, every 1% reduction in HbA1c was associated with a 14% reduction in risk of MI. The DCCT and UKPDS both compared a HbA1c level of approximately 7% with their intensive therapies with 9%

and 8% in their respective conventional groups. The more recent ACCORD and ADVANCE trials, which attempted to lower HbA1c levels with intensive therapy to even lower levels, achieving HbA1c of approximately 6.5%, compared with approximately 7.5%, have been unable to demonstrate a benefit of intensive glycemic management with regard to CVD outcomes. In fact, the ACCORD study was stopped prematurely due to excess mortality in the intensive group. The cause of the excess mortality is not clear. Consequently, the goal of maintaining glycemia as close to normal as is safely possible is to reduce microvascular and neurological complications but not CVD. A HbA1c target of <7% seems appropriate for most patients; this target may be individualized based on patient age and comorbidities.

HYPERTENSION

Three-quarters of patients with diabetes have hypertension. Microalbuminuria and proteinuria are often accompanied by difficult-to-control hypertension. Controlling blood pressure to <140/90 mm Hg reduces the risk of cardiovascular disease by 33–50% in patients with diabetes, and lower targets may be appropriate. The ACCORD blood pressure trial did not show a cardiovascular benefit of targeting systolic blood pressure <120 mm Hg compared to 135–140 mm Hg in patients with established diabetes and cardiovascular disease or CVD risk factors with creatinine <1.5 mg/dL. The event rate in the control group was half that expected. Blood pressure control is synergistic with glycemic control in reducing microvascular complications of diabetes, reducing the risk by 12% for every 10 mm Hg reduction in systolic blood pressure.

Blood pressure should be measured at every visit. Blood pressure targets should be lower in patients with nephropathy. The preponderance of evidence continues to support a blood pressure goal of <130/80 mm Hg for renal rather than cardiovascular indications, and it is very clear that pharmacological therapy is required to reduce blood pressure below 140/90 mm Hg to reduce the risk of all complications. Patients with diabetes frequently require at least two agents to lower blood pressure to current targets. Patients with persistent hypertension on more than four drugs should be screened for hyperaldosteronism, renal artery stenosis, and other causes of secondary hypertension.

LIPID MANAGEMENT

Patients with diabetes should be screened with an annual fasting lipid profile unless they have a low-risk lipid profile (low-density lipoprotein [LDL] <100 mg/dL, high-density lipoprotein [HDL] >50 mg/dL, and triglycerides <150 mg/dL), in which case screening can be performed less frequently. Classically, diabetic dyslipidemia is characterized by high triglyceride and low HDL cholesterol levels with variable LDL cholesterol. Nonetheless, the focus

of lipid management is LDL lowering, based on clinical trial data showing mortality benefits. Hyperglycemia can exacerbate hypertriglyceridemia, so fasting lipid levels should be repeated after HbA1c is better controlled.

All HMG CoA reductase inhibitors, or statins, have been associated with primary and secondary prevention of CVD death and MI in association with LDL cholesterol lowering. Although the largest absolute and relative risk reductions are seen in subjects with the highest baseline LDL cholesterol values, there is no lower limit of LDL beyond which benefit ceases to accrue.

The Heart Protection Study showed a 27% reduction in vascular event rate in patients with diabetes with a baseline LDL of <116 mg/dL assigned to simvastatin 40 mg. The CARDS trial showed a 35% relative risk reduction in primary prevention of CVD events in patients with diabetes with mean LDL cholesterol levels <118 mg/dL at study entry assigned to atorvastatin 10 mg. Consequently, the American Diabetes Association recommends that all patients with diabetes who have CVD, or who are older than 40 years and have one or more additional CVD risk factors, be prescribed a statin regardless of baseline lipid levels and that statins be considered for use in younger patients with several CVD risk factors. For patients with lipid levels above target, the treatment goal is LDL cholesterol <100 mg/dL.

The data for triglyceride lowering are more equivocal. Treatment with a fibrate, such as gemfibrozil, in patients with known CVD, one-quarter of whom also had diabetes, reduced the risk of cardiovascular death, nonfatal MI, and stroke by 22%. The ACCORD Lipid trial did not show a cardiovascular benefit of adding fenofibrate to simvastatin in patients with established diabetes and CVD or CVD risk factors. Consequently, the first steps for triglyceride lowering are lifestyle modification with a relatively low-carbohydrate, low-saturated fat diet and exercise to promote weight loss. Implementing tight glycemic control dramatically lowers triglyceride levels. Patients with triglycerides >500 mg/dL should be treated with fibrates to prevent pancreatitis. The addition of triglyceride-lowering medications to statins should be based on individual patient comorbidities.

ASPIRIN

Low-dose aspirin (75–162 mg/day) is associated with an approximately 30% reduction in risk of MI and 20% reduction in risk of stroke. Aspirin is recommended for patients with diabetes over 40 years of age with a history of CVD and those with additional CVD risk factors (hypertension, family history, smoking, hyperlipidemia, or microalbuminuria).

EXERCISE AND DIET

Thirty minutes of brisk walking daily reduces insulin resistance, lowers glucotoxicity, and improves cardiovascular health. Exercise sustains weight loss in combination with a calorie-restricted diet. These lifestyle measures are the foundation of all efforts to improve glycemia and overall health and prevent cardiovascular disease in type 2 diabetes. Referrals to a certified diabetes educator or nutritionist improve patient compliance with lifestyle modification and medication compliance. Group lifestyle interventions, such as the ones studied in the Diabetes Prevention Program and Look AHEAD studies, are now being recommended by many insurers and conducted in YMCAs, making this highly effective therapy accessible to more people.

SLEEP

Sleep apnea affects 30–50%, and possibly more, people with type 2 diabetes and is associated with worsening hypertension, glucose tolerance, and CVD risk.

CONCLUSION

Prevention and delay of diabetes complications require a multifaceted approach. All patients with diabetes benefit from glycemic control to reduce microvascular and neurological complications and, in type 1 diabetes, macrovascular complications. Control of glycemia, blood pressure, and lipids, maintenance of a normal weight, and smoking cessation positively interact to reduce the risk of microvascular and macrovascular complications. This principle was demonstrated in the Steno-2 trial, which randomly assigned 160 patients with type 2 diabetes and microalbuminuria to a multifactorial intervention using renin-angiotensin-aldosterone antagonists, statins, aspirin, and tight glycemic control or to conventional therapy. After 8 years of follow-up, the intervention group had a 50% reduction in death. One patient in the intensive group, versus six in the conventional group, progressed to ESRD. The intensive group had a 55% reduction in laser photocoagulation.

Notably, as in the non–clinical trial setting, many of the participants in the Steno-2 intensive group failed to achieve treatment targets. In NHANES data collected in 1999–2000, only 7.3% of adults with diagnosed diabetes achieved treatment targets of HbA1c <7%, blood pressure <130/80 mm Hg, and total cholesterol <200 mg/dL. The failure to achieve targets may be due in part to patient factors, such as depression, which has a higher prevalence in patients with diabetes and may decrease adherence to treatment. Diagnosis and management of depression in order to promote self-management behavior and improved overall health are additional facets of diabetes care. Additionally, factors related to the health care system may not support optimal diabetes management. Novel care strategies may be required in order to reduce the $116 billion in medical costs and $58 billion in disability, work loss, and premature mortality that diabetes costs society and to realize the benefits of prevention of complications for people with diabetes.

ADDITIONAL READING

CONSENSUS STATEMENTS/REVIEWS

American Diabetes Association. Standards of medical care in diabetes—2012. *Diabetes Care.* 2012;35:S11–S63.

Crandall JP, Knowler WC, Kahn SE, et al.; Diabetes Prevention Program Research Group. The prevention of type 2 diabetes. *Nat Clin Pract Endocrinol Metab.* 2008;4(7):382–93.

Hanas R, John G; International HbA1c Consensus Committee. 2010 consensus statement on the worldwide standardization of the hemoglobin A1c measurement. *Clin Chem.* 2010;56(8):1362–4.

Inzucchi SE. Clinical practice. Management of hyperglycemia in the hospital setting. *N Engl J Med.* 2006;355(18):1903–11.

Kashyap P, Farrugia G. Diabetic gastroparesis: What we have learned and had to unlearn in the past 5 years. *Gut.* 2010;59(12):1716–26.

Nathan DM, Buse JB, Davidson MB, et al.; American Diabetes Association; European Association for the Study of Diabetes. Medical management of hyperglycaemia in type 2 diabetes mellitus: A consensus algorithm for the initiation and adjustment of therapy. A consensus statement from the American Diabetes Association and the European Association for the Study of Diabetes. *Diabetologia.* 2009;52(1):17–30.

Ockrim Z, Yorston D. Managing diabetic retinopathy. *BMJ.* 2010;341: c5400.

SELECTED SEMINAL AND RECENT MAJOR CLINICAL TRIAL REPORTS

ACCORD Study Group. Effects of intensive glucose lowering in type 2 diabetes. *N Engl J Med.* 2008;358:2545–59.

Cushman WC, Evans GW, Byington RP, et al. Effects of intensive blood-pressure control in type 2 diabetes mellitus. *N Engl J Med.* 2010;362(17):1575–85.

Diabetes Control and Complications Trial Research Group. The effect of intensive treatment of diabetes on the development and progression of long-term complications in insulin-dependent diabetes mellitus. *N Engl J Med.* 1993;329(14):977–86.

Gaede P, Lund-Andersen H, Parving HH, Pedersen O. Effect of a multifactorial intervention on mortality in type 2 diabetes. *N Engl J Med.* 2008;358(6):580–91.

Ginsberg HN, Elam MB, Lovato LC, et al. Effects of combination lipid therapy in type 2 diabetes mellitus. *N Engl J Med.* 2010;362(17):1563–74.

Holman RR, Paul SK, Bethel MA, Matthews DR, Neil HA. 10-year follow-up of intensive glucose control in type 2 diabetes. *N Engl J Med.* 2008;359:1577–89.

UK Prospective Diabetes Study Group. Intensive blood-glucose control with sulphonylureas or insulin compared with conventional treatment and risk of complications in patients with type 2 diabetes (UKPDS 33). *Lancet.* 1998;352(9131):837–53.

UK Prospective Diabetes Study Group. Tight blood pressure control and risk of macrovascular and microvascular complications in type 2 diabetes (UKPDS 38). *BMJ (Clin Res ed.).* 1998;317(7160):703–13.

QUESTIONS

QUESTION 1. A 32-year-old Caucasian man presents with polyuria, polydipsia, and weight loss for 1 month. A random glucose level is 367 mg/dL. He has a family history of diabetes in both grandfathers, with onset in their 60s and treatment with oral agents. On exam, his pulse is 102 beats per minute, blood pressure is 126/72 without orthostatic changes. His height is 70 inches, and his weight is 160 lb (down from his usual weight of 170 lb), and current BMI is 23 kg/m². Physical examination reveals a muscular young man in no acute distress. The remainder of the exam is normal, including normal vibratory sensation. Laboratory values reveal Na 139, K 3.7, Cl 100, HCO_3 29.8 mmol/L, BUN 18, Cr 1.1, and glucose 267 mg/dL; microalbumin/creatinine ratio of 65 mg/g (nl <30 mg/g); HbA1c 10.6%; urine ketones trace.

Which of the following is the most appropriate next management step?

A. Start metformin
B. Start glyburide
C. Start insulin
D. Start an ACE inhibitor
E. Schedule an ophthalmologic exam in the next year

QUESTION 2. Intensive glycemic control in patients with long-standing type 2 diabetes has been demonstrated to result in all of the following EXCEPT:

A. Prevention of retinopathy
B. Prevention of end-stage renal disease
C. Prevention of neuropathy
D. Prevention of heart attack and stroke

QUESTION 3. A 64-year-old woman with type 2 diabetes and obesity presents for evaluation. She states that she is watching portion size and fat intake and walking 30 minutes per day. Medications include aspirin 81 mg/day, metformin 1000 mg twice daily, lisinopril/HCTZ 20/25 mg/day, calcium, and vitamin D. She has no drug allergies. On exam, pulse is 72, blood pressure is 128/70, and BMI is 34 kg/m². She is obese without central predominance, dorsocervical fat pad, or violaceous striae. Cardiopulmonary exam is normal. A liver edge is not appreciated. Skin is without lesions. Peripheral pulses are full, and sensation is intact to light touch and vibration, but ankle reflexes are absent. Fasting laboratory values include HbA1c 8.2%; total cholesterol 213 mg/dL; HDL 37 mg/dL; LDL 104 mg/dL; triglycerides 362 mg/dL; AST 56 U/L; ALT 63 U/L; Alk Phos 67 U/L; total bilirubin 0.3 mg/dL; creatinine 1.0 mg/dL.

In addition to addressing glycemic control, what is the most appropriate next management step?

A. Start simvastatin 20 mg daily
B. Start nicotinic acid extended release 500 mg at bedtime
C. Start gemfibrozil 600 mg twice daily

D. A and B
E. A and C

QUESTION 4. A 46-year-old woman with long-standing type 1 diabetes and hypothyroidism presents for follow-up. Diabetes complications include retinopathy, with focal photocoagulation in both eyes 6 months previously, nephropathy with proteinuria and creatinine 2.0 mg/dL, and peripheral neuropathy. She takes insulin, lisinopril 40 mg, HCTZ 25 mg, amlodipine 10 mg, and simvastatin 40 mg, as well as gabapentin, calcium, L-thyroxine, and vitamin D. Exam reveals a thin woman in NAD. Pulse is 80, blood pressure is 128/80, and BMI is 24 kg/m² and is notable for the absent vibratory and monofilament perception in her feet. HbA1c is 7.8%, total cholesterol is 140 mg/dL, HDL is 52 mg/dL, LDL is 87 mg/dL, and triglycerides are 236 mg/dL. What is the appropriate next management step?

A. Add extended release nicotinic acid
B. Add gemfibrozil
C. Add ezetimibe
D. Add aspirin

QUESTION 5. A 58-year-old African-American male has had type 2 diabetes associated with obesity for 5 years. Initially treated with metformin (850 twice per day), his HbA1c level decreased from 7.9% at diagnosis to 6.4%. He recently stopped smoking, and his weight increased from 212 to 232 (current BMI 33 kg/m²). The patient is treated with an ACE inhibitor with blood pressure measurements routinely <130/76. His LDL-cholesterol level is 96 with an HDL level of 48 mg/dL. Estimated GFR is 96 mL/min. The patient has recently noted polyuria, nocturia, and developed pruritus diagnosed as candidiasis. His most recent HbA1c is 10.8%.

In addition to topical therapy for his candidiasis, what is an appropriate next step?

A. Increase metformin to 1000 bid and titrate to 3 g per day
B. Add a sulfonylurea
C. Substitute a DPP-4 inhibitor for the metformin
D. Add a DPP-4 inhibitor to the metformin
E. Start a long-acting insulin in the evening

ANSWERS

1. C
2. D
3. A
4. D
5. E

52.

METABOLIC SYNDROME

Rajesh K. Garg

DEFINITION

Metabolic syndrome (MetS), also referred to as the insulin resistance syndrome or syndrome X, refers to a constellation of metabolic abnormalities that tend to cluster together and lead to a substantial increase in risk of atherosclerotic cardiovascular disease (CVD). Although manifestations of MetS have been recognized since the 1920s, it was first described as a syndrome by Gerald Reaven in 1988. The most commonly used definition of MetS in the United States is the one proposed by the National Cholesterol Education Program's Adult Treatment Panel III (NCEP ATPIII). The definition was first published in 2001 and then updated in 2004 (see table 52.1); however, there are other definitions as well (see table 52.2). Most definitions include insulin resistance (IR) or abdominal obesity as the essential criterion. The NCEP definition does not require the presence of IR or obesity as an essential criterion. However, most individuals diagnosed with MetS according to the NCEP definition are both obese and insulin resistant.

The reason for a myriad of definitions of MetS is the uncertainty about its pathogenesis. Whereas some experts consider IR to be the central abnormality in MetS, others consider visceral obesity to be the primary defect. The criteria for obesity itself are variable and depend on the population being studied. For example, in Asian populations, overweight is defined as a body mass index (BMI) of >23 kg/m^2 and obesity as BMI >25 kg/m^2, and central obesity is defined as waist circumference >80 cm for women and >90 cm in men. These cutoffs are based on data comparing Asians with white populations. For example, Asians with BMI >23 kg/m^2 have CVD risk factors equivalent to white people with BMI >25 kg/m^2.

PREVALENCE

According to third National Health and Examination Survey (NHANES III) completed during 1988–1994, 47 million Americans had MetS. The prevalence of MetS increases with age. In NHANES III data, whereas 6.7% of adults in age range 20–29 years had MetS, the prevalence was 43.5% in age range 60–69 years. There were also clear racial differences in the prevalence of MetS. Under NCEP criteria, Mexican Americans had the highest age-adjusted prevalence of MetS (31.9%). Prevalence among whites was 23.8%, among African Americans 21.6%, and among other racial/ethnic groups 20.3%. In combined populations age-adjusted prevalence was similar for men and women. However, African-American women had 57% higher prevalence than men, and Mexican-American women had 26% higher prevalence than men. Use of updated NCEP criteria will increase the prevalence in all groups by approximately 5%.

The prevalence of MetS is related to the prevalence of obesity. With increasing prevalence of obesity over the last few decades, the prevalence of MetS, especially among African-American women, has increased.

PATHOGENESIS

The original descriptions of MetS had implicated IR as the central defect. There are several features in favor of IR being the common pathophysiological defect in MetS. Insulin resistance can explain hyperinsulinemia, glucose intolerance, type 2 diabetes, hypertriglyceridemia, and low high-density lipoprotein (HDL) concentrations due to reduced action of insulin on carbohydrate and lipid metabolism. Insulin resistance is associated with decreased disposal of the ingested triglycerides due to decreased lipoprotein lipase activity. Moreover, there is an upregulation of very-low-density lipoprotein (VLDL) production from the liver. Insulin resistance decreases utilization of glucose in muscle and liver and increases hepatic gluconeogenesis, thus causing impaired glucose tolerance. Besides these metabolic effects, IR may lead to hypertension as a result of decreased endothelial nitric oxide (NO) bioavailability.

However, many experts consider obesity as the central pathophysiological abnormality and IR the consequence

Table 52.1 NCEP ATPIII DEFINITION OF METABOLIC SYNDROME

PRESENCE OF THREE OF THE FOLLOWING FIVE CRITERIA QUALIFIES FOR METABOLIC SYNDROME

Waist circumference >102 cm (40 in.) in men and >88 cm (35 in.) in women

Serum triglycerides ≥150 mg/dL (1.7 mmol/L)

Serum HDL cholesterol <40 mg/dL (1 mmol/L) in men and <50 mg/dL (1.3 mmol/L) in women

Blood pressure ≥130/85 mm Hg

Fasting plasma glucose (FPG) ≥100 mg/dL (5.6 mmol/L)

of obesity. Obesity is often associated with dyslipidemia. Obesity is also associated with hypertension due to vasoconstriction caused by reduced bioavailability of NO, which is inactivated by increased generation of reactive oxygen species. Obese subjects also have increased sympathetic tone and activation of the renin-angiotensin-aldosterone system. Excess adipose tissue also releases other products including cytokines and prothrombotic factors and is associated with low adiponectin. High tumor necrosis factor α (TNF-α) levels are present in adipose tissue as well as in plasma of obese individuals and can cause a proinflammatory state that is both insulin resistant and atherogenic. Elevated plasminogen activation inhibitor (PAI-1) levels in obesity contribute to a prothrombotic state, again increasing

the risk of atherosclerotic cardiovascular events. Low adiponectin levels that accompany obesity are associated with worsening of IR. Visceral obesity seems to be more important than generalized obesity. Excessive fatty acids released by visceral adipose tissue can create IR by making more fuel available to liver and muscle. Free fatty acids have also been shown to interfere with the insulin signaling pathway. Although visceral adipose tissue is more active in producing all these changes, the underlying mechanisms for the association between visceral obesity and MetS are not fully understood.

Isolating IR from obesity is difficult. Insulin resistance generally rises with increasing obesity; however, all obese individuals are not necessarily insulin resistant. Similarly, IR can be present in nonobese individuals. These observations suggest a role of genetic or environmental factors in determining IR. Whether a single underlying abnormality is responsible for clustering of the components of MetS remains unclear.

Insights into the mechanistic connection between MetS and its complications are still limited. The risks for CVD and diabetes are greater in individuals with MetS than in those with obesity alone. Presence of MetS is associated with higher levels of C-reactive protein (CRP) and PAI-1 than the presence of individual metabolic abnormalities. The greater the number of MetS components, the higher the levels of CRP and PAI-1. Inflammation may be the common link between MetS and its clinical consequences,

Table 52.2 COMPARISON AMONG VARIOUS DEFINITIONS OF METABOLIC SYNDROME

	NCEP	WHO	IDF	EGIR	AACE
Obesity	WC >102 cm in men; >88 cm in women	BMI >30 kg/m² and/or waist:hip ratio >0.9 in men, >0.85 in women	WC depends on ethnicity	WC ≥94 cm in men; ≥80 cm in women	BMI >25 kg/m² and/or WC: >102 cm in men, >88 cm in women
IR		Type 2 diabetes or impaired glucose tolerance or IR on insulin clamp studies		Fasting hyperinsulinemia	Clinical evidence of IR
Glucose	FPG >100 mg/dL		FPG >100 mg/dL	FPG >110 mg/dL	FPG >100 mg/dL or 2-hour OGTT >140 mg/dL
Blood pressure (mm Hg)	>130/85	≥140/90	>130/85	>140/90	>130/85
Triglyceride	≥150 mg/dL	≥150 mg/dL	≥150 mg/dL	≥178 mg/dL	≥150 mg/dL
HDL cholesterol	<40 mg/dL in men; <50 mg/dL in women	<35 mg/dL in men; <39 mg/dL in women	<40 mg/dL in men; <50 mg/dL in women	<40 mg/dL	<40 mg/dL in men; <50 mg/dL in women
Other		Microalbuminuria			
Criteria for diagnosis	Any 3	IR plus 2 others	Obesity plus 2 others	IR plus 2 others	IR or obesity plus 2 others

NOTES: NCEP, National Cholesterol Education Program; WHO, World Health Organization; IDF, International Diabetes Federation; EGIR, European Group for the study of Insulin Resistance; AACE, American Association of Clinical Endocrinologists; WC, Waist circumference; IR, Insulin resistance; FPG, Fasting plasma glucose; OGTT, Oral glucose tolerance test.

CVD and diabetes. Alternatively, a yet unrecognized common abnormality may be responsible for MetS as well as CVD and diabetes.

CLINICAL SIGNIFICANCE

The clinical significance of MetS has been questioned recently because multiple studies demonstrate that the risk for CVD in MetS is no greater than the cumulative risk associated with its individual components. Indeed, data from the San Antonio Heart Study and the Framingham Heart Study suggest that the Framingham Risk Score (FRS) is better than a diagnosis of MetS at predicting CVD. Framingham Risk Scoring takes into account other risk factors, for example, age, sex, serum total or LDL cholesterol, and smoking status in addition to the metabolic syndrome components. Therefore, FRS is a preferred method for CVD risk prediction. However, the presence of MetS in nondiabetic individuals is a strong predictor of their developing type 2 diabetes in future. In the Framingham Heart Study, individuals without type 2 diabetes mellitus at baseline had a fivefold increase in risk for developing diabetes if they had MetS as compared to people without MetS. Thus, based on these data, a diagnosis of MetS does not help in CVD risk prediction, but it may help in prediction of type 2 diabetes. However, a diagnosis of MetS may lead to a more aggressive CVD risk reduction.

MANAGEMENT OF METABOLIC SYNDROME

GENERAL CONSIDERATIONS

Management of the metabolic syndrome is aimed at reducing the risk of CVD and new-onset diabetes. In general the management strategy is based on targeting individual risk factors and is not different from that of a patient without MetS (table 52.3). Lifestyle interventions are the mainstay of therapy to reduce metabolic risk factors. Weight loss by modification of diet and increased physical activity is advised. A healthy lifestyle will help in reduction of all the components of MetS. However, drug therapy may be required in many patients to achieve the goals for individual risk factors. Framingham risk scoring is necessary to set the goals and to decide about drug therapy.

MANAGEMENT OF OBESITY IN METABOLIC SYNDROME

Abdominal obesity is the hallmark of MetS and is considered an essential component in many of its definitions as described above. There is no specific treatment for abdominal obesity. General weight loss reduces IR, lowers other risk factors including triglycerides and blood pressure, and raises high-density lipoprotein (HDL) cholesterol. Furthermore, weight loss decreases serum levels of CRP, TNF-α, and PAI-1 and is associated with a decrease in oxidative stress. Therefore, NCEP ATPIII guidelines recommend obesity to be the primary target of intervention in MetS. Weight loss should be achieved with dietary changes and increased physical activity. Nutrition counseling by a trained nutritionist is recommended. The dietary plan should be individualized by taking into account an individual's habits and sociocultural factors. Low-carbohydrate diets may be more successful in short-term weight loss; however, long-term weight loss is equivalent with various types of diets and depends more on total caloric intake. Increased unsaturated fat intake, as in the Mediterranean diet, may help to control dyslipidemia and cause better reduction in IR and inflammatory markers. It should be noted that most weight loss trials have been conducted for 1–2 years only, and even in this short period, participants have shown a gradual weight gain after an initial weight loss. Therefore, it is more important to improve eating habits in a sustainable way. Emphasis should be on eating regular meals and paying attention to portion sizes. Social support and stress management are also important to sustain weight loss.

The importance of a regular exercise regimen cannot be overemphasized. Thirty minutes of moderate-intensity

Table 52.3 MANAGEMENT OF METABOLIC SYNDROME

ABNORMALITY	RECOMMENDED TREATMENT
Obesity	Lifestyle interventions
Insulin resistance/glucose intolerance	Lifestyle intervention Optional metformin
Hypertension	Joint National Commission-7 guidelines
Hypertriglyceridemia	Fibric acid derivatives Nicotinic acid
HDL cholesterol	Nicotinic acid

physical activity on most days of the week is recommended for most adults. Higher levels of physical activity will be more beneficial in MetS. Physical activity does not have to be all at one time. Short multiple bouts of 10–15 minutes of exercise that accumulate to about 1 hour per day are a practical and effective strategy for weight control in MetS.

A realistic goal for weight reduction is to reduce body weight by 5–10% over a period of 6–12 months. Most data show a very significant reduction in CVD risk factors with a very small reduction in weight. After initial weight loss, long-term maintenance of new, lowered weight is extremely important.

REDUCTION OF INSULIN RESISTANCE WITH DRUG THERAPY

Some experts believe that IR plays a central role in causation of MetS and should be the primary focus of treatment. Although weight loss and increased physical activity reduce IR and should be the primary mode of therapy, drug therapy to reduce IR is also an option. Currently, biguanides (metformin) and thiazolidinediones (rosiglitazone and pioglitazone) are the available agents to reduce insulin resistance. Although these drugs are approved for use in type 2 diabetes mellitus, all three drugs have also been shown to decrease the incidence or delay the onset of type 2 diabetes. Metformin may be a more attractive option in MetS because it helps in weight loss, corrects dyslipidemia, and lowers blood pressure. However, its use in MetS has not been tested in clinical trials. Metformin reduced the incidence of type 2 diabetes in the diabetes prevention program and was associated with fewer CVD events in the United Kingdom Prospective Diabetes Study (UKPDS). The American Diabetes Association (ADA) recommends considering the use of metformin in prediabetic patients who have impaired fasting glucose as well as impaired glucose tolerance. Both rosiglitazone and pioglitazone reduce insulin resistance. In addition, pioglitazone also corrects dyslipidemia. However, both agents are associated with weight gain and a high risk of heart failure. Moreover, there are concerns about the association of rosiglitazone with increased CVD mortality. Overall, the risk-benefit profile of TZDs dictates against their use in MetS.

A new class of drugs called cannabinoid receptor antagonists are being developed for use in MetS. Originally, these drugs were developed for treatment of obesity because they have an appetite suppressant effect. Clinical trials with rimonabant, the first drug in this class, revealed a very impressive reduction in all components of MetS. Unfortunately, rimonabant is associated with risk of major depression and is not approved for use in the United States. The drug is available in Europe and many other countries. Other drugs of this class are in various phases of clinical trials and may soon become available.

TREATMENT OF DYSLIPIDEMIA IN METABOLIC SYNDROME

Fibric acid derivatives and nicotinic acid can lower triglycerides and increase HDL cholesterol. Some studies suggest a reduction in CVD endpoints with fibrates in patients with MetS. However, according to NCEP the primary goal of treatment is reduction of LDL cholesterol. Lowering triglycerides and raising HDL cholesterol are considered secondary goals of lipid therapy. Therefore, in most patients fibrates and/or nicotinic acid are used in combination with a statin. There are no clinical trials to show the benefits of this combination on CVD events. Nicotinic acid is more efficacious than fibrates in raising HDL cholesterol, but it can cause a rise in plasma glucose levels.

TREATMENT OF HIGH BLOOD PRESSURE

Guidelines for treatment of hypertension in MetS are the same as in the Seventh Joint National Commission (JNC7) guidelines for non-MetS patients. Lifestyle changes described above for weight loss also help reduce blood pressure. No specific class of antihypertensive drugs is recommended for use in patients with MetS. However, diuretics and beta blockers are known to worsen IR and cause dyslipidemia. Clinical trials with angiotensin-converting enzyme inhibitors and angiotensin receptor blockers have shown a reduction in IR and a decrease in incidence of type 2 diabetes. Therefore, these drugs may be more useful in patients with MetS. However, the majority of clinical trials indicate that the main reason for reduction in CVD events associated with antihypertensive drugs is lowering of blood pressure. Therefore, it is more important to use a drug that effectively lowers blood pressure.

TREATMENT FOR PROINFLAMMATORY AND PROTHROMBOTIC STATE

No specific drugs are available to control the proinflammatory and prothrombotic state in MetS. However, more and more drugs are being tested for these effects. Low-dose aspirin reduces CVD events, and its risk–benefit profile favors its use in patients with MetS. When otherwise indicated, drugs with demonstrated suppressive effects on inflammatory cytokines and prothrombotic factors should be preferably used in MetS.

UNUSUAL CONDITIONS ASSOCIATED WITH METABOLIC SYNDROME

Rare disorders such as lipodystrophy caused by single-gene mutations may be associated with MetS. However, for the general population, MetS is probably a polygenic disorder. MetS is being detected more and more often in HIV patients, where it may be due to side effects of protease-inhibitor drugs. Lipodystrophy and IR are also often present in these patients. Additionally, MetS is being increasingly recognized as a side effect of other commonly used drugs, for example, corticosteroids, antidepressants, antipsychotics, and antihistamines. All these drugs can cause weight gain and IR. In most clinical situations these drugs cannot be stopped in spite of their side effects. Therefore, special attention should be paid to control the metabolic abnormalities associated with their use.

CONCLUSION

There is lack of consensus on the definition, clinical significance, and management of MetS. A common underlying pathophysiological mechanism has not been identified. Obesity and/or IR seem to be the central defects and, therefore, the primary targets of therapy. With increasing prevalence of obesity, the prevalence of MetS is also increasing. Clinically, MetS predicts the risk of CVD similar to that predicted by combining the risks associated with individual abnormalities. Therefore, treatment guidelines include treatment of individual risk factors. Whether a diagnosis of MetS will lead to more aggressive risk reduction and improve clinical outcomes remains to be determined.

ADDITIONAL READING

Day C. Metabolic syndrome, or what you will: Definitions and epidemiology. *Diab Vasc Dis Res.* 2007;4(1):32–8.
Eckel RH, Grundy SM, Zimmet PZ. The metabolic syndrome. *Lancet.* 2005;365(9468):1415–28.
Grundy SM, Cleeman JI, Daniels SR, et al. Diagnosis and management of the metabolic syndrome: An American Heart Association/National Heart, Lung, and Blood Institute Scientific Statement. *Circulation.* 2005;112(17):2735–52.
Kashyap SR, Defronzo RA. The insulin resistance syndrome: Physiological considerations. *Diab Vasc Dis Res.* 2007;4(1):13–9.
Stern MP, Williams K, Gonzalez-Villalpando C, Hunt KJ, Haffner SM. Does the metabolic syndrome improve identification of individuals at risk of type 2 diabetes and/or cardiovascular disease? *Diabetes Care.* 2004;27(11):2676–81.
Tota-Maharaj R, Defilippis AP, Blumenthal RS, Blaha MJ. A practical approach to the metabolic syndrome: Review of current concepts and management. *Curr Opin Cardiol.* 2010;25(5):502–12.
Wannamethee SG, Shaper AG, Lennon L, Morris RW. Metabolic syndrome vs Framingham Risk Score for prediction of coronary heart disease, stroke, and type 2 diabetes mellitus. *Arch Intern Med.* 2005;165(22):2644–50.

QUESTIONS

QUESTION 1. Which one of the following is not included in the NCEP ATPIII diagnostic criteria of metabolic syndrome?

A. HDL
B. Blood Pressure
C. Glucose
D. LDL
E. Waist circumference

QUESTION 2. How many abnormal features are required for a diagnosis of metabolic syndrome according to NCEP ATPIII definition?

A. One
B. Two
C. Three
D. Four
E. Five

QUESTION 3. Metabolic syndrome is the strongest predictor for which of following conditions?

A. Myocardial infarction
B. Diabetes mellitus
C. Stroke
D. Heart failure
E. Renal failure

QUESTION 4. Which one of the following is the mainstay of the treatment of metabolic syndrome?

A. Lifestyle interventions
B. Insulin sensitizers
C. Anti-inflammatory drugs
D. Lipid-lowering drugs

QUESTION 5. The decision about drug therapy in metabolic syndrome depends on the following:

A. Number of abnormal components
B. CRP levels
C. Abnormal values of individual components
D. All patients should be treated with metformin

ANSWERS

1. D
2. C
3. B
4. A
5. C

53.

METABOLIC BONE DISEASES

Meryl S. LeBoff

Bone is a dynamic and complex organ that undergoes constant remodeling. It consists of an organic matrix (collagen and some noncollagenous proteins), minerals (calcium and phosphate in hydroxyapatite crystals), and water. Normally bone mass is maintained by a tight coupling of bone breakdown by osteoclasts followed by bone formation by osteoblasts. This chapter summarizes three metabolic bone diseases. Osteoporosis is characterized by a decreased bone mass with a normal mineral-to-matrix ratio and superimposed skeletal fragility and fractures; osteomalacia occurs when there is a reduced mineralization of the matrix; and Paget's disease is a disorder in which there is excessive, disorganized bone resorption and formation.

OSTEOPOROSIS

Osteoporosis is the most common metabolic bone disease. An estimated 50% of women and 25% of men aged 50 years and older will develop an osteoporotic fracture in their remaining lifetime. Fractures rise exponentially with age, with wrist fractures as the earliest sign of osteoporosis, followed by a dramatic rise in spine and hip fractures. Although only 25% of spine fractures are clinically evident without an x-ray, spine fractures lead to loss of height, kyphosis, abdominal distension, restrictive lung disease, and an increased risk of subsequent spine and hip fractures. Hip fractures are the most serious osteoporotic fractures. Approximately 50% of patients who sustain a hip fracture lose the ability to walk independently; an estimated 12–24% of women and 30% of men die within the first year. In the United States only 20% of patients who sustain a fragility fracture of the spine, hip, or arm are evaluated or treated for their osteoporosis. A fragility fracture is defined as a fracture occurring with minimal trauma such as falling from a standing height. Thus, despite the health consequences of osteoporosis and availability of effective treatments that reduce fracture risk, it is under-diagnosed and under-treated.

Peak bone mineral density (BMD) is achieved after puberty by age 25 years, after which bone loss ensues in both sexes. In women there is accelerated loss of bone for 5–8 years following menopause. Over a lifetime, women lose an estimated 50% of the bone in the spine and proximal femur and 30% of the bone in the appendicular skeleton; men lose two-thirds of these amounts. Thus, optimization and maintenance of peak bone mass may reduce the risk of fractures later in life. The advent of bone density testing using dual x-ray absorptiometry (DXA) makes it possible to quantify the amount of bone in the spine, hip, forearm, and total body with little radiation exposure. A BMD in a patient is compared with that of (1) age-matched controls to determine whether the BMD is diminished relative to an age-matched cohort (e.g., Z score, see figure 53.1) and (2) young-normal controls to assess whether there is a decrease in BMD from peak bone mass (T score). Low bone mass (osteopenia) is defined as a T score between –1.0 and –2.5. Osteoporosis is a T score of –2.5 or lower or osteopenia with a fragility fracture in an adult.

In the United States it is estimated that 40 million adults will have osteopenia, and 12 million will have osteoporosis. Although there is an inverse relationship between BMD and future fracture risk, more than half of fragility fractures occur in patients with osteopenia. This is because more adults have osteopenia than osteoporosis, and other clinically important factors contribute to the risk of fracture. The evaluation of patients for osteoporosis should include a careful history and physical examination to identify risk factors and secondary causes of osteoporosis, and a BMD. Secondary causes of osteoporosis are common and affect an estimated 40–65% of women and men.

Table 53.1 lists some of the secondary causes of low bone mass and osteoporosis. In each of these disorders bone loss results from a net increased bone resorption, deficient bone formation, or both. Supraphysiological levels of exogenous or endogenous (Cushing's disease/syndrome) glucocorticoids produce an early loss of trabecular bone with a smaller effect on cortical bone, resulting in a decrease in bone formation, an increase in bone resorption, and a negative calcium balance.

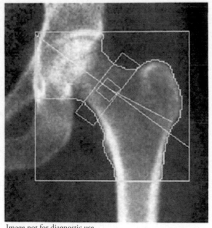

DXA Results Summary:

Region	Area (cm²)	BMX (g)	BMD (g/cm²)	T-score	PR (%)	Z-score	AM (%)
Neck	4.94	2.96	0.599	−2.2	71	0.0	99
Troch	10.86	6.89	0.634	−0.7	90	1.0	119
Inter	16.60	15.74	0.948	−1.0	86	0.7	114
Total	32.41	25.60	0.790	−1.2	84	0.7	112
Ward's	1.30	0.63	0.484	−2.1	66	0.8	124

Total BMD CV 1.0%

WHO Classification: Osteopenia

FRAX® *WHO Fracture Risk Assessment Tool*

10-year Fracture Risk[1]	Without Prior Fracture	With Prior Fracture
Major Osteoporotic Fracture	20%	28%
Hip Fracture	7.3%	9.8%

Reported Risk Factors:
US (Caucasian), Neck BMD-0.599, BMI=28.1, alcohol use

Image not for diagnostic use
96 x 95
NECK: 49 x 15
HAL: 102 mm

[1] FRAX® Version 3.01. Fracture probability calculated for an untreated patient. Fracture probability may be lower if the patient has received treatment.

Figure 53.1. DXA of the Hip. Bone mineral density is compared with the young adult mean at peak bone mass and age-matched controls. The *T*-score and *Z*-score are an index of the number of standard deviations compared with young-normal and age-matched controls, respectively.

Glucocorticoids produce a dose dependent rise in fracture risk, particularly at prednisone doses of 5 mg/day or higher; very high doses of inhaled corticosteroids can also lead to a decrease in bone mass. In long-standing hyperthyroidism or supraphysiological thyroid hormone replacement, the resulting accelerated bone turnover may produce bone loss, which can be detected by a very suppressed thyroid-stimulating hormone (TSH). A number of hypogonadal states (e.g., anorexia nervosa, athletic triad, or gonadal suppression) may result in bone loss and an early risk of fractures. In connective tissue disorders, the abnormal collagen is the basis for compromised skeletal integrity. Renal disease is associated with an increased risk of fractures that may result from osteoporosis, but this condition must be distinguished from aplastic bone disease, secondary hyperparathyroidism, or osteomalacia. Although rheumatoid arthritis affects only approximately 1% of the population, it is associated with an elevated fracture risk through multiple mechanisms.

Low BMD and increased fracture risk also occur in patients with a variety of gastrointestinal and hepatic disorders in association with a number of factors including malabsorption, nutritional deficiencies, and/or increased inflammatory markers. In patients with celiac disease, adherence to a gluten-free diet results in a reversal of the disease process and an increase in bone mass. As shown in table 53.1, a growing list of medications are associated with osteoporosis, including drugs that suppress endogenous sex steroid production (i.e., aromatase inhibitors), proton pump inhibitors, selective serotonin reuptake inhibitors, cyclosporine A or tacrolimus, and others.

The evaluation for secondary causes of osteoporosis is directed at identification of treatable disorders and includes the determination of serum calcium, 25-hydroxyvitamin D [25(OH)D], parathyroid hormone [PTH], and sensitive TSH levels (especially in adults on thyroid hormone); liver tests; complete blood count; possibly serum and urinary protein electrophoresis; and measurement of 24-hour urinary calcium and creatinine levels. Additional endocrinologic or neoplastic processes should be considered in patients with progressive bone loss and fractures and those in whom fragility fractures are uncommon, such as young adults, premenopausal women, and men younger than 60. Correction of the underlying cause of osteoporosis may result in improvements in bone.

Current guidelines recommend bone density testing of the spine and hip in women aged ≥65 and men aged ≥70; postmenopausal women with risk factors and men age 50 and older with clinical risk factors; adults in whom you are considering therapy for osteoporosis or need to monitor the response to therapy; and women discontinuing estrogen. In 1997 Medicare mandated coverage for BMD testing every 2 years in estrogen-deficient women; patients with radiologic evidence of low bone mass or a fracture; glucocorticoid-treated subjects; patients with primary hyperparathyroidism (forearm bone density also indicated here); and for monitoring the response to an approved osteoporosis treatment. DXA also provides a useful technique called vertebral fracture assessment for detecting spine fractures.

A new clinical tool, the FRAX® calculator, uses epidemiologic data from many countries to estimate fracture risk (http://www.shef.ac.uk/FRAX) among the large number

Table 53.1 CAUSES OF LOW BONE MASS AND/OR OSTEOPOROSIS

Endocrinological abnormalities:
  Glucocorticoid excess
  Thyroid excess
  Hypogonadism
  Anorexia
  Athletic triad
  Prolactinomas
  Hyperparathyroidism (primary or secondary)

Process affecting the marrow:
  Multiple myeloma
  Mastocytosis
  Leukemia
  Gaucher disease

Chronic kidney disease (CKD):
  Hypercalciuria

Gastrointestinal diseases:
  Postgastrectomy
  Primary biliary or alcoholic cirrhosis
  Inflammatory bowel disease

Connective tissue disorders:
  Osteogenesis imperfecta
  Homocystinuria
  Ehlers-Danlos syndrome

Rheumatologic disorders:
  Ankylosing spondylitis
  Rheumatoid arthritis

Immobilization:
  Paraplegia
  Space flight

Medications:
  Aromatase inhibitors
  Thiazolidine medications
  Proton pump inhibitors
  Serotonin-uptake inhibitors
  Anticonvulsants
  Heparin
  Methotrexate
  GnRH agonists
  Lithium
  Cyclosporine-A

of individuals with osteopenia. FRAX® incorporates risk factors and BMD in a model to predict the 10-year absolute fracture risk for a hip fracture or four osteoporotic fractures (hip, wrist, proximal humerus, and clinical spine fractures). Clinical risk factors incorporated in the FRAX® calculator released by the World Health Organization (WHO) include age, gender, parental history of a hip fracture, weight and height to calculate body mass index, a personal history of an osteoporotic fracture, rheumatoid arthritis, current smoking, current glucocorticoid use, alcohol use (>3 units daily), and secondary causes of osteoporosis (yes/no). Secondary causes specified in FRAX® include type 1 diabetes mellitus, osteogenesis imperfecta, hypogonadism, premature menopause, long-standing hyperthyroidism, malabsorption, and chronic liver disease. Several limitations to FRAX® are important for clinical decisions regarding treatment. On the assumption that secondary causes of osteoporosis lead to changes in BMD, entering a BMD in the FRAX® calculator removes the impact of the secondary cause on the absolute fracture risk. Many medical conditions and treatments that increase fracture risk are not included in FRAX®. With FDA approval, FRAX® output is available on bone density machines and is included in many BMD reports. Thus, use of FRAX® in conjunction with good clinical judgment holds the promise that the many women and men around the world with osteopenia who are at high risk of fracture will be identified and treated.

Risk-factor analysis and physical examination are essential in deciding which patients may benefit from therapy to prevent or treat osteoporosis. Therapy is recommended in patients with evidence of osteoporosis with a spine or hip fracture or a spine or hip T-score ≤−2.5. Using a cost–benefit analysis, the National Osteoporosis Foundation provided treatment thresholds (calculated by FRAX® using the United States database) for adults with a 10-year risk of major fracture of ≥20% or a hip fracture of ≥3%. Patients with osteopenia aged 50 years and older and/or with physician concerns about secondary causes of osteoporosis should also be considered for treatment. To reduce the high prevalence of osteoporotic fractures, lifestyle changes (e.g., smoking cessation, avoidance of excessive alcohol, and healthy weight maintenance), reversal of modifiable risk factors, and optimization of calcium and vitamin D intake should be implemented. If calcium intake from diet and supplements is inadequate to balance the daily calcium loss, bone loss ensues. Longitudinal studies show that supplemental calcium is modestly helpful in retarding bone loss. According to the Institute of Medicine (IOM) Report in 2011, children and adolescents between the ages of 9 and 18 years and pregnant women between the ages of 14 and 18 years require a total calcium intake of 1300 mg elemental calcium daily. Premenopausal women and men 19–50 years require 1000 mg/day, and women aged 51 years and older and men aged 71 and older require 1200 mg/day to prevent negative calcium balance. In the absence of underlying disorders of calcium homeostasis, these calcium intakes are generally safe. However, in the Women's Health Initiative (WHI), 1000 mg of supplemental calcium daily was associated with a 17% increased risk of kidney stones in postmenopausal women, and recent analyses showed an association between calcium supplements and increased risk of cardiovascular disease. Calcium carbonate is the most widely used supplement, containing 40% of elemental calcium by weight; it should be taken with food, as achlorhydric subjects cannot absorb it well on an empty stomach. Calcium citrate, which contains 24% elemental calcium, has enhanced bioavailability and is absorbed on an empty stomach or with reduced gastric acidity.

ROLE OF VITAMIN D

Vitamin D increases calcium absorption, and both calcium and vitamin D are important for skeletal health. Vitamin D is activated in the skin by sunlight or absorbed in the intestine and then converted to 25(OH)D in the liver. The 1,25-dihydroxyvitamin D [1,25(OH)$_2$D] metabolite is synthesized in the kidney from 25(OH)D through activation of the 1-hydroxylase enzyme, which is stimulated by hypophosphatemia, hypocalcemia, and PTH. New data indicate that 1,25(OH)$_2$D is also synthesized from 25(OH)D in many cells and then inactivated internally, resulting in important cellular effects on immune and other functions.

Low levels of vitamin D have previously been documented at all ages (children and adults) because of inadequate exposure to ultraviolet light, insufficient intake, use of sun block, increased skin pigment, obesity, or impaired absorption (biliary or gastrointestinal diseases). Nursing home residents, adults with hip fractures, patients with malabsorption, or those not exposed to ultraviolet light or on vitamin D supplements are at high risk for vitamin D deficiency. Mild vitamin D insufficiency may not cause symptoms, but it can contribute to low bone mass. Severe vitamin D deficiency causes osteomalacia (see below). In addition, vitamin D deficiency has been associated with impaired muscle function, increased risk of falls, and some malignancies (e.g., colorectal, breast, and prostate cancer); additional data are needed from randomized controlled trials to assess the benefit of vitamin D supplementation on these outcomes.

There is debate concerning the boundaries for vitamin D insufficiency and sufficiency. In the IOM report (2011), an inadequate level of vitamin D was recently defined as a 25(OH)D <20 ng/mL. The Endocrine Society practice guideline reported a sufficient 25(OH)D level for bone as a 25(OH)D ≥30 ng/mL. Studies of women hospitalized with hip fractures showed a substantial number of women with low vitamin D levels according to both thresholds. Data from prospective, placebo-controlled studies and a meta-analysis support the recommendation that patients should also have a minimum of 800 IU of vitamin D daily to reduce the risk of fractures, although more data are needed from randomized clinical trials using higher doses of vitamin D. The NIH-funded Vitamin D and Omega-3 Trial (VITAL) (1 U01 CA138962) is a large-scale, randomized, primary prevention trial testing 2000 IU/day vitamin D-3 (cholecalciferol) and/or 1 g/day omega-3 fatty acids versus placebo on cardiovascular disease and cancer endpoints among 20,000 men and women and, in ancillary studies, on fracture and other outcomes.

For osteoporosis prevention and treatment, individuals should be advised to consume adequate vitamin D and calcium and to participate in a regular exercise program (see table 53.2 for recommended dietary allowance of calcium and vitamin D). Dietary sources of calcium and vitamin D include milk and calcium-supplemented orange juice (300 mg calcium and 100 IU vitamin D/8 oz), fortified cereals, and cereal bars; vitamin D is also found in salt water fish, cod liver oil, and egg yolk. Multivitamins have previously contained 400 IU of vitamin D, with new preparations containing 500–1000 IU. Many calcium preparations also contain vitamin D. Approaches to restore very low levels of 25(OH)D level to a sufficient level with high doses of vitamin D-2 and close monitoring are shown in table 53.3. The goals of therapy for osteoporosis are to reduce bone resorption and to enhance bone formation. Weight-bearing and muscle-strengthening exercises may modestly increase BMD and reduce falls. In postmenopausal women a 2002 Cochrane Review of the effects of exercise on bone, aerobics, weight-bearing, and resistance exercises had positive effects on spinal BMD, and walking improved hip bone BMD. Strategies should also include implementation of balance training and fall prevention and other approaches (e.g., safe home, review of prescription medications, corrected vision).

Table 53.2 DIETARY REFERENCE INTAKES FOR CALCIUM AND VITAMIN D

LIFE STAGE GROUP	CALCIUM RECOMMENDED DIETARY ALLOWANCE (MG/DAY)	VITAMIN D RECOMMENDED DIETARY ALLOWANCE (IU/DAY)
9–18 years old	1300	600
19–50 years old	1000	600
51–70 year old	1000	600
51–70 year old females	1200	600
71+ years old	1200	800
14–18 years old, pregnant/lactating	1300	600
19–50 years old, pregnant/lactating	1000	600

SOURCE: Modified from IOM (2011).

Table 53.3 VITAMIN D REPLETION

25-(OH) VITAMIN D	RECOMMENDED TREATMENT DOSE
<10 ng/mL	Evaluation by a bone specialist.
<20 ng/mL	50,000 IU vitamin D-2 weekly for 8 weeks and then recheck level. Once sufficient level is reached, consider maintenance with 600–1000 IU of vitamin D-3 daily or 50,000 IU vitamin D-2 once or twice monthly as needed.

There are a number of FDA-approved (see table 53.4) and emerging therapies for the prevention and treatment of osteoporosis. Because ≤20% of patients with fragility fractures are treated for their underlying osteoporosis, it is critically important to initiate osteoporosis therapy to reduce subsequent fractures in these individuals.

HORMONE THERAPY

Estrogen replacement decreases bone resorption and increases BMD. Data from the large WHI show that oral conjugated estrogen plus progestin (Prempro™) or estrogen (Premarin™) alone decreased the risk of clinical

Table 53.4 OSTEOPOROSIS PREVENTION AND TREATMENT: FDA-APPROVED DRUGS

DRUG	DOSAGE	OSTEOPOROSIS INDICATIONS	EFFECTIVE IN FRACTURE REDUCTION (+/−) VERTEBRAL	HIP	NONVERTEBRAL
Estrogen	0.625 mg PO daily, variable-dose patches, gels, and creams	Prevention of PMO*	+	+	+
Selective estrogen receptor modulators Raloxifene (Evista™)	60 mg PO daily	Prevention and treatment of PMO*	+	−	−
Calcitonin (Miacalcin™, Fortical™) (Calcimar™)	200 IU intranasally daily 100 IU subcutaneously or intramuscularly every other day	Treatment of PMO* (>5 years past menopause)	+	−	−
Bisphosphonates Alendronate (Fosamax™)	70 mg PO once weekly	Prevention and treatment of PMO* and osteoporosis in men; Prevention and treatment of GIO†	+	+	+
Risedronate (Actonel™)	35 mg PO once weekly; 150 mg PO monthly	Prevention and treatment of PMO* and osteoporosis in men; Prevention and treatment of GIO†	+	+	+
Ibandronate (Boniva™)	2.5 mg PO daily, 150 mg PO once weekly, 3 mg IV every 3 months	Prevention and treatment of PMO*	+	−	−
Zoledronic Acid (Reclast™)	5 mg IV once yearly	Treatment of PMO*; In patients at high risk of fracture defined as a recent low-trauma hip fracture to reduce clinical fractures; GIO†	+	+	+
RANKL inhibitor Denosumab (Prolia®)	60 mg subcutaneously every 6 months	Treatment of PMO at high risk for fractures	+	+	+
PTH Teriparatide (Forteo™)	20 μg subcutaneously daily (for maximum of 2 years)	Treatment of PMO* and men with osteoporosis who are at high risk for fracture	+	NA	+

NOTES: *PMO, postmenopausal osteoporosis; †GIO, glucocorticoid-induced osteoporosis.
SOURCE: Modified from IOM (2011).

spine fractures by 35% and 38% and hip fractures by 33% and 39%, respectively. Estrogen and progestin, however, increased the risks of heart disease, stroke, pulmonary embolism, and breast cancer; the estrogen-alone arm raised the incidence of stroke. Women starting hormone therapy within 10 years of menopause, however, in more recent studies did not show an increased risk of cardiovascular disease. In a controlled study, very low doses of transdermal estradiol (0.014 mg/day) increased spine BMD by 2.6%. Hormone therapy for 2–3 years has been shown to prevent bone loss and fractures. Hormone therapy is very effective to control moderate or severe menopausal symptoms, although it is prudent to use the lowest dose for the shortest duration to control symptoms. Although hormone therapy is FDA-approved for the prevention of osteoporosis, the FDA recommends that nonestrogen medications be considered first.

Selective Estrogen Receptor Modulators

Selective estrogen receptor modulators (SERMs) are a class of drugs that bind to estrogen receptors and can selectively function as agonists or antagonists in different tissues. Raloxifene (Evista™) is approved by the FDA for the prevention and treatment of osteoporosis and prevention of invasive breast cancer; other SERMs are undergoing clinical investigation. A large, multicenter, randomized, placebo-controlled study of raloxifene treatment for 3 years increased BMD of the spine and hip by 2.6% and 2.1%, respectively, and reduced spine fractures by 55% in women without prevalent vertebral fractures, with no effect on wrist or nonspine fractures; the risk of deep vein thrombosis is similar to hormone therapy side effects and includes a small increase in leg cramps and hot flashes. Tamoxifen™, which has estrogen agonist-like effects on bone and the endometrium (including some cases of endometrial carcinoma), produces a small increase in BMD in postmenopausal women with a history of breast cancer, although it is associated with bone loss in premenopausal women.

Calcitonin

Calcitonin is an inhibitor of osteoclast-mediated bone resorption and is approved for the treatment of osteoporosis. Calcitonin nasal spray (200 IU/day) increases spinal BMD by only 1.0–1.5% and decreases spine fractures by 33% but not other fractures; recent studies show some improvements in measures of bone microarchitecture. Side effects of calcitonin include nausea, flushing, and rhinorrhea with the nasal preparation.

Bisphosphonates

Bisphosphonates are analogues of pyrophosphate that are adsorbed onto the hydroxyapatite of bone and inhibit bone resorption through various mechanisms; bisphosphonates reduce the depth of resorption pits and new bone remodeling, thereby producing positive bone balance. Oral preparations of bisphosphonates include alendronate, risedronate, and ibandronate, which increase spine and femoral neck BMD by 8% and 3.5%; 5.4% and 1.6%; and 5.7% and 2.4%, respectively. Table 53.4 shows the FDA-approved indications for bisphosphonate therapy and their antifracture effects. When choosing a bisphosphonate, data on the best available antifracture efficacy (in the absence of head-to-head comparisons) indicate that alendronate, risedronate, or intravenous zoledronic acid reduce spine, hip, and nonspine fractures. Alendronate decreases spine fractures by 47%, hip fractures by 51%, and nonvertebral fractures by 50%. Risedronate reduced the risk of new vertebral fractures by 41–49%, hip fractures by 40%, and nonvertebral fractures by 36% in 3 years, with reductions in spine fractures in the first year. In contrast, intermittent or daily-dose ibandronate decreased spine fractures by 50–62% in 3 years without an effect on nonspine fractures in the overall cohort. Once-yearly intravenous zoledronic acid decreased the incidence of clinical spine, hip, and nonspine fractures by 77%, 41%, and 25%, respectively, over 3 years. Alendronate currently has the lowest cost, as it is available in generic form; nongeneric preparations include vitamin D. Oral risedronate and ibandronate are available as a once-a-month therapy. A new form of oral risedronate (Atelvia) can be taken with food and without needing to sit upright pre and post dose. Zoledronic acid IV (5 mg infusion once a year) should be considered in patients with the poor compliance with oral bisphosphonates (>50% of patients stop oral therapy) and for patients with esophageal disorders, inability to sit or stand upright for 30 minutes, or intolerance to oral bisphosphonates. Zoledronic acid should also be considered in patients with a recent hip fracture (after 2 weeks to 90 days) or spine fractures, optimally after correction of vitamin D deficiency, with evidence to support efficacy of this treatment in secondary prevention of fractures and for prolonged survival. Bisphosphonates are excreted renally and should not be used for patients with a creatinine clearance <30–35 mL/min; for patient safety, the author's practice is to ensure an eGFR above this range, a sufficient 25(OH)D level >30–32 ng/mL, and normal calcium level before each zoledronic acid infusion.

Side effects of oral bisphosphonates include upper gastrointestinal symptoms and rare esophagitis. Bisphosphonate use has been associated with osteonecrosis of the jaws (ONJ), predominantly in cancer patients treated with bisphosphonates to reduce skeletal metastases. Although the true prevalence of ONJ is not known, the estimated prevalence is 1 in 10,000 to 1 in 100,000 patient-treatment years. The FDA implemented a "precaution" regarding ONJ for bisphosphonates. A low but significant risk of atrial fibrillation (AF) was reported with zoledronic acid, but in a recent review the FDA did not identify a risk of AF for this class of drugs. Cases of atypical femur fractures have been reported in bisphosphonate-treated subjects on longer-term therapy. Side effects of intravenous bisphosphonates including acute-phase reactions (e.g., flu-like syndrome, malaise, myalgias) may occur in approximately 10–30% of subjects after intravenous bisphosphonates but decrease with each subsequent infusion, and possibly with oral acetaminophen administration for 24 hours. A number of physicians consider discontinuation of alendronate after 5 years of use because of post-hoc data generated in patients (without severe osteoporosis) in the alendronate fracture extension trial. The study authors of that paper concluded that, although stopping alendronate for up to 5 years did not significantly increase fracture risk, women at high risk of clinical spine fractures may benefit from continued alendronate use. According to the 2011 FDA review more data are needed on long-term use of bisphosphonates and bisphosphonate holidays.

Parathyroid Hormone

Advances in the treatment of osteoporosis include the availability of the only anabolic agent, PTH, that enhances bone formation instead of suppressing bone resorption. Continuous secretion of PTH, as in hyperparathyroidism, results in bone loss (particularly in the forearm and hip). Intermittent PTH injections (daily), however, produce robust increases in bone mass and improve bone microarchitecture. PTH stimulates bone formation and remodeling through multiple mechanisms, with an early increase in markers of bone formation before bone resorption, with the development of an "anabolic window."

In a large, multicenter, randomized, placebo-controlled study in postmenopausal women, teriparatide (PTH_{1-34}) increased spinal BMD by 9.7% and femoral neck BMD by 2.8%, with a small decrease in the distal radial site that was similar to placebo-treated subjects. PTH (20 µg daily) reduced the risk of spine fractures by 65% and nonspine fractures by 53%. PTH also showed beneficial effects on bone in men and glucocorticoid-treated subjects. The biologically active fragment PTH_{1-34} has properties similar to the full-length intact PTH_{1-84}, which is being investigated and is approved for use in Europe.

Concurrent treatment with alendronate and PTH attenuates the anabolic action of PTH. Thus, it is important to stop a bisphosphonate before starting PTH therapy. Bisphosphonate therapy, however, should be started immediately on completion of PTH to consolidate the anabolic effects of PTH on bone.

Teriparatide (20 µg) is administered as a daily subcutaneous injection for up to 24 months, using a pen that contains a one-month supply (table 53.4). Side effects include transient redness at the injection site, headache, nausea, hypotension (rare), and mild hypercalcemia. Rodents treated with nearly life-long daily teriparatide have an increased risk of osteosarcoma. Teriparatide is FDA-approved for the treatment of postmenopausal women and men with osteoporosis at high fracture risk. Teriparatide has a black-box warning about the risk of osteosarcoma documented in rodents; an increased prevalence has not, to date, been observed in humans. For this reason, teriparatide should not be used in patients with Paget's disease, an elevated alkaline phosphatase, bone metastases, prior x-ray therapy, or hypercalcemia, or in children or young adults with open epiphyses. Alternative modes of administration of PTH such as a nasal spray of PTH_{1-34}, oral and transdermal preparation are under investigation.

Denosumab

The receptor activator of nuclear factor kappa B ligand (RANKL) is secreted by osteoblasts, binds to its RANK receptor on osteoclasts, and plays an important role in activation and proliferation of osteoclasts. A human monoclonal antibody to RANKL, denosumab, administered as a subcutaneous injection every 6 months inhibits osteoclastogenesis and leads to suppression of bone turnover, with a greater increase in BMD than placebo or alendronate. In 2010 denosumab was FDA approved for the treatment of postmenopausal osteoporosis in women at high risk for fracture. It has very recently also been approved for treatment of bone disease associated with breast and prostate cancer. The FDA included warnings and precautions regarding serious infections, skin reactions at the injection site, and ONJ. Because denosumab is contraindicated in hypocalcemia, a baseline calcium should be performed along with a dental exam prior to initiating therapy.

OTHER EMERGING OSTEOPOROSIS THERAPIES

Strontium ranelate is composed of two strontium atoms bound to ranelic acid that, when administered orally, is distributed in bone and both stimulates bone formation and inhibits bone resorption. Studies in humans show changes in markers of bone turnover consistent with these effects. In postmenopausal women with at least one spine fracture, 2 g of oral strontium ranelate compared with placebo increased BMD in the spine and femoral neck 14.4% and 8.3%, respectively; adjusting for the strontium content in the spine that affects the BMD measurement, the BMD actually increased 6.8% from baseline in the strontium-treated group and decreased 1.3% in the placebo group. In a subsequent large study of postmenopausal women with osteoporosis, followed for 3 and 5 years compared with placebo, strontium ranelate therapy led to a reduction in nonspine fractures of 16% and 15% and among high-risk women, a decrease of morphogenic spine fractures of 39% and 24% and hip fractures of 36% and 43%, respectively. Thus, strontium ranelate reduces fractures at multiple sites.

Side effects of strontium ranelate include diarrhea, nausea, and headache that improve over time and transient increases in creatinine kinase levels. More data are needed regarding other side effects such as venous thromboembolism, seizure, DRESS Syndrome and memory loss reported in some studies. Strontium ranelate is not currently approved for use by the FDA, but it has been in use clinically in Europe since 2004.

Other new therapies for osteoporosis under investigation include calcium-sensing-receptor antagonists, sclerostin inhibitors, integrin antagonists, and cathepsin-K inhibitors.

OSTEOMALACIA

Like osteoporosis, osteomalacia is a treatable disease and should not be overlooked. Osteomalacia develops from a deficiency of vitamin D, phosphate, or calcium and decreased incorporation of calcium and phosphate in the hydroxyapatite of bone (table 53.5). Reduced availability of vitamin D or abnormal metabolism of vitamin D with reduced 25(OH)D levels (in severe liver disease and nephrotic syndrome or with use of anticonvulsant drugs) and 1,25(OH)$_2$D levels (in chronic kidney disease) may produce osteomalacia. Osteomalacia is frequently manifested by generalized bone pain. In more pronounced cases, bony deformities (e.g., bowing in children), pseudofractures with radiolucent stress fractures perpendicular to the periosteum (located on the proximal, medial aspects of the long bone or pubic rami), osteopenia, or fragility fractures may occur. In vitamin D deficiency the calcium and phosphate levels are usually slightly decreased or in the low-normal range, with an upper-normal-range or elevated PTH level. An elevated serum alkaline phosphatase level also suggests a vitamin D deficiency.

Phosphate deficiency leads to osteomalacia most commonly in syndromes characterized by decreased renal phosphate conservation and increased fibroblast growth factor-23 (FGF-23). The familial X-linked hypophosphatemic vitamin D–resistant rickets in children or osteomalacia in adults usually presents with hypophosphatemia, a renal phosphate leak, and rachitic or osteomalacial changes, respectively, and an inappropriately normal or low-normal 1,25(OH)$_2$D level. Decreased renal tubular phosphate reabsorption is also a feature of oncogenic osteomalacia, associated largely with benign mesenchymal tumors, fibrous dysplasia, prostatic carcinoma, and rarely with other malignant tumors. Such patients typically present with hypophosphatemia, normocalcemia, muscle weakness, and inappropriately reduced 1,25(OH)$_2$D levels. Although many of these tumors are small and difficult to find, their removal results in complete resolution of this disorder. Generalized renal tubular disorders and inhibitors of mineralization are also associated with osteomalacia.

Vitamin D deficiency may be treated with physiological doses, but higher doses are effective in raising the serum 25(OH)D level (table 53.3). With intestinal malabsorption, very high doses of vitamin D (e.g., 50,000 IU several times a week) may be necessary until the underlying process is treated. In patients with disorders of renal tubular reabsorption (e.g., X-linked hypophosphatemic rickets/osteomalacia, oncogenic osteomalacia), phosphate therapy with 1,25(OH)$_2$D (to prevent an increase in PTH levels following phosphate) improves the bone healing. In chronic kidney disease 1,25(OH)$_2$D or vitamin D analogues are used; maintaining the serum calcium phosphate product under 55 is indicated. Reduction of phosphate absorption with phosphate binders should be provided.

Table 53.5 CAUSES OF OSTEOMALACIA AND RICKETS (IN CHILDREN)

Alteration in the Metabolism of Vitamin D
Reduced 25-hydroxyvitamin D: severe liver disease, nephrotic syndrome, anticonvulsant drugs
Reduced 1,25-dihydroxyvitamin D or altered action on target tissues: kidney disease, vitamin D-dependent rickets type I, vitamin D-dependent rickets type II
Phosphate Deficiency
Decreased phosphate availability: dietary deficiency, phosphate-binding antacid
Impaired intestinal phosphate absorption: pancreatic insufficiency, intrinsic bowel disease, short bowel syndromes
Decreased renal tubular phosphate reabsorption: familial: X-linked hypophosphatemic rickets/osteomalacia; osteomalacia, oncogenic osteomalacia
Generalized Renal Tubular Disorders, renal tubular acidosis, ureterosigmoidoscopy, carbonic anhydrase inhibitors (acetazolamide)
Miscellaneous mineralization defects
Inhibitors of mineralization: fluoride, bisphosphonates (e.g., etidronate), aluminum (e.g., TPN, CRF)
Hypophosphatasia

PAGET'S DISEASE

Paget's disease is a common bone disorder that affects 2% of the population over age 55. An estimated 15%–30% of patients have a family history of this disease, and some new gene mutations have been identified (e.g., in sequestosome gene and rank). Paget's disease is characterized by localized increased bone resorption by multinucleated osteoclasts and formation of disorganized, weakened woven bone. Although many patients are asymptomatic, the clinical signs and symptoms of Paget's disease include bone pain and increased warmth of affected bones, associated joint symptoms, skeletal deformities (e.g., bowing), pathologic fractures, increased cardiac output, hearing loss and other nerve compression, and rarely osteogenic sarcoma. The pelvis, sacrum, vertebrae, lower extremities, and skull are commonly involved sites. Although serum calcium and phosphorus levels are usually normal, with immobilization hypercalcemia can ensue. The serum total and bone-specific alkaline phosphatase levels, markers of bone formation and turnover, are usually elevated in patents with Paget's disease; in the absence of liver disease the total alkaline phosphatase is a good marker of disease activity. Urine and/or serum markers of bone resorption (N-telopeptide of type 1, C-telopeptide of type 1 collagen) may also be elevated in patients with Paget's disease, but they are not routinely measured. X-ray studies characteristically show enlarged bones, thickened cortices, and osteolytic, osteoblastic, and/or combined changes. Bone scans are useful to diagnose the overall disease activity and to determine whether there is localized monostotic or polyostotic disease. Treatment is very effective and is instituted for bone pain, neurological complications, hypercalcemia, increased cardiac output, or fractures. Other indications are directed at prevention of disease progression.

There are a number of effective oral and intravenous therapies for the treatment of Paget's disease, some of which produce sustained remissions (shown in table 53.6 [see www.paget.org]). Patients with Paget's disease should also be treated with calcium, vitamin D (see osteoporosis section above), and acetaminophen or nonsteroidal anti-inflammatory drugs for degenerative joint symptoms. Treatment for Paget's disease can now result in marked improvements in disease activity and symptoms and prolonged remissions.

ADDITIONAL READING

Black DM, Delmas PD, Eastell R, et al. Once-yearly zoledronic acid for treatment of postmenopausal osteoporosis. *N Engl J Med.* 2007;356(18):1809–22.

Cummings SR, San Martin J, McClung MR, et al. Denosumab for prevention of fractures in postmenopausal women with osteoporosis. *N Engl J Med.* 2009;361(8):756–65.

Dawson-Hughes B. A revised clinician's guide to the prevention and treatment of osteoporosis. *J Clin Endocrinol Metab.* 2008;93(7):2463–5.

Ettinger B, Black DM, Mitlak BH, et al.; Multiple Outcomes of Raloxifene Evaluation (MORE) Investigators. Reduction of vertebral fracture risk in postmenopausal women with osteoporosis treated with raloxifene: Results from a 3-year randomized clinical trial. *JAMA.* 1999;282(7):637–45.

Grover D, LeBoff MS. Osteoporosis/vertebral fractures. In Leslie J De Groot MD Ed., Android and Iphone APP, *Endocrinology and Endocrine Emergencies.* South Dartmouth, MA: Endocrine Education, Inc; 2011.

Holick MF, Binkley NC, Bischoff-Ferrari HA, et al. Evaluation, treatment, and prevention of vitamin D deficiency: an Endocrine Society clinical practice guideline. *J Clin Endocrinol Metab.* 2011;96(7):1911–30.

Institute of Medicine. *2011 Dietary Reference Intakes for Calcium and Vitamin D.* Washington, DC: The National Academies Press; 2011.

Jackson RD, LaCroix AZ, Gass M, et al. Calcium plus vitamin D supplementation and the risk of fractures. *N Engl J Med.* 2006;354(7):669–83.

LeBoff MS, Kohlmeier L, Hurwitz S, Franklin J, Wright J, Glowacki J. Occult vitamin D deficiency in postmenopausal US women with acute hip fracture. *JAMA.* 1999;281(16):1505–11.

McClung MR, Geusens P, Miller PD, et al.; Hip Intervention Program Study Group. Effect of risedronate on the risk of hip fracture in elderly women. *N Engl J Med.* 2001;344(5):333–40.

Neer RM, Arnaud CD, Zanchetta JR, et al. Effect of parathyroid hormone (1–34) on fractures and bone mineral density in postmenopausal women with osteoporosis. *N Engl J Med.* 2001;344(19):1434–41.

Office of the Surgeon General. *Bone Health and Osteoporosis: A Report of the Surgeon General.* Rockville, MD: U.S. Department of Health and Human Services, Public Health Service, Office of the Surgeon General; 2004.

Ross AC, Manson JE, Abrams SA, et al. The 2011 report on dietary reference intakes for calcium and vitamin D from the Institute of Medicine: What clinicians need to know. *J Clin Endocrinol Metab.* 2011;96(1):53–8.

Shane E, Burr D, Ebeling PR, et al. Atypical subtrochanteric and diaphyseal femoral fractures: Report of a task force of the American Society for Bone and Mineral Research. *J Bone Miner Res.* 2010;25(11):2267–94.

Siris ES, Lyles KW, Singer FR, Meunier PJ. Medical management of Paget's disease of bone: Indications for treatment and review of current therapies. *J Bone Miner Res.* 2006;21(Suppl 2):P94–8.

Tannenbaum C, Clark J, Schwartzman K, et al. Yield of laboratory testing to identify secondary contributors to osteoporosis in otherwise healthy women. *J Clin Endocrinol Metab.* 2002;87(10):4431–7.

Watts NB, Ettinger B, LeBoff MS. Perspective: FRAX™ Facts. *J Bone Mineral Res.* 2009;24(6):975–9.

QUESTIONS

QUESTION 1. A 50-year-old man with severe Crohn's disease presents with generalized bone pain and an elevated

Table 53.6 TREATMENT OF PAGET'S DISEASE

Injectable calcitonin, salmon

FDA-approved bisphosphonates: etidronate, pamidronate, tiludronate, alendronate,* risedronate,* zoledronic acid*

Nonsteroidal anti-inflammatory drugs (alleviate associated joint pain)

NOTE: *New potent bisphosphonates may produce sustained "remissions."

alkaline phosphatase. An x-ray of his proximal femurs shows bilateral pseudofractures indicative of osteomalacia. The most likely laboratory features compatible with this clinical picture would be:

A. High calcium and low parathyroid hormone (PTH) levels
B. Low phosphate and normal 25-hydroxyvitamin D levels
C. Low calcium and low PTH levels
D. Low phosphate and low 25-hydroxyvitamin D concentrations

QUESTION 2. A 78-year-old woman fell and was admitted to the hospital with a right femoral neck fracture. She has lost 4 inches in height, and she states that her mother had a hip fracture. She went through menopause at age 40. Her BMI is 18.

How should you evaluate her?

A. Orthopedic surgery, physical therapy, and fall prevention
B. Bone density test

C. Treatment of her osteoporosis
D. Evaluation for secondary causes of her osteoporosis
E. All of the above

QUESTION 3. The FRAX® calculator (http://www.shef.ac.uk/FRAX) incorporates risk factors in a model to predict the 10-year absolute fracture risk for a hip fracture or total fracture (hip, wrist, proximal humerus, and clinical spine fractures). This tool helps guide clinical decisions to treat a woman or man with:

A. A fragility fracture
B. Osteopenia
C. Osteoporosis
D. All of the above

ANSWERS

1. D
2. E
3. B

54.

ENDOCRINE BOARD REVIEW

Alexander Turchin and Ajay K. Singh

QUESTION 1. A 68-year-old man is being treated with heparin for pulmonary embolism. Four days after admission, he has sudden onset of severe abdominal pain and tenderness. He is found to have hyponatremia and hyperkalemia, and his hematocrit is 35%, as compared with 40% at the time of admission.

The most appropriate next step is to:

A. Measure serum aldosterone
B. Measure serum cortisol
C. Measure serum cortisol after administration of corticotropin (ACTH)
D. Measure urinary cortisol excretion
E. Start total fluid restriction at 1200 cc/24 hours

QUESTION 2. A 52-year-old woman is brought to the office after falling and striking her abdomen on the edge of a chair. She had abdominal pain soon thereafter, but it has subsided. She is normotensive. Physical examination is unremarkable except mild abdominal tenderness. Computed tomography (CT) of the abdomen reveals a 3-cm hypodense left adrenal mass. Biochemical studies (measurements of serum aldosterone, plasma renin activity, and plasma metanephrines and normetanephrines) are normal. The most appropriate next step is:

A. ACTH stimulation test
B. Measurement of serum cortisol after administration of 1 mg of dexamethasone at midnight
C. Measurement of urinary cortisol excretion
D. Repeat biochemical studies in 6 months
E. Repeat abdominal CT in 6 months

QUESTION 3. A 24-year-old veterinary student has had symptoms of hypoglycemia before breakfast for several months. Laboratory studies early one morning reveal the following:

Serum glucose 28 mg/dL
Serum insulin 65 μU/mL (normal 5–15)
Serum C-peptide 0.1 ng/mL (normal 0.5–3.0)
Serum cortisol 27 μg/dL (normal 8–25)
The most likely cause of these results is

A. Adrenal insufficiency
B. A non-islet-cell tumor
C. An insulinoma
D. Surreptitious administration of insulin
E. Surreptitious ingestion of glyburide

QUESTION 4. A 65-year-old woman is found to have hypercalcemia at the time of her annual examination. She has been well but admits to some weakness and fatigue and thinks that her memory may be declining. Her appetite is good, her weight is stable, and she has no history of nephrolithiasis or fracture. Her physical examination is normal.

Her serum calcium is 10.8 mg/dL (normal 8.6–10.5), parathyroid hormone (PTH) 52 pg/mL (normal 15–65), serum creatinine 0.7 mg/dL, and 25-(OH)-vitamin D 42 ng/mL (normal 30–60).

What is the most appropriate next step?

A. Bone densitometry
B. Measurement of urinary calcium
C. Referral to a surgeon for parathyroidectomy
D. Repeat measurements of serum calcium in 4 and 8 weeks
E. TcO_4-sestamibi parathyroid imaging

QUESTION 5. Repeat serum calcium concentration is 10.9 mg/dL. The sestamibi imaging study is normal. The most appropriate next step is

A. Bone densitometry
B. Measurement of serum alkaline phosphatase
C. Reevaluation in 3 months
D. Referral to a parathyroid surgeon
E. Treatment with alendronate (Fosamax)

QUESTION 6. A 56-year-old woman who has had diabetes mellitus for 10 years under good control on metformin 1000 mg twice a day and glyburide 5 mg twice a day is admitted to the hospital with pneumonia. Her hospitalization is complicated by sepsis, acute renal failure, and a stroke. Nasogastric tube is placed, and 24-hour enteral tube feeding is initiated. Her diabetes treatment:

A. Should remain the same
B. Should change to glargine (Lantus®) once daily
C. Should change to NPH three times a day
D. Should change to regular insulin every 6 hours
E. All scheduled medications should be stopped and sliding-scale lispro (Humalog®) insulin started

QUESTION 7. A 44-year-old woman has had weakness and nervousness for several months. She also has noted occasional palpitations and has lost 5 lb. Her pulse rate is 108 beats/min. She has mild eyelid retraction and a tremor of her hands but no thyroid enlargement or nodules. Her serum thyroid-stimulating hormone (TSH) concentration is 0.01 μU/mL (normal 0.4–4.0) and serum free thyroxine concentration is 2.0 ng/dL (normal 0.8–1.6). Her thyroid radioiodine uptake at 24 hours is 52% (normal 15–35) with diffuse pattern.

The next step is to:

A. Measure serum C-reactive protein
B. Administer ^{123}I radioiodine isotope
C. Administer ^{131}I radioiodine isotope
D. Start propylthiouracil
E. Start methimazole

QUESTION 8. A 32-year-old woman has had erratic menstrual periods since adolescence and amenorrhea for about 4 months. She has had mild facial hirsutism for more than 10 years. She recently gained about 5 lb and has had less energy than in the past. Her blood pressure and pulse rate are normal. She has mild facial hirsutism but no striae, central adiposity, or galactorrhea. Neurological examination is normal. Her prolactin is measured to be 52 ng/mL (normal 4–30), and pituitary magnetic resonance imaging (MRI) is normal.

The most appropriate next step is to order:

A. Ovarian ultrasonography
B. Head CT
C. Serum luteinizing hormone (LH)
D. Serum testosterone
E. Serum TSH

QUESTION 9. A 68-year-old woman was found unresponsive at home by her daughter. In the emergency department, her temperature was 103.2, oxygen saturation 70% on room air, blood pressure 90/40, and heart rate 115. When given oxygen she was sleepy but arousable. She was hospitalized and treated with intravenous fluids and antibiotics. On day 2 thyroid function tests (TFTs) were drawn because of persistent sinus tachycardia. TSH was 0.15 μU/mL (normal 0.5–5.0), and free thyroxine was 0.6 ng/dL (normal 0.8–1.6). The best next step is:

A. Pituitary MRI
B. Thyroid ultrasound
C. Thyroid ^{123}I scan and uptake
D. Initiate thyroxine 100 μg daily
E. Reevaluate in 4–6 weeks

QUESTION 10. A 75-year-old woman comes for a follow-up visit 2 years after initiating alendronate (Fosamax) for treatment of osteoporosis. She takes calcium 500 mg twice daily and vitamin D 800 units daily. She takes alendronate on Sunday mornings together with the rest of her medications. She walks a mile 5 days a week. Her 25(OH) D level is 32 ng/mL (normal). Two years ago her T score in left hip was –2.6. A week ago follow-up bone densitometry showed a 2% decrease in the left hip (non significant). The best next step is:

A. Ask her to skip the morning calcium on Sundays
B. Double her calcium dose
C. Double her vitamin D dose
D. Add raloxifene (Evista®)
E. Add teriparatide (Forteo®)

QUESTION 11. A 62-year-old man comes for follow-up of diabetes. He used to be treated with metformin 1000 mg bid and glipizide 10 mg bid, but 2 years ago glipizide was stopped and glargine (Lantus®) insulin started. He now takes 30 units of glargine at night. He wakes up from hypoglycemia two to three times a week, but his daytime glucose ranges between 150 and 220 mg/dL. His A1C is 7.5%. The best next step is:

A. Stop glargine and restart glipizide
B. Take glargine in the morning instead of at night
C. Decrease glargine and add a rapidly acting insulin before every meal
D. Stop glargine and start detemir (Levemir®) insulin at night
E. Ask him to eat a snack before going to bed

QUESTION 12. A 57-year-old woman is evaluated for severe hypertension resistant to treatment with three antihypertensive medications and hypokalemia. She is found to have aldosterone 24 ng/dL and plasma renin activity 0.2 ng/mL/hr. Plasma metanephrine and normetanephrine levels are normal. Abdominal CT shows multiple small nodules of <1 cm in both the left and right adrenal glands, but a 2-cm benign-appearing nodule in the right adrenal gland. The best next step is:

A. Abdominal MRI
B. Repeat the CT in 6 months
C. Refer to an experienced surgeon for right adrenalectomy
D. Adrenal vein sampling
E. 24-hour urine collection for aldosterone and creatinine

QUESTION 13. A 41-year-old man comes to your office complaining of progressive erectile dysfunction over the last several years. Evaluation shows testosterone 1200 pg/mL (nL 1800–6900) and prolactin of 73 ng/mL (normal 4–23), confirmed by dilution. Pituitary MRI shows a 2-cm suprasellar mass consistent with pituitary adenoma. He denies headaches; his neurological examination is normal, and visual fields are intact. Morning cortisol is 12 μg/dL. The best next step is:

A. Surgical resection of the tumor
B. Start bromocriptine (Parlodel®)
C. Start cabergoline (Dostinex®)
D. Start testosterone patch
E. Repeat pituitary MRI in 6 months

QUESTION 14. A 25-year-old man comes in for a routine physical. He had craniopharyngioma resection at the age of 12 and has been taking levothyroxine ever since. His current dose is 112 μg daily. Blood tests show TSH of 0.05 μU/mL (normal 0.5–5.0) and free thyroxine 0.8 ng/dL (normal 0.8–1.6). The best next step is:

A. Decrease levothyroxine to 88 μg daily
B. Increase levothyroxine to 125 μg daily
C. Radioactive iodine uptake
D. Pituitary MRI
E. Reevaluate in 6 months

QUESTION 15. A 71-year-old man returns to see you for follow-up of type 2 diabetes. He also has hypercholesterolemia, congestive heart failure, hypertension, remote history of pancreatitis, and osteoarthritis. His current medications include glipizide 10 mg twice daily and simvastatin 20 mg qhs. His hemoglobin A1c is 7.8%, and fasting blood glucose 130–150 mg/dL. The best next step is:

A. Start metformin 1000 mg daily
B. Start exenatide (Byetta) 5 μg SQ twice daily
C. Start sitagliptin (Januvia) 100 mg daily
D. Start pioglitazone (Actos) 15 mg daily
E. Start glargine (Lantus) insulin 15 units SQ qhs

ANSWERS

1. C. This man has adrenal insufficiency caused by bilateral adrenal hemorrhages. These hemorrhages are most likely to occur in patients being treated with heparin or warfarin, perhaps augmented by illness-induced stimulation of ACTH secretion and therefore increased adrenal blood flow and hormone secretion. The key clinical findings are abdominal pain and tenderness, hyponatremia, hyperkalemia, anemia, and also hypotension.

The diagnosis of acute adrenal insufficiency is best confirmed by measurements of serum cortisol before and 30 and/or 60 minutes after administration of ACTH. Both basal and stimulated serum cortisol values should be low in patients like this. Also, they can be treated with dexamethasone (or another glucocorticoid known not to be detected by the serum cortisol assay in use) immediately after the basal serum sample is collected. Measurements of basal serum cortisol alone (B) are not adequate for diagnosis of adrenal insufficiency because the values may be low as a result of an illness-related fall in serum cortisol-binding globulin. (Simultaneous measurements of basal serum cortisol and ACTH alone, if, respectively, low and high, should also confirm the diagnosis, but this simpler approach is not used widely because it takes up to a week to get the results of ACTH measurements in most hospitals.)

Decreased production of aldosterone, as manifested by a low serum aldosterone level (which could be detected by A) does not, in and by itself, predict a decreased production of cortisol. Decreased production of cortisol is a more serious condition and should be ruled out first. Urinary cortisol excretion (D) is not a reliable test for diagnosis of adrenal insufficiency. Fluid restriction will not treat hyponatremia due to adrenal insufficiency and is contraindicated for patients with an acute hemorrhage.

2. E. This woman has an adrenal incidentaloma—a finding common in her age group. Cushing syndrome is unlikely given normal blood pressure and normal physical examination. A 3-cm adrenal tumor would have been expected to produce enough cortisol to lead to noticeable physical findings. Therefore B and C, which test for Cushing syndrome, would be unnecessary. Hyperaldosteronism and pheochromocytoma have been excluded by physical examination and biochemical studies. It is uncommon for nonsecretory adrenal tumors to develop hormonal production later; therefore, repeating biochemical studies (D) is not recommended unless new symptoms or physical findings develop. Adrenal tumors, and particularly unilateral ones, do not usually cause adrenal insufficiency, and therefore an ACTH stimulation test (A) is not indicated.

The more important question is whether the incidentaloma is an adenoma or a carcinoma. Most 3-cm hypodense incidentalomas are benign, and the risk of carcinoma rises as size increases. It is impossible to distinguish benign and malignant adrenal tumors by biopsy, and hence, only their size and appearance on imaging studies are used when deciding whether to recommend surgical resection. Patients with adrenal incidentalomas that are ≥4–5 cm, whatever the appearance on imaging, are often advised to have surgery, as are patients whose lesions have a noticeable rate of growth. Therefore, a repeat CT (E) to ensure the size of the tumor is not increasing with time is in order.

3. D. This student is surreptitiously taking insulin. Low serum glucose and high serum insulin concentrations suggest insulin-induced hypoglycemia. These findings are compatible with an insulinoma (C), surreptitious injection of insulin (D), and surreptitious ingestion of glyburide (E). The low serum C-peptide concentration is strong evidence that the patient is taking insulin, rather than secreting it, because insulin and C-peptide are secreted in equimolar amounts by the beta cells of the pancreatic islets. Hypoglycemia is rare in patients with adrenal insufficiency (A), and a cortisol level of 27 μg/dL rules it out. Some non-islet tumors secrete insulin-like growth factor (IGF-2) (B), which can bind to and activate insulin receptors, thereby causing

hypoglycemia. These patients have low serum insulin and C-peptide concentrations.

Of note, C-peptide is a single chain of 31 amino acids (MW 3020), connecting the A and B chains of insulin in the proinsulin molecule. Unlike insulin, C-peptide has no known physiological function. C-peptide has a longer half-life than insulin (two to five times longer); thus, higher concentrations of C-peptide persist in the peripheral circulation, and these levels fluctuate less than insulin. Plasma C-peptide concentrations may reflect pancreatic insulin secretion more reliably than the level of insulin itself.

4. D. This woman probably has mild hypercalcemia caused by primary hyperparathyroidism. Her PTH levels, although normal, are inappropriately high for her mildly elevated calcium. However, the calcium elevation could also be transient or a laboratory error. We only have one measurement and otherwise normal laboratory parameters. Here it would be important to calculate the actual level of calcium, but we need the serum albumin concentration, which is not provided (Formula: Corrected total calcium [mg/dL] = (measured total calcium [mg/dL]) + 0.8 (4.4 − measured albumin [g/dL]). Measuring the calcium again would be reasonable. She has some symptoms, but whether they can be attributed to the hypercalcemia is debatable. Hypertension is not an important manifestation of hyperparathyroidism and usually does not improve after successful parathyroidectomy. Given the lack of a convincing constellation of findings, the probability of a spurious calcium elevation is reasonably high. Therefore, the most appropriate next step is to confirm it after a period of time (D) before proceeding to more expensive and/or invasive maneuvers. Patients like this with mild hypercalcemia and inappropriately high serum PTH concentrations should be asked if they are taking lithium or hydrochlorothiazide, either of which may cause parathyroid hyperplasia and mild hypercalcemia.

The symptoms are suspicious for primary hyperparathyroidism, but the serum PTH level is not elevated (the parathyroid hormone [PTH] level is typically 1.5–2 times the upper limit of the reference range). On the other hand, PTH is not suppressed either. A decreased serum phosphate level <2.5 mg/dL (0.81 mmol/L) may be seen in primary hyperparathyroidism, but the serum phosphate is not provided here. The other lab values are fine. The most sensitive and reliable technique is ^{99m}Tc sestamibi scanning because of its ability to produce a three-dimensional image that can be used for visual reference by the surgeon intraoperatively, albeit only after a diagnosis of primary hyperparathyroidism is made and the patient is referred to a surgeon.

5. A. The hypercalcemia is now confirmed, providing further evidence that the patient has primary hyperparathyroidism. The decision that has to be made now is whether the patient needs to be treated surgically. In absence of clear symptoms of hyperparathyroidism, the criteria for surgical intervention developed at the Third International Workshop on the Management of Asymptomatic Primary Hyperparathyroidism apply. According to these guidelines, asymptomatic patients with primary hyperparathyroidism should be referred for surgery if any of the following are true:

1. Calcium is ≥1.0 mg/dL above the upper limit of normal

2. Creatinine clearance <60 mL/min

3. Bone mass at the hip, lumbar spine, or distal radius is >2.5 standard deviations below the peak (T score <−2.5) and/or previous fragility fracture

4. Age <50 years

5. Follow-up is anticipated to be difficult

Bone densitometry (A) would help establish whether the patient meets these criteria. Sestamibi imaging studies are less than 100% sensitive, so a negative study does not rule out a parathyroid adenoma or hyperplasia. Treatment with a bisphosphonate (E) is a reasonable option if the patient has low bone density and is not a surgical candidate or declines surgery. Most patients with primary hyperparathyroidism have normal serum alkaline phosphatase concentrations (B) unless they have severe bone disease.

6. D. Enteral tube feedings have two characteristics important for treatment of hyperglycemia: (1) they provide an even caloric intake over the course of 24 hours, and (2) they can frequently be withdrawn suddenly, as in the case of the patient removing the tube or clinical deterioration. An antihyperglycemic regimen should conform to these constraints. Neither metformin nor glyburide (A) would be appropriate in the setting of an acute renal failure. Both glargine (B) and NPH (C) insulins have long half-lives and present a risk of hypoglycemia if tube feeding is withdrawn. The action of a dose of regular insulin (D) lasts for about 4–6 hours and thus presents a reasonable balance between the risk of hypoglycemia and an increased nursing workload if injections (of shorter-acting insulins) were to be administered more frequently. A sliding scale alone without scheduled insulin (E) is unlikely to control hyperglycemia in a patient with known diabetes.

Management of hyperglycemia in a hospitalized patient is important for practical reasons as well as for its potential impact on outcomes. This is reviewed in more detail elsewhere (Clement et al. *Diabetes Care.* 2004;27(2):553–91). The use of oral hypoglycemics in renal disease is discussed by Yale et al. (*J Am Soc Nephrol.* 2005;16[Suppl 1]:S7–10). Glyburide or glibenclamide is an oral antihyperglycemic drug of the sulfonylurea class. The sulfonylureas (glyburide, gliclazide, glipizide, glibenclamide, tolbutamide, and chlorpropamide) have increased potency as the renal function decreases and are contraindicated in severe renal failure. Furthermore, the long action of sulfonylureas and predisposition to hypoglycemia in patients not consuming their normal nutrition are relative contraindications. Metformin is contraindicated in renal failure because of the associated risk for lactic acidosis. Other risk factors for lactic acidosis in metformin-treated patients are cardiac disease, including congestive heart failure (CHF) hypoperfusion, old age, and chronic pulmonary disease. Furthermore, metformin has added side effects of nausea, diarrhea, and decreased appetite, all of which may be problematic during acute illness in the hospital.

7. E. This woman has clinical manifestations of hyperthyroidism caused by Graves disease. This diagnosis is confirmed by measurements of serum free thyroxine and TSH and radioiodine imaging. Thyroiditis is unlikely given the prolonged duration of symptoms and is ruled out by the increased radioiodine uptake by the thyroid. Thyroid nodular disease is ruled out by the diffuse uptake of radioiodine by the thyroid. No further diagnostic workup is necessary. Levels of C-reactive protein (A) are usually unchanged in patients with hyperthyroidism and do not have diagnostic value under the circumstances. The next step, therefore, is to consider treatment. In patients with Graves disease, unlike in those with hyperthyroidism caused by hyperactive thyroid nodules, long-term remission can frequently be induced by thioamides without long-term sequelae. On the other hand, radioiodine treatment with ^{131}I (C) commonly leads to hypothyroidism. It is therefore a second-line choice, particularly in patients with mild hyperthyroidism, such as this one. When radioiodine is used for treatment of hyperthyroidism, ^{131}I isotope is preferred to the ^{123}I isotope (B) because it emits a significant fraction of its radiation as beta-rays (electrons), which have a very short depth of penetration and will not affect any tissues beyond the thyroid that is taking up the iodine. Of the two thioamides, methimazole (E) is both more effective than propylthiouracil (D) and appears to have a lower frequency of some of the serious side effects, such as liver failure.

The choice between propylthiouracil and methimazole is also influenced by the U.S. Food and Drug Administration (FDA)'s boxed warning for propylthiouracil that states that propylthiouracil should be second-line therapy and reserved for use in patients who cannot tolerate other treatments, such as methimazole, radioactive iodine, or surgery.

8. E. The common causes of amenorrhea are pregnancy, hypothalamic amenorrhea, hyperprolactinemia, and ovarian disorders (in particular the polycystic ovary syndrome). Based on her history she may have polycystic ovary syndrome (PCOS), but recent acceleration of the symptoms and elevated prolactin point to the presence of another condition. Although it is not uncommon for patients with primary hyperprolactinemia to have a normal pituitary MRI, a workup for secondary causes, including primary hypothyroidism (E), is indicated. Other etiologies of elevated prolactin may include dopamine antagonists (e.g., antipsychotic medications), seizures, and stress. Head CT (B) will not provide significant additional information given a nor-

mal pituitary MRI. Ovarian ultrasonography (A) may or may not be abnormal even if the patient has PCOS and will not shed light on the secondary causes of hyperprolactinemia. Serum luteinizing hormone (C) will be suppressed in all patients with elevated prolactin, independent of the etiology. None of the secondary causes of hyperprolactinemia leads to abnormal testosterone levels in women (D).

For the diagnosis of PCOS, the European Society for Human Reproduction and Embryology (ESHRE) and the American Society for Reproductive Medicine (ASRM) require at least two of the following three features: oligo-ovulation or anovulation manifested as oligomenorrhea or amenorrhea, hyperandrogenism or hyperandrogenemia, and polycystic ovaries on ultrasonography. The elevated prolactin level does not favor PCOS. On the other hand, with hyperprolactinemia, women typically present with a history of oligomenorrhea, amenorrhea, or infertility and visual-field defects or headache (the latter because of the presence of a pituitary tumor). The galactorrhea is due to the direct physiological effect of prolactin on breast epithelial cells. In this patient, the prolactin level is not very high, and the pituitary MRI was normal. Although hypothyroidism is a possibility, facial hirsutism is unusual. The elevated prolactin level can be seen in hypothyroidism. Notably, prolactin elevation was found in 36% of patients with overt hypothyroidism and in 22% of patients with subclinical hypothyroidism (Hekimsoy et al. *Endocr J.* 2010 Oct 5.; Raber et al. *Clin Endocrinol (Oxf)*. 2003;58(2):185–91).

9. E. This woman had thyroid hormone levels measured while critically ill. Critical illness commonly results in a profile referred to as "sick euthyroid syndrome" in which TSH, thyroxine, and particularly triiodothyronine are all low. Although a similar profile can result from secondary hypothyroidism, the latter disease is much less common and therefore pituitary MRI (A) to look for pituitary lesions that could cause it is not indicated. There are no data that thyroxine supplementation (D) in the setting of acute illness improves outcomes. Neither thyroid ultrasound (B), which is expected to be normal, nor ^{123}I scan and uptake (C), which will likely be low/nonfocal, will provide specific information that will help make the diagnosis.

10. A. Calcium can decrease the absorption of alendronate and other bisphosphonates and thus their efficacy. Patients should not take calcium for at least several hours after the bisphosphonate (A). A daily calcium dose of 2000 mg (B) is excessive—1500 mg is recommended for postmenopausal women. Her vitamin D level is adequate, so additional vitamin D supplementation (C) is unlikely to be helpful. Neither raloxifene (D) nor teriparatide (E) has been shown to decrease the incidence of hip fractures and therefore would not be the first choice for treating a patient with a pronounced osteoporosis in the hip.

Alendronate is in a class of medications called bisphosphonates. The bisphosphonate class includes etidronate (Didronel®), ibandronate (Boniva®), pamidronate

(Aredia®), risedronate (Actonel®), tiludronate (Skelid®), and zoledronic acid (Reclast®). Bisphosphonates are used for treating osteoporosis (reduced density of bone that leads to fractures) and bone pain from diseases such as metastatic breast cancer, multiple myeloma, and Paget disease.

11. C. This man takes a large dose of basal (glargine) but no prandial insulin. His nighttime hypoglycemic episodes indicate that his glargine dose is too high. It therefore should be decreased, and rapid-acting (e.g., lispro or aspart) premeal insulin added to control his postprandial hyperglycemia (C). Given that his A1C is over 7% even on this large dose of glargine it is unlikely that replacing glargine with glyburide (A) would improve his glucose control. In most patients glargine provides 24-hour coverage so changing the time of administration (B) will not change insulin levels at night. Although detemir typically provides less than 24-hour coverage, administration of the same dose of detemir at bedtime (D) is likely to lead to hypoglycemic episodes for the same reason that glargine did. Eating a snack at bedtime (E) may improve the hypoglycemia, but it will not improve the postprandial hyperglycemia and will increase the average glucose levels/A1C, placing him at higher risk for complications.

INSULIN	ONSET	PEAK	EFFECTIVE DURATION
Humalog or lispro	15–30 min	30–90 min	3–5 hours
Novolog or aspart	10–20 min	40–50 min	3–5 hours
Apidra or glulisine	20–30 min	30–90 min	1–2½ hours

12. D. This patient has findings indicative of primary hyperaldosteronism. If a solitary adenoma is the source of the excess aldosterone, surgical resection is the recommended treatment. However, nonsecretory adrenal adenomas (incidentalomas) are common in this age group. Therefore, a finding of an adrenal adenoma in a patient with a biochemical picture of primary hyperaldosteronism is not sufficient to conclude that it is the source of aldosterone production. Referral for surgery (C) is therefore premature at this point. Adrenal vein sampling (D) is used in this situation to confirm that the excess aldosterone is coming from the adrenal vein on the same side as the nodule on CT. Abdominal MRI (A) could be helpful in identifying a pheochromocytoma, which has a bright signal on T2 but is not helpful for diagnostic workup of hyperaldosteronism. Urinary aldosterone excretion (E) has not been validated as a diagnostic test for hyperaldosteronism; if the biochemical diagnosis remains in question, salt suppression test should be used for confirmation. If adrenal vein sampling does not localize aldosterone production to the side of the adenoma, a follow-up CT in 6 months (B) is reasonable to ensure the adenoma is not increasing in size and thus suspicious for malignancy. However, treatment of hyperaldosteronism should not be postponed until then.

Primary hyperaldosteronism is characterized by increased aldosterone secretion from the adrenal glands, suppressed plasma renin activity (PRA), hypertension, and hypokalemia. Increased aldosterone excretion from the adrenals results primarily from either a unilateral aldosterone-producing adenoma or Conn syndrome (50–60% of cases) or bilateral adrenal hyperplasia (40–50% of cases). The PA/PRA ratio is 20 or greater with a PA 15 ng/dL or greater (this patient has a ratio of 120 and plasma aldosterone level of 24 ng/dL). Some would do a 24-hour urine aldosterone level after 3 days of salt loading as a confirmatory test. (A 24-hour aldosterone excretion rate of greater than 14 μg with a concomitant 24-hour urine sodium >200 mEq is diagnostic of primary hyperaldosteronism.) However, in this case a CT has already been done. The most likely diagnosis is an adenoma, but because of the multinodularity, adrenal venous sampling should be performed after CT scanning.

13. A. This man has a pituitary macroadenoma, elevated prolactin level, and low testosterone. Low testosterone could be due to the compression of the pituitary by the macroadenoma, suppression of gonadotrophs by elevated prolactin, or both. High prolactin is most likely caused by the tumor's compression of the pituitary stalk leading to decreased flow of dopamine from the hypothalamus. It is unlikely that the tumor itself produces prolactin because in that case prolactin levels would be expected to be much higher (hundreds or thousands of nanograms per milliliter). Consequently, treatment with dopamine agonists such as bromocriptine (B) or cabergoline (C) is not likely to affect the tumor. His macroadenoma is large, placing him at risk for future development of panhypopituitarism, optic chiasm compression, and severe headaches. It is therefore imperative that it be treated. Because dopamine agonists will not work, surgical resection is the only available option (A). Surgical referral should not be postponed (E) because of the nonnegligible risk of development of irreversible complications as this large tumor continues to grow. There is a possibility that his testosterone levels will improve after the tumor is resected and stalk compression has been relieved with consequent drop in prolactin levels, so the decision about testosterone supplementation (D) is best postponed until then.

14. B. This patient has postsurgical secondary hypothyroidism. His TSH level therefore cannot be used to assess his thyroid status. Low TSH is common in these patients and does not indicate that his levothyroxine dose should be lowered (A). Free thyroxine levels should be used to make the decision about thyroid hormone supplementation instead. Based on the low normal free thyroxine level, his levothyroxine dose should be increased (B). Sufficient information is available to make the decision now, and extended follow-up (E) is unlikely to change it. Imaging studies, including radioactive iodine uptake (C) or pituitary MRI, (D) will not be helpful.

In 20–40% of patient's with central hypothyroidism (low TSH, low normal free thyroxine) from a craniopharyngioma, there is direct compression or destruction of the hypothalamus and pituitary stalk, leading to growth hormone deficiency, TSH deficiency, ACTH deficiency, antidiuretic hormone deficiency, and luteinizing hormone or follicle-stimulating hormone deficiency. The correct treatment is to increase the levothyroxine to 125 μg daily (Curtis et al. *Pediatr Neurosurg.* 1994;21[Suppl 1]:24–7).

15. E. This man has poorly controlled diabetes. Further increase in glipizide dose is unlikely to lower his blood glucose significantly, and a new antihyperglycemic agent should be initiated. Metformin (A) is contraindicated in patients with heart failure because of increased risk for lactic acidosis. Acute pancreatitis has been reported in patients taking both exenatide (B) and sitagliptin (C), and these medications are therefore not recommended in patients with history of pancreatitis. Pioglitazone (D) can exacerbate CHF and is contraindicated in patients with this condition. Therefore, initiation of insulin, for example glargine (E), is the optimal therapeutic intervention for treatment of his hyperglycemia.

55.

ENDOCRINE SUMMARY

Graham T. McMahon

Classic disorders of the endocrine system result from states of excess or deficiency of hormones due to hyperfunction or hypofunction of the glands (table 55.1). Hypofunction can result from glandular destruction (e.g., tumor, infection, hemorrhage) or hormone biosynthetic problems. Hyperfunction usually results from a tumor or autoimmune stimulation. Some selected disorders that are covered during the course are noted, along with some of the diagnostic approaches. Resistance to hormones also plays a major role in disease—particularly in diabetes.

Diagnostically, if an endocrinologist suspects that a hormone is inappropriately low, he or she will try to stimulate it; if high, he or she will try to suppress it (table 55.2). Failure to rise or fall normally indicates either failure of the gland or unregulated hyperfunction. It is often possible to measure the level of the upstream hormone to determine the location (central [pituitary] or peripheral) of the problem. By going through this process, we capitalize on the presence of feedback loops. Similarly, treatments for endocrine disorders aim to replace the hormone in deficiency states (e.g., hypothyroidism) or to interfere with production in excess states (e.g., prolactinoma).

PITUITARY TUMORS

Pituitary tumors account for approximately 15% of all primary intracranial neoplasms. Proliferation of cells within the pituitary can cause hormonal excess syndromes or compress the pituitary resulting in hormonal deficiency. Pituitary tumors can expand and interfere with local anatomic structures such as the optic chiasm and cavernous sinuses.

PROLACTINOMA

Prolactin-secreting tumors account for the majority of functional pituitary tumors. More than 90% are small (<1 cm) benign tumors that do not increase in size.

Clinical Features

Hyperprolactinemia leads to galactorrhea in approximately 80% of affected women. High levels of prolactin interfere with the secretion of gonadotropin-releasing hormone from the hypothalamus, resulting in amenorrhea/oligomenorrhea, and infertility in women, and hypogonadism in men. Both men and women develop osteoporosis if hyperprolactinemia is left chronically untreated. Macroprolactinomas can enlarge by one-third or more during pregnancy.

Evaluation

Dopamine tonically inhibits prolactin release, so medications that interfere with dopamine are often associated with hyperprolactinemia. Phenothiazines, butyrophenones, metoclopramide, risperidone, monoamine oxidase inhibitors, tricyclic antidepressants, verapamil, and serotonin-reuptake inhibitors can all increase prolactin levels. Large pituitary tumors can compress the pituitary stalk and impair normal dopamine signaling, resulting in hyperprolactinemia. Chronic renal failure and severe primary hypothyroidism are also associated with hyperprolactinemia. Magnetic resonance imaging (MRI) of the pituitary is recommended when a patient has elevated prolactin levels and other causes of hyperprolactinemia have been excluded.

Treatment

Both cabergoline (which is typically given twice weekly) and bromocriptine (given twice daily) are effective in decreasing prolactin levels and reducing tumor size in >80% of patients. The goal of treatment in microadenomas is symptomatic relief in patients with galactorrhea and restoration of eugonadism and bone density. Both micro- and macroprolactinomas can be managed medically; surgery is required only rarely. Treatment is continued for at

Table 55.1 SELECTED ENDOCRINE HORMONES AND THEIR RELATED CLINICAL SYNDROMES

GLAND	HORMONE	STRUCTURE*	HYPERFUNCTION (DIAGNOSTIC STRATEGY)	HYPOFUNCTION (DIAGNOSTIC STRATEGY)
Anterior lobe of pituitary	Prolactin (PRL)	Protein (198)	Prolactinoma (prolactin levels high)	
	Growth hormone (GH)	Protein (191)	Acromegaly (IGF-1 levels, oral glucose tolerance test)	GH deficiency (Arg-GHRH stimulation test, or insulin tolerance test)
	Adrenocorticotropic hormone (ACTH)	Peptide (39)	Cushing disease (high ACTH and 24-hour urine free cortisol, failure to suppress on dex-supp test)	Central adrenal insufficiency failure to respond to ACTH stimulation test (no CRH-stim test)
Posterior lobe of pituitary	Antidiuretic hormone (ADH)(vasopressin)	Peptide (9)	SIADH (hyponatremia, exclude other causes)	Diabetes insipidus (become dehydrated on water deprivation test)
Thyroid gland	Thyroxine (T$_4$)	Tyrosine derivative	Hyperthyroidism (TSH low, uptake on scan high in Graves, low in thyroiditis) Thyroid nodule (TSH low, hot nodule on scan)	Hypothyroidism (TSH high)
	Calcitonin	Peptide (32)	Medullary carcinoma of the thyroid (aspirate, calcitonin level)	
Parathyroid glands	Parathyroid hormone (PTH)	Protein (84)	Hyperparathyroidism (calcium high, PTH normal or high, urinary Ca high)	Hypoparathyroidism
Adrenal cortex	Glucocorticoids (e.g., cortisol)	Steroids	Cushing syndrome (morning cortisol high after overnight dex suppression test, ACTH low)	Addison disease (cortisol fails to rise after stimulation with high-dose ACTH)
	Mineralocorticoids (e.g., aldosterone)	Steroids	Conn syndrome/hyperaldosteronism (high aldo/renin ratio)	Hypoaldosteronism (high renin, low aldo)
Adrenal medulla	Epinephrine/ Norepinephrine	Tyrosine derivative	Pheochromocytoma (metanephrines and urinary catecholamines and metanephrines high)	
Testes/Adrenal	Testosterone	Steroid	Hirsutism or virilization (high androgens, DHEAS)	Male hypogonadism (LH high, testo low)
Pancreas (Islets of Langerhans)	Insulin	Protein (51)	Insulinoma (insulin, C-peptide, endoscopic ultrasound) Type 2 diabetes (plasma glucose)	Type 1 diabetes (plasma glucose)
Kidney	Erythropoietin	Protein	Paraneoplastic syndrome	Anemia (Hct)
	Calcitriol	Steroid derivative		Hypovitaminosis D, secondary hyperparathyroidism (PTH, Ca)

NOTE: *Numbers within parentheses indicate the number of amino acids in the protein or peptide(s).

least 2 years in patients with microadenomas and generally given indefinitely in patients with macroadenomas. Macroadenomas that extend beyond the sella in women should generally be debulked surgically before pregnancy is attempted; pregnant women with macroprolactinomas are generally managed with bromocriptine throughout their pregnancy.

ACROMEGALY

Acromegaly is rare and develops when somatotropes proliferate and oversecrete growth hormone. These tumors tend

Table 55.2 CAUSE, DIAGNOSIS, AND TREATMENT OF HYPO AND HYPERFUNCTION

	SUSPECT HYPOFUNCTION	SUSPECT HYPERFUNCTION
Cause	Gland destruction Defective biosynthesis	Tumor/hyperplasia Autoimmune stimulation
Diagnose	Try to stimulate production	Try to suppress production
Treat	Replace the hormone	Interfere with the production of the hormone, or remove the gland

to grow slowly and insidiously and are rarely associated with plurihormonal polysecretion. Most of these tumors are >1 cm (i.e., are macroadenomas) at the time of presentation.

Clinical Features

The features of acromegaly are diverse and are generally related to somatic growth (acral enlargement, malocclusion, carpal tunnel syndrome), tissue enlargement (macroglossia, prostatic hypertrophy, left ventricular hypertrophy, sleep apnea, goiter), and metabolic interference (diabetes mellitus, hypertriglyceridemia, hypogonadism).

Evaluation

The biochemical diagnosis of acromegaly is made by confirming autonomous secretion of growth hormone during a 2-hour, 75-g oral glucose tolerance test. Nadir growth hormone levels in excess of 1 μg/L are consistent with the diagnosis, especially if the patient also has an elevated level of insulin-like growth factor-1 (IGF-1).

Treatment

Neurosurgical resection is the treatment of choice for most resectable pituitary tumors associated with acromegaly. Complications such as hypopituitarism and recurrence risk correlate with the size of the tumor. Medical treatments for acromegaly include somatostatin receptor ligands (octreotide and lanreotide), which suppress pituitary release of growth hormone, dopamine antagonists (cabergoline and bromocriptine are minimally effective), and use of a growth hormone receptor antagonist (pegvisomant). Radiotherapy is used for unresponsive tumors, but it is associated with high risk of panhypopituitarism. Levels of IGF-1 are used to monitor treatment efficacy.

OTHER PITUITARY DISORDERS

DIABETES INSIPIDUS

Central diabetes insipidus is a heterogeneous condition characterized by polyuria and polydipsia due to a deficiency of arginine vasopressin. In many patients it is caused by the destruction or degeneration of the neurons that originate in the supraoptic and paraventricular nuclei of the hypothalamus. The three main causes of diabetes insipidus (trauma/surgery, tumors, and idiopathic) account for approximately equal fractions of cases.

Clinical Features

Diminished or absent arginine vasopressin causes polyuria or polydipsia by diminishing the patient's ability to concentrate urine. These patients generally have severe nocturia and consume 3–20 liters of liquid daily. Nephrogenic diabetes insipidus is characterized by a decrease in the ability to concentrate urine due to a resistance to arginine vasopressin action in the kidney.

Evaluation

Diabetes insipidus is diagnosed when urine is inappropriately dilute (urine specific gravity of ≤1.005 and a urine osmolality <200 mOsm/kg) in a patient with a high serum osmolality (generally >287 mOsm/kg). Because many patients can maintain a normal osmolality with access to water, a water-deprivation test is often necessary to document the abnormality and exclude primary polydipsia. A vasopressin analogue can be given to patients at the end of a water deprivation test to exclude nephrogenic diabetes insipidus. Patients with central diabetes insipidus should undergo pituitary imaging with an MRI.

Treatment

Diabetes insipidus is treated with either subcutaneous, nasal, or oral preparations of vasopressin analogues and ready access to water.

LYMPHOCYTIC HYPOPHYSITIS

Lymphocytic hypophysitis is an uncommon autoimmune disease in which the pituitary gland is infiltrated by lymphocytes, plasma cells, and macrophages, usually causing impaired function. Lymphocytic hypophysitis is mainly associated with late pregnancy or the postpartum period, although it can occur in nonpregnant women, some of whom may be postmenopausal, and in men. This disorder may have an autoimmune origin, and it is associated with other autoimmune disorders, especially autoimmune thyroiditis. Tests for antinuclear antibodies and rheumatoid factor are often positive, and the erythrocyte sedimentation rate may be elevated. Headache, visual field impairment, and more rarely diplopia are due to extrasellar pituitary enlargement with optic chiasma compression and/or to invasion of cavernous sinuses. Deficiency of adrenocorticotropic hormone ((ACTH; resulting in secondary hypoadrenalism) is the earliest and most frequent endocrine manifestation. MRI usually demonstrates extrasellar symmetrical pituitary enlargement and loss of the posterior pituitary bright spot. Treatment is symptomatic with compressive effects reduced through treatment with high-dose corticosteroids (20–60 mg per day of prednisone) and/or surgical decompression. The prognosis for hormonal recovery is poor.

HYPOTHYROIDISM

Presentation of Hypothyroidism

Hypothyroidism affects about 2% of adult women and about 0.2% of adult men. Primary hypothyroidism refers to intrinsic thyroid failure and accounts for 99% of cases; secondary hypothyroidism refers to hypothyroidism that results from pituitary dysfunction. The most common cause of primary hypothyroidism in iodine-sufficient areas is chronic autoimmune (Hashimoto) thyroiditis. This is most common among older women and is generally permanent. Thyroidectomy, radioiodine treatment, and external radiation therapy are other frequent causes of hypothyroidism. Both iodine deficiency and excess can cause hypothyroidism. Iodine deficiency is a type of hypothyroidism associated with goiter. It is the most common cause of hypothyroidism worldwide but is quite uncommon in the United States, where iodine is added to salt. Acute administration of iodine suppresses thyroxine synthesis; however, patients recover their thyroid function after just a few days of treatment. Other drugs that cause hypothyroidism include antithyroid drugs (e.g., methimazole, propylthiouracil), amiodarone, lithium, and interferon-α.

Hypothyroidism can be transient when related to thyroiditis. Inflammation of the thyroid gland can be painful or entirely painless. Hypothyroidism occurring postpartum is one of the most common presentations of thyroiditis. Transient hypothyroidism lasts up to as long as 6 months, but the hypothyroidism will have resolved in a significant majority within 3 months.

Clinical Features

Patients with hypothyroidism can present with a variety of nonspecific symptoms. Some of the most common features include dry skin, cold intolerance, weight gain, constipation, menorrhagia, and fatigue. The clinical picture of hypothyroidism is now a good deal milder since screening became more common. The most common signs in patients with moderate to severe hypothyroidism include bradycardia, delayed ankle reflexes, periorbital puffiness, and coarse hair. The term myxedema refers to the appearance of the skin and subcutaneous tissues in a patient who is severely hypothyroid.

Evaluation

Patients with primary thyroid failure will have an elevated thyroid-stimulating hormone (TSH) level and low thyroxine concentration. Central hypothyroidism should be suspected if the TSH is normal or low and the thyroxine level is low. Patients receiving high-dose salicylates or phenytoin appear to have low TSH levels due to an assay artifact.

Treatment

Patients with an elevated TSH level should be treated with replacement thyroxine with a target TSH of between 1 and 2. Levothyroxine has a long half-life, and once-daily treatment results in a nearly constant serum thyroxine level. As a result of variations in the thyroxine content of individual formulations, reassessment of the adequacy of replacement is indicated if the formulation is changed. The mean replacement dose of thyroxine is 1.6–1.8 µg/kg (generally 75–112 µg/day in women and 125–200 µg/day in men). A lower dose should be initiated in the elderly and titrated upward as needed. Obese patients require doses that are approximately 20% higher. Drugs that interfere with the absorption of levothyroxine include cholesytramine calcium carbonate, and ferrous sulfate. Patients receiving estrogen replacement also require a higher dose of levothyroxine.

Combination replacement of liothyronine and levothyroxine is requested by some patients, but it is not supported by the balance of clinical trial data. If instituted, 25 µg of levothyroxine can be replaced with 5 µg of liothyronine. Desiccated thyroid, liothyronine alone, and other thyroid preparations are not recommended.

Transient hypothyroidism can be difficult to distinguish from Hashimoto thyroiditis. It is reasonable to attempt to reduce the dose of levothyroxine by 50% after approximately 3 months in patients who are suspected to have had transient hypothyroidism: if the TSH measured 6 weeks later rises, then the initial dose is reinstated; if the TSH is stable, then thyroxine can be withdrawn, and the TSH checked again.

Patients with an elevated TSH and a normal thyroxine level are most likely to have subclinical hypothyroidism. Testing for the presence of thyroid peroxidase antibody can be helpful in such patients, as it predicts the progression to permanent hypothyroidism. These patients should be monitored for the development of more severe hypothyroidism, or levothyroxine can be initiated at the outset.

Patients with central hypothyroidism should have their thyroxine dose titrated to the level of free thyroxine.

Hypothyroidism During Pregnancy

Levothyroxine requirements increase as early as the fifth week of gestation. Given the importance of maternal euthyroidism for normal fetal cognitive development, women with hypothyroidism should have their levothyroxine dose increased by approximately 30% as soon as pregnancy is confirmed. Thereafter, serum thyrotropin levels should be monitored, and the levothyroxine dose adjusted accordingly.

HYPERTHYROIDISM

Causes of Hyperthyroidism

Hyperthyroidism can be caused by an increased production of thyroid hormone (as in Graves disease or an autonomous nodule) or increased release of preformed thyroid hormone (as in thyroiditis). Hyperthyroidism can also be caused by overreplacement with exogenous thyroid hormone, ectopic hyperthyroidism, or by unregulated stimulation of the TSH receptor (as in trophoblastic disease or a TSH-secreting pituitary adenoma).

Clinical Features

The presentation of hyperthyroidism can be highly variable, especially in older people. Characteristic symptoms include anxiety, tremor, palpitations, heat intolerance, insomnia, oligomenorrhea, and weight loss despite an increased appetite. Typical signs include tachycardia, systolic hypertension, tremor, lid retraction, lid lag, warm skin, and hyperreflexia. The presence of a goiter will depend on the cause of the hyperthyroidism. A single palpable nodule or multiple nodules suggests an autonomous thyroid adenoma or a multinodular goiter as the source, respectively; a painful tender thyroid gland suggests granulomatous thyroiditis. Signs that are suggestive of Graves disease include goiter, thyroid bruit, exophthalmos, periorbital edema, and pretibial myxedema.

Evaluation

The diagnosis of hyperthyroidism is confirmed using biochemical testing of the thyroxine and TSH levels. An increased thyroxine level with a suppressed TSH characterizes overt hyperthyroidism. Patients with subclinical hyperthyroidism may have a normal thyroxine level and a suppressed TSH. Occasional patients demonstrate T_3 toxicosis with a normal thyroxine level and an elevated level of triiodothyronine. TSH-induced hyperthyroidism and thyroid hormone resistance, each characterized by an increased level of TSH, are very rare. An elevated thyroxine with a normal TSH level is usually attributed to abnormalities in thyroid-binding proteins in patients who are clinically euthyroid.

When the etiology of the hyperthyroidism is unclear, a thyroid radioiodine-uptake study can be performed. Graves disease is characterized by a high uptake, thyroiditis by a low uptake.

Treatment

Propylthiouracil and methimazole are the antithyroid drugs used in the United States. These agents are actively concentrated by the thyroid gland, and their primary effect is to inhibit thyroid hormone synthesis by interfering with thyroid peroxidase-mediated iodination of tyrosine residues in thyroglobulin, a critical step in the synthesis of thyroxine and triiodothyronine. Propylthiouracil also blocks the conversion of thyroxine to triiodothyronine within the thyroid and peripheral tissues, although the clinical importance of this function

is uncertain. No dose adjustment is needed in patients with renal or liver failure, among children or the elderly.

The usual starting dose of methimazole is 20 mg per day as a single daily dose, and the usual starting dose of propylthiouracil is 100 mg given three times a day. Following initial dosing, follow-up testing of thyroid function is suggested approximately every 6 weeks until the thyroid function tests normalize. Many patients can ultimately be controlled at a low dose. Testing frequency can be reduced to every 6 months over time. Following a discussion about the risk of relapse, antithyroid drugs can be withdrawn after 12–18 months to determine if ongoing treatment is required.

Cutaneous reactions to antithyroid drugs are quite common and usually mild. The drug should be discontinued in patients complaining of arthralgias, as this may be a presentation of a transient migratory polyarthritis associated with antithyroid drug use. The most feared side effect of antithyroid drugs is agranulocytosis. This complication occurs in approximately 1 in every 270 patients given antithyroid drugs. A baseline differential white cell count should be obtained before treatment is restarted and retested if fever or sore throat develops. The drug should be discontinued if the granulocyte count is <1000 per cubic millimeter. Hepatotoxicity and vasculitis (drug-induced lupus) are rare but well described.

Current treatments for Graves disease include antithyroid drugs, radioiodine, and surgery. Initial treatment usually includes an antithyroid drug such as methimazole 20 mg taken once daily. Beta blockers provide symptomatic relief, but their use is not universally recommended. For patients with more severe hyperthyroidism, iodine treatment can provide rapid relief of symptoms. A typical approach would be to prescribe 3 drops of saturated solution of potassium iodide three times daily for up to 10 days. Radioiodine can be given as primary treatment for patients with Graves hyperthyroidism, although many clinicians will wait until the first relapse before offering this approach. Hyperthyroidism can be exacerbated for a short time by radioiodine treatment. In patients with cardiac disease or in the elderly in whom such an exacerbation would be risky, pretreatment with antithyroid drugs can be useful. Surgery is usually reserved for patients with an obstructing goiter.

Hyperthyroidism associated with toxic thyroid adenomas can be treated with antithyroid drugs and a beta blocker. As these autonomous nodules do not resolve spontaneously, more definitive treatment is usually indicated after the initial symptoms have been controlled. Radioiodine is a preferred over surgery for most patients, but this is less likely to be effective in patients with large or multiple nodules.

Hyperthyroidism During Pregnancy

Women who develop hyperthyroidism while pregnant are at increased risk of spontaneous abortion, premature labor, stillbirth, and preeclampsia. Changes in thyroid hormone binding globulin (usually doubles), levels of human chorionic gonadotropin (that can mimic the actions of TSH), and endogenous physiology (altered TSH responsiveness) can complicate the biochemical assessment of thyroid function in pregnancy. As radioiodine is absolutely contraindicated during pregnancy, antithyroid drugs are the preferred treatment for pregnant women with hyperthyroidism. Propylthiouracil remains the preferred treatment for hyperthyroidism occurring during pregnancy. The dose should be minimized to prevent fetal hypothyroidism, as the drug does cross the placenta. Methimazole may be associated with congenital anomalies including aplasia cutis and choanal or esophageal atresia. Generally treatment is given to a point where mild hyperthyroidism is allowed to persist. Low thyroid function at birth is found in approximately half of neonates whose mothers received an antithyroid drug; ultimate intelligence has been demonstrated to be normal. Both methimazole and propylthiouracil are approved for nursing mothers by the American Academy of Pediatrics, although they do appear in breast milk in minute quantities.

THYROID NODULES

In the United States, between 4% and 7% of the adult population have a palpable thyroid nodule. Only 5% of these are malignant. Other causes of nodules include thyroid cyst, a colloid nodule, a focal area of thyroiditis, and benign follicular neoplasms. Nodules can be solitary or multiple. The risk of cancer is not lower when nodules are multiple, as was previously thought.

Evaluation

The history can provide useful prognostic information. Rapid growth, or the presence of a family history of thyroid carcinoma or multiple endocrine neoplasia (MEN) increases the risk that a nodule is cancerous. Risk increases more moderately if age is <20 years or >70 years, if the patient is male, if there is a history of head and neck irradiation, if the nodule is >4 cm, or if there are local symptoms such as dysphagia, hoarseness, or cough. High-risk signs include a hard nodule and the presence of regional lymphadenopathy.

A suppressed TSH level suggests a benign hyperfunctioning nodule. Hyperfunctioning nodules are so rarely malignant that if the TSH is suppressed, fine-needle aspiration (FNA) can be deferred. A normal or high TSH level does not obviate the need for further investigation. Ultrasonography can be performed in the office and increases the sensitivity and specificity the FNA result. Ultrasonography can detect high-risk features such as hypoechogenicity, microcalcifications, irregular margins, increased vascularity by Doppler, and evidence of local lymphadenopathy.

Patients undergoing FNA do not typically need to stop aspirin or anticoagulants. The procedure is safe and well tolerated. Each lesion >1 cm in size should be sampled with two to four passes of the needle.

Cystic nodules can be drained after any solid portion has been aspirated, although most recur; use of sclerosants such as ethanol and tetracycline has been disappointing.

Radionucleotide scanning uses ^{123}iodine, ^{131}iodine, or ^{99}mtechnetium-pertechnetate to detect whether a nodule is functioning. A scan can also determine whether a nodule is dominant within a multinodular or retrosternal gland. A scan cannot accurately determine the size of a thyroid nodule.

Treatment

Benign nodules can remain in situ. Repeat ultrasonography after 9–12 months to ensure that there has been no significant change in size is suggested. Levothyroxine suppression is no longer recommended, as TSH must be suppressed to <0.1 mU/L to effectively suppress nodular growth or formation, and suppression to this level is associated with an increased risk of bone loss and atrial fibrillation.

Follicular neoplasm may be benign or malignant, and cellular aspirates cannot distinguish these two. If the patient prefers, or if the nodule is cold on radionucleotide scanning, then excision is recommended.

Malignant nodules should be excised with a total thyroidectomy and usually require postoperative thyroid ablation with ^{131}iodine. Disease recurrence can be screened for using thyroglobulin measurements.

Nondiagnostic aspirates occur about 10% of the time. If a second sample is again nondiagnostic, then referral for surgical excision is appropriate.

THYROID CANCER

Papillary and follicular thyroid cancers account for approximately 75% and 10% of all cancers in the thyroid gland, respectively. Metastases and medullary and anaplastic cancers make up the balance of cases. The 10-year survivals are very different for these tumors, ranging from 98% for papillary, 92% for follicular, and 13% for anaplastic carcinoma.

Clinical Features

Most tumors are detected incidentally, or a nodule is palpated. High-risk features of a nodule include rapid growth, a family history of thyroid carcinoma or multiple endocrine neoplasia, age <20 years or >70 years, male gender, and a history of head and neck irradiation. Local symptoms such as dysphagia, hoarseness, or cough are worrisome.

Evaluation

Thyroid cancers are almost always diagnosed by FNA. Differentiated cancers are staged according to the TNM classification. In this classification all patients aged <45 years of age are stage 1 unless they have distant metastases (stage 2). For older patients, stage depends on size, presence, and laterality of lymph node involvement and whether distant metastases have been detected.

Treatment

Total thyroidectomy is the primary therapy for differentiated thyroid cancer, although unilateral lobectomy can be considered for tumors <1 cm. Regional neck dissection is indicated if a preoperative neck ultrasound shows evidence of adenopathy. Following surgery, most patients undergo radioiodine treatment to ablate any thyroid remnant so that serum thyroglobulin can be used as a tumor marker. High-risk patients undergo radioiodine scans (after withdrawal of replacement thyroxine and dietary iodine restriction) to determine the extent of any metastatic disease, and the uptake of iodine in these scans is used to dose therapeutic radioiodine. All patients are treated with levothyroxine to prevent symptomatic hypothyroidism and reduce potential thyrotropin stimulation of tumor growth. The target thyrotropin level is generally below or in the bottom half of the normal range; lower targets are used for advanced disease. Adjuvant external-beam radiotherapy and some chemotherapy are occasionally used for refractory cases.

Anaplastic thyroid cancer is almost always fatal. The cancer is generally treated surgically. If unresectable, some of these tumors respond to paclitaxel and external beam radiotherapy for local control.

OSTEOPOROSIS

Osteoporosis is a common problem ultimately afflicting half of all postmenopausal women and about a quarter of men. It is characterized by low bone mass and an increased risk of fracture. Fractures occur because of qualitative and quantitative deterioration in the trabecular and cortical skeleton. Bone quality cannot be measured clinically, but bone mineral density can be measured easily using bone densitometry.

Clinical Features

Osteoporosis is asymptomatic until fracture occurs. Vertebral fracture is the most common, and the majority are asymptomatic. Hip fracture and radial fractures are common.

Evaluation

Most fractures of the hip, wrist, and vertebral body with no occurrence of trauma are indicative of osteoporosis. On densitometry, osteopenia is defined as bone mass that is between 1 and 2.5 standard deviations below the mean peak bone mass of control population. Osteoporosis is defined as a bone mass value >2.5 standard deviations below the

peak bone mass of a control population. Generally the hip and spine are imaged. In postmenopausal white women, the relative risk of fracture is increased by a factor of 1.5 to 3 for each decrease of 1.0 in the T score. Densitometry also provides the deviation of bone mass from age-matched controls and reports this as a Z-score. The Z-score determines whether any bone loss is substantially greater than expected for age. A basic evaluation with low bone density comprises a biochemical profile, liver enzymes, alkaline phosphatase, 25-hydroxyvitamin D, and a complete blood count. Patients with low Z-scores should have evaluation for secondary causes of bone loss such as hyperparathyroidism, hyperthyroidism, and malabsorption. Markers of bone turnover (such as urinary N-telopeptide) can be useful in determining the need for treatment in equivocal cases.

Treatment

An optimal initial strategy for patients with low bone mass includes supplemental calcium (1200 mg) and vitamin D (400 to 800 IU daily, for postmenopausal women) when appropriate, weight-bearing physical activity (30 min at least three times per week), and smoking cessation counseling if needed. Patients with any of the following four criteria qualify for pharmacologic intervention

- History of hip or vertebral fracture
- Osteoporosis by densitometry
- Any fracture and osteopenia by densitometry
- Osteopenia by densitometry with a 10-year fracture risk in excess of 20% (risk calculator at http://www.shef.ac.uk/FRAX/)

Alendronate (70 mg orally once weekly) and risedronate (35 mg once weekly or 150 mg once a month) are given orally. Zolendronate 5 mg is given intravenously once a year. All have been shown to reduce hip and spine fracture risk. Ibandronate (150 mg once monthly by mouth) has not been shown to reduce hip fractures.

Gastrointestinal adverse effects of oral bisphosphonates are rare if administration instructions are followed. Hypocalcemia can complicate bisphosphonate treatment if vitamin D levels are not sufficient. Osteonecrosis of the jaw is a rare complication of bisphosphonate use, occurring once per 10,000 to 100,000 patient-years. Although most cases have been in cancer patients or in patients with multiple myeloma treated with intravenous bisphosphonates, rare cases have been noted in patients with postmenopausal osteoporosis taking oral bisphosphonates. Intravenous bisphosphonates lead to short-term flu-like symptoms.

Synthetic parathyroid hormone (PTH; teriparatide teriparatide) is available for daily subcutaneous use and increases bone mineral density and reduces fracture risk. It is generally reserved for patients with severe osteoporosis; treatment is limited to 24 months. Denosumab is an injectable medication used to manage patients who cannot tolerate or be treated with bisphosphonates, or who have severe osteoporosis.

Monitoring densitometry should generally be performed no more frequently than every 2 years.

HYPERCALCEMIA

Clinical Features

Patients with mild hypercalcemia (10.5–12 mg/dL) are often asymptomatic. Patients with more severe hypercalcemia can present with nonspecific symptoms that include nausea, anorexia, constipation, abdominal pain, bone pain, fatigue, polydipsia, and confusion. Calcium levels higher than 14 mg/dL are dangerous and can be lethal. Signs of hypercalcemia include dysrhythmias, hypertension, and a shortened QT-interval on an electrocardiogram.

Evaluation

The two most common causes of hypercalcemia are primary hyperparathyroidism and neoplastic disease, accounting for more than 90% of cases, and these can be discriminated on the basis of the serum parathyroid hormone level. Primary hyperparathyroidism has a relatively benign course. Osteoporosis and renal impairment are two important long-term consequences that drive early intervention. Parathyroidectomy is recommended for patients with an elevated parathyroid hormone and hypercalcemia who are less than the age of 50, if the calcium is >12.5 mg/dL, if there are renal stones, evidence of renal insufficiency, the Z-score on bone densitometry is <2, or urinary calcium excretion is particularly high. A preoperative parathyroid sestamibi scan can assist the endocrine surgeon and limit the extent of surgery. Intraoperative parathyroid hormone levels allow the surgeon to be confident of the procedure's success before surgical closure. Medical management of primary hyperparathyroidism with calcimimetics is currently limited to clinical trials.

Chronic renal failure generally causes hypocalcemia. If untreated, prolonged high phosphate and low vitamin D levels can lead to increased PTH secretion and subsequent hypercalcemia. This is termed tertiary hyperparathyroidism and can be managed surgically or medically.

Hypercalcemia of malignancy is usually symptomatic and can be severe. Solid tumors induce hypercalcemia by releasing parathyroid-hormone related protein (PTHrp), which mimics the action of endogenous parathyroid hormone. Bone destruction by metastatic disease or myeloma can also induce hypercalcemia, often in association with an elevated alkaline phosphatase level.

Vitamin D can induce hypercalcemia if taken in overdose or if there is excessive action of the 1-alpha-hydroxylase that creates the active form of vitamin D. This enzyme is hyperactive in patients with granulomatous disease such as sarcoidosis and responds well to treatment with glucocorticoids while the underlying disease is being treated. Consumption of large amounts of calcium or vitamin A can rarely lead to hypercalcemia.

Familial hypocalciuric hypercalcemia is an autosomal dominant condition caused by a mutation in the gene for the calcium receptor. Patients have an innocuous course characterized by mild to moderate hypercalcemia, normal or slightly elevated parathyroid hormone levels, and low urinary calcium excretion. These patients do not benefit from parathyroidectomy.

Treatment

Treatment of severe hypercalcemia includes emergent fluid repletion with saline and intravenous administration of bisphosphonates. Initially saline is given at 200–300 mL/hr and adjusted to maintain the urine output to 100–150 mL/hr. A loop diuretic can be added but is not always necessary and can lead to hypokalemia and hypomagnesemia. In the United States, pamidronate and zoledronate are bisphosphonates licensed for use in this indication. Zolendronate is preferred as it can be given over a shorter time (15 minutes as compared to 2 hours for pamidronate) and is more potent. Hypocalcemia occurs in up to 50% of patients treated with bisphosphonates for hypercalcemia of malignancy, although symptomatic hypocalcemia is rare. Calcitonin is characterized by good tolerability but poor efficacy in normalizing the serum calcium level. However, a major advantage of calcitonin is the acute onset of the hypocalcemic effect (reduction of 1–2 mg/dL within 6 hours), which contrasts with the delayed (approximately 2–4 days) but more pronounced effect of bisphosphonates. It is administered intramuscularly or subcutaneously every 12 hours at a dose of 4 IU/kg. Gallium nitrate is characterized by high efficacy and few adverse events apart from renal toxicity (10% of cases). However, data are very limited and further trials are necessary.

HYPOPARATHYROIDISM

Hypocalcemia results from inadequate parathyroid hormone, an insufficient supply of vitamin D, abnormal magnesium levels, or during metabolic circumstances such as sepsis or pancreatitis. Hypoparathyroidism is diagnosed when the parathyroid hormone level is inappropriately low in a patient with hypocalcemia and a normal magnesium level.

Clinical Features

Neuromuscular symptoms such as muscle cramping, circumoral numbness and tingling, and muscle twitching are the most typical presenting features of hypocalcemia. As calcium levels drop further, seizures, heart failure, bronchospasm, and laryngospasm can occur. Chronic hypocalcemia can lead to cataracts and basal ganglial calcification and has been associated with pseudotumor cerebri.

Hypoparathyroidism typically results from surgical intervention in the neck and occurs in up to 5% of total thyroidectomy surgeries. Parathyroid sufficiency generally requires a single remaining parathyroid gland. Parathyroid failure may also occur if the parathyroids accumulate iron (e.g., hemochromatosis) or copper (Wilson disease). Autoimmune destruction of the parathyroid glands is generally associated with the autoimmune polyendocrine syndrome type 1 (which incorporates at least two of the triad of Addison disease, hypoparathyroidism, and chronic mucocutaneous candidiasis). Early-onset hypoparathyroidism accompanying immunodeficiency characterizes the DiGeorge syndrome. Magnesium is essential for parathyroid hormone secretion, and both hyper- and hypomagnesemia can lead to hypocalcemia.

Evaluation

The corrected total calcium should be calculated (measured total calcium in mg/dL + 0.8 [4 – serum albumin in g/dL]) or ionized calcium measured. The laboratory evaluation should include measures of intact parathyroid hormone, 25-hydroxyvitamin D, phosphate, and magnesium.

Treatment

Patients with severe symptoms of hypocalcemia should be treated with intravenous calcium gluconate. Long-term management requires patients to receive calcium salts and a vitamin D metabolite, such as calcitriol. Each are titrated to obtain normal levels. Thiazides can be used to reduce hypercalciuria and prevent nephrolithiasis, particularly if the 24-hour urinary calcium level exceeds 250 mg. Parathyroid hormone repletion is not yet available for the treatment of hypoparathyroidism.

ADRENAL FAILURE

Acute adrenal failure can result from hemorrhage, tumor invasion, antifungal medications, acquired immunodeficiency syndrome, or infection that affects both adrenal glands. Addison disease refers to chronic adrenocortical insufficiency due to dysfunction of the entire adrenal cortex (incorporating glucocorticoid, mineralocorticoid, and sex steroid deficiency). Adrenal failure becomes symptomatic when approximately 90% of adrenal function has been lost.

Clinical Features

Patients in acute adrenal crisis present with nausea, vomiting, and vascular collapse. Abdominal or flank pain and fever may be present. Chronic adrenal failure presents insidiously with weakness, fatigue, anorexia, nausea, and weight loss. Examination may reveal both hyperpigmentation (resulting from the stimulant effect of adrenocorticotropin on melanocytes) and vitiligo (autoimmune destruction of melanocytes). Other examination features include decreased body hair owing to loss of adrenal androgens, a feature that is especially noteworthy in women.

Evaluation

Patients with acute adrenal failure will generally be hypotensive. Hyperkalemia and hyponatremia are indicators of mineralocorticoid deficiency. Eosinophilia and hypoglycemia may accompany adrenal crisis. A random cortisol level may be inappropriately low for a stressed patient. An adrenocorticotropin stimulation test generally comprises measurement of cortisol and aldosterone at baseline, intravenous injection of 250 µg of adrenocorticotropin, with aldosterone levels drawn at 30 minutes and cortisol levels drawn at 60 minutes. An aldosterone level that fails to increase by 5 ng/dL is indicative of abnormal mineralocorticoid function. The cortisol level should rise to >20 µg/dL and increase by at least 7 µg/dL from baseline to establish normal glucocorticoid function. Thyrotropin and thyroxine levels should be measured. Adrenal autoantibodies can be helpful to establish risk of other autoimmune conditions.

Treatment

Acute treatment comprises 50–100 mg of hydrocortisone administered intravenously. Clinical improvement should follow within 6 hours. Glucocorticoid repletion generally comprises hydrocortisone 15–25 mg daily in two to three divided doses, titrated to symptoms. Mineralocorticoid repletion should be initiated with fludrocortisone, generally 0.05–0.2 mg per day, titrated to blood pressure, potassium, and morning plasma renin activity. Patients should be provided with injectable glucocorticoids for emergency use such as during vomiting, diarrhea, trauma, and wear an emergency identification bracelet or necklace.

ADRENAL NODULES AND TUMORS

Adrenal masses are detected in approximately 3% of all abdominal computed tomography (CT) scans and in approximately 10% of all autopsies. When evaluating adrenal masses the clinician should consider whether the mass is malignant and whether it is hormonally active. The adrenal cortex can produce a variety of hormones and syndromes including cortisol (Cushing syndrome), aldosterone (Conn syndrome), androgens (virilization), and estrogens (feminization); the adrenal medulla generates catecholamines (pheochromocytoma).

Evaluation

Imaging features can help to determine the malignancy risk. High-risk features include irregular shape, diameter greater than 4 cm, high CT attenuation value (>10 Hounsfield units [HU]), and inhomogeneous enhancement after intravenous contrast. Metastatic disease from another source tends to cause bilateral disease and have a similar attenuation as the liver on T1 imaging, and a high T2 signal intensity. Benign nodules (that may be functional) tend to be round, homogeneous, and smaller (<4 cm) with low CT attenuation (<10 HU), and isointense with the liver on T1- and T2-weighted MRI imaging. Adrenal cysts, myelolipoma, and adrenal hemorrhage are usually readily distinguishable by their unique imaging characteristics.

Clinical Features

Pheochromocytoma can be suggested by the presence of hypertension (can be chronic or paroxysmal), a history of "spells," headache, palpitations, or pallor. Even in the absence of any symptoms, pheochromocytoma should always be excluded before proceeding to surgery as intraoperative risks of an unrecognized pheochromocytoma are high. Serum metanephrines are specific and sensitive providing the patient has not consumed/acetaminophen (Tylenol) in the prior 72 hours. Two consecutive 24-hour urinary collections for total metanephrines and catecholamines provide confirmatory evidence.

Primary aldosteronism is suggested by refractory hypertension and, occasionally, hypokalemia. An aldosterone-to-renin ratio >30 when the aldosterone is at least 10 ng/dL is suggestive. To obtain an interpretable result, patients must not be taking aldosterone receptor antagonists (such as spironolactone, eplerenone) or beta blockers. A suppressed renin in a patient taking an angiotensin-converting enzyme (ACE) inhibitor or angiotensin receptor blocker is highly suggestive of hyperaldosteronism.

Measures of androgens and estrogens are not routinely performed in the absence of suggestive symptoms or signs. Virilization is suggested by male-pattern baldness, deepening of the voice, and clitoromegaly in women. Feminization in men is suggested by gynecomastia, decreased libido, and loss of muscle strength.

PRIMARY ALDOSTERONISM

Primary aldosteronism resulting from an adrenal adenoma is a reversible cause of hypertension; it accounts for at least 10% of causes of resistant hypertension. These tumors are usually <2 cm in size and are benign; most adenomas are unilateral.

Clinical Features

Most patients are asymptomatic or have minimal symptoms. Headache may accompany severe hypertension. Polyuria, nocturia, and muscle cramps may accompany hypokalemia.

Evaluation

Spontaneous hypokalemia with metabolic alkalosis and a serum sodium level at the high end of the normal range or hypernatremia is common. Plasma renin activity is suppressed in almost all patients with untreated primary aldosteronism, and plasma aldosterone levels are elevated. A plasma aldosterone-to-plasma renin ratio >30 with a plasma aldosterone >20 ng/dL usually indicates primary aldosteronism. Aldosterone concentrations are uninterpretable in a patient on spironolactone. Diuretics, ACE inhibitors, and angiotensin receptor blockers can falsely elevate the plasma renin activity, leading to a lower aldosterone-to-plasma renin activity ratio; therefore, the presence of suppressed plasma renin activity in a patient treated with a diuretic or, especially, an ACE inhibitor or angiotensin receptor blocker is a strong predictor for primary hyperaldosteronism. The most definitive test in diagnosing primary aldosteronism is a nonsuppressed 24-hour urinary aldosterone excretion rate during a salt load (of at least 1 teaspoon of salt daily for 3 days). Patients over the age of 40 generally require adrenal vein sampling to avoid resecting an innocuous cortical adenoma.

Treatment

Patients with biochemical evidence of primary hyperaldosteronism and a unilateral adenoma on tomography can proceed to unilateral adrenalectomy. Patients with bilateral adrenal hyperplasia, and patients who either refuse or are not surgical candidates can be managed with spironolactone or eplerenone, with a program of salt restriction and regular aerobic activity.

PHEOCHROMOCYTOMA

Catecholamine-secreting tumors can result in a dramatic and life-threatening clinical syndrome. Most of these tumors arise from the adrenal medulla. Tumors arising outside of the adrenal gland are termed paraganglionomas. These tumors are rare, accounting for fewer than 1 per 1000 cases of hypertension.

Clinical Features

The classic triad includes episodic headache, palpitation, and diaphoresis. Spells may occur as infrequently as monthly or multiple times daily. Anxiety, nausea, tremor, chest and epigastric pain, and weight loss are other reported features. Patients with pheochromocytoma are typically hypertensive; approximately half of the patients will have episodic hypertension.

Evaluation

Because pheochromocytomas can occur in association with the multiple endocrine neoplasia type 2 syndrome and in von Hippel-Lindau syndrome, indications of these diagnoses should be sought.

Patients at low risk for pheochromocytoma can have the diagnosis excluded by measuring catecholamines and metanephrines in a 24-hour urine collection, a test with high specificity. High-risk patients can be screened with plasma metanephrines; acetaminophen must be avoided for 72 hours before this test is performed. Most patients with pheochromocytomas have urinary or plasma levels that are at least three to four times the upper limit of normal. Tricyclic antidepressants, levodopa, labetalol, ethanol, sotalol, amphetamines, buspirone, benzodiazepines, methyldopa, and chlorpromazine all increase catecholamines and should be avoided.

If the diagnosis is biochemically confirmed, imaging of the adrenals with MRI is recommended; these lesions are usually at least 3 cm in size. Pheochromocytomas are uniquely hyperintense on T2-weighted images. Nuclear medicine scanning with ^{123}I-metaiodobenzylguanidine or positron-emission tomography can be performed if MR/CT imaging is negative.

Treatment

Patients with pheochromocytoma should be managed by experienced hypertension specialists. Surgery is the treatment of choice and can be a high-risk procedure. Preoperative preparation generally combines alpha blockade (such as phenoxybenzamine, titrated to postural hypotension) with calcium-channel or beta blockers as needed. Some clinicians recommend metyrosine, but there is limited experience with this inhibitor of catecholamine synthesis. Perioperative crises are managed with nitroprusside. Surgical resection is prudent for malignant pheochromocytomas, although long-term survival is poor.

CUSHING SYNDROME

Chronically elevated glucocorticoid levels result in protean symptoms and signs that are common (such as obesity, hyperglycemia, and hypertension) and nonspecific (weakness, acne, edema, striae, headache, plethora). These features make the diagnosis of Cushing syndrome challenging. The hypercortisolemia of Cushing syndrome can originate in the adrenal or result from a pituitary adenoma or other tumor secreting adrenocorticotropin.

Clinical Features

The most common presenting feature is obesity of the face, neck, and abdomen that spares the extremities. Facial fat deposition can result in a "moon" face exacerbated by deposition of fat in the supraclavicular fat pads, which makes the neck appear shortened. These patients develop skin thinning, atrophy, and easy bruising. Striae typical of Cushing syndrome are typically purple in color, wide, and multiple, factors that help distinguish them from stretch marks associated with obesity. Women with Cushing disease may have signs of hyperandrogenism such as hirsutism. Proximal myopathy (usually described as difficulty rising from a seated position), psychiatric change (emotional lability, depression, and mild paranoia are common), and hypertension are often present at presentation. Other features associated with longer-standing or more severe hypercortisolemia include glucose intolerance, glaucoma, and osteopenia.

Evaluation

The first step in evaluating whether a patient may have Cushing syndrome is to elucidate any history of exposure to corticosteroids, including potent inhaled, injected, or topical steroids, or medroxyprogesterone acetate—a progestin with intrinsic steroid activity. Factitious Cushing syndrome accounts for <1% of all cases and is suggested by erratic and inconsistent results. In such cases, synthetic glucocorticoids can be assayed directly in the urine.

To establish hypercortisolemia, at least two 24-hour urine samples for free cortisol (and creatinine) should be obtained. Patients whose levels are greater than three times higher than the upper reference range can be assumed to have Cushing syndrome. Patients with equivocal values should be retested after a few weeks or be evaluated with further testing according to the clinical suspicion.

An overnight dexamethasone suppression test is also used as a screening test to diagnose hypercortisolemia. In this test, an 8 a.m. serum cortisol level is drawn after a 1-mg dexamethasone dose at 11 p.m.–midnight. Most normal patients should suppress their endogenous cortisol level to <2 μg/dL. A screening strategy that uses three consecutive late-evening salivary cortisols may ultimately replace these aforementioned tests. These can be performed by an ambulatory patient with minimal instruction. Reference ranges are laboratory specific.

Once the diagnosis of Cushing syndrome is secure, a source for the hypercortisolemia should be sought. Determining whether Cushing syndrome is ACTH-dependent or adrenal in origin requires accurate measurement of ACTH levels. Cortisol secretion can be deemed to be ACTH-independent if the ACTH is <5 pg/mL when the cortisol level is >15 μg/dL. Under the same circumstances the syndrome is very likely to be ACTH-dependent (Cushing disease) if the ACTH level is >15 pg/mL when the cortisol is at least 15 μg/dL; ACTH levels of between 5 and 15 pg/mL are less specific but usually indicate ACTH dependency. Patients with equivocal values should be reinvestigated.

Patients with ACTH-independent hypercortisolemia should undergo thin-slice CT of the adrenal glands to identify the responsible adenoma, carcinoma, or nodules.

Patients with ACTH-dependent hypercortisolemia should undergo further testing to discriminate between Cushing disease related to a pituitary adenoma and that related to ectopic ACTH secretion. Tumors recognized to secrete ACTH include small-cell cancer of the lung and bronchial and thymic carcinoids. Clinicians should resist the temptation to image the pituitary because 10% of the population have a structurally abnormal pituitary. Patients should instead undergo a high-dose dexamethasone suppression test, where 2 mg of dexamethasone is given every 6 hours for 2 days. This test capitalizes on the fact that ACTH-secreting pituitary adenomas retain some feedback responsiveness and often suppress their ACTH production when ambient glucocorticoid levels are high. Cortisol levels are reduced by >90% among 70% of those with Cushing disease. In the same study, by contradistinction, no patients with ectopically derived ACTH suppressed cortisol below 90% in response to this high-dose suppression test.

Petrosal sinus sampling using corticotropin-releasing hormone (CRH) stimulation is a final approach to confirming that ACTH is derived from the pituitary. Criteria for confirming the pituitary as the source of the ACTH include a ratio of ACTH between one side of the petrosal sinus and the peripheral plasma of >2, or a ratio >3 during infusion of CRH as compared with the level before infusion is begun. If one side has an ACTH level that is a multiple of 1.4 times or more the level on the opposite side, then the adenoma is highly likely to reside on that side. Patients with suspected ectopic ACTH should have an octreotide imaging performed with chest plain and tomographic images obtained as indicated.

Treatment

The goal of treatment of Cushing syndrome is the eradication of any tumor, suppression of cortisol levels to as low as possible, and avoidance of permanent hormone dependency. The treatment of choice for Cushing disease is transsphenoidal pituitary resection, irrespective of the size of the pituitary tumor. The more extensive the resection, the greater is the risk of permanent hypopituitarism. This may have particular implications for younger patients who have yet to start a family. Pituitary radiation can be provided to patients with unresectable or residual tumors, although this is associated with a high rate of hypopituitarism.

Adrenal tumors causing hypercortisolemia are best resected. Medical management of unresectable tumors, or patients with metastatic hormonally active adrenal cancer, is challenging because these malignancies are poorly responsive to adjuvant therapies. Patients may benefit from the use of mitotane, an adrenal poison. These patients must be given supplemental glucocorticoids in replacement doses to ensure they do not develop adrenal insufficiency during treatment. Patients with uncontrollable hypercortisolemia can benefit from adrenal steroid enzyme inhibitors such as ketoconazole or metyrapone. Experimental chemoradiotherapy or additional agents may be available as part of a clinical trial.

HIRSUTISM

Hirsutism refers to the appearance of excessive terminal hair that appears in a male pattern in women. Approximately 5% of women are hirsute. Hirsutism results from an interaction between the androgen level and the sensitivity of the hair follicle to androgen; as a result, androgen levels do not correlate well with the degree of hirsutism. Approximately one-half of women with hirsutism have the idiopathic condition.

Clinical Features

Clinical features that suggest one of the rare or more serious causes of hirsutism include abrupt onset, a presentation later in life, and progressive worsening. Symptoms and signs of virilization include frontal balding, acne, clitoromegaly, and deepening of the voice. Hair growth on the upper lip, chin, chest, abdomen, back, pubis, and legs should be assessed. Hirsutism should be distinguished from hypertrichosis, the appearance of generalized excessive hair growth that is genetically determined or follows treatment with glucocorticoids, phenytoin, or cyclosporine.

Evaluation

If hirsutism is moderate or severe, the plasma testosterone and free testosterone should be measured in the early morning (ideally, on days 4–10 of the menstrual cycle in cycling women).

Hyperandrogenism is most frequently related to the polycystic ovary syndrome, one of the most common hormonal disorders affecting women. The syndrome is diagnosed when the patient has at least two of chronic hyperandrogenism, oligo- or anovulation, and polycystic ovaries and other diagnoses are excluded. These patients often have menstrual irregularity, obesity, and evidence of insulin resistance (e.g., acanthosis nigricans). A pelvic ultrasound is not required for diagnosis. Additional testing may include a pregnancy test if the patient has amenorrhea. These patients should be evaluated for glucose intolerance and sleep apnea and often respond well to insulin sensitizers such as metformin or a thiazolidinedione. Spironolactone and oral contraceptives are frequently used to manage hirsutism in these patients.

Other causes of hyperandrogenism are unusual. Virilizing congenital adrenal hyperplasia is suggested by the premature growth of pubic hair and clitoromegaly and can be excluded by measuring the morning 17-alpha-hydroxy-progesterone level.

Cushing syndrome is suggested by the development of truncal obesity, moon face, buffalo hump, purple striae, or proximal muscle weakness (see chapter 48, this volume, on adrenal disorders). Hyperprolactinemia is suggested by the presence of galactorrhea and an elevated prolactin level. Acromegaly is suggested by the coarsening of facial features or by hand enlargement and confirmed by an elevated insulin-like growth factor-1 level.

Androgen-secreting tumors are very rare, but they should be considered among women with an acute presentation or who have very high levels of testosterone (>200 ng/dL). Such women should be evaluated with a level of dehydroepiandrosterone sulfate and an abdominal and pelvic ultrasound.

Idiopathic hirsutism is the most common diagnosis after these other disorders have been excluded by clinical or laboratory features.

Treatment

Hirsutism can be managed with cosmetic and hormonal therapy. It is useful to complete an objective assessment of the degree of hirsutism in advance of initiating treatment. The Ferriman-Gallwey score is one such scoring system.

Cosmetic approaches include bleaching, shaving, waxing, electrolysis, laser treatment, and the use of depilatory agents. Eflornithine hydrochloride cream can be used for facial hirsutism but must be used approximately 8 weeks before its efficacy can be determined.

Estrogen-progestin contraceptives suppress plasma testosterone levels and can reduce the need for shaving and slow the progression of hirsutism. Contraceptives with nonandrogenic progestins (e.g., Yasmin, Ortho-Cyclen, or Demulen 1–50) are preferred. Antiandrogens can be offered when hirsutism is moderate to severe. Spironolactone at high dose (50–100 mg twice a day) is effective in reducing hirsutism. Patients must be informed that spironolactone may be teratogenic and is generally not prescribed to women who are sexually active without an oral contraceptive. Hyperkalemia is rarely associated with spironolactone among women with normal renal function. Flutamide is an antiandrogen that is associated with hepatotoxicity and is not generally recommended for managing hirsutism. Cyproterone acetate is an antiandrogen that is available in Canada, Mexico, and Europe but not in the United States.

MALE HYPOGONADISM

Testosterone deficiency can result from disease of the testes or from pituitary or hypothalamic dysfunction. These causes can be distinguished by measuring the gonadotropins—luteinizing hormone and follicle-stimulating hormone.

Clinical Features

Intrauterine testosterone deficiency can result in micropenis and cryptorchidism, and when it occurs before puberty testosterone deficiency will result in incomplete maturation, a eunuchoid habitus, and reduced peak bone mass. When testosterone deficiency occurs after puberty, a decrease in libido and erectile function occur, with loss of sexual hair, muscle mass, and bone mineral density. Gynecomastia can be present.

Evaluation

The normal adult testis is approximately 4–6 cm in length or 20–25 milliliters in volume. The lower body segment (sole to pubis) should normally be no more than 2 cm longer than the upper segment (pubis to crown). Breast enlargement, small testes, and behavioral abnormalities suggest Klinefelter syndrome. Anosmia suggests Kallmann syndrome.

Total testosterone and sex-hormone–binding globulin concentrations should be measured in a morning sample with luteinizing hormone and follicle-stimulating hormone. Free testosterone measurements are generally unreliable. Semen analysis is appropriate if infertility is a primary concern.

Treatment

Testosterone treatment should be reserved for men with clinical symptoms and signs of hypogonadism accompanied by a subnormal testosterone concentration who have a normal prostate-specific antigen level. Testosterone esters can be given by intramuscular injection weekly or biweekly. Transdermal testosterone gels are available in sachets and a metered dose pump and are administered daily after showering; patients should be cautious about skin-to-skin transmission to a bed-partner. Testosterone patches are available but cause local irritation. The dose is titrated to a morning total testosterone level, drawn before the next dose. Clinicians should monitor for symptoms of benign prostatic hypertrophy, sleep apnea, and acne, and monitor prostate-specific antigen and hematocrit for erythrocytosis.

DIABETES MELLITUS

The prevalence of diabetes mellitus is increasing exponentially around the globe. The disease affects approximately 18 million Americans. Type 2 diabetes accounts for approximately 95% of all cases and is characterized by insulin resistance and hyperglycemia. Hyperinsulinemia occurs early in the disease but is not maintained indefinitely. Many patients ultimately require insulin to maintain glucose in the normal range. Because almost 80% of all patients with diabetes will die from cardiovascular complications, cardiovascular risk reduction is the primary target.

Clinical Features

Diabetes is diagnosed if there are symptoms of diabetes (polyuria, polydipsia, unexplained weight loss) and a random glucose of >200 mg/dL. A fasting glucose >126 mg/dL or a glucose of >200 mg/dL 2 hours after a 75-g glucose load are also diagnostic. Diagnostic use of the hemoglobin A1c (HbA1c) is not recommended. Screening every 3 years for diabetes is recommended for all patients who are overweight with risk factors and in everyone from the age of 45.

Hyperglycemia to meet the diagnostic criteria for diabetes (prediabetes) is categorized as either impaired fasting glucose (fasting glucose 100–125 mg/dL) or impaired glucose tolerance (glucose 140–199 mg/dL 2 hours after a 75-g glucose load). Diabetes can be prevented in patients with either of these conditions if patients lose weight and embark on an exercise program. Metformin reduces the incidence of diabetes in these high-risk patients by approximately 25%.

Evaluation

Secondary causes of diabetes should be considered when evaluating any patient with newly diagnosed hyperglycemia. Drugs that are associated with hyperglycemia such as glucocorticoids, antipsychotics, and some antiretrovirals should be reevaluated to determine if an alternative agent can be substituted safely. Genetic causes of diabetes should be excluded if a strong family history of diabetes is present or a typical phenotype (e.g., Down, Turner, or Klinefelter) is noted. Endocrinopathies such as Cushing syndrome, acromegaly, pheochromocytoma, hyperthyroidism, and others should be sought from the history and examination. Patients with diseases that affect the exocrine pancreas such as hemochromatosis, chronic pancreatitis, pancreatic malignancy, or cystic fibrosis are at high risk for diabetes; treatment of the underlying disease is often critical to reduce the rate of progression to insulin deficiency and to manage the hyperglycemia.

Treatment

Patients who are newly diagnosed with type 2 diabetes should be provided with a glucometer and testing instructions and referred for diabetes education and medical nutrition therapy. The optimal frequency of fingerstick glucose testing has not been determined. Smoking cessation and the benefits of exercise and weight loss should be emphasized. Targets of treatment are listed in table 55.3.

Table 55.3. TREATMENT GOALS FOR PATIENTS WITH DIABETES

TARGETS FOR PATIENTS WITH DIABETES	
HbA1c	<7%
Fasting glucose	90–130 mg/dL
Peak post-prandial glucose	<180 mg/dL
Blood pressure	<130/80 mm Hg
Urine microalbumin	<30 mg/day creatinine
Lipids	
LDL	<100 mg/dL*
HDL	>40 mg/dL

Daily low-dose aspirin therapy (age >40 or additional risk factors)
Annual foot examination
Yearly dilated eye examination by an ophthalmologist

NOTE: *<70 mg/dL if additional risk factors are present

For patients with type 2 diabetes requiring treatment, metformin remains the first-line agent of choice. Patients should be warned that early gastrointestinal side effects are not uncommon and should be tolerated if possible; these usually abate within 2 weeks. Metformin use is associated with cardiovascular risk reduction but cannot be used among patients with a creatinine above 1.5 mg/dL or among those who have severe chronic illnesses. Sulfonylureas are generally recommended as second-line agents because they are cost-effective. Short-acting sulfonylureas such as glipizide are preferred for their shorter half-life, especially among older patients. Thiazolidinediones such as pioglitazone or rosiglitazone are used as third-line agents or among patients with contraindications to first- and second-line drugs but have more limited efficacy; rosiglitazone has been associated with cardiovascular toxicity. More recent approaches to glycemic management include the use of glucagon-like peptide (GLP)-1 analogues, and inhibitors of dipeptidyl-peptidase-4 (DPP-4). GLP-1 analogues such as exenatide and liraglutide provide modest improvements in hemoglobin A1c and can contribute to weight loss in some patients; they are often used in the place of insulin in patients who are close to their hemoglobin A1c goal who may benefit from weight loss. DPP-4 inhibitors appear to be safe, but their efficacy is limited to a hemoglobin A1c drop of <0.7 percentage points.

For patients with type 2 diabetes who remain hyperglycemic despite two oral agents, insulin is a suitable choice. A typical starting dose of insulin is 0.3 units/kg. Insulin management should include a basal insulin (such as insulin glargine, detemir, or NPH) titrated to a fasting glucose of approximately 100 mg/dL. If the HbA1c remains elevated, shorter-acting insulins can be added incrementally, starting with a dose before the largest meal and then before other meals. The short-acting insulin dose can be titrated to a postprandial glucose level taken approximately 3 hours after a test meal. Patients in need of insulin treatment should be warned to check their glucose levels before driving.

Patients with type 1 diabetes require lifelong insulin treatment. Typically basal insulin is used with ultrashort-acting insulins given before each meal or snack. Patients with type 1 diabetes can be taught to count carbohydrates and how to calculate both correction and prandial insulin dosing. These patients should work with a diabetes team and can benefit from the convenience of insulin-pump therapy. Blood pressure, lipid, and renal, eye, and foot care guidelines are similar to those for patients with type 2 diabetes.

Preventing Complications

Blood pressure control is at least as important as glycemic control in reducing long-term cardiovascular disease incidence in patients with diabetes. Treatment with an ACE inhibitor is typically used first-line, with thiazide diuretics or calcium-channel blockers added as necessary. Alpha blockers should generally be avoided. Most patients require two to four antihypertensive agents to achieve a blood pressure of <130/80 mm Hg.

Urinary microalbumin levels should be assessed yearly. The presence of >30 mg of microalbumin per gram of creatinine is a risk factor for nephropathy and cardiovascular disease. ACE inhibitors and angiotensin receptor blockers should be titrated until the microalbumin level is suppressed below 30 mg/g creatinine.

Levels of low-density lipoprotein (LDL) above 100 mg/dL are associated with increased cardiovascular risk. Statins should be offered to such patients. Although ezetimibe effectively lowers LDL, there are no data suggesting that it prevents cardiovascular events. Hyperlipidemia in diabetes typically features hypertriglyceridemia and low levels of high-density lipoprotein (HDL). Though the latter can be treated with fibrates or niacin, there is little evidence that this treatment reduces cardiovascular risk.

GESTATIONAL DIABETES

Gestational diabetes (GDM) refers to any diabetes that is diagnosed during pregnancy. Screening is optimally performed at 24 to 28 weeks of gestation or earlier in high-risk women (positive family history, obesity, prior macrosomia). Diagnosis is suggested by a fasting glucose of >126 mg/dL, a random glucose of >200 mg/dL, or a glucose >140 mg/dL 1 hour after 50-g glucose load. Diagnosis during pregnancy is confirmed using a 3-hour glucose tolerance test using a 100-g glucose load. Criteria for a positive 3-hour glucose tolerance test include a fasting glucose of >95 mg/dL, a 1-hour sample >180 mg/dL, a 2-hour sample >155 mg/dL, or a 3-hour sample >140 mg/dL. Patients with gestational diabetes should be provided with nutritional counseling and a glucometer. Fasting glucose readings should be kept <90 mg/dL and 1-hour postprandial levels should be <120 mg/dL. A minority of women with GDM will require insulin therapy; usually insulin NPH and ultrashort-acting insulins

(lispro or aspart) are used. Oral agents are not routinely used to manage GDM: sulfonylureas are contraindicated in pregnancy, and safety data for metformin use are very limited.

HYPERGLYCEMIA IN THE HOSPITAL

Hyperglycemia during hospitalization is associated with significant increases in morbidity and mortality. Normalization of glucose has been shown to be beneficial among patients in medical and surgical intensive care units. In intensive care settings, intravenous insulin infusions are often recommended if glucose is >140 mg/dL and titrated thereafter to a glucose of <110 mg/dL. The patient can be transitioned to subcutaneous insulin when stable (e.g., extubated, off pressors) whether or not he or she is eating. If glucose control has been on target, many clinicians start with an insulin dose that is 80% of the previous day's total daily insulin use. Prescriptions should be written for basal, prandial, and correction doses.

ENDOCRINE SYNDROMES

MULTIPLE ENDOCRINE NEOPLASIA

MEN types 1, 2A, and 2B are rare genetic syndromes comprising multiple hormonally active tumors and some cancers (table 55.4).

Table 55.4 COMPONENTS OF THE MULTIPLE ENDOCRINE NEOPLASIA AND AUTOIMMUNE POLYENDOCRINE SYNDROMES

SYNDROME	MUTATION	COMPONENTS
Multiple Endocrine Neoplasia		
Type 1	MENIN	Primary hyperparathyroidism Pituitary tumors Enteropancreatic tumors
Type 2A	RET	Medullary thyroid cancer Pheochromocytoma Parathyroid hyperplasia Cutaneous lichen amyloidosis
Type 2B	RET	Medullary thyroid cancer Pheochromocytoma Mucosal neuromas Intestinal ganglioneuromas Marfanoid habitus
Autoimmune Polyendocrine Syndrome		
Type 1	AIRE	Primary adrenal insufficiency Hypoparathyroidism Mucocutaneous candidiasis
Type 2	Polygenic, HLA DR3	Primary adrenal insufficiency Autoimmune thyroid disease Type 1 diabetes mellitus

MEN-1

Hyperparathyroidism is the most common manifestation of MEN-1, caused by hyperplasia of multiple parathyroid glands. Penetrance is almost 100% by age 50 years. The second most common tumors are pancreatic polypeptide–producing pancreatic tumors. Gastrinomas occur in approximately 60% of patients with MEN-1 and are often metastatic at the time of diagnosis. Glucagonomas are rare. Prolactinomas are the most common of the pituitary tumors in patients with MEN-1, but acromegaly occurs in some 25% of patients. Other tumors that are reported to occur in patients with the MEN-1 syndrome include carcinoid tumors of the foregut, angiofibromas, lipomas, and benign adrenal adenomas.

MEN-2

Type 2A MEN accounts for almost 95% of cases of type 2 MEN. C-cell hyperplasia is a precursor for medullary thyroid cancer that arises multifocally and bilaterally. Pheochromocytomas occur in the third to fourth decade and are typically bilateral. Frank hyperparathyroidism is unusual. Patients suspected of MEN-2 should have testing for the *RET* germ line mutation and annual screening with plasma metanephrines. Prophylactic thyroidectomy with lymph node dissection is recommended in children younger than 5 years who have a *RET* germ line mutation in exon 16.

AUTOIMMUNE POLYENDOCRINE SYNDROME

Polyglandular autoimmune syndromes are constellations of multiple endocrine gland insufficiencies. These are extremely rare disorders and are usually apparent by early adolescence.

The order of appearance of components in autoimmune polyendocrine syndrome-type 1 is generally candidiasis, hypoparathyroidism, and then adrenal insufficiency. The screening antibody panel can include autoantibodies to 21-hydroxylase, 17-hydroxylase, thyroid peroxidase and thyroid-stimulating immunoglobulins, glutamic acid decarboxylase and islet cell antibodies, and parietal cell enzyme antibodies.

Autoimmune polyendocrine syndrome-type 2 is more common than type 1. Primary adrenal insufficiency is an obligatory component. Primary hypogonadism, celiac sprue, and myasthenia gravis can also complicate the presentation. The onset is generally in the fourth decade or later, with a female predominance.

ADDITIONAL READING

American Diabetes Association. Standards of Medical Care in Diabetes 2008. *Diabetes Care.* 2008;Suppl 1:S12–54.

Clarke N, Kabadi UM. Optimizing treatment of hypothyroidism. *Treat Endocrinol.* 2004;3(4):217–21. *Endocrinol Metab Clin North Am.* 2005;34(2):385–402.

Cozzi R, Baldelli R, Colao A, Lasio G, Zini M, Attanasio R; Italian Association of Clinical Endocrinologists (AME). AME position statement on clinical management of acromegaly. *J Endocrinol Invest.* 2009;32(6 Suppl):2–25.

Hegedus L. Clinical practice. The thyroid nodule. *N Engl J Med.* 2004;351(17):1764–71.

MacLean C, Newberry S, Maglione M, et al. Systematic review: Comparative effectiveness of treatments to prevent fractures in men and women with low bone density or osteoporosis. *Ann Intern Med.* 2008;148(3):197–213.

Melmed S. Acromegaly. *N Engl J Med.* 2006;355(24):2558–73.

Mikhail N, Cope D. Evaluation and treatment of primary hyperparathyroidism. *JAMA.* 2005;294(21):2700.

NIH state-of-the-science statement on management of the clinically inapparent adrenal mass ("incidentaloma"). *NIH Consens State Sci Statements.* 2002;19(2):1–25.

Ockrim Z, Yorston D. Managing diabetic retinopathy. *BMJ.* 2010;341:c5400.

Pearce EN, Farwell AP, Braverman LE. Thyroiditis. *N Engl J Med.* 2003;348(26):2646–55.

Reddy R, Hope S, Wass J. Acromegaly. *BMJ.* 2010;341:c4189.

Rosenfield RL. Hirsutism. *N Engl J Med.* 2005;353(24):2578–88.

Shoback D. Hypoparathyroidism. *N Engl J Med.* 2008;359(4):391–403.

Weetman AP. Graves' disease. *N Engl J Med.* 2000;343:1236–48.

SECTION 6

NEPHROLOGY AND HYPERTENSION

56.

ACUTE KIDNEY INJURY

Bradley M. Denker

Acute renal failure, now referred to as acute kidney injury (AKI), complicates 5–10% of general hospital admissions and is associated with increased morbidity and mortality and prolonged hospitalizations. The definition of AKI varies, but it is usually defined as an increase in serum creatinine concentration of 25–50% above the baseline, a decline in estimated glomerular filtration rate (eGFR) of 25–50%, or the need for renal replacement therapy. It is now recognized that changes in GFR are delayed manifestations of renal injury, and the development of urinary biomarkers may help to identify AKI earlier in the course of injury. The major causes of AKI in hospitalized patients include prerenal causes (~40%), postrenal causes (~5–10%), and intrinsic diseases affecting blood vessels, glomeruli, or tubules. Of the intrinsic causes, tubular disorders (acute tubular necrosis and acute interstitial nephritis) are the most common etiologies, accounting for 40–50% of all causes of AKI. Acute glomerulonephritis and vascular disorders are rare etiologies of AKI in hospitalized patients (<5%).

REGULATION OF GLOMERULAR FILTRATION

To understand mechanisms of renal injury, it is helpful to review the regulation of glomerular filtration. Figure 56.1A shows the arrangement of glomerular perfusion with afferent (inflow) and efferent (outflow) movement of blood to and from a single glomerulus. GFR through each glomerulus is determined by the pressure gradient across the glomerular basement membrane (P_{GC}), and total GFR is the sum of filtration from all individual glomeruli (~800,000/kidney). As shown in figure 56.1A, GFR is regulated by hormonal control of vascular tone in the afferent and efferent arterioles to maintain pressure across the glomerular basement membrane. Normally, GFR is maintained over a wide range of mean arterial pressures (figure 56.1B). GFR is preserved as mean systemic blood pressure falls by afferent vasodilation (more inflow; mediated by prostaglandins) and by efferent vasoconstriction (increased resistance thereby maintaining transcapillary pressure to maintain GFR; mediated by angiotensin II). Figure 56.1B shows the changes in GFR with falling mean arterial pressure (MAP) in control conditions (circles). GFR is maintained over a wide range of MAPs and does not significantly fall until MAP <80 mm Hg.

However, in the setting of angiotensin II inhibition (angiotensin-converting enzyme [ACE] inhibitor or angiotensin receptor blocker [ARB]), GFR begins to fall at higher mean arterial pressures (120 vs. 80) and falls much more significantly (figure 56.1B, squares). Figure 56.1A shows the loss of efferent vasoconstriction leading in lower GFR.

MECHANISMS OF REDUCED GLOMERULAR FILTRATION

POSTRENAL

Urinary outflow obstruction is a reversible cause of AKI that must be excluded early in the evaluation of AKI. Finding an obstruction by ultrasound not only identifies the cause of AKI, it also may reveal the anatomic etiology for the obstruction. This allows the management of the patient to be directed toward relief of the obstruction. However, the renal ultrasound may not reveal a dilated collecting system early in the course of obstruction, and with bulky pelvic tumors, the compression of the ureters may prevent dilation. Therefore, it is important to have a high index of suspicion for obstruction in these clinical scenarios even in the absence of hydronephrosis on ultrasound. In addition, obstruction in a single kidney (such as from a kidney stone) will not result in a significant change in GFR due to compensation from the remaining kidney. The finding of a severe reduction in GFR from obstruction must involve the outflow tract (such as prostate hypertrophy) or a bilateral process.

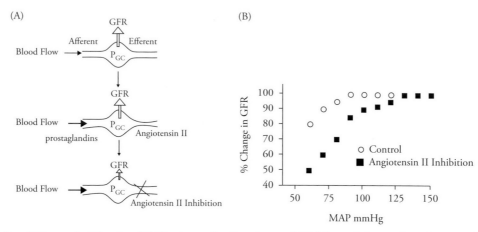

Figure 56.1. Autoregulation of Glomerular Filtration. (A) The glomerular filtration rate (GFR) for each glomerulus is determined by glomerular capillary pressure (P) and is represented by the open arrow. Total GFR is the sum of all individual glomeruli. The magnitude of blood entering the glomerulus through the afferent arteriole is shown by size of solid black arrow. With a drop in renal blood flow, GFR is preserved by afferent vasodilation (mediated by prostaglandins) and efferent vasoconstriction (mediated by angiotensin II). In the presence of angiotensin blockade, efferent vasoconstriction is inhibited, and GFR falls due to the decrease in PGC. (B) The changes in GFR from baseline as a function of mean arterial pressure (MAP). Open circles are control conditions. Black squares are in the presence of an angiotensin-converting enzyme inhibitor.

PRERENAL

The definition of prerenal AKI is any etiology of reduced renal perfusion resulting in a decreased GFR *without* intrinsic renal damage. By definition, prerenal AKI will resolve when adequate renal perfusion has been restored. The etiologies of prerenal AKI can be broadly divided into volume depletion, peripheral vasodilation, decreased cardiac output, intrarenal vasoconstriction, and impaired autoregulatory responses (material summarized in table 56.1). In clinical practice there are often multiple prerenal mechanisms contributing to the decreased GFR. For example, volume depletion in addition to decreased cardiac output or impaired autoregulatory response due to medications is a common combination of factors. In all causes of prerenal AKI, the renal compensatory mechanisms discussed above (afferent vasodilation and efferent vasoconstriction) are preserved, and GFR will be protected until compensatory mechanisms are overwhelmed.

Volume depletion is a common cause of prerenal AKI and can be seen with any fluid loss. These include blood loss from any site or protracted vomiting or diarrhea. Bleeding from the gastrointestinal tract or other locations can lead to prerenal AKI after approximately 5% of blood volume loss or after mean arterial pressure falls below 80 mm Hg. Other causes of volume depletion include severe insensible losses that occur with systemic skin reactions or burns and renal etiologies from the overuse of diuretics, uncontrolled hyperglycemia (osmotic diuresis), or with adrenal insufficiency.

Peripheral vasodilation leads to shunting of blood away from the renal circulation and contributes to decreased renal perfusion. This commonly occurs with certain medications (anesthetics, vasodilators) and is also a major feature of both the hepatorenal and sepsis syndromes. Other mechanisms of decreased renal perfusion can be seen with intrinsic cardiac disease (acute myocardial infarction, decompensated congestive heart failure, valvular abnormalities, arrhythmias), pulmonary processes (pulmonary emboli or pulmonary hypertension), or from renal artery stenosis (either when bilateral or occurring in a single kidney). Intrarenal vasoconstriction, especially on the afferent arteriole, also contributes to decreased perfusion and GFR in the sepsis and hepatorenal syndromes. Intrarenal vasoconstriction is also seen with the use of certain medications and hypercalcemia (see table 56.1).

Finally, hemodynamic AKI can result from impairment of the autoregulatory mechanisms. Nonsteroidal anti-inflammatory drugs (NSAIDs) inhibit prostaglandins and prevent compensatory vasodilation of the afferent arteriole (figure 56.1). ACE inhibitors and ARBs prevent angiotensin II actions on the efferent arteriole and block compensatory vasoconstriction necessary for maintaining GFR with reduced perfusion (figure 56.1). These are commonly used medications and are often taken simultaneously. Nevertheless, most patients will not suffer hemodynamic AKI until there is another perturbation of the system (i.e., mild volume depletion from a gastrointestinal source or more aggressive diuresis). As discussed above, inhibiting either the afferent or efferent compensation will make patients more susceptible to hemodynamic mechanisms of AKI, and inhibiting both afferent and efferent mechanisms further increases the risk.

INTRINSIC CAUSES OF AKI

The three anatomic structures that can be injured with intrinsic kidney injury are the renal tubules, the glomeruli, and blood vessels (table 56.2). Of these, the renal tubules are the most susceptible to acute injury. Although kidneys receive 25% of cardiac output, the enormous metabolic activity within the tubules renders the environment quite hypoxic. In the renal cortex, arterial oxygen tension is approximately 50 mm Hg, but it rapidly falls to 10 mm Hg

Table 56.1 PRERENAL MECHANISMS OF AKI

Intravascular Volume Depletion
Bleeding, poor oral intake, insensible losses (burns, exfoliative skin reactions) Gastrointestinal: vomiting, diarrhea Renal osmotic diuresis (hyperglycemia), overuse of diuretics, hypoadrenal

Peripheral Vasodilation
Antihypertension medications, pain medications, anesthetics, sepsis, anaphylaxis, hepatorenal syndrome

Decreased Cardiac Output
Myocardial: acute infarction, cardiomyopathy, decompensated congestive heart failure, pericardial effusion with tamponade, arrhythmias Pulmonary: acute pulmonary embolism, pulmonary hypertension

Intrarenal Vasoconstriction
Drugs (e.g., cyclosporine, amphotericin), hypercalcemia, vasopressors (norepinephrine, epinephrine), ionic contras, sepsis, hepatorenal syndrome

Impaired Autoregulatory Responses
Inhibition of afferent vasodilation: prostaglandin inhibitors (NSAIDs) Inhibition of efferent vasodilation: ACE inhibitors, ARBs

in the medulla. This normally hypoxic environment renders the renal tubules uniquely susceptible to any disruption in oxygen delivery.

Tubular Etiologies of AKI

Any etiology of prerenal AKI can lead to acute tubular injury, commonly referred to as ATN (acute tubular necrosis). The factors that determine whether the reduced GFR is prerenal or has produced tubular damage relate to the severity and duration of the injury. As discussed above, the response of the kidneys to restoration of perfusion is the most important consideration in distinguishing these possibilities. Volume-depleted patients must receive adequate volume resuscitation, but knowing whether intrinsic damage has occurred is important for anticipating the clinical course and prognosis of patients with acute renal failure. Numerous criteria can be utilized to help distinguish prerenal AKI from ATN, and these are summarized in table 56.3. All of these biochemical indicators reveal whether tubular function is intact (i.e., without injury). The appropriate renal response to volume depletion is to preserve sodium (by catecholamine and angiotensin II stimulation of sodium reabsorption in the proximal tubule) leading to concentrated urine with very low sodium (see table 56.3). In addition, filtered urea nitrogen is reabsorbed in the proximal tubule along with sodium. As a result, blood urea nitrogen (BUN) rises disproportionately to the rise in serum creatinine (creatinine is not reabsorbed but, rather, secreted), and the BUN/creatinine ratio often exceeds 20:1 with volume depletion. Although the BUN/creatinine ratio and the urine findings in table 56.3 are helpful for distinguishing prerenal AKI from ATN, they are often indeterminate.

Finally, the urinalysis can be helpful. With prerenal AKI, the urinary sediment is bland and may only reveal hyaline casts characteristic of concentrated urine, whereas ATN (tubular injury) is often associated with muddy brown casts (~85% of ATN presentations) and renal tubular epithelial cells reflecting dead/necrotic renal tubular epithelial cells shed into the urine.

In addition to hemodynamic insults resulting in ATN, the renal tubules are also susceptible to toxic injuries (see table 56.2). Again, this reflects the hypoxic metabolic environment and renal clearance for many of these compounds. Many etiologies of toxic ATN result from administered agents, but endogenous compounds liberated into the circulation such as myoglobin with rhabdomyolysis and free hemoglobin can also cause tubular injury. The clinical presentation and biochemical findings of toxin tubular injury are similar to what is described above for hemodynamic etiologies. However, a urinalysis showing strongly positive blood by dipstick and only a few red blood cells should prompt an investigation for myoglobin or free hemoglobin in the blood and urine (as seen with rhabdomyolysis and hemolysis, respectively).

Two other mechanisms of tubular injury are important causes of AKI. Interstitial nephritis (common) and intratubular obstruction (less common) must be considered in the evaluation of patients with AKI (table 56.2). Interstitial nephritis is most commonly allergic in origin and has been reported with virtually every category of medication and may *not* be associated with systemic manifestations (rash, eosinophilia). The kidneys can also be affected by interstitial infiltrates in infectious disorders, malignancy (lymphoma, leukemia), and autoimmune disorders (sarcoid, rheumatologic diseases). With allergic interstitial nephritis the cellular infiltrate is often mononuclear and not eosinophilic. As a result,

Table 56.2 INTRARENAL MECHANISMS OF AKI

Glomerular	A.	Nephrotic syndrome and AKI
		1. Minimal change disease with acute injury
		2. Collapsing glomerulopathy
		3. NSAIDs (acute interstitial nephritis plus membranous or minimal change disease)
	B.	Rapidly progressive glomerulonephritis
		1. Antiglomerular basement membrane disease
		2. Pauci-immune glomerulonephritis (often ANCA associated)
		3. Immune complex glomerulonephritis
		a. Low complement levels; lupus, postinfectious, cryoglobulinemia, poststrep. GN
		b. Normal complement levels; IgA nephropathy, Henoch-Schönlein purpura (HSP), fibrillary (immunotactoid GN)
Tubular	A.	Acute tubular necrosis
		1. All etiologies in table 56.1
		2. Toxic injury: ionic contrast, drugs (gentamicin), pigments (myoglobin)
	B.	Acute interstitial nephritis
		1. Medications, herbs, supplements
		2. Infectious: pyelonephritis, viral (CMV)
		3. Infiltrative: lymphoma, leukemia, sarcoidosis, Sjögren syndrome
	C.	Intratubular obstruction
		1. Drugs: acyclovir, sulfonamides, indinavir
		2. Crystals: oxalate, uric acid
		3. Protein: Bence-Jones protein with multiple myeloma
Vascular	A.	Thrombotic microangiopathy:
		1. TTP, HUS, antiphospholipid antibody syndrome
		2. Malignant hypertension, scleroderma, DIC
	B.	Vasculitis
		1. Small vessels: Pauci-immune glomerulonephritis (Churg-Strauss, Wegener granulomatosis/microscopic polyarteritis, hypersensitivity and cryoglobulinemia)
		2. Medium vessels: polyarteritis nodosa

a negative urine eosinophil count does not exclude drug-induced interstitial nephritis. With all etiologies of interstitial nephritis, the urinalysis will often have white blood cells, red blood cells, and may have white blood cell and red blood cell casts. Even in the absence of systemic manifestations, the clinical scenario will often suggest the diagnosis of interstitial nephritis (e.g., initiation of a new medication with development of AKI and abnormal urinalysis).

Another important mechanism of AKI results when crystals, drugs, or proteins precipitate within the renal tubules, resulting in intratubular obstruction. Often the patients at risk develop this complication in the setting of volume depletion and a concentrated urine. The hemodynamic consequences on GFR are identical to those of urinary obstruction at more distal sites, but intratubular obstruction will not be associated with hydronephrosis. Uric acid and oxalates are the most common crystals that precipitate within the tubules. Uric acid may precipitate in the tumor lysis syndrome, and oxalates with primary hyperoxalosis or ethylene glycol ingestion. Certain drugs (acyclovir, indinavir, methotrexate, sulfonamides) may precipitate if overdosed or administered to a volume-depleted patient, especially in the setting of pre-existing renal insufficiency. Occasionally the drug crystals can be identified on the urinalysis. Finally, paraproteins can precipitate within renal tubules, and this is most commonly seen in multiple myeloma and precipitated Bence-Jones proteins.

Glomerular Etiologies of AKI

Acute glomerulonephritis is a rare cause of acute kidney injury (table 56.2), but rapid diagnosis and treatment can prevent the development of end-stage renal disease. An overview of glomerular disease can found in chapter 61, and here the focus will be on disorders associated with AKI. Glomerular disease can be broadly divided into the nephrotic syndrome (>3.5 g of proteinuria/day, hypoalbuminemia, edema, hypercholesterolemia) and nephritic syndrome (hypertension, edema, azotemia, active urinary sediment with red blood cells, white blood cells, and cellular casts). Nephrotic syndrome is not usually associated with acute reductions in GFR. However, there are three clinical syndromes to consider in patients presenting with nephrotic syndrome and AKI. First, minimal change disease (normal glomeruli but podocyte foot process effacement on renal biopsy) in elderly or volume-depleted

Table 56.3 LABORATORY PARAMETERS USED TO DISTINGUISH PRERENAL AZOTEMIA FROM ACUTE TUBULAR NECROSIS

LABORATORY PARAMETER	PRERENAL AZOTEMIA	ACUTE TUBULAR DAMAGE
BUN/creatinine ratio	>20:1	10–15:1
Urine sodium (U_{Na}), meq/L	<20	>40
Fractional excretion of Na: $$FE_{Na} = \frac{U_{Na} \times P_{cr} \times 100}{P_{Na} \times U_{cr}}$$	<1%	>2%
Urine osmolality (mOsm/L H_2O)	>500	<350
Urine/plasma creatinine (U_{cr}/P_{cr})	>40	<20

patients can have coexisting ATN. Second, collapsing glomerulopathy (focal and segmental glomerulosclerosis with collapsed glomeruli on kidney biopsy) is associated with rapid declines in GFR and can lead to end-stage disease within months. This syndrome is often seen in HIV-positive patients, but it can also be seen in the absence of HIV disease. Finally, allergic reactions to NSAIDs are commonly associated with minimal change or membranous patterns of injury *in addition* to classical findings of allergic interstitial nephritis. As a result, these patients will often have AKI and a picture of allergic interstitial nephritis and nephrotic syndrome.

Acute glomerulonephritis or rapidly progressive glomerulonephritis (RPGN) can present as part of a systemic disease or may be renal limited. The presentation usually includes hypertension, AKI, and active urinary sediment. The hallmark of an active urinary sediment in acute glomerulonephritis is the presence of dysmorphic red blood cells and red blood cell casts. Red blood cell casts are not always visualized, but hematuria of renal origin (dysmorphic red blood cells) is nearly universal. Other cells and casts, especially white blood cells and casts can also be present. RPGN can develop through three major mechanisms. (1) Antiglomerular basement membrane antibody disease (GBM), also known as Goodpasture syndrome, may be associated with pulmonary hemorrhage. Rapid diagnosis and treatment with plasmapheresis and cytotoxic agents is imperative because renal recovery is rare when the creatinine reaches 5.8 mg/dL. (2) Pauci-immune etiologies of glomerulonephritis do not reveal immune complex staining or deposits on kidney biopsy and are often associated with antineutrophil cytoplasmic antibodies (ANCA). These disorders typically include Wegener granulomatosis, Churg-Strauss syndrome, and microscopic polyarteritis. (3) Immune complex diseases are typically divided into those with normal complement levels and those with hypocomplementemia. Systemic lupus erythematosus, postinfectious causes (streptococcal [group A] pharyngitis and subacute bacterial endocarditis are most common), and cryoglobulinemia are the most common etiologies of acute glomerulonephritis associated with low complement levels. These disorders are discussed in more detail in chapter 61. Other glomerular diseases that can present with AKI and do not include complement deposition are IgA nephropathy, the most common etiology of glomerulonephritis worldwide, Henoch-Schönlein purpura (HSP), and a less common deposition disease known as fibrillary or immunotactoid glomerulonephritis. Table 56.2 summarizes these disorders.

Vascular Etiologies of AKI

Damage to the renal microcirculation can mimic acute glomerulonephritis, although the pathologic pattern is distinct from other etiologies of acute glomerulonephritis. The glomerular capillary is uniquely susceptible to injury and is frequently a target of pathology even when other capillary beds are spared. Glomerular endothelial cells are disproportionately affected in systemic microangiopathies such as thrombotic thrombocytopenic purpura (TTP) and hemolytic uremic syndrome (HUS). In addition to systemic thrombocytopenia and evidence for intravascular hemolysis, these disorders are characterized by platelet microthrombi in glomerular capillary loops and thickened glomerular basement membranes. The occlusion of blood flow in the renal microcirculation leads to shearing of red blood cells and loss of GFR. Both TTP and HUS can present as primary diseases (such as diarrhea-associated *Escherichia coli* 0157 toxin-mediated), as a paraneoplastic syndrome in malignancy, or as complications of therapy with medications including cyclosporine, chemotherapy agents, or radiation therapy. Endothelial damage with a thrombotic microangiopathy is also seen in malignant hypertension, scleroderma crisis, and disseminated intravascular coagulation. Thrombotic microangiopathy can also be seen with antiphospholipid antibody syndrome associated with systemic lupus and as a complication of pregnancy. In all of these conditions the underlying renal pathophysiology is identical and therefore not distinguishable by kidney biopsy.

Vasculitis (table 56.2) of small arterioles can result in acute glomerulonephritis as described above. These are often ANCA associated and usually associated with Churg (DIC) Strauss (asthma, eosinophilia), Wegener granulomatosis (pulmonary or ENT involvement common), microscopic polyarteritis (similar to polyarteritis nodosa [PAN]), hypersensitivity (drug related), cryoglobulinemia (often seen with hepatitis B or C or paraprotein disease), or HSP. Vasculitis of medium-sized arteries as seen with PAN can result in AKI, but vasculitis of large arteries (giant cell and Takayasu arteritis) rarely results in renal failure.

COMMON SCENARIOS OF AKI IN HOSPITALIZED PATIENTS

AKI in hospitalized patients is often associated with complications of procedures performed in the course of evaluation and treatment of other disease processes. AKI that develops during a hospital course can often be anticipated. The two most common scenarios are postoperative AKI and radiologic imaging/intervention injuries.

POSTOPERATIVE AKI

There are numerous variables that increase the risk for AKI in patients undergoing surgical procedures. Any patient with pre-existing chronic renal disease is at higher risk, and the more severe the chronic kidney disease, the greater the risk for procedure-related AKI. Virtually all patients will have anesthesia-induced drops in blood pressure due to the vasodilatory action of anesthetic agents. This alone will not cause AKI in most settings, but if there is significant blood loss or larger drops in blood pressure for a prolonged interval, this can result in AKI. Certain medications taken prior to surgery including NSAIDs and ACE inhibitors or ARBs may interfere with normal renal autoregulatory mechanisms (as described above) and, when combined with anesthesia-induced drop in blood pressure, may lead to AKI. Other risk factors include the length of the procedure and the type of operation. Vascular and cardiac surgeries pose a higher risk, and large blood loss or the use of cardiopulmonary bypass also increases the risk of AKI. Finally, it is important to identify additional potential nephrotoxins administered during the surgery including antibiotics or irrigants (many of which are highly nephrotoxic if absorbed).

POSTINTRAVENOUS CONTRAST AND ANGIOGRAPHIC PROCEDURE AKI

There are two common mechanisms of AKI in the setting of intravenous contrast (see table 56.4). One results from renal toxicity related to contrast exposure (contrast nephropathy), and the other is atheroembolic syndrome resulting from mechanical disruption of cholesterol plaque during an angiographic procedure. Atheroemboli to the renal arteries can occur spontaneously, but they are usually associated with angiographic procedures through the femoral artery. The atheroembolic syndrome is often associated with a diffuse systemic reaction that can mimic an acute autoimmune disease and may include livido reticularis, fever, eosinophilia, hypocomplementemia, and AKI. On renal biopsy, cholesterol emboli may be visualized in the small intrarenal arteries. The course and prognosis of renal atheroembolic disease are variable. Some patients will recover, but others will progress to end-stage disease requiring renal replacement over the course of days to weeks because many of these patients had existing chronic kidney disease prior to

the procedure. Some patients exhibit a waxing and waning course in which GFR will worsen and improve over several weeks to months before stabilizing with reduced GFR.

Contrast nephropathy (table 56.4) is associated with increased creatinine 24–48 hours postcontrast exposure, and the usual course is for the creatinine to peak at 3–5 days and then begin to recover. Most patients will return to baseline creatinine, but there is likely a subclinical loss of GFR not reflected in the postprocedure baseline creatinine. Several studies have shown that developing contrast nephropathy is associated with increased morbidity and mortality in addition to longer hospital stays. The risk factors for developing contrast nephropathy are pre-existing renal disease, volume depletion at the time of exposure, dose and osmolality of the contrast agent, coexisting diabetes, coexisting congestive heart failure, and recent use of NSAIDs (table 56.4). Unlike atheroembolic disease that may not be preventable, the risk of contrast nephropathy can be reduced with pit-procedure interventions. Several studies have confirmed the benefit of intravenous hydration. Although exact regimens differ, the use of normal saline or sodium bicarbonate-based fluids is associated with a lower incidence of contrast nephropathy. Other medications such as the use of diuretics and mannitol have not been shown to be of benefit. Numerous studies and a recent meta-analysis have shown the benefit of treating high-risk patients with N-acetylcysteine (Mucomyst), an antioxidant, the day before and day of the procedure if possible.

MANAGEMENT OF AKI

Treatment of AKI depends on the etiology, but in most circumstances it is supportive (table 56.5). As described above, detecting hydronephrosis and urinary obstruction on ultrasound provides an etiology and therapeutic plan.

Table 56.4 SUMMARY OF CONTRAST NEPHROPATHY AND ATHEROEMBOLIC RENAL DISEASE

	CONTRAST NEPHROPATHY	ATHEROEMBOLIC DISEASE
Can occur spontaneously	No	Yes
Associated with angiography	Yes	Yes
Signs/symptoms	None	Fever, eosinophilia, livido reticularis, stigmata of emboli, low complements
Urinalysis/urine chemistry	Low FE_{Na}, bland sediment	Hematuria
Mechanism of injury	Afferent vasoconstriction (acute), tubular toxicity	Embolization of cholesterol crystals to small renal arterioles—acute inflammation
Course	Creatinine peaks at 3–5 days; returns to baseline	Variable; often waxes and wanes
Risk factors	CKD, volume depletion, dose and osmolality of contrast, diabetes, CHF, NSAIDs	Known vascular disease, procedure (renal angiography highest risk, but can be seen with any intervention)
Prevention	Intravenous fluids, N-acetylcysteine	None

Table 56.5 MANAGEMENT OF AKI

A. Prevention
    Avoid volume depletion, nephrotoxins, and hypotension in risk
        situations
    Use intravenous fluids and N-acetylcysteine in high-risk patients
        receiving contrast (CKD, diabetics)

B. Support care once AKI established
    a. Volume expansion—restrict Na, diuretics
    b. Hyponatremia—free water restriction
    c. Hyperkalemia—restrict, diuretics, Kayexalate
    d. Metabolic acidosis—bicarbonate administration
    e. Hyperphosphatemia—oral phosphate binders if possible,
        otherwise observe
    f. Hypocalcemia—replace calcium, consider vitamin D
    g. Nutrition—TPN or external feeds at @35 kcal/kg
    h. Anemia—GI prophylaxis, transfusions, DDAVP, estrogens
    i. dose all medications for GFR < 10 mL/min
    j. Avoid ACE inhibitors, ARBs, NSAIDs, and other nephrotoxic
        medications if possible (aminoglycosides)

C. Indications for renal replacement therapy
    a. Pericarditis
    b. Encephalopathy
    c. Refractory volume overload
    d. Hyperkalemia
    e. Refractory acidosis

Acute glomerulonephritis is often treated with immunosuppressive medications to reduce inflammation and lower the risk for scarring but requires a kidney biopsy for diagnosis. Most causes of AKI are either prerenal or tubular in origin. In straightforward prerenal AKI resulting from volume depletion, GFR will begin to improve within hours of restoring adequate circulatory volume. If there is a medication component contributing to hemodynamically mediated decreased GFR, then it may take longer for the pharmacologic effects to dissipate. In acute interstitial nephritis, stopping the offending medication will usually lead to resolution of the allergic reaction. However, in some circumstances treatment with steroids may be indicated, as they may shorten the duration of the renal injury. In ATN, there are no effective remedies once injury is established. Numerous interventions have been tried including atrial natriuretic peptide, diuretics, dopamine, and calcium channel blockers, but none of these has proven effective in human disease. Therefore, prevention of ATN, when possible, is the mainstay of therapy in high-risk situations. Surgical and radiographic procedures in addition to new medications are the main threats to renal function in hospitalized patients. Identifying patients at risk and employing preventive measures (such as avoiding nephrotoxins, use of hydration and Mucomyst with IV contrast) will reduce, but not eliminate, the risk of AKI.

Once AKI with tubular injury is established, the primary goal is to prevent additional renal injury and manage the complications of severely reduced GFR. Avoidance of volume depletion, hypotension, and exposure to nephrotoxins constitute the hallmarks of support. The natural history of ATN is to enter a maintenance phase that can persist for weeks to months depending on the severity of the injury. During this interval the GFR is usually <10 mL/min, and renal replacement therapy may be required. It is essential that all renally excreted medications be appropriately dosed for the low GFR in order to avoid additional injury. In most patients, tubular regeneration will occur and GFR will improve—but often not back to baseline levels. Once ATN is established, there is no proven role for dopamine, diuretics, calcium channel blockers, or atrial naturetic peptide in altering the natural history of the injury. Oliguric ATN (urine output <400 mL/day) is associated with a poorer prognosis than nonoliguric ATN, and nonoliguric patients are easier to manage. The use of diuretics may increase urine output in oliguric ATN, but it does not alter the prognosis and is not generally recommended.

The medical management of patients with AKI is focused on correcting the resulting metabolic disturbances. Volume overload may be managed with diuretics, but high doses of loop diuretics, often in combination with thiazide diuretics, are required to achieve an effective diuresis. The major metabolic disturbances are hyperkalemia and metabolic acidosis. If urine output is established with diuretics, potassium may be easier to manage. If hyperkalemia is acute and severe, then short-term interventions should be utilized (insulin/glucose, sodium bicarbonate, beta-agonists, and calcium). Kayexalate is effective with repeated doses, but acute dialysis may be required to manage life-threatening hyperkalemia. Metabolic acidosis may be managed with sodium bicarbonate, but the sodium load can contribute to volume expansion. Other electrolyte disturbances such as hyponatremia, hyperphosphatemia, hypocalcemia, and hypermagnesemia can usually be managed with conservative measures. In the ICU setting, nutritional requirements are high, and often this is provided through the use of total parenteral nutrition (TPN). Patients on TPN have large obligate fluid intake, and with oliguria intake may be limited. Platelet dysfunction and bleeding may be treated with DDAVP (increases release of von Willebrand factor), and/or estrogens, and patients should be protected from gastrointestinal bleeding with the use of proton-pump inhibitors.

Failure to control any of these factors may necessitate renal replacement therapy. The most common indications for dialysis are volume management, hyperkalemia, and acidosis. Uremic encephalopathy and pericarditis are two other important indications for dialysis. Although acute peritoneal dialysis has been used in the past, nearly all patients today are currently treated with intermittent hemodialysis or a continuous dialysis modality such as CVVH (continuous venovenous hemofiltration). Continuous modalities require specialized equipment, specially trained staff, and must be performed in an ICU setting. Although they are better tolerated than intermittent hemodialysis in hemodynamically unstable patients, to date, there are no data showing better outcomes with continuous modalities.

SUMMARY

Acute kidney injury is common in hospitalized patients and is associated with increased morbidity, mortality, and length of stay. The initial approach should be to rule out obstruction with an imaging study and look for other reversible causes of AKI. In addition, medications that interfere with autoregulation of GFR should be avoided in the acute setting. Although specific therapies for reversing acute tubular injury are currently lacking, the situations that place patients at high risk for ATN are well known and can be minimized by optimizing hemodynamics and medications. The most common high-risk scenario for AKI in hospitalized patients is in the setting of intravenous contrast for imaging studies. Intravenous hydration and the use of N-acetylcysteine can reduce the risk for AKI in this setting. Recognition and discontinuation of medications causing acute interstitial nephritis will help shorten the course of AKI. In those patients who have suffered acute tubular injury, the cornerstone of management is supportive: maintenance of hemodynamic stability and avoidance of nephrotoxins. Renal replacement therapy, usually by intermittent hemodialysis or a continuous therapy, is indicated when medical management is unable to address metabolic and/or volume complications.

ADDITIONAL READING

Arroyo V, Guevara M, Gines P. Hepatorenal syndrome in cirrhosis: Pathogenesis and treatment. *Gastroenterology.* 2002:122:1658.

Asif A, Epstein M. Prevention of radiocontrast-induced nephropathy. *Am J Kidney Dis.* 2004;44:12.

Brochard L, Abroug F, Brenner M, et al. An official ATS/ERS/ESICM/SCCM/SRLF statement: Prevention and management of acute renal failure in the ICU patient: An international consensus conference in intensive care medicine. *Am J Respir Crit Care Med.* 2010;181(10):1128–55.

Bouchard J, Macedo E, Mehta RL. Dosing of renal replacement therapy in acute kidney injury: Lessons learned from clinical trials. *Am J Kidney Dis.* 2010;55(3):570–9.

Denker BM, Brenner BM. Azotemia and urinary abnormalities. In Fauci AS, Braunwald E, Kasper DL, et al., eds. *Harrison's Principles of Internal Medicine.* 17th ed. (pp. 268–74). New York: McGraw-Hill; 2008.

Hricik DE, Dunn MJ. Angiotensin-converting-enzyme inhibitor-induced renal failure: Causes, consequences, and diagnostic uses. *J Am Soc Nephrol.* 1990;1:845.

Lameire N, Van Biesen W, Vanholder R. Acute renal failure. *Lancet.* 2005;365(9457):417–30.

Macedo E, Bouchard J, Mehta RL. Renal replacement therapy for acute renal failure. *Minerva Urol Nefrol.* 2009;61(3):189–204.

Miller TR, Anderson RJ, Linas SL, et al. Urinary diagnostic indices in acute renal failure: A prospective study. *Ann Intern Med.* 1978;89:47.

Rihal CS, et al., Incidence and prognostic importance of acute renal failure after percutaneous coronary intervention. *Circulation.* 2002;105(19):2259–64.

Shrier RW, Wang W, Poole B, Mitra A. Acute renal failure: Definitions, diagnosis. pathogenesis and therapy. *J Clin Invest.* 2004;114:5–14.

QUESTIONS

QUESTION 1. A 22-year-old male is seen in the emergency room for evaluation of acute renal failure. He explains that he has just finished running the Boston marathon. He complains of severe leg cramps. He tells you that his urine is light pink. He has no significant past medical history. He is not taking any medications. He denies recent alcohol consumption. His physical examination shows a blood pressure of 100/60 mm Hg, with a 15 mm Hg drop in his systolic pressure on standing, a heart rate of 110 beats per minute, and a temperature of 37.4°C. His JVP is 2–3 cm. He has clear lungs and a normal cardiovascular and abdominal examination. He has no edema. His skin turgor is reduced. Urinalysis reveals SG of 1020, pH 5.0, 4+ blood, rest negative. His urine sediment shows 0–2 hyaline casts but is otherwise negative.

The next step in management would be:

A. Obtain intravenous access and begin treatment with Ringer's lactate solution
B. Obtain intravenous access and begin treatment with isotonic saline
C. Arrange for an urgent renal ultrasound to investigate his hematuria
D. Administer N-acetylcysteine for his acute kidney injury
E. Arrange for an urgent renal biopsy

QUESTION 2. A 67-year-old man presents with a 1-week history of anorexia, nausea, lassitude, and pedal edema. He has history of long-standing hypertension, well controlled with hydrochlorothiazide and amlodipine. He has been taking fenoprofen for osteoarthritis of the hip for the past 3 months. Physical examination is notable for BP 157/93 mm with 2+ pitting edema. His urinalysis reveals protein 4+, 1+ blood, 2–4 RBCs and 15–20 WBCs per hpf, and occasional granular casts. Laboratories notable for BUN 93 mg/dL; Cr 7.8 mg/dL; Alb 2.9 g/dL; HCT 29%. ANCA (−), antinuclear (+) 1:40 titer, anti-dsDNA antibody level 0, 24-hour protein excretion 7.7 g. Renal ultrasound showed normal-sized kidneys bilaterally without obstruction. Three months previously his serum creatinine was 1.7 mg/dL. The nephrotic-range proteinuria and renal failure are most likely the result of:

A. Lupus nephritis
B. Multiple myeloma
C. Systemic small vessel vasculitis
D. Fenoprofen-induced nephrotic syndrome and interstitial nephritis
E. Renal vein thrombosis secondary to membranous nephropathy

QUESTION 3. A 52-year-old female presents to the emergency room with unstable angina. She is noted to have a

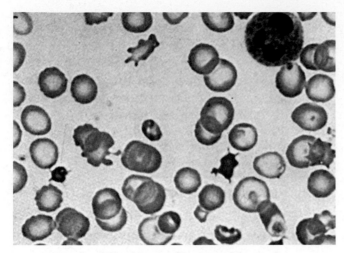

Figure 56.2. Peripheral Blood Smear of Patient in Question 4.

past medical history of mild chronic renal insufficiency (creatinine of 1.8 mg/dL). She is transferred to the coronary care unit, and therapy for her unstable angina is initiated. A cardiac catheterization is planned for the next day. Risk factors that would predispose this woman to contrast nephrotoxicity include all of the following except:

A. Diabetes mellitus
B. Pre-existing renal insufficiency
C. The volume of IV contrast utilized in the procedure
D. Presence of extracellular volume contraction
E. A history of coronary artery disease

QUESTION 4. A 57-year-old female with a history of mild hypertension presents with headache and a blood pressure of 240/140 mm Hg. She is alert and fully oriented and has experienced low grade fever over last 72 h. She has grade 4 papilledema on her funduscopic examination. The rest of the examination is unremarkable. Her labs are notable for a HCT of 22%, WBC is 6000, platelet count 95,000, sodium 138 meq/L, potassium 4.3 meq/L, chloride 102 meq/L, bicarbonate 22 meq/L, BUN 84 mg/dL, a serum creatinine of 4.5 mg/dL, calcium 11.2 mg/dL, phosphate 4.2 mg/dL, albumin 4.9 g/dL. PT and PTT are normal. Her urinalysis shows 1+ blood, 1+ protein. Her urine sediment shows: few RBCs/high powered field and no casts. She is admitted to the intensive care unit for treatment. Her peripheral smear is shown in figure 56.2.

What is the most likely diagnosis?

A. Acute kidney injury from hypertensive urgency
B. Thrombotic thrombocytopenia purpura/hemolytic uremic syndrome
C. Scleroderma renal crisis
D. Acute kidney injury from malignant hypertension
E. Disseminated intravascular coagulation

ANSWERS

1. B
2. D
3. E
4. D

57.

ELECTROLYTE DISORDERS

David B. Mount

SODIUM DISORDERS

Disorders of serum sodium concentration ([Na$^+$]) are caused by abnormalities in water homeostasis leading to changes in the relative ratio of Na$^+$ to body water. Water intake and circulating vasopressin (AVP) are the dominant mediators in the defense of serum osmolality (table 57.1); defects in one or both of these defense mechanisms cause most cases of hyponatremia and hypernatremia. AVP secretion and thirst are both activated by increases in serum osmolality. Circulating vasopressin then acts on renal, V2-type vasopressin receptors in the thick ascending limb of Henle and principal cells of the collecting duct, leading to renal retention of water (figure 57.1). Notably, volume status also modulates the release of AVP by the posterior pituitary, such that hypovolemia is associated with higher circulating levels of the hormone at each level of serum osmolality. Hypovolemia can thus be associated with hyponatremia due to retention of ingested free water in response to increased AVP. Similarly, in the setting of reduced "effective circulating volume" and impaired "arterial circulatory integrity," as seen in cirrhosis and heart failure, the associated neurohumoral activation leads to an increase in circulating AVP, predisposing to hyponatremia. These interactions among volume status, AVP release, and water homeostasis can lead to diagnostic confusion. A key concept in this regard is that the absolute serum [Na$^+$] conveys no diagnostic information as to the volume status of a given patient, with hyponatremia in particular occurring at all extremes of whole-body water and Na$^+$-Cl$^-$ content.

HYPONATREMIA

Diagnostic Approach

Hyponatremia, defined as a serum [Na$^+$] <135 mM, is a very common disorder, occurring in up to 22% of hospitalized patients. This disorder is almost always the result of an increase in circulating AVP and/or increased renal sensitivity to AVP, combined with an intake of free water. A notable exception is hyponatremia due to low solute intake, as in extreme vegan diets or "beer potomania," wherein urinary solute concentrations are inadequate to support the excretion of ingested free water; the reduced capacity for renal water excretion is easily overwhelmed in these patients, leading to water retention and hyponatremia.

The underlying pathophysiology for the typical exaggerated or "inappropriate" vasopressin response differs in patients with hyponatremia, as a function of their extracellular fluid volume. Hyponatremia is thus subdivided diagnostically into three groups, depending on clinical history and volume status, that is, hypovolemic, euvolemic, and hypervolemic hyponatremia (see figure 57.2). Notably, hyponatremia is frequently multifactorial, particularly when severe; clinical evaluation should examine all the possible causes for increased AVP, including nausea, pain, and drugs.

Laboratory investigation of a patient with hyponatremia should include a measurement of serum osmolality, to exclude "pseudohyponatremia" due to hyperlipidemia or hyperproteinemia. Serum glucose should also be measured. Serum [Na$^+$] falls by approximately 1.4 mM for every 100 mg/dL increase in glucose due to glucose-induced water efflux from cells; this form of hyponatremia resolves with normalization of serum glucose. Urine electrolytes and osmolality are particularly critical tests in the initial evaluation of hyponatremia. In particular, a urine [Na$^+$] <20 mM is consistent with hypovolemic hyponatremia in the clinical absence of a "hypervolemic" Na$^+$-avid syndrome such as congestive heart failure (see figure 57.2). Urine osmolality <100 mosmol/kg is suggestive of polydipsia. A urine osmolality >400 mosmol/kg indicates that AVP excess is playing a more dominant role, whereas intermediate values are more consistent with multifactorial pathophysiology (e.g., AVP excess with a component of polydipsia). Patients with hyponatremia due to decreased solute intake, as in "beer potomania," typically have urines with [Na$^+$] <20 mM and urine osmolality in the range of <100 to the low 200s. Finally, in the right clinical setting, thyroid, adrenal, and

Table 57.1 OSMOREGULATION VERSUS VOLUME REGULATION

	OSMOREGULATION	VOLUME REGULATION
What is sensed	Plasma osmolality	"Effective" circulating volume, arterial circulatory integrity
Sensors	Hypothalamic osmoreceptors	Carotid sinus Afferent arteriole Atria
Effectors	AVP Thirst	Sympathetic nervous system Renin-angiotensin-aldosterone system ANP/BNP AVP
What is affected	Urine osmolality Water intake	Urinary sodium excretion Vascular tone

NOTES: See text for details. AVP, arginine vasopressin; ANP, atrial natriuretic peptide; BNP, brain natriuretic peptide.
SOURCE: Rose BD, Black RM. *Manual of Clinical Problems in Nephrology*. Boston: Little Brown & Co, 1988.

pituitary function should also be tested; hypothyroidism and secondary adrenal failure due to pituitary insufficiency are important causes of euvolemic hyponatremia, whereas primary adrenal failure causes hypovolemic hyponatremia. Radiological imaging should also be considered, looking for a pulmonary or central nervous system (CNS) cause for inappropriate AVP secretion and hyponatremia.

Hypovolemic Hyponatremia

Hypovolemia causes marked neurohumoral activation, inducing systems such as the renin-angiotensin-aldosterone

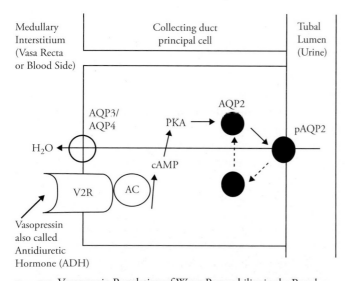

Figure 57.1. Vasopressin Regulation of Water Permeability in the Renal Collecting Duct. Vasopressin binds to the type 2 vasopressin receptor (V2R) on the basolateral membrane of principal cells, activates adenylyl cyclase (AC), increases intracellular cyclic adenosine monophosphatase (cAMP), and stimulates protein kinase A (PKA) activity. Cytoplasmic vesicles carrying aquaporin-2 (AQP) water channel proteins are inserted into the luminal membrane in response to vasopressin, thereby increasing the water permeability of this membrane. When vasopressin stimulation ends, water channels are retrieved by an endocytic process and water permeability returns to its low basal rate. The AQP3 and AQP4 water channels are expressed on the basolateral membrane and complete the transcellular pathway for water reabsorption. pAQP2, phosphorylated aquaporin-2.

axis (RAA), the sympathetic nervous system, and circulating AVP (see table 57.1). The increase in circulating AVP helps preserve blood pressure via vascular and baroreceptor V1A receptors and increases water reabsorption via renal V2 receptors; the latter effect can lead to hyponatremia in the setting of increased free water intake. Nonrenal causes of hypovolemic hyponatremia include GI (vomiting, diarrhea, tube drainage, etc.) and "insensible" loss of Na^+-Cl^- (sweating, burns, respiratory tract); urine $[Na^+]$ is typically <20 mM in these cases. These patients may be clinically classified as euvolemic, with only the reduced urine $[Na^+]$ to indicate the cause of their associated hyponatremia.

The *renal* causes of hypovolemic hyponatremia share an inappropriate loss of Na^+-Cl^- in the urine, leading to volume depletion; urine $[Na^+]$ is typically >20 mM (figure 57.2). The deficiency in circulating aldosterone can lead to hyponatremia in primary adrenal insufficiency and other causes of hypoaldosteronism; hyperkalemia and hyponatremia in a hypotensive and/or hypovolemic patient with high urine $[Na^+]$ should strongly suggest this diagnosis. Salt-losing nephropathies are characterized by impaired renal tubular function and thus a reduced ability to reabsorb filtered Na^+-Cl^-, leading to hypovolemia and neurohumoral activation. Typical causes include reflux nephropathy, interstitial nephropathies, postobstructive uropathy, medullary cystic disease, and the recovery phase of acute tubular necrosis. Diuretic therapy, particularly with thiazides, causes hyponatremia via a number of mechanisms, most prominently the diuretic-associated volume depletion. Increased excretion of an osmotically active nonreabsorbable or poorly reabsorbable solute can also lead to volume depletion and hyponatremia; important causes include glycosuria, ketonuria, and bicarbonaturia (e.g., in proximal renal tubular acidosis, where the associated bicarbonaturia leads to loss of Na^+). Finally, the syndrome "cerebral salt-wasting" is a rare cause of hypovolemic hyponatremia due to inappropriate natriuresis in association with intracranial disease; causative disorders include subarachnoid hemorrhage,

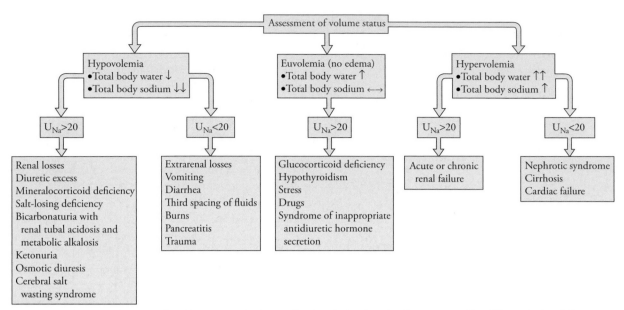

Figure 57.2. The Diagnostic Approach to Hyponatremia. See text for details. Reprinted with permission from Kumar S, Berl T. Diseases of water metabolism. In Schrier RW (ed.). *Atlas of Diseases of the Kidney,* Vol. 1. New York: Wiley; 1999.

traumatic brain injury, craniotomy, encephalitis, and meningitis. Distinction from the syndrome of inappropriate antidiuresis (SIAD) is difficult but critical for successful management because cerebral salt wasting will typically respond to aggressive Na+-Cl− repletion.

Hypervolemic Hyponatremia

Patients with hypervolemic hyponatremia develop an increase in total body Na+-Cl− that is accompanied by a proportionately *greater* increase in total body water, leading to a reduced serum [Na+]. Again, the causative disorders can be separated by the effect on urine [Na+], with acute or chronic renal failure uniquely associated with an increase in urine [Na+] (see figure 57.2); advanced renal insufficiency can reduce the ability to excrete free water, leading to hyponatremia. The pathophysiology of hyponatremia in the sodium-avid edematous disorders (congestive heart failure [CHF], cirrhosis, and nephrotic syndrome) is similar to that in hypovolemic hyponatremia, except that the "effective circulating volume" is decreased due to the specific etiologic factors, for example, cardiac dysfunction in CHF. Urine [Na+] is typically very low, that is, <10 mM; this Na+-avid state may be obscured by diuretic therapy, depending on the timing of sample collection, schedule, and choice of diuretics. The degree of hyponatremia is an indirect index of the associated neurohumoral activation (see table 57.1) and thus an important prognostic indicator in hypervolemic hyponatremia. Management consists of treating the underlying disorder (e.g., angiotensin-converting enzyme [ACE] inhibition in heart failure, Na+ restriction, diuretic therapy, and, when appropriate, H2O restriction). Vasopressin antagonists are effective in

normalizing hyponatremia associated with both cirrhosis and CHF however, conivaptan cannot be utilized in patients with chronic liver disease and cirrhosis.

Euvolemic Hyponatremia

SIAD is the most common cause of euvolemic hyponatremia (see table 57.2). Other causes include hypothyroidism and secondary adrenal insufficiency due to pituitary disease; whereas the deficit in circulating aldosterone in primary adrenal insufficiency causes *hypovolemic* hyponatremia, the predominant glucocorticoid deficiency in secondary adrenal failure leads to *euvolemic* hyponatremia. Common causes of SIAD include pulmonary disease (e.g., pneumonia, tuberculosis, pleural effusion) and CNS diseases (e.g., tumor, subarachnoid hemorrhage, meningitis); SIAD also occurs with malignancies, most commonly small-cell lung carcinoma, and drugs, most commonly selective serotonin reuptake inhibitors (SSRIs) (table 57.2).

The initial treatment of euvolemic hyponatremia should include treatment or withdrawal of the underlying cause, if feasible and appropriate. Water restriction to <1 L/day is a cornerstone of therapy but may be ineffective or poorly tolerated; thirst is also stimulated in these patients, at lower than the usual physiological osmolalities. Patients who fail to respond to water restriction can be treated with loop diuretics to inhibit the countercurrent mechanism and reduce urinary concentration, combined with oral salt tablets to replace diuretic-induced salt loss. Historically, oral demeclocycline has been used to treat SIAD that fails water restriction or furosemide/salt tablets; this agent is, however, associated with acute kidney injury, necessitating close follow-up of renal function. More recently, vasopressin

Table 57.2 CAUSES OF THE SYNDROME OF INAPPROPRIATE ANTIDIURESIS (SIAD)

MALIGNANT DISEASES	PULMONARY DISORDERS	DISORDERS OF THE CENTRAL NERVOUS SYSTEM	DRUGS	OTHER CAUSES
Carcinoma	Infections	Infection	Drugs that stimulate release of AVP or enhance its action	Hereditary (gain of function mutations in the vasopressin V2 receptor)
Lung	Bacterial	Encephalitis	Chlorpropamide	
Small cell	pneumonia	Meningitis	SSRIs	
Mesothelioma	Viral pneumonia	Brain abscess	Tricyclic antidepressants	
Oropharynx	Pulmonary abscess	Rocky mountain spotted	Clofibrate (Atromid-s, Wyeth)	Idiopathic
Gastrointestinal tract	Tuberculosis	fever	Carbamazepine (Epitol, Lemmon;	Transient
Stomach	Aspergillosis	AIDS	Tegretol Ciba-Geigy)	Endurance
Duodenum	Asthma	Bleeding and masses	Vincristine (Oncovin, Lilly;	exercise
Pancreas	Cystic fibrosis	Subdural hematoma	Vincasar, Pharmacia and Upjohn)	General
Genitourinary tract	Respiratory failure	Subarachnoid hemorrhage	Nicotine	anesthesia
Ureter	associated with	Cerebrovascular accident	Narcotics	Nausea
Bladder	positive-pressure	Brain tumors	Antipsychotic drugs	Pain
Prostate	breathing	Head trauma	Ifosfamide (Ifex, Bristol-Myers	Stress
Endometrium		Hydrocephalus	Squibb; Neosar, Pharmacia and	
Endocrine thymoma		Cavernous sinus thrombosis	Upjohn)	
Lymphomas		Other	Nonsteroidal anti- inflammatory drugs	
Sarcomas		Multiple sclerosis	MDMA ("ecstasy")	
Ewing sarcoma		Guillain-Barré syndrome	AVP analogues	
		Shy-Drager syndrome	Desmopressin (DDAVP, Rhone-	
		Delirium tremens	Poulenc Rorer; Stimate, Centeon)	
		Acute intermittent	Oxytocin (Pitocin, Parke-Davis;	
		porphyria	Syntocinon, Novartis)	
			Vasopressin	

NOTES: AIDS, the acquired immunodeficiency syndrome; SSRI, selective serotonin reuptake inhibitor; MDMA, 3,4-methylenedioxymethamphetamine ("Ecstasy").
SOURCE: Reprinted with permission from Ellison DH, Berl T. Syndrome of inappropriate antidiuresis. *N Engl J Med.* 2007;356:2064–72. Copyright 2007 Massachusetts Medical Society. All rights reserved.

antagonists have been shown to be safe and effective in normalizing serum [Na⁺] in SIAD.

Treatment of Hyponatremia

Three important considerations guide the therapy of hyponatremia. First, the presence and/or severity of symptoms determine the urgency of therapy. Patients with acute hyponatremia (table 57.3) present with symptoms that can range from headache, nausea, and/or vomiting, to altered mental status, seizures, obtundation, and/or death. Patients with chronic hyponatremia (present for >48 hours) are less likely to be symptomatic but may demonstrate subtle deficits in neuropsychological function, including gait abnormalities and an increased risk of falls. Chronic hyponatremia also increases the risk of bony fractures due to the increased risk of falls and to a hyponatremia-associated reduction in bone density. Second, patients with chronic hyponatremia are at risk for osmotic demyelination syndrome, typically central pontine myelinolysis, if serum [Na⁺] is corrected by >10–12 mM within the first 24 hours and/or by >18 mM within the first 48 hours. Brain cells in chronic hyponatremia reduce the intracellular concentration of organic osmolytes (creatine, betaine, glutamate, and taurine) to cope with hypo-osmolality; the intracellular *reaccumulation* of these solutes is attenuated and delayed after reestablishment of normal tonicity, leading to osmotic

demyelination in the setting of overly rapid correction of hyponatremia. Third, the response of the serum [Na⁺] to interventions such as hypertonic saline or vasopressin antagonists can be highly unpredictable, such that frequent monitoring of serum [Na⁺] (every 2–4 hours) is required during therapy with these measures.

Acute symptomatic hyponatremia can occur in several clinical settings (table 57.3). This syndrome is a medical emergency; a sudden drop in serum [Na⁺] can overwhelm the capacity of the brain to regulate cell volume, leading to massive cerebral edema. Notably, this may occur after relatively modest reductions in serum [Na⁺]. Premenopausal women are particularly prone to severe symptoms of acute hyponatremia; neurological consequences are comparatively rare in male patients. A critical and often overlooked complication is respiratory failure, which may be hypercapnic due to CNS depression or normocapnic due to neurogenic, noncardiogenic pulmonary edema; the associated hypoxia amplifies the impact of hyponatremic encephalopathy. Many of these patients develop hyponatremia from iatrogenic causes, including hypotonic fluids in the postoperative period, prescription of a thiazide diuretic, colonoscopy preparation, or intraoperative use of glycine irrigants. Polydipsia occurring with a cause of increased AVP may also cause acute hyponatremia, as with increased water intake in the setting of strenuous exercise (e.g., marathon-associated hyponatremia). The drug Ecstasy (3,4-methylenedioxymethamphetamine,

Table 57.3 CAUSES OF ACUTE HYPONATREMIA

Iatrogenic
    Postoperative; premenopausal women
    Hypotonic fluids with cause of ↑ vasopressin
    Glycine irrigant: TURP, uterine surgery
    Colonoscopy preparation
    Recent institution of thiazides

Polydipsia

MDMA ("Ecstasy") ingestion

Exercise induced

Multifactorial, e.g., thiazide and polydipsia

NOTES: MDMA, 3,4-methylenedioxymethamphetamine ("Ecstasy"); TURP, transurethral resection of the prostate.

Table 57.4 CAUSES OF DIABETES INSIPIDUS

Central Diabetes Insipidus
    Pituitary surgery
    Head trauma
    Tumors
    Cerebrovascular event or hypoxic encephalopathy
    Infections
    Idiopathic—?autoimmune
    Granulomatous disease—sarcoid, histiocytosis X
    Hereditary—autosomal dominant mutations in preprovasopressin/
        neurophysin, Wolfram syndrome

Nephrogenic Diabetes Insipidus
    Genetic
        X-linked: V2 vasopressin receptor
        Autosomal recessive/dominant: aquaporin-2
        Autosomal recessive: aquaporin-1 (proximal tubule and thin limb)
    Drug-induced, e.g., lithium, cisplatin, demeclocycline,
        ifosfamide, foscarnet
    Hypokalemia
    Hypercalcemia
    Infiltrating lesions, e.g., sarcoidosis, amyloidosis
    Cellular defect, e.g., after acute tubular necrosis

Gestational Diabetes Insipidus

MDMA) can also cause acute hyponatremia, rapidly inducing both AVP release and increased thirst.

Treatment of acute symptomatic hyponatremia should include hypertonic saline to acutely increase serum [Na$^+$] by 1–2 mM/hr to a total increase of 4–6 mM; this increase is typically sufficient to alleviate acute symptoms, after which corrective guidelines for chronic hyponatremia are appropriate (see below). A number of equations have been developed to estimate the required rate of hypertonic solution; one popular approach is to calculate a "Na$^+$ deficit," where the Na$^+$ deficit = $0.6 \times$ body weight $\times$ (target [Na$^+$] – starting [Na$^+$]). However, a major caveat is that the increase in serum [Na$^+$] can be highly unpredictable during treatment with hypertonic saline due to rapid changes in the underlying physiology; serum [Na$^+$] should be monitored every 2–4 hours, with appropriate adjustments in the rate of administered saline. In hypokalemic patients, K$^+$-Cl$^-$ replacement can also lead to an increase in serum [Na$^+$], given that serum [Na$^+$] is a function of exchangeable Na$^+$ *and* K$^+$, divided by whole body water; this phenomenon can also lead to an overly rapid correction in serum [Na$^+$] in chronic hyponatremia (see below). The administration of supplemental oxygen and ventilatory support can also be critical in acute hyponatremia in the event that patients develop acute pulmonary edema or hypercapnic respiratory failure. Intravenous loop diuretics will help treat acute pulmonary edema and will also increase free water excretion by interfering with the renal countercurrent multiplication system. It should be emphasized that vasopressin antagonists do *not* have a role in the management of acute hyponatremia.

The rate of correction should be comparatively slow in *chronic* hyponatremia (<10–12 mM in the first 24 hours and <18 mM in the first 48 hours), so as to avoid osmotic demyelination syndrome. Vasopressin antagonists are highly effective in SIAD and in hypervolemic hyponatremia due to heart failure or cirrhosis. Should patients overcorrect serum [Na$^+$] in response to vasopressin antagonists, hypertonic saline, or isotonic saline (in chronic hypovolemic hyponatremia), hyponatremia can be safely reinduced or stabilized

by the administration of the vasopressin *agonist* desmopressin (DDAVP) and the administration of free water, typically intravenous D5W.

HYPERNATREMIA

Hypernatremia is usually the result of a combined water and volume deficit, with losses of H$_2$O in excess of Na$^+$. Elderly individuals with reduced thirst and/or diminished access to fluids are at the highest risk of developing hypernatremia. Patients with hypernatremia may rarely have a central defect in hypothalamic osmoreceptor function, with a mixture of both decreased thirst and reduced AVP secretion; causes include primary or metastatic tumor, occlusion or ligation of the anterior communicating artery, trauma, hydrocephalus, and inflammation. More commonly, hypernatremia develops following the loss of water via renal or nonrenal routes, combined with a reduced intake of water. "Insensible losses" of water due to evaporation from the skin or respiratory tract may increase in the setting of fever, exercise, heat exposure, severe burns, or mechanical ventilation. Diarrhea is, in turn, the most common gastrointestinal cause of hypernatremia. Osmotic diarrhea and viral gastroenteritides typically generate stools with Na$^+$ and K$^+$ <100 mM, thus leading to water loss and hypernatremia; secretory diarrheas typically result in isotonic stool and hypovolemia +/– hypovolemic hyponatremia. Common causes of renal water loss include osmotic diuresis secondary to hyperglycemia, postobstructive diuresis, or drugs (e.g., mannitol); water diuresis per se occurs in central or nephrogenic diabetes insipidus (DI). The various causes of central and nephrogenic DI are listed in table 57.4. Nephrogenic DI is most commonly due to therapy with lithium, which inhibits the renal response to AVP and can cause chronic distal tubular injury. Gestational DI is a rare complication of pregnancy wherein increased activity of a placental protease with vasopressinase activity leads to reduced circulating AVP; DDAVP is an effective therapy, given its resistance to the enzyme. Finally, the ingestion or iatrogenic administration of excess Na$^+$ is a rare cause of hypernatremia, typically occurring with the IV administration of excess hypertonic Na$^+$-Cl$^-$ or Na$^+$-HCO$_3^-$.

Diagnostic Approach

The history should focus on the presence or absence of thirst, polyuria, and/or an extrarenal source for water loss, such as diarrhea. The physical exam should include a detailed neurological examination and assessment of the extracellular fluid volume; accurate documentation of daily fluid intake and daily urine output is also required. Laboratory investigation should include a measurement of serum and urine osmolality in addition to urine electrolytes. The appropriate response to hypernatremia and a serum osmolality >295 mOsm/kg is the excretion of low volumes (<500 mL/day) of maximally concentrated urine, >800 mOsm/kg. Should this be the case, then an extrarenal source of water loss is primarily responsible. Patients with hypernatremia often exhibit polyuria; should an osmotic diuresis be responsible, with excessive excretion of Na$^+$-Cl$^-$, glucose, and/or urea, then daily solute excretion will be >750–1000 mOsm/day (>15 mOsm/kg body water/day) (see figure 57.3). More typically, patients with hypernatremia and polyuria will have a predominant water diuresis, with excessive urination of hypotonic urine. Adequate differentiation between nephrogenic and central causes of DI, if not apparent from the clinical scenario, requires the measurement of the response in urinary osmolality to DDAVP combined with measurement of circulating AVP; patients with nephrogenic DI will fail to respond to DDAVP, with a high circulating AVP level. Notably, water deprivation testing is inappropriate in hypernatremic patients because they are already hypertonic (with adequate stimulus for AVP release). For patients with hypernatremia due to renal loss of water, it is critical to quantify *ongoing* daily losses, using the formula for electrolyte-free water clearance, in addition to calculating the baseline water deficit (the relevant formulas are discussed in table 57.5).

Treatment of Hypernatremia

The approach to the management of hypernatremia is outlined in table 57.5. As with hyponatremia, it is advisable to correct the water deficit slowly to avoid neurologic compromise, decreasing serum [Na$^+$] over 48–72 hours. Depending on the blood pressure or clinical volume status, it may be appropriate to initially treat with hypotonic saline solutions (one-fourth or one-half normal saline); blood glucose should be monitored in patients treated with large volumes of D5W, should hyperglycemia occur. Calculation of urinary electrolyte-free water clearance is helpful to estimate

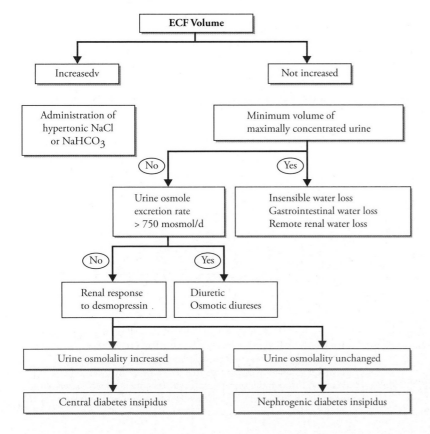

Figure 57.3. The Diagnostic Approach to Hypernatremia. See text for details. Reprinted with permission from Singer GG, Brenner BM. Fluid and electrolyte disturbances. In Fauci AS, Braunwald E, Kasper DL, et al. (cds.). *Harrison's Principles of Internal Medicine,* 17th ed. (pp. 274–84). New York: McGraw-Hill; 2008.

daily ongoing loss of free water in patients with nephrogenic or central DI (see table 57.5). Other forms of therapy may be helpful in selected cases of hypernatremia *after* normalization of the serum [Na$^+$] has been accomplished with free water repletion.

Patients with central DI may respond to the administration of intranasal DDAVP. Patients with nephrogenic DI due to lithium may reduce their polyuria with amiloride (2.5–10 mg/day) or hydrochlorothiazide (12.5–50 mg/day). These diuretics are thought to increase proximal water reabsorption and decrease distal solute delivery, thus reducing polyuria; amiloride may also decrease entry of lithium into principal cells in the distal nephron by inhibiting the amiloride-sensitive epithelial sodium channel (ENaC). In practice, however, most patients with lithium-associated DI are able to compensate for their polyuria by simply increasing their water intake. Occasionally nonsteroidal anti-inflammatory drugs (NSAIDs) have also been used to treat polyuria associated with nephrogenic DI, reducing the negative effect of local prostaglandins on urinary concentration; however, the nephrotoxic potential of NSAIDs typically limits their utility.

POTASSIUM DISORDERS

Potassium (K$^+$) is the major intracellular cation, and extracellular K$^+$ constitutes <2% of total-body K$^+$ content. In consequence, changes in the exchange and distribution of intra- and extracellular K$^+$ can lead to marked hypo- or hyperkalemia. Insulin, beta-2-adrenergic agonists, thyroid hormone, and alkalosis tend to promote K$^+$ uptake by cells, leading to hypokalemia. For example, hyperthyroid patients can present with hypokalemic periodic paralysis, with intermittent weakness accompanied by hypokalemia, hypomagnesemia, and hypophosphatemia; more common in males of Asian or Latin American origin, this disorder responds dramatically to the nonselective beta blocker propranolol, followed by treatment of the underlying thyroid disease. In contrast, acidosis, insulinopenia, or acute hyperosmolality (e.g., after treatment with mannitol) promote the *efflux* of K$^+$ from tissues, leading to hyperkalemia. A corollary is that massive necrosis and the attendant release of tissue K$^+$ can cause severe hyperkalemia, particularly in the setting of acute kidney injury and reduced excretion of K$^+$. Hyperkalemia due to rhabdomyolysis is thus particularly common because of the enormous store of K$^+$ in muscle; hyperkalemia may also be prominent in tumor lysis syndrome due to the efflux of K$^+$ from malignant cells.

Changes in body K$^+$ content are primarily mediated by the kidney, which reabsorbs filtered K$^+$ in hypokalemic, K$^+$-deficient states and secretes K$^+$ in hyperkalemic, K$^+$-replete states. Although K$^+$ is transported along the entire nephron, the principal cells of the connecting segment and cortical collecting duct play the dominant role in renal K$^+$ excretion. Apical Na$^+$ entry into principal cells via the amiloride-sensitive ENaC generates a lumen-negative potential difference, which drives passive K$^+$ exit through

Table 57.5 **MANAGEMENT OF HYPERNATREMIA**

Water Deficit
1. **Estimate total-body water (TBW): 50–60% body weight (kg) depending on body composition**
2. **Calculate free-water deficit: [(Na$^+$ − 140)/140] × TBW**
3. **Administer deficit over 48–72 hours**

Ongoing Water Losses
4. **Calculate free-water clearance, C$_e$H$_2$O:**

$$C_e H_2 O = V \left(1 - [U_{Na} \pm U_K / S_{Na}]\right)$$

where V is urinary volume, U$_{Na}$ is urinary [Na$^+$], U$_K$ is urinary [K$^+$], and S$_{Na}$ is serum [Na$^+$]

Insensible Losses
5. **~10 mL/kg per day: less if ventilated, more if febrile**

Total
6. **Add components to determine water deficit and ongoing water loss; correct the water deficit over 48–72 hours and replace daily water loss.**

SOURCE: Reprinted with permission from Mount DB. Electrolytes/acid-base. In Fauci A, Braunwald E, Kasper D, et al. (eds.). *Harrison's Manual of Medicine,* 17th ed. (pp. 3–21). New York: McGraw-Hill; 2009.

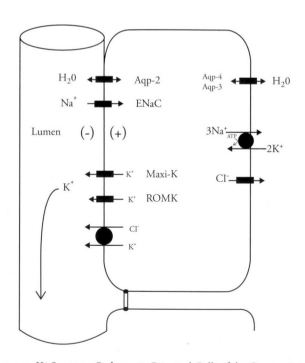

Figure 57.4. K$^+$ Secretory Pathways in Principal Cells of the Connecting Segment (CNT) and Cortical Collecting Duct (CCD). The absorption of Na$^+$ via the amiloride-sensitive epithelial sodium channel (ENaC) generates a lumen-negative potential difference, which drives K$^+$ excretion through the apical secretory K$^+$ channel ROMK (renal outer medullary K$^+$ channel). Flow-dependent K$^+$ secretion is mediated by an apical voltage-gated, calcium-sensitive maxi-K channel.

apical K^+ channels (see figure 57.4). Knowledge of this relationship is critical for the bedside understanding of potassium disorders. For example, decreased distal delivery of Na^+ in prerenal states reduces the lumen-negative potential difference and blunts the ability to excrete K^+, leading to hyperkalemia. Hyperkalemia is also a predictable consequence of drugs that directly inhibit ENaC, such as amiloride, triamterene, trimethroprim (in trimethoprim/sulfamethoxazole), and pentamidine. Aldosterone has a major influence on potassium excretion, increasing the activity of ENaC channels and thus amplifying the driving force for K^+ secretion across the luminal membrane of principal cells; abnormalities in the renin-angiotensin-aldosterone system can cause both hypo- and hyperkalemia.

HYPOKALEMIA

Hypokalemia, defined as a serum $[K^+]$ of <3.6 mM, occurs in up to 20% of hospitalized patients. Major causes of hypokalemia are outlined in table 57.6. Atrial and ventricular arrhythmias are the most serious consequences; patients with concurrent magnesium deficit and/or digoxin therapy are at increased risk of hypokalemia-associated arrhythmias. Other clinical manifestations include muscle weakness, which may be profound at serum $[K^+]$ <2.5 mM. If hypokalemia is sustained, patients may develop hypertension, polyuria, renal cysts, and renal failure.

The cause of hypokalemia is usually obvious from history, physical examination, and/or basic laboratory tests. However, persistent hypokalemia may require a more thorough evaluation (see figure 57.5). The history should focus on medications (e.g., laxatives, diuretics, antibiotics), diet and dietary habits (e.g., licorice), and symptoms that suggest a particular cause (e.g., periodic weakness, diarrhea). The physical examination should pay particular attention to blood pressure, volume status, and signs suggestive of specific hypokalemic disorders, for example, hyperthyroidism and Cushing syndrome. Initial laboratory evaluation should include electrolytes, blood urea nitrogen (BUN), creatinine, serum osmolality, Mg^{2+}, Ca^{2+}, a complete blood count, and urinary pH, osmolality, creatinine, and electrolytes. The presence of a non−anion gap acidosis suggests a distal, hypokalemic renal tubular acidosis or diarrhea; calculation of the urinary anion gap can help differentiate these two diagnoses. The urine anion gap is calculated as urine

Table 57.6 **CAUSES OF HYPOKALEMIA**

I. Decreased intake
  A. Starvation
  B. Clay ingestion
II. Redistribution into cells
  A. Acid-base
    1. Metabolic alkalosis
  B. Hormonal
    1. Insulin
    2. Beta-2-adrenergic agonists (endogenous or exogenous)
    3. Alpha-adrenergic antagonists
  C. Anabolic state
    1. Vitamin B-12 or folic acid administration (red blood cell production)
    2. Granulocyte-macrophage colony-stimulating factor (white blood cell production)
    3. Total parenteral nutrition
  D. Other
    1. Pseudohypokalemia
    2. Hypothermia
    3. Hypokalemic periodic paralysis
    4. Thyrotoxic periodic paralysis
    5. Barium toxicity
III. Increased loss
  A. Nonrenal
    1. Gastrointestinal loss (diarrhea)
    2. Integumentary loss (sweat)
  B. Renal
    1. Increased distal flow: diuretics, osmotic diuresis, salt-wasting nephropathies
    2. Increased secretion of potassium
      a. Mineralocorticoid excess: primary hyperaldosteronism, secondary hyperaldosteronism (malignant hypertension, renin-secreting tumors, renal artery stenosis, hypovolemia), apparent mineralocorticoid excess (hereditary, licorice, chewing tobacco, carbenoxolone), congenital adrenal hyperplasia, Cushing syndrome, Bartter syndrome, Gitelman syndrome
      b. Distal delivery of nonreabsorbed anions: vomiting, nasogastric suction, proximal (type 2) renal tubular acidosis, diabetic ketoacidosis, glue-sniffing (toluene abuse), penicillin derivatives
      c. Other: amphotericin B, Liddle syndrome, hypomagnesemia

SOURCE: Reprinted with permission from Mount DB. Electrolytes/acid-base. In: Fauci A, Braunwald E, Kasper D, et al. (eds.). *Harrison's Manual of Medicine,* 17th ed. (pp. 3–21). New York: McGraw-Hill; 2009.

[Na$^+$] plus urine [K$^+$] minus urine [Cl$^-$]. The ammonium ion NH$_4^+$ should be the major "unmeasured cation" in acidemic patients, such that the physiologically appropriate urinary anion gap (as in diarrhea with normal renal function) should be a *negative* value; patients with renal tubular acidosis or acidosis associated with renal insufficiency will have a *positive* value for the urine anion gap. Serum and urine osmolality are required for calculation of the transtubular K$^+$ gradient (TTKG), which should be <3 in the presence of hypokalemia (see also section discussing hyperkalemia below); urine from patients with "redistributive" hypokalemia (e.g., in thyrotoxic paralysis) will have a TTKG of <2–3, whereas urine from patients with renal potassium wasting will typically have a TTKG of >4. Further tests such as urinary Mg^{2+} and Ca^{2+}, urine diuretic screens, and/or plasma renin and aldosterone levels may be necessary in specific cases. The most common causes of chronic, diagnosis-resistant hypokalemia are Gitelman syndrome (hereditary hypokalemic alkalosis with hypomagnesemia and hypocalciuria), surreptitious vomiting, and diuretic abuse; each has

specific patterns of urine electrolytes. Urinary testing for diuretics may be positive in patients with diuretic abuse.

Treatment of Hypokalemia

Hypokalemia can generally be managed by correction of the underlying disease process or withdrawal of a causative medication combined with oral K$^+$-Cl$^-$ supplementation. However, hypokalemia is refractory to correction in the presence of magnesium deficiency, which should also be corrected when present; notably, renal wasting of both cations may be particularly prominent after renal tubular injury, for example, from cisplatin nephrotoxicity. If loop or thiazide diuretic therapy cannot be discontinued, a distal tubular K$^+$-sparing agent, such as amiloride or spironolactone, can be added to the regimen if otherwise appropriate and indicated. If hypokalemia is severe (<2.5 mmol/L) and/or if oral supplementation is not feasible or tolerated, intravenous K$^+$-Cl$^-$ can be administered through a central vein with cardiac monitoring and frequent measurement of serum [K$^+$]

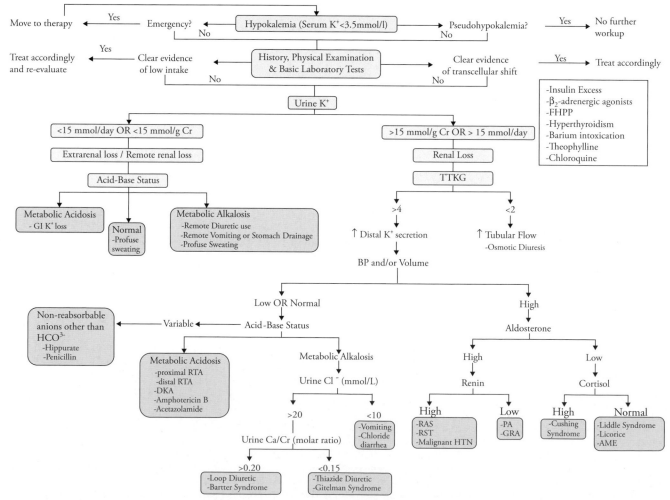

Figure 57.5. The Diagnostic Approach to Hypokalemia. See text for details. FHPP, familial hypokalemic periodic paralysis; GI, gastrointestinal; TTKG, transtubular potassium gradient; CCD, cortical collecting duct; BP, blood pressure; RTA, renal tubular acidosis; DKA, diabetic ketoacidosis; RAS, renal artery stenosis; RST, renin-secreting tumor; HTN, hypertension; PA, primary aldosteronism; GRA, glucocorticoid-remediable aldosteronism; AME, apparent mineralocorticoid excess. This figure was published in Mount DB, Zandi-Nejad K. Disorders of potassium balance. In Brenner BM (ed.). *The Kidney,* 8th ed. (pp. 547–87). Amsterdam: Elsevier; 2008. Copyright Elsevier 2008.

in an intensive care setting at rates that should not exceed 20 mmol/hr. Intravenous K⁺-Cl⁻ should always be administered in saline solutions rather than dextrose; the dextrose-induced increase in insulin can acutely exacerbate hypokalemia.

HYPERKALEMIA

Hyperkalemia is usually defined as a potassium level of 5.5 meq/L, occurring in up to 10% of hospitalized patients. Hyperkalemia is most frequently caused by a decrease in renal K⁺ excretion (see table 57.7). However, dietary K⁺ intake can have a major, rapid effect on serum [K⁺] in susceptible patients, for example, diabetics with hyporeninemic hypoaldosteronism and chronic kidney disease. Drugs that impact on the renin-angiotensin-aldosterone axis are also a frequent cause of hyperkalemia, particularly given recent trends to co-administer these agents, for example, spironolactone or eplerenone or angiotensin receptor blockers with an ACE inhibitor in cardiac and/or renal disease.

The first priority in the management of hyperkalemia is to assess the need for emergency treatment (electrocardiographic (EKG) changes and/or [K⁺] ≥ 6.5–7.0 mM). This should be followed by a comprehensive workup to determine the cause (figure 57.6). History and physical examination should focus on medications (e.g., ACE inhibitors, NSAIDs, trimethoprim/sulfamethoxazole), diet and dietary supplements (e.g., salt substitutes), risk factors for acute kidney failure, reduction in urine output, blood pressure, and volume status. Initial laboratory tests should include electrolytes, BUN, creatinine, serum osmolality, Mg^{2+}, Ca^{2+}, a complete blood count, and urinary pH, osmolality, creatinine, and electrolytes. A urine [Na⁺] <20 mM indicates that distal Na⁺ delivery may be a limiting factor in K⁺ excretion; volume repletion with 0.9% saline or treatment with furosemide may then be effective in reducing serum [K⁺] by increasing distal Na⁺ delivery. Serum and urine osmolality are required for calculation of the TTKG. The expected values of the TTKG are largely based on historical data, and are

Table 57.7 **CAUSES OF HYPERKALEMIA**

I. "Pseudo"-hyperkalemia
   A. Cellular efflux; thrombocytosis, leukocytosis, in vitro hemolysis
   B. Hereditary defects in red cell membrane transport
II. Intra- to extracellular shift
   A. Acidosis
   B. Hyperosmolality; radiocontrast, hypertonic dextrose, mannitol
   C. Beta-2-adrenergic antagonists (noncardioselective agents)
   D. Digoxin or ouabain poisoning
   E. Hyperkalemic periodic paralysis
   F. Lysine and epsilon-aminocaproic acid (structurally similar, positively charged)
III. Inadequate excretion
   A. Inhibition of the renin-angiotensin-aldosterone axis; ↑ risk of hyperkalemia when used in combination
     1. ACE-inhibitors
     2. Renin inhibitors; Aliskiren (in combination with ACE-inhibitors or ARBs)
     3. Angiotensin receptor blockers (ARBs)
     4. Blockade of the mineralocorticoid receptor; Spironolactone, eplerenone
     5. Blockade of the epithelial sodium channel (ENaC); Amiloride, triamterene, trimethoprim, pentamidine, nafamostat
   B. Decreased distal delivery
     1. Congestive heart failure
     2. Volume depletion
     3. NSAIDs, cyclosporine
   C. Hyporeninemic hypoaldosteronism
     1. Tubulointerstitial diseases; SLE, sickle cell anemia, obstructive uropathy
     2. Diabetes, diabetic nephropathy
     3. Drugs. NSAIDs, beta-blockers, cyclosporine
     4. Chronic kidney disease, advanced age
   D. Renal resistance to mineralocorticoid
     1. Tubulointerstitial diseases; SLE, amyloidosis, sickle cell anemia, obstructive uropathy, post-ATN
     2. Hereditary: pseudohypoaldosteronism type I: defects in the mineralocorticoid receptor or the epithelial sodium channel (ENaC)
   E. Advanced renal insufficiency with low GFR
   F. Primary adrenal insufficiency
     1. Autoimmune: Addison disease, polyglandular endocrinopathy
     2. Infectious: HIV, CMV, TB, disseminated fungal infection
     3. Infiltrative: amyloidosis, malignancy, metastatic cancer
     4. Drug-associated: heparin, low-molecular-weight heparin
     5. Hereditary; adrenal hypoplasia congenita, congenital lipoid adrenal hyperplasia, aldosterone synthase deficiency
     6. Adrenal hemorrhage or infarction; may occur in antiphospholipid syndrome

SOURCE: Reprinted with permission from Mount DB. Electrolytes/acid-base. In: Fauci A, Braunwald E, Kasper D, et al. (eds.). *Harrison's Manual of Medicine*, 17th ed. (pp. 3–21). New York: McGraw-Hill; 2009.

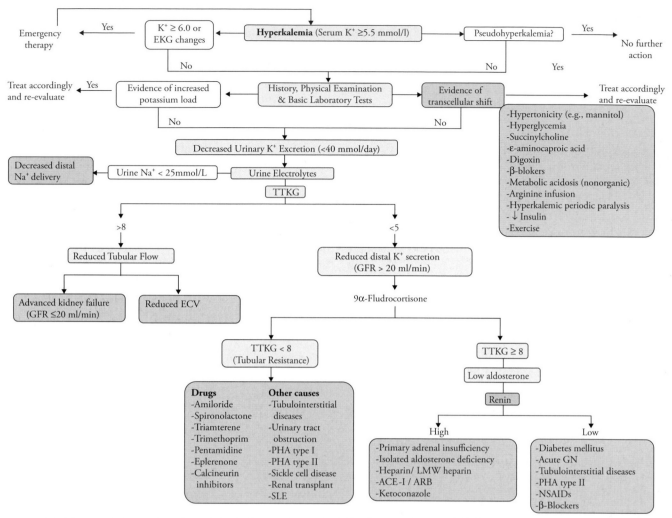

Figure 57.6. The Diagnostic Approach to Hyperkalemia. See text for details. EKG, electrocardiogram; TTKG, transtubular potassium gradient; CCD, cortical collecting duct; GFR, glomerular filtration rate; ECV, effective circulatory volume; acute GN, acute glomerulonephritis; HIV, human immunodeficiency virus; NSAIDs, nonsteroidal anti-inflammatory drugs; LMW heparin, low-molecular-weight heparin; ACE-I, angiotensin-converting enzyme inhibitor; ARB, angiotensin II receptor blocker; PHA, pseudohypoaldosteronism; SLE, systemic lupus erythematosus. This figure was published in Mount DB, Zandi-Nejad K. Disorders of potassium balance. In Brenner BM, ed. *The Kidney,* 8th ed. (pp. 547–87). Amsterdam: Elsevier; 2008. Copyright Elsevier 2008.

<3 in the presence of hypokalemia and >7–8 in the presence of hyperkalemia.

$$\mathbf{TTKG} = \frac{[K^+]_{urine} \times Osm_{serum}}{[K^+]_{serum} \times Osm_{urine}}$$

Treatment of Hyperkalemia

The most important consequence of hyperkalemia is altered cardiac conduction, with the risk of bradycardic arrest. Figure 57.7 shows the typical EKG patterns of hyperkalemia. EKG manifestations of hyperkalemia should be considered a true medical emergency and treated urgently. However, EKG changes of hyperkalemia are notoriously insensitive, particularly in patients with chronic kidney disease; given these limitations, patients with significant hyperkalemia

($[K^+] \geq 6.5$–7.0 mmol/L) in the absence of EKG changes should also be aggressively managed.

Urgent management of hyperkalemia includes a 12-lead EKG, admission to the hospital, continuous cardiac monitoring, and immediate treatment. Treatment of hyperkalemia (table 57.8) is divided into three categories: (1) antagonism of the cardiac effects of hyperkalemia; (2) rapid reduction in $[K^+]$ by redistribution into cells; and (3) removal of K^+ from the body. Treatment of hyperkalemia is summarized in tables 57.3–57.5. Kayexalate, an ion-exchange resin (sodium polystyrene sulfonate) that exchanges sodium for potassium in the GI tract, is frequently prescribed for the acute and chronic treatment of hyperkalemia. Kayexalate is almost invariably administered with sorbitol to prevent constipation. Unfortunately, the administration of Kayexalate with sorbitol has been associated

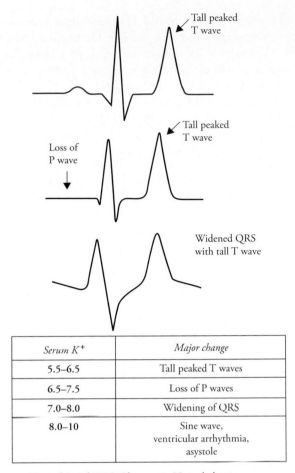

Serum K+	*Major change*
5.5–6.5	Tall peaked T waves
6.5–7.5	Loss of P waves
7.0–8.0	Widening of QRS
8.0–10	Sine wave, ventricular arrhythmia, asystole

Figure 57.7. Typical Serial EKG Changes in Hyperkalemia.

with intestinal necrosis, a rare but often fatal complication. In September 2009, FDA warned against co-administering Kayexalate with sorbitol due to the risk of intestinal necrosis. It should be emphasized that the onset of action of Kayexalate is at best 4–6 hours, so it has little impact on the acute management of hyperkalemia. Therefore, clinicians must carefully consider whether emergency treatment with Kayexalate is actually necessary for the treatment of hyperkalemia. However, there are settings where the risk–benefit analysis favors the administration of Kayexalate for treatment of hyperkalemia, for example, in oliguric renal failure without possibility of dialysis. Notably, single 30-g doses of Kayexalate are rarely effective, with repeated doses required for a substantial effect on serum [K+].

ADDITIONAL READING

Batlle DC, Hizon M, Cohen E, Gutterman C, Gupta R. The use of the urinary anion gap in the diagnosis of hyperchloremic metabolic acidosis. *N Engl J Med.* 1988;318:594–9.

Berl T. Impact of solute intake on urine flow and water excretion. *J Am Soc Nephrol.* 2008;19:1076–8.

Choi MJ, Ziyadeh FN. The utility of the transtubular potassium gradient in the evaluation of hyperkalemia. *J Am Soc Nephrol.* 2008;19:424–6.

Chung HM, Kluge R, Schrier RW, Anderson RJ. Clinical assessment of extracellular fluid volume in hyponatremia. *Am J Med.* 1987;83:905–8.

Ellison DH, Berl T. Clinical practice. The syndrome of inappropriate antidiuresis. *N Engl J Med.* 2007;356:2064–72.

Loh JA, Verbalis JG. Disorders of water and salt metabolism associated with pituitary disease. *Endocrinol Metab Clin North Am.* 2008;37:213–34.

Mohmand HK, Issa D, Ahmad Z, Cappuccio JD, Kouides RW, Sterns RH. Hypertonic saline for hyponatremia: Risk of inadvertent overcorrection. *Clin J Am Soc Nephrol.* 2007;2:1110–7.

Mount DB, Krahn TA. Hyponatremia: Case vignettes. *Semin Nephrol.* 2009;29:300–17.

Mount DB, Zandi-Nejad K. Disorders of potassium balance. In Brenner BM, ed. *Brenner and Rector's The Kidney* (pp. 547–87). Philadelphia: W. B. Saunders; 2008.

Perianayagam A, Sterns RH, Silver SM, et al. DDAVP is effective in preventing and reversing inadvertent overcorrection of hyponatremia. *Clin J Am Soc Nephrol.* 2008;3:331–6.

Sterns RH, Nigwekar SU, Hix JK. The treatment of hyponatremia. *Semin Nephrol.* 2009;29:282–99.

Sterns RH, Rojas M, Bernstein P, Chennupati S. Ion-exchange resins for the treatment of hyperkalemia: Are they safe and effective? *J Am Soc Nephrol.* 2010 May;21(5):733–5.

Table 57.8 **MANAGEMENT OF HYPERKALEMIA**

MECHANISM	THERAPY	DOSE	ONSET	DURATION	COMMENTS
Stabilize membrane potential	Calcium	10% Ca-gluconate, 10 mL over 10 min	1–3 min	30–60 min	Repeat in 5 min if persistent EKG changes; avoid in digoxin toxicity
Cellular K+ uptake	Insulin	10 U R with 50 mL of D50, if BS <250	30 min	4–6 hours	Can repeat in 15 min; initiate D10W IV at 50–75 mL/hr to avoid rebound hypoglycemia
	Beta-2 agonist	Nebulized albuterol, 10–20 mg in 4 mL saline	30 min	2–4 hours	Can be synergistic/additive to insulin; should not be used as sole therapy; use with caution in cardiac disease; may cause tachycardia/hyperglycemia
K+ removal	Kayexalate	30–60 g PO in 20% sorbitol	1–2 hours	4–6 hours	May cause ischemic colitis and colonic necrosis, particularly in enema form and postoperative state
	Furosemide Hemodialysis	20–250 mg IV	15 min Immediate	4–6 hours	Dependent on adequate renal response/function. Efficacy depends on pretreatment of hyperkalemia, the dialyzer used, blood flow and dialysate flow rates, duration, and serum to dialysate K+ gradient

SOURCE: Reprinted with permission from Mount DB. Electrolytes/acid-base. In: Fauci A, Braunwald E, Kasper D, et al [eds]. *Harrison's Manual of Medicine,* 17th ed. (pp. 3–21). New York: McGraw-Hill; 2009.

QUESTIONS

QUESTION 1. You admit a 40-year-old woman with a 1-week history of flu-like illness and profuse diarrhea. She has received 1.5 L of NS.

On exam, HR is 80 supine, 105 standing, Bp 110/70. JVP is seen at 5 cm.

Admission laboratory studies find Na^+ 121, K^+ 3.6, urine Na^+ 12, urine Osm 450.

Current labs (6 hours after admission to ER) find Na^+ 130, K^+ 3.5, urine Na^+ 18, urine Osm 300.

Which of the following therapies is the most appropriate?

A. Normal saline at 200 mL/hr
B. Normal saline with 40 mEq/L at 200 mL/hr
C. Conivaptan 40 mg load, then continuous infusion at 20 mg/day
D. D5W at 75 mL/hr
E. D5W at 75 mL/hr after 1 μg of DDAVP

QUESTION 2. Therapy with which of the following drugs is most likely to cause nephrogenic diabetes insipidus associated with acute renal insufficiency?

A. Foscarnet
B. Interferon-α
C. Acyclovir
D. Ganciclovir
E. Vincristine

QUESTION 3. A 20-year-old woman is brought to the emergency department with altered mental status. She had attended a "rave" in the South End of Boston the night PTA. She became drowsy at ~2 a.m. and vomited several times. At 8 a.m. she had a generalized seizure that lasted ~15 sec.

Exam: Unresponsive, HR 84, RR 16, BP 145/85. Heart sounds normal, clear chest, no peripheral edema. Head and neck WNL, no evidence of trauma.

Laboratory studies find Na^+ 121, creatinine 0.5, K^+ 3.6, uric acid 3.7, Cl^- 90, Osm 242.

Which of the following is the most likely cause of this syndrome?

A. Ecstasy-induced hyponatremia
B. Hyponatremia secondary to seizure
C. Occult brain tumor
D. Acute intracerebral bleed
E. Compulsive drinking

QUESTION 4. Which of the following measures is the single most appropriate management of this patient's hyponatremia (patient in question 3)?

A. IV infusion of conivaptan, the FDA-approved vasopressin antagonist
B. IV infusion of 3% saline
C. IV infusion of mannitol to reduce intracerebral edema
D. IV infusion of Lasix
E. Urgent neurosurgical consultation

QUESTION 5. A 32-year-old Hispanic man was admitted with weakness and a K^+ of 2.0. He was very healthy until 2 months PTA, when he developed intermittent leg weakness. He denies drug or laxative abuse, is on no medications.

FH: Mother has DM, one sister thyroid disease.

Exam: Temp 97.2, BP 176/96, HR 102, RR 16; otherwise exam WNL.

Lab studies found the following:

	ADMISSION:	5 MONTHS PTA
Na	139	143
K	2.0	3.8
Cl	105	107
HCO_3^-	26	29
BUN	11	16
Creatinine	0.6	1.0
Glu	145	136
PO_4	1.2	
Ca	8.8	8.8
Mg	1.3	1.9
Alb	3.8	

Which of the following studies is most likely to be diagnostic?

A. Serum PTH
B. Serum aldosterone
C. Serum insulin
D. Urine pH and urine electrolytes
E. Thyroid function studies

QUESTION 6. A 63-year-old man is admitted to the hospital for confusion, attributed to hepatic encephalopathy. You are asked to see him for evaluation of a low bicarbonate level. Physical exam reveals mild jaundice and ascites.

Laboratory studies found Na^+ 134, K^+ 5.4, Cl^- 110, ABGs 7.32/29/80/15, urine pH 6.0, urine Na^+ 2, HCO_3^- 14, AG 10.

Which of the following is the most likely cause of this patient's metabolic acidosis and hyperkalemia?

A. Excessive backleak of H^+ in the collecting duct
B. Diarrhea from lactulose
C. Impaired proximal bicarbonate reabsorption
D. Insufficient distal Na^+ delivery
E. Adrenal insufficiency

ANSWERS

1. E
2. A
3. B
4. B
5. E
6. D

58.

ACID–BASE DISTURBANCES

Julian L. Seifter

The regulation of acid–base balance in the body underlies the importance of pH in a variety of cellular and subcellular biological functions; for example, regulation of protein synthesis and intermediate carbohydrate metabolism are pH-sensitive processes. Clinically, this is apparent by the failure to grow normally in an acidemic environment and explains an increase in anaerobic glycolysis in alkalemia, due to an increase in a rate-limiting step of glycolysis phosphofructokinase-1. pH is important in numerous transport functions across membranes, such as increasing acid extrusion from cells when cellular pH drops. In general, cellular pH is lower than extracellular pH related to the electronegativity within cellular structures. The delivery of oxygen to tissues such as the brain and skeletal muscle is very much dependent on extracellular pH via the shift in the oxyhemoglobin dissociation curve.

SIGNS AND SYMPTOMS OF ACID–BASE DISORDERS

Many of the symptoms of acid–base disorders are neurological in nature. For example, patients who hyperventilate and develop respiratory alkalemia frequently feel light-headed and may even lose consciousness, related to a marked elevation in pH and decreased oxygen delivery to brain cells. Fortunately, the brain can compensate for acid–base disturbances in short order. Patients with metabolic acidosis may have insensitivity to sympathomimetic drugs, may note fatigue, dyspnea on exertion, and deep ventilatory excursions known as Kussmaul respiration. Nausea and vomiting are also frequent symptoms and may be attributed to uremia in the kidney failure patient.

DEFINITIONS

Abnormalities in blood pH are termed acidemia, that is a pH of <7.38, or alkalemia, that is, a pH of >7.42. These terms should be distinguished from abnormal processes that may be simultaneously present, known as respiratory or metabolic acidosis and respiratory or metabolic alkalosis (see table 58.1). Since an individual can have many processes leading to a single perturbation in blood pH in the acid or alkali direction, one must be able to single out those individual processes even if they are masked by other coinciding disturbances. The place to start in making these distinctions is from clues in the patient's history. Examples include vomiting, which most likely would suggest an alkalotic process; or voluminous diarrhea, which would be more likely to produce an acidotic rather than an alkalotic process, although the latter is possible. A patient with chronic lung disease might have chronic hypoventilation and respiratory acidosis, whereas a patient with chronic renal disease may be more prone to developing a metabolic acidosis. Because patients can have multiple processes, including more than one metabolic disturbance, it becomes necessary to try to recognize these independent disturbances that together may result in a blood pH that is normal, acidemic, or alkalemic.

A simple acid–base disturbance refers to a single process responsible for the disturbance, for example, a metabolic acidosis causing acidemia. Mixed disturbances indicate that more than one process contributes to the disorder; for example, one could have simultaneous metabolic acidosis and metabolic alkalosis completely negating the effect on pH, yet still important in terms of pointing to the patient's pathology. It is not enough to diagnose an acid–base problem without looking for underlying etiologies.

ANALYSIS OF ACID–BASE DISORDERS

It is common practice to utilize the carbon dioxide and bicarbonate determinations of arterial or venous blood when analyzing an acid–base problem. Arterial blood gas measurements include a direct measurement of pH and P_{CO_2} and a calculated value of bicarbonate. Venous measurements carefully collected in an anticoagulated tube and

pH	Pco$_2$/HCO$_3^-$	PRIMARY DISORDER
Acidemia	↓HCO$_3^-$	Metabolic acidosis
	↓Pco$_2$	Respiratory acidosis
Alkalemia	↑HCO$_3^-$	Metabolic alkalosis
	↓Pco$_2$	Respiratory alkalosis

free of ambient air are less invasive but do not usually give information about oxygenation, and it must be realized that the venous pH is typically 0.05 pH units more acid than arterial pH and venous Pco$_2$ is usually 6 mm Hg higher than corresponding arterial CO$_2$. These relationships may change in patients who are hypometabolic, hypothermic, or are in low cardiac output states.

The Henderson-Hasselbalch equation is a logarithmic expression of the overall chemical reactions between carbon dioxide in water, carbonic acid (H$_2$CO$_3$), and the bicarbonate concentrations. The determination of CO$_2$ in solution is approximated by the product of the measured Pco$_2$ and the solubility of carbon dioxide in aqueous media. The equation is as follows:

$$pH = pK + \log(HCO_3)/(0.03 \times Pco_2)$$

From this relationship it is evident that the pH is proportional to the ratio of HCO$_3$/Pco$_2$ rather than simply HCO$_3$ or Pco$_2$. A common error related to this is that the serum HCO$_3$ concentration measured on a routine blood without pH or Pco$_2$ would be equated to a particular acid–base problem. Thus, an elevated bicarbonate concentration does not by itself indicate alkalemia because it could also be a compensatory response to a respiratory acidosis with an elevated Pco$_2$ in the denominator. It should be noted that the compensatory process for a primary change in one of the variables, bicarbonate or Pco$_2$, is a change in the other variable in the same direction, tending to normalize the ratio and bringing the pH back toward normal.

COMPENSATIONS

Compensations refer to internal modifications, usually involving pulmonary or renal function, that help regulate body fluid pH. Such modifications are self-correcting: primary metabolic disorders result in respiratory compensation, and primary respiratory disorders lead to metabolic (renal) compensations. It follows that patients with severe lung disease may not be able to compensate adequately for metabolic disturbances, and patients with renal disease may not be able to compensate adequately for respiratory disorders. The compensations that we usually consider from the blood gas measurements involve afferent signaling from the peripheral blood as sensed by arterial chemosensors, triggering a central nervous system (CNS) medullary response to control ventilation. Patients with CNS disease may also not compensate normally for respiratory or metabolic disturbances.

An often overlooked phenomenon is that the pulmonary system mitigates the degree of respiratory disturbance as the kidneys are simultaneously correcting for that disturbance. For example, if alveolar air space disease decreases gas exchange, leading to retention of carbon dioxide, the increased CO$_2$ recognized in the carotid body chemosensor will send an afferent signal to the brainstem, which will then attempt to increase ventilation. This compensation may be inadequate, such that a continued elevation of carbon dioxide will pertain. The kidney will both increase bicarbonate reabsorption in its tubules and increase ammoniagenesis, allowing for more H$^+$ to be eliminated, accounting for the compensation of a respiratory acidosis. The limitation of this compensation will be the kidney's ability to generate ammonia.

The compensation for hyperventilation, in which more carbon dioxide is cleared by the lungs than is produced, will lead to a lower Pco$_2$ and elevated pH. The severity of this elevated pH will be worse acutely before compensatory factors emerge. The pulmonary response to the elevated pH and low Pco$_2$ is to signal the medullary centers of the brain to slow ventilation; yet, as in the respiratory acidosis setting, the respiratory response will be incomplete. The renal response related to a fall in Pco$_2$ is to decrease both bicarbonate reabsorption (resulting in an alkaline bicarbonate-rich urine) and ammonium excretion. Because the excretion of bicarbonate is less limited, it is often the case that chronic respiratory alkalosis accounts for the most complete compensation of the primary acid–base disturbances.

Metabolic disturbances require both renal and pulmonary responses to compensate and adapt to a change in pH. (Formulas used for calculating the appropriate degree of compensation are shown in table 58.2.) For example, a metabolic acidosis from diarrhea, resulting in acidemia and a low bicarbonate concentration, will stimulate the chemosensors signaling to the brain to initiate hyperventilation. This response will help bring the pH back toward normal, but it will fall short of complete compensation. Possible reasons for this include limitations on pulmonary function, but they could also be an energy-sparing adaptation that allows for a less severe degree of hyperventilation and use of respiratory muscles while the most dangerous drops in pH are avoided. The renal limitation for compensating for a metabolic acidosis has to do with physiological limits on the production of ammonia.

The compensation for metabolic alkalosis is probably the most incomplete for several reasons. From the renal point of view, compensation would allow for the excretion of bicarbonate. This will be limited by factors that develop in

Table 58.2 COMPENSATION FOR ACID–BASE ABNORMALITY

ABNORMALITY	ADJUSTMENT
Metabolic acidosis	expected P_{CO_2} = 1.5(HCO_3) + 8
Metabolic alkalosis	expected P_{CO_2} = 0.9(HCO_3) + 9
Acute respiratory acidosis	each increase in P_{CO_2} of 1, pH should decrease by 0.008
Acute respiratory alkalosis	each decrease in P_{CO_2} of 1, pH should increase by 0.008
Chronic respiratory acidosis	each increase in P_{CO_2} of 1, pH should decrease by 0.003
Chronic respiratory alkalosis	each decrease in P_{CO_2} of 1, pH should increase by 0.003

metabolic alkalosis that conserve bicarbonate and therefore limit the correction in pH. These factors include chloride depletion, decreases in glomerular filtration rate, volume depletion, potassium depletion, and hypercapnia, all of which enhance proximal bicarbonate reabsorption. This limitation may be beneficial to other electrolyte homeostasis, such as fluid retention and potassium conservation. From a respiratory compensatory point of view, severely elevated pH and bicarbonate concentrations will signal the chemosensors to cause medullary hypoventilation. When the P_{O_2} falls, it will stop this feedback mechanism.

Compensatory responses are usually complete in hours to days. The degree of compensation can be predicted only by empirical information. There is no physiological mechanism that would dictate the degree to which compensation will occur. Some important relationships have been determined experimentally. One such is the relationship between P_{CO_2} and bicarbonate concentration in metabolic acidosis. The Winter formula is:

$$P_{CO_2} = 1.5(HCO_3) + 8 \pm 2$$

When this calculation is carried through in a patient with metabolic acidosis, recognized as a fall in both pH and HCO_3 concentration, a comparison can be made between the calculated P_{CO_2} and the patient's P_{CO_2}. If the observed and calculated values for P_{CO_2} are similar, a primary metabolic acidosis causing the acidemia is suggested. However, as mentioned before, there could be a metabolic acidosis of greater magnitude and a simultaneous metabolic alkalosis such that the pH remains acid. The Winter equation reaches importance in establishing a mixed disturbance. If, for example, the P_{CO_2} observed was less than the P_{CO_2} calculated for a primary metabolic acidosis, a second condition lowering P_{CO_2} is suspected, and that would need to be a primary respiratory alkalosis. A simple approach to considering acid–base problems is depicted in table 58.3.

METABOLIC ACIDOSIS

Retention of acid consumes endogenous alkali stores, reflected by a fall in serum bicarbonate. However, serum bicarbonate, if at a stable level, is not in itself an indication of the achievement of external acid–base balance. For example, in some patients with chronic kidney disease or those with some form of renal-tubular acidosis, there is a daily retention of acid with a stable but low bicarbonate concentration. The acid is incorporated into bone mineral, liberating bicarbonate salts at the expense of bone disease. Metabolic acidosis may be the result of one or more of three processes: (1) the pathologic overproduction of endogenous acids, such as ketoacids and lactic acid or the consumption of exogenous substances such as methanol with an acidic

Table 58.3 GENERAL APPROACH TO AN ACID–BASE DISORDER

1. Is there acidemia or alkalemia?
   Acidemia pH <7.35
   Alkalemia pH >7.45

2. What is the *primary* process (metabolic or respiratory, acidosis or alkalosis)?
   [HCO_3] defines the metabolic component
   • Low (<20 mmol/L) = Metabolic acidosis
   • High (>33 mmol/L) = Metabolic alkalosis

   P_{CO_2} defines the respiratory component
   • Low (<35 mm Hg) = Respiratory alkalosis
   • High (>45 mm Hg) = Respiratory acidosis

3. Is there an appropriate compensatory response?
   • Remember the *direction* of compensation
   • Remember that compensation is almost never complete
   • Remember the Winter formula
     In a metabolic acidosis, the predicted P_{CO_2} is:
     $$(1.5 \times HCO_3^-) + 8 \pm 2$$

4. If this is an anion gap acidosis, are there other clues to a second *primary* process?
   Calculate the Delta anion gap/Delta HCO_3^- (*"delta-delta"*)
   • For every 1 meq/L of acid added to circulation, the serum bicarbonate should decrease by 1 meq/L, and the anion gap should increase by 1 meq/L
   • Thus, the Delta anion gap/Delta HCO_3^- should be 1.
   Delta AG/Delta HCO_3^-:

   1 Simple anion gap acidosis
   <1 Superimposed non-gap acidosis
   >1 Superimposed metabolic alkalosis

form (formic acid); (2) a failure of renal acid excretion and bicarbonate regeneration, as in kidney failure; and (3) loss of alkali stores, as in diarrhea or renal-tubular acidosis.

CLASSIFICATION OF METABOLIC ACIDOSES

The Anion Gap

Chemically, the classification to help arrive at a diagnosis is made by the use of the serum anion gap. The anion gap, which only reports the usual, routinely measured electrolytes, will yield a gap because normally circulating ions are not being directly measured and entered into the equation. If they were, there would be electroneutrality and, hence, no gap. The equation for the serum anion gap is as follows:

$$[Na] - [Cl + HCO_3] = AG$$

The usual normal contributor to the anion gap is circulating albumin, which accounts for about 10–12 meq/L or 2.5 meq/L per g/dL of albumin. When the actual number deviates from the normal anion gap, the presence of an unmeasured charged species is indicated. If the gap is higher than normal, there is an unmeasured anion such as lactate or salicylate. If the anion gap is lower than normal, either a low albumin state exists or there is the presence of an unmeasured cation, as in multiple myeloma.

A comparison may be made between the change in the anion gap from normal (the anion gap observed minus 12) to the change in bicarbonate concentration from normal (25 minus the bicarbonate). This entity, known as the "delta-delta," may help to determine a mixed disorder. Examples include a large increase in the anion gap without as large an increase in the change in the bicarbonate fall; such a finding might suggest the simultaneous presence of an anion gap metabolic acidosis and a metabolic alkalosis. Alternatively, the gap acidosis could be associated with a chronic respiratory acidosis, which would also tend to raise the bicarbonate concentration. Another example would be the observation of a change in bicarbonate concentration greater than the change in anion gap, as would be found in the setting of simultaneous anion gap metabolic acidosis and either a respiratory alkalosis or an additional hyperchloremic metabolic acidosis.

Causes of an anion gap metabolic acidosis are shown in table 58.4. In patients with chronic renal failure, sulfates, phosphates, and organic acid anions are poorly filtered and accumulate in the extracellular space. L-Lactic acidosis is another common cause, induced by either hypotensive shock, hypoxemia, or sepsis, but also by tumors, such as certain lymphomas, as well as drugs and toxic ingestions. Some drugs that can cause lactic acidosis include isoniazid and nucleoside reverse transcriptase inhibitors. Propylene glycol, used as the diluent for many drugs, including lorazepam, when given in high concentrations may metabolize to lactic acid. Metformin, used in treatment of diabetes, is more likely to cause lactic acidosis when used in the setting of poor renal function. In some patients with intestinal bacterial overgrowth, a condition known as D-lactic acidosis may develop as a result of the bacterial lactate dehydrogenase and the production of the nonphysiological isomer of lactic acid, D-lactic acid.

Salicylates are among other ingestions that may result in anion gap metabolic acidosis, particularly in overdose situations. Acetaminophen toxicity has increasingly been found to be a cause of acquired 5-oxyprolinuria. Methanol will cause a severe anion-gap acidosis with toxic acids including formic acid developing, and ethylene glycol, particularly ingested in antifreeze, will give organic acid anions. In some cases, it is useful to compare an anion gap and osmolar gap to support the suspicion of a toxic overdose. The calculated osmolarity is $2 \times [Na] + [glu]/18 + [BUN]/2.8 + [ethanol]/4.6$, where glucose, blood urea nitrogen (BUN) and ethanol concentrations are given as milligrams per deciliter. The measured osmolality is performed by freezing point depression in the laboratory. The difference between measured and calculated values should be normally <10 mM. If that value is exceeded, then the presence of a nonelectrolyte is suspected. If there is also an anion gap present, then the clinician should suspect substances such as methanol and ethylene glycol. The goal of therapy would be to prevent breakdown of the alcohols to the toxic acid anions. Treatments such as inhibitors of alcohol dehydrogenase and hemodialysis are frequently used.

Table 58.4 **CAUSES OF A HIGH-ANION-GAP METABOLIC ACIDOSIS**

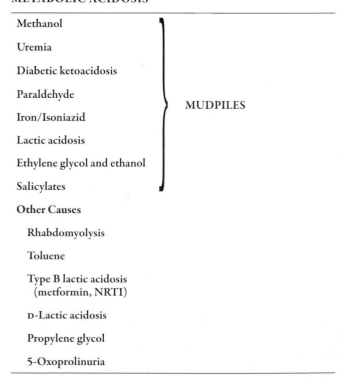

Methanol	
Uremia	
Diabetic ketoacidosis	
Paraldehyde	MUDPILES
Iron/Isoniazid	
Lactic acidosis	
Ethylene glycol and ethanol	
Salicylates	
Other Causes	
Rhabdomyolysis	
Toluene	
Type B lactic acidosis (metformin, NRTI)	
D-Lactic acidosis	
Propylene glycol	
5-Oxoprolinuria	

The "delta-delta," which is the relationship between the change in anion gap from normal and the change in the serum bicarbonate from normal, is expressed:

$$(AG - 12)/(25 - bicarbonate)$$

For example, if a patient with a normal serum albumin and an acidemia, had an anion gap of 32 meq/L and a serum HCO_3^- of 11 meq/L, the delta/delta would be 20/14. This value exceeds 1 and therefore suggests the presence of an additional metabolic alkalosis.

HYPERCHLOREMIC ACIDOSIS

In this group of disorders (table 58.5), the serum anion gap is normal because the fall in bicarbonate concentration is balanced by an increase in the chloride concentration instead of an unmeasured anion. The more common disorders are associated with hypokalemia, as in the following instances. In the case of watery diarrhea with large stool volumes, the loss of K^+ and Na^+ are accompanied either by HCO_3^- or by organic anions of bacterial origin. These losses may be excessive in small bowel disease or ileostomies—but also in the majority of colonic diarrhea cases. Several forms of renal tubular acidosis are also associated with losses of Na^+, K^+, and HCO_3^-, resulting in a relatively increased Cl^- concentration in the blood to compensate for the loss of HCO_3^-. These disorders are usually distinguished from each other by the medical history, but evaluation of urine electrolytes may be useful. Attention should be paid to the urinary anion gap:

$$UAG = (U_{Na} + U_K) - U_{Cl}$$

In the presence of a non–anion gap metabolic acidosis, if the value is greater than zero, an additional unmeasured anion is suggested. Assuming that this value does not represent an excreted anion, such as a ketoacid anion, then this finding suggests the absence of large amounts of the cation NH_4^+. NH_4^+ should be very elevated in patients whose acidosis originates from a nonrenal source because the kidney's capacity to generate NH_3 is preserved. Therefore, when the anion gap is positive, ammonium is low, and a renal source is suggested. When the anion gap is negative, that is, less than zero, it is assumed that the kidney is able to produce ammonia, and therefore a nonrenal source is suspected. In some situations a stool anion gap can be measured by measuring Na^+, K^+, and Cl^- in watery stool. If the stool anion gap is greater than the serum bicarbonate concentration, those losses will result in a hyperchloremic acidosis. In contrast, if the stool gap were less than the serum bicarbonate concentration, a metabolic alkalosis would be predicted.

Renal tubular acidosis (RTA) is an uncommon cause of metabolic acidosis in clinical practice Key features of types 1 and 2 RTA are shown in tables 58.6 and 58.7.

There are some forms of hyperchloremic acidosis that are associated with high potassium. When these conditions involve renal disorders, they are frequently termed type 4

Table 58.5 CAUSES OF NON-ANION-GAP ACIDOSIS

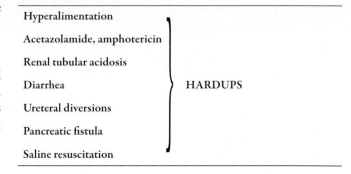

Hyperalimentation	
Acetazolamide, amphotericin	
Renal tubular acidosis	
Diarrhea	HARDUPS
Ureteral diversions	
Pancreatic fistula	
Saline resuscitation	

RTAs. Important disorders of the distal nephron at sites where both K^+ and H^+ are secreted and Na^+ is reabsorbed include the following conditions. Hypoaldosteronism with low plasma renins can be the result of renin antagonists, beta blockers, nonsteroidal anti-inflammatory drugs, or autonomic neuropathies as in diabetes and amyloidosis. Hypoaldosteronism with a high plasma renin suggests adrenal insufficiency or selective hypoaldosteronism. There are renal tubular disorders that are associated with elevations of both renin and aldosterone. Of particular importance when one notices a hyperkalemic hyperchloremic acidosis is to consider systemic disorders such as systemic lupus, myeloma, light chain disease, or sickle cell nephropathy. It is critical to exclude urinary tract obstruction. In all of these conditions the urinary anion gap will be positive, suggesting low ammonium excretion. There are other forms of hyperkalemic hyperchloremic acidosis that result from the ingestion or infusion of chloride salts, such as HCl, NaCl, KCl, $CaCl_2$, or arginine and lysine hydrochloride salts.

"More HCO_3^- is needed to treat a proximal than distal RTA. since the proximal disorder is associated with large clearance of HCO_3 as the serum HCO_3 is raised. It often requires very large quantities of bicarbonate salts, whereas in distal renal tubular acidosis, an amount of bicarbonate equal to the estimated acid load per day is all that is required to maintain acid–base balance. That amount is approximately 1–2 meq of H^+ per kilogram body weight per day.

Treatment of Metabolic Acidosis

In determining the amount of bicarbonate to treat metabolic acidosis, one can use the following formula:

$$Amount\ of\ HCO_3\ deficit =$$
$$(25 - [HCO_3]) \times [0.5] \times body\ weight.$$

The entire calculated value should not be given all at once; rather, after a third of the calculated value has been given, a recalculation should be made, and then reiteratively until the disturbance is corrected. In certain cases where the metabolic acidosis will resolve on its own, it may be particularly important not to give excessive bicarbonate replacement because an overshoot alkalemic state may develop.

Table 58.6 TYPE 1 RENAL TUBULAR ACIDOSIS (DISTAL)

Pathophysiology
  Distal tubule fails to excrete ammonium

Causes
  Autosomal dominant inherited disorder
  Acquired causes
  Systemic lupus erythematosus
  Sickle cell anemia
  Nephrocalcinosis-related disorders
  Hyperparathyroidism
  Medullary sponge kidney
  Medications and Toxins
  Amphotericin B
  Lithium
  Toluene

Clinical features
  Musculoskeletal weakness
  Recurrent nephrolithiasis

Labs
  Arterial blood gas (ABG)
  Non-anion-gap metabolic acidosis
  Urine pH
  Elevated >5.5 despite metabolic acidosis
  Serum potassium
  Low or normal
  Fractional excretion of bicarbonate
  FE-HCO$_3$ <5%: Distal RTA
  FE-HCO$_3$ >15%: Proximal RTA
  Assumes serum bicarbonate >20 meq/L

Management: bicarbonate supplementation
  Dose: 1–2 meq/kg/day
  Goal: Serum bicarbonate > 22 meq/L
  Correct hypokalemia

Table 58.7 TYPE 2 RENAL TUBULAR ACIDOSIS (PROXIMAL)

Pathophysiology
  Proximal tubule defect of bicarbonate reabsorption
  Results in bicarbonate wasting

Causes
  Medications
  Acetazolamide
  Fanconi syndrome
  Medullary cystic disease
  Multiple myeloma
  Nephrotic syndrome
  Renal transplantation

Clinical features
  Failure to thrive
  Growth retardation
  Vomiting
  Dehydration
  Lethargy

Labs
  Arterial blood gas
  Non-anion-gap metabolic acidosis
  Serum bicarbonate decreased
  Usually not lower than 15 meq/L
  Urine pH
  Exceeds 5.5 except in severe metabolic acidosis
  Fractional excretion of bicarbonate
  FE-HCO$_3$ exceeds 15% if serum bicarbonate >20 meq/L
  FE-HCO$_3$ <5% in distal RTA

Radiology: x-ray
  Children: rickets
  Adults: osteopenia

Management
  High dose bicarbonate supplementation
  Oral bicarbonate 10–25 meq/kg/day
  Observe for hypokalemia
  Treat osteomalacia in adults
    Vitamin D supplementation
    Calcium supplementation
  Treat rickets in children
    Vitamin D supplementation
    Sodium phosphate 1.6 g per day

This is especially true in seizure-induced lactic acidosis, in which the lactate may disappear through hepatic metabolism within an hour, and alkalinization of the patient may result in additional seizure activity. It should be recalled that in acute alkalinization, the ionized calcium concentration falls, so that any treatment with bicarbonate mandates attention to the serum calcium level to avoid tetany. Other complications of sodium bicarbonate treatment include extracellular volume expansion and hypernatremia.

METABOLIC ALKALOSIS

Metabolic alkalosis is recognized by the elevation of the serum bicarbonate concentration, and the compensatory hypoventilation results in an elevation of P_{CO_2}. [HCO$_3$] may be elevated either by exogenous alkali intake (e.g., HCO$_3$, citrate, acetate), or by gastrointestinal or renal losses of excessive acid or chloride-rich fluids. There must be both a source of new bicarbonate (generation) and stimuli to the kidney to maintain a new high level of bicarbonate (maintenance).

Maintenance of metabolic alkalosis is usually achieved by increased rates of proximal tubular HCO$_3$ reabsorption.

This is in turn related to extracellular volume depletion, primarily mediated by angiotensin II, hypokalemia, and hypercapnia. The second major element of maintenance is the presence of hyperaldosteronism.

CLASSIFICATION OF METABOLIC ALKALOSES
Chloride-Responsive

The chloride-responsive alkaloses are usually associated with volume depletion and loss of chloride-rich fluids from the body. Common disturbances include gastric alkalosis from vomiting and chloride-wasting diuretics such as furosemide and thiazides. Occasionally, diarrhea will result in high stool chloride, particularly in cases of villous adenoma of the colon and some infectious diarrheas including cholera. Renal chloride losses in Bartter and Gitelman syndromes behave in a similar fashion to those from loop and thiazide diuretics. Many of these volume-depleted states are associated with hyponatremia, high renin, and high aldosterone levels.

Chloride-Unresponsive

In these conditions, volume depletion is usually absent, and in fact hypertension may be the characteristic that brings the patient to attention. Most often, there is a primary increase in mineralocorticoids due to either adrenal adenomas or hyperplastic adrenal glands. Since the primary increase is in aldosterone, leading to volume expansion, renin levels are usually low. In unilateral renal artery stenosis, the increase in renin from the affected kidney leads to an increase in angiotensin II and then aldosterone, which promotes the sodium retention, potassium wasting, and acid wasting associated with the typical hypokalemic metabolic alkalosis. Finally, intrarenal disorders such as activating mutations of the epithelial sodium channel in the collecting duct or inhibition of the 11-beta-hydroxysteroid dehydrogenase will lead to the same peripheral picture of hypertension, hypokalemia, and alkalosis. In all of these conditions, the $[Na^+]$ in the blood may be elevated. In the Na channel-activating mutation (Liddle syndrome), both renin and aldosterone levels will be decreased. Licorice containing glycyrrhetic acid inhibits the dehydrogenase enzyme, allowing the normally present cortisol to activate the aldosterone receptor. There will be a high cortisol-to-cortisone ratio and low renin and aldosterone levels.

Except when diuretics or tubular disorders are the cause of renal chloride wasting, the chloride-responsive and -unresponsive types can be distinguished by evaluation of urinary chloride concentration. The chloride-responsive alkaloses are associated with a low urine chloride (<20 meq/L), whereas the chloride-unresponsive state will have high urine chlorides (>20 meq/L). Another distinction is that the chloride-responsive alkaloses will improve with infusion of saline, whereas the chloride-unresponsive states will not. In both cases a potential complication of saline infusion is a worsening of hypokalemia; in the first case, owing to the rapid excretion of bicarbonate, which will increase potassium excretion, and in the second case, owing to the increased Na^+ delivery to the aldosterone-acting site in the situation where aldosterone is not able to be suppressed.

A particular cause of metabolic alkalosis is seen in severe hypoalbuminemia. In this case, observed mostly in severely malnourished patients, the anion bicarbonate is increased as the anion of albumin is decreased. Chloride is low neither in the blood nor in the urine.

Some important facts in metabolic alkalosis include these:

1. Hypokalemia in vomiting is due to renal potassium wasting, which may be severe.

2. Treatment of alkalosis depends on adequate KCl as well as NaCl replacement.

3. Urine Na^+ may be high, despite volume depletion in the early stages of gastric alkalosis; the best indicator to support the volume-depleted state is the low urinary chloride.

4. Paradoxical aciduria is noted in the established phase of gastric alkalosis, as mechanisms to preserve volume and K^+ lead to increased HCO_3^- reabsorption and maintenance of metabolic alkalosis.

5. Respiratory compensation is not so predictable in metabolic alkalosis.

RESPIRATORY ACIDOSIS

Respiratory acidosis involves the primary retention of CO_2 through alveolar hypoventilation. The most common causes of respiratory acidosis are listed in table 58.8. The compensatory response by the kidneys is to generate new bicarbonate by the excretion of an increased amount of NH_4^+. A high P_{CO_2} also increases renal HCO_3 reabsorption to help maintain the compensatory response. A patient with kidney disease may not compensate well for respiratory acidosis. The pH is more acidic acutely as it takes days to achieve renal compensation which, though incomplete, significantly raises blood pH towards normal. The effects of hypercapnia include cerebral edema. A rapid drop in P_{CO_2}, as by ventilation, in a patient with compensated respiratory acidosis may result in posthypercapnic metabolic alkalosis as the P_{CO_2} falls more rapidly than the HCO_3. This may be managed either by slowly decreasing P_{CO_2} or by administration of adequate chloride salts to allow disposition of the $[HCO_3]$.

RESPIRATORY ALKALOSIS

In respiratory alkalosis, carbon dioxide elimination transiently exceeds production, leading to a decreased P_{CO_2}

Table 58.8 CAUSES OF RESPIRATORY ACIDOSIS

CNS depression
Trauma/infections/tumor
Cerebrovascular
Accidents
Drug overdose
Neuromuscular disorders
Myopathies
Thoracic disorders
   Hydrothorax
   Pneumothorax
   Lung disorder
   Bronchial obstruction
   Emphysema (chronic obstructive airway disease)
   Severe pulmonary edema

Table 58.9 CAUSES OF RESPIRATORY ALKALOSIS

| CNS disturbances |
| Psychogenic (anxiety) |
| Pregnancy |
| Hypoxia |
| Drug toxicity/overdose |
| Pulmonary disorders |
| Embolism |

and increased pH. As listed in table 58.9, causes include diseases of the central nervous system, fever, hypoxemia, anxiety, and pulmonary diseases. The compensatory decrease in HCO_3 reabsorption leads to the renal excretion of sodium bicarbonate and retention of chloride. The alkalemia is more severe acutely and can lead to headaches, nausea, vomiting, and even syncope or tetany. pH can approach normal in the chronic state, as in pregnancy. CNS effects of respiratory alkalosis include transient cerebral vasoconstriction. Metabolic effects of respiratory alkalosis include low phosphorus and high lactate levels, both related to increased cellular glycolytic activity.

POTASSIUM AND ACID–BASE BALANCE

The serum potassium in acid–base disorders is frequently associated with losses or gains of electrolyte-containing fluids. However, there are effects on the shift of K^+ from or into cells. Acidosis may raise potassium as potassium leaves cells, whereas alkalosis may decrease potassium as potassium enters cells. In general, metabolic disturbances have a greater effect on these distributions than do respiratory disturbances. Hyperchloremic acidosis has more effects to raise K than organic acidosis. But most importantly, the relationship of pH and potassium does not always hold. Look for other processes involving potassium, such as diarrhea, ketoacidosis, vomiting, and renal tubular acidosis.

ADDITIONAL READING

Frithsen IL, Simpson WM Jr. Recognition and management of acute medication poisoning. *Am Fam Physician.* 2010;81(3):316–23.

Kraut JA, Kurtz I. Toxic alcohol ingestions: Clinical features, diagnosis, and management. *Clin J Am Soc Nephrol.* 2008;3(1):208–25.

Kraut JA, Madias NE. Approach to patients with acid–base disorders. *Respir Care.* 2001;46(4):392–403.

Kraut JA, Madias NE. Serum anion gap: Its uses and limitations in clinical medicine. *Clin J Am Soc Nephrol.* 2007;2(1):162–74.

Kraut JA, Madias NE. Metabolic acidosis: Pathophysiology, diagnosis and management. *Nat Rev Nephrol.* 2010;6(5):274–85.

QUESTIONS

QUESTION 1. A 34-year-old man presents with chronic renal failure, complaining of dyspnea on exertion, fatigue, and nausea. HCT 28, pH 7.30, HCO_3 15, Pco_2 30. Which statement is true?

A. This patient has a simple metabolic acidosis due to failure to produce NH_3, with expected compensation.

B. This patient has a primary metabolic acidosis from chronic renal failure and a primary respiratory alkalosis from anemia.

C. The patient has an elevated anion gap metabolic acidosis with expected compensation.

D. This patient has a hyperchloremic metabolic acidosis from a renal tubular acidosis; one should consider myeloma.

E. The symptoms of dyspnea, fatigue, and nausea are from uremia and could not be from his acidemia.

QUESTION 2. A 54-year-old woman with Sjögren syndrome has polyuria (U_{osm} 200), hypokalemia, and hyperchloremic metabolic acidosis.

Expected urine electrolytes are:

A. Na 90, K 60,Cl 50
B. Na 50, K 60, Cl 110
C. Na 20, K 35, Cl 80
D. Na 25, K 35, Cl 20

QUESTION 3. Distinguishing features of proximal versus distal RTA in a 65-year-old man with hyperchloremic acidosis include all EXCEPT:

A. Less severe acidosis in proximal
B. Absence of bone demineralization in proximal
C. Presence of Fanconi syndrome in proximal
D. Hypokalemia worse after treatment in proximal
E. Less HCO_3 needed to treat a proximal RTA

QUESTION 4. A 79-year-old woman presents to the emergency department with a history of severe constipation, lethargy, and weakness. Past medical history is of chronic obstructive pulmonary disease (COPD), hypothyroidism, and osteoporosis. Her medications include Dulcolax, L-thyroxine, Tums, and Caltrate 600+D. On physical examination, she is drowsy and oriented only in place but not date. Her JVP is 6 cm, blood pressure 106/72 mm Hg with a heart rate of 98 beats per minute. Cardiovascular, lung, and abdominal examinations are unremarkable. Her neurological examination is nonfocal. She has mild reduction in skin turgor and no edema. Her electrolytes are as follows: Na 140 meq/L, K 3.9 meq/L, Cl 94 meq/L, CO$_2$ 37 meq/L, BUN 51 mg/dL, creatinine 2.4 mg/dL, glucose 110 mg/dL, Ca 13.8 mg/dL, serum albumin 3.4 mg/dL

The most likely diagnosis is:

A. Chronic respiratory acidosis from COPD
B. Metabolic alkalosis and milk-alkali syndrome
C. Paget disease

D. Adrenal insufficiency

E. Hyperthyroidism

QUESTION 5. A 78-year-old man presents to the emergency department with a 2-day history of confusion and bloody diarrhea. Blood chemistries drawn in the ED are as follows:

Na 138 meq/L, K 4.0 meq/L, Cl 104 meq/L, CO_2 16 meq/L, Cl 104 meq/L, serum creatinine 1.4 mg/dL, BUN 29 mg/dL, glucose 129 mg/dL.

With an appropriate physiological response (i.e., well-compensated state), his predicted P_{CO_2} should be, in mm Hg:

A. P_{CO_2} 32

B. P_{CO_2} 45

C. P_{CO_2} 16

D. P_{CO_2} 20

E. P_{CO_2} 55

ANSWERS

1. A
2. D
3. E
4. B
4. D
5. A

59.

DIALYSIS AND TRANSPLANTATION

J. Kevin Tucker

According to projections from the United States Renal Data Service (USRDS), >600,000 individuals in the United States will have end-stage renal disease (ESRD) by 2010. The leading cause of ESRD in the United State is diabetes, followed by hypertension. As the care of diabetic patients has improved, particularly in the area of cardiovascular disease, they are living through their cardiovascular complications long enough to develop ESRD. As a consequence, since the inception of the Medicare ESRD program. the dialysis population has gradually become older with increasing numbers of comorbid conditions. Renal replacement therapy in the form of hemodialysis or peritoneal dialysis may serve as a bridge to the best form of renal replacement, renal transplantation. The demand for suitable kidneys for transplantation far exceeds the supply, leaving many patients on dialysis for extended periods of time.

PREPARING THE PATIENT FOR RENAL REPLACEMENT THERAPY

Preparing a patient for renal replacement therapy requires a multidisciplinary team approach among the primary care provider, nephrologist, renal social worker, dietician, nephrology nurse educator, dialysis access surgeon, and the transplant surgeon. The primary care provider must ensure timely referral to the nephrologist when chronic kidney disease (CKD) is recognized so that appropriate diagnostic testing may be done and appropriate steps to retard progression may be taken. The social worker plays a critical role in helping patients to cope with the psychological impact of impending ESRD. Furthermore, patients with advanced chronic kidney disease often have financial and insurance issues, and the social worker's input on these issues is essential. The renal dietician helps patients to understand the importance of nutritional management in both the predialysis and the dialysis setting. As an example, dietary potassium restriction is an important element in treating the hyperkalemia associated with type 4 renal tubular

acidosis, which is common in patients with stages 4 and 5 CKD. The nephrology nurse educator, working in conjunction with the nephrologist, educates patients and their families regarding the various modalities of renal replacement therapy and helps patients make a well-informed decision regarding the most appropriate form of renal replacement. The dialysis access surgeon creates the vascular access for hemodialysis or places a peritoneal dialysis catheter if the patient chooses this modality for renal replacement. The access surgeon continues to follow the patient through the course of renal replacement therapy for any dialysis access-related issues. The transplant surgeon and transplant team should see the patient early for evaluation for renal transplantation. In some cases, if an appropriate living donor is available, the patient may be transplanted preemptively, thus avoiding completely the need for dialysis.

HEMODIALYSIS VERSUS PERITONEAL DIALYSIS

In the United States, only about 8% of incident dialysis patients choose peritoneal dialysis, whereas the numbers of patients choosing peritoneal dialysis in Canada, the United Kingdom, Europe, and Asia are proportionally higher. Peritoneal dialysis is underutilized in the United States for several reasons. First, incident dialysis patients are becoming older, and older patients are less likely to choose a home dialysis modality because they find the procedure technically challenging. Second, the expansion of ambulatory dialysis facilities across the United States has made hemodialysis readily accessible to most patients. When patients are adequately educated regarding the two modalities, more patients choose peritoneal dialysis.

Most patients are capable of successful treatment with either hemodialysis or peritoneal dialysis; however, there are some physical conditions that may limit a patient's choices. As an example, the patient with crippling rheumatoid arthritis and ESRD may not have the manual dexterity required to perform peritoneal dialysis. A patient who has had multiple abdominal surgeries may have abdominal adhesions that would impede solute transport across the peritoneal membrane, rendering peritoneal dialysis ineffective. The patient with an abdominal hernia needs to have it repaired prior to performing peritoneal dialysis. Similarly, there are physical limitations that make peritoneal dialysis the preferred dialytic modality. Severe congestive heart failure with chronic volume overload and chronic hypotension make volume removal (ultrafiltration) with hemodialysis difficult. The continuous nature of volume removal with peritoneal dialysis makes it better tolerated from a hemodynamic standpoint. Finally, patients who have been on hemodialysis for a number of years and have run out of vascular access sites may have to switch to peritoneal dialysis if transplantation is not imminent. Large body mass index or body habitus per se are no longer considered contraindications to peritoneal dialysis. The most recent Kidney Foundation's Disease Outcomes Quality Initiative (KDOQI) targets for adequacy of dialysis are generally achievable even in large patients.

Although most patients are suitable for hemodialysis or peritoneal dialysis, in some situations one modality may confer specific advantages. Residual renal function is an important determinant of survival in both hemodialysis and peritoneal dialysis. Patients who are treated with peritoneal dialysis maintain their residual renal function for longer periods than do patients who are treated with hemodialysis. (This residual renal function is also relied on more for total solute clearance with peritoneal dialysis than with hemodialysis.) A young patient newly diagnosed with ESRD is likely to need the full spectrum of renal replacement therapies, that is, hemodialysis, peritoneal dialysis, and transplantation over the course of his or her lifetime. Therefore, in a young patient it is logical to start with peritoneal dialysis as a bridge to transplantation while there is still excellent residual renal function. If the transplant fails and the patient has to return to dialysis 10–20 years later, the upper extremities are preserved for vascular access.

Most studies suggest that hemodialysis and peritoneal dialysis are equivalent with respect to long-term survival; however, peritoneal dialysis may offer a survival advantage within the first 2 years of dialysis. Randomized studies of survival with the two dialysis modalities are difficult to perform because of the importance of patient choice with respect to dialysis modality, thus limiting recruitment for such studies.

TECHNICAL ASPECTS
OF HEMODIALYSIS

Hemodialysis is a two-step process of removing solutes and fluid from the blood. The two processes are solute removal by *diffusion* and *convection* and fluid removal by *ultrafiltration*. Blood is removed through a vascular access—a fistula, graft, or catheter—and run through the dialysis circuit,

which includes an artificial kidney or dialyzer. By the principle of diffusion, solutes are removed from the blood, which is pumped through the dialyzer, and move down their concentration gradient into the dialysate compartment. The dialysate solution is lower in solute concentration and runs countercurrent through the dialyzer. A transmembrane pressure gradient is applied across the dialysis membrane, allowing the ultrafiltration of fluid. With ultrafiltration of fluid, some solutes are removed by convection.

In the United States hemodialysis is most commonly performed three times weekly. There is, however, increasing interest in more frequent forms of dialysis including daily home dialysis and nocturnal in-center hemodialysis. In the latter modality, patients are dialyzed for 6–8 hours overnight three times per week, whereas the usual time on hemodialysis is typically 3.5–4 hours. Data from the Frequent Hemodialysis Network Trial group indicate that when compared to conventional thrice-weekly hemodialysis, hemodialysis six times per week may confer advantages with respect to cardiac function, control of hypertension, and control of serum phosphate.

TECHNICAL ASPECTS OF
PERITONEAL DIALYSIS

Peritoneal dialysis utilizes the peritoneal membrane with its vast vascular supply as the dialysis membrane. A peritoneal dialysis catheter is placed surgically, usually at least 2 to 3 weeks prior to initiation of dialysis. Patients are trained to perform peritoneal dialysis in one of two ways: *continuous ambulatory peritoneal dialysis* (CAPD) or *automated peritoneal dialysis* (APD). In CAPD, dialysate is instilled into the peritoneal cavity through the peritoneal dialysis catheter (figure 59.1). The dialysate contains dextrose, which acts as the osmotic driving force for fluid removal. Solutes move across the peritoneal membrane down their concentration gradient into the dialysate compartment. At the end of a period of 4–6 hours, the patient drains the dialysate and instills fresh dialysate into the peritoneal cavity. In states of volume overload, the patient may remove more fluid at his or her own discretion by increasing the concentration of dextrose in the dialysate. In APD, the patient uses an automated device that assists in performing dialysis, usually overnight with a cycler. The cycler performs several exchanges overnight such that the patient most often does not have to perform manual exchanges during the day. Because of the convenience of APD, more patients in North America are choosing this peritoneal dialysis modality over CAPD.

VASCULAR ACCESS

Vascular access remains the Achilles heel of hemodialysis. Dialysis access complications are a major source of morbidity

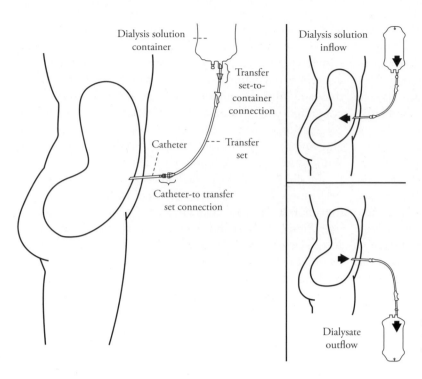

Figure 59.1. Continuous Ambulatory Peritoneal Dialysis (CAPD). In CAPD, dialysate is instilled into the peritoneal cavity through the peritoneal dialysis catheter.

Dialysis solution container

Transfer set-to-container connection

Catheter

Transfer set

Catheter-to transfer set connection

Dialysis solution inflow

Dialysate outflow

for ESRD patients and account for >$1 billion per year in health care expenditures.

The three primary types of hemodialysis access devices are the arteriovenous (AV) fistula, the arteriovenous graft, and the dialysis catheter. The native AV fistula (figure 59.2A) is the best and the preferred long-term dialysis access. It offers several advantages over the other hemodialysis access types: (1) It has the longest life. (2) Because it has no synthetic material, it rarely becomes infected. (3) It requires fewer interventions to maintain patency. The AV fistula is created by anastomosis of an artery to a vein, usually in the nondominant arm. The most commonly created fistulae are the radiocephalic (Brescio-Cimino) fistula at the wrist and the brachiocephalic fistula at the elbow. The vascular access surgeon may use preoperative venous mapping with ultrasound to determine the best site for fistula creation.

An AV fistula may require 2–3 months to mature, that is, to be of sufficient caliber such that it can be cannulated with two 16-gauge needles and support a blood flow through the dialysis circuit of 300–450 mL/min. Therefore, the patient with stage 4–5 CKD should be referred to the vascular access surgeon at least 6 months before the initiation of dialysis. KDOQI guidelines suggest that patients be referred for vascular access when the serum creatinine is >4 mg/dL or the glomerular filtration rate is <25 mL/min. The failure to refer the CKD patient for vascular access in a timely manner puts that patient at risk of starting dialysis with a catheter, which in and of itself carries a greater mortality risk than starting dialysis with an AV fistula. Patients with CKD should also be educated regarding the importance of preserving veins for vascular access. Venipuncture should be avoided in the nondominant arm in order to better preserve those veins for vascular access.

When the vasculature is not suitable for creation of an AV fistula based on physical examination or preoperative ultrasound venous mapping, the surgeon and nephrologist may decide that the best option is placement of an AV graft (figure 59.2B). The AV graft is created by interposing a synthetic material such as polytetrafluoroethane (PTFE)

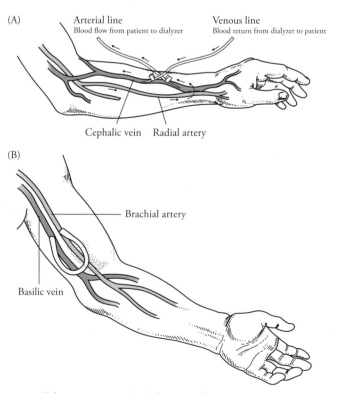

(A)

Arterial line
Blood flow from patient to dialyzer

Venous line
Blood return from dialyzer to patient

Cephalic vein   Radial artery

(B)

Brachial artery

Basilic vein

Figure 59.2 (A) Native AV Fistula. (B) AV Graft.

between the artery and the vein. The most commonly placed AV grafts are the straight graft between the radial artery and the basilic vein and the loop graft between the brachial artery and the basilic vein. AV grafts have the advantage of being suitable for dialysis within 2–3 weeks of creation. However, grafts thrombose more frequently than fistulae and require more interventions to remain patent, and even with interventions to maintain patency, most grafts last only about 2 years.

Dialysis catheters are generally reserved for patients who have no other vascular access options or for patients who require a catheter as a "bridge" until a fistula is mature. Dual-lumen cuffed catheters are placed in the internal jugular vein and tunneled through subcutaneous tissues, usually under ultrasound guidance. The subclavian vein should be avoided because of the risk of subclavian vein thrombosis, which renders the whole upper extremity unsuitable for future vascular access creation. Nontunneled, noncuffed catheters are often used in cases of acute kidney injury in which a short course of dialysis (1–2 weeks at most) is anticipated. These catheters may be placed at the bedside with ultrasound guidance in the internal jugular or femoral vein. If the patient needs a longer course of dialysis, the nontunneled, noncuffed catheter should be exchanged for a more permanent tunneled, cuffed catheter.

INFECTIONS COMPLICATIONS RELATED TO DIALYSIS ACCESS

Infectious complications are the second most common cause of mortality for patients with ESRD. ESRD patients may have impaired cellular and humoral immunity. Furthermore, hemodialysis and peritoneal dialysis catheters carry infection risks because they are foreign bodies.

Hemodialysis catheter infections occur at a rate of 2 to 5.5 per 1000 patient days. Catheter-related bacteremia should be suspected in any patient who has fever and/or shaking chills. Empirical antibiotic therapy to cover both Gram-positive and Gram-negative organisms should begin after blood cultures have been obtained. The "gold standard" treatment for hemodialysis catheter–related infections is to remove the catheter and to place a new tunneled catheter after the patient has been afebrile for 48 hours and surveillance blood cultures are documented as negative. This approach, however, may require that the patient remain in the hospital for several days and that the patient have a temporary (nontunneled, noncuffed) catheter placed for dialysis.

As an alternative approach to treating dialysis catheter–related bacteremia, some centers have successfully used the strategy of catheter exchange over a guidewire when there is no sign of a tunnel infection and the patient shows rapid clinical improvement with antibiotic therapy. Another treatment approach is to "lock" the infected catheter with an antibiotic solution in order to eliminate the layer of biofilm that adheres to the catheter surface.

Regardless of which treatment approach is used, the patient with catheter-related bacteremia warrants close monitoring for development of signs of a metastatic infection such as endocarditis, septic arthritis, osteomyelitis, discitis, or epidural abscess. These metastatic infections often are not clinically apparent for weeks to months following the episode of bacteremia. *Staphylococcus aureus* is the most virulent organism with respect to metastatic infections, and attempts at catheter salvage in cases of *S. aureus* bacteremia may lead to unacceptably high rates of metastatic infections.

The major infectious complication related to peritoneal dialysis is peritonitis. Peritonitis is one of the major causes of failure of the modality and transfer to hemodialysis.

Peritonitis may be asymptomatic, with the patient noticing only that the dialysate effluent is cloudy. When symptoms develop, they typically include abdominal pain, fever, nausea, and vomiting. The workup for peritonitis should include laboratory examination of the effluent for cell count, Gram stain, and culture. A cell count >100/µL with more than 50% PMNs is suggestive of peritonitis. Empirical antibiotics should be administered to cover both Gram-positive and Gram-negative organisms. Antibiotics may be administered intravenously or by the intraperitoneal route by adding them to the dialysis solution. If the cultures are positive for more than one organism, abdominal imaging and surgical consultation should be obtained because polymicrobial peritonitis is often associated with an intra-abdominal catastrophe such as a perforated viscus. Peritonitis with mycobacterium or fungus almost always mandates removal of the catheter because these organisms are very difficult to eradicate with antimicrobial therapy alone.

Nasal carriage of *S. aureus* is a major risk factor for exit-site infections, tunnel infections, and peritonitis with this organism. The application of an antibiotic cream to the exit site has been shown to reduce peritoneal dialysis infections. Mupirocin applied to the exit site daily reduces rates of *S. aureus* infections; however, it does not help with Gram-negative infections, particularly *Pseudomonas*. More recent data indicate that gentamicin cream applied to the exit site prevents peritoneal dialysis catheter–related infections from both Gram-positive and Gram-negative organisms.

ANEMIA MANAGEMENT

The anemia of chronic kidney disease usually becomes apparent before patients require renal replacement therapy. Although deficiency of the sialoglycoprotein erythropoietin (EPO) is an important cause of the anemia of CKD, numerous other factors play a role (table 59.1), including iron deficiency, chronic inflammation, occult blood loss,

Table 59.1 CAUSES OF EPO RESISTANCE

Iron deficiency

Infection

Chronic inflammation

Hyperparathyroidism

Occult blood loss

Malignancy

Folate and B-12 deficiencies

Hemoglobinopathies

Aluminum intoxication

and secondary hyperparathyroidism. The mainstays of treatment of anemia in dialysis patients are administration of EPO and intravenous iron. EPO is typically administered intravenously to hemodialysis patients and subcutaneously to peritoneal dialysis patients. Intravenous iron is given in the hemodialysis unit to maintain the transferrin saturation (serum iron/total iron binding capacity × 100%) at >20%. The administration of intravenous iron improves the bone marrow response to EPO and reduces the total amount of EPO required to maintain the hemoglobin at its target. Lower doses of EPO confer substantial cost savings to the health care system because EPO costs are a major expenditure for the ESRD program. Intravenous iron is available in several different preparations in the United States: iron sucrose (Venofer®), iron gluconate (Ferrlecit®), ferumoxytol (Feraheme®), and iron dextran. Iron dextran is used less commonly because of the risk of anaphylactic reactions associated with these preparations.

The recommended targets for hemoglobin in both CKD patients and dialysis patients have come under increased scrutiny since the publication of several studies showing that higher hemoglobins are associated with worse outcomes in both predialysis and dialysis patients. KDOQI suggests a target hemoglobin in the range of 11–12 g/dL for both nondialysis patient and dialysis patients who are receiving erythropoiesis-stimulating agents (ESAs). Regular (at least monthly) monitoring of the hemoglobin is imperative for any patient who is receiving an ESA in order to avoid potentially dangerous overcorrection of anemia.

BONE DISEASE AND MINERAL METABOLISM MANAGEMENT

Disordered mineral metabolism may begin in CKD patients as early as stage 2. Prompt evaluation and treatment of mineral disorders is important to prevent more severe complications by the time the patient requires renal replacement therapy. As the GFR goes below about 40 mL/min,

phosphorus levels begin to rise due to the diseased kidneys' inability to excrete it, and levels of vitamin 1,25-$(OH)_2D_3$ (calcitriol) begin to fall because of decreased levels of the enzyme 1-alpha-hydroxylase, which is present in renal tubular cells. The rise in serum phosphate levels and the fall in serum calcium both feed back on the parathyroid gland to increase production of parathyroid hormone (PTH). High levels of PTH lead to a condition of high bone turnover and resorption, osteitis fibrosa.

Dietary phosphate restriction is an important early step in preventing secondary hyperparathyroidism. In animal studies, a rise in PTH can be prevented by stringent dietary phosphate restriction. In CKD patients, particularly dialysis patients for whom malnutrition may already be an issue, phosphate binders are given with meals to control serum phosphate levels (table 59.2). Aluminum hydroxide is the most potent binder of dietary phosphorus but should not be used chronically because of the risk of aluminum toxicity. It may be used in short courses of 2–3 days for severe hyperphosphatemia. Calcium acetate and calcium carbonate are commonly used phosphate binders but carry the risk of causing hypercalcemia, especially when given with a vitamin D analogue. Sevelamer hydrochloride, sevelamer carbonate, and lanthanum carbonate are non–calcium-based binders that should be used preferentially when serum calcium levels are higher than target (see table 59.3). Sevelamer also has the advantage of lowering LDL cholesterol.

When PTH exceeds target despite dietary phosphate control, the next step is addition of an analogue of vitamin 1,25$(OH)_2D_3$, which acts to suppress PTH production. Vitamin D analogues used in the United States are calcitriol (Rocaltrol®), paricalcitol (Zemplar®), and doxercalciferol (Hectorol®). Serum calcium and phosphorus must be monitored with use of vitamin D analogues because they promote intestinal absorption of both calcium and phosphorus. Hypercalcemia is more likely to occur when

Table 59.2 PHOSPHATE BINDERS

BINDER	COMMENTS
Aluminum hydroxide	Potent risk of aluminum toxicity; use only for short courses in cases of severe hyperphosphatemia
Calcium carbonate	Cost effective; runs risk of high serum calcium when coupled with vitamin D analogue
Calcium acetate	Same as with calcium carbonate
Sevelamer hydrochloride	Non–calcium-based binder; preferred for patients with hypercalcemia; risk of metabolic acidosis
Sevelamer carbonate	No risk of metabolic acidosis
Lanthanum carbonate	Alternative non–calcium-based binder

Table 59.3 KDOQI TARGETS FOR BONE AND
MINERAL METABOLISM

Calcium	8.4–9.5 mg/dL
Phosphorus	3.5–5.5 mg/dL
Calcium × Phosphorus	<55 mg^2/dL^2
Parathyroid hormone	150–300 pg/mL

vitamin D analogues are used with a calcium-based phosphate binder. Vitamin D analogues are usually given intravenously to hemodialysis patients and orally to peritoneal dialysis patients. 25-OH-Vitamin D deficiency is also common in dialysis patients. Although it is likely to be beneficial to replete vitamin D in such patients because of the extraosseal effects of vitamin D, there are no data that show doing so is effective in treating secondary hyperparathyroidism.

More severe cases of hyperparathyroidism may not respond to vitamin D analogues but may respond to the calcimimetic agent cinacalcet (Sensipar®), which acts on the parathyroid glands' calcium-sensing receptor to inhibit PTH release. Gastrointestinal side effects and hypokalemia requiring supplemental calcium are common with cinacalcet, and it is considerably more expensive than vitamin D analogues. Parathyroidectomy should be considered for patients with musculoskeletal symptoms for whom medical therapy has not been effective.

EVALUATION OF THE PATIENT FOR KIDNEY TRANSPLANTATION

Medical evaluation of a potential kidney transplant recipient is important to ensure that the recipient is stable enough to undergo the surgical procedure without adverse perioperative, particularly cardiovascular, complications and that there are no unrecognized medical problems that may be adversely affected by immunosuppression, such as occult infections and occult malignancies. Given the prevalence of coronary artery disease and left ventricular dysfunction in patients with CKD particular attention should be paid to screening for coronary artery disease. Most transplant centers utilize pharmacologic stress testing followed by cardiac catheterization and revascularization if indicated. The timing of cardiac catheterization with respect to initiation of dialysis must be considered in patients being considered for preemptive transplantation. In such patients the dye load from cardiac catheterization may cause a steep enough decline in glomerular filtration rate such that dialysis must be initiated. Patients being considered for kidney transplantation should also be screened for viral infections including HIV, hepatitis B, hepatitis C, cytomegalovirus (CMV), and Epstein-Barr virus (EBV) as well as for syphilis. Although HIV is no longer considered an absolute contraindication to

renal transplantation, the viral load must be well controlled, and the transplant center should have expertise in managing this special transplant population. Patients with hepatitis C antibodies and positive titers for hepatitis RNA may need a pretransplant liver biopsy to determine the degree, if any, of underlying fibrosis or cirrhosis. The routine vaccination of dialysis patients against hepatitis B has greatly reduced the number of potential renal transplant recipients who are hepatitis B surface antigen positive. In the case of these patients who have evidence of active viral replication, antiviral therapy should be considered prior to kidney transplantation. CMV-naive recipients who receive a kidney from a CMV-positive donor are at greater risk for CMV-associated disease in the posttransplant setting. Similarly, an EBV-negative recipient who receives a transplant from an EBV-positive donor is at greater risk for posttransplant lymphoproliferative disorder (PTLD), especially if heavily immunosuppressed. Screening for occult malignancies generally follows age-appropriate guidelines for the general population. Female recipients should have a Pap smear and a mammogram if older than 40 years of age. Men should have a PSA if older than 50 years of age. All recipients over the age of 50 should have fecal occult blood testing with colonoscopy if positive.

Active malignancy, active infection, severe cardiovascular disease that makes the patient a high operative risk, and severe obesity are generally considered contraindications to transplantation. Psychiatric illness and medical noncompliance are often considered in the evaluation process. Psychiatric illness per se may be a contraindication if it interferes with the patient's ability to comply with the posttransplant regimen. Similarly medical noncompliance is a relative contraindication. There are many patients who have been noncompliant with dialysis and medications but fully compliant with posttransplant medications and follow-up.

TRANSPLANT MEDICATIONS

Transplant medications have revolutionized the field of transplant medicine such that acute rejection rates reported to the United States Renal Data System are now <10%. Newer medications are more specific and able to target differing parts of the immune system (table 59.4). Glucocorticoids remain an important part of many immunosuppression protocols, although there is increasing interest in steroid-free protocols. Glucocorticoids are also useful in treating acute rejection, usually as pulses of methylprednisolone at doses of 500–1000 mg/day for 3 days. The side effects of glucocorticoids are well known, including weight gain, diabetes, osteoporosis, osteonecrosis, myopathy, and cataracts.

Azathioprine has been used since the early days of transplantation, so there is much collective experience with this medication. It acts by inhibiting purine biosynthesis, thereby limiting lymphocyte replication. When used in conjunction

Table 59.4 DRUGS USED IN KIDNEY TRANSPLANTATION FOR IMMUNOSUPPRESSION

DRUGS	COMMENTS
Glucocorticoids	Block synthesis of cytokines including IL-2; side effects: weight gain, diabetes mellitus, cataracts, osteoporosis, osteonecrosis
Azathioprine	Imuran®: inhibits purine biosynthesis; side effects: bone marrow suppression; major interaction with allopurinol
Mycophenolate mofetil	CellCept®; selective effect on lymphocyte replication; side effects: bone marrow suppression and GI toxicity
Cyclosporine	Neoral® and others; calcineurin inhibitor; side effects: gingvial hyperplasia, hirsutism, hypertension
Tacrolimus	Prograf®; calcineurin inhibitor; side effects: diabetes mellitus, hypertension, neurotoxicity
Sirolimus	Rapamycin; mTOR inhibitor; side effects: hyperlipidemia and bone marrow suppression
Monoclonal antibodies	Basiliximab (Simulect®); Daclizumab (Zenapax®); block activated T cells expressing IL-2 receptor
Polyclonal antibodies	ATGAM and Thymoglobulin; nonspecifically block T cells

with allopurinol for the treatment of gout, severe bone marrow suppression may occur since azathioprine is partially metabolized by xanthine oxidase, the enzyme inhibited by allopurinol.

Mycophenolate mofetil (MMF) is a newer drug that has replaced azathioprine in many transplant centers' immunosuppression protocols. MMF inhibits inosine monophosphate dehydrogenase, the rate limiting enzyme in de novo purine biosynthesis, and its effect is relatively lymphocyte specific. The major toxicities of MMF are gastrointestinal—nausea, vomiting, and diarrhea—and bone marrow suppression.

There are two drugs that belong to the category of calcineurin inhibitors: cyclosporine and tacrolimus (FK 506). The calcineurin inhibitors inhibit synthesis of interleukin-2 (IL-2) and other molecules that are important for T-cell activation. Importantly, the calcineurin inhibitors are themselves nephrotoxic, and drug levels must be monitored. Because cyclosporine and tacrolimus are metabolized by the cytochrome P450 system, drugs that activate the P450 system may cause cyclosporine or tacrolimus levels to rise or fall (see table 59.5). Side effects related to cyclosporine include gingival hyperplasia, hypertension, hirsutism, neurotoxicity, and posttransplant diabetes mellitus. Tacrolimus has a similar side-effect profile, although it is thought to cause less hirsutism and is not generally associated with gingival hyperplasia. It is, however, more neurotoxic and more associated with posttransplant diabetes mellitus than cyclosporine.

Sirolimus is a macrolide antibiotic that blocks the proliferative response of T and B cells to cytokines. Sirolimus binds to the same intracellular protein to which tacrolimus binds, the FK binding protein, but it does not block calcineurin. Its mechanism of action is by inhibition of a kinase called the mammalian target of rapamycin (mTOR). The major side effects of sirolimus, in addition to bone marrow suppression, are hyperlipidemia and interstitial pneumonitis.

Antilymphocyte antibodies come in two forms: polyclonal antibodies and OKT3, a mouse monoclonal antibody raised against the CD3 receptor complex on human T cells. The polyclonal antibodies are raised in horses or rabbits by immunization with human lymphoid tissue. These antibodies are nonspecific immunosuppressive agents targeting all T cells. They may be used as induction immunosuppression or to reverse episodes of acute rejection.

Humanized or chimeric anti-IL-2 receptor antibodies have also been developed as induction immunosuppression for kidney transplant recipients. These drugs are more specific forms of immunosuppression because the full IL-2 receptor is expressed only on activated T cells.

INFECTIOUS POSTTRANSPLANT COMPLICATIONS

Infections occurring in the kidney transplant recipient differ depending on the time period posttransplant. Those

Table 59.5 DRUGS/SUBSTANCES THAT INCREASE AND DECREASE CYCLOSPORINE LEVELS

INCREASE	DECREASE
Diltiazem	Barbiturates
Verapamil	Phenytoin
Nicardipine	Carbamazepine
Amlodipine	Isoniazid
Ketoconazole	Rifampin
Fluconazole	
Erythromycin	
Clarithromycin	
Grapefruit juice	

infections occurring in the first month posttransplant are associated with the surgical procedure itself. These include surgical wound infections, infections related to vascular catheters, and urinary tract infections. General surgical procedures designed to minimize infections in the postoperative period, such as removing indwelling catheters as soon as feasible, help to minimize risk of these early infections. Prophylaxis with trimethoprim-sulfamethoxazole also may help to prevent urinary tract infections.

Within 1–6 months posttransplant, the risk of opportunistic infections increases. Infection with organisms such as CMV, EBV, *Pneumocystis carinii*, *Nocardia*, and *Listeria monocytogenes* may occur during this time period unless prevented by prophylaxis with antiviral drugs such as valganciclovir or antibacterial agents such as trimethoprim-sulfamethoxazole.

More than 6 months following transplantation the risk of opportunistic infections decreases as the amount of immunosuppression needed to maintain allograft function diminishes. Patients who require relatively high-dose immunosuppression during this time period because of poor allograft function or because of an episode of acute rejection are at higher risk and should remain on appropriate antimicrobial prophylaxis for longer periods of time. CMV infection is one of the more severe late infectious complications that may occur, particularly in patients who are heavily immunosuppressed. Those at highest risk are CMV-naive recipients who receive a kidney from a CVM-positive donor. Symptoms and signs of CMV disease include fever, malaise, leukopenia, and allograft dysfunction. The virus is best detected by specialized antigen assays or by PCR. Treatment involves reduction in immunosuppression and antiviral therapy with intravenous ganciclovir for 2–4 weeks followed by oral antiviral therapy for 2–3 months.

NONINFECTIOUS POSTTRANSPLANT COMPLICATIONS

There are a number of complications that are unique to transplant recipients. Diabetes mellitus, hypertension, and osteoporosis are common posttransplant complications, but their management generally relies on the same principles as for the general population.

Malignancies, particularly those of squamous epithelia, occur more frequently in transplant recipients. Transplant recipients, especially those treated with azathioprine, should be monitored for the development of skin cancers and should be advised to use sunscreen. Women should undergo annual Pap smears to screen for cervical dysplasia and cervical cancer.

Posttransplant lymphoproliferative disorder (PTLD) is a unique complication of transplantation that occurs in 1–5% of renal transplant recipients. Those at highest risk are EBV-negative recipients who receive a kidney from an EBV-positive donor and those recipients who have required high total doses of immunosuppression. The pathogenesis of the disorder involves the infection and transformation of B lymphocytes by EBV. These transformed B cells undergo polyclonal proliferation from which a malignant clone may emerge. PTLD may present with fever, night sweats, and lymphadenopathy. Extranodal involvement of the kidney may present as allograft dysfunction. Other sites of extranodal involvement include the GI tract, lungs, and the central nervous system. Treatment involves first reduction of immunosuppression followed by chemotherapeutic agents if the disease does not respond to reduction in immunosuppression alone.

Posttransplant erythrocytosis (PTE), defined as a hematocrit >51%, occurs in 10–15% of renal transplant recipients. It usually occurs only in the setting of good allograft function. The mechanism is not directly related to erythropoietin, as erythropoietin levels are not necessarily elevated in PTE. PTE can be managed by phlebotomy or by administering angiotensin-converting enzyme inhibitors or angiotensin-receptor blockers, both of which have been shown to be effective at reducing the hematocrit in this condition.

ADDITIONAL READING

Chan MR, Yevzlin AS. Tunneled dialysis catheters: Recent trends and future directions. *Adv Chronic Kidney Dis.* 2009;16(5): 386–95.

Fishbane S. Cardiovascular risk evaluation before kidney transplantation. *J Am Soc Nephrol.* 2005;16:843–5.

Gaston RS, Julian BA, Curtis JJ. Post-transplant erythrocytosis: An enigma revisited. *Am J Kidney Dis.* 1994;24:1.

Goodman WG. The consequences of uncontrolled secondary hyperparathyroidism and its treatment in chronic kidney disease. *Semin Dial.* 2004;17:209–16.

Konner K, Nonnast-Daniel B, Ritz E. The arteriovenous fistula. *J Am Soc Nephrol.* 2003:14:1669–80.

Mehrotra R, Marsh D, Vonesh E, Peters V, Nissenson A. Patient education and access of ESRD patients to renal replacement therapies beyond in-center hemodialysis. *Kidney Int.* 2005;68:378–90.

Muirhead N. Update in nephrology. *Ann Intern Med.* 2010;152(11): 721–5.

Pastan S. Bailey J. Dialysis therapy. *N Engl J Med.* 1998;338:1428–37.

QUESTIONS

QUESTION 1. A 23-year-old woman with diffuse proliferative lupus nephritis has progressed to stage 4 CDK despite aggressive treatment with cytotoxic agents. A recent kidney biopsy has shown advanced fibrosis. Her BMI is 30 kg/m². All of the following are true with respect to renal replacement options EXCEPT:

A. She should be educated regarding hemodialysis, peritoneal dialysis, and transplantation.

B. She should be encouraged to lose weight prior to renal transplantation.

C. Her obesity excludes her as a candidate for peritoneal dialysis.

D. She should be referred to a vascular surgeon for immediate creation of an AV fistula if her renal replacement choice is hemodialysis.

QUESTION 2. A 52-year-old man with ESRD secondary to diabetes is maintained on an immunosuppressive regimen of cyclosporine, mycophenolate mofetil, and prednisone. He develops posttransplant hypertension. Which of the following antihypertensive medications may affect cyclosporine levels?

A. Losartan
B. Enalapril
C. Amlodipine
D. Hydrochlorothiazide

QUESTION 3. A 65-year-old man with severe osteoarthritis develops ESRD from chronic NSAID use. He develops uremic symptoms and begins hemodialysis via a tunneled catheter. Within his first month of dialysis he develops *S. aureus* bacteremia, for which he is treated with intravenous vancomycin with rapid clinical improvement. One month later he has a swollen right knee with a palpable effusion. He has low-grade fever and malaise. His anemia does not respond to EPO. Which of the following statements is (are) true regarding the pathogenesis of this patient's constellation of findings?

A. Knee joint aspiration for cell count and culture is indicated.

B. Infection and inflammation may underlie this patient's EPO unresponsiveness.

C. Nasal carriage of *S. aureus* may be a risk factor for this patient's infection.

D. Attempted salvage of tunneled catheters in the setting of *S. aureus* infection carries an unacceptably high risk of metastatic infection.

E. All of the above.

QUESTION 4. A 30-year-old woman with ESRD presents to your practice for evaluation. In review of her laboratories, she is found to have a calcium of 10.5 mg/dL and a phosphorus of 6.7 mg/dL, and she is not on a phosphate binder. Each of the following would be an appropriate phosphate binder choice EXCEPT:

A. Sevelamer carbonate
B. Lanthanum carbonate
C. Calcium acetate
D. Sevelamer hydrochloride

QUESTION 5. A 30-year-old woman with ESRD secondary to type 1 diabetes receives a kidney transplant from a live donor. The donor is EBV positive, and the recipient is EBV negative. She has early rejection requiring treatment with high-dose steroids and a monoclonal antibody but recovers good allograft function. One year later she develops fever, night sweats, pulmonary infiltrates, and a pleural effusion. Pleural fluid cytology reveals a lymphocytic infiltrate that is suspicious for lymphoma. Which of the following is the most likely diagnosis?

A. Pseudomonas pneumonia
B. Rapamycin pneumonitis
C. Posttransplant lymphoproliferative disorder
D. *Pneumocystis carinii* pneumonia

ANSWERS

1. C
2. C
3. E
4. C
5. C

60.

SYSTEMIC COMPLICATIONS OF CHRONIC KIDNEY DISEASE

Mark E. Williams

The magnitude of the public health problem due to chronic kidney disease (CKD) in the United States is gaining recognition. More than 19 million adult Americans, or 11%, have CKD, the majority with stage 1–3 disease. Many of the complicating features traditionally described in the end-stage kidney patient (ESRD) population are increasingly being noted in chronic kidney disease patients. It is now understood that complications of CKD develop earlier in the course and lead to adverse outcomes in their own right. CKD thus becomes a systemic disorder as it progresses. The major complications of CKD to be discussed—hypertension, cardiovascular disease, anemia, and bone-mineral disorders—are consistently found and are to a degree independent of the primary cause of the kidney disease.

Complications of CKD are importantly associated with the level of kidney function (see figure 60.1) and tend to worsen as CKD progresses. Just as CKD generally progresses, so do its complications. In some cases evidence for complications can be detected before symptoms become manifest, whereas in others, the stage where the complication began may be difficult to determine. One measure of the impact is that all-cause hospitalization rates are three times higher in patients with CKD than in the general population, and the majority of hospitalizations among ESRD patients are for management of complications that began with CKD. Unfortunately, at all stages of CKD, death is more common than the need for initiation of dialysis. For patients who progress to ESRD, CKD complications will be clinically significant as risk factors for morbidity and mortality during renal replacement therapy: optimization of pre-ESRD care becomes a key to improved dialysis outcomes. As a result, guidelines such as the National Kidney Foundation's Kidney Disease Outcomes Quality Initiative (KDOQI) state in their action plan that evaluation and treatment of CKD complications should begin at stage 3, when the estimated glomerular filtration rate (GFR) is <60 mL/min/1.73 m².

HYPERTENSION

Management of hypertension remains the greatest CKD challenge because of its pervasiveness, management difficulty, and ultimate consequence to the patient. Three central issues are interrelated: how to achieve blood pressure targets, how to slow kidney progression, and how to reduce cardiovascular risks.

In the general population only two-thirds of hypertensive patients are actively treated, and less than a third are controlled to the traditional targets of <140/<90 mm Hg despite the fact that high blood pressure is the factor most responsible for patient deaths worldwide. Hypertension is even more challenging when accompanied by CKD: (1) high blood pressure is more prevalent and levels are higher as CKD becomes mores severe (figure 60.2); (2) poorly controlled hypertension, whether a cause or consequence of CKD, is an independent risk factor for kidney disease progression and cardiovascular complications; (3) current guidelines for hypertension control in patients with CKD recommend a goal of <130/<80 regardless of the degree of proteinuria; and, (4) CKD is associated with even less hypertension control than the general population. In the National Health and Nutrition Examination Survey (NHANES) analysis, 70% of those with elevated creatinine levels had hypertension, and three-quarters were being treated, but only 11% were reaching treatment goals. In the United States, levels of hypertension control in CKD patients rarely reach Joint National Committee 7 (JNC7) guidelines (Chobanian et al., 2003). The elderly and blacks are even more likely to have inadequate hypertension control. In addition to determining the appropriate blood pressure goals, studies have addressed the issue of whether systolic or diastolic pressure is more important. In the general U.S. population isolated systolic hypertension is the most common form of blood pressure elevation, and systolic pressure is more closely predictive of cardiovascular events than is diastolic pressure. Evidence also indicates that elevated systolic

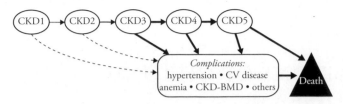

Figure 60.1. Chronic Kidney Disease Progression and Its Complications. CKD chronic kidney disease, stages 1–5, as designated by the NKF KDOQI guidelines. Risk of complications and death increase as kidney disease worsens. CKD-BMD chronic kidney disease, bone/mineral disorder. Reprinted by permission from Macmillan Publishers Ltd: Eknoyan G. Chronic kidney disease definition and classification: The quest for refinements. *Kidney Int.* 2007;72:1183. Copyright 2007.

blood pressure (>140 mm Hg) is the primary determinant of development and progression of nephropathy, especially in those over 55 years of age. Clinical practice guidelines are supportive of the importance of lowering systolic pressure in both diabetic and nondiabetic CKD patients.

The kidneys are considered the chief source of hypertension in CKD. Pathophysiology is complex, but the major factor in common kidney conditions such as glomerulonephritis, diabetic nephropathy, and hypertensive nephrosclerosis is sodium retention leading to volume expansion. Less obvious is a heightened vascular tone, attributed to vaso-

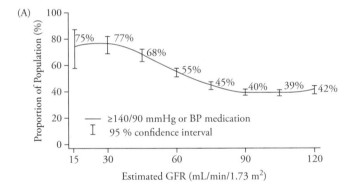

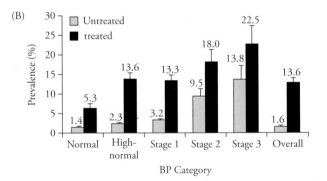

Figure 60.2. Prevalence of High Blood Pressure and Elevated Creatinine. (A) Prevalence of high blood pressure by level of GFR, from NHANES III. Values are adjusted to age 60 years. (B) Prevalence of elevated serum creatinine (vertical axis) according to hypertension category as defined by JNC VI guidelines, in treated and untreated individuals. Reprinted from National Kidney Foundation. K/DOQI Clinical Practice Guidelines for chronic kidney disease: Evaluation, classification, and stratification. *Am J Kidney Dis.* 2002;39(Suppl 1):S1–S266, with permission from Elsevier.

constrictive factors such as angiotensin and/or sympathetic activity.

It is now recognized by physicians that blood pressure reduction is critically important in preserving kidney function in hypertensive CKD patients. Uncontrolled hypertension is closely linked to CKD progression, especially in proteinuric conditions such as diabetic nephropathy, whereas control may be less beneficial in nonproteinuric disease, including hypertensive nephrosclerosis. It can also add end-organ hypertensive damage to any underlying kidney condition. The KDOQI guidelines for hypertension in proteinuric kidney disease derive from multiple treatment trials. Data suggest that tight blood pressure control reduces microalbuminuria, proteinuria, and decline in kidney function.

Current guidelines are also lacking confirmatory evidence from clinical trials in diabetic nephropathy. Few data are available on the benefit of tight blood pressure control in slowing progression of proteinuric diabetic CKD. No randomized trials directly support the systolic target of <130 mm Hg or the diastolic goal of <80 mm Hg, although a reduction in cardiovascular events was seen in the diabetic subgroup with a diastolic target of 80 mm Hg in the HOT trial. In summary, the current blood pressure targets are based on results from trials involving large numbers of CKD patients, although the <130/<80 goal has not been studied in a randomized diabetic CKD trial.

The third goal of antihypertensive therapy in CKD is to reduce cardiovascular risk. Hypertension is the dominant risk factor for cardiovascular disease (CVD) worldwide. In the general population epidemiologic studies have indicated a graded relationship of systemic pressure levels and cardiovascular disease and have indicated benefit when pressures are lowered to 140/90 mm Hg. The relevance of hypertension as an important risk factor for CVD in CKD is well established. Risks of morbidity and mortality for CV events in CKD are higher than for the general population at all stages of CKD. All patients with CKD are placed in the highest risk category for CVD. Nonetheless, interventional trials aimed at CVD risk reduction have included few CKD patients. In the absence of firm data on blood pressure levels and CVD risk in CKD, the KDOQI work group and others have extrapolated from available data to include CVD risk reduction in the adoption of the <130/<80 blood pressure goal.

The general approach to hypertension management in CKD patients is shown in table 60.1. All antihypertensive drugs can be used to lower blood pressure in CKD patients, but most patients will require a combination of several agents to reach the current targets. In determining the appropriate antihypertensive drug regimen in the CKD patient, the clinician must address (1) the degree of hypertension, (2) how to slow renal progression, and (3) CVD risk assessment. Most hypertensive CKD patients will require two or more

Table 60.1 GENERAL APPROACH TO HYPERTENSION MANAGEMENT IN CKD PATIENTS

1. Initial considerations in selecting therapy include the level of kidney impairment, the amount of proteinuria, the level of blood pressure, and the degree of cardiovascular risk.

2. Primary goal of therapy is to meet blood pressure target of <130/<80 mm Hg.

3. Secondary goals are to slow CKD progression and reduce cardiovascular disease risk.

4. Lifestyle modifications should be included in treatment recommendations.

5. ACEI/ARBs are preferred therapy for patients with proteinuria.

6. All classes of antihypertensive agents can be used in CKD hypertension.

7. Two or more antihypertensive drugs will typically be required to meet treatment goals.

8. Risk of adverse side effects will require frequent monitoring on a case-by-case basis.

drugs to achieve current targets. Whereas achieving target pressures is important for CDK patients, the initial agents should also be selected based on safety, tolerance, and renal/cardiovascular benefit.

Treatment recommendations are depicted in figure 60.3. All patients with hypertension by JNC7 criteria require drug therapy and healthy lifestyle interventions, such as restriction of dietary sodium (<100 mmol sodium = 2.4 g Na = 6 g NaCl), increased physical activity, weight loss (to <24 kg/m² females, <27 kg/m² males), and dietary alcohol restriction. These changes are appropriate for all CKD patients. However, data in hypertensive subjects indicate they are

seldom sustainable. The poor dietary habits of hypertensives in the United States have limited implementation of the dietary approach in the JNC7 guidelines. Of note, patients with systolic pressures >20 and diastolic pressures >10 mm Hg above goal should have combination therapy initially. There is no preferred initial therapy for nondiabetic UKD patients without proteinuria.

Blood pressure lowering with agents that block the renin-angiotensin system have consistently shown better kidney outcomes in large clinical trials than drugs that have other actions, and these should be used as first-line agents for reducing the progression of kidney disease. Both ACEIs

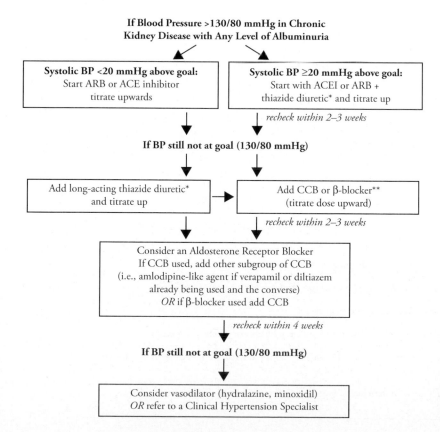

Figure 60.3. BP Treatment Algorithm for CKD Hypertensive Patients. *Hydrochlorothiazide or chlorthalidone. **Beta blockers should be preferred in cases of post–myocardial infarction, heart failure, or tachyarrhythmia. Modified from Nephrology Self-Assessment Program, 2006;5(5); and National Kidney Foundation. K/DOQI clinical practice guidelines on hypertension, antihypertensive agents in chronic kidney disease. *Am J Kidney Dis.* 2004;43:1–290.

and ARBs can improve kidney outcomes in adult CKD patients independent of their role in reaching BP goals. The KDOQI guidelines recommend ACEI or ARB therapy titrated to maximal tolerated doses for all hypertensive patients with diabetes or a urinary protein excretion over 200 mg/g creatinine in a random urine test. RAS blocking agents are known to reduce intraglomerular hypertension, improve the filtration barrier, and reduce proteinuria. Second drug choice in patients on ACEI/ARBs should be a diuretic, in order to counter volume expansion, add to the hypotensive effects of initial therapy, and help control hyperkalemia. There are no preferred secondary agents for nondiabetic CKD patients without proteinuria (spot urine total protein/creatinine <200 mg/g). Most patients will also require multiple interventions to prevent or ameliorate CVD, including smoking cessation, lipid-lowering therapy, and diabetes control.

ANEMIA

Anemia is a frequent CKD complication that, until recently, has received more attention in the ESRD patient. Anemia is highly prevalent in CKD before the development of ESRD and may affect up to 40% of CKD 4–5 patients not on dialysis. As CKD worsens, anemia becomes more likely and is associated with significant morbidity and mortality. Its detection and management with erythropoiesis-stimulating agents (ESAs), synthetic forms of erythropoietin that stimulate marrow red blood cell production, have led to clinical practice guidelines and have become an important quality indicator of improved patient outcomes. Key factors in CKD anemia management are listed in table 60.2.

Although the etiology of CKD anemia is multifactorial, it occurs predominantly because of reduced endogenous renal erythropoietin synthesis, leading to insufficient red cell production by the bone marrow. Reduced red cell survival and inhibitors of erythropoiesis may also contribute in advanced kidney failure. Other etiologies of anemia must be ruled out before it can be attributed to renal causes. For example, more than a third of anemic patients with moderate CKD may be found to be relatively or absolutely iron deficient. Deficiencies of vitamin B-6 or B-12 and the marrow-suppressive effects of secondary hyperparathyroidism may need to be considered. Diabetes is another clinical condition that may worsen CKD anemia. CKD anemia is classified as normocytic normochromic.

Mild anemia is usually asymptomatic, but clinical features in moderate cases include nonspecific tiredness, fatigability, cold intolerance, and reduced exercise tolerance. The initial evaluation should include a complete blood count, absolute reticulocyte count, serum ferritin, and serum transferrin saturation. Neither a bone marrow biopsy nor measurement of the serum erythropoietin level is normally required. Uncorrected, anemia is an independent risk factor for cardiovascular morbidity and mortality in ESRD. Observational studies indicate that anemia increases the risk of left ventricular hypertrophy and dysfunction and also of myocardial ischemia.

Optimal CKD anemia management must integrate use of ESAs and of iron, monitoring iron balance while avoiding iron deficiency or excess. Because erythropoiesis requires iron, most CKD patients who respond to ESAs will eventually develop a need for iron supplementation. Iron deficiency is the most common reason that patients fail to initiate or maintain a response to ESAs. Iron status should be assessed both before and during treatment of CKD anemia for prompt diagnosis and effective treatment of iron deficiency. Maintaining adequate iron stores can reduce the patient's ESA requirement, but multiple diagnostic

Table 60.2 KEY FACTORS IN CKD ANEMIA MANAGEMENT

1. ESA treatment should be initiated when hemoglobin <10.0 g/dL.

2. Recommended ESA starting doses are:
   Epoetin-alpha 10,000 U weekly or 20,000 U every other week
   Darbopoetin 45 μg/kg body weight weekly.

3. Hemoglobin therapeutic target range in CKD is 11–12 g/dL according to NKF KDOQI guidelines and 10–12 g/dL in FDA product labeling.

4. Use the lowest ESA dose needed to reach the hemoglobin target and avoid blood transfusions.

5. Maintaining hemoglobin targets over 13.0 g/dL increases the risk of life-threatening adverse events.

6. ESAs are contraindicated in patients with uncontrolled hypertension.

7. Hemoglobin levels should be followed weekly after initiation of therapy until levels are stable, then monthly.

8. Iron supplementation is recommended when serum ferritin is <100 ng/mL coupled with a TSAT (serum transferrin saturation) of <20%.

9. Common causes of ESA hyporesponsiveness are iron deficiency, bleeding, infection or other intercurrent illness, hospitalization.

laboratory tests may be required in CKD to determine iron status. The primary laboratory parameters used are serum ferritin and transferrin saturation. The single best test for iron deficiency is the serum ferritin. Ferritin, the indicator of tissue iron stores, is a reticuloendothelial system protein measurable in the circulation, after release from the tissues. The lower limit for normal ferritin in CKD patients should be 100 ng/mL; a lower value indicates iron deficiency. A low ferritin is a reliable measure of deficient stores. However, ferritin is an acute-phase reactant and may be falsely elevated into the normal or high range in the presence of infection, inflammation, or malignancy. The serum protein transferrin is used to transport iron from reticuloendothelial storage to the bone marrow for erythropoiesis. The calculated transferring saturation (TSAT) is a measure of circulating iron bound to transferrin. Low (<20%) transferrin saturation is a less specific measure of iron deficiency. A low serum iron is also expected but may lack specificity. Two other available measures of iron deficiency are a low reticulocyte hemoglobin content and an elevated level of soluble transferrin receptor.

The major cause of iron deficiency in non-CKD patients is occult or overt blood loss. In contrast, GI malabsorption of iron is uncommon in the non-CKD population, because hepcidin, a regulator of iron balance, is reduced in iron deficiency, allowing greater gastrointestinal iron absorption. In CKD patients, failure to reduce hepcidin, possibly because of impaired renal clearance, reduces iron absorption and makes iron balance more dependent on iron stores, which become depleted due to its utilization for red cell production. In addition to absolute iron deficiency, additional conditions involving iron balance include (1) functional iron deficiency, where liver and other iron stores are adequate but cannot be mobilized, TSAT is low (<20%), ferritin is normal to high normal (>100 ng/mL in CKD), and anemia improves with iron therapy; (2) inflammatory blockade, where laboratory parameters are similar but ferritin increases while saturation stays low in response to oral or even intravenous iron; and (3) iron overload, characterized by markedly elevated ferritin levels, a situation where intravenous iron should be avoided.

Anemic CKD patients with low transferrin saturation levels and normal or elevated serum ferritin levels are common problems. Studies cited in the 2006 KDOQI guidelines indicated that bone marrow iron could be low with ferritin levels even over 100 ng/mL. Recent data suggest that intravenous iron may be effective in optimizing the erythropoietin response in anemic ESRD patients with adequate FSA doses, low TSAT, and ferritin levels as high as 500–1200 ng/mL. However, the guidelines also discouraged use of intravenous iron when the serum ferritin was >500 ng/mL. Laboratory parameters should be checked initially then every 3 months in CKD patients, with additional testing after a course of intravenous iron or in patients no longer responsive to ESAs. The patient whose ferritin is elevated will need further evaluation with other lab studies and clinical assessment.

Adequate available iron is required to optimize the erythropoietic response to ESAs, and studies indicate that intravenous iron can reduce ESA requirements. In CKD, the route of administration for iron can be oral or intravenous. Although oral iron should be attempted, its efficacy will be limited by both impaired GI absorption and frequent GI intolerance. Intravenous iron (ferric gluconate, iron sucrose, or iron dextran), commonly given to ESRD patients but also available for CKD, can improve ESA responsiveness, but its use is limited by inconvenience, dosing protocols, cost, and perception of risk. When used, intravenous iron may be given as single or sequential doses. Because of insufficient data, the benefit of iron treatment to patients in CKD is viewed by KDOQI as a matter of opinion, not evidence.

ERYTHROPOIESIS-STIMULATING AGENTS

Nearly two decades since their introduction into clinical practice in 1989, ESAs have revolutionized the management of ESRD patients and, to a lesser extent, those with CKD. The current use of ESAs in as many as 20% of CKD patients derives from several studies showing an association between higher hemoglobin levels and physical functioning, exercise capacity, and quality of life in CKD/ESRD patients. Conversely, observational studies have also associated worsening anemia below a hemoglobin of 11 g/dL with greater mortality risk. Additional data regarding ESAs in ESRD have indicated a reduction in transfusion requirements and improved quality of life assessment. It was therefore unexpected when more recent randomized clinical trials showed that, should ESAs target higher hemoglobin levels, outcomes would actually worsen. The impact on the management of CKD anemia has been significant.

Current ESAs available in the U.S. are epoetin-alpha and darbopoetin. ESAs promote red blood cell production through the same mechanism as endogenous erythropoietin. Anemic CKD patients should be treated on an individualized basis, and hemoglobin checked every week until stable, then monthly (table 60.2).

ESA management has relied on guidelines from KDOQI and recommendations made by the FDA. The initial KDOQI guidelines (1997) recommended targeting a hemoglobin level of 11–12 g/dL, and, in 2006, the upper hemoglobin target was increased to 13 g/dL, with no distinction between ESRD and CKD patients. However, higher hemoglobin level with larger ESA doses might also carry increased risk in kidney patients. The extent to which CKD patients would benefit from higher achieved hemoglobin levels has been examined in recent trials. These trials have raised safety issues with using high doses of ESAs to target higher hemoglobin concentrations. The mechanism for these adverse effects is not incompletely understood, nor is it clear whether the ESA itself or the treatment hemoglobin level is responsible. In response to these data, the KDOQI guidelines in 2007 revised the target to 11–12 g/dL, and levels were not to exceed 13 g/dL.

Other common side effects seen in clinical trials of treated CKD-anemia patients include hypertension, infection, myalgias, headache, and rash. Hypertensive encephalopathy and seizures were noted in the initial FSA clinical trials in ESRD patients. New or worsening high blood pressure is a frequent complication of ESA use, and initiation or increased use of antihypertensive agents may be required. Patients with uncontrollable hypertension should avoid ESA use until blood pressure control is achieved. An extremely rare ESA side effect associated with hyporesponsiveness to the agents is pure red cell aplasia.

CARDIOVASCULAR DISEASE

Data from studies of the general population were the first to indicate that CKD amplifies cardiovascular disease (CVD) risk, by a remarkable factor of 2–4 (figure 60.4). The decline in CVD mortality in the general population has not benefited CKD patients, in whom it is the principal cause of mortality. Patients with CKD should be is considered in the "highest risk" group, not only for accelerated coronary disease, stroke, and all-cause cardiovascular mortality but also due to structural abnormalities such as ventricular hypertrophy, heart failure, and conduction system abnormalities. Cardiovascular risk is heightened in CKD whether it is manifested by minimally decreased estimated GFR or even by low levels of urinary albumin excretion. Patients with

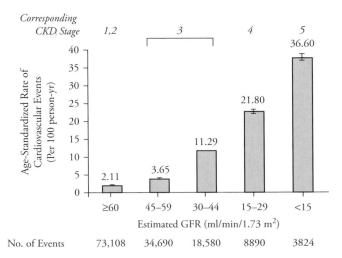

Figure 60.4. Rates of Cardiovascular Events According to Estimated GFR in the General Population. CKD stages are assigned per eGFR. The adjusted risk of cardiovascular events increased as eGFR decreased. Reprinted with permission from Go AS, Chertow GM, Fan D, et al. Chronic kidney disease and the risks of death, cardiovascular events, and hospitalization. *N Engl J Med.* 2004;351:1296–1395. Copyright 2007 Massachusetts Medical Society. All rights reserved.

minimal reduction in kidney function (at a GFR of about 75 mL/min) are at risk regardless of the cause of CKD, and the adjusted relative risk appears to be inverse to level of kidney function. Furthermore, recent data suggest that CVD is independently associated with further worsening of kidney function. Therefore, identification and treatment of premature CVD, including heart failure, myocardial infarction, angina, arrhythmias, and cerebrovascular/peripheral vascular disease, should be a high priority in CKD. Data to assess CVD risk should include estimated GFR and urinary albumin excretion, an electrocardiogram, serum glucose, fasting lipids, and height and weight to calculate the body mass index.

The CKD patient suffers from a multifactorial interplay of traditional and nontraditional CVD risk factors. CKD patients have a high prevalence of many traditional factors. Whether traditional risk factors work differently in CKD is not clear. However, it is accepted that increased CVD risk exceeds what established factors such as hypertension, diabetes, smoking, and dyslipidemias would contribute. The growing list of nontraditional factors including anemia, C-reactive protein, LPa, fibrinogen, and abnormal mineral metabolism interrelate in an environment of endothelial dysfunction, oxidative stress, vascular calcification, and inflammation.

Recent data suggest that for coronary events such as myocardial infarction, CKD patients are less likely to receive medical (aspirin, beta blockers) and coronary (thrombolytic therapy, percutaneous procedures) therapies, adding to the potential importance of prevention of CVD in CKD patients. The approach to CVD risk reduction in CKD involves (1) applying CVD strategies from the general population and (2) assessing the benefit of reducing specific risk factors (hypertension, lipid lowering) in patients affected by CKD. Studies of CVD risk reduction have generally excluded patients with elevated serum creatinine levels (although estimated GFRs in many cases were not normal in enrolled subjects). Clinical trial data testing therapies for risk factor reduction including hypertension, anemia, and dyslipidemia in CKD are limited. Regarding risk reduction, the cardiovascular effects of treating hypertension in the CKD population are as yet unproven. Use of blood pressure agents is in most cases an extrapolation from the general population (table 60.3). CKD patients have rarely been the focus of hypertension trials. Although other studies were unable to demonstrate any benefit of blood pressure reduction on cardiovascular events, the HOPE trial provided evidence that CKD patients might benefit more than others from blood pressure reduction. For stroke prevention, hypertension control is the most important strategy in CKD. Comparisons of the cardiovascular effects of different antihypertensive agents in CKD populations are insufficient. The KDOQI blood pressure target is <130/<80 mm Hg. Congestive heart failure trials in the general population have made beta blockers and

ACEI the cornerstones of therapy for congestive heart failure. ACEI may be used in CKD while monitoring closely for hyperkalemia or any acute rise in the serum creatinine from baseline. With regard to coronary interventions, it is known that CKD patients have higher restenosis rates after coronary angioplasty/stenting and greater risk of death following coronary bypass surgery.

In the general population with high low-density lipoprotein (LDL) levels, statins (hydroxymethyl glutaryl CoA reductase inhibitors) are effective for primary and secondary prevention of cardiovascular events. Evidence in favor of beneficial risk reduction in CKD is weak for lipid lowering, which must be added to the perception of the heightened risk of statins in CKD patients. Dyslipidemia in CKD is common and includes elevated lipoprotein remnants, lipoprotein a, and LDL-C. Most of the clinical trials on statins have excluded CKD patients. According to the KDOQI guidelines for management of dyslipidemias, the National Cholesterol Education Program guidelines apply to patients with CKD 1–4, and the initial drug therapy for high LDL should be statins; in patients with hypertriglyceridemia, gemfibrozil may be the fibrate of choice. Prescribed widely in the general population for prevention of vascular disease, statins were evaluated in the CARE trial of patients who had suffered a myocardial infarction and had hypercholesterolemia. The study excluded patients with proteinuria or significant creatinine elevations, but over one-third of the 4156 patients enrolled had a CrCl <75 mL/min. A subgroup analysis of those with CKD indicated that pravastatin reduced the incidence of future coronary events without more adverse events, even in those with diabetes or hypertension. About a quarter of patients in a subsequent pooled analysis of three studies (including CARE, the LIPID study, and the West of Scotland Coronary Prevention Study) had concomitant CKD, and their risk of CVD was increased by 1.26. Risk was reduced by pravastatin, with similar benefit in nondiabetic and diabetic patients. In the presence of CKD, statins may reduce inflammatory markers such as C-reactive protein, tumor necrosis factor, and interleukins. Given the high risk in CKD patients, statins are suggested for patients with an LDL over 100 ng/mL (a more aggressive target LDL of 70 has been suggested by some). Data on raising high-density lipoprotein (HDL) or lowering triglycerides are not available. Dosages of statins may need to be reduced. The role of antioxidant therapy in CVD remains to be defined.

It is likely that patients with CVD complicating CKD will require multiple sustained interventions, a strategy that may rely on the whole being greater than the sum of its parts. One model for multifactorial intervention is the STENO-2 study, which utilized not only combined but intensified therapy consistent with current American Diabetes Association guidelines (hypertension control, low-fat diet, glycemic control, statins/fibrates, ACEI/ARBs, smoking cessation) in diabetic patients with metabolic syndrome and microalbuminuria. After a mean of 7.8 years, intensive therapy lowered the risk of CVD by about 50%, consistent with additive effects of the individual therapies. Results from a 5.5-year observational follow-up, during which the risk factors for the two groups converged, indicated persistent cardiovascular risk reduction.

BONE AND MINERAL METABOLISM

No longer limited to secondary hyperparathyroidism and renal osteodystrophy, the CKD complication termed *mineral and bone disorder* (CKD-MBD) is now considered to be a broader, more complex syndrome of bone disease and systemic calcification (table 60.4). Mineral and bone disturbances are linked to morbidity and mortality in ESRD patients, but their impact on CKD outcomes is less well described. Renal bone disease in its various forms creates bone loss and fracture risk. Vascular calcification has emerged as a serious complication of CKD and contributes to cardiovascular disease. In addition, some data suggest

Table 60.3 IMPACT OF CARDIOVASCULAR DISEASE ON SELECTION OF ANTIHYPERTENSIVE AGENTS IN CKD PATIENTS

	CHF + SYSTOLIC DYSFUNCTION	POST-MI + SYSTOLIC DYSFUNCTION	POST-MI	ANGINA	HIGH RISK FOR CAD
Thiazide or loop diuretic	X				X
ACEI/ARBs	X	X			X
Beta-blockers	X	X	X	X	X
Calcium channel blockers				X	X
Aldosterone antagonists	X	X			

NOTES: CHF, congestive heart failure; MI, myocardial infarction; CAD, coronary artery disease; ACEI, angiotensin-converting enzyme inhibitors; ARBs, angiotensin receptor blockers.

Table 60.4 KEY FEATURES OF CKD-BMD DISORDER

1. Multisystemic disorder of bone and mineral metabolism

2. Interrelated derangements in phosphorus, parathyroid hormone, vitamin D, and calcium

3. Skeletal abnormalities of bone mineralization, strength, and turnover; fracture risk

4. Risk of vascular and other soft tissue calcifications

5. Deficiency of vitamin D a common problem

an association between CKD progression and a high calcium-phosphorus product. The current KDOQI targets for CKD-BMD are shown in table 60.5. However, studies have demonstrated that patients continue to lack laboratory evaluation or receive traditional therapies such as vitamin D analogues and phosphate binders in CKD.

Calcium, phosphorus, parathyroid hormone (PTH), and endogenous vitamin D are all implicated in CKD-MBD in a "perfect storm" that develops as kidney function worsens. At the center of the storm is excess PTH secretion attributed to phosphorus retention and inadequate production of 1,25-OH-D by the impaired kidneys. The reduction in 1,25-OH-D (calcitriol) worsens hypocalcemia, further stimulating parathyroid release. Eventually parathyroid gland hyperplasia occurs, adding to the "storm" when cell abnormalities such as reduction in the calcium-sensing receptor (by reducing the response to calcium) and the vitamin D receptor (by reducing responsiveness to endogenous vitamin D) occur. With therapies such as phosphate binders, vitamin D analogues, and calcimimetics, the CKD-MBD storm can be made "imperfect."

Compared to the general population, CKD patients are at increased risk for extraskeletal calcification. Vascular calcification is increasingly understood to be an active process, similar to bone mineralization, and not a passive process in which circulating calcium and phosphorus precipitate when levels are high. Mineral deposition in CKD involves phenotypic changes in vascular smooth muscle cells, converting them into osteogenic cell types whose secreted matrix tends to become mineralized. The cell conversion is initiated by several CKD factors including mineral imbalance and a direct effect of vitamin D. Mineral deposition is further worsened by deficiencies of endogenous calcification inhibitors. Particularly when inhibitors are deficient, elevated phosphorus levels play a key role. Clinically, the process is linked to calcification of atheromatous intimal plaques, which may occlude vessels or rupture, and to medial calcification, which is associated with vascular stiffening and coronary hypoperfusion. Noninvasive assessment of vascular calcification in CKD depends primarily on electron beam computed tomography (CT) imaging.

Because of its importance in the pathogenesis of CKD-MBD and the high morbidity and mortality associated with kidney failure, the need for aggressive phosphorus control is being given high priority (table 60.5). Because of the ceiling on renal phosphorus excretion in CKD (despite the phosphaturic actions of PTH and FGF-23), reducing dietary phosphorus intake is required to preserve neutral balance in moderate CKD. Limiting phosphorus intake to <1000 mg/day should be started when either the phosphorus or the parathyroid level is above the KDOQI target. (More severe phosphorus restriction would severely compromise dietary protein intake at the same time and should be avoided.) The limitations on reduced intake have led to alternative strategies to achieve the same balance through the use of phosphate binders taken with meals as CKD worsens. Selecting a phosphate binder requires attention to both efficacy and safety. The most common initial binder of choice (except when the serum calcium is >10.2 mg/dL) is calcium-based, including calcium carbonate and calcium acetate. However, recent studies have suggested a correlation between binder-related calcium intake and vascular calcification. The dose of elemental calcium should therefore be limited to 1500 mg/day. Calcium acetate in balance studies appears to bind more phosphorus. Compared to calcium-based binders,

Table 60.5 KDOQI GUIDELINES FOR TARGETS AND FREQUENCY OF MEASUREMENTS FOR CKD-BMD LABORATORY VALUES

CKD STAGE	EGFR (ML/MIN)	TARGET PHOSPHORUS (MG/DL)	TARGET CALCIUM (mg/dL)	TARGET PARATHYROID HORMONE (pg/mL)	LABORATORY FREQUENCY
3	30–59	2.7–4.6	"normal range for laboratory"	35–70	Calc phos 12 mos; PTH 12 mos
4	15–29	2.7–4.6	"normal range for laboratory"	70–110	Calc phos 3 mos; PTH 3 mo
5	<15 or dialysis	3.5–5.5	8.4–9.5	150–300	Calc phos monthly; PTH 3 mos

SOURCE: From National Kidney Foundation. K/DOQI clinical practice guidelines: bone metabolism and disease in chronic kidney disease. *American Journal of Kidney Diseases.* 2003;42(supp 4):S1–S201, with permission from Elsevier.

minimal effects on serum calcium have been found with sevelamer hydrochloride, a calcium-free binder, in several ESRD studies. Recent evidence suggests that progression of vascular calcification in prevalent as well as new dialysis patients may also be reduced with sevelamer compared to calcium-based binders. An effective alternative noncalcium binder option also reported to cause less hypercalcemia is lanthanum, a soft metallic rare earth element. Animal studies have raised concern about long-term accumulation of lanthanum in lungs, kidneys, and bones. In human ESRD, minimal but increased bone lanthanum content persisting after a year off lanthanum has raised further concerns. No benefits on vascular calcification or lipid levels have been shown. Issues regarding safety and tolerability of phosphate binders must be viewed in the context of known complications of uncontrolled hyperphosphatemia. Both sevelamer and lanthanum are significantly more expensive that calcium-based binders.

Vitamin D receptor activators are among the most widely used drugs in the CKD population. In dialysis patients, they improve bone mineral density and reduce histologic bone abnormalities. They may reduce CKD hospitalizations. Oral vitamin D analogues are applied in CKD not only to reach target parathyroid levels but also to correct vitamin D deficiency. Acting through dose-related receptor stimulation in the parathyroid chief cells, the hormone directly suppresses PTH release while also leading to calcium and phosphorus intestinal absorption. In dialysis patients and more recently CKD patients, administration of active D analogues has now been associated with survival improvement. However, a recent meta-analysis of 76 trials in various stages of CKD included only five trials directly comparing new vitamin D analogues with established ones. Vitamin D compounds did not consistently reduce parathyroid levels. Concerns that resulting hypercalcemia, hyperphosphatemia, and hypercalciuria could cause nephrocalcinosis and worsen kidney function in CKD may be diminished by using newer vitamin D analogues that have less hypercalcemic potential. However, no difference between traditional vitamin D and newer selective analogues has been proven. For secondary hyperparathyroidism (SHPT) KDOQI guidelines suggest starting vitamin D analogues when calcium is <9.5 and phosphorus <4.6 mg/dL. Calcitriol, a nonselective analogue, is started at 25 μg daily but may cause hypercalcemia at higher doses. Paracalcitol given intravenously has been widely used in hemodialysis patients, where it causes less hypercalcemia, and is now approved orally for CKD at a starting dose of 1 μg daily. Doxercalciferol may also have a lower incidence of hypercalcemia. Starting dose is 1 μg daily.

Low vitamin D levels my also contribute to CKD-MBD in advanced CKD, where low $1,25\text{-}(OH)_2D_3$ is expected due to impaired renal 1-hydroxylase levels. Black and diabetic patients are at increased risk. 25-OH-D, a measure of vitamin D stores, must also be assessed because of reduced solar exposure and poor daily intake as well as increased degradation to other metabolites in CKD. Vitamin D may play an important role in health beyond bone and mineral disorders, including potential benefits against autoimmune disease, cancer, and oxidative stress. Vitamin D stores should be checked on initial evaluation then annually in CKD 3–4 patients. Replacement should be based on 25-OH-D levels <30 ng/mL, while avoiding elevations in calcium/phosphorus or oversuppression of PTH.

RENAL OSTEODYSTROPHY

At the epicenter of the "perfect storm" of CKD-BMD is SHPT, a condition in which oversecretion of PTH is associated with increased parathyroid gland growth. In the normal feedback loop, PTH is secreted in response to hypocalcemia, mediated through the calcium-sensing receptor, and leads to increased bone resorption of calcium and renal calcium reabsorption and vitamin D synthesis, which in turn enhances intestinal calcium absorption. In advancing CKD, phosphate retention leads to a reciprocal fall in serum calcium, providing the fundamental stimulus to parathyroid release. The prevalence of hyperphosphatemia and hypocalcemia becomes significant in CKD stage 4, and the rise in parathyroid levels is commonly preceded by a decline in active vitamin D levels.

In addition to its vascular calcification effects, SHPT is associated with several types of renal osteodystrophy, which refers to abnormal bone morphology secondary to CKD. Although bone pain and fractures are infrequent in predialysis patients, morphologic bone abnormalities occur early; the majority of CKD 3–4 patients have histologic evidence of bone disease, mostly high turnover related to SHPT, including classic osteitis fibrosa cystica and mixed osteodystrophy. The risk of high-turnover bone disease increases with PTH levels. Decreased bone density on dual-energy x-ray absorptiometry (DEXA) screening in the spine, hips, and arms has also been related to PTH levels. Low-turnover forms, including adynamic bone disease and osteomalacia, were uncommon but may be increasing. The risk of fracture in CKD increases with worsening kidney function.

Advances in medical management of renal osteodystrophy can improve CKD-MBD to an "imperfect storm." Phosphate control with diet and binders improves $1.25\text{-}(OH)_2D_3$ deficiency. Vitamin D analogues, proven to inhibit PTH release before changes in serum calcium occur when given intravenously, can correct SHPT and prevent bone disease when given in CKD 3–4. KDOQI parathyroid target levels are above the normal range in order to maintain bone remodeling and avoid iatrogenic adynamic bone disease, which presents as fractures and hypercalcemia (table 60.5). The standard vitamin D therapy for vitamin D deficiency for CKD 3–4, ergocalciferol, can also achieve modest parathyroid suppression. Cinacalcet, a recently approved calcimimetic agent available for use in dialysis patients with SUPT, binds to the calcium-sensing receptor, increases cell sensitivity to extracellular calcium, and suppresses PTH production independent of vitamin D. The calcimimetic (30–180 mg once daily with food) also improved calcium/phosphorus parameters and reduced parathyroid levels by about one-third in CKD patients in short-term studies. Hypocalcemia may require supplemental calcium and vitamin D.

OTHER COMPLICATIONS AND MANAGEMENT

Dietary therapy is also important for the management of CKD complications. Available data provide only modest support, particularly in proteinuric conditions, to dietary protein restriction as an effective or practical means to slow kidney progression in CKD. The decision to prescribe a low-protein diet is supported more by experimental studies than clinical trials. It also has potential benefit to several CKD complications: possible improvement in blood pressure, attenuation of acidosis (by limiting endogenous acid production), improved hyperphosphatemia, benefit to the lipid profile (because meat and dietary sources are reduced), and, in advanced cases, avoidance of uremic symptoms. Protein malnutrition in CKD may result from protein degradation and loss of appetite. Metabolic acidosis begins to develop in CKD stages 3–4 as the capacity for renal ammonia excretion begins to decline and hydrogen ions are retained. Renal acidosis weakens bone structure as mineral is lost when bone acts as a buffer. Acidosis may be corrected by use of sodium bicarbonate or citrate salts as long as the patient is not taking aluminum-based phosphate binders. For hyperkalemic patients, renal potassium excretion can be increased by diuretics or fludrocortisones. Quality of life tends to decline as CKD progresses. CKD is often complicated by clinical wasting due to anorexia, protein malnutrition, loss of lean body mass, and increased basal metabolic rate, possibly related to buildup of proinflammatory cytokines during CKD progression. Because anorexia is combined with poor utilization of dietary nutrients, nutritional supplementation is usually ineffective. CKD is increasingly recognized as a risk factor for cognitive impairment. Results of cognitive testing indicate that CKD is associated with poor learning, reduced concentrating, and poor visual attention. In addition to the above complications, medical management of the CKD patient involves health maintenance. Preventative health measures are underutilized in CKD patients. CKD patients should be vaccinated against influenza, pneumococcal disease, and hepatitis B, screened annually for tuberculosis, and undergo cancer screening to include carcinoma of the prostate, colon/rectum, breasts, and cervix, as well as renal cell carcinoma. The current target glycated hemoglobin level for diabetic CKD patients is 7.0% or less.

ADDITIONAL READING

Chobanian AV, Bakris GL, Black HR, et al. The Seventh Report of the Joint National Committee on Prevention, Detection, Evaluation, and Treatment of High Blood Pressure: The JNC7 report. *JAMA.* 2003;289:2560–72.

Eknoyan G. Chronic kidney disease definition and classification: The quest for refinements. *Kidney Int.* 2007;72:1183.

National Kidney Foundation. K/DOQI clinical practice guidelines for chronic kidney disease: Evaluation, classification, and stratification. *Am J Kidney Dis.* 2002;39(Suppl 1):S1–S266.

National Kidney Foundation. K/DOQI clinical practice guidelines for management of dyslipidemias in patients with kidney disease. *Am J Kidney Dis.* 2003;41:I-IV,S1–91.

National Kidney Foundation. K/DOQI clinical practice guidelines for bone metabolism and disease in chronic kidney disease. *Am J Kidney Dis.* 2003;42(Suppl 3):S1–S202.

National Kidney Foundation. K/DOQI clinical practice guidelines on hypertension, antihypertensive agents in chronic kidney disease. *Am J Kidney Dis.* 2004;43:1–290.

National Kidney Foundation. KDOQI clinical practice guidelines and clinical practice recommendations for anemia in chronic kidney disease: 2007 Update of hemoglobin target. *Am J Kidney Dis.* 2007;50(Suppl 3):476–530.

Ryan TP, Sloand JA, Winters PC, Corsetti JP, Fisher SG. Chronic kidney disease prevalence and rate of diagnosis. *Am J Med.* 2007;120: 981–6.

QUESTIONS

QUESTION 1. Features of CKD bone and mineral disorders are known to include all EXCEPT:

    A. Positive phosphorus balance
    B. Reduction of cardiovascular risk with Cinacalcet
    C. Increased fracture risk
    D. Vitamin D deficiency is common
    E. Vascular calcification

QUESTION 2. For optimal CKD management:

    A. The best test of iron deficiency is the serum iron.
    B. Serum EPO level should be checked prior to initiation of ESAs.
    C. The major cause of iron deficiency is GI blood loss.
    D. Iron overload results in hyporesponsiveness to ESAs.
    E. None of the above.

QUESTION 3. CKD complications:

    A. Are independent of the level of kidney function
    B. Are symptomatic
    C. Do not depend on the primary cause of kidney disease
    D. Should be addressed in CKD stage 4
    E. None of the above

QUESTION 4. The hypertensive CKD patient who presents with systolic BP >20 and diastolic BP >10 mm Hg above goal should be initiated on:

A. Vasodilator
B. Combination therapy
C. Diuretic
D. ACEI
E. ARB

QUESTION 5. CVD risk is heightened in which CKD patients:

A. ESRD
B. Microalbuminuria
C. Nondiabetic
D. eGFR <75 mL/min
E. All of the above

ANSWERS

1. B
2. E
3. C
4. B
5. E

61.

HEMATURIA AND PROTEINURIA

Hasan Bazari

Hematuria and proteinuria are common problems encountered in medicine that may be benign conditions or be harbingers of severe systemic illness and require vigorous evaluation and treatment. This chapter is categorized into conditions that are defined by the presence of hematuria alone, conditions limited to proteinuria alone, or those in which proteinuria is combined with hematuria. The evaluation and therapy of conditions that combine both is dealt with in the latter part of the chapter.

HEMATURIA

Hematuria can be classified as microscopic or gross hematuria when there is visible blood and can present with or without symptoms. There are a number of causes of red urine without hematuria, including porphyria and many drugs such as phenazopyridine, rifampin, B-12, and phenytoin as well as food components in beets and blackberries. Microscopic hematuria is defined as two or more red blood cells per high-powered field (hpf), although there are many different definitions. The dipstick is used as the screening test for hematuria and needs to be confirmed with microscopy. The dipstick will test positive with both hemoglobin and myoglobin in the setting of hemolysis and rhabdomyolysis, respectively. There can be transient hematuria that is associated with vigorous exercise, intercourse, trauma, or menses. In these circumstances the evaluation should be repeated with appropriate instructions to the patient. Patients with persistent hematuria should be considered for evaluation, the approach to which is discussed below. The prevalence of microscopic hematuria varies based on the series from 0.11% to 16.1% based on the series and screening method used. In evaluating hematuria, the crucial determination is whether there is confidence in identifying hematuria as glomerular or nonglomerular. Hematuria can be identified as being more likely to be glomerular when there is accompanying proteinuria, hypertension that is new, renal insufficiency, the presence of acanthocytes or dysmorphic red

blood cells, or the presence of cellular casts, especially red blood cell casts. In the absence of clear indication of glomerular origin of hematuria a systematic evaluation should be undertaken. There have been valid arguments questioning the utility of screening and undertaking an exhaustive evaluation of hematuria.

Patients with documented glomerular hematuria, proteinuria, or renal insufficiency will require evaluation for glomerular causes of hematuria. These are categorized in table 61.1. The diseases include ANCA-associated vasculitis, anti–glomerular basement membrane (GBM) disease, hypocomplementemic immune complex vasculitis, and normocomplementemic systemic vasculitis. The antineutrophil cytoplasmic antibody (ANCA) associated vasculitis includes Wegner granulomatosis, microscopic polyangiitis, and pauci-immune crescentic glomerulonephritis. Anti-GBM disease, also known as Goodpasture syndrome, is often associated with pulmonary involvement, although it may be limited to just the kidneys. Hypocomplementemic immune complex glomerulonephritis includes poststreptococcal glomerulonephritis, systemic lupus erythematosus, cryoglobulinemia, hypocomplementemic vasculitis, membranoproliferative glomerulonephritis, subacute bacterial endocarditis, and visceral abscesses. The normocomplementemic immune complex glomerulonephritides include IgA nephropathy and Henoch-Schönlein purpura, both of which share the presence of IgA immune complexes as the major immune complexes. The serological evaluation should be the same whether there is presence of proteinuria or renal insufficiency.

The presentation of isolated hematuria may be asymptomatic or part of an evaluation for a complaint that may or may not be related to the hematuria. The causes can be categorized as glomerular or nonglomerular. Glomerular causes can include all of the diseases discussed in table 61.1. However, the absence of proteinuria, hypertension, and renal insufficiency makes it less likely that these conditions are responsible for the hematuria. There have been several series in which there have been biopsies of patients with no

Table 61.1 RAPIDLY PROGRESSIVE GLOMERULO-NEPHRITIS

- Anti-GBM disease
- Pauci-immune necrotizing glomerulonephritis
  – Wegener granulomatosis
  – Microscopic polyangiitis
  – Churg-Strauss syndrome

- Immune complex glomerulonephritis
  – Hypocomplementemic glomerulonephritis

  - Systemic lupus
  - Endocarditis
  - Cryoglobulinemia
  - Poststreptococcal glomerulonephritis
  - Membranoproliferative glomerulonephritis
  – Normocomplementemic glomerulonephritis
  – IgA nephropathy
  – Henoch-Schönlein purpura
  – Fibrillary glomerulonephritis

Table 61.2 NONGLOMERULAR GLOMERULONEPHRITIS

Transient: exercise
Renal

Nephrolithiasis, pyelonephritis, polycystic kidney disease, renal cell carcinoma, sickle cell disease or trait, transitional cell carcinoma, tuberculosis

Lower tract

Transitional cell carcinoma of the bladder, urinary tract infection, prostatitis, prostate cancer, ureteral stricture, schistosomiasis, nutcracker syndrome, Osler-Weber-Rendu syndrome

Urethral

other etiology for hematuria, who have undergone renal biopsies for no other etiology for hematuria. More than half of these patients had a normal kidney biopsy. Those with kidney disease had mainly had IgA nephropathy and thin basement membrane disease. The latter is a familial disorder with autosomal dominant inheritance and often represents the carrier state for autosomal recessive form of Alport syndrome as well as Alport syndrome, which is an X-linked recessive disease with uniform onset of end-stage renal disease in men and a variable but more benign clinical course in women. The mutations for Alports are in COL4A5, and those for the autosomal diseases in COL4A3 and COL4A4 genes. In some series the mutations in COL4A5 mostly cause Alport syndrome and thin basement membrane disease in a small minority. Other focal glomerulonephritides make up a small number of cases presenting as isolated hematuria. The longer the duration of the hematuria and familial nature of the disease may reflect a better prognosis and allow most patients to forgo a kidney biopsy.

Nonglomerular causes of hematuria can be classified anatomically as detailed in table 61.2. Upper sources of hematuria include sources from the kidney itself, including nephrolithiasis, pyelonephritis, renal call carcinomas, autosomal dominant polycystic kidney disease, medullary sponge kidney, renal pelvis and ureteral transitional cell carcinoma, hypercalciuria, hyperuricosuria, sickle cell trait and disease, tuberculosis, renal infarct, and papillary necrosis. Lower-tract sources include common benign conditions such as urinary tract infection, prostatitis, and urethritis as well as more malignant conditions such as bladder cancer and prostate cancer. Other conditions include ureteral strictures, schistosomiasis, and nutcracker syndrome with the left renal vein compressed between the aorta and the superior mesenteric artery, and retroaortic left renal vein. Other unusual causes of gross hematuria include hereditary hemorrhagic telangiectasia (HHT or Osler-Weber-Rendu syndrome) and loin pain–hematuria syndrome. Patients with

sickle cell trait can have gross hematuria from medullary ischemia. Rarely sickle cell trait can be associated with renal medullary carcinoma, which has a poor prognosis. The epidemiology of hematuria varies with age. In children there have been several large screening studies that have shown very rare instances of malignancies such as Wilms tumor. The incidence of malignancies is higher in patients with gross hematuria. Patients who are older than 40, and definitely those who are older than 50, have a higher prevalence of malignancies such as bladder cancer and warrant evaluation. Patients with macroscopic hematuria had an 18.9% prevalence of malignancy compared with a 4.8% prevalence of malignancy with microscopic hematuria in one series.

RISK FACTORS FOR MALIGNANCIES

In all patients with microscopic hematuria, about 5% will be found to have malignancies, predominantly transitional cell carcinoma of the bladder. The risk factors for malignancy include older age, cigarette smoking, occupational exposure to chemicals, leather manufacturing, rubber and tire manufacturing, phenacetin use, cyclophosphamide, mitotane, and aristolochic acid exposure. Gross hematuria is much more likely to be associated with a diagnosis of malignancy. Many patients with both bladder cancer and renal cell carcinoma will have gross hematuria at presentation.

EVALUATION OF HEMATURIA

HISTORY

The history should include the search for symptoms of stone disease, weight loss or flank pain, symptoms of systemic vasculitis, drug exposure, smoking, occupational exposure to aniline dyes in leather manufacturing, family history of hematuria, and kidney disease, as well as accompanying hearing loss. Radiation exposure, cyclophosphamide exposure, and analgesic use are all risk factors for the development of bladder and ureteral cancer. Bladder symptoms such as urinary urgency, dysuria, and frequency may reflect infection, inflammation, or malignancy. Use of anticoagulation may be important in the evaluation, but the diagnostic evaluation cannot be truncated based on the presence of a coagulopathy.

EXAMINATION

The blood pressure (BP) may be important if elevated. Findings of sinusitis, eye findings, arteriovenous (AV) malformations, rash, arthritis, pulmonary findings of consolidation, cardiac dysfunction, and the detection of palpable masses, and prostate tenderness or enlargement may all be clues to the etiology of hematuria.

LABORATORY EVALUATION

The laboratory evaluation should include a focused panel based on elements of the history and physical examination. The serum creatinine is important, as are the presence of anemia and coagulopathy.

Patients with suspected glomerular hematuria should have a panel of tests including antinuclear antibody, antineutrophil cytoplasmic antibody, anti–glomerular basement membrane antibody, C3 and C4 complements, cryoglobulins, blood cultures when indicated, anti-DNAse B or antistreptolysin O.

The urinalysis is crucial in the evaluation of proteinuria. The presence of proteinuria often points to a glomerular origin. The presence of dysmorphic red blood cells, especially the presence of acanthocytes, is also consistent with a glomerular source. Competency in the assessment of red cell morphology comes with experience but can streamline the evaluation of hematuria avoiding unnecessary tests with cost and risks such as computed tomography (CT) scans and cystoscopy. Red cell casts are pathognomonic for glomerular disease and will preclude the evaluation for a nonglomerular hematuria.

Patients with proteinuria on the dipstick should have a protein: creatinine ratio for quantification of the degree of proteinuria.

Urine cytology is crucial in patients who are older. The sensitivity of urine cytology is about 70%, but the specificity is close to 100%. There have been a small number of patients in whom all other tests may fail to reveal a source, but a positive cytology can lead to a diagnosis of bladder cancer. Urine cytology should be done in patients older than 40 years of age, and positive results pursued with cystoscopy as well as imaging studies.

IMAGING

Intravenous Urography

Intravenous urography (IVU) has been traditionally used in the evaluation of hematuria. The limitations of the study include the limitations of the sensitivity of the study and the inability of the study to distinguish solid and cystic lesions. The use of contrast may be an issue for patients with renal insufficiency. The use of IVU has waned with time, and both ultrasound and CT scan have become more the standard of care with sensitivity for CT above 90% and only 50% for intravenous urography. Kidney stones are better visualized with CT scan.

Ultrasound

Ultrasound has many advantages including ease of use and availability, lack of radiation, and lack of contrast exposure. Ultrasound may miss small lesions, with lesions smaller than 3 cm yielding a sensitivity of 80%. Ultrasound can miss ureteral lesions and stones in the collecting system. Ultrasound may be the preferred modality in patients who are at low risk for malignancies, in pregnancy, and in young patients who are at lower risk for malignancies.

CT Scan

Over the last few years, CT scanning has emerged as the best modality for imaging the genitourinary tract. A non-contrast CT scan is done for patients in whom a kidney stone is suspected as the cause of the hematuria based on the presentation. Following this, contrast-enhanced CT scan is performed to look for enhancing masses as well as delineation of the collecting system. The sensitivity for CT for the detection of ureteral stones is 100%. CT scan may also image the bladder and define lesions that cause ureteral or bladder deformities. This may preclude the need for cystoscopy in a younger patient population under age 40, where the incidence of bladder cancer is much lower. Nonetheless, the performance of cystoscopy would not be discouraged, as there are small numbers of patients in every series who have bladder cancer in their 20s. Multidetector CT scan was found in a large study to have a sensitivity of 64% and a specificity of 98% and had a higher accuracy compared with intravenous urography.

Retrograde Pyelogram

Retrograde pyelograms have largely been replaced by cystoscopy and cystourethroscopy which allow for both diagnostic biopsies and occasional therapeutic interventions on small lesions. There may be instances of hematuria where a retrograde pyelogram may need to be done.

Cystoscopy

Cystoscopy should be performed in all patients in whom there is a significant risk of bladder cancer. These include patients older than 40 years old, those with a smoking history, and those with significant exposure to carcinogens for the genitourinary tract such as aniline dyes and cyclophosphamide. Women have a lower incidence of bladder cancer, and there may be lower yield in the performance of cystoscopy.

Patients with gross hematuria have a higher likelihood of having a malignant lesion as the etiology and warrant a full evaluation including cystoscopy even at younger ages.

APPROACH TO THE PATIENT WITH HEMATURIA

The patient with a single episode of microscopic hematuria should be instructed to have a repeat evaluation and also be instructed to avoid heavy exertion prior to testing (figure 61.1). A single episode of microscopic hematuria in a high-risk patient or a single episode of gross hematuria in adults warrants evaluation. If the patient is low risk, the repeat urine testing is negative, and the evaluation ends. In those who have persistent microscopic hematuria, a single episode but with risk factors for bladder cancer, and those with a single episode of gross hematuria, there should be a comprehensive evaluation. Urine microscopy done by someone with experience in the identification of dysmorphic red cells in the urine may obviate the need for evaluation for a nonglomerular source of hematuria, as may the presence of proteinuria, abnormal renal function, or the presence of cellular casts. Gross hematuria is classically seen in certain forms of glomerulonephritis such as IgA nephropathy, poststreptococcal glomerulonephritis, and occasionally anti-GBM disease. Gross hematuria related to glomerulonephritis is often "tea" or "Coca-Cola" colored.

If there is evidence for glomerular disease, the workup typically involves serological evaluation followed by a decision to do a renal biopsy prior to the institution of therapy. Therapy may be instituted empirically prior to a biopsy in certain conditions where there is rapid decline in renal function or a serological test with a high degree of specificity such as an ANCA or anti-GBM test in the context of a high-probability clinical situation. In the presence of only microscopic hematuria and a negative serological evaluation, the decision to proceed with a kidney biopsy has to be individualized. There may be no specific diagnosis on the kidney biopsy in the majority of cases of patients with microscopic hematuria. Among those who do have a diagnosis, the majority have IgA nephropathy or thin basement membrane disease. The former is treated when it manifests with high-grade proteinuria, progressive renal deterioration, or rapidly progressive glomerulonephritis but not with just asymptomatic hematuria. Benign treatments such as fish oil and close monitoring of renal function as well for proteinuria are recommended for patients with mild IgA nephropathy. Thin basement membrane disease has been traditionally thought of as a benign disease with autosomal dominant inheritance. Many of these patients have mutations in the alpha-3 and -4 chains of type 4 collagen and represent the carrier state for the autosomal recessive form of Alport. The finding of thin basement membrane disease has also been reported with mutations in the alpha-5 chain, which is more traditionally associated with the X-linked Alport, the cause of Alport in 85% of patients. Thin basement membrane disease has also been associated with focal sclerosis is certain families, and caution needs to be exercised in prognosticating in a very young patient with no family history and thin basement membrane disease on kidney biopsy. Given that a renal biopsy incurs a small risk of significant bleeding, and the lack of therapeutic options and potential prognostic uncertainty for both IgA nephropathy and thin basement membrane

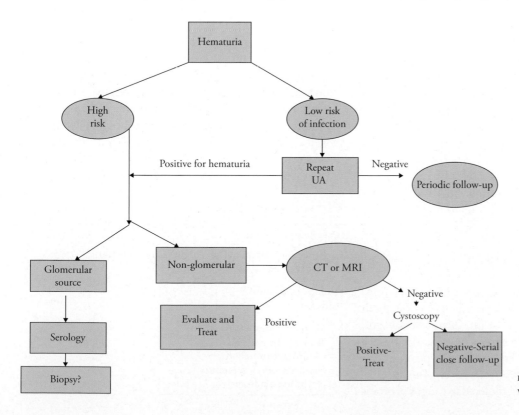

Figure 61.1. Approach to the Patient with Hematuria.

disease, it would be reasonable to discuss the risks and benefits with a patient prior to a decision to biopsy. Most patients are comfortable with close follow-up except under unusual circumstances. One setting in which a biopsy may be done with a lower threshold is in the transplant donor evaluation, in which there will be risk to the donor if donation occurs in the setting of intrinsic renal disease. In this circumstance a renal biopsy that is normal would allow for the organ donation to proceed if the remainder of the evaluation for hematuria is negative. There are reports of patients with thin basement membrane being organ donors after confirmation with a kidney biopsy. This is an area of uncertainty, and caution should be used, especially if there is not a benign family history and definitely in the young organ donor.

For those with no evidence for glomerular bleeding, the evaluation should include treatable conditions that may resolve the hematuria, specifically urinary tract infections. Those with documented infection should have a repeat urinalysis after treatment of the infection. If the hematuria resolves, no further evaluation is needed. The remainder should include some form of imaging with ultrasound or CT scan with less reliance on intravenous urography. The need for imaging has to be tempered with the likelihood of finding a treatable lesion. The probability of malignancy in children is exceedingly low. Routine screening for hematuria in children and adults who are asymptomatic is not recommended. In the presence of hematuria in children, if imaging is undertaken a renal ultrasound will provide sufficient information. In adults and especially those over 40 years old, those with risk factors for bladder cancer, and those with gross hematuria of nonglomerular origin, CT scan with and without contrast as well as cystoscopy should be done. Imaging of the bladder with CT scan will miss mucosal lesions, and cystoscopy also allows for biopsies to be obtained. Urine cytology is also recommended in high-risk patients, as it may occasionally detect the presence of lesions that are not found on initial cystoscopy and imaging, leading to further evaluation. Those with an extensive workup with a negative evaluation, low risk for malignancy, younger age, and only microscopic hematuria require no further evaluation. Patients with gross hematuria with a negative evaluation may warrant further evaluation such as angiography and do require close follow-up for lesions that may have been missed on the initial evaluation.

PROTEINURIA

Proteinuria is often an incidentally noted laboratory finding, and at other times the central finding of a critically ill patient. The kidney filters 180 L of ultrafiltrate a day, and the concentration of albumin in Bowman's space is about 1 mg/dL. Normal protein excretion is <150 mg per day with less than 10–20 mg of albumin excretion a day. The proteins that are filtered, which are lower-molecular-weight proteins

and some albumin, are reabsorbed for the most part in the proximal convoluted tubule, and most of the secreted proteins originate from the renal tubular epithelial cells and are called Tamm-Horsfall proteins.

CLASSIFICATION OF PROTEINURIA

Proteinuria can be classified as overt proteinuria or microalbuminuria, which is detected by radioimmunoassay, enzyme-linked immunosorbent assay, or nephelometry. The dipstick is sensitive to albumin but not to other proteins such as light chains. Low-level proteinuria that is not detectable by the dipstick may be clinically very significant. Microalbuminuria is the excretion of between 30 and 300 mg of albumin per gram of creatinine. Initially defined in the setting of type 1 diabetes mellitus (DM) as the earliest stage of diabetic nephropathy, it has become a marker of renal disease with prognostic significance for cardiovascular outcome, as have overt proteinuria and chronic kidney disease.

Classification of Overt Proteinuria

Proteinuria can be classified in the following categories (table 61.3):

1. Overflow proteinuria. The kidney may provide an innocent excretory function for low-molecular-weight proteins that are produced in abnormal quantities and are freely filtered and excreted. The most common cause of overflow proteinuria is in the setting of monoclonal gammopathies, in which excessive light chain production can lead to a number of renal manifestations including myeloma kidney with acute renal failure, amyloidosis, and light chain deposition disease with concurrent albuminuria and nephrotic syndrome as well as an isolated finding of Bence-Jones proteinuria with no renal manifestations. Another rarer cause of overflow proteinuria is lysozymuria in the setting of acute myelogenous leukemia. Light chains may not be detected as well as by the dipstick, and there will be a discrepancy between the dipstick and the quantitative measurement of proteinuria. Sulfosalicylic acid was used to detect

Table 61.3 **PROTEINURIA**

Overflow proteinuria
Bence-Jones or monoclonal light chain proteinuria
Lysozymuria
Tubular proteinuria
Albuminuria
Microalbuminuria
Transient proteinuria
Orthostatic proteinuria
Nonnephrotic albuminuria
Nephrotic syndrome

light chains in the past in the setting of an unimpressive dipstick test for proteinuria.

2. Tubular proteinuria. The protein excretion in patients with tubular injury main reflects failure of the proximal convoluted tubule to reabsorb filtered protein and some tubular secretion of protein. The quantity will be <1 g a day, and on electrophoresis these are mainly low-molecular-weight proteins.

3. Albuminuria.
   a. Microalbuminuria has been discussed above.
   b. Transient proteinuria. Transient excretion of small amount of albumin is common in certain acute settings including fever, pneumonia, exercise, and congestive heart failure. The proteinuria resolves with resolution of the acute illness. The total amount of protein seldom exceeds 1 g a day.
   c. Orthostatic proteinuria. Young patients with asymptomatic proteinuria should be evaluated for this condition in which there is predominantly proteinuria with upright position and not on recumbency. This is deemed to be a benign condition based on lack of renal pathology on biopsy and a benign course with long-term follow-up over decades. This condition may occasionally reflect the initial stage of a more serious renal lesion and hence should be followed closely.
   d. Nonnephrotic proteinuria. Proteinuria in the nonnephrotic range if not from overflow proteinuria can represent tubulointerstitial disease or glomerular disease. If the protein:creatinine ratio is >1, it is likely glomerular in origin. Patients with a ratio of <1 could have either a glomerular or a tubulointerstitial source for their proteinuria. Urine protein electrophoresis is useful in distinguishing between the two. In general for glomerular lesions, the degree of proteinuria reflects the extent of renal disease unless there is advanced chronic kidney disease.
   e. Nephrotic syndrome is defined by the excretion of >3.5 g of protein a day associated with hypertension, edema, hypoalbuminemia, and hyperlipidemia. The presence of nephrotic syndrome is usually clinically evident. The nephrotic syndrome can be associated with a hypercoagulable state.

Differential Diagnosis

The differential diagnosis of proteinuria is summarized in table 61.4 and includes the following:

1. Transient proteinuria: Fever, pneumonia, exercise, congestive heart failure.

2. Overflow proteinuria: Bence-Jones proteinuria, multiple myeloma, amyloidosis, lymphoma, Waldenstrom, monoclonal gammopathy of uncertain significance. Lysozymuria is seen with acute myelogenous leukemia.

Table 61.4 ETIOLOGY OF PROTEINURIA

Transient proteinuria	Fever, exercise, CHF
Overflow proteinuria	Myeloma, AML
Microalbuminuria	Diabetes mellitus
Orthostatic proteinuria	Usually benign
Tubular proteinuria	Acute kidney injury, interstitial nephritis
Glomerular proteinuria	All renal glomerular diseases
Nephrotic syndrome	Primary and secondary GN, familial
Nephritic syndromes	RPGN, indolent GN, familial and genetic

3. Microalbuminuria is seen in diabetes mellitus and hypertension as well as syndrome X. Diabetics should be screened yearly for type 2 DM and yearly starting at year 5 after onset for type 1 DM.

4. Orthostatic proteinuria can be idiopathic and benign or rarely an early manifestation of a primary renal disease. Patients need an appropriate laboratory evaluation and close follow-up.

5. Tubular proteinuria. These can be transient in the setting of acute tubular injury such as aminoglycoside- or cisplatinum-induced tubular injury as well as acute ischemic injury. The differential diagnosis of acute interstitial nephritis includes collagen vascular diseases such as systemic lupus and Sjögren as well as sarcoidosis and tubulointerstitial nephritis with uveitis (TINU) syndrome. Infections such as *Legionella* pneumonia, leptospirosis, and ehrlichiosis can cause acute interstitial nephritis. Bence-Jones proteins can induce tubular dysfunction and cause tubular proteinuria.

6. Glomerular proteinuria and nephrotic syndrome. This can be subclassified as either primary renal disease, genetic, or secondary to a systemic disease.
   a. Primary renal disease in adults includes membranous nephropathy, focal and segmental glomerulonephrosclerosis, minimal change disease, and membranoproliferative glomerulonephritis in order of frequency, although recent series have shown that focal segmental glomerulosclerosis (FSGS) may now be the leading cause of idiopathic nephrotic syndrome.
   b. Familial nephrotic syndrome with a number of mutations identified in podocyte proteins including nephrin, podocin, and alpha-actinin-4. These cause predominantly pediatric disease but are increasingly being recognized in adults as a cause of nephrotic syndrome.
   c. Secondary causes of nephrotic syndrome include:
      i. Malignancies with membranous nephropathy from solid tumors such as lung cancer. Hodgkin disease is associated with minimal change disease, membranous nephropathy from non-Hodgkin,

primary (AL) amyloidosis from myeloma or lymphoma, and secondary (AA) amyloidosis from renal cell carcinoma.

    ii. Drugs such as nonsteroidal anti-inflammatory drugs (NSAIDs) induce minimal change disease and focal sclerosis; captopril is associated with membranous nephropathy, and pamidronate is associated with focal sclerosis.

    iii. Infections associated with membranous nephropathy include hepatitis B, hepatitis C, malaria, syphilis, and schistosomiasis. Endocarditis, osteomyelitis, and tuberculosis with chronic infections can cause the AA form of amyloidosis.

    iv. Chronic inflammatory conditions such as familial Mediterranean fever lead to AA amyloidosis.

7. Nephritic diseases and rapidly progressive glomerulonephritis. These can classified in four categories:

    a. Anti-GBM disease with renal and pulmonary disease manifest as pulmonary hemorrhage, usually in smokers.

    b. ANCA-associated vasculitis with Wegner granulomatosis, microscopic polyangiitis, and Churg-Strauss syndrome. These all share pulmonary involvement, with asthma and eosinophilia being unique to Churg-Strauss syndrome. These diseases also have renal involvement, mononeuritis multiplex, arthritis, and skin lesions.

    c. Immune complex glomerulonephritis with low complements including systemic lupus, subacute bacterial endocarditis, cryoglobulinemia, membranoproliferative glomerulonephritis, and visceral abscess.

    d. Immune complex glomerulonephritis with normal C3 and C4. This includes IgA nephropathy and Henoch Shonlein purpura.

EVALUATION OF PROTEINURIA

The evaluation of patients with proteinuria starts with a careful review of the history and a meticulous physical examination. Central to the extent and pace of the evaluation are the quantification of the proteinuria, the presence of a nephritic component, and the level of accompanying renal function.

History

The history should review and look for features of systemic disease. Systemic lupus erythematosus, ANCA-associated vasculitis, and amyloidosis all may have distinct skin manifestations. Sinusitis can be seen in ANCA-associated vasculitis. Easy bruising is seen in amyloidosis. A careful history of drug intake, both prescribed and over-the-counter medications, may be useful in the evaluation of proteinuria. Nonsteroidal anti-inflammatory drugs are common causes of both proteinuria and renal insufficiency. A unique combination of interstitial nephritis with nephrotic syndrome secondary to minimal change disease is induced by NSAIDs. Systemic features of weight loss and constitutional symptoms may reflect an underlying malignancy. The history of abrupt onset of edema, foamy urine, and hypertension is often the initial and dramatic presentation of nephrotic syndrome. Intravenous drug use and high-risk sexual behavior can lead to infections such as HIV, hepatitis B, and hepatitis C, all of which are associated with renal involvement. A family history of renal disease may be a clue to Alport syndrome, especially if there is an X-linked inheritance pattern.

Physical Examination

The BP may be very elevated in certain forms of renal disease such as membranous nephropathy, whereas it tends to be less elevated in minimal change disease and HIV-associated nephropathy. The physical examination may reveal a classical rash of amyloidosis or systemic lupus, or there can be joint swelling, macroglossia, hepatosplenomegaly, or edema. Lymphadenopathy that is pathological may be a clue for an underlying lymphoma with a paraneoplastic nephrotic syndrome.

Laboratory Evaluation

The laboratory evaluation (table 61.5) includes the hematocrit, which may be low in certain systemic diseases, especially if the renal function is normal. The anion gap may be low with multiple myeloma. There may be evidence for a renal tubular acidosis or hypercalcemia with myeloma. The

Table 61.5 **EVALUATION OF HEMATURIA AND PROTEINURIA**

Hematocrit	ANA
Cr or eGFR	Complements C3 and C4
Anion-gap	Antineutrophil cytoplasmic antibody (ANCA)
Serum bicarbonate	Antiglomerular basement membrane antibody
Urinalysis and sediment	Cryoglobulins
Calcium	Hepatitis serology with hepatitis B surface antigen and antibody
Globulins	as well as hepatitis C antibody and viral RNA
Urine protein:Cr ratio	Antistreptolysin O or anti-DNAse B acute titers
Transaminases	
Viral hepatitis serologies when indicated urine eosinophils	
Urine *Legionella* antigen	
24-hour urine collection for proteinuria	
Split collection for orthostatic proteinuria	
Urine for Bence-Jones	

liver function tests may be abnormal with viral hepatitides. The lipids may be markedly elevated in patients with nephrotic syndrome in addition to hypoalbuminemia. The urinalysis is central in the evaluation of proteinuria. The urine protein dipstick is more sensitive to albumin than other proteins and therefore will underestimate the degree of Bence-Jones proteinuria. 1+ proteinuria is approximately 30 mg/dL, and 3+ is about 500 mg/dL. The presence of hematuria and leukocytes in the dipstick as well as examination of the urine sediment is crucial in the evaluation of the patient with proteinuria. Dysmorphic red blood cells and red cell casts are indicative of glomerular pathology. Granular and tubular cell casts suggest tubular injury. White cell casts are seen in cases of interstitial nephritis, which can be idiopathic as seen in TINU syndrome, in infections such as *Legionella* pneumonia, or in drug-induced allergic interstitial nephritis.

Twenty-four-hour urine collections used to be the cornerstone of quantifying proteinuria but have been replaced by the spot urine protein:creatinine ratio in large part because of inaccuracies in the 24-hour urine collection. The urine protein:creatinine ratio, which is the ratio of protein to creatinine, expressed as an mg/dL-to-mg/dL ratio, has been validated to be accurate in large studies. There have been arguments against its use based on the diurnal variation in protein excretion as well as variations in creatinine excretion based on dietary intake. There are patients in whom the evaluation will include a split 24-hour collection to evaluate for orthostatic proteinuria.

The next step in the evaluation of proteinuria is ensuring that the proteins are predominantly albumin in certain circumstances. Both overflow proteinuria with Bence-Jones proteins and tubular proteinuria can be detected by the urine immune electrophoresis looking for monoclonal light chains. The serum immune electrophoresis and urine for Bence-Jones allow diseases such as multiple myeloma and amyloidosis to be screened for. In amyloidosis there will be large amounts of albumin and light chains that are monoclonal in most patients. The newer serum free light chain assay allows for higher sensitivity in detecting monoclonal disorders.

Other serologies that may be obtained include the following:

- Antinuclear antibodies (ANA) when indicated and if appropriate more specific lupus tests such as anti-dsDNA
- *Complements C3 and C4*
- *Antineutrophil cytoplasmic antibody (ANCA)* in patients with a systemic vasculitis, especially if there is also pulmonary involvement.
- *Anti–glomerular basement membrane antibody* is essential in patients with an active sediment and often pulmonary involvement
- *Cryoglobulins*

- *Hepatitis serology with hepatitis B surface antigen and antibody as well as hepatitis C antibody and viral RNA if indicated.*
- *Anti-streptolysin O or anti-DNAse B* acute titers for the diagnosis of poststreptococcal glomerulonephritis.

Imaging

Imaging will often be done when appropriate to look for underlying systemic disorders such as malignancies, which may be the underlying cause for nephrotic syndrome. Both solid tumors and lymphomas can present with nephrotic syndrome, especially in the elderly. The malignancy is usually detected by a careful history and physical examination combined with age-appropriate screening for malignancies. An exhaustive evaluation for an underlying malignancy does not need to be undertaken for all cases of nephrotic syndrome.

Renal ultrasound will reveal congenital absence or hypoplasia of one kidney, which leads to focal sclerosis. Renal ultrasound may reveal hydronephrosis, and a voiding cystoureterogram (VCUG) may reveal reflux as the etiology for proteinuria especially in children.

Kidney Biopsy

Kidney biopsies are usually done under real-time ultrasound guidance with a severe complication rate of about 1–2% of significant bleeding requiring transfusion. Therefore, biopsies should be undertaken with a clear discussion of risks and benefits. The current indications for a percutaneous renal biopsy are rapidly progressive glomerulonephritis of unknown etiology with a negative serological evaluation, patients with nephrotic syndrome, patients with acute renal failure of uncertain etiology, patients with lupus nephritis to determine optimal therapeutic approach, and in patients with both hematuria and proteinuria. Consideration of renal biopsy in patients with <1 g of proteinuria per day and in patients with isolated hematuria has to be individualized. Patients with proteinuria of between 1 and 3.5 g/day may be considered for renal biopsy if they do not have far advanced chronic kidney disease and are candidates for aggressive management.

Therapy of Specific Renal Conditions

Therapeutic approaches are summarized in table 61.6 and include the following possibilities:

1. Transient proteinuria resolves spontaneously and requires no specific treatment.

2. Overflow proteinuria is fully evaluated, and treatment is of the underlying myeloma or lymphoma.

3. Microalbuminuria should be managed with angiotensin-converting enzyme (ACE) inhibitors and

Table 61.6 THERAPY OF PROTEINURIA

• Overflow proteinuria	• Treat myeloma if indicated
• Orthostatic or transient proteinuria	• No specific therapy needed
• Microalbuminuria	• BP control, ACEI/ARB therapy
• Proteinuria in nonnephrotic range	• ACEI/ARB +/− specific therapy
• Nephrotic syndrome	• ACEI/ARB +/− specific therapy
• RPGN	• Therapy tailored to diagnosis
• All patients	• BP control
	• Lipid management
	• ACEI/ARB use when proteinuria is present
	• Aldosterone antagonists for proteinuria
	• Modest protein restriction
	• Vitamin D therapy for deficiency
	• Anticoagulation for thrombosis

or angiotensin receptor blockers (ARBs) as well as BP control.

4. Patients with tubulointerstitial disease should have treatment for the underlying disorder including withdrawal of offending drugs. Multiple myeloma with myeloma kidney or cast nephropathy will need specific therapy.

5. Patients with albuminuria that is <1 g/day should have an extensive evaluation unless they have a commonly associated disorder such as diabetes mellitus, and the decision to biopsy will be influenced by the presence of hematuria, chronic kidney disease, hypertension, and age. Therapy should be undertaken only when a clear diagnosis is established.

6. Patients with proteinuria of between 1 and 3.5 g should have an evaluation including a renal biopsy unless they have a known diagnosis such as diabetes mellitus, have advanced chronic kidney disease, or are not candidates for aggressive therapy.

7. Patients with nephrotic syndrome should be evaluated unless they have a known etiology such as NSAID use or diabetes. Therapeutic considerations, stage of kidney disease, and risks of treatment need to be considered.

   a. Idiopathic nephrotic syndrome is treated with just steroids for minimal change disease and focal sclerosis and a combination of steroids and melphalan, mycophenolate, or cyclophosphamide for membranous nephropathy. Refractory cases of minimal change disease and focal sclerosis may be treated with steroids combined with mycophenolate or cyclophosphamide. Other considerations include IV IgG and cyclosporine.

   b. Secondary causes of nephrotic syndrome are treated with more disease specific approaches. Diabetic nephropathy is treated with the more general treatments for proteinuric renal disease detailed in the next section. Systemic lupus is treated based on the stage of disease after kidney biopsy with steroids and cyclophosphamide for more severe disease.

Amyloidosis of the AL variety, either primary or secondary to multiple myeloma, is treated with myeloma-directed therapy. Nephrotic syndrome secondary to malignancies is directed toward therapy of the malignancy. Withdrawal of drugs when there is a drug that can be implicated, consideration of biopsy if the proteinuria fails to abate, and treatment with steroids can be considered in the appropriate settings. HIV and hepatitis B and C–associated diseases are treated with antiviral therapy, and cases of rapidly progressive glomerulonephritis may be treated with steroids and cyclophosphamide.

8. Rapidly progressive glomerulonephritis is often treated empirically while a diagnostic evaluation is in progress, as delay in treatment may lead to irreversible renal dysfunction. In general, high-dose pulse steroids with intravenous cyclophosphamide at 2 mg/kg/day is often used in severe cases. Anti-GBM disease is additionally treated with plasma exchange. Subacute bacterial endocarditis is treated with just antibiotics and without immunosuppression. Cryoglobulinemia is treated with plasma exchange in the acute setting and immunosuppression with steroids and cyclophosphamide, but hepatitis C–associated cryoglobulinemia is ultimately treated with anti-HCV therapy with PEG-interferon and ribavirin.

GENERAL MANAGEMENT OF PROTEINURIA

All patients with proteinuria are managed with some common approaches:

1. *ACE inhibitors and ARBs* alone or in combination should be used as initial agents for renal protection. They have been shown to be effective in the earliest stages of chronic kidney disease with just microalbuminuria to advanced stage 4 chronic kidney disease. Hyperkalemia and acute rise in creatinine are the major limitations in addition to cough or angioedema as a side effect of ACE inhibitors.

2. *BP control.* BP control is essential in the management of patients with proteinuria and chronic kidney disease. The Joint National Committee 7 (JNC7) recommends a SBP <130 and DBP <80. The National Kidney Foundation recommends goals of SBP <125 and DBP <75 for patients with chronic kidney disease. Certain dug classes are more effective at controlling proteinuria than others. Dihydropyridine calcium channel blockers may increase proteinuria as opposed to beta blockers and nondihydropyridine calcium channel blockers.

3. *Protein intake.* Control of proteinuria to 0.7–0.8 g/kg/day was shown in the MDRD study to have a beneficial effect.

4. *Sodium intake and diuretic use.* Control of sodium intake and possible diuretic use become more important as the level of proteinuria increases: 80–120 mmol/day is the recommendation. Thiazide diuretics are used more for blood pressure control, and loop diuretics for control of edema. The combination of the two agents is powerful and may induce hypokalemia, metabolic alkalosis, and prerenal azotemia.

5. *Lipid control.* Lipid control is essential from two perspectives. Patients with microalbuminuria, proteinuria, and chronic kidney disease are at increased risk for cardiovascular disease and need meticulous management of risk factors. Patients with nephrotic syndrome tend to develop impressive hyperlipidemia, which increases the risk for cardiovascular disease and needs to be managed often with a combination of diet and several lipid-lowering agents.

6. *Aldosterone antagonists.* Aldosterone has effects on proliferation and scarring, and aldosterone blockade is being increasingly recognized as an important part of the treatment of proteinuria. Aldosterone blockade is correlated with control of proteinuria.

7. *Anticoagulation.* Patients with nephrotic syndrome are at risk for thromboembolic complications, especially patients with membranous nephropathy. Empirical anticoagulation of patients with severe membranous nephropathy is controversial. However, patients should be monitored for the development of renal vein thrombosis, deep venous thrombosis, and pulmonary emboli, all of which warrant anticoagulation until resolution of the nephrotic syndrome.

8. *Vitamin D deficiency.* Patients with nephrotic syndrome and those with renal insufficiency develop vitamin D deficiency, which should be evaluated for and treated with replacement.

ADDITIONAL READING

Chou R, Dana T. Screening adults for bladder cancer: A review of the evidence for the U.S. preventive services task force. *Ann Intern Med.* 2010;153(7):461–8.

Chugh A, Bakris GL. Microalbuminuria: What is it? Why is it important? What should be done about it? An update. *J Clin Hypertens (Greenwich).* 2007;9(3):196–200.

Jimbo M. Evaluation and management of hematuria. *Prim Care.* 2010;37(3):461–72, vii.

Kelly JD, Fawcett DP, Goldberg LC. Assessment and management of non-visible haematuria in primary care. *BMJ.* 2009;338:a3021.

Lambers Heerspink HJ, Brinkman JW, Bakker SJ, Gansevoort RT, de Zeeuw D. Update on microalbuminuria as a biomarker in renal and cardiovascular disease. *Curr Opin Nephrol Hypertens.* 2006;15(6):631–6.

Tu WH, Shortliffe LD. Evaluation of asymptomatic, atraumatic hematuria in children and adults. *Nat Rev Urol.* 2010;7(4):189–94.

QUESTIONS

QUESTION 1. A 22-year-old Chinese-American male presents with a complaint of red urine. He describes 2 days of a sore throat, low-grade fever, and a dry cough. He has no family history of renal disease. Urinalysis shows 1+ protein, 2+ blood, but is otherwise negative. His urine sediment examination shows 10–20 erythrocytes per high-power field, but no leukocytes or casts are present. A rapid throat swab (rapid antigen detection testing or RADT) is negative. His blood urea nitrogen (BUN) and serum creatinine level are 20 mg/dL and 0.8 mg/dL, respectively. Which one of the following is the most likely diagnosis?

A. Poststreptococcal glomerulonephritis
B. Nephrolithiasis
C. Transitional cell carcinoma of the bladder
D. IgA nephropathy
E. Urinary tract infection

QUESTION 2. A 52-year-old male patient presents with asymptomatic painless gross hematuria. He is completely asymptomatic. Risk factors for significant disease, such as a uroepithelial malignancy, include all of the following, EXCEPT:

A. Age >40 years
B. Smoking history
C. History of pelvic irradiation
D. History of occupational exposure to benzenes
E. A positive BTA Stat test

QUESTION 3. False-positive reactions of the urine dipstick for albuminuria have been reported in all of the following situations, EXCEPT:

A. Patients with an acid urine (pH of 5.0)
B. In a patient being treated with penicillin
C. If the dipstick is immersed too long
D. Presence of gross hematuria
E. In a patient being treated with a sulfonamide

QUESTION 4. A 45-year-old white male presents with massive lower extremity edema and foamy urine. On physical examination, he has a blood pressure of 132/84 mm Hg and heart rate of 72 beats per minute. He has 2+ to 3+ lower extremity edema. There is no rash. Laboratory data show 4+ for dipstick protein but was otherwise negative. His urine sediment examination shows fatty casts and an oval fat body cast but no cellular casts. His serum creatinine is 1.1 mg/dL. His serum albumin is 1.2 g/dL His complements are normal.

The most likely diagnosis is:

A. Henoch-Schönlein nephritis
B. Lupus nephritis
C. Membranous glomerulopathy
D. Membranoproliferative glomerulonephritis
E. Postinfectious glomerulonephritis

QUESTION 5. A 41-year-old African-American male with a history of hypertension and long-standing substance abuse presents to your urgent care clinic with generalized edema of 1 week duration. He says that he noticed progressive lower extremity edema and had been seen by your colleague in urgent care the previous week and started on furosemide, 40 mg twice daily. Past medical history of depression, hypertension for the past 5 years, and drug dependency. Medications: he is on atenolol 50 mg once daily and furosemide 40 mg twice daily. He is single, lives alone, and volunteers a history of long-standing intermittent cocaine abuse, heavy alcohol consumption (he says he quit 2 years ago), and tobacco consumption (1 pack per day for the past 25 years). Physical examination shows no acute distress and is remarkable for vital signs showing a temperature of 36.80°C, heart rate 73 beats per minute, respiratory rate of 20, and a blood pressure of 178/99 mm Hg. He has 4+ pitting edema to his knees. His urinalysis shows 4+ protein but is otherwise negative. His urine microscopy shows several fatty casts and one oval fat body. The most likely diagnosis is:

A. Minimal change disease
B. Membranous nephropathy
C. FSGS
D. Hypertensive nephrosclerosis
E. Membranoproliferative glomerulonephritis

ANSWERS

1. D
2. E
3. A
4. C
5. C

62.

PARENCHYMAL RENAL DISEASE

Mariam P. Alexander and Ajay K. Singh

Parenchymal renal disease can be considered anatomically under the headings of glomerular, tubular, tubulointerstitial, and vascular disease. Most patients present with a clinical syndrome of nephron injury. The clinical features of parenchymal renal disease frequently depend on the component of the kidney that is affected—for example, glomerulonephritis presents with worsened kidney function, hypertension, hematuria, proteinuria, and red cell casts. Tubulointerstitial nephritis presents with azotemia, pyuria and/or white cell casts.

SYNDROMES OF NEPHRONAL INJURY

ISOLATED GLOMERULAR HEMATURIA

This is defined as persistent microscopic hematuria with dysmorphic red blood cells, negative "dipstick" for proteinuria, normal serum creatinine concentration, and normal blood pressure. Common causes include IgA, hereditary nephritis, and thin basement membrane disease (figure 62.1).

ISOLATED NONNEPHROTIC PROTEINURIA

Isolated nonnephrotic proteinuria is defined as proteinuria >150 mg/dL (60% of which is usually albuminuria). Figure 62.2 depicts causes of functional and persistent proteinuria. A renal biopsy is rarely indicated in those with low-grade proteinuria (<500–1000 mg/day) if there is an absence of hematuria, absence of clinical or serological evidence of systemic disease that can cause a glomerulonephritis, and normal renal function (figure 62.2).

NEPHROTIC SYNDROME

The nephrotic syndrome is defined as heavy proteinuria (≥3.5 g/day/1.73 m² surface area), edema, hypoalbuminemia, and hyperlipidemia.

Causes of nephritic syndrome are shown (table 62.1). The most common causes of the nephrotic syndrome in adults are primary focal and segmental glomerulosclerosis and membranous glomerulonephritis. In children, the most common cause of nephrotic syndrome is minimal change disease. Selected causes of nephrotic syndrome are discussed below.

The nephrotic syndrome comprises heavy proteinuria (≥3.5 g/day/1.73 m² surface area), edema, hypoalbuminemia, and hyperlipidemia. In the absence of a systemic disease, it is quite likely that one of the three major causes of the idiopathic nephrotic syndrome is present: membranous nephropathy, minimal change disease, or primary focal and segmental glomerulosclerosis.

ACUTE NEPHRITIC SYNDROME

This is characterized by hematuria, red cell casts, azotemia, variable proteinuria, oliguria, edema, and hypertension. It is often caused by a systemic disease that requires a renal biopsy to establish its diagnosis and guide treatment. The classic example of this is acute postinfectious glomerulonephritis. Examples include systemic lupus erythematosus (SLE), microscopic polyangiitis, Wegener granulomatosis, and anti-glomerular basement membrane (GBM) disease.

UNEXPLAINED ACUTE KIDNEY INJURY

Most often the diagnosis is not based on a renal biopsy. Biopsy is indicated in those settings in which the diagnosis is uncertain, as may sometimes be the case with acute interstitial nephritis secondary to drugs.

IMPORTANT CAUSES OF NEPHROTIC SYNDROME

Minimal Change Disease

Minimal change disease (MCD), or nil disease, is a major cause of nephrotic syndrome in children and accounts for 15–20% of adult cases. The exact underlying cause of MCD is unclear. Accumulating evidence suggests that systemic

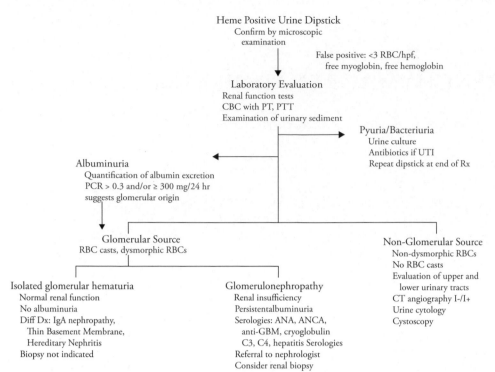

Figure 62.1. Hematuria Workup.

T-cell dysfunction results in the production of a glomerular permeability factor. This circulating factor directly affects the glomerular capillary wall, resulting in foot process fusion and marked proteinuria.

The abrupt onset of a nephrotic syndrome (glomerular proteinuria >3.5 g/day in an adult or >40 mg/hr/m² in a child, hypoalbuminemia, and edema) is the typical presentation of MCD. Hematuria and/or hypertension may be present in about 20% of cases. Renal function (as evaluated by either serum creatinine or estimated glomerular filtration rate [eGFR]) is

usually normal, but 15–30% of adults (usually over the age of 40 years) may present or develop acute kidney injury.

The renal pathology is characterized by minimal or absent glomerular abnormalities (figure 62.3). The most consistent observation is seen on electron microscopy: simplification of the visceral epithelial cells with widespread and diffuse effacement of the foot processes.

Treatment is with a trial of prednisone at 1 mg/kg/day. The response to steroids is usually dramatic. Treatment in children consists of prednisone, 60 mg/m²/day (maximum

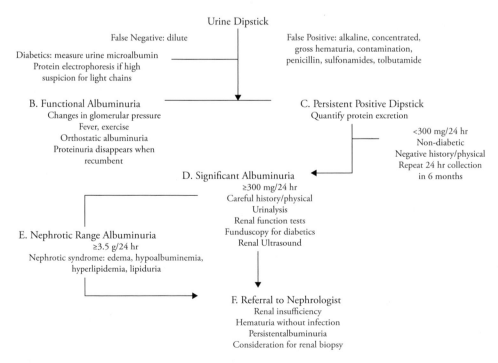

Figure 62.2. Proteinuria Workup.

Table 62.1 CAUSES OF NEPHROTIC SYNDROME

Primary Causes

Membranous
Focal segmental glomerulosclerosis (FSGS)
Minimal change disease
IgA

Secondary Causes

Medications
   e.g., gold, NSAIDs, interferon-α, heroin, Captopril

Allergens
   e.g., bee sting, pollen

Infections
   e.g., bacterial, viral, helminth

Cancer
   e.g., solid (lung, colon, stomach), leukemia, Hodgkin

Autoimmune diseases
   e.g., lupus nephritis

Metabolic diseases
   e.g., diabetes mellitus

Pregnancy
   e.g., preeclampsia

---

doses of 80 mg/m²/day) until a remission has been induced (or for 4 weeks, whichever is shorter) and then 35–40 mg/m² every other day for about 12 weeks followed by slow tapering. Adults with established MCD are treated with prednisone, 1 mg/kg/day until remission (or for 6 weeks, whichever is shorter) followed by slow tapering. Treatment is generally continued for about 8 weeks in children and 16 weeks in adults, with slow tapering thereafter. About 95% of children and about 90% of adults will respond with a complete remission of proteinuria with this initial regimen, earlier in children and later in adults. However, many patients (40–60%) will relapse, either during the tapering phase of treatment (steroid-dependent relapses) or weeks, months, or even years later. Intercurrent infections or allergies may trigger a relapse. Some patients have frequent relapses (>2 year) and require repeated courses of therapy.

Focal and Segmental Glomerulosclerosis

There are primary and secondary forms of focal and segmental glomerulosclerosis (FSGS). Primary FSGS is a clinicopathological diagnosis that is characterized by the absence of clinical or histological evidence of an antecedent glomerulonephritis, immune complex deposition, or systemic disease with glomerular involvement. The primary form of FSGS is due to podocyte injury of unknown cause.

The typical clinical presentation is with the insidious onset of nonnephrotic proteinuria or the nephrotic syndrome. Hypertension and reduction in estimated glomerular filtration rate (GFR) are common at the time of presentation. Urinary protein excretion may be very high, sometimes in excess of 20 g/day, and the proteinuria is nonselective, with a high fractional excretion of IgG (often >0.2). Serum complement components are normal.

It is important to differentiate primary from secondary forms of FSGS. A history of sub-nephrotic-range proteinuria, slower onset of symptoms, and predisposing factors such as obesity, renal mass loss, and chronic interstitial nephritis accompanied by typical biopsy findings are useful in making the diagnosis of secondary FSGS.

Renal biopsy findings of FSGS are variable because there are several histological variants. The most common abnormality(classical form of FSGS) is segmental sclerosis (figure 62.4). The collapsing variant, observed in

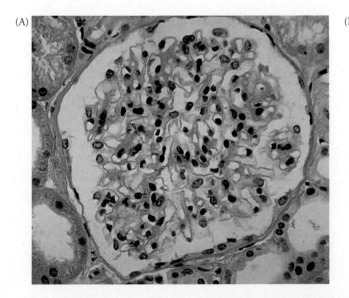

(A)

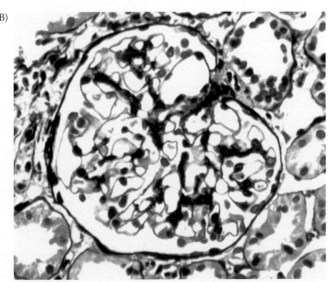

(B)

Figure 62.3. Normal Comparison (A) versus Minimal Change Disease (B). Photo courtesy of Dr. Helmut Rennke.

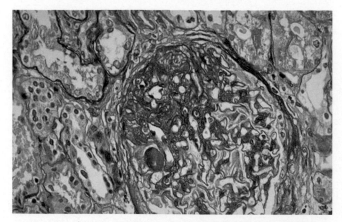

Figure 62.4. Focal Segmental Glomerulosclerosis. Photo courtesy of Dr. Helmut Rennke.

HIV-associated nephropathy, is less common and shows collapse and sclerosis of the entire glomerular tuft rather than segmental injury. On electron microscopy there is diffuse effacement of epithelial cell foot processes even in areas where there are no light microscopic abnormalities.

Unlike MCD, FSGS is generally resistant to steroid therapy. If steroids are used alone, oral prednisone in a dose of 1 mg/kg per day or 2 mg/kg every other day is given for 2–3 months with slow tapering over another 2–3 months. However, only about one-half of the patients respond to steroid therapy, and patients frequently need adjunctive therapy, such as cyclosporine (4–5 mg/kg/day for 3–6 months). Treatment resistance (lack of a complete or partial remission) is strongly associated with a high risk of progression to end-stage renal disease (ESRD), which may be very rapid if proteinuria is in excess of 15–20 g/day. Patients with FSGS may relapse after a complete or partial remission. A higher incidence of recurrence after transplantation is also present.

Membranous Glomerulopathy

Membranous nephropathy (MN) is among the most common causes of the nephrotic syndrome in nondiabetic adults over age 40 years. MN can be idiopathic (75–85% of adults), or secondary to hepatitis B antigenemia, autoimmune diseases, thyroiditis, malignancies, and the use of certain drugs such as gold, penicillamine, captopril, and nonsteroidal anti-inflammatory drugs. Only about 25% of children with MN have the idiopathic form.

MN may affect all age groups but has a peak incidence in the 40s and 50s. It has no racial predilection. At presentation, 60–70% of patients have the nephrotic syndrome with the remainder having subnephrotic proteinuria (<3.5 g/24 hours). Microscopic hematuria is common (30–40%), but macroscopic hematuria and red cell casts are rare. At presentation, most patients are not hypertensive (<20%), and most do not have renal insufficiency (<20%). In patients with severe nephrotic syndrome clinical manifestations of hypercoagulability may arise (deep venous thrombosis, pulmonary embolism, or renal vein thrombosis).

On renal biopsy the characteristic lesion on light microscopy is uniform, diffuse thickening of the GBM throughout all glomeruli in the absence of significant hypercellularity (figure 62.5). The thickness is due to subepithelial deposits with basement membrane response. The basement membrane encases the subepithelial deposits, resulting in "spike formation." There are four stages of evolution: Stage 1 is irregular subepithelial electron-dense deposits. When GBM material accumulates between deposits forming spikes it is stage 2. The basement membrane completely encircles the deposits (stage 3) and then incorporates it into the basement membrane (stage 4).

Treatment with glucocorticoids alone is insufficient therapy for membranous glomerulopathy. Recommended treatment is with a combination of steroids and alkylating agents cyclophosphamide or chlorambucil. The efficacy of mycophenolate mofetil for treatment of MN is unknown. Rituximab, an anti-CD20 monoclonal antibody, has been found efficacious in case series and case reports. Angiotensin blockade at high doses with either an angiotensin-converting enzyme inhibitor or an angiotensin receptor blocker should be used to treat hypertension and proteinuria The disease may recur in the renal transplant, but this is relatively uncommon (10–15%).

The prognosis of MN is very much a function of the quantity of proteinuria. Patients with nephrotic-range proteinuria, over 6 g for over 6 months, tend to pursue a progressive course. Young women with moderate proteinuria tend to do very well; older males fare less well. Spontaneous complete or partial remissions of proteinuria occur in about 40% of patients, usually within 3–5 years of diagnosis. Overall, at 20 years after diagnosis about one-third of patients will have developed ESRD, about one-third will be in remission, and about one-third will have varying levels of persisting proteinuria and renal function. Among

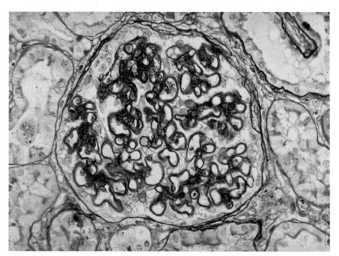

Figure 62.5. Membranous Glomerulopathy. Photo courtesy of Dr. Helmut Rennke.

those who undergo remission either spontaneously or with drugs, about 67% remain in remission, while the rest either have recurrent relapses without progression to renal failure (20%) or progress to renal insufficiency (13%).

NEPHRITIC SYNDROME

Glomerulonephritis is defined as acute inflammation of the glomerular compartment. Nephritis results from injury to one or more of the cell types or structures that comprise the glomerulus—endothelial, epithelial, or mesangial cells or the basement membrane. Injury can be categorized into several different pathological patterns, which are broadly grouped into nonproliferative or proliferative types. The etiology of these different types of nephritis can be either primary causes, i.e., ones that are intrinsic to the kidney, or secondary causes, which are associated with certain infections (bacterial, viral, or parasitic pathogens), drugs, systemic disorders (SLE, vasculitis), or diabetes (table 62.2). Serological testing for autoantibodies and evaluation of the pattern of hypocomplementemia are usually very helpful in the workup of patients (table 62.3). Ultimately, however, renal biopsy is often necessary to make a definitive diagnosis.

The nephritic syndrome is characterized by hematuria, red cell casts, azotemia, variable proteinuria, lipiduria, edema, and hypertension.

IMPORTANT CAUSES OF NEPHRITIC SYNDROME

Acute Diffuse Proliferative Glomerulonephritis (Postinfectious Glomerulonephritis, PIGN)

This syndrome is most commonly seen in children and less often in adults. Males are affected more frequently (M:F ratio 2:1). Presentation is either in a sporadic or epidemic form, 1–3 weeks after infection with nephritogenic strains of group A beta-hemolytic streptococcal infection (types 12, 4, 1, and 49) affecting the throat or 3–6 weeks after a skin infection. The delay in the renal symptoms after the throat or skin infection is related to the time period required to produce the antibodies that mediate the renal disease.

Clinical presentation is characterized by an abrupt onset of cola-colored urine, puffiness of face and eyelids, moderate proteinuria, and hypertension.

Laboratory investigations include elevated antistreptolysin O (ASLO) titer (in cases of skin infections, anti-DNAse-B and antihyaluronidase are more often positive), decreased C3 and CH50. Additional positive findings in PIGN include elevated ESR, dysmorphic RBCs in urine, and RBC casts. Reduction of C3 seldom persists for >8 weeks (an important finding to differentiate from membranoproliferative glomerulonephritis (MPGN), which shows a persistent decrease in complement levels). In children, with symptomatic management, 95% recover clinically within 2 months of onset and morphologically within 3 years, although a few may progress to chronicity.

Many other infections can produce postinfectious glomerulonephritis resembling poststreptococcal glomerulonephritis. These include, but are not limited to, *Mycoplasma pneumoniae*, cytomegalovirus (CMV), *Streptococcus* pneumonia, *Neisseria* meningitis, *Salmonella*, toxoplasmosis, diphtheroids, *Propionibacter* species, and *Staphylococcus aureus* and *albus*.

Renal pathology is characterized by global hypercellularity of endothelial and mesangial cells in the glomeruli and an increase in the mesangial matrix. There is abundant polymorphonuclear (PMN) cell infiltration within glomerular capillaries—this is often referred to as "exudative" glomerulonephritis. Occasional crescents may be present. Immunofluorescence shows a granular pattern of immune deposits—a "starry sky" pattern. Electron microscopy shows subepithelial "humps" and small subendothelial/mesangial deposits.

Treatment should be focused on eliminating the streptococcal infection with antibiotics and providing supportive therapy until spontaneous resolution of glomerular inflammation occurs. Even if the patient presents with AKI, short-term prognosis is good, and >95% of the children will recover from the initial episode. Immunosuppressive therapy and dialysis rarely are necessary. Adults with PIGN have a 60% chance of recovery. Persistent proteinuria is a sign of poor prognosis.

IgA Nephropathy or Berger Disease

In 1968 Berger and Hinglais described a group of patients with episodic macrohematuria, persistent microhematuria, and moderate proteinuria. Their kidney biopsies revealed a

Table 62.2 CAUSES OF NEPHRITIS

Primary Causes
Diffuse and global
Minimal change disease
Membranous nephropathy
Proliferative
Acute diffuse (endocapillary, postinfectious)
Mesangial (e.g., IgA)
Focal and segmental
Focal proliferative
Focal segmental

Secondary Causes
ANCA associated
e.g., Wegener
Antibody associated
Anti-GBM nephritis
Immune complex mediated
e.g., lupus nephritis

Table 62.3 HYPOCOMPLEMENTEMIA IN THE WORKUP OF GLOMERULAR DISEASE

PATHWAY	COMPLEMENT	DISEASE
Classical	Low C3, C4, CH50	Lupus nephritis Mixed essential cryo
Alternate	Low C3, Normal C4	Poststrep GN Postinfect GN SBE Shunt Hep B MPGN type 2
Reduced synthesis	Acquired Hereditary (C2 def)	Liver disease Lupus

focal proliferative glomerular lesion with IgA in the glomeruli. The acute form was characterized by Volhard and Fahr as a "synpharyngetic" episode (most often caused by *Staphylococcus aureus* and *albus*) of hematuria, usually without azotemia, edema, and hypertension.

IgA nephropathy (IgAN) has an estimated prevalence of 25–50 cases per 100,000 people (considered by some to be the most common form of glomerulonephritis worldwide). It is more common among Asian and Native American populations and rare in African Americans. All ages may be affected; however, IgAN is most prominent in the second and third decades (80% between 16–35 years). Males are affected more than females. Genetic predisposition is likely questionable because there are no consistent associations with human leukocyte antigen (HLA) except that HLA-B35 is more common in French patients. There are also rare cases described of a familial form of IgA nephropathy that is associated with deafness.

Gross hematuria is often the first presenting symptom 24–48 hours following a pharyngeal or gastrointestinal infection, vaccination, or strenuous exercise. Asymptomatic cases present with microscopic hematuria during a routine physical. There are a varied array of presentations—ranging form intermittent gross hematuria to persistent microhematuria. Constitutional symptoms (fever, muscle aches, malaise, fatigue, and flank/abdominal pain) often accompany the nephritis.

There are no specific tests short of a renal biopsy that are diagnostic of IgA nephropathy.

Although nonspecific, IgA levels may be elevated in >50% of patients. C3/C4 may be normal or even elevated in some patients. The typical pathologic finding is a focal or diffuse mesangioproliferative glomerulonephritis and diffuse mesangial IgA immune deposits on immunofluorescence (figure 62.6), which are deposited in a diffuse granular pattern located primarily within the mesangium.

There is no specific treatment for IgA nephropathy. Angiotensin-converting enzyme (ACE) inhibitors slow the progression of renal decline (some studies suggest that this more so particularly in patients with DD genotype of the ACE gene). Treatment with steroids has been used, and some studies suggest efficacy. However, the use of steroids remains controversial, and it is suggested that they may be more effective in IgA patients with nephrotic syndrome and minimal change disease. Treatment with fish oil is controversial; a meta-analysis suggests that patients at high risk of progression (male gender, hypertension, presence of microhematuria, presence of proteinuria, and renal insufficiency) may benefit. A combination of oral cyclophosphamide, dipyridamole, and low-dose warfarin has not demonstrated long-term benefits.

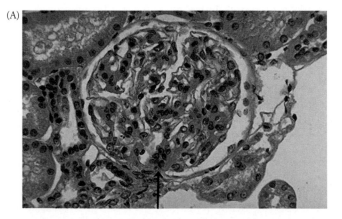
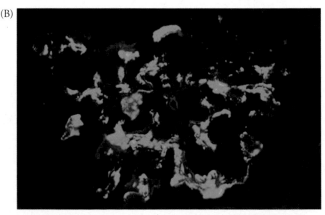

Figure 62.6. IgA Nephropathy. (A) Light microscopy. (B) IgA mesangial staining on immunofluorescence. Photo courtesy of Dr. Helmut Rennke.

Similarly, cyclosporine has not demonstrated benefit. Overall prognosis is that as many as 20–50% of the patients will eventually develop ESRD within 20 years' time. Markers for a worse prognosis are persistent hypertension, proteinuria, nephrotic syndrome, persistent microhematuria, old age, and male sex (present at initial presentation).

RAPIDLY PROGRESSIVE OR CRESCENTIC GLOMERULONEPHRITIS

The presentation is an abrupt-onset acute nephritis that is characterized by a rapid decline in kidney function (a doubling of serum creatinine or a 50% reduction in glomerular filtration rate within a 3-month period). Typically patients rapidly progress to renal failure within weeks. An accurate and urgent diagnosis is essential in these patients. A renal biopsy and checking of serologies—antineutrophil cytoplasmic antibody (ANCA), anti-GBM antibodies, antinuclear antibodies, anti-dsDNA antibodies, and complements—are essential. Renal biopsy reveals a crescentic glomerulonephritis.

FOUR CLASSES OF CRESCENTIC GN BASED ON PATHOGENETIC MECHANISMS

Four classes of crescentic glomerulonephritis are type 1 (anti-GBM positive), type 2 (immune complex disease; anti-GBM and ANCA negative), type 3 (pauci-immune; ANCA positive), and type 4 (double-antibody-positive disease, which has features of both types 1 and 3.

Anti-GBM Nephritis (Type 1)

Anti-GBM nephritis presents with rapidly progressive renal failure with hematuria and red cell casts. A presentation which includes dyspnea and hemoptysis (i.e., pulmonary hemorrhage) is termed Goodpasture syndrome. There is a bimodal distribution with the first peak at age 30 years and second peak at 60 years. In 20–60% of patients there is a prodrome of an upper respiratory tract infection that precedes

the disease. Patients usually have subnephrotic proteinuria (<3 g/24 hours), hematuria, a nephritic urinary sediment, and hypochromic microcytic anemia of the iron deficiency type. Hypertension is uncommon (20% of the patients). Risk factors for anti-GBM nephritis include a history of exposure to hydrocarbons, cigarette smoking, metallic dust, D-penicillamine, cocaine, and influenza A2 infections.

Anti-GBM nephritis is caused by the presence of anti-GBM autoantibodies that react with the noncollagenous domain of the alpha chain of type IV collagen. This collagen is expressed predominantly in the glomerular and pulmonary alveolar capillary basement membrane. Anti-GBM autoantibodies bind antigen after chronic insult of the GBM. This reaction induces activation of complement and leukocyte recruitment, resulting in necrotizing segmental proliferative glomerulonephritis, disruption of capillary walls, and eventually crescent formation.

The pathologic abnormalities are striking (figure 62.7). Light microscopy shows a diffuse crescentic glomerulonephritis with linear deposits of IgG1 and IgG4 along the GBM on immunofluorescence. (A similar immunofluorescence pattern is observed in biopsies of the alveolar basement membrane.)

The clinical course is that of rapid deterioration in renal function (days to weeks) frequently with the need for dialysis. A chest x-ray showing abnormal bilateral hilar and basilar interstitial shadowing would point strongly to associated pulmonary hemorrhage and a diagnosis of Goodpasture syndrome. Anti-GBM enzyme-linked immunosorbent assay (ELISA) can be used to detect circulating anti-GBM antibodies; the assay is specific for the NCI domain of the alpha-3 chain of type IV collagen. This antibody is detected in more than 90% of individuals with anti-GBM nephritis. The level of plasma creatinine is usually a good indication of the degree of progression. The gold standard for diagnosis is renal biopsy.

Without treatment, patients with anti-GBM nephritis and/or Goodpasture syndrome have a very poor prognosis. Most patients die of either severe renal or pulmonary complications. End-stage renal disease is not uncommon in

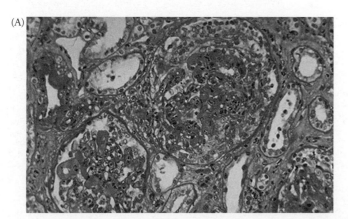

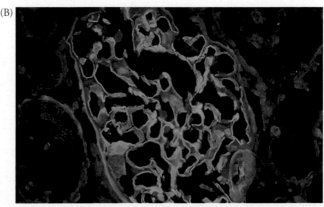

Figure 62.7. Anti-GBM Nephritis. (A) Light microscopy. (B) Linear IgG staining on immunofluorescence. Photo courtesy of Dr. Helmut Rennke.

patients who are oliguric, anuric, or with a plasma creatinine of >5–7 mg/dL. The goal of therapy is to suppress the formation of new antibodies and remove pre-existing antibodies. This strategy has decreased the death of these patients to less than 10% for 1-year survival. Therapy is plasmapheresis with plasma exchange for 2 weeks on consecutive days, prednisone, 1 mg/kg (after an initial methylprednisone pulse of 1 g/day for 3 consecutive days), and cyclophosphamide, 2–3 mg/kg orally once each day. Patients with rapidly progressive glomerulonephritis (RPGN) have a worse prognosis. The endpoint of treatment is when the anti-GBM antibodies are undetectable in the blood.

Lupus Nephritis (an Example of Type 2)

Renal involvement is frequently observed in patients with SLE. The overall prevalence of SLE is 4–250 cases per 100,000. Lupus nephritis (LN) predominantly affects women of childbearing age (M:F = 1:16 ratio); 85% of the patients will be younger than 55 years of age. SLE appears to be more common and to have more severe renal involvement in the African-American population. Forty to eighty-five percent of patients with SLE will have complications involving the kidney (LN), but the spectrum of renal disease (histological class) is highly variable. There is no clearly defined genetic pattern for predisposition to SLE. However, a significant percentage of family members of patients with SLE develop the disease (5–12%). In addition, there is evidence for a predisposing role of hormonal factors, including the strong predominance of women of childbearing age and the increased incidence of SLE in postmenopausal women taking estrogen. Other predisposing factors include exposure to sunlight, ultraviolet radiation, medications, and viral/bacterial exposure.

SLE can affect any organ system (table 62.4). Renal involvement often develops concurrently or shortly following

the onset of SLE and may follow a protracted course with periods of remission and exacerbations. A special rare subset of patients ("silent LN") have no clinical findings of renal involvement but will present with proliferative LN on biopsy. Transformation from one class to another is relatively frequent.

The diagnosis of SLE is often clinical with laboratory features. The American Rheumatism Association has developed criteria under which 4 of the 11 findings are required for a 96% sensitivity and specificity to diagnose SLE. The criteria encompass the following clinical and laboratory features: malar rash; discoid lupus; dermal disease; photosensitivity; oral or nasal ulcerations; nondeforming arthritis; serositis, including pleuritis and pericarditis; central nervous system disease, such as seizures or psychoses; hematologic involvement manifested by the presence of anemia, leukopenia, lymphopenia, or thrombocytopenia; immunologic markers of disease manifested by a positive lupus band test, a positive anti-DNA or anti-Sm antibody test, a false-positive Venereal Disease Research Laboratory (VDRL) test, or a positive antinuclear antibody reaction; renal involvement, defined as persistent proteinuria exceeding 500 mg daily (3+ on the dipstick), or the presence of cellular casts, consisting of erythrocyte, hemoglobin, granular, tubular, or mixed.

Serositis	Blood abnormalities	Malar rash
Oral ulceration	Renal involvement	Discoid rash
Arthritis	Antibodies	
Photosensitivity	Immunologic abnormalities	
	Nervous system	

Renal biopsy is often important for the treatment of patients with LN (figure 62.8). The International Society of Nephrology and Renal Pathology Society have classified LN. This classification has described more specific criteria to define the various classes of LN.

Table 62.4 **ORGAN INVOLVEMENT IN SLE**

Rash
- 50–60% of patients
- Butterfly rash on face, livedo reticularis, purpuric rash
- Associated patchy alopecia + oral ulceration (10%)

Arthralgia
- 75% of patients
- Usually nondeforming, usually several joints
- Hands, also other joints
- Associated myalgias and weakness

Heme
- 75% of patients
- Normochromic normocytic anemia, thrombocytopenia

CNS
- 30% of patients, 12% presenting feature
- Mood disorders, headache common
- Chorea, facial nerve palsies seizures, hemiparesis
- Frank psychosis/coma

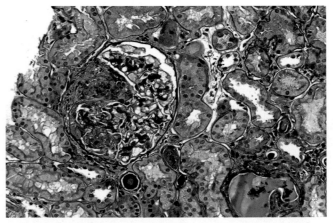

Figure 62.8. Lupus Nephritis Class IV. Light microscopy. Photo courtesy of Dr. Helmut Rennke.

Class I	**Minimal mesangial lupus nephritis**
	Normal glomeruli by light microscopy, but mesangial immune deposits by immunofluorescence

Class II	**Mesangial proliferative lupus nephritis**
	Purely mesangial hypercellularity of any degree or mesangial matrix expansion by light microscopy, with mesangial immune deposits. A few isolated subepithelial or subendothelial deposits may be visible by immunofluorescence or electron microscopy, but not by light microscopy

Class III	**Focal lupus nephritis**
	Segmental or global, endo- or extracapillary glomerulonephritis involving <50% of all glomeruli, with focal subendothelial immune deposits, with or without mesangial alterations. Lesions could be active or inactive.

Class IV	**Diffuse lupus nephritis**
	Segmental or global endo- or extracapillary glomerulonephritis involving ≥ 50% of all glomeruli, typically with diffuse subendothelial immune deposits, with or without mesangial alterations. This is divided into diffuse segmental when (IV-S) lupus nephritis ≥50% of the involved glomeruli have segmental lesions (<50% of tuft involvement) and diffuse global (IV-G) when glomeruli have global lesions (≥50% of tuft involvement). Lesions could be active or inactive.

Class V	**Membranous lupus nephritis**
	Global or segmental subepithelial immune deposits with or without mesangial alteration
	Class V lupus may occur in combination with class III or IV, in which case both will be diagnosed

Class VI	**Advanced sclerotic lupus nephritis**
	≥90% of glomeruli globally sclerosed without residual activity.

Class II disease carries a good prognosis, and treatment may not be indicated. It is difficult to speculate on the course and prognosis of class III patients because of its varied course. Often steroids and cytotoxic therapy are required. Patients with class IV require steroids and cytotoxic therapy. The standard of care in many hospitals for severe forms of class IV disease is three consecutive doses of pulse methylprednisone (1 g IV each day), followed by high-dose prednisone starting at 1 mg/kg/day and tapered over 3 months to approximately 10–30 mg/day. Adjunctive cytotoxic therapy is recommended. There is debate about whether oral or intravenous pulse cyclophosphamide should be given. In many centers, mycophenolic acid (MMF) is now preferred over cyclophosphamide because of its similar efficacy but lower adverse risk profile. MMF is also now preferred over azathioprine.

ANCA-Associated Vasculitis (Example of Type 3): Wegener Granulomatosis (Renamed as "Granulomatosis with Polyangiitis")

Vasculitis may affect the large, medium, or small blood vessels. Small-vessel vasculitis may be further classified as ANCA-associated or non–ANCA-associated vasculitis. ANCA-associated small-vessel vasculitis includes microscopic polyangiitis, granulomatosis with polyangiitis Churg-Strauss syndrome, and drug-induced vasculitis.

Granulomatosis with polyangiitis may occur at any age of life; peak incidence is in the fourth to sixth decade of life. Granulomatosis with polyangiitis is associated with increased titers of antineutrophil cytoplasmic antibodies. ANCA are directed against antigens present within the primary granules of neutrophils and monocytes. Whether the ANCA is the cause or an epiphenomenon remains controversial.

The clinical presentation of granulomatosis with polyangiitis is quite variable and ranges from a subclinical presentation with progressive involvement of the respiratory tract and mild renal findings to a more fulminant presentation with acute glomerulonephritis or RPGN.

Granulomatosis with polyangiitis predominantly affects respiratory tract, but vasculitic multisystemic involvement is not uncommon. Upper respiratory involvement includes sinusitis, tinnitus, and hearing loss with otic discharge and pain. Lower respiratory tract symptoms include cough with dyspnea progressing to hemoptysis and alveolar hemorrhage.

Multisystemic disease may include skin (e.g., papules, purpura), joints (arthralgias, arthritis), eyes (conjunctivitis, episcleritis), nervous system, the liver, the thyroid, the gallbladder, and the heart. The renal presentation varies from a rapidly progressive glomerulonephritis and renal failure to a more gradual decline in GFR with nonnephrotic-range proteinuria, hematuria, and red cell casts.

The key serologic abnormality is the presence of ANCA antibodies detected on indirect immunofluorescence or ELISA. Proteinase-3 (PR3)-ANCA cause a cytoplasmic pattern of staining (C-ANCA). Myeloperoxidase (MPO)-ANCA leads to a perinuclear (P-ANCA) pattern of staining. Between 88% and 96% of patients with granulomatosis with polyangiitis are ANCA positive, most commonly C-ANCA, but P-ANCA is also observed. The typical pathology on renal biopsy is a focal segmental necrotizing and crescentic glomerulonephritis. Vasculitis may involve the small and medium-size renal arteries, veins, and capillaries. Immunofluorescence shows a pauci-immune pattern (i.e., with little immunoglobulin deposition).

Untreated patients have a 1-year survival rate of 20–50%. The recommended initial treatment is methylprednisone (500 mg to 1000 mg IV daily for 3 consecutive days) followed by high dose oral prednisone (1 mg/kg/day) and oral cyclophosphamide (2 mg/kg/day, not to exceed 200 mg/day). Pulse intravenous cyclophosphamide is an acceptable alternative regime. Remission with corticosteroids and cyclophosphamide occurs in 85–95% of patients. IV cyclophosphamide with plasmapheresis may be better in patients with pulmonary hemorrhage or those who are critically ill. Azathioprine and rituximab have also been used in treatment.

ADDITIONAL READING

Beck LH Jr, Salant DJ. Glomerular and tubulointerstitial diseases. *Prim Care*. 2008;35(2):265–96.

Couser WG. Glomerulonephritis. *Lancet*. 1999;353(9163):1509–15.

Erwig LP, Rees AJ. Rapidly progressive glomerulonephritis. *J Nephrol*. 1999;12(Suppl 2):S111–9.

Hildebrandt F. Genetic kidney diseases. *Lancet*. 2010;375(9722): 1287–95.

Kodner C. Nephrotic syndrome in adults: Diagnosis and management. *Am Fam Physician*. 2009;80(10):1129–34.

Little MA, Pusey CD. Rapidly progressive glomerulonephritis: Current and evolving treatment strategies. *J Nephrol*. 2004;17(Suppl 8): S10–9.

Merrill JP. Glomerulonephritis (third of three parts). *N Engl J Med*. 1974;290(7):374–81.

Ortega LM, Schultz DR, Lenz O, Pardo V, Contreras GN. Review: Lupus nephritis: Pathologic features, epidemiology and a guide to therapeutic decisions. *Lupus*. 2010;19(5):557–74.

Orth SR, Ritz E. The nephrotic syndrome. *N Engl J Med*. 1998;338(17): 1202–11.

Walters G, Willis NS, Craig JC. Interventions for renal vasculitis in adults. *Cochrane Database Syst Rev*. 2008;3.

QUESTIONS

QUESTION 1. A 22-year-old woman is admitted with a diagnosis of Goodpasture syndrome. This diagnosis is confirmed by an ELISA and Western blot analysis demonstrating anti-GBM antibodies. A preliminary reading of the renal biopsy confirms the diagnosis of anti-GBM nephritis. Her serum creatinine is 3.2 mg/dL. Two weeks previously her serum creatinine was 0.7 mg/dL. Which of the following therapeutic options would be most appropriate for her:

A. Prednisone 60 mg/day for 1 month followed by a gradual weaning of her prednisone dose

B. Pulse methylprednisone accompanied by daily plasmapheresis with exchange, followed by high-dose oral prednisone coupled with cyclophosphamide, until her anti-GBM titer is undetectable

C. Pulse methylprednisone followed by high-dose oral prednisone coupled with cyclophosphamide until her anti-GBM titer is undetectable

D. Prednisone 60 mg/day plus cyclophosphamide, 3 mg/kg/day

E. Plasmapheresis alone

QUESTION 2. A 42-year-old woman presents to your office with a 4-week history of a petechial rash on her legs, gross hematuria, and edema. She relates a 2-year history of intermittent polyarthralgias. Physical examination is notable for mild periorbital edema. Vital signs show a blood pressure of 164/88 mm Hg and a heart rate of 66 beats per minute. Her lungs, cardiovascular examination, and abdominal examinations are normal. She has 3+ edema. Urinalysis shows 4+ blood, 4+ proteinuria, 1+ leukocytes. Urine sediment examination shows 15–20 dysmorphic red cells and 1 RBC cast per high-powered field. Her electrolytes are normal, BUN was 36 mg/dL, creatinine 1.8 mg/dL. Serological examination shows an ANA, ASLO, ANCA, and anti-GBM that are negative. Complements are normal. Skin biopsy showed a leukocytoclastic vasculitis. A renal biopsy is performed.

The most likely finding on the renal biopsy is:

A. A WHO class IV diffuse proliferative glomerulonephritis

B. A minimal change lesion

C. Glomeruli showing fibrinoid necrosis

D. Kimmelstiel-Wilson lesions with nodular glomerulosclerosis

E. A mesangial proliferative lesion

QUESTION 3. A 14-year-old patient presents with periorbital and lower extremity swelling approximately 10 days after complaining of a sore throat and feverishness that was diagnosed as strep throat. She has been treated with penicillin, and her throat symptoms and fever have cleared completely. Urine microscopy shows red cells and red cell casts. Complements show a low C3. The next step in management is to:

A. Pulse the patient with 1 g of methylprednisone for three consecutive doses and then 60 mg/day or oral prednisone tapered over 1 month.

B. Restart the patient on penicillin.

C. Treat the patient with oral prednisone (60 mg/day) tapered over 1 month.

D. Observe—the illness may resolve spontaneously.

E. Pulse the patient with methylprednisone, 1 g, for three consecutive doses and arrange for a 7-day course of daily plasmapheresis with plasma exchange.

QUESTION 4. A 22-year-old man presents with hematuria detected on a routine physical. He is completely asymptomatic. He tells you that he has had one prior episode of what he thinks was hematuria—during an upper respiratory infection 3 years previously he noticed pinkish urine—however, it resolved spontaneously. Past medical history, family history, and social history are all negative. Physical examination is normal. Urine dipstick is negative except for 2+ blood. Urine microscopy shows 5–10 red blood cells per high-powered field. ASLO, ANA, and ANCA titers are negative. Complements are normal.

The most likely diagnosis is:

A. Subclinical poststreptococcal glomerulonephritis

B. IgA nephropathy

C. Lupus nephritis

D. Alport syndrome

E. Thin basement membrane disease

QUESTION 5. A 24-year-old African-American office worker presents to her primary care provider with a 5-day history of feverishness, severe exhaustion, and painful and stiff joints in her hands and her feet. Past medical history is negative. Family history is notable for a maternal aunt who has a history of lupus. Physical examination shows a normal head and neck examination except for a mild malar flush. Vital signs reveal a blood pressure of 144/94 mm Hg, heart rate of 72 beats per minute, and a temperature of 37.8°C. Cardiac, lung, and abdominal examinations are normal. She has swollen joints in her hands and feet. There is 1+ lower extremity edema. Laboratory analysis shows 2+ blood and 4+ albumin on her urine dipstick. Urine microscopy shows 10–15 red blood cells per high-powered field and 1 red cell cast. Serum creatinine is 1.1 mg/dL, Blood urea nitrogen is 22 mg/dL. Electrolytes are normal. ANA is positive at 1:640, anti-dsDNA antibody titer is 650 U/L. Both C3 and C4 are low. The next step in management is:

A. Urgently refer the patient to a nephrologist for same-day pulse methylprednisone therapy and a renal biopsy.

B. Start the patient on 1.5 g twice daily of mycophenolate mofetil and prednisone 60 mg/day.

C. Start the patient on prednisone, 60 mg daily, and arrange for follow-up in 1 week's time.

D. Arrange for an urgent CT-guided renal biopsy.

E. Start the patient on prednisone 60 mg/day and urgently refer the patient to hematology for initiation for cyclophosphamide therapy.

ANSWERS

1. B
2. E
3. D
4. B
5. A

63.

CHRONIC KIDNEY DISEASE

Ajay K. Singh

Chronic kidney disease (CKD) is defined by the National Kidney Foundation (NKF) as either (1) a glomerular filtration rate (GFR) of <60 mL/min with or without kidney damage for 3 or more months or (2) the presence of kidney damage for 3 or more months demonstrated by pathologic abnormalities, markers of kidney damage (e.g., blood or urine composition), or imaging tests. In the United States it is estimated that CKD affects 7–10% of the adult population or 15–20 million individuals, although specific subgroups such as African Americans and Hispanics are at especially high risk. Chapter 60 in this section of the volume reviews the complications of CKD.

STAGING AND CLASSIFICATION OF CKD

CKD is staged by using glomerular filtration rate (GFR) categories. The NKF Kidney Disease Outcomes Quality Initiative (KDOQI) has classified CKD into five stages (see table 63.1). The strengths of the NKF KDOQI classification are its simplicity and its use of estimated GFR (eGFR) to classify CKD into different stages. The widespread adoption of the classification has resulted in a uniform system understood and applied worldwide. However, the NKF CKD classification does have several limitations. It stages the severity of kidney disease on the basis of GFR without incorporating other important parameters such as albuminuria. Two patients with similar GFR but with wide differences in the degree of proteinuria at baseline are likely to have very different prognoses. The patient with high-degree proteinuria is more likely to progress to end-stage renal disease. The NKF classification also leaves unaddressed the significance of reduced GFR below 60 mL/min/1.73 m^2 in certain subgroups, such as the elderly, the undernourished, and members of specific ethnic groups. For example, elderly individuals with reduced GFR may never develop end-stage renal disease. Patients with congestive cardiac failure may have a low GFR because of hemodynamic reasons but do not have any structural evidence of kidney disease, and

kidney function may normalize once the heart failure is treated. Furthermore, the NKF CKD criteria may not apply to some racial groups because their GFR may be lower than Western levels as a consequence of smaller stature, lower muscle mass, and/or vegetarianism.

More recently, the Kidney Disease Improving Global Outcomes group has proposed modifications to the NKF staging system by subdividing stage 3 of CKD into stage 3a representing mild-to-moderate CKD (GFR of 45–59 mL/min/1.73 m^2) and stage 3b representing moderate-to-severe CKD (GFR of 30–44 mL/min/1.73 m^2). In addition, each CKD stage is classified according to the degree of albuminuria: A1 representing optimum and high-normal albuminuria (<29 mg/g); A2 representing high degree of albuminuria (30–299 mg/g), and A3 representing very high and nephrotic (>300 mg of albumin/gram urinary creatinine. Greater levels of albuminuria and more advanced stage of CKD are associated with higher all-cause mortality, cardiovascular mortality and and progression to end-stage renal failure.

EPIDEMIOLOGY OF CKD

It is estimated that approximately 19 million individuals in the United States have CKD (table 63.2). Most individuals with CKD are people with earlier stages of CKD: there are estimated to be approximately 11.2 million individuals with stage 1 or 2 CKD—persistent albuminuria with normal or mildly decreased GFR (GFR<60 mL/min/1.73 m^2 or higher)—and about 8.3 million individuals with stage 3 CKD or worse (GFR <60 mL/min/1.73 m^2). Of those with stage 5 CKD, the number of individuals with kidney failure treated by dialysis and transplantation exceeded 300,000 in 1998, and although the prevalence is likely to demonstrate continued growth, recent data reported from the U.S. Renal Data System (USRDS) suggest that the incidence rate of end-stage renal disease (ESRD) (new cases of kidney failure) appears to have stabilized after 20 years of annual increase of 5% to 10% per year. (In the latest numbers from

Table 63.1 NKF CLASSIFICATION OF CKD

Stage 1	Kidney damage with normal or supranormal GFR, GFR ≥90
Stage 2	Kidney damage with mild reduction in GFR, GFR 60–89
Stage 3	Moderate reduction in GFR, GFR 30–59
Stage 4	Severe reduction in GFR, GFR 15–29
Stage 5	Kidney failure, GFR <15 or on dialysis

SOURCE: Reprinted with permission from K/DOQI clinical practice guidelines for chronic kidney disease: Evaluation, classification, and stratification. Kidney Disease Outcome Quality Initiative. *Am J Kidney Dis.* 2002;39(2) [Suppl 1]:S17–S31, with permission from Elsevier.

USRDS, the ESRD incidence rate was 338 per million with an annual increase of just 1%.)

SCREENING FOR CKD

Screening for CKD is cost-effective in high-risk populations, such as African Americans, Native Americans, Hispanics, and in patients with diabetes mellitus and hypertension. This is because kidney disease becomes symptomatic in the late stages of CKD, whereas therapeutic strategies such as angiotensin blockade and tighter blood pressure control are proven to be effective at earlier stages. Thus, early detection of CKD could potentially prevent ESRD in a significant proportion of high-risk patients. African Americans and Native Americans develop kidney failure at a fourfold higher rate than white Americans (953 and 652 cases per million in African Americans and Native Americans, respectively, compared to 237 per million among Caucasians). Patients with diabetes mellitus and hypertension and those with urine dipstick positive for protein have a higher risk of developing CKD. The NKF KDOQI guidelines for CKD recommend that all individuals should be assessed as part of routine health examinations to determine whether they are at increased risk for developing CKD. Individuals at high risk for kidney disease, particularly those with diabetes, hypertension, or a family history for these conditions and/or for kidney disease, should undergo formal testing. Such testing can be performed easily with a urinalysis, a first morning or a random "spot" urine sample for albumin or protein and creatinine assessment, and a serum creatinine level. The American Diabetes Association (ADA) recommends that for all type 2 diabetics at the time of diagnosis and all type 1 diabetics 5 years after initial diagnosis, an evaluation for microalbuminuria should be performed. If the dipstick is positive for either red or white blood cells, a microscopic analysis should be performed of the urinary sediment.

NKF KDOQI GUIDELINES FOR CKD SCREENING IN PATIENTS WITH HYPERTENSION

- Serum creatinine measurement for GFR estimation
- Protein-to-creatinine ratio in a first morning or random "spot" urine specimen
- Either dipstick testing or urine sediment examination for red blood cells or white blood cells
- In patients with hypertension found to have CKD
- Imaging of the kidneys, commonly by ultrasound
- Measurement of serum electrolytes (Na^+, K^+, Cl^-, HCO_3^-)

MEASUREMENT OF KIDNEY FUNCTION

USE OF SERUM CREATININE

Measurement of serum creatinine is currently the most widely utilized measure for the assessment of kidney function. However, the use of serum creatinine has several limitations (table 63.3). Because creatinine production is dependent on muscle mass, it needs to be interpreted cautiously among individuals with low muscle mass, among females, and in elderly patients. In patients with low muscle mass, the serum creatinine underestimates the degree of kidney function impairment, whereas among individuals with large muscle mass (such as body builders), the serum creatinine overestimates actual GFR. Another source of inaccuracy is the effect of noncreatinine chromogens when the alkaline picrate assay (Jaffe reaction) for creatinine is

Table 63.2 PREVALENCE OF CKD IN THE UNITED STATES BY CKD STAGE

STAGE	DESCRIPTION	GFR*	POPULATION (THOUSANDS)	PREVALENCE
1	Kidney damage with normal or supranormal GFR	≥90	5900	3.3%
2	Kidney damage with mild decrease in GFR	60–89	5300	3.0%
3	Moderate decrease in GFR	30–59	7600	4.3%
4	Severe decrease in GFR	15–29	400	0.2%
5	Kidney failure	<15	300	0.2%

NOTE: *GFR expressed in mL/min/1.73 m².

Table 63.3 LIMITATIONS OF SERUM CREATININE AS A MEASURE OF KIDNEY FUNCTION

Influence of muscle mass on creatinine generation	High-muscle-mass patients, higher serum creatinine (e.g., athletes, body builders) Low-muscle-mass patients, lower serum creatinine
Effect of creatinine secretion	Patients with CKD: greater proportion of creatinine is secreted than filtered
Medications blocking proximal secretion	Cimetidine Trimethoprim Probenecid

utilized. These factors include acetoacetate, cephalosporins, and high concentrations of furosemide. Modern versions of the Jaffe assay have reduced these effects by adjusting temperature, assay constituents, and various calibration settings.

Given these limitations with serum creatinine as a measure of actual GFR, the NKF KDOQI and the National Kidney Disease Education Program (NKDEP) have recommended the use of actual or, when this is unavailable, a prediction equation for estimating GFR. Since in most situations direct measurement of GFR is not feasible, a prediction equation to estimate GFR is the most practical and accurate method to assess kidney function. The modification of diet in renal disease (MDRD) and Cockcroft-Gault equations are now the most popular prediction equations to assess GFR in adults.

Recently, an isotope dilution mass spectroscopy (IDMS)-traceable MDRD equation (also known as the MDRD 3 equation) has been developed. In essence this is a modified MDRD equation used when creatinine values are generated from a laboratory that has calibrated its creatinine measurement to a set of creatinine standards. The MDRD 3 equation is as follows:

$$175 \times [SCr]^{-1.154} \times [Age]^{-0.203} \times [0.742 \text{ if patient is female}]$$
$$\times [1.21 \text{ if patient is black}]$$

PREDICTION EQUATIONS FOR GFR

Cockroft-Gault Equation

This prediction equation is commonly used in clinical practice. Its major limitations are these: (1) It has limited generalizability. This is because it was originally formulated to calculate the creatinine clearance in patients without kidney disease (Canadian males). It has not been widely validated in different populations and under different clinical situations. (2) The Cockroft-Gault (CG) equation tends to overestimate GFR, especially among patients with chronic kidney disease. This is because it utilizes serum creatinine to estimate creatinine clearance. The limitations of measuring creatinine clearance apply to the CG equation. Among patients with moderate to severe kidney disease, creatinine secretion as a proportion of total creatinine excretion increases, resulting in an overestimation of the creatinine

clearance. (3) Like the MDRD equation, the CG equation is inaccurate among individuals with normal or near-normal kidney function. (4) The CG equation uses weight, which frequently results in inaccuracies at extremes of weight and/ or when there is a measurement error in the assessment of weight. Despite these limitations CG remains popular, especially among pharmacists who utilize it for drug-dosing adjustments in patients with reduced kidney function.

Modification of Diet in Renal Disease

The MDRD Study GFR prediction equation was developed in 1999. The equation is based on 1628 nondiabetic subjects aged 18–70 years with renal insufficiency. The formula utilizes urea, creatinine, and albumin as well as demographics of age, gender, and race (black or white). If race is unavailable and white race is assumed, the GFR will be underestimated by 18% if the patient is black. This equation has been validated in American black and white racial groups. It has also been validated in diabetics, predialysis patients, and renal transplant recipients. Validation for other subgroups such as Asians, children, and the elderly still needs to be performed. In 2000 a simplified MDRD equation (MDRD 2) was made available. It is based on serum creatinine as the only laboratory value—in the absence of urea or albumin. The MDRD formula yields an eGFR normalized to 1.73 m^2 body surface area. Adjusting for body surface area is necessary when comparing a patient's eGFR with normal values or when determining the stage of CKD. However, an uncorrected eGFR may be preferred for clinical use in some situations, such as drug dosing.

The advantages of the MDRD equation over the CG equation are shown in table 63.4. However, there are several

Table 63.4 ADVANTAGES OF THE MDRD OVER CG EQUATION

Direct comparison of the MDRD and the Cockcroft–Gault (CG) equation demonstrates the MDRD equation to be superior for estimating GFR, particularly in the range GFR <60 mL/min/1.73m^2
More widespread validation of MDRD than CG (e.g., in various populations)
No requirement for additional information for MDRD (e.g., measurements of weight) beyond that already collected by pathology laboratories

Table 63.5 SITUATIONS IN WHICH THE MDRD EQUATION SHOULD BE USED CAUTIOUSLY

Populations in which the MDRD equation is not validated or in which validation studies have not been performed

Individuals with near-normal or normal kidney function

Severe malnutrition or obesity

Extremes of body size and age

Exceptional dietary intake (e.g., vegetarian diet or creatine supplements)

Disease of skeletal muscle, paraplegia

Rapidly changing kidney function

---

clinical situations in which caution should be applied in using the MDRD equation (table 63.5).

More recently, a new equation called the CKD-Epi equation has been proposed. This equation has less bias at high eGFRs and can be used to report eGFRs >60 mL/min/1.73 m². However, it has not been applied widely by clinical laboratories.

CLEARANCE BY RADIOLOGIC CONTRAST AGENTS AND RADIOACTIVE ISOTOPES

GFR can be calculated by the measurement of urinary or plasma clearances of isotopes or via images produced from a gamma camera. There are four different agents that are used in clinical practice: ^{125}I-iothalamate, ^{51}Cr-ethylenediaminetetraacetic acid, ^{99m}Tc-diethylenetriaminepentaacetic acid, and iohexol. These agents have been shown to correlate well with inulin clearance. They also have high precision in the setting of moderate to severe renal dysfunction. Inulin clearance is the gold standard for measurement of actual GFR because it is freely filtered and neither secreted nor reabsorbed by the kidney. However, it is not widely used in clinical practice largely for logistical reasons.

CREATININE CLEARANCE MEASUREMENT BY 24-HOUR URINE COLLECTION

Difficulties with 24-hour urine creatinine measurements include variations in urine collection (i.e., incorrect collections) and variations in the tubular secretion of creatinine. Studies have shown that in trained patients there can be up to a 14% variation in urine creatinine (Cr) quantity secondary to incorrect collection, and in untrained patients this can be as high as 70%. With regard to variations in tubular secretion, in patients with moderate to severe renal dysfunction, >50% of the urinary Cr can result from tubular secretion, thus leading to overestimation of the creatinine clearance by this method. In order to compensate for overestimation of GFR from tubular secretion of Cr

in the 24-hour urine collection, the collection can be performed after oral administration of cimetidine, an organic cation that is a known competitive inhibitor of creatinine secretion. Alternatively, the use of the mean of urea and creatinine clearance measurements calculated from 24-hour urine collections has been suggested. Creatinine clearance overestimates GFR because creatinine is both filtered by the glomerulus and to a lesser degree, secreted by the proximal tubule. On the other hand, urea underestimates GFR because it is both filtered and reabsorbed. The mean value of the creatinine and urea clearance more closely approximates the actual GFR in the setting of GFR measurements less than 15 mL/min/1.73 m².

CYSTATIN C

Cystatin C is a nonglycosylated basic protease inhibitor produced by nucleated cells at a constant rate, is freely filtered by glomeruli, and is completely metabolized after tubular reabsorption. Unlike creatinine, serum cystatin C level is not dependent on muscle mass and is not differentially expressed based on gender. GFR as estimated from the plasma cystatin C concentration has been found to correlate well with iothalamate GFR measurements in Pima Indians with diabetes mellitus (DM) and normal or supranormal GFR. Cystatin has greater sensitivity than Cr for small changes in GFR. Recent studies suggest that cystatin C may be a better indicator of predicting risk for cardiovascular disease than either serum creatinine or a GFR prediction equation.

MANAGEMENT OF CKD PROGRESSION

As a clinical syndrome CKD is characterized by progressive decline in kidney function such that the kidney's ability to adequately excrete waste products and to contribute to the constancy of the body's homeostatic functions is severely impaired. Mild CKD is asymptomatic, moderate CKD is frequently characterized by hypertension, anemia, and abnormalities in mineral metabolism, whereas advanced CKD is characterized by uremia. CKD may become relentlessly progressive as the damage to functioning nephrons leads to a maladaptive response among the remaining nephrons. The progressive decline in kidney function in individuals with CKD is variable and depends both on the cause of the underlying insult and on patient-specific factors. There is consensus that renal disease progression rates are heterogeneous both between different etiologies and within the same etiology. Thus, patients with polycystic kidney disease (PKD) may progress more slowly than patients with diabetic nephropathy; however, among patients with diabetic nephropathy there are patients who progress fast and others who progress hardly at all. Evidence also points to the importance of several factors in modulating kidney progression. These

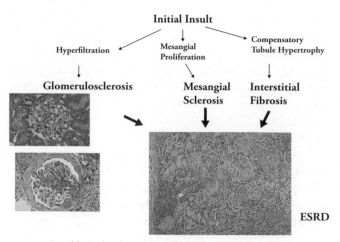

Figure 63.1. Possible Pathophysiological Processes Leading to Kidney Scarring.

include albuminuria, the presence of systemic hypertension, age, gender, genetic factors, and smoking. However, regardless of the initial insult, the end result from a pathology standpoint is a scarred end-stage kidney (figure 63.1).

End-stage renal disease is the term used to denote CKD requiring renal replacement therapy (dialysis or transplantation). The incidence of ESRD in the United States is approximately 268 cases per million population per year. However, ESRD is overrepresented among African Americans (829 per million population per year, as compared with 199 per million population per year among white Americans). The major causes of ESRD in the United States are diabetes mellitus (44%), hypertension (30%), glomerular disease (15%), polycystic kidney disease, and obstructive uropathy. Elsewhere in the world, where the incidence of diabetes mellitus has not reached epidemic proportions—for example in Europe and parts of the developing world—chronic glomerulonephritis (20%) and chronic reflux nephropathy (25%) are the commonest causes of ESRD.

CKD is usually asymptomatic when there is mild impairment in kidney function, whereas when GFR is markedly reduced, the patient is usually markedly symptomatic and may be severely disabled. In the early stages of CKD (stages 1 and 2 using the NKF KDOQI CKD stages), patients may present simply with an elevated serum creatinine and blood urea nitrogen (BUN) level but no symptoms. These individuals are usually unaware that they have any abnormalities in their kidney function, and they usually fail to register on the "radar screen" of their internists. However, even at this early stage insidious effects on target organs may become manifest. For example, patients may have mild to moderate hypertension, mild anemia, left ventricular hypertrophy, and subtle changes in bone structure from renal osteodystrophy. As kidney function gradually declines—with glomerular filtration rates reaching <30 mL/min, early features of uremia become evident. These include worsening or more difficult to control hypertension, extracellular volume expansion (manifest as edema and dyspnea), hyperkalemia and acidosis, anemia, and abnormalities in cognitive, psychological, and physical functions. Uremia reflects the accumulation of metabolic toxins, some characterized and others unknown, that influence the functioning of a variety of organ systems. The clinical presentation is often quite heterogeneous (figure 63.2) and is thought to reflect a variable balance between biochemical and endocrine deficiencies and excesses (figure 63.3). In this late stage, the need for renal replacement therapy is imminent, and dialysis and/or transplantation becomes inevitable in order to sustain life (table 63.6).

The indications for initiating renal replacement therapy include severe refractory abnormalities in biochemistry (severe hyperkalemia and acidosis), severe pulmonary edema, bleeding, metabolic encephalopathy, and the presence of pericarditis. Subtler but no less important indications include malnutrition and marked tiredness and lethargy.

Life expectancy for a 49-year-old patient with ESRD is, on average, approximately 7 years, lower than that for colon cancer and prostate cancer and one-quarter that of the general population. This reduction in life expectancy is

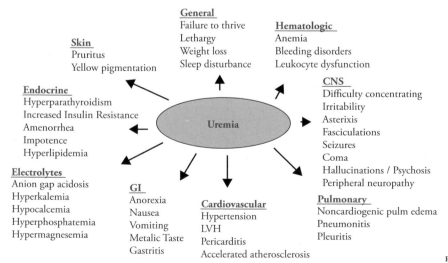

Figure 63.2. Clinical Manifestations of Uremia.

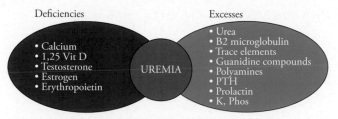

Figure 63.3. Biochemical and Endocrine Imbalances in Uremia.

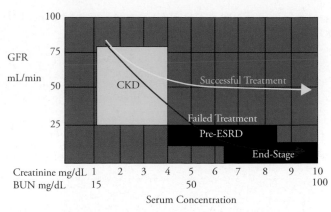

Figure 63.4. Schematic Showing Progression of Patients through the Stages of CKD.

largely attributable to cardiovascular complications. Nearly 50% of all deaths in patients with ESRD are due to cardiovascular causes. The risk is 17 times that of the general population. Remarkably, this gap is largest in young patients with end-stage renal disease. The risk factors for cardiovascular disease in individuals with chronic renal failure include, but are not limited to, the magnitude of the calcium-phosphorus product with its risk of coronary calcification, the presence of dyslipidemia, hypertension, hyperhomocysteinemia, and the presence of left ventricular hypertrophy (LVH). The clinical manifestations of cardiovascular disease in ESRD patients include LVH, left ventricular dilatation, diastolic dysfunction, macro- and microvascular disease, and abnormalities in autonomic function—increased sympathetic discharge and increased circulating catecholamine levels. Vascular disease may involve calcification of coronary vessels and valve disease. Indeed, calcification of the mitral valve annulus and the aortic valve cusps is common among ESRD patients.

KDOQI ACTION PLAN BY STAGE OF CKD

The NKF KDOQI group has released an action plan for management of patients with CKD as determined by stage of CKD. In stage 1 CKD these guidelines suggest the diagnosis and treatment of CKD, treatment of comorbid conditions, prevention of progression of renal disease, and CVD risk reduction. In stage 2 the issue of primary concern is that of estimating and managing renal disease progression. The focus in stage 3 disease is that of evaluating and treating

complications, whereas stage 4 CKD, the immediate predialysis stage, consists of preparation for renal replacement therapy. The management of stage 5 CKD is that of initiation and maintenance of renal replacement therapy. Thus, in addition to the task of diagnosing and treating the specific etiology of renal disease, the broad themes that govern early versus late renal disease management are those of prevention of progression in the early stages of CKD, management of complications beginning in the early stages and continuing throughout the follow-up of patients, and preparation for renal replacement in the later predialysis phase (figures 63.4 and 63.5).

It is important to appreciate that declining kidney function is associated with altered clearance of many drugs (e.g., aminoglycosides), as well as increased toxicity (e.g., iodinated contrast agents and phosphate based enemas). In addition, gadolinium exposure in patients with moderate-to-severe CKD may be associated with an increased risk of nephrogenic systemic fibrosis. Lastly, some drugs are contraindicated in patients with moderate-to-severe CKD (e.g., metformin, because of the risk of lactic acidosis).

There are three important elements to the management of progression in CKD patients.

Table 63.6 **INDICATIONS FOR INITIATION OF RENAL REPLACEMENT THERAPY**

- **Refractory hyperkalemia**
- **Acute pericarditis**
- **Fluid overload or pulmonary edema refractory to diuretics**
- **Encephalopathy**
- **Severe peripheral neuropathy**
- **Hypertension refractory to antihypertensive medications**
- **Severe uremic bleeding; clinically significant bleeding diathesis attributable to uremia**
- **Intractable nausea and vomiting**

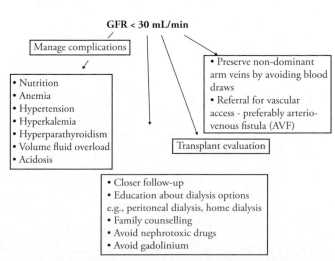

Figure 63.5. Management Strategies for Patients with More Advanced CKD.

Table 63.7 2003 NKF-KDOQI CLINICAL PRACTICE GUIDELINES FOR ANTIHYPERTENSIVE THERAPY RECOMMENDATIONS

Blood pressure measurement at each health care encounter

Target blood pressure of less than 130/80 for all patients with kidney disease, including those with diabetic kidney disease and nondiabetic kidney disease, regardless of degree of proteinuria, and in renal allograft recipients

Use of an ACE inhibitor/ARB in patients with diabetic kidney disease, and use of ACE inhibitor in nondiabetic kidney disease with proteinuria (spot U_p/U_{Cr} ratio of ≥200 mg/g), to retard progression of kidney disease, irrespective of the presence of hypertension

SOURCE: Reprinted with permission from K/DOQI Clinical Practice Guidelines on Hypertension and Antihypertensive Agents in Chronic Kidney Disease. © 2004 National Kidney Foundation, Inc.

The Use of Angiotensin Blockers to Protect the Kidney

Both landmark studies in animals by Brenner and colleagues as well as studies in humans support an independent role for angiotensin blockade in renoprotection. Angiotensin-converting enzyme (ACE) inhibitors or angiotensin receptor blockers (ARBs) can be used. It is important to titrate the dose of ACE inhibitor or ARB to maximal levels using reduction of proteinuria as the yardstick for efficacy. In addition, sodium restriction and diuretics in conjunction with ACE inhibitor/ARB therapy increase their antiproteinuric effects and should be used in an adjunctive fashion. (ACE inhibitors and ARBs are contraindicated in patients who are pregnant and in patients with a history of angioedema.) Currently, the use of dual blockade with both an ACE inhibitor and an ARB is not recommended because of a higher rate of adverse risk from dual blockade.

Control of Blood Pressure

The MDRD study demonstrated that patients targeted to MAP of 92 and 107 mm Hg had rates of decline of GFR of −3.56 and −4.10 mL/min/year, respectively, and that there was greater effect with increasing levels of albuminuria. This study, taken in conjunction with several other studies that have been published subsequently, suggests a key role for blood pressure reduction in retarding the progression of kidney disease. Indeed, a recent study suggests that this beneficial effect of controlling blood pressure on kidney disease

extends for a prolonged period of time. The 2003 NKF KDOQI clinical practice guidelines for antihypertensive therapy recommendations are shown in table 63.7.

With regard to adjunctive antihypertensive agents, the guidelines suggest diuretics followed by either beta blockers or calcium channel blockers in diabetic kidney disease as well as in nondiabetic albuminuric kidney disease. In patients with kidney disease in the absence of significant albuminuria, diuretics are the preferred agent, followed by ACEI, ARB, beta blocker, or calcium channel blocker. Finally, in recipients of renal allografts, the NKF KDOQI guidelines (table 63.8) recommend calcium channel blockade, diuretic therapy, and beta blockade, ACE inhibitor, or ARB.

Adjunctive Strategies in Retarding Progression

1. *Strict glycemic control.* The DCCT and UKPDS studies for type 1 and type 2 diabetics, respectively, have unequivocally demonstrated the benefits of tight glycemic control with a goal HbA1c of <7.0%.

2. *Protein restriction.* The KDOQI Guidelines for Nutrition in Chronic Renal Failure recommend restriction of protein intake to 0.8 g/kg/day in all patients with CKD, with further restriction to 0.6 g/kg/day in those with CrCl less than 25 mL/min. The guidelines also recommend a caloric intake of 30–35 kcal/kg/day.

3. *Smoking cessation.* Smoking has been implicated as a risk factor in the progression of kidney disease, particularly

Table 63.8 NKF KDOQI ANTIHYPERTENSIVE GUIDELINES FOR CKD PATIENTS

TYPE OF KIDNEY DISEASE	TARGET BLOOD PRESSURE (mm Hg)	PREFERRED AGENTS FOR CKD WITH OR WITHOUT HYPERTENSION	OTHER AGENTS TO REDUCE CVD RISK AND REACH BLOOD PRESSURE TARGET
Diabetic kidney disease	<130/80	ACE inhibitor or ARB	Diuretics preferred, then BB or CCB
Nondiabetic kidney disease with spot U_p/U_{Cr} ratio ≥200 mg/g	<130/80	ACE inhibitor	Diuretics preferred, then BB or CCB
Nondiabetic kidney disease with spot U_p/U_{Cr} ratio <200 mg/g	<130/80	No preference	Diuretics preferred, then ACI inhibitor, ARB, BB, CCB
Disease in the kidney transplant recipient	<130/80	No preference	CCB, Diuretic, BB, ACE inhibitor, ARB

SOURCE: Reprinted with permission from K/DOQI Clinical Practice Guidelines on Hypertension and Antihypertensive Agents in Chronic Kidney Disease. © 2004 National Kidney Foundation, Inc.

diabetic kidney disease. The postulated mechanisms of injury include a heightened risk of atherosclerosis, vascular occlusion, and reduction in renal blood flow. Smoking cessation is recommended in all patients.

4. *Management of obesity.* Obesity may result in an acquired resistance to the beneficial effects of inhibition of the RAS axis. Further, weight loss may facilitate the actions of ACE inhibition and/or angiotensin receptor blockade. In addition, obesity may induce certain renal diseases, such as focal segmental glomerulosclerosis, postulated to be due to a mechanism of hyperfiltration. Weight loss is recommended in CKD patients with a goal body mass index (BMI) of <25.

ADDITIONAL READING

Brenner BM. Retarding the progression of renal disease. *Kidney Int.* 2003;64(1):370–8.

Coresh J, Astor BC, Greene T, Eknoyan G, Levey AS. Prevalence of chronic kidney disease and decreased kidney function in the adult US population: Third National Health and Nutrition Examination Survey. *Am J Kidney Dis.* 2003;41(1):1–12.

Coresh J, Byrd-Holt D, Astor BC, et al. Chronic kidney disease awareness, prevalence, and trends among U.S. adults, 1999 to 2000. *J Am Soc Nephrol.* 2005;16(1):180–8.

Coresh J, Stevens LA. Kidney function estimating equations: Where do we stand? *Curr Opin Nephrol Hypertens.* 2006;15(3):276–84.

Coresh J, Stevens LA, Levey AS. Chronic kidney disease is common: What do we do next? *Nephrol Dial Transplant.* 2008;23(4):1122–5.

de Jong PE, Brenner BM. From secondary to primary prevention of progressive renal disease: The case for screening for albuminuria. *Kidney Int.* 2004;66(6):2109–18.

Johnson CA, Levey AS, Coresh J, Levin A, Lau J, Eknoyan G. Clinical practice guidelines for chronic kidney disease in adults: Part I. Definition, disease stages, evaluation, treatment, and risk factors. *Am Fam Physician.* 2004;70(5):869–76.

Levey AS, Astor BC, Stevens LA, Coresh J. Chronic kidney disease, diabetes, and hypertension: What's in a name? *Kidney Int.* 2010;78(1):19–22.

Levey AS, Eckardt KU, Tsukamoto Y, et al. Definition and classification of chronic kidney disease: A position statement from Kidney Disease: Improving Global Outcomes (KDIGO). *Kidney Int.* 2005;67:2089.

McClellan WM. Epidemiology and risk factors for chronic kidney disease. *Med Clin North Am.* 2005;89(3):419–45.

National Kidney Foundation. K/DOQI clinical practice guidelines for chronic kidney disease: Evaluation, classification and stratification. *Am J Kidney Dis.* 2002;39(Suppl 1):S1.

Stevens LA, Levey AS. Measurement of kidney function. *Med Clin North Am.* 2005;89(3):457–73.

Stevens LA, Padala S, Levey AS. Advances in glomerular filtration rate-estimating equations. *Curr Opin Nephrol Hypertens.* 2010;19(3):298–307.

Vassalotti JA, Stevens LA, Levey AS. Testing for chronic kidney disease: A position statement from the National Kidney Foundation. *Am J Kidney Dis.* 2007;50(2):169–80.

QUESTIONS

QUESTION 1. A 78-year-old African-American man is referred to the CKD clinic because of an apparently reduced estimated GFR (eGFR). He is otherwise healthy. Past medical history is notable for hypertension diagnosed by his primary care physician about 15 years ago. He has a mildly elevated cholesterol treated with atorvastatin. His blood pressure (BP) has been quite stable—in the 150–160/80–90 mm Hg range. He is status post a recent hip replacement that went well. He has no allergies. Medications include hydrochlorothiazide 50 mg/day, atorvastatin 10 mg qd. He is a former smoker. On physical examination he is a healthy looking obese man. His BP is 152/68 mm Hg and heart rate 72 bpm. Weight 120 kg JVP 8 cm. The rest of the examination is negative. The urinalysis reveals a specific gravity (SG) of 1015, pH 5.0, 3+ albumin, and is otherwise negative. The urine sediment is bland. His BUN and creatinine are 28 and 1.1 mg/dL, respectively.

All of the following statements are true EXCEPT:

A. Estimating his GFR using the Cockcroft-Gault equation will result in a gross overestimation of his actual GFR.

B. Evidence indicates that elderly black patients do not benefit from angiotensin blockade.

C. Management of his hypertension should include workup for the possibility of sleep apnea syndrome.

D. His black race and the presence of albuminuria place this patient at a higher risk of progression regardless of his eGFR.

E. His estimated eGFR will be approximately 20% higher than that of a similar white patient.

QUESTION 2. A 44-year-old man is seen in follow-up for management for his presumed ibuprofen-associated gastritis. Two weeks previously he was told to discontinue his ibuprofen, and the cimetidine was begun. He feels much better. Laboratory testing reveals that his serum creatinine is now 1.4 mg/dL, up from a baseline 6 months previously of 0.9 mg/dL. The patient's urinalysis on dipstick is negative, and the urine microscopy is bland. The most likely reason for the bump in serum creatinine is:

A. Ibuprofen-associated acute interstitial nephritis

B. Renal vasoconstriction from ibuprofen therapy

C. Ibuprofen-precipitated minimal change disease

D. Cimetidine-associated interstitial nephritis

E. Cimetidine-mediated inhibition of tubular creatinine secretion

QUESTION 3. A 44-year-old patient with type 2 diabetes mellitus develops microalbuminuria (22 μg albumin/g creatinine) on two separate measurements. Her blood pressure is 138/77 mm Hg. At this point you should:

A. Begin the patient on hydrochlorothiazide

B. Begin the patient on lisinopril

C. Begin the patient on lifestyle modifications; include a DASH diet and salt restriction

D. Begin the patient on a calcium channel blocker

E. Observe the patient and schedule a follow-up appointment in 3 months

QUESTION 4. You are asked to consult on a 62-year-old African-American male diabetic with nephropathy. Routine chemistry labs show a potassium of 6.2 meq/L. All of the following would be changes seen on the EKG compatible with hyperkalemia, EXCEPT:

A. Peaked T waves
B. Prolonged QRS
C. Flattened P wave
D. Sine-wave-appearing QRS complex
E. U wave

QUESTION 5. A 52-year-old African-American female presents to the emergency room with unstable angina. She is noted to have a past medical history of CKD (serum creatinine of 1.8 mg/dL). She is transferred to the coronary care unit, and therapy for her unstable angina is initiated.

A cardiac catheterization is planned for the next day. Her cardiologist asks you for an estimate of her risk of developing contrast nephrotoxicity. Which one of the following would be the closest estimate?

A. 60%
B. <5%
C. 20%
D. >80%
E. >95%

ANSWERS

1. B
2. E
3. B
4. E
5. C

64.

ESSENTIAL AND SECONDARY HYPERTENSION

Ajay K. Singh

Hypertension is one of the most common chronic diseases confronting humanity. The worldwide prevalence is estimated to be approximately 26%, or approximately 1 billion individuals. The World Health Organization estimates that high blood pressure causes one in every eight deaths, making hypertension the third leading source of mortality in the world. In the United States, the National Health and Nutrition Educational Survey (NHANES) survey reports an incidence of approximately 30% in individuals 18 years and older. The prevalence is higher in older individuals, non-Hispanic blacks, and women. Essential hypertension is the most prevalent hypertension type, affecting 90–95% of hypertensive patients.

DEFINITION OF HYPERTENSION

Systolic and diastolic hypertension in the general population are defined as a blood pressure (BP) of ≥140/≥90 mm Hg measured on at least three separate occasions. BP should be measured while seated in a quiet room with arm muscles relaxed. It is important to maintain the cubital fossa at heart level. A suitable size cuff should be used. It is recommended that the BP should be repeated if it is >140/90 mm Hg, and measurement should be in both arms.

The stages of hypertension, as defined by the Joint National Committee 7 (JNC7), are shown in table 64.1. (Newer guidelines [JNC8] will be available in 2011.) Individuals with a systolic BP of 120–139 mm Hg or a diastolic BP of 80–89 mm Hg should be considered as prehypertensive, and lifestyle modification initiated. Those with BPs in the range of 130/80 to 139/89 mm Hg have twice the risk of hypertension as those with lower values. The target BP for all patients with hypertension is <140/90 mm Hg (or 130/80 mm Hg in patients with hypertension and diabetes or chronic kidney disease). Key recommendations from JNC7 are shown in table 64.2. In addition to lifestyle modification, patients who fall into stage 1 hypertension should receive drug therapy, preferably with a thiazide-type diuretic.

Patients in stage 2 hypertension require more aggressive management. JNC7 guidelines recommend that stage 2 hypertension patients should be initiated on two antihypertensive agents, one of them a thiazide-type diuretic. Persistent hypertension is one of the risk factors for stroke, myocardial infarction, heart failure, and arterial aneurysm and is a leading cause of chronic kidney failure.

Although the prevalence of high blood pressure is high, there is a low awareness rate. Fifty-three percent of patients with hypertension are being treated with medications. Of those treated, 29% have their blood pressure <140/90 mm Hg. Data from several studies indicate that increasing awareness improves BP control.

PRIMARY HYPERTENSION

Primary or essential hypertension is defined as high blood pressure for which no medical cause can be found. About 90–95% of cases are termed primary hypertension. The etiopathogenesis of primary hypertension remains obscure, although various factors have been implicated; these include increased sympathetic nervous activity, genetic factors, mineralocorticoid excess, increased angiotensin II activity, reduced renal mass, race, salt sensitivity, and the presence of insulin resistance.

Hypertension is a major risk factor for cardiovascular disease, heart failure, stroke, left ventricular hypertrophy, and chronic kidney disease. For example, among 347,978 men screened for participation in the Multiple Risk Factor Intervention Trial, the risk of fatal stroke for those with systolic blood pressure over 180 mm Hg was about 15 times as high and the risk of fatal ischemic heart disease seven times as high as the rates among those with optimal blood pressure The optimal interval for screening for hypertension is not known. The 2007 United States Preventive Services Task Force (USPSTF) guidelines on screening for high blood pressure recommend screening every 2 years for persons with systolic and diastolic pressures below 120 mm Hg and 80 mm Hg,

Table 64.1 CLASSIFICATION OF HYPERTENSION*

Normal blood pressure: systolic <120 mm Hg and diastolic <80 mm Hg

Prehypertension: systolic 120–139 mm Hg or diastolic 80–89 mm Hg

Hypertension:

   Stage 1: systolic 140–159 mm Hg or diastolic 90–99 mm Hg
   Stage 2: systolic ≥160 mm Hg or diastolic ≥100 mm Hg

NOTE: * Isolated systolic hypertension is considered to be present when the blood pressure is ≥140/<90 mm Hg, and isolated diastolic hypertension is considered to be present when the blood pressure is <140/≥90 mm Hg.
SOURCE: The Seventh Report of the Joint National Committee on Prevention, Detection, Evaluation, and Treatment of High Blood Pressure (JNC7). National Institutes of Health, National Heart, Lung, and Blood Institute, U.S. Department of Health and Human Services, 2004.

---

respectively (normal BP in JNC7), and yearly for persons with a systolic pressure of 120–139 mmHg or a diastolic pressure of 80–89 mm Hg (prehypertension in JNC7).

Workup of hypertension should include a thorough history and physical examination and laboratory workup (table 64.3). Common and uncommon causes of secondary hypertension and clues to secondary causes of hypertension are shown in table 64.4.

MANAGEMENT OF HYPERTENSION

Treatment of hypertension should follow the broad outlines recommended by JNC7 (figure 64.1). Key recommendations derived from JNC7 are listed (table 64.2).

LIFESTYLE MODIFICATIONS

A recommended initial step is lifestyle modification. Components of lifestyle modification that have demon-

strated effectiveness in reducing blood pressure include the following:

- Weight reduction in patients who are obese to achieve a body mass index of 18.5–24.9

- A decrease in daily sodium intake to <2.4 g

- Regular aerobic physical activity of 30 minutes daily on most days of the week

- Moderation of alcohol consumption

- Smoking cessation

Additionally, patients should be encouraged to adopt a diet rich in fruits, vegetables, and low-fat dairy products, with reduced content of total and saturated fat modeled on the Dietary Approaches to Stop Hypertension (DASH). The DASH diet has been demonstrated to be beneficial in reducing elevated blood pressure levels, particularly when combined with low sodium intake.

Table 64.2 RECOMMENDATIONS FROM JNC7 FOR HYPERTENSION PREVENTION AND MANAGEMENT

In persons older than 50 years, systolic BP of more than 140 mm Hg is a much more important cardiovascular disease (CVD) risk factor than diastolic BP.

The risk of CVD, beginning at 115/75 mm Hg, doubles with each increment of 20/10 mm Hg; individuals who are normotensive (normal BP) at 55 years of age have a 90% lifetime risk for developing hypertension.

Individuals with a systolic BP of 120 to 139 mm Hg or a diastolic BP of 80 to 89 mm Hg should be considered as prehypertensive and educated about health-promoting lifestyle modifications to prevent CVD.

Thiazide-type diuretics should be used in drug treatment for most patients with uncomplicated hypertension, either alone or combined with drugs from other classes. Certain high-risk conditions are compelling indications for the initial use of other antihypertensive drug classes (ACE inhibitors, angiotensin-receptor blockers, beta blockers, and calcium channel blockers).

Most patients with hypertension will require two or more antihypertensive medications to achieve goal BP (<140/90 mm Hg, or <130/80 mm Hg for patients with diabetes or chronic kidney disease).

If BP is >20/10 mm Hg above goal BP, consideration should be given to initiating therapy with two agents, one of which usually should be a thiazide-type diuretic.

The most effective therapy prescribed by the most careful clinician will control hypertension only if patients are motivated. Motivation improves when patients have positive experiences with and trust in the clinician. Empathy builds trust and is a potent motivator.

SOURCE: The Seventh Report of the Joint National Committee on Prevention, Detection, Evaluation, and Treatment of High Blood Pressure (JNC7). National Institutes of Health, National Heart, Lung, and Blood Institute, U.S. Department of Health and Human Services, 2004.

Table 64.3 INITIAL LABORATORY WORKUP OF PATIENTS WITH HYPERTENSION

Urinalysis

Serum creatinine and/or blood urea nitrogen

Plasma potassium

Random blood glucose

Serum cholesterol, lipids, lipoprotein cholesterol

Hematocrit

Electrocardiogram

Serum uric acid

Chest x-ray

PHARMACOTHERAPY

JNC7 recommends that initial treatment in patients should be with a thiazide-type diuretic unless the patient has a coexisting compelling condition (see below) (figure 64.1). The thiazide diuretic (preferably chlorthalidone) could be given either alone or in combination with a drug from one of the other drug classes: angiotensin-converting enzyme (ACE) inhibitors, angiotensin receptor blockers (ARBs), beta blockers (BBs), or calcium channel blockers (CCBs). The beneficial effects of thiazides are supported by data obtained from the ALLHAT trial. Thiazide diuretics appear to be as effective as other antihypertensive agents and are the most cost-effective antihypertensives to date.

JNC7 emphasizes the importance of individualizing therapy by focusing on compelling conditions (table 64.5).

Table 64.4 SECONDARY CAUSES OF HYPERTENSION AND CLINICAL CLUES

Common
Intrinsic renal disease
Renovascular disease
Mineralocorticoid excess/aldosteronism
Sleep apnea
Uncommon
Pheochromocytoma
Glucocorticoid excess/Cushing disease
Coarctation of aorta
Hyper-/hypothyroidism
Clinical Clues For Secondary Hypertension
Young age
Family history of renal disease
Evidence of renal disease
Hypertension due to drugs
Episodes of sweating, headache, anxiety (pheochromocytoma)
Episodes of muscle weakness and tetany (hyperaldosteronism)

In patients with angina pectoris JNC7 recommends BBs or long-acting CCBs as first-line agents. Patients with acute coronary syndrome (unstable angina or myocardial infarction) should be initiated on BBs and ACE inhibitors. After myocardial infarction, BBs, ACE inhibitors, and aldosterone antagonists have been shown to be beneficial. In patients with heart failure JNC7 recommends ACE inhibitors and BBs. In patients with symptomatic ventricular dysfunction or end-stage heart disease, other agents such as BBs, ARBs, and aldosterone antagonists should be considered. In patients with diabetes mellitus JNC7 recommends thiazide-type diuretics, BBs, ACEIs, ARBs, and CCBs. In patients with chronic kidney disease (CKD) JNC7 recommends ACE inhibitors or ARBs. Adding in a loop diuretic should also be considered.

HYPERTENSION SYNDROMES

HYPERTENSION EMERGENCIES

A hypertensive emergency is a condition in which elevated blood pressure results in target organ damage to one or more of the following: the cardiovascular system, the kidneys, and/or the central nervous system. Hypertensive emergencies are potentially life-threatening and usually associated with blood pressures ≥180/120 mm Hg. Hypertensive urgency is defined as severely elevated blood pressure (i.e., systolic >220 mm Hg or diastolic >120 mm Hg) with no evidence of target organ damage. A hypertensive emergency requires immediate intervention and acute reduction in blood pressure to either reverse or attenuate further target organ damage. In contrast, the treatment of hypertensive urgency can be more deliberate.

Malignant Hypertension

Fewer than 1% of patients with essential hypertension develop malignant hypertension. The average age at diagnosis is 40 years, and men are affected more often than women. Risk factors for malignant hypertension include cigarette smoking, black race, medication nonadherence, and individuals with secondary hypertension. Prior to effective therapy, life expectancy was less than 2 years, with most deaths resulting from stroke, renal failure, or heart failure. With current therapy, including dialysis, the survival rate at 1 year is >90% and at 5 years is >80%. Malignant hypertension is characterized by severe hypertension with associated ophthalmological findings of retinal hemorrhages, exudates, and/or papilledema (figure 64.2). Renal involvement manifests clinically with azotemia and an abnormal urinalysis—presence of hematuria, proteinuria, and red cell casts (figure 64.3). Renal biopsy (if one is performed) usually demonstrates arteriosclerosis

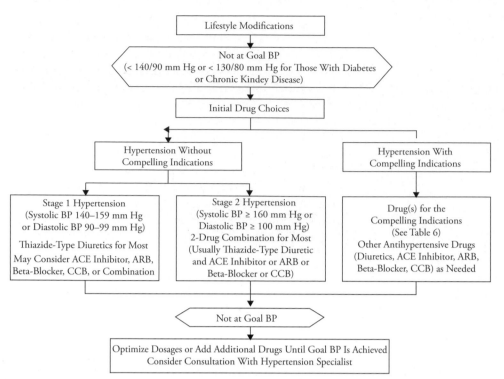

```
┌─────────────────────────────────┐
│      Lifestyle Modifications    │
└─────────────────────────────────┘
```

Not at Goal BP
(< 140/90 mm Hg or < 130/80 mm Hg for Those With Diabetes
or Chronic Kindey Disease)

Initial Drug Choices

Hypertension Without
Compelling Indications

Hypertension With
Compelling Indications

Stage 1 Hypertension
(Systolic BP 140–159 mm Hg
or Diastolic BP 90–99 mm Hg)

Thiazide-Type Diuretics for Most
May Consider ACE Inhibitor, ARB,
Beta-Blocker, CCB, or Combination

Stage 2 Hypertension
(Systolic BP ≥ 160 mm Hg or
Diastolic BP ≥ 100 mm Hg)
2-Drug Combination for Most
(Usually Thiazide-Type Diuretic
and ACE Inhibitor or ARB or
Beta-Blocker or CCB)

Drug(s) for the
Compelling Indications
(See Table 6)
Other Antihypertensive Drugs
(Diuretics, ACE Inhibitor, ARB,
Beta-Blocker, CCB) as Needed

Not at Goal BP

Optimize Dosages or Add Additional Drugs Until Goal BP Is Achieved
Consider Consultation With Hypertension Specialist

Figure 64.1. Algorithm for JNC7 Recommended Treatment of Hypertension.

and fibrinoid necrosis. Neurological presentations include occipital headaches, cerebral infarct, cerebral hemorrhage, or hypertensive encephalopathy. Hypertensive encephalopathy is a symptom complex comprising of severe hypertension, headache, vomiting, visual disturbance, mental status changes, seizure, and retinopathy with papilledema. Focal signs and symptoms are uncommon and may indicate another process, such as cerebral infarct or hemorrhage. Gastrointestinal symptoms are nausea and vomiting. Diffuse arteriolar damage can result in microangiopathic hemolytic anemia.

Patients with malignant hypertension are usually admitted to an intensive care unit for continuous cardiac monitoring and frequent assessment of neurological status and urine output. Blood pressure measurements should be measured in both arms. A rapid assessment for target organ damage is performed, both clinically and by a laboratory workup. The clinical workup must include a complete cardiac, neurological, and ophthalmoscopic examination. Hypertensive retinopathy is graded using the Keith-Wagner classification (table 64.6). Examination of the urine is also essential (see figure 64.1). Proteinuria and hematuria are common. Red cell casts may be seen on urine sediment examination. An intravenous line is essential for medications. The initial goal of therapy should be to reduce the mean arterial pressure by approximately 20–25% over the first 24–48 hours or the mean arterial pressure (MAP) to 110–120 mm Hg, whichever is higher. An intra-arterial line is helpful for continuous titration of blood pressure. Use of short-acting antihypertensive agents administered intravenously is recommended (table 64.7). The most widely used intravenous medications are nitroprusside, nitroglycerin, labetalol, and fenoldopam.

Hypertensive urgencies do not mandate admission to a hospital. The goal of therapy is to reduce blood pressure within 24 hours, and this can be achieved as an outpatient, frequently with orally administered medications.

Table 64.5 COMPELLING CONDITIONS AND JNC7 RECOMMENDED TREATMENTS

Heart failure	Thiazide, BB, ACEI, ARB, Aldo antagonist
Postmyocardial infarction	BB, ACE inhibitor, Aldo antagonist
High CAD risk	Thiazide, BB, ACE, CCB
Diabetes mellitus	Thiazide, BB, ACE, ARB, CCB
Chronic kidney disease	ACEI, ARB
Recurrent stroke prevention	Thiazide, ACE inhibitor

RESISTANT HYPERTENSION

The JNC7 defines resistant hypertension as failure to achieve goal BP (<140/90 mm Hg for the overall

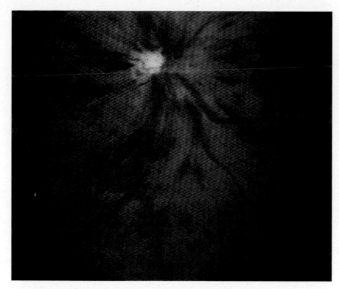

Figure 64.2. Fundoscopic Appearance of Hypertensive Retinopathy. The picture shows extensive flame shaped hemorrhages.

population and <130/80 mm Hg for those with diabetes mellitus or chronic kidney disease) when a patient adheres to maximum tolerated doses of three antihypertensive drugs including a diuretic. Resistant hypertension is present in 5% of patients with hypertension in a general practice setting, but it is much more common in specialty settings such as a renal clinic. An approach to resistant hypertension is shown in table 64.8. Because a suboptimal dosing regimen or inappropriate antihypertensive drug combination is the most common cause of resistant hypertension, the first step in management is to review the medication regimen. The most important interven-

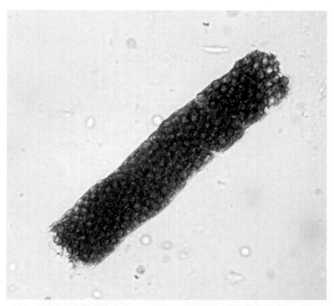

Figure 64.3. Typical Appearance of a Red Cell Cast in a Patient with Malignant Hypertension with Renal Thrombotic Microangiopathy.

tion is to target subtle or clinically apparent extracellular volume expansion by either adding a diuretic agent or increasing the dose of diuretic or changing the diuretic class based on kidney function. A thiazide diuretic is preferred if the patient's estimated GFR (eGFR) is >50 mL/min/1.73 m². Switching to a loop diuretic, such as furosemide or bumetanide is recommended once the eGFR falls <50 mL/min/1.73 m². In addition, the patient should be on a blocker of the RAS along with a calcium antagonist. Options for a fourth agent include a vasodilator, a beta blocker, or a peripheral alpha blocker. Adding a complementary calcium channel blocker (e.g., adding diltiazem to nifedipine XL) has also been recommended. On the other hand, dual blockade with both an angiotensin receptor blocker and an ACE inhibitor does not result in additive BP reduction and maybe harmful.

ENDOCRINE HYPERTENSION SYNDROMES

Endocrine hypertension includes the following disorders.

Primary Aldosteronism

Primary hyperaldosteronism is the most common form of endocrine hypertension. It affects 5–10% of all patients with hypertension. The two most common forms of primary aldosteronism are Conn syndrome—a single adrenal tumor produces excessive aldosterone, and bilateral adrenal hyperplasia—both adrenal glands are enlarged and cause hyperaldosteronism. Adrenal carcinoma is an extremely rare cause of primary hyperaldosteronism. Excessive aldosterone production by the adrenal glands leads to fluid retention, potassium loss manifest as mild to moderate hypokalemia, metabolic alkalosis, and hypertension. Initial workup should include electrolytes, serum aldosterone, and plasma renin activity (PRA). A significant elevation of the plasma aldosterone-to-renin ratio is to 30 (normal ratio is 4–10). If the plasma aldosterone concentration is >20 ng/dL and the ratio is >30, the sensitivity and specificity for primary aldosteronism are >90%. Confirmatory testing should and include either measurement of serum aldosterone level after 3 days of an unrestricted sodium diet and 1 hour of full recumbency, or measurement of 24-hour urinary aldosterone excretion, or an oral or intravenous salt-loading test with measurement of serum aldosterone level and PRA. Additional testing includes high-resolution, thin-slice (2–2.5 mm), adrenal computed tomography (CT) scanning with contrast, and adrenal venous sampling. Adrenal venous sampling probably has its greatest utility in the setting of either totally normal adrenal imaging despite biochemical evidence for primary aldosteronism or settings in which bilateral

Table 64.6 KEITH-WAGENER CLASSIFICATION FOR HYPERTENSIVE RETINOPATHY

INDICATION	DIURETIC	BB	ACE INHIBITOR	ARB	CCB	ALDOANT
			RECOMMENDED DRUGS			
Heart failure	•	•	•	•		•
Post-MI		•	•			•
High CAD risk	•	•	•		•	
Diabetes	•	•	•	•	•	
CKD			•	•		
Recurrent stroke prevention	•		•			

NOTES:
- Grade 1 – Mild arteriolar narrowing, tortuosity, irregular caliber with copper/silver wiring
- Grade 2 – Focal narrowing and arteriovenous nicking
- Grade 3 – Retinal hemorrhages (flame-shaped and blot hemorrhages), cotton wool spots, and hard exudates
- Grade 4 – Severe grade 3 plus papilledema

adrenal pathology is present on imaging. MRI is not superior to contrast-enhanced CT scanning for adrenal visualization. Bilateral adrenal hyperplasia is best treated with medications such as spironolactone or eplerenone. Surgery is the treatment of choice for the lateralizable variants of primary hyperaldosteronism.

Cushing Syndrome

Cushing syndrome is caused by prolonged exposure to elevated levels of either endogenous glucocorticoids or exogenous glucocorticoids. Cushing syndrome can be due to direct adrenal involvement (adrenal Cushing) or independent of adrenocorticotropic hormone (ACTH) secretion

(i.e., ACTH-independent). ACTH-dependent Cushing disease is either secondary to an anterior pituitary tumor (in approximately 80%) or to ectopic ACTH syndrome (table 64.9). Nonpituitary ectopic sources of ACTH include oat cell carcinoma, small-cell lung carcinoma, or carcinoid tumor. A more detailed discussion is provided in the endocrine section of this book (section 5, chapter 48).

Pheochromocytoma

This is a syndrome caused by tumors of the adrenal glands. Pheochromocytoma is rare. These tumors produce excessive amounts of epinephrine, norepinephrine, or other catecholamines. The classic triad of symptoms in patients with

Table 64.7 DRUGS COMMONLY USED FOR THE TREATMENT OF HYPERTENSIVE EMERGENCY

DRUG	DOSAGE	ONSET/ DURATION OF ACTION	POTENTIAL ADVERSE EFFECTS
Nitroprusside	0.25–10 µg/kg/min	Instant/1–2 min	Thiocyanate cyanide poisoning
Nitroglycerine	5–100 µg/min	1–5 min/3–5 min	Flushing headache, methemoglobin
Nicardipine	5–15 mg/hr	5–10 min/1–4 hr	Tachycardia, flushing
Hydralazine	10–20 mg	5–15 min/3–8 hr	Flushing, tachycardia
Enalapril	10–40 mg IM, 1.25–5 mg IV q6hr	20–30 min/6 hr	Hypotension, hyperkalemia
Fenoldopam	0.1–0.3 µg/kg/min	5 min/10–15 min	Flushing, headache, tachycardia
Labetalol	20–80 mg IV bolus every 10 min, 2 mg min IV infusion	5–10 min/3–6 hr	Heart block, ortho hypotension
Esmolol	200–500 µg/kg/min for 4 min, then 150–300 µg/kg/min	1–2 min/10–20 min	Hypotension
Phentolamine (α1 blocker)	5–15 mg IV	1–2 min/3–10 min	Tachycardia, flushing, headache

Table 64.8 APPROACH TO PATIENT WITH RESISTANT HYPERTENSION

- Measure BP accurately
  "Persons should be seated quietly for 5 minutes with feet on the floor and the arm supported at heart level."
  Cuff must be appropriately sized (cuff bladder must encircle 80% of the arm)
  Check both arms and a leg (or palpate pulses carefully)

- Consider "white coat hypertension" (WCH)
  Home and ambulatory BP monitoring (ABPM)

- Consider "pseudoresistance"
  Pseudohypertension (calcification of the arteries resulting in failure of the BP cuff to compress and occlude flow)
  Nonadherence (may account for up to 50% of resistant cases)
  Inadequate regimen
  Interfering medicines and substances also need to be considered
  - NSAIDs
  - Excessive alcohol, caffeine, or tobacco
  - Excessive salt intake
  - Oral contraceptives
  - Sympathomimetic agents (nasal decongestants, anorectic pills, cocaine, amphetamine-like stimulants)
  - Glucocorticoids
  - Anabolic steroids
  - Erythropoietin
  - Cyclosporine
  - Black licorice
  - Herbal supplements (e.g., ma huang and ginseng)

- Consider secondary causes
  Obstructive sleep apnea
  - Obesity (metabolic syndrome)
  - Endocrinopathies
    • Hyperaldosteronism, thyroid problems, pheochromocytoma
  - Kidney disease
    • Renal insufficiency and renal artery stenosis

a pheochromocytoma consists of episodic headache, sweating, and tachycardia. Patients with a pheochromocytoma have episodic or sustained hypertension. About 10% of these tumors are located outside the adrenal glands (extra-adrenal) in various locations in the body. Extra-adrenal pheochromocytomas are also known as paragangliomas. About 10% of the tumors are malignant. Pheochromocytomas may present as a part of multiple endocrine neoplasia (MEN) syndromes (table 64.10). MEN syndromes can involve other endocrine organs such as the parathyroid glands, the pituitary, the thyroid, as well as other organs such as the kidney, pancreas, or stomach. The MEN 2A and 2B syndromes, which are autosomally inherited, have been traced to germline mutations in the *ret* proto-oncogene. The *ret* proto-oncogene, located

Table 64.9 CAUSES OF CUSHING SYNDROME

ACTH-Dependent
Pituitary tumor (Cushing disease pituitary hypersecretion of ACTH)
Nonpituitary tumors (ectopic secretion of ACTH)
Nonhypothalamic tumors (ectopic secretion of corticotropin-releasing hormone [CRH] causing ACTH secretion)
Administration of exogenous ACTH (iatrogenic or factitious Cushing syndrome)
ACTH-Independent
Exogenous administration of glucocorticoids (iatrogenic or factitious Cushing syndrome)
Adrenocortical adenomas and carcinomas
Primary pigmented nodular adrenocortical disease (bilateral adrenal micronodular hyperplasia)
Bilateral ACTH-independent macronodular hyperplasia

Table 64.10 PHEOCHROMOCYTOMA SYNDROMES

SYNDROME	KEY CHARACTERISTICS
MEN 2A (Sipple syndrome)	Medullary thyroid carcinoma, hyperparathyroidism, pheochromocytomas, and Hirschsprung disease. >95% of cases of MEN 2A have mutations in the *ret* proto-oncogene
MEN 2B	Medullary thyroid carcinoma, pheochromocytoma, mucosal neurofibromatosis, intestinal ganglioneuromatosis, Hirschsprung disease, and a marfanoid body habitus; a germline missense mutation in the tyrosine kinase domain of the *ret* proto-oncogene
VHL disease	Pheochromocytoma, cerebellar hemangioblastoma, renal cell carcinoma, renal and pancreatic cysts, and epididymal cystadenomas; >75 germline mutations in a VHL suppressor gene on chromosome 3.8
Neurofibromatosis or von Recklinghausen disease	Congenital anomalies (often benign tumors) of the skin, nervous system, bones, and endocrine glands; only 1% of patients with neurofibromatosis have been found to have pheochromocytomas, but as many as 5% of patients with pheochromocytomas have been found to have neurofibromatosis

on chromosome 10, encodes a tyrosine kinase receptor involved in the regulation of cell growth and differentiation. Pheochromocytomas occur bilaterally in the MEN syndromes in as many as 70% of cases.

Other types of endocrine hypertension are shown in table 64.11.

HYPERTENSION IN THE ELDERLY

Hypertension is quite common in the elderly. Primary hypertension is the most common type, but common identifiable causes (e.g., renovascular hypertension) should be considered. In the elderly, systolic blood pressure (SBP) appears to be a better predictor of cardiovascular events than diastolic blood pressure. However, pseudohypertension and "white-coat hypertension" are common, and readings outside the office should be emphasized. Therapy should begin with lifestyle modifications. Starting doses for drug therapy should be lower than those used in younger adults; however, the goal of therapy is the same as with younger patients (<140/90 mm Hg), although an interim goal of SBP <160 mm Hg may be necessary. In the 2008 HYVET (Hypertension in the Very Elderly) trial, active treatment with perindopril was associated with a 30% reduction in the rate of fatal or nonfatal stroke, a 39% reduction in the rate of death from stroke, a 21% reduction in the rate of death from any cause, a 23% reduction in the rate of death from cardiovascular causes, and a 64% reduction in the rate of heart failure.

Table 64.11 ENDOCRINE SYNDROMES OF HYPERTENSION

TYPE OF SYNDROME	KEY CHARACTERISTICS
Familial hyperaldosteronism type I (also known as glucocorticoid-remediable aldosteronism)	Clinical: About 1% of cases of primary hyperaldosteronism. May be detected in asymptomatic individuals when screening offspring of affected individuals, or patients may present in infancy with hypertension, weakness, and failure to thrive due to hypokalemia. Genetics: Autosomal dominant with low frequency of new mutations. Presence of a hybrid or chimeric gene on chromosome 8q consisting of the regulatory region of the 11-beta-hydroxylase gene coupled to the coding sequence of the aldosterone synthase gene.
Familial hyperaldosteronism type II (FH-II, also known as pseudohypoaldosteronism type 2 or Gordon syndrome)	Clinical: Rare familial renal tubular defect characterized by hypertension and hyperkalemic metabolic acidosis in the presence of low renin and aldosterone levels. Genetics: Autosomal dominant. It is due to absent WNK1 or WNK4 kinase function in the distal nephron.
Liddle syndrome	Clinical: Early-onset severe hypertension, hypokalemia, metabolic alkalosis in the setting of low plasma renin and aldosterone, low rates of urinary aldosterone excretion, and a family history of hypertension. Genetics: Autosomal dominant disorder caused by hyperactivity of the amiloride-sensitive sodium channel (ENaC) of the principal cell of the cortical collecting tubule.
Apparent mineralocorticoid excess (AME)	Clinical: Presents with hypertension and hypokalemia. Genetics: Autosomal recessive disorder. Results from mutations in the *HSD11B2* gene, which encodes the kidney isozyme of 11-beta-hydroxysteroid dehydrogenase type 2.
Licorice ingestion	Clinical: Presents with hypertension and hypokalemia. Pathophysiology: Pseudoaldosteronism due to ingestion of certain types of licorice (usually black licorice).

HYPERTENSION IN PREGNANCY

Hypertension is the most common medical problem encountered during pregnancy, complicating 2–3% of pregnancies. Hypertension during pregnancy is an important source of both maternal and fetal morbidity, and of maternal mortality, especially in the developing world. Hypertensive disorders during pregnancy are classified into four categories by the National High Blood Pressure Education Program Working Group on High Blood Pressure in Pregnancy: (1) chronic hypertension, (2) preeclampsia-eclampsia, (3) preeclampsia superimposed on chronic hypertension, and (4) gestational hypertension (table 64.12).

CHRONIC HYPERTENSION

Chronic hypertension may be either essential or secondary. About 20–25% of women with chronic hypertension develop preeclampsia during pregnancy. In normal pregnancy women's mean arterial pressure drops 10–15 mm Hg over the first half of pregnancy. Most women with mild chronic hypertension (i.e., SBP 140–160 mm Hg, DBP 90–100 mm Hg) have a similar decrease in blood pressures and may not require any medication during this period. If maternal blood pressure rises to ≥160/100 mm Hg, however, drug treatment is recommended. The goal of pharmacologic treatment should be a DBP of less than 100–105 mm Hg and an SBP less than 160 mm Hg. Women with pre-existing end-organ damage from chronic hypertension should have a lower threshold for starting antihypertensive medication (i.e., >139/89) and a lower target BP (<140/90).

PREECLAMPSIA

The incidence of preeclampsia in the United States is estimated to range from 2% to 6% in healthy nulliparous women. Preeclampsia can be classified into mild, severe, and HELLP syndrome (table 64.13). Most cases (75%) are mild; 10% occur in pregnancies of less than 34 weeks' gestation. Risk factors for preeclampsia include nulliparity, age >40 years, a family history of preeclampsia, multiple gestations, chronic hypertension, antiphospholipid antibody syndrome, underlying renal disease, obesity, diabetes, and thrombophilia. Clues to differentiate preeclampsia from chronic hypertension include the presence of visual disturbances, such as scintillations and scotomata; the presence of new-onset headache—described as frontal, throbbing, or similar to a migraine headache; new-onset epigastric pain; and rapidly increasing or nondependent edema. (Edema is no longer included among the criteria for diagnosis of preeclampsia.)

Magnesium sulfate is the drug of choice for seizure prophylaxis in women with preeclampsia. Therapy is started at the beginning of labor or prior to cesarean section and continued 24 hours postpartum in most cases. The duration of postpartum therapy may be modified depending on the severity of the disease. Treatment is started by administering an IV loading dose of 4–6 g magnesium sulfate, followed by a maintenance dose of 1–3 g/hr. Management of hypertension in patients with preeclampsia is shown in table 63.14. Systolic blood pressure of 160 mm Hg or greater and/or diastolic pressure of 110 mm Hg or greater must be treated. The goal is to maintain the blood pressure around 140/90 mm Hg.

Management of Mild Preeclampsia

Because delivery is the only cure for a pregnancy complicated by mild preeclampsia; if the mother is >37 weeks, the fetus should be delivered. Vaginal delivery is the first choice, but with induction of labor regardless of cervical status; cesarean section should be performed based on

Table 64.12 **CLASSIFICATION OF HYPERTENSION IN PREGNANCY**

DISORDER	KEY CHARACTERISTICS
Chronic hypertension	BP ≥140/90 mm Hg before pregnancy or diagnosed before 20 weeks of gestation not attributable to gestational trophoblastic disease, or hypertension first diagnosed after 20 weeks of gestation and persistent after 12 weeks postpartum.
Preeclampsia/eclampsia	BP of 140/90 mm Hg or greater after 20 weeks of gestation in a woman with previously normal blood pressure and with proteinuria (≥0.3 g protein in 24-hour urine specimen). Eclampsia is defined as seizures that cannot be attributable to other causes in a woman with preeclampsia.
Superimposed preeclampsia (on chronic hypertension)	New-onset proteinuria (≥300 mg/24 hours) in a woman with hypertension but no proteinuria <20 weeks of gestation. A sudden increase in proteinuria or blood pressure, or platelet count less than 100,000, in a woman with hypertension and proteinuria before 20 weeks of gestation.
Gestational hypertension	BP of 140/90 mm Hg or greater for the first time during pregnancy. No proteinuria. BP returns to normal less than 12 weeks postpartum. Final diagnosis made only postpartum.

Source: National High Blood Pressure Education Program Working Group on High Blood Pressure in Pregnancy Hypertension

Table 64.13 PREECLAMPSIA SYNDROMES

PREECLAMSIA SYNDROME	KEY FEATURES
Mild preeclampsia	1. BP ≥140/90 mm Hg on two occasions, at least 6 hours apart 2. Proteinuria ≥1+ protein on random dipstick or ≥300 mg of protein in a 24-hour urine collection, or urine protein-creatinine ratio ≥0.3 as a criterion for proteinuria

Severe preeclampsia	Presence of preeclampsia plus >1 of following:
	  Systolic BP ≥160 mm Hg
	  diastolic BP ≥110 mm Hg (on two occasions at least 6 hours apart)
	  Proteinuria ≥5 g/24-h
	  Pulmonary edema
	  Oliguria (<400 mL in 24 h)
	  Persistent headaches
	  Epigastric pain and/or impaired liver function
	  Thrombocytopenia
	  Intrauterine growth restriction

HELLP syndrome (hemolysis, elevated liver enzyme, low platelets)	Form of severe preeclampsia
	  Hemolysis
	  Abnormal peripheral smear
	  Indirect bilirubin >1.2 mg/dL
	  Lactate dehydrogenase >600 U/L
	  Elevated liver enzymes (serum AST >70 U/L)
	  Low platelets/coagulopathy (platelet count <100,000/mm^3, elevated PT or aPTT, decreased fibrinogen, increased d-dimer)

SOURCE: National High Blood Pressure Education Program Working Group on High Blood Pressure in Pregnancy Hypertension.

Table 64.14 MANAGEMENT OF HYPERTENSION IN PREECLAMPSIA

MEDICATION	KEY ISSUES
Hydralazine	Hydralazine is a direct peripheral arteriolar vasodilator and, in the past, was widely used as the first-line treatment for acute hypertension in pregnancy. Hydralazine has a slow onset of action (10–20 min) and peaks approximately 20 min after administration. Hydralazine should be given as an IV bolus at a dose of 5–10 mg, depending on the severity of hypertension. It may be administered every 20 min up to a maximum dose of 30 mg. The side effects of hydralazine are headache, nausea, and vomiting. Importantly, hydralazine may result in maternal hypotension, which may subsequently result in a nonreassuring fetal heart rate tracing in the fetus.
Labetalol	Labetalol is a selective alpha blocker and nonselective beta blocker that produces vasodilatation and results in a decrease in systemic vascular resistance. The dosage for labetalol is 20 mg IV with repeat doses (40, 80, 80, and 80 mg) every 10 min up to a maximum dose of 300 mg. Decreases in blood pressure are observed after 5 min (in contrast to the slower onset of action of hydralazine) and results in less over-shoot hypertension than hydralazine. Labetalol decreases supraventricular rhythm and slows the heart rate, reducing myocardial oxygen consumption. No change in afterload is observed after treatment with labetalol. The side effects of labetalol are dizziness, nausea, and headaches. After achieving satisfactory control with IV administration, an oral maintenance dose can begin.
Calcium channel blockers	Calcium channel blockers act on arteriolar smooth muscle and induce vasodilatation by blocking calcium entry into the cells. Nifedipine is the oral calcium channel blocker that is used in the management of hypertension in pregnancy. The dosage of nifedipine is 10 mg po every 15–30 min with a maximum of 3 doses. The side effects of calcium channel blockers include tachycardia, palpitations, and headaches. Concomitant use of calcium channel blockers and magnesium sulfate is to be avoided. Nifedipine is commonly used postpartum in patients with preeclampsia for blood pressure control.
Sodium nitroprusside	Used in a severe hypertensive emergency, nitroprusside results in the release of nitric oxide, which subsequently results in significant vasodilation. Preload and afterload are then greatly decreased. The onset of action is rapid, and severe rebound hypertension may result. Cyanide poisoning may occur subsequent to its use in the fetus. Therefore, its use should be reserved for postpartum care or just before the delivery of the fetus.

standard obstetric criteria. If the mother is <37 weeks' gestation then the optimal management depends on gestational age and severity of the disease. The mother should be hospitalized and monitored carefully, antepartum testing (nonstress test [NST] and biophysical profile [BPP]) should be performed at admission and twice per week until delivery.

Management of Severe Preeclampsia

For severe preeclampsia diagnosed >34 weeks' gestation, delivery is most appropriate. Vaginal delivery is the first choice, and cesarean section should be based on routine obstetric indications. Women with severe preeclampsia who have nonreassuring fetal status, ruptured membranes, labor, or maternal distress should be delivered regardless of gestational age. For women <34 weeks' gestation, corticosteroids for fetal lung maturity should be administered. If a woman with severe preeclampsia is >32 weeks' gestation and has received a course of steroid, she should be delivered as well. Fetal monitoring should include daily nonstress test and ultrasonography performed to monitor for the development of oligohydramnios and decreased fetal movement. In addition, daily blood tests should be performed for liver function tests (LFTs), complete blood count (CBC), uric acid, and lactate dehydrogenase (LDH). Patients should be instructed to report any headache, visual changes, epigastric pain, or decreased fetal movement.

ECLAMPSIA

Eclampsia is defined as new onset of grand mal seizure activity and/or unexplained coma during pregnancy or postpartum in a woman with preeclampsia. Eclampsia and preeclampsia account for >60,000 maternal deaths each year worldwide. In developed countries, the maternal death rate has been reported as 0–1.8%.

Management of Eclampsia

The most important goals are to stabilize the patient, deliver the fetus after the patient has been stabilized, and prevent further seizure activity. Stabilization of the patient involves protection of the airway, oxygen therapy, and establishing intravenous access. Once the patient has been stabilized, that is, seizure activity has abated, or the comatose state is resolved, the fetus should be delivered. The patient and fetus should be very closely monitored, and the patient is induced. Delivery by the vaginal route is preferred. However, if vaginal delivery is associated with delay and/or fetal or maternal distress, then immediate cesarean section is preferred. Intrapartum complications include fetal growth retardation, nonreassuring fetal heart rate patterns, and placental abruption. Preeclamptic/

eclamptic pregnancies of <28 weeks' gestation are associated with a high rate of maternal mortality. Further seizure activity is possible but is generally prevented by administration of magnesium sulfate (4–6 g over 20 min as a loading dose followed by a maintenance dose of 1–2 g/hr as a continuous intravenous infusion); 90% of women will not have a recurrent seizure after treatment with magnesium sulfate, but if a second or recurrent seizures occur, then control with lorazepam or diazepam should be considered.

GESTATIONAL HYPERTENSION

Gestational hypertension refers to hypertension with onset in the latter part of pregnancy (>20 weeks' gestation) without any other features of preeclampsia and followed by normalization of the blood pressure postpartum. Of women who initially present with apparent gestational hypertension, about one-third develop the syndrome of preeclampsia. The main goal in working up patients with gestational hypertension is to exclude the possibility of preeclampsia. The pathophysiology of gestational hypertension is unknown, but in the absence of features of preeclampsia, the maternal and fetal outcomes are usually normal. Patient workup should include measurement of urine protein excretion, laboratory evaluation (for uric acid, liver function tests, platelet and coagulation factors, and kidney function), and fetal assessment. Unless blood pressure is >160/90 mm Hg no pharmacological treatment is indicated. No steroids need to be administered, and the pregnancy can proceed to term. Gestational hypertension may, however, be a harbinger of chronic hypertension later in life, and follow-up with a primary care physician is reasonable.

Table 64.15 **CAUSES OF RENOVASCULAR HYPERTENSION**

Major Causes
Atherosclerosis
Fibromuscular dysplasia
Minor Causes
Vasculitis (Takayasu arteritis)
Dissection of the renal artery
Thromboembolic disease
Renal artery aneurysm
Renal artery coarctation
Extrinsic compression
Radiation injury

Table 64.16 RISK FACTORS ASSOCIATED WITH RENOVASCULAR DISEASE

- Carotid artery disease
- Coronary artery disease
- Diabetes mellitus
- Hypertension
- Obesity
- Old age
- Peripheral vascular disease (vascular disease in the extremities, e.g., the legs)
- Smoking
- Familial history of AD or RAS

RENOVASCULAR HYPERTENSION

Renovascular hypertension (RVHT) denotes nonessential hypertension in which a causal relationship exists between anatomically evident arterial occlusive disease and elevated blood pressure. Pathophysiologically, RVHT reflects renin-angiotensin-aldosterone activation as a result of renal ischemia. RVHT is the most common type of secondary hypertension, accounting for 1–5% of patients with hypertension. Renal artery stenosis (RAS) is also being increasingly recognized as an important cause of chronic renal insufficiency and end-stage renal disease. Studies suggest that ischemic nephropathy from RAS may be responsible for 5–22% of advanced renal disease in all patients older than 50 years in the United States. The incidence of renovascular disease is bimodal: it is common in younger women and older men and is twice as common in white as in African-American individuals. Causes of RVHT are shown in table 64.15.

Major complications of RVHT include end-organ damage due to chronically uncontrolled hypertension (CAD, stroke, and progressive renal insufficiency).

Table 64.17 CLINICAL CLUES SUGGESTING THE POSSIBILITY OF RENAL ARTERY STENOSIS

- Difficult-to-control hypertension despite adequate medical treatment
- Hypertension with renal failure or progressive renal insufficiency
- Accelerated or malignant hypertension
- Severe hypertension (diastolic blood pressure >120 mm Hg) or resistant hypertension
- Hypertension with an asymmetric kidney
- Paradoxical worsening of hypertension with diuretic therapy

Table 64.18 WORKUP OF RENOVASCULAR DISEASE

- Serum creatinine and creatinine clearance
- 24-hour urine protein
- Urinalysis
- Measurement of plasma renin activity
- Ultrasound/duplex ultrasound
- Captopril renography
- CT angiography (spiral CT)
- Magnetic resonance angiography
- Renal arteriography/intra-arterial digital subtraction angiography (DSA), or carbon dioxide angiography

Risk factors for RHVT are shown in table 64.16. RVHT should be suspected in patients younger than 30 years or older than 50 years, those patients with symptoms of atherosclerotic disease elsewhere, and those with a negative family history of hypertension. Other clinical clues are shown in table 64.17.

Once patients are identified as being at higher risk of RAS, the choice of the best test for diagnosis is controversial. Options for the workup of RHVT are shown in table 64.18. Accurate identification of patients with correctable renovascular hypertension can be difficult with the use of standard noninvasive techniques because they provide only indirect evidence of the presence of renal artery lesions (e.g., sonography, CT angiography [CTA], magnetic resonance angiography [MRA]). On the other hand, invasive techniques with more accurate diagnostic potential can produce a worsening of renal function because of contrast toxicity and complications related to the procedure itself (e.g., arterial puncture, catheter-induced atheroembolism). When the history is highly suggestive and there is minimal risk for radiocontrast-mediated renal injury, conventional angiography or digital subtraction angiography is the appropriate initial test. In patients at risk of contrast nephropathy, a carbon dioxide angiogram should be considered. Alternatives to angiography include a MRA or duplex ultrasonography. However, patients with chronic kidney disease and an estimated GFR of <30 mL/min/1.73 m², MRA with gadolinium is contraindicated because of the potential risk for nephrogenic systemic fibrosis/nephrogenic fibrosing dermopathy (NSF/NFD).

Treatment of RVHT is still debated. All patients need medical therapy: treatment with antihypertensive drugs to optimize blood pressure control and risk-factor management—smoking cessation and hyperlipidemia treatment. In many patients blood pressure can be well controlled with calcium channel blockers, beta blockers, and many other classes of drugs. ACE inhibitors should be avoided in patients with bilateral RVD. However, in some patients blood pressure may be particularly difficult to control or may require multiple antihypertensive agents. In these patients percutaneous renal angioplasty or surgical revascularization should be considered. In patients with diffuse atherosclerosis, the complication rate with both surgery and angioplasty is relatively high. Medical therapy may be preferred to other treatments after a careful weighing of risks and benefits of the invasive intervention.

In those patients in whom intervention is necessary, angioplasty has become the procedure of choice. The patency rate after angioplasty is strongly dependent on the size of the vessel treated and the quality of inflow and outflow through that vessel. Previously, a solitary or transplanted kidney was considered a contraindication for renal angioplasty; however, this is no longer the case, and angioplasty is now considered the procedure of choice for treatment of RAS in these patients. Technical success is achieved in >90% of patients, and patency rates are 90–95% at 2 years for fibromuscular disease and 80–85% for atherosclerosis. Restenosis requiring repeat angioplasty has been reported in fewer than 10% of patients with fibromuscular disease and in 8–30% with atherosclerotic stenosis. Improvement in blood pressure control with fewer antihypertensive medications is achieved in 30–35% of fibromuscular lesions and in 50–60% of atherosclerotic lesions. Surgical revascularization is reserved for patients in whom the main renal artery appears completely occluded and in whom the surviving renal parenchyma is vascularized by collaterals. Surgical revascularization might also be used when an ostial stenosis is present with a buttressing atheroma on either side of the ostium. Several surgical options are available. The stenotic segment may be excised and the artery resutured directly onto either the aorta or surviving stump. A vein graft may be transplanted, or the kidney resected and reimplanted in the iliac fossa with the renal artery anastomosed to the iliac artery.

ADDITIONAL READING

Beckett NS, Peters R, Fletcher AE, et al. Treatment of hypertension in patients 80 years of age or older. *N Engl J Med*. 2008;358:1887–98.

Chobanian AV, Bakris GL, Black HR, et al.; National Heart, Lung, and Blood Institute Joint National Committee on Prevention, Detection, Evaluation, and Treatment of High Blood Pressure; National High Blood Pressure Education Program Coordinating Committee. The Seventh Report of the Joint National Committee on Prevention, Detection, Evaluation, and Treatment of High Blood Pressure: The JNC 7 report. *JAMA*. 2003;289(19):2560–72. Erratum in: *JAMA*. 2003;290(2):197.

Flack JM, Sica DA, Bakris G, et al.; International Society on Hypertension in Blacks. Management of high blood pressure in Blacks: An update of the International Society on Hypertension in Blacks consensus statement. *Hypertension*. 2010;56(5):780–800.

Hackam DG, Khan NA, Hemmelgarn BR, et al.; Canadian Hypertension Education Program. The 2010 Canadian Hypertension Education

Program recommendations for the management of hypertension: part 2—therapy. *Can J Cardiol*. 2010;26(5):249–58.

Jim B, Sharma S, Kebede T, Acharya A. Hypertension in pregnancy: A comprehensive update. *Cardiol Rev*. 2010;18(4):178–89.

Sarafidis PA, Bakris GL. Resistant hypertension: An overview of evaluation and treatment. *J Am Coll Cardiol*. 2008;52(22):1749–57.

Sarafidis PA, Bakris GL. State of hypertension management in the United States: Confluence of risk factors and the prevalence of resistant hypertension. *J Clin Hypertens (Greenwich)*. 2008;10(2):130–9.

Williams B. The changing face of hypertension treatment: Treatment strategies from the 2007 ESH/ESC hypertension guidelines. *J Hypertens Suppl*. 2009;27(3):S19–26.

QUESTIONS

QUESTION 1. A 39-year-old white male is seen in clinic for a routine physical. He is noted to have a BP of 160/95 mm Hg, a heart rate of 72 beats per minute, but his examination is otherwise unremarkable. You can diagnose hypertension if which of the following is true:

A. Two further BP readings are >140/90.
B. He has diabetes and a SBP >140.
C. He has SBP >120.
D. He has DBP >90.
E. You cannot officially diagnose hypertension.

QUESTION 2. A 52-year-old man presents with blood pressures consistently >150/90 mm Hg and a history of diabetes. You recommend to your patient:

A. An endocrine consultation
B. HCTZ 12.5 mg PO qd
C. HCTZ 50 mg PO qd
D. Lisinopril 40 mg PO qd
E. Metoprolol 25 mg PO bid

QUESTION 3. A 40-year-old woman who is G3/P2 and is at 34 weeks of gestation presents with a blood pressure of 210/110 mm Hg and a seizure. What is the best way to control her seizure?

A. A loading dose of phenytoin
B. Treatment with diazepam
C. Treatment with amobarbital sodium
D. A loading dose of magnesium sulfate

QUESTION 4. A 42-year-old man presents to you for management of his newly diagnosed hypertension. On several measurements in the clinic and at home his blood pressure has been documented in the 150–155/90–95 mm Hg range. He is on no medications except for tadalafil (Cialis) for erectile dysfunction (ED). His physical examination is normal. In light of his ED, which one of the following drugs would be least likely to cause ED?

A. Hydrochlorothiazide
B. Metoprolol

C. Clonidine

D. Lisinopril

QUESTION 5. A 25-year-old white female is diagnosed with fibromuscular disease as the cause for her hypertension. The most likely finding on her angiogram corresponding to this diagnosis will be:

A. An ostial lesion of her right renal artery

B. A string-of-beads appearance unilaterally in the proximal one-third of the right renal artery

C. A string-of-beads appearance bilaterally in the distal one-third of her renal arteries

D. Distal arterial disease in smaller intrarenal branch vessels

ANSWERS

1. A
2. D
3. D
4. D
5. C

65.

URINALYSIS

Kenneth Lim, Theodore I. Steinman, and Li-Li Hsiao

Urinalysis is an integral part of the initial evaluation of renal and urinary tract disease. It may also provide an indication of the presence of systemic disease affecting the kidneys. Analysis of the urine should consist of (1) examination of the physical properties of urine; (2) examination of the chemical properties by dipstick urinalysis; and (3) microscopic examination of the sediment. Techniques employed in the collection and laboratory handling of urine are of primary importance and may have significant bearing on results. A midstream specimen is required in men and women; however, in order to avoid contamination with vaginal secretions in women, the external genitalia should first be cleaned. Urine may also be collected via a bladder catheter or suprapubic bladder puncture. Examination of the urine should occur within 2 hours after collection. Delays of >2 hours result in the accumulation of ammonia from the breakdown of urea; the higher pH dissolves casts and promotes cell lysis causing inaccurate sediment examination. Refrigeration of specimens at +2°C to +8°C can preserve urine for up to 8 hours but may allow precipitation of phosphates or urates. Preservatives that can be used for the formed elements of urine include formaldehyde, glutaraldehyde, "cellFIX," and lyophilized borate-formate sorbitol powder.

PHYSICAL PROPERTIES

Important diagnostic information can be gained by visual inspection of the *physical* appearance of urine (tables 65.1 and 65.2).

CHEMICAL PROERTIES

SPECIFIC GRAVITY

Specific gravity defines the number and weight of dissolved particles and can be measured using an ionic reagent strip.

The urine specific gravity provides an indication of the amount of free water present in relation to the amount of solute. A low specific gravity may be seen in diabetes insipidus or following heavy water ingestion; a high specific gravity can occur with excess solute excretion (i.e., glycosuria) and volume contraction/dehydration. Abnormally high values can occur in the presence of hyperosmolar osmotic agents (i.e., contrast agents).

URINE PH

Urine pH can be evaluated in two ways: a dipstick with a mixed pH indicator detects urine pH between 5 and 8.5, although a pH meter with a glass electrode can provide a more accurate measurement and can detect a wider range of pH values. Urine is usually in the pH range of 4.5 to 7.8, but due to metabolic activity, it is normally slightly acidic (i.e., 5.5–6.5). Patients with metabolic acidosis, volume depletion, or those who consume large quantities of protein may present with a more acidic urine. Patients with renal tubular acidosis (particularly of the distal segment), infection with urea-splitting organisms (e.g., *Proteus*), and those consuming vegetarian diets may present with a more alkaline urine. Prolonged storage of urine with accumulation of ammonia from urea will also cause a high urine pH.

GLUCOSE

Glycosuria occurs when the filtered load of glucose exceeds the reabsorbing capacity of the tubules (i.e., 180–200 mg/dL). The dipstick test is dependent on the oxidation of glucose to gluconic acid and hydrogen peroxide by glucose oxidase. Hydrogen peroxide reacts with a chromogen, such as potassium iodide to produce a colored product. Glycosuria can be observed in diabetes mellitus, Cushing syndrome, liver and pancreatic disease, and Fanconi syndrome. False-positive results can occur in the presence of levodopa, following ingestion of sodium hypochlorite (bleach; this is an example of an oxidizing detergent), and hydrochloric acid.

Table 65.1 PHYSICAL PROPERTIES OF URINE: CLARITY AND COLOR

	PATHOLOGIC CAUSES	OTHER CAUSES
Cloudy/turbid	In presence amorphous calcium phosphate crystals (occurs only in alkaline urine), pyuria, chyluria, lipiduria, hyperoxaluria	Purine-rich foods (hyperuricosuria)
Discoloration		
Red	Hematuria, hemoglobinuria, myoglobinuria, porphyria	Beets, blackberries, rhubarb, phenolphthalein, rifampin (Rifadin)
Green or blue	Pseudomonal UTI, biliverdin	Amitriptyline, indigo carmine, IV cimetidine, IV Promerhazine, methylene blue, triamterene, propofol, motorcycle accident, intragastric balloon placement
Orange	Bile pigments	Phenothiazines, phenazopyridine
Brown or black	Bile pigments, melanin, methemoglobin	Cascara, levodopa, methyldopa, senna, blackwater fever, malaria infection from *Plasmodium falciparum*.
Yellow	Concentrated urine	Carrots, cascara

NOTES: UTI, urinary tract infection; IV, intravenous.
SOURCES: Hanno et al. *Clinical Manual of Urology*. 3rd ed. New York: McGraw-Hill, 2001; Simerville et al. *Am Fam Physician*. 2005; Crane et al. Chyluria. *Urology*. 1977;9:429; Bernante et al. *Obes Surg*. 2003;13:951; Blakey et al. *Pharmacotherapy*. 2000;20:1120; Bodenham et al. *Lancet*. 1987;2:740; Lepenies et al. *Nephrol Dial Transplant*. 2000;15:725.

False-negative results can occur in the presence of excess excretion of uric acid and ascorbic acid.

KETONES

Acetic acid is detected using a sodium nitroprusside or nitroferricyanide and glycine reaction. Ketones are most commonly detected in diabetic and alcoholic ketoacidosis. They can also be observed in pregnancy, carbohydrate-free diets, starvation, vomiting, and strenuous exercise. False-positive results can occur when levodopa metabolites, free sulfhydryl groups, or highly pigmented urine is present.

Table 65.2 PHYSICAL PROPERTIES OF URINE: ODOR

ODOR	PATHOLOGIC CAUSES
Pungent	Bacterial urinary tract infections, due to production of ammonia
Fruity or sweet	Diabetic ketoacidosis
Musty or mousy	Phenylketonuria
Sweaty feet	Isovaleric academia
Rancid butter or fishy	Hypermethioninemia
Fecal	Gastrointestinal-bladder fistulas
Sulfuric	Cystine decomposition
Other	Medications (e.g., penicillin) and diet (e.g., asparagus, coffee) may also cause different odors in urine.

PROTEIN

Urine dipstick tests provide an approximate quantification of urinary protein concentration on a scale of 0 to 4+ (table 65.3). The urine dipstick test is sensitive to albumin but less sensitive to low-molecular-weight proteins such as beta-2-microglobulins and immunoglobulin light chain proteins. Detection of protein by urine dipstick employs the use of tetrabromophenol blue dye impregnated on paper as a pH indicator. Urine dipstick does not detect positively charged light chains of immunoglobulins that may be detected by addition of sulfosalicylic acid. False-positive results may occur in the presence of highly alkaline urine that cannot be compensated by the dye's buffer. A lower threshold of approximately 10–20 mg/dL of urinary protein is required for detection by routine dipstick test. Quantitative methods such as 24-hour urine protein collection, spot urine protein-to-creatinine ratio, urinary albumin evaluation, or albumin-to-creatinine ratio is required for further evaluation of persistent proteinuria. Evaluation for glomerular

Table 65.3 INTERPRETATION OF RESULTS OF URINE DIPSTICK TEST FOR PROTEINURIA

0	Negative
Trace	15–30 mg/dL
1+	30–100 mg/dL
2+	100–300 mg/dL
3+	300–1000 mg/dL
4+	>1000 mg/dL

Table 65.4 DIFFERENTIAL DIAGNOSES OF PROTEINURIA

GLOMERULAR LESIONS

	SELECTIVE	NONSELECTIVE	OTHER CAUSES
Differential diagnoses	Minimal change disease (MCD)	Focal and segmental glomerulosclerosis, IgA nephritis, lupus nephritis, diabetic nephropathy	Polycystic kidney disease, pyelonephritis, rhabdomyolysis, hemoglobinuria, obstruction, vesicoureteral reflux, orthostatic, medications (i.e., chronic lithium exposure, analgesics, aminoglycosides), metabolic defects (i.e., oxalosis, cystinosis, hypercalcemia), trace metals (i.e., lead, mercury, cadmium).
Pathology	Predominantly albumin excretion which is relatively innocuous Interstitial infiltrates seldom develop despite heavy proteinuria	Variety of proteins found in urine, including immunoglobulins (i.e., IgG) and complement components C5 to C9 Complement proteins enter tubular fluid and cause complement-mediated injury resulting in tubulointerstitial inflammation	
Assessment	Urinary proteins can be assessed using selectivity indices, SDS-PAGE (sodium dodecyl sulfate polyacrylamide gel electrophoresis) and isoelectric focusing (IEF) These tests can be used to predict response to therapy.		

SOURCE: Woo K, Lau YK. *Singapore Med J.* 2001;42(8):385–9.

injury regardless of renal function should be made with proteinuria >2–3 g/day.

Differential diagnosis of proteinuria is provided in table 65.4. It can be classified as selective versus nonselective proteinuria. Orthostatic proteinuria generally occurs in patients <30 years with proteinuria typically <1 g/day. In suspected cases, an 8-hour overnight, supine urinary protein measurement should be <50 mg. The clinical approach to proteinuria identified on a screening should be tailored to identify existing renal damage and the potential for future injury to the kidney. A 24-hour urine protein collection together with serum creatinine should be obtained, together with microscopic examination of the urinary sediment.

Key Points in Proteinuria

- Urine dipstick test is most sensitive to albumin and less sensitive to low-molecular-weight proteins.

- False-positive results may occur in highly alkaline urine.

- Quantitative methods such as 24-hour urine protein collection, protein-to-creatinine ratio, or albumin-to-creatinine ratio should be considered for further evaluation of proteinuria.

- Random spot urine protein-to-creatinine ratio (PCR) accurately estimates 24-hour total protein measurement.

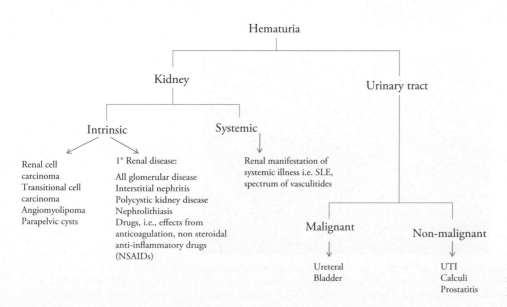

Figure 65.1. Common Differential Diagnoses for Hematuria.

Table 65.5 MICROSCOPIC EXAMINATION OF CELLS IN URINE

	ERYTHROCYTES (FIGURE 65.2)	LEUKOCYTES (FIGURE 65.3)	EPITHELIAL CELLS (FIGURE 65.4)
Normal morphology	Pale, biconcave disks Approximately 7 μm in diameter Normal RBCs that have been altered by varying osmolality of the urine should be distinguished from dysmorphic RBCs	Granular spheres Approximately 10–12 μm in diameter Nuclear details are usually well defined in fresh urinary specimens	Four epithelial cell types can be identified on microscopy of the urine sediment
Abnormal morphology and pathology	Isomorphic: regular in shape and contour—can be of glomerular or nonglomerular origin Dysmorphic: irregular in shape and contour—observed in glomerular disease Swollen (ghost) cells due to hyperosmolarity require identification under phase-contrast microscopy Shrunken (crenated) cells can be identified by spiked borders under light microscopy	Neutrophils: most frequently observed and indicative of UTI or any inflammatory condition in the upper and lower urinary tract or active proliferative glomerulonephritis False-positive results can occur frequently in young women due to contamination from genital secretions Eosinophils: can be a marker for acute allergic interstitial nephritis, various types of glomerulonephritis, prostatitis, chronic pyelonephritis or urinary schistosomiasis	Squamous epithelial cells: derived from shedding of the distal genital tract. Indicative of urine contamination from genital secretions when present in large amounts Transitional epithelial cells: bladder origin and can be a benign finding or reflect bladder irritation. Rarely, can be seen in large transitional cell malignancies Renal tubular epithelial cells: result from exfoliation of tubular epithelium seen in acute tubular necrosis, acute interstitial nephritis, and other tubular injury. Also found in glomerulonephritis

SOURCE: Birch et al. *Clin Nephrol.* 1983;20(2):78–84; Pollock et al. *Kidney Int.* 1989;36(6):1045–9; Pollock *Am J Med.* 1983;75(1B):79–84; Fogazzi et al. *J Nephrol.* 2005;18(6):703–10; Nolan et al. *N Engl J Med.* 1986;315(24):1516–9; Nolan and Kelleher. *Clin Lab Med,* 1988;8(3):555–65;Tetu. *Mod Pathol.* 2009;22 (Suppl 2):S53–9; Skoberne et al. *Am J Physiol Renal Physiol.* 2009;296(2):F230–41.

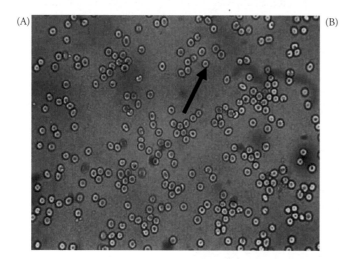

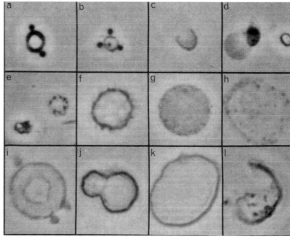

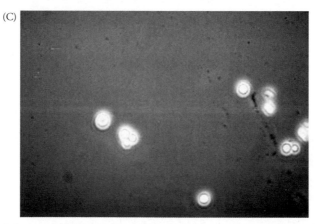

Figure 65.2. Erythrocytes in Urinary Sediments. (A) Isomorphic red blood cells which are uniformly round, biconcave, 7 μm in diameter, and have ample hemoglobin. These increased numbers are typically associated with lower urinary tract inflammation. ×400 magnification. (B) Dysmorphic RBC in urine sediment in glomerular hematuria. ×4000. (C) Erythrocytes under phase contrast—oil droplets.

- Sulfosalicylic acid (SSA) can be used for dipstick-negative proteinuria to detect positively charged light chains of immunoglobulins.
- Proteinuria is defined as >150 mg/day.
- Presence of proteinuria indicates renal injury (table 65.4).
- In orthostatic proteinuria, suspected cases should be confirmed by an 8-hour overnight urinary measurement demonstrating <50 mg/day.

BLOOD

The dipstick test is dependent on the pseudoperoxidase activity of hemoglobin. The dipstick test has a sensitivity range of approximately 91–100% with specificity ranging from 65% to 99%. It is more sensitive to free hemoglobin and myoglobin than to intact erythrocytes. Hemoglobin detected on dipstick may occur as a result of hematuria, intravascular hemolysis, or myoglobinuria that can be secondary to conditions such as rhabdomyolysis. A positive result may also occur with lysis of erythrocytes on standing, an alkaline pH, or a low relative density (especially <1.010). When the dipstick test for hemoglobin is positive, microscopic sediment examination should be performed to distinguish hematuria from other causes.

Hematuria is defined by three or more red blood cells per high-powered field. The presence of hematuria is always an abnormal finding and may result from renal or extrarenal causes (figure 65.1). The most benign form of hematuria is its appearance after vigorous exercise (in marathon runners), which disappears in 24–48 hours.

Key Points in Positive Dipstick for Blood

- Dipstick test is dependent on the pseudoperoxidase activity of hemoglobin.
- Dipstick test is more sensitive to free hemoglobin and myoglobin than to intact erythrocytes.
- It has sensitivity of 91–100% and specificity of 65–99%.
- Microscopic sediment examination should be performed in positive cases.
- Positive dipstick test may occur in hematuria, intravascular hemolysis, or myoglobinuria such as in rhabdomyolysis.
- Hematuria is defined as three or more red blood cells per high-powered field and is indicative of renal or extrarenal pathologies.

(A)

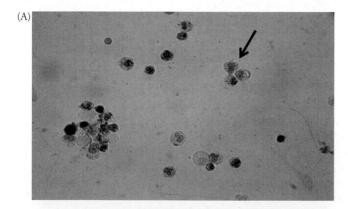

(B)

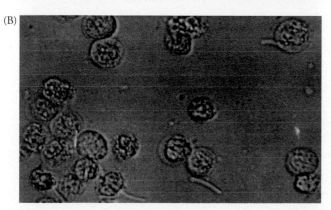

Figure 65.3. Leukocytes in Urinary Sediments. Polymorphonuclear leukocytes in which the lobed nuclei are readily evident (A, arrow and B). These increased numbers may be associated with lower urinary tract infection or with renal disease affecting either tubules, interstitium, or the glomerulus. ×400 magnification.

(A)

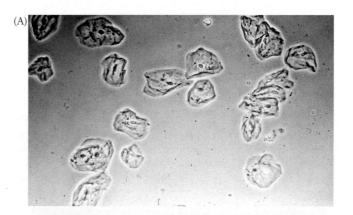

(B)

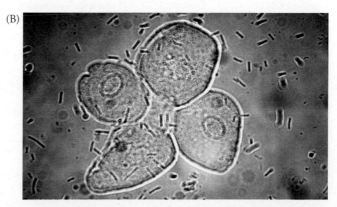

Figure 65.4. Epithelial Cells in Urinary Sediments. (A) Squamous epithelial cells. (B) Transitional epithelial cells in the presence of bacteria (arrow).

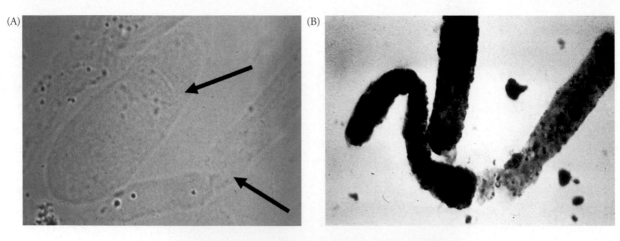

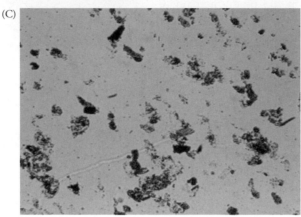

Figure 65.5. Hyaline and Granular Casts in Urinary Sediments. (A) Hyaline casts, best visualized under phase microscopy. (B) Granular casts. (C) Muddy brown casts in acute tubular necrosis (ATN) ×100.

Table 65.6 MICROSCOPIC EXAMINATION OF CASTS IN URINE

	PATHOLOGIC CAUSES AND DESCRIPTION
Hyaline (figure 65.5A)	Can be observed under normal conditions, in concentrated acidic urine and under various physiological states, including strenuous exercise, dehydration, and febrile disease. Large numbers are frequently seen in congestive heart failure and minimal change disease nephrotic syndrome.
Granular (figure 65.5B and 65.5C)	Formed from amalgamation of Tamm-Horsfall protein, debris of cells, and plasma proteins. Classification as finely or coarsely granular casts depends on how much digestion of debris has occurred within cast. Nonspecific causes and can be observed in a variety of glomerular or tubular diseases. In acute tubular necrosis, large numbers of "muddy brown" granular casts can be observed.
Waxy (figure 65.6A and 65.6B)	Opaque, formed from degeneration of hyaline, granular, and cellular casts. Can be detected by light microscopy. Observed in CKD and have been reported as frequent finding in rapidly progressive glomerulonephritis.
Fatty (figure 65.6C)	Formed by lipid droplets. Frequently are doubly refractile (Maltese crosses). Seen in nephrotic syndrome and mercury poisoning.
Red cell (figure 65.7A)	Active glomerular injury and is a finding that signifies serious glomerular disease. Characteristic of proliferative extra- and endocapillary necrotizing glomerulonephritis.
Leukocyte (figure 65.7B)	Reflects trapping of WBCs within a matrix of tubular proteins (must distinguish from WBCs appearing in clusters, which have no distinct borders). Observed in acute pyelonephritis, acute interstitial nephritis and other interstitial inflammatory processes. More frequent observation in glomerulonephritis than RBC casts and reflect the degree of inflammation.
Renal tubular epithelial (RTE) cell casts (figure 65.7C)	Typically observed in acute tubular necrosis, acute interstitial nephritis, and also less frequently in glomerular disorders.

SOURCE: Serafini-Cessi, F., N. Malagolini, and D. Cavallone. *Am J Kidney Dis*, 2003; 42(4): 658–76.

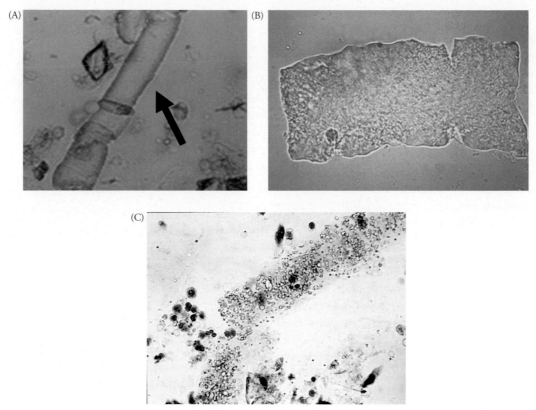

Figure 65.6 Waxy and Fatty Casts in Urinary Sediments. (A) Waxy casts (arrow) in chronic glomerular disease. (B) Broad waxy cast. (C) Fatty casts seen in ethylene glycol poisoning.

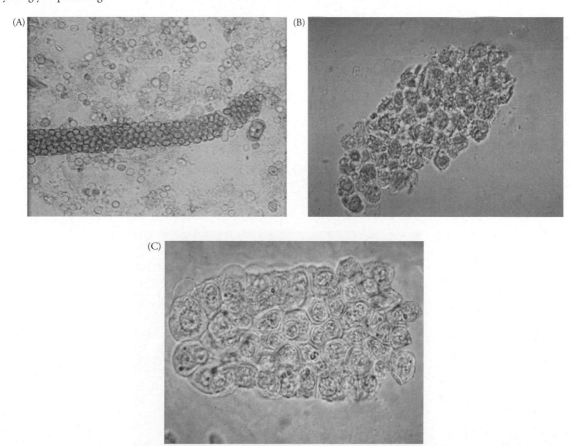

Figure 65.7 Red Blood Cell, White Blood Cell, and Tubular Epithelial Cell Casts in Urinary Sediments. (A) RBC cast. (B) WBC casts. Note that granular cytoplasm WBCs are 1.5–2 times larger than RBCs. (C) Renal tubular epithelial (RTE) cell casts. Note the elliptically located nucleus consistent with RTE cell cast.

LEUKOCYTES

The urine dipstick detects leukocyte esterase released from lysed neutrophils and is indicative of pyuria associated with glomerular and/or interstitial inflammation or lower urinary tract infection. The dipstick reagent strip should be allowed to stand for 1 minute before reading to detect significant pyuria accurately. False-positive results can occur with granulocyte lysis in long-standing urine or glomerular epithelial cells that can contaminate the specimen. False-negative results may occur with hyperglycemia, albuminuria, tetracycline, cephalosporins, and oxaluria.

Bacteria produce nitrites by the reduction of urinary nitrates that can be detected by urine dipstick. This process occurs in the presence of many Gram-negative and some Gram-positive organisms. False-negative results can occur in the presence of ascorbic acid and high specific gravity. They may also occur with low levels of urinary nitrate due to diet, prolonged storage of urine, and rapid transit of urine in the bladder. Urinary tract infection is more likely if both leukocyte esterase and nitrites are positive on dipstick examination. However, infection cannot be definitively ruled out if both tests are negative.

MICROSCOPIC EXAMINATION

Microscopic examination of the urine sediment is necessary for a complete urinalysis. The identification of cells, casts, crystals, lipids, and organisms can yield important diagnostic information. Examination of urinary sediment provides clues to diagnosis and management of renal or urinary tract disease and to detection of metabolic or systemic disease not directly related to the kidney.

CELLS

Erythrocytes, leukocytes, and epithelial cells are the three main types of cells found in urine in various pathologic conditions (see table 65.5; figures 65.2–65.4).

CASTS

The formation of casts occur when proteins, predominantly Tamm-Horsfall protein secreted by cells of the thick ascending limb of the loop of Henle, trap cells, fat, bacteria, and other inclusions. These amalgamations are then excreted in urine (table 65.6; figures 65.5–65.7).

(A)
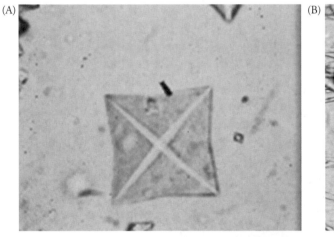

(B)
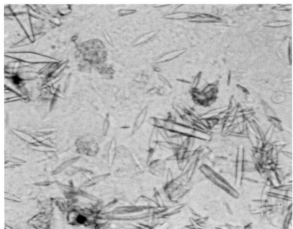

(C)
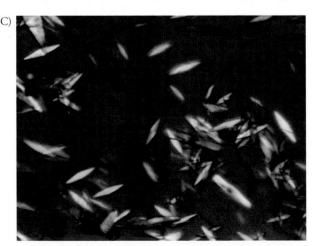

Figure 65.8. Calcium Oxalate Crystalluria. (A) Calcium oxalate dihydrate crystal. ×400. (B) Calcium oxalate monohydrate crystalluria in bright field. (C) Calcium oxalate monohydrate crystalluria in polarized field.

CRYSTALS

Many crystals observed in urine are present as artifacts due to the precipitation of normally dissolved substances at room temperature. Several different types of crystals can be identified based on their morphology, appearance under polarized light, and measurement of urine pH (see table 65.7; figures 65.8–65.11).

LIPIDS

Lipids may be identified free in the urine and within the cytoplasm of tubular epithelial cells or macrophages, where they are known as oval fat bodies. Oval fat bodies are seen in nephrotic syndrome (figure 65.12).

ORGANISMS

Bacteria are frequently observed in urine specimens due to nonsterile handling of urine and delays in examination (figure 65.13). Gram-negative streptococci and staphylococci can be distinguished by appearance under high-powered magnification. Gram-staining, culture, and in vitro testing against antibiotics can help guide pharmacological therapy in more complicated cases. Contaminants from genital secretions include organisms such as *Candida, Trichomonas vaginalis,* and *Enterobius vermicularis.*

URINALYSIS PATTERNS IN KIDNEY DISEASE

Urinalysis findings are most diagnostically useful when results from individual components of the test are considered together. In many cases certain combinations of urinary findings may be strongly suggestive of specific renal disorders.

HEAVY PROTEINURIA WITH FATTY CASTS OR BLAND SEDIMENT

Urinalysis demonstrating this combination of findings is suggestive of a glomerular lesion presenting as nephrotic

Table 65.7 MICROSCOPIC EXAMINATION OF CRYSTALS IN URINE

	DESCRIPTION
Calcium oxalate (figure 65.8)	Two types can be identified which precipitate at pH 5.4 to 6.7. Bihydrated (or Wedellite) crystals usually take bipyramidal appearance and do not polarize light. Monohydrated (or Whewellite) crystals may take ovoid, dumbbell, or ovoid shapes and do polarize light.
Uric acid (figure 65.9)	Found in acidic urine (pH ≤5.8). May be observed in various forms, including needle-shaped, rhomboid, rosettes, lemon-shaped, and four-sided "whetstones." Polychromatic appearance can be observed under polarizing light.
Calcium phosphate crystals and amorphous phosphates (figure 65.10)	Calcium phosphate crystals precipitate in alkaline urine (pH ≤7.0). Highly pleiomorphic crystals occur as prisms, rosettes and needles of various size and shape that polarize light intensely. Amorphous calcium phosphate crystals precipitate at a pH of ≤7.0 and produce a cloudy appearance to the urine. They do not polarize light. Appear as tiny particles, lack color and are identical to amorphous urates.
Triple phosphate or struvite (figure 65.10)	Take form of a "coffin-lid," as three- to six- sided prisms, and are found only in alkaline urine (pH ≤7.0). Composed of magnesium ammonium phosphate.
Cholesterol	Usually observed as flat particles with a corner notch. Transparent and often clumped together.
Cystine (figure 65.10)	Found as hexagonal plates that polarize light. Precipitate in acidic urine.
Crystals due to drugs (figure 65.11)	Sulfonamide crystals: observed as spheres or needles. Indinavir, a highly activated retroviral agent (HARRT) used in HIV: may cause birefringent plate and starburst structures, generally in association with impaired kidney function. Acyclovir crystals: needle-like in shape and demonstrate negative birefringence under polarized light. Sulfadizine crystals have a characteristic "shaves of wheat" appearance. Ampicillin crystals: take form a long, slender needle. Other drugs may cause transient crystalluria, including triamterene, and primidone. Some drugs (e.g., vitamin C) and toxins (e.g., ethylene glycol) may promote formation of monohydrated calcium oxalate crystals.

SOURCES: Burns, Finlayson. *Invest Urol.* 1980;18(2):174–7; Finch et al. *Clin Sci (Lond).* 1981;60(4):411–8; Fogazzi. *Nephrol Dial Transplant.* 1996;11(2):379–87; Perazella. *Am J Med.* 1999;106(4):459–65.

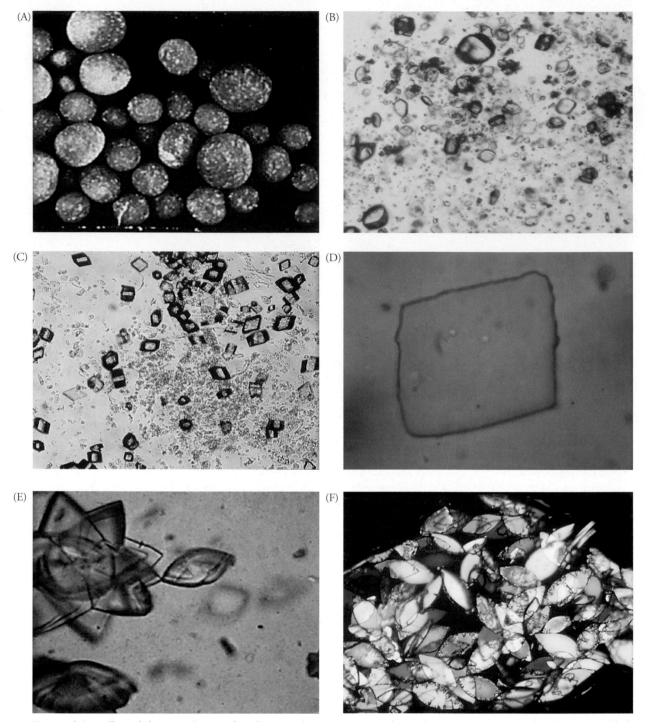

Figure 65.9. Uric Acid Crystalluria. (A) Uric acid stones. (B–E) Uric acid crystals in various forms: four-sided "whetstones" (B, C), rhomboid (D), lemon shape (E). (F) Uric acid crystals under polarized light.

syndrome (>3.5 g per day). The absence of cells or casts, denoted as bland sediment, often describes a noninflammatory glomerular disorder.

DYSMORPHIC RED BLOOD CELLS OR RED BLOOD CELL CASTS WITH PROTEINURIA

The constellation of dysmorphic red blood cells and/or red blood cell casts with proteinuria is characteristic of nephritic syndrome. The presence of red cell casts is indicative of active glomerular injury and is a finding that signifies serious glomerular disease. However, it should be noted that the absence of these findings does not exclude glomerulonephritis. The presentation of red blood cell casts and/or dysmorphic red cells in any patient regardless of renal function or proteinuria should always be followed by an evaluation for glomerular disease or renal vasculitis.

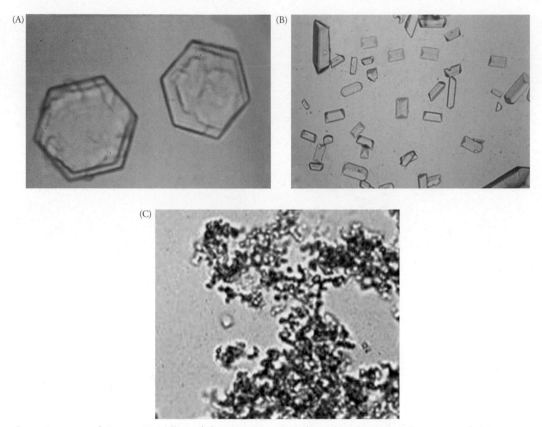

Figure 65.10. Amorphous, Struvite, and Cystine Crystalluria. (A) Cystine crystals are shaped like hexagons. Cystine crystals are quite rare. (B) Struvite crystals (triple phosphate) look like rectangles or coffin lids. (C) Amorphous phosphate crystals appear as aggregates of finely granular material without any defining shape.

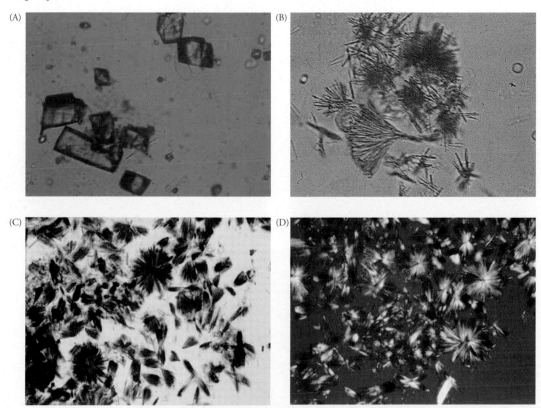

Figure 65.11. Microscopic Appearance of Drug-Induced Crystals. (A) Sulfonamide crystals are typically yellow in color and often resemble uric acid crystals. However, sulfa crystals are easily distinguished from uric acid by confirmatory tests. Sulfa crystals are readily soluble in acetone and exhibit a positive dextrine/sulfuric acid test ("old yellow newspaper" test). (B) Sulfadiazine crystals are a common finding with administration of trimethoprim-sulfadiazine. They are often seen as "sheaves of wheat" or radially striated spherules. (C) Indinavir crystalluria. (D) Indinavir crystals under polarized light.

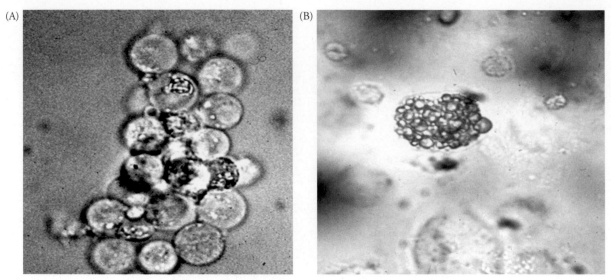

Figure 65.12. Lipids in Urinary Sediments. (A) Free fat in urine. (B) Oval fat body.

HEMATURIA WITH DYSMORPHIC RED BLOOD CELLS AND PYURIA

Various renal pathologies should be considered in patients with this combination of urinary findings. Differential diagnoses should include glomerular disease, tubulointerstitial nephritis, vasculitis, urinary obstruction, crystalluria, cholesterol embolization, and renal infarction.

ISOLATED HYALINE CASTS

Large numbers of isolated hyaline casts are almost always due to the presence of congestive heart failure. However, these casts can also be seen in minimal change disease, healthy individuals, concentrated acidic urine, and under various physiological states, including strenuous exercise, dehydration, and febrile disease. They are easily visualized under phase-contrast microscopy.

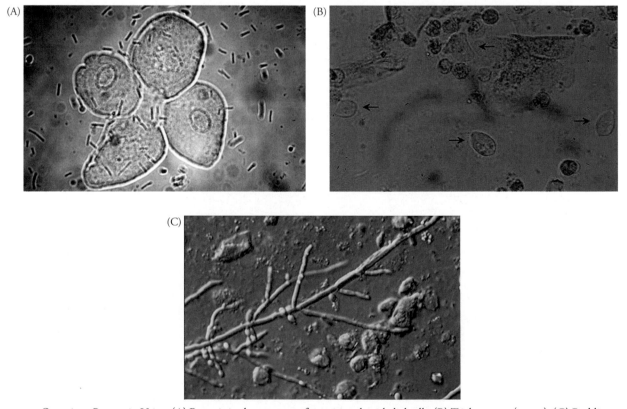

Figure 65.13. Organisms Present in Urine. (A) Bacteria in the presence of transitional epithelial cells. (B) Trichomonas (arrow). (C) Budding yeast.

ISOLATED HEMATURIA WITH MONOMORPHIC RED BLOOD CELLS

This combination of urinary findings is usually suggestive of crystalluria, nephrolithiasis, or malignancies of the genitourinary tract. In rare cases it may be suggestive of glomerular disease such as IgA nephropathy or thin basement membrane disease. However, dysmorphic red blood cells and red blood cell casts are usually present in these glomerular pathologies.

FREE TUBULAR EPITHELIAL CELLS, EPITHELIAL CELL CASTS, AND GRANULAR CASTS

In the presence of acute renal failure, this constellation of urinary findings is indicative of acute tubular necrosis as a result of ischemia and/or administration of a nephrotoxin. In hyperbilirubinemia, these cells and casts can be found stained with bile in the urinary sediment, and a serum bilirubin >10 mg/dL will help confirm the diagnosis.

FREE WHITE BLOOD CELLS, WHITE BLOOD CELL CASTS, GRANULAR CASTS, AND MILD PROTEINURIA

This constellation of urinary findings is indicative of tubulointerstitial disease, including pyelonephritis, drug-induced tubulointerstitial nephritis, and systemic disorders such as sarcoidosis.

ADDITIONAL READING

Echeverry G, Hortin GL, Rai AJ. Introduction to urinalysis: Historical perspectives and clinical application. *Methods Mol Biol.* 2010; 641:1–12.

Grossfeld GD, Litwin MS, Wolf JS, et al. Evaluation of asymptomatic microscopic hematuria in adults: The American Urological Association best practice policy—part I: Definition, detection, prevalence, and etiology. *Urology.* 2001;57(4):599–603.

Grossfeld GD, Litwin MS, Wolf JS, et al. Evaluation of asymptomatic microscopic hematuria in adults: The American Urological Association best practice policy—part II: Patient evaluation, cytology, voided markers, imaging, cystoscopy, nephrology evaluation, and follow-up. *Urology.* 2001;57(4):604–10.

Heitzmann L. *Urinary Analysis and Diagnosis by Microscopical and Chemical Examination.* New York: William Wood & Company; 1921.

Rabinovitch A. *Urinalysis and Collection, Transportation, and Preservation of Urine Specimens: Approved Guideline.* 2nd ed. NCCLS document GP16-A2. Wayne, PA: National Committee for Clinical Laboratory Standards; 2001.

Simerville JA, Maxted WC, Pahira JJ. Urinalysis: A comprehensive review. *Am Fam Physician.* 2005;71:1153–62.

ACKNOWLEDGMENTS

The authors wish to acknowledge and express their deepest gratitude to Dr. Wendy Brown, Chief of Nephrology, at VA Hospital, Chicago, IL and Dr. Robert Cohen at the Beth Israel and Deaconess Hospital, Boston, MA for their generosity in providing the figures used in this chapter.

QUESTIONS

QUESTION 1. A 62-year-old patient with type 2 diabetes mellitus is admitted to the hospital for evaluation of hemoptysis of 2-week duration and feeling of unsteadiness on his feet. He gives a history of gradually worsening dyspnea over the past 10 years. He has a cough productive of copious sputum during winter months and has had several prior "lung infections" during the winter months. He has noticed some general malaise, loss of appetite, and tiredness becoming worse recently. Medications used are metformin and Ventolin inhaler. Social history reveals moderate beer intake—one to two beers each night. Smoking history of 20–30 cigarettes/day for 40 years. He works as a janitor. Examination reveals mild dyspnea at rest. He is confused and agitated. Not cooperative. Blood pressure on admission is 168/92 mm Hg without orthostasis. HR 84 bpm. Lungs: scattered rhonchi; reduced right base air entry and dullness on percussion. He has no peripheral edema. Additional labs reveal:

- Urinalysis: SG 1.010, pH 5.0, rest negative
- Urine sodium 42 meq/L
- Urine osmolality 615 mOsm
- Electrolytes: Na 100, K 3.5, CO_2 30, Cl 72, BUN 5.0, creatinine 0.6, glucose 180, uric acid 2.6

All of the following statements are true *except*:

A. The patient's total body sodium is normal.
B. The calculated serum osmolality is approximately 200 mOsm/kg.
C. The patient has evidence of either inappropriate or appropriate ADH secretion.
D. The uric acid level seen in this patient is typical for a patient with SIADH.
E. Use of 3% hypertonic saline would be the best treatment at this point in this patient.

QUESTION 2. A 42-year-old woman presents to your office with a 4-week history of a petechial rash on her legs, gross hematuria, and edema. She relates a 2-year history of intermittent polyarthralgias. She is taking ibuprofen 600 mg twice daily for her joint pains. Physical examination is notable for mild periorbital edema, a BP of 164/88 mm Hg, HR 66 bpm, afebrile. Her lungs, cardiovascular examination, and abdominal examinations are normal. She has 3+ edema. Urinalysis shows a SG of 1.020, pH 5.0,

4+ blood, 4+ proteinuria, 1+ leukocytes, with the rest of the dipstick negative. Urine sediment examination shows 15–20 dysmorphic red cells. Her electrolytes are normal, BUN 36 mg/dL, creatinine 1.8 mg/dL. The most likely finding diagnosis is:

A. A proliferative glomerulonephritis
B. A minimal change lesion
C. Acute interstitial nephritis from the ibuprofen
D. Kimmelstiel-Wilson lesions with nodular glomerulo-sclerosis
E. Analgesic nephropathy from exposure to ibuprofen

QUESTION 3. A 67-year-old man presents with a 1-week history of anorexia, nausea, lassitude, and pedal edema. He provides a past history of long-standing hypertension, well controlled with hydrochlorothiazide and amlodipine. Medications: fenoprofen for osteoarthritis of the hip for the past 3 months. On physical examination the patient has a blood pressure of 157/93 mm Hg, a heart rate of 72 bpm, and a temperature of 97.8°F. His JVP is 8 cm, and he has normal cardiac and pulmonary examinations. He has 2+ pitting edema. Urinalysis shows a specific gravity of 1.017, protein 4+, 1+ blood, and negative for glucose. Microscopic examination of the sediment showed 2–4 erythrocytes and

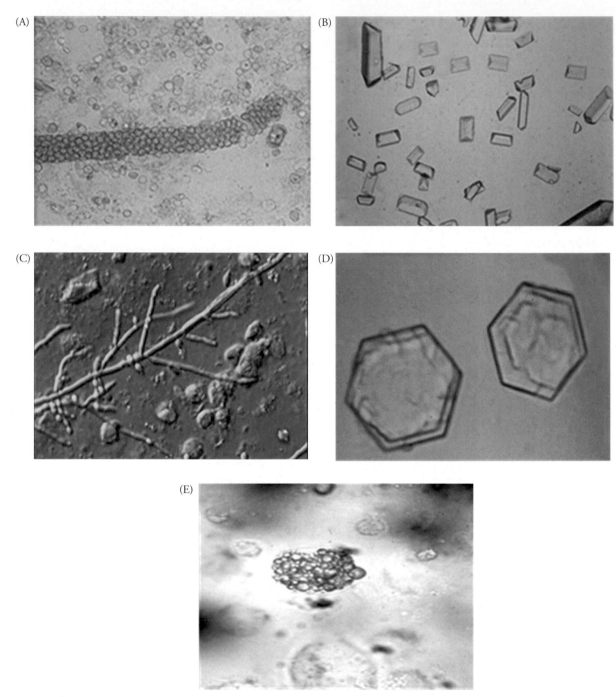

Figure 65.14. Figure for question 4

15–20 leukocytes/hpf, and occasional granular casts. BUN 93 mg/dL, Cr 7.8 mg/dL, Na 137, K 4.4, Cl 95, CO_2 21, Ca 9.2, Phos 7.8, UA 7.7 mg/dL, Alb 2.9 g/dL, HCT 29%. ANCA (–) Antinuclear (+) 1:40 titer, anti-dsDNA antibody level 0. 24-hour protein excretion 7.7 g. Renal ultrasound showed normal-sized kidneys bilaterally without obstruction. Three months previously his serum creatinine was 1.7 mg/dL. The nephrotic-range proteinuria and renal failure are most likely the result of:

A. Lupus nephritis
B. Multiple myeloma
C. Systemic small vessel vasculitis
D. Fenoprofen-induced nephrotic syndrome and interstitial nephritis
E. Renal vein thrombosis secondary to membranous nephropathy

QUESTION 4. Match the type of urine structure with its corresponding appearance from figure 65.14 (see picture):

1. Oval fat body
2. Red cell cast
3. Cystine crystal
4. Struvite crystal
5. Budding yeast

ANSWERS

1. B
2. C
3. D
4. E, A, D, B, C

66.

NEPHROLOGY BOARD REVIEW

Bradley M. Denker

QUESTION 1. A 50-year-old white male with a history of essential hypertension suffered two transient ischemic attacks without permanent neurological sequelae within the last 12 months. He is treated with lisinopril, 20 mg, and hydrochlorothiazide, 25 mg daily; office blood pressures (BP) are 140/85. A 24-hour ambulatory blood pressure monitor is obtained. Which of the following statements about 24-hour blood pressure monitoring is NOT TRUE?

A. Cardiovascular risk correlates better with elevated blood pressure on ambulatory monitoring than with office blood pressures.
B. Patients normally exhibit a nocturnal dip in blood pressure of at least 10%.
C. Higher ambulatory blood pressure monitoring strongly correlates with progressive renal disease and the development of end-stage kidney failure.
D. Dipping of nocturnal blood pressure correlates with the day–night difference in heart rate.
E. Ambulatory blood pressure monitoring can be used to distinguish true hypertension from "white coat" hypertension.

QUESTION 2. A 55-year-old African-American male comes to the emergency room complaining of 2 days of blurred vision, headaches, and nausea. He has a history of hypertension but ran out of his medications about 2 weeks ago. He is awake and alert. Blood pressure is 220/120 mm Hg with no orthostatic changes. Funduscopic exam shows bilateral hemorrhages and blurred optic disk margins. The remainder of the physical exam was notable only for an S4 gallop and the absence of edema. Laboratory studies revealed a creatinine of 2.5 mg/dL (was 1.2 6 months prior) and normal electrolytes. Which of the following therapies is most appropriate for initial management?

A. Sublingual nifedipine in the emergency room while awaiting an ICU bed
B. Intravenous enalaprilat
C. Intravenous nitroglycerin
D. Intravenous esmolol
E. Sodium nitroprusside

QUESTION 3. A 44-year-old white male with obesity (body mass index 32 kg/m^2), type II diabetes with hemoglobin A1c 8.4% on oral agents is found to have urinary microalbumin/creatinine of 112 µg/g is seen in your office for follow-up. His office blood pressure is 160/100 mm Hg, but he is convinced that these elevations are secondary to white coat hypertension. You ask him to obtain a home blood pressure cuff and confirm its accuracy. He returns with home blood pressure readings ranging from 135/85 to 160/90. In addition to lifestyle changes, which of the following antihypertensive strategies is recommended as initial therapy?

A. Hydrochlorothiazide 25 mg daily
B. Hydrochlorothiazide 50 mg daily with the addition of a beta blocker within 2 weeks
C. Lisinopril 10 mg daily and then titrate up to 40 mg to maximize BP effects
D. Lisinopril 10 mg daily plus hydrochlorothiazide 25 mg and titrate to maximize BP effects
E. Calcium channel blocker plus hydrochlorothiazide 25 mg

QUESTION 4. A 60-year-old black female is seen for the first time in many years. The family history is strongly positive for type 2 diabetes, and she is found to have a serum creatinine of 3.1 mg/dL, 1.5 g of protein/24 hours, and hemoglobin A1c of 8%. A renal ultrasound shows 11-cm kidneys with echogenic cortex. Which of the following statements about the use of an angiotensin-converting enzyme (ACE) inhibitor in this patient is true?

A. Since her renal failure is advanced, there is no benefit in delaying progression of her chronic kidney disease.
B. Evaluate serum creatinine and serum potassium 1 month after initiating therapy.
C. Evaluate serum creatinine and potassium 1–2 weeks after starting therapy and discontinue the drug if creatinine increases by 10% over baseline.
D. Evaluate serum creatinine and potassium 1–2 weeks after starting therapy, and discontinue the drug if

creatinine increases by 10% over baseline or serum potassium is 5.0 meq/L.

E. Evaluate serum creatinine and potassium 1–2 weeks after starting therapy, and discontinue the drug if creatinine increases by >30% over baseline or hyperkalemia (>5.4 meq/L) develops despite dietary counseling and the use of loop diuretics.

QUESTION 5. A 27-year-old man with AIDS is hospitalized with a cough, fever, and a pulmonary infiltrate on chest x-ray (CXR). Therapy is initiated with trimethoprim-sulfamethoxazole. On admission, the serum creatinine is 1.6 mg/dL, and blood urea nitrogen (BUN) is 21 mg/dL; on reexamination 3 days later, the serum creatinine is 2.2 mg/dL and blood urea nitrogen, 23 mg/dL. Results of urinalysis both on admission and 3 days later are normal. Urine output on day 3 is 1350 mL. The most likely cause of the increased creatinine is:

A. AIDS glomerulopathy
B. Trimethoprim-mediated decrease in creatinine secretion
C. Intratubular obstruction secondary to sulfonamide
D. Acute interstitial nephritis (AIN) caused by trimethoprim-sulfamethoxazole therapy
E. Acute tubular necrosis secondary to sepsis

QUESTION 6. A previously healthy 42-year-old man becomes ill with fever (temperature 38°C [100.4° F]), malaise, myalgias, and a sore throat. The next day, he describes gross hematuria and right flank pain. Urinalysis shows protein 3+ and RBC casts. His BUN is 42 mg/dL, and serum creatinine is 1.8 mg/dL. Electrolytes are within normal limits. Serological testing reveals normal complements, a normal IgA level, a 1:40 antinuclear antibodies (ANA) anti-DNA ab level of 0, and negative antistreptolysin O (ASLO), and antineutrophil cytoplasmic antibody (ANCA) titers. His anti-glomerular basement membrane (GBM) titers are also negative. Which of the following is the most likely diagnosis?:

A. World Health Organization (WHO) class IV lupus nephritis
B. IgA nephropathy
C. Rapidly progressive glomerulonephritis secondary to granulomatosis with polyangiitis (Wegener granulomatosis)
D. Goodpasture syndrome
E. Poststreptococcal glomerulonephritis

QUESTION 7. All of the following statements regarding torsemide are true, EXCEPT:

A. It has a bioavailability higher than that of furosemide.
B. Like furosemide, torsemide is a loop diuretic.
C. It has a shorter half-life than furosemide.
D. It does not accumulate in renal failure.
E. Torsemide is less ototoxic than furosemide.

QUESTION 8. A 61-year-old man with a past history of rheumatoid arthritis for 15 years and gold therapy for 12 years, with excellent control of his symptoms, presents with a 6-month history of edema. He is on no medications other than furosemide and gold salts. He denies nonsteroidal anti-inflammatory drug (NSAID) therapy in the recent past year. Physical examination showed a well-developed man in no acute distress. Blood pressure was 120/80. There was 4+ edema present. His serum creatinine is 1.0 mg/dL, a 24-hour urine sample shows 10 g of protein, and his serum albumin is 1.8 g/dL. Urinalysis shows 4+ albumin on dipstick but is otherwise negative with a bland urinary sediment. His treatment with gold salts is discontinued, but his proteinuria persists with a 24-hour urine showing 14 g/day. The most likely diagnosis is:

A. Membranous glomerulopathy secondary to gold
B. Idiopathic membranous glomerulopathy
C. Primary focal segmental glomerulosclerosis
D. Rheumatoid vasculitis

QUESTION 9. You are asked to consult on a 62-year-old African-American male with acute-on-chronic renal insufficiency secondary to diabetes mellitus ascribed to contrast nephrotoxicity. Routine chemistry labs show a potassium of 8.2 mg/dL. All of the following would be changes seen on the electrocardiogram (EKG) compatible with hyperkalemia, except:

A. Peaked T waves
B. Prolonged QRS
C. Flattened P wave
D. Sine-wave-appearing QRS complex
E. U wave

QUESTION 10. The most common type of kidney stone observed in the United States is:

A. Cystine stone
B. Triple phosphate stone
C. Struvite stone
D. Calcium oxalate stone
E. Uric acid stone

QUESTION 11. A 48-year-old male end-stage renal disease (ESRD) patient presents to the ED with a K = 7.8 meq/L and HCO_3 = 22. His EKG shows peaked T waves. Recommended initial treatment includes all of the following EXCEPT:

A. Calcium gluconate 10 mL, IV
B. Insulin 10 units and 1 amp of 50% dextrose
C. Albuterol nebulizer (10–20 mg)
D. IV bicarbonate 8.4%, 1–2 amps IV
E. Emergent dialysis

QUESTION 12. A 42-year-old male 8 days post–bone-marrow transplantation on treatment with FK506 (tacrolimus), among many other medications, is diagnosed with a type IV renal tubular acidosis. All of the following features would be compatible with this diagnosis except:

A. A urine pH of 5.0
B. The presence of hyperkalemia

C. A negative urine anion gap of –22

D. A serum bicarbonate of 18

E. A normal anion gap

QUESTION 13. The most common cause of mortality in patients in ESRD patients on chronic hemodialysis is:

A. Hyperkalemia

B. Infection

C. Cardiac disease

D. Severe acidosis

E. Acute GI bleeding

QUESTION 14. A 60-year-old man who has been previously in good health and on no medications develops the nephrotic syndrome. No systemic causes are identified, and serologic workup is completely negative. The most likely histologic lesion on renal biopsy is:

A. Light chain nephropathy

B. Membranous glomerulopathy

C. Myeloma kidney

D. Membranoproliferative glomerulonephritis

E. IgA nephropathy

QUESTION 15. A 26-year-old man is brought to the emergency department by paramedics after ingesting 200 tablets of 325-mg aspirin. On examination he is tachypneic (respiratory rate [RR] 28 breaths/min), heart rate 105 beats/min, blood pressure 130/74 mm Hg, and oxygen saturation 98% on room air. His salicylate concentration was 90.6 mg/dL. His initial arterial blood gases (ABGs) gave pH 7.49, P_{CO_2} 20 mm Hg, P_{O_2} 95 mm Hg, and bicarbonate 16 meq/L. His serum electrolytes initially are normal. He receives intravenous volume repletion with isotonic sodium bicarbonate and activated charcoal. However, within 1 hour of arrival to the emergency room the patient becomes delirious and has a generalized seizure. Two hours after arrival, salicylate concentration was 98.6 mg/dL.

The next best step is:

A. Oral N-acetylcysteine administration

B. Hemodialysis

C. Therapy with fomepizole

D. Repeat the dose of activated charcoal and induce vomiting with 30 mL of ipecac

E. Intubation and transfer to the ICU

ANSWERS

1. D. There is no association of nocturnal dipping with day-night differences in heart rate. The definition of hypertension on ambulatory blood pressure monitoring is defined based on the time of day:

A 24-hour average above 135/85 mm Hg

Awake average above 140/90 mm Hg

Asleep average above 125/75 mm Hg

Studied have confirmed elevated blood pressures on 24-hour monitoring correlate with left ventricular hypertrophy, progressive renal insufficiency and microalbuminuria, and cardiovascular and all-cause mortality. Similar associations are seen in patients who are nondippers (do not decrease asleep blood pressure by at least 10%).

2. E. Sodium nitroprusside is the drug of choice in this patient with end-organ damage and hypertensive emergency. It should only be used as initial therapy due to the potential accumulation of cyanide, especially with reduced FFR. There is no role for sublingual therapy in this situation. Intravenous esmolol is effective, especially in the setting of an aortic dissection, and intravenous nitrates are particularly useful in the setting of acute coronary ischemia. Intravenous enalaprilat should be avoided because the blood pressure response in malignant hypertension is variable and unpredictable. It should also be avoided in acute myocardial ischemia. Labetalol is also an excellent therapy but should be avoided in patients with heart failure or bronchospasm.

3. D. Current Joint National Committee 7 (JNC7) guidelines recommend that patients with stage 2 hypertension (>160 systolic or >100 diastolic) be treated with two drugs as initial therapy. This includes a diuretic (usually a thiazide) and either an ACE inhibitor or ARB or beta blocker or calcium channel blocker. However, for patients with kidney disease (as defined by microalbuminuria in this case), the second agent should be an ACE inhibitor or ARB. Target blood pressures in this population (chronic kidney disease or diabetes) should be <130/<80.

4. E. There is no contraindication to initiating therapy with an ACE inhibitor or ARB in this case, and the literature supports benefit in delaying progression even with advanced renal disease. Inhibition of the renin-angiotensin system will lead to reduced glomerular capillary pressure and decreased glomerular filtration rate (GFR). This is the mechanism of lower proteinuria and less glomerulosclerosis over time. The expected decline in GFR is up to 30%, and if it remains stable, the therapy can be continued. If creatinine rises >30%, an investigation into bilateral renal artery stenosis should be considered. The effects on potassium are variable. The drugs should not be discontinued with mild hyperkalemia, especially before attempts are made to minimize the increase with dietary counseling and the use of loop diuretics.

5. B. Trimethoprim-sulfamethoxazole is associated with an elevation in serum creatinine, no change in BUN, no evidence of acute renal failure (ARF) trimethoprim-sulfamethoxazole therapy results in inhibition of tubular secretion. Clinical syndromes include allergic interstitial nephritis with fever, rash, and eosinophilia induced by the sulfa moiety and hyperkalemia with salt wasting due to amiloride-like action of trimethoprim, and rarely, crystallization of sulfamethoxazole metabolite and renal stone formation

6. B. The synpharyngitic presentation of this clinical syndrome of acute glomerulonephritis coupled with normal serologies highly suggests a diagnosis of IgA nephropathy. Poststrep glomerulonephritis (GN) usually occurs approximately 2 weeks after the onset of a sore throat.

7. C. Torsemide is a loop diuretic. It has a higher bioavailability (80% vs. 50%) and longer $t_{\frac{1}{2}}$ than furosemide (3 hours vs. 1 hour). Metabolism mainly in liver; unaffected by renal function. Torsemide does not accumulate in ARF, and consequently, in patients with renal failure, torsemide is less ototoxic than furosemide. In a healthy person, 15–20 mg torsemide = 40 mg furosemide. In ARF, give torsemide 100 mg. This is bioequivalent to 200 mg of furosemide.

8. A. The other possibility is AA amyloid secondary to rheumatoid arthritis. However, this is less likely because the patient has no other clinical evidence suggestive of AA amyloidosis. Renal disease with RA includes:

- Membranous nephropathy
- Mesangial proliferative GN +/– IgA deposits
- Diffuse proliferative GN
- Necrotizing and crescentic GN (rheumatoid vasculitis)
- Amyloidosis
- Medication associated (gold, NSAIDs)

9. E. A flat T wave, prolonged QRS—if severe, as a sine wave—and peaked T waves may all be seen. A U wave is seen in patients with hypokalemia.

10. D. In the United States 75% of all kidney stones are calcium oxalate stones; 10–15% are uric acid stones; 15–20% struvite stones; and 1% cystine stones.

11. D. IV bicarbonate would not be necessary because the patient is not significantly hypobicarbonatemic. Further, IV bicarbonate takes several hours to have its effect.

Although a survey of 63 nephrology program directors advocated bicarbonate as first-line therapy (Iqbal et al. *N Engl J Med.* 1989 320(1):60–61), its role is in fact quite controversial. In animal studies IV bicarbonate has variable impact, whereas in human studies, infusion of $NaHCO_3$ 400–600 mmol over 16–24 hours resulted in a modest 0.6 mmol/L reduction in K at 4–6 hours and 1.6 mmol/L reduction at 16–24 hours. Elements in the acute treatment of severe hyperkalemia include:

- Profile risk in patient: absolute value of K, presence of EKG changes, rate of rise, ? other ions contributing to cell E_m, medications
- Stabilize myocardium: calcium gluconate, 10% solution, 10–20 cc IV bolus
- Shift K into cells: regular insulin, 10 units + 50 cc 50% dextrose, IV bolus; albuterol (5 mg/mL), 10–20 mg, nebulized over 10 min; sodium bicarbonate

- Remove K from body: Kayexalate; acute hemodialysis against a low-K bath

12. C. Type 4 RTA is characterized by a urine anion gap that is positive, and the urine pH is typically less than 5.5 with hyperkalemia. The metabolic acidosis is typically non–anion gap. These patients usually have either aldosterone resistance or deficiency.
For selective aldosterone deficiency:

With low renin—hyporeninemic hypoaldosteronism (e.g. diabetic nephropathy): prostaglandin synthesis inhibitors

With normal or high renin—normoreninemic hypoaldosteronism or hyperreninemic hypoaldosteronism in critically ill patients: ACE inhibitor, heparin therapy, cyclosporine

For aldosterone resistance:

In pseudohypoaldosteronism type I (infant's), pseudohypoaldosteronism type II (Gordon syndrome), or adult aldosterone hyporesponsiveness and renal insufficiency: spironolactone administration

13. C. Cardiac causes are the most common cause of death in ESRD patients on hemodialysis, accounting for approximately 50% of the all-cause mortality. Risk factors include left ventricular hypertrophy (LVH) (? from anemia vs. hypertension vs. volume overload), presence of hypertension (due to renal disease vs. sympathetic overactivity vs. volume overload). Underlying vascular disease is secondary to elevated lipids including homocysteine levels and increased coronary calcification.

14. B. The most common cause of a primary glomerular process in adults is membranous glomerulopathy (followed closely by focal segmental glomerulosclerosis). In children, the most common cause is minimal change disease.

15. B. Although this patient does not present with some of the common earliest signs and symptoms of toxicity—nausea, vomiting, diaphoresis, and tinnitus with or without hearing loss—he does manifest other central nervous system (CNS) presentations: hyperventilation, agitation, delirium, followed by convulsions (lethargy, stupor, and coma). A marked elevation in temperature is a sign of severe toxicity and typically preterminal condition. The hyperventilation and respiratory alkalosis are because salicylates stimulate the respiratory center in the brainstem. The respiratory alkalosis predominates initially, but ABGs may also reveal a mixed respiratory alkalosis and metabolic acidosis. Keys to management are (1) gastric decontamination with activated charcoal—this has shown to reduce the amount of active salicylate by 50–80%; (2) fluid replacement because salicylate toxicity can induce major fluid losses through tachypnea, vomiting, hypermetabolic state,

and insensible perspiration; (3) urinary alkalinization with sodium bicarbonate because this results in enhanced excretion of the ionized acid form of salicylate (urine pH must be maintained at 7.5–8.0); (4) hemodialysis or hemoperfusion. Extracorporeal therapy is indicated when patients manifest with renal failure, acute decompensated heart failure, CNS abnormalities, severe acid–base or electrolyte imbalance, hepatic compromise with coagulopathy, acute lung injury, and/or a salicylate concentration >100 mg/dL.

Dialysis can be used to treat overdoses of methanol, ethylene glycol, isopropanol, lithium, mannitol, theophylline, acetaminophen, and aspirin. Dialysis is not useful in treating benzodiazepines, digoxin, Dilantin, phenothiazines, and tricyclics.

67.

NEPHROLOGY SUMMARY

Ajay K. Singh and Kuyilan Karai Subramanian

This chapter comprises of a potpourri of topics that are important for the boards.

DIABETIC NEPHROPATHY

Diabetic nephropathy (DN) is the leading cause of end-stage renal disease (ESRD) in Western societies and accounts for approximately 50% of the patients on renal replacement therapy in North America. DN is responsible for approximately 20% of all deaths in patients younger than 40 years old. The prevalence of microalbuminuria is around 30–35% in both types of diabetes (DM). The risk factors for the development of DN include hyperglycemia, systemic hypertension, glomerular hypertension and hyperfiltration, proteinuria, cigarette smoking, hyperlipidemia, and gene polymorphisms affecting the activity of the renin-angiotensin-aldosterone axis. Other key facts are summarized in table 67.1.

CLINICAL FEATURES

Preclinically, patients may have asymptomatic glomerular hypertension and hyperfiltration causing an enlargement of the kidneys seen on ultrasound. With approximately 5 years of insult from glomerular hypertension and hyperfiltration, the kidneys start to develop microalbuminuria as an initial manifestation of the disease. Figure 67.1 shows an approximate timeline for the progression of diabetic nephropathy in predominantly untreated patients. The microalbuminuria is clinically undetectable to the conventional dipstick test. Nephrotic levels of proteinuria, hypertension, and progressive loss of renal function may develop after about 5–10 years of microalbuminuria. Diabetic nephropathy usually presents itself in patients 12–22 years after the clinical diagnosis of DM. The disease is progressive in nature and eventually leads to chronic renal failure and ESRD in a significant proportion of patients. The course of the patients with type 2 DM will vary depending on whether they present late or are diagnosed late.

Approximately 25% of type 2 diabetics have microalbuminuria at the time of diagnosis, and 3% of newly diagnosed type 2 DM have clinically apparent nephropathy. The majority of patients with type 2 DM have evidence of cardiovascular and hypertensive complications.

PATHOLOGY

Three cardinal features of renal pathology are basement membrane thickening, accumulation of mesangial matrix (with or without Kimmelstiel-Wilson nodules), and vascular disease (see figure 67.2 and table 67.2). In addition, there is frequently associated evidence of vascular disease. The renal pathologic changes are very similar in patients with type 1 or type 2 diabetic nephropathy. In approximately 20% of biopsies there is a superimposed glomerular lesion with diabetic kidney disease being present in the background.

DIAGNOSIS

Patients with diabetic nephropathy usually present with hyperglycemia, hypertension (systolic hypertension in particular), either microalbuminuria or proteinuria, and renal dysfunction. Microscopic hematuria may be seen

Table 67.1 KEY FACTS ON DIABETEIC NEPHROPATHY

Most common cause of ESRD in West
45% of all U.S. patients with ESRD
100,000 diabetics with ESRD in the United States
Costs approximate $10–16 billion/year
Mortality of diabetic with ESRD is higher than nondiabetic
Cardiovascular complications four- to eightfold higher in diabetic with renal disease than without renal disease

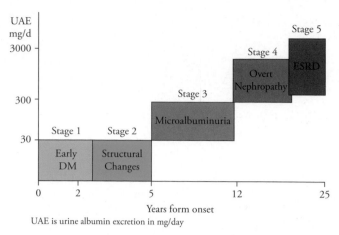

Figure 67.1. Approximate Rates of Progression in the Different Stages of Diabetic Nephropathy.

but is unusual. In approximately 10% of patients, red cell casts in the urine sediment have been reported. Patients will frequently have evidence of other complications of DM, such as retinopathy, peripheral vascular disease, and a sensory neuropathy. Patients with more advanced diabetes may have the Charcot foot (increased warmth, erythema, swelling, absence of pain in the lower extremity or foot), diabetic ulcers, skin disease including acanthosis nigricans—darkening and thickening of certain areas of the skin especially in the skin folds—or scleroderma diabeticorum—thickening of the skin on the back of the neck and upper back (figure 67.3).

TREATMENT AND PROGNOSIS

Treatment is summarized in table 67.3. Both the Diabetes Control and Complications Trial (DCCT) study for type 1 diabetics and the United Kingdom Prospective Diabetes Study (UKPDS) for type 2 diabetics demonstrate unequivocally that tight control of blood sugar (aiming for

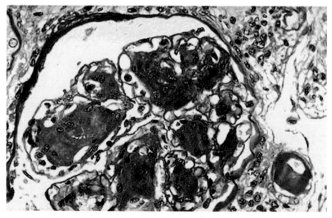

Figure 67.2. Diabetic Nephropathy. Picture shows the Kimmelstiel-Wilson lesions of nodular glomerulosclerosis, characteristic of diabetic renal disease. Courtesy of Helmut G. Rennke, MD.

a HbA1c of <7%) is associated with reduced micro- and macrovascular damage. Angiotensin-converting enzyme (ACE) inhibitors or angiotensin receptor blockers (ARBs) are drugs of choice as they control both systemic hypertension and intraglomerular hypertension by inhibiting the actions of angiotensin II on the systemic vasculature and renal efferent arterioles. ACE or ARBs inhibitors are effective in delaying the progression of the renal disease in patients with DM. Renoprotection coupled with blood pressure control are recommended to a target of <130/80 mm Hg (Joint National Committee 7 (JNC7) guidelines) using ACE inhibitors or ARBs as first-line therapy. However, more than one drug is needed to control blood pressure; consequently, diuretics, long-acting calcium channel blockers (CCBs), and beta blockers are reasonable adjuncts. Other important interventions in DN that should be considered are dietary protein restriction (0.8 g/kg/day of protein)—recommended by the American Diabetes Association, cessation of smoking, and control of lipids—a target low-density lipoprotein (LDL) of 100 mg/dL is recommended by the ATPIII/NCEP guidelines.

HYPERTENSIVE NEPHROPATHY/ NEPHROSCLEROSIS

Hypertension affects the majority of the U.S. population. By the age of 60 years, over 50% of the U.S. population will be hypertensive (defined as having a repeatedly elevated blood pressure of ≥140/90 mm Hg). The causes are many and include idiopathic or secondary factors. Secondary factors include renal disease, endocrine causes such as Cushing disease and hyperparathyroidism, hypercalcemia, and pheochromocytoma, and primary hyperaldosteronism. Vascular causes include renovascular disease. Hypertension can result from renal failure; studies suggest that in stage 4 CKD over 75% of patients have evidence of hypertension. Less commonly, renal failure can result from hypertension.

Renal disease due to chronic hypertension is seen primarily in the black population with a ratio of eight to one, but it can be observed in whites as well. Approximately 5% of patients have accelerated or malignant hypertension (diastolic pressure >120), which may be associated with renal failure and retinal hemorrhages and exudates, with or without papilledema.

CLINICAL FEATURES

Patients with renal disease secondary to hypertension usually describe a long antecedent history of hypertension that is evidenced by a slow rise in BUN and creatinine. Retinopathy and left ventricular hypertrophy will be present in a majority of these patients. Depending on the severity of the renal damage, there may be either microalbuminuria or

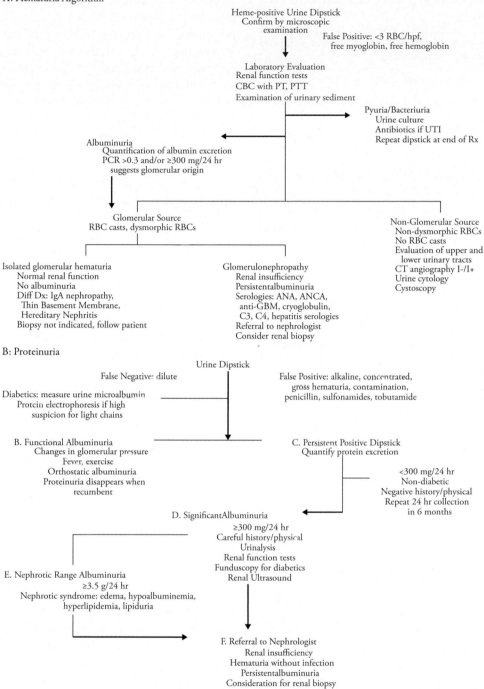

Hypocomplementemia in Glomerular Disease

PATHWAY	COMPLEMENT	DISEASE
Classical	Low C3, C4, CH50	Lupus nephritis Mixed essential cyto
Alternate	Low C3, Normal C4	Post-strep GN Post-infect GN SBE Shunt Hep B MPGN type 2
Reduced synthesis	Acquired	Liver disease
	Hereditary (C2 def)	Lupus

Figure 67.3. Diagnostic Workup Algorithm for Nephropathy.

Table 67.2 PATHOLOGICAL FEATURES OF DIABETIC NEPHROPATHY

Expansion of mesangial matrix with diffuse and nodular glomerulosclerosis (Kimmelstiel-Wilson nodules)

Thickening of glomerular and tubular BM

Arteriosclerosis and hyalinosis of afferent and efferent arterioles

Tubulointerstitial fibrosis

overt albuminuria. The risk for hypertensive renal disease is increased among individuals of black race, those with underlying renal disease, and those with chronically elevated blood pressure. Benign hypertensive nephrosclerosis is the most common clinical presentation.

PATHOGENESIS

The vascular response to hypertension is intimal thickening with medial hypertrophy and resultant luminal narrowing. This response minimizes the pressure variations in the arterioles and capillaries. With chronicity, the autoregulatory mechanisms of the arterioles fail, and vascular damage ensues. This results in increased permeability, platelet deposition, and deposition of hyaline-like material in the damaged vessels, leading to a permanent lesion of fibroelastic hyperplasia and fibrinoid necrosis. Often hyaline arteriolosclerosis accompanies these changes. Plasma renin, secreted by the kidney in the presence of vascular compromise, is markedly elevated. A self-perpetuating cycle of increasing angiotensin II/intrarenal vasoconstriction becomes established, leading to ischemia and renin

Table 67.3 TREATMENT STRATEGY FOR DIABETIC NEPHROPATHY

Lifestyle Changes
• Lose weight
• Stop smoking
• Low salt diet for BP control
Optimize Glycemic Control
• Benefit in both type 1 and type 2 patients
• Recommended: HbA1c <7.0%
Optimize Hypertension Management
• Goal blood pressure <130/80
• Use ACE inhibitors or ARB's, even if normotensive
• If intolerant of ACE inhibitors use ARBs or vice versa
Low-Protein Diet (Controversial)
• Protein restriction to 0.8 mg/kg/day once CKD develops

secretion. The influence of increased levels of vasoconstrictors (e.g., endothelin) and decreased levels of vasodilators (nitric oxide) may also contribute to vasoconstriction. Aldosterone levels are also elevated, and salt retention undoubtedly contributes to the elevation of blood pressure. The increased incidence in the black population is attributed to poorly defined environmental and genetic factors. Often hypertension in blacks is not associated with high renin secretion.

PATHOLOGY

Hypertensive nephropathy may involve the glomerulus, the vessels, and the tubulointerstitial tissue. In patients with advanced disease there may be marked nephron loss in the injured portions of the kidney with hypertrophic enlargement of the remaining segments. The entire glomerular tuft may be involved in a focal segmental fashion or a global segmental fashion. Tubular atrophy may be similar to ischemic type of renal injury. With severe disease, a chronic interstitial nephritis with hyperplastic arteriolitis (onion-skinning), fibrinoid necrosis of arterioles, and necrotizing glomerulitis is apparent.

DIAGNOSIS

A detailed history and the clinical presentation are usually sufficient for the diagnosis. In severe cases patients may have papilledema, retinopathy, encephalopathy, and cardiovascular abnormalities. Urinalysis may show nonnephrotic-range proteinuria. A renal biopsy is rarely indicated.

TREATMENT AND PROGNOSIS

Patients who present with hypertension should always be evaluated for reversible causes of hypertension. The goal of treatment is aimed at normalizing the blood pressure.

The target blood pressure based on JNC7 recommendations is ≤130/80 mm Hg. However, recent data point to a goal blood pressure of <140/90 for non-proteinuric hypertensive patients.

A similar goal is proposed in the National Kidney Foundation (NKF) guidelines on hypertension. The 2003 NKF Kidney Disease Outcomes Quality Initiative (KDOQI) clinical practice guidelines for antihypertensive therapy recommend:

• Blood pressure measurement at each health care encounter.

• Target blood pressure of <130/80 for all patients with kidney disease, including those with diabetic kidney disease and nondiabetic kidney disease, regardless of degree of proteinuria, and in renal allograft recipients.

- Use of an ACE inhibitor/ARB in patients with diabetic kidney disease, and use of ACE inhibitor in nondiabetic kidney disease with proteinuria (spot U_p/U_{cr} ratio of ≥200 mg/g), to retard progression of kidney disease, irrespective of the presence of hypertension.

- Adjunctive antihypertensive agents. NKF guidelines suggest diuretics followed by either beta blockers or calcium channel blockers in diabetic kidney disease as well as in nondiabetic proteinuric kidney disease (spot U_p/U_{cr} ratio of ≥200 mg/g). In patients with kidney disease in the absence of significant proteinuria, as defined by spot U_p/U_{cr} ratio of <200 mg/g, diuretics are the preferred agent, followed by ACE inhibitor, ARB, beta blocker, or calcium channel blocker. In recipients of renal allografts, calcium channel blockade, diuretic therapy, and beta blockade, ACE inhibitor, or ARB are recommended.

CYSTIC DISEASES OF THE KIDNEY

Simple renal cysts are common, occurring in 50% of patients older than 50 years of age.

The widespread use of ultrasonography (US) and computed tomography (CT) scan has led to an increased detection of simple cysts. Ultrasound criteria for the classification of simple renal cyst include (1) spherical or ovoid shape, (2) absence of internal echoes, (3) presence of a thin, smooth wall that is separate from the surrounding parenchyma, and (4) enhancement of the posterior wall, indicating ultrasound transmission through the water-filled cyst. If all of these criteria are satisfied and the patient is asymptomatic, no further evaluation of the cyst is necessary since the likelihood of a malignancy is very small. Symptomatic patients with the same ultrasound findings should undergo CT scanning with contrast. The gold standard for evaluating renal masses requires CT images <5 mm in thickness before and after contrast is given. The criteria for diagnosing a benign cyst on CT scan include (1) a homogeneous attenuation value near that of water, (2) no enhancement with intravenous contrast material, (3) no measurable thickness of the cyst wall, and (4) smooth interface with renal parenchyma. Magnetic resonance imaging (MRI) is typically used to evaluate patients with indeterminate lesions. MRI does not detect calcifications. The suspicion for malignancy should be raised if the benign criteria are not met, calcification is present within a cyst, or repeat studies show an enlarging lesion. CT scan has a sensitivity of 94% for detection of renal parenchymal masses, but MRI is statistically superior to CT scan in the correct characterization of benign lesions. If a cyst meets the criteria for being benign, periodic reevaluation is the standard of care. If the lesion is not consistent with a simple cyst, surgical exploration is recommended.

Acquired renal cystic disease occurs in as many as 90% of patients who receive dialysis for 5–10 years. The cysts develop as a consequence of chronic renal insufficiency and may be clinically apparent long before dialysis is instituted. Malignancy and metastases can develop in a small percentage of cases. Screening of all dialysis patients by renal US is recommended after 3 years of dialysis at 1- to 2-year intervals. Major clinical manifestations of acquired cystic disease include flank pain and hematuria in association with rupture of hemorrhagic cysts into the urinary tract or into the perinephric region. Cysts often resolve after successful renal transplantation.

AUTOSOMAL DOMINANT POLYCYSTIC KIDNEY DISEASE

Autosomal dominant polycystic kidney disease (ADPKD) is the most common renal hereditary disease, and that affects 1 in 400 to 1000 live births. ADPKD is usually recognized in adults between the third and fourth decades of life. Adult PKD causes renal insufficiency in 50% of individuals by the age of 70 years, and it accounts for 10% of dialysis patients in the United States. ADPKD is caused by a defective *PKD1* gene on chromosome 16p in 85% of cases. A positive diagnosis requires (1) at least two cysts (unilateral or bilateral) in patients younger than 30 years of age; (2) at least two cysts in each kidney in patients aged 30 to 59; or (3) four or more cysts in each kidney in patients over age 60. These age-specific data have been developed in reference to PKD1 patients. Pathology of ADPKD is characterized by massive enlargement of the kidneys secondary to cyst growth and development. The liver also contains cysts in about 40% of patients with ADPKD. Arterial aneurysms of the circle of Willis are found in about 10% of patients. Diagnosis by US is straightforward in advanced disease, but it may be less reliable in the early stages. CT scan and MRI are more informative, and genetic testing may be required when greater certainty is needed for ADPKD diagnosis.

MEDULLARY CYSTIC KIDNEY DISEASE

Medullary cystic kidney disease is a rare autosomal dominant cystic disease characterized by normal- to small-sized kidneys. When cysts are found, they are located at the corticomedullary junction and in the medulla. Diagnosis relies on clinical features with a thorough family history. CT scan is the most sensitive test for cyst detection. The first signs are inability to concentrate the urine and salt wasting, leading to polyuria and polydipsia. Medullary cystic disease progresses inevitably to ESRD by the age of 20–40 years. Transplantation is the treatment of choice.

MEDULLARY SPONGE KIDNEY

Medullary sponge kidney is usually not diagnosed before the fourth or fifth decade of life, when patients have secondary calcifications with passage of urinary stones or frequent urinary track infections. This is a benign disorder with incidence of 1 in 5000 in the general population. The diagnosis is made by intravenous urography, which shows irregular enlargement of the medullary and interpapillary collecting ducts bilaterally. There is no specific therapy for medullary sponge kidney disease. The patients should be advised to drink enough water in order to excrete over 2 L of urine a day. Patient's may benefit from a thiazide diuretic for hypercalciuria, allopurinol for hyperuricosuria, or potassium citrate for hypocitraturia.

RENAL CELL CANCER

Renal cell cancer occurs at a rate of 7.5 cases per 100,000 population annually. It accounts for >80% of renal malignancies in adults and occurs more frequently in men. Risk factors for renal cell carcinoma are smoking, chemicals such as cadmium and nitrosohydrocarbons, acquired cystic disease in ESRD, and von Hippel-Lindau disorder. Patients may present with hematuria, abdominal mass, flank pain, fever, weight loss, or varicocele, but many patients are asymptomatic until the disease is advanced. Laboratory findings include anemia or erythrocytosis, hepatic dysfunction, and hypercalcemia. CT scan with radiographic contrast is currently the most widely available, sensitive, and accurate nonoperative method available for making a presumptive diagnosis of renal cancer and its staging. MRI is used over CT scanning (1) when detecting tumors in regional lymph nodes and extension into the renal veins and inferior vena cava; (2) in patients with radiographic contrast allergy; and (3) when CT results are equivocal. For patients without distant metastases the treatment of choice is radical nephrectomy. The average survival of patients with metastases is only 6–9 months. Postoperative adjuvant radiation, hormonal therapy, and chemotherapy are not proven to prolong survival.

KIDNEY STONES

Kidney stone disease is a common cause of morbidity in the Western world. It affects 10–20% of the population and leads to hospitalization in 1 in 1000 individuals each year. In excess of 80% of kidney stones occur in white males. White males have a lifetime risk of stone formation approximating 20%. In contrast, the lifetime risk in white females is much lower—approximately 5–10%. There is also clear racial preponderance of stone disease among whites—blacks have an incidence rate of stone disease that is 25% that of whites. The peak age of onset for kidney stone formation is 20–30 years. However, there is a high recurrence rate—as high as 50% in 5 years among white males.

Kidney stones form in the renal tubule or collecting duct and arise when urine is supersaturated with insoluble materials. The nidus is usually a crystal or foreign object. Seventy-five percent of stones are primarily composed of calcium phosphate or calcium oxalate, 10–20% are struvite stones,

5% urate, and 1–2% cystine. Kidney stones can be found throughout the length of the urinary tract system. Symptoms depend on the type, location, and duration of kidney stones. Patients may be asymptomatic or have renal colic, hematuria, dysuria, frequency, or urinary tract infections. Symptoms associated with renal failure may arise when patients suffer from large staghorn calculi that impair renal function. The incidence and prevalence of kidney stones vary by region, age, sex, and race, but approximately 5% of American women and 12% of men will develop stones in their lifetime. The goals of management are to treat complications and symptoms, remove any stones, and prevent recurrences.

The clinical presentation varies depending on the location, size, and number of the stones. The majority of kidney stones occur in the upper tracts. The most common presentation is renal colic—the sudden onset of severe pain due to the presence of an obstructive renal or ureteral stone. Renal colic is typically spasmodic in character, lasting several minutes, typically localized to the flank, and often radiating down to the groin. Nausea and vomiting frequently accompany renal colic. Renal colic often occurs in the middle of the night or early morning while the patient is sedentary, and its severity has been described as akin to or worse than childbirth. The severity of pain is a common cause of patients coming to the emergency room. On the other hand, larger stones may present with painless obstruction or back pain. Stones that reach the ureterovesical junction often present with renal colic accompanied by urgency and frequency. Alternatively, stones that are located in the calyces may be completely asymptomatic. The general appearance of a patient with renal colic is of someone writhing in excruciating pain. Sometimes the patient presents with restlessness, and pacing about the room. The presence of fever usually heralds an accompanying urinary tract infection. Otherwise the physical examination may be completely negative. The laboratory evaluation should comprise a complete blood count, blood chemistries including measurement of urea (BUN) and creatinine, and a urinalysis. The presence of a urinary tract infection, particularly with pyelonephritis, will be associated with a leukocytosis. An elevated BUN and creatinine would suggest dehydration and/or the presence of an obstructing stone in a patient with a single kidney or bilateral obstructing stones. The urine usually demonstrates hematuria and pyuria. Assessment of urine pH is critical because an acid urine with a radiolucent stone will suggest a uric acid stone, whereas a very alkaline urine (pH >8.0) would suggest an infection with a urease-splitting organism (for example, *Proteus*, *Pseudomonas*, and *Klebsiella* species). The initial radiologic workup should comprise of a kidney-ureters-bladder (KUB) radiograph and an ultrasound or a noncontrast CT scan.

MANAGEMENT OF KIDNEY STONES

The management of kidney stones can be divided into the management of the acute stone episode, and if the stone is nonobstructing, management of the prevalent stone medically and/or surgically, and prevention of further stones. Management of the acute stone episode rests on optimal pain control using parenteral narcotic agents, hydration, and urologic consultation for potential removal of an obstructing stone. Medical management of a nonobstructing stone comprises increasing fluid intake to cause a urine output of >2 L/day, modification in diet, treatment targeted at changing urinary pH, and strategies to prevent further stones from forming. Surgical management depends on the size, location, and number of stones. Surgical options include extracorporeal shock wave lithotripsy (ESWL) and lithotripsy (percutaneous or transurethral). General rules of thumb are that cystine stones and calcium oxalate monohydrate stones are generally poorly broken up by ESWL, and percutaneous or transurethral lithotripsy for removal are favored. On the other hand, other calcium oxalate stones, struvite stones, and uric acid stones are generally amenable to ESWL, as well as to either percutaneous or transurethral routes for removal depending on the size and location of the stones.

ACUTE KIDNEY INJURY (ACUTE RENAL FAILURE)

Acute kidney injury (AKI) has replaced the use of the term "acute renal failure." AKI is defined as a reduction in renal function manifest by a rise in serum creatinine over a period of hours to days. AKI is frequently accompanied by dysregulation of extracellular fluid volume and electrolytes and marked increase in the retention of nitrogenous and nonnitrogenous waste products over a period of hours to weeks. Acute kidney injury may be oliguric (<400 mL/day) or nonoliguric (>400 mL/day). AKI can also be defined as an acute and sustained increase in serum creatinine of 0.5 mg/dL (44.2 μmol/L), if the baseline is <2.5 mg/dL (221 μmol/L), or an increase in serum creatinine >20% if the baseline is >2.5 mg/dL (221 μmol/L).

There have been several attempts to achieve consensus between intensivists and nephrologists on the definition of AKI. The Acute Dialysis Quality Initiative (ADQI) group published the RIFLE classification of AKI in 2004 based on three severity categories (risk, injury, and failure) and two clinical outcome categories (loss and ESRD) (table 67.4). The parameters assessed in the RIFLE classification are changes in serum creatinine level or glomerular filtration rate (GFR) or urine output (UO) from the patient's baseline. The baseline serum creatinine level and GFRs may not be readily available. Hence, the consensus committee recommends the use of the Modification of Diet in Renal Disease (MDRD) equation to estimate the patient's GFR/1.73 m². The proportional decrease in GFR is calculated from 75 mL/min per 1.73 m², the agreed-on lower limit of normal.

A modified RIFLE criterion schema has been proposed by the Acute Kidney Injury Network (AKIN). The AKIN diagnostic criteria and the classification/staging system (table 67.5) for AKI are an abrupt (within 48 hours) reduction in kidney function (currently defined as an absolute increase in serum creatinine of ≥0.3 mg/dL [≥26.4 μmol/L], a percentage increase in serum creatinine of at least 50% (1.5-fold from baseline), or a reduction in urine output (documented oliguria of <0.5 mL/kg per hour for >6 hours). The absolute increase in the serum creatinine levels (≥0.3 mg/dL) included in this diagnostic criterion is based on epidemiologic data demonstrating that changes in serum creatinine levels of 0.3–0.5 mg/dL are associated with increased mortality risk. In addition, the timeline of "within 48 hours" is deliberately included in the diagnostic criteria because of data demonstrating poorer outcomes within this period.

The causes of AKI may be prerenal (e.g., hypotension, arterial thrombosis), renal parenchymal (e.g., acute tubular necrosis or ATN, glomerulonephritis, tubulointerstitial nephritis), or postrenal (e.g., acute obstruction) (see table 67.6).

AKI IN THE HOSPITALIZED PATIENT

The prevalence of AKI has been reported to be approximately 1% of all hospital admissions in the United States. Major causes of hospital-acquired AKI include volume

---

Table 67.4 "RIFLE" CLASSIFICATION FOR AKI

Risk (R): Increase in serum creatinine level ×1.5 or decrease in GFR by 25%, or UO <0.5 mL/kg/h for 6 hours

Injury (I): Increase in serum creatinine level ×2.0 or decrease in GFR by 50%, or UO <0.5 mL/kg/h for 12 hours

Failure (F): Increase in serum creatinine level ×3.0, decrease in GFR by 75%, or serum creatinine level >4 mg/dL with acute increase of >0.5 mg/dL; UO <0.3 mL/kg/h for 24 hours, or anuria for 12 hours

Loss (L): Persistent AKI, complete loss of kidney function >4 weeks

End-stage kidney disease (E): Loss of kidney function >3 months

SOURCE: Reprinted with permission from Bellomo R, Ronco C, Kellum JA, et al. Acute renal failure—definition, outcome measures, animal models, fluid therapy and information technology needs: The Second International Consensus Conference of the Acute Dialysis Quality Initiative (ADQI) Group. *Crit Care.* 2004;8(4):R204–12.

Table 67.5 AKIN CLASSIFICATION/STAGING SYSTEM FOR AKI

STAGE	SERUM CREATININE CRITERIA	URINE OUTPUT CRITERIA
1	Increase in serum creatinine of more than or equal to 0.3 mg/dL ($\geq$26.4 μmol/L) or increase to more than or equal to 150% to 200% (1.5- to 2-fold) from baseline	Less than 0.5 mL/kg per hour for more than 6 hours
2[b]	Increase in serum creatinine to more than 200% to 300% (>2- to 3-fold) from baseline	Less than 0.5 mL/kg per hour for more than 12 hours
3[c]	Increase in serum creatinine to more than 300% (>3-fold) from baseline (or serum creatinine of more than or equal to 4.0 mg/dL [$\geq$354 μmol/L] with an acute increase of at least 0.5 mg/dL [44 μmol/L])	Less than 0.3 mL/kg per hour for 24 hours or anuria for 12 hours

NOTE: This classification is modified from RIFLE (Risk, Injury, Failure, Loss, and End-stage kidney disease) criteria. The staging system proposed is a highly sensitive interim staging system and is based on recent data indicating that a small change in serum creatinine influences outcome. Only one criterion (creatinine or urine output) has to be fulfilled to qualify for a stage. b200% to 300% increase = 2- to 3-fold increase. cGiven wide variation in indications and timing of initiation of renal replacement therapy (RRT), individuals who receive RRT are considered to have met the criteria for stage 3 irrespective of the stage they are in at the time of RRT.

SOURCE: Reprinted with permission from Mehta RL, Kellum JA, Shah SV, et al. Acute Kidney Injury Network: Report of an initiative to improve outcomes in acute kidney injury. *Crit Care.* 2007;11(2):R31.

depletion resulting in decreased renal perfusion, major surgery, septic shock, congestive cardiac failure, contrast nephropathy, and aminoglycoside antibiotics. Acute tubular necrosis (ATN) is identified as the most frequent clinicopathologic entity in hospital-acquired AKI followed by prerenal azotemia, acute-onset chronic renal failure, and urinary tract obstruction.

hemodynamic alterations, nephrotoxin administration, and prerenal factors. Sepsis and multiorgan failure remain the most common causes for AKI. AKI affects mostly the older and the severely and chronically ill patients admitted to the hospital. The overall in-hospital mortality rate among those with ICU-associated AKI is approximately 60% according to the BEST Kidney study.

AKI IN THE CRITICALLY ILL PATIENT

AKI occurs in 1–25% of patients admitted in critical care units. A multicenter cohort study focused on AKI occurring in the intensive care unit (ICU) reported sepsis as a major cause contributing to AKI, followed by

COMMUNITY-ACQUIRED AKI

Community-acquired AKI accounts for 1% of the hospital admissions in the United States, but no extensive community-based study on the epidemiologic trends in the United States have been conducted as yet. In developing countries

Table 67.6 CAUSES OF AKI

Prerenal
- Intravascular volume depletion: diarrhea, vomiting, hemorrhage, poor fluid intake, sepsis, and overdiuresis
- Decreased effective circulating volume to the kidneys: congestive cardiac failure, nephrotic syndrome, cirrhosis, or hepatorenal syndrome
- Renal hypoperfusion due to exogenous agents: ACE inhibitors, NSAIDs

Renal
- Acute tubular necrosis: ischemia
- Toxins: drugs (e.g., aminoglycosides), contrast agents, pigments (myoglobin or hemoglobin)
- Glomerular disease: RPGN, SLE, small-vessel vasculitis (granulomatosis and polyangiitis (Wegener's) or microscopic polyarteritis), Henoch-Schönlein purpura (immunoglobulin A nephropathy), Goodpasture syndrome
- Acute proliferative glomerulonephritis: endocarditis, poststreptococcal infection, postpneumococcal infection
- Vascular disease
  Microvascular disease: atheroembolic disease (cholesterol-plaque microembolism), TTP, HUS, HELLP syndrome (**H**emolysis, **E**levated **L**iver enzymes and **L**ow **P**latelets), or postpartum acute renal failure
  Macrovascular disease: Renal artery occlusion, severe abdominal aortic disease (aneurysm)
- Interstitial disease: Allergic reaction to drugs, autoimmune disease, systemic lupus erythematosus or mixed connective tissue disease, pyelonephritis, infiltrative disease (lymphoma or leukemia)

Postrenal
  Benign prostatic hypertrophy or prostate cancer, cervical cancer, retroperitoneal disorders, intratubular obstruction (crystals or myeloma light chains), pelvic mass or invasive pelvic malignancy, intraluminal bladder mass (clot, tumor, or fungal ball), neurogenic bladder, urethral strictures

AKI is recognized as the disease of the young and children in whom prerenal etiologies such as acute diarrheal illness are more common compared to the developed countries where AKI is more prevalent in the elderly. Falciparum malaria, HIV/AIDS, obstetric causes, dengue fever, snake bites, insect stings, botanical and chemical nephrotoxins, acute glomerulonephritis, hemolytic uremic syndrome, and alternative medical therapies are important etiological factors of AKI in the tropical clinical setting. Crush injury as a result of natural calamities such as earthquakes contributes to regional epidemics of AKI.

The patient with AKI usually presents with abnormal laboratory values and/or decreased urine output. A thorough history and physical examination are critical in evaluation. Key issues are (1) ascertaining a history suggestive of bladder outflow obstruction, for example, secondary to prostatism (e.g., nocturia, hesitation, and frequency of urination), assessment of any exposures to toxins or nephrotoxic medications (e.g., exposure to lead, ingestion of nonsteroidal anti-inflammatory drugs), and any systemic symptomatology suggesting an autoimmune etiology (e.g., arthralgias, arthritis, skin rash); (2) family history of diabetes or kidney disease; and (3) a physical examination focused on as the assessment of extracellular volume (edema, dry mucous membranes, hypertension, orthostatic hypotension, skin turgor), and detection of systemic process, such as an infection or an autoimmune process.

Urinalysis evaluation and microscopy of the urine sediment are essential in the workup of patients with AKI. Acute tubular necrosis is suggested by the presence of tubular cells, amorphous debris representing necrotic cells and deeply pigmented coarsely granular casts ("muddy brown"). Glomerulonephritis is suggested by the presence of red cells, particularly dysmorphic red cells and red cell casts. In acute tubulointerstitial nephritis, the presence of white cells, tubular epithelial cells, and white cell and/or tubular cell casts are typical. Examination of the urine should also include measurement of urine sodium, protein, and creatinine. In the workup of a patient suspected of glomerulonephritis, serologic testing, including measurement of complement fractions, and assays for antinuclear antibody (ANA), antineutrophil cytoplasmic antibody (ANCA), and antiglomerular antibody (anti-GBM) should be considered. Early evaluation with a renal ultrasound is essential in order to exclude urinary obstruction. Severe cases of acute tubular necrosis (ATN) and some forms of rapidly progressive glomerulonephritis (RPGN) (e.g., anti-GBM disease) may require a renal biopsy for diagnosis.

The management of AKI involves three broad approaches: (1) providing supportive care—fluid resuscitation or supporting blood pressure, instituting dialysis or continuous renal replacement therapy where indicated, and adjusting dose of medications that undergo renal excretion; (2) targeting the individual problem—for example, treating glomerulonephritis with steroids and cytotoxic immunosuppressive agents; and (3) treating complications of AKI—for example, volume overload with diuretics (the role of diuretics in AKI continues to be controversial).

ADDITIONAL READING

Alicic RZ, Tuttle KR. Management of the diabetic patient with advanced chronic kidney disease. *Semin Dial.* 2010;23(2):140–7.

Atkins RC, Zimmet P. Diabetic kidney disease: Act now or pay later. *Saudi J Kidney Dis Transpl.* 2010;21(2):217–21.

Coe FL, Evan AP, Worcester EM, Lingeman JE. Three pathways for human kidney stone formation. *Urol Res.* 2010;38(3):147–60.

Himmelfarb J, Ikizler TA. Acute kidney injury: Changing lexicography, definitions, and epidemiology. *Kidney Int.* 2007;71:971–6.

Kenny JE, Goldfarb DS. Update on the pathophysiology and management of uric acid renal stones. *Curr Rheumatol Rep.* 2010;12(2):125–9.

Muirhead N. Update in nephrology. *Ann Intern Med.* 20101;152(11): 721–5.

Pei Y, Watnick T. Diagnosis and screening of autosomal dominant polycystic kidney disease. *Adv Chronic Kidney Dis.* 2010;17(2): 140–52.

Waikar SS, Bonventre JV. Biomarkers for the diagnosis of acute kidney injury. *Nephron Clin Pract.* 2008;109(4):c192–7.

Waikar SS, Liu KD, Chertow GM. Diagnosis, epidemiology and outcomes of acute kidney injury. *Clin J Am Soc Nephrol.* 2008;3(3): 844–61.

Williams ME. Diabetic CKD/ESRD 2010: A progress report? *Semin Dial.* 2010;23(2):129–33. Epub 2010 Feb 22.

Worcester EM, Coe FL. Clinical practice. Calcium kidney stones. *N Engl J Med.* 2010;363(10):954–63.

SECTION 7

DIGESTIVE DISEASES AND DISORDERS OF THE PANCREAS AND LIVER

68.

ESOPHAGEAL DISEASES

John R. Saltzman

ESOPHAGEAL ANATOMY AND PHYSIOLOGY

In order to understand the disorders of the esophagus, it is important to understand its basic anatomy and physiology. The esophagus is a tubular muscular structure that extends from the pharynx to the stomach. The esophagus serves as a passage for the transport of food, prevents the regurgitation of food and gastric contents from the stomach, and allows for the venting of ingested air to decrease bloating. At the proximal and distal ends of the esophagus are sphincter muscles that help control esophageal function and, in a coordinated manner, allow for swallowing. At the proximal margin is the upper esophageal sphincter, which includes the inferior pharyngeal constrictor and cricopharyngeal muscles. The lower esophageal sphincter (LES) is a 2- to 4-cm-long high-pressure segment of smooth muscle that is tonically contracted at the distal margin of the esophagus and is located within the diaphragmatic hiatus.

The primary muscle layer of the esophagus (muscularis propria) is comprised of both skeletal and smooth muscle, depending on the location. In the proximal third of the esophagus, the muscularis propria is skeletal; in the lower two-thirds it is primarily smooth muscle. Acetylcholine is the mediator released by excitatory neurons; it controls contraction of muscles and esophageal peristalsis. Nitric oxide is released by neurons predominantly in the distal esophagus and serves in an inhibitory capacity on peristalsis and on lower esophageal sphincter tone.

THE SYMPTOMS OF ESOPHAGEAL DISEASE

Heartburn is the primary symptom of gastroesophageal reflux disease (GERD). Heartburn (also called pyrosis) is defined as a retrosternal burning discomfort that may radiate up toward the neck. Heartburn typically occurs in the postprandial period, especially after a high-fat or a large-volume meal. Postural changes, such as bending over, will often exacerbate symptoms. Relief of heartburn occurs with an upright position, swallowing of water or saliva, and by ingestion of antacids.

Regurgitation is the effortless appearance of gastric or esophageal contents in the mouth. In patients with severe GERD, regurgitation of bitter-tasting material occurs. This symptom may also occur in patients with esophageal obstruction from structural causes such as tumors or functional causes such as achalasia.

Water brash is a reflex induced by GERD that causes excessive salivation. Water brash is a distinct symptom that should not be confused with regurgitation.

Odynophagia is sharp, substernal pain with swallowing and usually due to erosive esophagitis. This is typically from an infectious or pill-induced esophagitis. Odynophagia is an unusual symptom of uncomplicated GERD, although it can occur in severe GERD.

Globus is the sensation of a lump or fullness in the throat that persists following swallowing. This sensation may be a manifestation of GERD.

Dysphagia is defined as the sensation of a delay of food during its passage from the mouth to the stomach. Patients may perceive of food as "sticking" or "getting caught" after swallowing. Complications of dysphagia include aspiration pneumonia and weight loss. Dysphagia can be categorized as oropharyngeal dysphagia, which is due to difficulty in initiating a swallow (transferring a food bolus from the hypopharynx to the esophagus), or as esophageal dysphagia, which is due to difficulty in transferring a food bolus through the esophagus. Oropharyngeal dysphagia is due to disorders of the pharynx, upper esophageal sphincter, and striated upper esophagus, whereas esophageal dysphagia is due to a structural defect or a neuromuscular disorder of the esophageal smooth muscle. Figure 68.1 shows the different types of dysphagia and the best tests to perform.

The most common cause of oropharyngeal dysphagia is neuromuscular dysfunction that disrupts the coordination of initial swallowing. Causes of oropharyngeal dysphagia

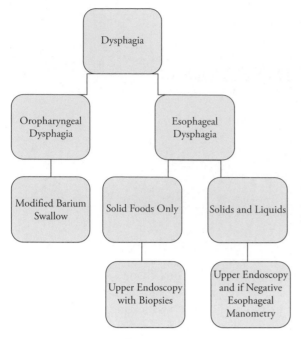

Figure 68.1. Algorithm for Classification and Evaluation of Dysphagia.

include cerebrovascular accidents, Parkinson disease, amyotrophic lateral sclerosis, and myasthenia gravis. Rare structural disorders that can cause oropharyngeal dysphagia include a Zencker's diverticulum (see esophageal structural abnormalities) and cervical osteophytes; these more commonly result in dysphagia to solids. The best test to detect an oropharyngeal source of dysphagia is a modified barium swallow with videofluoroscopy. This is often performed in collaboration with a speech pathologist at the time of the examination who can help identify abnormalities and direct specific swallow therapies.

The clinical history is important to distinguish the type and etiology of dysphagia. Oropharyngeal dysphagia is characterized by discoordination of swallowing, often accompanied by choking, gagging, nasal regurgitation, or coughing. These symptoms may be more prominent with liquids. Patients with dysphagia only to solids typically have esophageal dysphagia with a structural disorder of the esophagus such as a stricture (benign or malignant). These patients are best evaluated by an upper endoscopy to exclude structural lesions; if normal, biopsies from the mid- and distal esophagus should be obtained to exclude eosinophilic esophagitis (see inflammatory and infectious disorders), which can be present without an endoscopic abnormality. Patients with evidence of erosive esophagitis should be started on proton pump inhibitors, as acid reflux can cause motility abnormalities. Esophageal rings, such as a Schatzki's ring (see esophageal structural abnormalities) in the lower esophagus, often cause intermittent dysphagia to solids. The site where patients perceive food sticking is not entirely reliable, as when patients report an upper location, in about 30% of cases the site of obstruction is actually in the distal esophagus. Motility disorders of the esophagus, such as achalasia and scleroderma, are more likely to cause dysphagia to both solids and liquids. These conditions are best evaluated with an esophageal manometry study after an upper endoscopy has excluded a structural cause of dysphagia.

GASTROESOPHAGEAL REFLUX DISEASE

GERD is the most common and expensive digestive disease. GERD accounts for at least 9 million office visits to physicians in the United States each year, and annual direct costs for managing GERD exceed $10 billion. GERD is a chronic disorder that occurs as a result of the retrograde flow of gastroduodenal contents into the esophagus, resulting in a variable spectrum of symptoms.

Transient inappropriate relaxation of the lower esophageal sphincter is the predominant pathophysiological mechanism in the majority of patients (65%) with GERD. Relaxation of the LES occurs in response to swallowing or esophageal distension. Transient lower esophageal sphincter relaxation (TLESR) is a vagally mediated reflex that can be triggered by gastric distension. Transient lower esophageal sphincter relaxation is the main mechanism for reflux of gastric contents in normal persons. A chronically low LES pressure is the predominant GERD mechanism in patients with severe reflux disease.

Anatomic disruption of the gastroesophageal junction, commonly associated with a hiatal hernia, is another mechanism that contributes to the pathogenesis of reflux disease by impairing LES function and creating an intrathoracic reservoir of gastric contents. However, hiatal hernias are common and usually cause no symptoms.

Gastroparesis (delayed stomach emptying) is more common in patients with moderate to severe reflux disease and is an important factor in 10–15% of patients with GERD. Other gastric factors that contribute to GERD include increased gastric volume after meals and increased gastric pressure due to obesity. Increased gastric distention can cause an increase in TLESRs and volume of refluxate, particularly in GERD patients with large hiatal hernias. Reflux esophagitis is defined by esophageal mucosal lesions, whereas patients with GERD in the absence of mucosal damage have nonerosive or endoscopy-negative reflux disease.

EPIDEMIOLOGY

There is a significant variability in GERD worldwide with a weekly prevalence of symptoms in Western countries of 10–20% compared with <5% in Asia. GERD is a common disorder, and the prevalence of GERD in the United States appears to be increasing. In Western populations, 5–7% of healthy people describe having heartburn symptoms on a daily basis, 12–14% have symptoms at least once per week, and 15–25% report having heartburn at least once a month. Only one in four have discussed their symptoms with physicians. There appears to be no gender predominance of heartburn symptoms between men and women (except during pregnancy), although men tend to have more severe acid reflux (2–3:1) and Barrett's esophagus (3–10:1). For women, the prevalence of daily heartburn during pregnancy is at least 25%, mostly in the third trimester. Familial clustering of GERD has also been reported. There is a positive association between increasing body mass index and reflux symptoms, and even moderate weight gain can cause or exacerbate symptoms of reflux. This is, in part, a consequence of because inappropriate TLESR induced by obesity.

CLINICAL FINDINGS

The typical manifestations of gastroesophageal reflux disease are heartburn and regurgitation. Other symptoms of GERD include odynophagia, globus, and water brash. Symptoms can be aggravated by ingestion of direct irritants such as tomato sauce, spicy foods, coffee, tea, and alcohol. Certain foods, beverages, and behaviors will cause heartburn by reducing LES pressure. Fatty foods, peppermint, chocolate, caffeinated beverages, alcohol, and smoking can all lead to decreased LES pressure. Some medicines that can exacerbate GERD by lowering the LES pressure are listed in table 68.1.

Patients should be considered as having GERD if they have typical GERD symptoms twice a week or more for at least 4 to 8 weeks. "Alarm" signs in GERD that mandate testing are anorexia, dysphagia, odynophagia, anemia, gastrointestinal blood loss, weight loss, advanced age, or a family history of upper gastrointestinal cancer.

Table 68.1 MEDICATIONS THAT CAN CAUSE A DECREASE IN LES PRESSURE

Alpha-adrenergic antagonists

Anticholinergics

Antihistamines

Beta-adrenergic agonists, including inhalers

Calcium channel blockers

Diazepam

Estrogens

Narcotics

Progesterone

Theophylline

Tricyclic antidepressants

Extraesophageal symptoms are atypical manifestations of GERD, including noncardiac chest pain, asthma, cough, aspiration pneumonia, and laryngitis. Pathologic GERD can be found in up to 80% of patients with asthma. Atypical manifestations can occur in patients with or without typical symptoms of GERD.

Complications of GERD include the development of a stricture, gastrointestinal bleeding, Barrett's esophagus, and adenocarcinoma. Peptic strictures represent the progression of ongoing reflux with mucosal damage and secondary fibrosis.

DIAGNOSIS

Classic GERD can be diagnosed by a history of characteristic symptoms and the absence of alarm symptoms that is confirmed by a complete response to medical therapy. A meta-analysis that assessed the accuracy of normal-dose or high-dose proton pump inhibitors (PPIs) for 1–4 weeks in the diagnosis of GERD found a pooled sensitivity of 78% (95% CI 66–86%) and a specificity of 54% (44–65%) when ambulatory esophageal pH was used as a gold standard. Diagnostic testing is typically reserved for patients who fail to respond to a trial of adequate medical therapy or for patients who have alarm symptoms of GERD. The current diagnostic tests for GERD in patients who fail medical therapy or have alarm signs include upper endoscopy, ambulatory pH studies, and impedance testing.

Upper Endoscopy

Upper endoscopy involves the insertion of an endoscope through the mouth with direct inspection of the esophagus, stomach, and proximal duodenum. It can detect the extent and the severity of esophagitis as well as exclude the presence of other diseases such as tumors and peptic ulcers. The identification of esophagitis by upper endoscopy is highly specific (90–95%) for GERD but has a sensitivity of only around 50%. Two-thirds of GERD patients will have nonerosive reflux disease and thus negative findings of upper endoscopy. Upper endoscopy also allows evaluation for complications of GERD, such as strictures or Barrett's esophagus. If a patient has dysphagia and a stricture is detected, dilation of the stricture can be performed during the same procedure. Upper endoscopy is the test of choice in patients with alarm signs.

Intraesophageal Ambulatory pH Monitoring

Intraesophageal pH monitoring is the most accurate test to detect the presence of acid in the esophagus, with a sensitivity of about 85% and a specificity above 95%. It is most helpful in patients with difficult management problems or atypical presentations. Intraesophageal ambulatory pH monitoring typically is done by a probe that can record the distal esophageal pH continuously for 24 hours. The pH probe is passed transnasally to 5 cm above the manometrically determined LES. The data are collected by a battery-powered, beeper-sized device carried by the patient, who also records when meals are ingested and symptoms are experienced. This technique allows for correlation of symptoms with reflux episodes. Abnormal acid reflux episodes are defined as an esophageal pH below 4 for >4% of the total study duration. The discomfort associated with nasal probe placement prompted the development of a wireless pH monitoring system that allows for a wireless, pill-sized capsule to be attached to the distal esophageal mucosa. The wireless pH system allows for 48 hours of monitoring, compared to 24 hours of monitoring with a conventional pH probe, which may detect GERD in patients with day-to-day variability. The capsule detaches and is spontaneously passed within 2 weeks.

Esophageal pH testing should be used in a select minority of GERD patients for whom the information will influence management. Ambulatory esophageal pH monitoring can be performed on acid-suppressing medications in patients who have typical GERD symptoms but are unresponsive to therapy, to determine if additional medical or surgical therapy is indicated. Ambulatory esophageal pH monitoring is also helpful off acid-suppressing medications to determine if GERD is present in patients with atypical GERD symptoms, such as asthma or chronic cough. In the prefundoplication operative evaluation of GERD patients, ambulatory esophageal pH monitoring is also important to document the presence and severity of GERD, especially if the patient has nonerosive reflux disease.

Multichannel Intraluminal Impedance

The newest device to evaluate patients with GERD is the multichannel intraluminal impedance monitor that measures both acidic and nonacidic refluxates. This device measures the intraluminal impedance of the esophagus (a measure of the total resistance to current flow between two electrodes) and is capable of detecting both liquid and gas consistencies. The combination of measuring both acid and nonacidic reflux in the esophagus has several advantages over traditional pH testing. This test can be helpful in patients with both typical and atypical GERD who are refractory to therapy for acid reflux by assessing nonacid and/or nonliquid reflux. As this technology is new, further long-term studies are needed to understand the clinical role of multichannel intraluminal impedance monitoring.

MANAGEMENT

The goals of treatment for GERD are to eliminate symptoms, heal esophagitis, and prevent complications of GERD. Once a patient is in remission, the goal is to maintain symptom remission and prevent further tissue injury.

Lifestyle modifications are a cornerstone of the treatment of GERD, although not all are supported by clinical trials. Patients are instructed to avoid foods and beverages, such as high-fat and acidic foods, that can exacerbate symptoms of GERD. Avoidance of lying down for 3 hours after ingesting food may lessen reflux, as during this time period, food may remain in the stomach and contribute to reflux. Smaller and more frequent meals may also be useful for patients with GERD. Elevation of the head of the bed 6 inches with blocks underneath the head of the bed can also reduce reflux by using gravity to prevent reflux, although this is an unpopular intervention. The best position to reduce reflux when sleeping is to lie in the left lateral position. Other useful recommendations are to stop smoking and reduce weight, which can be critical to reducing or eliminating symptoms.

Medical treatment is with antacid and antisecretory agents. Over-the-counter antacids are taken at least twice a month by more than one-fourth of the U.S. population. Antacids, alginic acid, and baking soda provide temporary symptom relief by neutralizing refluxed acid. These agents are most useful for treating mild and infrequent reflux symptoms, typically induced by indiscretions in lifestyle. Prokinetic drugs such as metoclopramide and bethanechol can relieve symptoms of heartburn but are most appropriate in patients with delayed gastric emptying. Unfortunately these medications typically provide an incomplete response and have frequent side effects.

H_2-receptor antagonists inhibit the secretion of gastric acid by competitively blocking gastric parietal cell H_2 receptors. H_2 blockers are approximately 75% effective in patients with mild to moderate degrees of esophagitis. However, in patients with moderate to severe esophagitis, these medications are only 50% effective in healing esophagitis. Patients with nonerosive GERD are paradoxically often more difficult to treat than those with erosive GERD. Thus, H_2-receptor antagonists are appropriate in mild to moderate GERD. Of note, chronic H_2-blocker use may be associated with loss of efficacy and the development of tachyphylaxis.

Proton pump inhibitors (PPIs) act by blocking the hydrogen-potassium ATPase pump on the parietal cell apical surface. PPIs are more effective than H_2-receptor antagonists because they act on the final common pathway of acid secretion rather than on just one of the three receptors (histamine, acetylcholine, and gastrin) responsible for acid secretion. PPIs are effective in patients with mild GERD but are indicated as initial therapy in patients with moderate to severe GERD and in patients with complications of GERD, such as bleeding and strictures. Some patients with persistent nocturnal GERD despite twice-daily PPIs benefit from H_2-receptor antagonists taken at bedtime.

The timing of PPI use is important as PPIs are most effective when taken in a fasting state and are recommended to be ingested about 30 minutes before breakfast, when parietal cells have large numbers of active proton pumps. Side effects can occur in up to 3% of patients; the most common are headaches and diarrhea. There is potential for reduction of vitamin B-12 levels due to a decrease in protein-bound vitamin B-12 absorption with long-term PPI use, although this has not been seen clinically. Bacterial overgrowth of the small bowel can occur but rarely is significant unless there is also altered intestinal motility. The use of PPIs has been associated with marginally increased rates of community-acquired pneumonia, *Clostridium difficile* infection, hip fracture, and hypomagnesemia. PPIs may interact with some medications such as clopidogrel, although the clinical significance of this interaction is controversial.

Although most patients with GERD will be successfully managed with lifestyle modifications and medical therapy, some patients may have persistent symptoms despite treatment. Mechanical antireflux surgery can be employed in patients with a good clinical response to medical treatments who wish to discontinue medications, or in patients with established GERD who have persistent symptoms despite medical therapy. The most widely performed procedure is a laparoscopic Nissen fundoplication, with a symptomatic response rate of up to 90%. Complications following fundoplication include dysphagia, chest pain, gas-bloat syndrome, postoperative flatulence, and vagal nerve injuries leading to gastroparesis and diarrhea. The prevalence of these postoperative complications ranges between 5% and 20%.

CLINICAL COURSE AND PROGNOSIS

If a patient has responded to lifestyle changes and medical therapy with sustained symptom relief for 2–3 months, a trial of medication withdrawal should be attempted. If a patient is on a PPI, the dose can be reduced, it can be tapered to every other day, or the medication can be switched to an H_2-blocker. Most patients who are treated with H_2-blockers are on twice-daily medications and then can be tapered to a once-daily regimen. If a patient tolerates reduced medical therapy for 2 to 4 weeks without an increase in symptoms, the dosage can be further decreased, or the medication can be discontinued. The goal of long-term medical treatment is to provide the lowest level of medical therapy that effectively controls symptoms. However, if a patient experiences recurrent symptoms, the same medication that induces remission is usually required in the same dosage to maintain remission. For many patients, GERD is a chronic, relapsing disease with frequent symptom recurrence after medication withdrawal, thus requiring maintenance therapy. In nonerosive GERD, on-demand therapy can be a cost-effective alternative to maintenance treatment.

BARRETT'S ESOPHAGUS

The most important risk factor for the development of esophageal adenocarcinoma is Barrett's esophagus. It is estimated that patients with Barrett's esophagus have a 30- to 40-fold greater risk of esophageal adenocarcinoma than the general population. The development of a specialized columnar epithelium that replaces the normal squamous epithelium of the distal esophagus defines Barrett's esophagus. The pathophysiology of Barrett's esophagus involves GERD leading to reflux esophagitis with injury of the squamous epithelium. The injured epithelium heals with specialized columnar epithelium and intestinal metaplasia (required to diagnose Barrett's epithelium).

At the time of the initial diagnosis of Barrett's esophagus, approximately 8% of patients have adenocarcinoma. It is estimated that the risk of esophageal cancer is 0.12 to 0.5% per year in patients with known Barrett esophagus. Barrett esophagus shows a male-to-female ratio of 3–10:1, with an average age at the time of diagnosis of 55 years. Barrett esophagus is more likely to be found in patients with more severe GERD. It is estimated that 20% of patients with erosive esophagitis will develop Barrett's metaplasia, compared to 1% or less in unselected patients undergoing upper endoscopy.

There are no specific symptoms of Barrett's esophagus. Upper endoscopy with biopsy of the gastroesophageal junction is needed for the diagnosis of Barrett's esophagus. On upper endoscopy, Barrett's esophagus appears as tongues of salmon-colored mucosa (figure 68.2), and biopsies confirm the diagnosis. Current recommendations are for one-time screening upper endoscopy in patients who have long standing GERD (5 to 10 years) and those who are over the age of 50 years with GERD.

In patients who have Barrett's esophagus but no evidence of dysplasia, the upper endoscopy and biopsy should be repeated in 1 year. If Barrett's without dysplasia is confirmed, the interval can be lengthened to 2–5 years (most recommend 3 years). For low-grade dysplasia, once the histopatho-

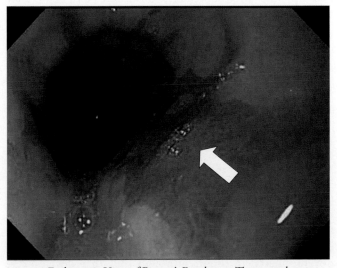

Figure 68.2. Endoscopic View of Barrett's Esophagus. The normal squamous epithelium of the esophagus appears white, and the Barrett's mucosa has a salmon color (arrow).

logic diagnosis is confirmed by review of the findings by a second expert pathologist, patients should undergo repeat endoscopy in 6 and 12 months for biopsy. If the low-grade dysplasia is stable, yearly surveillance endoscopies can be done or patients can undergo endoscopic ablation. In patients with Barrett's and high-grade dysplasia, the histopathologic diagnosis should also be confirmed by review of the findings by a second expert pathologist and a repeat endoscopy with multiple biopsies. If high-grade dysplasia is confirmed, one recommendation is to proceed with esophagectomy, as up to 30% of patients will have adenocarcinoma present at the time of surgical resection. An alternative strategy is to endoscopically resect or ablate the area. Endoscopies are then performed every 3 months, and surgery is done only if cancer is found.

In patients with either low- or high-grade dysplasia, a recent development in endoscopic treatment is radiofrequency ablation. In this endoscopic treatment method the lining of the esophagus is cauterized until mucosal sloughing occurs with subsequent regrowth of normal squamous esophageal mucosa. This treatment modality seems to eradicate low-grade dysplasia in over 90% of patients and high-grade dysplasia in about 80% of patients. Currently, new biomarkers are under investigation to attempt to improve the yield of surveillance in Barrett's esophagus and to reduce the sampling error associated with random biopsies.

The goals for treatment of patients with Barrett's esophagus are to eliminate the symptoms of GERD and prevent GERD complications. As patients with Barrett's esophagus tend to have more severe degrees of GERD, they may require high doses of medication or surgery to control their symptoms. Many patients are managed on PPIs to reduce the development of dysplasia, although the long-term benefits of this strategy have not been established in the literature. Antireflux surgery does not reduce the risk of adenocarcinoma in patients who have Barrett's esophagus, and continued surveillance of Barrett's esophagus after surgery is required, even if the surgery is successful and the patient is asymptomatic.

ESOPHAGEAL STRUCTURAL ABNORMALITIES

RINGS AND WEBS

The normal esophagus is about 20 mm in diameter, and patients rarely have difficulty swallowing when the luminal diameter is above 15 mm. Rings and webs are common structural abnormalities of the esophagus and can be found in up to 5% of the asymptomatic general population. These are commonly considered to be congenital or developmental in origin, although they may develop due to inflammatory conditions. Rings are circumferential narrowings of mucosa or muscle that are most common in the distal esophagus. Webs are partial narrowings that are always mucosal in origin and most common in the proximal esophagus. Rings and webs typically cause intermittent dysphagia to solids.

A common type of ring is the Schatzki's ring, which occurs at the junction of the esophagus and the stomach, is thin (<4 mm in thickness) and is associated with a hiatal hernia. Patients with ring diameters <13 mm are usually symptomatic, and those with a diameter between 13 mm and 20 mm may variably have symptoms. The cause of these rings is felt to be either congenital or associated with GERD. Patients who have symptoms should be treated with mechanical dilation at the time of upper endoscopy. Although dilation is effective, it is not uncommon for patients to have recurrent symptoms requiring additional dilations. Treatment with acid-suppressing medications after dilation may reduce the recurrence rate.

ESOPHAGEAL DIVERTICULA

The protrusion of a sac from the esophageal wall is an esophageal diverticulum. Esophageal diverticula can be of the upper esophagus, midesophagus, lower esophagus, and diffusely throughout the esophagus (intramural pseudodiverticulosis). Most esophageal diverticula are asymptomatic.

A Zencker's diverticulum is located just proximal to the upper esophageal sphincter, and although technically a hypopharyngeal diverticulum, it is often considered an esophageal diverticulum. These diverticula likely form in an area of weakness between the inferior constrictor and the cricopharyngeal muscles as a result of incomplete upper esophageal sphincter relaxation. Zencker's diverticula occur most commonly in elderly males. Patients with a Zencker's diverticulum may complain of dysphagia, halitosis, regurgitation of undigested food, throat discomfort, cough, and aspiration pneumonia. The diverticulum can fill with food that may be regurgitated when the patient lies down or bends over. The best test to detect a Zencker's diverticulum is a video barium swallow. Although small diverticula are often asymptomatic, symptomatic large diverticula should be treated. The standard procedure is a surgical cricopharyngeal myotomy, although recent advances have allowed for endoscopic treatment with incision of the septum between the esophagus and the diverticulum.

INFLAMMATORY AND INFECTIOUS DISORDERS

EOSINOPHILIC ESOPHAGITIS

Eosinophilic esophagitis is a chronic disorder that commonly presents in young adults between the ages of 20 and 40 years.

Patients typically present with dysphagia and often food impaction. This entity has been well described in children, but only recently has been recognized to occur in adults. It is also known as ringed, feline, allergic, or corrugated esophagus. Although the etiology is unknown, allergic conditions as well as GERD have been associated with eosinophilic esophagitis. Eosinophilic esophagitis is predominantly identified in males (80%).

The diagnosis is made by upper endoscopy and biopsy with endoscopic findings of mucosal fragility, multiple rings, white mucosal exudates, linear furrowing of the esophagus, and strictures (see figure 68.3). The diagnosis is confirmed by biopsies of the esophagus, which show eosinophils (>15–20 eosinophils per high-power field) in the esophageal mucosa more proximally than would be found in patients with GERD. It is important to exclude GERD by demonstrating a lack of clinical response to high-dose PPIs and by biopsy of both the gastroesophageal junction and more proximally in the esophagus.

The natural history of eosinophilic esophagitis is not entirely known in adults. Treatments have been primarily extrapolated from the pediatric experience with this disorder. Dietary and environmental triggers should be sought and should be eliminated if possible. The benefit of allergy testing and a food-elimination diet is not known, but referral to an allergist should be considered. Medical therapy is usually with topical corticosteroids such as fluticasone dipropionate (220 μg used without a spacer, swallowed twice daily), but leukotriene receptor antagonists and oral corticosteroids have also been shown to be helpful. Endoscopic dilation of the strictures may be needed, but the procedure must be done cautiously as the mucosa easily can tear, leading to perforation. The optimal duration of treatment is not known, as symptomatic relapses commonly occur after discontinuation of therapy, and long-term therapy may be required.

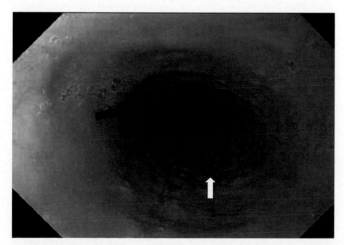

Figure 68.3. Endoscopic Appearance of Eosinophilic Esophagitis. Multiple rings (black arrows) and linear furrowing (white arrow) are seen.

PILL ESOPHAGITIS

There are many medications that are capable of injuring the esophagus. The most common medications that cause pill-induced esophagitis are listed in table 68.2 and include alendronate, antibiotics, aspirin, iron salts, nonsteroidals, potassium chloride, quinidine, and theophylline. More than 50% of pill-induced esophagitis is due to tetracycline and related medications, especially doxycycline. There are various mechanisms by which pills induce esophageal damage, including prolonged contact time with the esophageal mucosa and pill acidity. Commonly, pills get stuck at sites of anatomic narrowing, such as the arch of the aorta and the distal esophagus. Patients do not need to have esophageal anatomic disorders to develop pill esophagitis. Factors that increase the risk of pill esophagitis are advancing age, swallowing position, fluid intake, and pill size. Position may be the most important risk factor for esophageal injury, as medications ingested while supine with insufficient fluids may remain the in the esophagus for up to 90 minutes.

The symptoms of pill-induced esophagitis are chest pain and odynophagia, which can be quite severe and prolonged. Although the diagnosis is often a clinical one, upper endoscopy can confirm the diagnosis and exclude other causes. The endoscopic appearance of pill esophagitis is variable, including erosions, ulcerations, plaques, and strictures. The mainstay of treatment is to identify and avoid the offending drug. If possible, liquid forms of medication should be used. Medications should be administered with at least 15 mL of fluids, and patients should remain in the upright

Table 68.2 **MEDICATIONS THAT CAN CAUSE ESOPHAGITIS**

Alendronate
Antibiotics
Clindamycin
Doxycycline
Erythromycin
Penicillin
Tetracycline
Ascorbic acid
Aspirin
Iron salts
NSAIDs
Potassium chloride
Quinidine
Theophylline
Zidovudine

position for 30 minutes after swallowing pills. Symptom relief may occur with the use of topical anesthetics (e.g., viscous lidocaine) and coating the esophagus with antacids or sucralfate suspension.

INFECTIOUS CAUSES OF ESOPHAGITIS

Although esophageal infections are rare in normal hosts, infectious esophagitis is not uncommon in immunocompromised patients, including those who are posttransplant or on corticosteroids, and those with cancer on chemotherapy, diabetes, alcoholism, and HIV infection. Patients with infectious esophagitis typically have odynophagia, but may present with dysphagia, heartburn, fever, nausea, or bleeding. The three most common causes of infectious esophagitis are *Candida albicans*, cytomegalovirus (CMV), and herpes simplex virus (HSV). Less common infectious etiologies include Epstein-Barr virus, varicella-zoster virus, diphtheria, and primary HIV infection.

The most frequent cause of infectious esophagitis is *C. albicans*. Although *C. albicans* is normal oral flora, it can cause esophagitis in immunocompromised patients. In symptomatic patients with esophageal candidiasis, up to 75% will have oral thrush. The diagnosis is most accurately made by upper endoscopy showing white or yellow plaques, and brushings or biopsies showing hyphae and budding yeast. The diagnosis may also be clinically suspected and confirmed by a response to treatment. A commonly used antifungal treatment is a 14- to 21-day course of fluconazole (200 mg orally the first day followed by 100 mg per day). Alternative medications include itraconazole, voriconazole, and ketoconazole. Refractory disease may be treated by intravenous caspofungin or amphotericin.

Infection of the esophagus with CMV often occurs as part of a generalized gastrointestinal CMV infection in immunocompromised patients. Thus, the symptoms are quite variable and can be nonspecific. At upper endoscopy, there may be linear or deep ulcerations, and the diagnosis is confirmed from biopsies taken from the ulcer base. Biopsies should be sent for both histology and viral cultures. Treatment of CMV infectious esophagitis is with ganciclovir, valganciclovir, or foscarnet for at least 2 weeks and often also with a maintenance regimen until immune function improves.

HSV esophagitis can occur in both immunocompetent and immunocompromised hosts. In immunocompetent hosts, this usually is from reactivation of a latent infection, but may be from primary HSV. Upper endoscopy may show vesicles, which rupture to form ulcers with raised edges ("volcano-like"). The diagnosis is confirmed with biopsies from the edge of the ulcers, sent for both histology (showing multinucleated giant cells) and viral culture. Treatment is with a course of acyclovir given intravenously until the patient is able to tolerate oral therapy. Alternative therapies are foscarnet and famciclovir.

ESOPHAGEAL MOTILITY DISORDERS

Altered esophageal motility may occur due to primary motility disorders of the esophagus or secondary to systemic diseases. Motility disorders of the esophagus secondary to systemic diseases include scleroderma, diabetes mellitus, thyroid disease, amyloidosis, and other connective tissue diseases. Connective tissue disorders that may involve the esophagus include systemic lupus erythematosus, rheumatoid arthritis, Sjögren syndrome, mixed connective tissue disease, and inflammatory myopathies. The esophagus may also be affected by Behçet disease and cutaneous disorders including epidermolysis bullosa, bullous pemphigoid, cicatricial pemphigoid, pemphigus vulgaris, and lichen planus. The best test of esophageal motility is an esophageal manometry examination.

Esophageal manometry measures the pressure within the lumen of the esophagus with a nasal catheter. The principal use of this test is to diagnose primary esophageal motility disorders such as achalasia, diffuse esophageal spasm, or ineffective esophageal motility. Manometry is not indicated for the diagnosis and management of most patients who have GERD. However, the test is helpful in the preoperative assessment of esophageal motility in patients planned to undergo fundoplication surgery.

ACHALASIA

Achalasia is an esophageal motility disorder of unknown etiology characterized by both failure of LES relaxation and decreased or absent esophageal peristalsis. The incidence of achalasia is about 1 in 100,000, and it affects both sexes equally. It can occur at any age, but symptom onset is usually between the ages of 20 and 60. Achalasia occurs as a result of changes in Auerbach's plexus (the myenteric plexus located between the circular and longitudinal muscle layers), including inflammation, fibrosis, and loss of ganglion cells. This results in a loss of the postganglionic inhibitory neurons which contain both vasoactive intestinal polypeptide and nitric oxide. This leads to unopposed cholinergic stimulation, which causes high LES pressures and failure of LES relaxation. There is associated decreased or absent peristalsis, also due to the loss of nitric oxide. Chagas disease in Central and South America from *Trypanosoma cruzi* causes a similar denervation of the esophageal smooth muscle. As a result of immigration of persons chronically infected with Chagas disease, the incidence of this diagnosis is increasing in the United States.

Pseudoachalasia is the term for disorders that simulate the clinical appearance of achalasia. Tumors at the gastroesophageal junction are the main cause of pseudoachalasia and need to be excluded. Pseudoachalasia due to tumors is found in about 5% of patients diagnosed with achalasia.

The clinical manifestations of achalasia include dysphagia (both solid and liquid), regurgitation, chest pain, weight loss (often subtle), and aspiration pneumonia. Because the symptoms are slowly progressive and may start with dysphagia to solids only, most patients are symptomatic for years before seeking medical attention. Nocturnal regurgitation of solids occurs in about one-third of patients and may lead to pulmonary complications. Patients (especially those over the age of 60 years) with a rapid onset of symptoms (<6 months) and weight loss should be suspected of having pseudoachalasia. Chest pain is present in up to 50% of patients with achalasia, is more common in younger patients with earlier disease, and may last for hours. Weight loss occurs in up to 60%, and progresses with disease duration.

A barium swallow is the best initial test and characteristically shows a dilated esophagus with a smooth "bird's beak" narrowing of the gastroesophageal junction (figure 68.4). There will be a loss of primary peristalsis of the distal two-thirds of the esophagus with poor esophageal emptying, often with a dilated esophagus and an air–fluid level from retained food and secretions. Upper endoscopy should be done in all patients with careful inspection of the gastroesophageal junction to exclude pseudoachalasia due to tumors. The diagnosis of achalasia is confirmed by esophageal manometry showing decreased or absent LES relaxation, often with an elevated LES pressure and poor-to-absent esophageal peristalsis.

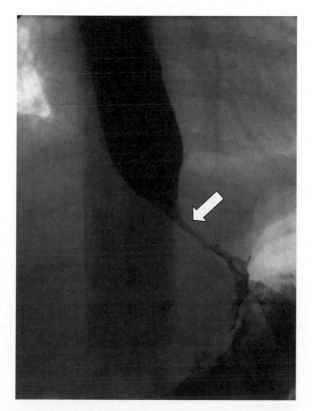

Figure 68.4. Barium Swallow Examination. Fluoroscopy shows a bird's beak smooth narrowing of the lower esophageal sphincter (LES) region (arrow) and a dilated esophagus in a patient with pseudoachalasia due to a gastroesophageal junction tumor.

Although there is no cure for achalasia, several treatments are available to relieve symptoms and improve esophageal emptying. Medications, including nitrates and calcium channel blockers, can reduce LES pressure and provide temporary relief of symptoms. However, the benefit of medical therapy is typically of short duration, and it is most commonly used as a temporizing agent before a more effective treatment. Endoscopic therapy consists of injection of botulinum toxin or pneumatic balloon dilation. The injection of botulinum toxin at the LES inhibits the release of acetylcholine from nerve terminals. It is effective in up to 85% of patients initially, but symptoms recur in over 50% of patients at 6 months. Although repeated injections of botulinum toxin can be given, this therapy is best for elderly patients and those at high surgical risk. Pneumatic dilation at endoscopy utilizes large balloons to disrupt the circular muscle of the LES. Patients have a good response in 50% to 93% of dilations, although about 30% of patients require repeat dilations. The main risk of pneumatic dilation is perforation of the lower esophagus due to the dilation. Because perforation can occur in 2–5% of patients treated with pneumatic dilation, patients treated by this method should be surgical candidates and have a barium swallow examination performed after the procedure to exclude this complication.

The most definitive therapy for achalasia is a surgical myotomy (Heller myotomy with surgical incision of the anterior LES). After laparoscopic surgical myotomy, a good response is found in 80–94% of patients. The development of GERD is a common complication of surgical myotomy, and some surgeons will also perform an antireflux procedure (fundoplication) at the same time as myotomy.

DIFFUSE ESOPHAGEAL SPASM

Diffuse esophageal spasm is a motility disorder characterized by the presence of more than 30% simultaneous and repetitive contractions in the esophageal body, which may be elevated in contraction amplitude. In contrast to achalasia, LES relaxation is normal, and normal esophageal peristalsis remains. Clinically, patients may complain of chest pain or dysphagia or both. On barium swallow, the classic appearance is a "cork-screw" esophagus. Medical treatment is usually not completely effective but is directed at relaxing the esophagus with calcium channel blockers or nitrates.

INEFFECTIVE ESOPHAGEAL MOTILITY

Ineffective esophageal motility is an esophageal motility disorder defined by low-amplitude esophageal contractions with a normal LES. This may result in increased esophageal exposure to acid and prolonged esophageal clearance times when recumbent. This is an increasingly recognized abnormality, especially in GERD patients with pulmonary symptoms.

NUTCRACKER ESOPHAGUS

Nutcracker esophagus is characterized by high-amplitude peristaltic contractions. It is often diagnosed in patients with noncardiac chest pain. It has recently been recognized to be a marker for increased visceral pain perception and not a primary esophageal motility disorder.

SCLERODERMA

Scleroderma is a syndrome caused by proliferation of connective tissue with fibrosis of multiple organs and a small-vessel vasculopathy. Gastrointestinal involvement occurs in >90% of patients, and esophageal involvement occurs in 70–80%. The effects of scleroderma on the esophagus include loss of esophageal peristalsis with eventual aperistalsis of the distal two-thirds of the esophagus and a very low or absent LES pressure. Esophageal symptoms of scleroderma include heartburn, regurgitation, and/or dysphagia, which may lead to esophagitis, strictures, and Barrett's esophagus. The combination of a patulous gastroesophageal junction along with esophageal aperistalsis with the inability to clear esophageal contents leads to severe and complicated reflux. Management of the esophageal manifestations requires aggressive medical therapy, stricture dilation (if needed), and surveillance for Barrett's esophagus. Surgical management of severe GERD with fundoplication must be carefully considered, as patients often have significant dysphagia postoperatively due to impaired peristalsis and the surgical tightening of the gastroesophageal junction.

ADDITIONAL READING

Arora AS. Management strategies for dysphagia with a normal-appearing esophagus. *Clin Gastroenterol Hepatol.* 2005;3:299–302.

Bohm M, Richter JE. Treatment of eosinophilic esophagitis: Overview, current limitations, and future direction. *Am J Gastroenterol.* 2008;103(10):2635–44.

Catarci M, Gentileschi P, Papi C, et al. Evidence-based appraisal of anti-reflux fundoplication. *Ann Surg.* 2004;239:325–37.

Francis DL, Katzka DA. Achalasia: Update on the disease and its treatment. *Gastroenterology.* 2010;139(2):369–74.

Furuta GT, Liacouras CA, Collins MH, et al.; First International Gastrointestinal Eosinophil Research Symposium (FIGERS) Subcommittees. Eosinophilic esophagitis in children and adults: A systematic review and consensus recommendations for diagnosis and treatment. *Gastroenterology.* 2007;133(4):1342–63.

Herbella FA, Patti MG. Gastroesophageal reflux disease: From pathophysiology to treatment. *World J Gastroenterol.* 2010;16(30):3745–9.

Horowitz M, Su YG, Rayner CK, Jones KL. Gastroparesis: Prevalence, clinical significance and treatment. *Can Gastroenterol.* 2001;15(21):805–13.

Hvid-Jensen F, Pedersen L, Drewes AM, Sørensen HT, Funch-Jensen P. Incidence of adenocarcinoma among patients with Barrett's esophagus. *N Engl J Med.* 2011 Oct 13;365(15):1375–83.

Kahrilas PJ, Shaheen NJ, Vaezi MF; American Gastroenterological Association Institute, Clinical Practice and Quality Management Committee. American Gastroenterological Association Institute technical review on the management of gastroesophageal reflux disease. *Gastroenterology.* 2008;135(4):1392–1413.

Lacy BE, Weiser K. Esophageal motility disorders: Medical therapy. *J Clin Gastroenterol.* 2008;42(5):652–8.

Moawad FJ, Veerappan GR, Wong RK. Eosinophilic esophagitis. *Dig Dis Sci.* 2009;54(9):1818–28.

Pace F, Antinori S, Repici A. What is new in esophageal injury (infection, drug-induced, caustic, stricture, perforation)? *Curr Opin Gastroenterol.* 2009;25(4):372–9.

Shaheen NJ, Sharma P, Overholt BF, et al. Radiofrequency ablation in Barrett's esophagus with dysplasia. *N Engl J Med.* 2009 May 28; 360(22):2277–88.

Sharma P. Clinical practice. Barrett's esophagus. *N Engl J Med.* 2009;3 61(26):2548–56.

Wang KE, Sampliner RE; Practice Parameters Committee of the American College of Gastroenterology. Updated guidelines for the diagnosis, surveillance and therapy of Barrett's esophagus. *Am J Gastroenterol.* 2008;103:788–97.

Zografos GN, Georgiadou D, Thomas D, Kaltsas G, Digalakis M. Drug-induced esophagitis. *Dis Esophagus.* 2009;22(8):633–7.

QUESTIONS

QUESTION 1. A 34-year-old male presents with intermittent dysphagia of solid foods for 3 years. He says that solid foods like chicken get stuck in the base of his throat, and he needs to vomit for relief of obstruction. He denies pain on swallowing with no difficulty swallowing liquids. He also denies heartburn, GI bleeding, and weight loss. Physical examination is normal. Endoscopy shows a ringed-like appearance of the esophagus with areas of linear furrows that are biopsied—pathology reveals an eosinophilic esophagitis. The next step in management should be:

A. Esophageal manometry
B. Initiate swallowed Fluticasone spray therapy
C. Referral to a surgery
D. Initiate omeprazole therapy
E. Botulinum toxin (Botox) injection of the lower esophageal sphincter

QUESTION 2. A 67-year-old woman complains of dysphagia, initially to solids, that has progressed over 3 months to both solids and liquids. She has no history of prior gastroesophageal reflux, and her only other medical problem is hypertension. Her only current medication is lisinopril. Her physical examination and routine blood tests are unremarkable. She undergoes a barium swallow, which shows a dilated esophagus with a bird's beak appearance of the gastroesophageal junction. The patient should next:

A. Be referred to a surgeon
B. Undergo an upper endoscopy examination
C. Be started on a calcium channel blocker
D. Have an esophageal manometry examination
E. Have a CT of the chest and abdomen

QUESTION 3. A 48-year-old woman with a long history of gastroesophageal reflux disease undergoes an upper endoscopy, which reveals several 2- to 3-cm strips of salmon-colored mucosa extending proximally from the gastroesophageal junction. Biopsies reveal Barrett's esophagus. *No dysplasia* is noted. Another endoscopy with biopsies 1 year later notes similar findings. What is the appropriate surveillance recommendation?

A. Biopsy of the Barrett's segment every 3–6 months
B. Biopsy of the Barrett's segment annually
C. Biopsy of the Barrett's segment every 3–5 years
D. Biopsy of the Barrett's segment every 10 years
E. No further surveillance is necessary

QUESTION 4. A 58-year-old presents with a 5-year history of progressive dysphagia for liquids and solids. She describes occasional nocturnal regurgitation of food. An UGI series reveals a dilated esophagus with beak-like narrowing at the level of the gastroesophageal junction. An upper endoscopy reveals no masses. Esophageal manometry is notable for high normal basal lower esophageal sphincter (LES) pressure, failure of the LES to relax with swallows, and esophageal body aperistalsis.

Appropriate management of her disease would include any of the following, EXCEPT:

A. Pneumatic dilation
B. Surgical resection of the distal esophagus
C. Surgical myotomy
D. Botulinum toxin injection

ANSWERS

1. B
2. B
3. C
4. B

69.

PEPTIC ULCER DISEASE

Tyler M. Berzin and Kenneth R. Falchuk

eptic ulcer disease (PUD) involves the stomach or duodenum and is a significant cause of morbidity and mortality both in the United States and worldwide, with a lifetime prevalence estimated at 5–15%. For a good part of the 20th century PUD was felt to be a condition related to stress and dietary factors. More recently, our understanding of PUD has been advanced by research into the role of gastric acid secretion and the benefits of various classes of antisecretory medications and, perhaps most importantly, in 1984, by Warren and Marshall, who identified *Helicobacter pylori* (*H. pylori*) as a pathogenic agent in this disease. Proton pump inhibitor (PPI) therapy and *H. pylori* eradication regimens have altered the natural history of what once was a chronic disease, and they have also reduced peptic ulcer complications, limiting the need for surgery.

PATHOPHYSIOLOGY

The formation of gastric and duodenal ulcers must be understood in light of the regulation of acid production and the normal gastrointestinal mucosal environment that protects against ulcer formation. The parietal cells of the gastric fundus and body are responsible for the majority of HCl secreted by the stomach. There are three major stimuli for parietal cell acid production: (1) acetylcholine secreted by the vagus nerve in the parasympathetic nervous system; (2) endocrine stimulation by gastrin from G cells in the gastric antrum; and (3) paracrine stimulation by local cells producing histamine. There are multiple overlapping negative feedback pathways through which decreased intraluminal pH in the stomach inhibits parietal cell HCl secretion.

Despite the acidity of the gastric lumen, where the pH drops below 2 during digestion, the epithelial linings of both the stomach and duodenum are protected by several factors. Mucous cells in the stomach secrete bicarbonate and a mucous gel rich in glycoprotein, creating a physical barrier and pH gradient between the acidic luminal interface and the more neutral epithelial surface environment. Duodenal

bicarbonate secretion is robust and helps normalize the pH of contents arriving from the stomach. Prostaglandin E may also play an important role in regulating the mucosal and epithelial microenvironment, as it appears to increase bicarbonate secretion, inhibit acid production, and regulate local blood flow.

CAUSES OF PEPTIC ULCER DISEASE

Peptic ulcers form when mucosal protective factors are overcome by a variety of mucosal aggressive factors, both endogenous and exogenous. Acid, pepsin, and bile are all potentially injurious to the mucosal lining of the gastrointestinal tract. Multiple abnormalities in the homeostatic regulation of gastric acid production have been implicated as potential contributors to PUD. These factors have included abnormal basal acid output, abnormal peak acid output (during meal ingestion), elevated serum gastrin level, and many others. Here we focus on two of the most important exogenous factors implicated in PUD, namely *H. pylori* infection and nonsteroidal anti-inflammatory drug (NSAID) medications, which exert direct toxic effects on the mucosa and disrupt mucosal protective factors. Zollinger-Ellison syndrome and other less-common conditions implicated in PUD are also reviewed.

HELICOBACTER PYLORI

Historical estimates have held that *H. pylori* was responsible for up to 90% of duodenal ulcers and up to 70% of gastric ulcers; however, the prevalence of *H. pylori* is decreasing in many parts of the developed world due to a number of factors including the emergence of effective *H. pylori* eradication regimens and improved sanitation. According to several recent studies in the United States, the prevalence of *H. pylori* among patients with PUD ranges from 35% to 60%. The prevalence of the infection tends to be highest in developing countries, with rates approaching 70–90% in the general population.

H. pylori is a helical Gram-negative rod primarily residing within the mucous layer of the stomach and occasionally attaching directly to gastric epithelial cells (either within the stomach or in other areas of the GI tract with gastric metaplasia). *H. pylori*'s mode of transmission is not well understood, but it may involve oral–oral or fecal–oral spread. The pathogenic steps in *H. pylori* infection may include disruption of the mucous barrier, bacterial production of ammonia (by the urease enzyme), elaboration of cytotoxins, and stimulation of local inflammatory responses. Multiple virulence factors have been identified in the *H. pylori* genome, including the genes *vacA* and *cagA*, which may induce numerous local effects including modulation of local inflammatory activity and direct epithelial cell damage. These virulence factors and others may play an important role in determining the clinical phenotype of *H. pylori* infection, which can vary widely.

In virtually all patients, *H. pylori* infection causes a chronic active gastritis, leading to a reduction in the acid-regulatory hormone somatostatin and a resulting increase in gastrin secretion and parietal cell acid production. Only a minority of infected patients develop PUD. In particular, *H. pylori* infection can lead to various patterns of gastritis, including antral-predominant gastritis (generally a high-acid-output state) and corpus-predominant atrophic gastritis (generally a low-acid-output state), as well as peptic ulcer disease, and gastric malignancies including gastric adenocarcinoma and mucosal associated lymphoid tissue (MALT) lymphoma (figure 69.1).

The reason *H. pylori* promotes ulcer formation in some individuals but not in others is not well understood. The mechanism by which *H. pylori* infection in the stomach can lead to ulcer formation in the duodenum is also the subject of intense investigation. It appears that the presence of gastric metaplasia in the duodenum allows local *H. pylori* colonization, triggering direct toxic effects and local inflammatory responses. Furthermore, *H. pylori* infection may lead to increased duodenal acidity due to modulation of gastrin and somatostatin secretion in the stomach.

NONSTEROIDAL ANTI-INFLAMMATORY DRUGS

After *H. pylori*, NSAIDs are the second most important etiologic factor in PUD. Common estimates are that up to one-quarter of patients using NSAIDs chronically (including aspirin) will develop duodenal or gastric ulcers. NSAID use is felt to correlate with a higher risk of bleeding complications and death in PUD. The injurious effects of NSAIDs are in part due to direct cytotoxic effects on epithelial cells, as well as inhibition of cyclo-oxygenase-1 (COX-1), with resulting reductions in prostaglandin production and bicarbonate and mucus secretion, and alterations in mucosal blood flow.

The risks of NSAID-induced ulcer formation and bleeding are greatest in patients with prior PUD and in patients using anticoagulant medications such as warfarin. In patients with NSAID-related PUD, cessation of NSAIDs is the optimal strategy to reduce the chance of ulcer recurrence. Among patients who require continuing NSAID therapy (including aspirin), misoprostol and PPIs have both been shown to decrease the risk of GI complications, although PPI therapy is preferred because of tolerability and ease of use. Recommendations vary regarding which NSAID users benefit most from concomitant PPI therapy. Generally, PPI cotherapy should be considered among NSAID users over 65 years old and should be strongly considered for patients on anticoagulation. For patients with prior PUD, *H. pylori* eradication

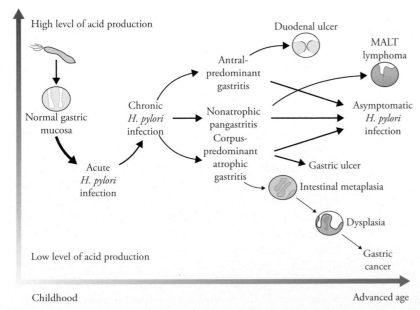

Figure 69.1. Natural History of H. pylori Infection. Reprinted with permission from Suerbaum S, Michetti P. Medical progress: *Helicobacter pylori* infection. *N Engl J Med.* 2002;347(15):1175–86. Copyright 2002 Massachusetts Medical Society. All rights reserved.

and continuing PPI cotherapy are mandatory if NSAIDs must be continued. COX-2–selective NSAIDs carry a smaller risk of GI ulceration, but the associated cardiac risk profile of COX-2 agents limits their practical usefulness. For patients requiring antiplatelet agents for cardiac disease, aspirin with PPI therapy has been shown to be associated with a lower risk of GI events than clopidogrel alone.

ZOLLINGER-ELLISON SYNDROME (GASTRINOMA)

The finding of severe peptic ulcer disease, particularly in the absence of obvious risk factors such as NSAID use or *H. pylori* infection, should trigger an evaluation for Zollinger-Ellison syndrome (gastrinoma). Zollinger-Ellison syndrome is rare, probably accounting for <1% of peptic ulcer disease. Multiple ulcers, severe gastroesophageal reflux disease, and malabsorption (leading to diarrhea and weight loss) are all classic findings of this syndrome, although many patients have peptic ulcer disease alone. Gastrinomas can occasionally be a feature of multiple endocrine neoplasia (MEN-1) syndrome and may therefore occur along with parathyroid and pituitary tumors.

If Zollinger-Ellison is suspected, a fasting serum gastrin level should be measured, preferably after a patient has discontinued acid-suppressive therapy for 7 days. Although a fasting gastrin level >1000 pg/mL is virtually diagnostic of Zollinger-Ellison, a moderately elevated gastrin level (>100 pg/mL at our institution) should be followed by a secretin-stimulation test, the provocative test of choice because of its high sensitivity. In Zollinger-Ellison syndrome, secretin causes an abnormal increase (of >200 pg/mL) in the serum gastrin level within minutes. Confirmatory testing then includes an octreotide scan (or *somatostatin receptor scintigraphy*), and an abdominal computed tomography (CT) scan or endoscopic ultrasound to localize the tumor, which is typically within the pancreas or duodenum in an anatomic region termed the *gastrinoma triangle*. Although PPI therapy may control acid hypersecretion, the risk of

malignancy (i.e., local metastatic spread) is such that gastrinomas must be resected when possible.

OTHER CAUSES OF GASTRODUODENAL ULCERS

Although NSAID ingestion and *H. pylori* infection are the two most common causes of peptic ulcer disease, numerous other conditions can contribute to ulcer formation (table 69.1). The term "peptic ulcer disease" specifically refers to ulceration occurring due to acid/pepsin exposure in the GI tract; however, we have also included other conditions that can cause gastroduodenal ulceration that may be mistaken for PUD (i.e., Crohn's disease and malignancy).

It is well known, although perhaps overstated, that gastric or duodenal ulcers can arise during critical illness. "Stress ulcers" are generally superficial and not a significant cause of major GI bleeding. The pathophysiology of stress ulcer formation is probably distinct from that of typical peptic ulcer disease and is thought to involve mucosal ischemia, hypoperfusion, and reperfusion. Historical terms have included *Cushing ulcers*, occurring in the setting of intracranial pathology, and *Curling ulcers*, occurring in burn patients. Known risk factors for stress ulcer formation include head trauma/neurosurgery, >30% burns, as well as mechanical ventilation and coagulopathy. Acid-suppression therapy with PPIs is indicated for stress ulcer prophylaxis in these specific settings. For the majority of patients hospitalized on general medical or surgical wards, however, stress ulcer prophylaxis is generally not necessary.

Corticosteroids are also frequently implicated in peptic ulcer formation; however, it is not clear that corticosteroid use alone increases the risk of PUD. Concomitant use of NSAIDs and corticosteroids, however, does seem to confer an increased risk of ulcer formation when compared to NSAID use alone. Other medications, including sirolimus and bisphosphonates, appear to be associated with PUD in some cases.

Chronic mesenteric ischemia can cause mucosal ulceration anywhere in the GI tract and should be a consideration in the evaluation of patients with nonhealing *H. pylori*–negative gastroduodenal ulcers. Advanced age, known atherosclerotic disease, and smoking are all risk factors for chronic mesenteric ischemia. Atherosclerotic disease of the GI tract may be clinically silent until two of the three major splanchnic vessels are involved because of the extensive collateral network within the GI vasculature.

Rare causes of gastric or duodenal ulcer formation include cocaine use (possibly due to vasoconstriction and/or thrombosis), herpes simplex virus and cytomegalovirus infections (largely in immunosuppressed patients), and Crohn's disease. Finally, gastric adenocarcinoma is always included in the differential diagnosis of gastric ulcers, and multiple endoscopic biopsies are mandatory to rule out malignancy in the setting of a nonhealing gastric ulcer.

Table 69.1 CAUSES OF GASTRIC AND DUODENAL ULCERS

NSAID use
H. pylori infection
Zollinger-Ellison syndrome
Critical illness (e.g., >30% burns, mechanical ventilation, brain injury)
Medications (corticosteroids, bisphosphonates, mycophenolate)
Ischemia
Cocaine use
Herpes simplex
Cytomegalovirus
Malignancy
Crohn's disease

CLINICAL PRESENTATION

Abdominal pain is a classic feature of peptic ulcer disease, but it is a highly nonspecific symptom. The abdominal pain of PUD is typically epigastric, nonradiating, and may occur in the postprandial period. Some patients will report improvement with antacid medications. Dyspepsia, a broader term that refers to a constellation of (usually epigastric) abdominal symptoms, including pain, bloating, and nausea, can be caused by a variety of disorders including PUD, nonulcer dyspepsia (symptoms in the absence of mucosal ulceration), pancreaticobiliary diseases, gastroesophageal reflux, and malignancy.

The three primary complications of peptic ulcer disease are hemorrhage, perforation, and obstruction. All three complications are occurring less frequently in the era of antisecretory therapy and *H. pylori* eradication; however, PUD remains the most common cause of significant upper-GI tract hemorrhage. Bleeding typically occurs when an ulcer in the stomach or duodenum erodes into a small or medium-sized blood vessel within the submucosa. Massive bleeding may be particularly likely in the rare circumstances when a posterior duodenal bulb ulcer penetrates the gastroduodenal artery or a gastric ulcer penetrates the left gastric artery. Melena (black tarry stool) is usually indicative of bleeding from the upper gastrointestinal tract (above the ligament of Treitz), and hematemesis may also occur. Massive upper-GI bleeding (typically >500 mL of blood loss) may also cause hematochezia (red blood in the stool). A number of clinical scoring systems exist, such as the Rockall score, that may predict outcome and mortality in PUD bleeding, although they are not consistently used in clinical practice. Most scoring systems identify advanced age, medical comorbidities, unstable hemodynamic status, and endoscopic findings of recent/active bleeding as the key features predictive of poor outcome. Appropriate triage to an intensive care unit, rapid resuscitation with fluid and blood products, proton pump inhibitors, and early endoscopic therapy are mainstays in the treatment of PUD with bleeding, a scenario in which mortality can approach 10%.

A peptic ulcer that erodes fully through the gastric or duodenal wall and into the peritoneum is termed a *perforating ulcer*. This is in distinction to the term *penetrating*, which implies erosion into adjacent organs (the pancreas, liver, etc.). The anterior wall of the duodenum and the lesser curvature of the stomach are the most common sites for perforation. Spillage of luminal contents into the peritoneum typically leads to severe abdominal pain due to peritonitis, which is accompanied by exquisite tenderness and abdominal rigidity on physical exam. Perforation can be confirmed by identifying subdiaphragmatic air on upright chest radiography or by identifying extraluminal air on abdominal CT scan. Urgent surgical intervention is mandatory.

Gastric outlet obstruction can occur either acutely or chronically in relation to peptic ulcer disease. Acute ulceration leading to edema within or near the pylorus or duodenal bulb can cause obstruction. Chronic ulceration with scarring can have similar effects. The typical symptoms of obstruction include nausea, vomiting, early satiety, and, in the chronic setting, weight loss. Physical exam may reveal distension and/or a succussion splash. Treatment of gastric outlet obstruction is initially supportive, including IV hydration, nasogastric tube decompression, and PPI therapy. Conservative therapy may be enough to relieve obstruction related to acute ulceration and edema in some cases, whereas obstruction due to chronic ulceration or scarring is more likely to require endoscopic dilation or surgery. The presence of gastric outlet obstruction mandates a thorough evaluation for malignancy with endoscopic biopsies.

DIAGNOSTIC EVALUATION OF PUD

In the absence of significant complications such as bleeding, perforation, or obstruction, the symptoms of peptic ulcer disease can be difficult to differentiate from other causes of abdominal pain or dyspepsia. If the history is highly suggestive of acid peptic disease (i.e., postprandial epigastric discomfort, alleviation with antacids, etc.), empirical acid-suppressive therapy with a PPI or H_2-receptor antagonist may be reasonable in patients who are under 55 years old in the absence of "alarm" features (table 69.2). *H. pylori* serology testing is also reasonable in this group of patients. Additional studies starting with upper endoscopy should be undertaken if symptoms do not subside with empiric therapy or if alarm symptoms are present.

TESTING FOR *HELICOBACTER PYLORI*

The first question to consider in discussing diagnostic tests for *H. pylori* is: who should be tested? Should all patients with dyspepsia be evaluated for *H. pylori*, or can specific subgroups of patients be identified for whom testing will yield the greatest benefit? The American College of Gastroenterology advocates a "test and treat" approach for *H. pylori* among certain patients who present with previously uninvestigated

Table 69.2 **ALARM FEATURES DURING EVALUATION OF DYSPEPSIA**

Weight loss
Anemia
Positive stool guaiac test
Early satiety
Dysphagia/odynophagia
Family history of GI cancer
Previous upper GI malignancy

Table 69.3 DIAGNOSTIC EVALUATION OF *H. PYLORI*

	COMMENTS
Noninvasive Testing	
Antibody serology	Inexpensive. Approximately 85% sensitive, 80% specific. May remain positive after eradication.
C^{13}- or ^{14}C-urea breath test	More expensive; >90% sensitivity and specificity. Can be used to document eradication.
Fecal antigen	Emerging option, limited data. Sensitivity/specificity similar to urea breath test. Can be used to document eradication, although may remain positive for >4 weeks.
Endoscopic Testing	
Histology	Approaching >95% sensitivity and specificity. The gold standard but requires appropriate biopsy sampling, tissue processing, experienced pathologist. Recent PPI or antibiotic use decreases sensitivity.
Rapid urease test	Can be >95% sensitive and specific, but results substantially impacted by PPI therapy. Can provide rapid diagnosis with commercially available kit.
Culture	Technically challenging and not widely available. Can provide information on antibiotic sensitivity.
PCR	Emerging option. Test characteristics include excellent sensitivity/specificity and information on antibiotic sensitivity.

dyspepsia. This approach is acceptable for patients under the age of 55 years and without "alarm" features (table 69.2). Noninvasive *H. pylori* testing (i.e., serology) is reasonable in this population, particular in regions where the prevalence of H.pylori is high. An alternative to the *H. pylori* test and treat approach in this group of patients is to begin with empirical antisecretory therapy (with H_2-receptor antagonist or PPI) and cessation of any NSAID use for 4 weeks, followed by *H. pylori* testing if symptoms persist. Endoscopy is indicated for persistent symptoms, for patients with alarm features, and in patients older than 55 years.

The most common noninvasive diagnostic tests for *H. pylori* are the *H. pylori* serology test and the urea breath test (table 69.3). The serologic test for antibodies against *H. pylori* is widely available and approximately 80% sensitive, but it cannot necessarily distinguish between active and prior infection. The urea breath test is more laborious and involves ingestion of radiolabeled urea, followed by measurement of the exhaled carbon isotope, which is released only in the presence of *H. pylori* urease activity. The urea breath test will only detect active *H. pylori* infection and may therefore be useful in order to document eradication. Fecal antigen testing for *H. pylori* is a third, emerging option that is only recently becoming widely available. The sensitivity and specificity of the fecal antigen test for initial diagnosis of *H. pylori* infection are similar to those of the urease breath test and serology. Furthermore, like the urease breath test, a positive fecal antigen test should generally reflect active infection; however, the test may remain positive for several weeks after *H. pylori* eradication therapy.

Histologic examination of mucosal biopsies obtained during endoscopy is considered the gold standard for evaluation of *H. pylori* infection with a sensitivity and specificity surpassing 95%. At least three biopsy samples are recommended for optimal sensitivity. Samples should be obtained from the stomach antrum and body. Biopsy samples can also

be assessed for *H. pylori* urease activity via a commercially available rapid urease test. The rapid urease test may be an excellent option if histologic processing and evaluation are not readily available. *H. pylori* culture is another diagnostic option and can provide information regarding antibiotic sensitivity; however, culturing the organism is technically challenging, and the sensitivity is generally lower than that of histologic examination. Polymerase chain reaction (PCR) tests are also being developed, which may have the advantage of very high sensitivity and specificity and may also provide important information regarding antibiotic sensitivity.

ENDOSCOPIC AND RADIOGRAPHIC EVALUATION

Esophagogastroduodenoscopy (EGD) is the diagnostic modality of choice for the investigation for dyspepsia in patients over 55 years old, for those with alarm symptoms (table 69.2), and for patients with dyspepsia that has persisted despite antisecretory therapy and/or the test and treat approach for *H. pylori*. Endoscopic evaluation provides several advantages over barium radiography and CT scan in the investigation of possible PUD. Endoscopy provides direct visualization of the mucosa, provides an opportunity for biopsy sampling of any abnormal findings and for *H. pylori* histology, and also provides an opportunity for intervention in the case of active ulcer bleeding. Nonbleeding ulcers may have endoscopic stigmata that suggest recent bleeding and increased likelihood of rebleeding. A clean-based ulcer (figure 69.2B) is less likely to rebleed than an ulcer with active bleeding at the time of initial endoscopic evaluation (figure 69.2A). Stigmata such as a nonbleeding visible vessel (figure 69.2C), an adherent blood clot, or a pigmented flat spot also predict a higher likelihood of recurrent bleeding. Among endoscopic findings of PUD,

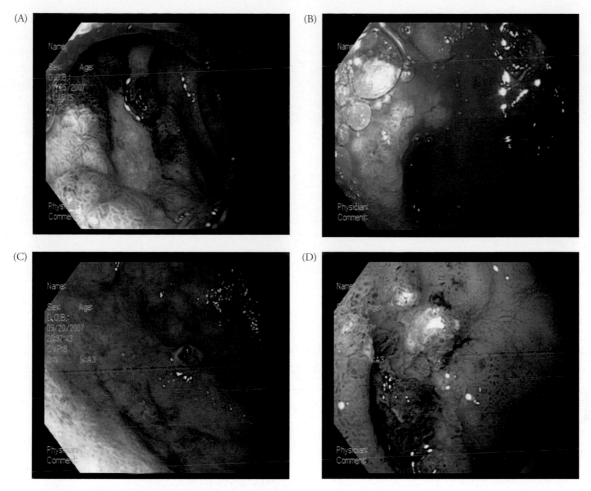

Figure 69.2. Duodenal Ulcer. (A) Clean-based duodenal ulcer with oozing blood. (B) Actively bleeding ulcer. (C) Visible vessel within base of large ulcer. (D) Duodenal ulcer after bipolar cautery therapy.

active bleeding during initial endoscopy predicts the highest rebleeding risk.

Repeat endoscopy is not required in the case of a duodenal ulcer if symptoms resolve with antisecretory therapy

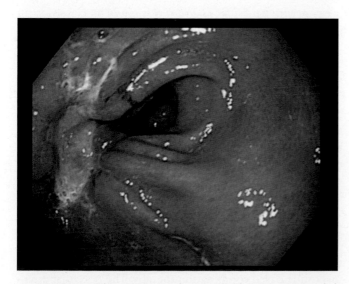

Figure 69.3. Gastric Ulcer. Large prepyloric gastric ulcer. Biopsies revealed adenocarcinoma.

and/or *H. pylori* eradication treatment. Gastric ulcers are managed differently because gastric malignancy can be mistaken for peptic ulcer disease (figure 69.3). The classic teaching is that gastric ulcers require at least seven biopsy specimens in order to effectively rule out malignancy, and many clinicians also recommend follow-up endoscopies to document complete healing of the ulcer. Although adequate biopsy sampling is mandatory, the cost-effectiveness of follow-up endoscopies for gastric ulcers is controversial, particularly in patients with clear risk factors for ulcer formation (e.g., NSAID use or *H. pylori* infection).

Upper gastrointestinal radiographs with barium (i.e., upper GI series) have excellent sensitivity for the identification of gastric and duodenal ulcers, but they are not frequently used in the investigation of PUD because of the advantages of endoscopic visualization and biopsy. Endoscopy has the added capability of identifying more subtle abnormalities, such as gastritis or erosions, that may cause symptoms but cannot be identified radiographically.

Upright chest radiograph is the initial test of choice if perforation is suspected, and many recommend a second plain film—either a supine abdominal film or left lateral decubitus film—for optimal detection of free air. Abdominal

CT and/or abdominal ultrasound can sometimes provide additional information if the suspicion for perforation remains high despite negative chest x-ray. Suspected gastric outlet obstruction can be evaluated initially by abdominal CT scan or upper endoscopy, but endoscopy remains mandatory early in the evaluation in order to obtain biopsies to evaluate for malignancy.

TREATMENT OF PEPTIC ULCER DISEASE

There are two arms in the treatment approach for peptic ulcer disease: (1) antisecretory therapy and *H. pylori* eradication to heal ulcers and prevent recurrence; and (2) medical, endoscopic, and surgical therapies to address the complications of peptic ulcer disease.

ANTISECRETORY THERAPY

PPIs and H$_2$-receptor antagonists are the mainstays of medical therapy for peptic ulcer disease. These two classes of antisecretory medications reduce parietal cell acid production and therefore increase gastric pH. Other medications, such as misoprostol (a prostaglandin), sucralfate, and antacids, are less effective at inducing ulcer healing, may require multiple doses per day, and no longer play a central role in the treatment of PUD.

Proton Pump Inhibitors

PPIs are the most effective class of medications for decreasing gastric acid secretion and inducing rapid healing of gastric and duodenal ulcers. PPIs directly inhibit HCl secretion by irreversibly inactivating the hydrogen-potassium ATPase on the parietal cell surface. The five PPI medications include pantoprazole, omeprazole, esomeprazole, lansoprazole, and rabeprazole. Of these, omeprazole and pantoprazole have been the most extensively studied.

For NSAID-induced gastroduodenal ulcers, one of the largest available studies has shown an ulcer healing rate (in the setting of ongoing NSAID use) of approximately 80% at 8 weeks with omeprazole 20 or 40 mg daily, compared to a 63% healing rate for ranitidine 150 mg twice daily. Without ongoing NSAID use, the healing rate at 8 weeks on PPI therapy approaches 90%. Similar data exist for other PPIs, and we tend to use the medications within this class interchangeably.

For bleeding peptic ulcers there is clear evidence to support a benefit for PPI therapy. An initial randomized placebo-controlled trial of oral omeprazole alone (i.e., *without* endoscopic therapy) for treatment of bleeding peptic ulcers demonstrated that the risk of continued bleeding or rebleeding was reduced from approximately 36% with placebo, to 11% in the oral omeprazole group. IV omeprazole given *before* endoscopy for upper GI bleeding appears to help initiate ulcer healing and reduces the need for endoscopic therapy for bleeding. Perhaps more importantly, a separate study on IV omeprazole given *after* endoscopic treatment of a bleeding ulcer reduced the rebleeding rate from 22% to 7%. The dosing strategy used in both major studies consisted of an 80 mg omeprazole IV bolus followed by an 8 mg/hr IV infusion for 72 hours.

After peptic ulcer bleeding or other complications have resolved, there is no clearly defined strategy to determine duration of oral PPI therapy. For large or bleeding ulcers, we typically recommend twice-daily PPI therapy for 4–6 weeks. For patients in whom ulcer recurrence appears likely (i.e., those with recurrent peptic ulcer disease or patients who must continue NSAID therapy), it may be reasonable to continue PPI therapy indefinitely.

H$_2$-Receptor Antagonists

The H$_2$-receptor antagonists, which include ranitidine, famotidine, cimetidine, and nizatidine, are also effective agents for inducing ulcer healing. This class of medications antagonizes the parietal cell histamine receptor, blocking one of the stimuli for parietal cell HCl secretion. H$_2$-receptor antagonists and PPIs are both reasonable first-line agents for mild dyspepsia and suspected ulcer disease or gastritis. H$_2$-receptor antagonists are not the preferred therapy in the setting of endoscopically identified significant ulcer disease or bleeding ulcers, because PPIs induce more rapid ulcer healing and reduce the chance of rebleeding.

H. PYLORI ERADICATION THERAPY

Eradication therapy is mandatory in all patients with peptic ulcer disease who are diagnosed with *H. pylori*. There is strong evidence to suggest that *H. pylori* eradication substantially reduces the risk of ulcer recurrence, including an initial trial that showed an 84% 1-year relapse rate in PUD patients with persistent *H. pylori* versus a 21% relapse rate in patients in whom *H. pylori* was eradicated. The recurrence rate is substantially lower now that *H. pylori* eradication regimens have become more effective using triple or quadruple antibiotic cocktails.

Several standard *H. pylori* eradication regimens are shown in table 69.4. The three standard regimens used in the United States have eradication rates that are approximately equivalent (~85%). We favor a twice-daily clarithromycin/amoxicillin/PPI combination for ease-of-use and tolerability. For penicillin-allergic patients, metronidazole is incorporated into the regimen in place of amoxicillin. The third combination in table 69.4, quadruple therapy with bismuth, may be particularly effective in two groups of patients: those with metronidazole-resistant *H. pylori* and those who have recurrent/persistent infection despite prior macrolide-based combination therapy. The potential disadvantage to bismuth quadruple therapy is the complicated

Table 69.4 SELECTED TREATMENT REGIMENS FOR *H. PYLORI*

REGIMEN	COMMENTS
Amoxicillin 1000 mg bid + Clarithromycin 300 mg bid + PPI bid (duration 10–14 days)	Typical first-line regimen, eradication rate ~85% in United States.
Metronidazole 500 mg bid + Clarithromycin 300 mg bid + PPI bid (duration 10–14 days)	Reasonable for PCN-allergic patients. Eradication rate ~85% in United States.
Bismuth subsalicylate 525 mg qid + Metronidazole 250 mg qid + Tetracycline 500 mg qid + PPI bid or H₂RA bid (duration 10–14 days)	Reasonable for PCN-allergic patients, eradication rate ~85% in United States. Complicated regimen. May be more effective for strains resistant to clarithromycin or metronidazole.

NOTE: bid, twice daily; qid, four times daily; PPI, proton pump inhibitor; PCN, penicillin; H₂RA, H₂-receptor antagonist.

(four times a day) dosing regimen. For all regimens, a 10- to 14-day treatment course is generally advocated, although there are emerging data in support of shorter duration of therapy. Continuation of PPI therapy after *H. pylori* eradication therapy for peptic ulcer disease is controversial, but mounting evidence suggests that eradication therapy is more important then maintenance PPI therapy in the prevention of ulcer recurrence.

ENDOSCOPIC TREATMENT OF PEPTIC ULCER DISEASE

Upper endoscopy is mandatory in nearly all patients with clinical evidence of upper GI bleeding. In the hemodynamically unstable patient with a suspected bleeding ulcer, every effort must be made to adequately resuscitate and stabilize the patient prior to attempting endoscopy. There are three primary therapeutic modalities in the endoscopic treatment of an actively bleeding peptic ulcer: epinephrine injection, placement of hemoclips, and cautery. Local epinephrine injection likely works in a temporizing fashion by causing tissue tamponade as well as vasoconstriction. Hemoclips and/or cautery are then used for more definitive treatment. Currently, the optimal endoscopic treatment for a bleeding ulcer consists of local epinephrine injection around the ulcer base, followed by the use of a second hemostatic method (hemoclip or cautery). Figure 69.2 shows a bleeding duodenal ulcer before (figure 69.2B) and after (figure 69.2D) endoscopic therapy with epinephrine injection and bipolar cautery.

As discussed previously, IV PPI therapy is clearly beneficial after endoscopic treatment of a bleeding ulcer. Biopsies for *H. pylori* are generally not obtained when an endoscopy is performed for hemostatic control of a bleeding ulcer; therefore, *H. pylori* serologic testing should be used to assess for infection. Although the identity of duodenal ulcers does not generally require biopsy confirmation, gastric ulcers may harbor malignancy (i.e., gastric adenocarcinoma, figure 69.3) and therefore must be evaluated carefully with multiple biopsy samples as described previously, either during the initial endoscopy or during a follow-up procedure.

SURGICAL TREATMENT OF PEPTIC ULCER DISEASE

The need for surgical intervention in peptic ulcer disease has fallen dramatically with the advent of potent antisecretory therapy and the identification of *H. pylori*. Elective surgeries to reduce acid secretion such as Billroth I or Billroth II antrectomy (or "subtotal gastrectomy") and truncal or selective vagotomies are now exceedingly rare. These surgeries reduce acid secretion either by removing the parietal cell mass (antrectomy) or by interrupting vagal stimulation of parietal cells (vagotomy).

Now, surgical management of peptic ulcer disease is focused primarily on the urgent treatment of ulcer perforation (typically at the anterior duodenal bulb and the lesser curvature of the stomach). Surgical intervention typically involves simple closure, omental patch, and/or ulcer excision, all of which may be performed laparoscopically.

Surgery is also a consideration when a bleeding peptic ulcer cannot be controlled endoscopically or with embolization by selective mesenteric angiography, in which case the bleeding ulcer can be oversewn. Finally, gastric outlet obstruction, which is a rare complication of peptic ulcer disease in the era of PPI therapy, is most commonly managed by antrectomy with gastrojejunostomy (Billroth II), with or without vagotomy. The gastroenterologist and surgeon must undertake a careful evaluation for malignancy in the setting of gastric outlet obstruction. In the future, pneumatic dilation by endoscopy may be a viable therapeutic option for gastric outlet obstruction caused by peptic ulcer disease.

ADDITIONAL READING

ASGE Standards of Practice Committee; Banerjee S, Cash BD, Dominitz JA, et al. The role of endoscopy in the management of patients with peptic ulcer disease. *Gastrointest Endosc.* 2010;71(4):663–8.

Chan FK, Ching JY, Hung LC, et al. Clopidogrel versus aspirin and esomeprazole to prevent recurrent ulcer bleeding. *N Engl J Med.* 2005;352(3):238–44.

Gralnek IM, Barkun AN, Bardou M. Management of acute bleeding from a peptic ulcer. *N Engl J Med.* 2008;359(9):928–37.

Kuroo MS, Yattoo GN, Javid G, et al. A comparison of omeprazole and placebo for bleeding peptic ulcer. *N Engl J Med.* 1997;336(15):1054–8.

Lau JY, Leung WK, Wu JC, et al. Omeprazole before endoscopy in patients with gastrointestinal bleeding. *N Engl J Med.* 2007;356(16):1631–40.

Lau JY, Sung JJ, Lee KK, et al. Effect of intravenous omeprazole on recurrent bleeding after endoscopic treatment of bleeding peptic ulcers. *N Engl J Med.* 2000;343(5):310–6.

Marshall BJ, Goodwin CS, Warren JR, et al. Prospective double-blind trial of duodenal ulcer relapse after eradication of *Campylobacter pylori. Lancet.* 1988;2(8626–8627):1437–42.

Marshall BJ, Warren JR. Unidentified curved bacilli in the stomach of patients with gastritis and peptic ulceration. *Lancet.* 1984;1(8390):1311–5.

Rockall TA, Logan RF, Devlin HB, Northfield TC Risk assessment after acute upper gastrointestinal haemorrhage. *Gut.* 1996;38(3):316–21.

Yeomans ND, Tulassay Z, Juhász L, et al. A comparison of omeprazole with ranitidine for ulcers associated with nonsteroidal anti-inflammatory drugs. Acid Suppression Trial: Ranitidine versus Omeprazole for NSAID-Associated Ulcer Treatment (ASTRONAUT) Study Group. *N Engl J Med.* 1998;338(11):710–26.

QUESTIONS

QUESTION 1. Which of the following statements is/are true regarding *Helicobacter pylori*?

A. *H. pylori* resides almost exclusively in areas of gastric epithelium.

B. Chronic *H. pylori* infection may be a risk factor for gastric adenocarcinoma and MALT lymphoma.

C. The prevalence of *H. pylori* is rising in most parts of the world.

D. A and B.

E. A, B, and C.

QUESTION 2. Which is the most sensitive and specific test for *H. pylori* infection?

A. *H. pylori* antibody serology

B. *H. pylori* fecal antigen testing

C. Histologic assessment of gastric biopsy specimen with at least three samples obtained

D. *H. pylori* culture of gastric biopsy specimen with at least three samples obtained

E. C and D

QUESTION 3. Which of the following should be a primary recommendation for patients with GI bleeding in the setting of NSAID use?

A. Cessation of NSAIDs if possible, initiation of PPI to promote rapid ulcer healing, and consideration of *H. pylori* testing

B. Cessation of NSAIDs if possible, initiation of H_2-receptor antagonist to promote rapid ulcer healing, and consideration of *H. pylori* testing

C. Administration of COX-2 inhibitors instead of nonselective NSAIDs

D. Evaluation for other risk factors for PUD including Zollinger-Ellison syndrome

E. None of the above

QUESTION 4. The optimal treatment of an actively bleeding duodenal ulcer is:

A. Endoscopic therapy with local therapy (cautery, hemoclipping, etc.) and administration of IV H_2-receptor antagonist

B. Endoscopic therapy with local therapy (cautery, hemoclipping, etc.) and administration of IV PPI

C. Endoscopic therapy with local therapy (cautery, hemoclipping, etc.) without need for antisecretory medication if hemostasis is achieved.

D. IV PPI administration, nasogastric lavage, and empirical *H. pylori* eradication

E. IV H_2-receptor antagonist administration and rapid referral to angiography or surgery

QUESTION 5. Which of the following endoscopic findings predicts a high risk of recurrent bleeding?

A. Visible vessel at ulcer base

B. Large size of ulcer (>2 cm)

C. Clean-based ulcer

D. Ulcer location in the duodenal bulb (proximal duodenum)

E. Ulcer location in greater curvature of stomach

ANSWERS

1. D
2. C
3. A
4. B
5. A

70.

DIARRHEA AND MALABSORPTION

Molly L. Perencevich and Robert S. Burakoff

DEFINITIONS

The objective definition of diarrhea is stool weight >200 g per day. The more common subjective definition is frequency of defecation that is greater than or equal to three stools per day combined with less-than-normal form and consistency. Diarrhea is also defined by duration. Acute diarrhea is defined as <2 weeks in duration, persistent diarrhea between 2 and 4 weeks, and chronic diarrhea more than 4 weeks in duration. In the United States most cases of acute diarrhea are due to infections and are self-limited. Noninfectious etiologies are more common in chronic diarrhea. The evaluation and general management of acute and chronic diarrhea are discussed in this chapter.

NORMAL INTESTINAL PHYSIOLOGY

Ten liters of fluid enter the jejunum daily with 2 L from food and drink and 8 L from luminal secretions (salivary, gastric, biliary, and pancreatic). Of this, 1 L enters the colon, and approximately 80–100 mL are ultimately excreted daily. This reflects the incredible reabsorptive capacity of the intestine. Diarrhea usually represents a 100-mL (or 1–2%) increase in fecal fluid. Many disorders that cause diarrhea do so by disrupting this physiology.

ACUTE DIARRHEA

ETIOLOGY

The most common causes of acute diarrhea are infective illnesses (90% of cases). Infective etiologies include viruses, bacteria, and protozoa (table 70.1). Noninfective causes include medications (table 70.2), poorly absorbed sugars (e.g., sorbitol), enteral feeding, ischemic colitis, and diverticulitis. Fecal incontinence and fecal impaction with associated leakage should also be considered in the evaluation of diarrhea.

EVALUATION

Figure 70.1 shows an algorithm for the evaluation of acute diarrhea. The history and physical exam can help you decide how much evaluation to pursue. Ninety percent of cases of acute diarrhea do not need diagnostic evaluation, as the majority of cases are mild and self-limited. However, there are several clinical features that require additional testing. These include:

- Grossly bloody diarrhea
- Profuse diarrhea leading to dehydration
- Duration >48 hours or more than six unformed stools during 24 hours
- Severe abdominal pain (especially if over the age of 50)
- Temperature greater than 38.5°C (101.3°F)
- Recent hospitalization or use of antibiotics
- Diarrhea in the immunocompromised or elderly

A detailed history about possible exposures can contribute to identifying the etiology of acute diarrhea. The following epidemiologic factors should be assessed:

- Travel
  - Traveler's diarrhea is caused most commonly by enterotoxigenic *Escherichia coli* and is found in endemic regions of Latin American, Africa, and Asia. Enteroaggregative *E. coli* is also a cause of traveler's diarrhea. Other pathogens commonly associated with travel include *Giardia Cyclospora* and *E. histolytica*.
  - Camping and backpacking in wilderness areas: *Giardia*.
  - Cruise ship: Norwalk virus.

Table 70.1 INFECTIOUS AGENTS THAT CAUSE DIARRHEA

Bacteria

- Preformed toxins: *Staphylococcus aureus, Bacillus cereus, Clostridium perfringens*
- *Salmonella* species: typhoidal *(S. typhi, S. paratyphi)* and nontyphoidal
- *Shigella* species
- *Campylobacter* species
- *Yersinia enterocolitica*
- *Escherichia coli*: enterotoxigenic (traveler's diarrhea), enterohemorrhagic (O157:H7), enteroinvasive, enteropathogenic,* enteroaggregative, and enteroadherent*
- *Vibrio cholerae*
- *Vibrio parahaemolyticus*
- *Clostridium difficile*
- *Aeromonas* species
- *Plesiomonas shigelloides*

Viruses

- Rotavirus*
- Calicivirus (including Norwalk virus)
- Adenovirus (serotypes 40 and 41)
- Cytomegalovirus (CMV)

Protozoa

- *Giardia lamblia*
- *Cryptosporidium parvum*
- Microsporidia
- *Cyclospora cayetanensis*
- *Isospora belli*
- *Entamoeba histolytica*

NOTES: * These pathogens tend to cause diarrhea more often in children than adults.

Table 70.2 MEDICATIONS THAT CAN CAUSE DIARRHEA

- Antibiotics
- Chemotherapeutic agents
- Anti-inflammatory agents: NSAIDs, 5-aminosalicylates, gold
- Antiarrhythmics: Quinidine, digoxin
- Antihypertensives: Beta blockers
- Antacids: Especially those containing magnesium
- Acid-suppressive medications: Proton pump inhibitors, histamine-2 receptor antagonists
- Colchicine
- Prostaglandins: Misoprostol
- Theophylline
- Antidepressants: Some SSRIs (citalopram, sertraline)
- Metformin
- Vitamin and mineral supplements

NOTE: NSAIDs, nonsteroidal anti-inflammatory drugs; SSRIs, selective serotonin reuptake inhibitors.

SOURCE: Schiller LR, Selling JH. In Feldman M, et al. (eds.), *Sleisenger & Fordtran's Gastrointestinal and Liver Diseases,* 7th ed. Philadelphia: WB Saunders, 2002.

- Food: Exposures include specific food items as well as outbreaks related to food handling.

  - Chicken: *Salmonella, Campylobacter,* and *Shigella.*
  - Undercooked hamburger, salad greens, bean sprouts: Enterohemorrhagic *E. coli* (0157:H7).
  - Fried rice: *B. cereus.*
  - Mayonnaise or creams: *S. aureus* and *Salmonella.*
  - Eggs: *Salmonella.*
  - Seafood (especially raw): *Vibrio* species and *Salmonella.*

- Immunocompromised states: This includes patients with primary immunodeficiency as well as acquired immunodeficiency (such as AIDS, malignancy, and immunosuppressive medications). In addition to common pathogens (which can cause more severe disease), these patients are also at risk of other opportunistic infections.

  - Opportunistic infections: *Mycobacterium* species, viruses (cytomegalovirus, herpes simplex virus), and protozoa *(Cryptosporidium, Isospora, Cyclospora,* Microsporidia).
  - Neutropenic patients are at risk of developing necrotizing enterocolitis (also called typhlitis), which is caused by invasion of enteric flora in the setting of mucosal injury.
  - Proctocolitis can be caused by agents transmitted per rectum such as *Neisseria, gonorrhea, Chlamydia, Treponema pallidum,* and herpes simplex virus.
  - Patients with hemochromatosis are at risk of infections with *Vibrio* species and *Yersinia.*

- Daycare: People who have children at a daycare or who work at a daycare are at increased risk of injections with *Shigella, Giardia, Cryptosporidium,* and rotavirus.

- Hospitalization or recent antibiotics: People with recent or current antibiotic use or exposure to healthcare facilities are at increased risk of *C. difficile* infection.

Symptoms can also contribute to determining the etiology of infectious diarrhea. Key symptoms to assess for include fever, nausea and vomiting, abdominal pain, quality of diarrhea (watery, bloody, mucoid), and quantity of diarrhea (volume, frequency). The clinical picture is often related to the pathophysiology of the organism, including the location of pathogen activity (small vs. large bowel; table 70.3) and the pathogenic mechanism (toxin production, adherent versus invasive organisms; table 70.4).

Infections of the small bowel often result in larger volume and less frequent diarrhea compared to infections of the colon, which usually result in more frequent and smaller-volume diarrhea. This is due to the greater absorptive capacity of the small intestine and reservoir capacity of the

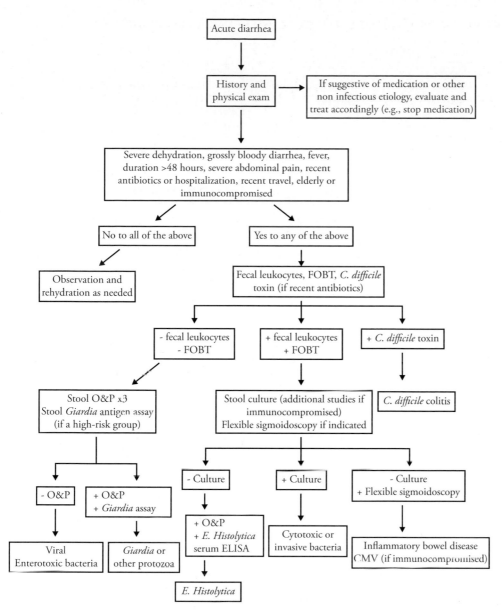

Figure 70.1. Algorithm for the Evaluation of Acute Diarrhea. FOBT, fecal occult blood test; O&P, ova and parasites; ELISA, enzyme-linked immunosorbent assay; CMV, cytomegalovirus. Modified from Sabatine MS (ed.). *Pocket Medicine: The Massachusetts General Hospital Handbook of Internal Medicine,* 3rd ed. Baltimore: Lippincott Williams & Wilkins, 2004.

distal colon. Diarrhea caused by pathogens involving the colon more often have blood and evidence of inflammation in the stool (which is described further in the next section). The pathogenic mechanisms listed in table 70.4 also correlate with symptoms. In general, pathogens whose mechanisms involve preformed toxins, enterotoxins, adherence to enterocytes, as well as most viruses tend to have a clinical picture with more vomiting and watery diarrhea. In comparison, pathogens that produce cytotoxins or are more invasive cause an inflammatory diarrhea with predominant abdominal pain, fever, and bloody diarrhea. Of note, unlike many other causes of inflammatory diarrhea, enterohemorrhagic *E. coli* (O157:H7) can present without a fever.

Several organisms have unique clinical syndromes and complications (table 70.5). Some organisms are more likely to cause significant dehydration or vomiting as well as gastrointestinal complications such as hemorrhagic colitis and

toxic megacolon. *Salmonella* has several clinical syndromes, including enteric (typhoid) fever, which is characterized by a prolonged fever in addition to gastrointestinal and other symptoms, gastroenteritis, bacteremia, and endovascular infections, localized infections (e.g., joints), and a carrier state. Enterohemorrhagic *E. coil* (O157:H7) and *Shigella* can cause hemolytic uremic syndrome. Several organisms are associated with reactive arthritis, including *Shigella, Salmonella, Yersinia, Campylobacter,* and *C. difficile.* This is an immune-mediated aseptic synovitis that usually occurs 1–3 weeks after onset of the diarrhea. The arthritis is usually asymmetrical, mono- or oligoarthritis of usually the large joints. There can also be enthesopathy, sacroiliitis, and dactylitis (sausage digits) of the extremities. *Campylobacter jejuni* is also associated with Guillain-Barré syndrome with onset usually within 3 months of diarrhea onset. Treatment with antibiotics does not prevent Guillain-Barré or reactive

Table 70.3 ASSOCIATION BETWEEN LOCATION OF INFECTION AND CLINICAL FEATURES

	SMALL BOWEL	COLON
Pathogens	*Vibrio cholerae* *Escherichia coli:* enterotoxigenic, enteropathogenic, enteroaggregative, and enteroadherent *Salmonella**# Rotavirus Calicivirus *Giardia lamblia* *Cryptosporidium*	*Shigella* *Escherichia coli:* enterohemorrhagic (O157:H7), enteroinvasive *Campylobacter** *Yersinia** *Clostridium difficile* Cytomegalovirus (CMV)* *Entamoeba histolytica*
Location of abdominal pain	Midabdomen	Lower abdomen, rectum
Volume of stool	Large	Small
Type of stool	Watery	Mucoid
Frequency of stool	Frequent	Very frequent
Visible blood in stool	Rare	Common
Fecal leukocytes	Rare	Common (except *E. histolytica*)

NOTES: *These pathogens can involve the small or large bowel, although most commonly affect the location under which they are listed. #*Salmonella typhi* and *S. paratyphi* act predominantly at the small bowel, while nontyphoidal *Salmonella* acts at both the small bowel and colon.

SOURCE: Hamer DH, Gorbach SL. In Feldman M, et al. (eds.): *Sleisenger & Fordtran's Gastrointestinal and Liver Diseases,* 7th ed. Philadelphia: WB Saunders, 2002.

Table 70.4 ASSOCIATION BETWEEN PATHOGENIC MECHANISM AND CLINICAL FEATURES

PATHOGENS	INCUBATION PERIOD	FEVER	NAUSEA, VOMITING	ABDOMINAL PAIN	DIARRHEA	BLOOD IN STOOL	FECAL LEUKOCYTES
Preformed bacterial toxins							
B. cereus, S. aureus	1–8 hours	–/+	+++	++	+++ (watery)	–	–
C. perfringens	8–16 hours	–/+	+++	++	+++ (watery)	–	–
Enterotoxin-producing Enterotoxigenic *E. coli, V. cholerae*	8–72 hours	–/+	++	++	+++ (watery)	–	–
Enteroadherent Enteropathogenic, enteroaggregative, and enteroadherent *E. coli; Giardia, Cryptosporidium*	1–8 days	–/+	+	++	++ (watery)	–	–
Cytotoxin-producing Enterohemorrhagic *E. coli* (O157:H7)	12–72 hrs	+	–/+	+++	++ (initially watery, quickly bloody)	+	+
C. difficile	1–3 days	+	–/+	+++	++ (usually watery, occasionally bloody)	+	+
Invasive organisms							
• Minimal inflammation: Rotavirus, Norwalk virus	1–3 days	+++	++	++	++ (watery)	–	–
• Variable inflammation: *Salmonella, Campylobacter, V. parahaemolyticus, Yersinia*	12 hrs–11 days	+++	–/+	++	++ (watery or bloody)	+	+
• Severe inflammation: *Shigella,* enteroinvasive *E. coli, E. histolytica*	12 hrs–8 days	+++	–/+	++++	++ (bloody)	+	+

SOURCES: Camilleri M, Murray JA. In Fauci AS, et al. (eds.), *Harrison's Principles of Internal Medicine,* 17th ed. New York: McGraw-Hill, 2008; Thielman NM, Guerrant RL. Acute infectious diarrhea. *N Engl J Med.* 2004;350:42.

Table 70.5 COMPLICATIONS ASSOCIATED WITH PATHOGENS CAUSING INFECTIOUS DIARRHEA

COMPLICATION	PATHOGENS
Dehydration	*V. cholera*, enterotoxigenic *E. coli*, rotavirus
Severe vomiting	Preformed toxins (*S. aureus*, *B. cereus*, *C. perfringens*), rotavirus, calicivirus
Hemorrhagic colitis	Enterohemorrhagic *E. coli* (O157:H), *Shigella*, *Salmonella*, *Campylobacter*, *V. parahaemolyticus*
Toxic megacolon, intestinal perforation	*Shigella*, enterohemorrhagic *E. coli* (O157:H7), *C. difficile*
Hemolytic-uremic syndrome	Enterohemorrhagic *E. coli* (O157:H7), *Shigella*
Reactive arthritis	*Shigella*, *Salmonella*, *Yersinia*, *Campylobacter*, *C. difficile*
Distant localized infections	*Salmonella*
Guillain-Barré syndrome	*Campylobacter*
Mimic of appendicitis	*Yersinia*
Erythema nodosum	*Yersinia*

SOURCE: Hamer DH, Gorbach SL. In Feldman M, et al. (eds.), *Sleisenger & Fordtran's Gastrointestinal and Liver Diseases*, 7th ed. Philadelphia: WB Saunders, 2002.

arthritis. *Yersinia* can have a clinical presentation that mimics acute appendicitis due to localization in the right lower quadrant, and onset can be more insidious than other causes of acute infectious diarrhea. It can also be associated with erythema nodosum as well as reactive arthritis.

Physical Exam

The physical examination is important to assess for degree of dehydration, fever, abdominal pain, and peritoneal signs, which will help guide evaluation and treatment.

Initial Laboratory Evaluation

A serum complete blood count, electrolytes, and renal function can be used to assess for evidence of inflammation, dehydration, and electrolyte depletion. These are helpful in assessing the severity of the diarrhea. Blood cultures can also be considered if a patient is sick and toxic appearing, especially if *Salmonella* is suspected, as it can often cause bacteremia and associated endovascular or localized infections.

Stool Studies

Samplings that test fecal leukocytes and occult blood are appropriate first steps. The standard method for assessment of fecal leukocytes is the Wright stain. However, there is variable sensitivity and specificity of the tests depending on processing and observer expertise. An alternative test is the fecal lactoferrin latex agglutination assay. Lactoferrin is a neutrophil product and therefore a marker of fecal leukocytes. This test has better sensitivity and specificity, but it is not widely available. Tables 70.3 and 70.4 above show the correlation between location and pathogenic mechanism to the presence of fecal blood and leukocytes. The presence of fecal leukocytes and occult blood often suggests a bacterial and inflammatory etiology for the diarrhea. Common bacterial etiologies include *Campylobacter*, *Salmonella*, *E. coli* O157:H7, *Shigella*, and *C. difficile*. The protozoa *E. histolytica* also causes an inflammatory diarrhea, although it often has relatively few fecal leukocytes.

If the stool is negative for fecal leukocytes and occult blood, and the patient is not severely ill, you can consider treating symptomatically for several days. The most likely etiology is either viral (more than 75%) or bacterial pathogens elaborating a preformed toxin or enterotoxin. Stool culture is positive in only up to 5% of these cases and is therefore not frequently informative. Diagnostic tests for viruses are not typically used. However, stool culture should be considered in several clinical settings:

- Patients with severe and bloody diarrhea. Stool cultures may have higher utility with cultures positive in 40–60% of cases.

- Immunocompromised patients.

- Sick patients with significant comorbidities.

- Patients with inflammatory bowel disease, in order to differentiate between infection and inflammatory bowel disease flare.

- Food handlers or concern for outbreak.

Routine culture usually includes *Campylobacter*, *Salmonella*, and *Shigella*. You may need to notify the lab to test for specific pathogens such as *E. coli* O157:H7 and *Yersinia*. A single specimen should be adequate for diagnosis as bacteria are shed continuously.

Additional stool testing should be done based on the clinical picture. If a patient has had a recent or current hospitalization or exposure to antibiotics within the past 3 months, a stool *C. difficile* toxin assay should be performed. If proctitis is suspected, a rectal swab can be done to assess for *Neisseria gonorrhea*, *Chlamydia*, and herpes simplex virus.

Testing stool for ova and parasites (O&P) is not indicated for most patients with acute diarrhea, but it should be performed in high-risk groups. These include:

- Community waterborne outbreak (*Giardia*, *Cryptosporidium*)

- Consumption of untreated water (*Giardia*)

- Exposure to daycare centers (*Giardia*, *Cryptosporidium*)

- Travel to endemic countries (*Giardia*, *Cryptosporidium*, *E. histolytica*)

- Men who have sex with men (*Giardia*, *E. histolytica*)

- Patients with AIDS (*Giardia*, *E. histolytica*, others)

- Bloody diarrhea with few or no fecal leukocytes (*E. histolytica*)

- Persistent diarrhea for greater than 14 days

As there is intermittent shedding of the pathogens (in contrast to bacteria), three specimens should be sent on consecutive days to evaluate for ova and parasites. Additional stool stains (acid-fast, trichrome) and antigen immunoassays can enhance detection of protozoa. For example, there is a stool antigen immunoassay for *Giardia* and a serum serologic test enzyme-linked immunosorbent assay [ELISA]) for *E. histolytica*.

Pathogens that should be reported to government agencies include *Salmonella*, *Shigella*, *E. coli* O157:H7, *V. cholera*, *Giardia*, and *Cryptosporidium*.

Radiological Evaluation

Radiological evaluation is rarely indicated unless the patient is severely ill or has symptoms of obstruction or peritonitis. X-rays and computed tomography (CT) scans can be used to assess for colitis, ileus, obstruction, toxic megacolon, and perforation.

Endoscopic Evaluation

Endoscopic evaluation is rarely needed in the evaluation of acute diarrhea, but it should be considered in several patient groups.

- Patients in whom the diagnosis of inflammatory bowel disease versus infectious diarrhea is not clear.

- Patients in whom the diagnosis of ischemic colitis is suspected but not clear.

- Immunocompromised or other high-risk patients should have endoscopy to evaluate for cytomegalovirus.

- Endoscopy can also be used to diagnose *C. difficile* infection by identification of pseudomembranous colitis, although this is used less frequently now with better toxin assays.

Flexible sigmoidoscopy is usually performed instead of colonoscopy in the evaluation of acute diarrhea, as it is usually adequate for diagnosis with decreased associated risks.

TREATMENT

Supportive Therapy

Rehydration is a principal part of supportive therapy for acute diarrhea. Oral rehydration can be very effective in many patients who are not severely dehydrated. The most effective oral solutions act on the glucose-sodium cotransporter, which remains intact in many diarrheal illnesses. The presence of glucose and salt allows the intestine to absorb water from the lumen. The World Health Organization (WHO)-recommended oral rehydration solution (ORS) is composed of 20 g glucose (or 40 g sucrose), 3.5 g sodium chloride, 2.5 g sodium bicarbonate, and 1.5 g potassium chloride per liter of water. The commercial over-the-counter WHO ORS (Rehydralyte) has 20% less sodium, so a larger volume is needed for rehydration. An alternative rehydration solution can be made with 4 tablespoons of sugar, one-half teaspoon salt, and one-half teaspoon baking soda added to one liter of water. There are also rice-based oral rehydration solutions (e.g., Cera-Lyte). Beverages intended for sweat replacement (e.g., Gatorade) do not have enough sodium and are not equivalent to ORS. However, they are often sufficient for mild cases in otherwise healthy people. Combinations of diluted fruit juices and salted broths can be used in a similar manner. Intravenous fluids (0.9% normal saline or lactated Ringer's) are often required in profoundly dehydrated patients.

Diet modification can also help with symptoms. In addition, adequate nutrition is important for regeneration of enterocytes. Boiled starches or cereals with salt, as well as the BRAT diet (bananas, rice, apple sauce, toast), are options. Because temporary postinfectious lactose malabsorption is common, a lactose-free diet is often helpful. In addition, avoiding alcohol, caffeine, and sugar substitutes may improve symptoms.

Other measures to improve symptoms include stopping any medications that are not necessary and may be contributing to the diarrhea (such as stool softeners) as well as adjustment of tube feeds (dilute to provide hydration, decrease rate, or add fiber) if relevant.

Antidiarrheal Agents

Antidiarrheal agents can be considered in patients with mild to moderate nonbloody diarrhea and no significant fevers. Antimotility agents that decrease peristalsis include loperamide and diphenoxylate atropine. Loperamide (Imodium) is usually dosed at 4 mg initially and then 2 mg after each loose bowel movement with a maximum of 16 mg per day for 2 days. Diphenoxylate atropine (Lomotil) is usually dosed at one to two tablets (up to 4 mg) up to four times per day for 2 days. It has central opiate and anticholinergic properties. Both agents can cause hemolytic uremic syndrome in patients infected with enterohemorrhagic *E. coli* (O157:H7). Bismuth subsalicylate (Kaopectate, Pepto-Bismol) is another antidiarrheal agent. It provides better symptom relief than placebo, but it is not as good as loperamide. The dose is two tablets or 30 mL every 30 min for eight doses. It also helps with symptoms of nausea. Probiotics (such as lactobacillus, acidophilus, *Saccharomyces boulardii*) have potential roles in the treatment of traveler's diarrhea and *C. difficile* colitis.

Empirical Antibiotic Therapy

Empirical antibiotic therapy has not been shown to have significant benefit in patients with mild community-acquired diarrhea in otherwise healthy patients, and it is not generally recommended in these cases. However, empirical antibiotic therapy is recommended in several patient populations:

- Severely ill immunocompetent patients with clinical features of fever, bloody diarrhea, dehydration, and more than eight stools per day or symptoms for longer than 1 week.

- Immunocompromised (AIDS, malignancy, transplant recipients) and elderly patients.

- Moderate to severe traveler's diarrhea (more than four stools per day, fever, blood or mucus in stool).

- *C. difficile* colitis.

Empirical antibiotics should be avoided in patients with suspected or documented infection with enterohemorrhagic *E. coli* because there is concern for increasing toxin production and risk of causing hemolytic uremic syndrome.

Fluoroquinolones are frequently used as empirical antibiotic therapy. Ciprofloxacin, 500 mg twice daily, levofloxacin, 500 mg once daily, and norfloxacin, 400 mg twice daily are typically used for 3–5 days. Alternative agents, especially if fluoroquinolone resistance is suspected, are azithromycin, 500 mg daily for 3 days, and erythromycin, 500 mg twice daily for 5 days. Fluoroquinolone resistance is of particular concern if *Campylobacter* is suspected; the high rate of resistance is thought to be related to widespread use of fluoroquinolones in poultry feeds. Empirical treatment for *C. difficile* and *Giardia* can be initiated if clinically suspected while physicians are awaiting confirmatory studies.

If an intestinal pathogen is identified, the appropriate antibiotic therapy should be initiated as outlined in table 70.6. Antibiotics are not generally recommended in enteric *Salmonella*, *Yersinia*, and *Campylobacter* infections unless the patient is severely ill, immunosuppressed, or has significant comorbidities. However, as bacteremia can occur in patients with *Salmonella* infections, patients who are at increased risk of seeding other sites (including patients older than age 50 and those who are immunosuppressed or have sickle cell disease, vascular grafts, artificial joints, or valvular heart disease) should receive antibiotics.

CHRONIC DIARRHEA

ETIOLOGY

The etiologies of chronic diarrhea are more diverse, and the evaluation often less clear. In developed countries the major causes of chronic diarrhea are irritable bowel syndrome, inflammatory disorders (inflammatory bowel disease), malabsorption syndromes (lactose intolerance, celiac disease), and chronic infections (especially in immunocompromised patients). In developing countries chronic infections (bacterial, mycobacterial, parasitic) are the most common causes of chronic diarrhea. Medications can also cause chronic diarrhea (table 70.2). In addition, fecal incontinence and fecal impaction with associated leakage should be considered in the evaluation of chronic diarrhea.

Chronic diarrhea can be characterized by pathophysiological mechanism as osmotic, secretory, inflammatory, steatorrheal (fatty), and dysmotility (table 70.7). Few etiologies cause diarrhea by one mechanism alone, and most cause diarrhea by several coexisting mechanisms.

Osmotic Diarrhea

Osmotic diarrhea is caused by the presence of poorly absorbed and osmotically active solutes that cause retention of water in the intestinal lumen. Electrolyte absorption is normal. It is characterized clinically by diarrhea that stops with fasting. There is often a large stool osmotic gap (the difference between the expected and calculated stool osmolarity) of >125 mOsm/kg (normal is <50 mOsm/kg). This gap reflects the nonelectrolyte substances that are causing the osmotic diarrhea. The stool osmotic gap is calculated by the following equation:

$$\text{Stool osmotic gap} = \text{stool osmolarity (usually 290)} - 2\,(\text{fecal }[Na^+] + [K^+])$$

The expected stool osmolarity is 290 mOsm/kg. Measurement of stool osmolarity is not routinely

	FIRST-LINE TREATMENT	ALTERNATIVE TREATMENT AND COMMENTS
Bacteria		
S. aureus, B. cereus, C. perfringens	Not needed	TMP/SMX only if severe
Salmonella • Enteric (typhoid) fever • Nontyphoidal salmonellosis	FQ for 5–7 days FQ for 3–7 days for gastroenteritis**#**; longer durations if other sites of infection	Check cultures for drug resistance, including nalidixic acid. Ceftriaxone, azithromycin, and TMP/SMX are alternatives.
Shigella	FQ for 3–5 days	Ceftriaxone, azithromycin, and TMP/SMX (if susceptible) are alternatives
Campylobacter	Macrolide for 5–7 days*	FQ is alternative (increasing FQ resistance)
Yersinia	FQ for 7–10 days*	TMP/SMX, doxycycline/aminoglycoside, and ceftriaxone are alternatives
Enterotoxigenic, enteroinvasive, enteropathogenic, enteroaggregative, and enteroadherent *E. coli*	FQ for 1–3 days	Azithromycin and TMP/SMX are alternatives
Enterohemorrhagic *E. coli* (O157:H7)	Not advised	Antibiotics should be avoided
V. cholerae	Doxycycline (single dose)	Ciprofloxacin or macrolides are alternatives
C. difficile	Oral metronidazole and/or vancomycin for 10–14 days	Stop offending antibiotics if possible. Treatment depends on severity
Viruses		
Rotavirus, calicivirus, adenovirus	No antibiotic therapy	
Cytomegalovirus	Ganciclovir or foscarnet for 3–6 weeks	Usually only in immunocompromised patients
Protozoa		
Giardia lamblia	Metronidazole for 7–10 days	Tinidazole and nitazoxanide are alternatives
E. histolytica	Metronidazole for 5–10 days	Followed by luminal amebicides (iodoquinol or paromomycin) to prevent recurrence
Cryptosporidium	Nitazoxanide for 3 days*	Paromomycin/azithromycin is an alternative. Difficult to treat. Immune reconstitution in patients with AIDS is helpful
Microsporidia	Albendazole for 3 months	Immune reconstitution in patients with AIDS is helpful.
Isospora, Cyclospora	TMP/SMX for 7–10 days	Ciprofloxacin is alternative. After treatment, patients with AIDS may benefit from maintenance therapy with TMP/SMX

NOTES: FQ, fluoroquinolones (ciprofloxacin, norfloxacin, or levofloxacin); TMP/SMX, trimethoprim/sulfamethoxazole.
* Antibiotics only if severe or if significant comorbidities.
# As *Salmonella* can cause bacteremia, endovascular infections, and other localized infections, patients who are at increased risk of seeding other sites (including patients older than age 50, immunosuppression, sickle cell disease, vascular grafts, artificial joints, and valvular heart disease) should receive antibiotics.
SOURCE: Thielman NM, Guerrant RL. Acute infectious diarrhea. *N Engl J Med.* 2004;350:43.

recommended because as colonic bacteria continue to metabolize carbohydrates, the fecal osmolarity increases, resulting in a falsely elevated stool osmotic gap.

Exogenous causes include ingestion of poorly absorbed ions (magnesium, sulfate, and phosphate) in the form of antacids and osmotic laxatives, as well as sugar substitutes and nonabsorbable fats that are designed to be poorly absorbed. Loss of a nutrient transporter, such as congenital disaccharide deficiencies (the most common of which is lactase deficiency, which affects up to 75% of non-Caucasians), leads to carbohydrate malabsorption and results in osmotic diarrhea. The bloating and gas symptoms that are common in lactose intolerance are due to fermentation of the nonabsorbed carbohydrate. Lactose intolerance can also be acquired for weeks to months after infectious gastroenteritis. Steatorrheal causes of diarrhea (as described below) also result in an element of osmotic diarrhea due to malabsorbed fat in the intestinal lumen.

Table 70.7 CAUSES OF CHRONIC DIARRHEA CATEGORIZED BY MECHANISM

Osmotic Causes

Ingestion of poorly absorbed agents
    Osmotic laxatives: Magnesium citrate, sodium phosphate, polyethylene glycol
    Nonabsorbed carbohydrates and fats: Sorbitol, lactulose, mannitol, Splenda, Olestra
    Lactase and other disaccharidase deficiencies: Congenital and postenteritis

---

Secretory Causes

Exogenous secretagogues
    Stimulant laxatives: Senna, Bisacodyl
    Dietary: Chronic ethanol ingestion, caffeine
    Medications: Prostaglandins, theophylline, colchicine

Endogenous secretagogues
    Bile acid diarrhea
        Postcholecystectomy
        Bile acid malabsorption: heal resection, ileal Crohn disease, small bowel bacterial overgrowth, fistula
    Hormone-producing tumors: Carcinoid (serotonin), VIPoma (VIP), medullary cancer of the thyroid (calcitonin), mastocytosis (histamine), gastrinoma (gastrin), colorectal villous adenoma (prostaglandin)
    Endocrine causes: Hyperthyroidism, Addison disease

Congenital electrolyte absorption defects: e.g., defective Cl/HCO_3 transporter causing congenital chloridorrhea
Loss of absorptive surface area
    Ileocecal resection
    Inflammatory bowel disease, microscopic colitis
    Colon carcinoma, lymphoma

Vasculitis
Partial bowel obstruction or fecal impaction
Idiopathic secretory diarrhea: Epidemic secretory (Brainerd) diarrhea, sporadic idiopathic secretory diarrhea
Dysmotility (rapid transit)

Steatorrheal (Fatty) Causes

Intraluminal maldigestion
    Pancreatic exocrine insufficiency
    Bile salt deficiency
        Decreased synthesis: liver disease, cholestasis
        Conjugation of bile salts: bacterial overgrowth
        Interruption of enterohepatic circulation: Ileal resection, active ileal Crohn disease

Mucosal malabsorption
    Celiac sprue, tropical sprue, Whipple disease, infections *(Mycobacterium avium-intracellulare, Giardia)*
    Small bowel bacterial overgrowth, short gut syndrome
    Abetalipoproteinemia: Inherited defect in chylomicron formation
    Medications: Colchicine, cholestyramine, neomycin

Inflammatory Causes

Inflammatory bowel disease (IBD): Crohn disease, ulcerative colitis
Microscopic colitis: Lymphocytic colitis, collagenous colitis
Immune-related mucosal diseases: Eosinophilic gastroenteritis, chronic graft-versus-host disease
Radiation colitis
Ischemic colitis
Diverticulitis
Infections
    Bacteria: *C. difficile, Mycobacterium tuberculosis, Yersinia*
    Ulcerating viral infections: cytomegalovirus, herpes simplex virus
    Invasive parasitic infections: *E. histolytica,* strongyloides
Malignancy: Colon cancer, lymphoma

(continued)

Table 70.7 *(Continued)*

Motility Causes

Systemic diseases: Diabetic autonomic neuropathy, hyperthyroidism, scleroderma
Irritable bowel syndrome (IBS), postinfectious IBS
Postvagotomy
Drugs (prokinetic)

SOURCES: Schiller LR, Selling JH. In Feldman M, et al. (eds.), *Sleisenger & Fordtran's Gastrointestinal and Liver Diseases,* 7th ed. Philadelphia: WB Saunders, 2002; Camilleri M, Murray JA. In Fauci AS, et al. (eds.), *Harrison's Principles of Internal Medicine,* 17th ed. New York: McGraw-Hill, 2008.

Secretory Diarrhea

Secretory diarrhea is caused by alterations in fluid and electrolyte transport across the intestinal mucosa resulting in increased intestinal secretion or decreased absorption. The hallmarks are that it is large-volume (>1 L per day), watery, and painless. It usually persists with fasting (although it can decrease with fasting if this decreases endogenous secretagogue production) and can occur at night. It also has a normal stool osmolar gap of <50 mOsm/kg.

Exogenous causes include stimulant laxatives, dietary secretagogues, and medications. Infection with *Vibrio* enterotoxins is also a classic cause of acute secretory diarrhea. Endogenous secretagogues include bile acids and hormones secreted by neuroendocrine tumors. Increased bile acid stimulation of colonic secretion can be caused by cholecystectomy (decreased bile acid storage) and bile salt malabsorption (caused by Crohn ileitis, small bowel resection, bacterial overgrowth, fistula). Hormone-producing tumors (such as carcinoid) cause secretory diarrhea by producing a variety of hormones (such as serotonin) that stimulate fluid secretion by intestinal epithelial cells. These tumors often have other associated symptoms (often systemic) related to the secreted hormones. Decreased intestinal surface area can result in inadequate fluid and electrolyte absorption resulting in a secretory diarrhea. This can occur with ileocecal resection as well as inflammatory or infiltrative processes of the mucosa (inflammatory bowel disease, microscopic colitis, colon carcinoma, and lymphoma). Rare congenital syndromes, such as congenital chloridorrhea, cause secretory diarrhea by lacking a specific transporter (in chloridorrhea it is the Cl^-/HCO_3^- exchanger). Other causes include vasculitis (ischemia or cytokines causing decreased absorption), partial bowel obstruction or fecal impaction (fluid hypersecretion), and rapid transit dysmotility disorders (reduced time for absorption). Last, idiopathic secretory diarrhea is a diagnosis given when no other etiology is found and the diarrhea is secretory. It can be epidemic (also called Brainerd diarrhea) or sporadic, and both forms tend to resolve within 2 years.

Steatorrheal Diarrhea

Steatorrheal (or fatty) diarrhea is due to fat malabsorption in the small intestine. The hallmarks include floating stool that is difficult to flush, greasy or foul-smelling stool, and associated weight loss and nutritional deficiencies related to malabsorption. The fat in the intestinal lumen causes a degree of osmotic diarrhea, so symptoms usually decrease with fasting. Qualitative evaluation of fecal fat is most commonly done with a Sudan III stain. The quantitative 72-hour stool collection while the patient is eating >100 g of fat per day is abnormal if there is >7 g of fat per day, but this method is rarely done due to difficulty in obtaining specimens and limited reproducibility. Stool steatocrit is the method more commonly used and has good correlation with quantitative fecal fat. This is performed by acidifying stool, which separates the fecal homogenate into lipid, water, and solid phases, allowing the lipid to be measured.

The causes of steatorrheal diarrhea are those that prevent intraluminal metabolism and absorption of fat. Intraluminal metabolism is disrupted by pancreatitic exocrine insufficiency and bile salt deficiency. pancreatic exocrine insufficiency is most commonly caused by chronic pancreatitis. Bile salt deficiency can be caused by decreased synthesis (liver disease), deconjugation of bile salts (bacterial overgrowth), or interruption of the enterohepatic circulation (Crohn ileitis, small bowel resection). Mucosal malabsorption can be caused by celiac disease, tropical sprue, Whipple disease, infections *(Giardia, Mycobacterium avium-intracellulare),* medications, and chronic mesenteric ischemia. Patients with mucosal malabsorption usually have larger-volume diarrhea because the triglycerides are still broken down to free fatty acids in the lumen, which causes increased diarrhea. In intraluminal maldigestion, the triglycerides remain intact, and stool volumes are smaller.

Inflammatory Diarrhea

Inflammatory diarrhea is caused by disruption of the integrity of the intestinal mucosa by an inflammatory process. The hallmarks of inflammatory diarrhea are mucoid and bloody stool combined with symptoms of abdominal pain, fever, and tenesmus. Stool examination is usually positive for blood (gross blood or fecal occult blood test positive) and fecal leukocytes. However, some etiologies (such as microscopic colitis) may not cause enough surface damage to cause significant blood or fecal leukocytes. The inflammatory process may also incite other mechanisms (fat malabsorption, secretory, dysmotility) that contribute to the diarrhea.

Etiologies of inflammatory diarrhea include inflammatory bowel disease (Crohn disease, ulcerative colitis), microscopic colitis, colonic ischemia, radiation-induced colitis, diverticulitis, eosinophilic gastroenteritis, chronic graft-versus-host disease, colorectal cancer, and chronic infections. Inflammatory bowel disease (IBD) can range from mild to severe symptoms, and can be associated with extraintestinal manifestations (oral ulcers, eye lesions, arthralgias, rash). Microscopic colitis includes lymphocytic and collagenous colitis. It is most common in middle age and in people taking nonsteroidal anti-inflammatory drugs (NSAIDs) and it presents with intermittent watery diarrhea. Macroscopic evaluation during colonoscopy is often normal, but the diagnosis is made by pathology. Eosinophilic gastroenteritis results from eosinophilic infiltration of the mucosa and is often associated with a peripheral eosinophilia. Chronic infections include *C. difficile*, invasive bacteria (*Yersinia, Mycobacterium tuberculosis*), ulcerating viruses (cytomegalovirus, herpes simplex virus), and invasive parasites *(E. histolytica, Strongyloides)*.

Dysmotility Diarrhea

Abnormal intestine motility can cause diarrhea. The hallmarks are a watery diarrhea, sometimes with associated cramping. Stool features are often similar to secretory diarrhea, but mild steatorrhea can occur due to malabsorption in the setting of rapid transit.

Abnormal bowel motility can be associated with other types of diarrhea (e.g., infection) as a secondary feature, but it can also exist as a primary etiology. Systemic causes of hypermotility include hyperthyroidism, carcinoid syndrome, and diabetic autonomic neuropathy. Medications (such as prokinetic agents) and vagotomy procedures also cause diarrhea due to hypermotility. The hypomotility caused by scleroderma results in bacterial overgrowth, which disrupts digestion and alters electrolyte transport, resulting in diarrhea. Irritable bowel syndrome (IBS) is characterized by abnormal motor and sensory function of the intestine and can manifest with intermittent diarrhea. It is also referred to as a functional diarrhea syndrome. The stools are often loose (not usually large volume), most often occur during the day and most commonly in the morning and after meals, and rarely occur at night. They can have a mucoid component and can be associated with abdominal cramping and urgency/straining. They generally do not have significant associated weight loss or metabolic abnormalities. Factors such as new-onset diarrhea in an older patient, weight loss, blood in the stool, and anemia or abnormal electrolytes argue against IBS. Ultimately, IBS is a clinical diagnosis for which the Rome III criteria can be used. The Rome III criteria include recurrent abdominal pain or discomfort at least 3 days per month in the last 3 months associated with two or more of the following: (1) improvement with defecation, (2) onset associated with a change in frequency of stool, (3) onset associated with a change in form of stool. Postinfectious IBS can also occur, often in patients who may have had mild IBS prior to the infection.

EVALUATION

History

The history is helpful in diagnosing the type and cause of chronic diarrhea.

- Duration of symptoms, rapidity of onset (abrupt, gradual), pattern (continuous, intermittent)
- Stool characteristics: watery, bloody, mucoid, oily; volume; frequency
- Associated symptoms: abdominal pain, fever, weight loss, fecal urgency and incontinence, bloating/flatulence
- Systemic symptoms related to IBD: arthralgias, mouth ulcers, eye symptoms, rash
- Epidemiological factors: travel, sick contacts
- Aggravation/mitigating factors: diet (dairy, alcohol, caffeine, artificial sweeteners), relationship of symptoms to eating and fasting, stress
- Past medical history: diabetes, hyperthyroidism, surgery, radiation therapy, coronary artery disease/peripheral vascular disease, immunosuppression, AIDS
- Medication history, including over-the-counter and herbals/supplements
- Sexual history (including anal intercourse), risk factors for HIV
- Family history: IBD, neoplasm, celiac disease
- Institutionalized/hospitalized: medications, tube feeding, fecal impaction, recent antibiotics, *C. difficile*

Physical Exam

The physical examination can provide information regarding the severity and etiology of chronic diarrhea. The abdominal exam is important to evaluate for abdominal pain as well as abdominal masses and hepatosplenomegaly. Scars suggest prior abdominal surgery. The anorectal exam should include sphincter tone, occult blood, and evaluation for perianal fistula or abscesses. Clinical exam features suggesting the degree of fluid and nutritional depletion should be evaluated (dehydration, wasting, anemia). Other organ systems should be evaluated for features such as skin rashes (dermatitis herpetiformis in celiac disease, erythema nodosum in ulcerative colitis), flushing (carcinoid), mouth ulcers (IBD, celiac), thyroid palpation (and other signs of hyperthyroidism), lymphadenopathy (lymphoma, HIV), and arthritis (IBD).

Initial Laboratory Evaluation

Initial laboratory evaluation is guided in part by the history and physical exam. Common initial serum tests include a complete metabolic panel with differential, electrolyte panel, total protein and albumin, thyroid function tests, and erythrocyte sedimentation rate (ESR)/C-reactive protein (CRP) Lab tests to evaluate for malabsorption include iron studies, vitamin B-12, calcium, magnesium, cholesterol, albumin, carotene, and prothrombin time to determine nutritional deficiency. Celiac serology with tissue transglutaminase antibodies should also be considered if clinically appropriate.

Stool Studies

Initial stool studies for chronic diarrhea include fecal occult blood testing, fecal leukocytes, and stool culture. In addition to inflammatory disorders, stool can be occult blood positive in small bowel lymphoma and celiac disease. If clinically appropriate, investigators can also consider *C. difficile* toxin, O&P (three samples), and stool assay for *Giardia* antigen.

Endoscopic Evaluation

Endoscopic evaluation is considered for many patients with chronic diarrhea. Flexible sigmoidoscopy is a reasonable initial test as it is often sufficient to diagnose and has fewer associated risks. However, colonoscopy is indicated in patients older than 50 years old (and who need colorectal screening), iron deficiency anemia, and suspected IBD (terminal ileum for Crohn disease) or microscopic colitis (10% of patients have histologic findings only in the right colon). Biopsies should be taken even if the mucosa appears normal in order to evaluate for microscopic colitis. Upper endoscopy with biopsy may be useful for the evaluation of celiac sprue, tropical sprue, IBD, *Giardia*, and other infections. Capsule endoscopy can also be used to evaluate the small bowel, especially for evidence of Crohn disease and small bowel tumors.

APPROACH TO EVALUATION BASED ON PATHOPHYSIOLOGICAL MECHANISM

If the diagnosis is not clear initially, it can help to categorize the diarrhea into one of the pathophysiological mechanisms described above (osmotic, secretory, steatorrheal, inflammatory, dysmotility), which can further guide evaluation

and treatment. Remember to assess for common problems that can often be overlooked, such as lactose intolerance, fecal incontinence, and medications. Figure 70.2 shows an algorithm for the evaluation of chronic diarrhea.

If the diarrhea appears to be *osmotic,* additional testing includes:

- Evaluation for lactose intolerance
  - Lactose breath testing or empirical lactose exclusion
  - Stool pH (<5.6 suggests carbohydrate malabsorption due to increased fermentation in the colon)

- Laxative screen (for inadvertent or secretogogues laxative use)

If the diarrhea appears to be *secretory,* additional testing includes:

- Evaluation for chronic infection (especially if immunocompromised)
  - Bacterial: routine stool culture, *Aeromonas, Plesiomonas*
  - Parasites: standard O&P, *Giardia* stool antigen, Microsporidia, *Cryptosporidium*

- Evaluation for structural etiology
  - Abdominal imaging and/or endoscopy with biopsy to evaluate the small bowel and colon for IBD and other mucosal diseases, intestinal lymphoma, and colorectal cancer. Imaging will also assess for pancreatic neoplasm. Colonoscopy will also assess for melanosis coli in the setting of frequent laxative use.
  - Mesenteric angiography computed tomography angiography (CTA)/magnetic resonance angiography (MRA) will assess for small intestinal ischemia.

- Evaluation for neuroendocrine endogenous secretegogues
  - Plasma peptides (e.g., VIP, gastrin, glucagon, calcitonin)
  - 24-hour urine collection for 5-HIAA
  - thyroid-stimulating hormone (TSH), adrenocorticotropic hormone (ACTH), cortisol stimulation

- Empirical treatment with bile-acid binding resin (cholestyramine)

If the diarrhea appears to be *steatorrheal,* additional testing includes:

- Qualitative examination of stool fat (as described previously)

- Evaluation of for small bowel bacterial overgrowth
  - Breath tests (lactulose, ^{14}C-xylose)
  - Small bowel aspirate and culture
  - Empirical trial of antibiotics for bacterial overgrowth can be considered

- Evaluation for mucosal abnormalities
  - Celiac sprue serology (antitissue transglutaminase)
  - Small bowel radiology and/or endoscopy with biopsy

- Evaluation for pancreatic insufficiency
  - magnetic resonance imaging (MRI)/magnetic resonance cholangiopancreatography (MRCP) can show evidence of chronic pancreatitis.
  - Secretin test: Exogenous secretin is used to stimulate the pancreas. Bicarbonate output is measured by aspiration of duodenal contents by ERCP. This is rarely performed due to being invasive and complicated. Secretin-enhanced MRCP is increasingly being used to evaluate pancreatic exocrine function.
  - Stool for fecal elastase and chymotrypsin: Noninvasive tests make them easier, but they are reliable only in moderate to severe pancreatic insufficiency.
  - A trial of pancreatic enzymes can be considered.

If the diarrhea appears to be *inflammatory*, additional testing includes:

- Evaluation for chronic infection (especially if immunocompromised)
  - Bacterial: routine stool culture, *Aeromonas, Plesiomonas Mycobacterium tuberculosis*
  - Parasites: standard O&P, stool *Giardia* antigen, *Microsporidia, Cryptosporidium*
  - Viruses: cytomegalovirus, herpes simplex virus

- Evaluation for structural etiology
  - Abdominal imaging and/or endoscopy with biopsy to evaluate the small bowel and colon for IBD and other mucosal diseases, intestinal lymphoma, and colorectal cancer

If the diarrhea appears to be due to *dysmotility,* additional testing includes:

- Evaluation for systemic etiology (hyperthyroidism, diabetes)

- Empirical treatment of IBS

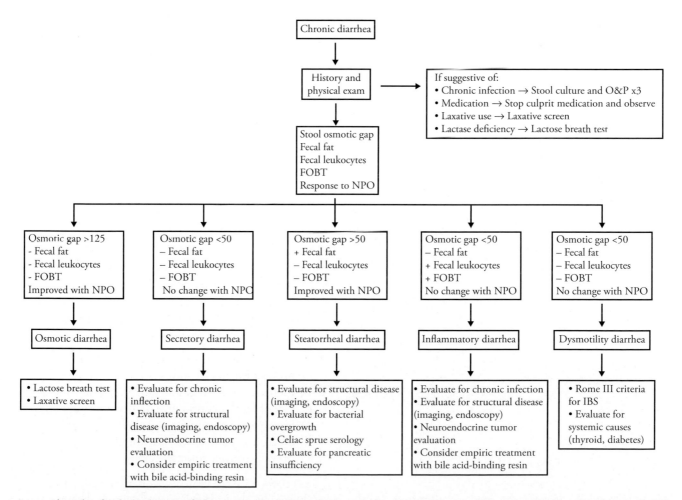

Figure 70.2. Algorithm for the Evaluation of Chronic Diarrhea. FOBT, fecal occult blood test; O&P, ova and parasites; NPO, nothing by mouth; IBS, irritable bowel syndrome. Modified from Sabatine MS (ed.). *Pocket Medicine: The Massachusetts General Hospital Handbook of Internal Medicine,* 3rd ed. Baltimore: Lippincott Williams & Wilkins, 2004.

TREATMENT

Treatment of chronic diarrhea depends on the etiology. If the underlying cause is reversible, such as stopping the culprit medication or treating an infection, the diarrhea should resolve with treatment. If the underlying cause is known but not reversible, treatment may improve the symptoms. Examples include a lactose-restricted diet in lactase deficiency, elimination of gluten from the diet in celiac disease, anti-inflammatory agents in IBD, cholestyramine for bile acid malabsorption, pancreatic enzyme replacement for pancreatic insufficiency, and octreotide for carcinoid syndrome. When the specific cause is not known but infection is not likely, antimotility agents can be used to relieve symptoms. Fiber supplements may improve stool consistency. Loperamide and diphenoxylate are often used for more mild cases. Tincture of opium, oral opioids, and octreotide can be used for more severe diarrhea. Probiotics are being evaluated, but no clear recommendations can be made at this point. For all patients, attention and treatment should also be focused on maintaining adequate hydration and replacement of electrolytes and fat-soluble vitamins if necessary.

ADDITIONAL READING

Bobo LD, Dubberke ER. Recognition and prevention of hospital-associated enteric infections in the intensive care unit. *Crit Care Med.* 2010;38(8 Suppl):S324–34.

Camilleri M. Chronic diarrhea: A review on the pathophysiology and management for the clinical gastroenterologist. *Clin Gastroenterol Hepatol.* 2004;2:198.

Donowitz M, Kokke FT, Saidi, R. Evaluation of patients with chronic diarrhea. *N Engl J Med.* 1995;332:725.

DuPont HL. Guidelines on acute infectious diarrhea in adults: The Practice Parameters Committee of the American College of Gastroenterology. *Am J Gastroenterol.* 1997;92:1962.

DuPont HL. Clinical practice. Bacterial diarrhea. *N Engl J Med.* 2009;361(16):1560–9.

Fine KD, Schiller LR. AGA technical review on the evaluation and management of chronic diarrhea. *Gastroenterology.* 1999;116:1464.

Grimwood K, Forbes DA. Acute and persistent diarrhea. *Pediatr Clin North Am.* 2009;56(6):1343–61.

Holtz LR, Neill MA, Tarr PI. Acute bloody diarrhea: A medical emergency for patients of all ages. *Gastroenterology.* 2009;136(6):1887–98.

Longstreth GF, Thompson WG, Chey WD, Houghton LA, Mearin F, Spiller RC. Functional bowel disorders. *Gastroenterology.* 2006;130:1480.

Musher DM, Musher BL. Contagious acute gastrointestinal infections. *N Engl J Med.* 2004;351:2417.

Thielman NM, Guerrant RL. Acute infectious diarrhea. *N Engl J Med.* 2004;350:38.

QUESTIONS

QUESTION 1. A 55-year-old man is admitted to the hospital for an elective removal of a cardiac pacemaker. Postremoval he develops a localized cellulitis at the incision site for which he is treated with intravenous antibiotics. On hospital day 3, the patient develops profuse watery diarrhea with leukocytosis and a low-grade fever. *Clostridium difficile* is the suspected cause of his diarrhea. What is the next best step in the management of this patient?

A. Send stool samples for *C. difficile* toxin analysis
B. Empirically begin metronidazole therapy
C. Empirically begin vancomycin therapy
D. Observe to see if the diarrhea is self-limited
E. Obtain a colonoscopy to evaluate for colonic pseudomembranes

QUESTION 2. A 22-year-old woman on a biking trip in Southern Spain drinks water from a fresh-water pond. Approximately 2 days later she develops a profuse watery, malodorous diarrhea, severe abdominal cramps, vomiting, and fatigue. The most likely diagnosis is:

A. *Clostridium difficile* infection
B. *Vibrio cholerae* cholera
C. Crohn disease
D. *Campylobacter jejuni* infection
E. *Giardia* infection

QUESTION 3. A 42-year-old man who presents to the emergency department with severe abdominal cramping and bloody stools is diagnosed on stool samples with an infection from enterohemorrhagic *E. coli* O157:H7. What should be the next step in management?

A. Vancomycin therapy
B. Supportive care but no antibiotic therapy
C. Treatment with ciprofloxacin
D. Obtain a colonoscopy to evaluate for colonic pseudomembranes
E. Levofloxacin therapy

QUESTION 4. An 88-year-old female nursing home resident with severe dementia is sent to the emergency department with a history of fecal impaction. The nursing home transfer note states that the patient has been complaining of abdominal distention, pain, and frequent small volume watery bowel movements. Manual disimpaction is performed. What would you recommend to the nursing home?

A. Start the patient on a regular dose of Dulcolax to prevent further episodes
B. Increase fluid intake and add fiber to the diet
C. Use of fecal incontinence diapers on a regular basis
D. Use of a positive-pressure rectal incontinence pad
E. Start the patient on an anticholinergic agent to prevent further colonic leaking

QUESTIONS 5. A 49-year-old woman traveling from Delhi to Chicago by air develops nausea, crampy abdominal pain, and watery diarrhea. She is a little dizzy on standing and has an increase in her heart rate with standing, but her blood pressure is 130/82 mm Hg. You are asked to evaluate the patient midflight. Limited examination is unremarkable except for some mild but diffuse abdominal tenderness. The best next step is to:

A. Ask the flight attendant if anyone on the plane has diphenoxylate and atropine (Lomotil) and start the patient on therapy immediately
B. Initiate oral hydration and observe the patient carefully
C. Administer acetaminophen for abdominal pain and observe the patient
D. Advise the patient to avoid eating, especially milk-containing foods
E. Recommend to the airline staff that the plane land immediately

ANSWERS

1. A
2. E
3. B
4. B
5. B

71.

INFLAMMATORY BOWEL DISEASE

Sonia Friedman

Inflammatory bowel disease (IBD) is a chronic inflammatory disease of the gastrointestinal tract that can affect any site from the mouth to the anus. The two major types of IBD are Crohn's disease (CD) and ulcerative colitis (UC).

EPIDEMIOLOGY

In North America, incidence rates range from 2.2 to 14.3 cases per 100,000 person-years for UC and from 3.1 to 14.6 cases per 100,000 person years for CD. Prevalence ranges from 37 to 246 cases per person-year for UC and from 26 to 199 cases per 100,000 person years for CD. IBD is slightly less common in Europe and rare in other areas except Israel, Australia, and South Africa. The highest mortality is during the first years of disease and in long-duration disease, due to the risk of colon cancer.

The peak age of onset of IBD is between 15 and 30 years. A second peak occurs between the ages of 60 and 80. The male-to-female ratio for UC is 1:1 and for CD is 1.1–1.8:1. UC and CD have a two- to fourfold increased frequency in the Jewish populations in the United States, Europe, and South Africa and occur more frequently in Ashkenazi than Sephardic Jews. The prevalence decreases progressively in non-Jewish, Caucasian, African-American, Hispanic, and Asian populations.

The effects of cigarette smoking are different in patients with UC and CD. The risk of UC in smokers is 40% that of nonsmokers, and former smokers have a 1.7-fold higher risk for UC than those who have never smoked. In contrast, smoking is associated with a twofold increased risk of developing CD. Appendectomy, especially before the age of 20, is protective against UC but increases the risk of CD. Oral contraceptive use may be associated with an increased risk of CD with an odds ratio in some studies of 1.4.

IBD runs in families. If a patient has IBD, the lifetime risk that a first-degree relative will be affected is about 10%. If both parents have IBD, the risk of a child developing it is about 36%. In twin studies, concordance of monozygotic twins for CD is 58%, and that for dizygotic twins is 4%. For UC, there is a concordance among monozygotic twins of 6% and no concordance in dizygotic twins. Anatomical site and clinical subtype of Crohn's disease is also concordant within families.

PATHOLOGY

ULCERATIVE COLITIS

UC is a mucosal disease that almost always involves the rectum and extends proximally to involve part or all of the colon. Forty to fifty percent of patients have disease limited to the rectum (proctitis) and rectosigmoid colon (proctosigmoiditis). Thirty to forty percent of patients have disease extending beyond the sigmoid but not involving the whole colon (extensive colitis), and 20% have a total or "pan" colitis. When the whole colon is involved, inflammation may extend 1–2 cm into the terminal ileum. This is called "backwash ileitis" and is probably of no clinical significance.

When the colon is mildly inflamed, the mucosa has a granular appearance. With more severe inflammation, the mucosa is edematous, erythematous, and hemorrhagic. Frank ulcerations are associated with fulminant colitis and are a warning sign that the patient requires urgent intervention to avoid perforation. In long-standing disease, inflammatory polyps (pseudopolyps) may be present as a result of epithelial regeneration. In remission the mucosa may appear normal, but in patients with many years of poorly treated inflammation, it appears atrophic and featureless, and the whole colon becomes narrowed and shortened.

CROHN'S DISEASE

CD can affect any part of the gastrointestinal tract from the mouth to the anus. Thirty to forty percent of patients have small bowel disease alone, 40–55% have disease involving both the large and small intestines, and 15–25% have colitis alone. In the 75% of patients with small intestinal disease, the terminal ileum is involved in 90%. Unlike UC, which almost always involves the rectum, the rectum is often spared in CD. CD is segmental with skip areas in the middle of diseased intestine. Perirectal fistulas, fissures, abscesses, and anal stenosis are present in one-third of patients with CD, particularly those with colonic involvement. Rarely, CD may also involve the liver or the pancreas.

Unlike UC, CD is a transmural process. Endoscopically, aphthous or small superficial ulcerations characterize mild disease; in moderate disease stellate ulcerations fuse longitudinally or transversely to demarcate islands of mucosa that are frequently histologically normal. This "cobblestone" appearance is characteristic of CD. As in UC, pseudopolyps can form in CD. Active CD is characterized by focal inflammation and formation of fistula tracts, and eventual fibrosis and stricturing of the bowel. Chronic and recurrent bowel obstructions are caused by a narrowing and thickening of the bowel. Projections of thickened mesentery, "creeping fat," encase the bowel and serosal and mesenteric inflammation promote fistula formation.

CLINICAL PRESENTATION

ULCERATIVE COLITIS

The clinical presentation of UC depends on the location of the disease. The major symptoms of UC are diarrhea, bleeding, tenesmus, passage of mucus, and crampy abdominal pain (table 71.1). Patients with proctitis alone tend to have bleeding and constipation because the stool is backed up behind an inflamed rectum. Patients with more extensive colitis have blood mixed with the stool or grossly bloody diarrhea. When the disease is severe, patients pass a liquid stool containing blood, pus, and fecal matter. Diarrhea is often nocturnal or postprandial and is almost always urgent. Although severe pain is not a predominant symptom, patients typically experience low-grade, crampy abdominal

Table 71.1 ULCERATIVE COLITIS: DISEASE PRESENTATION

	MILD	MODERATE	SEVERE
Bowel movements	<4 per day	4–6 per day	>6 per day
Blood in stool	Small	Moderate	Severe
Fever	None	<37.5°C mean	>37.5°C mean
Tachycardia	None	<90 mean pulse	>90 mean pulse
Anemia	Mild	>75% of normal	≤75% of normal
Sedimentation rate	<30 mm		>30 mm

pain relieved by defecation. Other symptoms in moderate to severe disease include anorexia, nausea, vomiting, fever, and weight loss.

The physical examination in patients with proctitis is significant for a tender anal canal and blood on rectal examination. With more extensive disease, patients have tenderness to palpation directly over the inflamed parts of the colon. Patients with a toxic colitis have severe pain and bleeding, and those with megacolon have hepatic tympany. Both may have signs of peritonitis if a perforation has occurred.

Complications

Only 15% of patients with UC present initially with severe disease. Massive hemorrhage occurs in 1% of patients, and treatment for the inflammation usually stops the bleeding. A colectomy is indicated if a patient requires more than 6–8 units of blood within 1–2 days. Toxic megacolon occurs when the transverse colon dilates to more than 5–6 cm and can occur in about 5–6% of attacks. It can be precipitated by electrolyte imbalances, prolonged bed rest, and narcotics. About 50% of acute colonic dilations will resolve with medical therapy alone, but the rest will require surgical intervention. Perforation is the most dangerous of complications, and the symptoms of peritonitis may be masked by high doses of glucocorticoids. The mortality rate for a perforated toxic megacolon is 15%. Rare patients may develop a toxic colitis with severe ulcerations that may perforate without first dilating. Colon strictures that form in patients with UC have a high probability of being malignant, and surgical resection should be performed if a colonoscope cannot be passed through the stricture.

Laboratory Findings

Active disease is associated with a rise in acute-phase reactants (C-reactive protein [CRP]), erythrocyte sedimentation rate (ESR), and platelet count and a decrease in hemoglobin. In severely ill patients, the serum albumin will fall quickly. Leukocytosis may be present but is not an indicator of disease severity. Stool cultures for bacterial pathogens, *Clostridium difficile* toxin, ova, and parasites should be performed. Diagnosis is based on negative stool examination and a sigmoidoscopy and biopsy, which reveal chronic active inflammation.

Endoscopic and Radiographic Findings

Sigmoidoscopy is used to assess disease activity. If the patient is not acutely flaring, a full colonoscopy is very helpful in assessing extent of disease. Pathology is also very helpful in grading disease activity. Colonoscopy is more useful than barium enema and computed tomography (CT) scanning in assessing extent and activity of UC.

CROHN'S DISEASE

CD usually presents as acute or chronic bowel inflammation and evolves to one of two disease phenotypes: a fibrostenotic-obstructing pattern or a penetrating fistulous pattern (table 71.2). Disease location and disease phenotype dictate treatment and prognosis.

Ileocolitis

The most common site of inflammation is the terminal ileum, and the most common presentation is a history of diarrhea, night sweats, gradual weight loss, and right lower quadrant pain. Pain is usually crampy and precedes and is relieved by defecation. It is uncommon to have frankly bloody diarrhea. Sometimes, the presentation will mimic acute appendicitis with significant right lower quadrant pain, a palpable mass, fever, and leukocytosis. Usually the fever is low grade; a high-grade fever suggests that an intra-abdominal abscess might be present. Because Crohn's disease has a more insidious onset than UC, symptoms may be ignored until they are severe, and 10–20% of body weight is often lost.

An inflammatory mass may be palpated in the right lower quadrant of the abdomen. This mass is composed of inflamed bowel, adherent and thickened mesentery, and enlarged abdominal lymph nodes. Extension of the mass can cause right ureter or bladder inflammation or obstruction of the right Fallopian tube in women. Edema, bowel wall thickening, and fibrosis of the bowel wall account for the radiographic "string sign" of a narrowed small bowel lumen.

With inadequate or no treatment, bowel obstruction can occur. Inflammation can cause edema of the bowel wall and intermittent pain and obstructive symptoms. The inflamed bowel wall will eventually scar down and form a stricture. In this scenario, obstruction is caused by impacted food or medication and can be resolved by intravenous fluids, nasogastric decompression, and bowel rest.

Table 71.2 **VIENNA CLASSIFICATION OF CROHN'S DISEASE**

Age at diagnosis
A1 <40 years
A2 ≥40 years

Location
L1 Terminal ileum
L2 Colon
L3 Ileocolon
L4 Upper gastrointestinal

Behavior
B1 Nonstricturing, nonpenetrating
B2 Stricturing
B3 Penetrating

Severe inflammation of the ileocecal area may lead to localized wall thinning with microperforation and fistula formation to the adjacent bowel, skin, bladder, or to an abscess cavity in the mesentery. Enterovesical fistulas usually present as dysuria or recurrent bladder infections or, less commonly, with pneumaturia or fecaluria. Enterocutaneous fistulas typically drain through abdominal surgical scars. Enterovaginal fistulas are rare and only occur in women who have had a hysterectomy. Patients present with dyspareunia or with a foul-smelling, often painful vaginal discharge.

Colitis and Perianal Disease

Patients present with low-grade fevers, abdominal pain, weight loss, crampy abdominal pain, and nonbloody diarrhea. Pain is caused by passage of stool through a narrowed and inflamed colon, and diarrhea can be partially due to rectal inflammation with decreased compliance. Toxic megacolon is rare in Crohn's colitis, as is gross bleeding. Stricturing in the colon occurs in 4–16% of patients and can cause symptoms of bowel obstruction. If a colonoscope cannot pass through the stricture, surgery is recommended because of the risk of a hidden colon cancer. Colonic disease may fistulize into the stomach or duodenum, causing feculent vomiting, or to the small bowel, causing diarrhea by short-circuiting of intestinal contents. Ten percent of women with Crohn's colitis will develop a rectovaginal fistula.

One-third of patients with Crohn's colitis develop perianal disease manifested by incontinence, large hemorrhoidal skin tags, anorectal fistulas, anal strictures, and perirectal abscesses. Not all patients with perianal disease will have evidence of colonic inflammation.

Jejunoileitis

Extensive Crohn's disease of the small intestine is associated with a loss of digestive and absorptive surface, resulting in malabsorption and weight loss. Patients will often have nutritional deficiencies including vitamin D, calcium, niacin, and vitamin B-12 deficiency and should be checked for these as well as for osteoporosis. Malabsorption can also cause hypoalbuminemia, hypomagnesemia, coagulopathy, and hyperoxaluria with nephrolithiasis in patients with an intact colon. Diarrhea is characteristic of active disease and is due to a combination of active inflammation, bacterial overgrowth from Crohn's strictures, and bile acid and occasionally fatty acid malabsorption due to extensive ileal disease.

Gastroduodenal Disease

Symptoms and signs of upper-gastrointestinal-tract disease include nausea, vomiting, epigastric pain, and an *Helicobacter pylori*–negative gastritis. Patients can present with a gastric outlet obstruction due to a stricture at the pylorus or in the duodenum. The second portion of the duodenum is more commonly involved than the duodenal bulb. Fistulas involving the stomach or duodenum can arise from the small or large bowel and do not necessarily signify the presence of upper-gastrointestinal-tract involvement.

Complications

Because CD is a transmural process, serosal adhesions develop that provide direct pathways for fistula formation. Free perforation is rare and occurs in 1–2% of patients, usually in the ileum or less commonly in the jejunum or as a complication of toxic megacolon. The peritonitis of free perforation may be fatal. Intra-abdominal and pelvic abscesses occur in 10–60% of patients and almost always require intravenous antibiotics and CT-guided drainage. Most patients will need eventual surgery to remove the offending bowel segment. Systemic glucocorticoids increase the risk of intra-abdominal and pelvic abscesses in Crohn's patients who have never had an operation. Other complications include bowel obstruction in 40%, severe perianal disease, malabsorption, and, rarely, massive hemorrhage.

Laboratory Findings

Laboratory abnormalities include an elevated ESR and CRP. Findings in more severe disease include a hypoalbuminemia, anemia, and leukocytosis. Stool ova and parasites, *Giardia* antigen, *C. difficile* toxin, and bacterial cultures should be negative.

Endoscopic and Radiographic Findings

Endoscopic features of Crohn's disease include rectal sparing, aphthous ulcerations, fistulas, and macroscopic and microscopic skip lesions. Colonoscopy allows examination and biopsy of the colon and terminal ileum. Wireless capsule endoscopy (WCE) allows direct visualization of the entire small bowel mucosa but cannot be used in the setting of a small bowel stricture. Capsule retention occurs in 4–6% of patients with established CD but in only <1% of patients with suspected CD. Early radiographic findings in the small bowel include thickened folds, aphthous ulcerations, and longitudinal ulcerations and transverse ulcerations. In more advanced disease, strictures, fistulas, inflammatory masses, and abscesses can be detected. The radiographic "string sign" represents long areas of circumferential inflammation and fibrosis, resulting in long segments of luminal narrowing. The segmental nature of CD results in long gaps of normal or dilated bowel between involved segments.

CT enterography is becoming the first-line test for evaluating Crohn's disease and its complications. It combines the improved spatial and temporal resolution of multidetector-row CT with large volumes of ingested neutral enteric contrast material to permit visualization of the entire small bowel and lumen. Unlike routine CT, which is used to detect the extraenteric complications of CD such as abscesses and fistulas, CT enterography clearly depicts the small bowel inflammation associated with Crohn's disease by displaying mural enhancement and thickening, engorged vasa recta, and perienteric inflammatory changes. Magnetic resonance imaging (MRI) is superior for visualizing pelvic lesions such as perirectal fistulas and ischiorectal abscesses.

Complications

Because Crohn's disease is a transmural process, serosal adhesions develop that provide pathways for fistula formation and reduce the influence of free perforation. Free perforation occurs in 1–2% of patients, usually in the ileum but occasionally in the jejunum or as a rare complication of toxic megacolon. The peritonitis of free perforation, especially colonic, may be fatal. Generalized peritonitis may also result from the rupture of an intra-abdominal abscess. Other complications include intestinal obstruction in 40% of patients, massive hemorrhage, which is rare, malabsorption, and severe perianal disease.

SEROLOGIC MARKERS

Several serologic markers may be used to differentiate between CD and UC and help to predict the course of disease. Two antibodies that can be detected in the serum of IBD patients are perinuclear antineutrophil cytoplasmic antibodies (pANCAs), largely to myeloperoxidase, and anti–*Saccharomyces cerevisiae* antibodies (ASCAs). pANCA positivity is found in about 60–70% of UC patients and 5–10% of CD patients; 5–15% of first-degree relatives of UC patients are pANCA positive, whereas only 2–3% of the general population is pANCA positive. pANCA may also identify specific disease phenotypes. pANCA positivity is more often associated with pancolitis, early surgery, pouchitis, or inflammation of the pouch after ileal pouch–anal anastomosis (IPAA), and primary sclerosing cholangitis. pANCA in CD is associated with colonic disease that resembles UC.

ASCA antibodies recognize mannose sequences in the cell wall mannan of *Saccharomyces cerevisiae*; 60–70% of CD patients, 10–15% of UC patients, and up to 5% of non-IBD controls are ASCA positive. Fifty-five percent of CD patients in a referral center population are seroreactive to outer membrane porin C (Omp C), and 50–54% of CD patients in a referral center population are positive for the I_2 antibody. The I_2 serologic response recognizes a novel homologue of the bacterial transcription-factor families from a *Pseudomonas fluorescens*–associated sequence.

Combining these diagnostic assays further improves their ability to diagnose Crohn's disease. In a referral population of patients with Crohn's disease, 85% of patients responded to at least one antigen (pANCA, ASCA, Omp C, and I_2); only 4% responded to all four. In addition, antigen positivity may help predict disease phenotype. ASCA positivity may be associated with an increased rate of early CD complications, Omp C–positive patients are more likely to have internal perforating disease, and I_2-positive patients are more likely to have fibrostenosing disease. Patients positive for I_2, Omp C, and ASCA are the most likely to have undergone small bowel surgery.

Cbir1 flagellin is an immunodominant antigen of the enteric microbial flora to which strong B-cell and CD4+ T-cell responses occur in colitic mice. Approximately 50% of patients with CD have serum reactivity to Cbir1, whereas UC have little or no reactivity to this flagellin. Anti-Cbir1 expression is associated with small bowel disease, fibrostenosing, and internal penetrating disease. Children with Crohn's disease positive for all four immune responses (ASCA+, Omp C+, I_2+, and anti-Cbir1+) may have a more aggressive disease phenotype with a shorter time of progression to internal perforating and/or stricturing disease.

DIFFERENTIAL DIAGNOSIS OF UC AND CD

UC and CD have similar features to many other diseases. As there is no key diagnostic test, a combination of clinical, laboratory, histopathologic, radiographic, and therapeutic observations are required. Once a diagnosis of IBD is made, distinguishing between UC and CD is difficult to impossible in 10–15% of cases. These are termed indeterminate

Table 71.3 DISEASES MISTAKEN FOR CROHN'S DISEASE

Infectious
Bacterial: *Salmonella*, *Shigella*, toxigenic *Escherichia coli*, *Campylobacter*, *Yersinia Clostridium difficile*, Gonorrhea, *Chlamydia trachomatis*
Mycobacterial: Tuberculosis, *Mycobacterium avium*
Parasitic: Amebiasis, *Isospora*, *Trichuris trichiura*, hookworm, *Strongyloides*
Viral: Cytomegalovirus, herpes simplex, HIV

Inflammatory
Appendicitis, diverticulitis, diversion colitis, collagenous/lymphocytic colitis, Behçet syndrome, solitary rectal ulcer eosinophilic gastroenteritis, neutropenic colitis, ischemic colitis, radiation colitis/enteritis, graft-versus-host-disease

Neoplastic, Drugs, and Chemicals
Nonsteroidal anti-inflammatories, phosphosoda, chemotherapy, lymphoma, lymphosarcoma, carcinoma of the ileum, familial polyposis, metastatic carcinoma

colitis. The diseases commonly mistaken for IBD are detailed in table 71.3.

INDETERMINATE COLITIS

There are some cases of IBD that cannot be recognized as either UC or CD and are called indeterminate colitis. Long-term follow-up over a period of years reduces the numbers of patients labeled indeterminate to about 10%. The disease course of indeterminate colitis is unclear, and surgical recommendations are difficult because about 20% of pouches in these patients will fail and eventually require an ileostomy. A multistage ileal pouch anal anastomosis (the initial stage consisting of a subtotal colectomy with Hartmann pouch) with careful histological evaluation of the resected specimen to exclude Crohn's disease is advised. Medical therapy is similar to UC and CD.

THE ATYPICAL COLITIDES

Two atypical colitides, collagenous colitis and lymphocytic colitis, have completely normal endoscopic appearances. Collagenous colitis has two main histological components: increased subepithelial collagen deposition and colitis with increased intraepithelial lymphocytes. Male-to-female ratio is 9:1, and most patients present in the sixth or seventh decade of life. The main symptom is chronic watery diarrhea and sometimes weight loss. Treatments are variable and range from sulfasalazine or Imodium and Lomotil to bismuth or glucocorticoids for refractory disease.

Lymphocytic colitis has features similar to collagenous colitis including age of onset and clinical presentation, but it has almost equal incidence in men and women and no subepithelial collagen deposition on pathologic section. However, intraepithelial lymphocytes are increased. Celiac disease should be excluded in all patients with lymphocytic colitis, as the frequency ranges from 9% to 27%. The treatment is the same as in collagenous colitis except for a gluten-free diet in patients with celiac disease.

Diversion colitis is an inflammatory process that arises in segments of the large intestine that are excluded from the fecal stream. Diversion colitis usually occurs in patients with ileostomies or colostomies when a mucous fistula or a Hartmann pouch has been created. Diversion colitis is reversible by surgical reanastomosis. Clinically, patients have mucous or bloody discharge from the rectum, and erythema, granularity, friability, and, in more severe cases, ulceration can be seen on endoscopy. There are areas of active inflammation with foci of cryptitis and crypt abscesses on histopathology. Crypt architecture is normal, and this differentiates it from UC. It may be impossible to distinguish it from CD. Short-chain fatty acid enemas will help in diversion colitis, but this treatment is difficult to tolerate, and the definitive therapy is surgical reanastomosis.

EXTRAINTESTINAL MANIFESTATIONS

IBD is associated with a variety of extraintestinal manifestations. Up to one-third of patients have at least one. Patients with perianal CD are at higher risk for developing extraintestinal manifestations than other IBD patients. The extraintestinal manifestations are detailed in table 71.4.

TREATMENT

5-ASA AGENTS

One of main therapies for mild to moderate UC and Crohn's colitis is sulfasalazine and the other 5-ASA agents (table 71.5). Although these agents are effective in inducing remission in UC and CD and maintaining remission

Table 71.4 EXTRAINTESTINAL MANIFESTATIONS

CATEGORY	CLINICAL COURSE	TREATMENT
Rheumatologic Disorders (5–20%)		
Peripheral arthritis	Asymmetric, migratory Parallels bowel activity	Reduce bowel inflammation
Sacroiliitis	Symmetric: spine and hip joints Independent of bowel activity	Steroids, injections, methotrexate, anti-TNF
Ankylosing spondylitis	Gradual fusion of spine Independent of bowel activity	Steroids, injections, methotrexate, anti-TNF
Dermatologic Disorders (10–20%)		
Erythema nodosum	Hot, red, tender, nodules/extremities Parallels bowel activity	Reduce bowel inflammation
Pyoderma gangrenosum	Ulcerating, necrotic lesions/ extremities, trunk, face, stoma Independent of bowel activity	Antibiotics, steroids, cyclosporine, infliximab, dapsone, azathioprine, intralesional steroids, thalidomide, NOT debridement or colectomy
Pyoderma vegetans	Intertriginous areas Parallels bowel activity	Evanescent; resolves without progression
Pyostomatitis vegetans	Mucous membranes Parallels bowel activity	Evanescent; resolves without progression
Metastatic Crohn's disease	Crohn's disease of the skin Parallels bowel activity	Reduce bowel inflammation
Sweet's syndrome	Neutrophilic dermatosis Parallels bowel activity	Reduce bowel inflammation
Aphthous stomatitis	Oral ulcerations Parallels bowel activity	Reduce bowel inflammation/topical Rx
Ocular Disorders (1–11%)		
Uveitis	Ocular pain, photophobia, blurred vision, headache Independent of bowel activity	Topical or systemic steroids
Episcleritis	Mild ocular burning Parallels bowel activity	Topical corticosteroids
Hepatobiliary Disorders (10–35%)		
Fatty liver	Secondary to chronic illness, malnutrition, steroid Rx	Improve nutrition, reduce steroids
Cholelithiasis	Patients with ileitis or ileal resection Malabsorption of bile acids, depletion of bile salt pool, secretion of lithogenic bile	Reduce bowel inflammation
Primary sclerosing cholangitis (PSC)	Intrahepatic and extrahepatic Inflammation and fibrosis leading to biliary cirrhosis and hepatic failure; 7–10% cholangiocarcinoma	ERCP/high-dose ursodiol lowers risk of colonic neoplasia

(continued)

Table 71.4 CONTINUED

Genitourinary Disorders (4–23%)		
Calculi	Calcium oxalate: following small bowel resection (colon intact)	Hydration, decrease diarrhea
	Uric acid: large ileostomy outputs	Hydration
Ureteral obstruction	Varies from minimal periureteral fibrosis to complete obstructive uropathy	Treatment varies

Other		
Thromboembolic disease (Clinical studies 1.3–6.4%; postmortem 39%)	Deep vein thrombosis, pulmonary embolus, cerebrovascular accidents, arterial emboli Correlates with classic risk factors for thrombosis	Anticoagulation/thrombolysis
Cardiopulmonary complications	Myocarditis, pleuropericarditis, endocarditis, airway disease, interstitial lung disease, necrobiotic parenchymal nodules, serositis	Treatment varies
Amyloidosis	Reactive to Crohn's disease (CD) diarrhea, constipation, renal failure	Treatment varies
Pancreatitis	Secondary to duodenal fistulas, ampullary CD, gallstones, PSC, medications (6-MP/AZA/5-ASA), autoimmune, primary CD of the pancreas	Treatment varies

Table 71.5 5-ASA PREPARATIONS

Oral 5-ASA Preparations			
PREPARATION	**FORMULATION**	**DELIVERY**	**DOSING (PER DAY)**
Azo-bond Sulfasalazine (500 mg) (Azulfidine)	Sulfapyridine-5-ASA	Colon	3–6 g (acute) 2–4 g (maintenance)
Olsalazine (250 mg) (Dipentum)	5-ASA-5-ASA	Colon	1–3 g
Balsalazide (750 mg) (Colazal)	Aminobenzoyl-alanine-5-ASA	Colon	6.75–9 g
Delayed-release Mesalamine (400, 800 mg) (Asacol)	Eudragit S (pH 7)	Distal ileum-colon	1.6–4.8 g (maintenance) 2.4–4.8 g (acute)
Mesalamine (1.2 g) (Lialda)	MMX mesalamine (SPD476)	Ileum-colon	2.4–4.8 g (acute)
Delayed and extended-release Mesalamine (0.375 g) (Apriso)	Intellicor extended-release mechanism	Ileum-colon	1.5 g (maintenance)
Sustained-release Mesalamine (250, 500, 1000 mg) (Pentasa)	Ethylcellulose microgranules	Stomach-colon	2–4 g (acute) 1.5–4 g (maintenance)
Rectal 5-ASA Preparations			
Mesalamine suppository (400, 500, 1000 mg) (Canasa)		Rectum	1–1.5 g (acute) 500 mg–1 g (maintenance)
Mesalamine enema (1, 4 g) (Rowasa)	60 mL, 100 mL suspension	Rectum-splenic flexure	1–4 g (acute) 1 g/day to 3 times/week (maintenance)

in UC, it is still unclear whether they have a role in maintaining remission in CD.

Sulfasalazine consists of 5-aminosalicylic acid joined to a sulfapyridine moiety. It is effective in treating mild to moderate UC and Crohn's ileocolitis and colitis, but its high rate of side effects limits its use. At the more effective, higher doses of 6–8 g per day, up to 30% of patients experience allergic reactions or intolerable side effects such as headache, anorexia, nausea, and vomiting that are attributable to the sulfa moiety. Many patients experience hypersensitivity reactions such as rash, fever, hepatitis, agranulocytosis, hypersensitivity, pneumonitis, pancreatitis, worsening of colitis, and reversible sperm abnormalities. Sulfasalazine can also impair folate absorption, and patients should be supplemented with folic acid.

Newer, sulfa-free aminosalicylate preparations deliver increased amounts of the pharmacologically active ingredient of sulfasalazine, 5-ASA or mesalamine, to the site of active bowel disease while limiting systemic toxicity. Sulfa-free aminosalicylate formulations include alternative azo-bonded carriers, 5-ASA dimmers, pH-dependent tablets, and continuous release preparations. Each has the same efficacy as sulfasalazine when equal concentrations are used. Balsalazide contains an azo-bonded mesalamine, the carrier molecule 4-aminobenzoyl-beta-alanine; it is effective in the colon. Asacol is an enteric-coated form of mesalamine, but it has a slightly different release pattern with the 5-ASA liberated at pH greater than 7. It disintegrates with complete breakup of the tablet in many different areas of the gut ranging from the small intestine to the splenic flexure. Some 50–75% of patients with mild to moderate UC and CD improve when treated with 2 g per day of 5-ASA. MMX mesalamine (Lialda) is a newer formulation of mesalamine that comes in capsules of 1.2 g. It can be given once or twice daily. The treatment effect is the same as that of Asacol at similar dosages.

Pentasa is another mesalamine formulation that uses an ethyl cellulose coating to allow water absorption into small beads containing the mesalamine. Water dissolves the 5-ASA, which then diffuses out of the bead into the lumen. The capsule disintegrates in the stomach, and the microspheres then disperse throughout the entire gastrointestinal tract from the small intestine to the distal colon in both fasted and fed conditions. Control trials of Pentasa and Asacol in active CD demonstrate a 40–60% clinical improvement or remission, but meta-analyses are inconclusive with regard to maintaining remission in CD.

Topical mesalamine enemas are effective in mild to moderate UC and CD. Clinical response occurs in up to 80% of UC patients with colitis distal to the splenic flexure. Mesalamine suppositories at doses of 500 mg twice a day are effective in treating proctitis.

GLUCOCORTICOIDS

The majority of patients with moderate to severe UC benefit from oral or parental glucocorticoids. Prednisone is usually started at doses of 40–60 mg per day for active UC that is unresponsive to 5-ASA therapy. Intravenous glucocorticoids may be administered as intravenous hydrocortisone 300 mg per day or methylprednisolone 40–60 mg per day in divided doses.

Topically applied glucocorticoids are also beneficial for distal colitis and may serve as an adjunct in those who have rectal involvement plus more proximal disease. Hydrocortisone enemas or foam may control active disease, although they have no proven role as maintenance therapy. These glucocorticoids are significantly absorbed from the rectum and can lead to adrenal suppression with prolonged administration.

Glucocorticoids are also effective for treatment of moderate to severe CD and induce a 60–70% remission rate compared to a 30% placebo response. Glucocorticoids play no role in maintenance therapy in either UC or CD. Once clinical remission has been induced, they should be tapered according to the clinical activity, normally at a rate of no more than 5 mg per week. They can usually be tapered to 20 mg a day within 4–5 weeks but often take several months to be discontinued altogether. The side effects are numerous including fluid retention, abdominal striae, fat redistribution, hyperglycemia, subcapsular cataracts, osteonecrosis, myopathy, emotional disturbances, and withdrawal symptoms. Most of these side effects, except for osteonecrosis, are related to the dose and duration of therapy.

Controlled ileal-release budesonide has been nearly equal to prednisone for ileocolonic CD with fewer glucocorticoid side effects. Budesonide is used for 2–3 months at a dose of 9 mg/day, then tapered. Budesonide 6 mg/day is effective in reducing relapse rates at 3–6 months but not at 12 months in CD patients with a medically induced remission.

ANTIBIOTICS

Despite numerous trials, antibiotics have no role in the treatment of active or quiescent UC. However, in pouchitis, which occurs in about one-third of UC patients after colectomy, an ileal pouch–anal anastomosis usually responds if treated with metronidazole or ciprofloxacin.

Metronidazole is effective in active inflammatory, fistulizing, and perianal CD. The most effective dose is 15–25 mg/kg per day used in three divided doses. It is usually continued for several months. However, side effects impair its use. They include nausea, metallic taste, and disulfiram-like reactions. Peripheral neuropathy can occur with prolonged administration over several months' time and, on rare occasions, is permanent despite discontinuation. Cipro, 500 mg twice a day, is also beneficial for inflammatory, perianal, and fistulizing CD. The side effects of ciprofloxacin include arthralgias and Achilles tendon rupture, and thus Cipro should be used long-term only with caution. These two antibiotics can be used as second-line drugs in active CD after 5-ASA agents and as first-line drugs in perianal and fistulizing CD. Rifaximin is a nonabsorbable antibiotic that has modest activity in CD.

AZATHIOPRINE AND 6-MERCAPTOPURINE

Azathioprine and 6-mercaptopurine (6-MP) are purine analogues commonly employed in the management of glucocorticoid-dependent IBD. Azathioprine is rapidly absorbed and converted to 6-MP, which is then metabolized to the active end product, thioinosinic acid, an inhibitor of purine ribonucleotide synthesis and cell proliferation. These agents also inhibit the immune response. Efficacy is seen at 6–12 weeks. Adherence can be monitored by monitoring the levels of 6-thioguanine nucleotides and 6-methylmercaptopurine, end products of 6-MP metabolism. Azathioprine, 2–2.5 mg/kg per day, or 6-MP, 1–1.5 mg/kg per day, have been employed successfully as glucocorticoid-sparing agents in up to two-thirds of CD and UC patients previously unable to be weaned from glucocorticoids.

Although these medications are usually well tolerated, pancreatitis can occur in up to 3–4% of patients; it usually occurs within the first month of therapy and is completely reversible after the drug is stopped. Other side effects of these drugs include nausea, fever, rash, and hepatitis. Bone marrow suppression, particularly leukopenia, is dose related and often delayed, necessitating regular monitoring of the complete blood count. Additionally, 1 in 300 individuals lacks thiopurine methyltransferase, the enzyme responsible for drug metabolism. An additional 11% of the population are heterozygotes with intermediate enzyme activity. Both are at increased risk of toxicity because of increased accumulation of thioguanine metabolites. Thiopurine methyltransferase (TPMT) phenotype can be checked to rule out a severe deficiency. In patients with intermediate activity, AZA/6-MP can be started at a third or a half of the usual dose. One meta-analysis demonstrated a fourfold risk of lymphoma in IBD patients on AZA/6-MP. No increased risk of solid organ tumors has been documented in IBD patients taking these medications long term.

METHOTREXATE

Methotrexate inhibits dihydrofolate reductase, resulting in impaired DNA synthesis. Intramuscular or subcutaneous methotrexate at 25 mg per week is effective in inducing remission and reducing glucocorticoid dosage, and 15 mg per week is effective in maintaining remission of CD. Potential toxicities include leukopenia and hepatic fibrosis, necessitating periodic evaluation of complete blood counts and liver enzymes. The role of liver biopsy in patients on long-term methotrexate is uncertain. Hypersensitivity pneumonitis is a rare but serious complication of therapy.

CYCLOSPORINE

Cyclosporine (CSA) alters the immune response by acting as a potent inhibitor of T-cell-mediated responses. Although CSA acts primarily via inhibition of IL-2 production from T-helper cells, it also decreases recruitment of cytotoxic T cells and blocks other cytokines including IL-3, IL-4, interferon-α, and tumor necrosis factor (TNF). It has a more rapid onset of action than 6-MP and azathioprine.

CSA is most effective given at 2–4 mg/kg per day in continuous infusion in severe UC refractory to intravenous steroids. In this scenario, about 80% of patients respond. CSA can be an alternative to colectomy, but the long-term success of oral CSA is not as dramatic. If patients are started on 6-MP or azathioprine at the time of discharge from the hospital, remission can be obtained. Intravenous CSA is effective in 80% of patients with refractory fistulas, but 6-MP and azathioprine must be used to maintain remission. Serum levels should be monitored and kept in a range of 200–400 ng/mL as measured by a high-performance liquid chromatography (HPLC) assay. The levels should be anywhere between 300 and 500 μg/mL as measured by monoclonal radioimmunoassay.

CSA has the potential for significant toxicity, and renal function should be frequently monitored. Hypertension, gingival hyperplasia, hypertrichosis, paresthesias, tremors, headaches, and electrolyte abnormalities are common side effects. Creatinine elevation calls for dose reduction or discontinuation. Seizures may complicate therapy especially if the patient is hypomagnesemic or if serum cholesterol levels are less than 120 mg/dL. Opportunistic infections, most notably *Pneumocystis carinii* pneumonia, have occurred with combination immunosuppressive treatment. Prophylaxis should then be given.

ANTI-TNF THERAPY

Infliximab, a chimeric monoclonal antibody directed against the proinflammatory cytokine tumor necrosis factor α, is approved by the U.S. Food and Drug Administration for use in moderate to severe Crohn's disease. Of active CD patients refractory to glucocorticoids, 6-MP, or 5-ASA, 65% will respond to intravenous infliximab (5 mg/kg); one-third will enter complete remission. Of the patients who experience an initial response, 40% will maintain remission for at least 1 year with repeated infusions of infliximab every 8 weeks. Infliximab is also effective in CD patients with refractory perianal and enterocutaneous fistulas, with a 68% response rate (50% reduction in fistula drainage) and a 50% complete remission rate. Reinfusion, typically every 8 weeks, is necessary to continue therapeutic benefits in many patients.

The development of antibodies to infliximab (ATI) is associated with an increased risk of infusion reactions and a decreased response to treatment. Patients who receive on-demand or episodic infusions rather than periodic (every 8 weeks) infusions are more likely to develop ATI. If infliximab is used episodically for flares, patients must use concomitant immunosuppression with AZA, 6-MP, or methotrexate in therapeutic doses to decrease the clinical consequences of immunogenicity of the chimeric antibodies. Moreover, prophylaxis with hydrocortisone before each infusion of infliximab will also decrease the formation of ATI. When the quality of response or the response duration to infliximab infusion decreases, this will be caused by high titers of ATI with formation of complexes and early elimination. Increase of the dosage administered to 10 mg/kg may restore the efficacy of the drug.

In the Crohn's disease and rheumatoid arthritis (RA) trials, six lymphomas were diagnosed for a follow-up of 4148 patient-years versus 0 for 691 placebo patient-years. All lymphomas occurred in patients treated with concomitant immunosuppression. Other morbidities of infliximab include acute infusion reactions, severe serum sickness, and increased risk of infections, particularly histoplasmosis and reactivation of latent tuberculosis. Rarely, infliximab has been associated with optic neuritis, seizures, and new-onset or exacerbation of clinical symptoms and/or radiographic evidence of central nervous system demyelinating disorders, including multiple sclerosis. It may exacerbate symptoms in patients with New York Heart Association functional class III/IV heart failure.

Infliximab has also shown efficacy in UC. In two large randomized, placebo-controlled trials, 37–49% of patients responded to infliximab, and 22% and 20% of patients were able to maintain remission after 30 and 54 weeks, respectively. Patients received infliximab at 0, 2, and 6 weeks and then every 8 weeks until the end of the study.

Recently, the fully human monoclonal antibody adalimumab (Humira) and the PEGylated humanized monoclonal antibody certolizumab pegol (Cimzia) have also been approved for the treatment of CD. Although adalimumab has been approved for Crohn's disease since February 2007, certolizumab pegol has only been approved since April 2008. Adalimumab is a recombinant human monoclonal IgG1 antibody containing only human peptide sequences and is injected subcutaneously. Adalimumab binds TNF-α and neutralizes its function by blocking the interaction between TNF and its cell surface receptor. Therefore, it seems to have a similar mechanism of action to infliximab but with less immunogenicity. Certolizumab is made up of the Fab' fragment of a humanized monoclonal antibody to TNF-α linked with two molecules of polyethylene glycol. Because it lacks the Fc portion of the antibody, certolizumab pegol only exerts its activity through binding to soluble TNF-α and cannot bind to cell surface receptors. Infliximab, adalimumab, and certolizumab all have about equal efficacy.

Although it has been approved for almost 2 years for the treatment of Crohn's disease, adalimumab is currently being studied for the treatment of UC and is expected to be successful. Finally, golimumab, another fully human monoclonal antibody that can be administered as either a subcutaneous injection or intravenous infusion is being investigated in both CD and UC.

INHIBITORS OF LEUKOCYTE ADHESION

Integrins are expressed on the surface of leukocytes and serve as mediators of leukocyte adhesion to vascular endothelium. α4-Integrin along with its β1 or β7 subunit interact with endothelial ligands termed adhesion molecules. Interaction between α4β7 and mucosal addressin cellular adhesion molecule (MAdCAM-1) is important in lymphocyte trafficking to gut mucosa. Natalizumab is a recombinant humanized IgG4 antibody against α4-integrin that has been shown to be effective in induction and maintenance of patients with Crohn's disease. It has been approved since February 2008 for the treatment of patients with Crohn's disease refractory or intolerant to anti-TNF therapy. The rate of response and remission at 3 months are about 60% and 40%, respectively, with a sustained remission rate of about 40% at 36 weeks. However, one patient died from progressive multifocal leukoencephalopathy (PML) associated with the JC virus in one of the clinical trials. An additional two cases were found in patients on natalizumab for multiple sclerosis (MS). This resulted in the withdrawal of natalizumab from the market for MS and from further development in other disease areas. On June 5, 2006, the FDA approved a Supplemental Biologics License Application (sBLA) for the reintroduction of natalizumab as monotherapy treatment for relapsing forms of MS. The reintroduction is under the auspices of a very tightly controlled pharmacovigilance program due to the previous cases of PML. As of June 2007, over 10,000 patients have received natalizumab for MS with no further reports of PML.

In December 2006, the sponsor filed a supplemental license application with the FDA for the treatment of Crohn's disease with natalizumab. On July 31, 2007, the Gastrointestinal Drugs and Drug Safety and Risk Management Advisory Committees of the FDA recommended the approval of natalizumab for the treatment of moderate to severe CD in patients who have failed or cannot tolerate available therapies. The FDA reapproved natalizumab in February 2008—but only under the TOUCH prescribing program. This program details strict criteria that doctors and patients must adhere to, including no concomitant immunomodulators, tapering of steroids by 6 months of treatment, signing of several consent forms, and a monthly check by the infusion nurses for signs and symptoms of PML. As of November 2008,

48,000 patients have been infused with natalizumab for both Crohn's and MS, and there have been a total of seven reported cases of PML. Only one patient with PML has had Crohn's disease.

NUTRITIONAL THERAPIES

Dietary antigens may act as stimuli of the mucosal immune response. Patients with active CD respond to bowel rest along with total enteral or total parenteral nutrition (TPN). Bowel rest and TPN are as effective as glucocorticoids for inducing remission of active CD but are not as effective as maintenance therapy. Enteral nutrition in the form of elemental or peptide-based preparations is also as effective as glucocorticoids or TPN, but these diets are not palatable. In contrast to CD, active UC is not effectively treated by either elemental diets or TPN. Medical therapies for IBD are shown in table 71.6.

SURGICAL THERAPY

Ulcerative Colitis

Nearly half of patients with extensive, chronic UC undergo surgery within the first 10 years of their illness. The indications for surgery are listed in table 71.7. Morbidity is about 20% in elective, 30% for urgent, and 40% for emergency proctocolectomy. The risks are mainly hemorrhage, sepsis, and neural injury.

The IPAA is the most frequent continence-preserving operation performed. Because UC involves only the mucosa, the mucosa of the rectum can be dissected out and removed down to the dentate line of the anus or about 2 cm proximal to it. The ileum is then fashioned into a pouch that serves as a neorectum. This pouch is then sutured circumferentially to the anus in an end-to-end fashion. If performed carefully, this operation preserves the anal sphincter and maintains continence. The overall operative morbidity is 10%, the major complication being bowel obstruction. Pouch failure necessitating conversion to permanent ileostomy occurs in 5–10% of patients. Some inflamed rectal mucosa is usually left behind, and endoscopic surveillance is necessary. Primary dysplasia of the ileal mucosa of the pouch has rarely occurred.

Patients with IPAAs usually have about six to eight bowel movements a day and one at night. The most frequent late complication of IPAA is pouchitis. In about one-third of patients with UC, this syndrome consists of increased stool frequency, watery stools, cramping, urgency, nocturnal leakage of stool, arthralgias, malaise, and fever. Although it usually responds to antibiotics, 3–5% of the time it is refractory to even immunomodulators or infliximab and requires pouch takedown.

Table 71.6 **MEDICAL MANAGEMENT OF IBD**

Distal UC
5-ASA (rectal and/or oral)
Glucocorticoid (rectal)
Glucocorticoid (oral)
Glucocorticoid (intravenous)
6-MP or azathioprine
Intravenous cyclosporine or infliximab
Extensive UC
5-ASA (oral and rectal)
Glucocorticoid (oral and rectal)
Glucocorticoid (intravenous)
6-MP or azathioprine
Intravenous cyclosporine or infliximab
Inflammatory CD
Sulfasalazine/antibiotics
Budesonide (ileal and right-sided colonic disease)
Prednisone
Intravenous glucocorticoid
6-MP/azathioprine
Methotrexate
Infliximab/adalimumab/certolizumab pegol
Natalizumab
Intravenous cyclosporine or tacrolimus
Fistulizing CD
Antibiotics
6-MP/azathioprine
Methotrexate
Infliximab/adalimumab/certolizumab pegol
Natalizumab
Intravenous cyclosporine or tacrolimus
Total parenteral nutrition (TPN)

Crohn's Disease

Most patients with CD require at least one operation in their lifetime. The need for surgery is related to duration of disease and site of involvement. Patients with small bowel disease alone have an 80% chance of requiring surgery; those with colitis alone have a 50% chance. The indications for surgery are shown in table 71.7.

Table 71.7 **INDICATIONS FOR SURGERY**

Ulcerative Colitis
Intractable disease
Fulminant disease
Toxic megacolon
Colonic perforation
Massive colonic hemorrhage
Extracolonic disease
Colonic stricture
Colon dysplasia or cancer

CD of Small Intestine
Stricture and obstruction unresponsive to medical therapy
Massive hemorrhage
Refractory fistula
Abscess
Malignancy

CD of Colon and Rectum
Intractable disease
Fulminant disease
Perianal disease unresponsive to medical therapy
Refractory fistula
Colonic stricture
Colon dysplasia or cancer

Small Intestinal Disease

CD is chronic and recurrent with no clear surgical cure, so as little intestine as possible is resected. For treating obstructive CD, the current surgical alternatives are resection or stricturoplasty. Resection of the diseased segment is the more frequently performed operation, and in most cases, primary anastomosis can be performed. If much of the small bowel has been resected and the stricture is short, a stricturoplasty can be performed. In this procedure a strictured area of intestine is incised longitudinally, and the incision is sutured transversely, thus widening the narrowed area. Complications include ileus, hemorrhage, fistula, abscess, leak, and restricture.

Colorectal Disease

Patients with CD with Crohn's colitis require surgery for intractability, fulminant disease, and anorectal disease. There are several alternatives available ranging from the use of a temporary ileostomy to resection of segments of diseased colon or even a total proctocolectomy. In 20–25% of patients with extensive colitis, the rectum is spared sufficiently to consider rectal preservation ("J-pouch" construction). Most surgeons believe that an IPAA is contraindicated in Crohn's with a high rate of pouch failure. Even though a diverting colostomy can help heal severe perianal disease or rectal vaginal fistulas, the disease recurs with reanastomosis. Often these patients require a total proctocolectomy and ileostomy.

CANCER IN INFLAMMATORY BOWEL DISEASE

The risk of neoplasia in chronic UC increases with duration and extent of disease. For patients with pancolitis, the risk of cancer rises 0.5–1% per year after 8–10 years of disease. This observed increase in cancer rates has led to the endorsement of surveillance colonoscopy with biopsies for patients with chronic UC as the standard of care. Annual or biennial colonoscopy with multiple biopsies has been advocated for patients with >8–10 years of pancolitis or 12–15 years of left-sided colitis and has been widely employed to screen and survey for subsequent dysplasia and carcinoma.

Risk factors for developing colorectal cancer in CD are a history of colonic (or ileocolonic) involvement and long disease duration. The cancer risks in CD and UC are probably equivalent for similar extent and duration of disease. A recent study that followed 259 patients with extensive Crohn colitis for 25 years reported a 25% chance of developing low-grade dysplasia (LGD), high-grade dysplasia (HGD), or cancer (CA) by the 10th surveillance exam and a 7% chance of developing flat HGD or CA by the 10th surveillance exam. There were 14 cancers found in this study: 3 on screening exam and 11 on surveillance exam or at surgery. Thus, the same endoscopic surveillance strategy used for UC is recommended for patients with chronic Crohn's colitis. A pediatric colonoscope can be used to pass narrow strictures in CD patients, but surgery should be considered in symptomatic patients with impassable strictures.

IBD patients are also at greater risk for other malignancies. Patients with CD may have an increased risk of developing non-Hodgkin lymphoma and squamous cell carcinoma of the skin. Although CD patients have a 12-fold increased risk of developing small-bowel cancer, this type of carcinoma is extremely rare.

ADDITIONAL READING

Abraham C, Cho JH. Inflammatory bowel disease. *N Engl J Med.* 2009;361(21):2066–78.

Arai R. Serologic markers: Impact on early diagnosis and disease stratification in inflammatory bowel disease. *Postgrad Med.* 2010;122(4):177–85.

Itzkowitz S, Present DH; Crohn's and Colitis Foundation of American Colon Cancer in IBD Study Group. Consensus conference: Colorectal cancer screening and surveillance in inflammatory bowel disease. *Inflamm Bowel Dis.* 2005;11(3):314.

Kornbluth A, Sachar DB; Practice Parameters Committee of the American College of Gastroenterology. Ulcerative colitis practice guidelines in adults. *Am J Gastroenterol.* 2004;99(7):1371.

Kulaylat MN, Dayton MT. Ulcerative colitis and cancer. *J Surg Oncol.* 2010;101(8):706–12.

Loftus EV. Clinical epidemiology of inflammatory bowel disease: Incidence, prevalence, and environmental influences. *Gastroenterology.* 2004;126:1504.

QUESTIONS

QUESTION 1. A 25-year-old female is referred to the gastroenterology clinic with a 6-month history of daily right lower quadrant pain, at least 8–10 loose bowel movements a day, and a weight loss of 15 lb over the past 6 months. She reports some low-grade fevers at home and increasing night sweats. She has difficulty tolerating many foods, including fresh fruits and vegetables, red meat, and milk products. She has just started a job teaching high school science and has missed too many days of work due to pain, fatigue, and urgent bowel movements.

Her physical exam is significant for a fever of 99.5°F, her blood pressure is 124/82, and her pulse is 96. Her lungs are clear, her heart rate and rhythm are regular, and her abdominal exam is significant for right lower quadrant pain to palpation. Her rectal exam is guaiac negative, and she has no perianal skin tags, fissures, or fistulas. Her hemoglobin is 10, her CRP is 7, and her white count is 9.6. Stool studies for ova and parasites are negative, stool *Giardia* antigen is negative, and stool for *C. difficile* and bacterial cultures are negative. Serologies are negative for celiac disease or thyroid abnormalities. Lactose breath test is negative for lactose intolerance.

The history, exam, and laboratory data are suspicious for Crohn's disease. What further studies should be done?

A. Small bowel series
B. Colonoscopy and biopsy
C. CT enterography
D. IBD serology 7 blood testing for ASCA IgA and IgG, anti-OmpC IgA, anti-CBir1, and pANCA

QUESTION 2. First, CT enterography is performed and reveals chronic thickening of the last 20 cm of the terminal ileum. Colonoscopy and biopsy are then performed. The colon is macroscopically and microscopically normal, and the terminal ileum is severely inflamed with deep ulcerations. Ileal biopsies reveal severe chronic active ileitis. What medical therapy should be started first?

A. Azathioprine

B. Infliximab/adalimumab/certolizumab pegol
C. Pentasa
D. Budesonide
E. Prednisone

QUESTION 3. The patient is given oral budesonide, 9 mg each morning. Symptoms worsen, and she now has severe right lower quadrant pain and fevers to 39.4°C. CT of the abdomen reveals a terminal ileal abscess. What should be done now?

A. Intravenous hydrocortisone
B. Surgical resection of the abscess and the terminal ileum
C. CT-guided abscess drainage and intravenous antibiotics
D. Stop budesonide and oral antibiotics at home

QUESTION 4. An 18-year-old man presents to the gastroenterology clinic with a 5-week history of bloody diarrhea. His symptoms started after eating a "bad" turkey sandwich, and he has had diarrhea mixed with blood each time he eats or drinks. He has lost 10 lb and is having crampy abdominal pain. Most recently, he has been waking up in the middle of the night to use the bathroom. He has been previously healthy with no history of NSAID use and no history of smoking. He has no family history of IBD or colon cancer.

On physical exam he is tachycardic at 102 and his BP is 105/82. His abdominal exam is significant for left-sided tenderness with no rebound. His rectal exam is negative for any fissures, skin, tags, or fistulas. His hemoglobin is 9.5, his sedimentation rate is 40, and his platelet count is 556. His temperature is 38°C. Stool bacterial cultures, ova and parasites and *C. difficile* are negative. Flexible sigmoidoscopy shows active inflammation, marked erythema, and contact bleeding to 30 cm and beyond the reach of the scope. Biopsies reveal moderate chronic active colitis.

What is the first line treatment for this patient?

A. Prednisone
B. A 5-ASA agent
C. Intravenous hydrocortisone
D. Azathioprine

QUESTION 5. Mesalamine at 2.4 g a day is given, and symptoms worsen. The dose is increased to 4.8 g a day and symptoms worsen still. What is the next step?

A. Prednisone
B. Intravenous hydrocortisone
C. Infliximab
D. Hydrocortisone enema BID

QUESTION 6. The patient starts prednisone at 40 mg a day. Within 24 hours, he is markedly better. He decreases the prednisone by 5 mg a week. When he reduces to 15 mg, some symptoms of diarrhea, blood, and abdominal cramps return. What is the next step?

A. Intravenous hydrocortisone
B. Azathioprine
C. Increase prednisone to 40 mg a day
D. Infliximab
E. Colectomy

1. C
2. B
3. C
4. A
5. A
6. B

72.

PANCREATIC DISEASE

Alphonso Brown and Steven D. Freedman

ACUTE PANCREATITIS

DEFINITION AND EPIDEMIOLOGY

Acute pancreatitis may be defined as the development of acute inflammation of the pancreas initially localized to the pancreatic parenchyma and interstitium. It is a fairly common condition with an annual incidence of the United States of 80 cases per 100,000 individuals. Within the United States, the annual cost of hospital facilities for the treatment of pancreatic diseases is approximately $3.6–6 billion a year. There is also an annual cost to society of $250 million per year in lost worker productivity associated with hospitalization.

PATHOGENESIS

The pathogenesis of early trigger events leading to acute pancreatitis is slowly being elucidated. The premature activation of pancreatic enzymes within the acinar cell is an early hallmark feature. This premature activation leads to the development of an inflammatory cascade within the acinar cell. Changes to the acinar cell, such as the rapid influx of calcium into the cytosolic space, are thought to facilitate the amplification of this inflammatory cascade within the pancreatic acinar cell. The other event that contributes to the pathogenesis is the retention of the activated pancreatic enzymes within the acinar cell; this results in a block in exocytosis and the colocalization of zymogens and lysosomal enzymes. The combination of premature activation of pancreatic proenzymes and intra-acinar retention of activated pancreatic enzymes results in initiation and amplification of interstitial and parenchymal pancreatic inflammation. The localized pancreatic inflammation can progress to systemic multiorgan failure. This manifestation of acute pancreatitis known as the systemic inflammatory response syndrome (SIRS) is responsible for the majority of the deaths associated with acute pancreatitis.

Interstitial edematous pancreatitis refers to acute pancreatitis in which the tissue remains viable and perfused.

Necrotizing pancreatitis refers to acute pancreatitis in which there is death of pancreatic tissue. Although it was originally thought that acute pancreatitis was due to premature activation of trypsin, it is now clear that the subsequent release of cytokines/chemokines leads to local and systemic inflammation.

Etiology

The most common causes of acute pancreatitis are listed in table 72.1. Within the United States gallstones and alcohol account for approximately 70% of the cases of acute pancreatitis. Biliary microlithiasis is a common cause of unexplained recurrent pancreatitis that may be overlooked. There are many drugs that may cause acute pancreatitis. Among some of the most common drug causes of acute pancreatitis are 5-aminosalicyclic acid agents, antiretroviral medications, sulfa drugs, thiazide diuretics, and angiotensin-converting enzyme (ACE) inhibitors. Although corticosteroids have been implicated in the genesis of acute pancreatitis, this is no longer thought to be the case. Although many other medicines have been described as causing acute pancreatitis, the drugs listed in table 72.1 are those that have the strongest association with the development of pancreatitis.

Variations in the anatomy of the pancreas have also been associated with the development of pancreatitis. Pancreas divisum is a common congenital abnormality of the pancreas found in 7% of the U.S. population. The problem in pancreas divisum is an incomplete or absence of fusion between the dorsal and ventral pancreatic ducts with the larger dorsal duct draining through the smaller minor papilla. Pancreatitis is thought to develop when there is drainage of the dorsal duct across a stenotic ampulla. There is controversy regarding whether having pancreas divisum truly is a risk factor for pancreatitis because the majority of individuals with pancreas divisum never develop the disease. Annular pancreas is a congenital pancreatic abnormality in which the pancreas encircles the duodenum. Pancreatic inflammation and edema

Table 72.1 CAUSES OF ACUTE PANCREATITIS

Gallstones
Alcohol
Hypertriglyceridemia
Medications
    5-Aminosalicylates
    Azathioprine
    6-Mercaptopurine
    Cimetidine
    Furosemide
    Isoniazid
    Metronidazole
    Valproic acid
    Tetracycline
    5-Mercaptopurine
    Alpha-methyldopa
    Estrogen-containing oral contraceptives
    Didanosine
    Salicylates
    Asparaginase

Hyperparathyroidism
Sarcoidosis
Scorpion bite
Organophosphate exposure
Sphincter of Oddi dysfunction
Cationic trypsinogen gene mutation
CFTR, SPINKI, or *PST1* gene mutation
Autoimmune
Cytomegalovirus
Coxsackievirus
HIV infection
Mumps
Malignancy
Cystic neoplasms
Pancreas divisum
Annular pancreas
Anomalous pancreatic-biliary junction
Idiopathic

during acute pancreatitis result in duodenal obstruction and the development of symptoms consistent with bowel obstruction.

High serum triglyceride levels can also result in acute pancreatitis when levels exceed 1000 mg/dL. Individuals with triglycerides levels >1000 mg/dL often have familial type V hyperlipidemia. When attempting to determine if acute pancreatitis is due to high serum triglycerides, it is important to measure triglyceride levels after the acute event since levels may be elevated due to pancreatitis itself. Hypercalcemia may also cause acute pancreatitis. Pancreatitis that occurs after endoscopic retrograde cholangiopancreatography (ERCP) is the most common iatrogenic cause. The incidence of this complication is approximately 4–6% at most centers. Individuals who undergo ERCP and sphincter of Oddi manometry have a 15–20% chance of developing iatrogenic pancreatitis.

Several infective agents have been implicated as causes of pancreatitis such as mumps. Motor vehicle trauma to the pancreas is the most common cause of pancreatitis in adolescents. Other etiologies include autoimmune diseases such as lupus and autoimmune pancreatitis, a condition in which there is a chronic lymphocyte-predominant inflammatory infiltrate involving the pancreas. Elevated serum IgG4 or increased rheumatoid factor titers are abnormal in up to 45% of patients with autoimmune pancreatitis.

Genetic mutations may also be responsible for the development of pancreatitis. This includes mutations in the cystic fibrosis transmembrane chloride channel (CFTR), which encodes for a chloride channel. The gene responsible for the development of hereditary pancreatitis has been identified as cationic trypsinogen, which, when mutated, results in the development of a mutated noncleavable form of trypsin that cannot be degraded. One of the adverse long-term sequelae of having hereditary pancreatitis is that carriers of the gene are at significantly increased risk of developing pancreatic adenocarcinoma.

SYMPTOMS

Acute pancreatitis classically presents with pain localized to the midepigastrium but may present in the right or left upper quadrants of the abdomen. This pain is often described by the patient as radiating to the back and is often accompanied by nausea, vomiting, and anorexia. In rare forms of acute pancreatitis such as autoimmune pancreatitis, there may be no abdominal pain. Other symptoms include fever, hypotension, and peritoneal signs. Grey-Turner's sign is bluish discoloration of the flanks resulting from pancreatitis-induced intra-abdominal hemorrhage. Cullen's sign is similar except the discoloration occurs around the periumbilical area. Both signs are rare and occur in <3% of cases of acute pancreatitis. The significance of Cullen's sign and Grey-Turner's sign is that they are associated with a mortality of as high as 35% when either sign is present.

DIAGNOSIS

The diagnosis of acute pancreatitis is a combination of at least two of the following: (1) severe upper-abdominal pain; (2) amylase and/or lipase levels greater than three times the upper limit of normal; (3) a dynamic contrast-enhanced computed tomography (CT) scan transabdominal ultrasound, or a magnetic resonance imaging (MRI) scan with gadolinium that shows evidence of pancreatic inflammation or necrosis.

DISEASE CLASSIFICATION

The majority of subjects with acute pancreatitis (approximately 80%) will have short-term resolution with a hospitalization lasting 3–4 days and a mortality <1%. Patients with severe disease are often hospitalized for weeks to months. Mortality of this group may be as high as 33%. Severe acute pancreatitis is defined by the Atlanta Criteria, which define "severe" as pancreatitis with any of the following coexisting conditions: multiorgan failure, greater than 33% necrosis of the pancreas by IV contrast CT or MRI, pancreatic pseudocyst, pancreatic ascites, or pancreatic pseudoaneurysm. Organ failure is defined as the occurrence of any of the following criteria occurring in the setting of acute pancreatitis: (1) serum creatinine sustained >2.0 mg/dL; (2) Po$_2$ < 60; (3) systolic blood pressure <90 mm Hg or >500 cc of GI blood loss within a 24-hour period. The development of organ failure within the first few days of an attack of acute pancreatitis is a poor predictor of outcome. Within the first week of acute pancreatitis the development of organ failure accounts for the majority of deaths. Beyond 2 weeks into an attack of pancreatitis, infected pancreatic necrosis is the leading cause of death.

SEVERITY STRATIFICATION

The need to rapidly determine which patients are at risk for developing severe acute pancreatitis has led to the development of several severity stratification systems. The most commonly used system is Ranson's criteria (table 72.2). One of the drawbacks of Ranson's criteria is that it takes 48 hours to obtain all of the data. The Acute Physiologic and Chronic Health Evaluation score (APACHE-II) evaluates 13 physiological parameters that can be measured at any time during the hospitalization. Studies have shown the APACHE-II to be a more acute predictor of severe outcome than Ranson's criteria. In general a Ranson's score >3 and an APACHE-II score >8 are considered to be indicative of poor prognosis and outcome.

A serum hematocrit >44 in subjects with acute pancreatitis was found to be an accurate predictor of severe acute pancreatitis and pancreatic necrosis. Other factors predictive of severe acute pancreatitis include a BMI >40 kg/m^2, an imaging study that shows the presence of a pleural effusion, elevated serum IL-6, or urinary trypsin. CT scanning is a very sensitive and readily available method for severity stratification in acute pancreatitis. CT scoring can be graded on a 10-point severity scoring system referred to as the Balthazaar scoring system. Despite its superior visualization properties and ready availability, CT may be contraindicated in individuals with renal dysfunction and acute pancreatitis. MRI with gadolinium is an alternative to CT scan that is as accurate as CT and does not have the possible renal toxicity. The disadvantage of MRI in severe acute pancreatitis is that patients may be too unstable to undergo an MRI scan.

TREATMENT

Treatment of acute pancreatitis is dependent on the etiology of the disease. Early management should focus on

Table 72.2 RANSON'S CRITERIA FOR ACALCULOUS PANCREATITIS

ON ADMISSION	48 HOURS AFTER ADMISSION
Age >55 yr	Decrease in HCT >10 points
WBC count >16,000/mm^3	Serum calcium <8 mg/dL
Glucose >200 mg/dL	Increase in BUN >5 mg/dL
LDH >350 IU/L	Base deficit >4 mmol/L
AST >250 U/L	Fluid deficit >6 L

identification and treatment of all reversible causes of acute pancreatitis.

Gallstone Pancreatitis

Detection of gallstone pancreatitis by transabdominal ultrasound should be performed early in subjects with suspected gallstone-induced pancreatitis. Additionally, biliary microlithiasis and sludge may cause pancreatitis in the absence of overt stones; magnetic resonance cholangiopancreatography (MRCP) may be attempted in cases where transabdominal ultrasound is limited due to bowel gas overlying the pancreas and gallbladder. If gallstone-induced pancreatitis is complicated by the development of cholangitis, then emergent ERCP with sphincterotomy should be performed prior to cholecystectomy. Several randomized trials have shown that in the setting of cholangitis, ERCP improves outcome.

Triglycerides usually do not cause pancreatitis unless the serum level exceeds 1000 mg/dL. Aggressive lipid-lowering agents once the pancreatitis has resolved are used to treat prevent further attacks. In severe cases, plasmapheresis has been used to remove excess triglycerides from the serum. Autoimmune pancreatitis may respond to treatment with high-dose steroids, Treatment is usually initiated at a starting dose of 40 mg of prednisone daily. Prednisone is weaned by 5 mg every 1–2 weeks.

Other Treatments

Analgesic Support

Patients with acute pancreatitis may require narcotic treatment for pain. The type of narcotics used and their duration are dependent on the patient and institutional prescribing practices.

Intravenous fluids are necessary because the majority of subjects with acute pancreatitis have severe third spacing. The majority of patients do not receive adequate fluid resuscitation. Careful monitoring of urine output and overall hemodynamic status should be monitored in subjects with severe acute pancreatitis. Central venous pressure (CVP) lines or Swan-Ganz catheterization may also be used to guide monitoring of hemodynamic status.

Antibiotics

The role of prophylactic antibiotic therapy in early acute pancreatitis remains controversial. There have been at least 10 studies evaluating the role of prophylactic antibiotic therapy in severe acute pancreatitis. Two recent meta-analyses show a slight mortality benefit for the early administration of prophylactic antibiotic therapy in severe acute pancreatitis. This is countered by a recent well-done randomized controlled trial that showed no mortality benefit after the prophylactic administration of antibiotics in severe acute pancreatitis. Thus, the precise role of prophylactic antibiotic therapy in severe acute pancreatitis remains controversial. There is currently no role for the administration of prophylactic antibiotics in mild interstitial edematous pancreatitis.

Pancreatic Rest

All subjects with acute pancreatitis should undergo bowel rest. The duration of pancreatic rest through withholding oral intake is dependent on the patient's recovery period. There currently are no definitive guidelines regarding when to restart oral nutrition and what should be the constituency of the nutrition. Most individuals will begin oral nutrition when symptoms are absent and they feel ready to eat.

Enteral Versus Parenteral Nutrition

Studies have shown a mortality and morbidity benefit when patients with severe pancreatitis are fed enterally beyond the ligament of Treitz compared to feeding with total parenteral nutrition (TPN). Subsequent studies have also showed that enteral feeding is safer and more cost-effective than TPN. Recently it has been shown that feeding via a gastrostomy tube may be as safe and efficacious as feeding beyond the ligament of Treitz. This question is currently being investigated in a multicenter randomized study.

Surgical Debridement

Surgical necrosectomy is indicated when infected necrosis is identified. Recently endoscopic and percutaneous approaches have shown promise as alternative debridement methods in select patients. Debridement of infected necrosis is usually delayed until 4–6 weeks into the course of the disease. Early debridement has been associated with poor outcomes.

Complications

Metabolic

Owing to the severe inflammation associated with acute pancreatitis, there are multiple metabolic complications that are common such as hyperglycemia, hypocalcemia, and hyperlipidemia. Treatment is usually supportive.

Pseudocysts

Pseudocysts are defined as fluid collections of fibrous and granulation tissue. Most pseudocysts develop 4–6 weeks after the development of severe acute pancreatitis. Only symptomatic pseudocysts should be treated. Treatment is by surgical endoscopic or radiological drainage depending on the location and local expertise.

Pancreatic Necrosis

The development of pancreatic necrosis occurs in 20% of cases of severe acute pancreatitis.

Multiorgan System Failure

Acute respiratory distress syndrome (ARDS) acute tubular necrosis, and other organ failure are treated supportively.

PROGNOSIS

The prognosis for severe acute pancreatitis remains poor with significant morbidity and mortality. For individuals with mild interstitial edematous pancreatitis, their prognosis is excellent.

CHRONIC PANCREATITIS

Chronic pancreatitis is defined as chronic inflammatory changes that may be patchy throughout the pancreatic gland. This typically results in chronic pain.

EPIDEMIOLOGY

The prevalence of chronic pancreatitis has been estimated to vary from 0.04% to 0.5% in the United States. The incidence of chronic pancreatitis in the United States is approximately 27.4 per 100,000.

ETIOLOGY

Although chronic alcohol abuse was thought to be the most common cause of chronic pancreatitis, in many patients there is no clear cause (idiopathic). There is no known minimal threshold level of alcohol ingestion that results in pancreatitis, but it has been reported that most individuals with chronic pancreatitis have 6 years of >150 g of ethanol consumption daily. Alcohol ingestion usually results in chronic calcific pancreatitis. Tropical pancreatitis is an idiopathic form of chronic pancreatitis typified by fibrocalcific disease and brittle diabetes. It is common in areas of Southeast Asia and Africa. The etiology remains unexplained. Recently it has been shown that greater than one-third of individuals with tropical pancreatitis have mutations in the *SPINK1* gene.

Genetic causes of chronic pancreatitis are similar to those seen in recurrent acute pancreatitis and include mutations in the genes encoding for *CFTR, PRSS1,* and *SPINK-1.* Chronic pancreatitis may result from repeated episodes of acute pancreatitis such as that seen in hypertriglyceridemia-induced pancreatitis.

PATHOGENESIS

The underlying mechanisms that lead to chronic pancreatitis remain unknown. Alcohol has been shown to cause chronic pancreatitis by direct toxic effects on the acinar cell. The remaining causes of damage to the pancreatic acinar cell occur due to a variety of mechanisms including increased oxidative stress, genetic abnormalities, tissue necrosis, and chronic obstruction or stricture formation.

DIAGNOSIS

Clinical Findings

The three main clinical findings associated with chronic pancreatitis are pain, steatorrhea, and diabetes. The onset of the time from the beginning of these symptoms is variable, but signs of exocrine failure manifest as steatorrhea or endocrine failure (diabetes mellitus) may occur 12–15 years after the onset of disease. Pain in chronic pancreatitis has been described as two variants. The first type is an intermittent pain syndrome with variable attacks of pain. This pain syndrome may eventually evolve into the second type—a constant severe debilitating pain syndrome. The reason for this transition is unclear but may relate to inflammatory changes in the celiac plexus neurons. The pain of chronic pancreatitis is very similar to that seen in acute pancreatitis. Approximately 20% of subjects with chronic pancreatitis do not develop pain and instead present with end-stage complications such as pancreatic steatorrhea and diabetes. Anorexia and weight loss are common findings in severe chronic pancreatitis.

LABORATORY TESTS

Lab Studies

Amylase and lipase levels do not correlate with disease activity in chronic pancreatitis and typically are normal. Other laboratory studies such as complete blood count (CBC) and liver function tests are typically normal. Pancreatic steatorrhea may be confirmed when a fecal elastase test demonstrates values <100 µg/g of stool.

Imaging

Imaging in acute pancreatitis is used to detect changes in the structure of the pancreas consistent with chronic pancreatitis. Standard x-ray imaging of the pancreas may reveal calcifications that are diagnostic for the disease. Pancreatic calcifications are seen in approximately 30% of patients with chronic pancreatitis. CT has a sensitivity that ranges from 70–90% and includes calcifications, pancreatic atrophy, and ductal dilation. MRI is as sensitive CT and has the added benefit of being able to evaluate the pancreatic ductal system, which can be further enhanced when secretin is administered to increase pancreatic ductal flow. ERCP is helpful in detecting abnormalities of the main pancreatic duct and the side branches. It does carry an increased risk of causing pancreatitis. Eridoscopic ultrasound (EUS) has emerged as a diagnostic tool for chronic pancreatitis. There are currently nine criteria used by EUS to diagnose chronic pancreatitis. The more criteria that are present, the higher the likelihood that a subject has chronic pancreatitis. It is unknown whether the absence of EUS features of chronic pancreatitis rules out the possibility of chronic pancreatitis in a given patient.

Functional Tests

The gold standard for the diagnosis of chronic pancreatitis is the endoscopic secretin pancreatic function test. In this test a tube is placed in the proximal duodenum, and pancreatic secretions are aspirated after the intravenous administration of secretin. The aspiration of the pancreatic fluid occurs every 15 minutes for 1 hour. The diagnosis of chronic pancreatitis is made when the peak bicarbonate level is <75 meq/L during the 60-minute collection period. The main strength of the endoscopic pancreatic secretin function test is its ability to confirm the diagnosis of chronic pancreatitis early in the course of disease when imaging tests are normal.

TREATMENT

Chronic pain can be difficult to manage. A comprehensive approach is recommended consisting of analgesics and the management of expectations including inability to work, insomnia, and depression. Agents that modulate visceral pain such as amitriptyline are sometimes used. We recommend that all subjects with chronic pancreatitis and chronic pain be managed through a dedicated pain center and a multidisciplinary management team.

Pancreatic Enzymes

Pancreatic enzymes have a dual role in the management of chronic pancreatitis. There is some evidence that pancreatic enzyme supplementation may decrease pain in chronic pancreatitis. However, a recent meta-analysis showed that there is no improvement in pain by administering pancreatic enzymes in chronic pancreatitis. Pancreatic enzymes are effective in the management of pancreatic steatorrhea. Enzymes are given with the initial ingestion of food with sufficient levels of lipase to prevent clinical signs of steatorrhea.

Endoscopic Therapy

Endoscopic therapy includes the placement of pancreatic stents, sphincterotomy, and endoscopic drainage of fluid collections. The ability to manage strictures and fluid collections endoscopically carries low morbidity and represents one tool for the management of chronic pancreatitis. However, the lack of randomized controlled trials for sphincterotomy or stenting in chronic pancreatitis patients without strictures prevents recommendation of these procedures. Celiac plexus blockade may be a short-term solution used for the treatment of chronic pain but typically lasts no more than 2–3 months.

Surgery

Surgical management of chronic pancreatitis may be considered when there is either a dilated pancreatic duct or extensive inflammatory or calcific disease localized to one area of the pancreas. A lateral pancreaticojejunostomy provides pain relief in 70% of patients when the duct is dilated >8 mm. Other surgical interventions such as distal pancreatectomy and modified Whipple procedures may be effective therapies. However, surgical resections may increase the risk of development of diabetes mellitus.

COMPLICATIONS

Pancreatic Pseudocyst

Unlike the pseudocysts seen in acute pancreatitis, of which 50% resolve spontaneously, pseudocyst development in chronic pancreatitis may result in cysts that do not spontaneously resolve and require drainage. Surgical, endoscopic, and radiological drainage procedures can be used to manage symptomatic pseudocysts. Rarely pseudocysts may form fistulas, become infected, or bleed.

Pancreatic Malignancy

Four percent of all patients with chronic pancreatitis will develop adenocarcinoma of the pancreas. The risk is increased threefold in smokers. Hereditary pancreatitis is associated with up to a 40% chance of developing adenocarcinoma by 70 years of age, especially if the gene is transmitted from the paternal side. Significant changes in symptoms, especially in older individuals, should prompt cross-sectional imaging to assess for malignancy.

PROGNOSIS

The long-term survival for patients with chronic pancreatitis remains limited with a 20-year survival of 40–50%. Early intervention and aggressive management may result in improved management of these patients.

PANCREATIC NEOPLASMS

The most common forms of pancreatic neoplasia that will be encountered by the practicing physician consist of the following broad categories: adenocarcinoma of the pancreas, cystic pancreatic neoplasms, and a variety of rare endocrine and neuroendocrine tumors of the pancreas.

Cystic neoplasms are the most common neoplasms of the pancreas. There has been a tremendous increase in the incidence of these lesions over the last several years. The increase can be attributed to the improved sensitivity of MRI and CT scans to detect small lesions of the pancreas. Cystic neoplasms may be classified into three principal types: serous cystadenomas, mucinous cystadenomas/carcinomas, and intraductal papillary mucinous neoplasms. Although the majority of pancreatic cystic neoplasms are benign, the mucin-containing neoplasms have the potential to develop into malignancy. Features that increase the risk of malignancy include the presence of mucin, cyst size >3 cm, dilation of the main pancreatic duct, and/or the presence of septations or lobularity. The presence of mucin plus one or more of these characteristics in an individual with a pancreatic cyst suggests that surgical resection be considered. In addition to these features, any symptoms that are caused by the presence of a cyst such as chronic abdominal pain, diarrhea, or obstructive jaundice also warrant surgical consideration. If the likelihood of malignancy of a cyst still cannot be determined despite evaluation of these features, an endoscopic ultrasound-guided fine-needle aspiration (FNA) can be performed. A cyst fluid CEA level of >192 mg/dL is associated with an 87% likelihood that the cyst is mucinous and may harbor malignancy. Mucin stains are usually performed on all cyst samples. FNA samples can also be sent for analysis of loss of heterozygosity and genetic mutations that are associated with increased malignant risk.

SEROUS CYSTADENOMAS

Serous cystadenomas have small centrally located multiseptated lesions cysts that usually have a central calcification and scar. They tend to occur almost exclusively in women and are usually found incidentally. Serous cystadenomas have almost no malignant potential, and the majority can be followed longitudinally with serial imaging. Treatment is recommended only for symptomatic lesions. Long-term prognosis is excellent.

MUCINOUS CYSTADENOMAS AND CYSTADENOCARCINOMAS

Mucinous cystadenomas and cystadenocarcinomas are generally large, peripherally located cysts that are septated. Peripheral calcification may also be present. These tumors tend to be slow growing and may harbor a solid or mass-like component. Although mucinous cystadenomas are not malignant, they are at high risk for malignant transformation. It may be extremely difficult to determine if a mucinous lesion is malignant by visual inspection. EUS-guided FNA of the lesion is not very sensitive, and surgical resection may be necessary to make the diagnosis and prevent malignancy. Prognosis after resection for localized noninvasive disease is excellent.

INTRAPAPILLARY MUCINOUS NEOPLASM

Intrapapillary mucinous neoplasms (IPMN) are mucous-secreting tumors originating in the main pancreatic duct or its side branches. Mucus plugging can lead to the development of acute pancreatitis by obstruction of pancreatic outflow. They are often discovered incidentally or as part of an evaluation for unexplained pancreatitis. A highly suggestive sign of these lesions is the presence of a patulous ampulla of Vater that is secreting large amounts of mucin.

NATURAL HISTORY, RECOMMENDED TREATMENT, AND PROGNOSIS

The natural history of these lesions is dependent on the extent of involvement of the pancreatic duct. Main-branch IPMN are more likely to develop into malignant lesions with a 30% prevalence of adenocarcinoma formation. Side-branch IPMN are slower growing than main-branch IPMN. They may also harbor malignancy at the time of detection, but the likelihood of this is much less than that of main-branch IPMN. Main-branch IPMN is treated with surgical resection: however this is dependent on localization of disease and the patient's surgical risk. Prognosis for resection of localized disease is excellent. Side-ranch IPMN is followed with MRCP generally on a 6- to 12-month basis with surgery prompted only when there is concern for malignant changes. Long-term prognosis after resection is excellent.

EXOCRINE NEOPLASMS OF THE PANCREAS

Adenocarcinoma of the exocrine pancreas is a highly lethal malignancy with a 1-year survival of <10%. Currently, it is the 11th most common cause of cancer seen in the United States and the fifth leading cause of cancer deaths in the United States. The lethal characteristics of the disease are due to the fact that early symptoms may be vague or absent. Low back pain that localizes to the midepigastrium and radiates to the back and weight loss are common presenting symptoms. A small percentage of individuals (<15%) will have new adult-onset diabetes mellitus develop as a presenting symptom. Other symptoms of pancreatic adenocarcinoma include unexplained pancreatitis and new-onset obstructive

jaundice. Risk factors for pancreatic cancer development include cigarette smoking, chronic pancreatitis, more than two first-degree relatives who developed pancreatic cancer, *BRCA-1* or *BRCA-2* mutation, mutations of the cationic trypsin gene or a history of the familial atypical mole melanoma nevus syndrome.

PATHOGENESIS

The pathogenesis of adenocarcinoma of the pancreas remains unknown; however, within recent years a neoplasia-carcinoma sequence has been described. According to this model pancreatic adenocarcinomas arise from the progression of normal pancreatic ductal epithelium through several dysplastic stages. These dysplastic areas are known as pancreatic intraepithelial neoplasia (Pan-IN). Pan-INs are graded by level of severity from 1 to 3. Pan-IN3 represents carcinoma in situ. Coincident with the progression through the Pan-IN stages, lesions destined to become pancreatic adenocarcinomas also begin to develop mutations in tumor suppressor genes. The most common mutation is the K-RAS gene which is found in at least 75% of adenocarcinomas of the pancreas.

DIAGNOSIS AND TREATMENT

The majority of pancreatic adenocarcinomas occur in the head of the pancreas (65%). Disease that occurs in the head of the pancreas is often diagnosed at an earlier stage because it usually leads to symptoms of jaundice and pancreatic outflow obstruction. Diagnosis may be confirmed with CT, MRI, endoscopic ultrasound, or ERCP. Each modality has its strengths, and the utility of each in the diagnosis of adenocarcinoma of the pancreas is a function of availability and local expertise. CA 19–9 levels >500 in the setting of a pancreatic mass is greater than 90% sensitive and specific for adenocarcinoma of the pancreas. Diseases such as cholangitis can produce false positives. CA19–9 levels in the 200–300 range when associated with an elevated CEA provide similar sensitivity and specificity. However, normal values of these markers do not rule out adenocarcinoma of the pancreas. The combination of CT imaging, laparoscopic evaluation, and laparoscopic ultrasound predicts resectability in >91% of cases.

Determinants of Resectability

The goal of the preoperative evaluation of pancreatic cancer is to determine if a malignancy is present and whether it is resectable. Findings indicative of unresectable disease are encasement of the superior mesenteric, celiac, or hepatic artery or veins by tumor or evidence of distant metastases. The goal of surgery is to remove all visualized disease and to have clear resection margins. If the disease is localized to the head of the pancreas, then generally a Whipple procedure is performed. Because of concerns with gastric emptying after a Whipple procedure, the pylorus-preserving Whipple procedure is frequently used. Although about 25% of subjects will develop delayed gastric emptying following the Whipple procedure, the majority will have resolution of their symptoms within 4–6 weeks. If the disease involves the body or tail, a distal pancreatectomy or subtotal pancreatectomy is performed.

Management of Unresectable Disease

Disease that is found to be unresectable is treated with palliative therapy including biliary stenting for malignant obstruction and surgery for duodenal obstruction. Weight loss is managed with a combination of pancreatic enzyme supplementation and supplemental feeding as indicated. Pain management consists of administration of analgesics including narcotics. Celiac plexus blockade has been shown to effectively palliate pain in subjects with pancreatic cancer involving the head of the pancreas. Tumors involving the body and tail of the pancreas have not shown as promising results.

PROGNOSIS AND TREATMENT

The 5-year survival rate for individuals who undergo successful surgical resection is approximately 10–30%. Studies of radiation therapy and chemotherapy alone have not shown any survival benefit in the management of pancreatic cancer. When radiation therapy and chemotherapy are used to treat individuals who have undergone surgical resection, there was a significant increase (23 vs. 11 months) in postresection survival rates. The drug gemcitabine was shown to improve the quality of life in subjects who receive it as part of a postresection regimen, although this treatment did not significantly improve mortality.

ADDITIONAL READING

Bradley EL 3rd. A clinically based classification system for acute pancreatitis. Summary of the International Symposium on Acute Pancreatitis. Atlanta, Ga, September 11–13. 1992. *Arch Surg.* 1993;128(5):586–90.

DiMagno MJ, DiMagno EP. Chronic pancreatitis. *Curr Opin Gastroenterol.* 2010;26(5):490–8.

Donahue TR, Reber HA. Pancreatic surgery. *Curr Opin Gastroenterol.* 2010;26(5):499–505.

Etemad B, Whitcomb DC. Chronic pancreatitis: Diagnosis, classification, and new genetic developments. *Gastroenterology.* 2001;120(3):682–707.

G o, VLW. Etiology and epidemiology of pancreatitis in the United States. In: Bradley EL III (ed.), *Acute Pancreatitis Diagnosis and Therapy* (pp. 238–9). New York: Raven Press, 1994.

Gupta K, Wu B. In the clinic. Acute pancreatitis. *Ann Intern Med.* 2010;153(9):ITC51–5; quiz ITC516.

Klein SD, Affronti JP. Pancreas divisum, an evidence-based review: Part I. Pathophysiology. *Gastrointest Endosc.* 2004;60(3):419–25.

Klein SD, Affronti JP. Pancreas divisum, an evidence-based review: Part II. Patient selection and treatment. *Gastrointest Endosc.* 2004;60(4):585–9.

Lara LP, Chari ST. Autoimmune pancreatitis. *Curr Gastroenterol Rep.* 2005;7(2):101–6.

Lowenfels AB, Sullivan T, Fioranti J, et al. The epidemiology and impact of pancreatic diseases in the United States. *Curr Gastroenterol Rep.* 2005;7(2):90–5.

Raraty MG, Connor S, Criddle DM, et al. Acute pancreatitis and organ failure: Pathophysiology, natural history, and management strategies. *Curr Gastroenterol Rep.* 2004;6(2):99–103.

Steer ML. Pathogenesis of acute pancreatitis. *Digestion.* 1997;58 Suppl 1:46–9.

QUESTIONS

QUESTION 1. You are asked to see a 42-year-old male who has suffered a first episode of pancreatitis. His pancreatitis was documented by a history of severe pain localized to the midepigastrum with radiation to the back and a serum lipase of 1500. He has no prior history of pancreatitis. He has no family history of pancreatic disease. Your preliminary evaluation reveals that he does not drink alcohol, has no gallstones, has normal triglycerides and electrolytes, and takes no medications. What do you recommend regarding his evaluation?

A. Perform an ERCP and evaluate him for ductal abnormalities.

B. Perform a cholecystectomy.

C. No further work-up is warranted at this time.

D. Perform an endoscopic ultrasound to look for evidence of a pancreatic mass.

E. None of the above.

QUESTION 2. A 35-year-old woman who has been in the hospital for 4 weeks with acute pancreatitis is about to be discharged. A CT scan obtained 3 days ago showed a 7-cm fluid collection in the head of the pancreas. The cyst was not present on a CT scan obtained at the onset of her admission. The official description by the radiology staff for the large fluid-filled mass is "pancreatic pseudocyst." The medical team is worried about sending her home with this large cyst in her pancreas. What do you recommend?

A. Contact the surgical team to arrange for surgical drainage of the cyst.

B. Discharge the patient and arrange for follow-up at a later date.

C. Schedule an endoscopic ultrasound in order to obtain a fine-needle aspiration of the cyst.

D. Check a CA 19–9 and reimage the abdomen in 6 weeks.

E. None of the above.

QUESTION 3. You are asked to see a 64-year-old male who has undergone a Whipple resection for newly diagnosed adenocarcinoma of the pancreas. The surgical resection margins were clear on subsequent evaluation, but evaluation of the lymph nodes revealed two nodes with evidence of adenocarcinoma. Which of the following therapies has been shown to have the greatest overall impact on patient quality of life?

A. Chemotherapy + radiation therapy + gemcitabine treatment
B. Chemotherapy + gemcitabine
C. Radiation therapy alone
D. Palliative decompressive bypass
E. Lymph node ablation + chemotherapy

QUESTION 4. A 50-year-old female is referred to you for evaluation of a newly diagnosed pancreatic cyst. The cyst was discovered during an evaluation for possible kidney stones. The patient has brought you a copy of her most recent MRI. On review you note that the cyst is 5.5 cm in size and has evidence of a few septations in the internal architecture. It is localized to the midbody of the pancreas. The main pancreatic duct is dilated to 10 mm behind the cyst but appears normal in the portion anterior to the cyst. She denies any history of known pancreatitis but has admitted to feeling full much earlier than she had in the past. She views her early satiety as a good thing and has been able to lose 15 lb in 2 months. What do you recommend?

A. CT scan of the abdomen
B. EUS and fine needle aspiration of the cyst.

C. Consideration for surgical resection
D. Repeat MRI scan in 6 months with close observation
E. None of the above

QUESTION 5. A 28-year-old male with a history of chronic abdominal pain and alcohol use is referred to you for evaluation. He reports that he developed constant pain about 3 years ago. The pain is severe and radiates to the back. He was once told that he might have chronic pancreatitis, but each time he goes to the emergency room he has normal serum lipase values and normal pancreatic cross-sectional imaging. Which of the following is the best method for investigating the patient's symptoms?

A. ERCP
B. Endoscopic ultrasound
C. Endoscopic pancreatic function test
D. MRCP with secretin
E. None of the above

ANSWERS

1. C
2. B
3. A
4. C
5. C

73.

LIVER DISEASE

Brian Hyett and Sanjiv Chopra

The proper evaluation of liver disease can present a challenge to the practicing clinician. Physicians are often faced with a confusing array of what are commonly referred to as "liver function tests." In fact, with the commonplace use of automated serum testing batteries, abnormal results are increasingly detected in asymptomatic persons. There are numerous examples of algorithms and flow diagrams designed with an aim toward aiding clinicians in completion of an adequate diagnostic valuation when faced with a particular set of abnormalities on liver function tests. However, a clearer understanding of these tests might be of greater value than such a systematic and regimented approach to the evaluation of liver disease.

An ideal liver function test would be one that could detect minimal liver disease, point to a particular liver function disorder, and be capable of reflecting the severity of the underlying problem. Because no such laboratory test exists, the term, liver function tests, generally refers to a group of serologic tests that evaluate different aspects of liver function; it is a term that is best utilized keeping in mind the clinical context and in conjunction with serial determinations to ascertain the evolution of the hepatic disorder. In addition, cholangiography, ultrasound, computed tomography (CT), magnetic resonance imaging (MRI), and histologic assessment (via liver biopsy) are often utilized to delineate the nature of the liver disease and as such may also be viewed in the broad context as tests of liver function.

SERUM TRANSAMINASES

Aspartate aminotransferase (AST), previously called serum glutamic oxaloacetic transaminase (SGOT), and alanine aminotransferase (ALT), previously called serum glutamic pyruvic transaminase (SGPT), are markers of hepatocyte injury. These enzymes transfer amino groups from aspartate and alanine to ketoglutaric acid. As liver cells are injured, their cell membranes become permeable, and enzymes leak into the systemic circulation. Therefore, elevations in aminotransferases suggest that liver cells are being injured. ALT is primarily localized to the liver but can originate from muscle. AST is in the liver as well, but it is also found on skeletal and cardiac muscle, the kidneys, and the brain. Thus, an isolated elevation of AST could be indicative of injury to one of these other organs.

Both AST and ALT are commonly utilized to assess liver function. Elevations in the thousands in the serum levels of AST, a mitochondrial enzyme, and ALT, a cytosolic enzyme, are encountered in acute viral hepatitis, acute drug- or toxin-induced liver damage, autoimmune hepatitis, Wilson disease, (hemolysis, elevated liver enzymes, and low platelets) syndrome, acute fatty liver of pregnancy, and ischemic hepatitis. The height of the elevation does not, however, correlate with extent of liver cell necrosis evident on liver biopsy and therefore has no predictive prognostic value. Rapidly decreasing transaminase levels together with a rising bilirubin level and prolongation of the prothrombin time (PT) predict a very poor prognosis.

In most of these conditions the transaminase levels usually return to normal over several weeks to months with resolution of the primary hepatic disorder. An exception is ischemic hepatitis, where the transaminase levels often return to normal within days as the hypotension or left ventricular failure is corrected or alleviated. The transaminase elevations are mild to modest in alcoholic hepatitis.

A common cause of transaminitis is medication-induced hepatic injury. Several drugs may cause raised liver enzymes. Common ones implicated frequently include nonsteroidal anti-inflammatory drugs, antibiotics, statins, antiepileptics, and antituberculosis drugs (see table 73.1). Several other medications and substances have also been implicated as injurious agents in liver disease (see table 73.2). Other causes of transaminitis include viral hepatitis, hemochromatosis and alpha-1-antitrypsin deficiency.

Characteristically, the ALT level is much higher than the AST, but this is variable in disease states, and patterns of their relationship are indicative of various conditions. For instance, in acute alcoholic hepatitis with cirrhosis, which has an inordinately high mortality. The AST and

Table 73.1 COMMONLY PRESCRIBED MEDICATIONS ASSOCIATED WITH TRANSAMINITIS

Nonsteroidal anti-inflammatory drugs
Antibiotics
Statins
Antiepileptic drugs
Antituberculous drugs

Table 73.3 ETIOLOGIES OF SERUM AMINOTRANS-FERASE LEVELS EXCEEDING 500 IU/L

Acute viral hepatitis
Drug or toxic liver injury
Ischemic hepatitis
Severe chronic active hepatitis
CBD stone
Acute Budd-Chiari and venoocclusive disease
Acute fatty liver of pregnancy and HELLP syndrome
Wilson disease

ALT are almost always <300 IU/L with an AST-to-ALT ratio greater than 2:1. Elevations greater than 500 IU in either transaminase level are unusual and signify a narrow differential diagnosis (see table 73.3). In patients with extrahepatic obstruction, both transaminase levels are almost invariably less than 1000 IU/L. One study of 140 patients with nonalcoholic steatohepatitis (NASH) confirmed by liver biopsy or alcoholic liver disease found a mean AST/ALT ratio of 0.9 in patients with NASH and 2.6 in patients with alcoholic liver disease. Within the population studied, 87% of patients with an AST/ALT ratio of 1.3 or less had NASH (87% sensitivity, 84% specificity). The severity of NASH as measured by the degree of fibrosis increased, as did the AST/ALT ratio. A mean ratio of 1.4 was found in patients with cirrhosis related to NASH. Wilson disease, a rare condition, can cause the AST/ALT ratio to exceed 4. Last, hepatic involvement with metastatic tumors, tuberculosis, sarcoidosis, and amyloidosis may cause a modest (up to threefold) rise in aminotransferases.

Significant elevations of transaminase levels have been noted in a few normal, healthy subjects while consuming a diet of conventional foods containing 25–30% of total calories as sucrose. False-positive elevations in AST levels

have been reported in patients receiving erythromycin estolate or *para*-aminosalicylic acid and during diabetic ketoacidosis, when the AST level has been determined by calorimetric assay. The opposite, that is, falsely lowered (sometimes absent) transaminases, has been observed in azotemic patients. AST activity increases significantly after hemodialysis, but the inhibitor does not appear to be urea. As for intrinsic changes in these enzymes, ALT has diurnal variation, may vary day to day, and may be affected by exercise. AST may be 15% higher in black men than white men at baseline. In addition, a study of Danish twins showed that genetic factors accounted for 33–66% of the variation in ALT in patients 73–94 years of age.

Although elevations in transaminase levels may be the first laboratory signal of liver disease (preicteric phase) or the only signal (anicteric hepatitis) to a physician, it is important to remember that significant liver damage may be present in a patient with normal levels of transaminases despite advanced liver disease (see table 73.4). This is well represented in a study of 22 NASH patients, in which there were almost twice as many patients with fibrosis progression than with regression (32% vs. 18%), yet progression of fibrosis occurred despite normalization of aminotransferase values and could not be confidently predicted by clinical or standard biological data. On the other hand, 1–4% of the asymptomatic population may have elevated serum liver chemistries.

"Unexplained" (normal liver biopsy results) elevations of both transaminase levels may have their basis in a primary muscle disorder, celiac sprue, thyroid disease, or adrenal insufficiency. Hence, obtaining serum for cortisol levels, tissue transglutaminase (TTG), thyroid-stimulating hormone (TSH), and creatine phosphokinase (CPK) is crucial to the complete workup of such patients (see table 73.5). Immediately after muscle injury, the AST/ALT ratio is generally greater than 3 but approaches 1 within a few days because of a faster decline in the serum AST. As for celiac sprue, one study of 140 consecutive patients with a comprehensive negative serologic workup and no significant pathology on biopsy found 13 patients (9.3%) with positive antigliadin and antiendomysial antibody tests and

Table 73.2 TYPES OF LIVER INJURY DUE TO POTENTIALLY INJURIOUS AGENTS (FROM UP-TO-DATE)

PREDICTABLE	IDIOSYNCRATIC	CAPABLE OF CAUSING CHRONIC DISEASE
17-Alpha alkyl steroids (2,6)	Methyldopa (1,3)	Methyldopa (1,3)
Acetaminophen (1)	Aspirin (1)	Isoniazid (1,3)
Ergot (10)	Phenytoin (1	Methotrexate (1,3,4)
Ethanol (1,2,3,4)	Halothane (1)	Nitrofurantoin (1,2,3)
Tetracycline (4)	Isoniazid (1,3)	Neoplasia
Vinyl chloride (6,7)	Chlordiazepoxide (1)	Vinyl chloride (6,7)
	Methotrexate (1,3,4)	Sex hormones (6,7,8,9)
	Nitrofurantoin (1,2,3)	
	Phenothiazines (1,2)	
	Phenylbutazone (1,2,5)	
	Sulindac (1,2)	
	Sulfonamides (1,2)	
	Valproic acid (1)	

NOTE: 1: hepatocellular necrosis; 2: cholestasis; 3: fibrosis; 4: steatosis; 5: granulomas; 6: peliosis hepatis; 7: angiosarcoma; 8: focal nodular hyperplasia; 9: hepatic adenoma; 10: ischemic necrosis.

Table 73.4 **UNDERLYING ETIOLOGIES FOR NORMAL OR ONLY MARGINALLY ELEVATED SERUM AMINO-TRANSFERASE VALUES DESPITE SIGNIFICANT LIVER DISEASE**

Chronic hepatitis C infection
Idiopathic genetic hemochromatosis
Nonalcoholic fatty liver disease
Patients receiving methotrexate

duodenal biopsies consistent with sprue. In most cases of sprue-induced transaminitis, the ALT and AST levels will normalize on a gluten-free diet.

ALKALINE PHOSPHATASE

Although alkaline phosphatase is used routinely as a marker of biliary injury, the physiological significance of the enzyme is not known. However, in vitro, alkaline phosphatase catalyzes the hydrolysis of phosphate esters in an alkaline environment. The hepatic isoenzyme is located on the luminal surface of the canalicular membrane. Obstruction of any part of the biliary tree results in increased synthesis of alkaline phosphatases, subsequent reflux of the enzyme into the hepatic sinusoids, and rise in serum level. Although patients with elevated alkaline phosphatases are often suspected of having a liver disorder, the possibility that serum alkaline phosphatase elevations stem from other organs (especially bone) should be considered given that as many as one-third of individuals with an elevated alkaline phosphatase levels have no evidence of liver disease.

Serum alkaline phosphatase originates from liver, bone, intestine, or placenta. Occasionally, patients with a malignant tumor may have elevations that are not caused by liver or bony metastases but instead are due to an isoenzyme. This molecule, referred to as Regan isoenzyme, is biochemically and immunologically indistinguishable from placental alkaline phosphatase and, in addition to being present in serum, can also be present in tumor tissue or in malignant effusion fluids. Women in the third trimester of pregnancy have elevated serum alkaline phosphatase due to an influx into blood of placental alkaline phosphatase. Individuals with blood types O and B who are ABH secretors and Lewis antigen-

Table 73.5 **CAUSES OF "UNEXPLAINED" ALT ELEVATIONS AND ASSOCIATED LABORATORY TESTING***

ISEASE	TESTING
Muscle disease/injury	CPK
Celiac sprue	TTG antibody
Adrenal insufficiency	cortisol
Thyroid dysfunction	TSH

NOTE: *Remember the mnemonic MCAT.

positive can have elevated serum alkaline phosphatase after ingesting a fatty meal due to an influx of intestinal alkaline phosphatase. There are reports in the literature of a benign familial occurrence of elevated serum alkaline phosphatase due to intestinal alkaline phosphatase. In one report, two-fold to fourfold elevations in serum alkaline phosphatase levels were reported in several members of a family. No bone or hepatic disorder was present in this family, who demonstrated the enzyme elevation in a pattern suggesting autosomal dominant inheritance. Alkaline phosphatase levels also vary with age: rapidly growing adolescents can have serum alkaline phosphatase levels that are twice those of healthy adults secondary to leakage of bone alkaline phosphatase into blood. The normal serum alkaline phosphatase gradually increases from age 40 to 65. For instance, the normal alkaline phosphatase for an otherwise healthy 65-year-old woman is >50% higher than that of a healthy 30-year-old woman.

Patients with cholestasis have increased levels of alkaline phosphatase. Markedly elevated levels of serum alkaline phosphatase are also found in patients with osteoblastic bone disorders or with cholestatic—both intrahepatic and extrahepatic—disease. Hence, in patients with jaundice, distinguishing intrahepatic cholestasis including primary biliary cirrhosis, granulomas in the liver from extrahepatic obstruction including stones, strictures, "silent" malignancies, and other possibilities, is not possible on the basis of the height of the serum alkaline phosphatase level. Patients with stage I or II Hodgkin disease, hypernephroma, congestive heart failure, myeloid metaplasia, peritonitis, diabetes, subacute thyroiditis, or uncomplicated gastric ulcer have been reported to have mild elevations in serum alkaline phosphatase levels that are probably stemming from the liver in the absence of overt liver involvement.

In the case of hypernephroma, cholestasis may be seen as part of a paraneoplastic syndrome. This is referred to as nephrogenic hepatic dysfunction syndrome or Stauffer syndrome. The cause is unknown but may relate to secretion of IL-6. Other rare causes of cholestasis with associated elevations in alkaline phosphatase include hyperthyroidism, amyloidosis, and benign recurrent intrahepatic cholestasis (BRIC or Summerskill-Walshe-Tygstrup) syndrome. Patients with Wilson disease often have normal or below-normal values despite transaminitis.

Although an elevation of the serum alkaline phosphatase level may be the first clue to hepatobiliary disease, the alkaline phosphatase level is normal on some occasions despite extensive metastatic hepatic deposits or complete bile duct obstruction. When alkaline phosphatase levels are markedly elevated, it is common practice to concurrently measure serum 5'-nucleotidase, gamma-glutamyl transpeptidase, or leucine aminopeptidase. In such instances, elevations of the levels of any of these three enzymes generally imply that the source of the elevated alkaline phosphatase

Table 73.6 COMMON CAUSES OF ELEVATIONS IN ALKALINE PHOSPHATASE

Complete or partial bile duct obstruction

Primary biliary cirrhosis (PBC)

Primary sclerosing cholangitis

Adult bile ductopenia

Certain drugs such as androgenic steroids and phenytoin and toxins associated with cholestasis

Infiltrative diseases including sarcoidosis, tuberculosis

Granulomatous diseases

Cancer metastatic to the liver and associated obstructive jaundice

Bile duct stricture

Liver allograft rejection

Infectious hepatobiliary diseases seen in patients with AIDS (e.g., cytomegalovirus or microsporidiosis and tuberculosis with hepatic involvement)

---

level is hepatobiliary and not bony. The most common causes of liver-related increases in alkaline phosphatase are outlined in table 73.6.

GAMMA-GLUTAMYL TRANSPEPTIDASE

Gamma-glutamyl transpeptidase (GGT) is found in hepatocytes and biliary epithelial cells. GGT is very sensitive for detecting hepatobiliary disease but lacks specificity. Elevated levels of serum GGT have been reported in a variety of clinical conditions, including myocardial infarction, pancreatic disease, renal failure, chronic obstructive pulmonary disease, diabetes, and alcoholism. High serum GGT values are also found in patients taking medications such as phenytoin and barbiturates and in the setting of alcohol use. In fact, a markedly elevated serum GGT level for several days often follows moderate alcohol ingestion. This has been used by many physicians to detect alcohol abuse in patients who underestimate or deny the ingestion of alcohol.

Medications such as phenytoin, carbamazepine, and barbiturates may also cause a mild rise in GGT. With other enzyme abnormalities, a raised GGT would support a hepatobiliary source. It would, for instance, confirm hepatic source for a raised alkaline phosphatase. An elevated GGT with raised transaminases and a ratio of AST to ALT of 2:1 or more would suggest alcohol-related liver disease. But other than conferring liver specificity to an elevated alkaline phosphatase and possibly being used in identifying patients with alcohol abuse, serum GGT offers no advantage over aminotransferases and alkaline phosphatase. In one prospective study that included 1040 inpatients, 13% had an elevated serum GGT activity; but only 32% had hepatobiliary disease.

In the remaining patients the elevated serum GGT may have been due to alcohol ingestion or medications, with subsequent rise in levels but without underlying liver disease.

5'-NUCLEOTIDASE

5'-Nucleotidase is found in the liver, intestines, brain, heart, blood vessels, and endocrine pancreas. Similar to alkaline phosphatase, this enzyme is located subcellularly to hepatocytes. Despite its wide distribution in various organs, serum levels of 5'-nucleotidase are thought to be secondary to hepatobiliary release by detergent action of bile salts on the plasma membranes of hepatocytes. Values are lower in children than in adults, rise gradually in adolescence, and reach a nadir as late as age 50. Elevations in serum 5'-nucleotidase are seen in conjunction with, and due largely to, the same causes of increased serum alkaline phosphatase. Studies suggest that serum alkaline phosphatase and 5'-nucleotidase are equally useful tests for demonstrating biliary obstruction or hepatic infiltrative lesions. Although values of the two enzymes are generally well correlated, the concentrations may not rise proportionately in individual patients. Thus, in selected patients, one enzyme may be elevated and the other normal.

Leucine aminopeptidase and 5'-nucleotidase levels may increase in normal pregnancy, whereas gamma-glutamyl transpeptidase levels do not. Unlike GGT, the predominant usefulness of the 5'-nucleotidase assay is its specificity for hepatobiliary disease. An increased serum 5'-nucleotidase concentration in a nonpregnant person suggests that a concomitantly increased serum alkaline phosphatase is of hepatic origin. However, because of the occasional dissociation between the two enzymes, a normal serum 5'-nucleotidase does not rule out the liver as the source of an elevated serum alkaline phosphatase.

BILIRUBIN

Bilirubin results from the enzymatic breakdown of heme. Unconjugated bilirubin is transported to the liver bound to albumin. It is water insoluble and cannot be excreted in urine. Conjugated bilirubin is water soluble and appears in urine. Within the liver it is conjugated to bilirubin glucuronide and is secreted into bile and the gut. The intestinal flora breaks it down into urobilinogen, some of which is reabsorbed and either excreted via the kidney into urine or excreted by the liver into the gastrointestinal tract. The remainder is excreted in the stool as stercobilinogen. Bilirubin production increases in hemolysis, ineffective erythropoiesis, resorption of a hematoma, and rarely in muscle injury. In all these cases the bilirubin is mainly in an unconjugated form. Conjugated hyperbilirubinemia characteristically occurs in parenchymal liver disease and biliary obstruction. The serum conjugated bilirubin level does not become elevated until the liver has lost at least one-half of its excretory capacity.

Liver disease predominantly impairs the secretion of conjugated bilirubin into bile. As a result, conjugated bilirubin is filtered into the urine, where it can be detected by a dipstick test. The finding of bilirubin in urine is a sensitive indicator of the presence of an increased serum conjugated bilirubin level. In many healthy people, the serum unconjugated bilirubin is mildly elevated, especially after a 24-hour fast. If this is the only liver function test abnormality and the conjugated bilirubin level and complete blood count are normal, this can be assumed due to Gilbert syndrome, with no further evaluation required. Gilbert syndrome is related to a variety of partial defects in uridine diphosphate- glucuronosyl transferase, the enzyme that conjugates bilirubin. Mild unconjugated hyperbilirubinemia (total bilirubin level <5 mg/dL) is seen not only in Gilbert disease but also in uncomplicated hemolytic disorders and congestive heart failure. Mild conjugated hyperbilirubinemia is a constant finding in Dubin-Johnson and Rotor syndromes. Conjugated hyperbilirubinemia of varying intensity is seen in a variety of liver disorders including acute viral, drug-induced, and toxin-induced hepatitis, shock liver, and metastatic disease to the liver (see table 73.7). Even in fulminant hepatitis, the liver is capable of conjugating bilirubin. The height of the serum bilirubin level is not useful in distinguishing intrahepatic cholestasis from extrahepatic obstruction. In fact, elevations in total serum bilirubin levels have been reported in patients with non–biliary tract sepsis. Although patients with fulminant hepatitis may be anicteric, the level of serum bilirubin is important prognostically in conditions such as alcoholic hepatitis, primary biliary cirrhosis, and halothane hepatitis. For instance, in primary biliary cirrhosis, elevations of >2.0 mg/dL in the total

Table 73.7 CAUSES OF ELEVATIONS IN SERUM BILIRUBIN WITH NORMAL ALT, AST, ALK PHOS

Unconjugated
1. Increased bilirubin production
• Hemolysis
• Ineffective erythropoiesis
• Blood transfusion
• Resorption of hematomas
2. Decreased hepatic uptake
• Gilbert syndrome
• Drugs—for example, rifampicin
3. Decreased conjugation
• Gilbert syndrome
• Crigler-Najjar syndrome
• Physiological jaundice of the newborn
Conjugated
1. Dubin-Johnson syndrome
2. Rotor syndrome

bilirubin level usually occur late in the course of the disease and imply a poor prognosis, whereas levels >10 mg/dL have been associated with 60% mortality in patients with halothane hepatitis.

When a patient has prolonged, severe biliary obstruction followed by the restoration of bile flow, the serum bilirubin level can decline rapidly for several days and then slowly return to normal over a period of weeks. The slow phase of bilirubin clearance results from the presence of delta-bilirubin, a form of bilirubin chemically attached to serum albumin 33. Because albumin has a half-life of 3 weeks, delta-bilirubin clears more slowly than bilirubin-glucuronide. Clinical laboratories can measure delta-bilirubin concentrations, but such measurements are usually unnecessary if the physician is aware of the delta-bilirubin phenomenon.

ALBUMIN AND GAMMA-GLOBULINS

Albumin is only one of many proteins that are synthesized by the liver. However, because it is easy to measure, it represents a reliable and inexpensive laboratory test for physicians to assess the degree of liver damage present in any particular patient. When the liver has been chronically damaged, the albumin may be low. This would indicate that the synthetic function of the liver has been markedly diminished. The serum albumin concentration is usually normal in chronic liver diseases until cirrhosis and significant liver damage are present. Albumin levels can be low in conditions other than liver diseases including malnutrition, some kidney diseases, and other rarer conditions.

Approximately 10 g of albumin is synthesized and secreted by the liver every day. With progressive liver disease, serum albumin levels fall, reflecting decreased synthesis. Albumin levels are dependent on a number of factors such as the nutritional status, catabolism, hormonal factors, and urinary and gastrointestinal losses. These should be taken into account when interpreting low albumin levels. Still, albumin concentration does correlate with the prognosis in chronic liver disease. Because two-thirds of the amount of body albumin is located in the extravascular, extracellular space, changes in distribution can alter the serum concentration. Albumin is synthesized by hepatic parenchymal cells and has a serum half-life of about 20 days. Hypoalbuminemia secondary to excessive loss of the protein is seen in patients with nephrotic syndrome or protein-losing enteropathy.

A rise in levels of globulins, primarily gamma-globulins, is frequently seen in patients with chronic hepatitis or cirrhosis. Elevations in IgA levels are common in alcoholic cirrhosis, and elevations in IgG levels are common in autoimmune chronic active hepatitis. Elevations in IgM levels are seen in primary biliary cirrhosis; of the immunoglobulins, only an elevation of the IgM fraction on immunoelectrophoresis has any significant specificity. Diminished levels of alpha-L-globulins due to deficient alpha-l-antitrypsin activity can be associated with chronic active hepatitis and cirrhosis in children and adults.

PROTHROMBIN TIME

The liver synthesizes blood clotting factors II, V, VII, IX, and X. The PT measures the rate of conversion of prothrombin to thrombin (requiring the above-mentioned factors) and reflects the synthetic function of the liver. The PT does not become abnormal until >80% of liver synthetic capacity is lost. This makes PT an insensitive marker of liver dysfunction. Still, abnormal PT prolongation may be a sign of liver dysfunction. Besides liver disease, the PT may be prolonged in vitamin K deficiency, warfarin therapy, liver disease, and coagulopathy. The prognostic utility of an elevated PT is exemplified by the 100% mortality reported in a study of patients with halothane hepatitis who had a prothrombin time greater than 20 seconds. Other clinically relevant aspects of coagulopathies include the necessity to correct these factor deficiencies in patients with significant bleeding and the fact that certain procedures such as liver biopsy are contraindicated in patients with a significant coagulopathy.

Because factor VII has a short half-life (6 hours), it is sensitive to rapid changes in liver synthetic function. Thus, PT is very useful for following liver function in patients with acute liver failure. Vitamin K is required for the gamma-carboxylation of the above-named factors. Hence, an elevated PT can result from a vitamin K deficiency. This deficiency usually occurs in patients with chronic cholestasis or fat malabsorption from disease of the pancreas or small bowel. A trial of vitamin K is a useful and well-established way to exclude vitamin K deficiency in such patients. The PT should improve within a few days if it is due to fat malabsorption but will not if secondary to intrinsic liver disease.

ANTIMITOCHONDRIAL ANTIBODY

Antimitochondrial antibody (AMA) is an autoantibody that is detected in the serum by a variety of methods. Mitochondrial antibodies are found in 0.8–1.6% of the general population, 6% of patients with cryptogenic cirrhosis, 10% of patients with chronic active hepatitis, and 85% to 90% of patients with primary biliary cirrhosis. The height of the AMA titer has no prognostic significance. The 10–15% of patients with PBC who are AMA negative have the same natural history of the disease as AMA-positive patients. Antimitochondrial antibodies are also found in a significant number of asymptomatic relatives of patients with primary biliary cirrhosis and chronic active hepatitis. Mitochondrial antibodies directed against a purported specific primary biliary cirrhosis antigen are believed to have high diagnostic relevance (most assays are 95% sensitive and 98% specific for PBC), and it has been stated that when such antibodies are not detected in the serum, a diagnosis of primary biliary cirrhosis should be made with caution and only after a careful period of clinical follow-up.

SERUM CERULOPLASMIN

Ceruloplasmin, a copper-containing glycoprotein, is an acute-phase reactant. Ninety-five percent of patients with Wilson disease have serum ceruloplasmin concentrations below 20 mg/dL. Ten percent of heterozygotes have low ceruloplasmin levels but remain healthy. Low concentrations may also be seen in patients with fulminant hepatitis unrelated to Wilson disease, nephrotic syndrome, and protein-losing enteropathies. Still, measurement of serum ceruloplasmin alone does not reliably establish or exclude the diagnosis. Further testing, usually urinary copper excretion, assessment for Kayser-Fleischer rings (figure 73.1), or liver biopsy, is required.

SERUM FERRITIN

Serum ferritin levels accurately reflect hepatic and total-body iron stores. Serum ferritin levels are low in iron deficiency and elevated in iron overload disorders such as genetic idiopathic hemochromatosis. Occasionally, normal levels of serum ferritin may be found in patients with precirrhotic hemochromatosis. Conversely, a very high level of serum ferritin may be present in patients who turn out not to have hemochromatosis. Serum ferritin levels may be elevated in the absence of iron overload in a variety of conditions (see table 73.8). Measurement of serum iron concentration, percentage transferring saturation, and serum ferritin level is the screening regimen currently recommended for idiopathic

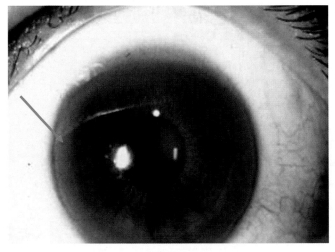

K-F Ring

Figure 73.1. Eye Findings in Wilson Disease; Kayser-Fleischer Ring.

Table 73.8 CAUSES OF ELEVATIONS IN SERUM FERRITIN

1. Idiopathic genetic hemochromatosis
2. Hepatocellular necrosis
3. Hodgkin
4. Leukemia
5. Hyperthyroidism
6. Uremia
7. Rheumatoid arthritis

Table 73.9 COMMON DISEASES ASSOCIATED WITH POSITIVE ANA

Hashimoto thyroiditis

Graves disease

Autoimmune hepatitis

Primary biliary cirrhosis

Autoimmune cholangitis

Pulmonary arterial hypertension

genetic hemochromatosis. Of note, cirrhosis is very unlikely in hemochromatosis if the patient is younger than 40 years old, has no hepatomegaly, has normal transaminases, and has a serum ferritin <1000.

ANTI-SMOOTH MUSCLE ANTIBODIES

Smooth muscle antibodies are directed against cytoskeletal proteins such as actin, troponin, and tropomyosin. They frequently occur in high titers in association with ANA. They are associated with autoimmune hepatitis and have been shown to occur in advanced liver diseases of other etiologies and in infectious diseases and rheumatic disorders. Although less prevalent than ANA, they are more specific, particularly when present in titers of 1:100 or more. Circulating anti–smooth muscle antibodies are also found in patients with chronic hepatitis C. The mean titer is generally higher in patients with autoimmune hepatitis.

ANTINUCLEAR ANTIBODY

ANAs are an often-utilized serologic marker of autoimmune disease and are present in several disorders (see table 73.9). These antibodies can also provide diagnostic and prognostic data concerning patients who have minimal symptoms or who have clinical features of more than one autoimmune disease. They are the most common circulating autoantibodies in autoimmune hepatitis. They are seen in both type 1 disease and rarely in type 2 disease. In most laboratories a titer of 1:100 or greater is considered positive. ANA may be the only autoantibody present or may occur in conjunction with anti–smooth muscle antibody. In one study the specific immunofluorescence patterns of ANAs did not distinguish clinical features of liver disease, although speckled patterns were associated with a younger age and greater aminotransferase activity, and multiple autoantibodies were frequently associated with each immunofluorescent pattern.

LACTATE DEHYDROGENASE

Serum lactate dehydrogenase comes from myocardium, liver, skeletal muscle, brain, or kidney tissue and red blood cells. Thus, an elevated serum lactate dehydrogenase value is nonspecific. Hepatic serum lactate dehydrogenase can be verified by isoenzymes. Increased lactate dehydrogenase levels are seen in patients with a variety of hepatobiliary disorders including acute viral or drug hepatitis, congestive heart failure, cirrhosis, and extrahepatic obstruction. Marked elevations in serum lactate dehydrogenase and alkaline phosphatase levels are highly suggestive of metastatic disease to the liver.

ULTRASOUND

Ultrasonography with Doppler flow studies presents a noninvasive, commonly utilized modality that provides valuable information regarding the appearance of the liver and blood flow in the portal and hepatic veins in cirrhosis and several other liver diseases. A study using high-resolution ultrasonography in cirrhotic patients (confirmed by biopsy or laparoscopy) found a sensitivity and specificity for cirrhosis of 91.1% and 93.5%, respectively, and positive and negative predictive values of 93.2% and 91.5%, respectively. Ultrasonography is the least expensive radiology study and does not pose the radiation exposure risks of other studies. Thus, it is appropriately the test of choice in the evaluation of liver and biliary tract disease in children and pregnant women. Ultrasonography also lacks the risk of nephrotoxicity from intravenous contrast seen in CT. Nodularity, irregularity, increased echogenicity, and atrophy are the ultrasonographic hallmarks of cirrhosis. It should be noted, however, that the absence of the above-mentioned features does not rule out cirrhosis.

Marked obesity and excessive intestinal gas can be limiting factors in obtaining good resolution of the images. Ultrasound examination of the liver will often identify mass lesions 1–2 cm in size in the hepatic parenchyma and do this independently of hepatic function. The nature of defects seen on technetium-99m sulfur colloid scanning—solid or cystic—can readily be ascertained, and ultrasound can thus facilitate guided aspiration of cysts or biopsy specimens of lesions. Ultrasonography is a useful procedure for detecting gallstones and confirming the presence of ascites, keeping in mind that study in the fasting state is important. Ultrasound is often used as the first test in the evaluation of patients with cholestatic jaundice. Dilated bile ducts can be readily seen on ultrasound examination in patients with mechanical extrahepatic biliary tract obstruction. Dilation of the bile ducts may not be evident if the obstruction is incomplete or intermittent or if it has been present for a short duration. Serial ultrasound examinations may provide clues in these circumstances. The common bile duct is frequently dilated following cholecystectomy. Hence, an enlarged duct in this situation does not necessarily signify ongoing biliary tract obstruction.

CT AND MRI

The predominantly used imaging tools other than ultrasonography in imaging the liver are CT and MRI. The goals of imaging patients with liver failure are to evaluate for cirrhosis and portal hypertension, to identify conditions that may complicate or preclude treatment, and to identify and stage tumor within the liver or extrahepatic malignancies. Continuous improvements in these imaging modalities over the past few years have expanded their role and improved their utility. At most centers, CT is the predominant tool in evaluating patients with advanced liver disease. Ultrasonography, MRI, and angiography maintain important screening and problem solving roles (see figures 73.2–73.4).

CT and MRI are quite accurate in depicting large hepatocellular carcinoma (HCC) lesions and complications such as portal or hepatic venous invasion or biliary ductal obstruction. Venous tumor thrombi, for example, are detected as vessel expansion, enhancing tumor thrombi, and contiguity with a parenchymal mass. Evaluations of potential liver donors and recipients are an equally important manifestation of CT and/or MRI. Common variants, including hepatic arterial anomalies, trifurcation of the portal veins, or large accessory or anomalous hepatic veins may preclude the use of a potential donor liver or may mandate alternate surgical approaches. Noninvasive imaging of the biliary tree of a potential living donor presents an ongoing challenge.

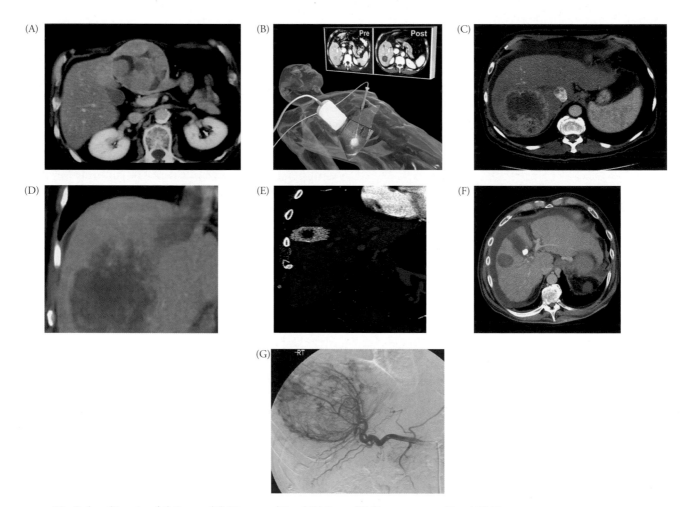

Figure 73.2. The Roles of Imaging. (A) Detect. (B) Diagnose. (C and D) Stage. (E) Plan treatment. (F and G) Treat.

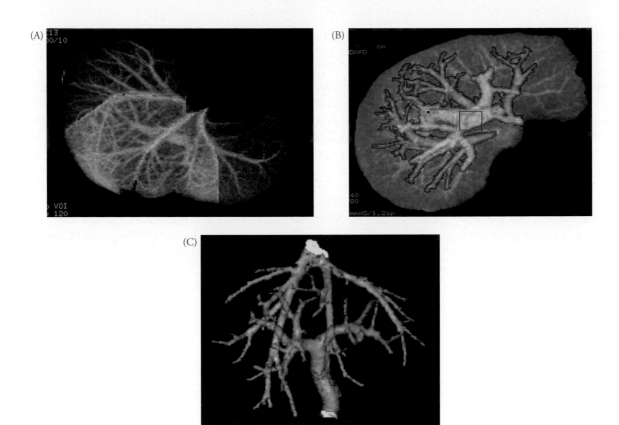

Figure 73.3. Contemporary CT Scanning Helps Plan Surgical Approach.

MR cholangiography has provided excellent depictions of the biliary tree, but experience with operative correlation is limited to small case series.

ENHANCED MAGNETIC RESONANCE CHOLANGIOGRAPHY

In routine magnetic resonance cholangiography (MRC), T2-weighted sequences in multiple planes depict the water content of bile in the biliary ducts and in the gallbladder. This represents a noninvasive method requiring no contrast agent.

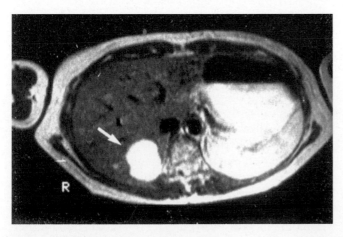

Figure 73.4. MRI Showing Hepatic Hemangioma.

However, due to limited resolution, MRC is not always conclusive. MRC is also sensitive to motion artifacts and does not provide any information on hepatobiliary function.

In recent years, several new liver-specific MR imaging contrast media have been utilized. Some of the agents are targeted to hepatocytes: gadobenate dimeglumine, Gd-BOPTA (MultiHance; Bracco Imaging, Milan, Italy), gadoxetic acid, Gd-EOBDTPA (Primovist; Schering, Berlin, Germany), and mangafodipir trisodium, Mn-DPDP (Teslascan; GE Healthcare, Chalfont St. Giles, United Kingdom). All these substances are to some extent eliminated by biliary excretion and may therefore be useful for investigating hepatobiliary function. In one head-to-head study, the earlier onset and longer duration of a high contrast between CHD and liver for Gd-EOB-DTPA facilitated examination of hepatobiliary excretion, concluding that Gd-EOB-DTPA may provide adequate hepatobiliary imaging within a shorter time span than Gd-BOPTA.

LIVER BIOPSY

Percutaneous needle biopsy of the liver is a commonly used, safe procedure that can be performed at the bedside. It often provides tissue diagnosis without resorting to general anesthesia and laparotomy, and most agree that it can be performed as an outpatient procedure provided facilities are available for short-term observation and hospitalization if necessary.

Indications for liver biopsy are outlined in table 73.10. Of note, liver biopsy provides no information regarding the site or nature of the obstructing lesion.

Contraindications for needle biopsy of the liver include uncooperative or comatose patients, hydatid cyst disease, hemangioma or angiosarcoma of the liver, right pleural disease or local infection at the proposed biopsy site, and significant coagulopathy. Providers usually will not perform a biopsy if a prolongation of the prothrombin time is >4 seconds over control, a partial thromboplastin time is <15 seconds over control, or a platelet count less than 75,000/mm³. Amyloidosis is not a contraindication unless the liver is very massively enlarged or there is an associated bleeding tendency. Liver biopsy is performed via percutaneous, transjugular, laparoscopic, open operative, or ultrasonography- or CT-guided fine-needle approaches. Before the procedure, a CBC with platelets and prothrombin time measurement should be obtained. Patients should be advised to refrain from consumption of aspirin and nonsteroidal anti-inflammatory drugs for 7–10 days before the biopsy to minimize the risk of bleeding.

The most common side effect is pain at the biopsy site or right shoulder, occurring in <5% of patients. Moderate to severe pain with or without hypotension usually manifests within the first 3 hours of the procedure. Serious bleeding occurs in <0.3% of patients, although asymptomatic subcapsular or intrahepatic hematomas are probably more common.

NONINVASIVE MARKERS OF FIBROSIS

Numerous investigators have examined noninvasive tests for assessing hepatic fibrosis. The two most widely investigated

Table 73.10 **INDICATIONS FOR LIVER BIOPSY**

Hepatocellular disease of uncertain cause
Unexplained hepatomegaly and/or splenomegaly
Hepatic filling defects demonstrated by radionuclide scanning US or CT scans
Chronic hepatitis
Fever of unknown origin
Alcoholic liver disease
Workup for hemochromatosis
Workup for Wilson disease
Workup for glycogen storage diseases
Assessment of portal hypertension
Staging of malignant lymphoma.
Workup for type I Crigler-Najjar syndrome

tools are the FibroTest (Biopredictive, Paris, France) and FibroScan (Echosens, Paris, France). The FibroTest is a composite of five serum biochemical markers (alpha-2-macroglobulin, apolipoprotein A1, haptoglobin, gamma-glutamyltranspeptidase, and bilirubin) associated with hepatic fibrosis. The FibroScan uses an ultrasound-based technique known as transient elastography to measure the speed of propagation of elastic waves through the liver. Both tests have been validated by multiple studies in various liver diseases. Limitations include their cost, failed validation, difficulty differentiating intermediate fibrosis stage, and the inability to exclude other conditions. Despite expert recommendations that these tests are not yet ready to fully replace liver biopsy, their use has become widespread.

ADDITIONAL READING

Batts KP. Iron overload syndromes and the liver. *Mod Pathol.* 2007;20 Suppl 1:S31–9.

Burke MD. Liver function. *Hum Pathol.* 1975;6:273–86.

Cohen JA, Kaplan MM. The SGOT/SGPT ratio—an indicator of alcoholic liver disease. *Dig Dis Sci.* 1979;24:835–8.

Combes B, Scheneker S. Laboratory tests. In: Schiff L, Schiff ER, eds. *Diseases of the Liver* (pp. 259–302). Philadelphia: JB Lippincott; 1982.

Davern TJ, Scharschmidt BF. Biochemical liver tests. In: Feldman M, Friedman LS, Sleisenger MH, eds. *Sleisenger & Fordtran's Gastrointestinal and Liver Disease: Pathophysiology, Diagnosis, Management.* 7th ed. (pp. 1227–38). Philadelphia: WB Saunders; 2002.

Fairbanks KD, Tavill AS. Liver disease in alpha 1-antitrypsin deficiency: A review. *Am J Gastroenterol.* 2008;103(8):2136–41.

Green RM, Flamm S. AGA technical review on the evaluation of liver chemistry tests. *Gastroenterology.* 2002;123:1367–84.

Kaplan MM. Alkaline phosphatase. *N Engl J Med.* 1972;286:200–2.

Kaplan MM. Understanding serum enzyme tests in clinical liver disease. In: Davidson CS, ed. *Problems in Liver Diseases* (pp. 79–85). New York: Stratton Intercontinental; 1979.

Triger DR, Charlton CAC, Ward AM. What does the antimitochondrial antibody mean? *Gut.* 1982;23:814–8.

Zimmerman l-U: Evaluation of the function and integrity of the liver. In: Henry JB, ed. Clinical Diagnosis and Management by Laboratory Methods (pp. 305–6). Philadelphia: WB Saunders; 1979.

QUESTIONS

QUESTION 1. A 62-year-old white male is referred for evaluation of a persistently elevated serum aminotransferase. His past medical history is notable for long-standing but well-controlled hypertension and hypercholesterolemia. He has been on amlodipine, 10 mg once daily, and atorvastatin, 20 mg once daily. He drinks two to three glasses of red wine on weekends. On examination, his blood pressure is 139/62 mm Hg, heart rate 78 beats per minute, he weighs 238 lb with a BMI of 32. His examination is otherwise normal.

His AST is 96 (was normal 2 years ago), ALT 109 (was normal 2 years ago), alkaline phosphatase 66, bilirubin 0.7, albumin 4.5, INR 1.1. CT scan of the abdomen shows low-density hepatic parenchyma. Which of the following is most likely causing this patient's elevated serum aminotransferase values?

A. Treatment with amlodipine
B. Nonalcoholic fatty liver disease
C. Treatment with atorvastatin
D. Primary biliary cirrhosis
E. Alcohol use

QUESTION 2. The treatment that you would recommend to the above patient would be:

A. Stop the amlodipine
B. Stop the atorvastatin
C. Weight loss
D. Observation only, no treatment
E. Complete abstinence from alcohol

QUESTION 3. A 29-year-old man presents with evidence of ascites and abnormal LFTs. He denies alcohol consumption but smokes (approximately one pack per day for the past 10 years). He has a history of emphysema diagnosed at the age of 22 years. All viral serologies are negative. His serum alpha1-antitrypsin levels is 72 mg/dL (reference range 100–300 mg/dL). A diagnosis of alpha-1-antitrypsin (AAT) deficiency is made. Which of the following phenotypes would most likely lead to this clinical presentation?

A. Pi MM
B. Pi SS
C. Pi ZZ
D. Pi MZ

QUESTION 4. A 39-year-old woman is found to have the following iron studies: serum iron 184, total iron binding capacity 250, serum ferritin 285 (normal 25–240). Her liver function tests are normal, and she is asymptomatic with a normal physical examination.

What is the next test that should be ordered?

A. Percutaneous liver biopsy
B. Serum B-12 and folate levels
C. Glucose tolerance testing
D. Gene testing for the hereditary hemochromatosis mutation
E. Abdominal CT scan with IV contrast

QUESTION 5. A 42-year-old gardener presents with an 8-month history of bullous lesions on the dorsum of his hands, his forearms, and his neck. He says that his urine is a port wine color. His physical examination is otherwise unremarkable. He reports drinking one to two six-packs of beer every week, and on laboratory examination he has a mildly elevated ALT (1.5 times normal). The most likely diagnosis is:

A. Bullous pseudoporphyria
B. Hydroa vacciniforme
C. Bullous systemic lupus erythematosus
D. Porphyria cutanea tarda
E. Epidermolysis bullosa acquisita

ANSWERS

1. B
2. C
3. C
4. D
5. D

74.

CIRRHOSIS

Chinweike Ukomadu and Ajay K. Singh

Cirrhosis is defined as a diffuse process characterized by fibrosis and conversion of normal architecture to structurally abnormal nodules. These regenerative nodules lack normal lobular organization and are surrounded by fibrous tissue. The word "cirrhosis" derives from Greek meaning *tawny* (the orange-yellow color of the diseased liver). René Laennec in 1819 coined the name cirrhosis to describe livers so diseased. The progression of liver injury to cirrhosis may occur over weeks to years. The chief complications are ascites, encephalopathy, and variceal bleeding.

Chronic liver disease and cirrhosis result in about 35,000 deaths each year in the United States. Cirrhosis is the ninth leading cause of death in the United States and is responsible for 1.2% of all U.S. deaths.

CAUSES OF CIRRHOSIS

The causes of cirrhosis are shown in table 74.1. The most common cause of cirrhosis in the United States is hepatitis C. Other common causes include alcohol and nonalcoholic fatty liver disease (NAFLD). Alcoholic liver disease once was considered to be the predominant cause of cirrhosis in the United States. Hepatitis C has emerged as the leading cause of both chronic hepatitis and cirrhosis. Many cases of cryptogenic cirrhosis appear to have resulted from NAFLD. When cases of cryptogenic cirrhosis are reviewed, many patients have one or more of the classical risk factors for NAFLD: obesity, diabetes, and hypertriglyceridemia. It is postulated that steatosis may regress in some patients as hepatic fibrosis progresses, making the histologic diagnosis of NAFLD difficult. Up to one-third of Americans have NAFLD. About 2–3% of Americans have nonalcoholic steatohepatitis (NASH), in which fat deposition in the hepatocyte is complicated by liver inflammation and fibrosis. It is estimated that 10% of patients with NASH will ultimately develop cirrhosis.

A poor correlation exists between histologic findings and the clinical picture. Some patients with cirrhosis are completely asymptomatic and have a reasonably normal life expectancy. Other individuals have a multitude of the most severe symptoms of end-stage liver disease and have a limited chance for survival.

CLINICAL FEATURES OF CIRRHOSIS

The clinical features of cirrhosis can be broadly attributed to decreased hepatic synthetic function (e.g., coagulopathy), decreased detoxification capabilities of the liver (e.g., hepatic encephalopathy), or portal hypertension (e.g., variceal bleeding) (figure 74.1).

Two important syndromes—hepatopulmonary syndrome (HPS) and portopulmonary hypertension (PPHTN)—may be observed in a minority of patients. In HPS, pulmonary arteriovenous anastomoses result in arteriovenous shunting. HPS is characterized by the symptom of platypnea (dyspnea that is relieved when lying down, and worsens when sitting or standing up). HPS is a potentially progressive and life-threatening complication of cirrhosis that can be detected most readily by echocardiographic visualization of late-appearing bubbles in the left atrium following the injection of agitated saline. Patients can receive a diagnosis of HPS when their PaO_2 is <70 mm Hg. Some cases of HPS may be corrected by liver transplantation. PPHTN has an unknown etiology. It is defined as the presence of a mean pulmonary artery pressure greater than 25 mm Hg in the setting of a normal pulmonary capillary wedge pressure. Patients who develop severe PPHTN may require aggressive medical therapy in an effort to stabilize pulmonary artery pressures and to decrease their chance of perioperative mortality in the setting of liver transplantation.

Hepatocellular carcinoma (HCC) occurs in 10–25% of patients with cirrhosis in the United States and most often is associated with hemochromatosis, alpha-1-antitrypsin deficiency, hepatitis B, hepatitis C, and alcoholic cirrhosis. HCC is observed less commonly in primary biliary cirrhosis and is

Table 74.1 CAUSES OF CIRRHOSIS IN THE UNITED STATES

Hepatitis C (26%)

Alcoholic liver disease (21%)

Hepatitis C plus alcoholic liver disease (15%)

Cryptogenic causes (18%)

Hepatitis B, which may be coincident with hepatitis D (15%)

Miscellaneous (5%)

Autoimmune hepatitis

Primary biliary cirrhosis

Secondary biliary cirrhosis (associated with chronic extrahepatic bile duct obstruction)

Primary sclerosing cholangitis

Hemochromatosis

Wilson disease

Alpha-1-antitrypsin deficiency

Granulomatous disease (e.g., sarcoidosis)

Type IV glycogen storage disease

Drug-induced liver disease (e.g., methotrexate, alpha-methyldopa, amiodarone)

Venous outflow obstruction (e.g., Budd-Chiari syndrome, veno-occlusive disease)

Chronic right-sided heart failure

Tricuspid regurgitation

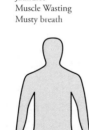

GENERAL
Jaundice
Muscle Wasting
Musty breath

PULMONARY
Pleural effusions
Interstitial edema
Hepatopulmonary
Syndrome (HPS).
Portopulmonary
hypertension
(PPHTH)

REPRODUCTIVE
Gynecomastia
Impotence
spider angiomata

GI
Hepatomegaly or
shrunken liver
Splenomegaly
Ascites

SKIN
Jaundice
Telangiectasias
Loss of axillary and pubic hair
Bruises
Caput medusae
Venous hum in epigastric region

CNS
Drowsiness
Confusion
Delirium
Personality changes
Hallucination
Asterixis

CARDIAC
Right heart failure
Cardiac fibrosis (cardiac cirrhosis)

HEMATOLOGIC
Easy bleeding
Bruises

HANDS/FINGERS
White nails
Disappearance of lunulae
Finger clubbing
Palmar erythema

BONES
Painful proliferative
Periostitis of long bones

Figure 74.1. Clinical Manifestations of Cirrhosis.

a rare complication of Wilson disease. Cholangiocarcinoma occurs in approximately 10% of patients with primary sclerosing cholangitis. Other conditions that appear with increased incidence in patients with cirrhosis include peptic ulcer disease, diabetes, and gallstones.

TREATMENT OF CIRRHOSIS

The management of cirrhosis consists of specific treatment for the underlying cause of cirrhosis and usually later for the inevitable complications of cirrhosis. Treatment of specific causes can be quite varied: for example, prednisone and azathioprine for autoimmune hepatitis, interferon and other antiviral agents for hepatitis B and C, phlebotomy for hemochromatosis, ursodeoxycholic acid for primary biliary cirrhosis, and penicillamine, trientine, and zinc for Wilson disease. Once cirrhosis develops, treatment is aimed at the management of complications such as ascites, hepatic encephalopathy, and variceal bleeding. Managing nutrition and pruritus are also important. Many patients complain of anorexia, which may be exacerbated by the mechanical effects of ascites on the GI tract. Patients frequently benefit from the addition of commonly available liquid and powdered nutritional supplements to the diet in order to ensure adequate calories and protein in their diets. Institution of a low-protein diet in the fear that hepatic encephalopathy might develop places the patient at risk for the development of profound muscle wasting. Zinc deficiency commonly is observed in patients with cirrhosis. Treatment with zinc sulfate at 220 mg orally twice daily may improve dysgeusia and can stimulate appetite. Furthermore, zinc is effective in the treatment of muscle cramps and is adjunctive therapy for hepatic encephalopathy. Pruritus is a common complaint in both cholestatic liver diseases (e.g., primary biliary cirrhosis) and noncholestatic chronic liver diseases (e.g., hepatitis C). Mild itching may respond to treatment with antihistamines. Cholestyramine is the mainstay of therapy for the pruritus of liver disease. Other medications that may provide relief against pruritus include ursodeoxycholic acid, ammonium lactate 12% skin cream (Lac-Hydrin, Westwood-Squibb Pharmaceuticals, Princeton, NJ), naltrexone (an opioid antagonist), rifampin, gabapentin, and ondansetron. Patients with severe pruritus may require institution of ultraviolet light therapy or plasmapheresis. Patients with chronic liver disease should also receive vaccination to protect them against hepatitis A. Other protective measures include vaccination against hepatitis B, pneumococci, and influenza.

PROGNOSIS OF CIRRHOSIS

Gauging prognosis in cirrhosis is important. Two scoring systems have been used (table 74.2). These are the

Table 74.2 CHILD-TURCOTTE-PUGH SCORING SYSTEM FOR CIRRHOSIS

CLINICAL VARIABLE	1 POINT	2 POINTS	3 POINTS
Encephalopathy	None	Stages 1–2	Stages 3–4
Ascites	Absent	Slight	Moderate
Bilirubin (mg/dL)	<2	2–3	>3
Bilirubin in PBC or PSC (mg/dL)	<4	4–10	10
Albumin (g/dL)	>3.5	2.8–3.5	<2.8
Prothrombin time: seconds prolonged or INR	<4 sec or INR<1.7	4–6 sec or INR 1.7–2.3	>6 sec or INR >2.3

NOTE: Child class A = 5–6 points, Child class B = 7–9 points, Child class C = 10–15 points.

Child-Turcotte-Pugh (CTP) system and the Model for End-Stage Liver Disease (MELD) scoring system. Epidemiologic work shows that the CTP score may predict life expectancy in patients with advanced cirrhosis. A CTP score of 10 or greater is associated with a 50% chance of death within 1 year. The MELD scoring system has been used to assess the relative severities of patients' liver diseases by liver transplant programs in the United States. MELD scores range from 6 to 40 points. The 3-month mortality statistics are associated with the following MELD scores: MELD score of <9, 2.9% mortality; MELD score of 10–19, 7.7% mortality; MELD score of 20–29, 23.5% mortality; MELD score of 30–39, 60% mortality; and MELD score of >40, 81% mortality.

COMPLICATIONS OF CIRRHOSIS

ASCITES

Ascites is defined as an accumulation of excessive fluid within the peritoneal cavity. Physiologically, it reflects total-body sodium and water excess, either as a consequence of perceived underfilling, or actual overfilling, or a combination of the two with some element of vasodilation. Ascites may be a complication of both hepatic and nonhepatic diseases. The most common causes of ascites in North America and Europe are shown in table 74.3.

Table 74.3 CAUSES OF ASCITES

Cirrhosis	85%
Mixed	8%
Heart failure	3%
Malignancy	2%
Tuberculosis	<1%
Pancreatic	<1%
Nephrotic	<1%

Currently the best way to classify ascites is to base it on the serum-ascites albumin gradient (SAAG). Ascites with a SAAG gradient of >1.1 g/dL is termed high-albumin-gradient or *portal hypertensive* ascites. In contrast, ascites with a SAAG gradient of <1.1 g/dL is known as low-albumin-gradient or *nonportal hypertensive* (table 74.4). (The SAAG is calculated by subtracting the ascitic fluid albumin value from the serum albumin value; it correlates directly with portal pressure. The specimens should be obtained relatively simultaneously. The accuracy of the SAAG results is approximately 97% in classifying ascites.) Another classification of ascites is based on its clinical severity. Thus, grade 1, mild, only visible on ultrasound; grade 2, detectable with flank bulging and shifting dullness; and grade 3, directly visible, confirmed with fluid thrill. In the past ascites was classified as transudative or exudative based on the ascitic protein level (exudative if ascites protein was >2.5 g/dL), but this is no longer a favored method of classification. Classic causes of transudative ascites are portal hypertension secondary to cirrhosis and congestive heart failure. Examples of exudative ascites include peritoneal carcinomatosis and tuberculous peritonitis.

Chylous ascites, caused by obstruction of the thoracic duct or cisterna chyli, most often is due to malignancy

Table 74.4 SERUM ASCITES ALBUMIN GRADIENT

HIGH (> 1.1 g/dL)	LOW (<1.1 g/dL)
Cirrhosis	Peritoneal CA
Alcoholic hepatitis	Tuberculosis
Heart failure	Pancreatitis
Massive liver mets	Bile leak
Fulminant liver failure	Nephrotic
Budd-Chiari	Lupus serositis

SOURCE: Reprinted with permission from Runyon BA, Montano AA, Antillon MR, et al. The serum-ascites albumin gradient is superior to the exudate-transudate concept in the differential diagnosis of ascites. *Ann Intern Med.* 1992;117:215–20.

(e.g., lymphoma) but occasionally is observed postoperatively and following radiation injury. Chylous ascites also may be observed in the setting of cirrhosis. The ascites triglyceride concentration is >110 mg/dL. In addition, ascites triglyceride concentrations are greater than those observed in plasma. Patients should be placed on a low-fat diet that is supplemented by medium-chain triglycerides. Treatment with diuretics and large-volume paracentesis may be required. Peritoneal diseases produce ascites with a SAAG of <1.1 g/dL (see table 74.2).

Clinical Features of Ascites

The key steps in the evaluation of ascites include acquiring a thorough history and physical, obtaining an ascitic fluid evaluation, and obtaining special tests. Clinically, ascites is suggested by the presence of abdominal distension, bulging flanks, shifting dullness, and elicitation of a "puddle sign" in patients in the knee-elbow position. A fluid wave may be elicited in patients with massive tense ascites. On physical examination the presence of vascular spiders, abdominal wall collaterals, and an umbilical nodule are useful in supporting the diagnosis of chronic liver disease as a cause of ascites. Paracentesis is routine for new-onset ascites, in patients on admission, and in patients who have a clinical deterioration. A diagnostic tap is performed with a 22-gauge 1.5-inch needle; whereas a therapeutic tap is performed with a 15- to 18-gauge needle. There is an approximate 1% complication rate with paracentesis. A popular option for the tap site is the left lower quadrant of the abdomen two fingerbreadths medial and cephalad to the anterior superior iliac spine. Special testing includes an abdominal ultrasound (ultrasound with Doppler can help assess the patency of hepatic vessels), cytology for peritoneal cancer, cardiac echo for suspected cardiac ascites, and tuberculosis (TB) smear and culture. Upper-GI endoscopy for screening of large varices is also an option. Factors associated with worsening of ascites include excess fluid or salt intake, malignancy, venous occlusion (e.g., Budd-Chiari syndrome), progressive liver disease, and spontaneous bacterial peritonitis (SBP).

Therapy for ascites should be tailored to the patient's needs. Options are shown in table 74.5. Some patients with mild ascites respond to sodium restriction or diuretics taken once or twice per week. Other patients require aggressive diuretic therapy, careful monitoring of electrolytes, and occasional hospitalization to facilitate even more intensive diuresis. The development of massive ascites that is refractory to medical therapy has dire prognostic implications, with only 50% of patients surviving 6 months.

Complications of Ascites

Spontaneous Bacterial Peritonitis
SBP is observed in 15–26% of patients hospitalized with ascites. The syndrome arises most commonly in patients whose low-protein ascites (<1 g/dL) contains low levels of complement, resulting in decreased opsonic activity. SBP appears to be caused by the translocation of GI tract bacteria across the gut wall and also by the hematogenous spread of bacteria. The most common causative organisms are *Escherichia coli, Streptococcus pneumoniae, Klebsiella* species, and other Gram-negative enteric organisms.

Classic SBP is diagnosed by the presence of neutrocytosis, which is defined as >250 polymorphonuclear (PMN) cells/mm³ of ascites in the setting of a positive ascites culture. Culture-negative neutrocytic ascites is observed more commonly. Both conditions represent serious infections that carry a 20–30% mortality rate.

The most commonly used regimen in the treatment of SBP is a 5-day course of cefotaxime at 1–2 g intravenously every 8 hours. Alternatives include oral ofloxacin and other intravenous antibiotics with activity against Gram-negative enteric organisms. Many authorities advise repeat paracentesis in 48–72 hours to document a decrease in the ascites PMN count to <250 cells/mm³ and to ensure the efficacy of therapy.

Once SBP develops, patients have a 70% chance of redeveloping the condition within 1 year. Prophylactic antibiotic therapy can reduce the recurrence rate of SBP to 20%. Some of the regimens used in the prophylaxis of SBP include norfloxacin at 400 mg orally every day 12 and trimethoprim-sulfamethoxazole at one double-strength tablet 5 days per week.

Therapy with norfloxacin at 400 mg orally twice per day for 7 days can reduce serious bacterial infection in patients with cirrhosis who have GI bleeding. Furthermore, it can be argued that all patients with low-protein ascites should undergo prophylactic therapy (e.g., with norfloxacin 400 mg/day PO) at the time of hospital admission, given the high incidence of hospital-acquired SBP.

Other Complications of Massive Ascites
Patients with massive ascites may experience abdominal discomfort, depressed appetite, and decreased oral intake. Diaphragmatic elevation may lead to symptoms of dyspnea. Pleural effusions may result from the passage of ascitic fluid across channels in the diaphragm.

Umbilical and inguinal hernias are common in patients with moderate and massive ascites. The use of an elastic abdominal binder may protect the skin overlying a protruding umbilical hernia from maceration and may help prevent rupture and subsequent infection. Timely large-volume paracentesis also may help to prevent this disastrous complication. Umbilical hernias should not undergo elective repair unless patients are significantly symptomatic or their hernias are irreducible. As with all other surgeries in patients with cirrhosis, herniorrhaphy carries multiple potential risks, such as intraoperative bleeding, postoperative infection, and liver failure because of anesthesia-induced reductions in hepatic blood flow. However, these risks become

Table 74.5 TREATMENT OPTIONS FOR DIURETIC-RESPONSIVE AND DIURETIC-RESISTANT ASCITES

CONVENTIONAL TREATMENT OPTIONS	KEY FEATURES
Abstinence from Alcohol	
Sodium restriction	First line of therapy Dietary sodium restriction <2000 mg sodium per day and for refractory ascites as much as <500 mg/day
Diuretics	Second line therapy Spironolactone (Aldactone) blocks the aldosterone receptor at the distal tubule. Dose 50–300 mg once per day. Alternative is eplerenone Furosemide (Lasix) may be used as a solo agent or in combination with spironolactone. Furosemide blocks sodium reuptake in the loop of Henle. Dosed at 40–240 mg per day in 1–2 divided doses. Avoid intravenous furosemide if possible because it may precipitate acute kidney injury (AKI). Starting doses: 100 mg/day spironolactone and 40 mg/day furosemide
Options for Diuretic-Resistant Ascites	
Large-volume paracentesis	Indicated when aggressive diuretic therapy is ineffective in controlling ascites (~5–10% of patients). Several large randomized, controlled trials have shown that repeated large-volume paracentesis (4–6 L) is safer and more effective for the treatment of tense ascites compared with larger-than-usual doses of diuretics. Procedure-associated risks include a 1% chance of significant abdominal-wall hematoma, 0.01% chance of hemoperitoneum, and a 0.01% chance of iatrogenic infection related to paracentesis. The only absolute contraindication to paracentesis is clinically evident fibrinolysis and disseminated intravascular coagulation. Controversy around whether to use salt-poor albumin (SPA) with a tap. One option is to reserve SPA for taps >5 L.
Vasopressin V2 receptor antagonist, e.g., Satavaptan	Improve diuresis and decrease the need for paracentesis in patients with diuretic-refractory ascites
Transjugular intrahepatic portosystemic shunt (TIPS)	A flexible metal prosthesis is used to bridge a branch of the hepatic and portal veins and is effective in reducing sinusoidal pressure. The procedure is performed percutaneously under radiologic guidance and obviates the need for surgery. It is recommended that coagulopathy (INR > 2 and platelet count < 50×10^9/L) be corrected first if indicated and that paracentesis be performed in patients with tense ascites prior to the procedure. Four randomized, controlled studies have compared TIPS with large-volume paracentesis in refractory ascites. All 4 studies showed better control of ascites with TIPS, but only one study showed a survival benefit. The rate of procedure-related complications is 10%, and of procedure-related mortality is 2%. Procedure-related complications include neck hematomas, hemobilia, puncture of the liver capsule causing intra-abdominal bleeding, and shunt occlusion. Absolute contraindications for TIPS insertion include serum bilirubin > 85 μmol/L (5 mg/dL), INR >2, functional renal disorder with serum creatinine >250 μmol/L (2.8 mg/dL), intrinsic renal disease with urine protein >500 mg/24 hours or active urinary sediment, grade III or IV hepatic encephalopathy, cardiac disease, portal vein thrombosis, noncompliance with sodium restriction, or the presence of carcinoma that is likely to limit the patient's lifespan to less than 1 year. Relative contraindications include dental sepsis, spontaneous bacterial peritonitis, and active infection (pneumonia or urinary tract infection).
Liver transplantation	Liver transplantation is the only definitive treatment for ascites and the only treatment that has been clearly shown to improve survival. Patients with cirrhosis who develop ascites should be assessed for possible liver transplantation because of their poor prognosis. Patients who develop renal dysfunction (GFR <50 mL/min) do much worse after liver transplantation (80% vs. 50% survival at 15 months) Other poor prognostic indicators include mean arterial pressure <82 mm Hg, urinary sodium excretion of <1.5 mEq/day, plasma norepinephrine levels of >570 pg/mL, poor nutritional state, presence of hepatomegaly, and serum albumin <25 g/L.

acceptable in patients with severe symptoms from their hernia. Urgent surgery is necessary in the patient whose hernia has been complicated by bowel incarceration.

Paracentesis in the Diagnosis of Ascites

Paracentesis is essential in determining whether ascites is caused by portal hypertension or by another process. Tests are listed in table 74.6. Ascites studies also are used to rule out infection and malignancy. Paracentesis should be performed in all patients with either new onset of ascites or worsening ascites. Paracentesis also should be performed when SBP is suggested by the presence of abdominal pain, fever, leukocytosis, or worsening hepatic encephalopathy. Some argue that paracentesis should be performed in all patients with cirrhosis who have ascites at the time of hospitalization, given the

Table 74.6 ASCITES TESTS

ROUTINE	OPTIONAL	SPECIAL
Cell count	Glucose	Cytology
Albumin	Lactate dehydrogenase	TB smear and culture
Culture	Gram stain	Triglycerides
Total protein		Bilirubin
		Amylase

significant possibility of asymptomatic SBP. Indeed, support for this includes the observation that the three most common signs of SBP, abdominal pain, fever, and leukocytosis, are seen in only 70% of persons with SBP.

Ascitic fluid with >250 PMN/mm³ defines neutrocytic ascites and SBP. Many cases of ascites fluid with >1000 PMN/mm³ (and certainly >5000 PMN/mm³) are associated with appendicitis or a perforated viscus with resulting bacterial peritonitis. Appropriate radiologic studies must be performed in such patients to rule out surgical causes of peritonitis. Lymphocyte-predominant ascites raises concerns about the possibility of underlying malignancy or tuberculosis. Similarly, grossly bloody ascites may be observed in malignancy and tuberculosis. Bloody ascites is seen infrequently in uncomplicated cirrhosis. A common clinical dilemma is how to interpret the ascites PMN count in the setting of bloody ascites. We recommend subtraction of 1 PMN for every 250 RBCs in ascites to ascertain a corrected PMN count.

The yield of ascites culture studies may be increased by directly inoculating 10 mL of ascites into aerobic and anaerobic culture bottles at the patient's bedside.

PORTAL HYPERTENSION

The normal liver has the ability to accommodate large changes in portal blood flow without appreciable alterations in portal pressure. Portal hypertension results from a combination of increased portal venous inflow and increased resistance to portal blood.

The portal hypertension of cirrhosis is caused by the disruption of hepatic sinusoids. However, portal hypertension may be observed in a variety of noncirrhotic conditions. Prehepatic causes include splenic vein thrombosis and portal vein thrombosis. These conditions commonly are associated with hypercoagulable states and with malignancy (e.g., pancreatic cancer).

Intrahepatic causes of portal hypertension are divided into presinusoidal, sinusoidal, and postsinusoidal conditions.

The classic form of presinusoidal disease is caused by the deposition of *Schistosoma* oocytes in presinusoidal portal venules, with the subsequent development of granulomata and portal fibrosis. Schistosomiasis is the most common noncirrhotic cause of variceal bleeding worldwide. *Schistosoma mansoni* infection is described in Puerto Rico, Central and South America, the Middle East, and Africa. *Schistosoma japonicum* is described in the Far East. *Schistosoma hematobium,* observed in the Middle East and Africa, can produce portal fibrosis, but more commonly it is associated with urinary tract deposition of eggs. The classic sinusoidal cause of portal hypertension is cirrhosis. The classic postsinusoidal condition is an entity known as veno-occlusive disease. Obliteration of the terminal hepatic venules may result from ingestion of pyrrolizidine alkaloids in comfrey tea or Jamaican bush tea and following the high-dose chemotherapy that precedes bone marrow transplantation.

Posthepatic causes of portal hypertension may include chronic right-sided heart failure, tricuspid regurgitation, and obstructing lesions of the hepatic veins and inferior vena cava. These latter conditions, and the symptoms they produce, are termed Budd-Chiari syndrome. Predisposing conditions include hypercoagulable states, tumor invasion into the hepatic vein or inferior vena cava, and membranous obstruction of the inferior vena cava. Inferior vena cava webs are observed most commonly in South and East Asia and are postulated to be due to nutritional factors.

Symptoms of Budd-Chiari syndrome are attributed to decreased outflow of blood from the liver, with resulting hepatic congestion and portal hypertension. These symptoms include hepatomegaly, abdominal pain, and ascites. Cirrhosis only ensues later in the course of disease. Differentiating Budd-Chiari syndrome from cirrhosis by history or physical examination may be difficult. Thus, Budd-Chiari syndrome must be included in the differential diagnosis of conditions that produce ascites and varices. A possible clue may come from the analysis of the ascetic fluid. The SAAG is usually greater than 1.1, but the ascitic fluid has a high protein content unlike that of cirrhotic ascites. Hepatic vein patency is checked most readily by performing an abdominal ultrasound with Doppler examination of the hepatic vessels. Abdominal computed tomography (CT) scan with intravenous contrast, abdominal magnetic resonance imaging (MRI), and visceral angiography also may provide information regarding the patency of hepatic vessels.

HEPATORENAL SYNDROME

This syndrome represents a continuum of renal dysfunction that may be observed in patients with cirrhosis and is caused by the vasoconstriction of large and small renal arteries and the impaired renal perfusion that results. The syndrome may represent an imbalance between renal vasoconstrictors and vasodilators. Plasma levels of a number of vasoconstricting substances are elevated in patients with cirrhosis and include angiotensin, antidiuretic hormone, and norepinephrine. Renal perfusion appears to be protected by vasodilators, including prostaglandins E$_2$ and I$_2$ and atrial natriuretic factor. Nonsteroidal anti-inflammatory drugs (NSAIDs) inhibit prostaglandin synthesis. They may potentiate renal vasoconstriction, with a resulting drop in glomerular filtration. Thus, the use of NSAIDs is contraindicated in patients with decompensated cirrhosis.

Most patients with hepatorenal syndrome are noted to have minimal histological changes in the kidneys. Kidney function usually recovers when patients with cirrhosis and hepatorenal syndrome undergo liver transplantation. In fact, a kidney donated by a patient dying from hepatorenal syndrome functions normally when transplanted into a renal transplant recipient.

Hepatorenal syndrome progression may be slow (type II) or rapid (type I). Type I disease frequently is accompanied by rapidly progressive liver failure. Hemodialysis offers temporary support for such patients. These individuals are salvaged only by performance of liver transplantation. Exceptions to this rule are the patients with FHF or severe alcoholic hepatitis, who spontaneously recover both liver and kidney function. In type II hepatorenal syndrome patients may have stable or slowly progressive renal insufficiency. Many such patients develop ascites that is resistant to management with diuretics.

Hepatorenal syndrome is diagnosed when a creatinine clearance <40 mL/min is present or when a serum creatinine >1.5 mg/dL, urine volume <500 mL/day, and urine sodium <10 mEq/L are present. Urine osmolality is greater than plasma osmolality. In hepatorenal syndrome, renal dysfunction cannot be explained by pre-existing kidney disease, prerenal azotemia, the use of diuretics, or exposure to nephrotoxins. Clinically, the diagnosis may be reached if central venous pressure is determined to be normal or if no improvement of renal function occurs following the infusion of at least 1.5 L of a plasma expander.

Nephrotoxic medications, including aminoglycoside antibiotics, should be avoided in patients with cirrhosis. Patients with early hepatorenal syndrome may be salvaged by aggressive expansion of intravascular volume with albumin and fresh frozen plasma and by avoidance of diuretics. Administration of oral prostaglandins may be beneficial, but this point is controversial. Use of renal-dose dopamine is not effective.

HEPATIC ENCEPHALOPATHY

Hepatic encephalopathy is a syndrome observed in some patients with cirrhosis that is marked by personality changes, intellectual impairment, and a depressed level of consciousness. The diversion of portal blood into the systemic circulation appears to be a prerequisite for the syndrome. Indeed, hepatic encephalopathy may develop in patients who do not have cirrhosis who undergo portocaval shunt surgery.

Clinical Features of Hepatic Encephalopathy

The symptoms of hepatic encephalopathy may range from mild to severe and may be observed in as many as 70%

of patients with cirrhosis. Symptoms are graded on the following scale:

Grade 0 - Subclinical; normal mental status, but minimal changes in memory, concentration, intellectual function, coordination

Grade 1 - Mild confusion, euphoria or depression, decreased attention, slowing of ability to perform mental tasks, irritability, disorder of sleep pattern (i.e., inverted sleep cycle)

Grade 2 - Drowsiness, lethargy, gross deficits in ability to perform mental tasks, obvious personality changes, inappropriate behavior, intermittent disorientation (usually for time)

Grade 3 - Somnolent but arousable, unable to perform mental tasks, disorientation to time and place, marked confusion, amnesia, occasional fits of rage, speech is present but incomprehensible

Grade 4 - Coma, with or without response to painful stimuli

Patients with mild and moderate hepatic encephalopathy demonstrate decreased short-term memory and concentration on mental status testing. Findings on physical examination include asterixis and fetor hepaticus.

Laboratory Abnormalities in Hepatic Encephalopathy

An elevated arterial or free venous serum ammonia level is the classic laboratory abnormality reported in patients with hepatic encephalopathy. This finding may aid in the assignment of a correct diagnosis to a patient with cirrhosis who presents with altered mental status. However, serial ammonia measurements are inferior to clinical assessment in gauging improvement or deterioration in patients under therapy for hepatic encephalopathy. No utility exists for checking the ammonia level in a patient with cirrhosis who does not have hepatic encephalopathy.

Some patients with hepatic encephalopathy have the classic but nonspecific electroencephalogram (EEG) changes of high-amplitude low-frequency waves and triphasic waves. EEG may be helpful in the initial workup of a patient with cirrhosis and altered mental status when ruling out seizure activity may be necessary.

CT scan and MRI studies of the brain may be important in ruling out intracranial lesions when the diagnosis of hepatic encephalopathy is in question.

Common Precipitants of Hepatic Encephalopathy

Some patients with a history of hepatic encephalopathy may have normal mental status when under medical therapy.

Others have chronic memory impairment in spite of medical management. Both groups of patients are subject to episodes of worsened encephalopathy. Common precipitants of hyperammonemia and worsening mental status are diuretic therapy, renal failure, GI bleeding, infection, and constipation. Dietary protein overload is an infrequent cause of worsening encephalopathy. Medications, notably opiates, benzodiazepines, antidepressants, and antipsychotic agents, also may worsen encephalopathy symptoms.

Nonhepatic causes of altered mental function must be excluded in patients with cirrhosis who have worsening mental function. A check of the blood ammonia level may be helpful in such patients. Medications that depress central nervous system function, especially benzodiazepines, should be avoided. Precipitants of hepatic encephalopathy should be corrected (e.g., metabolic disturbances, GI bleeding, infection, and constipation).

Lactulose is helpful in patients with the acute onset of severe encephalopathy symptoms and in patients with milder, chronic symptoms. This nonabsorbable disaccharide stimulates the passage of ammonia from tissues into the gut lumen and inhibits intestinal ammonia production. Initial lactulose dosing is 30 mL orally once or twice daily. Dosing is increased until the patient has 2–4 loose stools per day. Dosing should be reduced if the patient complains of diarrhea, abdominal cramping, or bloating. Higher doses of lactulose may be administered via either a nasogastric tube or rectal tube to hospitalized patients with severe encephalopathy. Other cathartics, including colonic lavage solutions, that contain polyethylene glycol (PEG) (e.g., Go-Lytely) also may be effective in patients with severe encephalopathy.

Neomycin and other antibiotics (e.g., metronidazole, oral vancomycin, paromomycin, oral quinolones) serve as second-line agents. They work by decreasing the colonic concentration of ammoniagenic bacteria. Neomycin dosing is 250–1000 mg orally two to four times daily. Treatment with neomycin may be complicated by ototoxicity and nephrotoxicity.

Rifaximin (Xifaxan, Salix Pharmaceuticals, Morrisville, NC) is a nonabsorbable antibiotic that received approval by the U.S. Food and Drug Administration (FDA) in 2004 for the treatment of travelers' diarrhea. Experience in Europe over the last two decades suggests that rifaximin can decrease colonic levels of ammoniagenic bacteria with resulting improvement in hepatic encephalopathy symptoms. Typical rifaximin dosing in European hepatic encephalopathy trials was two 200-mg tablets taken orally three times daily. Work is being done to determine if lower doses of the medication can effectively treat hepatic encephalopathy. One meta-analysis has suggested that rifaximin may be more effective than lactulose in the treatment of hepatic encephalopathy.

Other chemicals capable of decreasing blood ammonia levels are l-ornithine-l-aspartate (available in Europe) and sodium benzoate.

Low-protein diets were recommended routinely in the past for patients with cirrhosis. High levels of aromatic amino acids contained in animal proteins were believed to lead to increased blood levels of the false neurotransmitters tyramine and octopamine, with resulting worsening of encephalopathy symptoms. In our experience, the vast majority of patients can tolerate a protein-rich diet (>1.2 g/kg/day) including well-cooked chicken, fish, vegetable protein, and, if needed, protein supplements.

Protein restriction is rarely necessary in patients with chronic encephalopathy symptoms. Many patients with cirrhosis have protein-calorie malnutrition at baseline.

ADDITIONAL READING

Garcia-Tsao G, Bosch J. Management of varices and variceal hemorrhage in cirrhosis. *N Engl J Med.* 2010;362(9):823–32.

Ginès P, Schrier RW. Renal failure in cirrhosis. *N Engl J Med.* 2009;361(13):1279–90.

Ginès P, Cárdenas A, Arroyo V, Rodés J. Management of cirrhosis and ascites. *N Engl J Med.* 2004;350(16):1646–54.

Hou W, Sanyal AJ. Ascites: Diagnosis and management. *Med Clin North Am.* 2009;93(4):801–17, vii.

QUESTIONS

QUESTION 1. A 47-year-old woman is diagnosed with chronic hepatitis C. A liver biopsy shows grade 2/4 inflammation and stage 1/4 fibrosis. Which of the following is false regarding her management?

A. She can be treated with PEGylated interferon and ribavirin.

B. Obtain an US and AFP to screen for hepatocellular cancer.

C. There is no need to screen for esophageal varices given the low fibrotic content.

D. She should be vaccinated against hepatitis A and B if she is not immunoprotected.

QUESTION 2. A 42-yr-old man presents with new-onset ascites. Evaluation of the aspirate shows the following. Albumin of 3.6 g/dL, total protein of 7.0 g; cell count, 500 white blood cell (WBC) count with 95% lymphocytes. A serum albumin on the same day is 4.0 g/dL. Cultures of the ascitic fluid for bacteria and acid-fast bacilli are negative.

What is the best management option?

A. Treat with a third-generation cephalosporin for SBP

B. Institute low-salt diet and diuretics for cirrhotic ascites

C. Obtain a Doppler US to rule out Budd-Chiari syndrome

D. Perform a peritoneal biopsy

QUESTION 3. A 46-year-old Caucasian male is seen because of mildly elevated aminotransferases. ALT is 67 (nL 9–50), and AST is 49 (nL 7–45). Exam is remarkable for an enlarged liver, but otherwise there is no evidence of advanced liver disease. A subsequent evaluation shows the following: HbSAg, nonreactive; HCV antibody, nonreactive; ANA, negative; ASMA, negative; TSH, normal; Fe 250; TIBC 300; and ferritin 1200. CBC shows WBC of 5.6, HCT of 46, and platelet count of 190. A genetic test for hemochromatosis returns negative. What would you do next?

A. Obtain an MRI to quantify hepatic iron.
B. Perform a liver biopsy.
C. Tell him he has hemochromatosis and begin phlebotomy.
D. Repeat the genetic test.

QUESTION 4. Which of the following is true about spontaneous bacterial peritonitis (SBP)?

A. Ampicillin and gentamicin combination is first-line therapy for SBP.
B. The combination of antibiotic and albumin is superior to antibiotic alone for ascitic fluid sterilization.
C. Cultures in SBP usually grow multiple Gram-negative and Gram-positive organisms.
D. The risk of renal impairment can be reduced by treatment with antibiotics and albumin infusion.

QUESTIONS 5. A 54-year-old woman is seen because of fatigue and pruritus. She denies any prior medical issues and is taking no medications. Exam shows an enlarged liver. Laboratory data show the following: normal electrolytes, ALT 45 (9–50), AST 27 (7–45), alkaline phosphatase 860 (36–118), albumin is 3.4, total protein is 5.0, and cholesterol is 330. WBC is 4.6, HCT 38.0, and platelet count 120.

Which of the following serologic tests is most likely to be diagnostic?

A. Anti-smooth-muscle antibody
B. Antinuclear antibodies
C. Alpha-1-antitrypsin levels
D. Antimitochondrial antibodies

ANSWERS

1. B
2. D
3. B
4. D
5. D

75.

BOARD SIMULATION: GASTROENTEROLOGY

Muthoka L. Mutinga and Robert S. Burakoff

QUESTION 1. A 57-year-old woman presents with a 2-month history of pruritus and mild fatigue. Her skin examination reveals excoriations but no visible rash. Laboratory examination reveals an alkaline phosphatase elevated to three times normal, with otherwise normal liver biochemical tests. Her thyroid-stimulating hormone (TSH) is also elevated, and she has a positive antithyroid microsomal antibody test.

What is the most likely diagnosis, and what treatment is indicated?

    A. Primary sclerosing cholangitis; ursodiol
    B. Primary biliary cirrhosis; prednisone
    C. Primary sclerosing cholangitis; liver transplantation
    D. Primary biliary cirrhosis; ursodiol
    E. Congenital hepatic fibrosis; liver transplantation

QUESTION 2. A patient with persistent mild elevation of hepatic transaminases and a distant history of intravenous drug use is diagnosed with chronic hepatitis C (HCV), confirmed with a HCV RNA test. A liver biopsy is performed, and subsequently, treatment with Pegylated interferon and ribavirin is initiated.

Which of the following factors does NOT influence the chance of response to therapy?

    A. Viral genotype
    B. Quantitative HCV RNA level (viral load)
    C. Degree of hepatic transaminase elevation
    D. Duration of hepatitic C infection
    E. Degree of fibrosis noted on liver biopsy

QUESTION 3. A 55-year-old man presents with a 4-month history of intermittent, watery diarrhea, severe heartburn, and epigastric pain. He is diagnosed with four duodenal ulcers on endoscopic evaluation. He denies aspirin or non-steroidal anti-inflammatory drug (NSAID) use. Gastric antral biopsy testing for *Helicobacter pylori* bacteria is negative. His symptoms fail to respond to an acid suppression regimen consisting of omeprazole, 20 mg twice daily. A fasting serum gastrin level is 1850 pg/mL.

Which of the following is true of his likely diagnosis?

    A. The patient most likely has a somatostatinoma.
    B. Omeprazole may falsely lower serum gastrin levels.
    C. The tumor responsible for this disorder is most often located in the duodenum.
    D. The tumor responsible for this disorder is usually benign.
    E. The duodenal ulcers will not respond to any level of acid suppression therapy.

QUESTION 4. Which of the following is NOT an extraintestinal manifestation of Crohn disease?

    A. Sacroiliitis
    B. Uveitis
    C. Renal calculi
    D. Erythema nodosum
    E. Thyroiditis

QUESTION 5. A patient with cirrhosis due to alcohol abuse is found to have large esophageal varices on upper endoscopy. There is no history of prior upper gastrointestinal bleeding.

What is the appropriate therapy to prevent future variceal bleeding?

    A. Ursodiol
    B. Interferon
    C. Nonselective beta blocker
    D. Endoscopic sclerotherapy
    E. Proton pump inhibitor therapy (e.g., omeprazole)

QUESTION 6. Ascites is classified according to the serum ascites albumin gradient (SAAG), which is calculated by subtracting the albumin level in the ascites from that in the serum.

Which of the following conditions is associated with low gradient (SAAG <1.1 mg/dL ascites)?

    A. Budd-Chiari syndrome
    B. Cirrhosis due to hepatitis C
    C. Peritoneal carcinomatosis

D. Congestive heart failure

E. Acute alcoholic hepatitis

QUESTION 7. A 47-year-old woman presents with a 4-month history of watery diarrhea and 24-lb weight loss. Laboratory examination is notable for mild iron deficiency anemia and a low serum calcium level. Stool cultures and examination for ova and parasites are unremarkable. Thyroid laboratory testing is normal. A colonoscopy is performed, and the exam is normal, including inspection of the terminal ileum and histologic evaluation of random colon biopsies to assess for microscopic colitis. A tissue transglutaminase antibody is strongly positive.

Which of the following statements regarding this disorder is FALSE?

A. Dietary modification decreases the risk of small intestinal lymphoma.

B. This disease is more common in patients with diabetes mellitus.

C. This disease is seen most commonly in patients of Mediterranean background.

D. Small intestinal biopsies will reveal villous atrophy, crypt hyperplasia, and increased intraepithelial lymphocytes.

E. There is an association with autoimmune thyroid disease.

QUESTION 8. A 35-year-old woman is found to have abnormal results of iron studies on a routine physical examination. Her liver biochemical tests are normal, and her physical exam is unremarkable. She does not consume alcohol or over-the-counter medications or supplements. Her iron studies are as follows:

Serum iron 186

Total iron binding capacity (TIBC 255)

Serum ferritin 300 (normal 25–240)

What is the next test that should be ordered to facilitate the diagnosis?

A. Percutaneous liver biopsy

B. Serum B-12 and folate levels

C. Glucose tolerance testing

D. Gene testing for hereditary hemochromatosis

E. Abdominal computed tomography (CT) scan with intravenous contrast

QUESTION 9. Which of the following is NOT a feature of the hereditary nonpolyposis colon cancer syndrome (HNPCC)?

A. The mean age of first colon cancer is 40.

B. There is a predominance of distal colon cancers (distal to the splenic flexure).

C. The incidence of synchronous colon cancer is estimated to be nearly 20%.

D. There may be a family history of adenocarcinoma of the ovary, endometrium, or stomach.

E. The disorder is transmitted in an autosomal dominant fashion.

QUESTION 10. All of the following statements regarding hepatitis E are true EXCEPT:

A. The virus is endemic in India and Southeast Asia.

B. The clinical features of hepatitis E are similar to those of hepatitis A.

C. The virus is transmitted primarily via percutaneous blood exposure.

D. Hepatitis E is associated with a high rate of fulminant hepatic failure in pregnant women.

E. There is no effective vaccine available to prevent hepatitis E.

QUESTION 11. All of the following may be atypical manifestations of gastroesophageal reflux disease (GERD) EXCEPT:

A. Hoarseness

B. Chronic cough

C. Nocturnal asthma

D. Chronic diarrhea

E. Atypical chest pain

QUESTION 12. A 46-year-old man presents with a complaint of intermittent dysphagia for 10 years. He reports that food "sticks in my chest" approximately one or two times per month and that he needs to either wash down the bolus with water or regurgitate it. He has symptoms only with solid foods, primarily meat, rice, and bread. He has never had difficulty swallowing liquids. He has had no symptoms of odynophagia and has not experienced weight loss.

What is the most likely cause of his symptoms?

A. Schatzki's ring

B. Esophageal cancer

C. Achalasia

D. Diffuse esophageal spasms

E. Peptic stricture of the esophagus

QUESTION 13. All of the following are sequelae of *H. pylori* infection of the stomach, EXCEPT:

A. Gastric cancer

B. Atrophic gastritis

C. Gastric mucosa-associated lymphoid tissue (MALT) lymphoma

D. Duodenal adenocarcinoma

E. Duodenal ulcer

QUESTION 14. A 21-year-old presents for routine health examination. His family history is notable for colon cancer in his mother (age 45), maternal uncle (age 52), and maternal grandmother (age 56). The patient is asymptomatic, routine laboratory tests are normal, and the physical examination including a test for occult blood in the stool is unremarkable.

Which of the following represents appropriate recommendations for colorectal cancer screening for this patient?

A. Colonoscopy every 3–5 years beginning at age 40
B. Colonoscopy no less than every 10 years beginning at age 50
C. Colonoscopy every 2 years beginning at age 21, then annually beginning at age 40
D. Annual flexible sigmoidoscopy beginning at puberty

QUESTION 15. A 42-year-old man with a 15-year history of inflammatory bowel disease presents with new-onset jaundice, right upper quadrant pain, and fever. An ultrasound reveals a dilated common bile duct, and an endoscopic retrograde cholangiopancreatography (ERCP) reveals multiple strictures of the common bile duct (CBD) and intrahepatic bile ducts. A distal CBD stricture is dilated, and the patient's symptoms resolve, although his serum alkaline phosphatase remains persistently elevated at three times the upper limit of normal.

Which of the following statements regarding this disorder is TRUE?

A. This disorder is more common in Crohn disease.
B. Liver biopsy is the definitive diagnostic test for this disorder.
C. Ursodiol has been proven to be effective in treating this disorder.
D. The risk of cholangiocarcinoma is greatly increased in this disorder.
E. This disorder will not recur after liver transplantation.

QUESTION 16. An 86-year-old man develops abdominal cramps, watery diarrhea, and low-grade fever. Within 2 days his stools become bloody, and he feels weak and light-headed. He is seen in your office, and his exam is notable for a temperature of 100.8°F and mild orthostasis. His abdomen is diffusely tender, but no peritoneal signs are present. He has bloody stool in the rectal vault and a fine petechial rash on his lower extremities. Laboratory studies reveal a hematocrit of 27%, platelet count of 48,000, and creatinine of 3.5 mg/dL (his prior labs had been within the normal range).

Which of the following statements regarding this disorder is FALSE?

A. The hematologic and renal complications of this disorder are seen most often in young children and the elderly.
B. The illness is primarily transmitted through the ingestion of poorly cooked meat products.
C. Antibiotics are effective in preventing complications in this illness.
D. The diarrhea is usually self-limited.
E. The disease is caused by Gram-negative bacteria.

QUESTION 17. A 38-year-old landscaper presents with a 6-month history of bullous lesions on the dorsum of his hands, forearms and neck. His physical examination is otherwise unremarkable. He consumes 6–12 beers daily. On laboratory examination he has a mildly elevated ALT (1.5 times normal). He reports being rejected as a blood donor but is unsure why.

Which of the following statements about this patient and his condition is FALSE?

A. Abstinence from alcohol may improve his skin lesions.
B. He is likely to have evidence of chronic hepatitis C.
C. He is likely to have had a history of episodes of severe abdominal pain.
D. Phlebotomy is the accepted treatment for this disorder.

QUESTION 18. A 58-year-old woman is seen in your office with complaints of a 5-year history of progressive dysphagia for liquids and solids. She describes occasional nocturnal regurgitation of food. An upper GI series reveals a dilated esophagus with beak-like narrowing at the level of the gastroesophageal junction. An upper endoscopy reveals no mass or stricture, but there is some resistance to passage of the endoscope through the lower esophageal sphincter (LES), and some liquid and particulate residue is present in the esophagus despite confirmed preprocedure fasting. Esophageal manometry is notable for high normal basal LES pressure, failure of the LES to relax with swallows, as well as aperistalsis of the esophageal body.

Appropriate management of her disease would include any of the following, EXCEPT:

A. Pneumatic dilation
B. Surgical resection of the distal esophagus
C. Surgical myotomy
D. Botulinum toxin (Botox) injection of the lower esophageal sphincter

QUESTION 19. A 35-year-old woman presents with evidence of ascites and elevated hepatic transaminases. She does not drink alcohol. All viral serologic tests are negative. She is not overweight and has no history of autoimmune disorders. Of note, she has a history of emphysema diagnosed in her 20s despite absence of a history of tobacco use.

Which of the following phenotypes would most likely lead to this clinical presentation?

A. Pi MM
B. Pi SS
C. Pi ZZ
D. Pi MZ

QUESTION 20. A 39-year-old man presents with brisk hematochezia for 4 hours. In the Emergency Room his blood pressure is 92/62, and pulse is 100 beats/min in the supine position. Rectal examination reveals red blood and no palpable masses. Anoscopy is limited, revealing red blood in the rectal vault without a visible bleeding source of bleeding. His hematocrit is 33% (his baseline hematocrit 1 year ago was 45%). The platelet count and coagulation tests are normal. He denies aspirin or NSAID use and has had no recent upper gastrointestinal symptoms such as abdominal pain or nausea. A nasogastric tube is placed and yields clear fluid. He has no history of liver disease, abdominal or gastric surgery, or prior history of gastrointestinal bleed.

All of the following are possible causes of this patient's severe gastrointestinal hemorrhage, EXCEPT:

A. Colonic arteriovenous malformations (AVMs)
B. Duodenal ulcer
C. Internal hemorrhoids
D. Colonic diverticuli
E. Meckel diverticulum

QUESTION 21. A 35-year-old with Crohn disease presents to your office with complaints of intense epigastric pain of several hours' duration. He reports heavy alcohol use the night before. His medications include 6-mercaptopurine (6-MP) and Asacol (mesalamine). Laboratory tests are notable for amylase 700 U/L, lipase 1100 U/L, total bilirubin 2.5 mg/dL, direct bilirubin 0.5 mg/dL, AST 17 U/L, ALT 25 U/L, and alkaline phosphatase 72 U/L.
All of the following would be appropriate early steps in the management of this patient, EXCEPT:

A. Obtain abdominal ultrasound imaging
B. Arrange ERCP
C. Hold 6-MP and Asacol
D. Administer analgesics as needed for pain
E. Administer intravenous fluid and keep NPO

ANSWERS

1. D. Primary biliary cirrhosis (PBC) is a cholestatic liver disease most commonly affecting middle-aged women. It often presents with symptoms of fatigue and pruritus, although many patients are detected in the asymptomatic phase on routine laboratory testing. The typical early lab abnormality is an elevated alkaline phosphatase with otherwise normal liver biochemical tests. There is a close association between PBC and autoimmune thyroid disease and other autoimmune disorders. Ursodiol is currently the only treatment known to retard the progression of this disease, which, left untreated, will lead to end-stage liver disease requiring transplantation. Some experts are also using colchicine to limit fibrosis, and methotrexate in refractory cases, but the role of these medications is unproven.

Key point: Remember that the PBC is an autoimmune cholestatic liver disease and that ursodiol, a synthetic bile acid, is the treatment of choice. Also, PBC can be associated with other autoimmune disorders, most notably, autoimmune thyroid disease.

2. C. Combination therapy with pegylated interferon and ribavirin for chronic hepatitis C has been associated with an aggregate response rate of approximately 40–50% for patients with hepatitis C, genotype 1—the most prevalent genotype in the United States, accounting for 70% of patients with chronic hepatitis C. A sustained response to therapy is defined as absence of viremia 6 months after treatment is completed. Patients with such a response have a >90% chance of being virus negative at 5 years. Factors associated with an improved sustained response include female gender, viral genotypes 2 and 3, absence of fibrosis on biopsy, short duration of hepatitis C infection, and HCV RNA level <2 million copies/mL. The degree of hepatic transaminase elevation is not predictive of response to therapy.

Key point: Remember that hepatitis C genotype, viral load, degree of liver fibrosis, and duration of disease but *not* the level of transaminase elevation may influence the likelihood of antiviral response.

3. C. The findings of multiple duodenal ulcers, diarrhea, and a fasting serum gastrin of >1000 are highly suggestive of Zollinger-Ellison syndrome resulting from a gastrinoma of the gastrointestinal tract. Gastrinomas are most often located in the duodenum and pancreas, and most are malignant.

Interpretation of serum gastrin levels is complicated by the frequent use of proton pump inhibitors, which can falsely elevate gastrin levels, though not to the degree seen in Zollinger-Ellison syndrome. The ulcer diathesis will often respond to high-dose proton pump inhibitors (e.g., omeprazole, 40 mg twice daily), but the only definitive treatment is resection of the secretory tumor.

Key point: It is important to remember that a proton pump inhibitor (PPI) may raise serum gastrin above the normal range but usually only slightly above normal.

4. E. Crohn disease (and ulcerative colitis) can be associated with several extraintestinal manifestations that may result in significant morbidity and some mortality among certain groups of patients. Uveitis, sacroiliitis, and erythema nodosum are all autoimmune phenomena that frequently occur in patients with inflammatory bowel disease. Renal calculi are overly represented among patients with Crohn disease. These are usually calcium oxalate stones due to increased absorption of oxalate from the colon, often associated with steatorrhea. Thyroiditis is not clearly associated with Crohn disease.

Key point: Remember that joint involvement in IBD is usually characterized by asymmetric involvement of large joints.

5. C. Patients with portal hypertension and large esophageal varices benefit from prophylactic therapy to prevent gastrointestinal hemorrhage. Currently, pharmacologic prophylaxis with nonselective beta blockers (propranolol, nadolol, or timolol) is recommended. Endoscopic sclerotherapy

has been shown to be ineffective and possibly harmful when used for prophylaxis of variceal hemorrhage. Interferon, ursodiol, and acid inhibition therapy have not been shown to be effective in the prevention of variceal bleeding.

Key point: Remember that nonselective beta blockers (with or without oral nitrates) are the treatment of choice for primary prophylaxis of variceal bleeding.

6. C. The serum-ascites albumin gradient (SAAG) differentiates between ascites due to portal hypertension (formerly called transudative ascites) and that due to non–portal hypertensive states (formerly called exudative ascites) with 97% accuracy. Low-gradient ascites is seen in peritoneal carcinomatosis, tuberculous peritonitis, pancreatitis, and fungal infections of the peritoneum. The remaining answers are all associated with high-gradient ascites due to portal hypertension.

Key point: Remember that SAAG <1.1 is characteristic of ascites not related to portal hypertension, whereas a SAAG >1.1 is characteristic of ascites related to portal hypertension.

7. C. The constellation of symptoms, evidence of nutrient malabsorption, and positive tissue transglutaminase antibody are all consistent with a diagnosis of celiac sprue. This disorder primarily affects people of Northern European descent rather than those of Mediterranean ancestry. The disease is associated with both diabetes mellitus and autoimmune thyroid disease. The characteristic histologic features include flattening of the small intestinal villi (villous atrophy), deepening of duodenal crypts (crypt hyperplasia), and the presence of increased intraepithelial lymphocytes. Treatment involves elimination of gluten from the diet. Not only does this ameliorate symptoms, but there is some evidence suggesting that a gluten-free diet may decrease the risk of small intestinal lymphoma, which is seen with increased frequency in celiac disease.

Key point: Remember that gluten is present in barley, bulgur, couscous, farina, oats, rye, semolina, spelt, and wheat among others but is not present in arborio or basmati rice, beans, brown rice, cassava, corn, sweet potato, and others.

8. D. This patient's iron saturation is 73% (iron saturation = serum iron/TIBC). An iron saturation of >55% is suggestive of an iron overload syndrome, and this finding should initiate the workup for hereditary hemochromatosis. One might expect the serum ferritin to be higher in a patient with hemochromatosis; however, a 35-year-old female may lose enough blood from menstruation to keep her total body iron relatively low. The next test to obtain is the hemochromatosis genetic test (HFE gene analysis), which looks for the two most common mutations seen in hereditary hemochromatosis (the major mutation C282Y and minor mutation H63D). In a young, asymptomatic patient with normal liver function tests, a liver biopsy is not necessary. Phlebotomy therapy can be started on the basis of a positive genetic test alone, if iron overload is present. There is also no need to search for occult glucose intolerance

in the young patient without symptoms. CT scanning is not yet sensitive enough to determine the presence or degree of hepatic iron overload and should not be used to diagnose hemochromatosis.

Key point: Genetic testing for mutations of the HFE gene should be performed in people with elevated transferrin saturation and serum ferritin, and in first-degree family members of a known person with hereditary hemochromatosis.

9. B. Hereditary nonpolyposis colon cancer (HNPCC) is a syndrome characterized by an increased risk of colonic malignancy due to a defect in certain DNA mismatch repair genes that normally correct base-pair mismatches during DNA replication. The disorder is transmitted in an autosomal dominant fashion with high degree of penetrance. The mean age of presentation with cancer is 40. Synchronous colon cancer (a second colon cancer found at the time of the index colon cancer) is common, and there is a predominance of *proximal* tumors (60–80% are beyond/proximal to the splenic flexure). In some kindreds (called Lynch syndrome II), there is an increased incidence of other extracolonic malignancies including ovarian, endometrial, and gastric cancers.

Key point: In patients with HNPCC there is a predominance of tumors proximal to the splenic flexure.

10. C. Hepatitis E is a common cause of epidemic hepatitis in Africa and Asia and is seen in the United States primarily in returned travelers and immigrants from endemic areas. It is transmitted via the fecal–oral route and is associated with large outbreaks due to contaminated water systems. In general, it is a self-limited icteric illness with a similar clinical course to hepatitis A. An important exception to this generally benign course is the observation that pregnant women infected with hepatitis E have a high rate of fulminant hepatic failure, up to 25% in some series from India and Pakistan. There is currently no vaccine available for hepatitis E.

Key point: Remember that hepatitis E, much like hepatitis A, is transmitted via the fecal–oral route, does not cause chronic infection, and usually is associated with a benign course, except in pregnant women who are at increased risk of fulminant hepatitis.

11. The answer is D. In recent years, several clinical syndromes have been shown to be associated with gastroesophageal reflux disease. These include hoarseness and chronic laryngitis, chronic nonproductive cough, nocturnal asthma, and noncardiac chest pain. In such cases, the presence of acid reflux can be confirmed with a 24-hour intraesophageal pH monitor. Alternatively, an empirical trial of a proton pump inhibitor can be used, and symptomatic response can be assessed after 12 weeks of therapy. There is no association between simple gastroesophageal reflux and chronic diarrhea.

Key point: To prove an atypical manifestation is secondary to gastroesophageal reflux disease, an esophageal pH study must be performed.

12. A. This patient likely has a Schatzki's ring, a fibrous ring in the lower esophagus that causes intermittent obstructive symptoms. The key features of this disorder are intermittent dysphagia to solids with normal swallowing in between. Patients often report choking on meat or large pieces of bread and may need to regurgitate at times. Both esophageal cancer and a peptic stricture would result in progressive dysphagia for solids, whereas achalasia causes dysphagia for both solids and liquids early in its course. Esophageal spasms tend to present with episodes of chest pain and dysphagia. A Schatzki's ring is treated with endoscopic esophageal dilation, resulting in excellent relief of symptoms, though there is a small rate of recurrence.

Key point: A Schatzki's ring or peptic stricture is associated with dysphagia for solids, whereas an esophageal motility disorder is often associated with dysphagia for liquids and solids.

12. D. Infection with *H. pylori*, a Gram-negative urease-producing bacterium that colonizes the gastric mucosa, may lead to a variety of pathologic conditions. It is clearly associated with duodenal ulcer disease, and treatment of infection reduces the risk of ulcer recurrence by >80%. Chronic gastritis due to *H. pylori* can lead to atrophic gastritis and hypochlorhydria over decades. There is a clear relationship between chronic *H. pylori* infection and gastric adenocarcinoma, such that the WHO has declared *H. pylori* a class I carcinogen. There is also an interesting association between MALT lymphoma and *H. pylori*. Some studies have shown tumor regression after eradication of this organism. There is as yet no known association linking *H. pylori* infection with carcinoma of the small intestine.

Key point: Remember that chronic *H. pylori* infection can be associated with development of peptic ulcer disease, atrophic gastritis, gastric adenocarcinoma and gastric MALT lymphoma, but not duodenal carcinomas.

14. C. The history meets the criteria for HNPCC syndrome as follows: (1) three relatives with colorectal cancer (CRC)—one must be a first-degree relative of the other two; (2) one or more CRC cases occurring before the age of 50 years; (3) CRC involving at least two generations; (4) familial adenomatous polyposis (FAP) syndrome must be excluded.

Screening of family members in kindreds with HNPCC should consist of colonoscopy every 2 years beginning at age 21 until age 40, and annually thereafter. Genetic testing to identify mismatch repair gene mutations (e.g., *MSH2*, *MLH1*, and *MSH6*) is available.

Annual flexible sigmoidoscopy beginning at age 12 is recommended for screening in familial adenomatous polyposis syndrome. Genetic testing to identify APC gene mutations in this syndrome is also available.

Patients at moderate risk of colon cancer, such as those with a first-degree relative with adenomatous polyps or colon cancer at age <60 years should have screening colonoscopies performed every 3–5 years, beginning at age 40 years.

Colonoscopy no less than every 10 years, beginning at age 50 years, is recommended for patients at average risk for colorectal cancer.

Key point: Remember that screening of family members in kindreds with HNPCC should consist of colonoscopy every 2 years beginning at age 21 until age 40, and annually thereafter. In addition, genetic testing to identify mismatch repair gene mutations (e.g., *MSH2*, *MLH1*, and *MSH6*) is available.

15. D. This patient has primary sclerosing cholangitis (PSC), an inflammatory disorder of the biliary tree that leads to progressive stricturing of both small and large bile ducts, with recurrent bouts of cholangitis and eventual progression to biliary cirrhosis. It is strongly associated with inflammatory bowel disease. As many as 70–80% of patients with PSC have coexisting inflammatory bowel disease (ulcerative colitis, Crohn disease), although only 2.4–7.5% of patients with IBD will develop PSC. The diagnosis of PSC is made on ERCP. Liver biopsy has a low diagnostic yield. There is increasing evidence that ursodiol may be useful in this disorder, in a higher dose than that used for PBC, but this is not proven, and ursodiol is not universally recommended. Cholangiocarcinoma will develop in 7–15% of patients with PSC and is a common cause of mortality in these patients. Liver transplantation is effective in end-stage PSC, though there is some risk of recurrence in the transplanted liver.

Key point: PSC may be seen as a complication in both Crohn and ulcerative colitis. Total colectomy in ulcerative colitis will not result in resolution of PSC.

16. C. This patient has the hemolytic uremic syndrome (HUS), a sequela of infection with the Gram-negative bacterium, *Escherichia coli* O157:H7, the enterohemorrhagic *E. coli* strain. The disease is transmitted via poorly cooked meat products and begins as a syndrome of fever, abdominal cramps, and watery diarrhea. It progresses to frankly bloody diarrhea over a period of days and is generally self-limited. However, in very young children and in the elderly, a syndrome of renal failure, thrombocytopenia, and hemolytic anemia may develop, which may be fatal. Antibiotics have not been shown to prevent this complication; in fact, recent data suggest that antibiotic therapy may *promote* the development of HUS, and antibiotics are currently not recommended for the treatment of *E. coli* O157:H7 colitis.

Key point: Antibiotic therapy should be avoided in suspected cases of infection with *E. coli* O157:H7 because it promotes toxin release from the bacteria and can worsen the clinical outcome. Most people infected who develop illness with his strain of *E. coli* have a self-limited illness, but the young and elderly are more susceptible to develop HUS.

17. C. The patient has porphyria cutanea tarda (PCT), a disorder of heme breakdown and porphyrin metabolism. It is characterized by bullous lesions on sun-exposed areas that heal with scarring. Most patients with PCT have elevated liver biochemical tests, and many are found to have

chronic hepatitis C. In addition, there is a strong association with alcohol ingestion, and abstinence from alcohol may lead to a regression of the skin manifestations of PCT. The mainstay of treatment is phlebotomy, which greatly reduces iron stores and improves the lesions and liver abnormalities seen in PCT. Unlike acute intermittent porphyria, there is no abdominal pain syndrome associated with PCT.

Key point: Remember that, unlike acute porphyrias, PCT is not associated with abdominal and/or neurological symptoms. Also, many patients with PCT have chronic hepatitis C, iron overload, and many have a history of heavy alcohol use.

18. B. The patient has a classic history, imaging studies, and manometric findings for achalasia. Upper endoscopy is required to rule out causes adenocarcinoma of the proximal stomach or distal esophagus, which may mimic achalasia ("pseudoachalasia"). Achalasia is thought to result from progressive loss of ganglion cells within the myenteric plexus of the distal esophagus. Most patients present between the ages of 30 and 50 years. The most common presenting symptom is dysphagia. Initially the dysphagia occurs with solids, but then liquid dysphagia develops later in the clinical course. Other common symptoms include nocturnal regurgitation of undigested food and chest pain.

Resection of the distal esophagus is *not* a treatment for achalasia. Oral medical therapy for achalasia (e.g., isosorbide and nifedipine) is associated with rather poor symptom response (<50% response at 1 year). Botulinum toxin injections into the muscles of the LES are associated with approximately 60% response at 1 year, although repeated injections are often necessary. Balloon dilation has a better long-term response rate (60–90% at 1 year) but carries a risk of esophageal perforation (up to 4%). Surgical therapy includes open myotomy of the LES (>90% response at 1 year) and laparoscopic myotomy of the LES (90% response at 1 year). There is an approximately 10% incidence of postsurgical symptomatic reflux in these patients.

Key point: Achalasia is defined on manometry by high LES pressure with incomplete relaxation of the LES and aperistalsis in the body of the esophagus. One must remember that if the onset of dysphagia is of short duration, after the age of 50, with radiographic and manometric features of achalasia, one must rule out secondary achalasia due to either proximal gastric cancer or tumors in the mediastinum that invade the area of the lower esophageal sphincter.

19. C. This patient has alpha-1-antitrypsin deficiency. Alpha-1-antitrypsin is a protease inhibitor synthesized almost exclusively in the liver. It is responsible for inhibiting neutrophil-derived proteases, especially neutrophil elastase. There are over 75 different protease inhibitor (Pi) alleles. The normal alpha-1-antitrypsin phenotype is Pi MM. The most common pathologic phenotype causing both liver and lung disease is the Pi ZZ variant, in which serum alpha-l-antitrypsin activity level is <15% of normal. Pi SZ heterozygotes may rarely develop cirrhosis, whereas Pi MZ heterozygotes usually do not develop cirrhosis unless there is some other cofactor for liver disease such as heavy alcohol use or chronic viral hepatitis. The pathophysiology of liver injury is controversial but is hypothesized to be due to altered degradation of retained alpha-1-antitrypsin in the hepatocyte.

Key point: Remember that alpha-1-antitrypsin deficiency is an inherited disorder than can result in both liver and lung disease. Whereas the Pi MM phenotype is normal, the Pi ZZ phenotype results in the lowest level of alpha-1-antitrypsin and is the phenotype most commonly associated with cirrhosis.

20. C. Lower GI bleeding is severe and hemodynamically significant (e.g., resting tachycardia, postural hypotension) in 15% of patients. Approximately 15–20% of patients with severe, ongoing hematochezia and anemia have an upper GI source of bleeding. A nasogastric aspirate that is clear or nonbloody does *not* exclude an upper GI tract bleed unless bile is present. Meckel diverticulum is the most common cause of lower GI bleeding in children, although it may rarely cause lower GI hemorrhage in adults. Diverticular hemorrhage occurs in 3–5% of persons with colonic diverticuli. Bleeding from AVMs is usually subacute, although 15% of patients present with acute, massive hemorrhage. Hemorrhoids are not associated with massive lower GI bleeding in a patient without significant coagulopathy or portal hypertension.

Key point: A nasogastric aspirate that is clear or nonbloody does *not* exclude an upper GI tract bleed unless bile is present.

21. B. This patient has acute pancreatitis manifested by marked elevation of amylase and lipase. Alcohol is a common cause of acute pancreatitis. Patients with Crohn disease are at an increased risk for development of gallstones; these gallstones may lead to pancreatitis if they temporarily occlude the pancreatic duct outflow. Elevations of transaminases (ALT and AST), alkaline phosphatase, and bilirubin due to biliary obstruction are clues to a diagnosis of gallstone pancreatitis. Many drugs have been linked to acute pancreatitis such as 6-mercaptopurine (6-MP), azathioprine, hydrochlorothiazide (HCTZ), didanosine (ddI), and, rarely, Asacol, to name a few. Intravenous fluids, fasting (NPO), and narcotic analgesics are reasonable for initial management of pancreatitis. ERCP is indicated only in patients with severe gallstone pancreatitis (i.e., those with organ failure or significant necrosis) who fail to improve in their early hospital course, or in those with suspected ascending cholangitis. This patient's mild indirect hyperbilirubinemia with normal transaminases and alkaline phosphatase are suggestive of Gilbert syndrome—a benign, congenital condition resulting in impaired bilirubin conjugation—rather than an obstructive biliary process.

Key point: 6-MP and azathioprine can cause pancreatitis in 3% of patients and, if stopped immediately, rarely lead to severe pancreatitis and are unlikely to lead to chronic pancreatitis.

76.

REVIEW TOPICS IN GASTROENTEROLOGY AND HEPATOLOGY

Norton J. Greenberger

This chapter focuses on a potpourri of topics from liver disease that are popular subjects for the boards and that have not been covered in detail in the other chapters in this section.

PRIMARY BILIARY CIRRHOSIS

Primary biliary cirrhosis (PBC) is a slowly progressive cholestatic disease of the liver. The etiology is unknown; however, several lines of evidence point to an autoimmune mechanism, including the presence of autoantibodies, abnormalities in both cellular and humoral immunity, and the association with several other autoimmune diseases. The major pathology of this disease is a destruction of the small to medium bile ducts, which leads to progressive cholestasis and often end-stage liver disease. Key features of the disease are shown in table 76.1.

PBC is more common in women and those of northern European descent. Onset is usually in middle age (table 76.1), and one in four patients with PBC are discovered incidentally. Most patients develop symptoms over 5 to 20 years. The most common clinical presentation is with fatigue and pruritus. In the early stages of the disease the physical examination is normal, but later in its course, features consistent with cirrhosis and portal hypertension are common. There are several associated systemic abnormalities (see table 76.2).

The main laboratory findings with PBC are (1) liver function abnormalities—elevated aminotransferases including alanine aminotransferase (ALT), aspartate aminotransferase (AST), and alkaline phosphatase (ALP) and gamma-glutamyl transpeptidase (GGTP), and (2) antimitochondrial antibodies (AMAs)—AMAs are detected in 90–95% of patients with a specificity of 98% for PBC. AMAs target different components, mainly enzymes, in the mitochondria. The presence of anti-M2, anti-M4, anti-M8, and anti-M9 correlate with the severity of primary biliary cirrhosis.

There are four stages of PBC:

- Stage 1 (portal stage of Ludwig): Portal inflammation, bile duct abnormalities, or both are present.

- Stage 2 (periportal stage): Periportal fibrosis is present, with or without periportal inflammation or prominent enlargement of the portal tracts with seemingly intact, newly formed limiting plates.

- Stage 3 (septal stage): Septal fibrosis with active inflammation, passive paucicellular septa, or both are present.

- Stage 4 (cirrhosis): Nodules with various degrees of inflammation are present.

Treatment is summarized in table 76.1. The overarching goals of treatment are to slow the progression rate of the disease and to alleviate the symptoms. Liver transplantation appears to be the only life-saving procedure. Ursodeoxycholic acid (UDCA) is the major medication used to slow the progression of the disease. On the other hand, glucocorticoids, cyclosporine, methotrexate, colchicine, and azathioprine are unproven or do not alter the natural progression of PBC.

PRIMARY SCLEROSING CHOLANGITIS

Primary sclerosing cholangitis (PSC) is a chronic liver disease characterized by cholestasis with inflammation and fibrosis of the intrahepatic and extrahepatic bile ducts (table 76.3). The etiology is unknown; however, several lines of evidence point to an autoimmune mechanism, including the strong association with inflammatory bowel disease (IBD), and the presence of autoantibodies—antineutrophil cytoplasmic antibodies (ANCA), anticardiolipin (aCL) antibodies, and antinuclear antibodies (ANA). PSC may lead to cirrhosis of the liver with portal hypertension.

The mean age of onset is 40 years. In contrast to PBC there is a predilection for men. Approximately 75–90% of patients have IBD—mostly ulcerative colitis rather than

Table 76.1 KEY FEATURES OF PRIMARY BILIARY CIRRHOSIS

Description
- 95% patients are women
- Manifestations
  - Asymptomatic
  - Dermatologic
  - Pruritus
  - Hyperpigmentation
  - Musculoskeletal
  - Fatigue
  - Rheumatoid arthritis (10%)
  - Sjögren syndrome
  - Hypercholesterolemia
  - Xanthomatous peripheral neuropathy

Criteria for diagnosis
- Increased serum alkaline phosphatase 95%
- Positive antimitochondrial antibody 95%
- Liver biopsy—provides information on stage of disease, i.e., I–IV (cirrhosis)

Treatment
- Ursodeoxycholic acid, 13–15 mg/kg
- Meta-analysis trials—long-term >2 years
- Improvement in liver biochemical tests
- Reduction/delay in disease progression
- Possible improvement in transplant-free survival
- UDCA more effective in early disease
- Patient with advanced disease and complications should be referred for transplantation

Table 76.2 PRIMARY BILIARY CIRRHOSIS: ASSOCIATED SYSTEMIC ABNORMALITIES

- Pruritus
- Metabolic bone disease
- Hypercholesterolemia
- Malabsorption and steatorrhea
- Vitamin (fat soluble) deficiency: vitamins A, D, E, K
- Hypothyroidism (20% of patients)
- Anemia
- Xanthelasma in primary biliary cirrhosis

treat the symptoms and to prevent or treat the known complications. Liver transplantation is the only effective therapy and is indicated in end-stage liver disease.

HEPATITIS

Hepatitis refers to inflammation of the liver. The pathologic target is the hepatocyte (in contrast to cholangitis wherein the target is mostly biliary ductal cells). In hepatitis the predominant abnormality is with the aminotransferases (ALT and AST) rather than the alkaline phosphatase. Hepatitis can be acute or chronic (see table 76.4). Its causes can be either infectious or noninfectious. Infectious etiologies include viral, bacterial, fungal, and parasitic organisms. In the United States, viral hepatitis is most commonly caused by hepatitis A virus (HAV), hepatitis B virus (HBV), and hepatitis C virus (HCV). These three viruses can all result in an acute disease process with symptoms of nausea, abdominal pain, fatigue, malaise, and jaundice. HBV and HCV can also lead to chronic infection. Chronically infected liver may progress to cirrhosis and/or develop hepatocellular carcinoma.

AUTOIMMUNE HEPATITIS

Autoimmune hepatitis is characterized by progressive hepatocellular inflammation and necrosis, with progression to cirrhosis (table 76.5). Its etiology is unknown. However, as for PBC and PSC, several lines of evidence point to autoimmune mechanisms, including histopathologic evidence of cell-mediated immunity (hepatic histopathologic lesions composed predominantly of cytotoxic T cells and plasma cells), presence of autoantibodies (i.e., nuclear, smooth muscle, thyroid, liver), and association with other autoimmune diseases.

Autoimmune hepatitis mostly affects women (70–80%) and has a predilection for Caucasians of northern European ancestry with a high frequency of HLA-DR3 and HLA-DR4 markers. It has a bimodal distribution—10–30 years and 40–50 years. Autoimmune hepatitis clinical syndromes include acute hepatitis (fever, hepatic tenderness, and jaundice), chronic hepatitis (asymptomatic but with abnormal liver function tests (LFTs) and fatigue, pruritus,

Crohn disease. Clinical features in those patients who are symptomatic (20–40% are asymptomatic) include fatigue, jaundice, pruritus, and right upper quadrant pain.

The key laboratory findings are abnormal liver function tests. The most striking abnormality is the serum alkaline phosphatase, which is usually three to five times reference range values and cholestatic in nature (alkaline phosphatase fraction is liver disease in origin rather than bone disease in origin). The serum gamma-glutamyl transpeptidase level is also elevated. There is a modest increase in serum aminotransferase and bilirubin levels. Also seen are abnormalities on endoscopic retrograde cholangiopancreatography (ERCP) that include multiple strictures and dilations of the intrahepatic and extrahepatic biliary ducts.

As with PBC there are four stages of PSC:

- Stage 1: Portal hepatitis, degeneration of bile ducts with inflammatory cell infiltrate

- Stage 2: Extension of disease to periportal area with prominent bile ductopenia

- Stage 3: Septal fibrosis and necrosis

- Stage 4: Frank cirrhosis

PSC is a chronic progressive disease with no curative medical therapy. The goals of medical management are to

Table 76.3 KEY FEATURES OF PRIMARY SCLEROSING CHOLANGITIS (PSC)

Clinical features

- 75% of patients have inflammatory bowel disease (IBD) especially ulcerative colitis
- Asymptomatic with elevated serum alkaline phosphatase
- IBD patients with a persistently elevated serum alkaline phosphatase
- Jaundice with obstructive types liver tests (esp. men 30–40 years)
- Fatigue and pruritus
- Right upper quadrant abdominal pain, fever, chills, sweat

Criteria for diagnosis

- Demonstration of multifocal strictures and dilatation of intra-hepatic/extrahepatic bile ducts by MRCP or ERCP
- Liver biopsy supports the diagnosis with typical findings:
  - Include fibrosis with obliteration of small bile ducts and "onion skin pattern" stages I–IV (cirrhosis)
- Small duct PSC
  - Typical presentation but ERCP/MRCP exams do not show typical bile duct abnormalities but liver biopsy demonstrates characteristic histologic features
  - Delayed/reduced likelihood of disease progression and cholangiocarcinoma

Differential Diagnosis

- Cholangiocarcinoma develops in 8–15% of PSC patients
- Infection cholangiopathy (microsporidium, cryptosporidium) AIDS patients
- Autoimmune pancreatitis with bile duct stricturing

Complications

- Fatigue, pruritus, deficiency of fat soluble vitamins (A,D,E,K)
- Metabolic bone disease
- PSC increased risk of colon carcinoma patients with ulcerative colitis
- Cholangiocarcinoma—Difficult Dx—brush cytology ↑ Ca/9–9

Treatment

- No effective treatment; high-dose ursodeoxycholic acid (UDCA) 20 mg/kg → equivocal improvement in disease tests

Table 76.4 ACUTE VERSUS CHRONIC HEPATITIS

ACUTE HEPATITIS	CHRONIC HEPATITIS
Toxins (e.g., acetaminophen)	Toxins
Viral: A-E, CMV, EBV, HSV, VZV	Viral: B and C
	Metabolic: NAFLD
Auto immune hepatitis	Genetic
Vascular compromise	• Hemochromatosis
Fulminant Wilson disease	• Alpha-1-antitrypsin deficiency
	• Wilson disease
	Immune
	• Autoimmune hepatitis
	• Celiac sprue
	Vascular
	• Budd-Chiari syndrome
	• Right-sided heart failure
	• VOD

Phase 1—Viral replication:

Patients are asymptomatic during this phase. Laboratory studies demonstrate serologic and enzyme markers of hepatitis.

Phase 2—Prodromal phase:

Patients experience anorexia, nausea, vomiting, alterations in taste, arthralgias, malaise, fatigue, urticaria, and pruritus. Some develop an aversion to cigarette smoke.

Table 76.5 KEY FEATURES OF AUTOIMMUNE HEPATITIS

Spectrum of presentations

- Asymptomatic with abnormal liver tests
- Acute onset of jaundice
- Chronic liver disease with jaundice and hepatosplenomegaly
- Fulminant hepatic failure

Extrahepatic manifestations

- Thyroiditis
- Celiac sprue
- Hemolytic anemia
- Idiopathic thrombocytopenic purpura
- Ulcerative colitis
- Diabetes mellitus

Criteria for diagnosis

- Female sex
- Alkaline phosphatase/ALT or AST increase <1.5
- ANA, SMA, antiactin antibodies, LRM (+) >1:40
- (–) Test for antimitochondrial antibody
- (–) Test for drugs, viral hepatitis markers, alcohol history
- ↑ serum globulins >1.0–2.0 × normal
- Liver histology—interface hepatitis, lymphoplasmacytic infiltrate

Treatment

- Corticosteroids + azathioprine (steroid sparing) preferred Rx or corticosteroids alone if concerns about azathioprine, i.e., cytopenias, malignancy, thiopurine methyltransferase deficiency (TPMT)
- 85% of patients respond; indicators of poor response: Serum bilirubin does not decrease to <15 mg/dL after 2 weeks of treatment

and abdominal pain), or well-established cirrhosis. There are protean disease associations (table 76.6).

Autoimmune hepatitis is a treatable condition—with steroids and/or immunosuppressive agents (azathioprine). Without therapy, most patients die within 10 years of disease onset. Treatment with appropriate pharmacologic agents improves survival significantly.

INFECTIOUS CAUSES OF HEPATITIS

Hepatitis A (HAV), hepatitis B (HBV), hepatitis C (HCV), hepatitis D (HDV), and hepatitis E (HEV) cause 95% of cases of acute viral hepatitis observed in the United States. HCV is the most common cause of chronic hepatitis. The clinical stages or phases of disease with the viral hepatitides are listed below:

Table 76.6 AUTOIMMUNE HEPATITIS DISEASE ASSOCIATIONS

Hematologic complications
   Hypersplenism
   Autoimmune hemolytic anemia
   Coombs'-positive hemolytic anemia
   Pernicious anemia
   Idiopathic thrombocytopenic purpura
   Eosinophilia

Gastrointestinal complications
   Inflammatory bowel disease

Proliferative glomerulonephritis
Fibrosing alveolitis
Pericarditis and myocarditis
Endocrinologic complications
   Graves disease and autoimmune thyroiditis
   Juvenile diabetes mellitus

Rheumatologic complications
   Rheumatoid arthritis and Felty syndrome
   Sjögren syndrome
   Systemic sclerosis
   Mixed connective-tissue disease
   Erythema nodosum
Leukocytoclastic vasculitis
Febrile panniculitis
Lichen planus
Uveitis

When seen by a healthcare provider during this phase, patients are often diagnosed as having gastroenteritis or a viral syndrome.

Phase 3—Icteric phase:

Patients may note dark urine, followed by pale-colored stools.
In addition to the predominant gastrointestinal symptoms and malaise, patients become icteric and may develop right upper quadrant pain with hepatomegaly.

Phase 4—Convalescent phase:

Symptoms and icterus resolve.
Liver enzymes return to normal.

The key features of hepatitis A–E are listed in tables 76.7–76.12.

CHRONIC HEPATITIS

Chronic hepatitis is defined as inflammation of the liver that lasts at least 6 months. Common causes include hepatitis B and C viruses and drugs. Many patients are asymptomatic until the liver has become severely scarred.

Table 76.7 KEY FEATURES OF HEPATITIS A

- Single-stranded RNA virus.

- Causes mostly acute and occasionally relapsing episodes of hepatitis.

- Responsible for between 20% and 40% of acute hepatitis in the United States before immunization available.

- Fulminant liver failure is very rare but possible, particularly in setting of pre-existing chronic liver disease. At least one study has reported high mortality rates in the setting of chronic HCV infection.

- Transmission by the fecal-oral route with incubation period ranging from 2 to 8 weeks with an average of 4 weeks

- Presence of IgM antibodies to HAV signifies acute infection.

- IgG antibodies suggest prior infection or vaccination and thus immunoprotection.

- Postexposure treatment with IgG effective if given within 2 weeks.

- Postexposure IgG treatment does not decrease effectiveness of vaccination.

Table 76.8 KEY FEATURES OF HEPATITIS B

Double-stranded DNA virus
Cause of both acute and chronic hepatitis
Common disease, with an estimated worldwide prevalence of 350 million and 250,000 annual deaths. Most prevalent in Asia and sub-Saharan Africa

- 1.25 million cases in United States with 70,000 new infections/year

- 30% infections symptomatic, 70% subclinical

- 95% of adults recover, 3.5% of adults and 95% of children do not have an immune response adequate to clear the infection

- Modes of transmission are blood borne and sexual

Definitions
- Chronic hepatitis B—HBsAg (+) >6 months

- HBeAg (+) chronic hepatitis B—serum HBV-DNA >20,000 IU/mL

- HBeAg (–) chronic hepatitis B—serum HBV-DNA >2,000 IU/mL

- In both HBeAg (+) and HBeAg (–) chronic hepatitis there is intermittent or persistent ↑ALT/AST levels and liver biopsies show chronic hepatitis

- Inactive carrier state—HBsAg (+) >6 months

  – Serum HBV/DNA <20,000 IU/mL
  – Persistently normal ALT/AST
  – Liver biopsy shows absence of significant hepatitis (low necroinflammatory score)

Resolved hepatitis B—Previous known acute/chronic hepatitis B now HBsAg (–)

  – Undetectable serum HBV-DNA
  – HBsAg or HBsAb and HBcAb (+)

Chronic hepatitis can result in cirrhosis and portal hypertension. The differential diagnosis for chronic hepatitis is shown in table 76.3.

Table 76.9 INTERPRETATION OF HEPATITIS B SEROLOGIC TESTS

EXAMPLE MARKERS OF VIRAL HEPATITIS B TESTS

	HBsAG	HBsAB	HBcAB	INTERPRETATIONS
1	+	–	–	Acute viral hepatitis
2	+	–	–	Acute viral hepatitis Carrier (normal aminotransferases) Chronic hepatitis B (abnormal liver tests)
3	–	+	–	Remote infection immunization
4	–	+	–	Remote infection
5	+	+	+	Infection with more than one strain of hepatitis B (VDA, renal dialysis)
6	–	–	+	"Window phase" and hepatitis B Remote infection False positive

Table 76.10 KEY FEATURES OF HEPATITIS C

Previously known as non-A, non-B hepatitis, HCV is an RNA virus.

Approximately 1.8% of U.S. population is HCV antibody positive; 1.3% are HCV RNA positive. HCV RNA should be evaluated in HCV antibody-positive persons before a diagnosis is rendered.

Antibodies to HCV do not confer protective immunity.

Responsible for both acute (rare) and chronic (common) hepatitis.

Less than 20% of infected patients are symptomatic during acute infection.

The modes of transmission are both percutaneous and sexual. IV drug use is the most common mode of acquisition in the United States.

An estimated 80–85% progress to chronic hepatitis.

Extrahepatic manifestations:
- Cryoglobulinemia with palpable purpura, arthralgias, leukocytoclastic vasculitis, and glomerulonephritis.
- Porphyria cutanea tarda (PCT), a blistering rash most prominent in the sun-exposed areas of the body.

Variable natural history, but rate of fibrosis affected by alcohol intake.

HCV genotypes 1a and 1b are most common in the United States, but genotypes 2 and 3 are more easily treated with currently available therapies.

Progression to cirrhosis in 20–30% after 20 years.

HCV is currently the most common indication for liver transplantation in the United States.

Therapy for HCV is combination of interferon and ribavirin for 6 to 12 months.

PEGylated interferons plus ribavirin result in around a 55% sustained viral response.

Potential side effects of treatment are numerous and include fever, nausea, myalgias, depression, leukopenias, hemolytic anemia, and teratogenic effects.

WILSON DISEASE

Wilson disease is a rare autosomal recessive inherited disorder of copper metabolism. The condition is characterized by excessive deposition of copper in the liver, brain, and other tissues. The major physiological aberration is excessive absorption of copper from the small intestine and decreased excretion of copper by the liver. The genetic defect, localized to chromosome arm 13q, affects the copper-transporting adenosine triphosphatase (ATPase) gene (*ATP7B*) in the liver. Patients with Wilson disease usually present with liver disease during the first decade of life or with neuropsychiatric illness during the third decade. The diagnosis is confirmed by measurement of serum ceruloplasmin, urinary copper excretion, and hepatic copper content as well as the detection of Kayser-Fleischer rings. Key features are depicted in table 76.13.

NONALCOHOLIC FATTY LIVER DISEASE

Nonalcoholic fatty liver disease (NAFLD) is characterized by predominantly macrovesicular hepatic steatosis that occurs in individuals even in the absence of consumption of alcohol in amounts considered harmful to the liver. Patients who have the classic triad of obesity, type 2 diabetes

Table 76.11 KEY FEATURES OF HEPATITIS D

- A defective RNA virus that is dependent on coinfection with HBV
- Transmitted percutaneously or sexually
- May be transmitted with HBV (co-infection) or during active HBV (superinfection)
- Acute HDV may result in rapid progression in hepatitis leading to fulminant hepatitis

Table 76.12 KEY FEATURES OF HEPATITIS E (HEV)

- RNA virus
- Fecal–oral transmission
- Highest prevalence in Asia, Central America, Africa
- Clinical disease similar to hepatitis A
- Incubation period of 2 weeks to 2 months
- Fulminant hepatitis common during pregnancy with mortality rates reported at 15–25%
- Suspect in patients with acute hepatitis simulating hepatitis A but hepatitis A antibody (HAV-IgM) is negative
- Take careful travel history; hepatitis E found in Mexico, Egypt, South America, Pakistan, South Africa
- Check hepatitis E antibody (IgM) to confirm diagnosis

mellitus, and dyslipidemia (i.e., patients with the metabolic syndrome) are prone to develop NAFLD. The likelihood of having NAFLD is directly proportional to body weight. NAFLD is being increasingly recognized as a major cause of liver-related morbidity and mortality. Key features are shown in table 76.14.

ALCOHOLIC LIVER DISEASE

Alcoholic hepatitis is a syndrome of progressive inflammatory liver injury associated with long-term heavy intake of ethanol.

Table 76.13 KEY FEATURES OF WILSON DISEASE

Criteria for diagnosis

- Kayser-Fleischer rings, may also see sunflower cataracts
- ↓Serum ceruloplasmin <20 mg/dL (low predictive value)
- ↑Urine copper >100 μg/24-hr urine
- 25% need penicillamine challenge to have abnormal level
- Liver biopsy showing liver copper content >250 μg/g liver
- Usual age at presentation (5–40 years)

Special features

- Can present simulating autoimmune hepatitis
- Fulminant liver failure
- Release of copper causes Coombs'-negative intravascular hemolysis
- Rapidly progressive renal failure
- Coagulopathy unresponsive to vitamin K
- May show stigmata of advanced liver disease with markedly decreased serum albumin cholesterol, prolonged INR
- These patients require liver transplantation

Caveat

- Screen patients under age 40 with signs of chronic liver disease for Wilson disease.

Treatment: Lifelong therapy required

- Penicillamine—monitor urine copper excretion
- Trientine for patients unable to tolerate penicillamine
- Zinc has also been used for maintenance therapy

Table 76.14 KEY FEATURES OF NONALCOHOLIC FATTY LIVER DISEASE (NAFLD)

NAFLD spectrum includes steatosis, steatohepatitis, fibrosis, cirrhosis

75–80% of patients with "cryptogenic cirrhosis"

Patients with metabolic syndrome have a 75% likelihood of having steatohepatitis

Metabolic syndrome

- D = Dyslipidemia
- R = Insulin resistance
- O = Obesity
- P = Elevated blood pressure

Laboratory clues to Dx of NAFLD

- ↑ALT serum ALT/AST ratio >2:1 (opposite of alcoholic liver disease)

Treatment

- Weight loss
- Rx diabetes
- Rx hypercholesterolemia

Table 76.15 KEY FEATURES OF ALCOHOLIC LIVER DISEASE

Spectrum

- Asymptomatic (with abnormal liver tests) to steatohepatitis, severe alcoholic hepatitis, cirrhosis, liver failure

Peripheral manifestations

- Spider angiomata, palmar erythema, gynecomastia, parotid enlargement, Dupuytren's contractures, paucity axillary and pubic hair, testicular atrophy
- Triad of parotid enlargement, gynecomastia, and Dupuytren sign indicative of chronic alcohol use
- Decompensated cirrhosis
  - Jaundice
  - Ascites
  - Encephalopathy
  - Bleeding varices (can make a Dx of portal hypertension with triad of splenomegaly, ascites, ↑ venous collateral abdominal wall)

Can make a Dx of cirrhosis with two physical findings and two laboratory findings

- Ascites and asterixis
- Serum albumin <2.8 g/dL, INR >1.6

Laboratory abnormalities in alcoholic liver disease

- ↑AST
- ↑ALT : ALT ratio >3:1
- ↑MCV
- ↑GGTP

Treatment

- Prednisone and pentoxifylline may be transiently effective

It is characterized by a variable constellation of symptoms, which may include feeling unwell, hepatomegaly, ascites, and modest elevation of LFTs. Alcoholic hepatitis can vary from mild with only liver enzyme elevation to severe liver inflammation. Patients who are severely affected present with subacute onset of fever, hepatomegaly, leukocytosis, marked impairment of liver function (e.g., jaundice, coagulopathy), and manifestations of portal hypertension (e.g., ascites, hepatic encephalopathy, variceal hemorrhage). However, milder forms of alcoholic hepatitis often do not cause any symptoms. On histopathology, the liver exhibits characteristic centrilobular ballooning necrosis of hepatocytes, neutrophilic infiltration, megamitochondria, and Mallory hyaline inclusions. Steatosis (fatty liver) and cirrhosis frequently accompany alcoholic hepatitis. Key features are shown in table 76.15.

ADDITIONAL READING

Dienes HP, Drebber U. Pathology of immune-mediated liver injury. *Dig Dis.* 2010;28(1):57–62.

Hirschfield GM, Heathcote EJ, Gershwin ME. Pathogenesis of cholestatic liver disease and therapeutic approaches. *Gastroenterology.* 2010;139(5):1481–96.

Hu CJ, Zhang FC, Li YZ, Zhang X. Primary biliary cirrhosis: What do autoantibodies tell us? *World J Gastroenterol.* 2010;16(29): 3616–29.

Kaplan MM. Toward better treatment of primary sclerosing cholangitis. *N Engl J Med.* 1997;336(10):719–21.

Kaplan MM, Gershwin ME. Primary biliary cirrhosis. *N Engl J Med.* 2005;353(12):1261–73. Erratum *N Engl J Med.* 2006;354(3): 313.

Karlsen TH, Schrumpf E, Boberg KM. Update on primary sclerosing cholangitis. *Dig Liver Dis.* 2010;42(6):390–400.

Krawitt EL. Autoimmune hepatitis. *N Engl J Med.* 2006;354(1): 54–66.

Lamers MM, van Oijen MG, Pronk M, Drenth JP. Treatment options for autoimmune hepatitis: A systematic review of randomized controlled trials. *J Hepatol.* 2010;53(1):191–8.

Lee YM, Kaplan MM. Primary sclerosing cholangitis. *N Engl J Med.* 1995;332(14):924–33.

Lindor K. Ursodeoxycholic acid for the treatment of primary biliary cirrhosis. *N Engl J Med.* 2007;357(15):1524–9.

Powell LW. Overview: Liver disease and transplantation. *J Gastroenterol Hepatol.* 2009;24 Suppl 3:S97–S104.

Sinakos E, Lindor K. Treatment options for primary sclerosing cholangitis. *Expert Rev Gastroenterol Hepatol.* 2010;4(4): 473–88.

Spinzi G, Terruzzi V, Minoli G. Liver biopsy. *N Engl J Med.* 2001; 344(26):2030.

Strassburg CP. Therapeutic options to treat autoimmune hepatitis in 2009. *Dig Dis.* 2010;28(1):93–8.

SECTION 8

CARDIOVASCULAR DISEASE

77.

THE CARDIAC EXAM

Kenneth Lee Baughman

In this era of high technology and expensive testing, there is nothing more important than a good history and physical examination in the process of medical care. A focused cardiac history allows the clinician to establish a differential diagnosis. The physical examination is utilized not only as an overall assessment of the cardiovascular system but more specifically to pursue those diagnoses in the historical differential that can be confirmed or refuted by the physical findings. Critical physical examination findings are rarely uncovered unless the clinician is specifically probing for given physical examination characteristics and knows what would be expected in the face of disease. Only by applying skilled history and physical examination techniques can the clinician determine the rank order of the differential diagnosis and order those tests most likely to answer the question with the least inconvenience, pain, and cost to the patient.

GENERAL

The patient's general appearance is often overlooked. This can include the degree of discomfort the patient appears to be in, respiratory rate and labored breathing, and key physical examination findings that may direct more specific investigations. This might include dramatic jugular venous distension while in the seated position, suggesting a high right atrial pressure due to restrictive heart disease or constrictive pericarditis. It might also include a head bob or body titubations associated with severe aortic regurgitation. Patients with endocrinopathies often display characteristic facial and body habitus changes as seen in thyroid-related myxedema or adrenal gland dysfunctions and related Cushing syndrome. Similarly, patients with Marfan syndrome or Ehlers-Danlos syndrome have a typical morphologic appearance allowing recognition well before detailed examination begins. Finally, end-stage heart disease with overall cachexia colors not only the assessment of the nature of the heart disease and its severity but the prognosis for the patient.

Although this chapter concentrates on the cardiac examination, many clues to the cardiac diagnosis come from examination of other organs. In fact, by the time the skilled clinician listens to the heart, the probable heart disease diagnosis has already been established. We therefore begin our examination evaluating other organ systems that may give a clue to the cardiovascular diagnosis.

EYE EXAMINATION

Frequently findings in the eye suggest elevated cholesterol and other lipoproteins including xanthelasma, xanthoma, and arcus senilis. Xanthelasmas are yellow to orange plaques on the eyelids or medial canthus. Xanthomas are nodules or deposition of lipid-laden histiocytes, which may be evident around the eyes. Arcus senilis, or arcus cornealis, is a yellow-gray ring found in the outer periphery of the cornea. This is usually due to a deposit of fatty granules in the cornea. Other band keratopathies may be due to deposits such as copper in Wilson disease. Patients with sarcoidosis or other inflammatory conditions may have secondary iritis. Excessively blue sclera may be a clue to osteogenesis imperfecta or connective tissue disorders such as lupus erythematosus. Suffusion (beety redness and congestion) of the eyelids may be seen in individuals with excessively elevated hemoglobin levels. Proptosis (or exophthalmos) is a protrusion of one or both eyes. Although this may be familial or congenital and occasionally due to retro-orbital tumors, it is more typical bilaterally in thyroid disease (usually Graves disease). Ptosis of the lids is occasionally a feature of Kearns-Sayre syndrome, which is associated with muscular dystrophy.

Funduscopic examination of the eyes is also of benefit and is often overlooked despite the availability of ophthalmoscopes in most examination rooms. Funduscopic examination may reveal papilledema or bulging of the optic nerve compatible with elevated intracranial pressures and occasionally malignant hypertension. More frequent would be chronic changes of hypertension including atrioventricular (AV) nicking, and more severe forms of arterial hypertension include hemorrhage and exudates. Findings of neovascularization may be an indication of microvascular complications of diabetes. A Roth spot is a rounded white retinal spot with surrounding hemorrhage seen in bacterial endocarditis or hemorrhagic conditions. Hollenhorst plaques are atheromatous emboli that appear in the retinal arterioles and usually originate from the carotid arteries or great vessels. Each of the findings noted above may trigger more intensive investigation of suspected etiologies responsible for these physical characteristics.

ORAL CAVITY

The mouth should be examined in general to determine the size of the oropharynx and the degree of obstruction of the passageway by the tongue. Relatively narrow passageways, particularly in patients who are obese or have short squat necks, should trigger an assessment of obstructive sleep apnea. The high arched palate of an individual with Marfan syndrome can help confirm that diagnosis. The tongue and lips should be examined for central cyanosis, an indication of arteriovenous mixing in the heart, as opposed to peripheral cyanosis due to low cardiac output and/or central mixing. The tongue should be examined to ensure that it is not excessively large with dental indentations compatible with amyloidosis, or smooth related to iron deficiency anemia. Gingival decay is often an indicator of coronary artery disease and/or bacterial infection including endocarditis. The lips may also indicate capillary hemangiomas compatible with Osler-Weber-Rendu syndrome.

GENERAL SKIN EXAMINATION

The skin may be bronzed, particularly in non-sun-exposed areas, in individuals with hemochromatosis. Patients with amyloidosis display capillary fragility of the skin and will have "pinch purpura." In addition, individuals with amyloidosis who have had their heads in a dependent position (initially described after proctoscopy) may have periorbital purpura due to spontaneous capillary hemorrhage. Extensor tendons should be evaluated for tuberous xanthoma. These are often found in the extensor tendons in individuals with excess lipoproteins. The Achilles tendon is particularly advantageous as an area to examine, as are the extensor tendons on the hand. Tuberous xanthoma may also appear as lipid-laden plaques on any skin surface but particularly over the elbows. Patients with hyperthyroid myxedema have a doughy consistency to their skin and a unique lower extremity edema which is partially pitting but poorly responsive to diuresis. Patients with growth hormone excess-related acromegaly have similar edema as well as a doughy consistency to enlarged hands and feet. Striae are thin bands of skin that are initially red and transition to purple or white over time. These often appear in the abdomen or over the shoulders. These changes appear due to overextension of the skin or with metabolic syndromes such as Cushing. These changes may be seen in individuals who have had excessive weight loss or decrease in muscle mass (as in bodybuilders). Excessive laxity of the skin tissue along with features suggestive of Marfan syndrome may lead to the diagnosis of Ehlers-Danlos syndrome. Patients with scleroderma have virtually wrinkleless faces and tight skin over the digits, often with digital ulceration in the more advanced forms. Cyanosis of the periphery may be due to low cardiac output or right-to-left shunting in the heart. Characteristic findings are also seen in the peripheral embolic phenomenon associated with endocarditis. Osler nodes are tender and painful lesions, usually on the pads of the fingers and toes due to infected microemboli. Janeway lesions are nontender and raised hemorrhages, similarly from peripheral embolic phenomena.

SKELETON AND JOINTS

The general habitus of an individual with a connective tissue syndrome such as Marfan syndrome is characterized by excessive height and excessive arm span-to-height ratio. There is general hypermobility of joints, particularly fingers and elbows. Patients often have a straightened back and high arched palate. Less dramatic findings may be associated with myxomatous degeneration of the mitral valve (mitral valve prolapse) in the absence of a specific genetic abnormality of fibrillin. Patients who have suffered from rickets have bowed tibias, and those with Paget disease may have similar deformities and skeletal warmth due to excessive metabolic activity in the skeletal region affected. Findings of rheumatoid arthritis in the hands may signal the investigator to evaluate the patient for pericardial disease or accelerated atherosclerotic disease, as found in many individuals with long-standing inflammatory states. Inflammatory irritation of many joints (polyarticular) may be found in gout, pseudogout, or other inflammatory conditions such as sarcoidosis. Clubbing of the digits is expected in individuals with cyanotic congenital heart disease, advanced chronic obstructive pulmonary disease, or severe hepatic disease. This requires three features including loss of the unguophalangeal angle, appearance of a clubbed digit when viewed from above, and a soft spongy cuticle area compatible with increased capillary flow and activity.

THYROID GLAND

The thyroid gland should not be ignored. This can be examined with the ends of the examiner's digits addressing the thyroid from the front or with both hands from the back.

The examination is enhanced by having the patient swallow while the thyroid is examined, as some portions of the thyroid may fall below the clavicular margin at rest. General enlargement may be seen in inflammatory states including thyroiditis or Graves disease, and focal nodules may signal the potential for hyperactivity, hypoactivity, or thyroid malignancy.

JUGULAR VENOUS PRESSURE

The jugular venous pressure (JVP) can be accurately assessed by physical examination and clearly defines the right atrial pressure. The internal jugular vein is best utilized to assess the "phasic" character of the right atrial pressure as there are no valves between the right atrium and the right internal jugular vein. The external jugular vein, found lateral to the internal jugular vein, is a better measure of the mean right atrial pressure, as there are usually valves that dampen the phasic pressure. One must ensure that venous valves or other mechanical obstructions in the external jugular vein are not prohibiting an accurate assessment of the external jugular system. This is often the case in individuals who have indwelling cardiac fibrillators (ICD) or pacemakers on the side of the neck being examined. The internal jugular vein is located just to the lateral margin of the lateral head of the sternocleidomastoid muscle. In patients with markedly elevated JVP this is often missed as the clinician does not elevate the head of the patient's bed to a point where the meniscus of the internal jugular system is seen. One must think of the internal jugular vein as a direct manometer connected to the right atrium. The higher the right atrial pressure, the higher will be the column of blood in the jugular vein. The higher the column of blood in the jugular vein, the higher the patient's head must be elevated for the meniscus to be seen. Once the top of the meniscus is judged, the investigator should measure vertically from this plane to the midchest, the site of the mid right atrium. This distance in centimeters is equivalent to millimeters of mercury, after conversion for blood to mercury density. The assessment of the height of the right atrial pressure is critical in determining the patient's volume status or intrinsic disease of the right side of the heart or pulmonary system. Jugular veins that are mildly elevated may become more prominent with a hepatojugular reflux. In this maneuver the investigator applies gentle and persistent pressure for 15–30 seconds over the right upper quadrant. This compresses the liver and forces blood into the superior vena cava. If the right atrium is already volume overloaded, this excess blood will reflux into the superior vena cava and the JVP will rise. Positive hepatojugular reflux is an indication of borderline elevation of volume in the right side of the heart.

Specific waveforms are seen in the jugular venous tracing (particularly the internal jugular). These will include an A wave, due to right atrial contraction. This is followed by an x descent due to atrial relaxation and to the movement of the floor of the right atrium toward the apex in systole. There may be a C wave, due to a reflection on the venous system of the carotid, which lies adjacent to the vein in the vascular sheath in the neck. Next is the y descent due to tricuspid valve opening and a rapid decline in pressures of the right atrium during rapid ventricular filling. A V wave follows and is associated with a passive filling in the right ventricle and subsequently right atrium.

With inspiration, the JVP falls due to the negative intrathoracic pressure created in the chest. This negative intrathoracic pressure helps draw blood into the heart. If the patient has constrictive or restrictive heart disease, an increase in venous return will result in excessive volume to the right atrium, and the venous pressure will rise. This is termed a Kussmaul's sign and is seen in constrictive pericarditis, restrictive heart disease, or conditions of severe volume overload to the right side of the heart.

A giant A wave in the neck is due to atrial contraction against a stenotic or a closed tricuspid valve. The latter may occur due to ventricular premature contractions. A giant V wave or giant S wave in the neck replaces both the A and V wave and is seen in patients with significant tricuspid regurgitation. Prominent x and y descents are seen in individuals with constrictive heart disease.

The components of the venous pulse are timed by coordination with the carotid artery pulse. The investigator looks at the venous pulse wave form in the right neck while placing a finger gently on the carotid artery of the left neck. Waves that will rise before the carotid upstroke are A waves, waves that arise after the carotid upstroke are small V waves, and single waves that arise in the neck (giant V or S waves) are due to tricuspid regurgitation.

Most of what pulsates in the neck is venous as opposed to arterial. The venous pulsation is in the lateral part of the neck whereas carotid pulsations are quite medial, next to the trachea. One should be particularly astute to evaluate pulsating neck wave forms that "tickle the earlobes" and pulsate in coordination with arterial upstroke. This may be a subtle clue that the venous pressure is markedly elevated and stimulate the clinician to elevate the patient's head until a clear meniscus is seen and measurements are made. Occasionally, venous pulsations are more easily palpated than seen, and this should be correlated with the carotid pulsation, which is often much deeper, more central, and, in these instances, much lower in volume.

CAROTID ARTERY EXAMINATION

Carotid arteries are of importance to the examination as they are the arterial system closest to the heart. As with many physical findings, the investigator creates his or her own "data base" of normal examinations, allowing a more careful assessment of what is abnormal. The carotid arteries should be approached cautiously because some individuals may have carotid sinus sensitivity and examination of the carotids may result in asystole. One should listen to the carotids before touching them to determine whether or not there is evidence of a bruit to indicate carotid artery disease.

Patients with aortic stenosis have typically tardus and parvus carotid pulsations, typically a delay in rate of rise of the carotid and diminished fullness of the carotid pulsation. Patients with aortic stenosis often have thrills that are palpable in the carotid arteries and have transmitted murmurs from the aortic valve into the carotid system. Clearly, atherosclerotic carotid disease can mimic these findings, often a humbling experience to those attempting to discern the severity of an aortic valve problem. Patients with critical aortic stenosis often have an additional finding of an anacrotic shoulder to the upstroke of the carotid artery. On the other hand, patients with aortic regurgitation have bounding carotid arteries with a rapid upstroke and decline often described as "water hammer" or "pistol shot" in character. This may be associated with a patient's head bob or general body pulsation with each cardiac contraction. Patients with hypertrophic subaortic stenosis have a bifid and dynamic upstroke. This is characterized by a rapid rate of rise, a falloff in the upstroke, which is then replaced by a secondary rise. This is presumably due to midflow obstruction in the left ventricular outflow tract during systole.

Most common would be intrinsic carotid artery disease associated with stiff vessels and atherosclerosis. As carotid bruits are often faint, the patient and physician should suspend respiration while listening. One must differentiate a carotid systolic bruit from a venous hum, which is a continuous murmur due to flow through the internal jugular system and return to the thoracic cavity.

LUNG EXAMINATION

Before listening to the lungs, the chest cavity should be examined. Patients with congenital heart disease may have overdevelopment of the left or right chest. Additionally, the rate of respiration and the labor of breathing should be examined visually before listening. In addition, the examiner should always listen to the lungs before the patient takes a deep breath. Some murmurs have transmitted findings that are best heard without the background noise from inspiration. This includes pulmonic stenosis, which radiates from the anterior left sternal border to the left scapula posteriorly. Mitral regurgitation may radiate to the spine or to the top of the head. AV communication may also be heard in the lateral parts of the lungs compatible with congenital or acquired malformations. Coarctation of the aorta may also be heard in the area over the left chest, compatible with the area of narrowing. In addition to the features noted above, patients should be examined for evidence of chronic obstructive pulmonary disease as manifested by an increased chest diameter

and diminished diaphragm movement. Patients with connective tissue abnormalities may display pectus excavatum or pectus carinatum of the breast bone. This gives a caved-in or bird-like chest appearance, respectively. Once the lungs have been inspected and listened to for the above-noted abnormalities, percussion of the lung cavities should occur. This allows the investigator to determine whether or not there is an elevation of one or both of the diaphragms and whether or not they move normally with inspiration. This may indicate the presence of a pleural effusion, chronic airway disease, or diaphragm paralysis.

The typical cardiac findings in the lungs that are associated with congestive heart failure include rales. Rales reflect excess fluid in the lymphatic and alveolar system. Fine rales may be heard in individuals with interstitial lung disease, which can also be confused with congestive heart failure. Excessive fluid accumulation may result in peribronchial cuffing. This may be associated with audible wheezing due to airflow turbulence from edema of the medium-sized alveolar passageways. Pleural effusions are characterized by diminished or absent breath sounds associated with egophony. Egophony is a change in the quality of a whispered or spoken sound at the upper level of fluid accumulation in the lungs.

ABDOMINAL EXAMINATION

The abdomen should be inspected to determine whether or not there is ascites. This is evident by often tense distension of the abdominal cavity and a pear-shaped appearance. If there is less tense ascites, the investigator may be able to percuss the abdomen supine and laterally to assess the presence of "shifting dullness." The shifting dullness is the change in location of the fluid wave due to shifts either supine or left or right lateral decubitus position. The liver and spleen should be palpated. In the case of each of these organs, the investigator should begin the palpation low in the abdomen so as not to underestimate the size of the organ enlargement. One proceeds from the pelvic brim superiorly until a liver edge or spleen tip is felt. The liver or spleen is then percussed over the length of their dullness to determine the size of each organ. Occasionally, the spleen cannot be felt without deep inspiration. In more subtle instances of splenomegaly the investigator may percuss over the left lateral rib cage while the patient takes a deep breath. The change from clear to dullness indicates a spleen beneath the percussion site and can be used to determine the size of the organ. The liver should also be examined for pulsation. This is sometimes difficult to differentiate from chest wall movement in the case of active cardiac motion. Nonetheless, the investigator can place fingers on both sides of the liver edge and determine whether or not they are expanding. More frequently, however, the heel of the hand is placed against the presumed liver edge or thoracic cavity edge, and one determines a "push back" compatible with regurgitation. Pulsation of the liver is often seen in patients with severe tricuspid regurgitation. Patients with persistently elevated JVP and small livers must be evaluated for cardiac cirrhosis. The liver may also be a site for AV communication, and careful auscultation over the liver for continuous murmurs should be performed. The venous pattern over the abdomen or thorax should be assessed. Prominent veins may indicate obstruction of a more central venous conduit, often by tumor infringement.

PERIPHERAL ARTERIAL EXAMINATION

Every patient should be examined for the presence and quality of the carotid, brachial, radial, ulnar, femoral, popliteal, dorsal pedis, and posterior tibial arteries. The blood pressure should be assessed in both arms, and the femoral arteries should be auscultated for bruits. Palpation of the pulses demonstrates two distinct waves in most individuals. The first is a *percussion* wave compatible with blood flow through the artery, and the second a *tidal* wave. The tidal wave is formulated by a backflow of blood from the arterial column, usually associated with variations in peripheral resistance and more prominent in the elderly patients. The presence of pulse in each of the above-noted sites should be documented as well as its quality. Diminution or absence of pulses is usually associated with intrinsic disease of the arteries. This is most manifest in the lower extremities. If the pulse is not adequately felt, capillary refill should be assessed in the digits by compressing the nail bed and determining the rate of refill. Other evidence for peripheral arterial insufficiency should be looked for including loss of hair in the legs and ulcerations. These are particularly common in individuals with diabetes, who may have peripheral disease combined with peripheral neuropathy.

Pulse deficits may be found in coarctation or aortic dissections. Individuals with aortic coarctation have diminished lower extremity pulses and a dramatically increased brachial femoral arterial delay. Patients with significant aortic regurgitation have both Quincke's pulse and Duroziez's sign. Quincke's pulse is characteristic winking of the nail bed in the upper extremities. This is assessed by applying gentle pressure to the nail bed with the examiners finger milking approximately one-third of the color from the nail bed. A positive Quincke is characterized by a systolic blinking of the nail bed compatible with arterial expansion in systole. This is seen in individuals with wide pulse pressures, often aortic regurgitation, but also in sepsis, anemia, and hyperthyroidism. Duroziez's sign is assessed in the femoral arteries. The investigator places the diaphragm of the stethoscope over the femoral artery. Compression of the arterial pulse above the stethoscope will result in a systolic bruit. The investigator should compress the femoral artery until flow is virtually absent and then release pressure to establish a clear-cut systolic bruit. Individuals with aortic regurgitation will have not only a systolic bruit but a diastolic flow murmur as well. This excessive "to and fro" movement of the blood column is compatible with those conditions noted above, particularly aortic reflux.

Pulsus paradoxus should be assessed in individuals being considered for the diagnosis of pericardial tamponade. With normal inspiration there is an increase of flow of blood to the right heart and return of blood to the pulmonary circuit from the left atrium. This results in a right-to-left ventricular septal shift and removal of blood from the left atrium, respectively. These maneuvers decrease the amount of blood in the left ventricle, and therefore, with inspiration, the blood pressure may fall by up to 10–12 mm Hg. Excessive falls (>12 mm Hg) are seen in patients with pericardial tamponade as well as patients with severe chronic obstructive pulmonary disease or asthma (which would present with different physical examination features than those with pericardial disease). Evaluation of the pulsus paradoxus is difficult and done correctly by few clinicians. The clinician elevates the blood pressure cuff to above the level of the patient's systolic blood pressure. The cuff is then deflated exceedingly slowly. The operator determines the difference in systolic pressure from hearing an occasional systolic beat to every systolic beat. Only if the cuff is deflated slowly will this differentiation be evident. This is impossible to assess in individuals with irregular pulses such as atrial fibrillation or frequent ventricular premature contractions. Individuals with very marked pulsus paradoxus will have this evident by palpation of the major arteries, particularly the femoral and occasionally the brachial arteries.

Pulsus alternans is the appearance of a pulse with every other heart contraction. This finding is probably due to altered intracellular calcium handling in the myocardium. Therefore, every other heart contraction has enough contractility to manifest a peripheral pulsation. This is usually found in individuals with severe cardiomyopathy. It may be seen more rarely in individuals with a *swinging heart* in the face of massive pericardial effusion.

HEART INSPECTION

Before the heart is listened to, it must be inspected. The operator must evaluate both right and left ventricular activity and size. The patient's heart should in general be the same size as his or her fist. Therefore, the expected point of maximal impulse can be assessed by having the patient lay a clenched fist on his or her sternum. The tip of the lateral fist would indicate the expected point of maximal impulse. This can be assessed by inspection and/or by percussion to confirm the size of the heart.

The patient should be evaluated for right ventricular overload. This is best done by inspection of the lower sternum from the end of the bed or to the right of the patient, at the patient's body level. Excessive motion of the peristernal region is compatible with right ventricular overload unless the patient is thin with a small and vertically aligned heart, in which case this may be the left ventricular apex. The left ventricle should also be inspected. One must not underestimate the size of the left ventricle. Therefore, the clinician gazes laterally across the chest but extends the inspection to the midclavicular and midaxial region to ensure that the point of maximal impulse is not "over the horizon" of the chest wall.

The investigator should then palpate each ventricle. The right ventricle should be assessed by placing the palm of the right hand on the sternum while gently pressing the top of that hand with the left hand. A pushback is felt in the presence of right ventricular heaves. Occasionally, with less intense pressure one can feel extra components to this pushback, which usually represent palpable gallops. The left ventricular point of maximal impulse is assessed using the fingertips. The flattened right hand is extended to beyond the estimated point at which the maximal impulse is located. The fingers are then dragged back to the point of maximal impulse (PMI) to ensure that this is the site of maximal contraction.

The point of the left ventricular maximum impulse should be assessed. Patients with thick hearts including hypertrophic cardiomyopathy, aortic stenosis, or long-standing hypertension will have forceful contraction of the left ventricle. Patients with volume overload conditions, such as aortic and mitral regurgitation, will have a very active and often displaced point of maximal impulse. The activity of the PMI differentiates the volume overload conditions from cardiomyopathy, where the point of maximal impulse may be displaced but is inactive. If the point of maximal impulse is not easily felt, the patient should be rolled into the left lateral decubitus position, and the point of maximal impulse appreciated. Although this does not allow evaluation of the size of the heart, it does provide some indication of ventricular enlargement.

Occasionally in cases of severe mitral regurgitation there will be a left atrial heave. This is found superior to the right ventricular heave in systole. It is assessed by placing the heel of the hand on the high sternum and assessing the pushback. The heart should also be felt for thrills. Patients with aortic stenosis often have a thrill when over a 50 mm Hg gradient exists in the outflow tract. This would be present in the aortic region at the left sternal border.

Most underappreciated are palpable and audible gallops from the left ventricle. Fingertips on the point of maximal impulse should be able to trace the additional rise (S4) or fall (S3) of the gallop rhythm. If this is not appreciated visually, one can place a tongue blade or cotton swab over the PMI and visualize these extra movements of the point of maximal impulse signifying gallop rhythms. Once one has "timing" of the gallop, the fingers and ears are more apt to appreciate it. Recall that the gallops are pressure against the tympanic membrane and are not sounds such as S1 or S2.

Occasionally a double impulse at the point of maximal impulse will be seen in individuals who have aneurysms of the heart.

AUSCULTATION OF THE HEART

As noted in our general advice to the clinician, one rarely finds something on the examination that one does not to listen for. Therefore, if you suspect mitral stenosis you listen more closely to the intensity of the first heart sound and the interval sound between S2 and an opening snap or a diastolic rumble. If one is naive in the art of physical examination or is unclear as to what the patient might have, it is best to approach auscultation in a systematic fashion. This forces the clinician to listen to each component of the heart and determine whether or not it is abnormal and then to piece together the abnormalities into a picture compatible with a disease state.

One must listen for specific findings in certain locations. The aortic valve will be heard at the upper left sternal border. It is in fact best heard in the seated position. The pulmonic valve will be just to the left of the aortic valve and will usually be much less intense. The tricuspid valve sounds are always heard at the lower left sternal border. Mitral sounds are generally located at the apex but are transmitted widely across the precordium and back depending on the condition. In describing a murmur one must determine whether or not it is in systole or diastole, then what is the location (aortic, mitral, pulmonic, or tricuspid), and where does the murmur radiate.

The first heart sound is made of two components, the closure of the mitral and then the tricuspid valve. In some individuals where there is a delay in the closure, there may be two components of S1 heard. Tricuspid valve closures are usually soft and indistinct. The second heart sound is also due to closure of left- and right-sided valves, specifically the aortic and pulmonic valves. The sounds of closure of the aortic valve are usually twice that of the pulmonic valve because of the difference in diastolic pressure forcing the valves shut. Ejection clicks occur after the first heart sound and are usually related to the ejection of blood through a diseased valve or into an enlarged arterial circuit. This may be due to aortic or pulmonic valve or root disease. Mid- or late systolic clicks are also "sounds" that are typically heard in individuals with myxomatous degeneration of their mitral valves. This is due to the "wind in the sail"–like effect as the redundant valve balloons backward in systole. Third heart sounds are occasionally not gallops but are due to intra- or extracardiac noises. These may include

1. a pericardial knock as the heart expands in diastole and strikes the thickened pericardial surface.

2. a tumor plop may also occur in this time frame due to an atrial myxoma or clot dropping into the mitral apparatus in diastole.

An S3 gallop is created by rapid inflow into the left ventricle through the mitral valve. This may be physiologic in individuals with a great deal of blood flow (young and athletic) or in patients who have diminished blood flow and exceedingly weakened heart muscles (dilated cardiomyopathy). These "sounds" are pressures against your tympanic membrane or your fingertips and are not sounds like an S2 or an ejection click. An S4 gallop occurs just before S1 and is due to the rapid influx of blood with atrial systole into the left ventricle. This is usually seen in individuals with left ventricular hypertrophy of any etiology. Specific findings of note with cardiac sounds include the fixed splitting of an S2. This may occur with an atrial septal defect or patent foramen ovale. It is secondary to the lack of any change in the amount of blood being ejected from the left and right ventricles during systole with respiration, as there is equal filling of the ventricles in diastole with this condition. Wide splitting of the second heart sound may be seen in people with right bundle branch block, delayed emptying of the right ventricle due to right ventricular disease, or high pulmonary artery pressures. In normal inspiration the aortic and pulmonic closure sounds of S2 widen. This is caused by increased filling of the right ventricle and decreased filling of the left ventricle with inspiration. If there is a left bundle branch block, disease of the left ventricle, or increased pressure in the aorta, there may be paradoxical splitting of the second heart sound. In this instance the aortic valve and pulmonic valve increase in splitting does not occur, and there may be reverse splitting.

Increased intensity of the first heart sound is usually seen in conditions where the mitral valve remains open longer into diastole before systolic contraction forces it shut. If there is adequate contractility to the left ventricle, the valve will be shut briskly, like slamming a door. This is seen in mitral stenosis when the valve is still mobile and the high left atrial pressure keeps the valve open longer until systole forces it shut. The second heart sounds may also reflect changes in pressure. A very loud aortic component is often due to hypertension. A loud pulmonic closure sound usually reflects pulmonary hypertension and is often a key to determining this diagnosis.

SPECIFIC VALVULAR CONDITIONS

AORTIC STENOSIS

Aortic stenosis is characterized by a thickening of the aortic valve. This may be due to bicuspid aortic valve disease, but increasingly it is due to wear and tear in the tricuspid aortic valve in elderly patients. As our population ages, the number of people with systolic murmurs will increase. It is critical that the investigator be able to distinguish aortic sclerosis, due to age-related thickening of the aortic valve, from aortic stenosis. Although aortic sclerosis is usually benign, it may

result in aortic stenosis, and the transition may often be subtle. Signs of significant aortic stenosis include a delay in the peak of the systolic murmur, associated with an increased delay in the carotid upstroke. The later in systole the valve peaks, the more severe is the gradient across the valve. As the valve thickens, the aortic ejection click is often lost, and the aortic component of the S2 becomes less marked. While the murmur becomes progressively louder as the conditions worsens, once the ventricle begins to fail, the velocity of flow through the valve will diminish, and the murmur will become less evident. This will not, however, change the timing. Significant aortic stenosis should also be associated with a forceful point of maximal impulse and S4 gallop.

AORTIC REGURGITATION

Aortic regurgitation may be due to valvular heart disease (bileaflet disease, endocarditis) or aortic root disease as in Marfan syndrome or atherosclerotic dilation. The murmur of aortic reflux that remains close to the sternum is called a Proctor Harvey sign. This is usually indicative of aortic root disease. The murmur radiating to the apex is usually more compatible with valvular heart disease. These are not pure. With mild aortic regurgitation there is a sustained pressure difference across the aortic valve through diastole. Therefore, the murmur may be loud and prolonged. In severe aortic regurgitation, however, the aortic contents reflux into the left ventricle more rapidly. Therefore, the murmur may not be heard throughout all of diastole. In severe cases where the diastolic pressure in the aorta and the diastolic pressure in the ventricle are nearly the same (such as acute dissection), there may be no murmur. Patients with severe aortic reflux have peripheral findings including pistol-shot pulses, bounding carotids, and Quincke and Duroziez signs. Significant aortic regurgitation would be associated with a dynamic point of maximal impulse and a rapid diastole filling phase associated with an S3 gallop. Aortic regurgitation will often direct a jet against the anterior leaflet of the mitral valve. This may result in a diastolic "rumble," which can be confused with mitral stenosis.

MITRAL REGURGITATION

Mitral regurgitation has classically been thought of as a rheumatic process with a holosystolic murmur at the apex. In this condition the gradient of pressure between the left ventricle and left atrium is persistent throughout all of systole, resulting in the holosystolic nature of the murmur. Increasingly, however, mitral valve disease is not due to rheumatic heart disease but due to myxomatous degeneration. Myxomatous degeneration may often result in ruptured chordae tendineae or distinct prolapse of an anterior or posterior leaflet segment. Therefore, the pressure gradient is often not maintained through systole due to the amount of blood being regurgitated, and the radiation of the murmur is related to the direction of the blood flow jet. In patients with posterior mitral leaflet disorders, the posterior mitral leaflet is not able to close or coapt with the anterior leaflet, and the jet of blood will be ejected anteriorly. Therefore, posterior leaflet rupture would sound like a murmur radiating to the outflow tract and often is confused with aortic stenosis. Alternatively, an anterior leaflet defect would not be able to coapt with a posterior leaflet, and the blood would be directed posteriorly. This would be directed to the left atrium, which is adjacent to the spine. Therefore, the murmur would radiate up and down the spine and occasionally to the top of the head. Involvement of both leaflets will result in radiation of the murmurs in both directions. Significant mitral regurgitation is associated with volume overload of the left ventricle and an active point of maximal impulse often with filling gallops.

TRICUSPID REGURGITATION

Tricuspid regurgitation is often secondary to right ventricular volume and pressure overload and annular dilatation. This may be a reflection of chronic obstructive pulmonary disease or primary pulmonary hypertension but is usually caused by left-sided congestive heart failure. Tricuspid regurgitation is heard exclusively at the lower left sternal border. It does not radiate to any other site and is often subtle. In fact, the findings of a pulsatile jugular vein or pulsatile liver are much more sensitive and specific for tricuspid regurgitation than the murmur itself. With normal inspiratory volume shifts, a tricuspid regurgitant murmur may increase its intensity with inspiration. One must be careful to not have the patient take too deep a breath, which would separate your stethoscope from the patient's valve.

TRICUSPID STENOSIS

Occasionally because of an inflammatory condition such as carcinoid, the tricuspid valve can become regurgitant and stenotic. In the case of tricuspid stenosis, there is a soft diastolic murmur in the left sternal border location. This is usually thought to be present because of the JVP findings of a giant "A" wave.

PULMONIC STENOSIS AND REGURGITATION

Occasionally congenital heart disease will result in pulmonic stenosis or regurgitation and acquired diseases such as carcinoid may also affect the pulmonary valve as may endocarditis. Pulmonic stenosis is a systolic murmur, usually softer than aortic stenosis, which radiates from the left sternal border lateral to the aortic valve to the scapula. Pulmonic regurgitation may be found in any condition with pulmonary hypertension or pulmonary valve disease and is in a similar location, subtle, and in early diastole.

CONTINUOUS MURMURS

Continuous murmurs may be heard in any form of AV communication. The examiner is best advised to sharpen his or her auscultatory skills to appreciate the continuous murmur by listening over an AV fistula utilized for renal dialysis. Continuous murmurs are found when there is communication between the arterial and venous system. This might be in the presence of a patent ductus arteriosis, a coronary artery rupture into the heart, or other congenital conditions. Continuous murmurs may be heard associated with a venous hum and less frequently over peripheral or hepatic AV communications. A continuous murmur must be differentiated from the systolic and diastolic murmur that might combine the findings of aortic stenosis and regurgitation or pulmonic stenosis and regurgitation. These are distinct systolic and diastolic murmurs.

MITRAL STENOSIS

Mitral stenosis is found almost exclusively with rheumatic heart disease but is occasionally heard in patients with congenital heart disease. The typical sounds in mitral stenosis are an increased first heart sound, an increasingly loud pulmonic closure sound of S2, a shortened S2 opening snap interval, and a diastolic rumble persisting throughout the length of diastole, occasionally with presystolic accentuation. More significant mitral stenosis causes pulmonary hypertension as demonstrated by an increased pulmonic closure sound and evidence of right ventricular volume and pressure overload. In pure mitral stenosis the left ventricle is protected and therefore not enlarged. The S2 opening snap interval can be used to determine the height of the left atrial pressure. The higher the left atrial pressure, the more quickly the pressure will open the mitral valve in diastole, and therefore the S2 opening snap interval will shorten. A rumble is heard virtually exclusively at the apex and often requires exercise or auscultation in the left lateral decubitus position to identify it.

OTHER CONGENITAL HEART DISEASE MURMURS

ATRIAL SEPTAL DEFECT

Atrial septal defect findings are often subtle and are best characterized by fixed splitting of the second heart sound. There may be a flow murmur associated with diastolic flow through the tricuspid valve caused by left-to-right shunting. There may also be a systolic ejection murmur due to increased flow through the pulmonary outflow tract. There is no murmur generated from the defect itself.

VENTRICULAR SEPTAL DEFECT

The ventricular septal defect results in a nonholosystolic murmur at the left sternal border that usually does not radiate broadly. In cases where this is due to a muscular defect, the murmur can virtually disappear with Valsalva.

INNOCENT MURMUR

The clinician will spend a lifetime determining whether or not outflow murmurs are due to pathologic valvular heart disease or are innocent. Individuals with high flow through any valve can create enough turbulence to cause a murmur. This may be seen in individuals who are highly trained athletes or patients who are pregnant and have increased flow. Virtually all pregnant women will have aortic and/or pulmonic flow murmurs. The innocent murmur tends to be located near the sternum, is "vibratory," does not radiate, and is not associated with any other findings to suggest organic heart disease.

SIGNIFICANCE OF MURMURS

In determining the significance of a murmur one must determine if it is in systole or diastole. One must also determine its location and whether or not it is reflective of aortic, pulmonic, mitral, or tricuspid disease. Similarly, the radiation of the murmur and its duration will provide clues to whether or not it is innocent or due to organic heart disease.

The loudness of the murmur is also of interest but does not always correlate with the severity of the valvular problem. The murmur loudness has been traditionally determined on a scale of 1 to 6. Grade 1 is barely audible, grade 2 readily audible, grade 3 prominent but not loud, grade 4 loud but without a thrill, grade 5 very loud, and grade 6 can be heard without a stethoscope. Each murmur should be judged by its loudness. There is often a discrepancy between the loudness of the murmur and the severity of the problem, however. The patient with critical aortic stenosis and a poor ventricle may have a soft murmur but have both valvular and muscular problems. A patient with wide open aortic reflux and high left ventricle end-diastolic pressure may have no murmur or a soft murmur of aortic reflux but obviously a severe problem with valvular heart disease.

OTHER SOUNDS

PERICARDIAL RUB

Occasionally patients may present with chest pain and have a pericardial rub. A rub is generated by the epicardial and pericardial surfaces coming in contact during parts of the cardiac cycle. Traditionally the pericardial rub has three components. These are associated with blood movement in the left ventricle and include a systolic component during contraction, an early diastolic component in ventricular filling, and a late diastolic component with atrial filling. It is unusual for all three components to be heard. Before an investigator can abandon the diagnosis of pericardial disease, he or she should listen with the patient in the supine, left lateral decubitus, and sitting leaning forward positions. The positional nature of these sounds and the patient's complaints of pain usually help differentiate this diagnosis from others associated with valvular or myocardial disease.

MANEUVERS

Occasionally maneuvers are performed to enhance or differentiate murmurs. For instance, the best way to hear a murmur of aortic reflux is to have the patient lean forward, grip hands to increase outflow resistance, take a deep breath in, and then exhale. While the patient is holding his or her breath in expiration, you listen carefully for the aorta reflux. This allows the aorta to swing forward to the chest wall, increases afterload, and diminishes respiratory related interference with auscultation. This maneuver should also be done in any individual with a prosthetic heart valve to rule out aortic reflux or early valve degeneration if bioprosthetic.

Elevating the patient's legs increases preload or filling of the left ventricle. This may enhance murmurs on the right side of the heart and diminish murmurs such as hypertrophic cardiomyopathy on the left.

Inspirations (natural and not forced) may increase flow to the right side and enhance a murmur of tricuspid regurgitation or stenosis.

Exercise, such as sit-ups, is occasionally used to increase blood flow to enhance murmurs, particularly in mitral stenosis.

Squatting is occasionally utilized, particularly in congenital heart disease. Squatting is, however, a complex maneuver that simultaneously diminishes preload due to venous obstruction, increases afterload due to squatting, and is often complicated by an unusual position make auscultation difficult. Therefore, I tend not to perform the squat maneuver.

Valsalva can be performed to enhance under filling of the left heart and murmur of the idiopathic hypertrophic subaortic stenosis (IHSS). This is best done by placing the examiner's hand on the patient's abdomen. The patient is instructed to push back against the clinician's hand when the hand presses on the belly. While the hand is pressing the abdomen the murmur is auscultated to determine whether or not it is enhanced.

MURMUR OF HYPERTROPHIC CARDIOMYOPATHY

A patient who has a murmur that sounds like aortic stenosis in the aortic region and mitral regurgitation at the apex may have hypertrophic cardiomyopathy (HCM). This patient will have a mixed murmur and typically has a point of maximal impulse that is dynamic, active, forceful, and associated with an S4 gallop. Maneuvers such as the Valsalva maneuver may enhance the murmur. Similarly, these patients, if they are the one-third of those with HCM who have outflow obstruction, may have a bifid aortic pulse. As their hearts degenerate, the dynamic nature of their pulses and in fact the murmur itself may change.

PROSTHETIC HEART VALVES

Increasingly surgeons are using bioprostheses. These are not associated with distinct sounds until the valves degenerate, at which time they may show progressive signs of aortic stenosis or regurgitation. Mechanical valves (Starr Edwards, St. Jude, and Bjork Shilley) do create mechanical sounds when closed and opened. Therefore, dependent on the position in which they are located (aortic, mitral, or pulmonic) there may be an ejection sound into an aortic or pulmonic region or an opening sound in the mitral and tricuspid position. In the mitral and tricuspid position the S2 opening sound intervals can be used to judge the height of the atrial pressure. Each prosthetic valve, bioprosthetic or mechanical, will have a sewing ring. The sewing ring does create turbulence in the inflow or outflow area. Depending on the size of the prostheses (smaller are louder), there will be a systolic or diastolic flow murmur. This is most marked in the aortic position. Valves must be evaluated regularly to ensure that the closure and opening sounds remain crisp and clear. Evidence of excessive endothelial ingrowth into the mechanical prosthesis will result in diminished opening and closing sounds.

BLOOD PRESSURE

Assessing the blood pressure is a critical part of every cardiac physical examination. Specific guidelines have been addressed by the American Heart Association and should be followed. The patient should be seated comfortably, and the arm should be at the level of the heart. The patient should be quiet and calm before the pressure is taken. The cuff must be appropriate to the size of the patient's arm. The pressure in the cuff is elevated to above systolic pressure and deflated slowly. Phase 1 of the sounds is a tapping in systole. This is usually differentiated as systolic pressure. Phase 2 of the sound is a soft murmur of flow, phase 3 a louder murmur. Phase 4 represents a muffled deterioration of the murmur, and 5 is loss of the sound all together. The loss of the sound is usually termed diastole.

If the patient has difficult auscultation of the pressures due to low output or large arms, the arm can be raised above the head for a few seconds while the cuff is inflated. Then the arm is lowered, and the cuff is deflated as above. Associated with hand grip before auscultation, this may enhance the sounds in systole and diastole.

ADDITIONAL READING

Braunwald E, Lambrew CT, Rockoff SD, et al. Idiopathic hypertrophic subaortic stenosis: 1. A description of the disease based upon an analysis of 64 patients. *Circulation*. 1964;30:3–119.

Campbell M, Suzman SS. Coarctation of the aorta. *Br Heart J*. 1947;9: 185–212.

Chabetai R, Fowler NO, Guntheroth WG. The hemodynamics of cardiac tamponade and constrictive pericarditis. *Am J Cardiol*. 1970;26:480–9

Craige E. Phonocardiography in interventricular septal defects. *Am Heart J*. 1960;60:51–60.

Dexter L. Atrial septal defect. *Br Heart J*. 1956;18:209–25.

Ducas J, Magder S, McGregor M. Validity of the hepatojugular reflux and clinical test for congestive heart failure. *Am J Cardiol*. 1983;52:1299–303.

Fowler NO, Guase R. The cervical venous hum. *Am Heart J*. 1964; 67:135–6.

Harvey WP, Corrado MA, Perloff JK. Right sided murmurs of aortic insufficiency. *Am J Med Sci*. 1963;245:533–43.

Leathem A. Splitting of the first and second heart sounds. *Lancet*. 1954;267:607–14.

Sutton GC, Chatterjee K, Caves PK. Diagnosis of severe mitral regurgitation due to non-rheumatic chordal abnormalities. *Br Heart J*. 1973; 35:877–86.

Vancheri F, Gibson D. Relation of third and fourth heart sounds to blood velocity during left ventricular filling. *Br Heart J*. 1989;61:144–8.

QUESTIONS

QUESTION 1. A 68-year-old man with a long-standing history of hypertension and stable coronary disease complains of sudden severe acute chest pain radiating to his back. The emergency medical technicians measure blood pressure in both of his arms. The systolic pressure in his right arm is 98 mm Hg, and in his left arm it is 72 mm Hg. The most likely diagnosis is:

A. An acute myocardial infarction
B. Arterial thoracic outlet syndrome
C. Acute pulmonary embolism
D. Proximal dissection of his aorta
E. Acute pericarditis with cardiac tamponade

QUESTION 2. Which one of the following is the typical auscultatory finding in mitral valve prolapse?

A. An opening snap in diastole
B. A pericardial knock in diastolic
C. Mid- to late systolic click
D. A third heart sound (S3)
E. An early systolic click

QUESTION 3. Match the characteristic carotid pulsation with the cardiac disorder:

3.1. Jerky, with full expansion followed by sudden collapse (Corrigan's or water-hammer pulse)
3.2. Bifid carotid pulse with normal or delayed rise
3.3. Low amplitude and volume pulse with a delayed peak
3.4. Bounding and prominent pulse

A. Hypertension
B. Aortic stenosis

C. Aortic valve regurgitation

D. Combined aortic stenosis and regurgitation

QUESTION 4. Match the characteristic JVP abnormality with the cardiac disorder:

4.1. Steep x descent

4.2. Absent A waves

4.3. Prominent V waves

A. Atrial fibrillation

B. Cardiac tamponade

C. Tricuspid regurgitation

1. D
2. C
3.1. C
3.2. D
3.3. B
3.4. A
4.1. B
4.2. A
4.3. C

78.

ACUTE CORONARY SYNDROMES

Susan Cheng and Marc S. Sabatine

Acute coronary syndromes (ACS) are the result of acute myocardial ischemia occurring in the presence of coronary artery disease. The spectrum of ACS presentations includes unstable angina (UA), non–ST segment elevation myocardial infarction (NSTEMI), and ST segment elevation myocardial infarction (STEMI) (see table 78.1). UA is a clinical diagnosis that is made when a patient reports new anginal symptoms, crescendo angina, or angina at rest. Myocardial infarction (MI) is distinguished from UA by the presence of cardiac biomarker abnormalities, which reflect myocardial necrosis. A diagnosed MI may be either a STEMI or a non-ST elevation ACS (NSTE-ACS), depending on the absence or presence of ST segment elevation on the presenting electrocardiogram (ECG).

In total, ACS presentations account for over 2 million annual hospital admissions in the United States. Almost 1.4 million people suffer an ACS each year, of which 55% are new events, 31% are recurrent events, and 14% are silent events. Of all diagnosed MIs, approximately 30% are STEMI and 70% are NSTE-ACS events. Despite recent declines in associated mortality, coronary artery disease causes one out of every five deaths in the United States. Notably, half of MI-related deaths occur within the first hour, primarily due to ventricular dysrhythmias. Therefore, the presentation of ACS challenges the clinician to rapidly integrate key aspects of the history, physical examination, and diagnostic tests in order to diagnose correctly and manage effectively this potentially life-threatening condition.

PATHOPHYSIOLOGY

The pathophysiology underlying virtually all ACS is rupture or erosion of a vulnerable coronary atherosclerotic plaque. Vulnerable plaques usually cause only a moderate degree of stenosis, contain a soft atherogenic lipid core, and are covered by a thin cap that can easily rupture. Conversely, stable plaques tend to be larger, less lipid laden, and covered by a thick fibrous cap. Numerous factors contribute to plaque vulnerability, including inflammation and sheer stress. When a vulnerable plaque ruptures, the inner lipid-laden core is exposed to the bloodstream and activates multiple pathways leading to the rapid formation of a superimposed platelet- and fibrin-rich thrombus. This thrombus interrupts coronary blood flow, causing regional myocardial ischemia and, eventually if severe enough, infarction if not promptly treated with reperfusion therapies. Subtotal arterial occlusion typically manifests as NSTE-ACS, whereas total occlusion of a coronary artery often manifests as STEMI (table 78.1).

DIAGNOSIS

ACS is diagnosed by integrating key aspects of the history, examination, ECG, and cardiac biomarkers (table 78.2). During the evaluation of a patient with possible ACS, alternative cardiovascular and noncardiovascular causes of chest discomfort should always be entertained. In particular, conditions that can mimic ACS by presenting with chest pain and potentially ECG changes include aortic dissection (with or without coronary involvement), acute pericarditis, and pulmonary embolism.

CLINICAL PRESENTATION

ACS can occur at any time of day and may be triggered by physiological, physical, or emotional stress—or even the simple act of early morning awakening. Typical ACS symptoms include a substernal or left-sided chest discomfort, pain, or pressure that can radiate to the left arm, neck, or jaw. Accompanying symptoms may include dyspnea, nausea, vomiting, diaphoresis, lightheadedness, and palpitations. Women, older individuals, and diabetics are more likely to present with atypical symptoms as well as silent coronary attacks.

Table 78.1 SPECTRUM OF ACUTE CORONARY SYNDROMES

INCREASING SEVERITY OF ILLNESS

| DEFINITIONS | NON-ST SEGMENT ELEVATION ACS | | MYOCARDIAL INFARCTION |
	UNSTABLE ANGINA	NSTEMI	STEMI
Symptoms	New-onset angina (or equivalent); or Angina worse in frequency, duration, or intensity; or Angina at rest, usually <30 min		Angina (or equivalent) at rest, Usually >30 min
ECG	ST depressions; or TW inversions or flattening; or Normal-appearing ECG		ST elevation or equivalent
Biomarkers	Normal troponin	Elevated troponin	Very elevated troponin
Pathology	Subtotal coronary occlusion, more likely in the setting of multivessel disease with collaterals		Total coronary occlusion, more likely in the setting of single-vessel disease
	thrombus — plaque		thrombus — plaque
Treatment	Immediate medical therapy ± cardiac catheterization before discharge		Immediate medical therapy and immediate reperfusion (fibrinolysis or PCI)

PHYSICAL EXAMINATION

At baseline, coronary artery disease may be accompanied by signs of vascular disease in more accessible carotid or peripheral arterial beds with concomitant vascular bruits. At the time of an ACS, additional physical findings will vary depending on disease severity and associated complications. There can be an audible S4 due to impaired left ventricular (LV) compliance in the setting of myocardial ischemia. In an extensive MI, severe LV systolic dysfunction may be reflected by a palpable apical dyskinesis, soft S1, paradoxically split S2, and audible S3 in addition to classic signs of heart failure (jugular venous distension, rales, and edema). Frank cardiogenic shock can present with small volume pulses and a narrow pulse pressure in addition to classic signs of shock. Importantly, the degree of heart failure (HF) on examination portends a worse prognosis (see table 78.3).

Many ACS patients are hypertensive due to increased adrenergic stimulation. Conversely, hypotension suggests the presence of peri-MI complications, in which case the exam should focus on detecting the murmurs of mitral regurgitation or ventricular septal defect (often accompanied by a palpable thrill). Severe hypotension may also be part of the specific but insensitive triad for right ventricular (RV) infarct, which includes elevated jugular venous pressure (JVP) and clear lungs in addition to hypotension.

ELECTROCARDIOGRAM

The critical diagnostic test is the 12-lead ECG which allows the clinician to differentiate between NSTE-ACS and STEMI (or equivalent entities) and then to determine the most appropriate management (figure 78.1).

Table 78.2 THE LIKELIHOOD OF ACS BASED ON FEATURES OF HISTORY, EXAM, ECG, AND BIOMARKERS

	HIGH (ANY OF BELOW)	INTERMEDIATE (ANY OF BELOW)	LOW (MAY HAVE ANY OR ALL OF BELOW)
History	Chest or left arm pain like prior angina, history of CAD	Chest or left arm pain, age >70, male, diabetes	Atypical symptoms
Exam	Hypotension, HF, transient MR	Evidence of extracardiac atherosclerosis (PAD or CVD)	Pain reproduced on palpation
ECG	New STD (≥0.5 mm) or TWI (≥2 mm)	Old Q waves, old ST or T wave abnormal	TWF/TWI (in leads w/R waves) or normal
Cardiac biomarkers	Elevated Tn or CK-MB	Normal	Normal

Table 78.3 **KILLIP CLASSIFICATION FOR STEMI**

KILLIP CLASS	EXAMINATION	MORTALITY (30 DAYS)
1	No heart failure	6%
2	+S3 or basilar rales	17%
3	Pulmonary edema (rales >½ way up)	30–40%
4	Cardiogenic shock (systolic blood pressure (SBP) <90)	60–80%

In NSTE-ACS, a number of ECG patterns can be seen: ST-segment depressions, T-wave inversions, nonspecific ST- and T-wave changes, and occasionally no changes at all (table 78.1). Any ECG changes that come and go in timing with chest discomfort are often called "dynamic" and are highly suggestive of ischemia. The regionality of ECG changes in NSTE-ACS may correspond to but are not specific for the location of a coronary lesion.

In STEMI, the classic defining criteria include acute ST-segment elevations of 1 mm ST elevation in two contiguous limb leads, or 2 mm ST elevation in two contiguous

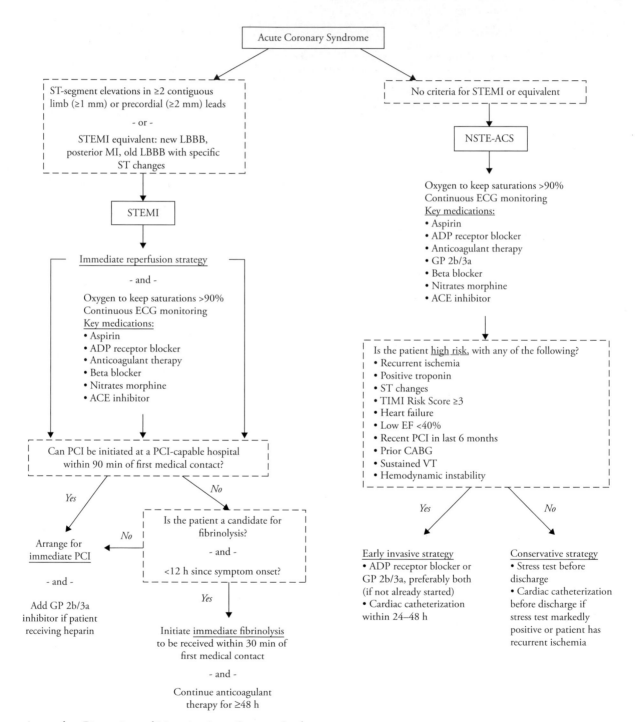

Figure 78.1. Approach to Diagnosing and Managing Acute Coronary Syndromes.

Table 78.4 LOCALIZATION OF STEMI

MYOCARDIAL REGION	ECG LEADS WITH ST ELEVATIONS	CORONARY ARTERY
Anteroseptal	V1–V4	Proximal LAD
Anterior	V3–V4	Mid-LAD
Apical	V5–V6	Distal LAD, LCX, or RCA
Lateral	I, aVL	LCX
Posterior	Posterior leads: V7–V9 (and ST depressions in V1–V2)	LCX
Inferior	II, III, aVF	RCA (~85%), LCX (~15%)
RV	V1–V2, R–V4	Proximal RCA

precordial leads. These criteria are not only specific for the location of a coronary lesion and the area of myocardium at risk (table 78.4), but they are also specific for the presence of an acute coronary occlusion in need of emergent reperfusion.

When there is clinical concern for a possible STEMI or STEMI-equivalent, a few situations benefit from more than the standard 12-lead ECG. For example, the suggestion of ST-segment elevations in the inferior leads (II, III, aVF) should prompt the placement of a right-sided lead (R-V4), which can show findings more specific for an RV infarct. The suggestion of ST-segment elevations in the inferior or high lateral leads (I, aVL) or reciprocal ST-segment depressions isolated to the right-sided precordial leads (V1, V2) should prompt the placement of posterior leads (V7, V8, V9), which can reveal findings more specific for a posterior infarction. Because of its posterior location, the left circumflex artery is the one coronary territory that may suffer a total occlusion despite a "silent" or apparently normal ECG.

A new left-bundle branch block (LBBB) is considered equivalent to a STEMI. The presence of an old LBBB typically interferes with the assessment of ST-segment changes. However, many would also consider an old LBBB with new ST deviations that are 1 mm concordant (in the same direction as the QRS) or 5 mm discordant (in the opposite direction from the QRS) as equivalent to STEMI.

Whereas ST-segment elevations typically represent injured myocardium, Q waves typically represent infarcted myocardium. Historically, the presence of pathologic Q waves in the distribution of a coronary territory on ECG was considered to reflect the presence of an old or recent transmural infarction. We now know that Q waves do not necessarily reflect the transmurality of an infarct. However, the development of Q waves still suggests the presence of less prominent collaterals, a larger infarct, a lower ejection fraction, and increased mortality.

CARDIAC BIOMARKERS

The diagnosis of MI can be made when cardiac biomarkers are elevated in combination with any of the following:

ischemic symptoms, ECG evidence of ischemia or recent infarct, and/or a new occlusive thrombus seen by coronary angiography. Moreover, the specific timing and pattern of cardiac biomarker elevation following the onset of myocardial ischemia offer prognostic as well as diagnostic information (figure 78.2). Notably, the absolute peak as well as the combination of time to peak and duration of elevation ("area under the curve") of cardiac-specific markers correspond to the extent of myocardial injury, subsequent myocardial dysfunction, and overall 1-year mortality.

Cardiac-Specific Markers

Detecting abnormally elevated cardiac-specific markers can facilitate early diagnosis of an acute MI and expedite management. Cardiac troponin I and T are proteins that originate from the cardiomyocyte apparatus and, therefore, are highly specific for cardiac injury when detected in the systemic circulation. Troponins start to rise within 3 hours of chest pain onset, peak within 24–48 hours, and return to baseline within 7–14 days (figure 78.2). Notably, troponin levels can be elevated in the setting of renal dysfunction; thus, interpretation must take this factor into account. However, in the appropriate clinical context, an elevated

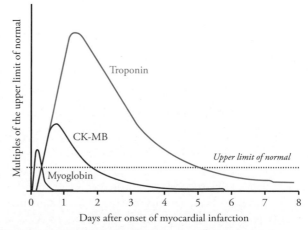

Figure 78.2. Appearance, Peak, and Duration of Cardiac Biomarker Elevations after Myocardial Infarction.

troponin in a patient with renal dysfunction remains a marker of poor prognosis.

Although elevations in total creatinine kinase (CK) correlate well with the extent of myocardial injury in ACS, the CK-MB isoenzyme is more specific to cardiac versus extracardiac muscle damage. CK-MB isoenzyme levels rise within 4 hours after acute injury, peak within 24 hours, and return to baseline within 48–72 hours (figure 78.2). Because CK-MB levels normalize more quickly than do troponins after an acute MI, serial CK-MB measures are more useful for the detection of post-MI ischemia and reinfarction, particularly following percutaneous coronary intervention (PCI).

Importantly, cardiac biomarkers may be negative very early in ACS (figure 78.2). However, the advent of highly sensitive cardiac troponin assays has improved the diagnostic accuracy of the troponin, increasing the sensitivity of a single sample at presentation from 70–75% to 90%. Moreover, among patients presenting within 3 hours of symptoms, the use of highly sensitive assays increases the sensitivity of a single measurement at presentation from 55% to 80–85%. Conversely, positive biomarkers may not always represent a typical ACS process. A number of non-ACS cardiac conditions can occasionally lead to myonecrosis and mildly elevated cardiac biomarkers: non-ACS coronary obstruction (e.g., spasm from Prinzmetal angina or cocaine, embolism, dissection, vasculitis); fixed atherosclerotic coronary disease with increased demand or decreased supply (e.g., tachycardia, hypovolemia, anemia, HF, aortic stenosis, or sepsis); and, other causes of myonecrosis (e.g., myocarditis, pulmonary embolism, cardiomyopathy, cardiac trauma, or subarachnoid hemorrhage).

TREATMENT

Early and appropriate risk stratification is essential for managing ACS. The critical decision point is the ECG: if ST-segment elevation (or its equivalent) is present, the patient should be treated with immediate reperfusion in addition to recommended medical therapies; if there is no ST-segment elevation (or equivalent), the patient should receive the same recommended medical therapies and then further risk stratification to decide if reperfusion should be pursued within the next 24–48 hours (figure 78.1).

BASIC MANAGEMENT

Any patient with suspected ACS should receive bed rest and continuous ECG monitoring to screen for ischemic and rhythm changes. Any patient diagnosed with a probable or definite ACS should be treated in a coronary care or step-down unit, depending on the severity of the ACS. Supplemental oxygen is recommended for the first 6 hours of ACS and then as needed to maintain an oxygen saturation >90%. In addition, a number of specific ACC/AHA recommended medications should be promptly administered (figure 78.1). The general goal of these therapies is (1) to counteract platelet and thrombin activity in the involved coronary artery, and (2) to improve the myocardial oxygen supply-demand mismatch caused by disrupted coronary blood flow.

Antiplatelet and antithrombin therapies are the foundation of medical treatment in ACS and should be administered at the time of initial evaluation.

- *Aspirin* will immediately and covalently modify cyclo-oxygenase-1 by acetylation, resulting in near-totally blocked thromboxane A_2 production by platelets, which halts thromboxane A_2-mediated platelet aggregation. Because aspirin has utility across the entire spectrum of ACS, it should be given immediately to all suspected ACS patients.

- *Adenosine diphosphate (ADP) receptor blockers* inhibit the P2Y12 platelet ADP receptor, thereby decreasing platelet activation and aggregation, and are indicated for all patients diagnosed with ACS. ADP receptor blockers include clopidogrel (currently the most widely used) and the third-generation agents prasugrel and ticagrelor. Clopidogrel (a prodrug that requires hepatic biotransformation into an active metabolite upstream) therapy at the time of presentation is frequently advocated. Clopidogrel is typically given with a loading dose (except for patients age >75 receiving fibrinolysis, in whom a loading dose should be avoided). As clopidogrel is an irreversible platelet inhibitor, it should be held 5 days prior to coronary artery bypass grafting (CABG) surgery. Prasugrel is a thienopyridine prodrug, like clopidogrel, but more quickly converted to its active metabolite. In contrast, ticagrelor has a completely different chemical structure, does not require metabolic activation, and is a reversible ADP receptor blocker.

- *Anticoagulant therapy* should also be given to all ACS patients. Several rapidly acting options exist including unfractionated heparin (UFH), the low-molecular-weight heparin enoxaparin, the highly selective Xa-inhibitor fondaparinux, and the direct thrombin inhibitor bivalirudin. Long-term oral anticoagulant therapy may also be indicated for concurrent LV thrombus, atrial fibrillation, or deep venous thrombosis.

- *Glycoprotein (GP) 2b/3a* inhibitors block the final common pathway of platelet aggregation and thereby complement the antiplatelet actions of aspirin and clopidogrel. There are currently three types of GP 2b/3a inhibitors in use: abciximab (fab fragment of a monoclonal antibody directed at the 2b/3a receptor), eptifibatide (a synthetic peptide), and tirofiban (a synthetic nonpeptide molecule). GP 2b/3a agents are reserved for higher-risk patients with MI, particularly in the setting of PCI.

Several anti-ischemic medications are available to help improve myocardial oxygen supply-demand mismatch:

- *Beta blockers* reduce heart rate, blood pressure, and contractility, which effectively decrease myocardial oxygen demand while also augmenting supply. In addition to relieving pain, beta blockers also reduce infarct size and prevent serious arrhythmias. Therefore, beta blockers should be started for even suspected ACS unless contraindicated (figure 78.1). The dosing goal of beta blockers is to control resting heart rate and blood pressure while relieving ischemic signs and symptoms. Nondihydropyridine *calcium channel blockers* (diltiazem or verapamil) may be considered as an addition or a substitute if beta blocker therapy is inadequate or contraindicated.

- *Nitrates* are vasodilators that relax coronary arteries and reduce cardiac afterload and preload, which lowers ventricular wall tension and oxygen demand. In addition, they improve bloodflow to the subendocardium and through collateral vessels. Therefore, nitrates should be used to treat chest discomfort and or symptoms of HF unless contraindicated (figure 78.1).

- *Morphine* is an analgesic with vasodilator properties and is recommended for refractory chest discomfort or the presence of HF unless contraindicated (figure 78.1). Anxiolytics may be used in addition to morphine to decrease anxiety in the acute setting.

In addition to the above therapies, certain additional medications can serve to optimize conditions affecting the vasculature and myocardium in the setting of an ACS. These medications effectively improve longer-term outcomes and can begin to offer benefit when started early, even within the first 24 hours:

- *Angiotensin-converting enzyme (ACE) inhibitors* block renin-angiotensin-aldosterone activity and, in doing so, reduce afterload and also prevent infarct expansion and remodeling. Therefore, ACE inhibitors should be given to all ACS patients with HF, LV dysfunction, or hypertension and considered in all patients without contraindications (figure 78.1). In this respect, *angiotensin receptor blockers* (ARBs) are likely equivalent and can be used as a substitute in cases of allergy to ACE inhibitors.

- *Statins* reduce recurrent events for all MI patients, likely through anti-inflammatory as well as lipid-lowering mechanisms. A high-dose statin can be started within the first 24 hours regardless of the patient's baseline lipid profile.

Medications to avoid in ACS include dihydropyridine calcium channel blockers (e.g., nifedipine) and empirical antiarrhythmics, which can increase mortality in the peri-MI setting.

MANAGEMENT OF STEMI

Rapid recognition of a STEMI is critical. The faster that normal flow can be restored to an occluded artery, the more myocardial necrosis can be prevented, and the more likely that at-risk myocardium will be salvaged, LV function preserved, and MI-related morbidity and mortality decreased. On diagnosing STEMI, therefore, reperfusion therapy should be performed immediately with concurrent administration of key adjunctive medical therapies (figure 78.1).

Emergent Reperfusion

The most important initial decision point in managing STEMI pertains to which method of emergent reperfusion to pursue. PCI is preferred if it can be initiated at a PCI-capable hospital within 90 min of the patient's first medical contact—even if rapid hospital transfer is required to achieve this time-sensitive goal (figure 78.1). If PCI cannot be initiated within 90 minutes, and <12 hours have passed since the onset of ischemic symptoms, then fibrinolysis should be administered within 30 minutes of first medical contact unless contraindicated (table 78.5). The benefit of fibrinolysis given >12 hours after symptom onset is less clear, but it is reasonable if there are ongoing ischemic symptoms and/or persistent ST-segment elevations without PCI availability.

Fibrinolysis

The fibrinolytic agents currently used to treat STEMI include streptokinase and the fibrin-specific agents alteplase (tPA), reteplase (rPA), and tenecteplase (TNK). Fibrin-specific agents are associated with lower mortality rates than streptokinase but also with a slightly higher risk of intracerebral

Table 78.5 CONTRAINDICATIONS TO FIBRINOLYTIC THERAPY

Absolute Contraindications
Any prior ICH
Intracranial neoplasm or AVM
Ischemic CVA within last 3 months
Suspected aortic dissection
Active internal bleed (except menses)
Significant close-head or facial trauma in last 3 months

Relative Contraindications
BP >180/110 or history of chronic severe hypertension
Any prior ischemic CVA, dementia, or other intracranial lesion
Recent trauma or internal bleed within 2–4 weeks
Major trauma or surgery in last 3 weeks
CPR
Noncompressible vascular punctures
Pregnancy
Active peptic ulcer disease
INR >2.0

hemorrhage. Concurrent antiplatelet and antithrombin therapies are required along with fibrinolysis to prevent reinfarction (figure 78.1).

Fibrinolysis offers a 50–85% success rate at opening the occluded artery within 90 minutes and is associated with a 20% mortality reduction in patients with STEMI or new LBBB. In fact, fibrinolysis given in the most timely fashion, prior to hospital arrival, is associated with an even further 17% mortality reduction. The magnitude of benefit is directly inverse to the time-to-treatment, where by far the greatest mortality reduction is seen when fibrinolytics are given within 1–3 hours of symptom onset. As more time passes, the mortality benefit progressively falls. Thus, fibrinolytics are recommended up to 12 hours after symptom onset; the benefit is less clear at 12–24 hours.

Fibrinolytics must be avoided in patients with absolute contraindications and given only with extreme caution in patients with relative contraindications (table 78.5). Notably, fibrinolysis poses an overall 5–6% risk of major bleed and an approximate 1% risk of intracranial hemorrhage. Patients at the highest risk for bleeding complications are older, lower in body weight, female, black, hypertensive, diabetic, with a history of stroke, and receiving excess heparinization or concurrent warfarin. Although age >75 years is not a contraindication to fibrinolysis, PCI is often favored in these patients.

Approximately 20–30% of patients receiving a fibrinolytic fail to reperfuse and subsequently have a high mortality rate. These patients should be referred for rescue PCI.

Percutaneous Coronary Intervention

In the setting of STEMI, the goal of PCI is to quickly determine the location of the acute thrombus by cardiac catheterization and then to mechanically recannulate the occluded coronary artery. Because PCI offers greater efficacy and safety than fibrinolysis when performed by skilled operators at high-volume centers, PCI is favored when both are available. Even transferring a patient to a primary PCI hospital may also be superior if it can be done to achieve PCI initiation within 90 minutes of first medical contact.

The major advantages of primary PCI over fibrinolysis are derived from its >90% success rate at opening an occluded artery while, at the same time, conferring much less bleeding risk. Compared to fibrinolysis, primary PCI for STEMI is associated with a 27% reduction in mortality, 65% reduction in reinfarction, 54% reduction in stroke, and 95% reduction in intracerebral hemorrhage.

Primary PCI for treating STEMI is especially more effective than fibrinolysis in the highest-risk patients presenting with HF, cardiogenic shock, or severe arrhythmias. For patients with post-MI cardiogenic shock, in particular, PCI should be performed <18 hours from the onset of shock whenever possible. PCI is also appropriate for patients with absolute or relative contraindications to fibrinolysis (table 78.5). However, the major limitations of PCI include the need for appropriate facilities, skilled/experienced personnel, and the timely availability of resources—all of which are more variable in practice than in clinical trials.

Immediate Medical Therapies for STEMI

Antiplatelet Agents

Aspirin remains the key antiplatelet therapy in STEMI, adding a 23% mortality reduction to the benefits of fibrinolysis. When given along with aspirin plus fibrinolysis, clopidogrel improves rates of infarct artery patency and even further decreases cardiovascular events and mortality without increasing risk of major bleed. For patients undergoing PCI, prasugrel may be favored over clopidogrel for reducing subsequent ischemic events. In addition to aspirin and an ADP receptor blocker, a GP 2b/3a inhibitor is also recommended to further reduce the risk for death and adverse outcomes in patients undergoing PCI.

Anticoagulants

Indirect anticoagulant therapy with UFH promotes vessel patency in STEMI when given in support of fibrinolytics. Compared to UFH, the low-molecular-weight heparin, enoxaparin, decreases risk of death or MI by 17%. Fondaparinux (a specific factor Xa inhibitor) is more effective than placebo in STEMI and appeared comparable to UFH. For STEMI patients receiving fibrinolysis, therefore, UFH or enoxaparin or fondaparinux is appropriate. For patients receiving primary PCI, UFH or enoxaparin (typically combined with a GP 2b/3a inhibitor) are reasonable choices. Alternatively, monotherapy with bivalirudin (a direct thrombin inhibitor), compared to UFH combined with a GP 2b/3a inhibitor, has been shown to lower mortality and bleeding. Fondaparinux, however, should be avoided in PCI patients given its risk for catheter thrombosis.

Anti-ischemics

Beta blockers given early are associated with decreased reinfarction by 22% and life-threatening arrhythmias by 15%. When appropriately administered, beta blockers are also likely to reduce all-cause death. Beta blockers should only be given orally, as opposed to intravenously, unless used to treat concurrent hypertension. As well, beta blockers should be avoided in patients with HF because they can precipitate cardiogenic shock. Nitrates may possibly offer a slight <5% mortality reduction in STEMI. By reducing preload and afterload, nitrates are effective at relieving ischemic symptoms and treating hypertension or HF. Morphine offers no mortality benefit but can help to relieve refractory ischemic symptoms.

Additional Therapies

Adding to the benefits of aspirin and beta blockers in STEMI, ACE inhibitors reduce mortality by 7% in the short term and 26% in the long term. The greatest benefit of ACE inhibitors is seen in patients with anterior MI, ejection fraction (EF) <40%, signs of HF, or a wall motion abnormality on imaging; ARBs appear roughly equivalent in this setting. Statins begin to offer benefit shortly after an acute MI and so can be started even before a lipid profile is obtained.

MANAGEMENT OF NON–ST SEGMENT ELEVATION ACUTE CORONARY SYNDROMES

NSTE-ACS presentations reflect an imbalance between myocardial oxygen supply and demand, typically as a result of a nonocclusive thrombus that has developed over a disrupted atherosclerotic plaque (table 78.1). NSTE-ACS can also result from dynamic coronary obstruction, conditions that involve increased oxygen demand in the setting of a fixed supply, or some combination thereof. Similar to STEMI, medical therapies for NSTE-ACS are aimed at counteracting thrombosis, improving supply–demand mismatch, and optimizing vascular and myocardial outcomes. However, because the coronary thrombus is typically nonocclusive, immediate reperfusion is not required (figure 78.1).

Because NSTE-ACS presentations encompass a wide range of disease severities with outcomes that vary accordingly, risk stratification is essential for appropriately tailoring therapy. Patients with NSTE-ACS who have a clinically high risk for adverse events are more likely than lower-risk patients to benefit from more aggressive interventions, such as early cardiac catheterization and use of a GP2b/3a inhibitor. Conversely, more aggressive interventions may cause more harm than good in lower-risk patients.

The TIMI and GRACE scoring systems are validated methods for identifying high- versus low-risk individuals. The TIMI risk score, in particular, has gained popularity for its ease of use at the bedside (table 78.6). In addition to a high GRACE or TIMI risk score, additional clinical features that identify high-risk patients with NSTE-ACS include age >75 years, accelerating symptoms >48 hours, postoperative state, EF <40%, ongoing or recurrent rest pain, hypotension, severe arrhythmias, pulmonary edema, ST-segment depressions >0.5 mm, and elevated cardiac biomarkers.

Immediate Medical Therapies for NSTE-ACS

Antiplatelets

As in STEMI, aspirin is the key antiplatelet agent in NSTE-ACS and provides a >50% reduction in death or reinfarction with the benefit starting within 1 day of treatment. The addition of clopidogrel to aspirin provides a further 20% reduction in cardiovascular death, MI, or stroke, with a reduction in ischemic events emerging within hours following treatment. For patients going on to PCI, there is an approximate 30% reduction in post-PCI ischemic events when clopidogrel is given prior to PCI rather than at the time of PCI. Therefore, upstream therapy with both aspirin and clopidogrel is advocated. Alternatively, in the setting of PCI, prasugrel reduces the risk of recurrent major adverse cardiovascular events compared with clopidogrel while conferring an increased risk of both nonsurgical and surgical bleeding. Similarly, in ACS patients treated with or without PCI, ticagrelor has been shown to lower the risk for recurrent major adverse cardiovascular events compared with clopidogrel, including cardiovascular mortality, while it slightly increases the risk of nonsurgical but not surgical bleeding.

GP 2b/3a inhibitors offer additional antiplatelet activity. The greatest benefit is seen in high-risk patients with positive troponins, a TIMI risk score ≥4, and/or who are going for PCI. Studies also indicate that patients considered at higher risk due to ST segment changes or diabetes are also much more likely than their counterparts to benefit from GP 2b/3a inhibitors. The timing of initiation of

---

Table 78.6 **THE TIMI RISK SCORE FOR NSTE-ACS, WITH FACTORS LISTED ACCORDING TO THE MNEMONIC "CARDIAC"**

Assign 1 Point for Each of the Following Factors, if Present
C Coronary artery disease, previously documented by angiogram as ≥50% stenosis
A Age ≥65
R Risk factors, ≥3 of the following: family history of CAD, hypertension, dyslipidemia, diabetes, smoking
D Deviation of the ST segments of ≥0.5 mm
I Ischemic pain occurring ≥2 times within the last 24 hours
A Aspirin taken within the last 7 days
C Cardiac biomarker elevation: troponin or CK-MB

Sum the Points (out of a Possible 7 Total) in Order to Determine Risk
The higher the total TIMI risk score, the higher the risk of combined outcome of death/MI/revascularization by 14 days: score 0–1, outcome risk 5%; score 2–3, risk 8–13%; score 4–5, risk 20–26%; score 6–7, risk 41%
Higher-risk patients derive greater benefit from LMWH, G2b/3a, and early invasive strategy

GP 2b/3a inhibitors remains controversial, with upstream therapy tending to reduce ischemic events at the cost of significantly higher bleeding.

Anticoagulants

Therapy with UFH, in addition to aspirin, appears to reduce death or MI by approximately a third compared to aspirin alone. Use of the low-molecular-weight heparin, enoxaparin, as compared with UFH further reduces ischemic events. Therefore, either UFH or enoxaparin is appropriate anticoagulant therapy in NSTE-ACS. Fondaparinux may be even more effective than enoxaparin at reducing mortality and is preferred in patients with an increased bleeding risk. Given its associated risk of catheter thrombosis, however, fondaparinux should be reserved for patients treated conservatively; otherwise, it should be supplemented with UFH when used around the time of PCI. Bivalirudin can be used in cases of heparin allergy—with outcomes results similar to that of indirect thrombin inhibitors—while not requiring concurrent GP 2b/3a therapy. Regardless of the chosen anticoagulant regimen, concomitant antiplatelet therapy, in the form of both aspirin and clopidogrel, should always be given as early as possible.

Anti-ischemics

Beta blockers are proven to prevent reinfarction and decrease mortality following any type of MI. In a threatening or evolving MI, beta blockers even slow progression to MI by 13%. Therefore, all NSTE-ACS patients should receive beta blocker therapy unless contraindicated (figure 78.1). A nondihydropyridine calcium channel blocker may help to alleviate ischemic symptoms if beta blocker therapy is inadequate or contraindicated. Although nitrates have no proven mortality benefit, they effectively improve signs and symptoms of ischemia and therefore should be given promptly when indicated. As with STEMI, morphine offers no known mortality benefit in NSTE-ACS but is also effective at relieving ischemic symptoms that are refractory to beta blockers and nitrates, although patients with refractory symptoms are best treated with urgent coronary angiography.

Additional Therapies

All NSTE-ACS patients with hypertension, diabetes, clinical HF, or low ejection fraction should receive an ACE inhibitor whenever possible. If not tolerated due to cough, the ACE inhibitor may be replaced by an ARB.

Although statins are best known for a marked approximate 30% long-term mortality reduction in CAD patients, starting intensive statin therapy early in the course of a hospitalization for ACS adds even more benefit. Initiating early therapy improves long-term treatment rates, and high-dose compared to moderate-dose therapy offers a 16% further reduction in cardiovascular events or coronary death. The

benefits of early statin therapy may be seen as early as 6 weeks following NSTE-ACS. Therefore, every patient should be on a high-dose statin within 24–96 hours of admission.

Cardiac Catheterization

There are two strategies for managing NSTE-ACS with respect to if and when to pursue cardiac catheterization (figure 78.1).

The *conservative strategy* can be applied to low-risk patients and involves treating with maximal medical therapy and then obtaining a low-level treadmill or pharmacologic stress test prior to discharge. Only those patients with recurrent ischemia (by symptoms and/or ECG changes) and patients with strongly positive stress tests are then referred for cardiac catheterization prior to discharge in order to define their coronary anatomy and then be treated by PCI or CABG as indicated.

The *early invasive strategy* involves routine cardiac catheterization within 24–48 hours of admission and concurrent PCI to treat high-grade lesions as needed; this strategy is indicated for all patients who are at high risk (figure 78.1). In high-risk patients, an early invasive strategy substantially reduces risk of recurrent MI or ischemia and modestly reduces mortality when compared to the conservative strategy. In low- to moderate-risk patients, the benefit of an early invasive strategy is less clear. In fact, an early invasive strategy may even increase the risk of adverse major outcomes among low-risk women, in particular.

COMPLICATIONS

Severe complications following MI are now much less frequent due to the success of modern reperfusion and adjunctive therapies. Nevertheless, they can still occur in the peri-MI period and particularly in patients who present late following a nonreperfused MI. The most severe post-MI complications—including shock, mechanical complications, and malignant dysrhythmias—are typically associated with STEMI rather than NSTE-ACS.

CARDIOGENIC SHOCK

When an acute MI is complicated by cardiogenic shock, the associated mortality rate approaches 90% but is reduced to 60% with contemporary interventions. Most cases of peri-MI cardiogenic shock are due to extensive LV dysfunction, which is almost always due to a large anterior infarction. Alternatively, shock can due to a severe right ventricular infarction, which occurs in up to 40% of patients with an inferior STEMI and often presents with the classic triad of hypotension, increased JVP, and clear lung fields. Peri-MI shock may also be due to mechanical complications of either anterior or inferior infarcts, typically in late-presenting patients who have sustained a large territory of myocardial damage.

Determining the cause of cardiogenic shock following MI is critical for determining the most appropriate management. To this end, the bedside echocardiogram and right-heart catheterization are useful diagnostic tools (table 78.7).

Mechanical Complications

Mechanical complications result from gross disruption of myocardial tissue and typically occur 1–2 days following a usually nonreperfused acute MI, at which time the infarcted myocardium is still inflamed and friable without having had the chance to heal and remodel in the face of increased demand and adrenergic stimulation. The most definitive treatment for mechanical complications is emergent surgical repair (table 78.7).

An acute *papillary muscle rupture* can occur within 2–10 days post-MI, usually following an inferior MI due to the posterior papillary muscle relying on single-vessel blood supply from this territory. Papillary muscle rupture causes acute mitral regurgitation and presents with sudden onset dyspnea, hypoxia, HF, and hypotension. The mitral regurgitation may not be audible on examination due to rapid equalization of the left atrial (LA) and LV pressures, but the diagnosis can be confirmed by echocardiogram suggested by or V waves in the pulmonary capillary wedge tracing on right heart catheterization.

Ventricular septal rupture causing an acute ventricular septal defect (VSD) can occur 1–20 days following either an anterior or inferior MI. An acute VSD usually presents with sudden-onset dyspnea and hypotension in addition to a pansystolic murmur and palpable systolic thrill. The diagnosis is confirmed by echocardiogram and/or right heart catheterization (table 78.7). If associated with an inferior MI, acute VSDs have a poorer prognosis because of the typically serpiginous nature of the rupture.

A *ventricular free wall rupture* can occur 2–14 days following an anterior or inferior STEMI. Elderly women are particularly at risk for free wall rupture, which can present as pseudoaneurysm, tamponade, sudden electromechanical dissociation, or death. Tamponade physiology may require immediate percutaneous pericardiocentesis prior to emergent surgery.

DYSRHYTHMIAS

Fortunately, widespread beta blocker use has reduced the frequency of life-threatening peri-MI *ventricular dysrhythmias*. Premature ventricular contractions (PVCs) are common in the first 24–72 hours and are usually asymptomatic and benign. Nonsustained ventricular tachycardia (defined as ≥3 sequential PVCs lasting for <30 sec) can be managed by treating any persistent ischemia, normalizing electrolytes, and uptitrating beta blocker therapy. Sustained and hemodynamically stable VT can be managed with beta blockade plus a trial of antiarrhythmics before consideration of defibrillation. Hemodynamically unstable VT or ventricular fibrillation (VF) should be treated with immediate defibrillation according to ACLS protocols.

Ventricular fibrillation predominantly occurs within the first 48 hours and is associated with an immediate

Table 78.7 DIAGNOSING AND TREATING CARDIOGENIC SHOCK FOLLOWING MI

| | | RIGHT HEART CATHETERIZATION | | | | |
	BEDSIDE ECHO	RA PRESSURE	WEDGE PRESSURE	CARDIAC OUTPUT	OTHER FINDINGS	TREATMENT
LV infarct/failure	Poor LV function	High	Very high	Very low	Loss of R voltage across anterior leads (on ECG)	Inotropes ± vasopressors, IABP or VAD, emergent reperfusion
RV infarct/failure	Dilated RV, poor RV function	Very high	Low	Very low	ST elevation in RV4-RV6 leads (on ECG)	Volume resuscitation (goal RA pressure 10–14 mm Hg) ± dobutamine, pulmonary vasodilators, emergent reperfusion
Papillary muscle rupture → MR	Severe MR	High	Very high	Very low	V waves in PCWP tracing (on RHC)	Diuretics, vasodilators, IABP, emergent surgery
Ventricular septal rupture	Septal defect	High	Very high	High	Step up of O₂ sat from RA to PA	Diuretics, vasodilators, inotropes, IABP, emergent surgery
Free wall rupture → Tamponade	Effusion and tamponade	Very high	Very high	Very low	Equalization of end-diastolic pressures (on RHC)	Fluid resuscitation ± inotropes, ± pericardiocentesis, emergent surgery
Pulmonary embolus	Dilated RV, poor RV function	Very high	Low	Low	PA diastolic pressure in excess of wedge	Anticoagulation, emergent fibrinolysis or thrombectomy

mortality of 20%. These patients often have sustained a larger infarct, have a lower ejection fraction, and have a higher incidence of HF. Peri-infarct VF always requires immediate defibrillation, along with beta blockade plus antiarrhythmic therapy with amiodarone, lidocaine, or procainamide while efforts are prioritized toward urgent reperfusion. Any hemodynamically unstable ventricular dysrhythmias (VT or VF) that are refractory to antiarrhythmic therapies should be considered for intra-aortic balloon pump (IABP) insertion in addition to urgent reperfusion. As well, any late-occurring ventricular dysrhythmias should prompt a full evaluation for recurrent ischemia.

In the aftermath following an MI, malignant ventricular arrhythmias are more likely to occur among individuals with sustained poor EF and particularly those who also have chronic heart failure or nonsustained ventricular arrhythmias. Therefore, placement of an internal cardiac defibrillator is recommended for individuals who have had an MI and a persistently low EF documented at least 6 weeks following the MI event.

Bradyarrhythmias are usually seen <24–48 hours following MI. At the time of an acute MI, symptomatic or advanced atrioventricular (AV) block can be treated with temporary pacing as attempts at reperfusion are made. Transcutaneous temporary pacing is arguably safer in the setting of fibrinolytic therapy, but transvenous temporary pacing is more effective in patients who have sustained large infarcts and may eventually require permanent pacing.

Sinus bradycardia or second-degree Mobitz I block (Wenckebach) can be seen in patients with inferior MI. These conditions typically resolve within 2–3 days and respond to atropine if associated with hypotension or ischemia. New Mobitz II block and third-degree (complete) heart block are usually associated with a large MI (anterior or inferior) and require temporary pacing. New bifascicular block or alternating right and left bundle branch block (BBB) also require temporary pacing because of the risk of progressing to complete heart block. Although it is relatively uncommon for patients presenting with MI to eventually need a permanent pacemaker, indications include unresolved severe sinus node dysfunction and second-degree Mobitz II block with BBB and third-degree block.

OTHER COMPLICATIONS

Pericarditis can follow any type of MI by 2–14 days and can present with chest discomfort, pericardial rub, and diffuse ST depressions and PR depressions on ECG. A more severe autoimmune pericarditis, also referred to as Dressler syndrome, with fever can manifest several weeks later. Post-MI pericarditis responds well to nonsteroidal anti-inflammatory agents, which can include high-dose aspirin. Anticoagulation should be avoided, if possible, to prevent intrapericardial bleed.

A left ventricular *aneurysm* is a noncontractile outpouching of thinned myocardium that can form in up to 5% of patients originally presenting with STEMI. Aneurysm formation typically occurs at least several days to weeks following a large transmural MI that is usually anterior in location. An anterior LV aneurysm can manifest with persistent anterior ST segment elevations on ECG. Once the diagnosis is confirmed by echocardiogram, long-term anticoagulation is recommended given the risk of associated mural thrombosis and systemic embolization.

SECONDARY PREVENTION

Care following any type of MI should include risk factor modification, long-term medications, and cardiac rehabilitation. Risk factor modification includes:

- Smoking cessation
- Blood pressure: goal <140/90 or <130/80 for patients with diabetes or chronic kidney disease
- Lipid control: goal low-density lipoprotein (LDL) <100 mg/dL (preferably <70 mg/dL)
- Exercise ≥30 min daily
- Weight optimization: goal body mass index (BMI) 18.5–24.9 kg/m², and goal waist circumference <40 in. for men and <35 in. for women
- Glucose control: goal HbA1c <7% for diabetics

  Long-term medications should include:
- Aspirin (at least 81 mg daily is recommended; even following PCI, long-term doses above 100 mg daily are likely not needed in the setting of concurrent ADP receptor blocker therapy)
- ADP receptor blocker therapy, ideally for ≥12 months (recommended uninterrupted duration of therapy depending on the type of treatment received for acute MI)
- Beta blocker therapy
- ACE inhibitor (or ARB) therapy for all patients with LV dysfunction, hypertension, diabetes, or chronic kidney disease
- Statin therapy

Aldosterone blockers are also recommend for patients without significant renal dysfunction or hyperkalemia and who are already on therapeutic doses of an ACE inhibitor or ARB, have an EF ≤40%, and have either symptomatic HF or diabetes. Warfarin is indicated in patients who have severe LV dysfunction (EF ≤30%) or an apical thrombus for at least 3 months following MI, although this has not yet been shown to offer a survival benefit. Recently, the addition of very low-dose anticoagulant therapy with the oral Xa inhibitor, rivaroxaban, to dual antiplatelet therapy with aspirin and clopidogrel has been shown to decrease mortality. All patients with CAD should receive an annual influenza vaccine. In addition, all CAD patients over age 65 should receive a pneumovaccine.

A program of exercise-based cardiac rehabilitation is recommended for all patients with CAD and may be particularly beneficial for those who have just had an MI. In conjunction with proven medical therapies for secondary prevention, cardiac rehabilitation may offer added benefit with regard to quality of life, exercise tolerance, and even mortality reduction.

ADDITIONAL READING

Anderson JL, Adams CD, Antman EM, et al. ACC/AHA 2007 guidelines for the management of patients with unstable angina/ non ST-elevation myocardial infarction: A report of the American College of Cardiology/American Heart Association Task Force on Practice Guidelines (Writing Committee to Revise the 2002 Guidelines for the Management of Patients with Unstable Angina/ Non ST-Elevation Myocardial Infarction): developed in collaboration with the American College of Emergency Physicians, the Society for Cardiovascular Angiography and Interventions, and the Society of Thoracic Surgeons; endorsed by the American Association of Cardiovascular and Pulmonary Rehabilitation and the Society for Academic Emergency Medicine. *Circulation*. 2007;116:e148–304.

Antman EM, Anbe DT, Armstrong PW, et al. ACC/AHA guidelines for the management of patients with ST-elevation myocardial infarction: A report of the American College of Cardiology/American Heart Association Task Force on Practice Guidelines (Committee to Revise the 1999 Guidelines for the Management of Patients with Acute Myocardial Infarction). *Circulation*. 2004;110:e82–292.

Antman EM, Hand M, Armstrong PW, et al. 2007 Focused Update of the ACC/AHA 2004 Guidelines for the Management of Patients with ST-Elevation Myocardial Infarction: A report of the American College of Cardiology/American Heart Association Task Force on Practice Guidelines, developed in collaboration with the Canadian Cardiovascular Society, endorsed by the American Academy of Family Physicians: 2007 Writing Group to Review New Evidence and Update the ACC/AHA 2004 Guidelines for the Management of Patients with ST-Elevation Myocardial Infarction, Writing on Behalf of the 2004 Writing Committee. *Circulation*. 2008;117:296–329.

Antman EM, Cohen M, Bernink PJ, et al. The TIMI risk score for unstable angina/non-ST elevation MI: A method for prognostication and therapeutic decision making. *JAMA*. 2000;284:835–42.

Chen ZM, Pan HC, Chen YP, et al.; COMMIT (ClOpidogrel and Metoprolol in Myocardial Infarction Trial) collaborative group. Early intravenous then oral metoprolol in 45,852 patients with acute myocardial infarction: Randomised placebo-controlled trial. *Lancet*. 2005;366:1622–32.

Gershlick AH, Stephens-Lloyd A, Hughes S, et al. Rescue angioplasty after failed thrombolytic therapy for acute myocardial infarction. *N Engl J Med*. 2005;353:2758–68.

Giugliano RP, White JA, Bode C, et al. Early versus delayed, provisional eptifibatide in acute coronary syndromes. *N Engl J Med*. 2009;360:2176–90.

Hazinski MF, Nolan JP, Billi JE, et al. Part 1: Executive summary: 2010 International Consensus on Cardiopulmonary Resuscitation

and Emergency Cardiovascular Care Science with Treatment Recommendations. *Circulation*. 2010;122:S250–75.

Keller T, Zeller T, Peetz D, et al. Sensitive troponin I assay in early diagnosis of acute myocardial infarction. *N Engl J Med*. 2009;361:868–77.

Mega JL, Braunwald E, Wiviott SD, et al. Rivaroxaban in patients with a recent acute coronary syndrome. *N Engl J Med*. 2012;366:9–19.

Mehta SR, Granger CB, Boden WE, et al. Early versus delayed invasive intervention in acute coronary syndromes. *N Engl J Med*. 2009;360:2165–75.

O'Donoghue M, Boden WE, Braunwald E, et al. Early invasive vs. conservative treatment strategies in women and men with unstable angina and non-ST-segment elevation myocardial infarction: A meta-analysis. *JAMA*. 2008;300:71–80.

Reichlin T, Hochholzer W, Bassetti S, et al. Early diagnosis of myocardial infarction with sensitive cardiac troponin assays. *N Engl J Med*. 2009;361:858–67.

Roger VL, Go AS, Lloyd-Jones DM, et al. Heart disease and stroke statistics 2011 update: A report from the American Heart Association. *Circulation*. 2011;123:e18–209.

Sabatine MS, Cannon CP, Gibson CM, et al. Addition of clopidogrel to aspirin and fibrinolytic therapy for myocardial infarction with ST-segment elevation. *N Engl J Med*. 2005;352:1179–89.

Stone GW, Witzenbichler B, Guagliumi G, et al. Bivalirudin during primary PCI in acute myocardial infarction. *N Engl J Med*. 2008;358:2218–30.

Wallentin L, Becker RC, Budaj A, et al. Ticagrelor versus clopidogrel in patients with acute coronary syndromes. *N Engl J Med*. 2009;361:1045–57.

Wiviott SD, Braunwald E, McCabe CH, et al; TRITON-TIMI 38 Investigators. Prasugrel versus clopidogrel in patients with acute coronary syndromes. *N Engl J Med*. 2007;357:2001–15.

QUESTIONS

QUESTION 1. A severe right ventricular infarct can typically present with the following features:

A. Normal JVP, clear lungs, hypotension, ST elevation in lead II

B. Elevated JVP, clear lungs, hypotension, ST elevation in lead III

C. Elevated JVP, clear lungs, hypertension, ST elevation in lead III

D. Depressed JVP, clear lungs, hypotension, ST elevation in aVF

E. Depressed JVP, rales halfway up the back, hypotension, ST elevation in II, III, and aVF

QUESTION 2. A 75-year-old woman with a history of long-standing hypertension, high cholesterol, diabetes, and former tobacco use arrives in the emergency department. She appears diaphoretic and is complaining of nausea. Her initial ECG shows 1.5 mm ST-segment elevations in leads III and aVF. The diagnosis is most likely:

A. Peptic ulcer disease

B. Appendicitis

C. Acute myocardial infarction most likely due to thrombotic occlusion of the RCA branch

D. None of the above

QUESTION 3. Which of the following factors is NOT associated with an added risk for adverse outcomes in a patient diagnosed with NSTE-ACS?

A. Presenting at age 70 years
B. Having a history of hypertension, high cholesterol, and diabetes
C. Having taken an aspirin every day for the prior 3 months
D. Having a prior history of pneumonia
E. Having ST-segment depressions of 0.5 mm in leads V5 and V6

QUESTION 4. Which of the following factors would disqualify a patient with STEMI from being eligible for fibrinolytic therapy?

A. Presenting within 2 hours of symptom onset
B. Presenting within 10 hours of symptom onset
C. Lack of resources to perform a PCI within 90 minutes of first medical contact
D. History of a 1-cm intracranial AVM diagnosed 9 months ago
E. Active menstruation

QUESTION 5. A 72-year-old woman presents with dyspnea, a blood pressure of 95/50, ST-segment elevations in V2 through V5, and bilateral pulmonary edema on chest x-ray. She becomes more hypotensive as well as progressively obtunded and requires intubation. Arrangements for emergent PCI are being made. A bedside echocardiogram shows a severely depressed ejection fraction, an extensive anterior wall motion abnormality, and mild mitral regurgitation. Which of the following medicines should be avoided in this patient?

A. Aspirin
B. Beta blocker
C. Unfractionated heparin
D. GP 2b/3a inhibitor
E. High-dose statin

ANSWERS

1. B
2. C
3. D
4. D
5. B

79.

VALVULAR HEART DISEASE

Christian T. Ruff and Patrick T. O'Gara

Valvular heart disease is frequently encountered in clinical practice. The prevalence of moderate to severe valvular heart disease in the United States is estimated to be 2.5% and increases significantly with age for both men and women. Whereas rheumatic disease remains a public health issue in many developing countries, degenerative diseases such as those associated with myxomatous replacement and degeneration predominate in industrialized countries. The physiological importance of valvular heart disease relates to its effects on cardiopulmonary performance. Symptom onset equates with a distinct change in natural history. The development of atrial fibrillation (AF), ventricular remodeling, hypertrophy, and/or pump dysfunction impacts long-term survival. Diagnosis is most commonly triggered by the appreciation of a heart murmur, following which a decision is made regarding the need for echocardiography for further assessment. Many heart murmurs are benign and need not prompt additional testing. Institution of medical therapy to ameliorate symptoms or prevent complications, such as the use of vitamin K antagonists for patients, should be coupled with an appraisal of the indications for surgical or percutaneous intervention. An integrated understanding of natural history based on the severity of the valve lesion within the context of individual patient comorbidities is the foundation for appropriate clinical decision making. We review here the major valve lesions; treatment and prevention of infective endocarditis are covered elsewhere.

MITRAL STENOSIS

ETIOLOGY AND PATHOLOGY

Two-thirds of all patients with mitral stenosis (MS) are women. MS is predominantly rheumatic in origin and rarely congenital. Often, there is coexistent mitral regurgitation (MR) and/or aortic valve disease. The incidence of MS has declined in developed nations due to a reduction in the incidence of streptococcal-mediated acute rheumatic fever, but it remains a major problem in developing nations. Less common causes include severe mitral annular calcification with leaflet involvement, a large left atrial myxoma, and congenital deformity of the valve apparatus.

The pathology of rheumatic MS involves thickening and scarring of the leaflets with fibrous tissue replacement and calcification. Fusion of the commissures and involvement of the subvalvular apparatus with fusion and foreshortening of the chordae tendineae result in a rigid, narrowed, funnel-shaped valve with a "fish mouth" appearance. The left atrium (LA) enlarges, and thrombi can develop with AF.

PATHOPHYSIOLOGY

In normal adults, the cross-sectional area of the mitral valve is 4–6 cm². Significant obstruction with alteration of hemodynamic function occurs when the orifice is 2 cm² (mild MS). Severe MS results when the mitral valve opening is reduced to 1.0 cm² or less. When MS becomes significant, LA pressure rises to maintain normal cardiac output. Chronically, this increase in LA pressure will lead to elevated pulmonary venous and arterial pressures, with a reduction in pulmonary compliance. Pulmonary artery hypertension results in right ventricular enlargement, and secondary tricuspid regurgitation (TR), and right-sided heart failure. Alternatively, the tricuspid valve may be primarily affected by the rheumatic process.

SYMPTOMS

The latent period between acute rheumatic carditis and the development of symptoms is variable, ranging from a few years to more than two decades. The initial symptoms are predominantly exertional dyspnea and fatigue, reflecting elevated LA/pulmonary artery wedge pressures and reduced cardiac output. Before the development of mitral valvotomy (see below), death usually occurred within 2–5 years from onset of symptoms. Symptoms are precipitated when a "stressor" causes LA pressures to rise acutely. Examples of such triggers include exercise, infection, anemia, rapid AF or other tachycardia, pregnancy, and thyrotoxicosis. As MS progresses, lesser degrees of stress can precipitate symptoms. Symptoms and signs of left-sided heart failure—orthopnea, paroxysmal nocturnal dyspnea, and pulmonary edema—can occur. Atrial arrhythmias, particularly AF, occur with increasing frequency as MS progresses. Pulmonary infections (bronchitis and pneumonia) are common, especially in the winter months. Systemic and pulmonary emboli (frequently from the enlarged atrial appendages of patients in AF) are an important cause of morbidity and mortality. Hemoptysis may occur with pulmonary infarction, pulmonary edema, pneumonia, or rupture of an engorged bronchial vein into the airway. With bronchial venous rupture, the sputum is bright red and not "blood tinged." Bleeding of this nature is very rare and usually subsides spontaneously.

PHYSICAL EXAMINATION

Inspection may be completely normal, but in some patients with severe MS a malar flush with pink/purplish telangiectasias may be observed. Patients in AF will have an irregular pulse. If severe pulmonary hypertension is present and the patient is in sinus rhythm, prominent *a* waves can be seen in the jugular venous waveform. Large *v* waves indicate TR. Palpation may reveal a parasternal lift due to an enlarged or pressure-overloaded right ventricle (RV). Stigmata of right-sided heart failure (hepatomegaly, ascites, peripheral edema) are observed with chronic, severe MS that has led to PA hypertension and RV decompensation. A loud first heart sound (S1) is heard in the early stages of the disease. Its intensity diminishes as the valve becomes more calcified and rigid. The intensity of the pulmonic component (P2) of the second heart sound (S2) increases as PA pressures rise. The opening snap (OS) is heard best when listening over the apex in the left lateral decubitus position in expiration and is followed by a low-pitched, rumbling, diastolic murmur. The time interval between S2 and the OS is inversely related to the height of the LA pressure. The OS fades as the valve becomes less pliable with time. Presystolic accentuation of the diastolic rumble can be appreciated in some patients in sinus rhythm but is not present once AF intervenes.

LABORATORY EVALUATION

The electrocardiogram (EKG) may show AF, a LA abnormality, or signs of RV hypertrophy. On chest roentgenogram (CXR), there may be straightening of the left-heart border and prominence of the pulmonary arteries. Kerley B lines are present when marked elevations in LA pressure result in chronic interstitial edema. Transthoracic echocardiography (TTE) is the most sensitive and specific noninvasive imaging test for the diagnosis and assessment of

MS. The evaluation should provide information regarding the morphologic appearance of the MV apparatus, peak and mean pressure gradients, MV area, presence of mitral regurgitation (MR) or other valvular pathology, estimated PA systolic pressure, and ventricular function. The findings can be used to determine suitability for percutaneous mitral balloon valvotomy (PMBV); left- and right-heart catheterization is useful when there is a discrepancy between the clinical and TTE findings.

TREATMENT

Prophylaxis for prevention of infective endocarditis (IE) is no longer recommended in the absence of a history of previous IE. Prophylaxis for secondary prevention of rheumatic fever should be provided according to current guidelines. Symptomatic patients benefit from oral diuretics and sodium restriction. If AF is present, beta blockers, nondihydropyridine calcium antagonists, and digitalis glycosides help provide rate control. Anticoagulation is indicated if AF is present and/or in any patient with a prior embolic event or known LA thrombus.

Mitral valvotomy can be performed surgically or percutaneously with a balloon and is indicated in symptomatic patients with isolated moderate to severe MS (valve area 1.5 cm^2 or 1.0 cm^2/m^2 body surface area). PMBV is also indicated in asymptomatic patients with moderate to severe MS and significant pulmonary hypertension (pulmonary artery systolic pressure >50 mm Hg at rest or >60 mm Hg with exercise). Ideal patients for PMBV have relatively mobile, thin leaflets without extensive calcification, subvalvular thickening, or significant MR, as assessed by TTE. An "echo score" derived from an integrated assessment of leaflet rigidity, thickening, calcification, and subvalvular disease provides a method to identify which patients would predictably benefit from a percutaneous approach. A score of ≤8 is considered favorable, and long-term results in appropriately selected patients are comparable to those achieved with surgery. A surgical approach (repair or replacement) is necessary in patients with significant MR (>2+) or persistent LA thrombus (table 79.1).

MITRAL REGURGITATION

ETIOLOGY AND PATHOLOGY

Mitral regurgitation (MR) is caused by a myriad of conditions that may affect the leaflets, annulus, chordae tendineae, papillary muscles, or subjacent left ventricular (LV) myocardium. They include myxomatous replacement, rheumatic disease, IE, cardiomyopathy with LV remodeling, ischemia, congenital anomalies, and degenerative calcification of the mitral annulus. MR results in progressive LA and LV enlargement, which, in turn, causes more MR.

Table 79.1 MANAGEMENT OF MITRAL STENOSIS

	Medical Management		
Rheumatic fever prophylaxis for appropriate patients			
Rate or rhythm control and anticoagulation for atrial fibrillation			
Diuretics and sodium restriction when indicated by dyspnea and heart failure			

Percutaneous Mitral Balloon Valvotomy (PMBV)		
Favorable valve morphology		Symptoms + MVA ≤1.5 cm²
		OR
Absence of left atrial thrombus	+	Asymptomatic + MVA ≤1.5 cm² + PASP >50 mm Hg at rest or >60 mm Hg with exercise
		OR
Absence of moderate/severe MR		Symptoms + MVA > 1.5 cm² + PASP > 50 mm Hg at rest or > 60 mm Hg with exercise

Mitral Valve Surgery (Repair or Replacement)		
Not a candidate for PMBV	+	Symptoms + MVA ≤ 1.5 cm²

PATHOPHYSIOLOGY

It is important to recognize the pathophysiological differences between acute and chronic MR. In acute severe MR, a significant volume load is delivered into an unprepared and relatively noncompliant LA, resulting in a significant rise in LA pressure and symptoms and signs of pulmonary edema. In chronic severe MR, the LA enlarges gradually, and its compliance characteristics are maintained. LA pressure does not rise precipitously, and the volume overload may be well tolerated for many years. Eventually, however, the LV dilates, and its contractile performance declines, leading to hemodynamic derangements and symptoms of heart failure. The natural history of the disease may be punctuated by AF or some other insult (chordal rupture, MI, IE, etc.) with more abrupt clinical deterioration (acute on chronic MR).

SYMPTOMS

Acute severe MR may develop in the setting of an acute MI, IE, or blunt chest wall trauma. Symptoms are related chiefly to the resultant pulmonary edema and include severe dyspnea, air hunger, restlessness, diaphoresis, and apprehension. Early symptoms with chronic severe MR include fatigue and decreased exercise tolerance due to the progressive reduction in forward cardiac output. Eventually, symptoms of pulmonary congestion will develop.

PHYSICAL EXAMINATION

With acute severe MR, the LV apical impulse is hyperdynamic but neither displaced nor enlarged. A left parasternal pulsation transmitted from systolic LA expansion may

be felt. The systolic murmur is of relatively short duration, decrescendo in its configuration, and of grade 3 or less intensity. It is best heard at the apex or toward the left lower sternal border. These characteristics derive from the rapid rise in LA pressure and the continued decline in the pressure gradient during the first half of systole. The murmur may not be audible in a ventilated patient with a large chest. In chronic severe MR, the LV impulse may be enlarged and displaced laterally. A loud S2 suggests pulmonary hypertension. The murmur may be holosystolic in timing and plateau in configuration. Radiation of the murmur reflects the direction of the MR jet. With central MR, the murmur typically radiates into the axilla. In patients with posterior leaflet prolapse or flail, the jet is directed anteriorly, and thus the murmur radiates to the base, where it may masquerade as aortic stenosis. Anterior leaflet prolapse or flail is associated with a posteriorly directed jet and a murmur that can be heard in the axilla or back. There is great individual variability. MV prolapse may be accompanied by a nonejection click, heard after the onset of the carotid upstroke. With severe MR, a short diastolic filling complex may be heard, comprising a third sound followed by a low-pitched murmur, and is attributable to enhanced, rapid LV filling. Bedside maneuvers are often employed to help identify a systolic murmur as mitral in origin. With hand grip and an increase in LV afterload, the MR murmur becomes louder. The click and murmur of MV prolapse move closer to S1 with rapid standing from a squatting position, as LV preload is abruptly decreased. With squatting, the click and murmur move away from S1, signifying the later onset of leaflet prolapse with increased LV preload. The midsystolic murmur associated with hypertrophic obstructive cardiomyopathy (HOCM) behaves in a similar fashion.

LABORATORY EVALUATION

EKG signs of LA enlargement should be sought in the presence of sinus rhythm. AF occurs commonly in patients with severe MR and often marks the onset of symptoms. In the acute setting, the EKG may show signs of an inferior or posterior MI. Increased LV voltage owing to eccentric hypertrophy is often observed in patients with chronic severe MR. The CXR may show evidence of LA or LV enlargement, depending on the clinical context and chronicity of the MR. With acute severe MR, there is often dense alveolar pulmonary edema despite a normal heart size. On rare occasion, the edema may be asymmetric and follow the course of the regurgitant jet into one or the other upper lobe pulmonary veins (right > left). Pulmonary venous redistribution and Kerley B lines are indicative of chronically elevated left-sided filling pressures. TTE is indicated to define the mechanism and severity of the MR, assess chamber sizes and ventricular function, and estimate PA pressures. The findings often dictate the timing of surgery. Serial TTE studies are an important component of longitudinal follow-up. Transesophageal echocardiography (TEE) may be needed for greater clarification of the anatomic and physiological findings in some patients. Three-dimensional TEE is usually reserved for intraoperative assessment and surgical planning. Cardiac MRI can be used to provide an accurate and semiquantitative assessment of MR severity in patients with suboptimal echocardiographic studies. Left- and right-heart catheterization is pursued when there is a discrepancy between the clinical and noninvasive findings. Routine coronary angiography prior to anticipated surgery can be performed invasively or using computed tomography (CT) techniques. The clinical context might also dictate the need for invasive angiography, as for example, with post-MI acute MR or chronic, ischemic MR.

TREATMENT

Surgery is required for treatment of acute severe MR (table 79.2). The type of operation is dictated by the anatomic findings and the presence or absence of coronary artery disease (CAD). Repair is preferred over replacement whenever possible given its more favorable effect on LV function, a lesser need for anticoagulation, and greater preservation of native valve tissue. Temporizing medical measures include diuretics for pulmonary congestion, sodium

Table 79.2 **MITRAL REGURGITATION: INDICATIONS FOR SURGERY**

Symptomatic patients with acute or chronic severe MR and EF >0.30
Asymptomatic patients with chronic severe MR and LV dysfunction
 (EF< 0.60 and/or LV end-systolic dimension ≥40 mm)
MV repair preferable to MV replacement when anatomically feasible

nitroprusside for rapid preload and afterload reduction, inotropic therapy as required, and intra-aortic balloon counterpulsation if needed. Management of chronic MR is focused on early identification of the indications for elective surgery in appropriate candidates, including onset of symptoms, LV ejection fraction (EF) ≤0.60, and/or LV end-systolic dimension ≥4.0 cm. Surgery is also reasonable in asymptomatic patients with PA hypertension or recent-onset AF. Some authorities advocate surgery for patients with severe MR who have none of these other indications provided there is a high likelihood of successful and durable repair in experienced hands. Vasodilators are not indicated in the absence of systemic hypertension or LV systolic dysfunction. Rhythm management is similar to that for patients with MS; anticoagulation is provided once AF intervenes. Treatment of angina for patients with ischemic MR follows standard principles.

MITRAL VALVE PROLAPSE

ETIOLOGY AND PATHOLOGY

Mitral valve prolapse (MVP) occurs in 1–2% of the general population with a female predominance and has a variable clinical course. The etiology is most often related to myxomatous replacement of mitral leaflet tissue. MVP occurs in patients with Marfan syndrome and similar connective tissue diseases but most often develops spontaneously. Two types of myxomatous change are described: fibroelastic deficiency (classic MVP) and Barlow disease, which refers to an extreme form of leaflet redundancy and billowing. Myomatous MV disease is by far the most common cause of MR for which surgery is required.

PATHOPHYSIOLOGY

Prolapse is defined by the superior displacement of one or both MV leaflets above the annular plane at end-systole. Lack of leaflet coaptation leads to MR, the severity of which can worsen with chordal rupture, flail, and/or annular dilatation. The MR is usually eccentric and directed opposite to the involved leaflet. With bi-1eaflet prolapse, the MR can be central or eccentric. Changes in LA and LV size and function then follow along the same course as expected for MR of other etiology.

SYMPTOMS

The clinical course is frequently benign. Patients may experience premature ventricular or atrial contractions and paroxysmal supraventricular (including PAF) and ventricular tachycardia, precipitating palpitations, lightheadedness, or syncope. Sudden death is very rare. Patients may report chest pain, although the mechanism is unclear.

A variety of other disorders have been associated with MVP, including migraine, stroke, transient ischemic attacks (TIAs), hypercoagulability, and panic, though a cause-and-effect relationship has not been consistently established. Many patients have hypermobile joints, thoracic spine disease, or inguinal hernias. IE can be the presenting illness.

PHYSICAL EXAMINATION

Classically, auscultation reveals a mid- to late systolic click murmur complex best heard at the lower left sternal border or apex. The changes in the timing of the click and murmur with standing and squatting as previously described are useful adjuncts to correct bedside diagnosis.

LABORATORY EVALUATION

The EKG is usually unremarkable but may show biphasic or inverted T waves in the inferior and apical leads. The diagnosis is confirmed with TTE, which also allows characterization of MR severity, ventricular function, and suitability for valve repair if indicated. TEE can provide superior visualization if needed for clinical decision making.

TREATMENT

Most patients do not require any specific therapy. Treatment of symptomatic arrhythmias may be required, and often beta blockers will be of use. Indications for MV repair are as discussed previously. Posterior leaflet repair is technically easier and more durable than anterior or bileaflet repair. The latter often requires construction of neochordae and/or chordal transposition. Posterior leaflet repair should be feasible in >95% of patients with this anatomy.

AORTIC STENOSIS

ETIOLOGY AND PATHOLOGY

Bicuspid aortic valve and its congenital variants (e.g., unicuspid valve) are now recognized as the most common causes of aortic stenosis requiring valve replacement surgery. Bicuspid disease is often familial and may be accompanied by aortic coarctation. Age-related calcific degeneration of a trileaflet valve is the second most common cause of AS. Rheumatic disease is rarely encountered in developed countries. Degenerative valve disease and atherosclerosis share several common risk factors, histopathologic characteristics, and pathogenetic traits. Some studies suggest that aggressive lipid reduction may retard the rate of progression of some forms of AS. In older adults with AS, the prevalence of significant CAD exceeds 50%.

PATHOPHYSIOLOGY

The obstruction to LV outflow produces a systolic pressure gradient between the LV and the aorta. Concentric LV hypertrophy develops gradually in response to the pressure overload and to normalize wall stress. Initially, cardiac output is preserved, and LV chamber dimensions are preserved. Diastolic performance is altered by the hypertrophy and interstitial fibrosis; LV diastolic pressure is increased. Ultimately, with unrelieved obstruction of sufficient magnitude, the LV pump failure occurs with dilation of the cavity and reduction in cardiac output. Severe AS is defined by a valve area of < 1.0 cm². In the presence of normal LV systolic function, severe AS is also characterized by a peak transvalvular jet velocity of ≥4 m/sec and mean valve gradient of ≥40 mm Hg.

SYMPTOMS/NATURAL HISTORY

Symptoms are rarely present until the valve obstruction is severe because of the ability of the hypertrophied LV to maintain a normal stroke volume. Although the rate of progression of AS varies among individual patients, longitudinal echocardiographic studies have suggested an average increase in mean gradient of 7 mm Hg/year and decrease in valve area of 0.1 cm²/year. Both the peak jet velocity and the severity of valve calcification are predictive of event-free survival. The cardinal symptoms of AS are exertional dyspnea, angina, and syncope. Although these symptoms are usually not apparent in patients with degenerative AS until the sixth to eighth decade, an insidious history of decreasing exercise tolerance and fatigue is often elicited, as may also be the case with younger patients with bicuspid disease. Symptoms or signs of more advanced left- or right-heart failure are ominous.

The natural history of untreated severe AS has been well documented. The average time to death from the onset of angina, syncope, and dyspnea are 5 years, 3 years, and 2 years, respectively. Heart failure and ventricular arrhythmias are the most common causes of death. Sudden death as the manifestation of severe AS in adult patients is very rare.

PHYSICAL EXAMINATION

The carotid or brachial artery pulse is characteristically reduced in amplitude and rises slowly to its peak (*pulsus parvus et tardus*), although arterial wall stiffening may mask this finding in the elderly. LV hypertrophy can be detected by a forceful, sustained apical impulse. A systolic thrill present at the base of the heart that tracks along the carotid arteries suggests significant stenosis. As AS progresses, LV systole is prolonged, moving the closure of the aortic valve (A2) closer to that of the pulmonic valve (P2). Eventually, A2 becomes inaudible and S2 single. Paradoxical splitting of S2 may also occur. An S4 is invariably present in sinus rhythm secondary to LV hypertrophy. An S3 signifies elevated LV end-diastolic pressures in a dilated ventricle. The murmur of AS is typically a loud (at least grade III/IV) diamond-shaped ejection murmur that begins after S1 and is heard best at the base of the heart in the right second intercostal space with radiation to the carotid arteries. It is important to note that in patients with severe stenosis and LV failure, the murmur may be soft and brief due to reduced transvalvular flow rates. A systolic ejection click is audible in many young patients with bicuspid disease. A diastolic murmur of aortic regurgitation signifies mixed disease.

LABORATORY EVALUATION

The EKG commonly shows LV hypertrophy with associated repolarization abnormalities ("LV strain pattern"). The chest may be unremarkable. Calcium in the region of the aortic valve should be assessed on the lateral film. Dilatation of the ascending aorta may signify aneurysm. Signs of aortic coarctation should be sought in young patients with bicuspid disease. TTE is essential in the diagnosis and management of AS. Leaflet number, morphology, calcification, and excursion are noted. Measurement of the trans-aortic valve velocity with pulsed wave Doppler can be used to estimate AS severity. LV size and function are important in clinical management, as is the presence or absence of concomitant ascending aorta dilatation. Left-heart catheterization and coronary angiography are routinely performed in older adult patients with severe AS referred for surgery or in patients with AS and symptoms of myocardial ischemia.

TREATMENT

The medical treatment is quite limited, and AS should be thought of as a surgical disease (table 79.3). As noted,

Table 79.3 **MANAGEMENT OF AORTIC STENOSIS**

Clinical Indicators of Severe Aortic Stenosis
Cardinal symptoms
• Exertional dyspnea
• Angina
• Syncope
Physical examination
• Carotid pulse weak with slow rise (pulsus parvus et tardus)
• Late-peaking diamond-shaped systolic murmur with single S_2
TTE
• Valve area <1.0 cm^2
• Mean gradient >40 mm Hg
• Jet velocity >4 m/sec
Indications for Aortic Valve Replacement
• Symptoms + severe AS
• Severe AS + undergoing CABG, surgery on aorta, or replacement of another valve
• Severe AS + LV dysfunction (EF <50%)

high-dose statin therapy may retard the rate of progression of calcific aortic stenosis, but data are limited. Patients with severe AS should be advised to avoid strenuous physical activity.

When heart failure is present, sodium restriction and the cautious administration of diuretics are indicated, but care must be taken to avoid volume depletion, which can cause a dangerous and potentially fatal decline in cardiac output. The critical management decision is the timing of surgical referral for aortic valve replacement (AVR). Surgery is indicated in symptomatic patients with severe AS (valve area 1.0 cm^2 or 0.6 cm^2/m^2). In asymptomatic patients with severe AS, surgery is indicated if LV dysfunction or aortic root dilation (>4.5 cm) are present. The operative risk is considerably higher, and long-term survival is diminished, in patients with significant LV dysfunction, so it is imperative to intervene before this advanced stage. Aortocoronary bypass grafting is performed with AVR in patients with coexisting coronary artery disease. AVR can be considered for treatment of moderate AS (valve area 1.0–1.5 cm^2) when surgery is perfumed for another indication (such as coronary artery bypass graft [CABG]. Percutaneous aortic balloon valvuloplasty is commonly performed in children and young adults with congenital AS and pliable valve leaflets without significant AR. It is not nearly as successful in adults because of high procedural morbidity and excessive rates of restenosis but may have a role as a temporary "bridge" to AVR in patients with significant comorbid conditions or shock.

AORTIC REGURGITATION

ETIOLOGY AND PATHOLOGY

Aortic regurgitation (AR) is caused by primary valve disease and/or as a consequence of aortic root disease. Valvular AR may be caused by congenital bicuspid aortic valve disease, myxomatous disease with prolapse, IE, or rheumatic disease. Aortic root disease leads to AR because of annular enlargement or deformation with subsequent impairment of leaflet coaptation. Causes of aortic root disease include hypertension, cystic medial degeneration (as seen with Marfan syndrome), inflammatory aortitis (ankylosing spondylitis, Reiter syndrome), and acute aortic dissection. Syphilitic aortitis is rarely seen in the current era.

PATHOPHYSIOLOGY

In acute severe AR, the unprepared LV operates on the steep portion of its diastolic pressure-volume relationship. LV diastolic pressure rises rapidly, and pulmonary edema follows. Forward LV stroke volume is compromised, and the heart rate increases to maintain cardiac output. The rate of rise of LV pressure dictates that the diastolic murmur is of short duration and relatively low intensity. With chronic AR, the LV undergoes compensatory dilatation and eccentric hypertrophy, which allow the preservation of a normal "effective" forward stroke volume, EF, and diastolic performance. Chronic AR is a state of excess preload and afterload. Eventually, afterload mismatch or preload exhaustion will occur to the extent that LV function will decline and symptoms develop.

SYMPTOMS

Patients with acute severe AR present with profound dyspnea, weakness, and signs of shock. Other symptoms or signs may provide clues as to the etiology of the AR, such as severe chest pain in patients with aortic dissection or fever and embolic phenomena in patients with IE. Patients with chronic AR may remain asymptomatic for years. Palpitations are common and usually attribute to isolated premature beats. Eventually, uncorrected chronic severe AR will lead to dyspnea as a manifestation of LV dysfunction. Anginal chest pain may occur in the absence of epicardial vessel atherosclerosis due to inadequate coronary driving pressure in the face of excess demand. Angina, orthopnea, and paroxysmal nocturnal dyspnea are all indicative of important LV compromise for which urgent intervention is warranted.

PHYSICAL EXAMINATION

The examination findings in acute severe AR are often subtle and can be easily missed. They include a soft S1 (due to premature close of the mitral valve); a short, soft, diastolic murmur and the absence of signs of severe diastolic runoff. The systolic blood pressure is not elevated, and the diastolic blood pressure does not reach the low levels seen with chronic AR. Thus, the pulse pressure in acute AR may not be appreciably widened. The eponymous findings in chronic AR have been the subject of many textbooks of cardiology. Classic findings include systolic hypertension, low diastolic pressure, a wide pulse pressure, and a rapid rise and fall of the arterial upstroke (Corrigan or water-hammer pulse). Lower extremity blood pressure is typically >10 mm Hg above the upper extremity blood pressure (Smith sign), and the magnitude of this difference may reflect the qualitative severity of the AR. Korotkoff sounds may be heard throughout full deflation of the blood pressure cuff (pistol shots), light pressure over the tips of the fingernails may cause systolic and diastolic blushing of the nail capillaries near their base (Quincke pulsation), or a diastolic bruit may be heard over the femoral artery as the pressure with which the diaphragm of the stethoscope is applied is gradually lessened (Duroziez sign). The carotid upstrokes may rarely be bisferiens (bifid). The second peak occurs prior to aortic valve closure. Palpation reveals a heaving, laterally displaced LV. The diastolic murmur of AR is typically high-pitched and decrescendo, heard best along the left sternal border,

especially when the patient is in the sitting position, leaning forward, at end-expiration. When the murmur is louder to the right of the sternum, aortic root disease should be suspected, as would also be the case with palpation of a pulsatile ascending aorta in the upper right parasternal area. The Austin Flint murmur in mid- to late diastole is better heard near the apex. It is created by an eccentric jet of AR striking the anterior MV leaflet. It can be distinguished from the diastolic murmur of MS on the basis of its response to vasodilators (decreases in intensity) and by the absence of other trappings of MS, such as an opening snap or atrial fibrillation. A systolic ejection click would suggest bicuspid valve disease. The examination should account for signs of underlying diseases such as Marfan syndrome (general appearance), IE (embolic phenomena, fever), or ankylosing spondylitis (bamboo spine).

LABORATORY EVALUATION

In chronic AR, there is EKG evidence of LVH and repolarization abnormalities. The CXR shows cardiomegaly with LV enlargement. The aorta may be ectatic or aneurysmal, though such changes may be difficult to discern. TTE is indicated to evaluate the mechanism of AR, quantitate its severity, assess LV size and systolic function, and examine the anatomy of the root and ascending aorta. If the aorta cannot be adequately visualized with TTE, then CT angiography, magnetic resonance imaging (MRI) or TEE should be performed, whenever there is suspicion of aortic pathology. Cardiac MRI can also provide excellent quantitation of AR severity. Cardiac catheterization with contrast aortography can provide supplemental information in difficult cases, but is now mainly employed to assess coronary anatomy preoperatively.

TREATMENT

Acute, severe AR is poorly tolerated, and appropriate patients should be evaluated for emergency surgery, the nature of which depends on the cause of the AR (table 79.4). Medical treatment of chronic AR should focus on blood pressure control to below 140/90 mm Hg, which can be difficult to achieve. The routine use of vasodilators to extend the compensated phase of asymptomatic AR is no longer considered strictly indicated. Indications for aortic

Table 79.4 **AORTIC REGURGITATION: INDICATIONS FOR SURGERY**

- **Symptoms + severe AR**
- **Asymptomatic + LVEF <0.50**
- **Asymptomatic with EF >0.50 and severe or progressive LV dilation (end-systolic dimension >25 mm/m² or end-systolic dimension >70 mm**
- **Moderate or severe AR and root or ascending aortic aneurysm requiring surgery**

valve replacement surgery in the chronic setting include onset of symptoms or the development of LV systolic dysfunction, defined by a resting EF that falls below the lower limit of normal for the noninvasive lab in which the patient is followed (usually 0.50). Progressive or severe LV dilatation despite preserved systolic function, approaching an end-diastolic dimension of 70–75 mm or an end-systolic dimension of 50 mm or 25 mm/m², is an additional consideration for surgery. Patients with root or ascending aortic disease with concomitant AR, especially those with bicuspid pathology or Marfan syndrome, are candidates for surgery once the maximal aortic dimension reaches or exceeds 4.5 cm. A valve-sparing root replacement procedure can often be accomplished in appropriately selected patients. Valve replacement is required for patients with deformed or calcified leaflets or enlarged annuli.

TRICUSPID STENOSIS

ETIOLOGY AND PATHOLOGY

Rheumatic heart disease is the most common cause of tricuspid stenosis (TS). In most patients, the valve pathology is mixed (TS/TR), and left-sided disease with MS is present.

PATHOPHYSIOLOGY

TS results in a diastolic pressure gradient between the right atrium (RA) and right ventricle (RV) that leads to systemic venous congestion. Cardiac output is compromised with relatively normal right ventricular and pulmonary artery pressures. The severity of concomitant MS is often underappreciated as the proximate valve lesion may mask the findings associated with the more distal valve lesion.

SYMPTOMS

Fatigue is frequent due to the low cardiac output. Systemic venous hypertension leads to peripheral edema, ascites, and hepatomegaly, which can cause significant discomfort.

PHYSICAL EXAMINATION

TS results in jugular venous distension with giant *a* waves and a slow *y* descent. Palpation and percussion of the abdomen may reveal hepatic enlargement and splenomegaly. In cases of severe hepatic congestion, cirrhosis can result in jaundice, ascites, and anasarca. Auscultation may reveal an opening snap of the tricuspid valve with a diastolic murmur heard best along the lower left sternal border. The murmur of TS is augmented during inspiration, which helps distinguish it from the murmur of MS. Most often, the auscultatory findings are dominated by valve disease.

LABORATORY EVALUATION

The EKG demonstrates RA enlargement or AF. The chest reveals a prominent RA. TTE is used to identify a thickened, rheumatic valve, measure the transvalvular gradient, and assess the severity of obstruction (tricuspid valve area) as well as the presence of any TR or left-sided disease.

TREATMENT

Medical therapy with salt restriction and diuretics helps relieve the symptoms of venous congestion. Surgery is recommended in symptomatic patients with moderate to severe TS (valve area <2.0 cm², mean transvalvular gradient >4 mm Hg). Valve repair/commissurotomy is preferable to replacement when feasible.

TRICUSPID REGURGITATION

ETIOLOGY AND PATHOLOGY

Tricuspid regurgitation (TR) may be primary or secondary. Primary causes include prolapse, Ebstein anomaly, carcinoid, and endocarditis. Secondary TR, which is much more common, is due to dilatation of the annulus from right ventricular enlargement in response to pulmonary artery hypertension of any etiology, cardiomyopathy, or primary pulmonic valve regurgitation.

PATHOPHYSIOLOGY

With tricuspid regurgitation, blood is ejected back into the RA during systole, resulting in the inscription of large *cv* waves in the RA pulse wave. Progressively severe TR leads to the ventricularization of the RA wave form. The RV becomes more dilated and volume overloaded.

Forward cardiac output is reduced, and atrial arrhythmias are common. Hepatic function may decline.

SYMPTOMS

Fatigue from a low cardiac output is frequent. Right-sided heart failure symptoms such as hepatomegaly, ascites, and peripheral edema predominate.

PHYSICAL EXAMINATION

Examination reveals elevation of the jugular venous pressure with prominent, systolic *cv* waves. Hepatomegaly, which may be pulsatile, ascites, and peripheral edema are common. Palpation of the heart reveals a parasternal RV lift. Auscultation is notable for a holosystolic murmur at the lower left sternal border that increases with inspiration (Carvallo's sign).

LABORATORY EVALUATION

The EKG may show signs of either RA enlargement or RVH. AF may be present. The CXR may demonstrate RA and RV enlargement. TTE is indicated to assess the mechanism of TR, quantify its severity, estimate PA pressures, examine RV size and function, and screen for the presence of left-sided heart disease.

TREATMENT

The treatment of TR depends in large measure on whether it is primary or secondary. On rare occasion, severe primary TR will necessitate valve repair or replacement if symptoms are not easily controlled with low-dose diuretic therapy. Often, the severity of secondary TR will diminish with successful treatment of the left-sided heart disease or pulmonary hypertension that caused it. In patients with mitral and tricuspid valve disease, intraoperative assessment of TR severity before and after MV surgery, with measurement of tricuspid valve annulus size, is required before a final decision is made regarding the need for concomitant tricuspid valve surgery.

PROSTHETIC VALVES

The major differences between mechanical and bioprosthetic (tissue) heart valve substitutes relate to durability and thrombogenicity. Mechanical valves are more durable and last longer but necessitate the use of lifelong anticoagulant therapy with vitamin K antagonists to prevent valve thrombosis and embolism. Bioprosthetic valves are less durable and prone to structural deterioration within 10–15 years of implantation but do not require anticoagulant therapy. The choice of heart valve substitute varies on an individual basis as a function of age, the desirability of future pregnancy, medical adherence, and lifestyle. In recent years, the pendulum has swung considerably in favor of tissue valve substitutes, primarily because of the problems associated with long-term anticoagulation. A tissue valve is generally recommended for patients over the age of 65 years. Younger patients who choose a tissue valve substitute in order to avoid anticoagulation must accept the need for reoperative surgery in the future. Antibiotic prophylaxis is indicated for any patient with a heart valve substitute or prior valve repair with ring annuloplasty.

ADDITIONAL READING

American College of Cardiology, American Heart Association Task Force on Practice Guidelines (Writing Committee to Revise the 1998 Guidelines for the Management of Patients with Valvular Heart Disease), Society of Cardiovascular Anesthesiologists, et al. ACC/AHA 2006 guidelines for the management of patients with valvular heart disease: A report of the American College of Cardiology/American Heart Association task force on practice guidelines (writing committee to revise the 1998 guidelines for the management of patients with valvular heart disease) developed in collaboration with the Society of Cardiovascular Anesthesiologists endorsed by the Society for Cardiovascular Angiography and Interventions and the Society of Thoracic Surgeons. *J Am Coll Cardiol.* 2006;48(3):e1–148.

Braunwald E. Valvular heart disease. In: Kasper DL, Braunwald E, Fauci AS, Hauser SL, Longo DL, Jameson JL (eds.). *Harrison's Principles of Internal Medicine.* 16th ed. New York: McGraw-Hill Medical Publishing Division; 2005: 1390.

Cheitlin MD, Armstrong WF, Aurigemma GP, et al. ACC/AHA/ASE 2003 guideline update for the clinical application of echocardiography—summary article: A report of the American College of Cardiology/American Heart Association task force on practical guidelines (ACC/AHA/ASE committee to update the 1997 guidelines for the clinical application of echocardiography). *J Am Coll Cardiol.* 2003;42(5):954–70.

Irwin RB, Luckie M, Khattar RS. Tricuspid regurgitation: Contemporary management of a neglected valvular lesion. *Postgrad Med J.* 2010;86(1021):648–55.

Foster E. Clinical practice. Mitral regurgitation due to degenerative mitral-valve disease. *N Engl J Med.* 2010;363(2):156–65.

Kurtz CE, Otto CM. Aortic stenosis: Clinical aspects of diagnosis and management, with 10 illustrative case reports from a 25-year experience. *Medicine (Baltimore).* 2010;89(6):349–79.

Otto CM, Bonow RO. Valvular heart disease. In: Libby P, Bonow RO, Mann DL, Zipes DP (eds.). *Braunwald's Heart Disease: A Textbook of Cardiovascular Medicine.* 8th ed. Philadelphia: Saunders; 2008: 1625.

Vahanian A, Baumgartner H, Bax J, et al. Guidelines on the management of valvular heart disease: The task force on the management of valvular heart disease of the European Society of Cardiology. *Eur Heart J.* 2007;28(2):230–68.

QUESTIONS

QUESTION 1. An asymptomatic 67-year-old man is referred by his primary care physician for evaluation of a heart murmur. He has not seen a physician regularly since he retired 10 years ago. He takes no medications.

The heart rate is 82 bpm, and blood pressure 147/85 mm Hg. Examination reveals an enlarged and laterally displaced LV impulse. A 3/6 holosystolic murmur is heard at the apex with radiation to the base. His jugular venous pressure is elevated. The rest of the examination is unremarkable.

EKG shows normal sinus rhythm with evidence of left atrial enlargement. TTE reveals thickening of the mitral valve with partial flail of the posterior leaflet. There is an anteriorly directed jet of severe mitral regurgitation. The left atrium and ventricle are dilated (LV end-systolic dimension 4.7 cm). Estimated LV EF is 40%.

Which of the following treatment strategies would you recommend?

A. Medical therapy with an ACE inhibitor with repeat echocardiogram in 6 weeks
B. No medical therapy but watchful waiting with close clinical follow-up for symptoms
C. Referral for mitral valve replacement
D. Referral for mitral valve repair
E. Medical therapy with a diuretic and exercise echocardiography

QUESTION 2. An 18-year-old woman is referred to you for evaluation of a heart murmur first heard during a routine preparticipation college athletic physical examination. She has no significant medical history and takes no medications. She trains 6 days a week for field hockey, including long runs, sprints, and weight training. She reports being short of breath at the end of sprints but denies chest pain, dizziness, or syncope. There is no family history of premature cardiac disease or sudden cardiac death.

Her pulse is 58 bpm, and her blood pressure is 100/65 mm Hg. Cardiac auscultation reveals an ejection click and a 2/6 crescendo-decrescendo systolic murmur at the second right interspace that intensifies in the beat following a premature beat. EKG shows sinus bradycardia and normal LV voltage.

Which of the following is the most likely diagnosis?

A. Bicuspid pulmonic stenosis
B. Hypertrophic obstructive cardiomyopathy
C. Bicuspid aortic stenosis
D. Mitral valve prolapse
E. Membranous aortic stenosis

QUESTION 3. A 22-year-old woman who recently emigrated from South Africa is referred from the high-risk obstetrics clinic. She has a history of rheumatic fever as a child and has known mitral stenosis. She is 24 weeks pregnant. She complains of palpitations and shortness of breath with activities of daily living. Her medications include metoprolol, furosemide, and digoxin.

Her pulse is irregularly irregular at a rate of 110–120 bpm, and her blood pressure is 94/66 mm Hg. Her venous pressure is approximately 12 cm H_2O. She has a parasternal lift. P2 is loud. There is an opening snap and a grade 3 mid-diastolic apical rumble with presystolic accentuation. She has 1+ bilateral lower extremity edema. Echocardiogram demonstrates severe mitral stenosis with mitral valve area of 1.0 cm^2 and a low echo score. There is minimal mitral regurgitation. Estimated pulmonary artery systolic pressure is 65 mm Hg.

Which of the following treatments would you recommend?

A. Continued medical management until delivery
B. Surgical mitral commissurotomy
C. Mitral valve replacement with a bioprosthesis
D. Percutaneous mitral balloon valvotomy
E. Mitral valve replacement with a mechanical prosthesis

QUESTION 4. A 31-year-old man is brought into the emergency department after a head-on motor vehicle accident. He was intubated in the field. Triage vital signs include a heart rate of 115 bpm and blood pressure of 86/60 mm Hg. General exam is notable for presternal bruising. Cardiac auscultation reveals a regular tachycardia with a summation gallop. Soft systolic and diastolic murmurs are heard along the upper left sternal border. EKG reveals sinus tachycardia. CT scan of the chest shows multiple rib fractures and pulmonary edema. There is no pericardial effusion.

A "stat" TTE is ordered. What is the most likely next step in the patient's management?

A. Placement of an intra-aortic balloon for temporary hemodynamic support
B. Mitral valve surgery
C. Aortic valve replacement
D. Placement of a left ventricular assist device

QUESTION 5. A 45-year-old man is referred to you from the orthopedics clinic for perioperative recommendations regarding anticoagulation in anticipation of elective anterior cruciate ligament repair. Two years ago he underwent bileaflet mechanical aortic valve replacement for a bicuspid aortic valve. His medical workup is also significant for hyperlipidemia. His only medications are warfarin and simvastatin. He has had no thromboembolic complications.

Which of the following strategies would you recommend?

A. Warfarin can be discontinued. It is only indicated for the first 3 months following mechanical aortic valve replacement in patients at low risk for thromboembolism.
B. Warfarin should be stopped 48–72 hours before the procedure and restarted 24 hours after the procedure. During the interruption, he should be bridged with intravenous unfractionated heparin until his INR returns to 2.0–3.0.
C. Warfarin should be stopped 48–72 hours before the procedure and restarted 24 hours after the procedure. During the interruption he should be bridged with aspirin 325 mg until his INR returns to 2.0–3.0.
D. Warfarin should be stopped 48–72 hours before the procedure and restarted 24 hours after the procedure. During the interruption he should be bridged with intravenous unfractionated heparin until his INR returns to 2.5–3.5.
E. Warfarin should be stopped 48–72 hours before the procedure and restarted 24 hours after the procedure with a goal INR 2.0–3.0. No bridging is necessary.

ANSWERS

1. D
2. D
3. D
4. C
5. B

80.

HEART FAILURE

Garrick C. Stewart and Gilbert H. Mudge, Jr.

DEFINITION AND EPIDEMIOLOGY

Heart failure is a complex clinical syndrome occurring in patients with an abnormality of cardiac structure or function that impairs the ability of the heart to fill with or eject blood. Patients with heart failure develop a constellation of symptoms (dyspnea and fatigue) and signs (edema and rales) that lead to frequent hospitalizations, poor quality of life, and a shortened life expectancy. Heart failure has also been defined as the failure of the heart to pump enough blood to meet the metabolic demands of the body, or the ability to do so only at elevated filling pressures. Congestive heart failure is the end stage for many cardiac diseases. Cardiomyopathy refers to any condition in which there is a structural abnormality of the myocardium itself.

The overall prevalence of heart failure in adults in developed countries is 2% and rises sharply with age. After age 40 years, the lifetime risk of developing heart failure for both men and women is one in five. Over 5 million Americans are living with heart failure, and it is a contributing factor in over 250,000 deaths each year. Heart failure accounts for over $35 billion in annual health care costs in the United States and remains the leading hospital discharge diagnosis in patients over 65 years old. Nearly half of all patients with heart failure have a preserved ejection fraction (>40–50%). As such, heart failure is now broadly categorized as heart failure with depressed ejection fraction (systolic failure) or heart failure with preserved ejection fraction (diastolic failure). Other common heart failure descriptors emphasize the physiology and tempo of clinical disease. This nomenclature includes left- or right-sided or biventricular, systolic or diastolic, forward or backward, high-output or low-output, and acute or chronic failure. Specific diagnostic schemes have been proposed for heart failure, such as the Modified Framingham criteria (table 80.1).

The most popular and durable classification scheme for the severity of heart failure is the New York Heart Association (NYHA) functional class (table 80.2). Functional class is assigned based on current symptom limitation, with changing functional classes over time. There is a strong relationship between NYHA class and mortality. A newer classification scheme is the American Heart Association (AHA)/American College of Cardiology (ACC) stages of heart failure (table 80.3). These stages emphasize the progressive nature of heart failure, from antecedent risk factors to the development of structural heart disease and the evolution of symptoms that may become refractory to medical therapies.

ETIOLOGY AND PRECIPITANTS OF HEART FAILURE

Underlying and precipitating causes of heart failure must be identified when caring for patients. Risk factors for heart failure development include hypertension, coronary heart disease, valvular disease (particularly aortic stenosis and mitral regurgitation), left ventricular hypertrophy, age, and diabetes. Studies estimate that coronary artery disease accounts for approximately two-thirds of heart failure in both men and women. Meanwhile 75% of patients with heart failure have a history of hypertension, many of whom have concurrent coronary disease. The cornerstone of heart failure prevention in the community is appropriate coronary risk factor reduction, blood pressure control, along with prevention of diabetes and the metabolic syndrome.

The progression of heart failure with reduced ejection fraction is mediated by cardiac remodeling and chamber enlargement accompanied by an obligatory reduction in ejection fraction, leading to a dilated cardiomyopathy. The causes of a dilated cardiomyopathy are listed in table 80.4. Potentially reversible causes of heart failure and cardiomyopathy include myocarditis, peripartum-, stress-, tachycardia-induced, and drug-induced cardiomyopathies. The most common cause of right heart failure is left heart failure.

Heart failure is a chronic progressive disease with relapsing and remitting symptoms. Periods of relative compensation can be punctuated by exacerbations marked by signs of congestion such as dyspnea and edema, often referred to as acute decompensated heart failure. Precipitants for

Table 80.1 DIAGNOSIS OF HEART FAILURE: MODIFIED FRAMINGHAM CRITERIA

MAJOR	MINOR
Elevated jugular venous pressure	Dyspnea on exertion
Pulmonary rales	Bilateral leg edema
Paroxysmal nocturnal dyspnea	Nocturnal cough
Orthopnea	Hepatomegaly
Third heart sound (S3 gallop)	Pleural effusion
Cardiomegaly on chest radiography	Tachycardia (>120 bpm)
Pulmonary edema on chest radiography	Weight loss >4.5 kg in 5 days
Weight loss >4.5 kg in 5 days in response to diuretic therapy for presumed heart failure	

NOTE: Diagnosis requires 2 major or 1 major and 2 minor criteria to be present and not attributed to another condition.
SOURCE: McKee PA, Castelli WP, McNamara PM, Kannel WB. The natural history of congestive heart failure: The Framingham study. *N Engl J Med.* 1971;285(26):1441–6.

heart failure exacerbation are myriad and can be attributed to patient behaviors such as dietary indiscretion (increased salt or excess fluid intake) or medication noncompliance (diuretics), disturbances in cardiac function (new atrial fibrillation or acute valvular dysfunction), or concurrent medical illness (pneumonia) (see table 80.5). For example, the sudden onset of pulmonary edema and heart failure 2–7 days after inferior myocardial infarction (MI) may be the result of papillary muscle rupture and acute mitral regurgitation.

PRESENTING FEATURES AND EVALUATION OF HEART FAILURE

SYMPTOMS

Heart failure has several characteristic symptoms that vary markedly among patients. The most common symptom of heart failure is shortness of breath (dyspnea), usually on exertion, related to elevated filling pressures transmitted to stretch receptors in the lungs or an inadequate cardiac output to meet the demands of the body during exercise. Orthopnea, dyspnea when lying down, is characteristic of left-sided heart failure and is often quantified as the number of pillows used at night. Paroxysmal nocturnal dyspnea may also be present with left heart failure with patients awakening at night and needing to sit on the edge of the bed or go to the window for fresh air. Periodic breathing (Cheyne-Stokes respiration) may be present in advanced heart failure and is marked by oscillations between rapid breathing and near apnea. Occasionally, heart failure patients may prefer to lie in the right lateral decubitus position, a condition known as trepopnea.

Fatigue and exercise intolerance are also cardinal symptoms of heart failure. Fatigue not only may be present with activity but often persists for hours or days after strenuous exertion. Symptoms of anorexia and abdominal discomfort, particularly in the right upper quadrant, are common in more advanced heart failure, especially in right heart failure. Other signs of heart failure include insomnia, cough, and depression. Last, a careful history must be taken for less obvious signs of sleep apnea (snoring, daytime somnolence), an important and underappreciated comorbid condition in many heart failure patients.

It must be emphasized that there is often discordance between the severity of symptoms at presentation and the objective degree of structural heart disease.

SIGNS

The physical exam provides important information about the nature of cardiac dysfunction, degree of volume overload, adequacy of cardiac output, and the presence of concurrent circulatory abnormalities such as pulmonary hypertension. Clues to the nature of cardiac dysfunction can be found by looking for signs of systemic illness affecting the heart (e.g., hyperthyroidism) and by auscultating for cardiac murmurs that reflect underlying structural heart disease (e.g., the systolic murmur of aortic stenosis).

Table 80.2 NEW YORK HEART ASSOCIATION FUNCTIONAL CLASS

Class I: No limitation of physical activity. Ordinary physical activity does not cause undue fatigue palpitation or dyspnea (shortness of breath).

Class II: Slight limitation of physical activity. Comfortable at rest, but ordinary physical activity results in fatigue palpitation or dyspnea.

Class III: Marked limitation of physical activity. Comfortable at rest, but less than ordinary activity causes fatigue palpitation or dyspnea.

Class IV: Unable to carry out any physical activity without discomfort. Symptoms of cardiac insufficiency at rest. If any physical activity is undertaken discomfort is increased.

SOURCE: The Criteria Committee of the New York Heart Association. *Nomenclature and Criteria for Diagnosis of Diseases of the Heart and Great Vessels.* 9th ed. (pp. 253–6). Boston: Little, Brown & Co; 1994.

Table 80.3 AHA/ACC STAGES OF HEART FAILURE

Stage A: At risk for heart failure but without structural heart disease or symptoms of heart failure

Stage B: Structural heart disease but without signs or symptoms of heart failure

Stage C: Structural heart disease with prior or current symptoms of heart failure

Stage D: Refractory heart failure requiring specialized intervention (e.g., mechanical circulatory assist devices, intravenous inotropes or vasodilators)

SOURCE: Hunt SA, Abraham WT, Chin MH, et al. 2009 focused update incorporated into the ACC/AHA 2005 Guidelines for the Diagnosis and Management of Heart Failure in Adults: A report of the American College of Cardiology Foundation/American Heart Association Task Force on Practice Guidelines: Developed in collaboration with the International Society for Heart and Lung Transplantation. *Circulation.* 2009;119(14):e391–479.

Gallop rhythms are best appreciated with the stethoscope bell placed at the cardiac apex, often with the patient in the left lateral decubitus position. An S3 gallop may be heard just after the second heart sound (S2). This third heart sound results from limitation of blood flow into the ventricle during early diastole, as in dilated cardiomyopathy or significant mitral regurgitation. The presence of an S3 is highly specific for a reduced ejection fraction and elevated left-sided filling pressure and has important prognostic significance. Patients with an S3 and asymptomatic left ventricular dysfunction are more likely to develop heart failure. Those with existing heart failure with an S3 gallop are more likely to be hospitalized for heart failure and have a higher mortality. Alternatively, an S4 gallop may be heard just before S1 and reflects a stiff ventricle responding to the atrial systolic contraction and thus is absent in atrial fibrillation. S4 gallops are common in conditions leading to a noncompliant ventricle and diastolic heart failure, such as chronic hypertensive heart disease, aortic stenosis, and hypertrophic cardiomyopathy.

Ventricular enlargement can be appreciated by palpation of the precordium. Signs of left ventricular enlargement include an enlarged point of maximal impulse displaced toward the midaxillary line, a sustained apical impulse, and even a palpable S3 gallop in severe heart failure. A holosystolic murmur of mitral regurgitation is often present in the setting of left ventricular enlargement. Pulsus alternans, an evenly spaced alternation of strong and weak peripheral pulses, can be present in severe left ventricular systolic heart failure. Signs of reduced cardiac output include depressed mental status, cool and clammy extremities, pallor, oliguria, distant heart sounds, resting tachycardia, narrow pulse pressure, and hypotension.

Signs of volume overload in heart failure include pulmonary congestion, elevated jugular venous pressure (JVP) and peripheral edema. Pulmonary congestion reflects evidence of left-sided heart failure. Pulmonary rales are often most prominent at the lung bases in heart failure and reflect an elevated pulmonary capillary wedge pressure leading to increased transudation of fluid from the blood pool to the interstitium and alveoli. Rales are more commonly heard in

Table 80.4 CAUSES OF DILATED CARDIOMYOPATHY

Ischemic heart disease

Infection
  Virus: CMV, HIV, hepatitis
  Bacteria: *Streptococcus* (rheumatic fever), typhoid fever, brucellosis
  Rickettsial disease
  Parasitic disease: Chagas disease
  Lyme disease

Depositional disease
  Amyloidosis
  Hemochromatosis

Toxins
  Alcohol
  Cocaine
  Amphetamines
  Cobalt

Medication-induced
  Adriamycin (doxorubicin)
  Cyclophosphamide
  Antiretrovirals

Endocrine disorders
  Hyper- or hypothyroidism
  Pheochromocytoma
  Acromegaly
  Diabetes mellitus

Nutritional deficiencies
  Thiamine
  Selenium

Neuromuscular disorders
  Duchenne muscular dystrophy
  Friedrich ataxia
  Myotonic dystrophy

Rheumatologic disease
  Systemic lupus erythematosus
  Scleroderma

Electrolyte abnormalities
  Hypophosphatemia
  Hypocalcemia

Miscellaneous
  Peripartum cardiomyopathy
  Tachycardia-mediated cardiomyopathy
  Sarcoidosis
  Familial cardiomyopathy
  Autoimmune myocarditis

acute or subacute decompensated heart failure. Rales may be absent in chronic heart failure despite elevated filling pressures because of increased lymphatic drainage and venous capacitance within the lungs. Pleural effusions (hydrothorax) can be present, often only in the right hemithorax, and are best appreciated by finding dullness to percussion and

Table 80.5 PRECIPITANTS OF HEART FAILURE EXACERBATION

Inadequate patient education

Excess salt and fluid intake

Concurrent medical illness (e.g., pneumonia, renal failure, thyroid disease)

Cardiac arrhythmias (atrial fibrillation/flutter, ventricular tachycardia)

Uncontrolled hypertension

Medication noncompliance

Acute myocardial ischemia

Worsening valvular heart disease

Anemia

---

reduced breath sounds at the bases. Severe chronic heart failure may produce cardiac cachexia.

Signs of right-sided heart failure include peripheral edema, increased abdominal girth from ascites, congestive hepatomegaly and splenomegaly, and an elevated JVP. The JVP reflects the filling pressure of the right atrium and is an important window into the heart. Serial assessment of the JVP may be singularly the most important physical finding in following patients with heart failure. The JVP is measured in centimeters from the right atrium, which by convention is located 5 cm below the manubriosternal angle. It is best appreciated using the internal jugular vein on the right side of the neck with the patient sitting at 45° with his legs horizontal. An abnormally elevated JVP is >10 cm. Manual compression of the right upper quadrant for >30 seconds can lead to a sustained elevation of JVP in states of volume overload, a sign known as hepatojugular reflux. The JVP normally goes down during inspiration because of negative intrathoracic pressure. However, an absence of a decrease or an increase in JVP during inspiration is known as Kussmaul's sign and reflects impaired right ventricular filling. Kussmaul's sign may be present in constrictive pericarditis, restrictive cardiomyopathy, and right ventricular infarction.

Secondary pulmonary hypertension is common in chronic left-sided heart failure and may significantly impair exercise tolerance. Physical signs of pulmonary hypertension include a loud P2, evidence of a murmur of pulmonic valve insufficiency (a high-pitched blowing, decrescendo diastolic murmur at the left second or third intercostal space, also known as a Graham-Steel murmur), and a palpable pulmonary tap at the left second intercostal space. Right-sided murmurs and sounds often increase with inspiration (Carvallo's sign) because of increased venous return to the right ventricle resulting in prolonged ejection time.

LABORATORY EVALUATION

The evaluation of a patient with new or suspected heart failure can be informed by several laboratory tests. Testing should include a complete blood count to assess for anemia, which can precipitate heart failure. Basic metabolic panel should be checked for renal function before initiation of diuretics or angiotensin-converting enzyme (ACE) inhibitors. Renal insufficiency is common in heart failure and often referred to as *the cardiorenal syndrome*, which may limit the ability to remove excess volume via the kidneys with diuretic therapy. Elevated liver function tests may reflect passive hepatic congestion or low cardiac output. Fasting glucose should be checked for the presence of underlying diabetes. When a dilated cardiomyopathy is present, its etiology may be discovered by assaying thyroid-stimulating hormone (thyrotoxicosis or hypothyroidism), iron studies (hereditary hemochromatosis), antinuclear antibodies (lupus), and HIV serology.

In states of elevated filling pressures, ventricular myocytes secrete a hormone called B-type natriuretic peptide, or BNP. Plasma concentrations are elevated in patients with both asymptomatic and symptomatic left ventricular dysfunction. BNP has been shown to be useful in distinguishing between heart failure from either systolic or diastolic dysfunction and pulmonary causes of dyspnea in the emergency room. Cutoff points for BNP have varied. In the emergency room setting BNP >100 pg/mL was highly sensitive for the diagnosis of heart failure, whereas a level >400 pg/mL improved specificity at the price of reduced sensitivity. A newer test for the N-terminal fragment of the BNP hormone (NT-proBNP) has been developed. NT-proBNP is elevated out of proportion to BNP in left ventricular dysfunction. However, several factors confound the routine use of BNP and NT-proBNP, including the fact that levels are lower in obese individuals and higher with those in renal failure. The utility of measuring natriuretic peptide levels in the diagnosis and monitoring of heart failure patients continues to evolve. Several other biomarkers have been used to assess prognosis in heart failure. For example, an elevated cardiac troponin after admission for acute decompensated heart failure is a marker of increased in-hospital mortality, but it is of little help in guiding therapy.

PREDICTORS OF PROGNOSIS

The literature would support many predictors of prognosis. These would include NYHA Classification, etiology, ejection fraction, serum sodium, comorbidities, concurrent coronary risk factors, a wide QRS duration, circulating neurohormonal levels (e.g., norepinephrine), and rhythm disturbances. However, once heart failure has become clinically overt, physiological parameters that assess the true impact on cardiac function are the better prognostic determinants. These would include resting heart rate, systolic blood pressure, cardiac output, and both pulmonary artery and pulmonary capillary wedge pressure. Formal cardiopulmonary testing to determine maximum oxygen uptake provides a quantitative assessment of functional capacity and important prognostic information about mortality in chronic heart failure. This is the best single prognostic determinant when cardiac transplantation or ventricular assist device therapy is being considered.

IMAGING AND HEMODYNAMIC ASSESSMENT

Chest radiography in suspected heart failure may reveal cardiomegaly, interstitial pulmonary edema, or pleural effusions. All patients with suspected heart failure should undergo routine electrocardiography to evaluate for the presence of arrhythmias, conduction disease, and chamber enlargement. Transthoracic echocardiography should be used in conjunction with the physical exam to determine the nature of underlying structural heart disease and to determine if left ventricular systolic function is preserved or reduced. The end-systolic and end-diastolic dimensions can be easily calculated and provide additional prognostic information. An end-diastolic diameter >7 cm portends a particularly dire prognosis. Cardiac magnetic resonance imaging is emerging as an important high-resolution tool to assess cardiac structure, function, and perfusion. Patients with risk factors or a history of coronary artery disease should undergo an evaluation for ischemia, either with coronary angiography or a myocardial perfusion study.

Invasive hemodynamic assessment can be used to measure filling pressures and calculate cardiac output. Right heart and pulmonary artery catheterization is performed using a Swan-Ganz pulmonary artery catheter. The catheter is balloon tipped and can be "wedged" into a branch of the pulmonary artery, creating a static column of blood to the left atrium and ventricle. The resulting pulmonary catheter wedge pressure provides a good estimate of left ventricular preload in the absence of significant pulmonary vascular disease, mitral stenosis, or tachycardia. A pulmonary artery catheter is important for distinguishing between cardiogenic pulmonary edema related to left heart failure (elevated wedge pressure >18 mm Hg) or acute respiratory distress syndrome (normal wedge). Patients whose pulmonary wedge pressure cannot be lowered below 25 mm Hg with aggressive medical therapies carry a poor prognosis. Routine use of pulmonary artery catheters to guide heart failure therapy has diminished after clinical trials failed to show a mortality benefit, while exposing the risk of infection, pulmonary infarction, and arrhythmia.

HEART FAILURE WITH REDUCED SYSTOLIC FUNCTION

PATHOPHYSIOLOGY

Heart failure often arises when acute adaptive mechanisms meant to compensate for some functional or structural cardiac abnormality become maladaptive. For example, in acute heart failure salt and water retention increases preload, vasoconstriction maintains perfusion to the vital organs, sympathetic stimulation augments cardiac output, hypertrophy unloads individual muscle fibers, and increased collagen production may reduce chamber dilatation. Over time these same mechanisms can impair cardiac performances. Salt and water retention produces pulmonary congestion and anasarca, vasoconstriction exacerbates pump dysfunction, sympathetic activation leads to increased mechanoenergetic inefficiency and ventricular remodeling, hypertrophy leads to deterioration and death of cardiac myocytes, and increased collagen production impairs cardiac relaxation. Long term, these maladaptive mechanisms alter energy metabolism, change in sarcomeric protein expression, resulting in abnormal excitation-contraction coupling, and leading to interstitial fibrosis and myocyte apoptosis. Activation of neurohormones like the renin-angiotensin-aldosterone system, the adrenergic nervous system, cytokines, and vasoactive peptides mediates and reinforces progressive remodeling and cardiac dysfunction. Fortunately, these same molecular pathways have been fruitful targets for the development of drug therapies for chronic heart failure.

ACUTE DECOMPENSATED HEART FAILURE

Treatment of acute decompensated heart failure involves stabilizing hemodynamics and ensuring tissue perfusion. All patients should be positioned upright, receive supplemental oxygen, and be ventilated adequately, often with the aid of noninvasive positive-pressure ventilation or endotracheal mechanical ventilation. Acute pulmonary edema may also be treated with vasodilators such as nitrates, which venodilate acutely, morphine, and furosemide, which produces net fluid loss through diuresis. Intravenous vasodilators such as nitroglycerin or sodium nitroprusside may be initiated along with intravenous loop diuretics either in bolus form or as a continuous drip. Beta blockade is contraindicated in patients with acute decompensated heart failure. Temporary use of intravenous inotropes (dobutamine or milrinone) or mechanical circulatory support may be required to augment cardiac output.

PHARMACOLOGIC TREATMENT CHRONIC HEART FAILURE

Diuretics

Pharmacologic therapy for chronic systolic heart failure has the goal of improving symptoms and prolonging survival.

Medical therapies may be divided into those that both improve mortality and reduce symptoms and those that only confer symptomatic benefit (see table 80.6). The most commonly used medications to relieve congestive symptoms are loop diuretics (furosemide, torsemide, bumetanide, ethacrynic acid), which promote net sodium and water loss by blocking sodium reuptake in the loop of Henle. Loop diuretics are available in both intravenous formulations for in-hospital use during acute exacerbations and oral forms for maintenance therapy. Despite their widespread use for symptomatic relief, loop diuretics have never been shown to confer a mortality benefit in chronic heart failure; such randomization probably cannot be done. Diuretic resistance may develop with chronic loop diuretic use. Resistance may be due to increased salt intake, modulation of sodium channels in the loop of Henle and distal convoluted tubule, and upregulation of the renin-angiotensin-aldosterone system. Thiazide diuretics such as chlorothiazide or metolazone may be added 30–60 minutes before loop diuretics for a synergistic response because they block sodium absorption in the distal nephron. Use of loop diuretics may also result in potassium loss, requiring the administration of a potassium-sparing diuretic such as triamterene or spironolactone. Another option for patients with diuretic resistance and refractory heart failure is bedside ultrafiltration, which can rapidly remove large fluid volumes through the peripheral veins without hemodynamic compromise.

ACE Inhibitors and Angiotensin Receptor Blockers

ACE inhibitors were the first class of medicines to show a mortality benefit in chronic heart failure after both MI and with nonischemic cardiomyopathies. They are the mainstay of therapy in both asymptomatic and symptomatic left ventricular dysfunction and should be used in all patients with left ventricular dysfunction unless contraindicated or not tolerated. ACE inhibitors are balanced arterial and venous vasodilators and block the deleterious remodeling effects of the renin-angiotensin system,

Table 80.6 PHARMACOLOGIC THERAPY FOR CHRONIC HEART FAILURE WITH REDUCED SYSTOLIC FUNCTION

IMPROVED MORTALITY	SYMPTOMATIC IMPROVEMENT ONLY
Beta-blockers	Loop diuretics
ACE-inhibitors	Digoxin
Angiotensin-receptor blockers (ARBs)	Nitrates
Aldosterone antagonists (spironolactone, eplerenone)	
Hydralazine/Isordil combination (African-American patients only)	

which is upregulated in heart failure. ACE inhibitors exhibit a class effect and should be titrated to a target dose with close monitoring of renal function because they often result in a drop in glomerular filtration rate in heart failure patients. Caution should be used in patients with baseline renal dysfunction or hyperkalemia, in whom ACE inhibitors may be contraindicated. A common side effect of ACE inhibitors is a dry cough, thought to be from an increase in circulating bradykinins. Angiotensin receptor blockers (ARBs) provide an alternative to heart failure patients intolerant to ACE-inhibitors because of cough. ARBs block angiotensin II receptors, which may be upregulated in patients with chronic ACE inhibition, and their concurrent use may prevent "ACE escape" by blocking downstream effects of angiotensin II. ARBs are well tolerated and indicated as first-line therapy in heart failure patients intolerant to ACE inhibitors because of cough. However, ARBs have a similar incidence of hyperkalemia, renal insufficiency, and hypotension. The evidence that ARBs should be added to patients already on ACE inhibition is less compelling.

Beta Blockers

Activation of the sympathetic nervous system in heart failure was first described in the 1960s, and circulating catecholamine levels correlate with disease severity and mortality. Early paradigms of heart failure focused on the acute compensatory nature of sympathetic activation with a reduced ejection fraction. The deleterious effects of chronic sympathoadrenergic activity were later proven after oral beta blocking convincingly reduced mortality in low-ejection-fraction heart failure patients. Long-term administration of beta blockers also prevents remodeling, attenuates fibrosis and hypertrophy, reduces arrhythmias, and improves functional status. Specific beta blockers shown to confer a mortality benefit in heart failure include carvedilol, extended-release metoprolol, and bisoprolol, but their relative efficacy has not been determined. Beta blockers should be used in all patients with stable, euvolemic heart failure and low ejection fraction and even in patients with asymptomatic left ventricular dysfunction. There are additive benefits to beta blockers and ACE inhibitors, although which drug to initiate first has been uncertain. Beta blockers should not be administered in the decompensated state when there is evidence for fluid accumulation. In general, beta blockers are started at a low dose while the patient is in hospital and uptitrated over several weeks after discharge. Patients should be monitored for signs of fatigue, bradycardia, and fluid retention, which may prompt adjustment of loop diuretic dosing.

Digoxin

Although the use of digitalis-based glycosides from the foxglove plant has been a mainstay of treating congestive heart failure since the 18th century, these agents were only recently subjected to the rigor of clinical trials. Digoxin has been shown to reduce heart failure hospitalizations and improve symptoms, but it does not improve mortality in chronic heart failure. Digoxin works by augmenting intracellular calcium levels and bolstering contractility while also reducing vagal input to the atrioventricular node. This combination of effects makes it an excellent drug for those heart failure patients with atrial fibrillation and a reduced ejection fraction. Digoxin use should be avoided in renal insufficiency. In heart failure digoxin is generally given at a low dose with serum levels maintained <1 mg/dL. Signs of digoxin toxicity include nausea, abdominal discomfort, yellow halo around lights, and heart block. Withdrawal of digoxin is often associated with worsening heart failure symptoms.

Aldosterone Antagonists

Spironolactone, an aldosterone receptor antagonist, is indicated for patients with class III/IV systolic heart failure (ejection fraction <35%) who are already on an ACE inhibitor and beta blocker. Spironolactone further inhibits the renin-angiotensin-aldosterone axis and attenuates remodeling and fibrosis in chronic heart failure. Eplerenone, a more selective aldosterone antagonist, has been shown to improve mortality in patients with postinfarction heart failure and ejection fraction <40%. Close monitoring of serum potassium and renal function must be undertaken after initiation of aldosterone antagonism. Great caution must be used with these agents in patients with renal dysfunction because of the risk of potentially fatal hyperkalemia. Low-dose aldosterone antagonists can be considered in such instances. Painful gynecomastia and galactorrhea may be seen in male patients on spironolactone, but these side effects are rare with eplerenone.

OTHER TREATMENTS

Venodilators such as long-acting nitrates may reduce congestive symptoms in some heart failure patients and may reduce chronic ischemia by lowering preload. Hydralazine and nitrates were the first vasodilators shown to improve heart failure survival, and they remain an effective alternative for patients who cannot be given an ACE inhibitor or ARB because of drug intolerance or renal insufficiency. This combination is also reasonable to consider in patients already taking an ACE inhibitor and beta blocker with persistent symptoms. In self-identified African-American patients, a fixed-dose combination of hydralazine and isosorbide dinitrate has been shown to confer a mortality benefit.

Electrolyte monitoring and supplementation constitute an important part of ongoing drug therapy for heart failure. For example, potassium depletion is common with diuretic use, whereas hyperkalemia may be seen with ACE

inhibitors, ARBs, aldosterone antagonists, and in renal insufficiency. In general, oral potassium supplements may be required to keep serum potassium levels between 4.0 and 5.0 mEq/L. Loss of magnesium and calcium is also common with chronic diuretic use.

Many nonpharmacologic measures are central to chronic heart failure therapy. Patient education regarding diet, medications, and fluid management is critical to prevent recurrent hospital admission and improve functional status. Patients with recurrent heart failure exacerbations should be told to have a salt-restricted diet (<2 g daily) and should adhere to an overall fluid restriction (often <2 L per day, or <64 oz). Daily weights should be measured each morning after voiding. If weight increases two pounds in a day or 5 pounds in 1 week, adjustment of diuretic dosing is indicated. Last, heart failure patients may benefit from an exercise program and cardiac rehabilitation, along with remote monitoring of their weight and vital signs.

There is no consensus that the presence of heart failure alone should be an indication for anticoagulation with warfarin therapy. But there is no question that such therapy is indicated in patients with heart failure and atrial fibrillation, or with comorbidities of transient cerebral ischemia, pulmonary embolism, venous thrombosis, recent anterior MI, or documented ventricular or atrial thrombosis.

Finally, for more advanced systolic dysfunction, intravenous inotropes or vasodilators may be initiated. Inotropes such as dobutamine, (beta-receptor agonist), dopamine (an alpha and beta agonist), or milrinone (a phosphodiesterase-3 inhibitor) increase myocardial contractility, stroke volume, and heart rate and modestly reduce afterload by vasodilatation, thereby augmenting cardiac output. Unfortunately, even as it improves perfusion, inotropic therapy can lead to malignant tachyarrhythmias and has never been shown to have a mortality benefit in either continuous or intermittent infusions. Pure vasodilators such as nitroprusside or nesiritide may also be used to reduce afterload and unload the failing ventricle. However, nitroprusside use is limited to a few days because of thyocyanate toxicity, and nesiritide may increase the risk of renal dysfunction.

MISHAPS OF MEDICAL THERAPIES

There are important mishaps in medical therapy that deserve emphasis. Nonsteroidal anti-inflammatory agents should be avoided if at all possible because they will promote excess sodium retention. Calcium channel blocking agents have negative inotropic effects and should not be considered in symptomatic heart failure. Oral drug absorption may be inadequate due to bowel edema or low cardiac output with reduced mesenteric blood flow. Recurrent heart failure may reflect inadequate afterload reduction, too much beta blockade, or inadequate diuresis; more often, it reflects inadequate patient education or noncompliance with and misunderstanding of complex medical regimens.

DEVICE-BASED THERAPIES

Heart failure patients with a reduced ejection fraction are six to nine times more likely to suffer sudden cardiac death than the general population. The mechanism of sudden cardiac death is ventricular tachycardia/fibrillation related to electrical instability of the myopathic heart. Implantable cardioverter defibrillators (ICDs) for the primary prevention of sudden death reduce overall mortality in symptomatic (NYHA Class II–III) heart failure patients with a reduced ejection fraction (<35%). ICDs also have a proven mortality benefit in patients after MI with an ejection fraction <30%. To be considered an ICD candidate, patients should be >40 days after MI or >3 months after percutaneous coronary intervention or coronary artery bypass graft (CABG). ICDs are also superior to medical therapy such as amiodarone for primary prevention of sudden cardiac death. All symptomatic heart failure patients should be optimized on medical therapy (particularly beta blockers and ACE inhibitors) for at least 3 months before ICD placement, for reverse remodeling may obviate the need for an ICD.

Many heart failure patients with a low ejection fraction often also have interventricular conduction delay, as manifest by a widened QRS complex (>120 msec) on electrocardiogram from either a bundle branch block or nonspecific conduction delay. This conduction delay creates dyssynchronous contraction of the left ventricle and can contribute to remodeling, mitral regurgitation, and symptoms of congestion. Class III–IV heart failure patients with reduced ejection fraction and conduction delay (QRS width >120–150 msec) may benefit from cardiac resynchronization therapy (CRT), also known as biventricular pacing. Pacemaker leads are placed in the right ventricule apex and the lateral free wall of the left ventricle via the coronary sinus to "resynchronize" contraction of both ventricles. This may lead to reverse remodeling, decreased mitral regurgitation, and a mortality benefit in select patients. Not every heart failure patient will respond to CRT. Prospectively identifying responders and nonresponders is an active area of research. Many patients eligible for ICD placement also meet criteria for resynchronization and are offered both therapies with a single device, known as CRTD.

Severe, refractory chronic heart failure (stage D or NYHA Class IV) or acute cardiogenic shock may require temporary or durable mechanical circulatory support. Traditionally this has taken the form of a temporary intra-aortic balloon counterpulsation pump. Although effective in reducing afterload and augmenting coronary perfusion, balloon pumps have a short lifespan (days to a few weeks), may lead to vascular compromise, including limb ischemia and renal failure, and can cause consumptive thrombocytopenia. Technological advances in recent years have led to the development of more durable implantable ventricular assist devices. These assist devices may be placed surgically or percutaneously. They directly augment cardiac output by creating a pump producing either pulsatile or nonpulsatile blood flow in parallel to the native ventricle. Such devices may be used as a bridge to cardiac transplantation, a bridge to cardiac recovery, or as a destination therapy for patients ineligible for transplant. The significant mismatch between donor heart availability and the expanding epidemic of advanced heart failure makes mechanical circulatory support a crucial, rapidly evolving therapy to extend life and improve symptoms in end-stage heart failure patients.

HEART FAILURE WITH PRESERVED SYSTOLIC FUNCTION

Heart failure with preserved ejection fraction (EF >40%), sometimes referred to a diastolic heart failure, is a disorder of impaired cardiac filling (diastole). Diastolic dysfunction is not synonymous with diastolic heart failure. Isolated diastolic dysfunction may occur in the absence of heart failure symptoms. Diastolic dysfunction can be seen in the elderly, particularly women, in patients with a history of hypertension, or concurrently in patients with systolic dysfunction. Patients with diastolic dysfunction often have an S4 gallop on exam and no evidence of ventricular dilatation. Diastolic function can be assessed noninvasively using echocardiography.

Nearly half of all heart failure patients have preserved systolic function. Etiologies of heart failure with preserved systolic function include chronic hypertension, hypertrophic cardiomyopathy, aortic stenosis with normal ejection fraction, ischemic heart disease, and restrictive cardiomyopathy. Women are more likely to be affected by diastolic heart failure than men. Diastolic heart failure from coronary ischemia is caused by increased myocardial stiffness produced from either a reduced supply related to epicardial coronary disease or an increased myocardial oxygen demand. Concentric left ventricular hypertrophy after years of hypertension may also contribute to diastolic heart failure because the stiff chamber cannot relax normally and its thickened walls can predispose to subendocardial ischemia. The presence of heart failure with severe aortic stenosis is an indication for aortic valve replacement. A common precipitant of heart failure in patients with diastolic dysfunction is atrial fibrillation. Atrial fibrillation is poorly tolerated because of the loss of the atrial kick, which is important for filling a stiff ventricle, and poor rate control with reduced diastolic filling time.

The evidence base for treating heart failure with preserved ejection fraction is regrettably small, in part because diastolic heart failure has only recently been considered a distinct entity and because of varying definitions of heart failure with preserved ejection fraction. No single pharmacologic agent has yet been shown to confer a mortality benefit in a randomized trial. Multiple ongoing clinical trials are addressing this important question. In general, diuretics are used to prevent volume overload. Hypertension is controlled, often with ACE inhibitors, angiotensin-receptor blockers, or dihydropyridine calcium channel blockers. Heart rate control is maintained, often with a beta blocker, to allow for adequate time for ventricular filling. When possible, patients should be maintained in sinus rhythm given the intolerance to atrial fibrillation.

HIGH-OUTPUT HEART FAILURE

Whereas most heart failure is characterized by a reduced cardiac output and elevated systemic vascular resistance, high-output failure is defined by a markedly elevated cardiac output and a low systemic resistance. This leads to ineffective blood volume and pressure, neurohormonal activation, and volume overload. There are several common etiologies of high-output heart failure, most notably systemic arteriovenous fistulas, thyrotoxicosis, and thiamine deficiency (table 80.7).

The physical exam in high-output heart failure reveals inappropriate-tachycardia and a venous hum over the jugular veins. Arterial examination is notable for signs of increased stroke volume, including a wide pulse pressure, bounding pulse with quick upstroke, and "pistol shot" sound heard over the femoral arteries. The extremities are often warm with evidence of vasodilatation. This must be carefully distinguished from aortic regurgitation, which is also characterized by increased stroke volume but also produces a diastolic murmur. Cardiac exam may reveal an enlarged point of maximal impulse from cardiomegaly and an S3 gallop from volume loading of the left ventricle.

The syndrome of high-output failure is markedly different from the temporary physiological increases in cardiac output seen with excitement, exercise, fever, and pregnancy. Although high-output states may be the sole cause of heart failure, the need to augment cardiac output transiently may trigger a heart failure exacerbation in patients with poor cardiac reserve from conditions such as valvular heart disease or underlying cardiomyopathy. The cornerstones of treatment for high-output heart failure are the identification and reversal of the underlying cause of the high-output state.

SPECIFIC CARDIAC DISORDERS PRESENTING WITH HEART FAILURE

MYOCARDITIS

Myocarditis represents a constellation of different cardiac diseases each marked by inflammation, usually triggered by an infection and autoimmune response. This inflammation may be focal or diffuse and involve any or all of the cardiac

Table 80.7 CAUSES OF HIGH-OUTPUT HEART FAILURE

Systemic arteriovenous fistulas (congenital or acquired)

Hyperthyroidism

Chronic anemia

Beriberi (vitamin B-1 or thiamine deficiency)

Dermatologic disorders (e.g., psoriasis)

Acromegaly

Paget disease of the bone

Cirrhosis

Renal disease (volume expansion)

Hyperkinetic heart syndrome

chambers. The gold standard for diagnosis is endomyocardial biopsy, although cardiac magnetic resonance imaging with gadolinium enhancement is increasingly being used to identify cases. In the developed world, viral infections such as coxsackievirus, adenovirus, and parvovirus B19 have been identified as the most common pathogens. However, a host of infectious agent can trigger myocarditis. For example, Chagas myocarditis from a parasitic infection with *Trypanosoma cruzi* is by far the most common cause of cardiomyopathy in Central and South American countries. A treatable and common form of myocarditis in the Northeastern United States is Lyme carditis from *Borrelia burgdorferi* infection. This form of myocarditis has a predilection for the conduction system and often leads to heart block requiring a temporary pacemaker, which usually resolves with a course of intravenous antibiotics such as ceftriaxone.

The spectrum of myocarditis can range from subclinical disease to fulminant myocarditis, in which cardiovascular collapse and death can occur shortly after a viral syndrome. Myocarditis, particularly postviral or lymphocytic myocarditis, may present as heart failure or a dilated cardiomyopathy. Often a viral prodrome may be recalled, although the development of cardiac dysfunction can lag considerably from the initial infectious insult. Myocarditis may also present with chest pain, often mimicking MI with ST segment changes, sudden cardiac death, or arrhythmias. In addition to volume overload, physical findings include a gallop rhythm signaling ventricular dysfunction, and a friction rub is suggestive of myopericarditis. Laboratory analysis may reveal a mildly elevated cardiac troponin. Treatment for myocarditis typically involves supportive care, monitoring for arrhythmias, avoidance of exercise, and pharmacologic therapy for heart failure. Targeted immunomodulating therapies have shown mixed results in speeding resolution of myocarditis and preventing development of dilated cardiomyopathy. There is no consensus as to the most appropriate immunosuppressive agent.

HYPERTROPHIC CARDIOMYOPATHY

Hypertrophic cardiomyopathy is a familial disorder inherited in an autosomal dominant fashion and is associated with both heart failure and sudden cardiac death. It produces significant left ventricular hypertrophy in the absence of conditions that increase afterload, such as aortic stenosis or long-standing hypertension. This disorder arises from mutations in genes coding for cardiac myocyte proteins, most commonly the beta-cardiac myosin heavy chain (40% of cases). Asymmetric septal hypertrophy can lead to obstruction of outflow from the left ventricle during systole as a result of dynamic narrowing of the outflow tract beneath the aortic valve and systolic anterior motion of the mitral valve. This condition is often referred to as hypertrophic obstructive cardiomyopathy (HOCM) or its previous name, idiopathic hypertrophic subaortic stenosis. Great care must be taken on physical examination to distinguish between hypertrophic cardiomopathy with dynamic outflow obstruction and valvular aortic stenosis (table 80.8). HOCM has several characteristic physical findings. These include a bifid carotid pulse, double apical impulse, and a systolic ejection murmur that increases with both valsalva maneuver and standing. These two maneuvers decrease left ventricular preload, thereby decreasing the diameter of the left ventricular outflow tract leading a louder murmur. Severe outflow obstruction can result in angina, syncope, and sudden death. Anything prompting a drop in preload must be avoided in HOCM, including the use of vasodilators and dehydration.

PERIPARTUM CARDIOMYOPATHY

Peripartum cardiomyopathy, also known as pregnancy-associated cardiomyopathy, is a rare but devastating cause of heart failure affecting mothers in the last month of pregnancy and up to 5 months postpartum. The incidence of peripartum cardiomyopathy has wide geographic variation, from 1:100 to 1:15,000 live births. Its cause is unknown, although may be related to inflammatory or autoimmune factors. Peripartum cardiomyopathy is characterized by an absence of other underlying cardiac disorder, symptoms of heart failure, and reduced systolic function on echocardiography. A number of risk factors for the development of peripartum cardiomyopathy have been identified, including older maternal age, multiparity, and African descent. Overall, treatment is similar to that of heart failure with low ejection fraction, including stabilizing hemodynamics and symptom relief. However, ACE inhibitors and ARBs are contraindicated in pregnancy and must never be given antepartum because of the risk of fetal renal failure, oligohydramnios, premature labor, and pulmonary hypoplasia. Hydralazine is the vasodilator of choice in this setting given its good safety profile. The overall 2-year mortality rate is 10%, but most women have complete recovery of their ejection fraction and a good prognosis. In women with peripartum cardiomyopathy who do not have normalization of their systolic function, subsequent pregnancy is particularly high risk and should be avoided.

STRESS CARDIOMYOPATHY

Reversible severe ventricular dysfunction has been reported after sudden episodes of emotional distress, neurological injury, or trauma. This stress cardiomyopathy has a predilection for creating wall motion abnormalities in the left ventricular apex and is also known as apical ballooning syndrome or takotsubo cardiomyopathy, after the shape of a traditional Japanese octopus pot. Chest pain and dyspnea are typical presenting features along with widespread T-wave inversions. Women are more likely to be affected than men. Cardiac catheterization is often required to rule out coronary ischemia. Marked improvement in ejection fraction in seen within a few days to 3 weeks of presentation. Plasma catecholamines are significantly elevated in this condition and may result in transient ventricular stunning. Traditional heart failure therapy is initiated, although patients may require a brief period of mechanical circulatory support until their myocardial function recovers.

CARDIAC AMYLOIDOSIS

Amyloidosis is a systemic disorder characterized by deposition of protein fibrils in the extracellular matrix. Amyloid protein can be produced as a result of a plasma cell dyscrasia, such as primary amyloid (AL, or light chain amyloid), mutations in the transthyretin gene (familial amyloid), or senile amyloid from wild-type transthyretin deposits. Amyloid protein infiltrating the myocardium produces a noncompliant, rubbery heart with frequent intracardiac thrombi and characteristic Congo red staining with green birefringence under polarized

Table 80.8 DISTINGUISHING HYPERTROPHIC OBSTRUCTIVE CARDIOMYOPATHY FROM VALVULAR AORTIC STENOSIS ON PHYSICAL EXAMINATION

	HYPERTROPHIC CARDIOMYOPATHY	AORTIC STENOSIS
Valsalva maneuver	Increased murmur	Decreased murmur
Standing	Increased murmur	Decreased murmur or no change
Passive leg elevation	Decreased murmur	Increased murmur or no change
Carotid pulsation	Brisk, often bifid	Parvus et tardus (weak and delayed)

light on biopsy. Amyloid cardiomyopathy is defined by myocardial or conduction system dysfunction, and the clinical course is largely determined by the nature of protein deposition. Cardiac involvement with AL amyloid has a rapid clinical progression, whereas familial or senile amyloid is associated with milder symptoms and a more indolent course.

The clinical presentation of amyloid heart disease is often dominated by signs of right heart failure, postural hypotension, and syncope, along with cardioembolic events such as stroke. The most common electrocardiographic finding is markedly low voltages in the limb leads. Echocardiography shows diastolic dysfunction, wall thickening, an increased echogenicity related to protein deposition, and the evolution of a restrictive cardiomyopathy. The presence of heavy proteinuria, hepatomegaly, orthostatic hypotension, and neuropathy along with heart failure provides diagnostic clues for systemic amyloidosis. Tissue diagnosis may be made from endomyocardial or fat pad biopsy. Treatment of cardiac amyloidosis is largely supportive. In general ACE inhibitors, calcium channel blockers, and digoxin should be avoided given their binding to amyloid protein and predilection for the development of hypotension. With the thrombotic risk, anticoagulation must be considered, particularly if atrial fibrillation is present.

RESTRICTIVE CARDIOMYOPATHY VERSUS CONSTRICTIVE PERICARDITIS

Restrictive cardiomyopathy is a disorder that produces a nondilated, rigid ventricle with normal wall thickness and preserved systolic function but with severely impaired ventricular filling. Constrictive pericarditis results from scarring and loss of elasticity of pericardial sac, leading to impaired filling of all four cardiac chambers. Both diseases may present with heart failure and a preserved ejection fraction. They must be carefully distinguished from each other because their treatment and prognosis are quite different.

A history of pericarditis, chest radiation, cardiac surgery, trauma, or a systemic disease affecting the pericardium (e.g., malignancy or tuberculosis) makes constrictive pericarditis more likely. A history of infiltrative disease (amyloidosis, hemochromatosis, or sarcoidosis) favors restrictive cardiomyopathy. Both conditions may have an elevated JVP with a prominent descent during diastole, and both may produce Kussmaul's sign. A pericardial knock can sometimes be heard in constrictive pericarditis. Both conditions generate low voltage on electrocardiography. Chest imaging with either computed tomography (CT) or magnetic resonance imaging (MRI) reveals a thickened pericardium in constrictive pericarditis.

In restrictive cardiomyopathy pericardial compliance is normal, and respiratory changes are transmitted to all chambers of the heart. However in constriction, because the pericardium shields the cardiac chambers but not the pulmonary vasculature from respirophasic pressure changes, venous filling of the right heart exceeds that of the left heart, and the interventricular septum bows to the left. Also, because all four chambers of the heart are within the constricted pericardium, there is equalization of end-diastolic pressure in all chambers on cardiac catheterization. Treatment of constrictive pericarditis involves excision of the pericardium (pericardiectomy). Treatment of restrictive cardiomyopathy is similar to that of other causes of diastolic heart failure, and its prognosis is poor, particularly in advanced cases when systolic function also becomes depressed.

COR PULMONALE

Cor pulmonale is a condition of dilatation and hypertrophy of the right ventricle leading to refractory right heart failure that is ultimately related to severe pulmonary hypertension resulting from diseases affecting the lung or its vasculature. Commonly patients will have a history of significant lung disease, such as severe emphysema, pulmonary fibrosis, and chronic hypoxemia, or may have a history of recurrent pulmonary thromboembolism. Presenting symptoms of cor pulmonale include fatigue, lethargy, angina in the absence of epicardial coronary disease, and right upper quadrant discomfort from hepatic congestion. Physical findings include peripheral edema, an elevated JVP, loud pulmonic component of the second heart sound (P2) from pulmonary hypertension, a right-sided S4 gallop from right ventricular hypertrophy, and plethora related to polycythemia. The electrocardiogram reveals signs of chronic right ventricular overload, including right atrial enlargement (P pulmonale), right axis deviation, R > S wave amplitude in V1, and incomplete right bundle branch block. Supplemental oxygen is the treatment of choice for cor pulmonale if chronic hypoxemia is the cause because it may reduce right heart failure symptoms along with polycythemia. Other treatments include diuretics, pulmonary vasodilators, digoxin, and even phlebotomy if the hematocrit is >55% to prevent hyperviscosity. In chronic obstructive pulmonary disease, the development of pulmonary hypertension and cor pulmonale portends a poor prognosis.

ADDITIONAL READING

Aurigemma GP, Gaasch WH. Clinical practice. Diastolic heart failure. *N Engl J Med.* 2004;351(11):1097–1105.

Braunwald E. Biomarkers in heart failure. *N Engl J Med.* 2008;358(20): 2148–59.

Dupree CS. Primary prevention of heart failure: An update. *Curr Opin Cardiol.* 2010;25(5):478–83.

Felker GM, O'Connor CM, Braunwald E; Heart Failure Clinical Research Network Investigators. Loop diuretics in acute decompensated heart failure: Necessary? Evil? A necessary evil? *Circ Heart Fail.* 2009;2(1):56–62.

Gheorghiade M, Follath F, Ponikowski P, et al.; European Society of Cardiology; European Society of Intensive Care Medicine. Assessing and grading congestion in acute heart failure: A scientific statement from the Acute Heart Failure Committee of the Heart Failure Association of the European Society of Cardiology and endorsed by the European Society of Intensive Care Medicine. *Eur J Heart Fail.* 2010;12(5):423–33.

Hunt SA, Abraham WT, Chin MH, et al. 2009 focused update incorporated into the ACC/AHA 2005 Guidelines for the Diagnosis and Management of Heart Failure in Adults: A report of the American College of Cardiology Foundation/American Heart Association Task Force on Practice Guidelines: developed in collaboration with the International Society for Heart and Lung Transplantation. *Circulation.* 2009;119(14):e391–479. Erratum *Circulation.* 2010;121(12):e258.

Jessup M, Brozena S. Heart failure. *N Engl J Med.* 2003; 348(20):2007–18.

McMurray JJ. Clinical practice. Systolic heart failure. *N Engl J Med.* 2010; 362(3):228–38.

Neubauer S. The failing heart—an engine out of fuel. *N Engl J Med.* 2007; 356(11):1140–51.

Nohria A, Mielniczuk LM, Stevenson LW. Evaluation and monitoring of patients with acute heart failure syndromes. *Am J Cardiol.* 2005;96(6A):32G–40G.

Sanz J, Fuster V. Update in cardiology. *Ann Intern Med.* 2010;152(12): 786–91.

QUESTIONS

QUESTION 1. A 78-year-old woman is admitted to the hospital with acute pulmonary edema. She has a history of moderately severe hypertension controlled with diuretics. Her physical examination reveals a heart rate of 110 beats/min and blood pressure of 170/90 mm Hg. Crackles are heard over both lung fields to the level of the mid scapulae. Neck veins are distended to 6 cm H$_2$O. A dynamic left ventricular impulse is inferolaterally displaced. Heart sounds are brisk and accompanied by a prominent fourth heart sound but no murmurs. Her electrocardiogram is remarkable only for left ventricular hypertrophy, a small left ventricular cavity size, and hyperdynamic wall motion. In addition to diuretic therapy, the best long-term therapy for this patient would be:

A. Digoxin and arterial vasodilator
B. Digoxin and long-acting nitrates
C. A beta blocker
D. An arterial vasodilator alone
E. Long-acting nitrates alone

QUESTION 2. All of the following are true about BNP, EXCEPT:

A. Levels increase with age.
B. Levels increase with renal failure.
C. Levels increase with obesity.
D. Levels decrease with treatment (e.g., carvedilol, spironolactone).
E. Levels are lower in heart failure with preserved EF.

QUESTION 3. All of the following are correct statements about aldosterone antagonism, EXCEPT:

A. Should be considered in most patients with heart failure and EF <40%.
B. Potassium and renal function should be measured frequently (at 1 week, 1 month, and periodically thereafter).
C. Contraindicated in hyperkalemia (K >5.5), advanced renal insufficiency (CrCl <30–50 cc/min, Cr >2.5 mg/dL).
D. Be cautious in the elderly, those with diabetes, and concomitant use of CYP3A4 inhibitors (eplerenone).
E. Spironolactone is superior to eplerenone post MI.

QUESTION 4. Match the stages of heart failure with the appropriate characteristics of the stage:

4.1 Stage A
4.2 Stage B
4.3 Stage C
4.4 Stage D

A. Structural heart disease with prior or current symptoms
B. Structural heart disease but w/o signs or symptoms of HF
C. Refractory HF requiring specialized interventions
D. At high risk for HF but no structural heart disease

ANSWERS

1. C
2. C
3. E
4.1. D
4.2. B
4.3. A
4.4. C

81.

PERICARDIAL DISEASE

Leonard S. Lilly

The pericardium is a two-layered sac that surrounds the heart. It is composed of an outer stiff fibrous coat (the *parietal pericardium*) and a thin inner membrane that is adherent to the external surface of the heart (the *visceral pericardium*). The visceral pericardium reflects back at the level of the great vessel origins to form the inner lining of the parietal layer. The space between these two layers normally contains 15–50 mL of serous pericardial fluid, which permits the heart to contract in a minimum-friction environment. The major diseases of the pericardium are acute pericarditis, cardiac tamponade, and constrictive pericarditis.

ACUTE PERICARDITIS

ETIOLOGY

Although many conditions can lead to acute pericardial inflammation (see table 81.1), >90% of cases are postviral or of unknown (idiopathic) origin. Since most instances of idiopathic pericarditis are likely due to undetected viral infection, the two are considered equivalent illnesses. The most commonly implicated viruses are coxsackie and echovirus strains. Less frequently cytomegalovirus (CMV), mumps, Epstein-Barr virus, varicella, rubella, parvovirus, and HIV are causal. The presence of such infections could be confirmed by polymerase chain reaction (PCR) amplification of DNA obtained from pericardial fluid, but that is uncommonly undertaken, as management decisions would not typically be affected.

Tuberculosis (TB) is only rarely encountered as a cause of pericarditis in industrialized countries today. However, it remains an important etiology in immunocompromised patients and in less-developed regions of the world. In Africa, TB is the most common etiology of pericardial disease in patients with HIV.

Pyogenic bacterial pericardial infections (e.g., staphylococci, pneumococci, streptococci) are also rare but may arise from spread of pneumonia, rupture of a perivalvular abscess, or from hematogenous seeding.

Pericarditis after myocardial infarction (MI) presents in one of two forms. The "early" type occurs 1–3 days after a transmural MI and arises from extension of myocardial inflammation to the adjacent pericardium. With the advent of acute revascularization therapies in MI (fibrinolysis and percutaneous coronary interventions), this form of pericarditis has become uncommon. The "delayed" form of post-MI pericarditis, termed *Dressler syndrome*, arises in some patients weeks or months following an acute MI and is thought to be of autoimmune origin, resulting from exposure to antigens released from necrotic myocardial cells. A similar syndrome, *postpericardiotomy pericarditis*, may occur weeks following cardiac surgical procedures.

Uremic pericarditis occurs in 6–10% of patients with chronic renal failure, and its development correlates with blood urea nitrogen levels. Pericarditis also develops by an unknown mechanism in up to 13% of patients already on chronic dialysis therapy.

Neoplastic pericarditis and effusions result most often from metastatic spread or local invasion by carcinoma of the lung, breast, or lymphoma. Gastrointestinal carcinomas and melanoma are less common causes. Primary pericardial tumors are very rare.

Radiation-induced pericarditis arises from prior therapeutic mediastinal irradiation. Its incidence correlates with the cumulative radiation dose and volume of cardiac exposure. Such injury may cause acute symptomatic pericarditis soon after the radiation is delivered, or instead it may result in fibrosis that first manifests as constrictive pericarditis many years later.

Pericardial involvement is common in collagen vascular diseases, presumably on an autoimmune basis. Up to 25% of patients with rheumatoid arthritis, 40% of those with systemic lupus erythematosus, and 10% of individuals with progressive systemic sclerosis experience clinical manifestations of acute pericarditis in the course of their systemic disease.

Drug-induced pericarditis has been reported with many pharmaceutical agents, either by inducing a lupus-like syndrome (e.g., hydralazine, procainamide, isoniazid,

Table 81.1 CAUSES OF ACUTE PERICARDITIS

"Idiopathic"

Infectious

    Viral, tuberculosis, pyogenic bacteria, fungi

Following myocardial infarction

    Early form

    Dressler syndrome

Postpericardiotomy

Uremia

Neoplastic

Radiation-induced

Collagen vascular diseases

Drug-associated

phenytoin, methyldopa) or on an idiosyncratic basis (e.g., minoxidil, anthracycline derivatives, cyclophosphamide, sulfa drugs).

CLINICAL FEATURES

Common symptoms of acute pericarditis include low-grade fever and chest pain. The discomfort is typically of sudden onset, intense, and located in the retrosternal and left precordial regions; it may radiate to the neck and left trapezius ridge. It can be differentiated from the discomfort of myocardial ischemia by its sharp, pleuritic, and positional character. It tends to be worse when lying supine and improves with sitting and leaning forward. Chest pain may not occur at all when inflammation develops slowly, such as in some patients with pericarditis due to TB, rheumatoid arthritis, neoplastic disease, radiation therapy, or uremia.

The predominant physical finding in acute pericarditis is a scratchy pericardial friction rub. It is of high frequency and heard best at end-expiration with the diaphragm of the stethoscope applied to the lower left sternal border as the patient leans forward. In its full form it consists of three components that correspond to phases of cardiac movement: ventricular contraction, ventricular relaxation, and atrial contraction. The rub can be transient, or only one or two components may be heard.

The electrocardiogram (EKG) in acute pericarditis (figure 81.1) is abnormal in >90% of patients and passes through four stages:

Stage 1: Diffuse, concave upward ST elevation in most leads, with the exception of aVR, often accompanied by PR-segment deviation opposite to the direction of the P wave (i.e., PR *depression* in lead II and PR *elevation* in lead aVR).

Stage 2: (Several days later): ST segments return to baseline.

Stage 3: Generalized T-wave inversion develops.

Stage 4: (Weeks or months later): ST segment and T waves have returned to baseline; no Q-wave development.

Individuals with the common EKG variant known as *early repolarization* display baseline ST elevations that can mimic stage 1 pericarditis. However, in distinction to those with early repolarization, the height of the ST segment in acute pericarditis tends to be >25% of the height of the T wave.

Blood studies reveal systemic inflammation (leukocytosis, elevated erythrocyte sedimentation rate, and C-reactive

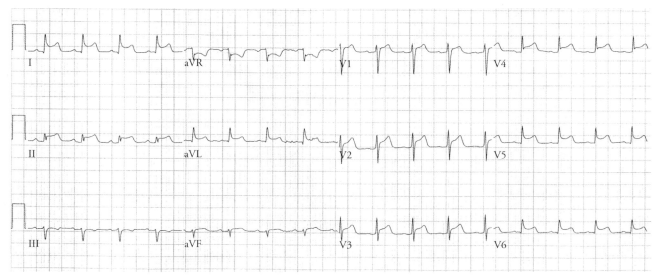

Figure 81.1. Twelve-Lead Electrocardiogram of Stage I Pericarditis. Diffuse ST segment elevation is present.

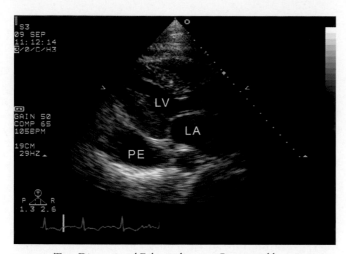

Figure 81.2. Two-Dimensional Echocardiogram. Parasternal long-axis view, demonstrating a posterior pericardial effusion (PE). LV, left ventricle, LA, left atrium.

protein) and often minor elevation of cardiac-specific troponins. The latter is a reflection of inflammation extending to the neighboring myocardium but does not predict an adverse outcome.

Most patients with acute pericarditis have no or only a small pericardial effusion, and chest radiography is frequently normal. However, if a large effusion (>250 mL) has accumulated, the cardiac silhouette becomes symmetrically enlarged. Echocardiography is a much more sensitive technique for the detection of pericardial effusion, as it can identify a collection of as little as 15 mL (see figure 81.2). A small effusion is identified as an echo-free space posterior to the left ventricle (LV). Larger effusions wrap around laterally and, if more than approximately 250 mL have accumulated, anterior to the heart as well.

Additional testing may be useful when specific etiologies of pericarditis are suspected, such as purified protein derivative (PPD) skin testing for TB, serologic testing (e.g., antinuclear antibodies) for collagen vascular diseases, mammography or chest CT for screening of breast and lung cancers, respectively. Even when a pericardial effusion is present, pericardiocentesis is not recommended in uncomplicated cases as the diagnostic yield is low and rarely affects management. It should be reserved for patients with large effusions or those with evidence of cardiac chamber compression (see below).

MANAGEMENT

There is a scarcity of randomized clinical trials in the management of pericardial diseases, and therefore therapy is generally empirical. Idiopathic or postviral pericarditis is a self-limited condition that tends to improve spontaneously within 1–3 weeks. The immediate goals of therapy are to reduce pericardial inflammation and relieve symptoms. Nonsteroidal anti-inflammatory drugs (NSAIDs) are first-line therapy (e.g.,

ibuprofen 600–800 mg tid or aspirin 650 mg qid). If symptoms do not respond promptly, useful adjuncts include colchicine (1 mg PO bid on first day, then 0.5 mg bid), a brief course of narcotic analgesics, or as last resort, a short regimen of corticosteroids (e.g., prednisone 60 mg PO × 2 days, then tapered off over 1 week). Although symptoms do respond promptly to steroids, patients who receive them are more prone to relapses. Hospitalization is appropriate for patients with high fever, large pericardial effusions, or in whom an etiology other than idiopathic/postviral is suspected.

Aspirin is the preferred anti-inflammatory agent for patients with pericarditis *early* after myocardial infarction, as other NSAIDs may impair healing of infarcted tissue. Patients with *delayed* post-MI pericarditis (Dressler syndrome) or postpericardiotomy pericarditis characteristically respond promptly to standard NSAID regimens, which can be used with less reservation at that later phase. Tuberculous pericarditis requires prolonged, multidrug, antituberculous therapy. Purulent pericarditis mandates aggressive antibiotic therapy and often catheter drainage of the pericardium. Pericarditis due to uremia is treated with initiation or intensification of dialysis. Forms of pericarditis associated with collagen vascular diseases respond to therapy directed against the underlying disorder, often including NSAID or glucocorticoid therapy. Drug-associated pericarditis responds to cessation of the offending agent. Neoplastic pericarditis is indicative of advanced-stage cancer, and therapy is usually palliative; if tamponade is present, drainage of pericardial fluid can be temporarily life saving (see below).

Recurrent pericarditis develops in up to 30% of patients after an initial episode. Recurrences are less frequent in patients who receive colchicine as part of the original treatment program. Recurrent pericarditis often responds to a renewed course of NSAID or colchicine therapy; refractory cases may require glucocorticoids, usually with a very slow taper (>1 month) to prevent additional occurrences. A recent report of a small number of patients showed benefit of intravenous immunoglobulin in suppressing symptoms of chronic idiopathic pericarditis.

Two serious complications may follow acute pericarditis: cardiac tamponade and chronic constrictive pericarditis.

CARDIAC TAMPONADE

Cardiac tamponade is characterized by the accumulation of pericardial fluid under sufficient pressure to compress and impair filling of the cardiac chambers. As a result, cardiac output declines substantially, which can lead to hypotensive shock and death.

ETIOLOGY

Any cause of acute pericarditis can lead to tamponade physiology, but the most common etiologies are neoplastic, idiopathic, and uremic pericarditis. Tamponade can also result from acute hemorrhage into the pericardial sac, for example, following chest trauma, as a complication of a proximal aortic dissection, bleeding after cardiac surgery, or myocardial perforation during percutaneous cardiac procedures.

PATHOPHYSIOLOGY

Because the pericardium is a relatively stiff structure, the sudden introduction of even a small volume of fluid into the pericardial space (as with acute hemorrhage) can lead to life-threatening cardiac chamber compression. However, when effusions accumulate more gradually, the parietal pericardium may physically stretch over time and accommodate larger volumes (>1 L) before hemodynamic compromise occurs.

In tamponade, the surrounding tense effusion limits ventricular filling and causes the diastolic pressure of each cardiac chamber to become elevated and equal to the high pericardial pressure. The right side of the heart is more susceptible to external compression than the left side because of its normally lower pressures. Thus, impaired right-sided chamber filling is one of the earliest signs of tamponade. Because the compressed chambers cannot accommodate normal venous return, systemic venous pressures rise. Limitation of early diastolic ventricular filling across the tricuspid valve is responsible for blunting of the normal *y* descent in the right atrial and systemic venous pressure tracings. Concurrently, the reduced diastolic ventricular filling decreases stroke volume and forward cardiac output.

The high pericardial pressure in tamponade exaggerates the relationship of normal ventricular interdependence: the volume of one ventricle can expand only when the size of the other decreases by the same amount. This principle applies to respiratory variations in ventricular filling. In normal individuals inspiration expands the right ventricle, shifts the interventricular septum toward the left, and thus slightly reduces LV filling and output over the next several beats. This results in a normal small inspiratory decline in systolic blood pressure. In cardiac tamponade the situation is amplified because the ventricles share a common, reduced space. Therefore, there is greater inspiratory reduction of LV output and blood pressure, and this is thought to be responsible for *pulsus paradoxus* (an inspiratory decrease in systolic BP >10 mm) in this condition.

CLINICAL FEATURES

Cardiac tamponade should be suspected when a patient with pericarditis or chest trauma develops signs and symptoms of systemic vascular congestion and decreased cardiac output. The patient may describe shortness of breath and chest discomfort; tachypnea and tachycardia are common. Other key physical findings are (1) hypotension with pulsus paradoxus, (2) jugular venous distension (with absence of the *y* descent), and (3) muffled heart sounds and inability to palpate the point of maximum cardiac impulse due to the surrounding effusion. Of note, pulsus paradoxus may not appear when coexisting conditions impede respiratory alterations in LV filling, including LV dysfunction, aortic regurgitation, and atrial septal defects. Conversely, pulsus paradoxus *may* appear in situations other than tamponade that cause large alterations in intrathoracic pressure, including acute and chronic pulmonary disease, and in some patients with constrictive pericarditis (see below).

The EKG typically demonstrates sinus tachycardia as well as low limb-lead voltage if a large effusion has accumulated. *Electrical alternans* (alternating height of the QRS complex in sequential beats—see figure 81.3) is uncommon but highly suggestive of a large effusion, as it results from shifting of the mean electrical axis as the heart swings from side to side within the large pericardial volume.

Echocardiography is the most useful noninvasive technique to evaluate for tamponade physiology. It can identify the presence, volume, and location of pericardial effusion and assess its hemodynamic significance. Sensitive and specific signs of tamponade include early diastolic collapse of the right ventricle (more specific) and cyclical compression of the right atrium (more sensitive). It is less common to observe cyclical indentation of the left atrium or LV, except in patients with loculated effusions that compress those chambers, as may occur after cardiac surgery. Other echocardiographic findings reflect the abnormal pathophysiology: distension of the inferior vena cava and exaggerated reciprocal respiratory variations in mitral and tricuspid diastolic Doppler velocities. Although these echocardiographic abnormalities are suggestive, it is the clinical characteristics of the patient that determine whether tamponade is present and dictate the aggressiveness of therapeutic interventions.

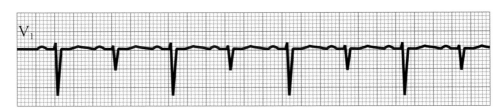

Figure 81.3. Electrocardiogram (EKG) Rhythm Strip Demonstrating Electrical Alternans. The depth of the QRS complex alternates from beat to beat as the heart swings within a large pericardial effusion, causing the mean electrical axis to shift back and forth.

MANAGEMENT

Although intravenous volume infusion may transiently improve blood pressure, the only effective management of cardiac tamponade is removal of the offending pericardial effusion. This is initially performed by closed pericardiocentesis, ideally in a cardiac catheterization laboratory, where the intracardiac hemodynamics can be monitored to confirm the diagnosis and assess the effect of fluid removal. The pericardiocentesis needle is usually inserted via a subxiphoid approach (to avoid piercing a coronary or internal mammary artery), often aided by echocardiographic guidance. A catheter is then threaded into the pericardial space and connected to a transducer for pressure measurement. Another catheter is inserted percutaneously into the right side of the heart and simultaneous recordings of intrapericardial and intracardiac pressures are compared. In tamponade, the pericardial pressure is elevated and is equal to the diastolic pressure in each cardiac chamber. In addition, the right atrial pressure tracing demonstrates blunting of the normal y descent, as described in the pathophysiology section above.

Following successful pericardiocentesis, the pressures in the cardiac chambers should decline as the pericardial pressure returns to normal. A pericardial catheter is often left in place for 1–2 days to allow more complete fluid drainage. For diagnostic purposes, pericardial fluid analysis should include blood counts, cytology and bacterial, fungal, and mycobacterial cultures, although the diagnostic yield of culture of pericardial fluid for *Mycobacterium tuberculosis* is low. If TB is suspected, a more rapid diagnosis from the pericardial fluid can be accomplished by polymerase chain reaction or by the finding of an elevated level of adenosine deaminase (>30 U/L in TB).

Open surgical drainage (via a subxiphoid approach) may be necessary for recurrences of cardiac tamponade or if hemodynamically significant loculated effusions are present. A surgical approach also allows acquisition of pericardial biopsies to aid in diagnosis when the cause of the effusion remains occult. For example, biopsy increases the diagnostic yield for *M. tuberculosis* to 80–90%. The creation of a pericardial window allows continuous drainage of pericardial fluid into the pleural space and prevents further recurrences of tamponade (e.g., for malignant effusions).

CONSTRICTIVE PERICARDITIS

Constrictive pericarditis is characterized by the development of abnormal pericardial rigidity that markedly impairs filling of the cardiac chambers.

ETIOLOGY

Any cause of acute inflammation can result in thickening, fibrosis, and calcification of the pericardium over time. The

Table 81.2 **ETIOLOGIES OF CONSTRICTIVE PERICARDITIS (*N* = 163)**

Postviral/idiopathic	46%
Post–cardiac surgical	37%
Prior mediastinal irradiation	9%
Miscellaneous (e.g., collagen vascular disease, tuberculosis)	8%

SOURCE: Bertog SC, Thambidorai SK, Parakh K, et al. Constrictive pericarditis: Etiology and cause-specific survival after pericardiectomy. *J Am Coll Cardiol.* 2004;43:1445–52.

most common conditions responsible for constrictive pericarditis in the United States are prior idiopathic/postviral pericarditis, cardiac surgery, mediastinal radiation therapy exposure, and connective tissue disorders (table 81.2). In developing countries, TB remains an important cause.

PATHOPHYSIOLOGY

In patients who have developed constrictive pericarditis, the rigid pericardium surrounding the heart impairs normal filling and causes elevation and equalization of diastolic pressures within the cardiac chambers. In the earliest phase of diastole (just after the mitral and tricuspid valves open), the ventricles actually begin to fill quite briskly because atrial pressures are typically elevated. However, as soon as the ventricles fill to the limit imposed on them by the surrounding rigid pericardium (still in early diastole), filling abruptly ceases. As a result, back pressure causes the systemic venous pressure to rise, leading to signs of right-sided heart failure. The subsequent reduced LV filling impairs stroke volume and cardiac output. Typically, systolic function of the ventricles is preserved in constrictive pericarditis. However if the inflammatory and scarring process has extended to the myocardium, contractile dysfunction may also contribute to the clinical presentation and limit the effectiveness of therapeutic pericardiectomy.

CLINICAL FEATURES

Clinical findings in constrictive pericarditis typically develop insidiously over a period of months to years. Symptoms of right-sided heart failure are common, including peripheral edema and increased abdominal girth due to hepatomegaly and ascites. Symptoms of left-sided congestion, such as exertional dyspnea and orthopnea, are less common. Late in the disease, signs of reduced cardiac output become manifest, including cachexia, muscle wasting, and fatigue.

Other findings are notable on examination. The jugular veins typically show marked elevation with two prominent descents during each cardiac cycle (x and y descents, as described below), creating a distinctive filling and collapsing pattern that is often evident from across the room. Unlike normal individuals (and those with cardiac tamponade) the degree of jugular venous distension fails to decrease, or may increase further, with inspiration (*Kussmaul sign*). The latter reflects the inability of the heart to accommodate the increased venous return that occurs with inspiration. On cardiac examination, an early diastolic high-pitched "knock" at the left lower sternal border or at the apex may be present. It results from the sudden cessation of ventricular filling in early diastole.

Pulsus paradoxus is found in the minority of patients with constrictive pericarditis. When present, its mechanism is different from that in cardiac tamponade and relates to failure of transmission of intrathoracic pressure to the cardiac chambers because of the surrounding rigid pericardium. Since inspiration in patients with constriction lowers the pulmonary venous pressure, but not left-sided heart pressures, the drive of blood from the pulmonary veins to the left atrium is reduced. Less LV filling translates to a decline in cardiac output and systolic pressure during inspiration.

The EKG generally displays only nonspecific ST and T-wave abnormalities, but atrial arrhythmias such as atrial fibrillation are common. The chest radiograph shows a normal or mildly increased cardiac silhouette. In some patients with chronic constriction (particularly those with TB pericarditis), calcification of the pericardium is present and can be best visualized at the right heart border on the lateral view. Echocardiography may demonstrate a thickened pericardium, but this is often difficult to appreciate on standard transthoracic imaging. Other echo findings include abrupt cessation of ventricular filling and a shuddering motion of the interventricular septum in early diastole, dilatation of the inferior vena cava, and characteristic Doppler abnormalities that reflect abbreviated diastolic ventricular filling: rapid deceleration of the early diastolic mitral inflow "E" wave velocity and reduction of the late diastolic inflow "A" wave velocity. With the decline in left-sided filling during inspiration (as described in the previous paragraph), there is an accompanying fall (>25%) in the mitral inflow "E" wave velocity, shifting of the interventricular septum to the left, and a reciprocal increase in tricuspid valve inflow velocity. Cardiac magnetic resonance (MR) and computed tomography (CT) scans are superior to echocardiography is assessment of pericardial anatomy. Pericardial thickness is usually increased at >2 mm in patients with constrictive pericarditis, although a minority of patients with proven constriction have normal thickness.

At cardiac catheterization, the characteristic findings of constrictive pericarditis are: (1) elevation and equalization of the diastolic pressures of each of the cardiac chambers; (2) the right atrial pressure tracing shows a prominent *y* descent (in distinction to the blunted *y* descent in cardiac tamponade); (3) The right and left ventricular pressure tracings show a diastolic dip and plateau configuration ("square root sign") as shown in figure 81.4, representing unimpeded early diastolic relaxation followed by abrupt

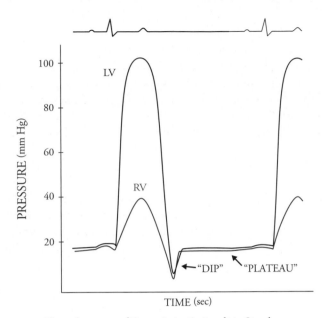

Figure 81.4. Hemodynamics of Constrictive Pericarditis. Simultaneous recordings of right (RV) and left (LV) ventricular pressures show elevation and equalization of the diastolic pressures, accompanied by an abnormal "dip and plateau" configuration.

cessation of diastolic filling as soon as ventricular volumes reach the limit imposed by the constricting pericardium. These hemodynamic findings may be masked in patients with intravascular volume depletion but can then be uncovered by infusion of an intravenous saline bolus in the catheterization laboratory.

The clinical presentation and hemodynamic findings of constrictive pericarditis can closely resemble those of restrictive cardiomyopathy (e.g., as caused by cardiac amyloidosis), another uncommon condition that impairs diastolic filling of the heart. It is important to distinguish these entities, as treatment approaches to them are very different. Although an endomyocardial biopsy may be necessary (biopsy results are normal in constrictive pericarditis and usually abnormal in the restrictive cardiomyopathies), the distinction can usually be made by less invasive means, as summarized in table 81.3. In distinction to constrictive pericarditis, patients with restrictive cardiomyopathy often have increased ventricular wall thickness, normal pericardial thickness, evidence of at least mild systolic dysfunction and pulmonary hypertension, and sluggish relaxation even at the very earliest phase of diastole.

MANAGEMENT

The patient with a fairly acute presentation of constrictive physiology (e.g., soon after cardiac surgery with near-normal pericardial thickness) may improve over a period of weeks to months with anti-inflammatory therapy. The only effective management of patients with the more common chronic pericardial constriction is complete surgical removal of the pericardium. A successful operation requires

	CONSTRICTIVE PERICARDITIS	RESTRICTIVE CARDIOMYOPATHY
Physical examination		
Kussmaul sign	Common	May be present
Pericardial knock	May be present	Absent
Pulmonary rales	Uncommon	Common
Electrocardiogram	Nonspecific ST and T-wave abnormalities	Low limb-lead voltage in infiltrative diseases
Chest x-ray		
Pericardial calcification	May be present	Absent
Echocardiography		
Thickened pericardium	Present	Absent
Thickened myocardium	Absent	Present (may be "speckled")
Exaggerated variation in transvalvular velocities	Present	Absent
Doppler tissue imaging at mitral annulus (represents LV relaxation rate at earliest phase of diastole)	Normal (> 8 cm/sec)	Reduced (< 8 cm/sec)
CT or MRI		
Thickened pericardium	Usually	Absent
Cardiac catheterization		
Equalized RV and LV diastolic pressures	Yes	LV often > RV by more than 3–5 mm Hg
Elevated PA systolic pressure	Uncommon	Common
Effect of inspiration on systolic pressures	Discordant: LV↓, RV↑	Concordant: LV↓, RV↓
Endomyocardial biopsy	Normal	Usually abnormal (e.g., amyloid)

NOTE: LV, left ventricle; PA, pulmonary artery; RV, right ventricle.

wide resection of the pericardial layers and is technically highly challenging. Even in very experienced hospitals, the operative mortality rate is >6%. After surgery, the majority of patients note symptomatic relief immediately. In others, presumably those with associated myocardial stiffness or fibrosis, improvement may be more delayed over a period of months. Patients with constriction due to viral/idiopathic pericarditis have the best outcomes after surgery, whereas results are less favorable in those with radiation-associated constriction.

EFFUSIVE-CONSTRICTIVE PERICARDITIS

Some patients with pericardial disease have features that reflect a combination of cardiac tamponade physiology *and* constrictive pericarditis. Such individuals typically present with pericardial effusion and symptoms, signs, and intracardiac pressure findings typical of tamponade. However, after the pericardial effusion is removed, the elevated intracardiac pressures do not fall to normal, and the hemodynamics of constrictive pericarditis supervene, with a prominent *y* descent in the right atrial pressure tracing and a "dip and plateau" configuration of the ventricular diastolic pressures. This syndrome is termed effusive-constrictive pericarditis, and the most common inciting etiologies are prior idiopathic/postviral pericarditis, mediastinal radiation

therapy, and neoplastic and tuberculous pericardial disease. Surgical pericardiectomy is usually required for full relief of symptoms.

ADDITIONAL READING

Bertog SC, Thambidorai SK, Parakh K, et al. Constrictive pericarditis: Etiology and cause-specific survival after pericardiectomy. *J Am Coll Cardiol.* 2004;43:1445–52.

ESC Committee for Practice Guidelines. Guidelines on the diagnosis and management of pericardial diseases, executive summary. *Eur Heart J.* 2004;25:587–610.

Grizzard JD, Ang GB. Magnetic resonance imaging of pericardial disease and cardiac masses. *Cardiol Clin.* 2007;25:111–40.

Imazio M, Bobbio M, Cecchi E, et al. Colchicine in addition to conventional therapy for acute pericarditis: Results of the COlchicine for acute PEricarditis (COPE) Trial. *Circulation.* 2005;112:2012–6.

Imazio M, Brucato A, Mayosi BM, et al. Medical therapy of pericardial diseases: Part I: Idiopathic and infectious pericarditis. *J Cardiovasc Med.* 2010;11(10):712–22.

Jiamsripong P, Mookadam F, Oh JK, Khandheria BK. Spectrum of pericardial disease: Part II. *Expert Rev Cardiovasc Ther.* 2009;7(9):1159–69.

Khandaker MH, Espinosa RE, Nishimura RA, et al. Pericardial disease: Diagnosis and management. *Mayo Clin Proc.* 2010;85(6):572–93.

Mookadam F, Jiamsripong P, Oh JK, Khandheria BK. Spectrum of pericardial disease: Part I. *Expert Rev Cardiovasc Ther.* 2009;7(9):1149–57.

Pande AN, Lilly LS. Pericardial disease. In: Solomon SD, ed. Essential Echocardiography (pp. 191–208). Totowa, NJ: Humana Press, 2007.

Roy CL, Minor MA, Brookhart MA, Choudhry NK. Does this patient with a pericardial effusion have cardiac tamponade? *N Engl J Med.* 2007;297:1810–18.

QUESTIONS

QUESTION 1. A 45-year-old previously healthy woman presents to the emergency department with fever, pleuritic chest pain, and a pericardial friction rub. The electrocardiogram shows sinus tachycardia, diffuse ST elevations, and PR-segment depression in lead II. Echocardiography demonstrates a small posterior pericardial effusion without cardiac chamber compression. Which of the following is correct?

    A. Glucocorticoid therapy is indicated to prevent progression of the effusion.

    B. The electrocardiogram will likely return to normal within 48 hours.

    C. Ventricular dysrhythmias are common in this setting.

    D. The relapse rate is >15%.

    E. Kussmaul sign is an expected physical finding.

QUESTION 2. A 56-year-old man presents to a physician's office with exertional dyspnea, marked jugular venous distention with prominent *x* and *y* descents, and peripheral edema. Pulsus paradoxus is not present. He has a history of Hodgkin disease 18 years earlier, treated with chemotherapy and mediastinal radiation therapy. He is admitted to the hospital, and right-sided heart catheterization is performed as part of the diagnostic workup. Selective hemodynamics are listed in the table:

CHAMBER	PRESSURE (mm Hg)	NORMAL (mm Hg)
Right atrium (mean)	16	≤8
Right ventricle	30/17	≤30/8
Pulmonary wedge (mean)	16	≤10

Which of the following statements is true?

    A. Pericardiocentesis should be performed urgently.

    B. Therapy should include a diuretic, ACE inhibitor, and a beta blocker.

    C. CT scan would be more helpful than echocardiography in confirming the diagnosis.

    D. Sinus bradycardia is likely present.

    E. Prior chemotherapy is likely responsible for these findings.

QUESTION 3. Which of the following statements about effusive-constrictive pericarditis is correct?

    A. Removal of pericardial fluid by pericardiocentesis normalizes the right atrial pressure.

    B. Uremia and drug-induced pericarditis are among the most common causes.

    C. Presenting physical findings resemble chronic constrictive pericarditis more than cardiac tamponade.

    D. Glucocorticoid therapy is curative in most cases.

    E. Resolution of this condition most often requires total pericardiectomy.

QUESTION 4. The following physical findings are typical of cardiac tamponade EXCEPT:

    A. Sinus tachycardia

    B. Jugular venous distension

    C. Kussmaul sign

    D. Inspiratory fall in systolic blood pressure >10 mm Hg

    E. Tachypnea

QUESTION 5. Each of the following statements regarding the EKG in acute pericarditis is true EXCEPT:

    A. The majority of patients demonstrate EKG abnormalities.

    B. Global ST-segment elevation is typical in early pericarditis.

    C. T-wave inversions develop before the ST elevations return to baseline.

    D. PR-segment deviation (opposite to the P-wave direction) is present in most cases.

    E. Sinus tachycardia is common.

ANSWERS

1. D
2. C
3. E
4. C
5. C

82.

ARRHYTHMIAS

Murali Chiravuri and Usha B. Tedrow

In the normal heart the sinoatrial (SA) node serves as the principal pacemaker and determines the heart rate. The SA node consists of groups of pacemaker cells marked by their ability to spontaneously depolarize and are located at the junction of the right atrium and the superior vena cava. The blood supply to the SA node is variable with the sinus nodal artery arising from the right coronary artery in 60% percent of cases and from the left circumflex artery in 40% of cases. Following depolarization of the SA nodal cells, the signal traverses the atrium before arriving at the atrioventricular (AV) node. The AV node is marked by its ability to delay impulse propagation, which allows for coordinated contraction of the atria and ventricles. The AV nodal artery arises from the right coronary artery in 90% of cases and from the left circumflex artery in 10% of cases. After exiting the AV node, the impulse is transmitted through the bundle of His, the right and left bundle branches, and ultimately exits the terminal Purkinje fibers of the conduction system into the myocardium near the apex of the heart.

The autonomic nervous system plays an important role in modulating the function of the cardiac conduction system. The SA and AV nodes are innervated by both the sympathetic and parasympathetic systems. Acetylcholine released by parasympathetic neurons decreases the rate of pacemaker depolarization, suppresses conduction, and increases the refractory period, whereas norepinephrine has the reverse effect.

BRADYARRHYTHMIAS

SINUS NODE DYSFUNCTION

Sinus Bradycardia: The normal sinus heart rate is between 60 and 100 beats per minute (bpm), but there may be wide variation in resting heart rate between individuals. For example, well-trained athletes may have significant vagal tone that results in a resting asymptomatic bradycardia. Sinus bradycardia may be caused by intracardiac processes

such as local ischemia and infiltrative disease, as well as extracardiac conditions such as hypothyroidism, hypothermia, stroke, and periods of enhanced vagal tone such as that seen during vasovagal syncope. It is important to exclude drug effects as an etiology for sinus bradycardia. Sinus pauses >3 seconds are considered abnormal and warrant intervention especially if the patient is symptomatic with these pauses.

Tachycardia Bradycardia Syndrome: This syndrome is marked by the presence of sinus or other bradycardia alternating with rapid supraventricular tachycardias (SVTs), most often atrial fibrillation. Medical control of the rapid arrhythmia is often limited by worsening bradycardia. Symptoms including light-headedness and syncope are most often caused by the bradycardia or by offset pauses. Offset pauses refer to a pause that occurs in the context of conversion of atrial fibrillation or flutter to sinus rhythm.

Sinoatrial Exit Block: Sinoatrial exit block occurs when impulse propagation out of the SA node is impaired. First-degree sinoatrial exit block involves delayed but present conduction out of the SA node and so cannot be diagnosed on the surface electrocardiogram (EKG). Second-degree sinoatrial block is marked by intermittent block out of the SA node and resultant dropped P waves on the EKG. Third-degree sinoatrial block, which involves complete block of sinus impulses out of the SA node manifests simply as complete sinus arrest on the surface EKG.

Diagnosis and Treatment

The principal goal of evaluation and treatment of sinus bradycardia is symptom alleviation, and the asymptomatic patient rarely warrants intervention. Symptomatic patients with documented sinus bradycardia or sinus arrest may not require further testing. In the symptomatic patient with suspected SA nodal dysfunction, maneuvers such as carotid sinus massage (CSM) and Holter or other noninvasive monitoring may prove useful. Electrophysiological testing does allow for functional testing of the SA node and more importantly can provide functional characteristics of atrial, AV nodal, and infranodal conduction as well. However in the modern era, this testing typically adds little to the information obtained from a patient's symptoms and cardiac monitoring.

Once all correctible conditions such as hypothyroidism have been addressed and all potentially causative drugs have been stopped, the mainstay of treatment for sinus node dysfunction is the implantation of a permanent pacemaker. Although a single-chamber atrial pacemaker may suffice, there is often concern of concomitant disease in other more distal parts of the conduction system, and so dual-chamber pacemakers are frequently implanted for symptomatic sinus node disease.

ATRIOVENTRICULAR CONDUCTION DISORDERS

Conduction disorders may occur at the level of the atrium, AV node, His bundle, or the infra-Hisian conduction system. Furthermore, impulse conduction may be prolonged, intermittent, or completely absent. Besides drugs and normal degenerative processes, there are several disease states that can cause AV conduction disease. These include myocardial ischemia, congenital AV block, cardiac surgery, infiltrative cardiomyopathies, myocarditis, Lyme carditis, and metabolic derangements among others. Furthermore, there are a number of neuromuscular diseases including myotonic muscular dystrophy, Erb's dystrophy, and Kearns-Sayre syndrome that are marked by progressive conduction disease and AV block.

First-degree AV block: First degree AV block is characterized by a prolonged PR interval (>200 ms) but a preserved 1:1 relationship between the atria and ventricles. The site of conduction delay cannot be ascertained from the surface EKG, but the absence of bundle branch block or a wide QRS does make an infra-Hisian site less likely.

Second-degree AV block, Mobitz type 1: Also referred to as Wenckebach block, this rhythm is marked by a progressive lengthening in the PR interval followed by a dropped QRS. Due to a progressive decrease in the rate of PR prolongation, careful analysis also reveals a shortening of the R-R interval prior to the dropped beat. The site of block is most often the AV node, although infranodal Wenckebach block may occur as well.

Second-degree AV block, Mobitz type 2: In this situation the PR interval remains constant, but there is intermittent conduction from the atria to the ventricles, often in a fixed ratio. Mobitz type II block most often occurs below the AV node at either the level of the His bundle or more commonly, in the infra-Hisian region. The majority of patients with this type of block show some form of bundle branch block reflective of underlying conduction disease.

Third-degree AV block: In complete heart block, no atrial impulses reach the ventricle. The escape rhythm often provides clues to the site of block. The presence of a narrow complex escape rhythm suggests block at the level of the AV node and less frequently at the level of the His bundle. A wide complex escape rhythm most often signifies infra-Hisian block.

Diagnosis and Treatment

The surface EKG remains the mainstay of diagnosis for AV block. It is important to note that in the setting of 2:1 block, it is not possible to differentiate between Wenckebach and Mobitz type II block. However, the presence of Wenckebach in another portion of the EKG or improvement of block with heightened adrenergic tone or with atropine are suggestive of Wenckebach block. Another important point is the differentiation of complete heart block from AV dissociation that occurs when the ventricular rate exceeds the atrial rate in the context of normal AV conduction.

First-degree AV block rarely warrants treatment except for the rare cases when the patient is symptomatic with a pacemaker syndrome-like constellation of symptoms. Vagolytic maneuvers such as exercise and atropine should decrease the PR interval if the AV node is the site of delay, whereas exacerbation by these maneuvers or underlying bundle branch disease may reflect an infranodal site of delay. Treatment of patients includes cessation of nodal blocking agents and only rarely is a pacemaker indicated. Likewise, Wenckebach block rarely requires treatment unless the patient suffers from symptomatic bradycardia or if there is a concern for rapidly progressive AV conduction disease as seen in certain neuromuscular diseases. In contrast, second-degree AV block without an identifiable and reversible etiology warrants consideration for a dual-chamber pacemaker.

The presence of newly diagnosed complete heart block or Mobitz type II block requires immediate attention. The initial assessment should evaluate the clinical and hemodynamic status of the patient; the escape rhythm should be carefully analyzed. Hemodynamic instability, prior syncope, symptomatic escape bradycardia, wide complex escape rhythms, heart rates <40 bpm and pauses >3 seconds all warrant consideration of a temporary pacing wire after transcutaneous pads have been placed. Additionally if the patient is remote from potential permanent pacemaker implantation, a temporary pacing wire should also be strongly considered. When all reversible causes have been addressed, the definitive treatment is pacemaker implantation.

SUPRAVENTRICULAR TACHYARRHYTHMIAS

TACHYARRHYTHMIAS INVOLVING THE SINUS NODE

Most tachycardias emanating from the sinus node are physiological in nature and reflect a high catecholaminergic state due to exercise, stimulants, stress and/or extracardiac stressors such as anemia, hypoxia, fever, hyperthyroidism, and hypovolemia.

Inappropriate sinus tachycardia (IST): This refers to a condition characterized by an elevated resting sinus rate and often an exaggerated sinus response to exertion. The etiology of this condition is unclear but is felt to be exacerbated by abnormal autonomic tone.

Postural orthostatic tachycardia syndrome (POTS): This syndrome occurs primarily in otherwise healthy young women marked by postural orthostatic symptoms including light-headedness and weakness on standing without hypotension but with an abnormal postural increase in sinus rate.

Sinus node reentry: Sinus node reentry refers to a reentrant tachycardia within the sinus node that cannot be distinguished from a regular sinus tachycardia on the surface EKG. However, this tachycardia is often marked by a sudden "jump" in heart rate followed by a return to the previous sinus rate.

Diagnosis and Treatment

The diagnosis of a sinus tachycardia is made by analyzing the P-wave morphology on the surface EKG and ideally, comparing it to a baseline EKG without arrhythmia. The P-wave and QRS morphology should be identical, although the patient may have a rate-related bundle branch block resulting in an altered QRS morphology. It is imperative to first rule out a secondary or physiological cause for the sinus tachycardia. Beta-blocker treatment is often effective with IST, and the goal of treatment with POTS is maintenance of intravascular volume with oral fluids, salt, and fludrocortisone. Ablative therapy of the sinus node can be considered in refractory and highly symptomatic patients but often does not lead to symptomatic improvement.

FOCAL ATRIAL TACHYCARDIA

Focal atrial tachycardia refers to an atrial tachycardia that originates outside of the SA node. The mechanism of these tachycardias may involve reentry, automaticity or triggered activity. Atrial tachycardias may originate from the right or left atrium. The most common sites of origin in the right atrium are the tricuspid annulus, the crista terminalis, and the os of the coronary sinus. By far the most common site of origin of left atrial tachycardias is the myocardial junction of pulmonary veins and the left atrial antrum.

Diagnosis and Treatment

The rates of atrial tachycardia can vary from 100–250 bpm. Careful analysis of the P-wave morphology often reveals differences from the native P-wave morphology, although atrial foci close to the SA node may be indistinguishable. Atrial tachycardias are often marked by sudden onset and equally sudden termination as opposed to sinus tachycardia, which tends to show more graduated acceleration and deceleration.

The first line of symptomatic atrial tachycardia is rate control with either beta blockers or calcium channel blockers, such as verapamil or diltiazem. In those patients with refractory symptoms despite medical treatment, catheter ablation is indicated. In those patients who have failed ablation or who are poor candidates for ablation, class III agents such as amiodarone and sotalol or class 1C agents such as flecainide can be used provided that the patient has been deemed suitable for such drugs.

ATRIAL FLUTTER

Common atrial flutter is due to a large macroreentrant circuit with a wavefront revolving around the tricuspid annulus. Atrial rates are typically between 240 and 300 bpm, most often with 2:1 conduction to the ventricles, resulting in a ventricular rate of 150 bpm. Concerns include rate control, rhythm control and anticoagulation due to risk of potential thromboembolic events, similar to atrial fibrillation, discussed below.

Diagnosis and Treatment

In typical counterclockwise atrial flutter, the wavefront proceeds up the atrial septum and down the right atrial free wall. P waves are negative in the inferior leads, positive in V1, and negative in V6. The circuit can also revolve in the clockwise direction, giving rise to positive P waves in the inferior leads and a negative deflection in V1. Re-entry is dependent on conduction through the cavo-tricuspid isthmus bounded by the tricuspid valve annulus, inferior vena cava, eustachian ridge, and coronary sinus os. Other atrial tachycardias can mimic atrial flutter, and in patients with prior atrial surgery or ablation, common atrial flutter may have an atypical EKG appearance. Rate control of atrial flutter is often quite challenging, owing to the regular repetitive flutter circuit. Beta blockers, calcium channel blockers, and digoxin are all reasonable choices but often may result in only a limited degree of rate control. Cardioversion and catheter ablation are reasonable options.

Catheter ablation is performed by placing a series of radiofrequency lesions across the cavo-tricuspid isthmus, creating a line of conduction block. Success is achieved in >95% of patients, and recurrences are less frequent than in those managed with antiarrhythmic drug therapy.

Approximately 20–30% of patients also have atrial disease that leads to atrial fibrillation in the next 20 months. A history of atrial fibrillation and depressed ventricular function increase the risk of subsequent atrial fibrillation.

ATRIAL FIBRILLATION

Atrial fibrillation (AF) is the most common supraventricular arrhythmia in the United States, and its prevalence increases with age. AF is an important risk factor for stroke and is a cause of increased mortality and hospitalizations in patients with heart failure. Sleeves of myocardium extending along the pulmonary veins are often important sites for the initiation of AF. Atrial scarring due to stretch and inflammation also plays a role in the substrate for maintenance of AF. The resulting arrhythmia is exceedingly rapid (>400 bpm) and disorganized in the atrium. The AV node is bombarded with these rapid signals and produces a somewhat slower, irregularly irregular ventricular response. Patients can have episodes that start and stop on their own (*paroxysmal*), and episodes that require medical intervention for termination (*persistent*). AF that is refractory to medical intervention to achieve sinus rhythm is termed *chronic*.

Diagnosis and Treatment

AF on surface EKG consists of an irregular baseline without clear P waves discernible and an irregularly irregular ventricular response. Therapy is directed at rate control, rhythm control, and anticoagulation.

Rate control can be achieved with beta blockers, calcium channel blockers, and digoxin. In cases where rate control cannot be achieved with medication, an AV junction ablation with permanent pacemaker implantation can be considered. In this case, the atria remain fibrillating, and the patient becomes pacemaker-dependent due to iatrogenic heart block.

Reasons to restore sinus rhythm include symptomatic intolerance of the arrhythmia, or a rare or first episode. Rhythm control can be achieved with antiarrhythmic drugs or catheter ablation. It is important to note that among patients with symptomatically tolerated AF, a difference in mortality or stroke risk has not been demonstrated when patients are randomized to a rate control or rhythm control strategy. For those with structurally normal hearts appropriate for rhythm control, the sodium channel blockers flecainide and propafenone can be reasonable. For those with structural heart disease, amiodarone is the most effective, but the potassium channel blockers sotalol and dofetilide can be reasonable options. Catheter ablation is 80–90% effective in maintaining sinus rhythm in patients with paroxysmal AF, but success rates fall to 50–60% among those with more persistent arrhythmia.

The risk of thromboembolic stroke in patients with AF is in the range of 6% per year and is further increased by about 40% in patients who also have heart failure. Long term anticoagulation with warfarin is indicated in those with a CHADS2 score of 2 or higher (one point each for congestive heart failure, hypertension, age >75 years, diabetes, and two points for a prior stroke or transient ischemic attack). In the acute setting, all patients with persistent arrhythmia lasting >48 hours merit short-term anticoagulation with a heparin or direct thrombin inhibitor as appropriate with a bridge to warfarin anticoagulation for a minimum of 6 weeks.

AV NODAL REENTRY

Atrioventricular node reentrant tachycardia (AVNRT) is the most common of the so-called paroxysmal supraventricular tachycardias. It presents as a narrow complex tachycardia unless there is concurrent rate-related aberrancy. The most common symptoms are palpitations, dizziness, shortness of breath, and chest pain. This arrhythmia can occur at any age but most often manifests itself in young adulthood.

The anatomic AV node consists of a compact portion and adjoining lobes. In patients with AV nodal reentry the lobe that extends along the tricuspid annulus toward the coronary sinus likely forms a functional pathway for slow conduction. The typical functional fast pathway demonstrates rapid conduction and has a long refractory time, whereas the slow pathway conducts slowly but has a shorter refractory period.

During normal sinus rhythm, conduction typically proceeds down the fast pathway. If an appropriately coupled atrial premature beat occurs, the impulse can block in the fast pathway but can still conduct down the slow pathway (due to the shorter refractory period of the slow pathway). The impulse then can find the fast pathway recovered for conduction, and a reentry circuit can continue.

Diagnosis and Treatment

The diagnosis of AVNRT is based on the symptom history and documentation of suggestive SVT on a surface EKG or on a recording monitor such as a Holter monitor. Typical "slow-fast" AVNRT in which antegrade conduction occurs over the slow pathway and retrograde conduction occurs over the fast pathway is characterized by near simultaneous atrial and ventricular activation. The P-wave is often buried in the QRS complex but can sometimes be seen immediately after the QRS complex. This may manifest as a R-R' on lead V1. In the atypical "fast-slow" form of AVNRT however, retrograde atrial activation is delayed and may be difficult to differentiate from other SVTs such as AVRT and atrial tachycardias.

Treatment is primarily centered on patient stability and symptom relief. In the acute setting, evaluation must focus on the clinical status of the patient. Hemodynamic instability, syncope, respiratory compromise, and/or angina warrant acute termination with adenosine or cardioversion. In the stable patient, vagal maneuvers and carotid sinus massage may be attempted. Medical therapy includes beta blockers and nondihydropyridine calcium channel blockers. The asymptomatic patient with rare occurrences and self-termination with vagal maneuvers may not warrant any daily treatment. Catheter ablation allows for definitive treatment of AVNRT in the patient with incomplete control with medications or in those patients who do not wish to take medications. There is a small but present risk (0.8%) of complete heart block during AVNRT ablation that requires implantation of a pacemaker.

ACCESSORY PATHWAY-DEPENDENT TACHYCARDIA

In the normal heart, the only electrical connection between the atria and ventricles is the AV node and His-Purkinje system. However in some individuals there exist additional pathways for impulse conduction that are referred to as accessory pathways. These pathways may conduct in the antegrade direction, retrograde direction, or both. Sinus conduction proceeding over the accessory pathway results in a delta wave and a short PR interval (<120 msec), referred to as a Wolf-Parkinson-White (WPW) pattern (figure 82.1). When this pattern is associated with arrhythmias, it is referred to as WPW syndrome. Accessory pathways are most often found in individuals with structurally normal hearts, but there is a significantly higher incidence of accessory pathways in certain conditions such as Ebstein's anomaly.

Regular tachycardia that utilizes an accessory pathway is referred to as atrioventricular reentrant tachycardia (AVRT).

Except in the rare instances of multiple accessory pathways, the circuit involves the atria, ventricles, AV node, and the accessory pathway. When the impulse travels anterograde down the AV node and back up the accessory pathway, it is referred to as orthodromic reentrant tachycardia (ORT); whereas when the impulse travels anterograde down the accessory pathway and back up the AV node, it is referred to as antidromic reentrant tachycardia (ART). ORT is manifested by a narrow complex tachycardia whereas ART, which is maximally preexcited, is a wide complex tachycardia. Of note, given that the atria and ventricles are integral parts of the tachycardia circuit, there is an obligatory 1:1 AV relationship in any form of AVRT. Tachycardia that persists in spite of evident variable conduction to the atria or ventricles effectively rules out AVRT.

Diagnosis and Treatment

The presence of a WPW pattern on a surface EKG reveals the presence of an accessory pathway, although the mere presence of an accessory pathway does not imply that AVRT has or will occur, and furthermore, it may be an innocent bystander in the context of another underlying tachycardia mechanism. The absence of a delta wave does not rule AVRT, as the accessory pathway may be far from the sinus node and/or may only conduct in the retrograde direction, that is, a concealed accessory pathway.

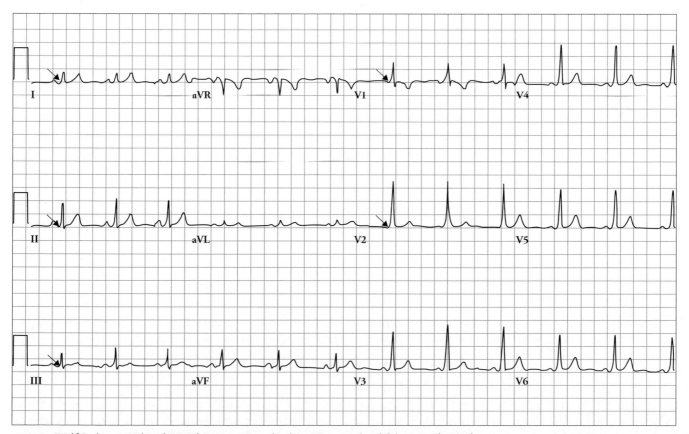

Figure 82.1. Wolf-Parkinson-White (WPW) Pattern. Note the short PR interval and delta waves (arrows).

The primary concern with WPW is the possibility of developing atrial fibrillation rapidly conducting over the accessory pathway leading to a rapid ventricular response and possibly ventricular fibrillation (VF). Risk factors for sudden death in WPW include prior atrial fibrillation, rapidly conducting pathways or multiple pathways, and a history of rapid SVT or syncope. An electrophysiological (EP) study can risk stratify the conduction characteristics of an accessory pathway and thereby determine the suitability of catheter ablation of the accessory pathway. In the case of a high-risk pathway, the patient may be placed on a sodium-channel-blocking drug to stabilize him or her until an EP study can be performed. Furthermore, as in the case of AVNRT, nodal-blocking agents can be used as first-line therapy in AVRT with concealed accessory pathways, but more definitive treatment is achieved with catheter ablation of accessory pathways.

JUNCTIONAL TACHYCARDIA

The normal AV junctional escape rate is 40–60 bpm but an accelerated junctional rhythm with rates between 70 and 130 bpm may occur, most often in the context of irritability of the AV junction. Junctional ectopic tachycardia may be due to conditions such as recent cardiac valvular surgery, myocardial ischemia, digitalis toxicity, or myocarditis. Rarely primary junctional automaticity can occur in isolation.

It is important to recognize that the entity paroxysmal junctional reciprocating tachycardia (PJRT), a slow long RP tachycardia, is a bit of a misnomer, actually resulting from a slowly conducting posteroseptal accessory pathway. This entity is an important cause of a tachycardia-induced cardiomyopathy in pediatric patients and is responsive to catheter ablation.

Diagnosis and Treatment

The diagnosis of junctional tachycardia is made by the observation of QRS morphology identical to that seen during sinus rhythm but with AV dissociation or evidence of retrograde P waves. True junctional ectopic tachycardia typically resolves as the inciting condition improves.

VENTRICULAR ARRHYTHMIAS

There are several features of ventricular tachycardia (VT) that should be considered during evaluation. It is of course important to initially look for clues that the wide complex tachycardia is not supraventricular in origin (see figure 82.2). The occurrence of three or more ventricular beats is termed nonsustained VT (NSVT) unless it lasts for >30 seconds, in which case it is referred to as sustained ff. The rates of VT are generally >120 bpm. A ventricular rate <110 bpm is referred to as an accelerated idioventricular rhythm (AIVR). VT with a single QRS morphology is referred to as monomorphic VT, whereas polymorphic VT

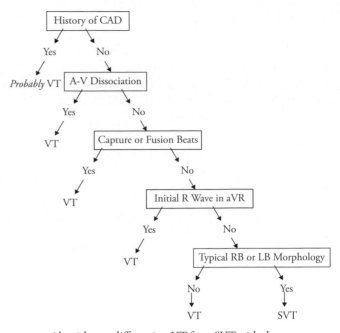

Figure 82.2. Algorithm to differentiate VT from SVT with aberrancy. A-V dissociation refers to independent atrial and ventricular activity. Capture beats refer to regularly conducted supraventricular beats during ventricular tachycardia while fusion beats refer to a QRS morphology that is a combination of the ventricular tachycardia and a supraventricular beat conducted down the conduction system.

is characterized by a constantly changing QRS morphology. Following the acute stabilization of the patient, it is critically important to ascertain the cardiac history and cardiac function of a patient with VT as this information alone can point to the underlying etiology of the arrhythmia.

SYNDROMES ASSOCIATED WITH VENTRICULAR ARRHYTHMIAS AND SUDDEN CARDIAC DEATH

Brugada Syndrome: This syndrome is an autosomal dominant syndrome characterized by EKG abnormalities and predisposition to ventricular arrhythmias. The primary mode of diagnosis is the EKG, which may show ST elevations in the anterior precordial leads in the context of a structurally normal heart. Occasionally these findings may be concealed and can be elicited with a class IC agent such as flecainide. Risk factors for sudden cardiac death (SCD) include an abnormal EKG pattern and a history of syncope. Given the lack of effective medications for this syndrome, the treatment is often prophylactic implantable cardioverter-defibrillator (ICD) placement.

Long QT Syndrome: The long QT syndrome is characterized by a prolonged QT interval and T wave abnormalities on the surface EKG. These patients are at increased risk of torsades de pointes, and the most common clinical presentation is palpitations or syncope. There are several genes that have been identified that can result in long QT syndrome, most affecting potassium and sodium channels in the heart. Sympathetic activation has been noted to correlate with cardiac events, and so beta blockers have some role in the management of this disease, although the residual risk of sudden cardiac death in many is sufficient to warrant ICD placement. Of note, in those cases where bradycardia or pause-dependent arrhythmias are noted, an increased programmed pacing rate on the ICD may prove beneficial.

Arrhythmogenic Right Ventricular Dysplasia: This refers to a genetic disorder characterized by fatty replacement of myocardial tissue primarily involving the right ventricle, resulting in ventricular arrhythmias. Given the right ventricular origin, the ventricular arrhythmias commonly have a left bundle branch block (LBBB) configuration, and the baseline EKG may show ST and T wave abnormalities in the anterior precordial leads. The condition often declares itself with palpitations, syncope, or sudden cardiac death, and symptoms are often exacerbated with exercise. The primary mode of diagnosis is with imaging technologies such as cardiac magnetic resonance imaging (MRI). Although medical therapy and VT ablation may suppress VT and improve symptoms, prophylactic ICD placement is warranted to prevent SCD.

Cardiomyopathies

Dilated and hypertrophic cardiomyopathies are associated with an increased risk of developing ventricular arrhythmias. Patients with a hypertrophic cardiomyopathy are at increased risk when they have a family history of cardiac death, a personal history of syncope, and have more severe forms of hypertrophy and outflow tract gradients in which case an ICD may be indicated. Patients with dilated cardiomyopathies are also at increased risk of ventricular arrhythmias and SCD, particularly if they suffer significant left ventricular dysfunction. These arrythmias are often scar related. ICD placement has been shown to be beneficial for primary prevention of SCD when the ejection fraction (EF) is <35%.

IDIOPATHIC VENTRICULAR TACHYCARDIA

Monomorphic VT that occurs in the context of a structurally normal heart is referred to as idiopathic ventricular tachycardia.

Outflow tract tachycardia: Also known as repetitive monomorphic VT, this form of VT most often originates from the right ventricular outflow tract (RVOT) and less frequently from the left ventricular outflow tract (LVOT). RVOT tachycardias manifest with a left bundle morphology and an inferior axis on the surface EKG. These tachycardias are often catecholamine sensitive, and adenosine may terminate them.

Fascicular ventricular tachycardia

Also referred to as idiopathic left ventricular tachycardia (ILVT), this tachycardia typically originates from the midseptal or inferoapical region of the left ventricle. The left posterior fascicle is most often involved in the tachycardia circuit. The surface EKG pattern is characteristically a right bundle morphology with a superior axis.

Diagnosis and Treatment

Idiopathic ventricular tachycardias are rarely life-threatening. Medications and catheter ablation are often able to suppress the arrhythmia, and an ICD is not indicated for these patients. Outflow tachycardias often respond to beta blockers and verapamil and, in refractory cases, to class III agents such as amiodarone and sotalol. Catheter ablation is increasingly being used to treat outflow tachycardias as the success rates are high with relatively low procedural risks. ILVT is characterized by its sensitivity to verapamil both for acute treatment and for chronic suppression. As with outflow tract VT, catheter ablation is increasingly being considered as front-line therapy given the high success rates and low risks involved.

ISCHEMIC VENTRICULAR TACHYCARDIA

Coronary artery disease (CAD) is the most common cause of ventricular tachycardia. Ventricular arrhythmias including polymorphic VT and VF can occur during active ischemia or during an acute coronary syndrome. However, monomorphic ventricular tachycardia typically occurs in the context of an existing myocardial scar that acts as a substrate for ventricular reentry. Scarring associated with CAD is often transmural but spares an endocardial rim of myocardial tissue that survives through direct diffusion from the intracavitary blood pool.

Diagnosis and Treatment

A wide complex tachycardia in a patient with CAD should be assumed to be VT until proven otherwise. VT that is clinically unstable should be promptly treated with DC cardioversion. When treating clinically "stable" VT however, medications such as lidocaine, amiodarone, and less frequently procainamide can be used in the acute setting. It is important to rule out active ischemia as a trigger for ventricular arrhythmias in the context of an ischemic substrate. Options for the chronic treatment of ischemic VT include medical therapy, ablation, and ICD implantation. If the EF is preserved, then the only role for an ICD lies in secondary prevention. However, if the EF is impaired then an ICD may be indicated for primary prevention of SCD. Drug therapy is often effective in treating ventricular tachycardia. The most common agents used to treat ischemic VT include beta blockers and the class III agents including amiodarone, although the class IA and class IB agents such as quinidine and mexiletine, respectively, also often prove useful. For the patient with medication refractory VT or in the patient with drug intolerance, VT ablation is an option that often provides excellent results.

BUNDLE BRANCH REENTRY

Bundle branch reentry (BBR) tachycardia refers to a specific form of VT that utilizes the endogenous conduction system as the circuit. Typical BBR tachycardia occurs in the context of a significantly dilated left ventricular cardiomyopathy with baseline left bundle branch (LBB) block and prolonged His to ventricle conduction times. The tachycardia is typically initiated by a premature ventricular contraction that is blocked retrograde in the right bundle but travels up the left bundle and down the now excitable right bundle to complete the circuit. BBR tachycardia can manifest the same QRS morphology as the baseline QRS morphology as it uses the His-Purkinje system as part of the circuit.

POLYMORPHIC VENTRICULAR TACHYCARDIA

Polymorphic VT (PMVT) is characterized by a continuously varying QRS morphology. Polymorphic VT is classified based on whether it occurs with a normal or prolonged QT interval at baseline.

PMVT in the context of a normal baseline QT interval may occur with underlying coronary ischemia. It may also occur in a structurally normal heart as a sporadic phenomenon or a part of a familial syndrome referred to as *catecholaminergic polymorphic VT* (CPVT). This syndrome is marked by sudden-onset PMVT or VF that typically occurs in a hyperadrenergic state. Medications, particularly digitalis are associated with multiform ventricular tachycardias, classically the bidirectional VT marked by an alternating LBBB/RBBB morphology. In the event that no reversible etiology is found, or if the arrhythmia persists after correction of an identifiable cause, an ICD may be indicated.

ADDITIONAL READING

Patel, A, Markowitz, SM. Atrial Tachycardia: mechanisms and management. *Expert Rev Cardiovasc Ther.* 2008;6(6): 811–22.

Goldberger, ZD, Rho, RW, Page, RL. Approach to the diagnosis and initial management of the stable adult patient with a wide complex tachycardia. *Am J Cardiol.* 2008;101(10):1456–66.

Hood, RE, Shorofsky, SR. Management of arrhythmias in the emergency department *Cardiol Clin.* 2006;24(1):125–33.

Goldenberg, I, Moss, AJ. Long QT syndrome. *J Am Coll Cardiol.* 2008;51(24):2291–2300.

Aronow, WS. Etiology, pathophysiology, and treatment of atrial fibrillation: part 1. *Cardiol Rev.* 2008;16(4):181–88.

Latif, S, Dixit, S, Callans, DJ. Ventricular arrhythmias in normal hearts. *Cardiol Clin.* 2008;26(3):367–80.

Andrikopoulos G, Tzeis S, Vardas PE. Technical advances in electrophysiology. *Heart.* 2011 Feb;97(3):237–43.

Kalin A, Usher-Smith J, Jones VJ, Huang CL, Sabir IN. Cardiac arrhythmia: a simple conceptual framework. *Trends Cardiovasc Med.* 2010 Apr;20(3):103–7.

QUESTIONS

QUESTION 1. Palpitations followed by syncope develop suddenly in a 16-year-old boy with known Wolff-Parkinson-White syndrome. In the emergency room the patient is alert when supine with a blood pressure of 85/50 mm Hg, but is nearly syncopal if he tries to sit up. A rhythm strip demonstrates a wide QRS tachyarrhythmia at 260 beats/min.

The best initial treatment is:

A. Intravenous procainamide
B. Intravenous verapamil
C. Intravenous dopamine
D. Electrical cardioversion
E. Intravenous digoxin

QUESTION 2. A 45-year-old man is noted to have an irregular pulse on elective physical examination. He is asymptomatic and unaware of his condition. His EKG demonstrates normal sinus rhythm with normal intervals and QRS morphology. Occasional unifocal premature ventricular contractions are noted on a rhythm strip. Echocardiography is performed with no demonstrable abnormalities of valves, chamber size, or pump function. A 24-hour ambulatory monitoring records 8542 isolated, but multiform, premature ventricular contractions, 842 couplets, and two 3-beat runs of ventricular tachycardia. After 48 hours of quinidine therapy, the number of premature ventricular contractions is reduced in half, no couplets are noted, and only a single triplet is observed. You are asked to provide an additional opinion by the family physician. After obtaining a history and examining the patient you recommend one of the following:

A. Discontinuing quinidine
B. Maintaining quinidine
C. Adding digoxin
D. Replacing the quinidine with propanolol

QUESTION 3. All of the following are indications for an ICD, EXCEPT:

A. History of VT/VF arrest
B. Nonsustained VT with inducible VT at EP study with EF <30% (MADIT I)
C. Brugada syndrome
D. EF <35% and NYHA class II/III heart failure (SCD HeFT)
E. Newly diagnosed nonischemic cardiomyopathy

ANSWERS

1. D
2. D
3. E

83.

CARDIOVASCULAR DISEASE PREVENTION

Jonathan D. Brown and Jorge Plutzky

Atherosclerotic cardiovascular disease (CVD) remains the leading cause of death in the developed world, causing approximately 600,000 fatalities annually in the United States. For classification purposes CVD is typically subcategorized into four groups: (1) coronary heart disease (CHD), (2) cerebrovascular disease, (3) peripheral arterial disease (PAD), and (4) aortic disease including aortic aneurysm and aortic dissection. Of these, nearly half of all cardiovascular deaths arise directly from CHD, manifested as acute myocardial infarction (MI)/sudden cardiac death or heart failure, with cerebrovascular disease causing an additional 20% of CVD deaths. Recent advances have helped to identify key risk factors that contribute directly to the initiation and progression of CVD.

This chapter focuses on how cardiovascular risk factors contribute to the initiation and progression of coronary heart disease (CHD). Cardiovascular risk factors are currently grouped into *traditional* and *nontraditional* types. *Traditional risk factors* include hyperlipidemia (or dyslipidemia), tobacco use, hypertension, diabetes mellitus, age, male gender, and family history, all of which have been linked to CHD, an association substantiated through multiple large prospective population studies. The categories can be further subdivided into *modifiable* and *nonmodifiable factors*: with dyslipidemia, tobacco use, hypertension, and diabetes comprising the former. In spite of their undeniable diagnostic and prognostic value, a portion of the population lacking these traditional risk factors remains at significant residual risk for CHD. As a result, there has been a major effort to identify novel factors that might help assess CHD risk within the population. These so-called nontraditional/novel factors include high sensitivity C-reactive protein (hsCRP), homocysteine, lipoprotein (a), and soluble adhesion molecules including s-ICAM and fibrinogen. Other candidate risk factors are frequently raised in the literature. The role of nontraditional factors in assessing patient risk for CHD is an evolving process that requires larger prospective clinical trials for validation and assessment of causality. Our discussion here centers on traditional risk factors in CHD management and treatment.

HYPERLIPIDEMIA/DYSLIPIDEMIA

NORMAL LIPID METABOLISM

The lipid component of blood has emerged as one of the most important, potent, and modifiable risk factors for CHD. Three distinct lipid/lipoprotein molecules are routinely measured in the blood: cholesterol, triglyceride, and fatty acids; phospholipids comprise another critical, but biologically distinct type of lipid possessing a phosphate functional group are not routinely quantified in the clinical laboratory. The average range for total cholesterol and triglyceride in plasma is based on population assessment of their distribution: total cholesterol: 100–200 mg/dL, triglyceride: 50–150 mg/dL. These ranges are often referred to as "normal values" although what truly constitutes a normal level of these molecules continues to evolve.

The hydrophobic nature of these lipids renders them insoluble in the blood stream and requires that they be packaged into larger hydrophilic lipoproteins—complex macromolecules composed of a mix of protein, cholesterol and specific lipids. Lipoproteins are further subfractionated based on charge and mass into five major groups: chylomicron (formed from intestinal absorption of dietary triglyceride), very-low-density lipoprotein (VLDL), intermediate-density lipoprotein (IDL), low-density lipoprotein (LDL), and high-density lipoprotein (HDL). Each lipoprotein fraction is composed of different quantities of cholesterol, triglyceride, and phospholipids; chylomicron and VLDL contain the highest triglyceride content, LDL and HDL carry predominantly cholesterol, and HDL also contains significant phospholipid. Triglycerides are three fatty acids attached to a monoacylglycerol backbone. Lipoproteins are also enriched with specific apolipoproteins ("apo-") that provide structural integrity for these particles, participate in determining metabolism, and serve as ligands for specific cellular receptors that facilitate lipoprotein particle removal from the circulation. Examples of apolipoproteins include apolipoprotein B, apolipoprotein E, and apolipoprotein CIII. LDL and VLDL are rich in apoB content. HDL is predominantly comprised of apoA-I and apoA-II. Chylomicrons contain apoE, whereas apoCII and CIII are important constituents of both chylomicrons and VLDL. In the case of LDL, apoB is a crucial protein that binds to the LDL receptor expressed on the surface of hepatocytes, leading to LDL clearance by the liver. As discussed below dysfunction of these proteins can lead to clinically relevant dyslipidemias.

The liver integrates systemic lipid metabolism beginning with dietary chylomicron uptake from the portal circulation followed by lipoprotein synthesis, packaging, and secretion into the circulation, in particular of VLDL, and ending finally with lipoprotein clearance and excretion of unused or excess lipid through the hepatobiliary system. Once formed, circulating lipoprotein content (cholesterol and triglyceride content) is significantly remodeled in peripheral tissues and in the bloodstream by cell-associated enzymes including lipoprotein lipase (LPL), hepatic lipase (HL), and endothelial lipase (EL), as well as circulating plasma enzymes including CETP (cholesterol ester transfer protein) and PLTP (phospholipid transport protein). Fundamental often overlooked concepts include the facts that lipoprotein particles, even within a specific type of particle, that is, VLDL or LDL or HDL, represent a range of different particles and that lipoproteins are in communication with one another. For example, during its transit through the circulation, VLDL undergoes metabolism and gradually loses its triglyceride content as fatty acids are hydrolyzed off by LPL, ultimately leaving behind a VLDL remnant that is enriched in cholesterol. As their names imply, both CETP and PLTP transfer cholesterol and phospholipids between LDL and HDL. The recycling process mediated by HDL lipoprotein is termed "reverse cholesterol transport" and removes atherogenic lipid from the artery. This system's net effect is to shuttle lipid derived from tissues and the artery wall back to the liver for excretion or recycling. A simple definition of dyslipidemia is a total cholesterol, LDL cholesterol, or triglyceride greater than the 90th percentile for the general population, or an HDL cholesterol below the 10th percentile for the general population. Clinically significant dyslipidemias that increase CHD risk can result from defects in any component within these pathways of lipoprotein synthesis, remodeling, or clearance.

THE CHOLESTEROL HYPOTHESIS

As a risk factor for predicting and treating CHD, the relationship between plasma lipid levels and atherosclerosis,

the "cholesterol hypothesis," is rooted in observations made by the German pathologist Rudolf Virchow during the 19th century, in which he identified that human atheroma contains cholesterol crystals. This hypothesis has now gained widespread acceptance based, in part, on several cross-sectional studies consistently demonstrating a graded positive association between plasma cholesterol levels and CHD frequency and mortality. As one example, in the Seven Countries Study, investigators found a continuous risk in CHD mortality in the population beginning at approximately 7% risk for a total cholesterol level of 200 mg/dL rising to 30% with cholesterol levels of 300 mg/dL. Importantly, this relationship was evident around the world and independent of other known risk factors such as hypertension and cigarette smoking. An earlier study by the Lipid Research Council found a similar relationship in which patients without known CHD and total cholesterol >240 mg/dL experienced a doubling of CVD mortality rate from approximately 2.5 to 5 per 1000 patient years. Based on data derived from the Framingham Heart Study, the lifetime risk of total CHD (all clinical manifestations) at age 40 years with a cholesterol ≥240 mg/dL is 57% in men and 33% in women, as compared to 31% in men and 15% in women with cholesterol level <200 mg/dL. This increased risk spans across all ages of adulthood, such that a 70-year-old with total cholesterol ≥240 mg/dL carries a 10-year risk for CHD of 28% in men and 29% in women, compared to 18% and 5% if total cholesterol is <200 mg/dL.

These data are important to consider from the standpoint of primary prevention given that approximately two-thirds of first major coronary events occur in persons ≥65 years. Moreover, these data combine with the evidence that atherosclerosis begins early in adulthood to have argued for earlier intervention and lower thresholds for treatment. One such group receiving increased attention in terms of primary prevention and CVD risk are women, many of whom will manifest CHD primarily in the postmenopausal period, although risk factors may have been driving risk much before this. Taken together, these data have led to a major shift in preventive cardiology over the last decade, moving away from notions of secondary and primary prevention, which are inherently artificial, and focusing more on relative risk that is independent of prior history. A major contributor to this risk is LDL cholesterol.

LDL CHOLESTEROL

Defining a causal relationship between cholesterol and CHD has required a deeper understanding of the aforementioned biochemical pathways involved in cholesterol and triglyceride metabolism as well as more refined tools for measuring cholesterol fractions in the blood. Brown and Goldstein's seminal work defining the LDL receptor

(LDLr) as the major protein responsible for hepatic clearance of circulating LDL, as well as the identification of LDLr loss of function mutations in patients who develop severely accelerated CHD (see discussion below on familial hypercholesterolemia), has provided confirmatory experimental evidence for the hypothesis that LDL cholesterol, specifically, contributes causally to atherosclerosis and CHD. LDL cholesterol and the oxidatively modified LDL particle directly promote atherogenesis through a variety of mechanisms including: (1) reduced bioavailability of nitric oxide leading to endothelial dysfunction and altered vascular tone; (2) increased macrophage uptake of lipid and formation of the foam cell within the artery wall; (3) increased expression of inflammatory cytokines that amplify proinflammatory cell recruitment within the atherosclerotic plaque; and (4) increased platelet aggregation.

In addition to oxidation of LDL, the particle size/concentration may impact the risk of atherosclerosis. Epidemiologic data suggest that small, dense LDL may impose a significantly increased risk for CHD. This has been shown in case-control trials in which patients with MI have smaller LDL particle size. It is important to recognize that patients with secondary disorders such as obesity and metabolic syndrome/diabetes mellitus often have small, dense LDL particles that may promote their CHD risk. Although dense LDL is a marker of a more atherogenic lipid profile, the routine measurement of particle size is not recommended by ATPIII guidelines for initial risk stratification of dyslipidemias. In fact, patients with elevated triglyceride values usually have increased small, dense LDL. Guideline recommendations for calculating levels of "non-HDL" as a secondary target for treatment are in effect an effort to generate a measure of apoB-containing particles and smaller, dense LDL that may persist after LDL has been controlled and may be further incorporated into the new adult treatment program guidelines (ATPIV) expected soon.

The strong association between LDL and CHD risk is further substantiated by the consistent risk reduction in CHD events in patients treated with LDL-lowering therapy. In particular, primary prevention trials with HMG CoA reductase inhibitors (statins) have demonstrated significant reductions in CHD events in patients across a broad spectrum of plasma cholesterol levels (see table 83.1). Based on these and other randomized prospective clinical trial data, the current cholesterol guidelines target LDL cholesterol as the primary treatment goal for lipid lowering in CHD risk modification. The clinical decision to treat is guided by the total cholesterol and LDL cholesterol levels along with the presence of additional traditional CHD risk factors such as hypertension, low HDL, age, gender, tobacco use, diabetes mellitus, or family history.

MONOGENIC DISORDERS CAUSING HYPERLIPIDEMIA/DYSLIPIDEMIA

The growing evidence connecting plasma lipids and CHD risk as well as the realization that lipid disorders and accelerated atherosclerosis cluster in families generated interest in classification systems of lipid abnormalities in the larger population. Frederickson, Levy, and Lees first categorized systematically dyslipidemias using measurements of cholesterol and triglyceride coupled with lipoprotein patterns after separation by electrophoresis. This classification included five types of hyperlipoproteinemia: type I—elevation of chylomicrons; type II—elevation of LDL; type IIb—combined elevation of LDL and VLDL; type III or broad beta disease—elevation of remnant lipoproteins; type IV—elevated VLDL; and type V—elevation of both chylomicron and VLDL. Recent identification of specific gene defects that cause lipoprotein disorders has partially supplanted this lipoprotein phenotype classification. Abnormalities of plasma cholesterol are now viewed as primary disorders arising from monogenetic defects in specific lipid metabolism pathways or as secondary disorders resulting as a consequence of systemic diseases including diabetes mellitus, hypothyroidism, nephrotic syndrome, or obesity among others.

Table 83.1 **PRIMARY PREVENTION LIPID LOWERING TRIALS**

TRIAL	PATIENT (N)	CHD RISK FACTORS	DURATION (YRS)	DRUG	LDL-C BASELINE	LDL-C CHANGE	MAJOR CORONARY EVENTS	CORONARY MORTALITY
WOSCOPS	6595	3+	4.9	Pravastatin	192	−26%	−31%	−33%
AFCAPS/TexCAPS	6605	<2	5	Lovastatin	150	−25%	−37%	NS
ASCOT/LLA	10305	3+	3.3	Atorvastatin	131	−33%	−21%	−.36% (fatal/nonfatal MI)
HHS	4081	1+	5	Gemfibrozil	Non-HDL-C >200 mg/dL		−34%	NS
WHO Cooperative	10,577		9	Clofibrate				+25% (total mortality)

LDL-C, low-density lipoprotein cholesterol, HDL-C, high-density lipoprotein cholesterol

Disorders of Low-Density Lipoprotein

Familial Hypercholesterolemia

Familial hypercholesterolemia (FH) is a genetic disorder of LDL cholesterol metabolism inherited in an autosomal dominant manner. The defect localizes to the LDLr gene with over 800 distinct mutations now described involving major gene rearrangements, gene deletions, point mutations, insertion of premature stop codons and mutations of the LDLr promoter that affect transcription of the LDLr gene. The connection between FH and disruption of the LDLr gene provides strong independent evidence for a causal relationship between LDL and CVD. Patients with dysfunctional or absent LDLr cannot effectively clear LDL from the plasma, thereby leading to marked elevations in circulating LDL and accumulation of cholesterol in the artery wall. There is a gene dose response in the phenotype such that homozygous and heterozygous mutation carriers manifest different severity of disease. Homozygous FH occurs with a prevalence of 1:1 million in the population. In homozygotes there are two mutant alleles (compound heterozygotes containing a distinct mutation on each allele also occur and lead to a homozygous phenotype). These patients are characterized by the degree of relative LDLr function: mutations are classified as *negative* if there is <2% LDLr activity or *defective* if there is 2–25% LDLr activity. Typically, total plasma cholesterol levels are >500 mg/dL and can rise as high as 1200 mg/dL. As a consequence of these extreme elevations in plasma cholesterol, patients develop characteristic clinical manifestations including cutaneous xanthomas, tendinous xanthomas in typical locations including the Achilles tendon or along metacarpophalangeal joints, as well as corneal arcus—all representing abnormal deposition of cholesterol in the skin, tendons, and around the iris of the eye. Progressive accumulation of cholesterol within the coronary arteries incites atherogenesis and promotes severe, accelerated CHD, typically manifesting in the first two decades of life with MI or angina. Epidemiologically, a strong positive association between LDLr mutations and premature CHD exists, reflecting this heightened propensity for atherosclerosis. Heterozygous FH occurs with a frequency of 1:500 in the population and presents a more varied phenotypic picture. Due to the single mutant allele only approximately 30–40% of these patients develop tendinous or cutaneous xanthomas. Often there will be a family history of hypercholesterolemia and CHD, and these patients typically manifest CHD later in the fourth decade of life. Treatment includes aggressive multidrug pharmacologic therapy aimed at lowering LDL cholesterol including high potency statins, inhibitors of intestinal cholesterol absorption, and niacin. When these modalities fail to reduce LDL cholesterol, FH patients can be treated with LDL apheresis—a form of plasma ultrafiltration that removes LDL from the plasma.

Familial Ligand-defective Apolipoprotein B

Although the molecular characterization of LDLR mutations provided key mechanistic insight into the FH phenotype, another population of patients with FH-like features were noted to have LDL particles that did not bind with high affinity to the LDL receptor. This group manifested a disease phenotype similar to a heterozygous FH carrier, but they possessed a defect in the LDL particle itself. Subsequent work identified a point mutation causing an arginine to glutamine (R3500Q) amino acid substitution in the apolipoprotein B gene product (APOB), the major protein constituent of LDL that is required for LDLr-mediated clearance of LDL in hepatocytes. This mutation significantly reduces LDL lipoprotein binding to its cognate receptor. Subsequent analysis has identified at least one other missense mutation in the APOB gene that affects LDL binding to the LDL receptor. This disease also transmits in an autosomal dominant fashion. The frequency of heterozygous familial ligand-defective apolipoprotein B (FDB) ranges between 1:500 and 1:700. Moreover, because the penetrance of the mutant APOB allele is not 100%, FDB patients typically manifest less severe overall disease including 20–25% lower LDL cholesterol compared with FH patients and have a slightly lower risk of CHD as compared to FH patients with LDLR mutations.

PCSK9

Until 2003 only the two autosomal dominant defects described above had been linked to hereditary hyperlipidemia. A third autosomal dominant disorder of LDL cholesterol metabolism had previously been mapped to chromosome 1p. Investigators have now identified that this novel locus involves the proprotein convertase subtilisin/kexin type 9 gene (PCSK9). This convertase is a serine protease synthesized by hepatocytes and secreted into the circulation that degrades hepatic LDL receptors. Interestingly, the missense mutation identified encodes for an activating mutation of the enzyme, thereby promoting excessive degradation of the LDLr in the liver. As a consequence, LDL cholesterol levels are elevated due to an inability to clear the lipoprotein through receptor-mediated endocytosis. Phenotypically, patients develop less severe disease compared with FH patients. Conversely, a population of patients harboring *inactivating* mutations of PCSK9 has been discovered. These patients' LDL cholesterol levels are well below the lower limit of the population and have a markedly reduced risk of CHD over their lifetime, without evidence of other abnormalities or untoward effects of low cholesterol. The larger role of PCSK9 in treatment of dyslipidemia awaits further elucidation of how this pathway influences cholesterol levels in the general population.

Abetalipoproteinemia

This is a rare, autosomal recessive disorder affecting the gene for microsomal triglyceride transfer protein (MTTP). Only approximately 100 cases are described worldwide, and the disease is more common in males. MTTP is a heterodimeric protein that plays a central role in beta-lipoprotein assembly, which includes LDL, VLDL, and chylomicron lipoproteins. As a consequence of this defect these patients cannot absorb dietary fats, leading to developmental problems associated with inadequate nutrition and vitamin deficiencies. Typically patients present during infancy with gastrointestinal symptoms including vomiting, diarrhea, abdominal bloating, and steatorrhea as well as failure to thrive due to intestinal malabsorption of lipids. Additional symptoms are related to vitamin A, vitamin E, and vitamin K deficiencies including sensory disturbances, ataxia, movement disorders, muscle weakness, and hematologic problems including anemia and abnormal clotting. Treatment requires a diet low in long-chain triglycerides (>18 carbons) in favor of short- and medium-chain triglycerides. Fat-soluble vitamin and iron supplements are also required.

Disorders of Triglyceride-Rich Lipoproteins: Chylomicron and VLDL

Normal fasting plasma triglyceride levels range between 50 and 100 mg/dL and can rise markedly following a lipid-laden meal when they are absorbed and packaged into chylomicrons for delivery to the liver. The role of plasma triglycerides as a risk factor for CHD independent from elevated LDL cholesterol and low HDL cholesterol has been difficult to prove, in part due to the frequent association of high triglycerides with high LDL and/or low HDL (especially in the diabetic population). A recent report analyzing two nested case control studies derived from the prospective studies Reykjavik and ERIC calculated an adjusted odds ratio for CHD of 1.76 and 1.58 for patients with triglyceride levels in the top third of log-triglyceride levels as compared with the bottom third. An additional meta-analysis of 27 prospective studies found a similar odds ratio of 1.72 for risk of CHD in patients with elevated triglycerides. In addition to CHD, severe elevations in triglyceride (>600 mg/dL) can cause pancreatitis necessitating preemptive treatment for some patients irrespective of their CHD risk. Factors contributing to elevated circulating triglycerides include genetic disorders (discussed below), as well as secondary factors including obesity, diabetes mellitus/metabolic syndrome, nephrotic syndrome, hypothyroidism, significant alcohol use, physical inactivity, and certain medications including estrogen replacement, tamoxifen, beta blockers, and immunosuppressives such as glucocorticoids and cyclosporine.

Familial Hypertriglyceridemia

Familial hypertriglyceridemia is an autosomal dominant disorder characterized by moderate elevations in plasma triglycerides (typically 200–500 mg/dL) and marked postprandial hypertriglyceridemia. This disorder is often accompanied by insulin resistance, obesity, diabetes mellitus, and

hypertension. The abnormality arises due to hepatic overproduction of VLDL, but specific gene defects have not yet been identified. The prevalence of this disorder ranges between 1:50 and 1:100, but it is highly heterogeneous, likely reflecting multiple defects in triglyceride metabolism.

Familial Hyperchylomicronemia (Buerger-Gruetz Syndrome)

This rare, type I hyperlipoproteinemia arises from loss of LPL function (mutations in ApoCII, a cofactor for LPL enzymatic function have also been described) and occurs with a worldwide prevalence of 1:1 million. Over 60 mutations in the LPL gene have been identified. As a consequence of LPL inactivity these patients cannot hydrolyze triglyceride from chylomicrons, leading to extreme elevations in this lipoprotein. Fasting triglycerides can reach >1000 mg/dL. Plasma will appear lipemic, and a chylomicron band usually appears on the top surface of the plasma if allowed to stand at 4° overnight. This degree of triglyceride elevation leads to recurrent pancreatitis and eruptive xanthomas in patients. Homozygous carriers often present in childhood with failure to thrive secondary to nutritional abnormalities. This syndrome can also be associated with xerostomia, xerophthalmia, and behavioral changes. Treatment requires avoidance of long-chain dietary fats and alcohol.

Disorders of High-Density Lipoprotein

In contrast to positive associations between LDL cholesterol and CHD, multiple epidemiologic studies have consistently identified an inverse relationship between HDL cholesterol level and CHD risk such that patients with elevated HDL cholesterol exhibit protection from atherosclerosis and CHD. The mechanism for this inverse relationship remains an active area of research. The failure of a recent clinic trial studying a novel drug designed to raise HDL levels points to the challenges in targeting this component of the cholesterol pathway.

Tangier Disease

HDL particles, which begin as lipid-poor disks, acquire cholesterol in the tissue or from transfer of cholesterol from LDL to HDL as mediated by plasma enzymes including PLTP and CETP, ultimately leading to the formation of mature lipid/cholesterol rich spherical HDL. ApoAI is the major acceptor protein for the initial cholesterol loading of the HDL particle. Efflux of cell-derived cholesterol requires specific transporters termed ATP binding cassette (ABC) transporters consisting of a large family of membrane proteins that facilitate lipid trafficking between cells and the plasma. At the molecular level, Tangier disease (TD) occurs due to mutations specifically in the ABCA1 transporter function that result in the inability of macrophages and keratinocytes to efflux cholesterol to nascent plasma HDL particles. This markedly impairs HDL formation in the plasma compartment resulting in low plasma levels of total HDL. The defect was originally described in a proband from Tangier Island located in the Chesapeake Bay, Maryland. Inheritance is autosomal recessive. Less than 100 reported cases have been found worldwide, but >50 mutations in the ABCA1 gene have since been identified to date. HDL cholesterol levels are less than the 5th percentile of the normal population. On physical exam, patients with homozygous TD demonstrate enlarged, orange tonsils, and hepatosplenomegaly. A closely related disorder called familial hypoalphalipoproteinemia (FHA) also maps to the ABCA1 gene, but it is inherited in an autosomal dominant fashion. Phenotypically these patients resemble TD patients. On account of phenotypic variability of heterozygous carriers of ABCA1 mutations, the association between low HDL in this group and CHD has been mixed. On balance, variation in the ABCA1 gene appears to confer an increased risk of CHD, and certainly low HDL is one of the most common findings in the plasma lipid panel from patients with known CAD. Individual mutations may ultimately influence the strength of these associations. As an illustration of this effect a recent analysis derived from three different population studies in Copenhagen examined heterozygous carriers for four ABCA1 mutations and did not identify increased susceptibility for ischemic heart disease compared with nonmutation carriers—adjusted hazard ratio 0.67. The reason for this finding in spite of low HDL levels is not known, but it may reflect low levels of either total or atherogenic LDL cholesterol or the phenotypic variability associated with these genetic disorders. Despite these questions, low HDL cholesterol levels remain an important risk factor for CHD in the general population, and developing therapies to raise plasma HDL cholesterol remains a major goal in the field of cardiovascular disease prevention.

A general table regarding expected changes in lipids in response to various pharmacologic agents is provided (table 83.2).

Table 83.2 LIPID MANAGEMENT: PHARMACOTHERAPY

THERAPY	TC	LDL-C	HDL-C	TG
Statins	19–37%	25–50%	4–12%	14–29%
Ezetimibe	13%	18%	1%	9%
Bile acid sequestrants	10%	10–18%	3%	Neutral
Nicotinic acid	10–20%	10–20%	14–35%	30–70%
Fibrates	19%	4–8%	11–13%	30%

TC, total cholesterol, LDL-C, low-density lipoprotein cholesterol, HDL-C, high-density lipoprotein cholesterol, TG, triglycerides.
Changes shown are general approximations; results may differ depending on the specific agents employed.

NONTRADITIONAL RISK FACTOR: HIGH-SENSITIVITY C-REACTIVE PROTEIN (HS-CRP)

Treatment of hyperlipidemia has a clear role in reducing risk of CHD in patients with elevated cholesterol. However, half of MIs and strokes occur in patients who have LDL cholesterol levels below recommended treatment guidelines. Inflammatory biomarkers, such as hs-CRP provide additional risk stratification. In the case of hs-CRP, elevated levels predict future vascular events independently of LDL cholesterol level, thereby improving global risk classification approaches. The utility of hs-CRP as a "target" of treatment to lower risk of CHD was recently supported in a randomized, placebo-controlled, primary prevention trial called JUPITER. This study enrolled patients with average cholesterol (LDL cholesterol ≤130 mg/dL) and an elevated hs-CRP ≥2.0 mg/L to treatment with rosuvastatin (20 mg) or placebo with a primary endpoint of first major cardiovascular event or confirmed death from cardiovascular causes. The trial was terminated early due to a significant reduction in the primary end point in patients treated with rosuvastatin. The hazard ratio was 0.56 for this primary endpoint and was statistically significant across all subgroups including first MI, stroke, or revascularization for unstable angina. Although LDL cholesterol remains the primary goal of therapy, these data raise critical questions regarding the potential use of hs-CRP to risk stratify patients with intermediate risk. JUPITER did not include an arm of the study treating patients with low LDL and low CRP based on prior subgroup analyses, suggesting that such patients do not benefit from statin therapy.

HYPERTENSION

Blood pressure follows a normal Gaussian distribution in the population, which has made concepts of "normal" and "abnormal" more difficult to define within a large population. However, based on significant epidemiologic data, most hypertension societies, including the Joint National Committee on Prevention, Detection, Evaluation, and Treatment of High Blood Pressure (JNC) define hypertension as a level of ≥140/90 mm Hg (NHLBI 2004). More recently, the JNC has changed the category of "high-normal" to a new category of "prehypertension" due to a greater appreciation of the benefits of early detection and intervention to prevent CHD and the continuous risk of developing hypertension over adulthood (table 83.3). In fact, the Framingham Heart Study (FHS) estimates that individuals who are normotensive at age 55 have a 90% lifetime risk for developing high blood pressure. Importantly, either the systolic or diastolic component is sufficient for a diagnosis, and the higher of the two measurements determines the diagnosis, CHD risk, and the aggressiveness of treatment. Hypertension is the most common primary diagnosis in America (35 million office visits with this as a primary diagnosis), but current blood pressure control rates are well below 50%. Approximately 30% of patients are actually completely

Table 83.3 JNC 7 CLASSIFICATION OF HYPERTENSION

BP CLASSIFICATION	SBP mm Hg	DBP mm Hg	LIFESTYLE CHANGE
Normal	<120	and < 80	Encourage
Pre-hypertension	120–139	or 80–89	Yes
Stage I hypertension	140–159	or 90–99	Yes
Stage II hypertension	≥160	or ≥ 100	Yes

unaware that they have hypertension. As a risk factor, the relationship between blood pressure and all cardiovascular disease including CHD, stroke, and heart failure, as well as kidney disease is continuous, consistent, and independent of other risk factors. It is also important to realize that hypertension rarely occurs in isolation from other risk factors. According to FHS only approximately 20% of patients have isolated hypertension. More commonly hypertension is associated with other metabolic abnormalities that may contribute to the degree of blood pressure elevation including hyperlipidemia, metabolic syndrome, and cigarette smoking use through catecholamines surges. Regardless of the cause, in adults in the age group 40–70 years, every increment in 20 mm Hg of SBP or 10 mm Hg DBP doubles the risk of CVD across the entire spectrum of blood pressure from 115/75 to 185/115—with ischemic coronary disease the most common organ damage associated with hypertension. *SBP is more strongly associated than DBP in these outcomes.*

Recent analysis of the National Health and Nutrition Education Survey (NHANES) database has found that the number-needed-to-treat (NNT) to prevent a cardiovascular death was 273 for patients with stage I hypertension and 34 for patients with stage II hypertension if a 12 mm Hg reduction in SBP is achieved over a 10-year period. In patients with multiple cardiac risk factors the number need to treat dropped to 27 and 12, respectively, for a similar reduction in SBP. Thus, an important way to integrate hypertension into the composite cardiovascular risk assessment is to consider the degree of hypertension, the presence of other cardiac risk factors, and evidence of target organ damage such as ischemic heart disease or heart failure. The association between hypertension and CHD is further strengthened from multiple prospective clinical trials that have demonstrated a consistent reduction in CHD risk with even modestly successful treatment of hypertension. These studies have compared various classes of antihypertensive therapies including renin-angiotensin axis inhibitors, beta blockers, calcium channel blockers, thiazide diuretics, and all lead to a 20–25% relative risk reduction in CHD events.

CIGARETTE SMOKING

A strong association between cigarette smoking and atherogenesis has been observed for many years but was directly assessed in the Atherosclerosis Risk in Communities (ARIC) study. The study included over 10,000 patients who had carotid artery intimal-medial thickness measured (CIMT)—a well-validated noninvasive metric of arterial atherosclerosis burden. In current smokers there was an associated 50% increase in progression of atherosclerosis as compared with nonsmokers on CIMT. Importantly the progression rates were similar between current and former smokers, suggesting that some of the effects of smoking may not be reversible after cessation. Mechanistically, smoking is associated with several pathophysiologic effects that likely promote atherosclerosis including: (1) elevation in LDL and triglyceride and reduced HDL; (2) activation of the sympathetic nervous system leading to increases in blood pressure, heart rate, and coronary vasoconstriction; (3) prothrombotic effect through inhibition of tissue plasminogen activator release from endothelium and increased tissue factor expression; (4) endothelial dysfunction including impaired endothelium dependent relaxation secondary to oxidative stress and reduced bioavailability of nitric oxide; (5) increased inflammation as noted by increases in CRP levels and fibrinogen; and (6) elevations in homocysteine, which may also promote endothelial dysfunction.

Smoking is an important independent risk factor for developing CHD. The incidence of MI is increased sixfold in women and threefold in men who smoke 20 cigarettes or more per day as compared with people who never smoked. Even more, cigarette smoking increases cardiovascular mortality, with an adjusted hazard ratio of 1.63 in one study. In patients with established CHD who continue to smoke after angioplasty there is a greater relative risk of death (1.76) and MI (2.08). In the SOLVD trial studying patients with left ventricular dysfunction, smoking significantly increased all cause mortality (relative risk 1.41) as well as incidence of death, recurrent heart failure requiring admission, or MI (relative risk 1.39). This association between smoking and CHD risk is further strengthened when considered in concert with data revealing the cardiovascular benefits of smoking cessation. Among patients without known CHD, smoking cessation has been associated with a cardiac event rate reduction ranging from 7% to 47%. The cardiac risks associated with smoking are reduced quickly after cessation. In addition, a recent meta-analysis of several prospective studies of patients who have had an acute coronary syndrome with prior CHD found that the relative risk for mortality was 0.64 (CI 0.58–0.71) in smokers who quit (n = 5659), compared with those who continued to smoke (n = 6944). An important smoking subgroup is the diabetic population. In patients with diabetes mellitus smoking increases the risk for microvascular and macrovascular complications. Specifically, there is a dose-dependent effect of smoking in diabetic women for risk of CHD: RR 1.7 for 1–15 cigarettes/day up to 2.68 for >15 cigarettes/day. There is a similar cigarette dose response with respect to mortality in female diabetic patients. Diabetics who smoke have increased risk for neuropathy and are more likely to progress to end-stage renal disease. Taken together, these data establish smoking as an important, independent risk factor for the development of CHD and identify a critical lifestyle intervention that can dramatically reduce cardiovascular disease both as primary and secondary CHD prevention.

DIABETES MELLITUS

Diabetes mellitus continues to increase in prevalence throughout the world and is a major, independent risk factor for CHD as well as other morbidity including renal disease and microvascular disease. The epidemiologic data for this association are persuasive. As an example, the Framingham Heart Study (FHS) found that the presence of type 2 diabetes mellitus (T2D) doubled the age-adjusted risk for cardiovascular disease in men and tripled it for women. Another study, the Multiple Risk Factor Intervention Trial (MRFIT) found in the 5163 male patients who reported taking medication for DM2, 9.7% died from CVD over a 12-year period, compared with 2.6% mortality rate among the 342,815 men who were not taking medications for T2D. A landmark study examined the 7-year incidence of fatal/non-fatal MI in diabetics versus nondiabetic patients with or without a history of prior MI. In patients without diabetes, the 7-year event rate was 18.8% for those with a prior MI and 3.5% in those without prior history. Importantly, in patients with diabetes mellitus, the 7-year incidence of MI was 45% in those who had a prior MI and 20.2% in patients without a prior history of MI. When comparing these two populations, the event rate was similar between nondiabetics who already had known CHD and diabetics with no previous history of CHD (18.8% vs. 20.2%). The National Cholesterol Education Program has embraced this key concept that diabetes mellitus should be viewed by the clinician as a CHD "risk equivalent" when assessing global cardiovascular risk, thereby relegating diabetics to a high-risk group even in the absence of overt heart disease. Although this discussion focused on type 2 diabetes, the relative risk for cardiovascular disease is even greater for patients with type 1 diabetes mellitus. In the FHS, the cumulative CHD mortality was 35% by age 55 in type 1 diabetes compared with 8% and 4% in nondiabetic men and women, respectively. Collectively these data establish the strong, positive association between diabetes mellitus

and CHD. The mechanisms for such interactions between diabetes and CHD are complex and varied.

Yet, despite this impressive CHD risk association, the goal of reducing macrovascular disease in patients with diabetes has remained a challenge, specifically with regard to glycemic control and cardiovascular outcomes. Several randomized placebo-controlled trials have demonstrated that aggressive glycemic control can significantly reduce the risk of microvascular diabetic complications including retinopathy as well as nephropathy. Although trends in these trials suggest a potential CVD benefit, no large, prospective antihyperglycemic therapy studied to date has been able to demonstrate significant reductions in CHD events in the patient with type 2 diabetes. CVD benefit has been demonstrated with metformin in a subgroup of patients with obesity (UKPDS). Pioglitazone, a member of the PPAR-gamma–acting thiazolidinedione drug class, has been shown to reduce coronary atherosclerosis and decreased a secondary endpoint of CVD, although a multifactorial primary endpoint did not show a difference (PROactive). In patients with type 1 diabetes, cardiovascular benefits with insulin treatment were not evident until some 20 years of follow-up data were obtained (DCCT-EDCT), raising questions if similar-length studies are needed in order to uncover benefit in type 2 diabetes. With regard to other concomitant risk factors including tobacco use, hypertension, and hyperlipidemia, however, patients with diabetes derive a substantial benefit from therapies targeting these factors. This explains why diabetes mellitus shifts the goals of antihypertensive and lipid-lowering therapy toward a more aggressive strategy, in fact treating patients with diabetes as if they have known CHD. At the moment, the most impressive data in reducing CVD risk in patients with diabetes come from a multipronged approach at improving all known risk factors (Steno-2).

ADDITIONAL READING

Grundy SM, Cleeman JI, Merz CN et al. Implications of recent clinical trials for the National Cholesterol Education Program Adult Treatment Panel III guidelines. *Circulation* 2004; 110(6):763.

Hegele RA. Familial Hypercholesterolemia. *N Engl J Med.* 2007; 356:1779.

Mazzone T, Chait A, Plutzky J. Lancet. Cardiovascular disease risk in type 2 diabetes mellitus: insights from mechanistic studies. 2008 May 24;371(9626):1800–9.

Ridker PM, Brown NJ, Vaughan DE et al. Established and emerging plasma biomarkers in the prediction of first atherothrombotic events. *Circulation* 2004;109:25 Suppl 1:IV6–19.

Ridker PM, Danielson E, Fonseca FAH et al. Rosuvastatin to prevent vascular events in men and women with elevated C-Reactive Protein. *NEJM* 2008;359:2195.

Rosamond W, Flegal K, Friday G et al. Heart Disease and Stroke Statistics – 2007 Update: A Report from the American Heart Association Statistics Committee and Stroke Statistics Committee. *Circulation* 2007; 115:e69.

Scott IA. BMJ Evaluating cardiovascular risk assessment for asymptomatic people. 2009; 338:a2844.

Mora S, Musunuru K, Blumenthal RS. The clinical utility of high-sensitivity C-reactive protein in cardiovascular disease and the potential implication of JUPITER on current practice guidelines. *Clin Chem.* 2009 Feb;55(2):219–28.

QUESTIONS

QUESTION 1. A 21-year-old white male comes to you for his first primary care visit. He is asymptomatic and has no past medical history. He informs you that he has been a smoker since the age of 16 and smokes one to two packs per day. Physical examination is normal. All of the following statements are correct, EXCEPT:

  A. You assess the patient's willingness to quit smoking.
  B. You advise the patient to stop smoking.
  C. You develop a plan for smoking cessation and arrange follow-up.
  D. You provide counseling, review pharmacologic therapy, and prescribe him nicotine gum and referral to a formal cessation program.
  E. None of the above since this is his first visit seeing you.

QUESTION 2. The strongest predictor of CV risk is:

  A. Low HDL
  B. Low apolipoprotein A1
  C. Apolipoprotein B
  D. Triglycerides
  E. C-reactive protein

QUESTION 3. All of the following statements regarding hormone therapy and selective estrogen-receptor modulators (SERMs) are correct, EXCEPT:

  A. Use of estrogen plus progestin is associated with a small but significant risk of CHD and stroke.
  B. Use of estrogen without progestin associated with a small but significant risk of stroke.
  C. Use of all hormone preparations should be limited to short-term menopausal symptom relief.
  D. Use of a selective estrogen receptor modulator (raloxifene) does not affect risk of CHD or stroke but is associated with an increased risk of fatal stroke.
  E. Hormone therapy and selective estrogen-receptor modulators (SERMs) should be used for the primary or secondary prevention of CVD.

QUESTION 4. All of the following statements from the AHA/ACC Guidelines for Secondary Prevention for Patients with Coronary and Other Atherosclerotic Vascular Disease: 2006 Update are correct, EXCEPT:

  A. The blood pressure goal should be <140/90 mm Hg or <130/80 if diabetes or chronic kidney disease.
  B. For all patients start dietary therapy (<7% of total calories as saturated fat and <200 mg/d cholesterol).
  C. The exercise goal for all patients should be 30 minutes 7 days/week, minimum 5 days/week.
  D. Goal Hb A1c in all patients should be <6%.
  E. ACE inhibitors should be used in all patients with LVEF <40%, and those with diabetes or chronic kidney disease indefinitely, unless contraindicated.

ANSWERS

1. E
2. C
3. E
4. D

ADULT CONGENITAL HEART DISEASE

Yuli Y. Kim, Michael J. Landzberg, and Anne Marie Valente

Historically, individuals with complex congenital heart disease rarely lived past childhood. Due to tremendous advances in diagnosis and treatment, now 85–90% of children born with congenital heart disease will survive into adulthood. Estimates suggest that over 1 million adults with congenital heart disease currently live in the United States. The number of adults with congenital heart disease (ACHD) is growing by approximately 5% each year. The majority of these patients do not appear to be followed by ACHD specialists. Therefore, it is essential that all physicians familiarize themselves with the unique clinical presentations of these patients, including the anatomy, physiology, and natural history in order to facilitate proper management and referral.

In 2001 the 32nd Bethesda Conference attempted to address the changing profile of adults living with congenital heart disease by developing guidelines for resource allocation. The model for delivery of care focuses on classification of congenital heart defects into different levels of complexity (see table 84.1), with referral to specialized adult congenital centers for increasing levels of complexity. In this chapter, we focus on several of the more common congenital heart lesions in each of these groups.

SIMPLE LESIONS

ATRIAL SEPTAL DEFECT

An atrial septal defect (ASD) is a communication between the atria and is one of the most common congenital heart defects. There are several types of ASD (see Figure 84.1), the most common of which is a secundum ASD, a defect in the region of the fossa ovalis. Primum ASD are located near the crux of the heart, sinus venous defects involve a deficiency between the posterior wall of the right atrium or superior vena cava and are associated with anomalous pulmonary venous drainage, and coronary sinus septal defects are very rare defects that involve unroofing of the septum between the coronary sinus and the left atrium. Defects that are large may lead to presentation in childhood, however many ASDs are not discovered until adult life when patients present with exercise intolerance, atrial arrhythmias, and dyspnea. In young adults, the dominant interatrial shunt is from left-to-right because left atrial pressure and both inflow and outflow resistances exceed those in the right atrium.

The degree of subsequent left-to-right shunting determines the amount of right heart volume overload and is dictated by the size of the defect as well as the diastolic properties of the heart. Pulmonary vascular disease leading to pulmonary hypertension develops in 5–10% of patients with untreated ASD, although this development may not be solely attributable to increased left-to-right flow. Clinical presentation, physical exam findings, and laboratory features are summarized in table 84.2.

In the past, adult survivors with uncorrected ASD were demonstrated to have reduced life expectancy. More recently, data suggest increased risk of atrial fibrillation and increased occurrence of symptomatic respiratory issues prompting hospitalization in patients not treated with surgery despite ASD significance. Therefore, persons with ASD and a significant shunt (evidence of otherwise unexplainable right heart dilation +/− Qp/Qs >1.5:1) should be offered closure.

Secundum ASD can often be closed percutaneously. Surgical closure is required for primum ASD, sinus venosus defects, and coronary sinus septal defects. The long-term prognosis after correction for patients younger than 25 years is comparable to that of the general population. Patients corrected at an older age, particularly those over 40, have decreased comparable long-term survival and experience higher rates of comorbidities including atrial arrhythmias and right heart failure.

VENTRICULAR SEPTAL DEFECT

A ventricular septal defect (VSD) is a communication between the ventricles and is the most common congenital anomaly seen in children; it may be an isolated defect or associated with complex cardiac disease. Several classification

Table 84.1 ADULT CONGENITAL HEART DISEASE LESIONS BY SEVERITY

Simple Complexity

Isolated congenital aortic valve disease
Isolated congenital mitral valve disease (e.g., except parachute valve, cleft leaflet)
Isolated patent foramen ovale or small atrial septal defect
Isolated small ventricular septal defect (no associated lesions)
Mild pulmonary stenosis
Previously ligated or occluded ductus arteriosus
Repaired secundum or sinus venosus defect without residua
Repaired ventricular septal defect without residua

Moderate Complexity

Aorto-left ventricular fistulae
Anomalous pulmonary venous drainage, partial or total
Atrioventricular canal defects (partial or complete)
Coarctation of the aorta
Ebstein anomaly
Infundibular right ventricular outflow obstruction of significance
Ostium primum atrial septal defect
Patent ductus arteriosus (not closed)
Pulmonary valve regurgitation (moderate to severe)
Pulmonary valve stenosis (moderate to severe)
Sinus of Valsalva fistula/aneurysm
Sinus venosus defect
Subvalvar or supravalvar aortic stenosis (except HCM)
Tetralogy of Fallot
Ventricular septal defect with
  • Absent valve or valves
  • Aortic regurgitation
  • Coarctation of the aorta
  • Mitral disease
  • Right ventricular outflow tract obstruction
  • Straddling tricuspid/mitral valve
  • Subaortic stenosis

Severe Complexity

Conduits, valved or nonvalved
Cyanotic congenital heart (all forms)
Double-outlet ventricle
Eisenmenger syndrome
Fontan procedure
Mitral atresia
Single ventricle (also called double inlet or outlet, common or primitive)
Pulmonary atresia (all forms)
Pulmonary vascular obstructive diseases
Transposition of the great arteries
Tricuspid atresia
Truncus arteriosus/hemitruncus
Other abnormalities of atrioventricular or ventriculoarterial connection not included above (i.e., criss-cross heart, isomerism, heterotaxy syndromes, ventricular inversion)

Adapted from the 32nd Bethesda Conference [1]
Reprinted from Warnes CA, Liberthson R, Danielson GK, et al. Task Force 1: the changing profile of congenital heart disease in adult life. JACC 2001; 37(5): 1170–1175, with permission from Elsevier.

systems exist for defining VSD. Figure 84.2 illustrates the location of various VSDs, which may be classified as membranous (conoventricular), muscular, conal septal (subpulmonary), or atrioventricular (AV) canal type.

The size and location of the VSD, and the relative resistances in the pulmonary and systemic vasculature, are determinants of hemodynamic significance. Accordingly, left-to-right shunting at the ventricular level leads to volume overload to the left-sided chambers. Rarely, excessive flow to the pulmonary vasculature over time may result in changes that can eventually lead to elevated pulmonary vascular resistance with reversal of flow (Eisenmenger syndrome [ES], see below). Clinical presentation, physical exam findings, and laboratory features are summarized in table 84.3.

Some VSDs become smaller over time and may close spontaneously, particularly those in the membranous and

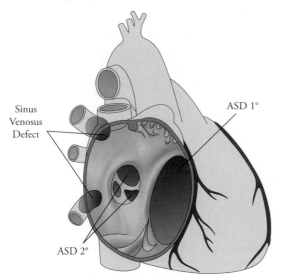

Figure 84.1. Anatomic Types of Interatrial Communications (see text for description). Atrial septal defect (ASD) 1° denotes primum ASD; ASD 2° denotes secundum ASD.

muscular septum. However, moderate or large VSD should be offered closure if there are symptoms of congestive heart failure, a significant left-to-right shunt (Qp:Qs >1.5:1), evidence of significant left ventricular volume overload or significant aortic regurgitation associated with conol spetal VSD. Closure of a VSD in the setting of ES can result in right ventricular failure and sudden death and is therefore contraindicated.

The outcome of patients with small VSD (without pulmonary hypertension or evidence of left ventricular volume overload) that do not require closure is generally excellent. However, 25-year survival rates correlate to size of the VSD, with decreased survival found in those with larger shunts. For those who have undergone closure with normal

pulmonary arterial pressures, life expectancy is normal whereas those with pulmonary hypertension at the time of repair have decreased survival. Complications may include endocarditis, arrhythmias, and aortic insufficiency for both repaired and unrepaired patients.

PULMONARY STENOSIS

Right-sided outflow tract obstruction can occur at various levels, including *valvar* (at the level of the pulmonary valve), *supravalvar* (above the level of the pulmonary valve), or *subvalvar* (either at the infundibular or subinfundibular level). Pulmonary stenosis (PS) may be associated with various genetic disorders including Noonan and Alagille syndromes. Hemodynamically significant PS can lead to right ventricular (RV) pressure overload with ensuing RV hypertrophy and failure. Clinical presentation, physical exam findings, and laboratory features are summarized in table 84.4.

The natural history of valvar PS is quite favorable with survival comparable to that of the general population. With mild valvar PS (Doppler peak instantaneous gradient <30 mm Hg by echocardiography), there is little progression of disease, and these patients can be followed without intervention. Based on natural history studies that did not include clearly defined criteria for either intervention or close follow-up, intervention remains recommended for individuals with severe PS. In the presence of symptoms, peak instantaneous Doppler gradient >50 mm Hg, and less-than-moderate pulmonary insufficiency, percutaneous balloon valvuloplasty is considered the procedure of choice for repair of valvar PS in the absence of hypoplastic annulus. Surgical repair using commissurotomy is indicated for more complex lesions, and valve replacement may be necessary if there is significant

Table 84.2 **ATRIAL SEPTAL DEFECT**

ANATOMY	CLINICAL PRESENTATION	PHYSICAL EXAM	LABORATORY FEATURES
Ostium secundum (65–75%): defect in the region of the fossa ovalis	Dyspnea Palpitations TIA, stroke (uncommon) Right heart failure	Wide, fixed split S2 RV lift Pulmonary ejection murmur at 2nd left intercostal space Prominent P2 if pulmonary hypertension is present	Chest radiography: - right heart dilatation depending on degree of shunt - enlarged central pulmonary arteries with increased vascular markings
Ostium primum (15–20%): within the spectrum of atrioventricular canal defect—associated with cleft mitral valve			EKG: - RSR' in V1 or complete RBBB - RAD for secundum and LAD for primum - 1st degree AVB suggests primum but can be seen in older patients with secundum
Sinus venosus (5–10%) - deficiency of the posterior wall of the atrium, SVC or IVC - anomalous pulmonary venous drainage			
Coronary sinus septal defect: deficiency of wall between coronary sinus septum and LA—often associated with left SVC			

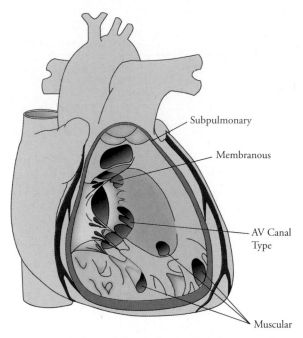

Figure 84.2. Anatomic Types of Ventricular Septal Defects. Muscular denotes defects in the muscular septum; AV Canal Type denotes defects in the inlet septum; Membranous denotes defects at the junction between the infundibular septum and muscular septum that may be confined to the membranous portion (perimembranous defects) or be associated with malalignment of the infundibular septum (conoventricular defects); Subpulmonary denotes defects in the outlet septum (also referred to as conal septal or supracristal defects).

Subpulmonary

Membranous

AV Canal
Type

Muscular

accompanying pulmonary insufficiency. Patients who have undergone surgical pulmonary valvotomy in childhood have excellent survival, however many will require re-intervention in adulthood.

MODERATE LESIONS

COARCTATION OF THE AORTA

Aortic coarctation is most commonly a discrete narrowing in the aortic isthmus just distal to the left subclavian artery and can be considered a diffuse arteriopathy.

A bicommissural aortic valve is present in >50% of subjects with aortic coarctation, and it may be associated with additional left-sided obstructive lesions (Shone's syndrome) and VSDs. Intracranial aneurysms, typically small and of unclear clinical significance, may be present in approximately 10% of people with aortic coarctation. There is a high prevalence of aortic coarctation in patients with Turner syndrome.

Hemodynamically, the increased afterload due to obstruction of flow from the left ventricle is associated with significant hypertension in the aorta and branch vessels proximal to the coarctation site and may be associated with systemic ventricular dysfunction, vessel aneurysm formation, and effects of premature atherosclerosis. Distal to the coarctation, there is diminished flow, and collaterals may develop to supplement areas of relative hypoperfusion. Clinical presentation, physical exam findings, and laboratory features are summarized in table 84.5.

In normals, the aortic pulse should be transmitted at equal speed and intensity from the left ventricle to the radial and femoral pulses that are approximately equidistant from the left ventricle. In patients with significant aortic coarctation, pulse wave propagation is both slowed and diminished distal to the coarctation, thereby delaying and diminishing femoral pulse relative to radial pulse. Standard practice dictates that all pulses should be checked at least once in the evaluation of all patients with systemic hypertension to rule out significant aortic coarctation.

Significant coarctation has previously been defined as a peak-to-peak gradient of 20 mm Hg across the stenosis as determined in the catheterization laboratory, although few data support this relatively arbitrary cut point that has been used to signify risk of sequelae. Several factors need to be considered in selecting the most appropriate method for repair including age, anatomy of the transverse and descending aorta, history of prior repair, and institutional expertise. Stent implantation became a treatment option in the early 1990s and may be appropriate in adults and adult-size adolescents. Balloon angioplasty with or without stent implantation is the accepted treatment approach

Table 84.3 **VENTRICULAR SEPTAL DEFECT**

ANATOMY	CLINICAL PRESENTATION	PHYSICAL EXAM	LABORATORY FEATURES
Perimembranous (80%)	Dyspnea Exercise intolerance Palpitations	Holosystolic murmur with smaller defects louder and higher pitched Diastolic rumble of increased mitral flow in case of large shunt Laterally displaced apical impulse in case of large shunt Prominent P2 if pulmonary hypertension is present	Chest radiography: - usually normal - cardiomegaly due to left atrial and left ventricular enlargement in case of significant shunt
Muscular (5–20%)			
Conal Septal (subpulmonary) (8–10%)—often associated with aortic insufficiency			EKG: - usually normal - LVH and left atrial enlargement in case of significant shunt
AV canal type (inlet) (5–8%)			

Table 84.4 PULMONARY STENOSIS

ANATOMY	CLINICAL PRESENTATION	PHYSICAL EXAM	LABORATORY FEATURES
Dome-shaped: narrow central opening with mobile valve; pulmonary artery usually dilated	Generally asymptomatic if mild or moderate; with severe: - dyspnea - chest pain - fatigue - palpitations - presyncope - cyanosis (if associated with a PFO or ASD)	Jugular venous waveform with prominent "a" wave RV lift at left sternal border Widely split S2, reduced or absent P2 Late-peaking systolic ejection murmur at LUSB Systolic ejection click that decreases with inspiration	Chest radiography: - typically normal unless RV failure present - RV and RA enlargement - dilated central PA - oligemic lung fields with severe PS EKG: - usually normal - RAD, RVH, RAE if severe PS
Dysplastic: thickened and poorly mobile			

in recurrent coarctation with good acute and intermediate outcomes.

In a past era of few medical therapies for systemic hypertension or heart failure, untreated patients with aortic coarctation had poor survival with an estimated mortality of 75% by 46 years of age and median age of death of only 31 years. Causes of death were related to uncontrolled hypertension, congestive heart failure, infective endocarditis, aortic rupture or dissection, and cerebral hemorrhage. Today, adult survivors after aortic coarctation intervention remain at risk for premature coronary and cerebrovascular disease, persistent hypertension, aortic aneurysm, and recoarctation. Those who have undergone surgical repair have a 20-year survival rate of 84%.

TETRALOGY OF FALLOT

Tetralogy of Fallot (TOF) is the most common cyanotic congenital cardiac defect in adults. This conotruncal anomaly results from anterior deviation of the infundibular septum and is characterized by (1) right ventricular tract outflow obstruction, (2) VSD, (3) overriding aorta, and (4) right ventricular hypertrophy.

The clinical presentation of unrepaired patients with TOF depends largely on the amount of right ventricular outflow tract obstruction, which is a major determinant in the amount of right-to-left shunting across the VSD. Thus, patients with TOF and minimal obstruction may have little if any cyanosis and can remain unrecognized until later in life. The surgical strategies for TOF repair have evolved over time. Adults who were operated on in the late 1950s and 1960s may have first undergone palliation with a systemic-to-pulmonary artery shunt (examples including central Waterston and Pott's shunts, and the more controlled classic and modified Blalock-Taussig shunts) to augment pulmonary flow prior to a complete repair. More recently, primary repair has been established that involves a right ventricular outflow tract patch or conduit with removal of infundibular-level obstruction and any additional muscle bundles, and VSD closure.

Clinical presentation, physical exam findings, and laboratory features are summarized in table 84.6.

For adults with TOF who survive either unrepaired or are status-post palliative shunt only, a relatively well-balanced situation must be present. These patients need to be monitored for progressive right ventricular outflow tract

Table 84.5 AORTIC COARCTATION

ANATOMY	CLINICAL PRESENTATION	PHYSICAL EXAM	LABORATORY FEATURES
Discrete: shelf-like stenosis of the aortic isthmus usually distal to the origin of the LSCA	Dependent on the severity of the obstruction Headache Epistaxis Dizziness Lower extremity claudication Abdominal angina Intracranial hemorrhage	Upper extremity or right arm hypertension BP differential between upper-lower extremities Brachial-femoral delay in pulse Prominent, nondisplaced apical impulse Soft systolic murmur at LUSB radiating to interscapular area	Chest radiography: - cardiomegaly - "E" or "reverse 3" sign from dilated LSCA proximal to and post-stenotic dilation distal to coarctation site - rib-notching from collaterals - enlarged ascending aorta may be seen with BAV
Diffuse: tubular hypoplasia of aorta		Loud A2 Systolic ejection click and mid-systolic murmur if bicuspid AV	EKG: - LVH
Associations: - BAV (70%) - intracranial aneurysm (10%) - VSD - Shone's complex - Turner syndrome		Continuous murmur between the scapulae or over the thorax from collaterals	

Table 84.6 TETRALOGY OF FALLOT

ANATOMY	CLINICAL PRESENTATION	PHYSICAL EXAM	LABORATORY FEATURES
RVOT obstruction VSD RVH Overriding aorta	If unrepaired: - dyspnea - palpitations - heart failure - endocarditis	Cyanosis, clubbing if unrepaired though severe cyanosis, squatting uncommon Diminished radial pulse on side of previous BT shunt RV lift RV outflow murmur at LUSB Single S2 Diastolic PR murmur at LUSB VSD murmur if residual lesion or patch leak	Chest radiography: - depends on prior surgical interventions - "boot-shaped" heart from RVH - right-sided aortic arch may be seen - pulmonary vasculature depends on relative blood flow to pulmonary bed
Associated with: - right-sided aortic arch (~25%) - secundum ASD (15%) - left SVC (5%) - anomalous origin of left anterior descending coronary artery from the right aortic sinus (10%) - 22q11 microdeletion including DiGeorge syndrome	If repaired: - often asymptomatic - dyspnea - exercise intolerance - palpitations - right heart failure - sudden death	Holosystolic murmur of TR at LLSB	EKG: - RVH - RBBB in prior repair - atrial and ventricular arrhythmias

obstruction, right heart failure, cyanosis, paradoxical emboli, and arrhythmias. In the postrepair patient, management is focused on residual lesions, their location, and severity—including pulmonary regurgitation, branch or more distal pulmonary artery stenosis, presence of aortopulmonary collaterals, aortic dilatation, aortic regurgitation, VSD patch leak, recurrent right ventricular outflow tract obstruction, and right ventricular outflow tract aneurysm.

Despite repair, adults with TOF require life-long follow-up due to potential for right-sided heart failure, aortic dilatation with resultant aortic insufficiency, left-sided heart dysfunction, and atrial and ventricular arrhythmias. Sudden cardiac death in adults with TOF has been well studied, with identification of several electrical and mechanical markers of increased risk.

EBSTEIN'S ANOMALY

Ebstein's anomaly is an abnormality of the tricuspid valve and right ventricular sinus. Failure of delamination of the septal and posterior leaflets of the tricuspid valve results in apical displacement of the tricuspid valve annulus. An associated ASD or patent foramen ovale is found in 80–94% of cases, with less frequent association with concomitant mitral regurgitation and left ventricular myocardial abnormalities. The hemodynamic consequences of the Epstein's anomaly are right ventricular dysfunction and tricuspid valve regurgitation. The right atrium acts as a passive reservoir for this regurgitant flow and progressively dilates. Clinical presentation, physical exam findings, and laboratory features are summarized in table 84.7. The natural history of this lesion varies from early presentation with shock to adult survival, depending on the degree of tricuspid valve

involvement, right ventricular dysfunction, and the presence and type of arrhythmias.

Patients with Ebstein's anomaly are at risk for arrhythmias and sudden cardiac death. The dilated right atrium creates a substrate for supraventricular tachyarrhythmias, and accessory pathways are common in these patients with Wolff-Parkinson-White syndrome found in 10–25%. As survival trends improve for these adults, the profile of noted arrhythmias increasingly includes potential for atrial fibrillation and flutter, as well as ventricular tachycardia and fibrillation.

Medical management consists of congestive heart failure treatment as appropriate. Catheter ablation of accessory pathways or supraventricular arrhythmias should be performed in these patients or at the time of surgical repair. Surgical correction should be considered for patients with decreased exercise tolerance, worsening heart failure symptoms despite medical therapy, intractable arrhythmias, progressive right ventricular dysfunction, and/or cyanosis. Surgical goals include optimization of right ventricular function, elimination of tricuspid regurgitation, and relief from cyanosis. The tricuspid valve may be repaired, although typically in older adults may have to be replaced in addition to closure of an interatrial communication.

SEVERE LESIONS

TRANSPOSITION OF THE GREAT ARTERIES

Transposition of the great arteries (TGA) is a form of atrioventricular concordance with ventriculoarterial discordance (each great artery arises from the incorrect ventricle). The most common form of TGA is referred to as D (dextro)

Table 84.7 EBSTEIN'S ANOMALY

ANATOMY	CLINICAL PRESENTATION	PHYSICAL EXAM	LABORATORY FEATURES
Apical displacement of the septal and often the posterior leaflet of the tricuspid valve Adherence of the septal and posterior leaflets to the underlying myocardium Dilation of the "atrialized" portion of the right ventricle Redundant, "sail-like" anterior leaflet	Varies depending on severity and associated lesions Asymptomatic if mild Cyanosis (if associated PFO or ASD) Dyspnea Fatigue Right heart failure Palpitations Paradoxical embolization Sudden death	Cyanosis If associated PFO or ASD Clubbing Variable jugular venous pulsations: Widely split S2 Musical Holosystolic murmur	Chest radiography; "globe-shaped" heart with clear lung fields
Associated with: ASD/PFO (80–94%) "Physiologically corrected" loop-TGA WPW (10–25%)			EKG: tall broad P waves of RAE incomplete or complete RBBB 1st-degree atrial arrhythmias

looped-TGA, in which all of the deoxygenated blood returns to the right atrium, right ventricle, and then back to the body through the aorta (figure 84.3). This creates systemic and pulmonary circulations that run "in parallel" (rather than in series) and is incompatible with life unless there is some type of communication between the two vascular circuits (ASD, VSD, or ductus arteriosus). Immediately after this physiology is recognized, if there is not an adequate mixing lesion, an emergent atrial septostomy or definitive repair may be performed.

The adult patient with TGA has almost invariably undergone prior surgical repair. The atrial switch repair (Senning or Mustard procedure) was pioneered in the 1960s. In these repairs systemic and pulmonary venous blood is redirected at the atrial level such that systemic venous (deoxygenated) blood is directed to the LV and travels out the pulmonary artery while pulmonary venous (oxygenated) blood returns to the RV and is ejected out the aorta. The arterial switch procedure was more recently introduced. In this repair, the great arteries are removed, and the pulmonary artery is connected to the right ventricle with its branches draped over the aorta (LeCompte maneuver), which has been connected to the left ventricle. Clinical presentation, physical exam findings, and laboratory features are summarized in table 84.8.

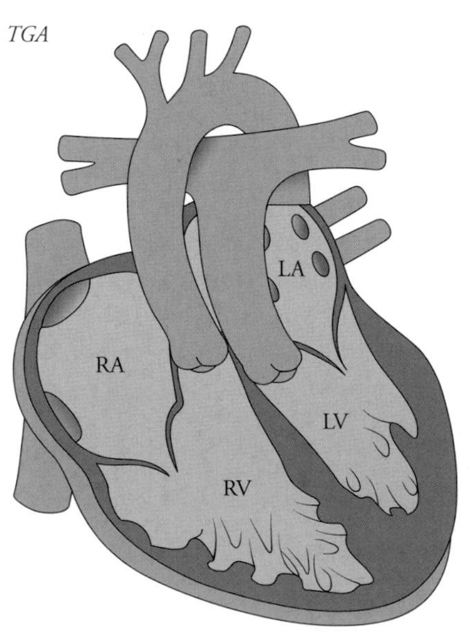

The long-term complications of these adult patients are dictated by the type of surgery they underwent in childhood. Patients who have undergone atrial switch repair have a systemic right ventricle that can progressively dilate and fail with concomitant tricuspid regurgitation. Congestive heart failure is the most common cause of death in this population. After atrial switch for TGA, 25-year survival approaches 75–90% (less so with an associated VSD or Mustard procedure). Later-term sequelae include arrhythmia (both tachy- and bradyarrhythmias), venous baffle obstruction, baffle leaks, and sudden cardiac death.

An alternative surgical procedure for patients with D loop TGA, VSD, and pulmonary stenosis is the Rastelli procedure, which allows the left ventricle to be the systemic ventricle. This procedure involves VSD patch closure which routes the left ventricle to the aorta and places a right ventricular to pulmonary artery conduit with oversewing of the native stenotic pulmonary valve. Long-term complications from this procedure include subaortic stenosis, conduit obstruction, residual VSD patch leak, and arrhythmias.

Patients who have undergone arterial switch procedures need to be monitored for supravalvar pulmonary artery stenosis, neoaortic dilation, and ensuing regurgitation. These patients must also be monitored for signs and symptoms of coronary ischemia as the coronary arteries are translocated at the time of the surgical correction.

Figure 84.3 Transposition of the Great Arteries. The aorta arises anteriorly from the right ventricle; the pulmonary artery arises posteriorly from the left ventricle.

Table 84.8 COMPLETE TRANSPOSITION OF THE GREAT ARTERIES

ANATOMY	SURGICAL REPAIR	CLINICAL PRESENTATION AND PHYSICAL EXAM	LABORATORY FEATURES
Ventriculo-arterial discordance	Atrial switch: - baffle synthetic material (Mustard) or native atrial tissue (Senning) - pulmonary venous blood → RV → aorta - systemic venous blood → LV → PA	Atrial switch: - exercise intolerance - heart failure - palpitations - pre-syncope or syncope - RV heave - holosystolic murmur of TR - prominent S2 at 2nd ICS	Chest radiography: - narrow mediastinum - normal pulmonary vascularity unless pulmonary hypertension present - RV-PA conduit calcification in Rastelli patients

Associated with:
- VSD (40–45%)
- LVOT (subpulmonary) obstruction (25%)
	Arterial switch:
	- great arteries are transected and reanastomosed to the appropriate ventricle
	- coronary arteries are removed and reimplanted
		Arterial switch:
		- usually asymptomatic diastolic murmur of AI if present
			EKG:
			Atrial switch
			  - ectopic or junctional
			  - RAD
			  - RVH
			Arterial switch:
			  - RVH suggests development of pulmonary stenosis

	Rastelli (for VSD + PS): - VSD patch closure directing LV blood across the VSD to the aorta. - PV is oversewn - valved conduit from the RV to PA	Rastelli: - palpitations - syncope - dyspnea - pulmonic ejection murmur of conduit flow often present; increasing harshness or thrill should lead to evaluation for conduit obstruction	Rastelli: - RBBB - may develop CHB

SINGLE VENTRICLE AND FONTAN CIRCULATION

The term *single ventricle* encompasses a wide spectrum of morphologies but is generally defined as one in which systemic venous and pulmonary venous blood enter a functionally single ventricle through a common atrioventricular connection. Common anomalies that fall under this definition include tricuspid atresia, hypoplastic left heart syndrome, double-inlet left ventricle, and heterotaxy syndromes. It is a rare form of congenital heart disease estimated to have an incidence of 54 cases per million live births.

The hemodynamics of the univentricular heart depend on a variety of factors including obstruction to systemic or pulmonary outflow, obstruction to inflow, the presence of an interatrial communication, anatomy and nature of venous return, relative systemic and pulmonary vascular resistances, and AV valve regurgitation. The physiology of the single ventricle is unique in this degree of pulmonary and systemic circulation interdependence.

Patients with unrepaired single ventricles have a poor prognosis with early mortality in childhood or adolescence, although some patients with double inlet left ventricles and transposed great arteries with a relatively well-balanced circulation can survive well into adulthood. Therefore, most patients encountered in adulthood have had prior surgical palliation which is usually performed in multiple stages culminating in the Fontan operation. Clinical presentation, physical exam findings, and complications are summarized in table 84.9.

The survival of patients after the lateral tunnel Fontan procedure is 91% at 10 years. Some patients present with decreased exercise tolerance and increasingly recurrent atrial arrhythmias. Adults with Fontan physiology are at risk of multiple organ dysfunction, including hepatic disease, renal dysfunction, and vascular issues. These patients have a unique physiology that predisposes them to many potential complications (including plastic bronchitis and protein-losing enteropathy) and require regular close care by a team of congenital specialists.

EISENMENGER SYNDROME

ES is the clinical phenotype of an extreme form of pulmonary arterial hypertension associated with congenital heart disease. Over time, in a left-to-right shunt, excessive flow to the pulmonary bed increases pulmonary vascular resistance that eventually results in reversal of the shunt, creating bidirectional or right-to-left flow. Although the classic form of the disease was initially used to describe the long-term consequences of a VSD, it can occur with any congenital defect with an initial left-to-right shunt. With advances in the early diagnosis and management of congenital heart disease, the incidence of ES has declined, although it is still seen in older patients and occasionally in younger patients—particularly in those from developing

Table 84.9 SINGLE VENTRICLE AND FONTAN CIRCULATION

ANATOMY	SURGICAL PALLIATION	CLINICAL PRESENTATION	LATE COMPLICATIONS FOLLOWING FONTAN

Tricuspid atresia
DILV
Hypoplastic left
  heart syndrome
Heterotaxy
  syndromes
	Modified BTS: subclavian artery to ipsilateral
	  PA to improve pulmonary blood flow
		After Fontan:
		- mostly NYHA functional
		  class I–II
		- usually no murmur
		- elevated, non-pulsatile jug-
		  ular venous waveform
		- single S2
			- Atrial tachyarrhythmia
			- Sinus node dysfunction
			- Thromboembolic events
			- Hepatic dysfunction
			- Protein losing enteropathy
			- Fontan pathway obstruction or leaks
			- Obstruction in RA to PA
			  anastomosis
			- Heart failure

	Bidirectional superior cavopulmonary
	  anastomosis (Glenn):
	- SVC to PA
	- usually with takedown of a previously
	  placed systemic to PA shunt
		Unpalliated patients:
		- cyanosis
		- erythrocytosis
		- bleeding diathesis
		- thromboembolic events
		- iron deficiency
		- hyperviscosity
		- stroke
		- cerebral abscess
		- renal dysfunction
		- gallstones, and cholecystitis
		- gout
		- hypertrophic
		  osteoarthropathy
			- Plastic bronchitis
			Cyanosis may be due to:
			- shunting through a surgically
			  created fenestration
			- shunting through a residual atrial
			  communication
			- pulmonary arteriovenous
			  malformations
			- systemic venous collateralization
			  with connection to a pulmonary
			  vein or pulmonary venous atrium
			- reopening of systemic veins to pul-
			  monary venous atrium
			- pulmonary pathology

	Total cavopulmonary anastomosis (Fontan):
	- IVC to PA by intraatrial lateral tunnel or
	  extracardiac conduit—pulmonary blood
	  flow is usually achieved passively, without
	  the assistance of a ventricular pumping
	  chamber		

countries—where these therapies are not readily available. The natural history of ES is variable, and although a cause of significant morbidity, many patients survive 30 years or more after the onset of the syndrome. Clinical presentation, physical exam findings, and laboratory features are summarized in table 84.10.

ES is a multiorgan disease process. Medical care recommendations have included sustaining adequate hydration, avoiding and treating anemia including iron supplementation when appropriate, oxygen supplementation, which may improve symptoms (but overall benefit is controversial), and anticoagulation (although this remains

Table 84.10 EISENMENGER SYNDROME

ANATOMY	CLINICAL PRESENTATION	PHYSICAL EXAM	LABORATORY FEATURES

Causes
- VSD
- ASD
- AV canal defect
- PDA
- aorto-pulmonary window
- truncus arteriosus
- surgically created
  systemic-to-pulmonary
  artery shunts
	Fatigue
	Exercise intolerance
	Dyspnea
	Syncope
	
	Complications:
	  Hyperviscosity symptoms
	    (headache, altered mentation,
	    blurred vision, paresthesia)
	  Bleeding
	  Thromboembolic events, stroke
	  Arrhythmias
	  Heart failure
	  Sudden death
	  Infections (endocarditis, cerebral
	    abscess, pneumonia)
	  Gout
	  Gallstones and cholecystitis
	  Renal dysfunction
	  Hypertrophic osteoarthropathy
		Cyanosis
		Clubbing
		Prominent v wave on jugular
		  venous examination
		Right parasternal heave
		Loud P2
		Holosystolic murmur of TR
		Signs of heart failure (edema,
		  ascites, hepatosplenomegaly)
			Laboratory:
			- erythrocytosis
			- iron deficiency
			- thrombocytopenia
			- hyperuricemia
			- elevated conjugated bilirubin
			
			Chest radiography:
			- dilated central PA
			- reduced vascularity not common
			
			EKG:
			- RVH
			- RAE
			- atrial arrhythmias

controversial due to in vitro predisposition to bleeding and occurrence of clinical hemoptysis, which has frequently been associated with pulmonary vascular thrombosis). Elevation of hematocrit above that considered appropriate for degree of cyanosis can be managed in *symptomatic* patients by hydration alone, or by performing phlebotomy with isovolumic replenishment; routine phlebotomy in the asymptomatic adult with ES is contraindicated. Cautious optimization of iron stores has been demonstrated to improve quality of life and functional performance in iron deficient adults with ES. Endocarditis prophylaxis is warranted as are yearly flu shots and Pneumovax vaccination. Pregnancy is sufficiently high risk to both the mother with ES and fetus and is, therefore, counseled against in strongest fashion. Contraception for women with ES who are of child-bearing age is typically recommended, avoiding use of estrogen if possible. Contraceptive and pregnancy termination counseling are considered standard of care. The risks and benefits of pregnancy termination as contrasted to attempted completion of pregnancy to and beyond term must be addressed and indivualized in any ES patient who contemplates childbirth, or who presents pregnant.

There is a growing body of evidence to suggest that the effects of pulmonary vascular changes in adults with ES are modifiable. Selective pulmonary vasodilators such as bosentan or sildenafil may not only be safe, but they likely are beneficial in this population. Select patients may be candidates for combined heart lung transplantation or preferably lung transplantation with concomitant repair of the intracardiac defect, if feasible. Timing of these interventions may be difficult because of the relatively long-term survival of these patients after the onset of the disease process.

SUMMARY

The general internist and cardiovascular specialist face increasing numbers of adults with moderate and more complex congenital heart disease in their practices. Epidemiologic review suggests that such affected individuals present with substantive medical as well as cardiovascular needs.

This chapter provides an overview of the most general cardiovascular issues faced by adults with congenital heart disease. Care providers are urged to establish continuous relationships with regional ACHD centers of excellence so as to (1) establish optimal communication and care planning for each ACHD patient they encounter, and (2) to ensure access to care review as specific or more novel issues arise.

ADDITIONAL READING

Attie F, et al. Surgical treatment for secundum atrial septal defects in patients >40 years old. A randomized clinical trial. *J Am Coll Cardiol.* 2001;38(7):2035–42.

Celermajer DS, et al. Ebstein's anomaly: presentation and outcome from fetus to adult. *J Am Coll Cardiol.* 1994;23(1):170–6.

Cohen MS, Wernovsky G. Is the arterial switch operation as good over the long term as we thought it would be? *Cardiol Young.* 2006;16 Suppl 3:117–24.

Earing MG, et al. Long-term follow-up of patients after surgical treatment for isolated pulmonary valve stenosis. *Mayo Clin Proc.* 2005; 80(7):871–6.

Galie N, et al. Bosentan therapy in patients with Eisenmenger syndrome: a multicenter, double-blind, randomized, placebo-controlled study. *Circulation.* 2006;114(1):48–54.

Gatzoulis MA, et al. Risk factors for arrhythmia and sudden cardiac death late after repair of tetralogy of Fallot: a multicentre study. *Lancet.* 2000;356(9234):975–81.

Ghai A, et al. Left ventricular dysfunction is a risk factor for sudden cardiac death in adults late after repair of tetralogy of Fallot. *J Am Coll Cardiol.* 2002;40(9):1675–80.

Hayes CJ, et al. Second natural history study of congenital heart defects. Results of treatment of patients with pulmonary valvar stenosis. *Circulation.* 1993;87(2 Suppl):I28–37.

Kidd L, et al. Second natural history study of congenital heart defects. Results of treatment of patients with ventricular septal defects. *Circulation.* 1993;87(2 Suppl):I38–51.

Mackie AS, et al. Health care resource utilization in adults with congenital heart disease. *Am J Cardiol.* 2007;99(6):839–43.

Murphy JG, et al. Long-term outcome after surgical repair of isolated atrial septal defect. Follow-up at 27 to 32 years. *N Engl J Med.* 1990;323(24):1645–50.

Nollert G, et al. Long-term survival in patients with repair of tetralogy of Fallot: 36-year follow-up of 490 survivors of the first year after surgical repair. *J Am Coll Cardiol.* 1997;30(5):1374–83.

O'Laughlin MP, et al. Use of endovascular stents in congenital heart disease. *Circulation.* 1991;83(6):1923–39.

Oliver JM, et al. Risk factors for aortic complications in adults with coarctation of the aorta. *J Am Coll Cardiol.* 2004;44(8):1641–7.

Qureshi AM, et al. Acute and intermediate outcomes, and evaluation of injury to the aortic wall, as based on 15 years experience of implanting stents to treat aortic coarctation. *Cardiol Young.* 2007;17(3):307–18.

Schwartz ML, et al. Long-term predictors of aortic root dilation and aortic regurgitation after arterial switch operation. *Circulation.* 2004;110(11 Suppl 1):II128–32.

Stamm C, et al. Long-term results of the lateral tunnel Fontan operation. *J Thorac Cardiovasc Surg.* 2001;121(1): 28–41.

Steele PM, et al. Isolated atrial septal defect with pulmonary vascular-obstructive disease—long-term follow-up and prediction of outcome after surgicalcorrection. *Circulation.* 1987;76(5):1037–42.

Warnes CA, et al. ACC/AHA 2008 Guidelines for the management of adults with congenital heart disease: A report of the American College of Cardiology/American Heart Association task force for practice guidelines for the management of adults with congenital heart disease. *J Am Coll Cardiol.* 2008.

Warnes CA, et al. Task force 1: the changing profile of congenital heart disease in adult life. *J Am Coll Cardiol.* 2001;37(5):1170–5.

QUESTIONS

QUESTION 1. A 44-year-old woman is referred to you for a murmur heard on routine physical exam. On further questioning, she relates that she has noted increased exercise intolerance over the past 3 years but thought it was because she was "getting older." She has no past medical history and is on no medications. On physical exam, the pulse is 76 and regular, blood pressure 136/78, and oxygen saturation is 99% on room air. The jugular venous pressure

(JVP) is estimated to be 10 cm H_2O. On palpation there is mild lift at the lower left sternal border. The rate is regular with a widely split S2 that varies minimally with respiration. There is a systolic ejection murmur heard at the left upper sternal border.

The rest of the exam is unremarkable. The lesion she most likely has is:

A. Tetralogy of Fallot
B. Atrial septal defect
C. Ventricular septal defect
D. Patent ductus arteriosus

QUESTION 2. A 32-year-old woman is being seen for a new patient evaluation. She does not know her exact diagnosis but tells you she had a "hole in my heart" that was repaired when she was around 2 years old. She was told that she was fixed and has not seen a doctor since childhood. On review of systems, she mentions that she gets frequent palpitations but no presyncope or syncope. On physical exam the blood pressure is 112/68, pulse is 72, and oxygen saturation is 98% on room air. You note a right thoracotomy scar, as well as a midline sternal scar. The radial pulse in her right arm is palpable but diminished. The JVP is not elevated. On palpation, there is a right ventricular lift. There is a harsh II/VI systolic ejection murmur at the left upper sternal border with a palpable thrill. In the same location, there is a short II/IV diastolic murmur creating a to-and-fro sound. The rest of the physical exam is unremarkable. On EKG, you note a right bundle branch block with a QRS duration of 176 ms. The most likely diagnosis is repaired:

A. Tetralogy of Fallot
B. Ventricular septal defect
C. Atrial septal defect
D. Patent ductus arteriosus

QUESTION 3. A 24-year-old man is seen in your office for hypertension. His blood pressure in the office is 180/90 in the right arm and 176/86 in the left arm. There is a loud S2 and diminished femoral pulses. He mentions frequent headaches and some fatigue in his legs with exercise. All of the following are associated with this lesion EXCEPT:

A. Intracranial aneurysms
B. Continuous murmurs heard between the scapulae

C. Differential cyanosis
D. Bicuspid aortic valve
E. Risk of premature coronary artery disease

QUESTION 4. Match the following congenital heart lesions to an associated genetic disorder:

1. Turner syndrome	A Tetralogy of Fallot
2. Down syndrome	B. Pulmonary stenosis
3. DiGeorge syndrome	C. Primum ASD
4. Noonan syndrome	D. Aortic coarctation

QUESTION 5. A 36-year-old man with an unrepaired ventricular septal defect comes for routine follow-up. He is originally from Haiti and moved to the United States 5 years ago and you have been following him ever since. On exam, his blood pressure is 110/54, pulse is 90, and oxygen saturation is 72%, which is his baseline. His exam is notable for mild perioral cyanosis and digital clubbing. His cardiac exam is notable for prominent v wave component of the jugular venous pulsation. There is a right ventricular lift and a laterally displaced apex. S1 is single with a widely split S2. The P2 component is prominent.

There is a II/VI holosystolic murmur at the left lower sternal border. The liver is prominent and pulsatile, felt approximately 3 cm below the costal margin. There is 1+ pitting edema in the lower extremities. His hematocrit is 70%. All of the following are potential complications:

A. Iron deficiency anemia
B. Gout
C. Hyperviscosity syndrome
D. Cerebral abscess
E. All of the above

ANSWERS

1. B
2. A
3. C
4.1 D
4.2 C
4.3 A
4.4 B
5. E

85.

PERIPHERAL VASCULAR DISEASE

Mark A. Creager

Atherosclerosis is a systemic disorder with regional manifestations in the heart, limbs, brain, and other organs. Advances in vascular biology, diagnostic imaging, pharmacotherapeutics, and intervention have provided physicians with greater opportunities to evaluate and manage patients with atherosclerotic vascular diseases. This chapter reviews several of these peripheral vascular diseases, including peripheral artery disease, abdominal aortic aneurysm, and carotid artery disease.

PERIPHERAL ARTERY DISEASE

Peripheral artery disease (PAD) is defined as the presence of a stenosis or occlusion in the aorta or arteries of the limbs. It is usually caused by atherosclerosis, although there are other causes of limb arterial occlusive disease. The aorta and iliac arteries are involved in approximately 25%, the femoral and popliteal arteries in 80–90%, and the tibial and peroneal arteries in 40–50% of patients. Most patients have stenoses or occlusions in more than one segment. Patients with PAD have an increased risk of cardiovascular and cerebrovascular events, including death, myocardial infarction, and stroke due to concomitant coronary and cerebral atherosclerosis. In addition, compromised blood flow to the legs may cause leg discomfort, limit functional capacity, impair quality of life, or jeopardize the viability of the limb. Therefore, the clinician should be cognizant of the clinical characteristics of PAD and knowledgeable about the diagnostic tests and treatment strategies available to manage these patients.

EPIDEMIOLOGY OF PAD

PAD is prevalent in approximately 4–5% of the adult population, affecting 8–10 million persons in the United States. As with other manifestations of atherosclerosis, the prevalence of PAD increases with age and is present in 15–20% of persons over the age of 65 years. Prevalence is greater in African Americans than non-Hispanic Caucasians and less in Hispanics and Asians. Modifiable risk factors for PAD include diabetes mellitus, cigarette smoking, hypercholesterolemia, and hypertension. Diabetes increases the relative risk of PAD by approximately fourfold, cigarettes by two- to threefold, and hypertension by 1.5-fold. For each 10 mg/dL increase in total cholesterol, there is a 10% increased risk of PAD. Elevated homocysteine levels are associated with a twofold risk of PAD. The prevalence of PAD is also increased in patients with insulin resistance, as occurs in patients with metabolic syndrome. Inflammatory biomarkers, such as C-reactive protein (CRP) and vascular cell adhesion molecule (VCAM) predict the future development of PAD. One population-based survey of primary care practices detected PAD in 29% of high-risk patients characterized by an age of 70 years or greater or by the use of cigarettes or a history of diabetes in those aged 50–69 years.

CLINICAL MANIFESTATIONS OF PAD

The cardinal symptom of PAD is intermittent claudication. This is typically described as an ache, cramp, pain, or feeling of fatigue in the affected leg, which occurs during walking and is relieved within 10 minutes of walking cessation. It usually occurs in the calf but may affect the buttocks, thigh, or foot, depending on the location of the occlusive lesions. Some patients have leg pain that is atypical for claudication in that it may not be reproducible with walking or may not resolve promptly at rest. Patients with PAD also have impaired walking ability, characterized by slow walking speed and decreased distance as well as altered balance, even in the absence of claudication. Patients with severe PAD may experience pain in the foot or toes at rest. This occurs when the blood supply to the foot does not meet the resting metabolic demands of the tissue and is termed critical limb ischemia. This pain may be worsened by leg elevation and may improve by dependency. Often, these patients dangle their feet over the bed at night for pain relief. Patients with critical limb ischemia also develop painful fissures and ulcers on the feet, which may progress to necrosis and gangrene.

Approximately 50% of patients with PAD have claudication, 33% have atypical symptoms or functional limitations, and 1–2% have critical limb ischemia; 50% are asymptomatic as detected by noninvasive tests in population-based studies.

The vascular examination to identify PAD should include measurement of blood pressure in each arm, auscultation for bruits in the abdomen and at each groin, and careful palpation of the arm and leg pulses, especially the femoral, popliteal, posterior tibial, and dorsalis pedis arteries. The legs should be inspected for muscle atrophy and skin abnormalities including peripheral cyanosis, pallor or dependent rubor, decreased temperature, and ulcers or necrotic lesions.

There are causes of PAD other than atherosclerosis, and the clinician should be aware of these, particularly in patients with atypical demographic characteristics, such as age <40 years or unusual location of symptoms or findings. These disorders include vasculitis, such as thromboangiitis obliterans, Takayasu arteritis, giant cell arteritis, atheroembolism, fibromuscular dysplasia, popliteal aneurysm, popliteal entrapment syndrome, cystic adventitial disease, coarctation of the aorta, vascular tumor, iliac artery syndrome of the cyclist, pseudoxanthoma elasticum, trauma, and radiation-induced arteriopathy.

DIFFERENTIAL DIAGNOSIS

The differential diagnosis of leg pain includes lumbosacral spine disease such as spinal canal stenosis and herniated discs, peripheral neuropathy, arthritis of the hip or knee, venous claudication, compartment syndrome, muscle spasms or cramps, and restless leg syndrome. A careful history and physical examination are usually sufficient to exclude these other causes of leg symptoms. For example, patients with spinal canal stenosis often experience pain with standing as well as walking and observe relief when they flex their trunk, as when leaning forward on a shopping cart. This symptom is often termed pseudoclaudication. Patients with arthritis have abnormal joint examinations including decreased range of motion and pain with joint maneuvers, joint swelling, or tenderness. Those with venous claudication often have a history of venous disease and marked leg swelling. Restless leg syndrome is particularly bothersome at night and characterized by frequent involuntary leg movement. As many of these problems occur in the elderly, it is not uncommon for patients to have more than one problem that causes leg symptoms, including both PAD and spinal canal stenosis, or PAD and osteoarthritis of the hip or knee.

NONINVASIVE DIAGNOSTIC TESTS

There are a variety of noninvasive diagnostic tests that are useful for confirming or excluding the diagnosis of PAD (see table 85.1). These are broadly characterized as physiological tests and imaging tests. The physiological or

Table 85.1 DIAGNOSTIC TESTS FOR PERIPHERAL ARTERY DISEASE

- Ankle brachial index
- Segmental pressure measurements
- Pulse volume recordings (PVR)
- Exercise stress testing
- Duplex ultrasonography
- Magnetic resonance angiography (MRA)
- Computed tomographic angiography (CTA)

hemodynamic tests include the ankle brachial index (ABI), segmental limb pressures, pulse volume recordings (PVR), and treadmill exercise testing with post exercise ABI. Noninvasive imaging studies include duplex ultrasonography, magnetic resonance angiography (MRA), and computed tomographic angiography (CTA).

The ABI is the ratio of the systolic pressure measured at the ankle over the dorsalis pedis or posterior tibial artery to the systolic pressure measured on the arm at the brachial artery. ABI can be measured as part of an office visit or in a vascular laboratory. The test uses sphygmomanometric cuffs placed over the right and left brachial arteries and each ankle. A Doppler probe is used to auscultate the brachial, posterior tibial, and dorsalis pedis arteries. The cuffs are sequentially inflated to suprasystolic pressure and then deflated. Systolic pressure is determined by the onset of flow as detected by the Doppler probe. For each leg, the higher of the dorsalis pedis or posterior tibial pressure is used for the numerator of the equation, and the higher of the left and right brachial artery pressure is used for the denominator. The normal ABI is 1.0–1.3. This is because systolic pressure in the arm and leg should be the same or slightly higher in the leg because of pulse wave amplification. Recognizing that there may be some variability of blood pressure over time as sequential measurements are obtained, an ABI of 0.9 or less is considered diagnostic of PAD. This criterion has approximately 95% specificity and sensitivity for significant stenoses when compared with angiography.

Segmental limb pressure measurements are similar in concept to the ABI; however, they require a greater number of cuffs that are placed along the thigh and calf of each leg. As with the ABI, these cuffs are inflated to suprasystolic pressure and then deflated, and the onset of systole is detected by a Doppler probe placed over the dorsalis pedis or posterior tibial artery at the ankle. Pressure differences of 10–20 mm Hg between cuffs provide insight into the location of significant stenoses in each leg.

PVR use plethysmographic principles to detect the change in the volume of a segment of a limb with each pulse. These use air-filled cuffs or strain gauges to obtain a graphic depiction of the pulse volume waveform along the thigh, calf, ankle, and metatarsal segments of each leg. The normal pulse volume waveform looks like a blood pressure wave with a rapid upstroke and downstroke that contains a dicrotic notch. In the presence of a stenosis proximal to the detector cuff the wave form becomes altered and is characterized by a delayed upstroke and decreased amplitude, analogous to the *pulsus tardus et parvus* of the carotid artery in patients with aortic stenosis.

A treadmill exercise test with measurement of postexercise ABI is used to assess a patient's walking capacity and detect PAD if the resting ABI is not diagnostic, yet the symptoms are highly suggestive of PAD. Immediately following maximal treadmill exercise, the patient is placed in a supine position and the ABI is measured. Normally, the rise in blood pressure that occurs with exercise is the same in the arm and the legs; therefore, there is no change in the ABI. However, if there is a significant flow-limiting stenosis affecting a leg artery, the ankle pressure does not rise as much as the arm pressure during exercise. Indeed, the ankle pressure frequently falls because the stenosis prevents flow augmentation to accommodate the dilated resistance vessels in the exercising extremity. Therefore, the postexercise ABI decreases, typically by more than 20%.

Color-assisted duplex ultrasonography enables both anatomic localization of the stenosis and assessment of its severity. An ultrasound probe is used to scan the arteries of the leg from the groin to the ankle. Gray-scale and color imaging are used to detect plaque and sites of flow turbulence. Interrogation of the arteries with pulsed Doppler permits measurement of blood flow velocity and is used to determine the significance of a stenosis. Normally, blood flow is laminar as depicted by a homogeneous color display, and there is consistency in velocity along the artery. A heterogeneous color display indicative of turbulence or acceleration of flow and a twofold or greater increase in velocity indicates the presence of a 50% or greater stenosis.

Magnetic resonance angiography (MRA) is used to provide anatomic definition of the aorta and peripheral arteries, particularly to assist planning of revascularization procedures. The sensitivity and specificity of gadolinium-enhanced MRA each exceed 90% for detection of significant stenoses when compared with conventional contrast angiography. An important benefit is that there is no ionizing radiation with MRA. An important potential limitation is gadolinium-associated nephrogenic systemic fibrosis in patients with renal insufficiency. Other limitations include the presence of a pacemaker, implantable cardioverter-defibrillator, morbid obesity, and claustrophobia precluding placement in an MRI scanner.

CTA uses iodinated contrast and multidetector CT scanners to image and define the anatomy of the aorta and peripheral arteries, particularly to plan revascularization in appropriate patients. Images can be displayed in three dimensions and rotated to optimize visualization. The sensitivity and specificity of contemporary CTA compared with conventional contrast angiography are >90%. The advantage of CTA is that it can be used in patients with metal clips or pacemakers. The disadvantages of CTA include exposing the patient to ionizing radiation and the risks associated with iodinated radiocontrast.

PROGNOSIS OF PAD

There are two important outcome categories that should be considered when managing patients with PAD: (1) cardiovascular events, such as myocardial infarction, stroke, and death; and (2) limb morbidity, including disabling claudication, critical limb ischemia, and limb loss. The risk of an adverse cardiovascular event is increased two- to fivefold in patients with PAD compared to age-matched groups without PAD.

Over a 5-year period approximately 15–30% of patients with PAD will experience a nonfatal myocardial infarction or stroke, and 15–30% will die, most from a cardiovascular event. The risk of myocardial infarction, stroke, or cardiovascular death in patients with PAD is similar to that of patients with coronary artery disease. All-cause mortality rate is inversely related to the ABI. In a meta-analysis of 16 cohort studies including 48,294 subjects and 480,325 person-years of follow-up, the hazard ratio for all-cause mortality for persons with an ABI <0.6 was over 4.0 compared with a reference group of persons whose ABI was 1.1 to 1.2 (figure 85.1). The prognosis is worst in patients with critical limb ischemia, of whom 20% die within 6–12 months.

The severity of intermittent claudication remains stable in most patients. Approximately 20% develop worsening claudication over 5 years, and 1–2% progress to critical limb ischemia annually. Of patients with critical limb ischemia, over 30% may ultimately undergo amputation, and only 50% are alive with two limbs 1 year after diagnosis.

TREATMENT OF PAD

The goals of treatment for PAD are to reduce the risk of adverse cardiovascular outcomes, improve functional capacity and quality of life, prevent progression of disease, and maintain limb viability. Risk-factor modification and antiplatelet therapy are used to prevent myocardial infarction, stroke, and cardiovascular death (table 85.2), and pharmacotherapy and selective use of revascularization strategies are used to improve symptoms and to preserve limbs.

Risk factor modification is indicated in patients with PAD as it is for other manifestations of atherosclerosis. Guideline statements support smoking cessation, lipid lowering, and blood pressure and glucose control. Patients with PAD who smoke cigarettes should be advised to stop smoking and offered smoking-cessation interventions. Statin therapy reduces the risk of myocardial infarction, stroke,

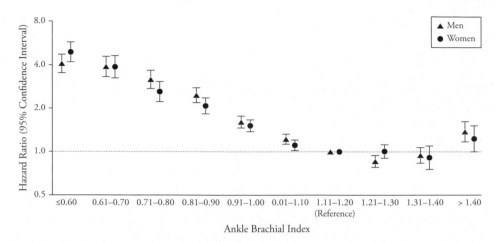

Figure 85.1. Ankle Brachial Index (ABI) and Mortality. Association of ABI with all-cause mortality in a meta-analysis of 16 cohort studies including 48,294 subjects and 480,325 person-years of follow-up. Reprinted with permission from Fowkes FG, Murray GD, Butcher I, et al. Ankle brachial index combined with Framingham Risk Score to predict cardiovascular events and mortality: A metaanalysis. *JAMA.* 2008;300(2):197–208. Copyright 2008 American Medical Association. All rights reserved.

and cardiovascular death in patients with PAD, as it does in patients with coronary artery disease. Therefore, statin therapy should be administered to patients with PAD to achieve a target LDL cholesterol of <100 mg/dL. Antihypertensive therapy reduces the risk of myocardial infarction, stroke, heart failure, renal insufficiency, and cardiovascular death. Any antihypertensive therapy drug that substantially lowers blood pressure may exacerbate symptoms, but it is more important to protect the patient from the systemic complications of hypertension. Both angiotensin-converting enzyme inhibitors and angiotensin receptor blockers reduce myocardial infarction, stroke, and death in patients with atherosclerosis, including those with PAD, and beta-adrenergic blockers are indicated in patients with myocardial infarction, congestive heart failure, and several cardiac arrhythmias and can be used in patients with PAD. In a meta-analysis of 11 randomized controlled trials, beta-adrenergic blocker therapy did not worsen claudication in patients with PAD. Antihypertensive therapy should be administered to hypertensive patients with PAD to achieve target blood pressure according to guidelines, which is less than 130/80 mm Hg in patients with diabetes or renal insufficiency or less than 140/90 mm Hg in others.

Table 85.2 **PAD RISK-REDUCTION THERAPIES**

- **Lifestyle modifications**
  ≥30 Minutes moderately intense physical activity daily
  Weight maintenance/reduction
- **Smoking**
  Complete cessation
- **Diabetes mellitus**
  HbA1c <7.0%
- **Dyslipidemia**
  LDL <100 mg/dL, modify HDL and TG
- **Hypertension**
  BP <140/90 mm Hg or <130/80 mm Hg in patients with diabetes
- **Antiplatelet therapy**

Optimal control of glucose in patients with diabetes reduces microvascular complications, such as nephropathy and retinopathy, but the data supporting optimal glucose control to reduce complications of atherosclerosis are less compelling. Recent studies have found no benefit, and possible harm, in lowering glycosylated hemoglobin less than 6.5%. Current guidelines recommend that patients with PAD be treated with glucose-lowering therapies to reduce the hemoglobin A1c to <7% in order to reduce microvascular complications and potentially improve cardiovascular outcomes. In light of newer studies, these recommendations will need further clarification.

Antiplatelet therapy reduces cardiovascular events in patients with atherosclerosis. The Antithrombotic Trialists' Collaboration reported a meta-analysis of 195 trials comprising 135,640 high-risk patients with cardiovascular or cerebrovascular disease and found that antiplatelet therapy reduced the risk of myocardial infarction, stroke, and cardiovascular death by 22% compared with placebo. Among the 42 trials of 9214 patients with PAD in this analysis, antiplatelet therapy reduced the risk of cardiovascular events by 22%. Two recent trials and a meta-analysis raised doubts about the efficacy of aspirin, particularly in patients with asymptomatic PAD. The Aspirin for Asymptomatic Atherosclerosis trial found that aspirin did not reduce vascular events in asymptomatic patients who did not have established cardiovascular disease but had an abnormal ABI detected at screening. Similarly, the Prevention of Arterial Disease and Diabetes (POPADAD) study found no benefit of aspirin in asymptomatic PAD subjects with diabetes. The CAPRIE study compared the efficacy of aspirin to the thienopyridine derivative, clopidogrel, in patients with acute myocardial infarction, recent ischemic stroke, or established PAD. Overall, clopidogrel reduced myocardial infarction, stroke, or cardiovascular death by 8.7% compared with aspirin. Among the subgroup of patients with

PAD, clopidogrel reduced the risk of cardiovascular events by 23.8%. Subsequently, the CHARISMA study compared the combination of aspirin and clopidogrel to aspirin alone in patients with established cardiovascular disease and those at risk for cardiovascular disease. There was no benefit of dual antiplatelet therapy over aspirin alone on the primary endpoint of myocardial infarction, stroke, or cardiovascular death. A post hoc analysis found that dual antiplatelet therapy reduced the risk of cardiovascular events in patients with established coronary artery disease, cerebrovascular disease or PAD by 12%, but it tended to increase these events in patients with multiple risk factors. Current guidelines recommend antiplatelet therapy to reduce the risk of myocardial infarction, stroke, or vascular death in patients with PAD. Aspirin, in daily doses of 75–325 mg, is recommended as a safe and effective antiplatelet therapy. Clopidogrel, 75 mg per day, is recommended as an effective alternative antiplatelet therapy to aspirin.

Treatment of symptomatic PAD is indicated to improve functional status, alleviate discomfort, and preserve limb function and viability. Treatment for intermittent claudication includes exercise rehabilitation and pharmacotherapy, such as cilostazol. The principal treatment of disabling claudication and critical limb ischemia is revascularization.

Exercise, particularly walking, improves walking distance in patients with claudication. A meta-analysis of studies that compared the efficacy of supervised exercise rehabilitation with no exercise found that peak walking distance increased by 120%, and the distance walked to the onset of claudication increased by 180%. Supervised exercise programs typically involve three to five sessions of treadmill or track walking per week for durations of 35–50 minutes per session for 3–6 months. There is little evidence that home-based exercise programs are effective. Potential mechanisms accounting for exercise-related improvement in walking distance include upregulation of angiogenic growth factors and collateral blood vessel development, enhancement in endothelium-dependent vasodilation, improved hemorheology, increased oxidative capacity of leg skeletal muscle, and better walking biomechanics.

There are only two drugs approved by the Food and Drug Administration for use in patients with intermittent claudication: pentoxifylline and cilostazol. Pentoxifylline is a methylxanthine derivative purported to improve hemorheology through a decrease in blood viscosity and improvement in red blood cell deformability. Several small studies have reported that pentoxifylline causes modest increases in walking distance, approximating 25%, and some have found no efficacy. Cilostazol is a phosphodiesterase III (PDE3) inhibitor that increases levels of cyclic adenosine monophosphate (cAMP), causes vasodilation, and inhibits platelet aggregation. The mechanism by which it improves claudication symptoms, however, is not known. Meta-analyses of multiple clinical trials have found that cilostazol increases maximal walking distance by approximately

40–50%. Cilostazol is contraindicated in patients with congestive heart failure, since other PDE3 inhibitors have been associated with increased mortality rates in these patients. Nutritional supplements, antioxidant vitamins, and chelating agents are not effective therapies for intermittent claudication. Therapeutic angiogenesis with a variety of angiogenic growth factors and cell-based therapies is under investigation.

Revascularization is indicated to treat patients with persistent, lifestyle-limiting claudication despite maximal medical therapy, and those with critical limb ischemia manifest as rest pain, nonhealing ulcer, or gangrene. The two options for revascularization are: (1) endovascular reconstruction including percutaneous transluminal angioplasty (PTA) and stents, and (2) open surgical reconstruction. The location, severity, and characteristics of the stenosis determine the feasibility and long-term success rates of endovascular interventions. The highest success rates are with short-segment stenoses in the iliac arteries. Iliac PTA and stenting is associated with 1-year patency rates of approximately 90% and 3-year patency rates of approximately 70%. PTA with or without stenting of the superficial femoral artery is associated with 60–70% 1-year patency rates and approximately 50% 3-year patency rates, depending on the length and severity of the lesion. Open surgical reconstruction includes aortoiliac/aortofemoral reconstruction, femoropopliteal bypass, and femorotibial or peroneal bypass, depending on the location of the lesions. Inflow disease affecting the aorta and iliac arteries is typically repaired prior to surgical treatment of outflow disease affecting the infrainguinal arteries, such as the superficial femoral, popliteal, tibial, and peroneal arteries. Aorto-bifemoral bypass is a durable operation with 5-year patency rates of approximately 85–90%. The 5-year patency rates for femoral-popliteal bypass depend on whether vein or synthetic material such as polyfluoroethylene (PTFE) is used for the bypass conduit and whether the distal anastomosis is placed above or below the knee. For example, 5-year assisted patency rates for an above-knee femoral-popliteal bypass using autogenous vein is approximately 75–80%, and 3-year patency rate for a femoral-tibial bypass graft using PTFE is approximately 25%. Operative mortality rates for aortobifemoral bypass and infrainguinal bypass procedures at high-volume academic centers approximate 1–3%.

ABDOMINAL AORTIC ANEURYSMS

An aortic aneurysm is a pathological expansion of the aorta. The normal diameter of the infrarenal abdominal aorta is 2 cm. An abdominal aortic aneurysm (AAA) is usually designated when the diameter of the abdominal aorta is >3.0 cm. However, this does not account for variations in body size. Thus, an alternative definition is when there is a

50% or greater increase in the diameter of a segment of the abdominal aorta relative to the proximal normal segment.

The pathophysiology of AAA formation differs from the intimal proliferative process that occurs in atherosclerotic occlusive conditions such as PAD. AAA formation involves inflammatory mediators and proteolytic degradation of the elastin and collagen fibers by matrix metalloproteinases. Subsequent weakening of the adventitia and media leads to aneurysmal disease by decreasing the aortic tensile strength, leading ultimately to aortic expansion and rupture.

EPIDEMIOLOGY OF AAA

The prevalence of AAA is greater in men than women and the prevalence increases with age. AAA occurs in approximately 3.5% of males and 1% of females over the age of 50 years. AAA develop less often in African Americans than in Caucasians. The annual incidence of AAA is approximately 40–50 per 100,000 men and 7–12 per 100,000 women. AAA accounts for over 15,000 deaths annually in the United States.

A history of AAA affecting a first-degree relative is associated with an approximate twofold risk of having an AAA. A personal history of cigarette smoking increases the odds of AAA by 3.6-fold. Other risk factors include hypertension and hypercholesterolemia. For reasons that are not known, the risk of AAA is less in patients with diabetes. The risk of AAA rupture is related to the diameter of the aorta. The 5-year rupture rate is <2% for AAA <4 cm, 25% for those 5.0–5.9 cm, 35% for those 6.0–6.9 cm, and 75% for those 7.0 cm. Also rupture risk is increased by 4.5-fold in women compared with men and twofold in smokers compared with nonsmokers. Elevated blood pressure confers a more modest risk for rupture.

CLINICAL PRESENTATION

Most AAAs are asymptomatic. Occasionally an AAA will cause epigastric, lower back, or abdominal pain. AAAs are occasionally diagnosed when a pulsatile abdominal mass is detected on physical examination. Physical examination is accurate in diagnosing AAA in approximately 50% of patients in whom it is present. More often, AAA is an incidental finding when abdominal imaging is performed for an unrelated reason. Ruptured AAA is a catastrophic event in which the patient presents in extreme distress or dies from circulatory collapse.

DIAGNOSIS OF AAA

Imaging techniques are used to confirm the diagnosis of AAA. These include ultrasound, computed tomographic (CT) imaging, magnetic resonance imaging (MRI), and conventional contrast aortography. A plain x-ray may raise suspicion of an AAA if calcification along the wall of the

dilated aorta is seen. Ultrasonography accurately determines the anterior-posterior, transverse, and longitudinal dimensions of an AAA. It is the most commonly used and least expensive method for diagnosing AAA. Its sensitivity for AAA ≥3.0 cm is virtually 100%. CTA is the preferred imaging modality for preoperative definition of aortic aneurysms. CTA can define the proximal and distal extension of AAA. It is especially useful when determining the feasibility of placement of an aortic endograft because it provides anatomic information such as the size and angulation of the neck as well as the relationship of the AAA to branch arteries. MRI and gadolinium-enhanced magnetic resonance angiography (MRA) are also used to characterize AAA. MRA can determine the diameter, proximal and distal extent of an AAA, and its relationship to branch arteries. As is the case with CTA, MRA is an accurate method to define aortic anatomy prior to placement of an aortic endograft. Contrast angiography is performed less frequently than the noninvasive imaging modalities because it is invasive, and it uses potentially nephrotoxic radiocontrast material. It is useful to define branch vessel anatomy and the longitudinal extent of aortic aneurysm. However, contrast angiography does not always provide accurate information about the diameter of an AAA, because it does not visualize the wall of the aneurysm, and lumen size may be misinterpreted if there is thrombus present.

POPULATION-BASED SCREENING FOR AAA

The United States Preventive Services Task Force has recently recommended one-time screening with ultrasonography of men ages 65–75 years who have ever smoked but against screening for women (U.S. Preventive Services Task Force, 2005). Guidelines from the American College of Cardiology, American Heart Association, and other professional organizations recommend ultrasound screening of men 60 years of age or older who are either the siblings or offspring of patients with AAA and of men who are 65–75 years of age who have ever smoked. These recommendations are based, in part, on several large studies. The Multicentre Aneurysm Screening Study (MASS) randomized 68,000 men between the ages of 65–74 years to ultrasound screening or no screening (Multicentre Aneurysm Screening Study Group 2002). There was a 42% reduction in the risk of AAA-related mortality among patients invited for screening compared to patients in the nonscreening group. Three other randomized clinical trials confirmed these findings.

MANAGEMENT OF AAA

Guidelines recommend repair of AAA >5.5 cm in diameter to eliminate the risk of rupture (table 85.3). In patients with symptomatic AAA, repair is indicated regardless of diameter. Surveillance by ultrasound or CT imaging

Table 85.3 ABDOMINAL AORTIC ANEURYSM: RECOMMENDATIONS FOR REPAIR

- Patients with infrarenal or juxtarenal AAA ≥5.5 cm in diameter should undergo repair to eliminate the risk of rupture.

- Patients with infrarenal or juxtarenal AAA 4.0–5.4 cm in diameter should be monitored by ultrasound or CT scans every 6–12 months to detect expansion.

- For AAA <4.0 cm in diameter, monitor by ultrasound every 2–3 years.

- In patients with symptomatic aortic aneurysms, repair is indicated regardless of diameter.

every 6–12 months is recommended for AAA 4.0–5.4 cm in diameter to detect expansion, and ultrasound surveillance every 2–3 years is recommended for AAA <4.0 cm in diameter. AAA that increase in size by 1 cm or more over 1 year should also be repaired. The recommendations to monitor AAA 4.0–5.4 cm and repair AAA >5.5 cm are based on two large randomized clinical trials, the United Kingdom Small Aneurysm Trial and the Aneurysm Detection and Management trial. In each trial patients were randomized to undergo early elective open surgery or to ultrasound surveillance, and follow-up was approximately 4.5 years. There was no difference in all-cause mortality among patients randomized to either management in both trials.

No medical therapies have been proven to reduce the risk of AAA expansion or rupture. Optimal control of blood pressure and lipids is indicated to reduce the risk of adverse cardiovascular events, as for patients with other manifestations of atherosclerosis. Long-term treatment with beta-adrenergic blocking agents has not been shown to reduce rate of AAA expansion. Doxycycline reduces matrix metalloproteinase production and reduces aneurysm expansion in experimental models; its efficacy in humans is not established.

Surgical repair of AAA entails endoaneurysmorrhaphy with intraluminal graft placement via an anterior transperitoneal or retroperitoneal approach. Prosthetic grafts used for AAA repair are typically made of Dacron or PTFE. A straight tube graft confined to the abdominal aorta is used in approximately 50% of patients. A bifurcated graft with extension to the iliac arteries is used in most other cases if there is calcification of the aortic bifurcation or concurrent aneurysmal involvement of the iliac arteries. Operative mortality rates range from 1.4% to 6.5%. Complications include myocardial infarction, congestive heart failure, pulmonary insufficiency, renal insufficiency, ischemic colitis, atheroembolism, and wound infections.

Endovascular repair of AAA is an alternative to open surgical repair in approximately 50% of patients. The feasibility of endovascular repair is based on anatomic features of the AAA. The procedure involves the placement of an aortic stent graft under fluoroscopic guidance. The stent graft is placed above and below the AAA into the distal abdominal aorta as a tube graft or into each of the iliac arteries as a bifurcated graft, depending on the aortic anatomy and extent of the AAA. Several trials have compared open surgery with endovascular repair for AAA. Short-term outcomes, including mortality, blood loss, and pulmonary complications were less in patients undergoing endovascular repair compared with conventional surgery. However, long-term follow-up of 2–4 years found that survival was equivalent in the two groups. A study of matched cohorts of Medicare beneficiaries undergoing endovascular or open surgical repair of AAA found that laparotomy-related complications, such as bowel obstruction or abdominal wall hernia, occurred more frequently in patients who had conventional surgery than among those who had endovascular repair.

An important complication of endovascular repair of AAA is endoleak, which is defined as persistent flow within the aneurysm sac. Endoleaks increase the potential for aneurysm expansion and rupture. Therefore, patients undergoing endovascular repair of AAA require long-term surveillance with CT scans. Patients with comorbid conditions that affect operative risk do not necessarily benefit from endovascular repair of AAA. One study found no deterrence in 4-year survival between endovascular repair and no intervention in patients considered unfit for open surgical repair.

CAROTID ARTERY DISEASE

The left and right internal carotid arteries originate at the bifurcation of their respective common carotid arteries, and course along the anteromedial aspect of the neck. The internal carotid artery enters the cranium through its canal in the petrous portion of the temporal bone, ultimately joining the Circle of Willis where it gives off the middle and anterior cerebral arteries. The most common cause of carotid artery disease is atherosclerosis. Ischemic stroke results from a mural thrombosis at a site of atherosclerotic plaque leading to artery-to-artery atheroembolism or to occlusive thrombus. Less common causes of carotid artery disease include Takayasu arteritis, giant cell arteritis, fibromuscular dysplasia, dissection, and radiation-induced arteriopathy.

EPIDEMIOLOGY

Over 700,000 strokes occur annually in the United States. Approximately 80% of all strokes are ischemic, and extracranial internal carotid artery stenosis accounts for 15–30% of these. Other causes of ischemic stroke include: intracranial atherosclerosis, lacunar infarction, thromboembolism, and atheroembolism. The risk of a recurrent ischemic stroke is 3–10% by 30 days and 5–14% by 1 year. Mortality rates at 30 days and 1 year are 8–12% and 15–25% respectively.

Approximately 30–50% of stroke survivors have partial or complete dependence, and approximately one-third experience cognitive decline or dementia.

Significant carotid artery disease, in which there is a stenosis >50%, is present in approximately 7–9% of men and 5–7% of women 65 years of age or older. Risk factors for carotid artery atherosclerosis include age, hypertension, hypercholesterolemia, diabetes, and cigarette smoking. Patients with carotid artery disease often have other manifestations of atherosclerosis and have a high risk of adverse cardiac events, such as myocardial infarction and death. The most important predictor of stroke among patients with carotid artery disease is the severity of the stenosis. The 5-year risk of ipsilateral stroke if carotid stenosis is 70% is approximately 11–12% for asymptomatic patients and over 25% for symptomatic patients.

CLINICAL PRESENTATION

Most patients with carotid artery disease are asymptomatic. Symptoms include transient ischemic attacks (TIA) and stroke. Symptoms of a TIA last <24 hours, and usually less than 15 minutes. Symptoms of a stroke typically persist and are a reflection of a fixed neural deficit. The neurological symptoms that result from carotid artery disease are focal and typically confined to the territory of the ipsilateral middle cerebral artery. These include contralateral hemiparesis, contralateral hemisensory loss, ipsilateral monocular visual defects, and aphasia.

Carotid artery disease may be detected by a vascular examination that includes auscultation of the neck for bruits. Approximately 4% of asymptomatic adults have a carotid bruit, and these patients have a threefold increased risk of ischemic stroke. Neck auscultation for carotid bruits should be performed in patients with neurological symptoms that suggest involvement of the middle cerebral artery territory subserved by the internal carotid artery. In addition, a complete neurological examination can indicate the location of an ischemic stroke in symptomatic patients. Signs of an ischemic stroke in the distribution of the right internal carotid artery/middle cerebral artery include: left hemiparesis, left hemisensory loss, left neglect, and abnormal visual-spacial abilities. Signs of an ischemic stroke in the left internal carotid artery/middle cerebral artery distribution include: right hemiparesis, right hemisensory loss, and aphasia.

DIAGNOSIS OF CAROTID ARTERY DISEASE

Diagnostic tests used to detect carotid artery stenosis include: duplex ultrasonography, MR angiography, CT angiography, and conventional contrast angiography (table 85.4). Color-assisted duplex ultrasonography can accurately assess the presence and severity of the stenosis. An ultrasound probe is used to scan the cervical portion of the common, internal, and external carotid arteries. Gray-scale and color imaging are used to detect plaque and sites of flow turbulence. The pulsed Doppler velocity is used to determine the severity of a stenosis. Several criteria have been proposed to quantify the severity of stenosis based on the systolic velocity. For example, one set of criteria uses a cutpoint of 230 cm/sec as the threshold for detecting ≥70% stenosis and 125 cm/sec as the cutpoint for identifying 50% stenosis. MRA visualizes the cervical portion of the carotid arteries. When performed in conjunction with an MRA of the brain, it can also provide information about intracranial vascular anatomy. The sensitivity and specificity of contrast-enhanced MRA exceed 90% for detection of significant stenoses when compared with contrast angiography. However, MRA may overestimate the severity of stenosis. CTA uses iodinated contrast to evaluate the carotid arteries. An advantage of CTA in patients suspected of having an ischemic stroke is that extracranial and intracranial arteries supplying the brain can be imaged in the same examination. Calcification may obscure the stenosis and limit the assessment of its severity. The sensitivity and specificity of CTA compared with conventional contrast angiography for 70–99% stenosis are 85% and 93%, respectively, and for occlusion they are 97% and 99%, respectively. Contrast angiography remains the gold standard for assessment of carotid artery stenosis, but it is used primarily for evaluation and management of carotid stenosis during endovascular procedures.

TREATMENT OF CAROTID ARTERY DISEASE

Treatment of carotid artery disease includes (1) medical therapies to reduce atherosclerosis progression and decrease the risk of stroke and other adverse cardiovascular events and (2) revascularization in selected circumstances to reduce the risk of ipsilateral ischemic stroke. Medical therapies include risk factor modification and antiplatelet drugs. Revascularization strategies include carotid endarterectomy and carotid artery stenting.

Medical treatment for carotid artery disease is comprised of lipid-lowering drugs, optimal blood pressure control, smoking cessation, glycemic control, and antiplatelet therapy. Statins reduce the risk of stroke in patients with

Table 85.4 **DIAGNOSTIC TESTS FOR CAROTID STENOSIS AND STROKE**

- **Carotid stenosis**
  Duplex ultrasonography
  MR angiography
  CT angiography
  Conventional angiography

- **Stroke**
  CT imaging
  MR imaging

coronary artery disease and in patients with cerebrovascular disease. Treatment with statins reduces stroke risk by over 20%. The Stroke Prevention by Reduction of Cholesterol Levels (SPARCL) study demonstrated a significant effect of high-dose statin in decreasing recurrent stroke, first major cardiovascular event, or need for revascularization in patients who had a prior stroke or TIA. Antihypertensive treatment reduces the risk of first stroke by 35–40%, although this is not specific for patients with carotid artery disease. In patients with prior stroke or transient ischemic attack, antihypertensive therapy reduces the risk of another stroke by 25%. It is possible that aggressive blood pressure lowering would cause symptoms in patients with a significant carotid artery stenosis. Although patients with diabetes are at increased risk for stroke, there is insufficient evidence to support the notion that optimal glucose control reduces the risk of stroke. Recent clinical studies failed to find a benefit on cardiovascular endpoints when the hemoglobin A1c was lowered to less than 6.5%.

Antiplatelet agents are indicated for the treatment of patients with carotid artery disease. Available antiplatelet therapies include aspirin, combination aspirin and extended release dipyridamole, and clopidogrel. The choice of agent depends, in part, on whether the antiplatelet therapy is used for primary prevention of stroke in a patient with carotid artery disease or for secondary prevention of recurrent ischemic stroke. In the Antithrombotic Trialists Collaboration, antiplatelet therapy reduced the risk of stroke, myocardial infarction, and cardiovascular death by 22% in patients with cerebrovascular disease. In the total population of the CAPRIE trial, clopidogrel reduced the risk of myocardial infarction, stroke, or vascular death compared with aspirin. However, there was no significant difference in outcome between aspirin and clopidogrel in the subgroup of patients with recent ischemic stroke. In MATCH, the combination of aspirin and clopidogrel was no more effective in preventing recurrent stroke than clopidogrel alone. In the CHARISMA trial, stroke risk was not different between the group treated with the combination of clopidogrel and aspirin compared with aspirin alone. In the ESPS-2 and the ESPRIT trials, the combination of sustained release dipyridamole and aspirin, compared with either agent alone, caused a greater reduction in the incidence of a second stroke. In the PRoFESS trial, the risk of recurrent stroke was not different between the group receiving combination treatment with aspirin and extended release dipyridamole and the group receiving clopidogrel. In the Warfarin Aspirin Recurrent Stroke Study, warfarin was no more effective than aspirin in preventing recurrent ischemic stroke or death, but it was associated with a higher risk of bleeding.

Carotid revascularization can be accomplished by either carotid endarterectomy or carotid artery stenting. Carotid artery endarterectomy is considered the standard of care for symptomatic patients with significant carotid artery stenosis. Carotid artery stenting is an alternative to carotid

endarterectomy in selected patients, particularly with significant comorbidities or whose anatomy adversely affects the risk of carotid endarterectomy.

There are several trials that support the use of carotid endarterectomy for symptomatic patients with significant stenoses. Both the North American Symptomatic Carotid Endarterectomy Trial (NASCET) and the European Carotid Surgery Trial (ECST) found that carotid endarterectomy reduces the risk of ipsilateral stroke in patients with symptomatic hemodynamically significant carotid artery stenosis, particularly 70% or greater compared with optimal medical therapy. In NASCET, the 30-month risk of ipsilateral stroke was 36% in the medical group and 9% in the carotid endarterectomy group. At the time of these trials, which were reported over 15 years ago, optimal medical therapy was primarily an antiplatelet drug. Carotid endarterectomy is also indicated for asymptomatic patients with significant, 70% or greater, carotid artery stenosis, although the evidence is less compelling. The Asymptomatic Carotid Artery Study (ACAS) and the MRC Asymptomatic Carotid Surgery Trial (ACST) reported 5-year risks of stroke or death of approximately 11–12% with optimal medical therapy and deferred surgery, and approximately 5–6.5% 5-year risks with immediate surgery. The 30-day risk of stroke or death associated with carotid endarterectomy approximates 3%, depending on the patient's age and comorbid conditions and whether the patient is symptomatic or asymptomatic.

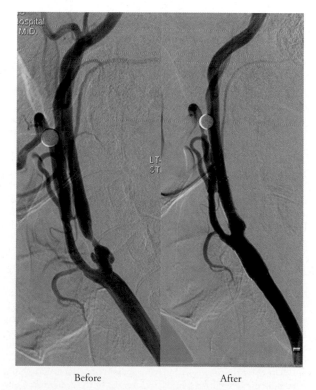

Before   After

Figure 85.2. Stenting of Carotid Arteries. Angiographic appearance of the left carotid artery of a patient with severe bilateral carotid artery stenoses, before and after carotid artery stenting.

Carotid artery stenting offers advantages over carotid endarterectomy since it does not require anesthesia, and recovery time is shorter (figure 85.2). Several registries and trials have found that outcomes with carotid artery stenting and carotid endarterectomy are comparable in certain conditions. The SAPPHIRE study compared carotid artery stenting with the use of an embolic protection device to carotid endarterectomy in high-risk patients, defined as clinically significant cardiac disease, severe pulmonary disease, contralateral carotid occlusion, recurrent stenosis after endarterectomy, or age >80 years. Two studies, EVA-3S and SPACE, reported that adverse outcomes occurred more frequently with carotid artery stenting than with carotid endarterectomy, but lack of operator experience and limited use of distal protection devices may confound interpretation of these studies. The National Institutes of Health sponsored Carotid Revascularization Endarterectomy versus Stenting Trial (CREST) randomized patients with symptomatic and asymptomatic carotid artery stenosis to carotid artery stenting or carotid endarterectomy. There was no difference in the primary composite outcome of stroke, myocardial infarction, or death between the two treatment groups after a median follow-up period of 2.5 years.

ADDITIONAL READING

Brott TG, Halperin JL, Abbara S, et al. 2011 ASA/ACCF/AHA/AANN/AANS/ACR/ASNR/CNS/SAIP/SCAI/SIR/SNIS/SVM/SVS Guideline on the Management of Patients with Extracranial Carotid and Vertebral Artery Disease: Executive Summary: A Report of the American College of Cardiology Foundation/American Heart Association Task Force on Practice Guidelines, and the American Stroke Association, American Association of Neuroscience Nurses, American Association of Neurological Surgeons, American College of Radiology, American Society of Neuroradiology, Congress of Neurological Surgeons, Society of Atherosclerosis Imaging and Prevention, Society for Cardiovascular Angiography and Interventions, Society of Interventional Radiology, Society of NeuroInterventional Surgery, Society for Vascular Medicine, and Society for Vascular Surgery. *Circulation*. 2011;124:489–532.

Goldstein LB, Bushnell CD, Adams RJ, et al; on behalf of the American Heart Association Stroke Council, Council on Cardiovascular Nursing, Council on Epidemiology and Prevention, Council for High Blood Pressure Research, Council on Peripheral Vascular Disease, and Interdisciplinary Council on Quali. Guidelines for the Primary Prevention of Stroke. A Guideline for Healthcare Professionals from the American Heart Association/American Stroke Association. *Stroke*. Stroke, 2011; 42: 517–84.

Hiratzka LF, Bakris GL, Beckman JA, et al.; American College of Cardiology Foundation/American Heart Association Task Force on Practice Guidelines; American Association for Thoracic surgery; American College of Radiology; American Stroke Association; Society of Cardiovascular Anesthesiologists; Society for Cardiovascular Angiography and Interventions; Society of Interventional Radiology; Society of Thoracic Surgeons; Society for Vascular Medicine. 2010 ACCF/AHA/AATS/ACR/ASA/SCA/SCAI/SIR/STS/SVM Guidelines for the diagnosis and management of patients with thoracic aortic disease: Executive summary: A report of the American College of Cardiology Foundation/American Heart Association Task Force

on Practice Guidelines, American Association for Thoracic Surgery, American College of Radiology, American Stroke Association, Society of Cardiovascular Anesthesiologists, Society for Cardiovascular Angiography and Interventions, Society of Interventional Radiology, Society of Thoracic Surgeons, and Society for Vascular Medicine. *Anesth Analg.* 2010;111(2):279–315.

Hirsch AT, Haskal ZJ, Hertzer NR, et al. ACC/AHA 2005 guidelines for the management of patients with peripheral arterial disease (lower extremity, renal, mesenteric, and abdominal aortic): Executive summary a collaborative report from the American Association for Vascular Surgery/Society for Vascular Surgery. Society for Cardiovascular Angiography and Interventions, Society for Vascular Medicine and Biology, Society of Interventional Radiology, and the ACC/AHA Task Force on Practice Guidelines (Writing Committee to Develop Guidelines for the Management of Patients With Peripheral Arterial Disease) endorsed by the American Association of Cardiovascular and Pulmonary Rehabilitation; National Heart, Lung, and Blood Institute; Society for Vascular Nursing; TransAtlantic Inter-Society Consensus; and Vascular Disease Foundation. *J Am Coll Cardiol.* 2006;47(6):1239–1312.

Kent KC. Endovascular aneurysm repair—is it durable? *N Engl J Med.* 2010;362(20):1930–1.

Olin JW, Allie DE, Belkin M, et al.; ACCF/AHA/ACR/SCAI/SIR/SVM/SVN/SVS 2010 performance measures for adults with peripheral artery disease. A Report of the American College of Cardiology Foundation/American Heart Association Task Force on Performance Measures, the American College of Radiology, the Society for Cardiac Angiography and Interventions, the Society for Interventional Radiology, the Society for Vascular Medicine, the Society for Vascular Nursing, and the Society for Vascular Surgery (Writing Committee to Develop Clinical Performance Measures for Peripheral Artery Disease). *Vasc Med.* 2010;15(6):481–512.

U.S. Preventive Services Task Force. Screening for abdominal aortic aneurysm: Recommendation statement. *Ann Intern Med.* 2005;142(3):198–202.

Weintraub NL. Understanding abdominal aortic aneurysm. *N Engl J Med.* 2009;361(11):1114–6.

White C. Clinical practice. Intermittent claudication. *N Engl J Med.* 2007;356(12):1241–50.

QUESTIONS

QUESTION 1. A 60-year-old man reports that he is experiencing cramping in his left calf after walking approximately three blocks. The cramp resolves after resting for 5 minutes. The symptom has been occurring for 6 months. Past history is notable only for hypertension. He smokes 1–2 packs of cigarettes each day. His only medication is metoprolol. His blood pressure is 138/86 mm Hg, heart rate is 64 bpm. The right femoral, popliteal, dorsalis pedis, and posterior tibial pulses are palpable. The left femoral pulse is palpable, but the left popliteal, dorsalis pedis, and posterior tibial pulses are not palpable.

Which one of the following treatments is indicated to improve his symptoms?

A. Clopidogrel
B. Discontinue metoprolol
C. Reduce the number of cigarettes smoked
D. Supervised exercise rehabilitation
E. Left iliac artery stent

QUESTION 2. A 63-year-old active woman is being seen for the first time by her new primary care physician. She has no specific complaints. She has hypertension and type 2 diabetes mellitus. She walks 2 miles each day for exercise. Her medications include lisinopril, simvastatin, and metformin. Her blood pressure is 134/78 mm Hg. Her right and left posterior tibial and dorsalis pulses are not palpable. Total cholesterol is 220 mg/dL, HDL cholesterol is 43 mg/dL, triglycerides are 250 mg/dL, and glycosylated hemoglobin is 6.9%.

Which one of the following diagnostic tests is indicated to plan further therapy?

A. Ankle brachial index
B. Magnetic resonance angiography
C. Computed tomographic angiography
D. Treadmill exercise tolerance test
E. Duplex ultrasound of the legs

QUESTION 3. A computed tomographic examination of the abdomen and pelvis, performed to evaluate episodic abdominal pain, detected an infrarenal abdominal aortic aneurysm with a maximal diameter of 4.6 cm. Which of the following interventions is indicated at this time?

A. No intervention
B. Beta-adrenergic blocker
C. Angiotensin receptor blocker (ARB)
D. Placement of an endograft
E. Open surgical repair

QUESTION 4. A 72-year-old man presents to the emergency room after a 15-minute episode of right arm weakness. The symptom has resolved. A left carotid bruit is heard. His past medical history includes an inferior myocardial infarction, hypercholesterolemia, and hypertension. He is a former smoker. His medications include aspirin, atorvastatin, atenolol, and hydrochlorothiazide. A duplex ultrasound of his carotid arteries detects an 80% stenosis of the left internal carotid artery. The next most appropriate treatment for this patient is:

A. Dipyridamole
B. Clopidogrel
C. Heparin
D. Carotid-subclavian artery bypass
E. Carotid endarterectomy

QUESTION 5. Which one of the following treatments has been shown to reduce the risk of recurrent ischemic stroke?

A. Atorvastatin
B. Cilostazol
C. Folic acid
D. Glyburide
E. Tissue plasminogen activator

ANSWERS

1. D
2. A
3. A
4. E
5. A

86.

EKG REFRESHER

Anju Nohria

The term electrocardiogram had its origins over 100 years ago when it was introduced in 1893 by Willem Einthoven at a Dutch Medical Society meeting. Einthoven subsequently received the Nobel Prize for developing the EKG. The standard 12-lead EKG was introduced in 1942. Despite the emergence of many tools to evaluate cardiac structure and function, the EKG remains an important, if not the most important, test. The EKG is crucial for interpretation of cardiac rhythm, conduction system abnormalities, and for the detection of myocardial ischemia. The EKG is also important in the workup of valvular heart disease, cardiomyopathy, pericarditis, and hypertensive disease. Last, the EKG detects electrolyte and metabolic abnormalities that may affect the heart, including disorders of potassium, calcium, and magnesium, and can be used to monitor drug treatment (specifically antiarrhythmic therapy).

At its very basic, the EKG is a plot of voltage measured by the leads on the vertical axis against time on the horizontal axis. The electrodes are connected to a galvanometer that records a potential difference. The needle (or pen) of the EKG is deflected a given distance depending on the voltage measured. The EKG waves are recorded on special graph paper, which is divided into 1-mm² gridlike boxes. Each 1-mm (small) horizontal box corresponds to 0.04 seconds (40 msec), with heavier lines forming larger boxes that include five small boxes and hence represent 0.20-second (200-msec) intervals (at the usual paper speed of 25 mm/sec). Vertically, the EKG graph measures the height (amplitude) of a given wave or deflection, as 10 mm (10 small boxes) equals 1 mV with standard calibration.

EKG FUNDAMENTALS

The normal rate and intervals (Surawicz and Knilans, 2008) are shown in figure 86.1, and the mean QRS axis in the frontal plane (Surawicz and Knilans, 2008) is given in figure 86.2.

Although it is rarely important to calculate the exact axis, recognition of an abnormal axis is important. This can be accomplished by looking at the net area under the QRS curves in leads I, aVF, and II (table 86.1).

A normal EKG is shown in figure 86.3. Incorrect lead placement can produce a number of variant configurations (Surawicz and Knilans, 2008). For example, with *right–left arm lead reversal*, there is a negative P wave with negative QRS complexes in leads I and aVL (figure 86.4B), although the precordial leads are unaffected. With *arm–leg lead reversal*, there is a far-field signal in one of the bipolar leads (II, III, or aVF) that records the signal between the right and left legs. This is seen as a lack of signal in that lead except for tiny QRS complexes (figure 86.4C).

P WAVE ABNORMALITIES

Under normal circumstances (Surawicz and Knilans, 2008), atrial activation starts in the sinus node and spreads radially through the right atrium, interatrial septum, and left atrium. The P wave axis in the frontal plane is therefore directed inferiorly and leftward and is between 0° and 75°. The P wave is always upright in I and II and inverted in aVR. It is usually also upright in III and aVF but may be biphasic or flat. It can be biphasic in V1 and V2, with the first part reflecting right atrial depolarization and the second part reflecting left atrial depolarization. The normal P wave has a duration <0.12 seconds and an amplitude ≤2.5 mm.

RIGHT ATRIAL ENLARGEMENT

In right atrial enlargement (RAE) (figure 86.5A), the P wave is tall and peaked in lead II (>0.25 mV), or the positive deflection in lead V1 or V2 is ≥0.15 mV. RAE is commonly seen with cor pulmonale, pulmonary hypertension, and congenital heart disease.

LEFT ATRIAL ENLARGEMENT

In left atrial enlargement (LAE) (figure 86.5B), the P wave in lead II may be broad (≥0.12 sec) or notched (peak-to-peak interval > 0.04 sec), or the P wave in V1 has a negative component that occupies more than one small box. LAE

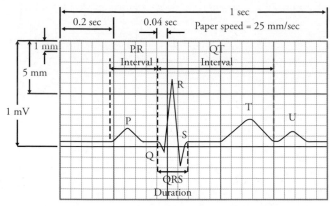

Figure 86.1. *Normal Rate and Intervals.* Provided regular rhythm, heart rate = 1500/# of small boxes between two consecutive R waves or 300/# of large boxes between two consecutive R waves; Heart rate = 60–100 bpm; PR = 0.12–0.20 sec; QRS ≤ 0.12 sec; QTc (QT/√RR) ≤ 0.45 sec in men and ≤ 0.47 sec in women. *Source*: Reproduced with permission from Walker HK et al. Clinical methods: The history, physical and laboratory examinations, 1990.

is commonly seen in mitral valve disease, hypertension, or other causes of left ventricular hypertrophy (LVH).

CARDIAC CONDUCTION ABNORMALITIES

In normal cardiac conduction, the electrical impulse is generated in the sinus node and spreads through the atria to the atrioventricular (AV) node (Surawicz and Knilans, 2008). In the AV node conduction slows, allowing time for the atria to contract before ventricular activation occurs. After the impulse passes through the AV node, it is conducted rapidly to the ventricles through the bundle of His, bundle branches, distal Purkinje fibers, and the ventricular

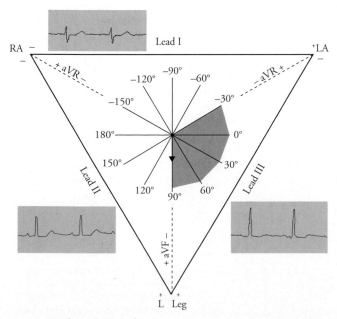

Figure 86.2. Einthoven's Triangle.

Table 86.1 CALCULATION OF THE QRS AXIS IN THE FRONTAL PLANE

AXIS	LEAD I	aVF	LEAD II
Normal (0° to +100°)	+	+	
Normal Variant (0° to –30°)	+	–	+
LAD (–30° to –90°)	+	–	–
RAD (>100°)	–	+	
R superior axis (–90° to +180°)	–	–	

myocardial cells to allow synchronized contraction of the right and left ventricles.

Atrioventricular Conduction Abnormalities

First-Degree AV Block
First-degree AV block (figure 86.6A) represents an increase in AV nodal conduction time and is defined as prolongation of the PR interval (>0.20 msec) with a 1:1 AV ratio. Isolated first-degree AV block usually has no clinical consequences and does not require treatment.

Second-Degree AV Block
Second-degree AV block is diagnosed when there is intermittent failure of one or more of the atrial impulses to conduct to the ventricles. Second-degree AV block is divided into Mobitz type I (Wenckebach) and Mobitz type II block.

In Mobitz type I block (figure 86.6B), the P-P interval is constant. There is progressive prolongation of the PR interval and shortening of the R-R interval, leading to a nonconducted P wave. The R-R interval containing the nonconducted P wave is <2 (P-P) interval. If Mobitz type I block is accompanied by a narrow QRS complex, the block is usually located in the AV node. If it is associated with a wide QRS, the block may occur in the AV node (75%) or infranodally (25%) within the His bundle or one of the bundle branches. Because it is usually localized to the AV node, it does not progress to complete heart block and does not require treatment unless the patient is symptomatic.

Mobitz type II block (figure 86.6B) is characterized by sinus rhythm with intermittent nonconducted P waves. The PR interval in conducted beats is constant, and the R-R interval containing the nonconducted P wave is exactly 2(P-P) interval. In most instances Mobitz type II block is associated with a wide QRS complex, and the block is located below the His bundle. In a smaller proportion of cases, Mobitz type II block is associated with a narrow QRS complex, and the block is located within the His bundle or less commonly within the AV node. Patients with Mobitz type II block may be asymptomatic or may experience lightheadedness or syncope depending on the ratio of conducted to non-conducted P waves. Because the block is generally distal to the His

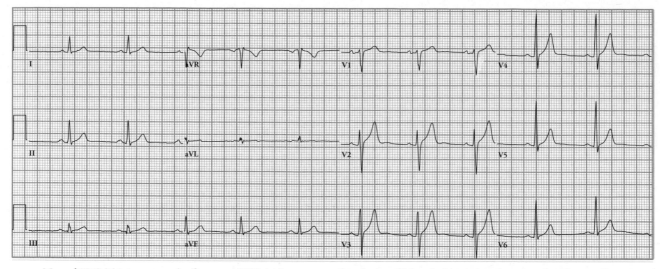

Figure 86.3. Normal EKG. This is an example of a normal EKG; its features are within the specified normal range, based on a large healthy population sample.

bundle, it can progress to complete heart block and usually requires treatment with pacemaker insertion.

Third-Degree AV Block

Third-degree AV block (figure 86.6C) or complete heart block is characterized by failure of the atrial impulses to reach the ventricles. In third-degree AV block, the atrial rate is usually greater than the ventricular rate because ventricular conduction is taken over by a subsidiary pacemaker, either within the AV node (junctional escape) or within the Purkinje fibers (ventricular escape). If the subsidiary pacemaker is located within the AV node, the QRS complex is narrow and the ventricular rate is usually between 40 and 60 beats per minute (bpm). If the subsidiary pacemaker is located within the Purkinje fibers, the QRS complex is wide, and the ventricular rate is usually <40 bpm. Third-degree AV block, especially when associated with a wide QRS, carries a poor prognosis and should be treated with a pacemaker.

AV Dissociation

AV dissociation is present when there is independent activation of the atria and ventricles from different pacemakers. Although third-degree AV block is a form of AV dissociation, AV dissociation can also occur in the presence of intact AV nodal conduction. In this case, the rate of ventricular activation, either from the AV node (junctional tachycardia or accelerated junctional rhythm) or from the ventricle (ventricular tachycardia or accelerated ventricular rhythm), exceeds the rate of atrial activation leading to AV block. This is in contrast to third-degree AV block where the atrial rate is usually greater than the ventricular rate. Occasionally, there can be simultaneous activation of the ventricle from two separate pacemakers (fusion complex) or premature activation of the ventricle by an anterograde supraventricular impulse (capture complex) that can also help exclude third degree heart block.

Intraventricular Conduction Abnormalities

If the QRS duration is >0.12 seconds, there is usually an abnormality of ventricular conduction.

Right Bundle Branch Block

In right bundle branch block (RBBB), the electrical impulse from the bundle of His does not conduct along the right bundle branch but proceeds normally down the left bundle branch (figure 86.7). Thus, the interventricular septum and left ventricle (LV) are depolarized in a normal fashion, and the right ventricle (RV) is depolarized later by means of cell-to-cell conduction that occurs from the interventricular septum and LV to the RV. This delayed and slower activation of the RV is manifest in the EKG by the following criteria (Surawicz and Knilans, 2008):

1. QRS duration ≥0.12 seconds

(A) Normal ECG   (B) Arm lead reversal   (C) Arm–leg lead reversal

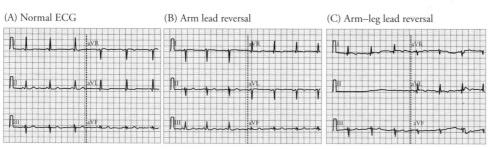

Figure 86.4. Incorrect Lead Placement. The figure depicts a normal EKG (A) and the alterations in limb lead appearance with incorrect lead placement (B and C).

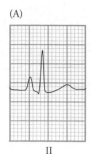
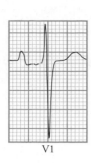
(A)

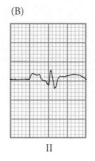
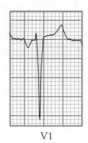
(B)

II   V1   II   V1

Figure 86.5. Atrial Enlargement. Panel A shows right atrial enlargement with tall P waves in II and V1. Panel B shows left atrial enlargement with broad and notched P waves in II and a large inverted secondary component of the P wave in V1.

2. A secondary R wave (R≠) in the right-sided precordial leads, with R≠ greater than the initial R wave (rsR≠ or rSR≠ pattern in V1 and V2)

3. A wide S wave in the QRS complex of left-sided leads (I, V5, and V6)

4. Delay in the onset of the intrisicoid deflection in the right precordial leads (R peak time in V1) >0.05 seconds.

RBBB may be present in patients with hypertension, rheumatic heart disease, acute and chronic cor pulmonale, myocarditis, cardiomyopathy, degenerative disease of the conduction system, congenital heart disease, Brugada syndrome, Kearns-Sayre syndrome, ventricular pre-excitation, after cardiac surgery, and rarely in patients with coronary artery disease. The prognosis depends on the underlying disease, ranging from benign in those who have a RBBB after cardiac surgery to potentially fatal in those with Brugada syndrome.

Incomplete Right Bundle Branch Block

Incomplete right bundle branch block is often seen with RV hypertrophy (RVH) and is diagnosed when the waveforms are similar to RBBB but with QRS duration <0.12 seconds. Occasionally, an rSr≠ pattern is present in V1 as a normal variant. However, in this case, the r≠ is usually smaller than the initial r wave.

Left Bundle Branch Block

Left bundle branch block (LBBB) (figure 86.8) occurs when there is interruption of conduction in the main left bundle branch or simultaneous disease in the anterior and posterior fascicles of the left bundle branch. The impulse then travels from the AV node down the His bundle and right bundle branch to the RV and then from the RV to the interventricular septum and LV through myocardial cell to cell conduction. This delayed and slower LV activation leads to the following EKG features (Surawicz and Knilans, 2008):

1. QRS duration ≥0.120 seconds

2. Broad, monophasic R wave in left-sided leads I, aVL, V5, and V6

3. Absence of Q waves in I, V5, and V6

4. Delay in peak R time (intrinsicoid deflection) >0.06 seconds in V5 and V6

5. Wide, deep S waves in the right precordial leads (V1–V3)

LBBB is most often present in patients with hypertensive heart disease, coronary artery disease, and dilated cardiomyopathy. Because the left bundle branch receives a dual blood supply from the left anterior descending artery and right coronary artery, its blockade usually implies an extensive

(A)

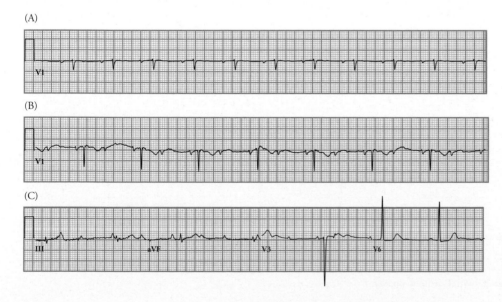

(B)

(C)

III   aVF   V3   V6

Figure 86.6. Atrioventricular Conduction Abnormalities. Panel A depicts first-degree AV block with PR >200 msec. Panel B depicts second-degree AV block. Because the ratio of conducted P waves is 2:1, it is not possible to differentiate between Mobitz I and Mobitz II block. Panel C depicts complete heart block with no AV communication and atrial > ventricular rate.

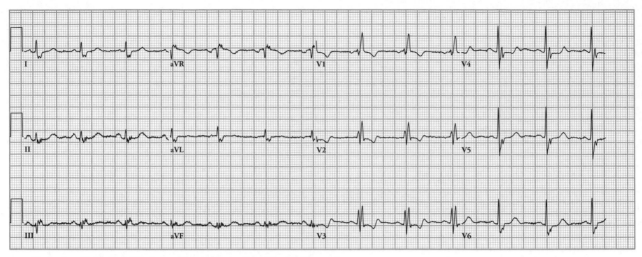

Figure 86.7. Right Bundle Branch Block in a Patient Status Post-Cardiac Transplant.

lesion in patients with coronary artery disease. LBBB can also be seen in patients with aortic stenosis, degenerative disease of the conduction system, and in some cases of rheumatic heart disease involving the LV. Presence of a LBBB in patients with LV systolic dysfunction confers a poor prognosis (Hardarson et al., 1987).

Incomplete Left Bundle Branch Block

Incomplete LBBB is often seen with LVH and is diagnosed when the waveforms are similar to LBBB but with QRS duration <0.12 seconds.

Hemiblocks

The left bundle branch is divided into two divisions: the anterior and posterior fascicles. The anterior fascicle supplies the anterior and lateral walls of the LV, and the posterior fascicle supplies the inferior and posterior walls of the LV. Normally, after leaving the bundle of His, the impulse travels simultaneously down both fascicles, resulting in synchronous contraction of the LV. However, if the anterior fascicle is diseased (left anterior hemiblock, LAHB), the impulse

travels down the posterior fascicle, activating the inferior and posterior walls before the anterior and lateral walls, causing asynchronous contraction of the LV. Conversely, if the posterior fascicle is diseased (posterior hemiblock, LPHB), the impulse travels down the anterior fascicle, activating the anterior and lateral walls before the inferior and posterior walls. The etiologies for LAHB and LPHB are similar to those for complete LBBB. However, isolated LAHB is much more frequent than isolated LPHB.

In LAHB, the late QRS vectors are shifted leftward and superiorly and are manifest by the following EKG criteria (Surawicz and Knilans, 2008): left axis deviation (−30° to −90°); qR complex in I and aVL (lateral leads) and rS complex in II, III, aVF (inferior leads); and normal or prolonged QRS duration.

In LPHB, the late QRS vectors are shifted rightward and inferiorly and are manifest by the following EKG criteria (Surawicz and Knilans, 2008): right axis deviation (+90° to +180°); a deep S wave in I (left-sided lead) and Q waves in II, III, and aVF (inferior leads); and normal or prolonged QRS duration.

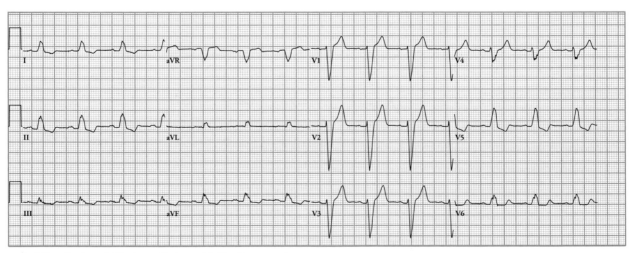

Figure 86.8. Left Bundle Branch Block in a Patient with Cardiomyopathy.

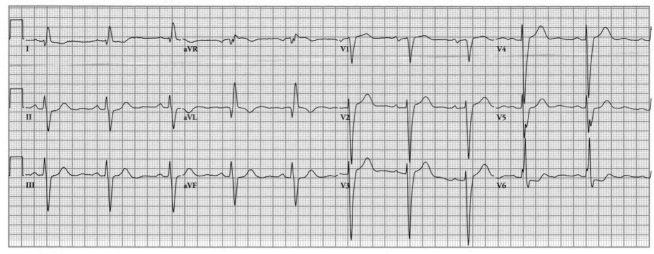

Figure 86.9. Left Ventricular Hypertrophy in a Patient with Long-standing Hypertension.

Bifascicular Block

Bifascicular block is present when there is either (1) simultaneous RBBB and LAHB, (2) simultaneous RBBB and LPHB, or (3) simultaneous LAHB and LPHB (Surawicz and Knilans, 2008). Patients with RBBB and either fascicular block tend to have additional disease within the conduction system and may progress to complete heart block.

Trifascicular Block

Trifascicular block is present when there is disease in the right bundle branch and in both fascicles of the left bundle branch, resulting in complete heart block.

VENTRICULAR HYPERTROPHY

LEFT VENTRICULAR HYPERTROPHY

The EKG criteria for diagnosing left ventricular hypertrophy (LVH) (figure 86.9) derive mainly from the increased LV mass, which results in exaggeration of the leftward and posterior QRS forces. Furthermore, the increased thickness of the LV wall prolongs the time needed for LV depolarization and thus may increase the QRS duration. Because depolarization is prolonged, repolarization is often abnormal, resulting in ST-T abnormalities. The increased LV mass can also result in subendocardial ischemia, further compounding the ST-T abnormalities. If present, the ST segment and T wave are directed opposite to the dominant QRS waveform (Surawicz and Knilands, 2008).

There are several EKG criteria for the diagnosis of LVH (Hsieh et al., 2005). However, for practical purposes, voltage criteria alone are most often used to diagnose LVH (table 86.2). The sensitivity of LVH diagnosed by EKG criteria in the general population above the age of 65 years is very low compared to echocardiography as the gold standard (5.9% to 25.8%) (Casiglia et al., 2008). Furthermore, the sensitivity increases with age and decreases with female gender and obesity (Casiglia et al., 2008; Levy et al., 1990). However, the specificity is very high (>90%) for all the voltage criteria outlined in table 86.1, and the presence of LVH by EKG criteria predicts increased cardiovascular mortality (Hsieh et al., 2005).

LVH is seen mostly in patients with pressure overload secondary to hypertension, aortic stenosis, or coarctation of the aorta. However, it can also be seen in conditions of volume overload such as mitral regurgitation, aortic insufficiency, and patent ductus arteriosus.

RIGHT VENTRICULAR HYPERTROPHY

Because the EKG vectors reflect the dominant LV, an increase in RV mass affects the EKG in proportion to the

Table 86.2 COMMONLY USED EKG VOLTAGE CRITERIA FOR LEFT VENTRICULAR HYPERTROPHY

NAME	CRITERIA
Cornell voltage	R in aVL + S in V3 >25 mm (men) and >20 mm (women)
Sokolow-Lyon voltage	S in V1 + R in V5 or V6 ≥35 mm; R in aVL ≥11 mm R in aVF ≥20 mm R in V5 or V6 ≥26 mm
Lewis index	(R in I + S in III) – (R in III + S in I) ≥17 mm
Minnesota code 3.1	R in V5 or V6 >26 mm R in either I, II, III, or aVF >20 mm R in aVL >12 mm
Gubner and Ungerleider	R in I and S in III ≥22 mm
Sum of 12 leads	Sum of max R and S amplitude in each of the 12 leads ≥179 mm

SOURCE: Reprinted from Hsieh BP, Pham MX, Froelicher VF. Prognostic value of electrocardiographic criteria for left ventricular hypertrophy. *Am Heart J.* 2005;150:161–7, with permission from Elsevier.

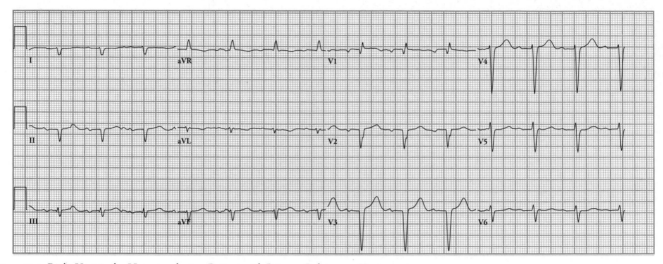

Figure 86.10. Right Ventricular Hypertrophy in a Patient with Primary Pulmonary Hypertension.

extent of RVH (figure 86.10). Because lead V1 is most proximal to the RV, it is most sensitive to the changes in RV mass. The right-sided leads may show increased voltage, delayed activation, and abnormalities in repolarization with RVH. The following EKG criteria can be used to diagnose RVH (Surawicz and Knilans, 2008):

1. Right axis deviation (>110°); or

2. R/S ratio >1 in V1 (in the absence of a posterior myocardial infarction or RBBB); or

3. R wave ≥7 mm in V1 (not the R≠ in RBBB); or

4. rSR≠ in V1 with R≠ >10 mm; or

5. S wave ≥7 mm in V5 or V6; or

6. RBBB with right axis deviation (exclude RBBB with LPHB if RAE present or if repolarization abnormalities seen in right-sided leads).

RVH is usually the result of conditions such as mitral stenosis, chronic cor pulmonale, or congenital heart disease.

COMBINED VENTRICULAR HYPERTROPHY

Combined ventricular hypertrophy (Surawicz and Knilans, 2008) is usually manifested as LVH with right axis deviation or with RAE.

MYOCARDIAL INFARCTION/ISCHEMIA

PRIOR TRANSMURAL OR Q WAVE INFARCTION

In a transmural infarction, the area of myocardial necrosis becomes electrically silent. The remaining vectoral forces tend to point away from this area, and thus an electrode facing the area of infarction records a negative deflection (Q wave) during depolarization. The specificity of the EKG for the diagnosis of transmural myocardial infarction is greatest when the Q waves occur in two or more contiguous leads or lead groupings (table 86.3) (Thygesen et al., 2007). In general, a Q wave is considered pathologic when it has a duration ≥0.03 seconds and an amplitude >25% of the following R wave (Surawicz and Knilans, 2008). Because the posterobasal portion of the LV is difficult to see on the standard 12-lead EKG, a posterior infarction is usually recognized through reciprocal changes in the anterior leads (figure 86.11). In patients without RVH, this is usually reflected by an initial R wave duration ≥0.04 seconds in V1–V2 with a R/S ratio ≥1 (Thygesen et al., 2007).

ACUTE MYOCARDIAL INFARCTION

Tall and peaked T waves (hyperacute T waves) in at least two contiguous leads (figure 86.12) provide an early sign of

Table 86.3 **LEAD GROUPS FOR LOCALIZATION OF MYOCARDIAL INFARCTION**

LOCATION OF INFARCTION	EKG LEADS
Septal	V1, V2
Anteroseptal	V1–V4
Anterolateral	I, aVL, V4–V6
Lateral	I, aVL, V5, V6
Inferior	II, III, aVF
Posterior	V3R, V4R and/or wide R wave in V1

SOURCE: Reprinted with permission from Thygesen et al. Universal definition of myocardial infarction. *Circulation.* 2007;116:2634–53.

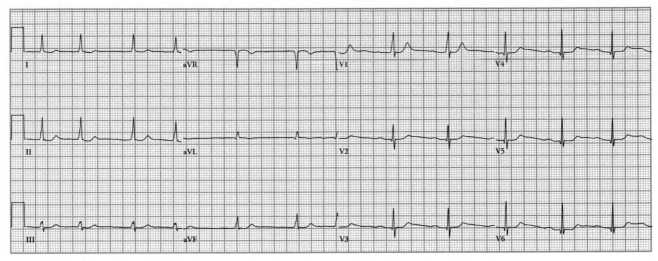

Figure 86.11. Old Posterior Myocardial Infarction.

myocardial infarction that may precede ST segment elevation (Thygesen et al., 2007). New ST segment elevation at the J point in two or more contiguous leads is more specific than ST segment depression in localizing the site of myocardial ischemia or necrosis (Thygesen et al., 2007) (figures 86.13, 86.14, 86.15). ST segment elevation ≥2 mm in men and ≥1.5 mm in women for V2–V3 and/or ST segment elevation ≥1 mm in all other leads is considered pathologic (Thygesen et al., 2007). Reciprocal ST segment depression is often seen in the opposite leads. In patients with inferior ST elevation (II, III, aVF), ST depression >1 mm in leads V1 and V2 suggests a concomitant posterior infarction (Zimetbaum and Josephson, 2003). Conversely, ST elevation >1 mm in V1 in association with ST elevation in II, III, and aVF suggests a right ventricular infarction. In this instance it is recommended to record right precordial leads because ST elevation >1 mm in V4R with an upright T wave in that lead is the most sensitive EKG sign for a right ventricular infarction (Zimetbaum and Josephson, 2003). ST elevations usually resolve within 2 weeks of a myocardial infarction, and persistence of ST elevation over longer periods of time should raise the possibility of a ventricular aneurysm (Surawicz and Knilans, 2008).

The diagnosis of acute myocardial infarction is difficult in the presence of a LBBB. In this setting, comparison with a previous EKG may be helpful. Concordant (i.e., in the same direction as the QRS vector) ST segment depression

≥1 mm in V1, V2, or V3 or in II, III, or aVF and elevation of ≥1 mm in V5 can indicate myocardial ischemia in the presence of a LBBB (Zimetbaum and Josephson, 2003). Extremely discordant ST deviation (>5 mm) is also suggestive of myocardial ischemia in the presence of a LBBB (Zimetbaum and Josephson, 2003).

In the presence of a pre-existing RBBB, new ST elevation or Q waves should suggest myocardial infarction (Thygesen et al., 2007).

It is important to note that ST segment elevation is not limited to acute myocardial infarction: other conditions such as an early repolarization pattern, LVH, coronary vasospasm, acute pericarditis, acute pulmonary embolus, hyperkalemia, and Brugada syndrome can present with ST segment elevation in association with other characteristic features (Wang et al., 2003).

The presence of conduction abnormalities (varying forms of heart block or bundle branch block) with acute myocardial infarction may lead to a poor prognosis (Zimetbaum and Josephson, 2003). The right coronary artery supplies the sinus node in 60% of people, the AV node in 90% of people, and the bundle of His via its AV nodal branch. Thus, sinus bradycardia or varying degrees of AV block can occur after an inferior myocardial infarction due to heightened vagal tone, and these are usually transient in nature. Complete heart block accompanied by a wide QRS escape rhythm in the presence of an inferior myocardial infarction may signify block below the AV node and impaired collateral circulation to an occluded left anterior descending artery (Zimetbaum and Josephson, 2003). The right bundle branch is supplied primarily by septal perforators from the left anterior descending artery and may receive collaterals from the right coronary or left circumflex arteries. The left anterior fascicle is supplied solely by septal perforators from the left anterior descending artery and is particularly susceptible to ischemia. The proximal portion of the posterior

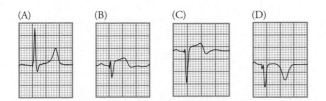

Figure 86.12. ST-T Changes During an Acute Myocardial Infarction. Initial tall hyperacute T waves (A) are followed by ST elevations (B). The T waves may begin to invert before the ST segment returns to baseline (C) and remain inverted after the ST segment normalizes (D).

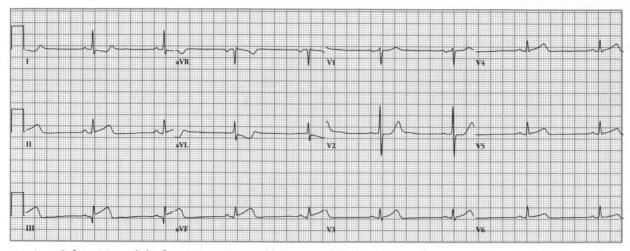

Figure 86.13. Acute Inferior Myocardial Infarction in a 56-Year-Old Woman with Epigastric Discomfort.

fascicle receives blood from the AV nodal branch of the right coronary artery and the septal perforators of the left anterior descending artery, and the distal portion receives blood from the anterior and posterior septal perforating arteries. Unlike inferior myocardial infarction, the presence of conduction abnormalities in association with an anterior myocardial infarction indicates proximal left anterior descending artery occlusion and necrosis of the conduction system. Anterior myocardial infarction can be associated with the development of Mobitz type II block, complete heart block, RBBB, LAFB, or, rarely, LPFB. The presence of bifascicular block, with or without PR prolongation, increases the risk of complete heart block (Zimetbaum and Josephson, 2003).

MYOCARDIAL ISCHEMIA

Myocardial ischemia can present as abnormally tall T waves, symmetric and deep inverted T waves ≥1 mm, horizontal or down-sloping ST depression ≥0.5 mm, nonspecific ST and T wave abnormalities, pseudonormalization of abnormal T waves, or the presence of QT prolongation in conjunction with one or more of the ST-T abnormalities described above (Surawicz and Knilans, 2008; Thygesen et al., 2007). Unlike ST elevation and Q waves, ST-T abnormalities are not specific for localizing the area of myocardial ischemia (Thygesen et al., 2007). The EKG findings of myocardial ischemia can be seen in a variety of conditions including intracranial bleeding, electrolyte disturbances, pericarditis, myocardial disease, pulmonary embolus, spontaneous pneumothorax, myocardial contusion, ventricular hypertrophy, ventricular conduction defects, drug effects, and following tachycardia (Surawicz and Knilans, 2008). These EKG changes should therefore be interpreted in the appropriate clinical context.

ELECTROLYTE ABNORMALITIES

HYPERKALEMIA

Hyperkalemia (figure 86.16) initially causes acceleration of the terminal phase of repolarization. As the serum K⁺ exceeds 5.5 meq/L, the T waves become tall and peaked.

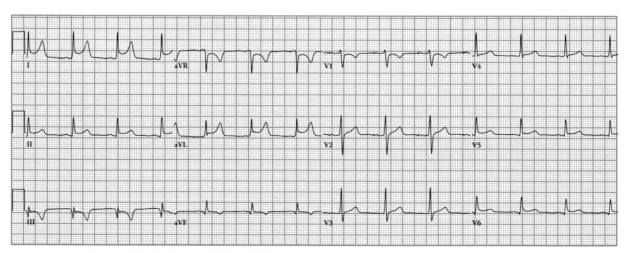

Figure 86.14. Acute Lateral Myocardial Infarction in a 38-Year-Old Smoker.

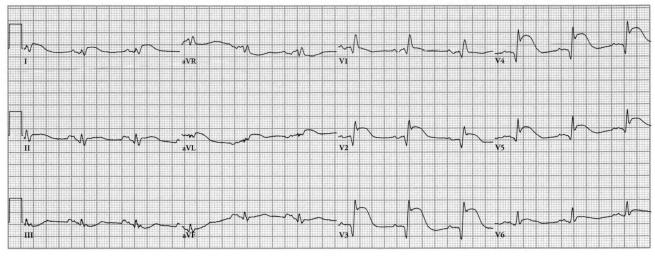

Figure 86.15. Acute Anterior and Lateral Myocardial Infarction in a 62-Year-Old Man with Hypertension and Hyperlipidemia.

Hyperkalemia reduces the resting transmembrane potential, leading to decreased sodium influx and slowing of intra-atrial and intraventricular conduction. Because the atrial myocardium is more sensitive to hyperkalemia, P wave flattening and PR prolongation often occur before changes in the QRS complex are seen. As the serum potassium concentration increases, the P wave becomes wider and eventually disappears (K+ >8 meq/L). Widening of the QRS complex is usually seen at K+ >6.5 mEq/L. This differs from the QRS widening seen in bundle branch blocks in that both the initial and terminal portions of the QRS complex are affected and wide S waves are seen in the left precordial leads. When the serum K+ exceeds 10 meq/L, ventricular depolarization becomes exceedingly slow such that portions of the ventricular myocardium undergo repolarization before depolarization is complete. Thus, as the QRS complex widens further, it blends with the T wave, giving a sine wave appearance. At serum K+ > 12–14 meq/L, ventricular asystole or ventricular fibrillation can be seen. With severe hyperkalemia, ST segment elevation resembling a pseudoinfarction pattern may occasionally be present (Surawicz and Knilans, 2008; Wald, 2006).

HYPOKALEMIA

Hypokalemia increases the resting membrane potential and the duration of the action potential (figure 86.17). In particular, it increases the duration of the refractory period. The typical EKG findings of hypokalemia are seen in 78% of people with a serum K+ <2.7 meq/L but may be seen once K+ falls below 3.5 meq/L. These include decreased T wave amplitude, ST segment depression ≥0.5 mm, and prominent U waves (>1 mm or taller than the T wave in the same lead). Severe hypokalemia can lead to ventricular dysrhythmias including ventricular tachycardia, ventricular fibrillation, and torsades de pointes. It can also lead to increased automaticity of ectopic atrial pacemakers and can be associated with paroxysmal atrial tachycardia, multifocal atrial tachycardia, atrial fibrillation, and atrial flutter (Surawicz and Knilans, 2008; Wald, 2006). The incidence

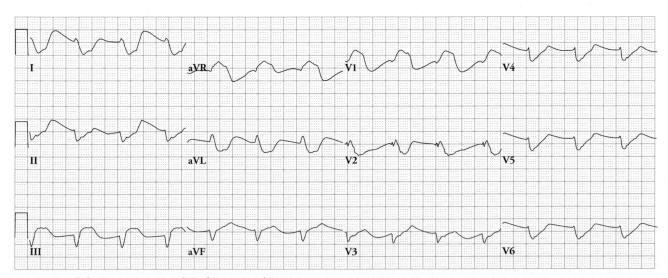

Figure 86.16. Hyperkalemia in a Patient with End-Stage Renal Disease.

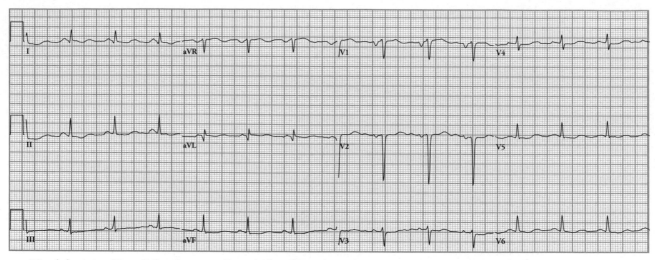

Figure 86.17. Hypokalemia in a Heart Failure Patient on Furosemide and Metolazone.

of both atrial and ventricular arrhythmias in the presence of hypokalemia is increased in patients receiving digitalis therapy (Surawicz and Knilans, 2008).

HYPERCALCEMIA

Hypercalcemia shortens the plateau phase of the action potential and decreases the effective refractory period, thus shortening the ST segment (figure 86.18). This is manifest on the EKG as a shortened QTc interval. The relationship between serum calcium levels and the QTc interval is not linear. The QTc interval is inversely proportional to serum Ca^{2+} up to a level ≤16 mg/dL. At Ca^{2+} >16 mg/dL, the T wave widens, and the QTc interval begins to normalize. Rather than the QTc interval, the QaTc interval (the interval from the beginning of the QRS complex to the apex of the T wave) is more closely correlated with serum Ca^{2+} concentrations, and a QaTc interval <0.27 seconds is seen in >90% of

patients with hypercalcemia (Surawicz and Knilans, 2008; Wald, 2006). Cardiac arrhythmias are uncommon in hypercalcemia (Surawicz and Knilans, 2008).

HYPOCALCEMIA

Hypocalcemia prolongs the duration of the plateau phase of the action potential and increases the effective refractory period, resulting in lengthening of the ST segment (figure 86.19). This is manifested on the EKG as prolongation of the QTc interval. Although the QTc duration is proportional to the extent of hypocalcemia, it rarely exceeds 140% of normal. A QTc duration >140% of normal suggests that an additional electrolyte abnormality is present and a QU interval is probably being measured (Surawicz and Knilans, 2008; Wald, 2006). Cardiac arrhythmias are uncommon in patients with hypocalcemia (Surawicz and Knilans, 2008).

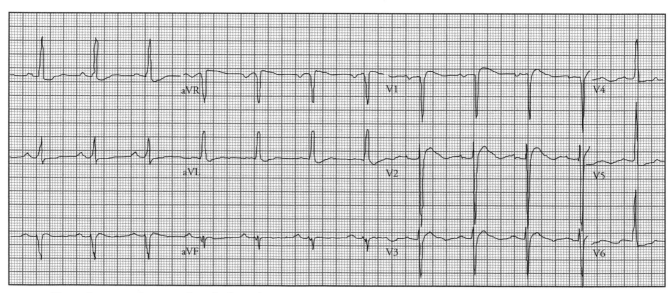

Figure 86.18. Hypercalcemia in a Patient with Multiple Myeloma.

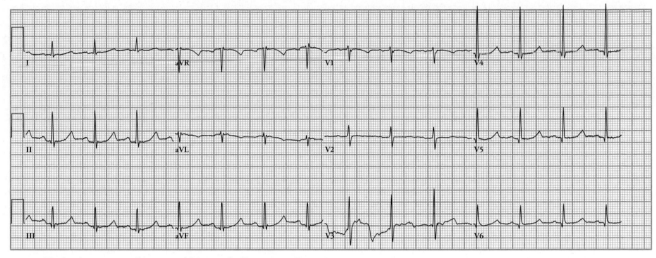

Figure 86.19. Hypocalcemia in an Intoxicated Man in the Emergency Room.

DRUG-INDUCED EKG CHANGES

ACQUIRED LONG QT SYNDROME

Several drugs lengthen cardiac repolarization and prolong the QTc interval. This prolongation of the QTc interval can result in a pause-dependent polymorphic ventricular tachycardia or torsades de pointes. Agents that are generally accepted to have risk of causing torsades de pointes are listed in table 86.4. Some of these agents (class Ia and III antiarrhythmics, terfenadine, erythromycin, cisapride, etc.) directly block sodium and potassium channels, resulting in repolarization abnormalities. Other drugs such as phenothiazines and haloperidol prolong the action potential. Other drugs not included in Table 86.4 may prolong the QTc but have not been clearly associated with torsades de pointes (e.g., alfuzosin, atazanavir, foscarnet, ranolazine), although others such as the azoles inhibit the hepatic cytochrome P-450 enzyme and decrease the metabolism of some QTc-prolonging agents, thus potentiating their effects. An extensive list of these agents can be found at http://www.torsades.org. Older age, female gender, impaired renal and hepatic function, structural heart disease, and slow heart rate can also facilitate drug-induced QTc prolongation. Patients with suspected or diagnosed congenital long QT syndrome are particularly susceptible to these drugs.

Table 86.4 DRUGS WITH INCREASED RISK OF TORSADES DE POINTES

Cardiac drugs
Quinidine, disopyramide, procainamide, sotalol, ibutilide, azimilide, dofetilide, amiodarone, phenylamine, bepridil

Noncardiac drugs
Arsenic trioxide, astemizole, chloroquine, cisapride, droperidol, halofantrine, haloperidol, levomethadyl, macrolides, methadone, pentamidine, phenothiazines, probucol, terfenadine, tricyclic anti-depressants, sparfloxacin

SOURCE: Arizona Center for Education and Research on Therapeutics.

A QTc duration >0.45 seconds in men and >0.47 seconds in women is considered abnormal. Although these cutoffs are somewhat arbitrary, in general a QTC >0.5 seconds should be considered a contraindication for using drugs that prolong cardiac repolarization (Van Mieghem et al., 2004).

DIGITALIS TOXICITY

Digitalis has both direct and indirect effects on the heart. It exerts its direct actions via inhibition of the sarcolemmal Na^+,K^+-ATPase pump and its indirect actions via baroreceptor sensitization and increased vagal tone. In therapeutic doses, digitalis decreases the automaticity of the sinus node, slows conduction at the AV node, and shortens the ventricular refractory period. The effects on ventricular repolarization are responsible for the characteristic ST-T changes seen in patients on digitalis therapy. These include a decrease in T wave amplitude, shortening of the QT interval, ST segment depression, and an increase in the U wave amplitude. The most typical finding is sagging of the ST segment such that the first part of the T wave is dragged down, making the T wave biphasic or negative (figure 86.20) (Surawicz and Knilans, 2008).

Given the narrow therapeutic range of digitalis, clinical manifestations of toxicity have been reported in as many as 23% of people taking digitalis (Beller et al., 1971). The hallmark of digitalis-induced cardiac toxicity is increased automaticity with concomitant conduction delay. Although, no single dysrhythmia is always present, premature ventricular beats (often multifocal and in a bigeminal or trigeminal pattern), various degrees of AV block, paroxysmal atrial tachycardia with block, atrial fibrillation with block, junctional tachycardia, and bidirectional ventricular tachycardia are common (Kelly and Smith, 1992). Both hyper- and hypokalemia potentiate digitalis-induced arrhythmias, and hypokalemia should be corrected in patients presenting with digitalis-induced ventricular tachycardia (Kelly and Smith, 1992). Even though a serum digitalis concentration >2 ng/mL is considered

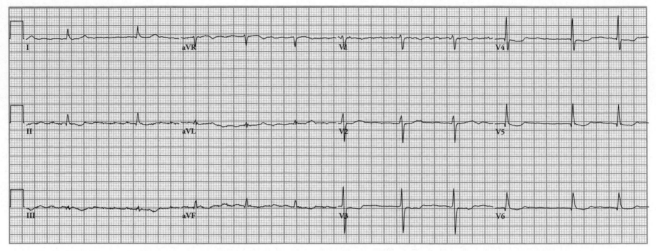

Figure 86.20. Typical ST Changes in Patient with Atrial Fibrillation and on Digitalis Therapy.

supratherapeutic, it does not correlate well with toxicity in every patient. Recognition of arrhythmias, withdrawal of drug therapy, and close monitoring are usually sufficient. However, in some cases with life-threatening arrhythmias, administration of the F(ab) fragment of antidigoxin antibodies may be warranted (Kelly and Smith, 1992).

TRICYCLIC ANTIDEPRESSANT POISONING

The primary mechanism for tricyclic antidepressant cardiac toxicity is fast sodium channel blockade resulting in an increase in the duration of the action potential and refractory period as well as slowing of AV conduction. The EKG changes include prolongation of the PR, QRS, and QT intervals, nonspecific ST-T abnormalities, AV block, right axis deviation of the terminal 0.04 seconds of the QRS complex (T 40 msec axis), and the Brugada pattern (downsloping ST elevation in V1–V3). Sinus tachycardia is the most common arrhythmia due to the anticholinergic effects of tricyclic antidepressants. However, AV block with unstable ventricular arrhythmias or asystole can also be seen. Life-threatening arrhythmias and death usually occur within 24 hours of toxic ingestion. A QRS duration >0.1 seconds predicts seizure activity, and a QRS duration >0.16 seconds predicts the development of ventricular arrhythmias. Alkalinization of blood with sodium bicarbonate is recommended in patients with a QRS duration >0.1 seconds because it helps dissociate the tricyclic antidepressant from the fast sodium channels and also improves the gradient for sodium entry into the cell (Thanacoody and Thomas, 2005).

MISCELLANEOUS CONDITIONS

CHRONIC OBSTRUCTIVE PULMONARY DISEASE

In chronic obstructive pulmonary disease (COPD), hyperinflation of the lungs leads to flattening of the diaphragm and clockwise rotation of the heart along its longitudinal axis. Thus, there is a rightward shift in the P and QRS axes in the frontal plane. Posterior displacement of the QRS forces and insulation of the heart by the hyperinflated lungs also lead to diminished QRS voltage in the limb leads and in V5–V6. Evidence of P-pulmonale is commonly seen in patients with COPD. The presence of both P wave and QRS changes increases the specificity of the EKG for COPD (Surawicz and Knilans, 2008).

ACUTE PULMONARY EMBOLISM

The EKG is relatively insensitive for the diagnosis of acute pulmonary embolus because 26% of patients with severe PE have no EKG abnormalities (Sreeram et al., 1994). The EKG findings in acute pulmonary embolus relate to acute dilatation of the RV. This is associated with clockwise rotation of the heart along its longitudinal axis and RV conduction delay. Although the SI, QIII, and TIII criteria have been classically described, they are present in only 11–50% of patients with acute pulmonary embolus (Van Mieghem et al., 2004). The presence of at least three of the following EKG criteria was able to accurately diagnose RV strain secondary to acute pulmonary embolus in approximately 75% of patients with a clinical suspicion of pulmonary embolus (Sreeram et al., 1994). These include (1) incomplete or complete RBBB; (2) S waves in I and aVL >1.5 mm; (3) transition zone shift in the precordial leads to V5; (4) Q waves in III and aVF but not in II; (5) QRS >90° or indeterminate; (6) limb lead voltage <5 mm; and (7) T wave inversion in III and aVF or in V1–V4 (figure 86.21).

ACUTE PERICARDITIS

The EKG changes in pericarditis (figure 86.22) are produced by an injury current caused by inflammation of the pericardial surface, including the atria (PR depression) and the ventricles (ST elevation) (Surawicz and Knilans, 2008). The evolutionary change of the EKG in pericarditis can be divided into four stages (Surawicz and Knilans, 2008):

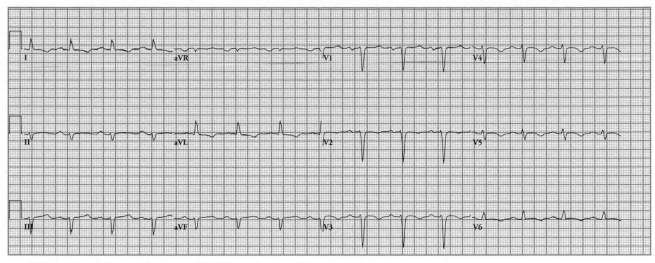

Figure 86.21. Thirty-Year-Old Man with Protein C Deficiency and Acute Pulmonary Embolus.

Stage 1: Diffuse PR depression and ST elevation (except for PR elevation and ST depression in aVR) with either normal T waves or T waves with increased amplitude

Stage 2: Isoelectric ST segments with upright T waves

Stage 3: Symmetric and inverted T waves

Stage 4: Normalization of the EKG

The EKG changes in pericarditis are differentiated from those in patients with ischemic heart disease by the diffuse nature of the ST elevation, abnormal relationship of the PR segment to the baseline (TP segment), and return of the ST segments to baseline prior to the occurrence of T wave changes.

HYPOTHERMIA

Hypothermia is defined as a core body temperature <35°C (95°F). As the body temperature falls, there is progressive slowing of the sinus rate and prolongation of the PR and QTc intervals. The most typical EKG finding is the Osborn or J wave, also known as the "camel hump" sign (figure 86.23). The J wave is an extra deflection at the junction of the terminal QRS complex and the beginning of the ST segment. The J wave is consistently found at body temperatures <25°C, and the amplitude of the J wave increases as body temperature declines. Tremor artifact is commonly seen in patients with hypothermia and is felt to be secondary to shivering. Atrial fibrillation is present in 50–60% of cases and appears at a body temperature <29°C. In severe hypothermia, bradycardia, asystole, and ventricular fibrillation can also occur (Surawicz and Knilans, 2008; Wald, 2006).

CENTRAL NERVOUS SYSTEM DISORDERS

Subarachnoid and intracerebral hemorrhages commonly produce EKG abnormalities. These are felt to be the result of

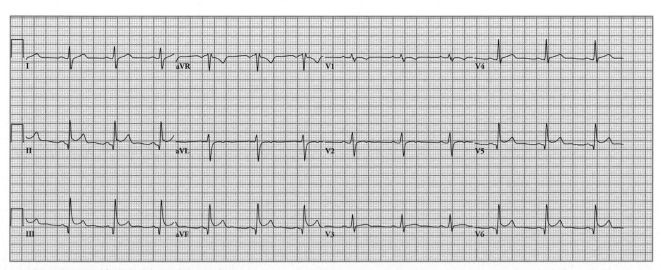

Figure 86.22. A 24-Year-Old Man with Viral Pericarditis.

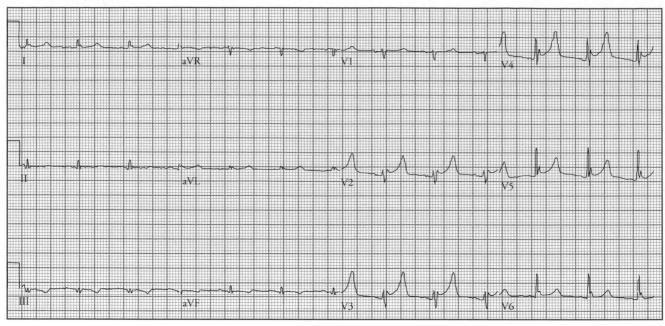

Figure 86.23. *A 45-Year-Old Homeless Man with Hypothermia. Source*: Reproduced with permission from the American College of Cardiology. Mason JW, Froelicher VF, Gettes LS. ECG-SAP III 2001.

increased sympathetic stimulation, which affects ventricular repolarization. The most common EKG findings are large, upright or deep, symmetrically inverted T waves, prolongation of the QRS complex, and prominent U waves (figure 86.24). ST segment elevation or depression, mimicking myocardial ischemia, may also occur. Diffuse ST elevations such as those seen in pericarditis can also be present. In some cases, abnormal Q waves suggestive of myocardial infarction may also be seen. Rhythm disturbances may also occur (Surawicz and Knilans, 2008).

ATRIAL SEPTAL DEFECTS

In atrial septal defects, there is left-to-right shunting of blood at the atrial level with volume loading and dilatation of the right atrium and right ventricle. Patients may present with sinus rhythm or atrial fibrillation (figure 86.25). First-degree AV block is commonly present, with a higher incidence in primum defects compared to secundum defects. Some patients may show evidence of right atrial enlargement. An rSR' pattern in lead V1 with a QRS duration <0.11 seconds representing right ventricular outflow tract hypertrophy is seen in the majority of patients with either primum or secundum defects. The frontal plane QRS axis is the most helpful differentiating factor between primum and secundum atrial septal defects. In primum atrial septal defect, there is abnormal left ventricular conduction, and the QRS axis is shifted to the left. Conversely, in secundum atrial septal defect, the QRS axis is shifted to the right (Surawicz and Knilans, 2008).

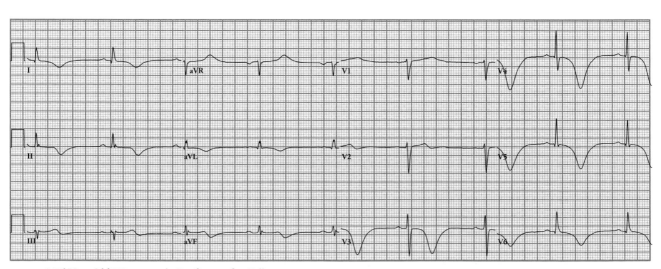

Figure 86.24. A 76-Year-Old Woman with Confusion after Fall.

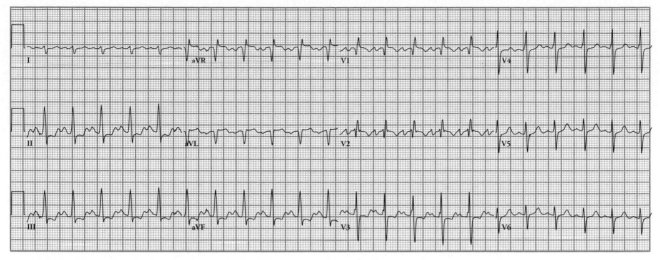

Figure 86.25. A 62-Year-Old Man with New-Onset Atrial Fibrillation and Right-Sided Heart Failure with Secundum Atrial Septal Defect.

DEXTROCARDIA

Dextrocardia is described as malposition of the heart in the right side of the chest. Lead I is the most telling lead in dextrocardia because the P wave, QRS complex, and T wave are inverted in this lead. Leads aVR and aVL are reversed, as are leads II and III. Lead aVF is unaffected. In the precordial leads, the usual placement of V1–V6 shows decreasing R wave amplitude. A repeat EKG with reversal of the left and right arm electrodes and placement of the precordial leads in the equivalent positions on the right chest, results in a normal-looking EKG (Surawicz and Knilans, 2008).

ADDITIONAL READING

Beller GA, Smith TW, Abelmann WH, Haber E, Hood WB Jr. Digitalis intoxication. A prospective clinical study with serum level correlations. *N Engl J Med.* 1971;284:989–97.

Casiglia E, Schiavon L, Tikhonoff V, et al. Electrocardiographic criteria of left ventricular hypertrophy in general population. *Eur J Epidemiol.* 2008;23:261–71.

Hardarson T, Arnason A, Eliasson GJ, Palsson K, Eyjolfsson K, Sigfusson N. Left bundle branch block: Prevalence, incidence, follow-up and outcome. *Eur Heart J.* 1987;8:1075–9.

Hsieh BP, Pham MX, Froelicher VF. Prognostic value of electrocardiographic criteria for left ventricular hypertrophy. *Am Heart J.* 2005;150:161–7.

Kelly RA, Smith TW. Recognition and management of digitalis toxicity. Am J Cardiol. 1992;69:108G–18G; disc 118G–9G.

Levy D, Labib SB, Anderson KM, Christiansen JC, Kannel WB, Castelli WP. Determinants of sensitivity and specificity of electrocardiographic criteria for left ventricular hypertrophy. *Circulation.* 1990;81:815–20.

Mason J (ed.). *Electrocardiography self-assessment program.* Bethesda, MD: American College of Cardiology, 2001.

Sreeram N, Cheriex EC, Smeets JL, Gorgels AP, Wellens HJ. Value of the 12-lead electrocardiogram at hospital admission in the diagnosis of pulmonary embolism. Am J Cardiol. 1994;73:298–303.

Surawicz B, Knilans T (eds.). *Chou's electrocardiography in clinical practice: Adult and pediatric.* Philadelphia: WB Saunders. Company, 2008.

Thanacoody HK, Thomas SH. Tricyclic antidepressant poisoning: Cardiovascular toxicity. *Toxicol Rev.* 2005;24:205–14.

Thygesen K, Alpert JS, White HD, et al. Universal definition of myocardial infarction. *Circulation.* 2007;116:2634–53.

Van Mieghem C, Sabbe M, Knockaert D. The clinical value of the EKG in noncardiac conditions. *Chest.* 2004;125:1561–76.

Wald DA. EKG manifestations of selected metabolic and endocrine disorders. *Emerg Med Clin North Am.* 2006;24:145–57, vii, 2006.

Wang K, Asinger RW, and Marriott HJ. ST-segment elevation in conditions other than acute myocardial infarction. *N Engl J Med.* 2003;349:2128–35.

Walker HK, Hall WD, Hurst JW. *Clinical methods: The history, physical, and laboratory examinations.* Chicago: Butterworth-Heinemann, 1990.

Zimetbaum PJ, Josephson ME. Use of the electrocardiogram in acute myocardial infarction. *N Engl J Med.* 2003;348:933–40.

87.

BOARD SIMULATION: CARDIOLOGY

Eldrin Foster Lewis

The American Board of Internal Medicine (ABIM) is focused mainly on management strategies. Cardiology represents the largest proportion of questions on the examination. The clinical symptoms and the clinical settings are very important. Thus, patients presenting to the emergency room or in the field with an acute process are more likely to have a major clinical event as compared to those patients presenting for routine clinical visits. The stem is important as well when interpreting electrocardiograms. There may be opportunities to narrow down choices to two best answers. These questions are not necessarily the format that you may see on the ABIM examination. Typical areas covered include acute coronary syndrome management, atrial fibrillation, valvular disease, vascular disease (e.g., aortic dissection), chronic heart failure management, arrhythmias, hypertension, and pre-operative assessments.

QUESTIONS

QUESTION 1. A 65-year-old female presents to clinic for follow-up after an acute myocardial infarction (MI) 2 months ago. She denies chest pain, dyspnea, or palpitations. She stopped smoking at the time of her myocardial infarction. On HR physical exam, her blood pressure BP was 152/94, heart rate 70 beats/min, and respiratory rate was 16 breaths/min. The exam was notable for a II/VI systolic murmur at the apex with a diffuse apical impulse, clear lungs, and no jugular venous distension. Electrocardiogram (EKG) revealed NSR and Q waves in V1–V3 with 1 mm ST elevations. Labs include sodium 142, blood urea nitrogen (BUN) 12, creatinine 0.8, erythrocyte sedimentation rate (ESR) 24, white blood cells (WBCs) 8.2, and hematocrit 41%. What is the most likely diagnosis?

A. Anterior wall myocardial infarction
B. Pericarditis
C. Dressler syndrome
D. Ventricular aneurysm
E. Right heart failure

QUESTION 2. A 79-year-old woman presents to the emergency room with progressive dyspnea, ascites, lower extremity edema, easy bruisability, and hoarseness. She has been previously healthy with a prior history of cholecystectomy in distant past. Exam reveals jugular venous distension, right-sided S3, and II/VI holosystolic murmur at apex. Echocardiogram demonstrates severe left ventricular hypertrophy (LVH), and EKG reveals sinus tachycardia and low voltage. All are true statements *except*:

A. Angiotensin-converting enzyme (ACE) inhibitors have been demonstrated to improve survival.
B. Hypertension is not a common cause.
C. An endomyocardial biopsy is recommended.
D. Prognosis is usually poor.
E. Heart transplantation may be beneficial.

QUESTION 3. A 62-year-old female with a history of lymphoma received radiation therapy in addition to chemotherapy with Adriamycin 9 years ago. She now presents to her primary care office with worsening dyspnea and right-sided heart failure signs. She has no traditional cardiac risk factors. Examination reveals a BP 100/75, HR 85, prominent *x* descent with venous distension, nonpalpable impulse, ascites, and 3+ edema. Echocardiogram reveals EF of 55% with septal bounce with no regional wall-motion abnormalities. Which of the following statements is *not* true?

A. Radiation therapy can cause valvular disease.
B. Cardiac magnetic resonance imaging (MRI) can be helpful in characterizing this disease.
C. The patient is not at significant risk for coronary artery disease.
D. Kussmaul's sign can be present in both conditions.
E. Ventricular interdependence is both sensitive and specific for constrictive pericarditis.

QUESTION 4. A 53-year-old woman with a history of smoking 3 years ago, hypertension, and diabetes mellitus presents to your office for routine visit. Fasting lipid profile reveals total cholesterol 230, high-density lipoprotein (HDL) 51, low-density lipoprotein (LDL) 131, and triglycerides 140. In addition to diet modifications, routine exercise, and blood pressure control, what would you do to manage this patient?

A. Refer for exercise test and start statin if positive
B. Start simvastatin 10 mg nightly
C. Reassure her that she is at target cholesterol goals
D. Start atorvastatin 80 mg nightly
E. Start niacin 1 g daily with aspirin

QUESTION 5. A 76-year-old woman presents to your office with 1 week of intermittent palpitations without associated symptoms. EKG reveals new-onset atrial fibrillation with heart rate of 82 beats/min and BP 128/84 with an otherwise unremarkable physical exam. All are false statements EXCEPT:

A. Restoration of sinus rhythm reduces risk of stroke compared with rate control and anticoagulation.
B. Patient can be treated with aspirin alone.
C. Warfarin should be started to reduce risk of stroke.
D. The combination of aspirin and clopidogrel is equivalent to warfarin.
E. Patient can be cardioverted now and complete 4 weeks of warfarin.

QUESTION 6. A 29-year-old woman who is 31 weeks pregnant presents to emergency room with mild dyspnea on exertion. Examination reveals BP 110/70, HR 95, clear chest, jugular venous pressure 7 cm water, and III/VI holosystolic murmur at apex. Echocardiography confirms moderate mitral regurgitation. She has no evidence of pulmonary hypertension. Management option includes which of the following?

A. Start low-dose furosemide
B. Arrange for emergent delivery of fetus
C. Plan mitral valve repair prior to delivery
D. Left and right heart catheterization
E. Proceed with pregnancy with close follow-up

QUESTION 7. A 61-year-old woman presents to the emergency room with chest pain and vague back pain. She has a history of diet-controlled hypertension and hypothyroidism. Physical examination is notable for unequal arterial pulsations of the upper extremities, BP 90/60, and HR 110 beats/min. Unequal arterial pulsations are commonly found in each of the following disorders EXCEPT:

A. Aortic dissection
B. Supravalvular aortic stenosis
C. Subvalvular aortic stenosis
D. Subclavian artery stenosis
E. Takayasu disease

QUESTION 8. A 62-year-old man presents to the emergency room following a motor vehicle accident in which he was wearing a seatbelt. He describes the onset of palpitations while driving and awakens finding himself on the side of the road. Past medical history notable for myocardial infarction 6 years ago and hypertension. Physical exam is remarkable

for mild facial lacerations. What is the most likely cause of this event?

A. Ventricular tachycardia
B. Epilepsy
C. High-degree atrioventricular (AV) block
D. Neurocardiogenic syncope
E. Hysterical fainting

QUESTION 9. A 63-year-old man presents to the emergency room with pleuritic chest pain and mild hypoxia after returning from a trip to Germany. Examination reveals a positive Homans, sign in the left leg. Among the following tests, which one is not compatible with a pulmonary embolism?

A. Normal chest x-ray
B. O_2 saturation of 94%
C. Normal perfusion lung scan
D. Normal electrocardiogram
E. Brain natriuretic peptide (BNP) of 440 pg/mL

QUESTION 10. A 58-year-old woman with history of ischemic dilated cardiomyopathy with left ventricular ejection fraction (LVEF) 25% presents to your office with increasing fatigue. She was started on carvedilol 3 weeks ago, and it was titrated upward. She denies chest pain, palpitations, or orthopnea but noted worsening dyspnea without a change in her weight. Medications include lisinopril 40 mg daily, carvedilol 25 mg twice daily (maximal doses), and furosemide 20 mg daily. Vital signs include BP of 110/76, pulse of 66/min, and respirations of 16/min. Physical exam demonstrated no jugular venous distension at 45 degrees with clear chest exam, no audible S3 or S4 gallop, and no peripheral edema. EKG revealed normal sinus rhythm with nonspecific ST-T-wave changes and IVCD with QRS duration of 110 msec. BNP is 700 pg/mL. What is the next best step?

A. Refer for cardiac resynchronization therapy
B. Refer for cardiac transplantation
C. Increase furosemide
D. Reduce dose of carvedilol
E. Start digitalis

QUESTION 11. A 71-year-old woman presents for a routine clinical visit for a physical. Her exam is notable for a BP of 124/60, HR 77 beats/min, splitting of the second heart sound. Which statement regarding splitting of the second heart sounds is NOT true?

A. Paradoxical splitting of S2 is expected in patients with a RV paced rhythm.
B. Delayed closure of the pulmonic valve with inspiration contributes to physiological splitting.
C. Fixed splitting of S2 is present with an ostium secundum atrial septal defect.
D. Severe pulmonary hypertension is associated with an accentuated P2.
E. Right bundle branch block is associated with paradoxical splitting of S2.

QUESTION 12. A 59-year-old man presents to the emergency room with systolic blood pressure of 224 mm Hg and diastolic blood pressure of 110 mm Hg. All of the following findings are characteristics of a hypertensive crisis EXCEPT:

A. Retinal hemorrhages
B. Microangiopathic hemolytic anemia
C. Azotemia and proteinuria
D. Normal mental status
E. All are characteristics of hypertensive crisis

QUESTION 13. Which anti-arrhythmic drug is associated with photosensitivity?

A. Verapamil
B. Procainamide
C. Amiodarone
D. Lidocaine
E. None of the above

QUESTION 14. A 66-year-old man with hypertension, diabetes, hypercholesterolemia, and prior prostate cancer presents to your office prior to a planned dental extraction and root canal. He is asking for antibiotics. Which of the following is an indication for endocarditis prophylaxis in this setting?

A. Previous bacterial endocarditis
B. Isolated secundum atrial septal defect
C. Mitral valve prolapse
D. Cardiac defibrillator
E. All of the above

QUESTION 15. You were called to the emergency room to see a 58-year-old woman presenting with hoarseness, worsening fatigue, new dyspnea, 14-lb weight gain, and lower extremity edema. Common cardiac findings in patients with hypothyroidism include each of the following EXCEPT:

A. Decreased blood pressure
B. Decreased heart rate
C. Pericardial effusion
D. Decreased cardiac output
E. Prolonged QT interval on the electrocardiogram

QUESTION 16. A 63-year-old male who had not seen a doctor in 10 years presents to clinic for a routine visit. He takes no medicines and denies allergies or past medical history. He noticed his BP was 170/100 at a drug store 3 weeks ago, which prompted the visit. He has tried decreasing salt intake. Exam demonstrates BP 166/106, HR 76, AV nicking, and loud S2. Routine labs and EKG are normal. What is the next appropriate step?

A. Atenolol
B. Further lifestyle change and recheck BP in 4–6 weeks
C. Captopril
D. Hydrochlorothiazide
E. Stress test

QUESTION 17. A 58-year-old male with history of hypertension presents to the emergency room with acute chest pain radiating to back with hypotension and a new, large left effusion on chest x-ray. Systolic blood pressure is different in the two arms. Appropriate steps in management include:

A. Treat with sodium nitroprusside
B. Start a loop diuretic
C. Surgical repair for distal dissection
D. Surgical repair for proximal dissection
E. Narcotics for pain relief

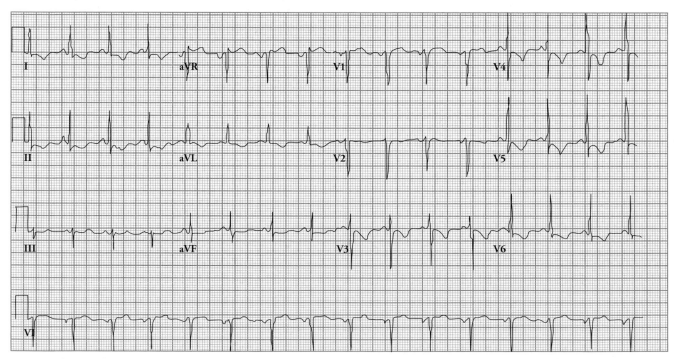

Figure 87.1. Electrocardiogram for Patient in Question 19.

QUESTION 18. Each of the following is a contributing factor to the development of essential hypertension EXCEPT:

A. Obesity
B. Alcohol consumption
C. Salt intake
D. Cigarette smoking
E. Lack of exercise

QUESTION 19. A 71-year-old woman with long-standing hypertension, diabetes, and 60 pack-year smoking history presents to the emergency room with 3 hours of new-onset chest pain radiating to the left arm with diaphoresis, nausea, and dyspnea. Physical exam was notable for HR of 89 beats/minute, BP of 133/70 mm Hg, clear lungs and 1/6 systolic murmur at the apex. Electrocardiogram is depicted in Figure 87.1 (baseline EKG is normal). The patient was given three sublingual nitroglycerin tablets over 20 min without improvement in symptoms. Which of the following statements is *false*?

A. Fibrinolytic therapy should not be used routinely in this population.
B. Clopidogrel can be used in patients who have hypersensitivity to aspirin.
C. This patient could be treated with abciximab as a conservative strategy for management of non–ST elevation myocardial infarction/unstable angina.
D. If the chest pain persists, you should proceed with diagnostic angiography with plan for intervention.
E. This patient should be admitted to the hospital for further management

QUESTION 20. A 64-year-old man is scheduled for right hip replacement. He presents to your clinic for pre-operative assessment. He has a past medical history of hypercholesterolemia, hypertension, benign prostate enlargement, and coronary artery disease with a stent placement in the left anterior descending artery 2 years ago due to angina with single vessel disease. He exercises daily by walking 2 miles without limitations or symptoms. What is the best option for pre-operative management?

A. Perform a stress test (standard Bruce protocol) without imaging to risk stratify prior to surgery.
B. Proceed to surgery without further testing.
C. Perform a pharmacologic stress test with imaging to risk stratify prior to surgery.
D. Perform a stress test (standard Bruce protocol) with echocardiography to risk stratify prior to surgery.
E. Repeat coronary angiography.

ANSWERS

1. D. This is a common problem faced by the clinician and is frequently asked on the boards. These are all post-MI complications (table 87.1). Persistent ST elevation after an acute MI is classically described in patients with a left ventricular aneurysm, although it can be the result of a large infarct as well. Left ventricular aneurysms more commonly occur after occlusion of a vessel in which there was not adequate collateral blood supply and thus are not as common in multivessel coronary disease. An acute anterior wall MI is less likely given the stable clinical presentation in the outpatient clinic and lack of chest pain, although silent injury may occur in some patient populations. Pericarditis is often associated with pleuritic chest pain often radiating to the ridge of the trapezius, and the EKG often has diffuse PR depression and ST elevation, although one can see regional pericarditis in situations such as post-bypass surgery. The pain can occur between 1 day and 6 weeks post-MI and can be difficult to distinguish from recurrent angina. Dressler syndrome is associated with pain, fever, elevated sedimentation rate and white blood cell count, generalized malaise, and pericardial effusion. It typically occurs 1–8 weeks post-MI. The lack of jugular vein distension (JVD), ascites, peripheral edema, and right ventricle (RV) heave decreases the likelihood of right heart failure.

2. A. This patient has amyloid heart disease. Amyloidosis is due to protein deposition, which can affect many organs. Once there has been a significant infiltration, clinical manifestations typically occur. The discordance of the left

Table 87.1 TYPICAL POST-MYOCARDIAL INFARCTION COMPLICATIONS

CHARACTERISTIC	VENTRICULAR SEPTUM	FREE WALL	PAPILLARY MUSCLE
Incidence	1–3% without reperfusion therapy 0.3% with fibrinolytic therapy 3.9% in cardiogenic shock	0.8–6.2% No change with fibrinolytic therapy	~ 1% (postero-medial > anterolateral)
Time course	Bimodal peak; within 24 hours and 3–5 days (range 1–14 days)		
Clinical manifestations	Chest pain, dyspnea, hypotension	Angina, pleuritic chest pain, hypotension, sudden death	Abrupt onset of dyspnea, pulmonary edema, hypotension
Physical findings	Harsh holosystolic murmur, thrill, S3, loud S2, RV/LV failure, cardiogenic shock	JVD (29%), pulsus paradoxus (47%), pulseless electrical activity, cardiogenic shock	Soft murmur, pulmonary edema, cardiogenic shock

SOURCE: Antman et al. (2004).

ventricle (LV) wall thickness on echocardiography with low voltage on EKG is highly suggestive of an infiltrative process. Rapid increase of LV wall thickness over the years also suggests an infiltrative process. Patients commonly have hoarseness and bruisability due to amyloid deposits. They develop a restrictive physiology and can develop massive right-sided heart failure, including ascites. Atrial fibrillation is common due to electromechanical uncoupling, and thrombus formation is a concern. These patients typically have a poor prognosis (median survival ~6 months post–onset of symptoms); however, there are some variants with better prognosis, which is the rationale for a workup, including an endomyocardial biopsy. Hypertension is a cause of LV hypertrophy, which is not the case in this patient. ACE inhibitors have not been tested in large randomized trials in patients with amyloid cardiomyopathy. There should be cautious use of vasodilators given the autonomic dysregulation that may be present in these patients. Digitalis should be avoided given the propensity for digitalis toxicity. Heart transplant can be offered in highly selected patients with isolated cardiac amyloidosis and is often followed by a stem-cell transplant to prevent recurrent amyloid depositions in the transplanted heart.

3. C. This patient is at risk for a cardiomyopathy due to Adriamycin exposure, and there can be a delay in the development of LV dysfunction, especially in younger patients. Echocardiography excludes this etiology. Radiation exposure places her at risk for coronary artery disease (CAD), constrictive pericarditis, restrictive cardiomyopathy, and valvular disease. Classically, patients develop CAD approximately 10 years post–radiation exposure and have a unique pattern with stenosis in the ostia of the major coronary arteries, possibly due to more intense radiation exposure in these areas. Her right-sided heart failure symptoms suggest restrictive versus constrictive physiology. Cardiac magnetic resonance imaging (MRI) can be helpful, as well as echocardiography with Doppler interrogation, chest computed tomography (CT) to evaluate pericardial thickness, and cardiac catheterization (gold standard). Table 87.2 details findings in these conditions.

4. B. Given her diabetes mellitus, this patient is at high risk, and thus her LDL and total cholesterol levels are not at target. For all patients with hypercholesterolemia, it is recommended to exercise and modify diet to improve lipid profile. However, there are some patient populations that should receive pharmacologic therapy. The ATP III LDL-C guidelines take into consideration the risk of the patient to establish target goals and interventions. Patients with established coronary heart disease (CHD) or who have a CHD risk equivalent (i.e., diabetes mellitus, peripheral arterial disease, abdominal aortic aneurysm, carotid disease, two or more risk factors with 10-year risk of >20%) are considered high risk (see table 87.3). Risk factors includes smoking, hypertension, HDL <40 mg/dL, family history of early CAD, and older age (males ≥45, females ≥55). Based on PROVE-IT, patients with an acute myocardial infarction could be treated with atorvastatin, 80 mg nightly. Generic drugs are available for other secondary prevention as well as for primary-prevention patients. Niacin is good to raise HDL. Exercise testing is not required to decide on statin use.

5. C. There is no difference in stroke risk with the two treatment strategies, possibly due to undetected paroxysmal atrial fibrillation (AF) and lack of anticoagulation in the patients managed with anti-arrhythmic drugs. Antithrombotic therapy is recommended for patients with atrial flutter as for those with AF and should be used in all patients except those with lone AF or contraindications. Decision regarding aspirin versus warfarin is based on thromboembolic complications risk, bleeding risk, and risk of potential contraindications for therapy (e.g., recurrent falls). The ACTIVE study recently was stopped early due to worse outcomes in patients with AF randomized to aspirin + clopidogrel compared to warfarin. Warfarin

Table 87.2 CONSTRICTIVE PERICARDITIS VERSUS RESTRICTIVE CARDIOMYOPATHY

CONSTRICTIVE PERICARDITIS	RESTRICTIVE CARDIOMYOPATHY
Pericardial resistance in later 2/3 of diastole	Intrinsic abnormality of diastolic function
Elevation and equalization of diastolic pressures	Normal LVEDV but increased diastolic pressure
Prominent "X" and "Y" descent	"Y" descent blunted relative to "X"
Right ventricular dip and plateau	Right ventricular and left ventricular diastolic dip and plateau
Decreased intracardiac volume, SV, CO	Equalization of diastolic filling pressures
Inspiratory augmentation of VR blunted	Blunted respiratory variation in trans-valvular flows
Kussmaul's sign	Kussmaul's sign may be present
Pulsus paradoxus uncommon (33%)	Pulsus paradoxus in some
Ventricular discordance	Ventricular concordance

SOURCE: Goldstein (2004).

Table 87.3 **NCEP GUIDELINES FOR LIPID MANAGEMENT**

RISK CATEGORY	LDL GOAL	INITIATE TLC	CONSIDER DRUG THERAPY
High risk: CHD* or CHD risk equivalents (10-year risk 20%)	100 mg/dL (optional goal: 70 mg/dL)	100 mg/dL	100 mg/dL (consider <100 mg/dL)
Moderately high risk: ≥2 risk factors (10-year risk 10% to 20%)	130 mg/dL	130 mg/dL	130 mg/dL (consider 100–129 mg/dL)
Moderate risk: 2+ risk factors (10-year risk 10%)	130 mg/dL	130 mg/dL	160 mg/dL
Lower risk: 0–1 risk factor	160 mg/dL	160 mg/dL	190 mg/dL (consider 160–189 mg/dL)

SOURCE: Grundy et al. (2004).

should be used for (1) patients with mechanical heart valves, (2) patients at high risk of stroke (prior stroke, transient ischemic attack [TIA], systemic embolism, or history of rheumatic mitral stenosis), and (3) patients with more than one moderate risk factor (i.e., age ≥75 years, hypertension, heart failure, heart failure, LVEF ≤35% or fractional shortening ≤25%, and diabetes mellitus). Aspirin (81–325 mg daily) is recommended as an alternative to vitamin K antagonists in low-risk patients or in those with contraindications to oral anticoagulation.

6. E. This patient is near term and does not have a load-bearing valvular lesion. Valvular heart lesions associated with high maternal and/or fetal risk during pregnancy include severe aortic stenosis with or without symptoms, aortic insufficiency with New York Heart Association (NYHA) functional class III–IV symptoms, mitral stenosis with NYHA functional class II–IV symptoms, severe mitral regurgitation with NYHA functional class III–IV symptoms, aortic and/or mitral valve disease resulting in severe pulmonary hypertension (pulmonary pressure >75% of systemic systolic blood pressure), aortic and/or mitral valve disease with severe LV dysfunction (LVEF <40%), mechanical prosthetic valve requiring anticoagulation, and aortic insufficiency in Marfan syndrome.

7. C. Typical causes of unequal pressures in upper extremities include diseases affecting the subclavian artery (e.g., subclavian artery stenosis), aortic dissection due to selective dissection, Takayasu disease, and supravalvular stenosis, as this may affect the direction of blood flow preferentially toward the innominate artery and right arm resulting in higher pressures. Aortic stenosis or subvalvular stenosis would not preferentially affect flow of blood, and coarctation of aorta is usually distal to the left subclavian artery and would not cause of unequal pressures in upper extremities. Given the physical exam findings, a thoracic aortic dissection should be excluded urgently.

8. A. Given the prior MI, this patient is at risk for scar formation, and ventricular tachycardia is the most likely cause of syncope. Syncope is a common presentation caused by diverse problems. The patient's history can be helpful in understanding the likely cause of syncope. Cardiac syncope

is manifested by rapid onset without aura, clear sensorium afterward, and a history of CAD and/or LV dysfunction. Bradyarrhythmias should be considered in patients with a history of conduction disease or heart transplant. Neurological syncope is often preceded by aura and has a clouded sensorium with incontinence, tongue biting, and/or seizure activity. Hysterical fainting is not accompanied by change in pulse, blood pressure, or skin color. These patients experience paresthesias of hands/face, hyperventilation, dyspnea, and signs of anxiety. Neurocardiogenic syncope is the underlying etiology of approximately 50% of cases. Precipitants include emotional distress, fear, decreased venous response, and pain.

9. C. Pulmonary embolism (PE) can be fatal, and quick diagnosis is imperative. The clinical presentation can be quite variable. Sinus tachycardia is one of the more common findings on EKG, occurring in over 90% of patients. Nonspecific T-wave changes and precordial T-wave inversions may occur in 70% of patients. The "S1Q3T3" pattern is specific, but it occurs quite infrequently, approximately 28% of cases. Chest x-ray abnormalities are common but very nonspecific. It is not uncommon to see a normal chest x-ray in PE patients, occurring in 12% of patients. Hypoxemia is common but not ubiquitous in PE patients, and pulse oximetry <95% is associated with increased risk of death and/or respiratory failure. Even in a large PE with hypotension, patients can have normal oxygen saturation at the time of presentation, especially in younger patients. Classic findings of an arterial blood gas (which is not necessary usually) include hypoxemia, respiratory alkalosis, and hypocapnia. BNP values tend to range from 100 to 500 pg/mL, likely due to right ventricular wall tension, and are associated with worse outcomes. Cardiac troponin can be mildly elevated as well due to right ventricular myocyte loss. A perfusion scan has an excellent negative predictive value. Thus, a normal perfusion scan practically excludes a significant PE. PE CT scans are now being done, and the resolution of the chest CT scanner is most important in determining the negative predictive value of this modality.

10. D. This patient likely did not tolerate such a rapid up titration of beta blockade and likely had a decreased cardiac

output. Beta blockers are recommended therapy for chronic heart failure patients and should be initiated in those who can tolerate it, even during a hospitalization, if there is no evidence of congestion; however, this class should be initiated at low doses and increased *slowly*. Cardiac output, and even LVEF, may decrease in the early course of treatment with beta blockers. Other acute complications include bradycardia, fatigue, bronchospasm, fluid retention/decompensated heart failure, hypotension, and dizziness. Over the next 3 months, patients often have improved symptoms, less fatigue, improved LVEF, and better drug tolerance. There are no signs of fluid retention on physical examination. An isolated BNP is of limited clinical utility, as many patients have persistently elevated BNP values, and does not necessarily mean volume overload. If the BNP increased over 2 weeks from 80 to 700 pg/mL, this would support volume retention. There are no definitive data for the routine use of BNP-guided therapy. Digitalis should not be initiated until patient remains symptomatic despite multiple classes of medicines with known survival benefit. Cardiac transplantation may be considered, but I would wait until therapy is optimized. The QRS duration is not prolonged enough to warrant cardiac resynchronization.

11. E. This is a question that enables deductive reasoning, which may be a possibility on the boards. Given that RV pacing has similar physiology to left bundle branch block, these cardiac sounds may be similar. Thus, answers A and E do not seem to be compatible. Increased filling during inspiration delays the closure of the pulmonic valve and thus P2. A soft S2 is associated with valvular stenosis, and loud S2 is associated with high afterload as may be evident with pulmonary or systemic hypertension. Fixed splitting of the S2 is associated with an atrial septal defect. A widened splitting, but not fixed, is associated with a right bundle branch block. Paradoxical splitting is associated with left bundle branch block or right ventricular pacing.

12. D. Normal mental status can be present during a hypertensive crisis. Hypertensive encephalopathy can be associated with confusion, irritability, headaches, stupor, neurological deficits, seizures, and coma. It is caused by a sudden rise in blood pressure, which results in acute damage to blood vessels, but is not always present with malignant hypertension. It could also be caused by failure of cerebral autoregulation causing excess cerebral blood flow and damage to the wall leading to increased vascular permeability.

Clinical features include renal insufficiency with proteinuria, hematuria, azotemia, microangiopathic hemolytic anemia, heart failure, nausea, and vomiting.

13. C. Drug toxicities of commonly used medicines are important for the boards and for clinical practice. Amiodarone can result in photosensitivity, which is why patients are encouraged to wear sunblock. Typically, patients experience a bluish-gray discoloration of their nose. Amiodarone can also cause acute hypersensitivity pneumonitis or (chronically) pulmonary fibrosis. Pulmonary

function test should be checked at least annually. Drug-induced hepatitis, hypothyroidism, hyperthyroidism, and corneal deposits (nearly all patients but without visual disturbances) are other side effects with amiodarone. Verapamil causes constipation, skin reaction, and gingival hyperplasia. Procainamide has gastrointestinal side effects and is dose dependent but can also cause fever, agranulocytosis, Raynaud, and systemic lupus. Lidocaine results in perioral numbness, diplopia, seizures, cholestatic jaundice, hyperacusis, and slurred speech.

14. A. The guidelines for subacute bacterial endocarditis (SBE) prophylaxis changed in 2007 given the paucity of data about routine antibiotic use that may outweigh the benefit of preventing such rare infections. Thus, fewer patients require antibiotics with the current guidelines. Previous bacterial endocarditis remains as a reason for SBE prophylaxis. Other indications include prosthetic cardiac valves or prosthetic material in a valve repair, unrepaired complex cyanotic heart disease, surgically corrected systemic shunts or conduits, cardiac transplant patients with valvulopathy, repaired congenital heart disease with residual defects or prosthetic device/patch that will not endothelialize, and completely repaired congenital heart disease within 6 months of a prosthetic material that will endothelialize. SBE prophylaxis can be given to the patients above who will undergo dental procedures that require manipulation of gingival tissue or periapical teeth or involve perforation of the oral mucosa. Amoxicillin is standard drug choice; ampicillin/cefazolin or ceftriaxone are intravenous options, and cephalexin/clindamycin/clarithromycin/azithromycin are options for penicillin-allergic patients.

15. A. This patient has hypothyroidism. Classic cardiac effects of this disorder include decreased heart rate and cardiac output and increased systolic blood pressure as a result of increased systemic vascular resistance. The LVEF can decrease, and this is a cause of heart failure. Other findings include pericardial effusion, increased low-density lipoprotein and triglyceride levels, and hyponatremia due to production of antidiuretic hormone. Hyperthyroidism is associated with increased heart rate, cardiac output, stroke volume, and systolic blood pressure. Systemic vascular resistance falls, and atrial fibrillation is common. Heart failure can occur as a result of hyperthyroidism as well.

16. D. Hydrochlorothiazide is the best choice because the first-line therapy for hypertension tends to be a diuretic, although this is somewhat controversial. It is a cost-effective strategy for hypertension control; nevertheless, 3.5 classes of medicines are required to optimize blood pressure control. One can tailor the choice of drugs to the patient population. As an example, ACE inhibitors could be used in patients with diabetes, heart failure, prior myocardial infarction with left ventricular dysfunction, and chronic kidney disease. Beta blockers may be used in patients with prior documented acute coronary syndrome or myocardial infarction. Secondary causes of hypertension are uncommon and

should be considered in special circumstances. Stress test is not required to determine treatment of hypertension.

17. D. The pleural findings and differential blood pressure suggest a proximal dissection of the thoracic aorta. Surgical repair for proximal dissection is the best option given the high mortality rate with this condition. Stabilization and pain relief can be done as a bridge to surgery, but they should not be the sole option. The combination of sodium nitroprusside and a beta blocker is good to reduce blood pressure and wall stress, but sodium nitroprusside should not be used in isolation. Distal dissections are often present in older patients with coronary artery disease and do not require urgent surgery. A loop diuretic should not be used, as the patients may be preload dependent if there is pericardial effusion from the dissection.

18. D. Cigarette smoking is a recognized risk factor for vascular disease. Inhalation causes an acute rise in systemic blood pressure and can cause vasoconstriction. However, it is not a contributor to chronic hypertension. Four major contributors to essential hypertension include obesity, excessive salt intake, excessive alcohol intake, and lack of exercise.

19. C. Abciximab (IIb/IIIa receptor antagonist) should only be used if an invasive strategy with planned percutaneous intervention will be followed. Another IIb/IIIa receptor antagonist (eptifibatide or tirofiban) can be used in the conservative strategy of management of USA/NSTEMI. The patient is high risk and would require admission to the hospital for either an early invasive strategy or conservative management with serial cardiac enzymes. Patients with refractory symptoms or recurrent symptoms after stabilization should proceed with diagnostic catheterization, especially given this patient's likelihood of coronary artery disease.

20. B. This is a common scenario on board exams. Given the patient's excellent exercise capacity and asymptomatic status, there is no need for further risk stratification. Treatment of single-vessel disease with angioplasty/stents is not indicated in an asymptomatic patient; thus, repeat angiography is not necessary. Pharmacologic stress tests should be performed in patients who are unable to exercise, and imaging is not required for patients with interpretable EKGs.

ADDITIONAL READING

Antman EM, Anbe DT, Armstrong PW, et al. ACC/AHA guidelines for the management of patients with ST-elevation myocardial infarction: A report of the American College of Cardiology/American Heart Association Task Force on Practice Guidelines (Committee to Revise the 1999 Guidelines for the Management of Patients with Acute Myocardial Infarction). *Circulation.* 2004;110(9):e82–292.

Goldstein JA. Cardiac tamponade, constrictive pericarditis, and restrictive cardiomyopathy. *Curr Problems Cardiol.* 2004;29(9):503–67.

Grundy SM, Cleeman JI, Merz CN, et al. Implications of recent clinical trials for the National Cholesterol Education Program Adult Treatment Panel III guidelines. *Circulation.* 2004;110(?):227–39.

88.

CARDIOLOGY: SUMMARY

Elliott M. Antman

It is estimated that almost 81 million Americans (one out of every three adults) have some form of cardiovascular disease (CVD). Thus, it is commonplace for practitioners of internal medicine to encounter patients with CVD in their daily office and hospital practices. It is not only the high prevalence of CVD that commands the attention of clinicians but also the fact that CVD currently is the leading cause of death in the United States, accounting for about one out of every three deaths. From an epidemiologic perspective, it is noteworthy that CVD death rates increase sharply with increasing age and are greater in men versus women as well as in black patients versus white/Hispanic patients. In addition to the gender and ethnic disparities in CVD that contemporary physicians face, we are in the midst of an epidemic of obesity in the industrialized world that threatens to partially offset many of the dramatic advances in management of CVD.

PRIMARY PREVENTION

The critical, initial step in managing CVD involves risk stratification to frame therapeutic strategies for primary prevention in at-risk individuals. Key terms in this regard are the *absolute risk* of CVD, which is the risk of developing CVD during a given period of time (e.g., 10 years), and *attributable risk,* which refers to the difference in the incidence of CVD between persons who have and have not been exposed to a CV risk factor. Since ischemic heart disease (IHD) is the most common form of CVD and accounts for about one-half of the deaths due to CVD, primary prevention strategies have focused on identification of risk factors for IHD and development of algorithms for IHD risk prediction. Investigators from the Framingham Heart Study developed the Framingham Cardiovascular Risk Score (figure 88.1), which incorporates demographic information (gender, age), the blood pressure, key laboratory findings including total, low-density lipoprotein (HDL) and high-density lipoprotein (HDL) cholesterol, and the presence or absence of diabetes and cigarette smoking. Separate score sheets have been developed for men and women to establish the 10-year risk of developing CHD (figure 88.1).

Comparable algorithms have been developed in Europe and published as the European Society of Cardiology Coronary Risk Chart. In general, patients with at least a 10% estimated risk of IHD over the next 10 years are candidates for behavioral and pharmacologic preventive therapies. The National Cholesterol Education Program published the Adult Treatment Panel III that provides recommendations for LDL targets (table 88.1) and algorithms for initiation of therapeutic lifestyle changes and pharmacologic interventions (figure 88.2). Table 88.2 summarizes the various preventive strategies for apparently healthy patients as well as those with clinically apparent vascular disease who are therefore in need of secondary prevention.

ATHEROSCLEROTIC VASCULAR DISEASE

Atherosclerosis is a generalized vascular disorder that may result in flow limitations in the coronary, cerebrovascular, and peripheral vascular beds, producing myocardial ischemic events (angina pectoris/acute coronary syndrome), stroke, and claudication/critical limb ischemia, respectively (figure 88.3).

Patients with exertional symptoms of myocardial ischemia (angina pectoris or anginal equivalent such as dyspnea on exertion) are likely to be suffering from IHD and generally warrant a stress test to assess their symptoms (see figure 88.4). Once the diagnosis of IHD is confirmed, management involves a combination of pharmacotherapeutic interventions to decrease demand ischemia, minimize risk factors, and minimize the development of thrombotic events. A guide to decision-making regarding coronary revascularization is shown in figure 88.5.

Disruption of a lipid-laden plaque in an epicardial coronary artery exposes tissue factor and oxidized LDL to the

(A) Step 1

Age		
Years	LDL Pts	Chol Pts
30-34	−1	[−1]
35-39	0	[0]
40-44	1	[1]
45-49	2	[2]
50-54	3	[3]
55-59	4	[4]
60-64	5	[5]
65-69	6	[6]
70-74	7	[7]

Step 2

LDL - C		
(mg/dl)	(mmol/L)	LDL Pts
<100	<2.59	−3
100–129	2.60–3.36	0
130–159	3.37–4.14	0
160–190	4.15–4.92	1
≥190	≥4.92	2

Cholesterol		
(mg/dl)	(mmol/L)	Chol Pts
<160	<4.14	[−3]
160–199	4.15–5.17	[0]
200–239	5.18–6.21	[1]
240–279	6.22–7.24	[2]
≥280	≥7.25	[3]

Step 3

HDL-C			
(mg/dl)	(mmol/L)	LDL Pts	Chol Pts
<35	<0.90	2	[2]
35–44	0.91–1.16	1	[1]
45–49	1.17–1.29	0	[0]
50–59	1.30–1.55	0	[0]
≥60	≥1.56	−1	[2]

Step 4

Blood Pressure					
Systolic (mm Hg)	Diastolic (mm Hg)				
	<80	80–84	85–89	90–99	≥100
<120	0[0] pts				
120–129		0 [0] pts			
130–139			1 [1] pts		
140–159				2 [2] pts	
≥160					3 [3] pts

Note: When systolic and diastolic pressures provide different estimates for point scores, use the higher number

Step 5

Diabetes		
	LDL Pts	Chol Pts
No	0	[0]
Yes	2	[2]

Step 6

Smoker		
	LDL Pts	Chol Pts
No	0	[0]
Yes	2	[2]

Step 7

Adding up the points	
Age	_____
LDL-C or Chol	_____
HDL-C	_____
Blood Pressure	_____
Diabetes	_____
Smoker	_____
Point total	_____

Key	
Color	Relative Risk
green	Very low
white	Low
yellow	Moderate
rose	High
red	Very high

(determine CHD risk from point total)

Step 8

CHD Risk			
LDL Pts Total	10 Yr CHD Risk	Chol Pts Total	10 Yr CHD Risk
<−3	−1%		
−2	2%		
−1	2%	[<−1]	[2%]
0	3%	[0]	[3%]
1	4%	[1]	[3%]
2	4%	[2]	[4%]
3	6%	[3]	[5%]
4	7%	[4]	[7%]
5	9%	[5]	[8%]
6	11%	[6]	[10%]
7	14%	[7]	[13%]
8	18%	[8]	[16%]
9	22%	[9]	[20%]
10	27%	[10]	[25%]
11	33%	[11]	[31%]
12	40%	[12]	[37%]
13	47%	[13]	[45%]
≥14	≥56%	[≥14]	[≥53%]

(compare to average person your age)

Step 9

Comparative Risk			
Age (Years)	Average 10 Yr CHD Risk	Average 10 Yr Hard* CHD Risk	Low** 10 Yr CHD Risk
30–34	3%	1%	2%
35–39	5%	4%	3%
40–44	7%	4%	4%
45–49	11%	8%	4%
50–54	14%	10%	6%
55–59	16%	13%	7%
60–64	21%	20%	9%
65–69	25%	22%	11%
70–74	30%	25%	14%

* Hard CHD events exclude angina pectoris

** Low risk was calculated for a person the same age, optimal blood pressure, LDL-C 100–129 mg/dL or cholesterol 160–199 mg/dl, HDL-C 45 mg/dL for men or 55 mg/dL for women, non-smoker, no diabetes

Risk estimates were derived from the experience of the Framingham Heart Study, a predominantly Caucasian population in Massachusetts, USA

Figure 88.1. Coronary Heart Disease (CHD) Score Sheet. Sheet for calculating 10-year CHD risk according to age, total cholesterol (TC) (or low-density lipoprotein cholesterol [LDL-C]), high-density lipoprotein cholesterol (HDL-C), blood pressure, diabetes, and smoking. Use of the LDL-C categories is appropriate when fasting LDL-C measurements are available. (A) Score sheet for men based on the Framingham experience in men 30–74 years old at baseline. Average risk estimates are based on typical Framingham subjects, and estimates of idealized risk are based on optimal blood pressure, TC of 160–199 mg/dL (or LDL of 100–129 mg/dL), HDL-C of 45 mg/dL, no diabetes, and no smoking. (B) Score sheet for women based on the Framingham experience in women 30–74 years old at baseline. Average risk estimates are based on typical Framingham subjects, and estimates of idealized risk are based on optimal blood pressure, TC of 160–199 mg/dL (or LDL of 100–129 mg/dL), HDL-C of 55 mg/dL, no diabetes, and no smoking. Pts = points. Reprinted with permission from Wilson PW, D'Agostino RB, Levy D, et al. Prediction of coronary heart disease using risk factor categories. *Circulation.* 1998;97:1837–47.

(B) Step 1

Age		
Years	LDL Pts	Chol Pts
30–34	–9	[–9]
35–39	–4	[–4]
40–44	0	[0]
45–49	3	[3]
50–54	6	[6]
55–59	7	[7]
60–64	8	[8]
65–69	8	[8]
70–74	8	[8]

Step 2

LDL - C		
(mg/dl)	(mmol/L)	LDL Pts
<100	<2.59	–2
100–129	2.60–3.36	0
130–159	3.37–4.14	0
160–190	4.15–4.92	2
≥190	≥4.92	2

Cholesterol		
(mg/dl)	(mmol/L)	Chol Pts
<160	<4.14	[–2]
160–199	4.15–5.17	[0]
200–239	5.18–6.21	[1]
240–279	6.22–7.24	[2]
≥280	≥7.25	[3]

Step 3

HDL-C			
(mg/dl)	(mmol/L)	LDL Pts	Chol Pts
<35	<0.90	5	[5]
35–44	0.91–1.16	2	[2]
45–49	1.17–1.29	1	[1]
50–59	1.30–1.55	0	[0]
≥60	≥1.56	–2	[–3]

Step 4

Blood Pressure					
Systolic (mm Hg)	Diastolic (mm Hg)				
	<80	80–84	85–89	90–99	≥100
<120	–3 [–3] pts				
120–129		0 [0] pts			
130–139			0 [0] pts		
140–159				2 [2] pts	
≥160					3 [3] pts

* Note: When systolic and diastolic pressures provide different estimates for point scores. Use the higher number

Step 5

Diabetes		
	LDL Pts	Chol Pts
No	0	[0]
Yes	4	[4]

Step 6

Smoker		
	LDL Pts	Chol Pts
No	0	[0]
Yes	2	[2]

Figure 88.1. (continued)

(Sum from steps 1–6)

Step 7

Adding up the points	
Age	_____
LDL-C or Chol	_____
HDL-C	_____
Blood Pressure	_____
Diabetes	_____
Smoker	_____
Point total	_____

Key	
Color	Relative Risk
green	Very low
white	Low
yellow	Moderate
rose	High
red	Very high

(determine CHD risk from point total)

Step 8

CHD Risk			
LDL Pts Total	10 Yr CHD Risk	Chol Pts Total	10 Yr CHD Risk
≤–2	1%	[≤–2]	[1%]
–1	2%	[–1]	[2%]
0	2%	[0]	[2%]
1	2%	[1]	[2%]
2	3%	[2]	[3%]
3	3%	[3]	[3%]
4	4%	[4]	[4%]
5	5%	[5]	[4%]
6	6%	[6]	[5%]
7	7%	[7]	[6%]
8	8%	[8]	[7%]
9	9%	[9]	[8%]
10	11%	[10]	[10%]
11	13%	[11]	[11%]
12	15%	[12]	[13%]
13	17%	[13]	[15%]
14	20%	[14]	[18%]
15	24%	[15]	[20%]
16	27%	[16]	[24%]
≥17	≥32%	[≥17]	[≥27%]

(compare to average person your age)

Step 9

Comparative Risk			
Age (Years)	Average 10 Yr CHD Risk	Average 10 Yr Hard* CHD Risk	Low** 10 Yr CHD Risk
30–34	<1%	<1%	<1%
35–39	<1%	<1%	1%
40–44	2%	1%	2%
45–49	5%	2%	3%
50–54	8%	3%	5%
55–59	12%	7%	7%
60–64	12%	8%	8%
65–69	13%	8%	8%
70–74	14%	11%	8%

* Hard CHD events exclude angina pectoris

** Low risk was calculated for a person the same age, optimal blood pressure, LDL-C 100–129 mg/dL or cholesterol 160–199 mg/dl, HDL-C 45 mg/dL for men or 55 mg/dL for women, non-smoker, no diabetes

Risk estimates were derived from the experience of the Framingham Heart Study, a predominantly Caucasian population in Massachusetts, USA

passing bloodstream, setting in motion platelet adhesion/ activation/and aggregation as well as initiation of the coagulation cascade. The patient presents with ischemic discomfort, and the 12-lead EKG is used to stratify the patient to the unstable angina/non–ST elevation myocardial infarction (UA/NSTEMI) versus ST-elevation myocardial infarction (STEMI) end of the acute coronary syndrome (ACS) spectrum (figure 88.6). Biomarkers detected in the peripheral circulation aid in the diagnosis of myocardial infarction; the cardiac-specific troponins (T and I) are the preferred markers of MI at present.

Antiplatelet therapies (aspirin, thienopyridines, glycoprotein [GP] IIb/IIIa inhibitors) and anticoagulant therapies (unfractionated or low-molecular-weight heparin, direct thrombin inhibitors, factor Xa inhibitors) are used across the ACS spectrum. Similarly, percutaneous coronary interventions involving balloon angioplasty and deployment of coronary stents (bare metal and drug-eluting) are now used across the ACS spectrum. Urgent reperfusion of the totally occluded coronary artery is needed in STEMI patients to prevent myocardium that is ischemic ("at risk") from progressing to necrosis

Table 88.1 UPDATED NCEP/ATP III GUIDELINES

RISK CATEGORY	LDL-C GOAL (mg/dL)
Very high risk defined as CVD and one or more of: • Diabetes mellitus • Multiple major risk factors • Poorly controlled risk factors • Metabolic syndrome • Patients with acute coronary syndrome	<100 Optional <70
High risk: • CHD or CHD risk equivalent	<100
Moderately high risk: • Two or more risk factors • Framingham score 10–20%	<130 Optional <100
Moderate risk: • Two or more risk factors • Framingham score <10%	<130
Low risk: 0–1 risk factors	<160

SOURCE: Modified from Davidson M. Pharmacologic therapy for hypertriglyceridemia and low HDL: Rationale for combination therapy. In: Antman EM (ed.), *Cardiovascular Therapeutics: A Companion to Braunwald's Heart Disease.* 3rd ed. (p. 516) Philadelphia: WB Saunders/Elsevier; 2007.

(i.e., limitation of infarct size). Reperfusion for STEMI can be accomplished with fibrinolytic agents, but the preferred approach at present is primary PCI, provided it can be implemented in a timely fashion (<90 min from contact with the medical system) by an experienced operator and team.

Algorithms for management of patients presenting with UA/NSTEMI and STEMI are shown in figures 88.7 and 88.8. Once patients recover from an ACS event, they should be treated with the secondary prevention measures outlined in table 88.2. Patients with an ACS event should be evaluated for evidence of important vascular disease in other beds such as cerebrovascular (carotid disease) and peripleural vascular (abdominal aortic aneurysm, lower extremity PAD) (figure 88.3).

HEART FAILURE

It is estimated that about 5 million patients in the United States have heart failure (HF). Contemporary concepts of heart failure focus on four stages (figure 88.9). Just as with CHD risk factors, the first two HF stages (A and B) do not involve clinical presentations with symptomatic HF, but rather describe the risk factors that predispose to the development of HF. Stage A involves conditions that put a patient at risk of HF (e.g., IHD, hypertension [HTN], diabetes mellitus [DM]) but without evidence of impaired left ventricular (LV) function, hypertrophy, or chamber distortion. Asymptomatic patients with CVH and/or impaired

LV function are classified as Stage B. Patients with current or past symptoms of HF in the setting of underlying structural heart disease are classified as Stage C. Those patients who remain symptomatic despite the treatments applied for Stages A–C are classified as Stage D and are candidates for advanced treatment strategies. Clinicians should view this classification scheme as complementary to the NYHA functional classification, which predominantly provides an assessment of the severity of symptoms for patients in Stages C and D.

Clinical presentation with HF should be viewed as a syndrome that may have as its cause disorders of the myocardium, endocardium, epicardium, or pericardium. Patients vary widely in the likelihood of developing symptomatic HF for a given degree of underlying heart disease and also vary in their ability to exercise for the same degree of measured CV dysfunction. An important additional concept is the progressive nature of HF in many patients, typically characterized by a change in the geometry and structure of the LV as a consequence of activation of endogenous neurohormonal systems.

Therapeutic strategies for HF begin with treatment of the underlying risk factors and early initiation of drugs to inhibit the renin-angiotensin-aldosterone system (RAAS). Once symptoms appear, therapies should be expanded to include diuretics, digitalis, and in selected patients biventricular pacing systems. Evidence exists that the risk of sudden cardiac death (SCD) can be decreased by the implantation of implantable cardioverter-defibrillators (ICDs), although ICDs should not be conceived of as treatment for the HF syndrome itself. Finally, advanced therapies ranging from circulatory support devices to surgical procedures and heart transplantation are options that should be considered in refractory patients.

The stages of HF and therapeutic recommendations are summarized in figure 88.9.

VALVULAR HEART DISEASE

The reservoir of patients with rheumatic mitral stenosis has diminished markedly in the United States, leaving mitral regurgitation (MR) and aortic valve disease (stenosis, regurgitation) as the major valve lesions internists are likely to encounter.

Medical management of patients with MR and aortic regurgitation (AR) centers around afterload reduction to minimize the amount of regurgitation and lessen the chance of development of LV systolic dysfunction. Serial echocardiograms are obtained to monitor for evidence of significant progressive LV enlargement, which serves as an indication for valve surgery even in the asymptomatic patient. Although valve replacement is typically performed in patients with severe AR, contemporary surgical techniques for severe MR emphasize mitral valve repair rather than replacement, to

Table 88.2 GUIDE TO CVD RISK REDUCTION

RISK FACTOR	APPARENTLY HEALTH PATIENTS	SECONDARY PREVENTION
Smoking cessation	Complete cessation	Complete cessation
Hypertension	<140/90 mm Hg	<130/80 mm Hg for patients with diabetes or chronic kidney disease
High cholesterol	LDL-C <160 mg/dL if patient has 0–1 other risk factors, * <130 mg/dL if two or more risk factors; also HDL-C >40 mg/dL and TG <200 mg/dL	Primary goal: LDL-C ≤100 and preferably ≤70 mg/dL. Secondary goal: HDL-C >40 mg/dL and TG <200 mg/dL
Physical inactivity	30 min of moderate physical activity on most, if not all, days of the week.	30 min of moderate physical activity on most, if not all, days of the week
Weight	BMI <25 kg/m², waist circumference <40 inches for men and <35 inches for women; at a minimum, no increase in weight	BMW <25 kg/m², waist circumference <40 inches for men and <35 inches for women; at a minimum, no increase in weight
Glucose control		Goal: HbA1c <7%. First-step therapy: weight reduction and exercise Second-step therapy: oral hypoglycemic agents Third-step therapy: insulin
Menopause	Combined estrogen plus progestin should not be used to prevent CVD in postmenopausal women	Combined estrogen plus progestin should not be used to prevent CVD in postmenopausal women
Antioxidants	Antioxidant supplements should not be used to prevent CVD	Antioxidant supplements should not be used to prevent CVD
Psychosocial	Evaluate for depression/anxiety disorders. Assess structural/functional support.	Evaluate for depression/anxiety disorders. Assess structural/functional support.
Antiplatelet agents		Aspirin, 75–162 mg/day; Clopidogrel, 75 mg/day for at least 1 month after BMS and at least 1 year after DES; long-term therapy (e.g., 1 year) after UA/NSTEMI and STEMI.
RAAS inhibition		ACE inhibitors or ARBs for patients with LVEF ≤40% and those with hypertension, diabetes, chronic kidney disease
Beta blockers		For all patients who have had an ACS or LV dysfunction with or without HF symptoms
Influenza vaccination		All patients with CVD should have an annual influenza vaccination
NSAIDs		Avoid if possible but use stepped care approach† if required to control musculoskeletal symptoms

NOTES: * Risk factors include age (men ≥45 years, women ≥55 years or postmenopausal), smoking, hypertension, diabetes, family history of congestive heart disease in first-degree relative, and HDL-C <40 mg/dL. If HDL-C ≥60 mg/dL, subtract one risk factor. BMI, body mass index; BP, blood pressure; HDL-C, high-density lipoprotein cholesterol; LDL-C, low-density lipoprotein cholesterol; TG, triglycerides.

SOURCES: Modified from: (1) Meadows J, Danik JS, Albert MAA. Primary prevention of ischemic heart disease. In: Antman EM (ed.), *Cardiovascular Therapeutics: A Companion to Braunwald's Heart Disease,* 3rd ed. (pp. 208–9). Philadelphia: WB Saunders/Elsevier, 2007; (2) Antman EM, Hand M, Armstrong PW, et al. 2007 focused update of the ACC/AHA 2004 Guidelines for the Management of Patients with ST-Elevation Myocardial Infarction. *Circulation.* 2008;117:296–329; (3) Anderson JL, Adams CD, Antman EM, et al. ACC/AHA 2007 guidelines for the management of patients with unstable angina/non ST-elevation myocardial infarction: A report of the American College of Cardiology/American Heart Association Task Force on Practice Guidelines (Writing Committee to Revise the 2002 Guidelines for the Management of Patients With Unstable Angina/Non ST-Elevation Myocardial Infarction). *Circulation.* 2007;116:e148–304.

† See Antman EM, Bettett JS, Daugherty A, Furberg C, Roberts H, Taubert KA. Use of nonsteroidal anti-inflammatory drugs: An update for clinicians: A scientific statement from the American Heart Association. *Circulation.* 2007;115:1634.

The stepped care approach to NSAIDs involves the following treatment options in the order listed if the preceding steps are inadequate for controlling the patient's symptoms.

1. Acetaminophen, aspirin, tramadol, narcotic analgesics (short term in appropriately selected patients)
2. Nonacetylated salicylates
3. Non–COX-2-selective NSAIDs
4. NSAIDs with some COX-2 activity
5. COX-2-selective NSAIDs

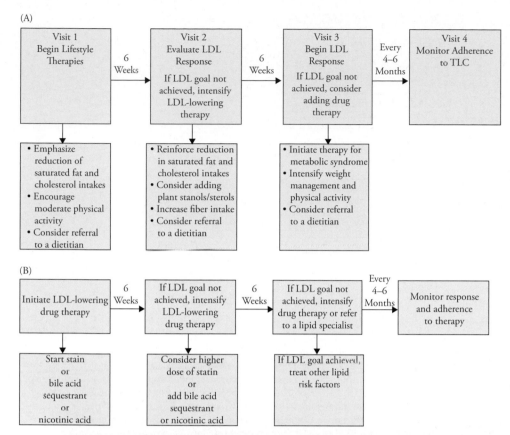

Figure 88.2. Algorithm for the Treatment of Hypertension. ACEI, angiotensin-converting enzyme inhibitor; ARB, angiotensin receptor blocker; BB, beta-adrenergic receptor blocker; CCB, calcium channel blocker. Modified from Chobanian AV, Bakris GL, Black HR, et al, for the National High Blood Pressure Coordinating Committee. Seventh report of the Joint National Committee on Prevention, Detection, Evaluation, and Treatment of High Blood Pressure. *Hypertension.* 2003;42:1206–52. From Krousel-Wood M, Materson BJ, Whelton PK. Initial evaluation and approach to the patient with hypertension. In: Antman EM (ed.). *Cardiovascular Therapeutics: A Companion to Braunwald's Heart Disease,* 3rd ed. (p. 572). Copyright Elsevier, 2007, p. 572. Reprinted with permission.

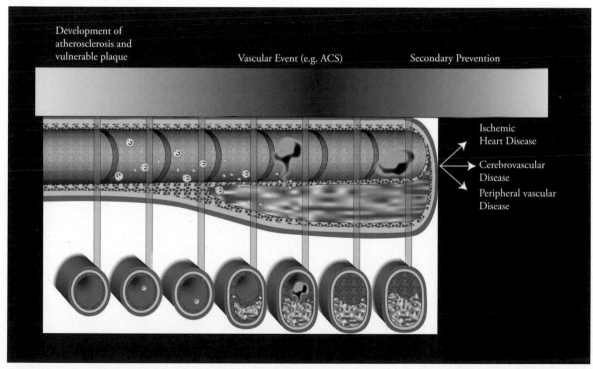

Figure 88.3. Acute Coronary Syndromes. The longitudinal section of an artery depicts the "timeline" of atherogenesis from a normal artery to lesion initiation and accumulation of extracellular lipid in the intima, to the evolution to the fibrofatty stage, to lesion progression with procoagulant expression and weakening of the fibrous cap. An acute coronary syndrome develops when the vulnerable or high-risk plaque undergoes disruption of the fibrous cap; disruption of the plaque is the stimulus for thrombogenesis. Thrombus resorption may be followed by collagen accumulation and smooth muscle cell growth. Following disruption of a vulnerable or high-risk plaque, patients experience ischemic discomfort resulting from a reduction of flow through the affected epicardial coronary artery. The flow reduction may be caused by a completely occlusive thrombus or subtotally occlusive thrombus. Modified with permission from Libby. *Circulation* 2001;104:365–72, Hamm, Bertrand, Braunwald. From: From Antman EM, Braunwald E. ST-elevation myocardial infarction: pathology, pathophysiology, and clinical features. In: Libby P, Bonow RO, Mann DL, Zipes DP (eds.), Braunwald's Heart Disease: A Textbook of Cardiovascular Medicine. 8th ed. Philadelphia, Saunders/Elsevier, 2008, p. 1210.

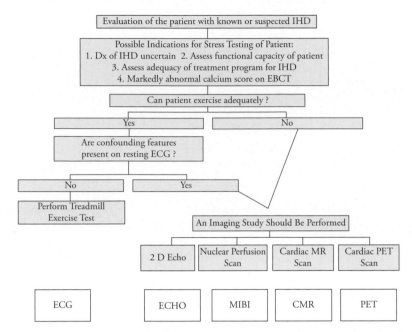

Figure 88.4. Evaluation of the Patient with Known or Suspected Ischemic Heart Disease. Shown here are an algorithm for identifying patients who should be referred for stress testing and the decision pathway for determining if a standard treadmill exercise with EKG monitoring alone is adequate. A specialized imaging study is necessary if the patient cannot exercise adequately (pharmacologic challenge is given) or if there are confounding features on the resting EKG (symptom-limited treadmill exercise may be used to stress the coronary circulation). Evaluation of the patient's symptoms, exercise capacity, and hemodynamic response is supplemented by EKG monitoring and specialized imaging procedures. IHD, ischemic heart disease; EBCT, electron beam computed tomography; EKG, electrocardiogram; MR, magnetic resonance; PET, positron emission tomography; ECHO, echocardiography; MIBI, methoxyisobutyl isonitrite; CMR, cardiac magnetic resonance. Reprinted with permission from Antman E, Selwyn AP, Braunwald E, Loscalzo J. Ischemic heart disease. In: Fauci AS, Kasper DL, Longo DL, et al. (eds.). *Harrison's Principles of Internal Medicine,* 17th ed. (pp. 1517–8). New York: McGraw-Hill, 2008.

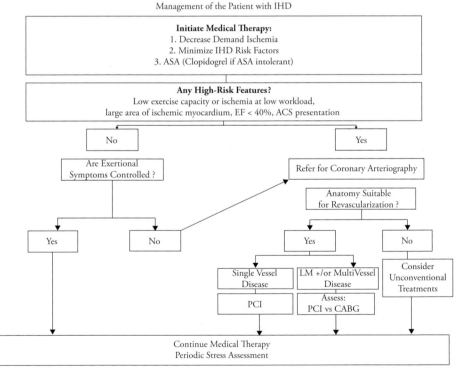

Figure 88.5. Algorithm for Management of the Patient with Ischemic Heart Disease. All patients should receive the core elements of medical therapy as shown at the top of the algorithm. If high-risk features are present, as established by the clinical history, exercise test data, and imaging studies, the patient should be referred for coronary arteriography. Based on the number and location of the diseased vessels and their suitability for revascularization, the patient is treated with either a percutaneous coronary intervention (PCI), coronary artery bypass graft (CABG) surgery, or should be considered for unconventional treatments. See text for further discussion. IHD, ischemic heart disease; ASA, aspirin; EF, ejection fraction; ACS, acute coronary syndrome; LM, left main. Reprinted with permission from Antman E, Selwyn AP, Braunwald E, Loscalzo J. Ischemic heart disease. In: Fauci AS, Kasper DL, Longo DL, et al. (eds.). *Harrison's Principles of Internal Medicine,* 17th ed. (p. 1525). New York: McGraw-Hill, 2008.

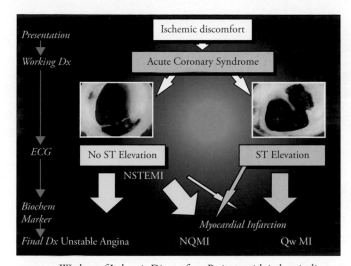

Figure 88.6. Workup of Ischemic Discomfort. Patients with ischemic discomfort may present with or without ST-segment elevation on the electrocardiogram (EKG). Of patients with ST-segment elevation, most ultimately develop a Q-wave MI (QwMI), whereas a few develop a non-Q-wave MI (NQMI). Patients who present without ST-segment elevation are suffering from either unstable angina or a non–ST-segment elevation MI (NSTEMI), a distinction that is ultimately made on the presence or absence of a serum cardiac marker such as CK-MB or a cardiac troponin detected in the blood. Most patients presenting with NSTEMI ultimately develop a NQMI on the EKG; a few *may* develop a QwMI. The spectrum of clinical presentations ranging from unstable angina through NSTEMI and STEMI are referred to as the acute coronary syndromes. Dx, diagnosis; NQMI, non-Q-wave myocardial infarction; QwMI, Q-wave myocardial infarction; CK-MB, MB isoenzyme of creatine kinase. Modified from *The Lancet.* 2001;358:1533–8; Davies. *Heart.* 2000;83:361–6; Antman EM, Anbe DT, Armstrong PW, et al. ACC/AHA American College of Cardiology Web Site, 2006. From Antman EM, Braunwald E. ST-elevation myocardial infarction: pathology, pathophysiology, and clinical features. In: Libby P, Bonow RO, Mann DL, Zipes DP (eds.). *Braunwald's Heart Disease: A Textbook of Cardiovascular Medicine.* 8th ed. (p. 1210). Copyright Elsevier, 2008,. Reprinted with permission.

minimize perioperative LV chamber enlargement from loss of the tethering action of the chordae tendineae and papillary muscles. Severe aortic stenosis is not a condition that can be managed and requires valve replacement.

Surgical replacement of a heart valve can be performed with either a bioprosthesis (preferred in elderly patients because of the lack of need for anticoagulation and less concern about need for repeat replacement resulting from prosthetic dysfunction) or a mechanical prosthesis (preferred in younger patients because of much lower risk of repeat replacement for prosthetic dysfunction, but requires anticoagulation to prevent thrombosis). Patients with a prosthetic heart valve should receive antibiotic prophylaxis against endocarditis when they undergo dental procedures.

CARDIAC ARRHYTHMIAS

The management of cardiac arrhythmias has undergone a major change with fewer patients treated with antiarrhythmic drugs and more being treated with ablation procedures and/or device implantation. Although antiarrhythmic

drugs were developed with the goals of decreasing the frequency of arrhythmias and, in the case of life-threatening arrhythmias, minimizing the risk of mortality, these goals in large part have not been met. Antiarrhythmic drugs

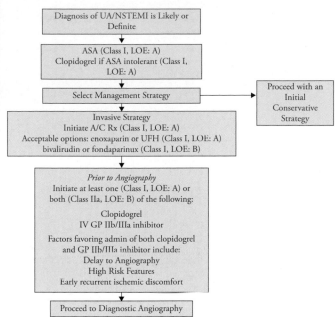

Figure 88.7. Algorithms for Management of Patients with UA/NSTEMI. (A) Initial invasive strategy. When multiple drugs are listed, they are in alphabetical order and not in order of preference. Evidence exists that GP IIb/IIIa inhibitors may not be necessary if the patient received a preloading dose of at least 300 mg of clopidogrel at least 6 hours earlier (Class I, Level of Evidence B for clopidogrel administration) and bivalirudin is selected as the anticoagulant (Class IIa, Level of Evidence B). ASA = aspirin; GP = glycoprotein; IV = intravenous; LOE = level of evidence; UA/NSTEMI = unstable angina/non–ST-elevation myocardial infarction; UFH = unfractionated heparin. (B) Initial conservative strategy. When multiple drugs are listed, they are in alphabetical order and not in order of preference. ASA = aspirin; EF = ejection fraction; GP = glycoprotein; IV = intravenous; LOE = level of evidence; LVEF = left ventricular ejection fraction; UA-NSTEMI = unstable angina/non–ST-elevation myocardial infarction; UFH = unfractionated heparin. (C) Management after diagnostic angiography. Evidence exists that GP IIb/IIIa inhibitors may not be necessary if the patient received a preloading dose of at least 300 mg of clopidogrel at least 6 hours earlier (Class I, Level of Evidence B for clopidogrel administration) and bivalirudin is selected as the anticoagulant (Class IIa, Level of Evidence B). An additional bolus of UFH is recommended if fondaparinux is selected as the anticoagulant. For patients in whom the clinician believes coronary atherosclerosis is present, albeit without any significant, flow-limiting stenoses, long-term treatment with antiplatelet agents and other secondary prevention measures should be considered. ASA = aspirin; CABG = coronary artery bypass graft; CAD = coronary artery disease; GP = glycoprotein; IV = intravenous; LD = loading dose; PCI = percutaneous coronary intervention; pre angio = before angiography; UA-NSTEMI = unstable angina/non–ST-elevation myocardial infarction; UFH = unfractionated heparin. Reprinted from Anderson JL, Adams CD, Antman EM, et al. ACC/AHA 2007 guidelines for the management of patients with unstable angina/non ST-elevation myocardial infarction: A report of the American College of Cardiology/American Heart Association Task Force on Practice Guidelines (Writing Committee to Revise the 2002 Guidelines for the Management of Patients with Unstable Angina/Non ST-Elevation Myocardial Infarction). *J Am Coll Cardiol.* 2007;50:e46–8, with permission from Elsevier.

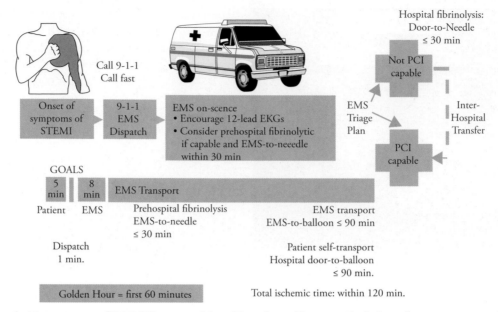

Figure 88.8. Options for Transportation of STEMI Patients and Initial Reperfusion Treatment Goals. Reperfusion in patients with STEMI can be accomplished by pharmacological (fibrinolysis) or catheter-based (primary PCI) approaches. The overarching goal is to keep total ischemic time within 120 min (ideally within 60 min) from symptom onset to initiation of reperfusion treatment. Within this context, the following are goals for the medical system based on the mode of patient transportation and the capabilities of the receiving hospital:
- Medical System Goals: EMS Transport (Recommended):
- If EMS has fibrinolytic capability and the patient qualifies for therapy, prehospital fibrinolysis should be started within 30 min of arrival of EMS on the scene.
  - If EMS is not capable of administering prehospital fibrinolysis and the patient is transported to a non-PCI-capable hospital, the door-to-needle time should be within 30 min for patients for whom fibrinolysis is indicated.
  - If EMS is not capable of administering prehospital fibrinolysis and the patient is transported to a PCI-capable hospital, the EMS arrival-to-balloon time should be within 90 min.
  - If EMS takes the patient to a non-PCI-capable hospital, it is appropriate to consider emergency interhospital transfer of the patient to a PCI-capable hospital for mechanical revascularization if:
  – There is a contraindication to fibrinolysis.
  – PCI can be initiated promptly within 90 min from EMS arrival-to-balloon time at the PCI-capable hospital. EMS Arrival→Transport to non-PCI-capable hospital→Arrival at non-PCI-capable hospital to transfer to PCI-capable hospital→Arrival at PCI-capable hospital-to-balloon time = 90 min.
  – Fibrinolysis is administered and is unsuccessful (i.e., "rescue PCI").

- Patient Self-Transport (Discouraged):
- If the patient arrives at a non-PCI-capable hospital, the door-to-needle time should be within 30 min of arrival at the emergency department.
- If the patient arrives at a PCI-capable hospital, the door-to-balloon time should be within 90 min.
- If the patient presents to a non-PCI-capable hospital, it is appropriate to consider emergency interhospital transfer of the patient to a PCI-capable hospital if:
  – There is a contraindication to fibrinolysis.
  – PCI can be initiated within 90 min after the patient presented to the initial receiving hospital or within 60 min compared with when fibrinolysis with a fibrin-specific agent could be initiated at the initial receiving hospital.
  – Fibrinolysis is administered and is unsuccessful (i.e., "rescue PCI").

The medical system goal is to facilitate rapid recognition and treatment of patients with STEMI so that door-to-needle (or medical contact-to-needle) for initiation of fibrinolytic therapy can be achieved within 30 min or door-to-balloon (or medical contact-to-balloon) for PCI can be achieved within 90 min. These goals should not be understood as "ideal" times but rather the longest times that should be considered acceptable for a given system. Systems that are able to achieve even more rapid times for treatment of patients with STEMI should be encouraged. Note "medical contact" is defined as "time of EMS arrival on scene" after the patient calls EMS/9-1-1 or "time of arrival at the emergency department door" (whether PCI-capable or non-PCI-capable hospital) when the patient transports himself/herself to the hospital. EMS indicates emergency medical system. PCI, percutaneous coronary intervention; STEMI, ST-elevation myocardial infarction. Source: Antman et al. (2007).

have complex effects on both the heart and extracardiac tissues (figure 88.10). In many patients they either are ineffective in controlling the arrhythmia and/or produce unacceptable toxicity. Noteworthy exceptions to the dismal track record of antiarrhythmics are (1) the complementary role of beta blockers to device therapy in patients

with IHD and life-threatening ventricular arrhythmias and (2) the utility of beta blockers and calcium channel blockers for controlling the speed of the ventricular rate in atrial fibrillation.

The common forms of paroxysmal supraventricular tachycardia are AV nodal reentrant tachycardia, atrioventricular

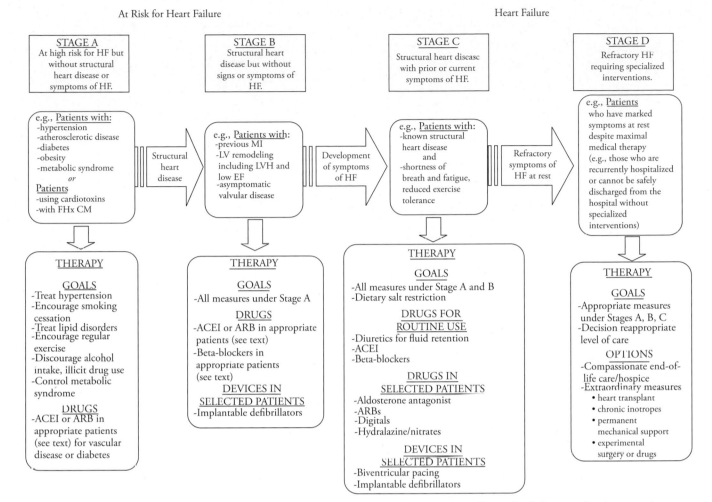

At Risk for Heart Failure   **Heart Failure**

STAGE A
At high risk for HF but without structural heart disease or symptoms of HF.

STAGE B
Structural heart disease but without signs or symptoms of HF.

STAGE C
Structural heart disease with prior or current symptoms of HF.

STAGE D
Refractory HF requiring specialized interventions.

e.g., Patients with:
-hypertension
-atherosclerotic disease
-diabetes
-obesity
-metabolic syndrome
        or
Patients
-using cardiotoxins
-with FHx CM

→ Structural heart disease →

e.g., Patients with:
-previous MI
-LV remodeling including LVH and low EF
-asymptomatic valvular disease

→ Development of symptoms of HF →

e.g., Patients with:
-known structural heart disease
        and
-shortness of breath and fatigue, reduced exercise tolerance

→ Refractory symptoms of HF at rest →

e.g., Patients who have marked symptoms at rest despite maximal medical therapy (e.g., those who are recurrently hospitalized or cannot be safely discharged from the hospital without specialized interventions)

THERAPY

GOALS
-Treat hypertension
-Encourage smoking cessation
-Treat lipid disorders
-Encourage regular exercise
-Discourage alcohol intake, illicit drug use
-Control metabolic syndrome

DRUGS
-ACEI or ARB in appropriate patients (see text) for vascular disease or diabetes

THERAPY

GOALS
-All measures under Stage A

DRUGS
-ACEI or ARB in appropriate patients (see text)
-Beta-blockers in appropriate patients (see text)

DEVICES IN SELECTED PATIENTS
-Implantable defibrillators

THERAPY

GOALS
-All measures under Stage A and B
-Dietary salt restriction

DRUGS FOR ROUTINE USE
-Diuretics for fluid retention
-ACEI
-Beta-blockers

DRUGS IN SELECTED PATIENTS
-Aldosterone antagonist
-ARBs
-Digitals
-Hydralazine/nitrates

DEVICES IN SELECTED PATIENTS
-Biventricular pacing
-Implantable defibrillators

THERAPY

GOALS
-Appropriate measures under Stages A, B, C
-Decision reappropriate level of care

OPTIONS
-Compassionate end-of-life care/hospice
-Extraordinary measures
  • heart transplant
  • chronic inotropes
  • permanent mechanical support
  • experimental surgery or drugs

Figure 88.9. Stages in the Development of Heart Failure: Recommended Therapy by Stage. FHx CM indicates family history of cardiomyopathy; ACEI, angiotensin-converting enzyme inhibitors; and ARB, angiotensin receptor blocker. Reprinted from Hunt SA, Abraham WT, Chin MH, et al. ACC/AHA 2005 guideline update for the diagnosis and management of chronic heart failure in the adult: A report of the American College of Cardiology/American Heart Association Task Force on Practice Guidelines (Writing Committee to Update the 2001 Guidelines for the Evaluation and Management of Heart Failure). *J Am Coll Cardiol.* 2005;46:1–82, with permission from Elsevier.

reentrant tachycardia, and atrial tachycardia. The most common arrhythmia that internists are likely to see is atrial fibrillation (AF).

Clinicians should distinguish a first-detected episode of AF, whether or not it is symptomatic or self-limited, recognizing that there may be uncertainty about the duration of the episode and about previous undetected episodes. AF is considered recurrent when a patient has had two or more episodes. If the arrhythmia terminates spontaneously, recurrent AF is designated paroxysmal; when sustained beyond 7 days, AF is designated persistent. First-detected AF may be either paroxysmal or persistent AF. The category of persistent AF also includes cases of long-standing AF (e.g., >1 year), usually leading to permanent AF.

Contemporary approaches to AF are designated *rhythm control* (where efforts are made to suppress recurrences of AF) and *rate control* (where AF is accepted as the underlying rhythm and efforts are made to slow the ventricular rate while chronic anticoagulation with warfarin to an International Normalized Ratio (INR) 2–3 is used to reduce the risk of

cerebrovascular embolism). A common problem encountered in clinical practice is the decision to initiate anticoagulation in patients for whom cardioversion is planned as part of a rhythm control strategy. Figure 88.11 provides an algorithm to guide the decision making in such circumstances.

Although internists need to maintain familiarity with the diagnosis and management of ventricular arrhythmias, it should be emphasized that contemporary treatment strategies largely involve ablation and implanted devices—approaches that mandate a close working relationship with invasive electrophysiologists. An algorithm for selecting patients for referral for implantation of an ICD for primary or secondary prevention of SCD is shown in figure 88.12.

CONGENITAL HEART DISEASE IN THE ADULT

The most common congenital heart defects that internists are likely to encounter in practice are septal defects (atrial

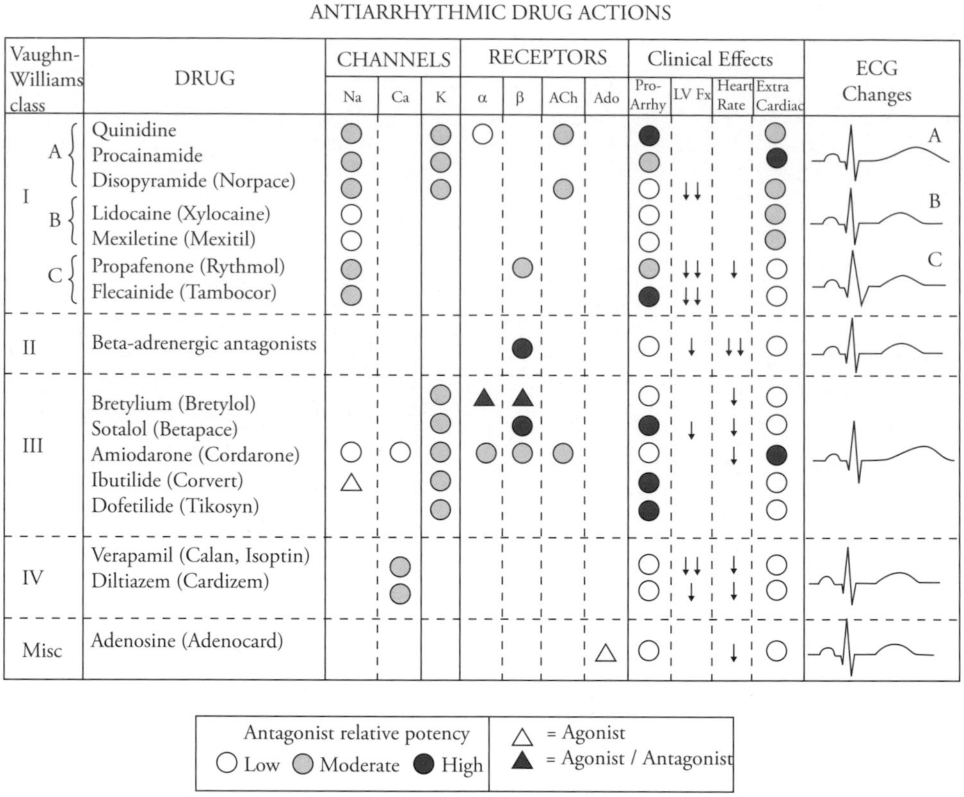

Vaughn-Williams class	DRUG	CHANNELS			RECEPTORS				Clinical Effects				ECG Changes
		Na	Ca	K	α	β	ACh	Ado	Pro-Arrhy	LV Fx	Heart Rate	Extra Cardiac	
I A	Quinidine	◐		◐	○		◐		●			●	A
I A	Procainamide	◐		◐					●			●	
I A	Disopyramide (Norpace)	◐		◐			◐		○	↓↓		◐	
I B	Lidocaine (Xylocaine)	○							○			◐	B
I B	Mexiletine (Mexitil)	○							○			◐	
I C	Propafenone (Rythmol)	◐				◐			◐	↓↓	↓	○	C
I C	Flecainide (Tambocor)	●							●	↓↓		○	
II	Beta-adrenergic antagonists					●			○	↓	↓↓	○	
III	Bretylium (Bretylol)			◐	▲	▲			○		↓	○	
III	Sotalol (Betapace)			◐		●			●	↓	↓	○	
III	Amiodarone (Cordarone)	○	○	◐	◐	◐	◐		○		↓	●	
III	Ibutilide (Corvert)	△		◐					●			○	
III	Dofetilide (Tikosyn)			◐					●			○	
IV	Verapamil (Calan, Isoptin)		◐						○	↓↓	↓	○	
IV	Diltiazem (Cardizem)		◐						○	↓	↓	○	
Misc	Adenosine (Adenocard)							△	○		↓	○	

Antagonist relative potency: ○ Low ◐ Moderate ● High
△ = Agonist ▲ = Agonist / Antagonist

Figure 88.10. Drug Classification System. This is a modification of the Sicilian Gambit drug classification system and includes designation by the Vaughan Williams system. The sodium channel blockers are subdivided into the A, B, and C subgroups based on their relative potency. The targets of antiarrhythmic drugs are listed across the top in columns. These targets are the ion channels—sodium, calcium, and potassium—and the receptors, alpha-adrenergic, beta-adrenergic, cholinergic (ACh), and adenosinergic (Ado). The next columns show a comparison of the clinical actions of the drugs, including proarrhythmic potential (Proarrhy), effect on left ventricular function (LV FX), effects on heart rate (Heart Rate), and potential for extracardiac side effects (Extra Cardiac). The electrocardiographic tracings indicate the changes that are caused by usual dosages of the drug: PR interval, QRS interval, and QT interval. The drugs are listed in rows with their brand names shown in parentheses. The symbols in the table indicate the relative potency of the drugs as agonists or antagonists. The solid triangle indicates the biphasic effects of bretylium to initially release norepinephrine and act as an agonist and subsequently to block further release and act as an antagonist of adrenergic tone. The number of arrows and their directions indicate the magnitude and direction, respectively, of the effect of the drugs on heart rate and left ventricular function (i.e., inotropy). From Woosley RL, Shirazi F. Arrhythmias/conduction disturbances. In: Antman EM (ed.). *Cardiovascular Therapeutics: A Companion to Braunwald's Heart Disease*, 3rd ed. (p. 434). Copyright Elsevier, 2007. Reprinted with permission.

septal defect [ASD], ventricular septal defect [VSD]), tetralogy of Fallot, transposition of the great arteries, and coarctation of the aorta. With improvements in management early in life, *many* individuals with hypoplastic left heart syndrome are now surviving into adulthood. Patients with congenital heart disease frequently will have undergone one or more cardiac surgical procedures, either palliative or for repair of a defect (table 88.3). Advances in catheter-based techniques have led to the percutaneous placement of devices (e.g., clamshell occluder for ASD) in many patients with congenital heart disease.

Communications between the systemic and pulmonary circulations may result in left-to-right and/or right-to-left shunting of blood. Because of the finite possibility of right-to-left shunting in patients with predominant left-to-right shunting, filters should be placed in intravenous lines to trap particulate matter. Patients with right-to-left shunting may develop cyanosis of the skin and mucous membranes

with clubbing of the nailbeds, an increase in erythrocyte mass/blood volume, renal dysfunction, diminished exercise capacity, and increased risk of cerebrovascular accidents as well as cognitive impairment.

Patients with unrepaired cyanotic congenital heart disease, those within 6 months of a completely repaired defect with prosthetic material or devices (surgically or percutaneously placed), and those with repaired defects but who have a residual defect at the site of or adjacent to a prosthetic patch or device are at risk for endocarditis and should receive antibiotic prophylaxis at the time of dental procedures.

Pulmonary arterial hypertension (PAH) may develop in familial and nonfamilial (idiopathic) forms. PAR is also seen secondary to a variety of rheumatological disorders, congenital heart defects with large left-to-right shunts, chronic thromboembolic disease, interstitial lung disease, and a range of lesions that result in left atrial hypertension.

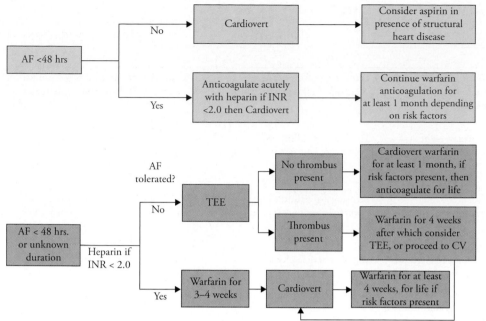

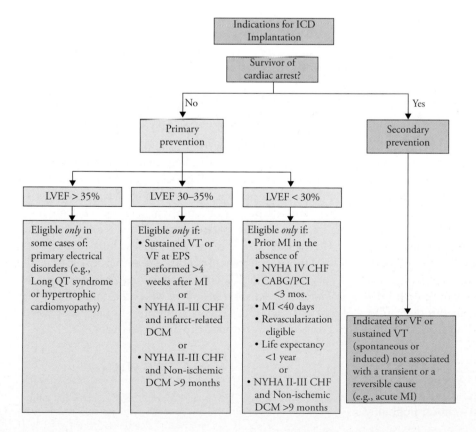

Figure 88.11. Algorithm for Anticoagulant Therapy Pericardioversion. From Zimetbaum P, Falk RH. Atrial fibrillation. In: Antman EM (ed.). *Cardiovascular Therapeutics: A Companion to Braunwald's Heart Disease,* 3rd ed. (p. 497). Copyright Elsevier, 2007. Reprinted with permission.

Current models of idiopathic PAH (iPAH) suggest there are abnormalities in the endothelial, nitric oxide, and prostacyclin pathways that result in inflammatory triggers. This has led to the introduction of endothelin receptor antagonists, exogenous nitric oxide, phosphodiesterase type 5 inhibitors, and prostacyclin derivatives as therapeutic approaches to iPAH.

PERICARDIAL DISEASE

Acute pericarditis is characterized by chest pain, a friction rub, and diffuse PR-segment/ST-T-wave abnormalities on the EKG. It is important to distinguish the chest pain of pericarditis from that of myocardial ischemia. A useful distinguishing feature is the fact that pericardial discomfort

Figure 88.12. Algorithm for Indications for ICD Implantation. CABG/PCI, coronary artery bypass graft/percutaneous coronary intervention; CHF, congestive heart failure; DCM, dilated cardiomyopathy; ICD, implantable cardioverter-defibrillator; LVEF, left ventricular ejection fraction; MI, myocardial infarction; NYHA, New York Heart Association; VF, ventricular fibrillation; VT, ventricular tachycardia. From Arora R, Frisch DR, Kadish AH. The role of implantable cardioverter-defibrillators in primary and secondary prevention of sudden cardiac death. In: Antman EM (ed.). *Cardiovascular Therapeutics: A Companion to Braunwald's Heart Disease,* 3rd ed. (p. 469). Copyright Elsevier, 2007.

Table 88.3 SURGICAL APPROACHES TO TETRALOGY OF FALLOT

NAME	PROCEDURE	INDICATION	LONG-TERM COMPLICATIONS
Palliation			
Black-Taussig shunt	Anastomosis of divided sub-clavian artery to right or left pulmonary artery	Tetralogy of Fallot, single ventricle/pulmonary stenosis	Pulmonary vascular disease, pulmo-nary artery distortion, ventricular volume overload, decreased ventricu-lar function
Waterston shunt	Ascending aorta to right pulmonary artery anastomosis	Tetralogy of Fallot, single ventricle/pulmonary stenosis	Pulmonary vascular disease, pulmo-nary artery distortion, ventricular volume overload, and decreased ventricular function
Potts shunt	Ascending aorta to right pulmonary artery anastomosis	Tetralogy of Fallot, single ventricle/pulmonary stenosis	Pulmonary vascular disease, pulmo-nary artery distortion, ventricular volume overload, and decreased ventricular function
Classic Glenn anastomosis	Superior vena cava to right pul-monary artery anastomosis	Single-ventricle physiology	Pulmonary arteriovenous malforma-tions, cyanosis
Bidirectional Glenn	Superior vena cava to right pulmonary artery anastomosis, pulmonary arteries in continuity	Single-ventricle physiology	Cyanosis
Repair			
Mustard procedure	Atrial baffle	D-transposition of the great arteries	Arrhythmias, decreased systemic right ventricular function, baffle leak, baffle obstruction, abnormal atrial volume conduction
Senning operation	Atrial baffle	D-transposition of the great arteries	See Mustard procedure
Rastelli operation	Intraventricular repair and right ventricle-to-pulmonary artery conduit	D-transposition of the great arteries/ventricular septal defect/left ven-tricular outflow tract obstruction	Conduit obstruction, myocardial dysfunction, arrhythmia
Fontan procedure	Atriopulmonary or total cavopulmonary connection for separation of systemic and pulmonary circulations	Tricuspid atresia, single-ventricle physiology	Arrhythmia, thrombus, protein-losing enteropathy, atrial distortion and abnormal volume conduction, baffle leak
Ross operation	Aortic valve replacement with native pulmonary valve, pulmonary homograft	Aortic stenosis, aortic regurgitation	Pulmonary regurgitation, homograft obstruction, aortic regurgitation

SOURCE: Modified from Martucci G, Mullen M, Landzberg MJ. Care for adults with congenital heart disease. In: Antman EM (ed.), *Cardiovascular Therapeutics: A Companion to Braunwald's Heart Disease*, 3rd ed, (p. 733). Philadelphia: WB Saunders/Elsevier, 2007.

frequently radiates to the trapezius muscle(s), whereas this is not seen with ischemic discomfort. Pericarditis typically responds to treatment with nonsteroidal anti-inflammatory drugs (NSAIDs), possibly with colchicine supplementation. Efforts should be made to avoid corticosteroids in acute peri-carditis because of the risk of precipitating a pattern of recur-rent episodes of pericarditis over an extended period of time.

Pericardial effusions typically do not require drainage unless there is suspicion of tamponade, an underlying infec-tion, or malignant invasion of the pericardium. Pericardial drainage can be accomplished by percutaneous pericardio-centesis, subxiphoid or balloon pericardiotomy, or an open surgical procedure.

Constrictive pericarditis may develop following cardiac trauma/surgery, infection (e.g., tuberculosis), or malignant invasion (e.g., neoplasms of the lung and breast) or may be idiopathic. Imaging studies such as echocardiography,

computed tomography (CT), and magnetic resonance imaging (MRI) scans may be helpful in identifying the pres-ence of a thickened, scarred pericardium. Pericardectomy is the definitive treatment for hemodynamically compromis-ing constrictive pericarditis, but symptomatic relief and nor-malization of cardiac pressures may take several months.

In addition to the conditions discussed above, internists should also be aware that pericardial disease can be seen in a vari-ety of general medical conditions including infections, myocar-dial infection, radiation treatment where the port involves the heart, renal failure, myxedema, connective-tissue disorders, and as a consequence of exposure to drugs and toxins.

ADDITIONAL READING

Anderson JL, Adams CD, Antman EM, et al. ACC/AHA 2007 guide-lines for the management of patients with unstable angina/non

ST-elevation myocardial infarction: A report of the American College of Cardiology/American Heart Association Task Force on Practice Guidelines (Writing Committee to Revise the 2002 Guidelines for the Management of Patients with Unstable Angina/Non ST-Elevation Myocardial Infarction) *Circulation.* 2007;116:e148–304.

Antman EM, Anbe DT, Armstrong PW, et al. ACC/AHA guidelines for the management of patients with ST-elevation myocardial infarction: A report of the American College of Cardiology/American Heart Association Task Force on Practice Guidelines (Committee to Revise the 1999 Guidelines for the Management of Patients with Acute Myocardial Infarction). *Circulation.* 2004;110:e82–292.

Antman EM, Bettett JS, Daugherty A, et al. Use of nonsteroidal anti-inflammatory drugs: An update for clinicians: A scientific statement from the American Heart Association. *Circulation.* 2007;115:1634–42.

Antman EM, Braunwald E. ST-Segment Elevation Myocardial Infarction. In Fauci AS, Kasper DL, Longo DL, et al. (eds.), *Harrison's Principles of Internal Medicine.* 17th ed. (pp. 1532–44). New York: McGraw-Hill; 2008.

Antman EM, Hand M, Armstrong PW, et al. 2007 focused update of the ACC/AHA 2004 Guidelines for the Management of Patients with ST-Elevation Myocardial Infarction. *Circulation.* 2008;117:296–329.

Antman EM, Loscalzo J. Ischemic Heart Disease. In: Fauci AS, Kasper DL, Longo DL, et al. (eds.) *Harrison's Principles of Internal Medicine.* 17th ed. (pp. 1514–27). New York: McGraw-Hill; 2008.

Chobanian AV, Bakris GL, Black HR, et al. The seventh report of the Joint National Committee on Prevention, Detection, Evaluation, and Treatment of High Blood Pressure: The JNC 7 report. *JAMA.* 2003;289:2560–72.

Executive summary of the third report of the National Cholesterol Education Program (NCEP) Expert Panel on Detection, Evaluation, and Treatment of High Blood Cholesterol in Adults (Adult Treatment Panel III). *JAMA.* 2001;285:2486–97.

Fuster V, Ryden LE, Cannom DS, et al. ACC/AHA/ESC 2006 Guidelines for the Management of Patients with Atrial Fibrillation. *Circulation.* 2006;114:e257–354.

Humbert M, Sitbon I, Simonneau S. Treatment of pulmonary arterial hypertension. *N Engl J Med.* 2004;351:1425–36.

Maisch B, Seferovic PM, Ristic AD, et al. Guidelines on the diagnosis and management of pericardial diseases executive summary: The Task Force on the Diagnosis and Management of Pericardial Diseases of the European Society of Cardiology. *Eur Heart J.* 2004;25:587–610.

Musco S, Conway EL, Kowey PR. Drug therapy for atrial fibrillation. *Med Clin North Am.* 2008;92:121–41, xi.

Rosamond W, Flegal K, Furie K, et al. Heart disease and stroke statistics—2008 update: A report from the American Heart Association Statistics Committee and Stroke Statistics Subcommittee. *Circulation.* 2008;117:e25–146.

Smith SC, Jr., Allen J, Blair SN, et al. AHA/ACC Guidelines for Secondary Prevention for Patients with Coronary and Other Atherosclerotic Vascular Disease: 2006 update. *Circulation.* 2006;113:2363–72.

Wilson W, Taubert KA, Gewitz M, et al. Prevention of infective endocarditis. *Circulation.* 2007;116:1736–1754.

Zipes DP, Camm AJ, Borggrefe M, et al. ACC/AHA/ESC 2006 Guidelines for Management of Patients with Ventricular Arrhythmias and the Prevention of Sudden Cardiac Death. *Circulation.* 2006;114:e385–484.

SECTION 9

NEUROLOGY

89.

THE SCREENING NEUROLOGICAL EXAMINATION

Galen V. Henderson

The neurological examination is not challenging or complex. It does have many components and includes a number of skills that can be mastered only through repetition of the same techniques on a large number of individuals with and without neurological disease. Please remember that the purpose of the examination is to simply localize the lesion. Based on patient history alone, 80% of lesion locations should be known, and then a very specific neurological examination is performed to confirm the location. The examination is the less time consuming of the two parts of the patient's neurological evaluation.

KNOWLEDGE OF EXAMINATION BASICS ESSENTIAL FOR ALL CLINICIANS

There is no single, universally accepted sequence of the examination that must be followed, but most clinicians begin with assessment of mental status followed by the cranial nerves, motor system, sensory system, coordination, and gait (see table 89.1). If this is not how the information is obtained, it is usually how the examination is documented. Whether the examination is basic or comprehensive, it is essential that it be performed in an orderly and systematic fashion to avoid errors and serious omissions. Thus, the best way to learn and gain expertise in the examination is to choose one's own approach and practice it frequently and do it in the same exact sequence each time.

The detailed description of the neurological examination that follows describes the most commonly used parts of the examination, with a particular emphasis on the components that are considered most helpful for the assessment of common neurological problems. Each section also includes a brief description of the minimal examination necessary for adequate screening for abnormalities in a patient who has no symptoms suggesting neurological dysfunction. A screening examination can be performed in 3–5 minutes in the office.

MENTAL STATUS EXAMINATION

The mental status examination starts as soon as the physician begins observing and talking with the patient. If there is a history that raises any concern for abnormalities of higher cortical function or if cognitive problems are observed during the interview, then detailed testing of the mental status is indicated.

The Montreal Cognitive Assessment (MoCA) is a standardized screening examination of cognitive function that is extremely easy to administer and takes a few minutes to complete. MoCA was designed as a rapid screening instrument for mild cognitive dysfunction. It assesses different cognitive domains: attention and concentration, executive functions, memory, language, visuoconstructional skills, conceptual thinking, calculations, and orientation. Time to administer the MoCA is approximately 10 minutes. The total possible score is 30 points; a score of 26 or above is considered normal.

Individual elements of the mental status examination can be subdivided into level of consciousness, orientation, speech and language, memory, fund of information, insight and judgment, abstract thought, and calculations.

Level of consciousness is the patient's relative state of awareness of the self and the environment; it ranges from fully awake to comatose. Since this chapter pertains to office practice, this will not be discussed in greater detail.

Orientation is tested by asking the person to state his or her name, location, and time (day of the week and date).

Speech is assessed by observing articulation, rate, rhythm, and prosody (i.e., the changes in pitch and accentuation of syllable and words).

Calculation ability is a test of attention and is assessed by having the patient carry out a computation that is appropriate to the patient's age and education (e.g., serial subtraction of 7 from 100 or 3 from 20; or word problems involving simple arithmetic). If that is too difficult for the patient, we have the patient spell the word "WORLD" forward and then backward. Or, have the patient count from 20 to 1 without errors.

Table 89.1 LOCALIZATON OF FOREBRAIN LESIONS

SITE	FINDINGS
Left frontal lobe	Anterior aphasia (Broca, transcortical motor), aphemia Ideomotor apraxia Decreased voluntary rightward saccades, left gaze preference Right hemiparesis, increased deep tendon reflexes and Babinski sign
Right frontal lobe	Motor neglect of the left world Ideomotor apraxia Decreased voluntary leftward saccades, right gaze preference Right hemiparesis, increased deep tendon reflexes, and Babinski sign
Bilateral frontal lobes	Perseveration, impersistence, stimulus-bound responses Impaired executive functions—planning, sequencing, judgment, insight, abstract reasoning Impaired motor (Luria) sequencing Snout, root, grasp, and palmomental reflexes Gegenhalten (paratonic rigidity)
Orbitofrontal	Disinhibition, aggressive impulsivity Anosmia Memory disturbance
Frontal convexity	Abulia—akinetic mutism Incontinence "Magnetic" gait
Midline frontal	Bilateral leg weakness Behavioral changes (cingulated gyrus)
Left parietal	Right cortical sensory loss (astereognosis, agraphesthesia, decreased two-point discrimination) Anomic aphasia, transcortical sensory aphasia, dysgraphia, dyscalculia, left-right disorientation, finger agnosia Right inferior quadranopsia
Right parietal	Left cortical sensory loss (as above) Left-sided neglect, anisognosis, constructional apraxia, dressing apraxia Left inferior quadranopsia
Left temporal lobe	"Posterior" aphasia (Wernicke's aphasia, transcortical sensory) Conduction aphasia Amnesia for verbal material (usually bilateral lesions) Right superior quadranopsia
Right temporal lobe	Dysprosody, amusia, nonverbal auditory agnosia Amnesia for nonverbal material (usually bilateral lesions) Left superior quadranopsia
Bilateral temporal lobes	
Medial	Amnesia
Perisylvian	Cortical deafness, auditory agnosia
Occipital lobes	
Left	Contralateral homonymous hemianopsia (macular sparing) Cortical blindness
Parieto-occipital	Alexia without agraphia (requires a lesion of the splenium of corpus callosum)
Temporo-occipital	Balint syndrome (simultanagnosia, optic ataxia, ocular apraxia)—impaired visuospatial localization Visual agnosia (including prosopagnosia, color agnosia, achromatopsia) Visual amnesia Confusional state
Thalamus	Agitated confusional state Decreased level of consciousness Amnesia Aphasia (transcortical sensory) Hemisensory loss Cerebellar ataxia
Basal ganglia	Parkinsonian syndrome Aphasia (transcortical motor) Hyperkinetic syndromes (e.g., hemiballismus with subthalamic nucleus infarction

Language is assessed by observing the content of the patient's verbal and written output, response to spoken commands, and ability to read. A typical testing sequence is to ask the patient to name successively more detailed components of clothing, a watch or a pen; repeat the phrase "No ifs, ands, or buts"; follow a three-step, verbal command; write a sentence; and read and respond to a written command.

Memory should be analyzed according to three main time scales: (1) immediate memory can be tested by saying a list of three items and having the patient repeat the list immediately, (2) short-term memory is assessed by asking the patient to recall the same three items 5 and 15 minutes later, and (3) long-term memory is evaluated by determining how well the patient is able to provide a coherent chronologic history of his or her illness or personal events.

CRANIAL NERVE EXAMINATION: BRAINSTEM LESIONS

The cranial nerves (CN) are best examined in numerical order, except for grouping together CN III, IV, and VI because of their similar function (see table 89.2).

CN I (OLFACTORY)

With eyes closed, ask the patient to sniff in alternating nostril a mild stimulus such as toothpaste, deodorant, or coffee.

This is very commonly abnormal in Parkinson disease or in inferior frontal lobe disease such as a brain tumor.

CN II (OPTIC)

Check visual acuity (with eyeglasses or contact lens correction) using a Snellen chart or similar tool. Test the visual fields by confrontation, that is, by comparing the patient's visual fields to your own. Individual eye fields should be tested. Face the patient at a distance of approximately 2–3 ft and place your hands at the periphery of your visual fields in the plane that is equidistant between you and the patient. Instruct the patient to look directly at the center of your corresponding eye or face and to indicate when and where he or she sees one of your fingers moving. Beginning with the two inferior quadrants and then the two superior quadrants, move your index finger of the right hand, left hand, or both hands simultaneously and observe whether the patient detects the movements. A single small-amplitude movement of the finger is sufficient for a normal response. Focal perimetry and tangent screen examinations should be used to map out visual field defects fully or to search for subtle abnormalities. Optic fundi should be examined with an ophthalmoscope, and the color, size, and degree of swelling or elevation of the optic disk noted, as well as the color and texture of the retina. The retinal vessels should be checked for size, regularity, arterial-venous nicking at crossing points, hemorrhage, exudates, and so forth.

Table 89.2 LOCALIZATION OF BRAINSTEM LESIONS

SITE	FINDING
Midbrain	
Tectum and Pretectum	Parinaud syndrome—large pupils with near-light dissociation, convergence-retraction nystagmus, impaired upgaze, eyelid retraction
	Abnormal pupils—midrange, unequal, irregularly shaped, impaired vertical eye movements
	Anterior INO
	Skew deviation
	Decreased arousal
	Nuclear CN III lesions (including bilateral ptosis and superior rectus deficits)
Tegmentum	Nuclear CN IV lesions (contralateral superior rectus deficits)
Central peduncles	Weber syndrome (ipsilateral CNIII, contralateral hemiparesis)
Red nucleus	Benedikt syndrome (ipsilateral CN III, contralateral tremor)
Ascending cerebellar fibers	Claude syndrome (ipsilateral CN III, contralateral cerebellar ataxia)
Pons	
Tegmentum	Ipsilateral gaze palsy ("wrong way eyes")
	Intranuclear ophthalmoplegia
	One and a half syndrome
	Skew deviation
	CN V, VI, VII, and VIII lesions
Basis pontis	Contralateral hemiparesis
	Contralateral ataxia
	Dysarthria
Medulla	
Lateral	Wallenberg syndrome (ipsilateral CN V, ipsilateral Horner syndrome, contralateral loss of pain and temperature below the neck [spinothalamic tract], vertigo, ipsilateral nystagmus, ipsilateral CN IX and X deficits, skew deviation)
Medial	Ipsilateral CN XII deficit, contralateral hemiparesis, contralateral medial lemniscus dificit (joint position and vibration)

CN III, IV, VI (OCULOMOTOR, TROCHLEAR, ABDUCENS)

Describe the size and shape of pupils and reaction to light and accommodation (i.e., as the eyes converge while following your finger as it moves toward the bridge of the nose). To check extraocular movements, ask the patient to keep his or her head still while tracking the movement of the tip of your finger. Move the target slowly in the horizontal and vertical planes; observe any paresis, nystagmus, or abnormalities of smooth pursuit (saccades, oculomotor ataxia, etc.). However, in practice it is typically more useful to determine whether the patient describes diplopia in any direction of gaze; diplopia of neurological origin should almost always resolve with one eye closed.

CN V (TRIGEMINAL)

Examine sensation within the three territories of the branches of the trigeminal nerve (ophthalmic, maxillary, and mandibular) on each side of the face. As with other parts of the sensory examination, testing of two sensory modalities derived from different anatomic pathways (e.g., light touch and temperature) is sufficient for a screening examination. Testing of other modalities, the corneal reflex (combination of CN V for sensory and CN VII for motor), and the motor component of CN V (jaw clench—masseter muscle) is indicated when suggested by the history.

CN VII (FACIAL)

Look for facial asymmetry at rest and with spontaneous movements. Test eyebrow elevation, forehead wrinkling, eye closure, smiling, and cheek puff. Look in particular for differences in the lower versus upper facial muscles; weakness of the lower two-thirds of the face with preservation of the upper third suggests an upper motor neuron lesion, whereas weakness of an entire side suggests a lower motor neuron lesion.

CN VIII (VESTIBULOCOCHLEAR)

Check the patient's ability to hear a finger rub or whispered voice with each ear. Further testing is not usually warranted. To determine whether the hearing loss is sensorineural or conductive, Rinne or Webber testing can be done.

CN IX, X (GLOSSOPHARYNGEAL, VAGUS)

Observe the position and symmetry of the palate and uvula at rest and with phonation ("aah"). The pharyngeal ("gag") reflex is evaluated by stimulating the posterior pharyngeal wall on each side with a sterile, blunt object (e.g., tongue blade), but the reflex is often absent in normal individuals. It has been estimated that 10% of patients as they become older, lose the ability to have a gag. This usually has no clinical implication in the awake patient.

CN XI (SPINAL ACCESSORY)

Check shoulder shrug (trapezius muscle) and head rotation to each side (sternocleidomastoid) against resistance.

CN XII (HYPOGLOSSAL)

Inspect the tongue for atrophy or fasciculations, position with protrusion, and strength when extended against the inner surface of the cheeks on each side. When the tongue is protruded, if there is weakness, it points to the side of weakness.

MOTOR EXAMINATION

The motor examination includes observations of muscle appearance, tone, strength, and reflexes. Although gait is in part a test of motor function, it is usually evaluated separately at the end of the examination.

APPEARANCE

Inspect and palpate muscle groups under good light and with the patient in a comfortable and symmetric position. Check for muscle fasciculations, tenderness, and atrophy or hypertrophy. Involuntary movements may be present at rest (e.g., tics, myoclonus, choreoathetosis), during maintained posture (pill-rolling tremor of Parkinson disease), or with voluntary movements (intention tremor of cerebellar disease or familial tremor).

TONE

Muscle tone is tested by measuring the resistance to passive movement of a relaxed limb. In the upper limbs tone is assessed by rapid pronation and supination of the forearm and flexion and extension at the wrist. In the lower limbs, while the patient is supine the examiner's hands are placed behind the knees and rapidly raised; with normal tone the ankles drag along the table surface for a variable distance before rising, whereas increased tone results in an immediate lift of the heel off the surface. Decreased tone is most commonly due to lower motor neuron or peripheral nerve disorders. Increased tone may be evident as spasticity (resistance determined by the angle and velocity of motion; corticospinal tract disease), rigidity (similar resistance in all angles of motion; extrapyramidal disease), or paratonia (fluctuating changes in resistance; frontal lobe pathways or normal difficulty in relaxing). Cogwheel rigidity, in which passive motion elicits jerky interruptions in resistance, is seen in parkinsonism.

STRENGTH

Testing for pronator drift is an extremely useful method for screening upper-limb weakness. The patient is asked to hold both arms fully extended and parallel to the ground with eyes closed. This position should be maintained for approximately 10 seconds; any flexion at the elbow or fingers or pronation of the forearm, especially if asymmetric, is a sign of potential weakness. Muscle strength is further assessed by having the patient exert maximal effort for the particular muscle or muscle group being tested. It is important to isolate the muscles as much as possible, that is, hold the limb so that only the muscles of interest are active. It is also helpful to palpate accessible muscles as they contract. Grading muscle strength and evaluating the patient's effort is an art that takes time and practice. Muscle strength is traditionally graded using the following scale:

0 = no movement

1 = flicker or trace of contraction but no associated movement at a joint

2 = movement with gravity eliminated

3 = movement against gravity but not against resistance

4− = movement against a mild degree of resistance

4 = movement against moderate resistance

4+ = movement against strong resistance

5 = full power

However, in many cases it is more practical to use the following terms:

Paralysis = no movement

Severe weakness = movement with gravity eliminated

Moderate weakness = movement against gravity but not against mild resistance

Mild weakness = movement against moderate resistance

Full strength

Noting the pattern of weakness is as important as assessing the magnitude of weakness. Unilateral or bilateral weakness of the upper-limb extensors and lower-limb flexors (pyramidal weakness) suggests a lesion of the pyramidal tract; bilateral proximal weakness suggests myopathy; and bilateral distal weakness suggests peripheral neuropathy.

REFLEXES

Those that are typically assessed include the biceps (**C5**, C6), brachioradialis (C5, **C6**), and triceps (**C7**, C8) reflexes in the upper limbs and the patellar or quadriceps (**L3**, L4) and Achilles (**S1**, S2) reflexes in the lower limbs. The patient should be relaxed, and the muscle positioned midway between full contraction and extension. Reflexes may be enhanced by asking the patient to voluntarily contract other, distant muscle groups (Jendrassik maneuver): for example, the patellar reflex is tested by hooking the flexed fingers of the two hands together and attempting to pull them apart. For each reflex tested, the two sides should be tested sequentially, and it is important to determine the smallest stimulus required to elicit a reflex rather than the maximum response. Reflexes are graded according to the following scale:

0 = absent

1 = present but diminished

2 = normoactive

3 = exaggerated

4 = clonus

SENSORY EXAMINATION

Evaluating sensation is usually the most unreliable part of the examination, because sensation is subjective and is difficult to quantify. In the compliant and discerning patient, the sensory examination can be extremely helpful for the precise localization of a lesion. With patients who are uncooperative or lack an understanding of the tests, it may be useless. The examination should be focused on the suspected lesion. For example, in spinal cord, spinal root, or peripheral nerve abnormalities, all major sensory modalities should be tested while looking for a pattern consistent with a spinal level and dermatomal or nerve distribution. In patients with lesions at or above the brainstem, screening the primary sensory modalities in the distal extremities along with tests of cortical sensation are usually sufficient.

The five primary sensory modalities—light touch, pain, temperature, vibration, and joint position—are tested in each limb. Light touch is assessed by stimulating the skin with single, very gentle touches of the examiner's finger or a wisp of cotton. Pain is tested using a new pin, and temperature is assessed using a metal object (e.g., tuning fork) that has been immersed in cold and warm water. Vibration is tested using a 128-Hz tuning fork applied to the distal phalanx of the great toe or index finger just below the nailbed. By placing a finger on the opposite side of the joint being tested, the examiner compares the patient's threshold of vibration perception with his or her own. For joint position testing, the examiner grasps the digit or limb laterally and distal to the joint being assessed; small 1- to 2-mm excursions can usually be sensed. The Romberg maneuver is primarily a test of proprioception. The patient is asked to stand with the feet as close together as necessary to maintain balance while the

Table 89.3 LOCALIZATION OF CEREBELLAR LESIONS

SITE	FINDING
Cerebellar hemisphere	Ipsilateral ataxia (intention tremor, dysdiadochokinesia, dysmetria)
Midline	Gait ataxia with widened base
	Truncal titubation
	Dysarthria (ataxic speech)
Vestibulocerebellum	Abnormal eye movements, skew deviation, hypo-, and hypermetric saccades, micro and macro square wave jerks, breakdown of smooth pursuit movements, opsoclonus,
	Contralateral head tilt (cerebellopontine angle tumor)

eyes are open, and the eyes are then closed. A loss of balance with the eyes closed is an abnormal response.

Cortical sensation is mediated by the parietal lobes and represents an integration of the primary sensory modalities; testing cortical sensation is meaningful only when primary sensation is intact. Double simultaneous stimulation is especially useful as a screening test for cortical function; with the patient's eyes closed, the examiner lightly touches one or both hands and asks the patient to identify the stimuli. With a parietal lobe lesion, the patient may be unable to identify the stimulus on the contralateral side when both hands are touched. Other modalities relying on the parietal cortex include the discrimination of two closely placed stimuli as separate (two-point discrimination), identification of an object by touch and manipulation alone (stereognosis), and the identification of numbers or letters written on the skin surface (graphesthesia).

COORDINATION EXAMINATION: CEREBELLUM OR ITS BRAINSTEM CONNECTIONS

Coordination refers to the orchestration and fluidity of movements. Even simple acts require cooperation of agonist and antagonist muscles, maintenance of posture, and complex servomechanisms to control the rate and range of movements. Part of this integration relies on normal function of the cerebellar and basal ganglia systems. However, coordination also requires intact muscle strength and kinesthetic and proprioceptive information. Thus, if the examination has disclosed abnormalities of the motor or sensory systems, the patient's coordination should be assessed with these limitations in mind (table 89.3).

Rapid alternating movements in the upper limbs are tested separately on each side by having the patient make a fist, partially extend the index finger, and then tap the index finger on the distal thumb as quickly as possible. In the lower limb, the patient rapidly taps the foot against the floor or the examiner's hand. Finger-to-nose testing is primarily a test of cerebellar function; the patient is asked to touch his or her index finger repetitively to the nose and then to the examiner's outstretched finger, which

moves with each repetition. A similar test in the lower extremity is to have the patient raise the leg and touch the examiner's finger with the great toe. Another cerebellar test in the lower limbs is the heel-knee-shin maneuver; in the supine position the patient is asked to slide the heel of each foot from the knee down the shin of the other leg. For all these movements, the accuracy, speed, and rhythm are noted.

GAIT EXAMINATION

Watching the patient walk is the most important part of the neurological examination. Normal gait requires that multiple systems—including strength, sensation, and coordination—function in a highly integrated fashion. Unexpected abnormalities may be detected that prompt the examiner to return, in more detail, to other aspects of the examination. The patient should be observed while walking and turning normally, walking on the heels, walking on the toes, and walking heel-to-toe along a straight line. The examination may reveal decreased arm swing on one side (corticospinal tract disease), a stooped posture and short-stepped gait (parkinsonism), a broad-based unstable gait (ataxia), scissoring (spasticity), or a high-stepped, slapping gait (posterior column or peripheral nerve disease), or the patient may appear to be stuck in place (apraxia with frontal lobe disease).

ADDITIONAL READING

Brazis PW, Masdeu JC, Biller J. *Localization in Clinical Neurology.* Philadelphia: Lippincott Williams & Wilkins, 2007.

Samuels MA, Ropper AH. *Samuels's Manual of Neurologic Therapeutics.* Philadelphia: Lippincott Williams & Wilkins, 2010.

QUESTIONS

QUESTION 1. A 65-year-old white male with a history of type 2 diabetes mellitus and hypertension who was recently diagnosed with sciatica presents to the emergency department with 2 days of progressive difficulty in walking and worsening back pain radiating down to his left leg. Examination shows depressed reflexes and reduced strength in both of his legs. He has saddle paresthesia. His toes are downgoing. His rectal tone is reduced. The most likely diagnosis is:

A. Stroke
B. Sciatica
C. Cauda equina syndrome
D. Acute back pain
E. Spinal abscess

QUESTION 2. A 55-year-old male presents with 1 day of blurred vision and a history of a curtain coming down causing him to transiently lose vision in his right eye. He denies any headache, weakness, or other symptoms. On examination he has a blood pressure of 154/88 mm Hg, heart rate of 72 beats/min, and is alert and oriented. Neurological examination is unremarkable with normal cranial nerves, motor function, and sensory function. What is his most likely diagnosis?

A. Right brainstem stroke
B. Cluster headache
C. Bell's palsy
D. Amaurosis fugax
E. Carotid artery dissection

QUESTION 3. A 74-year-old male presents to the emergency department with left-sided weakness. His examination shows normal cranial nerve examination, no facial droop, and weakness of his left arm and leg, 3/5 strength with ataxia of limb. He keeps asking whether he is. Where is his lesion?

A. Middle cerebral artery
B. Anterior cerebral artery
C. Posterior cerebral artery
D. Basilar artery
E. Carotid artery

ANSWERS

1. C
2. D
3. A

90.

STROKE

Galen V. Henderson

Stroke remains a major healthcare problem. It is estimated that there are >700,000 incident strokes in the United States each year, resulting in >160,000 deaths annually, with 4.8 million stroke survivors alive today. Although there was a 60% decline in stroke mortality over the 29-year period between 1968 and 1996, the rate of decline began to slow in the 1990s and has plateaued in several regions of the country. Despite an overall 3.4% fall in per capita stroke-related mortality between 1991 and 2001, the actual number of stroke deaths rose by 7.7%. Stroke ranks as the country's third leading cause of death. Stroke incidence may be increasing. From 1988 to 1997, the age-adjusted stroke hospitalization rate grew 18.6% (from 560 to 664 per 100,000), while total stroke hospitalizations increased 38.6% (from 592,811 to 821,760 annually). In 2004 the cost of stroke was estimated at $53.6 billion (direct and indirect costs), with a mean lifetime cost estimated at $140,048.

Stroke is also a leading cause of functional impairments, with 20% of survivors requiring institutional care after 3 months and 15%–30% being permanently disabled. Stroke is a life-changing event that affects not only the person who may be disabled but the entire family and other caregivers as well. Utility analyses show that a major stroke is viewed by more than half of those at risk as being worse than death. Despite the advent of treatment of selected patients with acute ischemic stroke with intravenous tissue-type plasminogen activator and the promise of other acute therapies, effective prevention remains the best treatment for reducing the burden of stroke.

Primary prevention is particularly important because >70% of strokes are first events. As discussed in the evidence-based guideline-supported sections that follow, high-risk or stroke-prone individuals can now be identified and targeted for specific interventions for primary prevention and some information regarding secondary prevention treatments and emergency management of ischemic stroke.

RECOMMENDATIONS FOR PRIMARY AND SECONDARY PREVENTION OF ISCHEMIC STROKE

ASSESSING THE RISK OF A FIRST STROKE

Each individual patient should have an assessment of his or her stroke risk The use of a risk-assessment tool such as the Framingham Stroke Profile should be considered, as these tools can help identify individuals who could benefit from therapeutic interventions and who may not be treated based on any individual risk factor.

Genetic Causes of Stroke

Referral for genetic counseling may be considered for patients with rare genetic causes of stroke. There remain insufficient data to recommend genetic screening for the prevention of a first stroke.

Cardiovascular Disease

Persons with evidence of noncerebrovascular atherosclerotic vascular disease (coronary heart disease, cardiac failure, or intermittent claudication) are at increased risk of a first stroke. Treatments used in the management of these other conditions (e.g., platelet antiaggregants) and as recommended in other sections of this guideline can reduce the risk of stroke.

Hypertension

Regular screening for hypertension (at least every 2 years in adults and more frequently in minority populations and the elderly) and appropriate management, including dietary changes, lifestyle modification, and pharmacological therapy by summarized by the Joint National Committee 7 (JNC7), are recommended.

Cigarette Smoking

Abstention from cigarette smoking and smoking cessation for current smokers are recommended. Data from cohort and epidemiological studies are consistent and overwhelming. Avoidance of environmental tobacco smoke for stroke prevention should also be considered. The use of counseling, nicotine products, and oral smoking-cessation medications has been found to be effective for smokers and should be considered.

Diabetes

It is recommended that hypertension be tightly controlled in patients with either type 1 or type 2 diabetes (the JNC7 recommendation of <130/80 mm Hg in diabetic patients is endorsed) as part of a comprehensive risk-reduction program. Treatment of adults with diabetes, especially those with additional risk factors, with a statin to lower the risk of a first stroke is recommended. Recommendations to consider treatment of diabetic patients with an angiotensin-converting enzyme (ACE) inhibitor or angiotensin receptor blocker (ARB) are endorsed.

Atrial Fibrillation

Anticoagulation of patients with atrial fibrillation who have valvular heart disease (particularly those with mechanical heart valves) is recommended. Antithrombotic therapy (warfarin or aspirin) is recommended to prevent stroke in patients with nonvalvular atrial fibrillation based on assessment of their absolute stroke risk and estimated bleeding risk while considering patient preferences and access to high-quality anticoagulation monitoring. Warfarin International Normalized Ratio [INR] 2.0–3.0 is recommended for high-risk (>4% annual risk of stroke) patients (and for most moderate-risk patients according to patient preferences) with atrial fibrillation who have no clinically significant contraindications to oral anticoagulants.

Other Cardiac Conditions

Various practice guidelines recommend strategies to reduce the risk of stroke in patients with a variety of cardiac conditions. These include the management of patients with valvular heart disease, unstable angina, chronic stable angina, and acute myocardial infarction (MI). Strategies to prevent postoperative neurological injury and stroke in patients undergoing surgical revascularization for atherosclerotic heart disease are discussed in detail in the recently published coronary artery bypass graft surgery guidelines. It is reasonable to prescribe warfarin for post–ST-segment–elevation patients with MI and left ventricular (LV) dysfunction with extensive regional wall-motion abnormalities, and warfarin may be considered in patients with severe LV dysfunction with or without congestive heart failure.

DYSLIPIDEMIA

National Cholesterol Education Program III (NCEP III) guidelines for the management of patients who have not had a cerebrovascular event with elevated total cholesterol, or with elevated non-high-density lipoprotein (HDL) cholesterol in the presence of hypertriglyceridemia, are endorsed. It is recommended that patients with known coronary heart disease (CHD) and high-risk hypertensive patients even with normal low-density lipoprotein (LDL) cholesterol levels be treated with lifestyle measures and a statin. The use of lipid-lowering therapy in diabetic patients is specifically addressed in the diabetes section of this guideline. Suggested treatments for patients with known CHD and low HDL cholesterol include weight loss, increased physical activity, smoking cessation, and possibly niacin or gemfibrozil.

ASYMPTOMATIC CAROTID STENOSIS

It is recommended that patients with asymptomatic carotid artery stenosis be screened for other treatable causes of stroke and that intensive therapy of all identified stroke risk factors be pursued. The use of aspirin is recommended unless contraindicated because aspirin was used in all of the cited trials as an antiplatelet drug except in the surgical arm of one study, in which there was a higher rate of MI in those who were not given aspirin. Prophylactic carotid endarterectomy is recommended in highly selected patients with high-grade asymptomatic carotid stenosis performed by surgeons with <3% morbidity/mortality rates. Patient selection should be guided by an assessment of comorbid conditions and life expectancy, as well as other individual factors, and be balanced by an understanding of the overall impact of the procedure if all-cause mortality is considered as one of the endpoints, and it should include a thorough discussion of the risks and benefits of the procedure with an understanding of patient preferences. Carotid angioplasty–stenting might be a reasonable alternative to endarterectomy in asymptomatic patients at high risk for the surgical procedure. However, given the reported periprocedural and overall 1-year event rates, it remains uncertain whether this group of patients should have either procedure.

SICKLE CELL DISEASE

It is recommended that children with sickle cell disease (SCD) be screened with transcranial Doppler (TCD) ultrasound starting at 2 years of age. It is recommended that transfusion therapy be considered for those at elevated stroke risk. Although the optimal screening interval has not been established, it is reasonable that younger children and those with TCD velocities in the conditional range should be rescreened more frequently to detect development of high-risk TCD indications for intervention. Pending further studies it is reasonable to continue transfusion even in those whose TCD velocities revert to normal. Magnetic resonance imaging (MRI) and MR angiography (MRA) criteria for selection of children for primary stroke prevention using transfusion have not been established, and these tests should not be substituted for TCD. Adults with SCD should be evaluated for known stroke risk factors and managed according to the general guidelines in this chapter.

POSTMENOPAUSAL HORMONE THERAPY

It is recommended that postmenopausal hormone therapy (with estrogen with or without a progestin) not be used for primary prevention of stroke. The use of hormone replacement therapy for other indications should be informed by the risk estimate for vascular outcomes provided by the reviewed clinical trials. There are not sufficient data to provide recommendations about the use of other forms of therapy such as selective estrogen receptor modulators.

DIET AND NUTRITION

A reduced intake of sodium and increased intake of potassium are recommended to lower blood pressure in persons with hypertension (class I, level of evidence A), which may thereby reduce the risk of stroke. The recommended sodium intake is ≤2.3 g/day (100 mmol/day), and the recommended potassium intake is ≥4.7 g/day (120 mmol/day). The DASH diet, which emphasizes fruit, vegetables, and low-fat dairy products and is reduced in saturated and total fat, also lowers blood pressure and is recommended. A diet that is rich in fruits and vegetables may lower the risk of stroke and may be considered.

PHYSICAL INACTIVITY

Increased physical activity is recommended because it is associated with a reduction in the risk of stroke. Exercise guidelines as recommended by the Centers for Disease Control (CDC) and the National Institutes of Health (≥30 min of moderate-intensity activity daily) as part of a healthy lifestyle are reasonable.

OBESITY AND BODY FAT DISTRIBUTION

Epidemiological studies indicate that increased body weight and abdominal fat are directly associated with stroke

risk. Weight reduction is recommended because it lowers blood pressure and may thereby reduce the risk of stroke.

METABOLIC SYNDROME

Management of individual components of the metabolic syndrome, including lifestyle measures and pharmacotherapy as recommended in the National Cholesterol Education Program ATP III and the JNC7 as reviewed in other sections of this guideline, are endorsed. Lifestyle management should include exercise, appropriate weight loss, and proper diet. Pharmacotherapy may include medications for blood pressure lowering, lipid lowering, glycemic control, treatment of microalbuminuria or proteinuria, and antiplatelet therapy (e.g., aspirin) according to the individual circumstance and risk. It is not known whether agents that ameliorate aspects of the insulin resistance syndrome are useful for reducing stroke risk.

ALCOHOL ABUSE

Reduction of alcohol consumption in heavy drinkers through established screening and counseling methods as outlined in the U.S. Preventive Services Task Force Update 2004 is endorsed. For those who consume alcohol, a recommendation of no more than two drinks per day for men and one drink per day for nonpregnant women best reflects the state of the science for alcohol and stroke risk.

DRUG ABUSE

Successful identification and management of drug abuse can be challenging. When a patient is identified as having a drug addiction problem, referral for appropriate counseling may be considered.

ORAL CONTRACEPTIVES

The incremental risk of stroke associated with use of low-dose oral contraceptives (OC) in women without additional risk factors appears low, if it exists. It is suggested that OC be discouraged in women with additional risk factors (e.g., cigarette smoking or prior thromboembolic events). For those who elect to assume the increased risk, aggressive therapy of stroke risk factors may be useful.

SLEEP-DISORDERED BREATHING

Sleep-disordered breathing (SDB) is associated with stroke risk. Questioning bed partners and patients, particularly those with abdominal obesity and hypertension, about symptoms of SDB and referral to a sleep specialist for further evaluation as appropriate may be useful, especially in the setting of drug-resistant hypertension.

MIGRAINE

There are insufficient data to recommend a specific treatment approach that would reduce the risk of first stroke in women with migraine, including migraine with aura.

HYPERHOMOCYSTEINEMIA

Recommendations to meet current guidelines for daily intake of folate (400 µg/day), B-6 (1.7 mg/day), and B-12 (2.4 µg/day) by consumption of vegetables, fruits, legumes, meats, fish, and fortified grains and cereals (for nonpregnant, nonlactating individuals) may be useful in reducing the risk of stroke. There are insufficient data to recommend a specific treatment approach that would reduce the risk of first stroke in patients with elevated homocysteine levels.

ELEVATED LIPOPROTEIN(A)

Although no definitive recommendations about lipoprotein (a) [Lp(a)] modification can be made because of an absence of outcome studies showing clinical benefit, treatment with niacin (extended-release or immediate-release formulation at a total daily dose of 2000 mg/day as tolerated) can be considered because it reduces Lp(a) levels by approximately 25%. Further recommendations must await the results of prospective trials utilizing niacin and statins in subjects stratified for Lp(a) concentration and apo(a) isoform subtypes.

ELEVATED LIPOPROTEIN-ASSOCIATED PHOSPHOLIPASE A$_2$

No recommendations about Lp-PLA$_2$ modification can be made because of an absence of outcome studies showing clinical benefit with reduction in its blood levels.

HYPERCOAGULABILITY

There are insufficient data to support specific recommendations for primary stroke prevention in patients with a hereditary or acquired thrombophilia.

INFLAMMATION

Currently, no evidence supports the use of high-sensitivity C-reactive protein (hs-CRP) screening of the entire adult population as a marker of general vascular risk. Aggressive risk-factor modification is recommended for patients at high risk for stroke given exposure to traditional risk factors regardless of hs-CRP level. In agreement with AHA/CDC guidelines, hs-CRP can be useful in considering the intensity of risk-factor modification in those at moderate general cardiovascular risk on the basis of traditional risk factors (class IIa, level of evidence B).

INFECTION

Data are insufficient to recommend antibiotic therapy for stroke prevention on the basis of seropositivity for one or a combination of putative pathogenic organisms. Future studies on stroke risk reduction based on treatment of infectious diseases will require careful stratification and identification of patients at risk for organism exposure.

ASPIRIN

Aspirin is not recommended for the prevention of a first stroke in men. The use of aspirin is recommended for cardiovascular (including but not specific to stroke) prophylaxis among persons whose risk is sufficiently high for the benefits to outweigh the risks associated with treatment (a 10-year risk of cardiovascular events of 6–10%). Aspirin can be useful for prevention of a first stroke among women whose risk is sufficiently high for the benefits to outweigh the risks associated with treatment.

RECOMMENDATION FOR ANTIPLATELET AGENTS IN SECONDARY PREVENTION OF STROKE

1. For patients with noncardioembolic ischemic stroke or transient ischemic attack (TIA), antiplatelet agents rather than oral anticoagulation are recommended to reduce the risk of recurrent stroke and other cardiovascular events.

2. Aspirin (50–325 mg/day) monotherapy, the combination of aspirin and extended-release dipyridamole, and clopidogrel monotherapy are all acceptable options for initial therapy.

3. The combination of aspirin and extended-release dipyridamole is recommended over aspirin alone.

4. Clopidogrel may be considered over aspirin alone on the basis of direct-comparison trials, and if patient is allergic to aspirin, clopidogrel is reasonable.

5. The addition of aspirin to clopidogrel increases the risk of hemorrhage. Combination therapy of aspirin and clopidogrel is not routinely recommended for ischemic stroke or TIA patients unless they have a specific indication for this therapy (i.e., coronary stent or acute coronary syndrome).

6. For patients who have an ischemic cerebrovascular event while taking aspirin, there is no evidence that increasing the dose of aspirin provides additional benefit. Although alternative antiplatelet agents are often considered for noncardioembolic patients, no single agent or combination has been well studied in patients who have had an event while receiving aspirin.

RECOMMENDATION FOR STATINS IN SECONDARY PREVENTION OF STROKE

1. Ischemic stroke or TIA patients with elevated cholesterol, comorbid coronary artery disease, or evidence of an atherosclerotic origin should be managed according to NCEP III guidelines, which include lifestyle modification, dietary guidelines, and medication recommendations.

2. Statin agents are recommended, and the target goal for cholesterol lowering for those with CHD or symptomatic atherosclerotic disease is an LDL-C level of <100 mg/dL. An LDL-C <70 mg/dL is recommended for very-high-risk persons with multiple risk factors.

3. On the basis of the SPARCL trial, administration of statin therapy with intensive lipid-lowering effects is recommended for patients with atherosclerotic ischemic stroke or TIA and without known CHD to reduce the risk of stroke and cardiovascular events.

4. Ischemic stroke or TIA patients with low HDL cholesterol may be considered for treatment with niacin or gemfibrozil.

ASSESSMENT OF ISCHEMIC STROKE PATIENT IN THE EMERGENCY DEPARTMENT

RECOMMENDATIONS FOR EMERGENCY DEPARTMENT

1. An organized protocol for the emergency evaluation of patients with suspected stroke is recommended. The goal is to complete an evaluation and to decide treatment within 60 minutes of the patient's arrival in an emergency department. Designation of an acute stroke team that includes physicians, nurses, and laboratory/ radiology personnel is encouraged. Patients with stroke should have a careful clinical assessment, including neurological examination.

2. The use of a stroke rating scale, preferably the National Institutes of Health (NIH) Stroke Scale, is recommended. Hospitals (i.e., administration) must provide the necessary resources to use such a scale.

3. A limited number of hematologic, coagulation, and biochemistry tests is recommended during the initial emergency evaluation.

4. Patients with clinical or other evidence of acute cardiac or pulmonary disease may warrant chest x-ray.

5. An electrocardiograph (EKG) is recommended because of the high incidence of heart disease in patients with stroke.

6. Most patients with stroke do not need a chest x-ray as part of their initial evaluation.

7. Most patients with stroke do not need an examination of the cerebrospinal fluid. The yield of brain imaging is very high for detection of intracranial hemorrhage. The clinical course of subarachnoid hemorrhage or acute central nervous system infections usually is distinct from that of ischemic stroke. Examination of the cerebrospinal fluid may be indicated for evaluation of a patient with a stroke that may be secondary to an infectious illness.

RECOMMENDATIONS REGARDING EARLY DIAGNOSIS

Brain imaging remains a required component of the emergency assessment of patients with suspected stroke. Both CT and MRI are options for imaging the brain, but for most cases and at most institutions, CT remains the most practical initial brain imaging test. A physician skilled in assessing CT or MRI studies should be available to examine the initial scan. In particular, the scan should be evaluated for evidence of early signs of infarction. Baseline CT findings, including the presence of ischemic changes involving more than one third of a hemisphere, have not been predictors of responses to treatment with recombinant tissue plasminogen activator (rtPA) when the agent is administered within the 3-hour treatment window. Information about multimodal CT and MRI of the brain suggests that these diagnostic studies may help in the diagnosis and treatment of patients with acute stroke. Imaging of the intracranial or extracranial vasculature in the emergency assessment of patients with suspected stroke is useful at institutions providing endovascular recanalization therapies. The usefulness of vascular imaging for predicting responses to treatment before intravenous administration of thrombolytic agents has not been demonstrated.

RECOMMENDATIONS REGARDING NEUROVASCULAR IMAGING

1. Imaging of the brain is recommended before initiating any specific therapy to treat acute ischemic stroke.

2. In most instances, CT will provide the information to make decisions about emergency management.

3. The brain imaging study should be interpreted by a physician with expertise in reading CT or MRI studies of the brain. Some findings on CT, including the presence of a dense artery sign, are associated with poor outcomes after stroke.

4. Multimodal CT and MRI may provide additional information that will improve diagnosis of ischemic stroke.

5. Nevertheless, data are insufficient to state that, with the exception of hemorrhage, any specific CT finding (including evidence of ischemia affecting more than one-third of a cerebral hemisphere) should preclude treatment with rtPA within 3 hours of onset of stroke.

6. Vascular imaging is necessary as a preliminary step for intra-arterial administration of pharmacological agents, surgical procedures, or endovascular interventions.

7. Emergency treatment of stroke should not be delayed in order to obtain multimodal imaging studies.

8. Vascular imaging should not delay treatment of patients whose symptoms started <3 hours ago and who have acute ischemic stroke.

GENERAL SUPPORTIVE CARE AND TREATMENT OF ACUTE COMPLICATIONS

Most of the recommendations about general acute management are based on limited data. Some of the aspects of acute management may never be tested in clinical trials, whereas other aspects of treatment, such as the best strategy for treatment of hyperglycemia or arterial hypertension, likely will be clarified by ongoing or future clinical research. Pending such trials, many of the suggestions that follow are based on consensus and thus are grade C recommendations.

RECOMMENDATIONS

1. Airway support and ventilatory assistance are recommended for the treatment of patients with acute stroke who have decreased consciousness or who have bulbar dysfunction causing compromise of the airway.

2. Hypoxic patients with stroke should receive supplemental oxygen. It is generally agreed that sources of fever should be treated and antipyretic medications should be administered to lower temperature in febrile patients with stroke. Medications such as acetaminophen can lower body temperature modestly, but the effectiveness of treating either febrile or nonfebrile patients to improve neurological outcomes is not established.

3. General agreement supports the use of cardiac monitoring to screen for atrial fibrillation and other potentially serious cardiac arrhythmias that would necessitate emergency cardiac interventions. It is generally agreed that cardiac monitoring should be performed during the first 24 hours after onset of ischemic stroke.

4. The management of arterial hypertension remains controversial. Data to guide recommendations for treatment are inconclusive or conflicting. Many patients have spontaneous declines in blood pressure during the first 24 hours after onset of stroke. Until more definitive data are available, it is generally agreed that a cautious approach to the treatment of arterial hypertension should be recommended.

5. Patients who have elevated blood pressure and are otherwise eligible for treatment of rtPA may have their blood pressure lowered so that their systolic blood pressure is ≤185 mm Hg and their diastolic blood pressure is ≤110 mm Hg before lytic therapy is started. If medications are given to lower blood pressure, the clinician should be sure that the blood pressure is stabilized at the lower level before treating with rtPA and maintained below 180/105 mm Hg for at least the first 24 hours after intravenous rtPA treatment. Because the maximum interval from stroke onset until treatment with rtPA is short, many patients with sustained hypertension above recommended levels cannot be treated with intravenous rtPA. It is generally agreed that patients with markedly elevated blood pressure may have their blood pressure lowered. A reasonable goal would be to lower blood pressure by approximately 15% during the first 24 hours after onset of stroke. The level of blood pressure that would mandate such treatment is not known, but consensus exists that medications should be withheld unless the systolic blood pressure is >220 mm Hg or the diastolic blood pressure is >120 mm Hg. It is generally agreed that the cause of arterial hypotension in the setting of acute stroke should be sought. Hypovolemia should be corrected with normal saline, and cardiac arrhythmias that might be reducing cardiac output should be corrected. It is generally agreed that hypoglycemia should be treated in patients with acute ischemic stroke. The goal is to achieve normoglycemia. Marked elevation of blood glucose levels should be avoided. Evidence from one clinical trial indicates that initiation of antihypertensive therapy within 24 hours of stroke is relatively safe. Thus, it is generally agreed that antihypertensive medications should be restarted at approximately 24 hours for patients who have pre-existing hypertension

and are neurologically stable unless a specific contraindication to restarting treatment is known. Evidence indicates that persistent hyperglycemia (>140 mg/dL) during the first 24 hours after stroke is associated with poor outcomes, and thus it is generally agreed that hyperglycemia should be treated in patients with acute ischemic stroke. The minimum threshold described in previous statements likely was too high, and lower serum glucose concentrations (possibly >140–185 mg/dL) probably should trigger administration of insulin, similar to the procedure in other acute situations accompanied by hyperglycemia. Close monitoring of glucose concentrations with adjustment of insulin doses to avoid hypoglycemia is recommended. Simultaneous administration of glucose and potassium also may be appropriate. Nonhypoxic patients with acute ischemic stroke do not need supplemental oxygen therapy. Data on the utility of hyperbaric oxygen are inconclusive, and some data imply that the intervention may be harmful. Thus, with the exception of stroke secondary to air embolization, this intervention is not recommended for treatment of patients with acute ischemic stroke.

6. Although data demonstrate the efficacy of hypothermia for improving neurological outcomes after cardiac arrest, the utility of induced hypothermia for the treatment of patients with ischemic stroke is not established. At the present time, insufficient evidence exists to recommend hypothermia for treatment of patients with acute stroke.

INTRAVENOUS THROMBOLYSIS

Intravenous administration of rtPA is the only FDA-approved medical therapy for treatment of patients with acute ischemic stroke. Its use is associated with improved outcomes for a broad spectrum of patients who can be treated within 3 hours of stroke onset. Earlier treatment (i.e., within 90 min) may be more likely to result in a favorable outcome. Later treatment, at 90–180 minutes, also is beneficial. Patients with major strokes (NIHSS score >22) have a very poor prognosis, but some positive treatment effect with rtPA has been documented. Because the risk of hemorrhage is considerable among patients with severe deficits, the decision to treat with rtPA should be made with caution. Treatment with rtPA is associated with symptomatic intracranial hemorrhage, which may be fatal. In the original NINDS trials, the risk of symptomatic bleeding was approximately 6%. The use of anticoagulants and antiplatelet agents should be delayed for 24 hours after treatment due to the increased risk of cerebral hemorrhage.

RECOMMENDATIONS

1. Intravenous rtPA (0.9 mg/kg, maximum dose 90 mg) is recommended for selected patients who may be treated within 3 hours of onset of ischemic stroke. Physicians should review the criteria used in the NINDS trial to determine the eligibility of the patient.

2. Besides bleeding complications, physicians should be aware of the potential side effect of angioedema that may cause partial airway obstruction.

3. A patient whose blood pressure can be lowered safely with antihypertensive agents may be eligible for treatment, and the physician should assess the stability of the blood pressure before starting rtPA.

4. A patient with a seizure at the time of onset of stroke may be eligible for treatment as long as the physician is convinced that residual impairments are secondary to stroke and not a postictal phenomenon.

5. The intravenous administration of streptokinase for treatment of stroke is not recommended.

6. The intravenous administration of ancrod, tenecteplase, reteplase, desmoteplase, urokinase, or other thrombolytic agents outside the setting of a clinical trial is not recommended.

INTRA-ARTERIAL THROMBOLYSIS

RECOMMENDATIONS

1. Intra-arterial thrombolysis is an option for treatment of selected patients who have major stroke of <6 hours' duration due to occlusions of the middle cerebral artery (MCA) and who are not otherwise candidates for intravenous rtPA.

2. Treatment requires the patient to be at an experienced stroke center with immediate access to cerebral angiography and qualified interventionalists. Facilities are encouraged to define criteria to credential individuals who can perform intra-arterial thrombolysis.

3. Intra-arterial thrombolysis is reasonable in patients who have contraindications to use of intravenous thrombolysis, such as recent surgery.

4. The availability of intra-arterial thrombolysis should generally not preclude the intravenous administration of rtPA in otherwise eligible patients.

ANTICOAGULANTS

RECOMMENDATIONS

1. Urgent anticoagulation with the goal of preventing early recurrent stroke, halting neurological worsening, or improving outcomes after acute ischemic stroke is not recommended for treatment of patients with acute

ischemic stroke. Urgent anticoagulation should not be used in lieu of intravenous thrombolysis for treatment of otherwise eligible patients.

2. Urgent anticoagulation is not recommended for patients with moderate to severe strokes because of an increased risk of serious intracranial hemorrhagic complications.

3. Initiation of anticoagulant therapy within 24 hours of treatment with intravenously administered rtPA is not recommended.

ANTIPLATELET AGENTS

RECOMMENDATION

1. The oral administration of aspirin (initial dose is 325 mg) within 24–48 hours after stroke onset is recommended for treatment of most patients.

2. Aspirin should not be considered a substitute for other acute interventions for treatment of stroke, including the intravenous administration of rtPA.

3. The administration of aspirin as an adjunctive therapy within 24 hours of thrombolytic therapy is not recommended.

4. The administration of clopidogrel alone or in combination with aspirin is not recommended for the treatment of acute ischemic stroke.

5. Outside the setting of clinical trials, the intravenous administration of antiplatelet agents that inhibit the glycoprotein IIb/IIIa receptor is not recommended.

DEFINITION OF TIA

The distinction between TIA and ischemic stroke has become less important in recent years because many of the preventive approaches are applicable to both groups. Stroke and TIA are pathogenetic mechanisms; prognosis may vary, depending on their severity and cause; and definitions are dependent on the timing and degree of the diagnostic evaluation. By conventional clinical definitions, if the neurological symptoms continue for >24 hours, a person has been diagnosed with stroke; otherwise, a focal neurological deficit lasting <24 hours has been defined as a TIA. With the more widespread use of modern brain imaging, many patients with symptoms lasting <24 hours are found to have an infarction.

The most recent definition of stroke for clinical trials has required either symptoms lasting >24 hours or imaging of an acute clinically relevant brain lesion in patients with rapidly vanishing symptoms. The proposed new definition of TIA is a "brief episode of neurological dysfunction caused by a focal disturbance of brain or retinal ischemia, with clinical symptoms typically lasting less than 1 hour, and without evidence of infarction." TIAs are an important determinant of stroke, with 90-day risks of stroke reported as high as 10.5% and the greatest stroke risk apparent in the first week.

Ischemic stroke is classified into various categories according to the presumed mechanism of the focal brain injury and the type and localization of the vascular lesion. The classic categories have been defined as large-artery atherosclerotic infarction, which may be extracranial or intracranial; embolism from a cardiac source; small-vessel disease; other determined cause such as dissection, hypercoagulable states, or sickle cell disease; and infarcts of undetermined cause. The certainty of the classification of the ischemic stroke mechanism is far from ideal and reflects the inadequacy or timing of the diagnostic workup in some cases to visualize the occluded artery or to localize the source of the embolism.

Recommendations for evaluation and treatment are the same as for stroke.

STROKE SYNDROMES

There are four broad categories of stroke, defined by their respective cerebrovascular distributions.

1. MCA stroke is the most common type of stroke. The MCA supplies most of the outer convex brain surface, nearly all the basal ganglia, and the posterior and anterior internal capsules. The neurological sequelae are diverse. MCA strokes are commonly associated with contralateral hemiparesis or hemiplegia, eye deviation toward the side of the MCA infarct, contralateral hemianopia, and contralateral hemianesthesia. Other manifestations include agnosia (inability to recognize people or objects), receptive or expressive aphasia, neglect (e.g., patients with visual neglect often have difficulty naming objects presented on the affected side), inattention, and autonomic dysfunction (e.g., excessive contralateral sweating).

2. The anterior cerebral arteries serve the most medial portions of the frontal lobes and the superior medial parietal lobes. The two anterior cerebral arteries arise from the internal carotid artery. Consequently, anterior cerebral artery strokes result in loss of frontal lobe function with disinhibition and speech perseveration, primitive reflexes (e.g., grasping, sucking reflexes), altered mental status, impaired judgment, contralateral weakness (greater in legs than arms), contralateral cortical sensory

deficits, gait apraxia (impaired initiation of movement and shuffling of feet), and urinary incontinence.

3. The posterior cerebral artery (PCA) supplies parts of the midbrain, subthalamic nucleus, basal nucleus, thalamus, mesial inferior temporal lobe, and occipital and occipitoparietal cortices. A PCA stroke resulting in unilateral infarction produces homonymous hemianopia. Sparing of the macula is encountered frequently in infarction of the occipital lobes due to PCA occlusion. Bilateral infarctions of the occipital lobes produce varying degrees of cortical blindness depending on the extent of the lesion. Patients often exhibit Anton syndrome, a state in which they fervently believe they can see when they cannot. Patients may describe objects that they have not seen previously in exquisite detail, completely in error and oblivious to that error. Another intriguing phenomenon is blindsight. Although cortically blind, patients can respond to movement or sudden lightening or darkening of their environment. Additional manifestations include visual agnosia (lack of recognition or understanding of visual objects or constructs), altered mental status, disorders of reading (alexia, dyslexia), disorder of color vision (achromatopsia, dyschromatopsia), and impaired memory.

4. Vertebrobasilar artery occlusions cause a wide variety of cranial nerve, cerebellar, and brainstem deficits. The vertebrobasilar arterial system perfuses the medulla, cerebellum, pons, midbrain, thalamus, and occipital cortex. Occlusion of large vessels in this system usually leads to major disability or death. The disability is multisystem dysfunction (e.g., quadriplegia or hemiplegia, ataxia, dysphagia, dysarthria, gaze abnormalities, cranial neuropathies). A hallmark of posterior circulation stroke is that there are crossed findings: ipsilateral cranial nerve deficits and contralateral motor deficits. This is contrasted to anterior stroke, which produces only unilateral findings.

One category of strokes, namely, lacunar strokes, do not have a geographic distribution per se because these result from occlusion of the small, perforating arteries of the deep subcortical areas of the brain. The infarcts are generally from 2 to 20 mm in diameter. The most common clinical syndrome is that of pure motor, pure sensory, and ataxic hemiparetic strokes. Lacunar infarcts commonly occur in patients with small vessel disease, such as diabetes and hypertension. Because lacunar strokes are usually small and well—they do not lead to impairments in cognition, memory, speech, or level of consciousness.

ADDITIONAL READING

Acker JE III, Pancioli AM, Crocco TJ, et al. Implementation strategies for emergency medical services within stroke systems of care: A policy statement from the American Heart Association/American Stroke Association Expert Panel on Emergency Medical Services Systems and the Stroke Council. *Stroke.* 2007;38(11):3097–3115.

Adams RJ, Albers G, Alberts MJ, et al. Update to the AHA/ASA recommendations for the prevention of stroke in patients with stroke and transient ischemic attack. *Stroke.* 2008;39(5):1647–52.

Easton JD, Saver JL, Albers GW, et al. Definition and evaluation of transient ischemic attack. A scientific statement for healthcare professionals from the American Heart Association/American Stroke Association Stroke Council; Council on Cardiovascular Surgery and Anesthesia; Council on Cardiovascular Radiology and Intervention; Council on Cardiovascular Nursing; and the Interdisciplinary Council on Peripheral Vascular Disease. *Stroke.* 2009;108:192–218.

Goldstein LB, Adams R, Becker K, et al. Primary prevention of ischemic stroke: A guideline from the American Heart Association/American Stroke Association Stroke Council: Cosponsored by the Atherosclerotic Peripheral Vascular Disease Interdisciplinary Working Group; Cardiovascular Nursing Council; Clinical Cardiology Council; Nutrition, Physical Activity, and Metabolism Council; and the Quality of Care and Outcomes Research Interdisciplinary Working Group: The American Academy of Neurology affirms the value of this guideline. *Stroke.* 2006;37(6):1583–1633.

Guiraud V, Amor MB, Mas JL, et al. Triggers of ischemic stroke: A systematic review. *Stroke.* 2010;41(11):2669–77.

Hassoun HT, Malas MB, Freischlag JA. Secondary stroke prevention in the era of carotid stenting: Update on recent trials. *Arch Surg.* 2010;145(10):928–35.

Stinear C. Prediction of recovery of motor function after stroke. *Lancet Neurol.* 2010;9(12):1228–32.

Wu TC, Grotta JC. Stroke treatment and prevention: Five new things. *Neurology.* 2010;75(18 Suppl 1):S16–21.

QUESTIONS

QUESTION 1. A 68-year-old man who is a heavy smoker presents with acute-onset vertigo, nystagmus, dysphagia, and a droop his right upper eyelid with an associated constricted right pupil.

The most likely diagnosis is:

A. Acute labyrinthitis
B. Benign paroxysmal positional vertigo
C. Lateral medullary infarction
D. Cluster headache ("Horton's headache")

QUESTION 2. A 74-year-old female with long-standing history of hypertension presents with a 1-day history of loss of fluency. Her daughter, who lives with her, says that her mother misses words in her sentences and garbles up what she's trying to say. She thinks her mother doesn't notice anything to her right and keeps knocking into furniture. She also describes her as being inattentive. On examination the patient has mild right-sided weakness that is worse in the arms. No left-sided deficits. No cranial nerve deficits.

What is the most likely diagnosis?

A. Subarachnoid hemorrhage
B. Basilar artery occlusion
C. Lacunar infarction
D. Left middle cerebral artery occlusion
E. Posterior cerebral artery occlusion

QUESTION 3. All of the following are typical of anterior cerebral artery strokes, EXCEPT:

A. Expressive aphasia
B. Altered mental status,
C. Contralateral weakness (greater in legs than arms)
D. Contralateral cortical sensory deficits
E. Urinary incontinence.

QUESTION 4. A 72-year-old normotensive woman realizes suddenly that she cannot see to her left and that her left hand tingles. Two years previously she had a stroke, which left her right arm and right leg weak. The family reports that during the past year she has become unreliable in daily responsibilities and often forgets people's names. CT scan shows a recent, well-circumscribed homogencous right parietal-temporal hemorrhage; an old, slit-like cavity in the left medial frontal lobe under the cortex; and moderate ventricular dilatation and cortical sulcal widening.

The most likely diagnosis is:

A. Hemorrhage into a brain tumor
B. Cerebral amyloid angiopathy
C. Embolization of cardiac origin with hemorrhagic infarction
D. Multiple cerebral aneurysms
E. Recurrent head trauma

QUESTION 5. A 76-year-old woman with mitral valve disease and chronic atrial fibrillation becomes suddenly confused while playing bridge with her friends. She is awake and alert, and her motor function appears intact and symmetric. She speaks in long sentences unconnected to the card game or the questions asked of her. She uses many word substitutions and nonsense words. She appears unable to understand questions put to her by friends.

The most likely diagnosis is:

A. Acute psychotic break
B. Transient global amnesia
C. Dominant hemisphere stroke
D. Nondominant hemispherc stroke
E. Digitalis toxicity

ANSWERS

1. C
2. C
3. A
4. B
5. C

91.

DEMENTIA

Andrew E. Budson and Daniel C. Sacchetti

ementia is a decline of cognitive function that eventually impairs the ability to carry out everyday activities. Dementia affects approximately 4–5 million people in the United States to varying degrees. Only approximately 1 in 100 individuals <65 years are thought to be affected by dementia, but this proportion reaches as many as one in three individuals age >85 years. There are a number common causes of cognitive impairment that are reviewed in this chapter (see table 91.1).

ALZHEIMER DISEASE

Alzheimer disease (AD) is defined as a neurodegenerative disease of the brain characterized by a clinical dementia with prominent memory impairment and specific pathology including senile plaques and neurofibrillary tangles. AD causes approximately 90% of dementia cases either alone or as part of a mixed dementia. The overall prevalence in the community is estimated at about 10% in population-based studies. AD increases with age; 5–10% of individuals age >65; 50% of those age >85. AD is the fourth leading cause of death (after heart disease, cancer, and stroke) and accounts for more than 100,000 deaths per year.

OVERVIEW

AD has a typical onset from age 60–100 years. The average patient lives approximately 10 years from diagnosis until death (average range 4–12 years). The Mini-Mental State Examination (MMSE) declines approximately 2 to 3 points per year on average in AD. The risk factors are depicted in table 91.2. Notably, AD is not part of normal aging. Age is the primary risk factor for AD. The family history is also an important risk factor: a first-degree relative with AD increases the risk of developing AD approximately fourfold. There is a genetic predisposition: late-onset AD has been associated with the APOE

E4 allele on chromosome 19. Early-onset familial AD has been associated with mutations of the amyloid precursor protein, presenilin 1, and presenilin 2 on chromosomes 21, 14, and 1, respectively. Other risk factors include female gender and head trauma that is associated with loss of consciousness or posttraumatic amnesia, and low educational attainment (more education reduces the risk of AD, possibly by creating a "cognitive reserve" that delays the onset of clinical symptoms). Strokes do not cause Alzheimer pathology, but they may contribute to cognitive dysfunction in patients who already have Alzheimer pathology. Small vessel ischemic strokes are common in aging in the white matter, basal ganglia, and thalamus.

AD is pathologically defined by both intraneuronal neurofibrillary tangles and extracellular amyloid beta-peptide senile plaques leading to severe neuronal loss. The pathophysiology is attributable both to the direct loss of cortical neurons and also to neuronal loss in the nucleus basalis of Meynert, resulting in reduced acetylcholine. Other important gross pathologic features include a brain weight reduced by approximately 200–300 g, atrophy of hippocampus and of temporal, parietal, and frontal cortex, and cerebral amyloid angiopathy—often found in blood vessels—leading to small hemorrhages.

CLINICAL PRESENTATION

AD typically presents first with memory loss, followed by word-finding, visuospatial, and frontal/executive dysfunction. Patients cannot remember new information, become disoriented, and show poor judgment and problem-solving skills. Behavioral problems such as irritability, exacerbation of premorbid personality traits, and aggression often develop later. Patients continue to lose function until they require round-the-clock care, usually in a long-term care facility. Although depression and anxiety were once thought to be a common cause of memory loss, it is now clear that these symptoms are common in the early stages of AD, making it likely that an elderly patient with depression and memory

Table 91.1 COMMON CAUSES OF COGNITIVE IMPAIRMENT

Alzheimer disease

Mild cognitive impairment

Dementia with Lewy bodies

Other parkinsonism syndromes

    Progressive supranuclear palsy

    Corticobasal degeneration

Vascular dementia

Frontotemporal dementia

---

loss has early AD. The two most commonly used criteria for AD are from the DSM IV-TR and the National Institutes of Neurological and Communicative Disorders and Stroke-Alzheimer's Disease and Related Disorders Association (NINCDS-ADRDA); new criteria were published in 2011 from the National Institute on Aging (NIA) and the Alzheimer's Association; see table 91.3 for key elements. Commonly used neuropsychological tests include these:

- Mini-Mental State Examination (MMSE)
- Mini-Cog
- Montreal Cognitive Assessment (MoCA)
- Blessed Dementia Scale (BDS)
- Consortium to Establish a Registry for AD (CERAD) battery

WORKUP

Laboratory studies that should be performed in working up AD include measurement of both vitamin B-12 level and thyroid-stimulating hormone (TSH) (both are essential). Other studies such as Lyme titer or rapid protein reagin (RPR) should be included if clinically indicated.

STRUCTURAL IMAGING

Computed tomography (CT) or magnetic resonance imaging (MRI) scan usually demonstrates atrophy of hippocampus,

Table 91.2 RISK FACTORS IN ALZHEIMER DISEASE

Aging

Family history

Genetic predisposition

Female gender

Low education

Head trauma

Stroke

Table 91.3 COMMON ELEMENTS FOR AD DIAGNOSIS

- Dementia: a progressive decline in cognition and function from the patient's previous level of functioning
- A progressive decline in memory and at least one other major area of cognition, such as language or executive function
- No disturbance of consciousness such as a delirium or acute confusional state
- The decline in function cannot be explained by another medical or brain disease

---

anterior temporal, and parietal lobes. However, AD cannot be either ruled in or ruled out by such atrophy. Most older adults show mild or moderate small vessel ischemic disease; this does *not* mean they have vascular dementia. Structural imaging is also important to rule out other etiologies such as large strokes, tumors, hemorrhages, and hydrocephalus.

FUNCTIONAL IMAGING

Fludeoxyglucose positron emission tomography (FDG-PET) or Tc99 single proton emission CT (SPECT) demonstrates temporal and parietal dysfunction. Functional imaging is not indicated in routine patients in whom AD is suspected, and it is not sensitive or specific enough to distinguish very mild AD from normal aging. However, functional imaging is helpful when (1) a diagnosis of AD seems clear, but the patient is young (65 years of age or less); and (2) when the patient is clearly demented, but it is not clear whether it is due to AD or another dementia such as frontotemporal or dementia with Lewy bodies. New types of functional imaging scans, such as those that image amyloid directly, are being developed.

STAGES OF AD

- *Very mild:* a slight but definite decline in memory, and sometimes word-finding; fully oriented; slight impairments in judgment and problem solving, community affairs, and home life and hobbies; typically able to prepare simple meals and can usually be on their own for few days without getting into trouble; MMSE 24–27.

- *Mild:* noticeable declines in memory and often word finding, interfering with everyday activities; shows some disorientation to time and place; judgment and problem solving are moderately impaired; unable to function independently in community affairs; cannot perform complicated hobbies and household tasks but may still be able to perform simple ones; able to perform personal care tasks such as brushing teeth, changing clothes, and bathing, although may need reminding to do these activities; patient usually safe to be on his or her own for a few hours but may forget to eat, take medications, bathe, and change clothes if left alone for a few days; MMSE 16–26.

Table 91.4 STAGES OF ALZHEIMER DISEASE

Very mild	• Slight decline in memory • Fully oriented • Slight impairments in problem solving and judgments • Can still function in day-to-day life without any problems
Mild	• Noticeable decline in memory to the point it interferes with activities • Slight disorientation to time and place • Cannot perform complex tasks or hobbies • Able to maintain personal care alone, but not for several days
Moderate	• Memory loss is severe • Ability to learn new material is significantly impaired • Severe impairment in problem solving and judgment • Cannot function independently • Should not be left alone
Severe	• Memory is severely impaired, and only fragments remain • Patient needs constant maintenance and attention • No independent activities are possible • Patients usually need care in a long-term facility

Table 91.5 OTHER CAUSES OF COGNITIVE IMPARIMENT

Encephalitis

Traumatic brain injury

Concussion

Stroke

Hypoxic-ischemic injury

Cardiopulmonary bypass

Subdural or epidural hematoma

Intracerebral hemorrhage

Seizure disorder

Temporal lobe surgery

Multiple sclerosis

Infections (including HIV)

Psychiatric disorders

Medication side effects

Hypoglycemia

Delirium secondary to a medical disorder

Sleep disorders

Hyper-/hypothyroidism

Other endocrine disorders

B-12 and other vitamin deficiencies

Lyme disease

Neurosyphilis (rare)

Wernicke-Korsakoff syndrome

• *Moderate:* memory loss is severe with only remote and/or very important memories retained; almost all new material is rapidly lost; disorientation to time and place are common; judgment and problem solving show severe impairment; only simple hobbies and household tasks can be maintained; patient appears well enough to be taken to activities outside the home; there is no pretense of independent function; assistance is needed in personal care activities such as dressing and hygiene, and urinary incontinence often develops; patient should not be left alone due to potential issues of wandering, incontinence, and safety; MMSE 6–17.

• *Severe:* memory is severely impaired, and only fragments of memory remain; patient is typically only oriented to self; judgment and problem solving are not possible; patient appears too ill to be taken to activities outside the home, and the patient is not capable of pursing hobbies or performing household tasks; patient requires help with all aspects of personal care and is frequently incontinent of both urine and feces; patient is usually managed in a long-term care facility; MMSE 0–10.

These stages of AD are summarized in table 91.4.

DIFFERENTIAL DIAGNOSIS

Nondementia causes of cognitive impairment are listed in table 91.5. The most common disorders to be confused with AD are the following other degenerative dementias:

• *Frontotemporal dementia:* If the patient showed personality changes or problems with behavior, language, judgment, or reasoning first and foremost, then a frontotemporal dementia should be considered.

• *Dementia with Lewy bodies:* If there is any evidence of parkinsonism and/or visual hallucinations and visual misperceptions, dementia with Lewy bodies should be considered.

• *Progressive supranuclear palsy and corticobasal degeneration* should also be considered if there is parkinsonism.

• *Vascular dementia* should be considered if there are many large strokes or severe small ischemic disease on the CT or MRI scan. However, if the history and cognitive exam suggest AD, then the patient most likely has a mixed dementia, AD plus vascular disease.

Table 91.6 PHARMACOLOGICAL TREATMENT FOR AD

| Cholinesterase inhibitors |
| Donepezil (Aricept) |
| Galantamine (Razadyne) |
| Rivastigmine (Exelon) |
| NMDA antagonists |
| Memantine (Namenda) |

TREATMENT OF AD

Anticholinergic medications should be avoided. Currently only symptomatic therapy is available (see table 91.6), and there are no proven disease-modifying therapies. The overarching goal of therapy is to modulate neurotransmitters—either acetylcholine or glutamate. Delaying the onset of disease and/or slowing the rate of progression with medical therapy is currently not possible; studies suggest these medications can, however, "turn the clock back" on AD symptoms for 6–12 months provided they are continued. The standard medical treatment for Alzheimer disease includes cholinesterase inhibitors (ChEIs): donepezil (Aricept), galantamine (Razadyne), and rivastigmine (Exelon). The partial NMDA antagonist memantine (Namenda) is believed to work by improving the signal-to-noise ratio of glutamatergic transmission at the NMDA receptor, although its clinical effects may also be related to its activity as a dopamine agonist. Cholinesterase inhibitors are FDA approved for mild, moderate, and severe AD, whereas memantine is FDA approved for moderate to severe AD.

MILD COGNITIVE IMPAIRMENT

Because degenerative diseases such as AD progress over years, patients with such disorders must have gone through a prodromal stage prior to obvious clinical manifestations of their disorder. The term mild cognitive impairment (MCI) is used to indicate patients who are presumed to be in this prodromal stage. Patients with MCI show abnormal cognition but do not meet criteria for dementia. MCI is usually divided into amnestic versus nonamnestic, and single versus multiple domains of impairment, leading to four common types (see table 91.7).

The incidence of MCI has been reported to be 1–6% per year, with the prevalence ranging from 3% to 22% in individuals >65 years of age, and rising with increasing age. About 70% of patients with a diagnostic label of MCI convert to AD or another dementia at a rate of about 10–15% per year (compared to 1–2% of the general population). The risk factors are similar to those for AD or other underlying disorder. Because MCI is not a specific disease, the pathology and pathogenesis depend on the etiology causing the cognitive impairment. The main difference between MCI and AD is that the decline in cognition is not yet to the point where it interferes with daily life.

CLINICAL PRESENTATION

The chief clinical manifestation is memory and/or other cognitive loss by patient and/or informant. By neuropsychological testing, the memory and/or other cognitive impairment is greater than what one would expect adjusted for age and education. However, general cognitive function is essentially normal. Insight is often preserved. Activities of daily living are also largely preserved. The patient is not demented.

WORKUP

Laboratory workup for MCI is similar to that for AD.

STRUCTURAL IMAGING

As in AD, structural imaging studies are necessary to evaluate for the presences of large strokes, tumors, hemorrhages, hydrocephalus, the extent of small vessel ischemic disease, and other such pathology. MCI attributable to cerebrovascular disease is often called vascular cognitive impairment (VCI). These patients typically show moderate to severe small vessel ischemic disease.

Table 91.7 COMMON TYPES OF MILD COGNITIVE IMPAIRMENT (MCI)

	AMNESTIC (MEMORY IMPAIRED)	NONAMNESTIC (MEMORY *NOT* IMPAIRED)
Single domain (only one impairment)	Amnestic MCI single domain • Only slight memory impairment	Nonamnestic MCI single domain • Single nonmemory cognitive impairment
Multiple domain (several impairments)	Amnestic MCI multiple domain • Slight memory and other cognitive impairments	Nonamnestic MCI multiple domain • Multiple nonmemory cognitive impairments
Likely etiology	Alzheimer disease	Other (cerebrovascular disease, non-Alzheimer neurodegenerative diseases)

FUNCTIONAL IMAGING

FDG-PET and Tc99 SPECT are neither sensitive nor specific enough to detect and/or determine the underlying etiology in a patient with MCI; they are not recommended.

DIFFERENTIAL DIAGNOSIS

The differential diagnosis of MCI is quite broad, as it includes everything from normal aging to mild forms of all dementia types. Common disorders that can cause MCI include:

- AD
- Cerebrovascular disease
- Other dementias
- Normal aging
- Depression and other psychiatric disorders
- Disorders that cause a static encephalopathy (encephalitis, head injury, subdural fluid collection, stroke)
- Medical disorders (e.g., renal failure)

TREATMENT

There are currently no FDA-approved treatments for patients with MCI. However, studies have shown that patients with amnestic MCI are improved by donepezil (Aricept); thus, treatment with donepezil or another cholinesterase inhibitor for patients with amnestic MCI is appropriate. Patients with MCI are often anxious and depressed because of their awareness of their cognitive deficits and benefit from a selective serotonin reuptake inhibitor (SSRI) medication such as sertraline (Zoloft).

DEMENTIA WITH LEWY BODIES (INCLUDING PARKINSON DISEASE DEMENTIA)

Dementia with Lewy bodies (DLB) is a neurodegenerative disease characterized clinically by a dementia, visual hallucinations, and parkinsonism. Dementia with Lewy bodies is the same as Parkinson disease dementia (same clinical picture in late stages, same pathology)—the only difference being that the initial symptoms are cognitive (dementia) in the former and motor (Parkinsonism) in the latter.

DLB accounts for up to 15% of cases of dementia (often mixed with AD). It is the second most common degenerative disease in the older adult after AD. The combination of dementia, parkinsonism, and visual hallucinations leads to nursing home placement and death earlier than in AD. Risk factors include age and male gender. The pathology is one of neurodegeneration associated with abnormal alpha-synuclein

metabolism and formation of intracellular Lewy bodies in various brain regions including brainstem, basal forebrain, limbic regions, and neocortical regions. The pathophysiology is attributable both to the direct loss of neurons and also to neuronal loss in brainstem centers that produce neurotransmitters, including the substantia nigra (producing dopamine) and the nucleus basalis of Meynert (producing acetylcholine). The key differences from AD are these:

- Parkinsonism (although up to 25% of patients do not present with parkinsonism)
- Visual hallucinations
- Similar cognitive testing, but dementia with Lewy bodies patients may show relatively greater impairment on measures of attention and less impairment in memory.

DIFFERENTIAL DIAGNOSIS

When considering a diagnosis of dementia with Lewy bodies, one should determine whether the patient's dementia would be best characterized by that diagnosis alone, AD alone, or both (table 91.8). If the patient meets criteria for both dementias, then the patient has a mixed dementia: dementia with Lewy bodies plus AD.

FEATURES OF DLB

- Dementia
- Parkinsonism
- Visual hallucinations
- Fluctuating cognition
- REM sleep behavior disorder
- Neuroleptic sensitivity

WORKUP

The laboratory workup of DLB is very similar to the workup of AD or MCI.

STRUCTURAL IMAGING

There are no features of dementia with Lewy bodies that are commonly observed on structural imaging.

FUNCTIONAL IMAGING

FDG-PET and Tc99 SPECT often show occipital dysfunction. Functional imaging is not necessary for the straightforward patient. Research into imaging of the dopamine transporter system by either SPECT or PET using specialized tracers is currently being developed.

- **Essential for a diagnosis**
  Dementia.
  Impairment in attention, executive function, and visuospatial ability are often prominent. Memory impairment may or may not be prominent initially.

- **Core features** (two are sufficient for a diagnosis of probably dementia with Lewy bodies, one for a possible diagnosis.)
  Fluctuating cognition (pronounced variations in attention and alertness)
  Visual hallucinations (recurrent, well formed, detailed, of people and/or animals)
  Spontaneous features of parkinsonism

- **Suggestive features** (one or more plus one core feature allows a probable diagnosis; one or more without any core features allows a possible diagnosis.)
  Rapid-eye-movement (REM) sleep behavior disorder
  Severe neuroleptic sensitivity
  Low dopamine transporter uptake in basal ganglia demonstrated by SPECT or PET imaging

- **Supportive features** (commonly present but have not proven to have diagnostic specificity)
  Repeated falls
  Transient unexplained loss of consciousness
  Orthostatic hypotension
  Reduced occipital activity and generalized low uptake on SPECT/PET perfusion scan

- **A diagnosis of dementia with Lewy bodies is less likely:**
  In the presence of clinically significant cerebrovascular disease noted on exam or radiology study.
  If parkinsonism only appears for the first time at a stage of severe dementia.
  In the presence of any other disorder sufficient to account for some or all of the clinical picture.

SOURCE: Adapted from McKeith et al., Dementia with Lewy bodies: Diagnosis and management: Third report of the DLB consortium. *Neurology.* 2005;65:1863–72.

TREATMENT

Anticholinergic medications should be avoided. The cholinesterase inhibitor rivastigmine (Exelon) has been approved for Parkinson disease dementia, which as discussed above is the same as dementia with Lewy bodies. The motor symptoms of parkinsonism are generally best treated with levodopa (along with carbidopa, usually referred to as Sinemet) in low dose. Successfully treating hallucinations is difficult, and pharmacologic treatment should be initiated when hallucinations become threatening or otherwise problematic. Only atypical neuroleptics should be used, such as quetiapine (Seroquel) at bedtime, because traditional neuroleptics such as haloperidol (Haldol) are highly likely to cause worsening parkinsonism. (Note black box warning: neuroleptics are not approved for dementia-related use in elderly patients; increased deaths due to cardiovascular or infectious events.) As in AD and MCI, depression and anxiety are common in patients with mild dementia with Lewy bodies and preserved insight; if these symptoms are present, an SSRI such as sertraline (Zoloft) is helpful.

OTHER PARKINSONISM SYNDROMES

PROGRESSIVE SUPRANUCLEAR PALSY (PSP)

This is a neurodegenerative disease of the brain due to the accumulation of hyperphosphorylated tau protein isoforms in the brain. It has a prevalence of 5 per 100,000. The main features of PSP include, slowing or other abnormality of vertical eye movements (supranuclear palsy), postural instability with falls, axial rigidity, frontal lobe signs and symptoms, and difficulty swallowing and eventually talking (pseudobulbar palsy).

Early cognitive and affective symptoms may include irritability, irascibility, apathy, introversion, and depression. Inappropriate sexual behavior may also be present. The patient may complain of visual symptoms including blurred vision, difficulty focusing, dry eyes, photophobia, and double vision. The gait, sometimes described as that of a drunken sailor, becomes more abnormal as the disease progresses. Impulsiveness may lead to suddenly rising from sitting, increasing risk of falls. Fractures and bruises are common due to falls. The "sloppy eating" that is frequently observed with PSP is attributable to the combination of loss of dexterity, swallowing difficulties, and difficulty looking down at the plate of food. In the severe stages the patient is typically confined to a wheelchair, and more severe chewing and swallowing difficulties, drooling, coughing, spluttering, and choking are common. Death is usually due to aspiration pneumonia.

There are no FDA approved treatments for progressive supranuclear palsy. Symptomatic treatments that are worth trying include levodopa or carbidopa (Sinemet), and memantine or amantadine.

CORTICOBASAL DEGENERATION

Corticobasal degeneration (CBD) is defined as a neurodegenerative disease of the brain characterized by asymmetric cortical dysfunction, often affecting motor control of a limb, along with cognitive dysfunction, rigidity, a jerky postural tremor, myoclonus, dystonia, and a gait disorder. Like progressive supranuclear palsy, it is caused by the accumulation of hyperphosphorylated tau isoforms.

OVERVIEW AND CLINICAL FEATURES

CBD has a prevalence of about 2 per 100,000. The most characteristic feature is that of asymmetric limb dysfunction. Other common signs and symptoms include useless limb, focal apraxias, sensory symptoms including numbness and tingling, rigidity, a jerky postural tremor, myoclonus, dystonia, speech disturbance, executive dysfunction, and behavioral disorder. Over time the affected limbs become more rigid, such that rapid movements such as pronation/supination and alternating finger tapping become impaired. Eventually even passive stretch may not be possible. The dementia of CBD differs from that of AD: whereas in AD medial temporal lobe dysfunction is most prominent, leading to memory difficulties, in CBD frontal and parietal dysfunction are common, thus leading to difficulties with executive function, visuospatial function, language, and praxis.

TREATMENT

There are no FDA-approved treatments for corticobasal degeneration. Antidepressants should be used to treat depression, which is often present. Dystonia may be relieved with botulinum toxin. Clonazepam may be helpful for myoclonus.

VASCULAR DEMENTIA/VASCULAR COGNITIVE IMPAIRMENT

Vascular dementia (VaD) can be defined as occurring concurrently with AD or other dementia etiologies or as a pure vascular dementia. If the patient shows no signs of any other etiology of his or her cognitive impairment, we would describe him or her as having a pure vascular dementia. If the patient has a neurodegenerative disease (such as AD) and has the average amount of cerebrovascular disease that a nondemented, non–cognitively impaired older adult has, we would describe him or her as simply having that neurodegenerative disease (such as AD). If the patient has a neurodegenerative disease (such as AD) and has a greater-than-average amount of cerebrovascular disease such that it is highly likely that the cerebrovascular disease is making a significant contribution to the patient's dementia, then we would describe him or her as having a mixed dementia and would then further specify, for example, a mixed dementia of AD plus vascular dementia.

OVERVIEW

Patients classified as mixed dementia of cerebrovascular disease plus a neurodegenerative disease probably make up 10–15% of all dementias. Pure vascular dementia occurs on the order

Table 91.9 **RISK FACTORS FOR VASCULAR DEMENTIA AND VASCULAR COGNITIVE IMPAIRMENT**

Cardiovascular
    Clinical strokes or transient ischemic attacks (TIAs)
    Hypertension
    Atrial fibrillation
    Coronary artery disease
    Atherosclerosis
Metabolic
    Diabetes
    Increased cholesterol
Habits
    Smoking
Demographics
    Old age
    Low educational attainment

of 1–5% of all dementias. The prognosis varies depending on etiology and severity. Risk factors are depicted in table 91.9. The pathology is variable. Cognitive impairment and dementia can occur in a variety of ways, with etiologies including large cortical strokes, small vessel ischemic disease, lacunar infarcts, and other etiologies. These different types of cerebrovascular disease can cause a variety of different types of signs and symptoms depending on where the damage occurs.

- Small vessel ischemic disease (subcortical ischemic vascular disease) attributable to two processes, lipohyalinosis and microemboli.

- Multi-infarct dementia (cortical vascular dementia, poststroke) typically due to multiple cortical strokes most commonly caused by large emboli.

- Strategic infarct dementia due to a focal lesion (or lesions), often quite small, that damages a brain region that is critical for cognitive brain function; the lesions are typically lacunar infarcts or embolic strokes, although hypertensive hemorrhages can also damage these regions.

- Cerebral amyloid angiopathy (CAA) caused by deposits of beta-amyloid in the media of small to medium arteries in the leptomeninges and superficial cortex, particularly in the parieto-occipital, temporoparietal, and sometimes frontal regions; it is more common in patients with AD.

- Others such as hypoperfusion, hemorrhages, and rare genetic disorders such as CADASIL.

VaD differs from AD in the following ways:

- VaD can affect any number of brain regions at any time with varying severity.

- Stepwise progression is common.

- Frontal/executive system dysfunction is common.

- Focal neurologic signs are common.

CLINCAL FEATURES

The typical symptoms of the different types of VaD are shown in table 91.10. The signs and symptoms depend on both the type of cerebrovascular disease and the particular brain structures affected. The finding of sudden, as opposed to gradual, symptoms is key. Signs of strokes or TIAs are usually present.

DIFFERENTIAL DIAGNOSIS

- AD and other neurodegenerative diseases
- Multiple sclerosis
- Vasculitis
- Systemic lupus erythematosus

WORKUP

The laboratory workup of VaD is very similar to the workup of AD or other forms of dementia.

STRUCTURAL IMAGING

Structural imaging is key to making a diagnosis of VaD. In order to make a diagnosis of pure vascular dementia or vascular cognitive impairment there needs to be sufficient cerebrovascular disease present on the CT or MRI scan to explain the degree of cognitive impairment. To make a diagnosis of a mixed dementia, with vascular dementia as a contributing factor, there must be more cerebrovascular disease present on the CT or MRI scan than may be commonly present in an older adult without cognitive impairment.

Table 91.10 TYPICAL SYMPTOMS OF VASCULAR DEMENTIAS

Small vessel ischemic disease	• Frontal subcortical dysfunction leading to difficulties in attention • Disrupted gait—"frontal gait" • Incontinence • Pseudobulbar symptoms
Multi-infarct dementia	• Poor attention • Aphasia • Disinhibition • Hemiparesis • Impairment of vision and other sensory modalities
Strategic infarct dementia	• Poor attention • Slurred speech (dysarthria) • Aphasia • Hemiparesis • Incontinence • Impaired coordination
Cerebral amyloid angiopathy	• Often first present with signs of AD • Visual disturbances • Wernicke's aphasia • Word finding difficulties • Visuospatial impairments

FUNCTIONAL IMAGING

Functional imaging is helpful only in excluding neurodegenerative diseases such as AD or frontotemporal dementia.

TREATMENT

The treatment of VaD is targeted to reduction of stroke risk factors. Although there are no FDA-approved medications for VaD, studies suggest both cholinesterase inhibitors and memantine provide significant benefit.

FRONTOTEMPORAL DEMENTIA

Frontotemporal dementia (FTD) is defined as dementia attributable to neurodegeneration of the frontal and/or temporal lobes, with or without Pick bodies. There are three primary variants: (1) frontal variant (Fv-FTD), (2) temporal variant (Tv-FTD), and (3) primary progressive aphasia (PPA)

OVERVIEW

FTD accounts for 20% of patients with early-onset dementia (age <65), approximately 2–5% of all dementias. FTD typically develops at a younger age (35–75) than AD. Its duration ranges, depending on the variant, from 2 to 20 years for Fv-FTD, 3 to 15 years for Tv-FTD, and 4 to 12 years for PPA. The median survival is 6–8 years. The pathology is characterized by neuronal loss and gliosis due to tau inclusions, ubiquitin-positive inclusions, neuronal intermediate-filament inclusions, and/or microvacuolar degeneration. Pick bodies may or may not be present. There is atrophy of frontal and/or temporal lobes. The atrophy can be asymmetric and also affect basal ganglia. The differences from AD are depicted in table 91.11 and include the following:

- Earlier onset.
- Behavioral symptoms, instead of memory loss, predominate early in the disease.
- Atrophy of frontal and/or temporal lobes.

Table 91.11 FRONTOTEMPORAL DEMENTIA VERSUS AD

FUNCTION	ALZHEIMER DISEASE	FRONTOTEMPORAL DEMENTIAS
Memory	Impaired early	Variable
Personality	Withdrawn, less confident	Apathetic, disinhibited
Social skills	Preserved early on	Early deterioration
Language	Fluent with normal output	Decreased output

SOURCE: Solomon PR, Budson AE. Alzheimer's Disease. *Clin Symposia.* 2003;54(1):1–44.

Table 91.12 CLINICAL FEATURES OF FRONTOTEMPORAL DEMENTIAS (FTDs)

Frontal variant FTD (Fv-FTD)	• Uninhibited, socially inappropriate behavior • Lacks awareness/concern for behavior • Loss of concern about personal appearance and hygiene • Loss of empathy • Mental rigidity • Impaired insight • Impaired judgment and planning • Stereotyped, ritualistic behavior • Memory relatively spared
Temporal variant FTD (Tv-FTD)	• Loss of memory for words • Anomia • Impaired word comprehension • Impaired person recognition • Personality changes
Primary progressive aphasia (PPA)	• Reduced speech rate • Repetition impaired • Phonologic and grammatical errors • Comprehends words

• Frontal variants maintain relatively good orientation to time and place, have relatively intact memory, and do not become geographically disoriented.

• Temporal variants show much more impairment in naming and language comprehension due to temporal lobe atrophy.

• Primary progressive aphasia is characterized by effortful speech, phonologic and grammatical errors, reading and writing difficulty, and progressive loss of speech.

DIFFERENTIAL DIAGNOSIS

• AD

• Corticobasal degeneration

• Progressive supranuclear palsy

• Dementia with Lewy bodies

• VaD

Characteristics of FTD are summarized in table 91.12.

WORKUP

Laboratory workup for FTD is similar to that for AD.

STRUCTURAL IMAGING

Structural imaging is usually normal early in disease. Lobar atrophy may or may not be seen in frontal lobes (Fv-FTD) and/or temporal lobes (Tv-FTD). Primary progressive aphasia may show left-sided perisylvian atrophy.

FUNCTIONAL IMAGING

Once the disease is established FDG-PET and Tc99 SPECT typically show frontal (Fv-FTD) and/or anterior temporal (Tv-FTD) or left perisylvian (primary progressive aphasia) dysfunction.

TREATMENT

There are currently no FDA-approved treatments for FTD. Treatment is supportive, including SSRIs and atypical neuroleptics (such as risperidone) to reducing unwanted behavioral symptoms. (Note black box warning: neuroleptics are not approved for dementia-related use in elderly patients; increased deaths due to cardiovascular or infectious events.)

ADDITIONAL READING

Budson AE, Price BH. Memory dysfunction. *N Engl J Med*. 2005;352: 692–9.

Budson AE, Kowall NW. *The Handbook of Alzheimer's disease and other dementias*. Wiley-Blackwell; 2011.

Budson AE, Solomon PR. *Memory Loss: A Practical Guide for Clinicians*. Philadelphia: Saunders Elsevier; 2011.

Graff-Radford NR. *Neurology Clinics: Dementia*. Philadelphia: Saunders Elsevier; 2007.

Growdon JH, Rossor MN. *The Dementias 2*. Philadelphia: Butterworth Heinemann Elsevier; 2007.

Jack CR, Albert MS, Knopman DS, et al. Introduction to the recommendations from the National Institute on Aging and the Alzheimer's Association workgroup on diagnostic guidelines for Alzheimer's disease. *Alzheimers Dement*. 2011;7:257–62.

Mayeux R. Clinical practice. Early Alzheimer's disease. *N Engl J Med*. 2010;362(23):2194–2201. Erratum *N Engl J Med*. 2010;363(12): 1190.

Mesulam MM. *Principles of Behavioral and Cognitive Neurology*. New York: Oxford University Press; 2000.

Querfurth HW, LaFerla FM. Alzheimer's disease. *N Engl J Med.* 2010; 362(4):329–44.

Solomon PR, Budson AE. Alzheimer's disease. *Clin Symposia.* 2003; 54(1):1–44.

QUESTIONS

QUESTION 1. An 82-year-old woman is brought by her daughter for evaluation of memory loss. The patient's daughter describes her mother as having trouble with short-term memory. She dates this as starting approximately 2 years back. She says that her mother complains of dizziness and unsteadiness on her feet. She is moody but some times seems depressed. She has developed urinary incontinence over the past 3 months. Past medical history of long-standing hypertension, diabetes mellitus, and peripheral vascular disease. On the MMSE, the patient scored 19/30 with abnormal clock drawing. On the Geriatric Depression Scale (GDS), the patient scored 3/15. Her brain MRI shows evidence of severe small vessel ischemic disease in frontal and parietal white matter, as well as pons and cerebellum.

The most likely diagnosis is:

A. Alzheimer disease
B. Vascular dementia
C. Creutzfeldt-Jakob disease
D. Huntington disease
E. Lewy body dementia

QUESTION 2. What criterion is required for the diagnosis of Alzheimer disease?

A. Disturbances in consciousness
B. Changes in personality
C. Static loss of memory function
D. Impairment of two areas of cognition
E. Agitation

QUESTION 3. All of the following are suggestive of dementia with Lewy bodies (DLB), *except*:

A. Fluctuations in cognitive function with varying levels of alertness and attention
B. Visual hallucinations
C. Parkinsonian motor features
D. Auditory hallucinations
E. REM sleep behavior disorder

ANSWERS

1. B
2. D
3. D

92.

NEUROLOGY BOARD SIMULATION

Galen V. Henderson

QUESTIONS

QUESTION 1. A 22-year-old male is evaluated in the emergency department after 12 hours of sudden onset of moderate neck pain followed by vertigo, ataxia, slurred speech, and difficulty swallowing. His medical history is unremarkable, and he is not taking any medications. Physical examination shows left ptosis, anisocoria with the left pupil smaller than the right, nystagmus, left-sided dysmetria, and decreased pain and temperature sensation on the left side of the face and right side of the body. computed tomography (CT) scan of the brain is normal.

What is the most appropriate test?

A. Repeat CT of the brain in 24 hours
B. Carotid ultrasound
C. Magnetic resonance imaging (MRI) MR angiography (MRA) of the brain and neck
D. Lumbar puncture

QUESTION 2. A 32-year-old male is evaluated for what he calls a "sinus headache." The headache occurs two or three times per month and is accompanied by facial pressure and occasional rhinorrhea. Resting in a dark quiet room gives minor relief. The symptoms resolve in 1 or 2 days regardless of treatment. He has tried multiple varieties of decongestants and antihistamines without success. Acetaminophen-aspirin-caffeine preparations provide minimal relief. He is currently symptomatic. On examination, the patient is pale and moderately distressed. Temperature is 37.1°C, pulse rate is 84/min, respiration rate 16/min, and blood pressure is 132/75 mm Hg. His face is tender on palpation.

What is his most likely diagnosis?:

A. Cluster headache
B. Migraine without aura
C. Sinus headache
D. Tension headache

QUESTION 3. A 70-year-old man is evaluated for a 9-month history of progressive gait disturbance. For the same period of time, he has noticed numbness and tingling in his hands and an occasional "electric shock" sensation into his arms and down his spine when he bends his neck. Examination show normal mental status and cranial nerves. Upper extremity strength is normal except for mild 4/5 weakness of the intrinsic muscles of his hands. Lower extremity strength is 4/5. There is vibratory loss in the hands and from the knees down. Reflexes are 2+ in the biceps bilaterally, with 3+ in the triceps and knee jerks, with sustained clonus in the ankles. An extensor planar response is present bilaterally. Gait is very stiff and narrow based, and his legs tend to "scissor" over each other as he walks forward.

Which of the following is the most likely diagnosis?

A. Parkinson disease
B. Lumbar spinal stenosis
C. Normal-pressure hydrocephalus
D. Cervical spondylotic myelopathy

QUESTION 4. A 70-year-old woman with a history of diabetes mellitus is admitted to the ICU after surgical repair of a small bowel perforation associated with peritonitis. After treatment of the sepsis, she cannot be weaned from the ventilator. Physical examination revels severe generalized weakness with sparing of cranial nerve function. Reflexes are absent, and the sensation is decreased to light touch in the distal upper and lower extremities. Cerebrospinal fluid protein concentration is normal

What is the most likely diagnosis?

A. Vasculitic neuropathy
B. Guillain-Barré syndrome
C. Diabetic lumbosacral polyradiculopathy
D. Critical illness polyneuropathy

Question 5. A 32-year-old woman is evaluated for a 2-week history of weakness of the right arm and left leg. The initial symptom was acute right wrist drop associated with sensory loss in a radial nerve distribution and severe pain. One week later, she developed similar symptoms in the left peroneal nerve distribution. The patient has systemic lupus erythematosus, and her medications include prednisone and hydroxychloroquine.

Which of the following is the most likely diagnosis?

A. Guillain-Barré syndrome
B. Toxic neuropathy
C. Motor neuron disease
D. Vasculitic neuropathy
E. Lyme disease

QUESTION 6. A 59-year-old man has been incontinent of urine eight times in the past 3 months. He complains of urgency and cannot inhibit micturition. His family notes that his gait has become hesitant and his thinking has slowed. He had a single episode of subarachnoid hemorrhage 2 years ago treated by clipping of an aneurysm. Medical history is otherwise unremarkable. Neurologic examination shows decreased spontaneity but good memory and normal use of language; a small-stepped, shuffling gait; and bilateral extensor plantar reflexes.

The most likely diagnosis is:

A. Normal-pressure hydrocephalus
B. Alzheimer disease
C. Cervical spondylitic myelopathy
D. Diabetic neuropathy
E. Parkinson disease

QUESTION 7. Ten days ago, a 22-year-old man had an inoculation of tetanus toxoid in his right arm after removal of a splinter. He now has severe pain in the right shoulder and right arm and paresthesias in the right hand. Physical examination shows severe weakness of muscles around the right shoulder girdle and absence of the right biceps reflex. Passive range of movement of the shoulder is normal. Sensory examination is normal, and other reflexes in the arms and legs are normal.

The most likely diagnosis is:

A. Brachial neuritis
B. Herniated C-7 disk
C. Epidural cervical spinal abscess
D. Cervical spinal cord tumor
E. Rotator cuff injury

Question 8. A 60-year-old man with a long history of back pain recently began feeling weakness and tingling in his legs when he walks more than a half a block. The symptoms disappear when he sits. He has no symptoms when doing bicycling-like exercises supine on his bed even after 30 minutes. Except for an absent left ankle reflex, neurological examination is normal. Foot and femoral pulses are normal.

The most likely diagnosis is:

A. Aortic atherosclerosis with claudication
B. Polyneuropathy
C. Herniated lumbar L-5 disc

D. Lumbar spinal stenosis
E. Cervical spondylitic myelopathy

QUESTION 9. A 25-year-old previously healthy man is found unconscious in his apartment. There is no evidence of trauma. On examination, he is responsive to voice and painful stimulation. There is no evidence of meningeal irritation. The pupils are 3 mm and unreactive. There are no inducible eye movements by the doll's eye maneuver or irrigation of a tympanic membrane with ice water. The blood pressure is 90/70 mm Hg, and the pulse rate is 54/min. Respiratory function is depressed.

The most likely diagnosis is:

A. Sedative drug overdose
B. Subarachnoid hemorrhage
C. Intracranial mass
D. Brainstem stroke
E. Narcotic overdose

QUESTION 10. A 35-year-old woman who had a renal transplant 4 years ago for renal failure due to membranous glomerulonephritis is hospitalized because of progressive right homonymous hemianopia. She has been treated with prednisone and cyclosporine. A test for the human immunodeficiency virus is negative. CT scan of the brain shows, in the left occipital lobe, a large low-density lesion that spares the cortical gray matter. There is no mass effect and no contrast enhancement. There are also similar smaller lesions throughout the white matter.

The most likely diagnosis is:

A. Multiple sclerosis
B. Glioma
C. Embolic stroke
D. Progressive multifocal leukoencephalopathy
E. Primary central nervous system lymphoma

QUESTION 11. A 70-year-old woman is hospitalized with aspiration pneumonia. She has had difficulty walking over the past 3–4 years. She now frequently falls and has been using a walker for 1 year. Her speech is unintelligible and she has poor vision. She was briefly treated with carbidopa-levodopa without improvement. On physical examination, she looks anguished, has difficulty with down gaze, and is severely dysarthric. She is rigid throughout but more so in the neck and has moderate bradykinesia and impaired gait and postural reflexes.

What is the most likely diagnosis?

A. Parkinson disease
B. Progressive supranuclear palsy
C. Normal-pressure hydrocephalus
D. Amyotrophic lateral sclerosis

QUESTION 12. A 50-year-old woman is evaluated for a 2-day history of headache and progressive sleepiness. She was diagnosed with breast adenocarcinoma 5 years ago and has received lumpectomy, breast radiation therapy, and chemotherapy with cyclophosphamide, methotrexate, and doxorubicin. The tumor recurred 1 year ago, and she has metastases to the liver, lung, and bone. Her medications include morphine sulfate and tamoxifen. On examination, she is afebrile, drowsy but can follow simple commands symmetrically with all four extremities. The pupils are 4 mm, symmetric, and reactive. She has mild bilateral papilledema. There is mild neck stiffness. CT of the head with and without contrast shows communicating hydrocephalus with no abnormal enhancement.

What is the most likely diagnosis?

A. Pseudotumor cerebri
B. Leptomeningeal carcinomatosis
C. Superior sagittal sinus thrombosis
D. Fungal meningitis

QUESTION 13. Four years after having lumpectomy and radiation treatment for breast carcinoma, a 45-year-old woman develops pain and weakness of the left leg that spreads over a period of 1 week to involve the right leg. She also has local back pain in the midthorax and a circumferential band-like sensation. In the past day, she has become incontinent of urine after brief urgency, and her genitalia are numb. The patient weighs 160 kg (352 lb). Reflexes are 3+ with unsustained ankle and knee clonus; toes are extensor and the legs occasionally jerk into a flexed posture.

The most likely diagnosis is:

A. Intramedullary metastasis
B. Epidural metastasis
C. Carcinomatous meningitis
D. Metastasis to the sagittal sinus
E. Radiation necrosis of the spinal cord

QUESTION 14. A 55-year-old male is evaluated in the emergency department after awakening with vertigo, ataxia, and headache. He has hypertension and stable angina, and his medications are aspirin, a beta blocker, and a statin. On examination, his blood pressure is 170/90 mm Hg. Physical examination reveals bidirectional nystagmus and gait ataxia. CT scan of the brain is normal. Examination on the following day reveals intractable hiccups, bidirectional horizontal nystagmus, normal strength, and dysmetria of the right upper and lower extremities.

Which of the following is the most likely diagnosis?

A. Ménière disease
B. Cerebellar infarction
C. Vestibular migraine
D. Benign positional vertigo
E. Vestibular neuronitis

QUESTION 15. A 23-year-old mechanic caught his hand in a vise. Two weeks later he developed a severe, constant ache in his hand. The hand becomes pale with some cyanotic mottling, feels cold and sweaty, and movement is limited.

The most likely diagnosis is:

A. Carpal tunnel syndrome
B. Occlusion of the ulnar artery
C. Psychophysiological disorder
D. Complex regional pain syndrome
E. Acute brachial plexus neuritis (Parsonage-Turner syndrome)

QUESTION 16. A 30-year-old man is evaluated for a 1-month history of episodes during which he is suddenly unable to speak. He has had five episodes; the last three were during the past week. There are no warnings preceding episodes, and they last 20–30 seconds. During the episodes, the patient has twitching of the right side of his face; on one occasion the twitching progressed to involve the right arm. The patient states that he is fully aware of his surroundings during the episodes and has no other symptoms. He has no significant medical history and takes no medications. Physical examination is normal.

Which of the following is the most likely diagnosis?

A. Transient ischemic attack
B. Frontal lobe seizure
C. Hemiplegic migraine
D. Hypoglycemia

QUESTION 17. A 60-year-old woman is transferred to a chronic facility 8 weeks after a cardiac arrest. The arrest occurred when she was at a restaurant and suddenly lost consciousness. When EMS arrived minutes later, she was found to be in Vfib arrest and was successfully cardioverted to normal sinus rhythm. Since her cardiac arrest, she has remained unresponsive, without any response to commands; 3 weeks after the arrest, she began to have the return of normal sleep–wake cycles.

On examination, he has a tracheostomy in place but is not on the ventilator and breathes well spontaneously. She occasionally yawns. Pupils are equal and reactive to light. Her eyes are open; she has spontaneous conjugate movements of her eyes to either side but does not appear to track objects or look at the examiner. She flexes her arms to noxious stimuli but has no evidence of any purposeful or voluntary response to visual, auditory, or tactile stimulation

Which of the following is the most appropriate description of this patient's condition?

A. Permanent vegetative state
B. Persistent vegetative state
C. Minimally consciousness state
D. Locked-in syndrome
E. Brain dead

QUESTION 18. A 75-year-old man is evaluated for dizziness. He feels light-headed when he stands and has fainted twice in the last year. He has a sense of imbalance with occasional falls that has developed insidiously over the past 3 years. He also has urinary incontinence, constipation, and impotence.

On examination, blood pressure is 130/80 mm Hg with a pulse rate of 80/min while lying down and a blood pressure of 80/50 mm Hg with no change in pulse rate standing up. There is impairment in fine motor movements bilaterally and in gait and balance. There is mild rigidity but no tremor. Deep tendon reflexes are brisk and symmetric, and extensor plantar response is present bilaterally.

What is the most likely diagnosis?

A. Systemic amyloidosis
B. Progressive supranuclear palsy
C. Multiple system atrophy
D. Vitamin B-12 deficiency
E. Parkinson disease

QUESTION 19. A 55-year-old man is evaluated for a 5-month history of progressive right foot drop and slurred speech. Physical examination reveals tongue weakness associated with tongue fasciculations and atrophy and a positive jaw jerk. The right leg is weak and atrophic with fasciculations. He has ankle clonus and an extensor plantar response. The sensory examination is normal.

What is the most likely diagnosis?

A. Cervical spondylosis
B. Myasthenia gravis
C. Spinal muscular atrophy
D. Amyotrophic lateral sclerosis

QUESTION 20. A 50-year-old man is evaluated for a 6-month history of progressive proximal muscle weakness, myalgias, fatigue, and distal paresthesias. He also has constipation and mild hoarseness. He has a history of obesity, hyperlipidemia, and hypertension. Medications include lovastatin and lisinopril.

Physical examination confirms the presence of hip and shoulder girdle weakness. Reflexes are normal, although the relaxation phase is delayed. Creatine kinase level is 12,000 U/L.

Which of the following is the most appropriate for this patient?

A. Remove the statin
B. Muscle biopsy
C. Thyroid-stimulating hormone assay
D. Electromyography
E. Acetylcholine receptor antibody titer

ANSWERS

1. C. This patient has had an ischemic stroke. The symptoms and signs involve multiple cranial nerves and crossed sensory deficits and cerebellar ataxia, which all localize to the left lateral medulla and cerebellum. The vascular territory is the posterior inferior cerebellar artery which is the major branch of the vertebral artery. The normal CT rules out a cerebral hemorrhage and may not be sensitive enough to visualize an early stroke in the posterior fossa. Because the patient is young, the most likely etiology is that he has had an arterial dissection of the vertebral artery, which usually causes pain in the posterior head or neck, Horner syndrome (miosis and ptosis), dysarthria, dysphagia, and decreased pain and temperature sensation of the face and contralateral body, dysmetria, ataxia, and vertigo. Carotid ultrasounds are rarely helpful in the evaluation of patients with posterior circulation syndromes. Lumbar puncture is used to evaluate suspected subarachnoid hemorrhage in the patient who has a severe headache and normal CT scan. These localized signs would be atypical for a subarachnoid hemorrhage.

Key points: Vertebral artery dissections typically presents with neck or head pain, Horner syndrome, dysarthria, dysphagia, decreased pain and temperature sensation, dysmetria, and ataxia and vertigo. MRA is a sensitive diagnostic test for vertebral artery dissections as a cause of stroke.

2. B. This patient presents with typical symptoms of migraine headache. Those symptoms include worsening of the headache with movement, limitation of activities, and requiring absence of light and sound. Although some of the autonomic features are present (congestion/rhinorrhea), the headache is not a cluster type because it last longer than 180 minutes. In addition, although not part of the absolute for cluster headache, patients with cluster headache prefer to be mobile because resting causes worsening of the pain. The patient does not have the secondary headache of sinus infection because of the lack of fever or discolored nasal discharge. Although sinus symptoms are not formal criteria for migraine, they are quite common and can complicate the diagnosis. Tension-type headache can be ruled out because of the disabling characteristic of the headache and the presence of both phono- and photophobia.

Key point: Migraine headache without aura includes worsening of headache with movement, limitation of activities, and phonophobia and photophobia.

3. E. The patient has bilateral weakness and vibratory loss in the hands and legs as well as bilateral upper motor neuron findings including spastic gait. These finding are most consistent with a cervical spinal cord process. The historical finding of a Lhermitte's sign, an electric shock-like sensation that occurs with neck flexion, is a helpful historical clue to the presence of a cervical spinal cord problem. The progressive nature of the symptoms suggests a compressive lesion, which can occur in this age group due to cervical spondylosis.

Lumbar spinal stenosis would not explain the upper extremity symptoms or the spasticity seen in the patient. Multiple sclerosis can present as a progressive spinal cord syndrome but would be unusual in this age group. Normal-pressure hydrocephalus presents as a shuffling "magnetic" gait as if the feet are glued to the floor, unlike the spastic gait of this patient. Amyotrophic lateral sclerosis is a purely motor syndrome that affects both the lower and upper motor neurons. The condition can cause weakness and spasticity but would not explain the sensory symptoms or signs in this patient.

Key points: Lhermitte's sign, an "electric shock" sensation down the neck, back, or extremities with flexion of the neck, is a helpful clue to cervical spinal cord disease. Cervical spondylosis is a chronic disorder of degenerative changes of the vertebrae, ligaments, and discs that may narrow the spinal canal and can cause cervical spinal cord compression.

4. D. Critical illness polyneuropathy is characterized by generalized or distal flaccid paralysis, depressed or absent reflexes, and distal sensory loss with relative sparing of cranial nerve function. The cause is unknown, but it usually occurs after admission to the intensive care unit, and the predisposing risk factors are sepsis and/or multiorgan failure or the use of paralytics. Cerebral spinal fluid protein is normal in this disorder.

Guillain-Barré syndrome is associated with weakness and respiratory failure that usually begins before admission to the intensive care unit and is usually preceded by a viral infection. Cranial nerves are frequently affected, and cerebrospinal fluid (CSF) protein concentration is usually elevated within 1 week and can be useful in distinguishing this disorder from critical illness polyneuropathy. Vasculitic and lumbosacral diabetic neuropathy are not associated with respiratory failure.

Key points: Critical illness polyneuropathy is a common cause of failure to wean from a ventilator in a patient with associated multiorgan failure and sepsis. Critical illness polyneuropathy is characterized by generalized distal flaccid paralysis, depressed or absent reflexes, and distal sensory loss with sparing of cranial nerve functions.

5. D. Vasculitic neuropathy, also called mononeuritis multiplex, involves damage to at least two mononeuropathies and is associated with pain, weakness, or sensory loss. Having common diseases such as polyarteritis nodosa, rheumatoid arthritis, systemic lupus erythematosus, or diabetes mellitus places patients at higher risk of developing the disease. Toxic neuropathies, Guillain-Barré syndrome, and motor neuron disease usually do not present as individual mononeuropathies and are not associated with pain.

Key points: Mononeuritis multiplex, vasculitic neuropathy, is a painful asymmetric asynchronous sensory and motor peripheral neuropathy involving isolated damage to at least two separate nerve areas. Mononeuropathy multiplex syndromes can be distributed bilaterally, distally and proximally, throughout the body.

6. A. Patients with normal-pressure hydrocephalus exhibit the classic triad of gait difficulties, urinary incontinence, and mental decline. It is often misdiagnosed as Parkinson disease (parkinsonism, tremor, rigidity), Alzheimer disease (primary cognitive disorder with memory disorders), and senility due to its chronic nature and its presenting symptoms. Although the exact mechanism is unknown, normal-pressure hydrocephalus is thought to be a form of communicating hydrocephalus with impaired CSF reabsorption at the arachnoid villi. Cervical spondylitic myelopathy usually affects arms and legs, and the patient may have a spastic gait. Diabetic neuropathy is a length-dependent neuropathy that predominately affects the longest nerves; therefore, the distal lower extremities are affected first.

Key point: Normal-pressure hydrocephalus exhibits the classic triad of gait difficulties, urinary incontinence, and mental decline.

7. A. Brachial neuritis is characterized by severe shoulder and upper arm pain followed by marked upper arm weakness. The temporal profile of pain preceding weakness is important in establishing a prompt diagnosis and differentiating acute brachial plexus neuritis from cervical radiculopathy. MRI of the shoulder and upper arm musculature may reveal denervation within days, allowing prompt diagnosis. Electromyography conducted 3–4 weeks after the onset of symptoms can localize the lesion and help confirm the diagnosis. Treatment includes analgesics and physical therapy, with resolution of symptoms usually occurring in 3–4 months. Patients with cervical radiculopathy present with simultaneous pain and neurologic deficits that fit a nerve root pattern. This differentiation is important to avoid unnecessary surgery for cervical spondylotic changes in a patient with a plexitis.

Key point: Brachial neuritis is characterized by severe shoulder and upper arm pain followed by marked upper arm weakness.

8. D. Lumbar stenosis (spinal stenosis) is a condition whereby either the spinal canal (central stenosis) or vertebral foramen (foraminal stenosis) becomes narrowed. If the narrowing is substantial, it causes compression of the nerves, which causes the painful symptoms of lumbar spinal stenosis. The most common cause of lumbar spinal stenosis is degenerative arthritis. Patients with spinal stenosis may or may not have back pain, depending on the degree of arthritis that has developed. Pressure on spinal nerves can result in pain in the areas that the nerves supply. The pain may be described as an ache or a burning feeling. It typically starts in the area of the buttocks and radiates down the leg. The pain down the leg is often called "sciatica." As it progresses, it can result in pain in the foot. As pressure on the nerve increases, numbness and tingling often accompany the burning pain, although not all patients will have both burning pain and numbness and tingling. Studies of the lumbar spine show that leaning forward can actually increase the space available for the nerves. Many

patients may note relief when leaning forward and especially with sitting. Pain is usually made worse by standing up straight and walking. Some patients note that they can ride a stationary bike or walk leaning on a shopping cart. Walking more than 1 or 2 blocks, however, may bring on severe sciatica or weakness. With aortic atherosclerosis with claudication, leaning forward will not make a difference.

Key point: Lumbar spinal stenosis is secondary to degenerative joint disease. Pressure on spinal nerves can result in pain in the areas that the nerves supply and can be relieved by leaning forward, as in leaning against a cart or riding a bicycle.

9. D. Patient is responsive to voice and stimulation and has no eye movements with the cold caloric examination. This localizes to the brainstem and is consistent with a locked-in syndrome. Patients with the locked-in syndrome are conscious because of intact cortical and upper brainstem function but are quadriplegic and can communicate only by moving their eyes vertically or blinking. The locked-in syndrome is caused by lesions of the base of the pons. Sedative drug overdose or narcotic would not give such a focal examination. Patient presenting with subarachnoid hemorrhage

Key point: Vascular lesions in the pons may cause the patient to be "locked-in" (intact consciousness, quadriparesis with abnormal caloric responses and vertical gaze intact).

10. D. Progressive multifocal leukoencephalopathy is characterized by progressive damage to the white matter of the brain at multiple locations. It occurs almost exclusively in people with severe immune deficiency, such as transplant patients on immunosuppressive medications, patients receiving certain kinds of chemotherapy, or AIDS patients. There is no enhancement with CT or MRI imaging of the brain.

For primary central nervous system lymphoma, neuroimaging reveals solitary lesions that are most commonly located supratentorially in the white matter of the frontal or parietal lobes or in the subependymal regions, but the lesions may also involve the deep gray matter. CT scans usually show high attenuation, probably because of high cellularity, and virtually all lesions show homogeneous contrast enhancement. On MRI, B-cell primary CNS lymphoma lesions are clearly delineated masses that appear isointense to hypointense on T1-weighted images and mostly hypointense on T2-weighted images. Nearly all lesions show homogeneous enhancement with contrast material. A classic presentation is the lesion that crosses the corpus callosum in a butterfly pattern. The time course is not appropriate for a brain tumor or stroke. The imaging and time course are not consistent with multiple sclerosis.

Key point: Progressive multifocal leukoencephalopathy is characterized by progressive damage to the white matter of the brain at multiple locations in patients with severe immune deficiency/suppression medication and does enhance on CT/MRI imaging of the brain.

11. B. Parkinsonism with early gait and balance involvement, vertical gaze palsy, severe dysarthria, and dysphagia suggests progressive supranuclear palsy. Lack of responsiveness of early gait and balance impairment to dopaminergic medications and lack of asymmetry make Parkinson disease unlikely. The lack of the classic triad of gait impairment, cognitive decline, and urinary incontinence makes normal-pressure hydrocephalus unlikely. Amyotrophic lateral sclerosis presents with weakness, muscle atrophy, and fasciculations, which are not present in this case.

Key points: Progressive supranuclear palsy is characterized by parkinsonism with early gait and balance involvement, vertical gaze palsy, and severe dysarthria and dysphagia. Normal-pressure hydrocephalus is characterized by the classic triad of gait impairment, cognitive decline, and urinary incontinence.

12. B. Leptomeningeal spread occurs in 5–15% of systemic carcinomas. It may present as a cranial neuropathy or spinal polyradiculopathy. Occasionally, it can present with confusion due to seizures, diffuse brain infiltration, or communicating hydrocephalus from obstruction of the arachnoid granulations. A chronic infectious meningitis could present in a similar fashion but is less likely because the patient is not severely immunocompromised.

Neither superior sagittal sinus thrombosis nor pseudotumor cerebri is associated with hydrocephalus. In this patient, the most appropriate next step to establish the diagnosis is a lumbar puncture to evaluate for malignant cells. Sometimes several lumbar punctures are required before a positive cytologic diagnosis is documented. MRI of the neuronal axis with contrast would be more likely to document leptomeningeal enhancement but is not a sensitive tool.

Key point: Leptomeningeal spread of the systemic carcinoma manifests as cranial neuropathy or spinal polyradiculopathy or as encephalopathy diffuse brain infiltration or communicating hydrocephalus.

13. C. Epidural metastases are very common in patients with advanced cancer. The tumor reaches the epidural space via contiguous spread from adjacent vertebral body metastases or, less commonly, from direct extension of tumor through the intervertebral foramina from adjacent tissue. Back pain is the herald symptom of epidural metastases, occurring, on average, many weeks to months prior to any neurological damage—that is, pain occurs long before there is any direct compression of the spinal cord. Carcinomatous meningitis usually presents with either confusion or cranial neuropathies and tends not to be painful. Lesions of the sagittal sinus will cause headache, papilledema, and, in severe cases cerebral hemorrhage and cerebral edema Radiation necrosis of the spinal cord will tend to be a painless myelopathy and affecting both extremities equally.

Key point: Epidural metastases are seen in patients with advanced cancer from direct extension of tumor through the intervertebral foramina from adjacent tissue. Back pain is the herald symptom of epidural metastases.

14. B. This patient presents with the classic signs of an ischemic or hemorrhagic cerebellar stroke, which are vertigo, headache, and ataxia. Although a CT scan can exclude hemorrhage, infarcts in the posterior fossa may not be well visualized early. His deterioration the following day with signs of brainstem compression (altered level of consciousness and intractable hiccups) indicates a dire situation, and urgent neurosurgical decompression is required. Peripheral vertigo may be result of many disorders of the ear including vestibular neuronitis, benign positional vertigo, and vestibular migraine acoustic neuroma and Ménière disease, but none of these causes unilateral limb ataxia, dysarthria, or hiccups. Headache may accompany vestibular migraine but is not a feature of the other peripheral disorders.

Key point: Classic symptoms of cerebellar stroke are headache, vertigo, and ataxia.

15. D. Complex regional pain syndrome (CRPS) is a chronic pain condition. The key symptom of CRPS is continuous, intense pain out of proportion to the severity of the injury that gets worse rather than better over time. CRPS most often affects one of the arms, legs, hands, or feet. Often the pain spreads to include the entire arm or leg. Typical features include dramatic changes in the color and temperature of the skin over the affected limb or body part, accompanied by intense burning pain, skin sensitivity, sweating, and swelling. The etiology of CRPS is not clear. In some cases the sympathetic nervous system plays an important role in sustaining the pain. Another theory is that CRPS is caused by a triggering of the immune response, which leads to the characteristic inflammatory symptoms of redness, warmth, and swelling in the affected area.

Carpal tunnel syndrome causes pain in the palm of the hand and weakness in the distribution of the median nerve. Occlusion of the ulnar artery usually will not cause our patient's symptoms because of the vascular compensation provided by the radial artery. Psychophysiological disorders would not explain the color change and change in temperature of the skin over the affected limb. Acute brachial plexus neuritis presents as pain and weakness of the upper shoulder or upper back. Distal hand function and sensation are usually not affected.

Key points: CRPS is a chronic pain condition that is continuous, intense pain out of proportion to the severity of the injury, which gets worse rather than better over time, and the extremity has changes in skin color and temperature over the affected area.

16. B. The patient most likely has partial seizures of the frontal lobe. The clinical presentation of partial seizures depends on their neuroanatomic location. In this case the seizures originate in Broca's language area and spread to the primary motor cortex. Frontal seizures are usually brief and without aura or postictal confusion. With the recent onset of seizures, brain scanning with an MRI should be done

to rule out space-occupying lesions or other pathology. Transient attack, hemiplegic migraine, and hypoglycemia can cause focal neurological deficits but would not cause twitching of the arm and face.

Key points: Frontal seizures are brief and are usually not associated with an aura or postictal confusion. The manifestation of partial seizures depends on their neuroanatomic location.

17. D. In this patient, severe cerebral anoxia from her cardiac arrest caused severe diffuse hemispheric cortical injury with relative preservation of brainstem function, leading to the development of a vegetative state. A vegetative state is a clinical condition of complete unawareness of self or the environment, accompanied by sleep–wake cycles and preservation of brainstem and hypothalamic functions. The term persistent vegetative state is defined as a vegetative state present 1 month after acute nontraumatic or traumatic brain injury. The permanent vegetate state is a vegetative state present 3 months after nontraumatic brain injury and 12 months after traumatic injury. The diagnosis of a vegetative state should be made only after careful observation of the patient for any signs of awareness or purposeful responsiveness.

In contrast to a vegetative state, in which here is no evidence of consciousness, in the minimally conscious state there is severely altered consciousness with minimal but definite behavioral evidence of awareness of the self or the environment. Patients with the locked-in syndrome are conscious because of intact cortical and upper brainstem function but are quadriplegic and can communicate only by moving their eyes vertically or blinking. The locked-in syndrome is caused by lesions of the base of the pons.

Brain death is the complete absence of all hemispheric or brainstem function including absence of respiratory drive.

Key points: Severe cerebral anoxia from cardiac arrest can cause severe diffuse cerebral hemispheric cortical injury with relative preservation of brainstem function, leading to the development of a vegetative state. A vegetative state is a condition of complete awareness of self or the environment, accompanied by sleep–wake cycles and preservation of brainstem and hypothalamic function.

18. C. This patient has evidence of dysautonomia (orthostatic hypotension, neurogenic bladder, constipation, and impotence), gait-predominant parkinsonism, and corticospinal tract sign. This constellation of symptoms is consistent with multiple system atrophy. Multiple system atrophy with prominent dysautonomia is commonly referred to as Shy-Drager syndrome.

Parkinson disease is usually asymmetric at onset, more commonly associated with tremor, and does not have prominent gait and balance involvement in the beginning of the disease. Parkinson disease can be associated with dysautonomia, but this usually occurs late in the disease and is not as pronounced. Vitamin B-12 deficiency can present with cognitive impairment, pyramidal signs, and peripheral neuropathy, but dysautonomia is not part of the clinical presentation. Progressive supranuclear palsy manifests itself with parkinsonism, vertical gaze palsy, and corticospinal signs but not dysautonomia. Parkinsonism is not part of the presentation of systemic amyloidosis.

Key point: Multiple system atrophy is characterized by orthostatic hypotension, neurogenic bladder, constipation, and impotence, with gait-predominant parkinsonism and corticospinal tract signs.

19. D. Amyotrophic lateral sclerosis is an acquired neurodegenerative disorder involving the cortical motor neurons in the frontal lobe, resulting in upper motor neuron sign (hyperreflexia, spasticity, extensor plantar responses) and the anterior horn cells in the spinal cord causing lower motor neuron signs/symptoms (atrophy, fasciculations, and weakness). Affected patients typically present with slowly progressive distal asymmetric muscle weakness associated with muscle atrophy and fasciculations. As a result of upper motor neuron degeneration in the frontal lobe, extensor plantar responses and pathologic hyperreflexia (ankle clonus) are also present.

Spinal muscular atrophy is a genetic disorder of children or young adults affecting only the anterior horn cells and therefore is not characterized by the pathologic hyperreflexia or extensor plantar response. Myasthenia gravis is a neuromuscular junction disorder that can cause dysarthria and dysphagia. The treatment is with acetylcholinesterase inhibitors, which may case fasciculations. Myasthenia gravis, however, does not cause upper motor neuron signs, and weakness is typically proximal and symmetric. Cervical spondylosis can cause a combination of upper motor neuron signs due to spinal cord compression and lower motor neuron signs due to nerve root compression; however, it is not associated with dysarthria and tongue weakness/fasciculations.

Key points: Amyotrophic lateral sclerosis is characterized by pathologic hyperreflexia, spasticity, and extensor plantar responses along with atrophy, fasciculation, and weakness. Muscle weakness in ALS usually begins distally and asymmetrically in the upper or lower extremities and may be limited initially to the bulbar muscles, resulting in dysarthria and dysphagia.

20. B. Hypothyroid myopathy is characterized by proximal muscle weakness, muscle hypertrophy, myalgias, and paresthesias. The physical examination is remarkable for the phenomenon of "myoedema," which can be elicited by percussion of the muscle with the reflex hammer as well as a delay in the relaxation phase of the muscle stretch reflex. Hypothyroid myopathy is usually associated with creatine kinase levels 10–100 times the upper limit of normal limits. Therefore, many patients with hypothyroid myopathy are inappropriately referred for electromyography or muscle biopsy before obtaining thyroid function tests.

Although myasthenia gravis can cause proximal muscle weakness and fatigue, it is not associated with myalgias, paresthesias, or muscle enzyme elevations.

Key points: Hypothyroid myopathy is characterized by muscle pain, cramps, stiffness, fatigue, and paresthesias. In hypothyroid myopathy, creatine kinase levels may be 10–100 times normal levels, but thyroid function tests should be performed before electromyography or muscle biopsy.

93.

NEUROLOGY SUMMARY

Tracey A. Cho, Emily Choi, James D. Berry, and Aneesh B. Singhal

Diseases of the brain, spinal cord, nerve, and muscle pose unique diagnostic and management challenges. The signs and symptoms of different neurological diseases often overlap, can mimic non-neurological diseases, can be transient in nature yet portend ominous outcome, and sometimes do not localize to a particular anatomical location. The diagnosis may not be apparent even with advanced imaging or other investigations. Brain imaging frequently reveals incidental abnormalities that further complicate management decisions. The frequent lack of a firm diagnosis, the relative paucity of established treatment options, and the chronic nature of many neurological diseases make management especially difficult. Nevertheless, careful history taking that focuses on establishing the *anatomical location* and the *temporal nature* of the disease process, combined with knowledge of the basic anatomy of the nervous system, makes it possible in most instances to decipher the various nervous system diseases. In this chapter we provide a general approach to diagnosis and briefly summarize the evaluation and management of specific neurological diseases and neurological emergencies that are more relevant to the practicing general physician or medical internist.

EVALUATION OF WEAKNESS

The symptom of weakness has a daunting list of differential diagnoses, ranging from neurological (e.g., diseases of the brain or spinal cord involving the corticospinal tract or supplemental motor pathways, diseases of the neuromuscular junction, motor nerves, and muscle), to non-neurological (e.g., asthenia from endocrine disturbances, electrolyte imbalance, and depression). Recognition of the three major types and patterns of neurological weakness (upper motor neuron, lower motor neuron, and myopathic weakness; table 93.1) can simplify history taking and help direct the examination toward localizing the anatomical site of the lesion. The patient should be asked about the circumstances during which the weakness is noted, the

onset, duration, and fluctuant nature of symptoms, associated sensory change, and the types of movements that are most impaired. Difficulty rising from squatting position or lifting objects over the head suggest proximal muscle weakness from neuromuscular causes; inability to open jars or stand on toes can suggest a distal process; sudden unilateral weakness suggests a vascular lesion (stroke) affecting the corticospinal tract; frequent falls could implicate paraparesis from a spinal cord lesion. Pharyngeal weakness is suggested by symptoms of difficulty with swallowing. Acute onset or rapidly progressive weakness should be worked up acutely (with particular regard for the 3-hour "window" for administration of IV tissue plasminogen activator (tPA) in the case of stroke and the 12- to 24-hour "window" for surgery in spinal cord compression), weakness with subacute onset should be worked up efficiently, and weakness with a chronic course should be worked up in due time provided respiratory muscle weakness is not apparent and there is no pharyngeal weakness that may increase the risk for aspiration pneumonia.

EVALUATION OF SENSORY SYMPTOMS

Sensory symptoms may arise from lesions in the peripheral nerve, or centrally in the sensory pathways, from the dorsal columns and spinothalamic tracts as they traverse the spinal cord and brainstem, to the thalamus, internal capsule, and cortical regions of the brain. The sensory system is notoriously difficult to evaluate because the physician needs to rely on patient perceptions not only for the history but also during the examination. For this reason it is important to evaluate for objective sensory loss toward the primary modalities of sensation (touch, pinprick, joint position, and vibratory sense) and carefully evaluate for "cortical" sensory changes such as graphesthesia and loss of two-point discrimination. The neurological history should focus on defining the *type* of sensory symptom (paresthesia, pain, allodynia, numbness, etc.) and the *pattern* of sensory loss, which depends on the onset,

Table 93.1 KEY FEATURES OF WEAKNESS

FEATURE	UPPER MOTOR NEURON	LOWER MOTOR NEURON	MYOPATHIC WEAKNESS
Muscle bulk	Normal (disuse atrophy may develop later)	Decreased	Variable
Muscle tone	Increased (except during the acute phase of central lesions)	Decreased	Decreased
Pattern of weakness	Upper extremity: extensor > flexor Lower extremity: flexor > extensor	Distal > proximal Segmental	Proximal
Deep tendon reflexes	Brisk +/− Clonus	Diminished or absent	Normal or diminished
Fasciculations	None	Present	Absent
Plantar reflex	Extensor	Flexor	Flexor

location, duration, progression, and associated symptoms. Common patterns of sensory loss include hemisensory change (brain or brainstem pathology or cervical spine disease if face is spared), spinal level (myelopathy), dermatomal (radiculopathy), stocking–glove (peripheral neuropathy), nerve distribution (mononeuropathy), and confluent nerve distributions (mononeuropathy multiplex). Trigeminal neuralgia (tic douloureux) causes excruciating paroxysms of stabbing facial pain. Recent medication and habit changes should be investigated (even something as simple as a change in hand position during computer use can contribute to compression neuropathies). Accompanying weakness and changes in deep tendon reflexes may help to localize the lesion, for example, distal symmetric sensory loss, associated with distal weakness, loss of muscle tone, and decreased tendon reflexes would suggest a peripheral motor-sensory neuropathy.

EVALUATION OF VISUAL SYMPTOMS

The most common visual symptoms resulting from neurological disorders include double vision (diplopia) and loss of vision, which could be localized to one or both eyes. For diplopia it is important to ascertain whether the double vision disappears with closure of either eye (monocular diplopia usually results from non-neurological causes such as lens dislocation), and the effect of horizontal and vertical eye movements on the degree of double vision. The examination should include observation of smooth pursuit to each of the cardinal directions of gaze, watching for misalignment of the eyes and noting the position in which it is most prominent. Associated features such as retro-orbital pain should raise suspicion of inflammation or a compressing brain aneurysm; associated hemiparesis would suggest a central lesion such as midbrain or pontine stroke; associated pain, eye redness, and chemosis suggest a local inflammatory lesion secondarily affecting the extraocular nerves or muscles that control eye movement; and associated ptosis or proximal muscular weakness would raise question of neuromuscular junction disorders such as myasthenia gravis.

Similarly, for visual loss it is essential to inquire whether the symptoms were localized to one eye or both eyes and to distinguish visual hemifield defects from unilateral loss of vision. Unilateral loss of vision suggests a prechiasmal lesion such as demyelinating diseases of the optic nerve (multiple sclerosis) or retinal or ocular ischemia (internal carotid artery stenosis, giant cell arteritis). Bilateral acute loss of vision usually localizes to the occipital-parietal lobes and can result from ischemia (cardiac arrest, top-of-the-basilar embolus, cerebral vasoconstriction syndromes), brain edema (hypertensive encephalopathy), or demyelinating diseases. Hemi–visual field loss (hemianopia) usually implicates postchiasmal lesions localizing to the lateral geniculate nucleus or occipital or temporal lobe from diseases such as stroke or brain tumor. Other visual symptoms include mild ptosis with miosis (components of the Horner syndrome, commonly resulting from carotid artery dissection) and positive visual phenomena such as scintillations and fortification spectra associated with unilateral headaches in patients with migraine.

COMMON NEUROLOGICAL CONDITIONS

SEIZURES

A seizure is defined as "a transient occurrence of signs and/or symptoms due to abnormal excessive or synchronous neuronal activity in the brain." Seizures can be primary or idiopathic (epilepsy) or secondary to head trauma, infection, stroke, metabolic insults, brain tumors, and other etiologies. *Epilepsy* is a brain disorder characterized by recurrent idiopathic seizures, often with specific underlying genetic abnormalities, and by the neurobiological, cognitive, psychological, and social consequences of recurrent seizures. In patients with epilepsy, seizures can be precipitated by minor factors (viral infection, lack of sleep, etc.) but are not referred to as provoked or secondary seizures. Seizures will affect about 5% of people at least once during their lifetime.

Among these, a smaller percentage will develop epilepsy. The prevalence of epilepsy in developed countries is about 5 per 1000.

Seizures can be classified as partial or generalized, with subtypes within each group (table 93.2). Focal seizures may spread to involve the entire brain (secondary generalization), whereas generalized seizures involve the entire brain from their onset and may have their genesis in the thalamus.

The most common differential diagnoses for seizures include syncope, nonepileptic seizures (also referred to as pseudoseizures or psychogenic seizures), panic attacks, migraine, dystonia, cataplexy, and nonepileptic myoclonus (e.g., after cardiac arrest). History taking should focus on distinguishing seizures from their mimics and, further, on characterizing the type of seizures because medical treatment is dependent on the subtype. Features that favor the occurrence of a bona fide seizure include the presence of incontinence, tongue biting, loss of awareness, adventitious movements, vocalizations, preceding aura, and a prolonged postictal confusional state. The examiner should carefully assess for possible provoking factors (drug intoxication or withdrawal, head trauma, meningitis/encephalitis, severe metabolic disturbance) and inquire about similar prior events, including febrile seizures in childhood and any personal or family history of seizure. For patients with a known seizure disorder, a full medication history should be obtained, including current medications and their doses, recent compliance, past antiepileptic medications and any allergies or adverse reactions, recent emotional and physical stressors such as lack of sleep, change in eating patterns, illness, or surgery. Additionally, it is important to know if the semiology of the current event is similar to or distinct from that of past seizures and if the patient has ever suffered from status epilepticus in the past. Medical and neurological physical exam should be performed to rule out ongoing or intermittent seizure, to uncover any signs of infection, trauma, drug intoxication, or other concurrent illness, and to rule out any neurocutaneous syndrome with a thorough skin exam. Vital signs, emergent blood glucose measurement, and clinical status should be observed carefully until the patient has returned to a baseline mental status.

Diagnostic evaluation after a first seizure should be directed at uncovering precipitating factors. Blood glucose, complete serum chemistries, liver function tests, complete blood count, arterial blood gas when appropriate, serum and urine toxicology, levels of any antiepileptic drugs being taken for psychiatric or pain disorders, urinalysis and culture, chest x-ray, electrocardiogram (EKG), and lumbar puncture, when indicated, to rule out inflammation or infection of the central nervous system (CNS) should all be performed. The workup for epileptic patients presenting with seizures of their typical semiology but increased duration or frequency is similar, although lumbar puncture is not indicated without compelling evidence for a CNS infection. It is not uncommon for a patient to be brought to the emergency department for a typical seizure that has occurred in public, and if reliable, these patients need not be reinvesti-

Table 93.2 CLASSIFICATION OF SEIZURES (INTERNATIONAL LEAGUE AGAINST EPILEPSY)

SEIZURE SUBTYPE	DEFINITION
GENERALIZED	**INVOLVE BOTH HEMISPHERES FROM ONSET**
Tonic	Generalized stiffening of the body with loss of consciousness.
Tonic-clonic (grand mal)	Stiffening of the body followed by alternating flexion and extension with loss of consciousness.
Clonic	Alternating flexion and extension without initial tonic phase with loss of consciousness.
Myoclonic	Sudden onset, brief muscle activation often described as a "body jerk." Consciousness may be preserved.
Atonic	Sudden onset loss of tone, causing the clinical entity called "drop attacks," typically with a loss of consciousness.
Absence (petit mal)	Staring episodes without loss of consciousness, but with loss of attention and lack of responsiveness lasting seconds, often associated with eye fluttering.
PARTIAL	**BEGIN FOCALLY**
Simple partial	Limited area of cortex involved causing no change in consciousness, and provoking signs and symptoms correlating to the area of cortex involved including alterations in sensation, language, or psyche, or localized movements, often tonic or clonic in nature.
Complex partial	Semiology is similar to simple partial seizures, but with impairment of consciousness either from onset or in the course of the event (suggesting a larger area of cortex is involved).
Complex partial with secondary generalization	Semiology is similar to complex partial seizures, but during the course of the event, there is spread to involve both hemispheres, causing bilateral symptoms.

gated for etiology. In the absence of persistent neurological deficit, history of trauma, or clinical suspicion for intracranial abnormality, acute imaging of the brain with computed tomography (CT) or magnetic resonance imaging (MRI) is not required and can be arranged on an outpatient basis. Otherwise, it should be done as a part of the acute evaluation. The yield of CT or MRI after a first unprovoked seizure is about 10%, identifying disorders such as stroke, tumor (figure 93.1), or neurocysticercosis. MRI is more sensitive than CT and is the preferred imaging modality if available. Serum prolactin may help differentiate nonepileptic seizure from an epileptic seizure if drawn within 30 minutes of the event and compared to the patient's baseline. Prolactin can rise after syncope and cannot be used to differentiate seizure from syncope. It is rarely used in practice because of its temporal and diagnostic limitations.

The first decision in treatment of epilepsy is whether an antiepileptic drug (AED) is necessary. For many causes of provoked seizures such as alcohol withdrawal or other

metabolic disturbances, treatment should be directed at the underlying process, and an AED is not necessary. In the case of symptomatic etiologies with possible structural changes—such as tumor, stroke, or head trauma—an AED is usually initiated and continued for at least a year. For those patients with recurrent seizures or a seizure in the setting of a clear irreversible cause, AED treatment should be initiated. In patients with a single unprovoked seizure of unknown cause, other factors may weigh in the decision to start treatment. The presence of risk factors such as an abnormal electroencephalogram (EEG), family history, abnormal neurological exam, presentation with status epilepticus, and postictal Todd's paralysis argue for treatment. Social factors such as the ability to drive or work may also contribute to the decision. Apart from AED treatment, patients should be instructed to avoid any factors that clearly precipitate their seizures, such as sleep deprivation, alcohol, or stress. They should also be advised to refrain from activities during which a seizure could lead to injury of themselves or others, including driving, operating heavy machinery, working at a height, or swimming or bathing alone. Each state has different regulations regarding driving, and the patient should be directed to the appropriate governing body.

In terms of choosing an AED, many factors contribute to the first-line choice for each patient, including the subtype of seizure, age of the patient, side effects, comorbid illnesses, and drug interactions (table 93.3). In general, certain agents have been shown to be more effective controlling partial or secondarily generalized seizures, including carbamazepine, valproic acid, phenytoin, and many of the newer agents, especially lamotrigine and oxcarbazepine. For primarily generalized epilepsies, first-line agents include valproic acid, lamotrigine, topiramate, levetiracetam, and zonisamide. Ethosuximide has efficacy specific to absence seizures. Pregnancy poses a particular problem for epilepsy treatment, as all AEDs are at least potentially teratogenic. Valproic acid and carbamazepine in particular should be avoided. This must be balanced with the adverse effects on the fetus of hypoxia from severe seizures. In women who require AED treatment for seizure control, the medication is usually continued at the lowest effective dose. Folic acid supplementation should be administered to help protect against neural tube defects.

The risk of recurrence after a first seizure of any kind ranges from 25% to 80% depending on other risk factors. Prognosis depends on many factors, including age, specific epilepsy syndrome, underlying lesions, and response to AED treatment. In general about 80% of patients will have a remission or good control with AED treatment. Most of the remaining 20% with poor control despite multiple AEDs and/or surgery are comprised of patients with infantile spasms or seizures related to a severe underlying lesion.

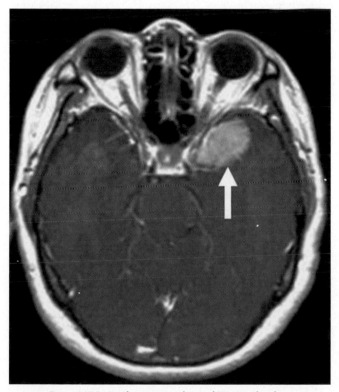

Figure 93.1. Brain MRI. Axial contrast-enhanced T1-weighted image showing an extra-axial enhancing mass consistent with a benign meningioma, in a patient with seizures. The role of EEG in the acute diagnosis of seizure is limited to the diagnosis of status epilepticus. However, in patients with a first unprovoked seizure, a follow-up EEG will reveal a significant abnormality in approximately 30% of cases. This is helpful to confirm the diagnosis of seizure and may help to predict recurrence. Patients with an abnormal EEG have a 50% chance of recurrence, about twice as likely as those with a normal EEG. In patients with no interictal epileptiform abnormalities, multiple EEGs can increase the negative predictive value for further seizure episodes to over 90%. Finally, the EEG can help distinguish among seizure subtypes, thus guiding specific treatment and prognosis.

Table 93.3 CATEGORIES OF ANTICONVULSANTS

Blockers of repetitive activation of sodium channel	Phenytoin, carbamazepine, oxcarbazepine, lamotrigine, topiramate
Enhancer of slow inactivation of voltage-gated sodium channel	Lacosamide, rufinamide
GABA-A receptor enhancers	Phenobarbital, benzodiazepines, vigabatrin, tiagabine, gabapentin and topiramate
Glutamate modulators	Topiramate, lamotrigine, felbamate
T-type calcium channel blockers (voltage-gated calcium channel)	Ethosuximide, valproate
N-type and L-type calcium channel blockers	Lamotrigine, topiramate, zonisamide, valproate
H-current modulators	Gabapentin, lamotrigine
Blockers of unique binding sites	Gabapentin, levetiracetam
Carbonic anhydrase inhibitors	Topiramate, zonisamide

HEADACHE

Headache is the most common neurological symptom in the outpatient setting. The 2004 International Classification of Headache Disorders Revision II (ICHD-II) classifies all headaches as either primary or secondary disorders. Primary headaches fit a recognized pattern with typical characteristics, and an underlying disease state is not the cause of the headache. Subcategories of primary headache disorders include migraine, tension headache, cluster and trigeminal autonomic type headaches, and other primary headaches. Table 93.4 shows the management of the common types of primary headache disorders. Secondary headache disorders are ones that result from an underlying process, which can be vascular, hemorrhagic, neoplastic, CSF-pressure related, substance use or withdrawal induced, inflammatory, or infectious. Table 93.5 shows the key features of the most

Table 93.4 COMMON PRIMARY HEADACHE DISORDERS

TYPE	CHARACTERISTIC	MANAGEMENT
Migraine – with aura – without aura – complicated	+/– visual, sensory aura; throbbing; usually unilateral; photophobia, phonophobia; onset over minutes to 1 hour; +/– nausea/emesis; identifiable triggers; improves with sleep; duration up to 24 hours.	*Abortive*: NSAIDs, acetaminophen, trigger avoidance, triptans, +/– ergots as outpatient; IV antiemetics, IV ergots as inpatient. *Prophylactic*: For headaches >1/week. *First line*: propranolol, topiramate; *Second line*: tricyclic antidepressants, calcium channel blockers, valproic acid (effective but limiting SE profile); *Third line*: gabapentin.
Tension-type headache	Constant; occipital predominance radiating frontally; bilateral; worse with emotional stress; worse later in day; duration up to days; +/– scalp tenderness.	*First line*: NSAIDs, acetaminophen, lifestyle change. *Second line*: occipital steroid injections, cervical muscle or frontalis Botox injections.
Primary thunderclap headache	Sudden onset; severe; maximal in severity at onset.	Urgent CT/MR with vascular imaging to exclude secondary causes such as ruptured cerebral aneurysm
Cluster	Sudden onset; unilateral; stabbing; orbital/supraorbital/temporal; occur in clusters with periods of quiescence between; +/– seasonal prevalence; at least one unilateral symptom of nasal congestion, sclera injection, tearing, facial/orbital edema, ptosis, myosis.	*Abortive*: oxygen, ergotamine. *Prophylactic* (used during a cluster): *First line*: oral prednisone (60 mg × 3 days, then taper). *Second line*: propranolol; lithium.
Trigeminal neuralgia	Stabbing/lancinating paroxysms of pain to a trigeminal distribution; unilateral symptoms; identifiable triggers.	*First Line*: Carbamazepine (start 200 mg bid or lower to avoid SE, titrate to max 600 mg bid). *Second line:* phenytoin, gabapentin, baclofen. *Surgical*: If MRI reveals vascular loop, surgery or radiosurgery may resolve symptoms.

Table 93.5 COMMON SECONDARY HEADACHE DISORDERS

EMERGENT CAUSES OF HEADACHE	CHARACTERISTIC HEADACHE FEATURES	FOCAL NEUROLOGICAL SIGNS	INITIAL DIAGNOSTIC WORKUP
Subarachnoid hemorrhage	Sudden onset, maximal at onset, bilateral, +/− throbbing, worst headache of life, +/− nausea	Confusion, depressed arousal, seizures, +/− focal motor/sensory/cranial nerve deficits	Noncontrast head CT, lumbar puncture, cerebral angiography (CT, MR, and/or catheter)
Intracranial hemorrhage	Worsening over hours, often with nausea, +/− throbbing	Focal neurological signs are present on exam. +/− confusion, +/− depressed arousal.	Noncontrast head CT, +/− brain MRI
Mass lesion	Gradual worsening over days or weeks, worst when recumbent, intermittent or constant, +/− lateralizing pain	Focal neurological signs are invariably present but may be subtle. Frontal lesions produce less deficits	Brain MRI with and without contrast, +/− CT initially (depending on availability of MRI)
Meningitis/encephalitis	Worsening over hours or days, often occipital with neck pain.	Nuchal rigidity, fever. Confusion/depressed arousal only in encephalitis	Lumbar puncture, noncontrast head CT prior if neurologic exam is not normal.
Carotid or vertebral dissection	Sudden onset, vertex pain is classic for carotid, occipital pain for vertebral, +/− preceding neck pain	Carotid: contralateral weakness, numbness, neglect, dysarthria. Vertebral: visual field deficit, dysarthria, incoordination, gait difficulty, nausea	Noncontrast head CT, noninvasive angiography (MRA/CTA), brain MRI with T1 fat saturated images.
Temporal arteritis	Lateralized frontal headache worse when chewing. May be retro-orbital. Progressive over days to weeks. Patients >50 years old.	Jaw claudication, visual dimming or transient monocular blindness, temporal tenderness, weight loss, fever, optic disk pallor	ESR, brain CT or MRI to rule out structural cause.
Acute angle closure glaucoma	Onset over hours, may be precipitated by dilated pupil exam, retro-orbital or orbital pain	Injected eye, decreased visual acuity in affected eye, often mydriasis	Occular pressure measurement.

common causes of secondary headaches and their initial management.

With a 10–18% prevalence of migraine, and 20–30% prevalence of tension-type headache in the general population, the vast majority of headaches are benign. However, headache can also be symptomatic of potentially ominous etiologies, leading to concern on the part of both the physician and the patient that a secondary etiology of headache may be overlooked without brain imaging. With proper history taking and a thorough neurological exam, and a basic understanding of the differential diagnosis for headache, these concerns can be waylaid. Guidelines for imaging in patients with headache are presented in table 93.6. Note that imaging is usually not indicated in patients with primary headache disorders such as migraine or tension-type headache who have a normal neurological examination.

ISCHEMIC STROKE

Stroke is defined as an acute neurological event secondary to ischemia or hemorrhage. Ischemic stroke results from ischemia of brain tissue secondary to either thrombosis or emboli to the cerebral vessels. Stroke ranks as the second leading cause of death worldwide, and approximately 795,000 people have new or recurrent stroke each year in the United States. On average, every 40 seconds someone in the United States has a stroke. Risk factors for stroke include age, hypertension, hyperlipidemia, smoking, diabetes, hypercoagulable states, cardiac arrhythmias such as atrial fibrillation, cardiomyopathy, and presence of a cardiac thrombus, among many others. Primary ischemic stroke and transient ischemic attacks (TIAs) conveniently divide into four subtypes: (1) large artery atherothrombotic (15%); (2) embolic (57%; cardiac, ascending aorta, or unknown source); (3) small vessel lacunar (25%); and (4) other (3%), such as arterial dissection, venous sinus occlusion, and arteritis. The symptoms of stroke are variable, depending on the vascular territory affected (table 93.7).

Patients presenting with symptoms of stroke should be admitted or referred to the nearest hospital for emergent care. Emergency management should include evaluation of the hemodynamic and respiratory stability of the patient with vital signs and brief clinical history and neurological exam including an assessment of the National Institutes of Health (NIH) stroke scale score. Brain imaging should be performed as soon as possible to determine the extent of the infarction and exclude mimics such as brain hemorrhage (figure 93.2).

The time of onset should be determined, and a neurologist should be consulted emergently for evaluation

Table 93.6 GUIDELINES FOR BRAIN IMAGING IN PATIENTS WITH HEADACHE

Emergent neurological imaging recommended	"Thunderclap" headache with abnormal neurological examination findings
Neurological imaging recommended to determine safety of lumbar puncture	Headache accompanied by signs of increased intracranial pressure Headache accompanied by fever and nuchal rigidity
Neurologic imaging should be considered	Isolated "thunderclap" headache
	Headache radiating to neck
	Temporal headache in an older individual

	New-onset headache in patient who
	  − is HIV positive
	  − has a prior diagnosis of cancer
	  − is in a population at high risk for intracranial disease

	Headache accompanied by abnormal neurologic examination findings, including papilledema or unilateral loss of sensation, weakness, or hyperreflexia
Neurological imaging not usually warranted	Migraine and normal neurological examination findings
No recommendation (some evidence for increased risk of intracranial abnormality)	Headache worsened by Valsalva maneuver, wakes patient from sleep, or is progressively worsening
No recommendation (insufficient data)	Tension-type headache and normal neurological examination results

SOURCE: Guidelines developed by the U.S. Headache Consortium, the American Academy of Neurology, the American College of Emergency Physicians, and the ACR.

and to determine eligibility for IVtPA, which is U.S. FDA approved for administration within 3 hours after stroke symptom onset. The dose of tPA is 0.9 mg/kg, 10% administered as a bolus and the remaining 90% by intravenous infusion over 1 hour. Contraindications to intravenous tPA include a stroke greater than one-third territory on noncontrast CT, evidence for brain hemorrhage, head trauma, prior history of intracerebral hemorrhage, rapidly resolving or minimal deficits, suspicion of subarachnoid hemorrhage, recent trauma or surgery within the prior 15 days, active internal bleeding or recent gastrointestinal bleeding, recent lumbar puncture or noncompressive arterial puncture within 7 days, bleeding diathesis (INR >1.7, PT >5, PTT >40, platelets <100, or known bleeding diathesis), uncontrolled hypertension (systolic blood pressure >185 or diastolic blood pressure >110 mm Hg despite medications), and seizures at onset. Patients receiving IV tPA should ideally be admitted to an intensive care unit for at least 24 hours for close monitoring of neurological status and blood pressure. Anticoagulation, arterial puncture, and antiplatelet agents should be avoided for 24 hours. A follow-up head CT scan should be obtained at 24 hours or earlier if there is a change in neurological examination. If the patient remains stable, he or she may be transferred to the floor for further diagnostic evaluation and management.

In academic or tertiary stroke centers, acute stroke treatment strategies also include intra-arterial approaches such as the administration of intra-arterial tPA or mechanical clot retrieval using FDA-approved devices such as the MERCI catheter or the Penumbra device. Patients with hemispheric

stroke symptoms presenting within 8 hours after symptom onset, or brainstem symptoms presenting within 24 hours after symptom onset, may be eligible. A facility with these capabilities should be contacted for consideration of transfer and assistance with medical management while the patient is en route.

Brain MRI using diffusion-weighted imaging has high sensitivity and specificity (over 95%) for ischemic stroke. The further diagnostic evaluation should be based on the suspected underlying pathophysiology. For example, vascular imaging should be performed using CT-angiography, MR-angiography, catheter angiography, or vascular ultrasound (carotid Duplex imaging) for suspected artery-to-artery stroke from carotid artery atherosclerosis or dissection. Cardiac evaluation using EKG, transthoracic or transesophageal ultrasound, and Holter monitoring is indicated for suspected cardioembolic stroke. Blood tests such as protein C, protein S, antithrombin III levels, and antiphospholipid antibodies, may be indicated in young individuals with cryptogenic stroke. Erythrocyte sedimentation rate and C-reactive protein levels may be obtained on suspicion of underlying malignancy, bacterial endocarditis, or cerebral vasculitis, with additional infectious or inflammatory workup as indicated. Further, a lipid panel and homocysteine and lipoprotein-a levels should be considered to assess vascular risk.

Treatment with an antiplatelet agent (aspirin, clopidogrel, aspirin-dipyridamole combination) or an anticoagulant agent such as warfarin, if indicated, should be initiated within 24 hours after admission. Prophylaxis against deep vein throm-

Table 93.7 COMMON STROKE SYNDROMES

DISTRIBUTION	SYMPTOMS
Middle cerebral artery	Weakness and sensory loss of contralateral face, arm, and leg, dysarthria, global aphasia in dominant hemisphere, apraxia and neglect in nondominant hemisphere, homonymous hemianopia, gaze deviation toward the lesion.
Anterior cerebral artery (ACA)	Contralateral leg weakness and sensory loss. If both ACAs involved, may have bilateral paraparesis, abulia, and urinary incontinence.
Ant. choroidal	Contralateral hemiplegia, hemihypesthesia, homonymous hemianopia.
Posterior cerebral artery	*P1: Precommunal PCA.* Infarction often involves P1 perforators to the midbrain, subthalamic, and thalamic signs. *Midbrain Syndromes:* Claude syndrome: 3rd nerve palsy + contralateral ataxia. Weber syndrome: 3rd nerve palsy + contralateral hemiplegia. Benedict syndrome: 3rd nerve palsy, contralateral ataxia, hemiplegia. *Thalamic Syndromes:* Dejerine–Roussy syndrome: Contralateral hemisensory loss. Artery of Percheron: Paresis of upward gaze and drowsiness and abulia. Coma, unreactive pupils, bilateral pyramidal signs. *P2: Postcommunal PCA.* Cortical temporal and occipital lobe signs. Hemianopia with macular sparing. Visual agnosia for faces, objects, mathematical symbols, and colors. Medial temporal lobe and hippocampal involvement can cause a disturbance in memory. Patients can also develop recognizable syndromes such as alexia without agraphia, peduncular hallucinosis (visual hallucinations of brightly colored scenes and objects), Balint syndrome (optic ataxia, ocular apraxia, visual inattention, and simultagnosia), Anton syndrome (denial of blindness), and palinopsia (persistence of the visual image).
Basilar	Somnolence, ptosis, disorders of ocular movement, paralysis of vertical gaze, convergence retraction nystagmus; pseudoabducens palsy, skew deviation, lid retraction, facial weakness, hearing loss, nystagmus, hemiplegia
SCA	Ipsilateral cerebellar ataxia, unstable gait, vertigo
AICA	Horizontal and vertical nystagmus, vertigo, nausea, vomiting. Ipsilateral facial paralysis. Paralysis of conjugate gaze to the side of the lesion. Ipsilateral deafness, tinnitus, cerebellar ataxia, Horner syndrome, impaired facial sensation. Contralateral pain and temperature sensation in the body.
PICA	Ipsilateral facial numbness, numbness to pain in the contralateral body. Ipsilateral ataxia. Gait instability. Nausea, vertigo. Horner syndrome.
Lacunar infarcts	Hemisensory loss and hemiparesis: Thalamocapsular Pure hemisensory loss: Thalamus Pure motor hemiparesis: Internal capsule, corona radiata, basis pontis Dysarthria/clumsy hand: Genu of the internal capsule, basis pontis Ataxic hemiparesis: Pons, midbrain, internal capsule

bosis with subcutaneous low-molecular-weight heparin, and the prompt evaluation of swallow function with implementation of measures to prevent aspiration pneumonia, are important. Patients should be evaluated by physical, occupational, and speech therapy if they have persistent deficits. If there is significant carotid stenosis (either moderate or severe) on vessel imaging, and depending on the surgical risk, the patient may be considered for carotid endarterectomy or stenting. The decision to use antiplatelets or anticoagulants for stroke prevention depends on the underlying pathophysiology; in general, warfarin is used only for high-risk cardiac sources such as atrial fibrillation, left ventricular thrombus, cardiomyopathy, and prosthetic heart valves. Stroke prevention therapy with cholesterol-lowering agents (statins), antihypertensive medications (preferably thiazide diuretics and angiotensin-converting enzyme inhibitors), or antidiabetic agents may be initiated if indicated as per the latest national treatment guidelines. After patients have been medically stabilized, if they exhibit persistent

deficits and cannot be cared for at home, they should be considered for inpatient rehabilitation or a nursing facility. Stroke unit care, prevention of acute poststroke complications, appropriate stroke preventive medications, and rehabilitation constitute the mainstay of therapy for ischemic stroke. With these measures, from 1995 to 2005, the stroke death rate has fallen to 29.7%, and the actual number of stroke deaths has declined 13.5%.

INTRACEREBRAL HEMORRHAGE

Intracerebral hemorrhages (ICHs) can be classified based on location (parenchymal, subdural, epidural, subarachnoid) or underlying etiology (primary hypertensive or secondary to ruptured berry aneurysms, vascular malformations, neoplasms, cerebral venous sinus thrombosis, blood dyscrasias, coagulopathies, etc.). Symptoms can vary depending on the location within the brain or spinal cord and may include coma or altered sensorium, weakness, sensory loss,

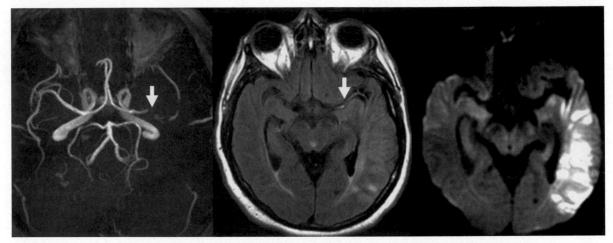

Figure 93.2. Brain MRI in Ischemic Stroke. Head MR angiography (left panel, axial three-dimensional time-of-flight image) shows an abrupt cutoff of the left middle cerebral artery (arrow). Fluid-attenuated inversion recovery sequence axial image (FLAIR, middle panel) shows hyperintensity in the middle cerebral artery (arrow), consistent with acute thrombus or slow flow within this artery; the surrounding brain parenchyma is hyperintense from early ischemic change. Axial diffusion-weighted image (DWI, right panel) shows hyperintense signal consistent with infarction.

aphasia, visual field deficits, headache, vomiting, and ataxia. The onset is typically acute, although symptom onset may be subacute, for example, with subdural hematomas or in patients with underlying brain tumor.

Hypertensive ICHs are commonly located in the basal ganglia, thalamus (figure 93.3), pons, and cerebellum. Chronic hypertension results in lipohyalinosis of small blood vessels, vessel wall weakening, and eventual rupture. Clinical examination may reveal clues to the location, for example, downward eye deviation with thalamic hemorrhage, deep coma with pinpoint pupils in pontine ICH, and severe headache, vomiting, nystagmus, and ataxia with cerebellar ICH. Space-occupying effects lead to raised intracranial pressure with consequent signs of brain herniation.

Lobar ICH (figure 93.4) can be hypertensive, although the most common cause is *cerebral amyloid angiopathy* (CAA), which is frequently associated with Alzheimer dementia. A sensitive antemortem marker of CAA is

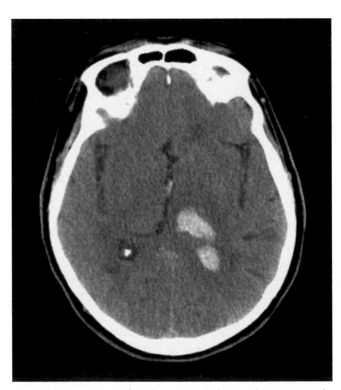

Figure 93.3. Hypertensive Left Thalamic Hemorrhage with Intraventricular Extension.

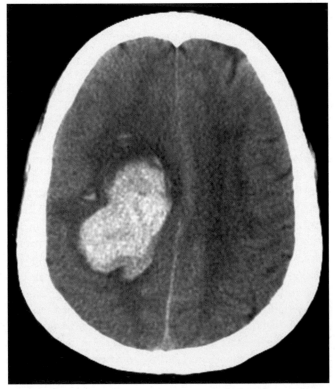

Figure 93.4. Parenchymal Brain Hemorrhage in the Right Frontal Lobe. Lobar hemorrhages usually result from underlying congophilic amyloid angiopathy.

the presence of multiple cerebral microhemorrhages on advanced MRI techniques (gradient-echo or susceptibility-weighted imaging). Location of these MRI lesions in the cortical-subcortical junction favors the diagnosis of CAA; deep lesions in the basal ganglia and thalamus favor a diagnosis of hypertensive vasculopathy. Because of their superficial location in the sensorimotor cortex, CAA-associated hemorrhages frequently manifest as a spell of numbness "marching" across the limb. In patients with severe CAA and prior ICH, it is reasonable to avoid antiplatelets and anticoagulants to reduce the risk of hemorrhage.

Subarachnoid hemorrhage (SAH) can be spontaneous, such as from ruptured berry aneurysms, or induced by head trauma. Aneurysmal SAH carries a high morbidity and mortality: it affects younger individuals, and of those who arrive to the hospital alive, the mortality rate within the first month is 45%. Among survivors, more than half are left with major deficits. Saccular aneurysms commonly occur at the terminal internal carotid artery, the middle cerebral artery bifurcation, top of the basilar artery, anterior communicating artery, and posterior communicating artery (figure 93.5). Mycotic aneurysms occur more distally. The rupture risk is higher with larger aneurysms (greater than 6–7 mm) and certain locations (e.g., top of the basilar). Common symptoms include sudden, severe headache, loss of consciousness, and neck stiffness. Delayed neurological consequences of SAH include rerupture, hydrocephalus, stroke from vasospasm, and hyponatremia from cerebral salt-wasting. Treatment of aneurysmal SAH includes prompt surgical clipping or endovascular coiling, treatment of raised intracranial pressure, and "triple H" (hypertension, hemodilution, and hypervolemic) therapy for cerebral

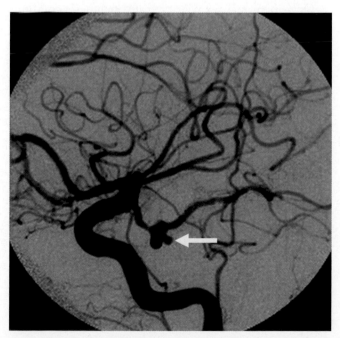

Figure 93.5. Cerebral Angiogram. Lateral projection, showing a saccular aneurysm in the posterior communicating artery (arrow).

vasospasm. Nimodipine, a centrally acting calcium channel blocker, has been shown to improve outcome.

ICH may result from ruptured *vascular malformations* such as cavernous angiomas, arteriovenous malformations, and dural arteriovenous fistulas. Treatment of the underlying using surgical, neurointerventional, or radiation approaches are warranted to reduce the risk for rebleeding and, in certain situations, to prevent initial hemorrhage. The most common *neoplasms* associated with ICH include cerebral metastases from melanoma, thyroid, renal cell, lung, and breast carcinomas, choriocarcinoma, and primary brain tumors—glioblastoma multiforme (adults) and medulloblastoma (children).

If an ICH is suspected, a plain head CT scan should be acquired urgently. Many centers perform acute arterial imaging with CT angiography, MR angiography, or catheter angiography to assess for underlying vascular lesions. Venous studies should be considered because cerebral venous sinus thrombosis can manifest with hemorrhage and brain edema. The goals of medical therapy are to control blood pressure to normal levels, reverse any coagulopathy by administering vitamin K or fresh frozen plasma, and reduce elevated intracranial pressure using mannitol or hypertonic saline. A neurosurgical consultation should be obtained for consideration of surgical evacuation, treatment of the underlying condition, or managing intracranial pressure by placing an intracranial bolt or ventricular drain. Surgical evacuation is controversial in hemispheric ICH; however, cerebellar ICHs are typically evacuated if there is risk for hydrocephalus or brainstem compression. At least in the initial stages, ICH patients are best managed in specialized neuro-intensive care units. Once they are medically stable, such tests should be performed to evaluate for underlying causes. The presence of acute blood sometimes makes it difficult exclude underlying causes such as brain tumors, in which case a brain MRI should be repeated after a few weeks.

GUILLAIN-BARRÉ SYNDROME

Guillain-Barré syndrome (GBS) is an acute polyradiculopathy characterized by areflexia, rapidly progressive ascending motor weakness, and, to a lesser degree, sensory loss and paresthesias of the extremities. Autonomic instability and diffuse back pain are common. GBS has many variants including the axonal, demyelinating, and the Miller-Fisher variant with ophthalmoplegia, ataxia, and descending motor weakness. Symptoms typically progress over days, peak at 3–4 weeks, and in most cases regress over a few weeks. Up to 30% develop respiratory weakness requiring mechanical ventilation, and 70% develop autonomic involvement leading to fluctuations in heart rate and blood pressure, loss of sweating, and urinary retention. Such patients should be admitted to an intensive care unit for monitoring or respiratory and hemodynamic support. Forced vital capacities

(FVC) and negative inspiratory force (NIFs) should be checked at least three times a day until the patient clearly shows no signs of progression.

GBS has been associated with *Campylobacter jejuni*, HIV, *Mycoplasma* pneumonia, *Haemophilus influenzae*, and Epstein-Barr and hepatitis virus infections. The differential diagnosis is broad and includes chronic inflammatory demyelinating neuropathy (CIDP), porphyria, diphtheria, heavy metal toxicity (arsenic, thallium, organophosphates, lead), vasculitis, myopathy, neuromuscular diseases such as myasthenia or botulism, Lyme disease, polio, tick paralysis, West Nile virus, and even basilar artery thrombosis. A workup should be undertaken to evaluate for infections and to rule out mimics. Electromyography (EMG) and nerve conduction studies are often normal in the initial stages but show typical findings of demyelinating radiculopathy after 8–10 days. Characteristic findings on cerebrospinal fluid examination are albuminocytological dissociation—elevated protein levels with mild pleocytosis.

Treatment options include a course of intravenous immune globulins or plasmapheresis. The benefit is greatest if the treatment is initiated earlier in the course of the disease, particularly within 2 weeks of symptom onset. In patients with facial and eye closure weakness, corneal dryness should be prevented. General measures such as narcotics for pain control and prophylaxis against deep vein thrombosis and pressure ulcers are important. GBS has an incidence of 1–2 per 100,000 per year. Ultimately, 2–5% of individuals die from complications, 70–80% will have a complete recovery by 1–2 years, and 20% will be left with residual weakness. There is a 3% incidence of recurrence. Factors associated with poor outcome include a fulminant course with maximum symptoms within 7 days, respiratory failure, autonomic imbalance, the axonal variant, low motor amplitude on neurophysiology studies, and age >60 years.

MYASTHENIA GRAVIS

This disorder of the neuromuscular junction is caused by antibodies against the postsynaptic acetylcholine receptor (AChR). It has an incidence rate of 10–20 per million per year affecting all age groups, and a bimodal age distribution with peaks in the second to third (female predominance) and sixth to eighth (male predominance) decades. There is a non-Mendelian genetic predilection with first-degree relatives of patients having a 1000-fold greater risk of developing MG. Approximately 65% of cases are associated with thymic hyperplasia, and 10% of myasthenics have a thymoma. Congenital myasthenic syndromes are less common and are due to genetic mutations affecting components of the neuromuscular junction rather than autoimmune causes.

Symptoms of myasthenia gravis include ptosis, diplopia, dysarthria, dysphagia, weakness of the neck, shoulder, or facial muscles, overall fatigue, weakness of the extremities, and respiratory failure in severe cases. Essentially any muscle may be affected, but sensory function is spared. Symptoms often fluctuate and are usually worse at night or after significant use. Muscle weakness can worsen with infections, stress, surgery, trauma, and several common medications including beta blockers, procainamide, lidocaine, quinidine, aminoglycosides, tetracycline, ciprofloxacin, clindamycin, phenytoin, lithium, trimethadione, chloroquine, D-penicillamine, and magnesium. Myasthenic crisis develops in 20% of patients and has a mortality of 4–8%. The differential diagnosis includes Lambert-Eaton syndrome associated with lung cancer, GBS, CIDP, botulism, cholinergic toxicity, motor neuron disease, thyroid disease, vasculitis, organophosphate poisoning, mitochondrial myopathy, muscular dystrophy, and skull-base tumors.

The diagnostic workup should include serum electrolytes, creatinine kinase, antinuclear antibodies, thyroid panel, antithyroid antibodies, and levels of AChR and MuSK (muscle-specific kinase) antibodies. AChR antibodies are detectable in approximately 85% of myasthenia patients but in only 50% with weakness of ocular muscles only. MuSK antibodies are present in approximately 40% of patients who are AChR-antibody negative. Edrophonium (Tensilon), a short-acting anticholinesterase, may be administered to look for signs of rapid improvement. Side effects of edrophonium include salivation, nausea, diarrhea, fasciculations, syncope, and bradycardia; thus, atropine should be ready for intravenous administration. EMG with repetitive nerve stimulation should be obtained, looking for a decremental response. Single-fiber EMG may reveal increased jitter. Chest CT should be obtained to evaluate for thymoma.

Outpatient management typically includes a combination of acetylcholinesterase inhibitors, often pyridostigmine, and steroid therapy. Weakness may worsen with initiation of steroid therapy; thus, steroids should be initiated with caution. Other immunosuppressive medications, such as azathioprine, mycophenolate mofetil, cyclophosphamide, cyclosporine, and tacrolimus, are sometimes used in more refractory cases. Thymectomy may be considered in patients younger than 60 and is recommended if a patient has a thymoma. Patients presenting with myasthenia crisis—worsening weakness with the risk of respiratory failure or death—should be admitted to the intensive care unit for close respiratory and hemodynamic monitoring. Intubation should be considered for forced vital capacity below 15 cc/kg and negative inspiratory force below −20. Peripheral oxygen saturations are not sensitive markers for impending respiratory failure because patients will often develop hypercarbia before hypoxia. Medical therapy should be initiated with the assistance of a neurologist and typically includes plasma exchange or intravenous immune globulins, steroids, and pyridostigmine. Precipitants such as specific medications should be removed and infections promptly treated.

PERIPHERAL NEUROPATHIES

Peripheral neuropathy affects up to 10% of the general population, with incidence increasing with age. Peripheral nerves carry both afferent (sensory input traveling to the CNS) and efferent (motor and autonomic output from the CNS) information. Afferent fibers consist of large myelinated fibers (vibration and position sense, tendon reflexes) and small unmyelinated fibers (pain and temperature sense). Efferent fibers also include large myelinated axons (motor information to muscles) and small unmyelinated nerves (autonomic output). As such, sensory symptoms, both positive and negative, are common manifestations, and muscle weakness and autonomic dysfunction are also frequently attributed to neuropathy.

Peripheral neuropathies follow common patterns including mononeuropathy, mononeuropathy multiplex, and polyneuropathy. Polyneuropathies can be further divided into predominantly motor, sensory, mixed sensorimotor, and autonomic neuropathies. Compression or vascular compromise may affect the entire nerve and result in a mononeuropathy. Axonal degeneration typically results in a symmetric length-dependent polyneuropathy involving both large and small fibers. The peripheral nerve is vulnerable to a multitude of toxic, vascular, and metabolic insults, and the nerve fibers are dependent on the cell body for nutritional support and regeneration. Thus, the longest fibers are often the first and most severely affected by axonal injuries. Demyelination typically affects the large-diameter sensory (vibration and position sense, tendon reflexes) and motor fibers. This usually occurs in a segmental pattern causing mononeuropathy or polyneuropathy affecting both proximal and distal nerves. Diabetes mellitus is the most common risk factor for *length-dependent peripheral neuropathy*, followed by alcoholism, nonalcoholic liver disease, malignancy, chronic renal disease, and family history.

Carpal tunnel syndrome is the most common *mononeuropathy* caused by compression of the median nerve by the flexor retinaculum in the wrist. It affects 0.1–4% of the population, with a female-to-male ratio of 3:1. Symptoms include forearm pain, paresthesias in the lateral 3½ fingers on the palmar aspect of the hand, and weakness with thumb abduction, opposition, and flexion. Symptoms are often worse at night. On exam there may be weakness, sensory loss in the distribution described above, atrophy of the thenar eminence, and a positive Tinel sign (symptoms elicited by tapping on the wrist) or Phalen sign (flexion of the wrist for at least 30 sec reproduces symptoms). Nerve conduction studies can establish the diagnosis (figure 93.6). In mild or early cases of CTS, conservative therapy may be initiated with wrist splints to be worn at night and avoiding repetitive movements, typing, or treating other predisposing conditions. Physical therapy and anti-inflammatory medications may be helpful. Steroid injections may be considered but typically offer only temporary relief. For refractory cases despite conservative therapy or if there is weakness or atrophy of muscles, the patient may benefit from carpal tunnel release surgery. *Meralgia paresthetica* is a sensory mononeuropathy caused by compression of the lateral femoral cutaneous nerve at the inguinal ligament or in the pelvis. Predisposing factors include obesity, tight belts, pregnancy, diabetes, abdominal or pelvic masses, or prolonged sitting. Symptoms include numbness, burning, or paresthesias in the anterolateral thigh. Treatment is aimed at relieving the compression, such as wearing looser clothing, belts, or holsters to modify compressive forces, weight loss, injection of local anesthetics, and steroids. Tricyclics, other medications targeted at relieving neuropathic pain such as Neurontin or pregabalin, and topical anesthetics may be considered as well. *Peroneal neuropathy* at the fibular neck is the most common lower extremity mononeuropathy. Lumbosacral and cervical radiculopathy are common, with incidence increasing with age. *Brachial* and *lumbosacral plexopathy* are rare but important causes of sensory and motor symptoms in the upper and lower extremity, respectively.

On examination, it is important to look for lymphadenopathy, organomegaly, musculoskeletal changes, or joint abnormalities such as atrophy, pes cavus, or hammer toes, abnormalities of the tonsils or oropharynx, skin, hair, and nail changes, and skin rash. As with all neurological disorders, a careful history and focused examination are essential in narrowing the long list of possibilities to a handful of diagnoses. The initial laboratory workup should include complete blood counts, erythrocyte sedimentation rate, serum electrolytes, liver and renal function tests, hemoglobin A1c, thyroid studies, vitamin B-12 levels, serum protein electrophoresis with immunofixation, and tests for infections such as Lyme or HIV as appropriate. Genetic tests may be indicated for suspected hereditary neuropathies. Further evaluation with electrophysiological studies, including EMG and nerve conduction studies, is indicated to confirm the presence of a neuropathy, provide precise localization, and further characterize the nature of the underlying nerve pathology, for example distinguishing between an axonal versus a demyelinating process. In cases where a diagnosis is unclear, and particularly if the there is suspicion for vasculitis or amyloidosis, a sural nerve biopsy may be useful. Small fiber neuropathy may be demonstrated on skin biopsy.

Treatment of peripheral neuropathy is directed at the underlying cause, when possible. This may include tight glucose control in diabetes, removal of toxins or offending drugs, thyroid or vitamin B-12 replacement, or treatment of systemic inflammatory or infectious conditions. Symptomatic treatment is typically directed at controlling neuropathic pain. Several antiepileptic and antidepressant medications have shown benefit in this regard, particularly gabapentin, pregabalin, amitriptyline, and duloxetine. Other options include opiate medications such as tramadol and nonpharmacologic treatment such as acupuncture. The prognosis for peripheral neuropathy depends on the underlying cause, severity, and

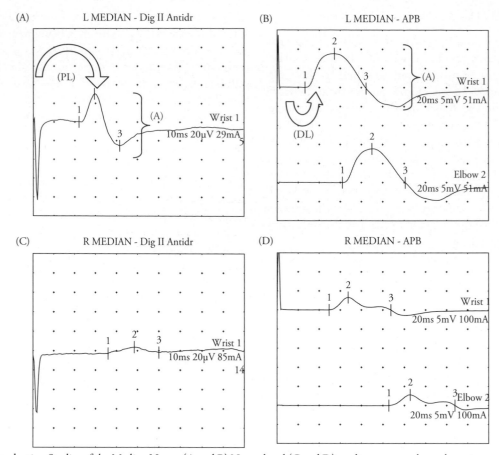

Figure 93.6 Nerve Conduction Studies of the Median Nerve. (A and B) Normal and (C and D) median neuropathy at the wrist as seen in carpal tunnel syndrome. (A) Sensory nerve action potential (SNAP) to digit 2 with normal amplitude (A) and peak latency (PL). (B) Compound muscle action potential (CMAP) to abductor pollicis brevis with normal amplitude (A) and distal latency (DL). (C) SNAP amplitude reduction and peak latency prolongation. (D) CMAP amplitude reduction and distal latency prolongation. Figure courtesy of James Berry.

chronicity. In general, axonal neuropathies have a poorer prognosis for recovery than demyelinating. If an offending agent is removed early enough, permanent neuropathy may sometimes be avoided. In many cases, however, the damage is permanent, and treatment must focus on symptom control and prevention of complications such as ulcers.

DEMENTIA, DELIRIUM, AND OTHER COGNITIVE IMPAIRMENTS

Dementia is defined as an acquired and persistent impairment in memory, plus at least one other cognitive domain (reasoning, spatial processing, language, or executive function), to an extent that daily functioning is compromised. In general, dementing illnesses are subacute to chronic, associated with underlying structural changes in the brain, and irreversible. *Mild cognitive impairment* (MCI) is a recent subjective memory complaint and corroborative evidence, with otherwise preserved cognitive function and daily functioning. The prevalence of MCI has been estimated at 12–15% of people aged 65 and over. Approximately 12% of people with MCI will progress to Alzheimer dementia within 1 year, and 50% will do so within 5 years. It should be noted that dementia and MCI do not cause alteration in

level of consciousness (LOC) and do not fluctuate rapidly (these are the hallmarks of *encephalopathy*). Distinguishing dementia or MCI from subacute encephalopathy in the acute hospital setting can be challenging. Furthermore, the two often coexist because of the increased susceptibility of patients with dementia to encephalopathy. For this reason, the evaluation of dementia should generally be deferred to the outpatient setting in an otherwise healthy patient.

The dementias can be classified by their predominant anatomical localization (subcortical vs. cortical), by their potential reversibility, or by etiology. For the internist, it is most useful to consider several broad categories based on etiology. *Neurodegenerative* disorders involve pathological processes that are specific to the brain, including Alzheimer disease (AD), dementia with Lewy bodies (DLB), and the frontotemporal dementias (FTD). *Vascular dementia* (VD) occurs in patients with cerebrovascular disease and clinical or subclinical infarcts. These two groups comprise the major irreversible dementias. *Reversible or treatable causes* of cognitive decline include chronic alcoholism, vitamin B-1 or B-12 deficiency, hypothyroidism, renal or liver failure, infections such as HIV, Lyme disease, chronic meningitis, and neurosyphilis, chronic subdural hematoma, normal-pressure hydrocephalus, brain tumors, paraneoplastic limbic encephalitis, toxic exposure to various drugs and heavy metals, depression (pseudodementia), and recurrent nonconvulsive seizures.

Delirium, encephalopathy, or *acute confusional state*, is a syndrome characterized by a fluctuating alteration in level of consciousness (LOC) and cognition. Cognition can be altered in a variety of ways, including the presence of illusions, hallucinations, delusions, and/or the loss of orientation, memory, language skills, ability to perform calculations, or reason. A feature that distinguishes encephalopathy from psychosis is that the latter does not affect the LOC. Much encephalopathy can be explained by acute medical illness, seizure, encephalitis, acute demyelination, stroke, recent surgery, systemic infection, electrolyte imbalances, hypoglycemia, pain, or medication effects or withdrawal, particularly in the elderly population. *Herpes simplex virus* (HSV) is a dreaded but uncommon cause of encephalitis that tends to cause a prodrome of subtle behavioral changes, low-grade fever, and finally acute mental status changes, alteration in consciousness, focal neurological deficits, and seizures. Whereas initial cerebrospinal fluid examination will reveal pleocytosis, the diagnosis of herpes simplex encephalitis rests on the detection of viral DNA in the cerebrospinal fluid. Brain imaging might show changes in the temporal lobes (figure 93.7). Hemorrhage is a commonly memorized but late-occurring event in HSV encephalitis and should not be relied on for diagnosis. Antiviral therapy (intravenous acyclovir) is the mainstay of treatment.

The *workup of dementia* begins with a complete history, during which corroborative information from close friends or family is critical, as the patient may not be able to provide an accurate history. Defining the onset, duration, and severity of symptoms, family history, and social habits including alcohol, tobacco, and drug use can often point to the correct diagnosis. Gradual progressive memory impairment as the initial presenting symptom is suggestive of AD. Prominent behavioral changes, such as inappropriate social conduct, point to FTD. Stepwise worsening in a patient with vascular risk factors typifies VD. Early visual hallucinations and fluctuations in alertness are often associated with DLB. Physical exam may reveal other important clues to the correct diagnosis. Whereas AD typically involves motor symptoms only later in the disease process, FTD is associated with rigidity and possibly amyotrophic lateral sclerosis. DLB features prominent parkinsonian signs, such as tremor, rigidity, bradykinesia, and shuffling gait. Patients with VD may have focal signs from stroke. Diagnostic testing in dementia is aimed at uncovering any reversible etiology. Investigations should include a thyroid function test, a vitamin B-12 level, and a neuroimaging test (preferably MRI) to assess for structural causes such as chronic subdural hematoma, normal-pressure hydrocephalus, or brain tumor. Lumbar puncture and EEG could be considered. Patients should be screened for depression, which can accompany or mimic dementia (pseudodementia). Formal neuropsychological testing can sometimes help to differentiate specific dementias, but these are usually obtained and interpreted through a memory disorders specialist.

AD is the most common form of dementia, affecting up to 4.5 million Americans and comprising 60–80% of cases of dementia. Aging is the most important risk factor, with prevalence increasing rapidly above age 65, when 1–2% of the population has AD. By age 75, 15% are affected, and the prevalence is as high as 30–40% among people aged 85 and over. In addition to aging, family history is an important risk factor, as 20% of patients with AD have first-degree relatives also affected. The underlying pathology in AD involves excessive accumulation of extracellular

(A)

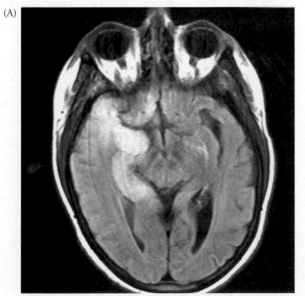

(B)

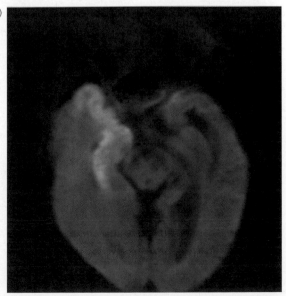

Figure 93.7. HSV-1 Encephalitis on MRI. (A) Fluid-attenuated inversion recovery (FLAIR) and (B) diffusion-weighted imaging (DWI) MRI sequences demonstrating abnormal signal in the right medial temporal lobe in a patient with HSV-1 encephalitis.

amyloid plaques consisting of abnormal beta-amyloid and intracellular neurofibrillary tangles consisting of hyperphosphorylated tau protein, especially in the temporal cortex and hippocampus. Over time, accumulation of plaques and tangles leads to neuronal death and atrophy, first in the temporal lobes and cholinergic system and later more globally (figure 93.8). Clinically, AD presents with progressive short-term memory impairment. As the disease worsens, patients develop difficulties with language (especially word finding) and visuospatial function. Daily functions such as driving, managing finances, and housekeeping suffer. Patients often become agitated or confused in unfamiliar settings. Despite these changes, comportment (routine behavior and superficial conversation) is preserved. Later in the disease, patients may develop gait difficulties, delusions, hallucinations, impaired judgment, behavioral difficulties, and seizures.

The mainstay of disease-modifying treatment is cholinesterase inhibitors, which have been shown to have a modest effect in slowing the rate of cognitive decline in AD. No clinical improvement is to be expected with their use. Donepezil, rivastigmine, and galantamine are all approved for use in mild to moderate AD, and donepezil is also approved for moderate to severe disease. The benefit of cholinesterase inhibitors in VD and DLB remains uncertain. Common side effects include nausea, vomiting, diarrhea, anorexia, and weight loss, which can be minimized by taking the drug with meals. Given the modest efficacy of cholinesterase inhibitors in symptomatic treatment, their use should be weighed against side effects and costs. Memantine, an NMDA-receptor antagonist, is approved for use in moderate to severe AD with benefits similar to those seen in the cholinesterase inhibitors. Side effects include dizziness, confusion, and hallucinations, but in general it has fewer side effects than cholinesterase inhibitors. Symptomatic pharmacologic treatment could include a selective serotonin reuptake inhibitor for depression or an atypical antipsychotic for psychotic symptoms (although recent data about increased mortality in elderly patients argue in favor of thorough explanation of the risk with the patient's health care proxy). The use of tricyclic antidepressant medications for sleep is limited by their anticholinergic effects, which can cause acute confusion and worsen AD symptoms.

After AD, the three most common causes of dementia include VD, DLB, and FTD. Their typical presenting symptoms, signs, and imaging findings are juxtaposed to those of AD in table 93.8. Parkinson disease (PD) is relatively common and is frequently associated with depression and dementia. Rare disorders producing dementia include Creutzfeldt-Jacob disease, Wilson disease, vitamin E deficiency, and Wernicke-Korsakoff syndrome. Although different dementias can present and progress somewhat differently, supportive care is critical and largely similar. Patient safety should be emphasized, as should that of the caretaker. Violent outbursts can be embarrassing to relatives. Support services in the home, adult care services, and finally placement in appropriate care settings should be actively arranged for caregivers by the treating physicians. As in pediatrics, anticipatory guidance should be a mainstay of visits so that caregivers will understand new challenges that might well lie ahead. Services that might be helpful to families include occupational and physical therapy, social work, financial planners, homemakers, visiting nurses, adult day care providers, and eventually, chronic nursing facilities or palliative care and home hospice providers.

(A)
(B)

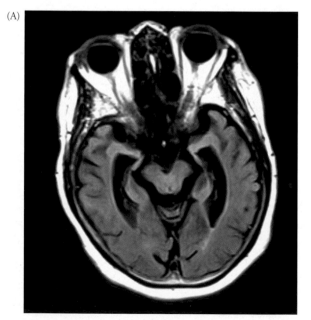
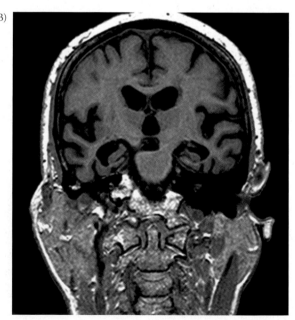

Figure 93.8. Alzheimer Disease on MRI. (A) FLAIR and (B) magnetization-prepared rapid gradient echo (MPRAGE) MRI sequences demonstrating prominent medial temporal lobe atrophy with enlargement of ventricles in a patient with moderate Alzheimer disease.

Table 93.8 CHARACTERISTICS OF THE FOUR MAJOR DEMENTIAS

DISEASE	EARLY SYMPTOMS	EARLY SIGNS	TYPICAL TEST RESULTS	UNDERLYING DISORDER
Alzheimer disease (AD)	Short-term memory loss precedes language difficulty (word searching often discovered only on direct questioning of family)	Delayed recall affected first. Later, word generation, spatial orientation, long-term memory	MRI/CT: Atrophy in the temporal > parietal lobes	Amyloid precursor protein is cleaved aberrantly, leading to accumulation of amyloid plaques. Hyperphosphorylated tau causes tangles.
Dementia with Lewy bodies (DLB)	Visual hallucinations and sleep disorder often precede bradykinesia and tremor	Waxing/waning signs of loss of executive function; parkinsonism (bradykinesia, tremor, cogwheel rigidity); REM sleep disorder.	MRI/CT: Posterior parietal and occipital atrophy.	Synuclein accumulation into cytoplasmic inclusions known as Lewy bodies appears to be the etiology of DLB.
Vascular dementia (VD)	Stepwise progression of memory deficits and focal neurological signs	Slowed cognition, stepwise deterioration with plateaus between. Focal neurological deficits are typically present due to symptomatic ischemic strokes.	MRI/CT: Marked white matter disease, evidence of prior strokes (cortical and/or subcortical). Stroke workup may reveal cause of ischemic strokes.	Evaluate for stroke risk factors including hypertension, hyperlipidemia, atrial fibrillation, hyperhomocysteinemia, malignancy, inflammatory disease.
Frontotemporal dementia (FTD)	Behavioral changes include apathy, depression, disinhibition, poor social demeanor, reduced executive functioning, and aphasia. Primary progressive aphasia may reveal expressive language deficits only	Frontal release signs (grasp, suck, snout, glabellar, palmomental reflexes), Luria testing deficits, poor social skills, abulia, aphasia, gaze palsy (progressive supranuclear palsy), limb apraxia/alien hand (corticobasilar degeneration)	MRI/CT: Atrophy of the frontal and temporal lobes	A number of distinct entities are associated with or cause frontotemporal dementias: parkinson-plus syndromes (CBD, PSP); amyotrophic lateral sclerosis/FTD complex is rare but described; FTD with parkinsonism is also well described

PARKINSONISM, TREMOR, AND OTHER MOVEMENT DISORDERS

Movement disorders are motor syndromes characterized by a paucity or slowness of movement or abnormal involuntary movement. A major challenge is to correctly classify the abnormal movement (table 93.9). The examination of movement disorders is largely observational: watch the patient in repose, while performing prespecified actions including limb positioning, writing, moving rapidly and repetitively, standing from a chair, walking, and performing any action that the patient feels will bring out the symptom. It is important to determine whether the movement can be voluntarily suppressed. A thorough exam of muscle tone, strength, reflexes, cranial nerves (especially eye movements), sensation, and gait should follow. Essential tremor and parkinsonism, including PD, are by far the most common movement disorders seen in the outpatient clinic.

Parkinsonism is a syndrome consisting of all or some of the following cardinal features: resting tremor, bradykinesia (slowed movements), rigidity (increased tone on passive movements), and postural instability (imbalance and tendency to fall). The term includes idiopathic PD and the so-called parkinsons-plus syndromes such as dementia with Lewy-bodies (DLB), multiple systems atrophy (MSA), progressive supranuclear palsy (PSP), and corticobasal degeneration (CBD). After AD, idiopathic PD is the second most common neurodegenerative disease. It has a prevalence of 0.3% of the population and an incidence rate of approximately 15 new cases per 100,000 person-years, with rates in men two to three times that for women. As for AD, the risk increases with age, with prevalence of 1% among those older than 60 and 3.5% in those over 85 years; only 4% are diagnosed under age 50. Although most cases are sporadic, 25% of patients with PD have a first-degree relative with PD, and earlier age of onset is associated with genetic causes.

Distinguishing PD from other forms of parkinsonism can be challenging, especially early in the course when cardinal signs may be lacking. A definite diagnosis of PD requires the presence of at least two cardinal features (rest tremor, bradykinesia, rigidity). Other features that are more typical for PD include unilateral onset, rest tremor, and persistence of asymmetry throughout the course. Supportive evidence may also be found in a positive response to treatment with dopamine replacement therapy: PD patients usually show a response to levodopa at a dose of 300–600 mg total daily dose, whereas a lack of response to levodopa, symmetrical onset, and lack of tremor should raise suspicion for an alternate diagnosis. Other red flags include early falls, prominent dysautonomia, and rapid progression. In atypical cases, MRI is useful to exclude structural causes of symptoms such as infarcts, tumor, or normal-pressure hydrocephalus. Routine MRI is typically normal in PD. *Essential tremor* is distinguished from PD by symmetrical intention tremor,

Table 93.9 COMMON TYPES OF ABNORMAL MOVEMENTS

MOVEMENT	DESCRIPTION
Tremor	Involuntary, rhythmic movement at a joint with oscillation of a specific frequency and amplitude. Description should include frequency, amplitude, and subtype. Subtypes include: Rest tremor (prominent in repose) Action tremor (prominent with use or positioning of limb) Intention tremor (an action tremor that worsens as the limb nears its target) Rubral tremor (near continuous, with action > rest tremor)
Bradykinesia	Slowness of movement causing hypophonia, reduced eye blink and arm swing, micrographia, festination of gait.
Chorea	Involuntary, irregular, arrhythmic, complex movements flowing from one muscle group to another. Often incorporated by patient into a voluntary movement.
Athetosis	Slow, sinuous movements, typically of the distal extremities.
Dystonia	Sustained muscle contraction. Examples include torticollis and writer's cramp.
Myoclonus	Brief, asymmetric, arrhythmic muscle contraction. Often referred to as a jerk. Can be single, multiple, or continuous. Can be focal or generalized.
Asterixis	Sudden loss of sustained tone in muscle.
Tic	Brief, stereotyped, repetitive movement, can be suppressed voluntarily, often associated with Tourette disease.

although less commonly it may be unilateral or present at rest. Bradykinesia and rigidity are lacking, and essential tremor is often improved by alcohol. As it may be inherited in an autosomal dominant pattern, family history is helpful. Involvement of the head is atypical for PD but may be seen in essential tremor in isolation or in conjunction with a hand tremor.

The foundation of treatment for PD is symptomatic management. As there are no proven disease-modifying (neuroprotective) treatments for PD, the timing of initiating symptomatic treatment depends on the disease burden and patient preference. The most effective medication remains levodopa, especially for bradykinesia and rigidity. It is typically administered with carbidopa in the form of Sinemet to reduce systemic metabolism. The most common side effects early on include nausea and drowsiness. These may sometimes be avoided by starting with a low dose and gradually escalating, as well as taking the medication with meals. Most patients taking levodopa will eventually develop dyskinesias (unwanted involuntary movements) or motor fluctuations (wearing off between doses). These can sometimes be delayed by initiating treatment with a dopamine agonist, either ropinirole (Requip) or pramipexole (Mirapex). Although they are associated with fewer dyskinesias and motor fluctuations, they are also less effective and more prone to side effects of somnolence, hallucinations, and leg edema. Generally, dopamine agonists should be considered in younger patients (<65 years) to prolong time to levodopa initiation, and older patients should receive levodopa in order to avoid the cognitive side effects of dopamine agonists. For younger patients with tremor predominance, anticholinergic agents such as trihexyphenidyl (Artane) and benztropine (Cogentin) may be useful, but they should be avoided in older patients or those with cognitive deficits. Management should also address nonmotor symptoms such as REM-sleep behavior disorder, depression, fatigue, and autonomic symptoms such as constipation, sexual dysfunction, and orthostatic hypotension. Essential tremor can be effectively treated with propranolol or primidone. For both PD and essential tremor, advanced refractory disease may improve with implantation of a deep brain stimulator in the subthalamic nucleus or globus pallidus in selected patients (figure 93.9).

Life expectancy is not altered in patients with essential tremor. The life expectancy of patients with PD depends on the age of onset but generally ranges between 9 and 11 years shorter than the normal population. Prominence of bradykinesia and rigidity at onset, as well as older age of onset, are associated with more rapid progression of motor symptoms. Conversely, tremor predominance is associated with a slower progression. Dementia, which occurs in 30–40% of patients with PD and is more common in those without tremor predominance, is associated with earlier nursing home placement and decreased survival. It should be emphasized that most patients progress slowly and remain functional for many years with appropriate symptomatic treatment.

MULTIPLE SCLEROSIS AND OTHER DEMYELINATING DISEASES

Multiple sclerosis (MS) is an autoimmune disease of unknown etiology that results in destruction of central myelin. The

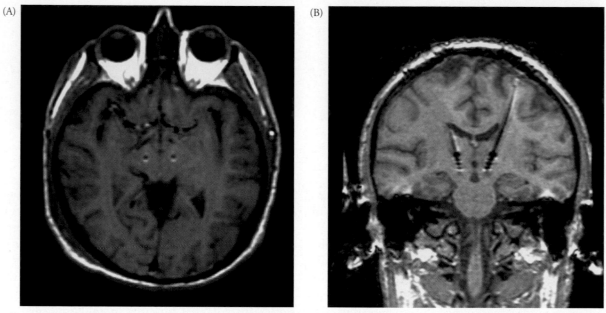

Figure 93.9. Deep Brain Stimulation for Parkinson Disease. (A) Axial T1 and (B) coronal spoiled gradient recalled acquisition (SPGR) MRI sequences demonstrating deep brain stimulator electrodes terminating in the bilateral subthalamic nuclei in a patient with advanced idiopathic Parkinson disease.

hallmarks of MS are demyelinating brain or spinal cord lesions that are separated in space and time *and* the exclusion of other potential causes of similar symptoms. The mean age of onset is 30 years of age. Onset before age 10 or after age 50 years should raise suspicion for an alternate diagnosis. There are apparent geographic disparities in MS prevalence, with rates highest in Europe, Australia, New Zealand, Canada, and the northern United States. This may be explained in part by racial differences in susceptibility, with the highest incidence rates among white populations. Prevalence rates also increase from southern to northern latitudes. Evidence suggests that increased sun exposure and supplemental vitamin D reduce the risk of developing MS. In the United States, the prevalence of MS is 1 per 1000. As with other autoimmune diseases, women are affected more than men (2:1 to 3:1). Genetic factors also play a role in the risks for MS. Approximately 20% of patients with MS have a relative also affected. Siblings of MS patients have a 3–5% risk of developing MS.

There are several patterns of disease in MS. In relapsing remitting MS (RRMS), patients have distinct attacks with without progression between relapses. Approximately 85–90% of cases present with this course, with onset typically in the late 20s. Most patients with RRMS will eventually develop disease progression with or without relapses, constituting secondary progressive MS (SPMS). In a small percentage of patients with primary progressive MS (PPMS), disease begins with a progressive course, typically at an older age than RRMS.

Less common forms of CNS demyelination include *acute disseminated encephalomyelitis* (ADEM) and *neuromyelitis optica* (NMO). ADEM is typically preceded by a viral infection or other immune stimulus such as vaccination and results in a typically monophasic illness of variable severity. It is more common in children but may occur in adults as well. NMO, also called Devic disease, is sometimes classified as a subtype of MS. It is characterized by optic neuritis and transverse myelitis simultaneously or in close succession. Typically, the brain is not clinically or radiographically affected. The spinal lesions tend to be more severe than in MS, and optic neuritis is often bilateral.

In the absence of any definitive test for MS short of brain biopsy, the diagnosis is based on clinical criteria, including symptoms, signs, and ancillary testing. Definite diagnosis requires two or more attacks and objective clinical evidence of two or more lesions. Attacks may be any clinical syndrome likely to result from CNS white matter inflammation and lasting at least 24 hours, including optic neuritis, transverse myelitis, and brainstem syndromes (table 93.10). MRI has become an essential tool in making the diagnosis. Brain MRI sequences should include axial and sagittal fluid attenuated inversion recovery (FLAIR), T2, and axial T1 pre- and postcontrast. Imaging the entire spinal cord with T2 and T1 pre- and postcontrast sequences may also reveal a subclinical lesion. MRI typically reveals multifocal T2 hyperintensities, most commonly located in the periventricular white matter, corpus callosum, and centrum semiovale (figure 93.10). The lesions are usually ovoid and situated perpendicular to the ventricles or corpus callosum. In the spinal cord, MS lesions are characteristically incomplete and rarely extend more than one or two spinal levels. Acutely, brain or spinal lesions may be enhancing on T1 postcontrast sequences. Later in the disease course, these lesions may become prominently hypointense on T1 images, and cortical atrophy may become apparent.

Table 93.10 TYPICAL PRESENTING SYMPTOMS IN MS

Sensory symptoms in limbs	Diplopia
Visual loss	Gait ataxia
Motor weakness	Sensory symptoms in face
Lhermitte sign (radiating electrical sensation with neck flexion)	Uhthoff phenomenon (worsening in hot ambient temperature)
Vertigo	Fatigue

Because many other process can lead to T2 hyperintensities on MRI, these changes must be interpreted in the setting of consistent clinical data and typical patterns.

When patients present with an initial demyelinating event but do not meet criteria for MS (so-called clinically isolated syndrome or CIS), MRI can help predict the risk for progression to clinically definite MS. Those with an abnormal MRI have a risk for developing MS anywhere from 56% to 88%, whereas those with a normal MRI have a 20% risk. Adjunct studies include cerebrospinal fluid studies, which may reveal intrathecal production of oligoclonal immune globulins, and visual evoked potential studies, which may reveal slowed conduction suggestive of prior optic neuritis. Although these tests may be suggestive of MS, they are far less predictive than MRI.

The four agents currently approved as first-line treatment in RRMS are glatiramer acetate (Copaxone, SC daily), interferon-β1a (Avonex, IM weekly), interferon-β1a (Rebif, SC TIW), and interferon-β1b (Betaseron, SC QOD). All have been shown to delay the progression to MS in patients with CIS and high-risk MRI and to reduce the frequency and severity of attacks in RRMS. Although there is little evidence that these agents reduce long-term accumulated disability, most neurology guidelines recommend use of these disease-modifying therapies for definite MS and strongly consider their use in patients with CIS and a high-risk MRI. For *refractory RRMS*, there are two other FDA-approved agents: natalizumab (Tysabri) and mitoxantrone (Novantrone). Both have significant potential toxicities, notably the small but real risk of progressive multifocal encephalopathy (PML) with natalizumab and bone marrow suppression with mitoxantrone. For *primary or secondary progressive MS*, there are no convincingly effective treatments. Options include pulse methylprednisolone, mitoxantrone, cyclophosphamide, azathioprine, and methotrexate. For *acute exacerbations*, there is some evidence that high-dose methylprednisolone (1 g IV daily for 3–5 days) may shorten the course of an attack without changing the overall course of the disease. Thus, for minor symptoms such as nonpainful paresthesias or mild weakness, steroid treatment is not indicated. Although a small percentage of patients with MS will have disease characterized as benign (i.e., no subsequent relapse) or malignant (rapid progression to disability), the usual

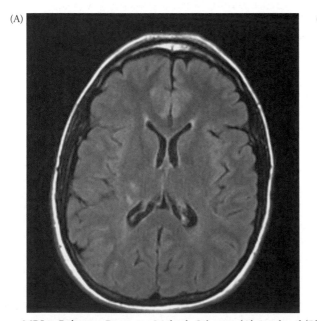
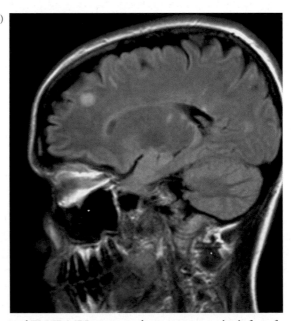

Figure 93.10. MRI in Relapsing Remitting Multiple Sclerosis. (A) Axial and (B) sagittal FLAIR MRI sequences demonstrating multiple foci of increased T2 signal, including lesions arranged perpendicular to the ventricles, in a patient with relapsing remitting multiple sclerosis.

course is slowly progressive. According to one recent large study, the median time from diagnosis to requiring a cane for ambulation is 28 years. Life expectancy is on average approximately 7 years less than the normal population but obviously varies with disease severity.

DIZZINESS AND VERTIGO

Dorland's dictionary defines *dizziness* as impairment in spatial perception and stability. The terms unsteadiness, feeling of faintness, light-headedness, unsteadiness, motion intolerance, imbalance, floating, or a tilting sensation are often used interchangeably to describe dizziness. The estimated overall incidence of dizziness, vertigo, and imbalance is 5–10%, and, as one would expect, is estimated to be much higher (at 40%) for those patients aged >40 years. Vertigo is a common subtype of dizziness and reflects an illusion of movement—a sense that the patient or the patient's surroundings are spinning or moving. Subjective vertigo is the term used to describe the patient's sense that he or she is spinning, whereas objective vertigo describes the patient feeling still but of objects appearing to move around him or her.

The causes of dizziness can be divided into peripheral and central causes (table 93.11). Approximately 40% of all cases of dizziness are from peripheral vestibular dysfunction, 10% from CNS lesions, 15% reflect a psychiatric disorder, 25% presyncope/dysequilibrium, and 10% nonspecific dizziness. Key clinical features of dizziness that suggest a peripheral cause include moderate or severe symptoms that are recurrent and worsened by changes in position. Positional nystagmus is typical. The nystagmus is characterized by a latent period before onset of approximately 2 to 20 seconds; the nystagmus usually lasts <1 minutes and has fatigability. In contrast, central causes of dizziness are suggested by the presence of continuous mild nonpositional

Table 93.12 **CAUSES OF VERTIGO**

- Ear disease
- Toxic conditions (alcohol, food poisonings)
- Postural hypotension
- Infectious disease
- Cervicogenic
- Disease of the eye or brain
- Psychological

vertigo with vertical nystagmus with no latent period and that lasts >1 minute and is nonfatiguing. Because central causes are frequently secondary to brainstem or cerebellar ischemia, additional brainstem characteristics may be present, including diplopia, autonomic symptoms, nausea, dysarthria, dysphagia, or focal weakness.

The most common causes of vertigo are shown in table 93.12. Causes of peripheral dizziness and key characteristics are shown in table 93.13. The most common cause of central dizziness is migraine, frequently referred to as vestibular migraine or migraine-associated dizziness. Other central causes include demyelination, acoustic tumors (figure 93.11), and brainstem or cerebellar vascular lesions (table 93.14).

Workup for dizziness, especially with a goal of distinguishing peripheral from central causes, includes standard

Table 93.11 **CAUSES OF DIZZINESS**

Peripheral

- Benign paroxysmal positional vertigo (BPPV) or canalithiasis—50%
- Vestibular neuronitis (labyrinthitis)—25%
- Meniere disease—10%
- Trauma
- Drugs (e.g., aminoglycosides)

Central

- Vertebrobasilar insufficiency—50%
- Multiple sclerosis
- Drugs (anticonvulsants, alcohol, hypnotics

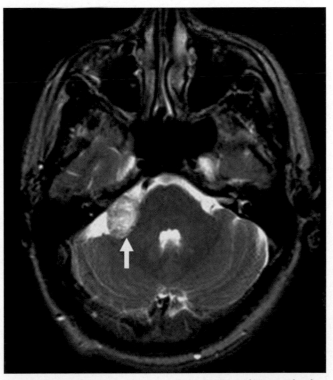

Figure 93.11. MRI of Acoustic Neuroma. Brain MRI, axial T2-weighted image, showing an acoustic neuroma (arrow).

Table 93.13 KEY CAUSES OF PERIPHERAL DIZZINESS

Benign Paroxysmal Positional Vertigo (BPPV)

- Brief moderate to severe recurrent episodes—lasts less than 1 min, self-limited, responds poorly to antivertigo drugs
- Associated with head position
- Gradually diminishes over a month or two
- No hearing loss
- Latency or delayed onset of clinical presentation
- Positive test for positioning nystagmus (using Nylen-Barany maneuver, also known as the Dix-Hallpike test)
- Caused by canalithiasis (otoconia floating in the endolymph) or cupulolithiasis (otoconia adherent to cupula)
- Posterior canal most commonly affected (90% of cases)
- Most effective treatment is canalith repositioning from the affected canal to the vestibular (using maneuvers)
- Medications not effective in treatment of BPPV

Vestibular Neuronitis

- Paroxysmal, single attack of vertigo, a series of attacks, or a persistent condition that diminishes over 3–6 weeks.
- May be associated with nausea, vomiting, and previous upper respiratory tract infections.
- Generally no auditory symptoms
- Associated with nystagmus
- Caused by inflammation of the vestibular nerve, thought to result from a reactivation of herpes simplex virus that affects the patient's vestibular ganglion and vestibular nerves (prodromal upper respiratory tract illness may or may not be present)

Cervicogenic Vertigo

- History of neck trauma and muscle spasm
- Limited cervical range of movement
- Positive chair rotation test (Fitz-Ritson)
- Patients may complain of dysequilibrium (tilt) more than rotational vertigo
- Overstimulation of upper cervical proprioceptors
- May overlap with BPPV or Ménière disease

Meniere Disease

- Sudden and recurrent (paroxysmal) attack of severe vertigo (fourth leading cause)
- Low-tone hearing loss, which may progress to severe hearing loss
- Low-tone tinnitus and sense of fullness in the ear
- Bilateral involvement in about 25% of patients
- Ménière disease etiology can be hereditary, autoimmune, infectious, or idiopathic
- >80% of patients respond to conservative therapy with salt restriction and diuretics. Other options: corticosteroids, given orally or intratympanically; intratympanic gentamicin (chemical labyrinthectomy), and surgery (shunting the endolymphatic sac).

blood tests, imaging (head CT, MRI/MRA), audiometry, and several specialist tests. Electronystagmography (ENG) is performed by a neurologist and is beyond the scope of the current chapter. However, briefly, a standard ENG test battery consists of three parts: oculomotor evaluation, positioning/positional testing, and caloric stimulation of the vestibular system.

Most cases of dizziness do not require referral. Criteria for referral include (1) severe vertigo that is disabling; (2) ataxia out of proportion to vertigo; (3) vertigo lasting

Table 93.14 CENTRAL CAUSES OF DIZZINESS

Migraine

- Women > men
- Motion intolerance/sickness
- Vestibular symptoms usually dissociated from headaches but may occur as an aura or as part of headache
- Treatment of migraine-associated vestibulopathy is the same as treatment of migraine
- Eliminate trigger factors

Vertebrobasilar Insufficiency Tias

- Sudden onset of dizziness with resolution of symptoms within 24 hours without residual subjective symptoms or objective signs
- Associated focal neurological symptoms of isolated or combined brainstem symptoms such as dizziness, diplopia, or weakness, headache
- Presence of associated risk factors (e.g., hypertension, diabetes mellitus, coronary artery disease)

Multiple Sclerosis (MS)

- Vertigo as presenting feature occurs in <10% with MS; dizziness or vertigo occurs at some point in the course in a third of patients
- Onset is usually at 20–40 years of age
- Episodes begin over hours to a few days and last weeks to months
- Associated typical symptoms include optic neuritis, ocular motor dysfunction, trigeminal neuralgia, sensorimotor deficits, myelopathy, ataxia, and bladder dysfunction
- Few patients present with hearing loss due to brainstem involvement
- Cause is recurrent, inflammatory central nervous system demyelination due to underlying autoimmune disorder

longer than 4 weeks; (4) changes in hearing; (5) presence of vertical nystagmus; (6) presence of focal neurological signs; and (7) systemic or psychiatric disease.

ADDITIONAL READING

Chong DJ, Bazil CW. Update on anticonvulsant drugs. *Curr Neurol Neurosci Rep.* 2010;10(4):308–18.

Huff JS, Fountain NB. Pathophysiology and definitions of seizures and status epilepticus. *Emerg Med Clin North Am.* 2011;29(1):1–13.

Kaski D, Seemungal BM. The bedside assessment of vertigo. *Clin Med.* 2010;10(4):402–5.

Kutz JW Jr. The dizzy patient. *Med Clin North Am.* 2010;94(5): 989–1002.

Loder E. Triptan therapy in migraine. *N Engl J Med.* 2010 Jul 1;363(1): 63–70.

Louis ED. Clinical practice. Essential tremor. *N Engl J Med.* 2001;345(12): 887–91.

Mayeux R. Clinical practice. Early Alzheimer's disease. *N Engl J Med.* 2010;362(23):2194–2201. Erratum *N Engl J Med.* 2010;363(12): 1190.

Nutt JG, Wooten GF. Clinical practice. Diagnosis and initial management of Parkinson's disease. *N Engl J Med.* 2005;353(10): 1021–7.

Post RE, Dickerson LM. Dizziness: A diagnostic approach. *Am Fam Physician.* 2010;82(4):361–9.

Querfurth HW, LaFerla FM. Alzheimer's disease. *N Engl J Med.* 2010;362(4):329–44.

Ropper AH, Gorson KC. Clinical practice. Concussion. *N Engl J Med.* 2007;356(2):166–72. Erratum *N Engl J Med.* 2007;356(17):1794.

Samuels MA. Update in neurology. *Ann Intern Med.* 2007;146(2): 128–32.

Scheuer ML, Pedley TA. The evaluation and treatment of seizures. *N Engl J Med.* 1990;323(21):1468–74.

SECTION 10

GENERAL INTERNAL MEDICINE

PREOPERATIVE EVALUATION AND MANAGEMENT BEFORE MAJOR NONCARDIAC SURGERY

Adam C. Schaffer and Sylvia C. W. McKean

There are more than 10 million major noncardiac surgical procedures performed in the United States per year, and this number is expected to grow as the population ages. The problem of perioperative cardiac events among patients undergoing noncardiac surgery is significant. The estimated risk of myocardial infarction (MI) in patients undergoing noncardiac surgery is 1.1% among unselected patients and 3.1% among patients at elevated risk of cardiac disease. The task of the internist providing preoperative evaluation of patients is not to provide medical "clearance." Instead, the role of the internist is, in addition to answering any specific questions posed by the requesting physician, to provide a thorough assessment of the patient's cardiovascular and other risks for the procedure. This risk assessment can assist in the balancing of risks and benefits that influences whether the surgeon decides to go forward with the procedure. The consulting internist must also provide specific suggestions regarding further testing that may be indicated for preoperative risk stratification and, most importantly, recommendations for measures that can be taken to mitigate the identified risks.

RISK ASSESSMENT

The most widely used index for assessing cardiac risk for major noncardiac surgery is the Revised Cardiac Risk Index (RCRI) developed by Lee, Goldman, et al. (1999). This index was designed to predict which patients were at elevated risk for major cardiac complications (defined as myocardial infarction, pulmonary edema, ventricular fibrillation or primary cardiac arrest, and complete heart block) from nonemergent noncardiac surgery. The factors in the RCRI (table 94.1) were derived based on 2893 patients age ≥50 years undergoing nonemergent noncardiac surgeries and were validated in a second patient cohort. The rates of major cardiac complications increase with the number of RCRI risk factors that are present. The rate is 0.5% for patients with zero risk factors, 1.3% for patients with one

risk factor, 4% for patients with two risk factors, and 9% for patients with ≥3 risk factors.

ACC/AHA GUIDELINES ON PERIOPERATIVE CARDIOVASCULAR EVALUATION AND CARE FOR NONCARDIAC SURGERY

The current American College of Cardiology/American Heart Association Guidelines on Perioperative Cardiovascular Evaluation and Care for Noncardiac Surgery (hereafter ACC/AHA Guidelines), released in 2007, provide a systematic approach to the preoperative evaluation of patients (figure 94.1). Pursuant to the ACC/AHA Guidelines Fleisher et al., 2007), as part of the history, physical, and review of the patient's data, the consultant needs to first ascertain whether there are any active cardiac conditions that require treatment prior to nonemergent surgery. These include unstable coronary syndromes (such as unstable or severe angina or MI within the last 30 days), decompensated heart failure (including New York Heart Association [NYHA] class IV or new onset), significant arrhythmias (including third-degree AV block, symptomatic ventricular arrhythmias, uncontrolled supraventricular arrhythmias, or symptomatic bradycardia), or severe valvular disease (including severe aortic stenosis, defined as a mean pressure gradient >40 mm Hg or aortic valve area <1.0 cm², or symptomatic mitral stenosis).

After it has been determined whether there are active cardiac conditions that require treatment prior to surgery, the risk of the surgery and the functional capacity of the patient need to be considered. The ACC/AHA Guidelines use a different definition of what constitutes high-risk surgery than was used in the RCRI derivation. High-risk surgery, as defined in the ACC/AHA Guidelines, is vascular surgery, including aortic or other major vascular procedures, as well as peripheral vascular surgery. Surgeries such as orthopedic surgery, nonvascular intraperitoneal and intrathoracic

Table 94.1 REVISED CARDIAC RISK INDEX (RCRI)

RISK FACTOR	DEFINITION
1. High-risk type of surgery	Intraperitoneal, intrathoracic, or suprainguinal vascular procedures
2. Ischemic heart disease	History of MI, positive stress test, current cardiac CP, nitrate usage, EKG with pathologic Q waves
3. History of congestive heart failure	History of CHF, pulmonary edema, or PND; rales or S3 on exam; chest x-ray with pulmonary edema
4. History of cerebrovascular disease	History of transient ischemic attack or stroke
5. Insulin therapy for diabetes	
6. Preoperative serum creatinine >2.0 mg/dL	

SOURCE: Reprinted with permission from Lee et al. (1999).

surgery, and head and neck surgery are all considered intermediate risk. Procedures such as breast surgery and endoscopic surgery are considered low risk.

Patients undergoing low-risk procedures can generally go to the OR without further testing regardless of their functional capacity. For patients undergoing procedures that are not low risk, the ACC/AHA Guidelines recommend that the patients' functional capacity be determined based on the history. The current threshold is defined as being able to achieve ≥4 METs (metabolic equivalents) of activity without cardiac symptoms, although this threshold may be raised in the future. A functional capacity of 4 METs corresponds to climbing a flight of stairs with a bag of groceries, walking 3.5 mph briskly on a level surface,

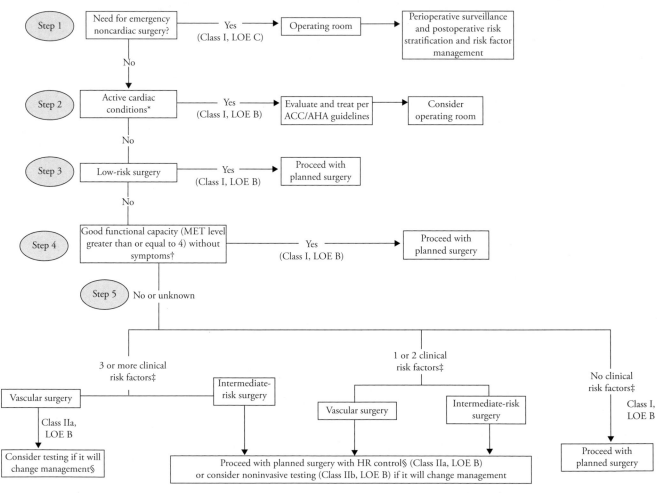

Figure 94.1. Cardiac Evaluation and Care Algorithm for Noncardiac Surgery. From ACC/AHA 2007 Guidelines. Reprinted with permission from Fleisher et al. (2007).

or sweeping the sidewalk. Instruments such as the Duke Activity Status Index provide a scale of different activities to help establish a person's functional capacity. Patients with a functional capacity of ≥4 METs can go to the OR without the need for additional testing.

Among patients with a functional capacity of <4 METs, further management is determined by the patient's risk factors as well as the risk of the procedure. The previous ACC/AHA Guidelines from 2002 used a system of three different levels of clinical predictors. This approach has been abandoned in favor of a simplified scheme in which the applicable clinical risk factors mirror the RCRI risk factors discussed above (history of ischemic heart disease, heart failure, cerebrovascular disease, diabetes mellitus, and renal insufficiency). An exception is high-risk surgery, which is integrated into the algorithm separately rather than considered a risk factor.

The ACC/AHA Guidelines state that, among patients who have a functional status of <4 METs, those with no risk factors can proceed directly to surgery. Those with one or two risk factors will generally proceed to surgery without additional testing unless noninvasive testing would alter management of the patient. The Guidelines suggest that patients with three or more risk factors undergoing vascular surgery be seriously considered for noninvasive testing prior to surgery. However, even in these patients, noninvasive testing should be obtained only if it will change management, which will depend on the assessed risk of the patient, the risk of the procedure, and the urgency of the procedure. In general in the absence of ongoing active cardiac conditions, the vast majority of patients will not require noninvasive testing prior to surgery, because trials of noninvasive testing and/or revascularization versus medical management prior to surgery have not shown a benefit to an interventional preoperative strategy. Patients with risk factors for cardiac disease should generally have their heart rates controlled with beta blockers (see discussion on beta blockers several sections below).

STUDIES OF PREOPERATIVE TESTING AND REVASCULARIZATION

Three key trials of preoperative strategies are the DECREASE-II trial, the CARP trial, and the DECREASE-V pilot study.

THE DECREASE-II TRIAL

This trial, by Poldermans et al. (2006), included about 1500 patients who were undergoing abdominal aortic or lower extremity arterial surgery. Patients categorized as intermediate risk were randomized to either a preoperative stress test or no stress test. Patients whose stress tests showed extensive ischemia were considered for revascularization, if feasible.

All patients received beta blockers, with a goal heart rate of 60–65 bpm.

Results

With a composite endpoint of cardiac death and nonfatal MI at 30 days, the intermediate-risk patients who got stress tests prior to surgery did no better than those who did not get stress tests. The rate of the composite endpoint among the patients who got stress tests was 2.3%, compared to 1.8% among the patients who did not receive stress tests ($p = 0.62$). Revascularization of the intermediate-risk patients with extensive ischemia also did not appear beneficial, although the number of patients in this group was too small to draw firm conclusions. In addition, those patients with lower heart rates had fewer cardiac events. Thus, the results of this trial suggest that it is not advantageous to have intermediate-risk patients undergo preoperative stress tests in patients who are receiving beta blockers.

THE CARP TRIAL

This trial, by McFalls et al. (2004), examined whether revascularization prior to surgery is beneficial in a population of patients undergoing vascular surgery. In this trial 510 patients who were considered at elevated cardiac risk, and who therefore had already undergone diagnostic cardiac catheterization, were eligible for enrollment only if their cardiac catheterization showed ≥70% coronary stenosis. Exclusion criteria included stenosis of the left main coronary artery, left ventricular ejection fraction (LVEF) <20%, or severe aortic stenosis. Enrolled patients were randomized to revascularization or no revascularization prior to surgery, with the rate of perioperative beta-blocker use similar in both groups, at around 85%. Among the patients who were revascularized, 59% underwent percutaneous coronary intervention (PCI), and 41% underwent coronary artery bypass graft (CABG).

Results

There was no significant difference in the outcomes between the revascularization and no-revascularization groups, who had similar MI rates at 30 days (11.6% in the revascularization group vs. 14.3% in the no revascularization group; $p = 0.37$). The two groups also had similar 30-day death rates and long-term outcomes. In this group of patients undergoing vascular surgery, all of whom had angiographically proven coronary artery disease (CAD), preoperative revascularization did not improve outcomes.

THE DECREASE-V PILOT STUDY

This trial, by Poldermans et al. (2007), sought to study a group at higher risk than the population enrolled in the

CARP trial. This pilot study included 101 patients undergoing major vascular surgery, who had at least three cardiac risk factors and whose stress tests showed extensive stress-induced ischemia. These patients were then randomized to either revascularization or no revascularization prior to surgery. Of the patients who were revascularized, 65% underwent PCI, while 35% underwent CABG. All patients received beta blockers, which were titrated to a goal resting heart rate of 60–65 bpm. Among those patients randomized to revascularization, 67% had three-vessel CAD (compared with 35% in the CARP trial).

Results

There was no significant difference in the incidence of the primary outcome—which was a composite of 30-day all-cause death and nonfatal MI—between the two groups, at 42.9% in the revascularization group versus 32.7% in the no revascularization group ($p = 0.30$). Although this was a pilot study, and so may have been underpowered, it corroborates the findings in the CARP study that, even among patients with documented CAD, preoperative revascularization does not appear to offer significant benefit. Pathophysiologically, the failure of preoperative revascularization to confer benefit in patients with known CAD undergoing vascular surgery raises the possibility that coronary lesions other than the flow-limiting ones that are addressed with revascularization may be causing perioperative events in these patients.

The results of these three studies helped shape the current ACC/AHA Guidelines, in which it is recommended that, in the absence of an active cardiac condition, patients be considered for preoperative noninvasive testing primarily under the narrow circumstances of high-risk patients undergoing high-risk vascular surgery—and then only when the results of the noninvasive testing would alter management.

REVASCULARIZATION PRIOR TO SURGERY AND MANAGEMENT AFTER REVASCULARIZATION

Revascularization prior to surgery requires careful management of the time period between revascularization and surgery and of patient's antiplatelet therapy. For patients who undergo balloon angioplasty without a stent, at least 2–4 weeks should elapse prior to surgery so that the vessel may heal. In patients who receive bare-metal stents, surgery should be delayed 4–6 weeks to allow for some endothelialization of the stent, but it should ideally occur before 12 weeks, which is the point at which the risk of restenosis is higher. Dual antiplatelet therapy (aspirin and clopidogrel) should be continued for at least 4 weeks after implantation of bare-metal stents. Even after 4 weeks, when clopidogrel may be stopped, aspirin should ideally be continued

perioperatively, subject to the surgeon's assessment of the bleeding risk.

With drug-eluting stents, the risk of stent thrombosis persists for a longer period than with bare-metal stents, and so a longer duration of dual antiplatelet therapy is indicated. Aspirin and clopidogrel should be continued for at least 12 months after implantation of a drug-eluting stent. Increasingly, some cardiologists are recommending dual antiplatelet therapy be continued beyond 12 months in patients with drug-eluting stents. Aspirin should be continued perioperatively, even after the 12-month period during which clopidogrel is required. Of course, the surgeon's assessment of the bleeding risk from aspirin, or aspirin and clopidogrel, needs to be considered in weighing whether to continue these agents perioperatively after revascularization. However, given the potentially severe consequences of stent thrombosis, premature discontinuation of aspirin and clopidogrel should be avoided if at all possible. If it is felt to be absolutely necessary to prematurely discontinue clopidogrel due to the surgical bleeding risk, then aspirin should be continued perioperatively, and the clopidogrel should be restarted as soon as possible.

These same time frames dictate which preoperative revascularization technique should be used. If the surgical bleeding risk is such that the surgery cannot be done with aspirin and clopidogrel, then if the surgery needs to happen in 14–29 days, balloon angioplasty should be used; if the surgery needs to happen in 30–365 days, then a bare-metal stent should be used; if the surgery needs to happen in >365 days, then a drug-eluting stent should be used. Aspirin should be continued perioperatively, if at all possible, even after the period is reached when clopidogrel may be stopped.

BETA BLOCKERS

Perioperative beta blockade appears to be of benefit among selected patients who are at elevated risk of perioperative cardiac events. The strongest indications for perioperative beta blockers are in patients who are already on them for an appropriate indication, especially patients with ischemia, as beta-blocker withdrawal perioperatively can be harmful. Patients in whom preoperative testing has demonstrated ischemia and who are undergoing vascular surgery also have a clear indication for beta blockers.

Lindenauer et al. (2005) performed a retrospective cohort study that examined the benefit of perioperative beta blockade, stratifying patients based on the RCRI risk factors. The primary outcome used was in-hospital death. This study found that beta blockade was helpful only among patients at elevated cardiac risk. Patients with zero RCRI risk factors showed harm from beta blockers. Clear benefit was seen among patients with three or more RCRI risk factors.

Included among the recommendations regarding perioperative beta blockade from the ACC/AHA Guidelines are that beta blockers are "probably recommended" in patients with coronary heart disease, or those with two or more clinical risk factors, undergoing intermediate-risk or vascular surgery. Vascular surgery is considered the highest-risk surgery by the ACC/AHA Guidelines, and so beta blockers are also reasonable in patients undergoing vascular surgery with one or more risk factors. When giving beta blockers perioperatively, it is not enough that they be "on board," as the benefit is greatest with a relatively low resting heart rate (figure 94.2), as long as hypotension is avoided. Thus, patients should have their beta blockers titrated to try to achieve a low-normal heart rate (i.e., in the 60bpm).

THE POISE TRIAL

Designed to address the lack of a large randomized controlled trial (RCT) of perioperative beta blockers, the PeriOperative ISchemic Evaluation (POISE) Trial enrolled 8351 patients undergoing noncardiac surgery with at least one cardiac risk factor. Patients were randomized to either placebo or controlled-release metoprolol (CR metoprolol), 100 mg orally 2–4 hours prior to surgery, a postoperative dose of CR metoprolol based on heart rate and blood pressure, and then 200 mg of CR metoprolol orally daily for the next 30 days.

Results

The patients who received the CR metoprolol had a lower rate of the primary outcome—a composite of cardiovascular death, nonfatal MI, and nonfatal cardiac arrest—than the placebo group (5.8% in the CR metoprolol group versus

6.9% in the placebo group; $p = 0.04$). However, the total mortality was higher in the CR metoprolol group (3.1%) than in the placebo group (2.3%) ($p = 0.03$). This higher mortality in the CR metoprolol group appears to have been driven by a higher rate of stroke in the CR metoprolol group (1.0%) than in the placebo group (0.5%) ($p = 0.005$).

There is controversy over what lessons should be drawn from the POISE trial. The authors of the trial argue that combining the POISE trial with other perioperative beta-blocker trials leads to the same conclusions, and therefore, we should reconsider current recommendations regarding perioperative beta-blocker use. However, it is very possible that the unfavorable total mortality outcome in the beta-blocker group in the POISE trial was due to the large dose of beta blockers being given so close to the beginning of surgery. Given the results of the POISE, it may be preferable to start beta blockers days or weeks, rather than hours, before surgery and to use lower starting doses that should be titrated up judiciously, in order to achieve a low-normal heart rate while avoiding hypotension.

THE DECREASE-IV TRIAL

This trial by Dunkelgrun et al. (2009) examined the effect of beta blockers in patients at intermediate cardiovascular risk undergoing noncardiovascular surgery. Patients, all of whom were beta blocker naive, were randomized to receive placebo ($n = 533$) or the beta blocker bisoprolol ($n = 533$), started a median of 34 days prior to surgery and titrated to a heart rate of 50–70 bpm.

Results

The primary endpoint, a composite of 30-day cardiac death and nonfatal MI, was reached in 2.1% of patients in the beta-blocker group versus 6.0% in the placebo group ($p = 0.002$). This trial also included a statin arm, which did not show a significant benefit, and a combined beta blocker and statin arm, which did not appear significantly better than beta blockers alone. Thus, this trial, unlike the POISE trial, was able to show a clear benefit to perioperative beta blockers started about a month prior to surgery and titrated to a goal heart rate of 50–70 bpm.

To summarize some conclusions that can be drawn about the use of beta blockers perioperatively:

- In patients who are taking beta blockers as outpatients for an appropriate indication, the beta blocker should be continued perioperatively, as beta-blocker withdrawal can be detrimental.

- In patients with known cardiac ischemia, such as has been demonstrated in preoperative stress testing, beta blockers should be used perioperatively in patients undergoing intermediate- and high-risk surgery.

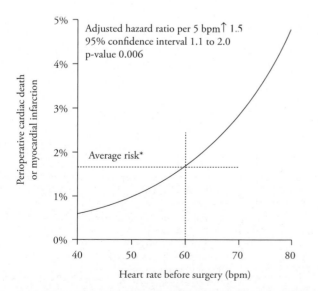

Figure 94.2. Relationship Between Perioperative Cardiac Events and Heart Rate before Surgery. From the DECREASE-II trial. Reprinted from Poldermans et al. (2005), with permission from Elsevier.

- In patients with at least three cardiac risk factors, and probably in those with at least two cardiac risk factors, especially if they are undergoing intermediate- and high-risk surgery, it is reasonable to use perioperative beta blockers.

- In patients in whom perioperative beta blockers are indicated, it is important to achieve a low-normal heart rate, but care needs to be taken to avoid hypotension that could lead to stroke or other adverse event. It is preferable to start beta blockers weeks to months prior to surgery, if possible.

OTHER MEDICATIONS TO DECREASE PERIOPERATIVE CARDIOVASCULAR RISK

STATINS

Statins have been shown in a number of retrospective studies to decrease perioperative cardiac events. The population examined in many of these studies was vascular surgery patients, so it is in this patient population that the data favoring a benefit from statins perioperatively are greatest. An RCT of statins in vascular surgery patients (Schouten et al., 2009) found a significant benefit from the perioperative use of statins (begun a mean of 37 days prior to surgery). Patients receiving statins (n = 250) had a postoperative cardiac ischemia rate of 10.8%, compared to 19.0% in the placebo group (n = 247) (p = 0.01). The statin group also had a significant reduction in death from cardiac causes or MI. Therefore, consistent with ACC/AHA Guidelines, statins should be continued in patients who are already taking them, and it is reasonable to use them in patients undergoing vascular surgery as well.

ALPHA-2 AGONISTS

The data on the perioperative use of alpha-2 agonists, such as clonidine, are limited. In one RCT involving 190 patients at elevated cardiac risk who received clonidine (orally and transdermally) perioperatively, there was a decrease in the incidence of myocardial ischemia in the clonidine group (14%) versus the placebo group (31%) (p = 0.01). However, at this time, clonidine should be considered a second-line agent, to be used only when other agents are either ineffective or contraindicated, in which case it may be considered in patients at elevated cardiac risk.

CALCIUM CHANNEL BLOCKERS

Perioperative calcium channel blockers have only been tested in small trials. A meta-analysis of these trials concluded that calcium channel blockers, especially diltiazem, reduced

ischemia and supraventricular tachycardias. However, the ACC/AHA Guidelines make no recommendations regarding their use.

PULMONARY RISK FACTORS AND RISK REDUCTION

Although less studied in the literature than perioperative cardiac complications, perioperative pulmonary complications can be a significant cause of morbidity. In one series, postoperative pulmonary complications developed in 3.4% of patients undergoing noncardiac surgery at Veterans Affairs hospitals. Postoperative pulmonary complications that contribute to this morbidity include pneumonia, respiratory failure requiring mechanical ventilation, bronchospasm, and atelectasis. A clinical guideline by Smetana et al. (2006) evaluated the literature on pulmonary risk factors for noncardiothoracic surgery and identified a number of risk factors for which there was good evidence. These risk factors fall into the three categories of patient-related risk factors, procedure-related risk factors, and laboratory tests (table 94.2). In one risk prediction model the most important risk factor was the type of surgery, with those surgeries that were closest to the diaphragm generally conferring the highest pulmonary risk.

The strategies to reduce perioperative pulmonary complications that have the most evidence behind them are those aimed at lung expansion, including incentive spirometry and deep breathing exercises. Other interventions that may be useful include use of spinal instead of general anesthesia, use of laparoscopic instead of open procedures, and avoiding long-acting neuromuscular blockading agents during surgery. Using nasogastric tubes only when clearly needed may also be useful in decreasing perioperative pulmonary complications. The data on the effect of preoperative smoking cessation are mixed. One study found that reducing smoking 6–8

Table 94.2 PULMONARY RISK FACTORS

PATIENT-RELATED	PROCEDURE-RELATED	LABORATORY TEST
Advanced age (>60 years old)	Aortic aneurysm repair	Albumin level <3.5 g/dL
ASA class ≥ II	Thoracic surgery	
CHF	Abdominal surgery	
Functional dependence (total or partial)	Upper abdominal surgery	
	Neurosurgery	
	Prolonged surgery	
COPD	Head and neck surgery	
	Emergency surgery	
	Vascular surgery	
	General anesthesia	

SOURCE: Smetana et al. (2006).

weeks before surgery decreased postoperative morbidity, though an effect on pulmonary complications could not be demonstrated. However, other studies have found that quitting or reducing smoking right before surgery might not be beneficial and may even be detrimental. Thus preoperative smoking cessation should occur at least 2 months prior to surgery.

PERIOPERATIVE MANAGEMENT OF THE DIABETIC PATIENT

Diabetics are at elevated risk for cardiovascular and other complications in the perioperative setting. Indeed, diabetes requiring insulin therapy is one of the RCRI risk factors. In addition to being a risk factor for cardiovascular events, inadequately controlled diabetes increases the risk for postoperative infections. No guidelines exist on exactly what the target blood glucose should be in perioperative patients. The American Diabetes Association recommends random blood glucose levels be kept <180 mg/dL and premeal blood glucose levels be kept <140 mg/dL in hospitalized patients who are not critically ill. One study of patients in the SICU compared intensive insulin therapy with a goal blood glucose of 80–110 mg/dL to conventional insulin therapy with a goal blood glucose of 180–200 mg/dL. Among patients in the SICU for >5 days, those patients in the intensive insulin therapy arm had a significant mortality benefit compared to those patients in the conventional insulin therapy arm.

Few data exist regarding the best perioperative glycemic management practices. The overriding principle is that patients who are type 1 diabetics must not go without basal insulin because of the risk of diabetic ketoacidosis. Sliding scale insulin alone in type 1 diabetics is not adequate. For patients undergoing minor procedures who are taking long-acting insulin (e.g., Lantus), a conventional approach is to have the patients take one-half their morning dose of insulin and have them receive an IV infusion of 5% dextrose at 100 mL/hr while they are NPO. Patients who are undergoing long or complicated procedures will generally require an IV insulin infusion to achieve glycemic control perioperatively.

Perioperative IV insulin therapy may be given as separate simultaneous infusions of insulin and glucose. Alternatively, infusion of a single bag containing both insulin and glucose (and usually also potassium) may be given. Patients receiving IV insulin require very frequent monitoring of their blood glucose levels, which should be checked at least hourly at the beginning of therapy. When transitioning the patient from IV insulin back to subcutaneous insulin, if using short-acting subcutaneous insulin, it should be given 1–2 hours prior to stopping the insulin infusion. If using intermediate- or long-acting subcutaneous insulin, it should be given 2–3 hours prior to stopping the insulin infusion.

BACTERIAL ENDOCARDITIS PROPHYLAXIS

The most recent guidelines on this matter, released by the AHA in 2007, have significantly narrowed the number of patients and clinical situations in which antibiotic prophylaxis to prevent bacterial endocarditis is indicated. Only the highest-risk patients undergoing certain procedures are now recommended to receive prophylaxis. Patients considered at highest risk include those who have a prosthetic cardiac valve, previous infective endocarditis, certain types of congenital heart disease, or cardiac transplantation recipients with valvular abnormalities. The procedures for which the highest-risk patients should receive prophylaxis include dental procedures involving gingival manipulations, respiratory procedures involving any incision or biopsy, and procedures involving infected skin. It is no longer recommended that patients with conditions such as mitral valve prolapse receive endocarditis prophylaxis. Moreover, endocarditis prophylaxis is no longer recommended for gastrointestinal or genitourinary procedures. The recommended regimen for antibiotic prophylaxis for dental procedures is ampicillin or, in penicillin-allergic patients, clindamycin, azithromycin, or clarithromycin.

GLUCOCORTICOIDS IN SURGICAL PATIENTS

Among patients taking exogenous glucocorticoids, who therefore may have adrenal suppression, the stress of surgery may lead to clinically significant adrenal insufficiency. This adrenal insufficiency may be manifested by hypotension and shock, although symptoms may be more nonspecific, such as abdominal pain. Laboratory abnormalities associated with adrenal insufficiency include hyponatremia and eosinophilia. Concern about the stress of surgery precipitating adrenal insufficiency has led to the use of perioperative glucocorticoid coverage, also referred to as *stress-dose steroids*. The incidence of perioperative adrenal insufficiency in surgical patients taking exogenous glucocorticoids is low, occurring less than 1% of the time, with some estimates as low as 0.01%. However, given the potentially serious consequences of perioperative adrenal insufficiency, and the fact that it is preventable, internists providing perioperative consultation need to be attentive to this issue.

According to recommendations made by Axelrod (2003), patients taking 5 mg of prednisone per day or less (or its equivalent) are unlikely to have adrenal suppression and so generally do not need perioperative glucocorticoid coverage, although they should be continued on their usual dose of glucocorticoids. Patients taking at least 20 mg of prednisone (or its equivalent) are likely to have adrenal suppression and so should receive perioperative glucocorticoid coverage. Adrenal suppression from exogenous

Table 94.3 PERIOPERATIVE GLUCOCORTICOID COVERAGE

MAGNITUDE OF SURGICAL STRESS	RECOMMENDED PERIOPERATIVE GLUCOCORTICOID COVERAGE		DURATION
	HYDROCORTISONE	METHYLPREDNISOLONE	
Minor (e.g., inguinal herniorrhaphy)	25 mg/day	5 mg/day	1 day
Moderate (e.g., total joint replacement)	50–75 mg/day	10–15 mg/day	1–2 days
Major (e.g., involves cardiopulmonary bypass)	100–150 mg/day	20–30 mg/day	2–3 days

Steroid doses are total mg/day IV. Hydrocortisone is generally divided every 8 hours, and methylprednisolone every 4–6 hours.
SOURCES: Salem et al. (1994); Axelrod (2003).

glucocorticoids may last as long as a year, so patients who previously have been on high-dose glucocorticoids should be considered for perioperative glucocorticoid coverage. Inhaled glucocorticoids and high-potency topical glucocorticoids may exert a systemic effect and cause adrenal suppression, and so patients taking these forms of steroids should also be considered for perioperative glucocorticoid coverage. Any patient who is taking exogenous glucocorticoids and who has a cushingoid appearance should be given perioperative glucocorticoid coverage.

The most widely cited regimen for perioperative glucocorticoid coverage is based on the recommendations of Salem et al. (1994; see table 94.3).

In cases in which the likelihood of adrenal suppression is unclear (e.g., patients unsure of how much glucocorticoids they are taking), or if there is a desire to avoid perioperative glucocorticoid coverage because of concern about side effects, an adrenocorticotropin hormone (ACTH) stimulation test may be performed. Patients are given synthetic ACTH (cosyntropin), 250 μg IV or IM, and then a plasma cortisol level is measured at 30 minutes and 60 minutes after administration. A plasma cortisol level >18 μg/dL at either time point suggests the patient does not have significant adrenal suppression, and so extra perioperative glucocorticoid coverage is not necessary. Plasma cortisol values <18 μg/dL after an ACTH stimulation test mean the patient may have adrenal suppression and so she or he should receive perioperative glucocorticoid coverage.

ADDITIONAL READING

Axelrod L. Perioperative management of patients treated with glucocorticoids. *Endocrinol Metab Clin North Am*. 2003;32(2):367–83.

Bauer SM, Cayne NS, Veith FJ. New developments in the preoperative evaluation and perioperative management of coronary artery disease in patients undergoing vascular surgery. *J Vasc Surg*. 2010;51(1):242–51.

Dunkelgrun M, Boersma E, Schouten O, et al. Bisoprolol and fluvastatin for the reduction of perioperative cardiac mortality and myocardial infarction in intermediate-risk patients undergoing noncardiovascular surgery: A randomized controlled trial (DECREASE-IV). *Ann Surg*. 2009;249(6):921–6.

Fleisher LA, Beckman JA, Brown KA, et al. ACC/AHA 2007 guidelines on perioperative cardiovascular evaluation and care for noncardiac surgery. *Circulation*. 2007;116(17):e418–99.

Fleisher LA, Beckman JA, Brown KA, et al. 2009 ACCF/AHA focused update on perioperative beta blockade incorporated into the ACC/AHA 2007 guidelines on perioperative cardiovascular evaluation and care for noncardiac surgery: A report of the American College of Cardiology Foundation/American Heart Association task force on practice guidelines. *Circulation*. 2009;120(21):e169–76.

Hoeks S, Flu W-J, van Kuijk J-P, Bax J, Poldermans D. Cardiovascular risk assessment of the diabetic patient undergoing major noncardiac surgery. *Best Pract Res Clin Endocrinol Metab*. 2009;23(3):361–73.

Lee TH, Marcantonio ER, Mangione CM, et al. Derivation and prospective validation of a simple index for prediction of cardiac risk of major noncardiac surgery. *Circulation*. 1999;100(10):1043–9.

Lindenauer PK, Pekow P, Wang K, Mamidi DK, Gutierrez B, Benjamin EM. Perioperative beta-blocker therapy and mortality after major noncardiac surgery. *N Engl J Med*. 2005;353(4):349–61.

McFalls EO, Ward HB, Moritz TE, et al. Coronary-artery revascularization before elective major vascular surgery. *N Engl J Med*. 2004;351(27):2795–2804.

POISE Study Group. Effects of extended-release metoprolol succinate in patients undergoing non-cardiac surgery (POISE trial): A randomised controlled trial. *Lancet*. 2008;371(9627):1839–47.

Poldermans D, Bax JJ, Schouten O, et al. Should major vascular surgery be delayed because of preoperative cardiac testing in intermediate-risk patients receiving beta-blocker therapy with tight heart rate control? *J Am Coll Cardiol*. 2006;48(5):964–9.

Poldermans D, Schouten O, Vidakovic R, et al. A clinical randomized trial to evaluate the safety of a noninvasive approach in high-risk patients undergoing major vascular surgery: The DECREASE-V Pilot Study. *J Am Coll Cardiol*. 2007;49(17):1763–9.

Salem M, Tainsh RE Jr., Bromberg J, Loriaux DL, Chernow B. Perioperative glucocorticoid coverage. A reassessment 42 years after emergence of a problem. *Ann Surg*. 1994;219(4):416–25.

Schouten O, Boersma E, Hoeks SE, et al. Fluvastatin and perioperative events in patients undergoing vascular surgery. *N Engl J Med*. 2009;361(10):980–9.

Smetana GW, Lawrence VA, Cornell JE. Preoperative pulmonary risk stratification for noncardiothoracic surgery: Systematic review for the American College of Physicians. *Ann Intern Med*. 2006;144(8):581–95.

QUESTIONS

QUESTION 1. You are asked by the surgery service to perform preoperative evaluations. Which of the following patients has the strongest indication for a preoperative stress test, based on the ACC/AHA Preoperative Evaluation Guidelines?

A. A 74-year-old female has a history of CVA, atrial fibrillation, and diabetes mellitus for which the patient takes metformin. She is being admitted for a partial colectomy to treat localized colon cancer. Her EKG shows atrial fibrillation, at a rate of 88 bpm, with no ischemic changes.

B. A 67-year-old female with a history of baseline serum creatinine of 1.7, diabetes mellitus for which the patient takes insulin glargine and prandial regular insulin, osteoarthritis, and a history of a DVT in the postoperative setting 3 years ago. She is admitted for a right knee arthroplasty. Her EKG shows normal sinus rhythm at a rate of 78 bpm, with an isolated Q wave in lead III.

C. A 75-year-old male with a history of CVA, CHF, diabetes mellitus for which the patient takes NPH insulin and prandial regular insulin. He is admitted for a fem-pop bypass. His EKG shows normal sinus rhythm at a rate of 89 bpm, with Q waves in leads II, III, and aVF.

D. A 78-year-old male with a history of atrial fibrillation, CHF, and baseline serum creatinine of 1.8. He is admitted for a fem-pop bypass. His EKG shows atrial fibrillation with a rate of 89 bpm and a Q wave in lead III.

E. A 69-year-old female with a history of CHF, MI, osteoarthritis, and diabetes mellitus for which the patient takes NPH insulin and prandial regular insulin. She is undergoing a left knee arthroplasty.

QUESTION 2. You are seeing patients for preoperative evaluation at the request of the surgery service. In which of the following patients is a beta blocker NOT indicated?

A. A 67-year-old male has a history of hypertension, for which he takes atenolol. He has no history of coronary artery disease. He is admitted for a right total hip arthroplasty after suffering a right femoral head fracture due to a mechanical fall.

B. A 65-year-old female with a history of ischemic heart disease and diabetes mellitus, for which she is on insulin, is admitted for a fem-pop bypass.

C. A 74-year-old male with a history of hypertension, for which he takes hydrochlorothiazide, who 2 years ago underwent exercise myocardial perfusion imaging showing mild-moderate reversible inferior ischemia. The patient, who has not been revascularized, is admitted for a partial colectomy.

D. A 69-year-old female with a history of diabetes mellitus for which she takes glyburide, atrial fibrillation (adequately rate controlled on diltiazem), hypertension, and osteoarthritis, is admitted for a left knee arthroplasty.

E. A 62-year-old female with a history of hypertension, chronic kidney disease with a baseline serum creatinine of 2.2 mg/dL, and CVA, who 2 years ago underwent exercise myocardial perfusion imaging showing mild-moderate irreversible inferior perfusion defect, is admitted for a left nephrectomy.

QUESTION 3. A 68-year-old male with a history of hypertension, diabetes mellitus on insulin glargine, and CVA, 9 months ago presented with chest pain after minimal exertion. At that time, he underwent a cardiac catheterization with placement of a drug-eluting stent in the left circumflex coronary artery. Since then, he has been chest pain–free. He is now admitted with a left femur fracture after a mechanical fall, for which he is scheduled to undergo a left hip arthroplasty. His medications include aspirin, clopidogrel, atenolol, and lisinopril. You are consulted for preoperative evaluation. You advise that the patient's beta blocker should be continued. What is the most appropriate additional recommendation to offer at this time?

A. The patient's aspirin should be continued, but it is appropriate to stop the clopidogrel to decrease the perioperative bleeding risk.

B. The patient should not undergo the surgery without a preoperative pharmacologic myocardial perfusion imaging test.

C. It is appropriate to stop both the aspirin and the clopidogrel to decrease the perioperative bleeding risk.

D. The patient should not undergo the surgery without first getting a preoperative resting echocardiogram.

E. The patient should be continued on both the aspirin and clopidogrel perioperatively if at all possible.

QUESTION 4. A 64-year-old female with a history of COPD, hypertension, myocardial infarction 3 years ago, and osteoarthritis is seeing you for a preoperative evaluation 5 days before a scheduled left hip arthroplasty due to severe osteoarthritis and pain in her left hip that limits her mobility. She is an active smoker, consuming 1 pack/day of cigarettes. Current medications include tiotropium inhaled daily, albuterol/Atrovent inhaler as needed for wheezing, atenolol, and simvastatin. She has never had pulmonary function testing. The patient reports that she does not have dyspnea with her limited mobility, and she has not had any exacerbations of her COPD requiring medical attention in the last year. What perioperative recommendation is most appropriate regarding her pulmonary status?

A. She should not undergo elective surgery until she has pulmonary function tests to establish the severity of her COPD.

B. She should stop smoking immediately.

C. She should stop her atenolol to prevent beta-blocker-induced bronchospasm.

D. She should start prednisone to help control her COPD perioperatively.
E. She should continue on the tiotropium and be given nebulized albuterol/Atrovent for any evidence of wheezing.

QUESTION 5. A 47-year-old female with a history of systemic lupus erythematosus, for which she has been on prednisone, 10 mg orally daily for the last year, also with history of a lower GI bleed and hypertension, has had chronic left hip pain, and has been diagnosed with osteonecrosis of the femoral head. Conservative therapy has been ineffective, and she is now scheduled for a left total hip arthroplasty. Which of the following perioperative recommendations regarding glucocorticoids in this patient is most appropriate?

A. She does not need any glucocorticoids perioperatively.
B. She should continue her home dose of glucocorticoids perioperatively.

C. She should receive 50 mg of hydrocortisone IV every 8 hours the day before, the day of, and then the day after surgery, after which she should continue her home dose of glucocorticoids.
D. She should only receive glucocorticoids if hypotension or other evidence of acute adrenal insufficiency develops.
E. She should undergo an ACTH stimulation test, and only if it indicates adrenal suppression should the patient receive perioperative glucocorticoid coverage beyond her usual glucocorticoid dose.

ANSWERS

1. C
2. D
3. E
4. E
5. E

95.

BASIC PRINCIPLES OF EPIDEMIOLOGY AND BIOSTATISTICS

Julie E. Buring and I-Min Lee

In reviewing past questions from the Boards, we clearly see that there are a small number of selected areas of epidemiological and biostatistical principles that are most frequently addressed: screening for disease control (including sensitivity, specificity, and predictive value of a screening test and bias in the interpretation of the results); measurement of data (including measures of disease frequency [incidence, prevalence] and measures of association [relative risk, attributable risk, number needed to treat]); and the interpretation of data (including types of epidemiological studies and the roles of chance, bias, and confounding in the interpretation of the findings). In this chapter, we review these topics in the context of specific clinical questions. The principles summarized are drawn extensively from the textbook *Epidemiology in Medicine* (Hennekens and Buring, 1987), and this book should be consulted for further examples. There are a number of other introductory-level epidemiology and statistical sources that can also be utilized, and these are listed at the back of this chapter.

Screening for Disease Control

Question 1:

One hundred women over the age of 50 received mammograms at a mobile breast cancer screening unit. Twenty-seven women had findings suspicious for malignancy on the mammogram; 19 of these women were confirmed as having breast cancer by biopsy. One woman had a negative mammogram but in the subsequent year developed breast cancer and is assumed to have had the disease at the time of screening. What is the sensitivity of the mammogram? The specificity? And the predictive value of a positive screening test?

VALIDITY AND YIELD OF A SCREENING TEST

Screening refers to the application of a simple, inexpensive test to asymptomatic individuals in order to classify them as likely or unlikely to have a particular disease. A disease is appropriate for screening if (1) it is serious, (2) its preclinical prevalence is high among the population screened, and (3) treatment given while the disease is asymptomatic is more beneficial than treatment given after symptoms develop. In addition, a valid screening test must be available. The validity of screening test is defined by its ability to correctly classify those who have preclinical disease as screening-test positive (measured by the sensitivity of a screening test) and those who do not have preclinical disease as screening-test negative (measured by the specificity of the screening test). Finally, the yield, or the number of cases detected by the screening program, is considered using the positive predictive value or the probability that a person actually has the disease if he or she tests positive on the screen.

Table 95.1 presents the data from Question 1 in the form of a 2 × 2 table, summarizing the relationship between the results of the screening test (mammography) and the "true" presence of the disease as assessed by the results of the appropriate subsequent diagnostic test (breast biopsy). Sensitivity can then be calculated as the probability of screening positive if the disease is truly present and specificity as the probability of screening negative if the disease is truly absent. In this example the sensitivity of the mammography is 19/20 or 95%, meaning that of those who were found to have breast cancer at biopsy, 95% of them tested positive on the mammogram; and the specificity, 72/80 or 90%, meaning that of those who were negative for breast cancer on biopsy, 90% tested negative on the screening mammogram. Finally, of those who tested positive on the mammogram, their predictive value of a positive test, or their probability of being diagnosed with breast cancer on biopsy was 19/27 or 70%.

WHAT INFLUENCES THE SENSITIVITY, SPECIFICITY, AND PREDICTIVE VALUE?

The sensitivity and specificity of a given screening test are in part dependent on where we are in our biological capabilities of identifying preclinical stages for a given disease and our

Table 95.1 CHARACTERISTICS OF A SCREENING TEST: SENSITIVITY, SPECIFICITY, AND PREDICTIVE VALUE

	Breast Cancer		
	Yes	No	
Positive	19	8	27
Mammogram			
Negative	1	72	73
	20	80	100

$$\text{Sensitivity} = \frac{\text{test positive}}{\text{disease positive}} = \frac{19}{20} = 95\%$$

$$\text{Specificity} = \frac{\text{test negative}}{\text{disease negative}} = \frac{72}{80} = 95\%$$

$$\text{Predictive value of a positive test} = \frac{\text{disease positive}}{\text{test positive}} = \frac{19}{27} = 70\%$$

technological abilities to develop a good screening test, but they can also be affected by what is called the criterion of positivity, that is, the cutoff value that is used to define an "abnormal" screening test. Lowering this criterion or making it less stringent—that is, setting the criterion of positivity for a screening for hypertension, for example, as a single systolic blood pressure of 120 mm Hg—will increase the sensitivity of the screening test and decrease the false negatives because everyone with hypertension will be picked up by the screen. But it will also lower the specificity of the test and increase the false positives in that many normotensive people will screen positive using this criterion. Similarly, raising the criterion or making it more stringent—that is, setting the criterion for positivity to 160 mm Hg—will mean that a higher proportion of those with hypertension will test negative on the screening test (decreased sensitivity and increased false negatives), but more individuals who are truly normotensive will screen negative (increased specificity and decreased false positives). The predictive value of a positive test is only slightly affected by changes in the sensitivity and specificity of the test, but it can be increased primarily by effecting an increase in the underlying prevalence of the preclinical disease in the screened population by, for example, targeting the screening program to a group at higher risk of developing the disease by nature of their risk factor profile (such as, in the case above, screening those over the age of 65).

BIAS IN THE INTERPRETATION OF SCREENING RESULTS

In evaluating the effectiveness of a screening program—that is, whether the screening program is effective in reducing morbidity or mortality from the disease—the screened and unscreened populations need to be comparable with respect to all other factors affecting the course of the disease besides the screening program itself. One source of bias that is of particular importance in the interpretation of the results of a screening program is *lead time bias* related to the amount of time by which the diagnosis of the disease has been advanced as a direct result of the screening program. Since screening is applied to asymptomatic individuals, every case picked up by screen is diagnosed earlier than if the diagnosis had been based on waiting for clinical symptoms to develop, and if that estimate of lead time is not taken into account when comparing mortality outcomes between screened and unscreened groups, survival from diagnosis may appear to be longer for the screened group only because the diagnosis was made earlier in the course of disease. Lead time bias can be addressed by comparing the age-specific death rates in the screened and non-screened groups rather than by comparing the length of survival from diagnosis to death.

Measurement of Data: Measures of Disease Frequency and Measures of Association

Question 2:

For each statement below, choose the measure of disease frequency that best describes each disease frequency:

Prevalence

Incidence

Standardized morbidity ratio

Age-specific measure

Age-adjusted measure

1. At the initial study examination, 17 persons per 1000 had evidence of coronary heart disease.

2. At the initial study examination, 31 persons aged 45–62 had evidence of coronary heart disease per 1000 persons examined in this age group.

3. At the initial study examination, men and women had the same prevalence of coronary heart disease, after controlling for differences in age between the groups.

4. During the first 8 years of the study, 45 persons developed coronary heart disease per 1000 persons who entered the study free of disease.

5. Among heavy smokers the observed frequency of angina pectoris was 1.6 times as great as the expected frequency during the first 12 years of the study.

MEASURES OF DISEASE FREQUENCY

It is necessary for any epidemiological investigation to be able to quantify the occurrence of disease by measuring the number of affected individuals given the size of the source population and the time period during which the data were collected, allowing the direct comparison of disease frequencies in two or more groups of individuals. The measures of disease frequency most frequently used are incidence and prevalence. As shown in table 95.2, prevalence represents a snapshot of the status of the population at a point in time and is calculated as the number of existing cases of a disease divided by the size of the total population at that specified time. Incidence, on the other hand, represents the development of disease and is calculated as the number of new cases of a disease that developed during a specified period of time divided by the population at risk of being a new case of the disease. The measures of disease frequency can be calculated for the population as a whole or can be specific to a particular category or subgroup of the population such as an age-specific or gender-specific frequency. When two or more populations are being compared, these measures can also be adjusted for baseline differences between the populations, such as an age- or gender-adjusted frequency, or the observed cases in a population can be compared to the number of cases that would be expected based on previous experience or another population (standardized morbidity ratio).

Thus, the correct answers for Question 2 would be:

1. At the initial study examination, 17 persons per 1000 had evidence of coronary heart disease: PREVALENCE

2. At the initial study examination, 31 persons aged 45 to 62 had coronary heart disease per 1000 persons examined in this age group: AGE-SPECIFIC PREVALENCE

3. At the initial study examination, men and women in the study had the same prevalence of coronary heart disease, controlling for differences between the groups with respect to age: AGE-ADJUSTED PREVALENCE

4. During the first 8 years of the study, 45 persons developed coronary heart disease per 100 persons who entered the study free of disease: INCIDENCE

5. Among heavy smokers, the observed frequency of angina pectoris was 1.6 times as great as the expected frequency during the first 12 years of the study: STANDARDIZED MORBIDITY RATIO

Calculation of Measures of Disease Frequency

Question 3:

At the beginning of 2007, 800 people diagnosed with diabetes lived in a city that had a midyear population estimated at 10,000. During that year, 200 new cases of diabetes were diagnosed in the city, and 40 people died of complications of diabetes.

1. What was the incidence per 1000 of diabetes during 2007?

2. What was the prevalence per 1000 of diabetes on January 1, 2007?

3. What was the prevalence per 1000 of diabetes on December 31, 2007?

4. What was the mortality per 1000 from diabetes during 2007?

5. If the prevalence of diabetes in 2000 was less than the prevalence of diabetes in 2007, could this be due to a change in the incidence rate, a change in the duration of the disease, or both?

The definitions given in table 95.2 provide the information needed to calculate each of the individual measures of incidence and prevalence. With regard to their interrelationship, prevalence—the proportion of the population that has a disease at a point in time—depends on both the rate of development of new disease during the period of time (incidence) as well as the duration of the disease from onset to termination (such as cure or death). Thus, a change in prevalence from one population to another or one time period to another can reflect a change in incidence, a change in the duration of the disease, or both.

Table 95.2 MEASURES OF DISEASE FREQUENCY IN EPIDEMIOLOGICAL STUDIES

$$\text{PREVALENCE} = \frac{\text{number of existing cases at a point in time}}{\text{total population}}$$

$$\text{INCIDENCE} = \frac{\text{number of new cases during a period of time}}{\text{population at risk}}$$

$$\text{STANDARDIZED MORBIDITY RATIO} = \frac{\text{observed number of cases}}{\text{expected number of cases}}$$

MEASURES OF DISEASE FREQUENCY CAN BE:

category-specific (i.e., age-specific)
category-adjusted (i.e., age-adjusted)

Thus, the answers to Question 3 would be:

1. Incidence of diabetes during 2007 = 200/10,000 = 20/1000

2. Prevalence of diabetes on January 1, 2007 = 800/10,000 = 80/1000

3. Prevalence of diabetes on December 31, 2007 = (800 + 200 − 40)/10,000 = 96/1000

4. Mortality from diabetes in the population during 2007 = 40/10,000 = 4/1000

5. If the prevalence of diabetes in 2000 were less than the prevalence of diabetes in 2007, this could be due to a change in the incidence rate, a change in the duration of the disease, or changes in both.

MEASURES OF ASSOCIATION

Whereas the calculation of appropriate measures of disease frequency is the basis for the description and the comparison of populations, it is also efficient and informative to combine the two frequencies being compared into a single summary parameter that estimates the association between the exposure and the risk of developing the outcome. This can be accomplished by calculating either the ratio of the measures of disease frequency for the two populations, which indicates how much more likely on a relative scale one group is to develop a disease than another, or the difference between the two measures of disease frequency, which indicates on an absolute scale how much greater the frequency of disease is in one group compared with the other. These two measures of association are referred to as the *relative risk* and the *attributable risk*.

The relative risk (RR) estimates the magnitude of the association between the exposure and disease and represents the likelihood of developing the outcome in the exposed group relative to those who are not exposed. Defined as the ratio of the incidence in the exposed group (Ie) divided by the corresponding incidence of disease in the nonexposed (Io) group, the relative risk is a measure of the strength of the association between the exposure and the disease. If there is no association between the exposure and disease, that is, under the null hypothesis, the relative risk will equal 1. Values >1 indicate that those who are exposed have an increased risk of developing the outcome, and values less than one, a decreased risk.

The attributable risk (AR) provides information about the absolute effect of the exposure or the excess risk of disease in those exposed compared with those nonexposed. The measure is defined as the difference between the incidence rates in the exposed and nonexposed groups, calculated as Ie − Io. If there is no association between the exposure and the disease, that is, under the null hypothesis, the attributable risk will equal 0. Assuming there is a causal relationship between the

Table 95.3 MEASURES OF ASSOCIATION IN A COHORT STUDY OR RANDOMIZED TRIAL: RELATIVE RISK, ATTRIBUTABLE RISK, AND NUMBER NEEDED TO TREAT

Death from Coronary Heart Disease

	Yes	No	
Statin	200	1800	2000
Placebo	300	1700	2000
	500	3500	4000

$$\text{Relative Risk (RR)} = \frac{\text{Incidence (exposed)}}{\text{Incidence (nonexposed)}} = \frac{200/2000}{300/2000} = 0.67$$

$$\text{Attributable Risk (AR)} = \text{Incidence (exposed)} - \text{Incidence (nonexposed)}$$
$$= \frac{200}{2000} - \frac{300}{2000} = -0.05$$

$$\text{Number Needed to Treat} = \frac{1}{\text{AR}} = \frac{1}{0.05} = 20$$

exposure and the disease and that the attributable risk is >0, its value indicates the number of cases of the disease among the exposed that can be attributed to the exposure itself, or alternatively, the number of cases of the disease among the exposed that could be eliminated if the exposure were eliminated. As such, the attributable risk is useful as a measure of the public health impact of a particular exposure.

The attributable risk can also be expressed as a percentage, calculated as AR% = AR/Ie × 100, in order to estimate the proportion of the disease among the exposed that is attributable to the exposure, or the proportion of the disease in that group that could be prevented by eliminating the exposure. In addition, for clinical purposes, the number needed to treat (NNT) to prevent one case of the outcome can be calculated, as the inverse of the absolute value of the attributable risk, or NNT = 1/AR.

The RR and AR provide very different but complementary types of information. The RR is a measure of the strength of the association between an exposure and disease and provides information that can be used to judge whether a valid observed association is likely to be causal. In contrast, the AR provides a measure of the public health impact of an exposure, assuming that the association is one of cause and effect.

Calculation of Measures of Association

Question 4:

A randomized trial was conducted of a new statin drug to assess its potential benefit on death from coronary heart disease. A total of 4000 patients were entered into the study, 2000 allocated to the active statin and 2000 to placebo. Of the 2000 assigned to the statin, 200 of these died from coronary heart disease in the 5-year median duration of follow-up; of the 2000 assigned to placebo, 300 died from coronary heart disease. What is the magnitude of the association between the statin and death from coronary heart disease? What is the potential public health impact of this drug? What is the number needed to treat to prevent one coronary heart disease death?

Table 95.3 presents the 2 × 2 table summarizing the randomized trial data from Question 4. The RR, calculated as the incidence of the outcome (dying from coronary heart disease) in the exposed (those assigned to statin) divided by the incidence in the nonexposed (those assigned to placebo), is 200/2000 divided by 300/2000 or 0.67. This means that those assigned to the statin had 67% of the risk, or 33% less risk (1 − 0.67), of dying from coronary heart disease during this period than those assigned to placebo. The AR, calculated as the incidence in the exposed minus the incidence in the nonexposed, is 200/2000 − 300/2000 or −0.05. This means that if statins are causally related to the prevention of coronary heart disease mortality, 5 per 100 of the coronary heart disease deaths in the placebo group could have been prevented by use of this statin. Taking the inverse of this attributable risk, 1/0.05, provides the number needed to treat, or 20, indicating that we would need to treat 20 patients with this statin over 5 years (the median duration of follow-up) to prevent one death from coronary heart disease.

Overview of Epidemiological Study Designs and the Interpretation of Study Results

Question 5:

A study was undertaken to evaluate the relationship between maternal smoking during pregnancy and low birth weight. A total of 350 mothers of low-birth-weight babies and 400 mothers of normal-weight babies were interviewed. Of the mothers of low-birth-weight babies, 200 reported smoking during the pregnancy, and 200 of the mothers of normal-weight babies also reported such a history. What kind of study design was this? What is the observed magnitude of the association between smoking and birth weight? Is the observed association a valid one?

WHAT KIND OF STUDY DESIGN WAS THIS?

There are a number of specific analytic study designs that can be used to evaluate an association between an exposure and disease, the choice depending on the particular research question as well as logistics and feasibility. The first broad classification is whether the investigation is an observational or an intervention study, and this depends on the role of the investigator in the study. In observational studies (either case-control or cohort), as the name suggests, the investigator observes the natural course of events in terms of who is exposed or not, and who develops the study outcome,

without intervening in any way. In an intervention study the investigators themselves allocate the exposure—there is not self-selection of the exposure on the part of the participants.

There are two basic types of observational studies: case-control and cohort. As shown in table 95.4, in a case-control study, participants are selected into the study based on their disease status: a group of those with the disease (cases) are compared to those without the disease (controls) with respect to the proportions in each group with the exposure of interest. In contrast, in a cohort study, participants are selected into the study based on the presence or absence of the exposure of interest and followed for the development of the outcome in each exposure group. An intervention study, also called a clinical trial, is a type of cohort study in that participants are identified by their exposure status and followed for the development of the outcome, but the distinguishing feature of the trial is that the exposure of each participant is allocated by the investigator. In a cross-sectional survey, the presence or absence of both exposure and disease is assessed at the same point in time, making it often difficult to distinguish whether the exposure preceded the development of the disease or whether the presence of the preclinical or early stages of the disease affected the individual's exposure level. In an observational or intervention study, the time sequence is more clearly identifiable.

Based on these definitions, Question 4 is describing a case-control study, in that mothers of babies who are low weight at birth (cases) are being compared to mothers of babies who are normal weight at birth (controls) with respect to the exposure of interest (maternal smoking during pregnancy). If the association between low birth weight and maternal smoking during pregnancy had been studied by classifying women as smokers or nonsmokers at the time of their first prenatal visit and correlating the smoking histories with subsequent birth weight, this would have been a cohort study design. An interventional study assigning individuals to a harmful exposure such as smoking cannot be ethically conducted, but a trial could have been designed assigning participants to two different approaches to the cessation of smoking during the pregnancy, for example, and then comparing subsequent birth weights. In a cross-sectional study, the investigators would have assessed the birth weights of newborns and assessed the smoking patterns of the mothers at the same point in time, that is, at the time of the birth. There would be no way, however, to assess whether the smoking pattern at the time of the birth was reflective of the pattern of smoking at earlier times in the pregnancy, which could be of more etiological interest.

WHAT IS THE MAGNITUDE OF THE ASSOCIATION BETWEEN THE EXPOSURE AND THE OUTCOME?

Table 95.5 presents the 2 × 2 table summarizing the data from Question 4. Because this example is a case-control study in which participants are selected on the basis of the

Table 95.4 OVERVIEW OF EPIDEMIOLOGICAL STUDY DESIGNS

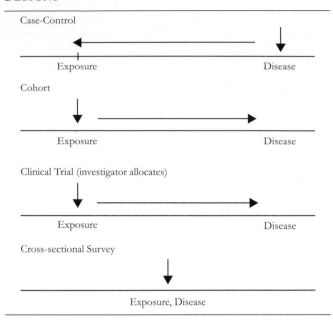

outcome under study, it is not possible to calculate directly the rate of development of the outcome given the presence or absence of the exposure. Thus, the formulas presented earlier in table 95.3 for the calculation of the RR and AR in a cohort study or randomized trial cannot be used in a case-control study. An estimate of the RR, however, can be made by calculation of the odds ratio (OR), which is the ratio of the odds of exposure among the cases to that of the controls (OR = ad/bc). In this case, the OR would be 1.3, which is interpreted as a RR and indicates that mothers who smoked during pregnancy had a 30% increased risk of low-birth-weight babies compared to mothers who did not smoke during pregnancy. In addition, because the incidence rates cannot be directly calculated, the AR can also not be calculated in a case-control study. However, an

Table 95.5 MEASURES OF ASSOCIATION IN A CASE-CONTROL STUDY: ODDS RATIO AND ATTRIBUTABLE RISK PERCENTAGE

		Birth Wight	
		Low	Normal
Smoking	Yes	200 (a)	200 (b)
	No	150 (c)	200 (d)
		350	400

$$\text{Odds Ratio (OR)} = \frac{ad}{bc} = \frac{200\,(200)}{200\,(150)} = 1.3$$

$$\text{Attributable Risk \% (AR\%)} = \frac{OR-1}{OR} = \frac{1.3-1}{1.3} = 23.1\%$$

estimate can be made of the AR%, calculated as: AR% = (odds ratio − 1)/odds ratio. In the example, this would be AR% = (1.3 − 1)/1.3 or 23.1%, indicating that if smoking causes low birth weight, 23% of low-birth-weight babies among smoking mothers would be due to the fact that they smoked, or could be eliminated if smoking were eliminated.

IS THIS OBSERVED ASSOCIATION VALID?

To determine if an association observed in a study is valid, we need to rule out three alternative explanations for the findings: the role of chance, the role of bias, and the role of confounding (table 95.6). Chance refers to that fact that any observed association can be due to sampling variability or the luck of the draw because inferences about the entire population are being drawn from the results of a sample. This is measured by a test of statistical significance and its resultant *p*-value. A result can also be judged to be due to bias or a systematic error in the measurement of the association between the exposure and the disease. And finally, the results can be due to confounding, baseline differences between the groups that are associated with the exposure and are independently associated with the disease, and in themselves could be responsible totally or in part for the association seen. These three explanations must always be examined before one can conclude that the association seen in a study represents a valid, or true relationship between the exposure and the disease.

Question 5a:

In comparing the difference in percentage of maternal smoking between mothers with and without a low-birth-weight baby, the *p*-value is found to be 0.2. The correct interpretation of the result is:

1. the null hypothesis is rejected.

2. the difference is statistically significant.

3. the difference occurred by chance.

4. the difference is compatible with the null hypothesis.

5. sampling variability is an unlikely explanation of the difference.

Table 95.6 ASSESSING THE VALIDITY OF AN EPIDEMIOLOGICAL STUDY

Is the association due to the play of CHANCE? Assess through tests of statistical significance and the resultant p-value.

Is the association due to the role of BIAS? Evaluate the potential for systematic error in the way the data were obtained or reported.

Is the association due to the effects of CONFOUNDING? Assess and control for effects of baseline differences between the groups that are associated with the outcome under study and that could be responsible for the observed association.

The *p*-value is the probability that the observed data, or data more extreme, would occur due to the effects of chance alone, given that there is truly no difference or association between the two groups (the null hypothesis). By convention in the medical literature, the cutoff for statistical significance is at the $p = 0.05$ level. Thus, if the *p* value is <0.05—that is, we would see the results we observed in our study by chance alone, given the null hypothesis that there is truly no association between the exposure and the disease, <1 out of 20 times—we reject the null hypothesis and conclude that the observed difference is statistically significant at the 0.05 level. Conversely, if $p \geq 0.05$—that is, we would see the observed results at least 1 time out of 20 given that there is no association between the exposure and the disease—we cannot reject the null hypothesis, and we conclude the difference is not statistically significant at the 0.05 level. The level of the *p* value does not mean that the observed association is due to chance or that chance is ruled out—it is only a measure of the likelihood that chance is or is not a likely explanation of the findings.

Thus, in Question 5a, because the *p* value is >0.05, the null hypothesis cannot be rejected, the difference is not statistically significant at the 0.05 level, and sampling variation is not an unlikely explanation of the data. It does not mean that the observed difference was due to chance, but it does mean that the difference is compatible with the null hypothesis of no association (answer 4).

Question 5b:

It was suggested that mothers of low-birth-weight babies who smoked would tend to deny such an activity due to feelings of guilt. Moreover, it was also observed that mothers of low-birth-weight babies tended to be younger than the mothers of the normal-weight children, and smoking rates are known to be higher in younger women in this population. These scenarios would be examples of the effects of:

1. chance

2. selection bias

3. recall bias

4. confounding

What effect would each of these scenarios have on the observed relative risk: result in an underestimate of the true relative risk, an overestimate, or be the same as the true relative risk?

The tendency of a mother of a low-birth-weight baby to deny her smoking history is an example of recall bias, which is the tendency of those who are affected to remember their experiences differently than those who are not similarly affected. In this case, the denying by mothers of low-birth-weight children of their smoking exposures during pregnancy would result in an underestimate of the true harmful association of smoking and birth weight. The fact that younger mothers are more likely to smoke and that, independently of smoking, younger mothers are more likely to have low-birth-weight babies, is an example of a confounding variable. If the confounding effect of age of the mother is not controlled, it could appear that smoking is more harmful to the birth weight of the baby than it may actually be (an overestimate of the true effect) because of the mixture of the effects of smoking with the young age of the mother, which in itself will result in a higher rate of low-birth-weight babies.

In epidemiological research, the interpretation of studies must always remain a matter of judgment based on all available evidence. However, this framework of alternative explanations that must be considered—evaluating the roles of chance, bias, and confounding—allows us an approach to judging the validity of a study and thus allows us to begin to consider the next step, which is whether the association observed is in fact one of cause and effect.

ADDITIONAL READING

Dawson B, Trapp RG, Trapp R. *Basic and Clinical Biostatistics*. New York: McGraw-Hill Medical; 2004.

Evidence-Based Medicine Working Group. *Users' Guides to the Medical Literature: A Manual for Evidence-Based Clinical Practice*. 2nd ed. New York: Mc-Graw Hill Professional; 2008.

Fletcher RW, Fletcher SW. *Clinical Epidemiology: The Essentials*. 4th ed. Philadelphia, PA: Lipincott Williams & Wilkins; 2005.

Friedman GD. *Primer of Epidemiology* 5th ed. New York: McGraw-Hill Medical; 2003.

Glantz SA. *Primer of Biostatistics*. New York: McGraw-Hill Medical; 2005.

Hennekens CH, Buring JE. *Epidemiology in Medicine*. Boston: Little, Brown and Company; 1987.

Rothman KJ. *Epidemiology: An Introduction*. New York: Oxford University Press; 2002.

Straus SE, Richardson WS, Glasziou P, Haynes RB. *Evidence-Based Medicine: How to Practice and Teach EBM*. 3rd ed. Edinburgh: Churchill Livingstone; 2005.

96.

CONTRACEPTION

Jane S. Sillman

The general internist needs to be up to date in contraception management. Each year nearly half of all pregnancies in the United States are unintended. Counseling about contraceptive options, provision of a back-up method, and information about emergency contraception can decrease the risk of unintended pregnancy. This chapter focuses on the aspects of contraception emphasized in Medical Knowledge Self-Assessment Program (MKSAP) 14: hormonal contraception, use of barrier methods, intrauterine devices, and emergency contraception.

EFFICACY OF CONTRACEPTIVE METHODS

The best method of contraception is one that is medically appropriate for the patient and that the patient is satisfied with and uses consistently. Effectiveness is measured by failure rates within the first year in two ways: (1) failure rate with perfect use—the percentage of women who become pregnant during the first year of use when they use the method perfectly; and (2) failure rate with typical use—the percentage of women who become pregnant during the first year of use, including those who use the method perfectly and those who do not. The typical use failure rate is the relevant rate to use when educating new-start patients (table 96.1).

HORMONAL CONTRACEPTION

Hormonal contraception is available as combined contraception with an estrogen and a progestin and as progestin-only contraception. Combined contraceptives are available as pills, patches, and vaginal rings. Progestin-only contraceptives are available as pills, injections, and implants.

COMBINED CONTRACEPTION

There are many combined oral contraceptive pills (OCPs) available. The estrogen in the pills is ethinyl estradiol, in doses of 35, 30, or 20 µg, depending on the pill. Each pill also contains one of seven different progestins. The progestins differ in androgenicity in laboratory studies, but these differences do not translate into differences in clinical side effects. All of the combined contraceptives suppress production of a woman's own androgens. All of the combined contraceptives decrease free testosterone, decrease the conversion of testosterone to its active form, dihydrotestosterone, and all improve acne. Combined contraceptive pills increase the risk of deep vein thrombophlebitis (DVT). This risk is mainly due to the dose of the estrogen. The risk of DVT is greater in pills with 50 µg of ethinyl estradiol than in pills with 20–35 µg. The type of progestin may slightly influence DVT risk. Some studies show a twofold greater risk of DVT with combined contraceptive pills containing the progestin desogestrel. This translates into an increase in absolute risk of 1–2 cases of DVT/10,000 women-years of use. As other studies do not show this increase in risk, and the absolute increase, if valid, is small, the American College of Obstetrics and Gynecology and the FDA do not recommend switching current users of pills containing desogestrel to other products. It is important to remember that the risk of DVT with an oral contraceptive pill is less than the risk of DVT during pregnancy (table 96.2). Patients who are carriers of the factor V Leiden mutation are at higher risk of DVTs at baseline, and their risk is increased further if they take an OCP. However, routine screening for this mutation is not recommended. Instead, the clinician should take a careful family history, inquiring about unexplained DVTs and pulmonary emboli in family members. It is appropriate to test women who have a strong family history.

There is a trend toward prescribing combined contraceptive pills with the lowest dose of ethinyl estradiol, 20 µg. These lowest-dose pills have equal efficacy to the pills with 30 and 35 µg of ethinyl estradiol. They are less likely to cause the estrogenic side effects of nausea and breast tenderness. It is possible but not proven that DVT risk is less with a 20-µg pill than with a 35-µg pill. There is also a trend toward prescribing monophasic pills. These are pills with the same daily dose of estrogen and progestin in each active pill. Patients

Table 96.1 EFFICACY OF CONTRACEPTIVE METHODS

METHOD	% OF WOMEN WITH UNINTENDED PREGNANCY IN FIRST YEAR OF USE	
	TYPICAL USE	PERFECT USE
No method	85	85
Cervical cap with spermicide		
Parous women	32	26
Nulliparous women	16	9
Diaphragm with spermicide	16	6
Condom	15	2
OCP	8	0.3
Transdermal patch	8	0.3
Vaginal ring	8	0.3
DMPA injection	3	0.3
IUD		
Copper	0.8	0.6
Levonorgestrel	0.1	0.1
Female sterilization	0.5	0.5
Male sterilization	0.15	0.10

SOURCE: Hatcher et al. (2005).

can use monophasic pills continuously, taking an active pill every day and omitting the placebo pills. Continuous use is gaining in popularity as growing numbers of women choose to decrease the frequency of their menstrual periods. Generic formulations of combined contraceptive pills are appropriate choices as they have equivalent efficacy to the brand-name pills and are about half the price.

Weight may decrease OCP efficacy. In a case-control study from the University of Washington, the risk of pregnancy more than doubled in patients with a body mass index (BMI) >27.3 (OR 2.2). As OCPs are so effective, this translated into a low absolute risk of pregnancy of 2–4 pregnancies/100 women-years of use (Holt et al., 2005). To maximize the effectiveness of OCPs in overweight women,

Table 96.2 RISKS OF DVT

	RISK OF DVT DEEP VEIN THROMBOSIS
No OCP, oral contraceptive pills	4–8/100,000 women per year
OCP	10–30/100,000 women per year
Pregnancy	60/100,000 women per year

NOTE: The risk of DVT with an OCP is less than with pregnancy.
SOURCE: Adapted from Hatcher et al. (2005).

it is reasonable to prescribe a pill with 35 µg of ethinyl estradiol and to advise patients to take the pill at the same time every day in order to maintain a consistent blood level. It is important to educate overweight women about these data and to discuss alternative contraceptive methods.

There are more than 50 studies on the relationship between OCPs and breast cancer. Most experts believe that OCPs have little, if any, effect on the risk of developing breast cancer.

The World Health Organization has medical eligibility criteria for starting contraceptive methods. Contraindications to combined OCPs include smoker older than age 35, uncontrolled hypertension, history of DVT or pulmonary embolus, known thrombogenic mutations, history of coronary artery disease or stroke, migraine with aura, personal history of breast cancer, and breast-feeding within the first 6 weeks.

There are different ways to start OCPs. The "quick start" is the current method of choice because it leads to better compliance in the first 6 months. The quick start method means that the patient starts taking her OCPs on the day that she gets her prescription, regardless of where she is in her menstrual cycle. She needs to use a back-up method, condoms, for the first week. Another option is the "first day" start, beginning the OCPs on day 1 of the menstrual period. The first day start does not require use of a back-up method. Finally, patients can use the "Sunday start," beginning the OCP on the Sunday of the week of the menstrual period. The advantage of the Sunday start is that withdrawal bleeding should be completed by the weekend. The Sunday start requires use of a backup method for the first week.

Continuous use of OCPs means daily use of the active OCPs, omitting the placebos. Monophasic pills are the formulations recommended for continuous use. Over time, continuous use can lead to amenorrhea. Patients on continuous use may have increased spotting, but this decreases over time. There are several indications for continuous use of OCPs. Patient convenience is a reasonable indication. Many patients prefer not to have a monthly menstrual period because of travel, work, or other personal reasons. Continuous use can be very helpful for the patient with menstrual migraines, migraines triggered by the drop in estrogen levels at the onset of the menstrual period. With continuous use, estrogen levels remain steady, and the frequency of menstrual migraines may significantly decrease. Continuous use of OCPs is also helpful for patients with dysmenorrhea and patients with endometriosis. Eliminating the menstrual period eliminates the pain that patients with dysmenorrhea and endometriosis experience at the time of menstruation. Patients with polycystic ovarian syndrome have consistent suppression of their androgen production, which can potentially lead to more improvement in acne.

Physicians are currently recommending continuous use for up to 1 year. The FDA approved the first year-long continuous use OCP in May, 2007. This pill contains 20 µg of ethinyl estradiol and 90 µg of levonorgestrel. A recent study of this pill and the return of menses found that 99% of participants had menses or pregnancy within 90 days of stopping the pill (Davis et al., 2008). Physicians can prescribe any monophasic pill this way.

The transdermal patch contains 20 µg of ethinyl estradiol and 150 µg of norelgestromin. The patient applies one patch per week for 3 weeks at rotating sites, and she will have a menstrual period during the fourth week. A recent study found that serum levels of estrogen were 60% higher with the patch than with a comparable OCP with 35 µg of ethinyl estradiol and the progestin, norgestimate (van den Heuvel et al., 2005). This finding led to concerns that the patch might be associated with a higher risk of DVT. At present, studies show conflicting results. Two studies comparing the patch with a 35-µg OCP with norgestimate showed equivalent risks of DVT (Jick et al., 2006, 2007). However, one study showed a twofold increase in DVT risk with the patch versus this comparable OCP: 41 versus 18 DVTs/100,000 women-years (Cole et al., 2007).

It is important to weigh the patch's advantages and disadvantages. The patch has several advantages. Studies show that users are more compliant with the patch than with OCPs, probably because they need to remember to do something only once a week. The patch is also excellent for continuous use. Patients who want to eliminate their menstrual periods simply continue to apply a patch once a week. There are also clear disadvantages to the patch. The most concerning disadvantage is the high serum estrogen level and possible increase in DVT risk with the patch. Another limitation is that the patch is less effective in women weighing 198 pounds or more.

The vaginal ring is a flexible, soft ring that releases 15 µg of ethinyl estradiol and 120 µg of etonogestrel, the active form of desogestrel, daily. The patient inserts the ring into the vagina and removes it after 3 weeks in order to have a menstrual period during the fourth week. The vaginal ring has some compelling advantages. It exposes patients to lower serum levels of estrogen and progestin than the pills and patch. There is some evidence that compliance is better with the ring than with pills. The ring user just needs to remember to insert the ring and remove it once a month. The ring is excellent for continuous use as it suppresses ovulation for 35 days. For continuous use the patient inserts the ring on the first day of the month, and simply inserts the next ring on the first day of the next month. One disadvantage of the ring is that it causes vaginal irritation in some women.

PROGESTIN-ONLY CONTRACEPTION

A World Health Organization (WHO) case-control study in 1988 showed that there was no increase in DVT, stroke, or MI with progestin-only pills. It is safe to use progestin-only contraception in pill, injectable, and implant formulations in women with contraindications to estrogen.

Injectable formulations of progestin-only contraception are widely used and highly effective. Depot medroxyprogesterone acetate (DMPA) provides contraception for up to 13 weeks. The dose is 150 mg given IM every 12 weeks, within the first 5 days of the menstrual period. Advantages of DMPA include its high efficacy. Studies show that teenagers on DMPA are less likely to become pregnant than teenagers on OCPs or the patch. DMPA leads to decreased blood loss, with amenorrhea in 50% of users after 1 year. DMPA can also lead to decreased dysmenorrhea, but this is an off-label indication for its use. Disadvantages of DMPA include irregular bleeding, weight gain, and delayed return of fertility. Fertility returns on average after 10 months, but it can be delayed for up to 2 years in some patients.

DMPA is associated with a decrease in bone density. This finding led to a black box warning from the FDA stating that women who use DMPA may lose significant bone density that may not be completely reversible and that DMPA should be used longer than 2 years only if other birth control methods are inadequate. Subsequent studies of the relationship of DMPA and bone density have been reassuring. An initial 3-year prospective study in users aged 18–21 and 14–18 showed that although bone density decreased on DMPA, the losses were reversible, and bone density returned to baseline 1 year after discontinuing DMPA (Scholes et al., 2005). The Society for Adolescent Medicine guidelines state: (1) appropriate patient selection is important; (2) patients on DMPA should take calcium 1300 mg and vitamin D 400 IU and exercise daily; (3) bone density testing is not routinely indicated; and (4) duration of use need not be restricted to 2 years. A recent large study of 3500 women, ages 18–44 showed complete recovery of bone mineral density 2–3 years after cessation of DMPA regardless of ethnicity, duration of use (up to 10 years), and age during use (Rosenberg et al., 2007).

A new lower dose of DMPA is now available for subcutaneous injection every 12 weeks. This 104-mg dose is equally efficacious. The advantages of this lower dose include: (1) less weight gain, (2) no effect on bone density, and (3) potential for women to self-inject at home. The disadvantages are that the low dose is currently more expensive and is not yet widely available.

The etonogestrel implant, Implanon, is effective for 3 years. It is a single rod implant 4 cm long and 2 mm in diameter, the size of a matchstick. It releases 60 µg of etonogestrel daily. It is placed under the skin of the upper arm with a 19-gauge disposable preloaded inserter. Clinicians must complete a training program on its insertion and removal. Advantages include decreased dysmenorrhea, high continuation rate in clinical trials, and easier insertion and removal than prior formulations with multiple implants. Disadvantages include unpredictable, irregular menstrual bleeding.

BARRIER METHODS

Condoms act as a mechanical barrier and are highly effective in protecting against HIV, gonorrhea, chlamydia, herpes simplex virus (HSV), and HPV. Patients with any concerns about sexually transmitted infections (STIs) should use condoms. Dual use of a condom plus another method of contraception such as the OCP significantly reduces the risk of both pregnancy and STIs. Physicians should no longer recommend spermicide-coated condoms. The spermicidal condom can be irritating to the vagina, provides no additional protection against pregnancy or STIs, is more expensive, and has a shorter shelf life. The advantages of condoms include decrease in the risk of HIV and other STIs. The main disadvantage is that the condom may break or fall off. It is important to educate patients who use condoms about emergency contraception and to provide them with access information and/or a prescription.

There are several barrier methods for women. The diaphragm is a latex device filled with spermicide and placed over the cervix. Advantages of the diaphragm are that it reduces the risk for cervical STIs and for cervical dysplasia. Disadvantages are that it requires fitting by a clinician, patients often do not use it, leading to a failure rate with typical use of 16%, and it is associated with an increased risk of urinary tract infections. The cervical cap, a smaller device, fits over the cervix and is filled with spermicide. Advantages, compared to the diaphragm, are that it is nonlatex and associated with less risk of urinary tract infection. Disadvantages are that it requires fitting by a clinician, may be hard for patients to insert, and is associated with a failure rate with typical use of 32% in parous women and 16% in nulliparous women. Lea's shield is a reusable cervical barrier used with spermicide. Its advantage is that one size fits all. It requires a prescription but does not require an office visit and is available from Planned Parenthood or online for $65. Its disadvantages are that the failure rate with typical use is 15%, and it is associated with an increased risk of urinary tract infections.

INTRAUTERINE DEVICES

Intrauterine devices (IUDs) are popular worldwide and are slowly increasing in use in the United States. Their advantages are that (1) they are highly effective—as effective as tubal sterilization; (2) they are safe. IUDs are associated with a small risk of pelvic inflammatory disease within the first 30 days after insertion (1/1000), thought to be related to ascension of bacteria during insertion. They are not associated with an increased risk of tubal infertility; (3) they are long lasting; (4) they provide quickly reversible contraception and are easily removed; (5) they are associated with the highest level of user satisfaction (99%); and (6) although they have a high up-front cost, they are highly cost-effective over their duration of use. For example, the levonorgestrel IUD costs up to $500 as a one-time cost and provides 5 years of contraception. In contrast, OCPs cost about $30 per month, for a 5-year cost of $30 × 12 months × 5 years of $1800. The disadvantages of IUDs include requiring a clinician visit for insertion. The American College of Obstetrics and Gynecology recommends that nulligravid and multiparous women at low risk for STIs who want long-term, reversible contraception are good candidates for IUDs.

There are two IUDs available in the United States. The intrauterine copper contraceptive is approved for 10 years of use. It works mainly as a spermicide. It causes a sterile inflammatory reaction in the endometrium that leads to sperm death. The copper ions also inhibit sperm motility, making it less likely that sperm will reach the fallopian tubes. The copper IUD does increase menstrual blood loss and therefore can increase dysmenorrhea. The levonorgestrel IUD is approved for 5 years of use. It initially releases 20 μg/day of levonorgestrel. This release falls to 14 μg/day after 5 years. Levonorgestrel causes cervical mucus to become thicker so sperm cannot enter the upper reproductive tract. It also causes atrophy of the endometrium, which prevents implantation. Its atrophying effect leads to a decrease in menstrual blood loss. By 1 year, up to 20% of users have amenorrhea.

EMERGENCY CONTRACEPTION

Emergency contraception is the use of any method to prevent pregnancy after intercourse. None of the current methods can cause an abortion, and none can disrupt an implanted pregnancy. There are three methods in current use: high-dose progestin-only pills (Plan B), combined oral contraceptive pills, and insertion of the copper intrauterine device. The copper IUD is most effective, followed by the progestin-only pills, and then the combined oral contraceptive pills (table 96.3).

Emergency contraception pills work in several ways to prevent pregnancy. They inhibit ovulation, decrease sperm migration, and increase the ova's resistance to fertilization. Use of high-dose progestin-only pills (Plan B) is the best option. Plan B consists of two pills of levonorgestrel 0.75 mg/pill. This progestin-only method causes less nausea and vomiting and has higher efficacy than the combined OCP method. It is the best choice for patients with any contraindications to estrogen. In addition, its dosage schedule is the simplest. The patient takes one dose of 1.5 mg levonorgestrel (both of the 0.75-mg pills) at one time, as soon as possible after the episode of intercourse. This method can be used for up to 5 days after intercourse. Efficacy decreases as the time from intercourse increases.

Combined OCPs can also be used for emergency contraception. The most effective pills are those with levonorgestrel or norgestrel as the progestin. Pills with norethindrone are slightly less effective. The method consists of two large doses of OCPs taken 12 hours apart. The first dose should be taken as soon as possible. The second dose should be 12 hours later and needs to be completed by 5 days after intercourse.

Each dose must contain at least 100 μg of ethinyl estradiol and either 1 mg of norgestrel or 0.50 mg of levonorgestrel. For example, a patient using her standard OCP with

Table 96.3 EMERGENCY CONTRACEPTION EFFICACY

METHOD	IF 1000 WOMEN HAVE INTERCOURSE	
	# PREGNANT	% REDUCTION
No Rx	80	—
Combined OCP	20	75
Plan B	10	88
IUD	1	99

20 µg of ethinyl estradiol and 0.1 mg of levonorgestrel will need to take five pills for the first dose and another five pills for the second dose. This high dose of estrogen causes nausea in 50% of patients and vomiting in 25%. To prevent this, patients should take an antiemetic 1 hour before the first dose. Meclizine, two 25-mg tablets, is a useful choice because its long duration of action covers both doses.

The copper intrauterine device should be inserted within 5 days of intercourse. It can be inserted up to 8 days after intercourse if ovulation is known to have occurred 3 or more days after the unprotected sex. In order to be effective it must be inserted before implantation has occurred. It prevents pregnancy by acting as a spermicide and preventing implantation. In the United States this method is used primarily in women who plan to continue to use the IUD for ongoing contraception. The levonorgestrel IUD is not effective as a method of emergency contraception.

The FDA approved over-the-counter access to Plan B in August, 2006. Plan B is available over the counter for women who are 18 or older who go to a participating pharmacy. The woman needs to show a photo ID as proof of age. Plan B costs $26–40 and can be bought online. Women who are 17 or younger need a prescription for Plan B. Women can find a local participating pharmacy by going to the emergency contraception web site, www.ec-help.org.

ADDITIONAL READING

Casey PM, Cerhan JR, Pruthi S. Oral contraceptive use and the risk of breast cancer. *Mayo Clin Proc.* 2008;83:86–91.

Cole JA, Norman H, Doherty M, Walker AM. Venous thromboembolism, myocardial infarction, and stroke among transdermal contraceptive system users. *Obstet Gynecol.* 2007;109:339–46.

Darney P, Patel A, Rosen K, Shapiro LS, Kaunitz AM. Safety and efficacy of a Single-rod etonogestrel implant (Implanon): Results from 11 international clinical trials. *Fertil Steril.* 2009;91:1646–53.

Davis AR, Kroll R, Soltes B, Zhang N, Grubb GS, Constantine GD. Occurrence of menses or pregnancy after cessation of a continuous oral contraceptive. *Fertil Steril.* 2008;89:1059–63.

Fantasia HC. Options for intrauterine contraception. *J Obstet Gynecol Neonat Nurs.* 2008;37:375.

Hatcher RA, Trussell J, Nelson AL, Cates Jr. W, Stewart FH, Kowal D. *Contraceptive Technology,* 19th ed. New York: Ardent Media; 2007.

Holt VL, Scholes D, Wicklund KG, Cushing-Haugen KL, Daling JR. Body mass index, weight, and oral contraceptive failure risk. *Obstet Gynecol.* 2005;105:46–52.

Jick SS, Kaye JA, Li L, Jick H. Further results on the risk of nonfatal venous thromboembolism in users of the contraceptive transdermal patch compared to users of oral contraceptive containing norgestimate and 35 microg of ethinyl estradiol. *Contraception.* 2007;76:4–7.

Jick SS, Kaye JA, Russmann S, Jick H. Risk of nonfatal venous thromboembolism in women using a contraceptive transdermal patch and oral contraceptives containing norgestimate and 35 ug of ethinyl estradiol. *Contraception.* 2006;73:223–8.

Kaunitz AM. Hormonal contraception in women of older reproductive age. *N Engl J Med.* 2008;358:1262.

Kaunitz AM, Arias R, McClung M. Bone density recovery after depot medroxyprogesterone acetate injectable contraception use. *Contraception.* 2008;77:67–76.

Legro RS, Jaimey GP, Kunselman AR, et al. Effects of continuous versus cyclic oral contraception: A randomized controlled trial. *J Clin Endocrinol Metab.* 2008;93:420–429.

Rosenberg L, Zhang Y, Constant D, et al. Bone status after cessation of use of injectable progestin contraceptives. *Contraception.* 2007;76:425–31.

Sanfilippo J, Downing D. Emergency contraception: When and how to use it. *J Family Pract.* 2008;Suppl S3.

Scholes D, LaCroix AZ, Ichikawa LE, Barlow WE, Ott SM. Change in bone mineral density among adolescent women using and discontinuing depot medroxyprogesterone acetate contraception. *Arch Pediatr Adolesc Med.* 2005;159:139–44.

van den Heuvel MW, van Bragt AJM, Alnabawy AKM, Kaptein MCJ. Comparison of ethinylestradiol pharmacokinetics in three hormonal contraceptive formulations: the vaginal ring, the transdermal patch and an oral contraceptive. *Contraception.* 2005;72:168–74.

White KO. Update on contraception. *Semin Reprod Med.* 2010; 28(2):93–94.

Yranski PA. Gamache ME. New options for barrier contraception. *J Obstet Gynecol Neonat Nurs.* 2008;37:384.

Zieman M, Hatcher RA, Cwiak C, Darney PD, Creinin MD, Stosur HR. *A Pocket Guide to Managing Contraception.* Tiger, GA: Bridging the Gap Foundation; 2010.

QUESTIONS

QUESTION 1. A 20-year-old woman is evaluated for dysmenorrhea that has worsened over the past 2 years. Her periods are regular and last for 5–6 days. She sometimes misses work because of her dysmenorrhea. Ibuprofen and naproxen have not helped her pain. She is not currently sexually active. Her pelvic exam is normal.

Which of the following is the most appropriate treatment for this patient?

A. Oral contraceptives
B. Depot medroxyprogesterone acetate (DMPA)
C. Meclofenamate
D. Magnesium
E. Tramadol

QUESTION 2. A 40-year-old woman wants to discuss contraceptive options. She and her husband have been using condoms but are having problems with condom breakage. She does not want additional children. She has heavy periods. She had a DVT after a long car ride 2 years ago.

Which of the following is the safest and most effective way to prevent pregnancy in this patient?

A. Oral contraceptive pill
B. Topical contraceptive patch
C. Diaphragm
D. Levonorgestrel intrauterine device

QUESTION 3. A 26-year-old woman had intercourse last night. Her partner was using a condom, and the condom broke. She usually takes an OCP with 0.15 mg desogestrel and 30 μg of ethinyl estradiol in each pill but forgot to take them for the past three nights. She is calling you for advice.

What is the most appropriate way to provide her with emergency contraception?

A. Teach her how to use her own OCPs for emergency contraception
B. Insert the copper IUD
C. Help her obtain Plan B
D. Insert the levonorgestrel IUD
E. Treat her with Ovrette, progestin-only pills

ANSWERS

1. A
2. D
3. C

BOARD SIMULATION: WOMEN'S HEALTH

Caren G. Solomon

QUESTIONS

QUESTION 1. A 32-year-old woman, G1P1, comes in for a visit 6 months postpartum. She is fatigued and has lost few of the 30 lb she gained during pregnancy. She takes a multivitamin, no other medications.

On physical examination, weight is 150 lb, height is 5'2". The thyroid feels slightly enlarged, without nodules, and is nontender.

Her complete blood count (CBC) is normal. The thyroid-stimulating hormone (TSH) level is 24 mIU/L.

Which of the following is *true*?

A. Subacute thyroiditis is the most likely diagnosis.
B. This condition is likely to recur following subsequent pregnancies.
C. TPO antibodies are likely to be negative.
D. You should wait for spontaneous resolution rather than treating with thyroxine.
E. She should have a thyroid ultrasound.

QUESTION 2. A 28-year-old woman comes to establish care. She has a long history of oligomenorrhea and hirsutism and was diagnosed by her gynecologist with polycystic ovary syndrome (PCOS). Records indicate normal prolactin and TSH levels, normal level of fasting 17-OH progesterone, and slightly elevated total testosterone level. Last menstrual period was 4 months ago, which is not unusual for her. She takes no medications.

On examination, weight is 160 lb, height 5'3". Blood pressure is normal. There is slight terminal hair growth in the moustache and sideburn distribution, above her umbilicus, and around her nipples. Pelvic exam is limited by body habitus but appears to be within normal limits.

All of the following are true EXCEPT:

A. This condition is associated with increased risk for glucose intolerance or diabetes.
B. Risk for endometrial hyperplasia or cancer is increased.
C. The finding of polycystic ovaries on pelvic ultrasound is highly sensitive and specific for the diagnosis.

D. Luteinizing hormone (LH) levels are not required to make the diagnosis.
E. Spironolactone may be useful in treatment of associated hirsutism.

QUESTION 3. A 48-year-old woman reports irregular menstrual cycles for the past year. Her last menstrual period was 9 weeks ago. She has been having hot flashes for the past 2 years, and they are interfering with sleep. She is healthy, without significant past medical history.

There is no family history of blood clots or breast cancer.

She takes no medications.

Physical exam is unremarkable; blood pressure is normal, and she has a normal pelvic exam and breast exam.

Which of the following statements is *false*?

A. An follicle-stimulating hormone (FSH) level should be checked to confirm menopause.
B. A low-dose oral contraceptive pill could be considered.
C. A history of deep venous thrombosis would be a contraindication to the use of postmenopausal hormone therapy.
D. Hot flushes are associated with an increase in skin temperature.

QUESTION 4. This patient decides at first to take nothing for her symptoms but returns a year later with persistent hot flashes and no menses for the past 6 months. She is interested in hormone replacement therapy.

Physical exam is normal.

Mammogram is negative.

Which of the following statements is *false*?

A. Hormone replacement therapy (HRT) is associated with increased risk for gallstones.
B. HRT increases the risk for deep venous thrombosis/pulmonary embolism.
C. Progestins may have negative effects on mood.
D. Vaginal bleeding is rare after the first 3 months on combined hormone replacement.
E. HRT increases the risk for stroke.

QUESTION 5. A 24-year-old woman complains of irregular menstrual cycles. She reports a 30-lb weight gain over the past 3 years, which she has attributed to a sedentary job. She takes no medications.

On exam, she is 180 lb, height 5'6". She has mild hirsutism and acne on the face and back. Abdomen is obese, with pale striae.

Diagnoses consistent with this presentation include all of the following EXCEPT:

A. Late-onset congenital adrenal hyperplasia
B. Polycystic ovary syndrome
C. Cushing disease
D. Turner syndrome
E. Androgen-secreting tumor

QUESTION 6. A 62-year-old woman comes to establish primary care. She is status postmenopause at age 52 and has never been on HRT.

History is notable for right tibia fracture while skiing 10 years ago and hypertension.

She takes hydrochlorothiazide 25 mg daily.

She smokes cigarettes, ½ pack/day. She does not drink alcohol. She swims regularly for exercise.

There is no family history of hip fracture.

On physical examination, her weight is 114 lb, height 5'4". Blood pressure is 128/80 mm Hg. The rest of the exam is unremarkable.

Risk factors for osteoporosis in this woman include all of the following EXCEPT:

A. Postmenopausal status
B. Cigarette smoking
C. Her weight
D. Her prior fracture
E. Use of hydrochlorothiazide

QUESTION 7. All of the following statements are true for the management of this patient EXCEPT:

A. She should take in 1200 mg calcium daily.
B. Drinking 2 cups of milk daily will give her adequate vitamin D.
C. Weight-bearing exercise is recommended.
D. Calcium carbonate supplements should be taken with meals.
E. Swimming would not be expected to increase her bone density.

QUESTION 8. You order a bone density of the spine: *T*-score is −2.6; *Z*-score is −1.1. All of the following are true EXCEPT:

A. She has osteoporosis.
B. Osteoarthritis of spine could falsely increase her bone density.
C. Her *Z*-score compares her to young normal women.
D. Bone mineral density (BMD) is the single best predictor of fracture.

E. This *Z*-score would not suggest the need for a workup for secondary causes of osteoporosis.

QUESTION 9. You discuss with her recommendations regarding calcium, vitamin D, weight-bearing exercise, and encourage her to stop smoking. You also recommend antiresorptive therapy. Which of the following statements is *true*?

A. Raloxifene therapy would be expected both to improve bone density and to reduce hot flashes.
B. Calcitonin reduces risk for hip fracture.
C. Neither alendronate nor risedronate may be taken with food.
D. Raloxifene does not increase risk for blood clots.
E. Routine dental work should be deferred in patients taking bisphosphonates.

QUESTION 10. A 48-year-old woman who has been your patient for several years comes in complaining of constipation and abdominal pain. She has seen two outside gastroenterologists for these complaints in the past year and has had colonoscopy, barium enema, endoscopy, and abdominal CT scan, all negative.

She has been well except for a fracture of the radius in a fall down the stairs the preceding year.

She is married, without children.

Exam is remarkable only for ecchymoses on the back and right arm.

You should:

A. Repeat a colonoscopy at your institution.
B. Ask her whether she has ever been hurt or threatened in her relationship.
C. Ask her generally about how she is doing, but avoid asking directly about domestic violence.
D. Call her husband and discuss the situation with him.

QUESTION 11. A 37-year-old woman comes for evaluation of a lump she discovered in the left breast 1 month earlier. She is G1P1, status postmenarche at age 14. She has regular menses monthly, last menstrual period (LMP) was last week. She drinks 4 cups of coffee daily.

Family history is negative for breast cancer. Her mother has fibrocystic breast disease.

On physical examination, she is well appearing. There is a 1.5-cm mass palpable in the left breast upper outer quadrant, which is slightly tender to palpation. There is no axillary adenopathy. You order a mammogram, which is negative.

Which of the following would be the most appropriate next step?

A. Reassure her. No intervention is indicated.
B. Schedule repeat mammogram in 4–6 months.
C. Tell her to stop coffee and other caffeine intake and return in 4–6 months for reexamination.

D. Order an ultrasound; if this is negative, no further workup is required.

E. Order an ultrasound; referral should be made for biopsy unless the lump is consistent with a simple cyst.

QUESTION 12. A 30-year-old G0P0 with a 10-year history of Type 1 DM is interested in becoming pregnant. She has history of nonproliferative retinopathy. Her last eye exam was 2 years ago. She checks blood sugars once daily.

Medications include NPH 20 U/Regular 8 U qAM and NPH 10 U at night. She also takes a prenatal vitamin.

Her blood pressure is 124/80 mm Hg; the rest of the examination is unremarkable.

Labs: HbA1c 9.0, creatinine 1.3 mg/dL. There is trace protein on urine dipstick.

All of the following would be recommended prior to conception EXCEPT:

A. An angiotensin-converting enzyme inhibitor should be started to minimize progression of renal disease in pregnancy.

B. She should increase her frequency of blood sugar monitoring.

C. She should be referred to ophthalmology.

D. Blood sugar control should be tightened to achieve a normal hemoglobin A1c.

E. She should have a prescription for glucagon.

QUESTION 13. A routine Pap smear in a 42-year-old woman shows atypical cells. She is in a monogamous relationship and has had normal Pap smears in previous years. Which of the following would be most appropriate?

A. Treat empirically with doxycycline and repeat Pap in 3 months.

B. This is a normal finding in a perimenopausal woman and does not require follow-up.

C. Endometrial sampling should be done to exclude endometrial cancer.

D. Perform human papilloma virus (HPV) testing for high-risk subtypes.

QUESTION 14. A 32-year-old woman, G1P0, 16 weeks pregnant, presents with palpitations and weight loss. Her pulse is 110. She has lid lag but no appreciable exophthalmos. The thyroid gland is symmetrically enlarged to about 1½ times normal size. TSH is <0.05 mIU/L, T_4 is 22.

All of the following are true EXCEPT:

A. PTU can be used in the first trimester of pregnancy.

B. A thyroid uptake should be performed to confirm the diagnosis.

C. A beta blocker could be used for symptoms.

D. Thyroid-stimulating immunoglobulins (TSI) would likely be elevated.

E. This condition is likely to improve with treatment over the course of pregnancy.

Question 15. A 22-year-old woman, G0P0, comes for contraceptive counseling. All of the following are true EXCEPT:

A. The risks associated with use of oral contraceptive pills (OCPs) outweigh the benefits for women with a history of coronary heart disease or stroke.

B. OCP use is associated with a reduced risk for ovarian cancer.

C. Intrauterine device (IUD) use is not associated with an increased risk of infertility in monogamous women.

D. Currently used OCPs are associated with a twofold increase in breast cancer risk.

QUESTION 16. You are paged by a 32-year-old woman who is worried about pregnancy after having had unprotected intercourse 36 hours prior. Her LMP was 16 days ago. Which of the following is *true*?

A. Loestrin (20 μg EE), 2 now and 2 more in 12 hours, is appropriate for use as emergency contraception.

B. Levonorgestrel, 1.5 mg as a single dose, is appropriate for use as emergency contraception.

C. It is too late to use emergency contraception.

D. Emergency contraception is not warranted at this time in the cycle.

QUESTION 17. A 32-year-old woman G1P0, pregravid body mass index (BMI) of 28 kg/m², 28 weeks of gestation, has a high glucose level (160 mg/dL) after 50 g glucose loading test. Oral glucose tolerance test results are consistent with gestational diabetes. Which of the following is *false*?

A. She is at increased risk for cesarean section.

B. Glyburide has been used safely in managing gestational diabetes.

C. Risk for diabetes outside of pregnancy is no greater than for a woman with uncomplicated pregnancy.

D. She should be referred to a nutritionist.

E. Treatment to reduce glucose levels reduces the risk for serious perinatal complications.

QUESTION 18. Acceptable Pap screening approaches for women over age 30 include:

A. Annual Pap

B. Pap every 2 to 3 years after three consecutive normal Paps

C. Combined Pap and HPV; if both normal repeat at 3 years

D. All of the above

ANSWERS

1. B. This patient has lymphocytic (or painless) thyroiditis, a condition that is reported to follow 2–16% of pregnancies. This condition is characterized by an initial hyperthyroid phase (within 6 months postpartum, lasting up

to 2 months) due to leakage of thyroid hormone from an inflamed thyroid gland, followed by a hypothyroid phase (typically occurring up to 10 months postpartum, and lasting 3–6 months), and then, in most cases, return to euthyroidism. Often the hyperthyroid phase is not appreciated clinically, and the patient presents with hypothyroidism. TPO antibodies are characteristically positive, and recurrence is common following subsequent pregnancies. Symptomatic hypothyroidism should be treated with thyroxine, which should not be required for >6 months unless the patient has developed permanent hypothyroidism (rare immediately, although it is well described over long-term follow-up). Thyroid ultrasound may be useful in the evaluation of a thyroid nodule but is not indicated in the evaluation of thyroiditis. Subacute thyroiditis is a painful inflammation of the thyroid that often is described following upper respiratory infection (URI).

2. C. PCOS affects approximately 5% of women of reproductive age and is clinically diagnosed by the combination of chronic anovulation and androgen excess (clinical manifestations and/or biochemical excess) not explained by another endocrine disorder (such as late-onset congenital adrenal hyperplasia, hyperprolactinemia, androgen-secreting tumor.) Although a polycystic appearance of the ovaries is generally present, this has also been noted in up to a quarter of women without other features of PCOS, and this finding is considered neither sufficient nor necessary for the diagnosis. LH levels are also typically elevated (with increased LH/FSH ratio), but this is also not considered a necessary finding for the diagnosis and need not be routinely measured.

A clear association has been observed between PCOS and insulin resistance, and studies have documented an increased prevalence of glucose intolerance and diabetes in affected women, even independent of associated obesity, which is common but not always present in affected women. Dyslipidemia is also more common in PCOS than in normally cycling women. Affected women also have increased risk for endometrial hyperplasia and cancer. There are reports of increased risks for hypertension, coronary heart disease, gestational diabetes, and gestational hypertension in these women also, although these have been less well substantiated. Treatment approaches include the oral contraceptive pill (to protect the uterus from unopposed estrogen stimulation, regulate cycles, and treat hirsutism), intermittent medroxyprogesterone (to protect the uterus), and spironolactone (to treat hirsutism). Insulin sensitizers (metformin, thiazolidinediones) have been reported to improve insulin sensitivity, reduce androgen levels, improve cycle regularity, and to induce ovulation in this condition.

3. A. Menopause is strictly defined as cessation of menses for ≥12 months, but menopausal symptoms often begin well before menses cease. Changes in cycle pattern also commonly precede amenorrhea. A high FSH is characteristic of menopause, but checking FSH levels is not indicated routinely; FSH level is an unreliable indicator of impending menopause in the perimenopausal woman. Hot flushes are common as women near or reach menopause; about 50% of women will experience them in the 2 years around cessation of menses, and up to 20% of women experience them in their 40s even while cycles are still regular. Flushes are experienced as a feeling of warmth and are associated with a measurable increase in skin temperature. Therapy with estrogen is very useful for hot flushes. In the woman who is still having menses, and without contraindications to OC use, the low-dose OCP can be useful for control of cycles and symptoms. Hormone replacement therapy remains a useful approach to symptoms in a woman without contraindications who is no longer menstruating, although the plan should be for short-term rather than indefinite use. However, a history of venous thromboembolism is a contraindication to its use. (Among other contraindications to use are a history of breast cancer, coronary heart disease, unexplained vaginal bleeding, and active liver disease.)

4. D. As above, estrogen is very useful for treatment of hot flushes; even low doses (e.g., conjugated equine estrogen 0.3 mg) may be sufficient to control symptoms. In a woman with an intact uterus, a progestational agent should routinely be given with estrogen for protection of the uterus. (Endometrial hyperplasia was reported in one-third of women treated with estrogen alone for 3 years; PEPI study, JAMA, 1995.) Adverse effects of HRT must be considered. Side effects of estrogen include nausea, headache, and heavy bleeding, whereas progestins may have adverse effects on mood and may cause breast tenderness. Bleeding is common on combined estrogen/progestin therapy. Bleeding is usually predictable on cyclical regimens, although unpredictable intermittent bleeding is common the first several months on daily combined regimens. After a year of combined daily HRT, the majority of women will be amenorrheic, but duration of bleeding tends to be longer in women who are closer to menopause. CEE/medroxyprogesterone (Prempro) increases risks for DVT/PE, breast cancer, stroke, gallstones, and dementia (in women 65 years or older). Coronary events were increased early after initiation of Prempro in randomized trials of secondary prevention (HERS, JAMA, 1998; overall there was no coronary benefit over 4+ years) and among women generally without history of heart disease (WHI, JAMA, 2002; NEJM, 2003). Thus, HRT is not indicated for the prevention of coronary disease.

5. D. Possible causes of irregular cycles and signs of androgen excess (hirsutism, acne) include polycystic ovary syndrome, late-onset congenital hyperplasia, Cushing syndrome, and androgen-secreting tumor. Turner syndrome (XO karyotype) is a cause of primary amenorrhea and is associated with other characteristic features, including short stature, failure to develop

secondary sexual characteristics, and somatic abnormalities (e.g., webbed neck, shield-like chest); androgen excess is not a feature of this syndrome.

6. E. Risk factors for osteoporosis include age, estrogen deficiency, cigarette smoking, lean body habitus, personal history of fracture, family history of osteoporosis in a first-degree relative, excessive alcohol intake, physical inactivity, Caucasian race, and inadequate intake of calcium. A history of dementia, falls, or frailty also increases fracture risk. Although some medications (e.g., glucocorticoids) increase risk for osteoporosis, hydrochlorothiazide reduces urinary calcium excretion and has been associated with reduced fracture risk.

7. B. Approaches that are recommended to optimize bone health include adequate intake of calcium (1200 mg recommended daily in a postmenopausal woman), and vitamin D (400 to 800+ IU daily). The following each contain about 300 mg calcium: 8 oz milk, 8 oz yogurt, 1.5 oz cheese. As most women do not take in four servings of such calcium sources daily, supplements are often recommended. Calcium carbonate (e.g., in Tums, Os-Cal, Caltrate) is reportedly better absorbed with meals, whereas calcium citrate (e.g., Citracal) can be taken at any time; the latter is better tolerated by some women but is also more expensive. Vitamin D is added to milk, but only 100 IU per 8-oz serving. A standard multivitamin will provide 400 IU vitamin D daily; there are several combined calcium/vitamin D supplements (e.g., Caltrate D, Citracal D) as well as over-the-counter vitamin D supplements that can be taken alternatively or additionally. Weight-bearing exercise is recommended. Swimming is not associated with an increase in bone density.

8. C. In interpreting bone density results, the *T*-score represents a comparison with "peak" bone density of young normal women, and the *Z*-score represents a comparison with age-matched women. The *T*-score is used to make the diagnoses of osteopenia (*T*-score between −1 and −2.5 standard deviations below peak) or osteoporosis (*T*-score < −2.5 standard deviations below peak). The *Z*-score may be used to identify women more likely to have secondary causes of osteoporosis; a *Z*-score below −2 suggests bone loss out of proportion for age. Osteophytes or a compression fracture may falsely elevate bone density readings, and such affected areas should be deleted from analysis.

9. C. Several medications have been approved for the treatment of osteoporosis; these include estrogen, raloxifene (a selective estrogen receptor modulator), bisphosphonates (alendronate, risedronate. ibandronate (oral) and zoledronic acid (IV infusion)), teriparatide (recombinant human PTH) (injection), and, more recently, denosumab (an inhibitor of RANK ligand, a regulator of osteoclasts) (injection). Estrogen therapy improves hot flashes, but raloxifene does not and may, on the contrary, worsen them. Both of these increase risk for blood clots. Data indicate a significant reduction in breast cancer risk in women treated with raloxifene. Hip fracture has not been shown to

be reduced in women treated with calcitonin or raloxifene, whereas bisphosphonates have been shown to significantly reduce hip fracture risk. Bisphosphonates must be taken on an empty stomach first thing in the morning without eating for 30 minutes to facilitate absorption; once-a-week formulations of alendronate and risedronate (and a once-monthly formulation of ibandronate) make compliance easier for many patients. Osteonecrosis of the jaw has been reported among patients taking bisphosphonates; the majority of reports of this complication have been in patients using high doses intravenously for metastatic bone disease, although there are scattered reports among patients taking these agents for osteoporosis. Routine dental care should not be withheld in patients taking bisphosphonates. Also of concern are reports of atypical femur fractures associated with bisphosphonate use, although this complication likewise appears rare.

10. B. The possibility of domestic violence should be considered in all women, regardless of background. Gastrointestinal complaints are common in these women. Unexplained fractures or bruising are more obvious clues, but there are often no outward signs, and abuse may be psychological rather than physical. It is recommended that all women be screened with a straightforward question asking about any history of being hurt or threatened; certainly screening is warranted in the case described.

11. E. A palpable breast mass requires further evaluation regardless of patient age or mammogram results. Although coffee has been associated with fibrocystic breast disease, a palpable discrete mass should not be attributed to this or other benign etiologies without appropriate workup. Ultrasound would be the next step; biopsy would be indicated for findings other than a simple cyst in this woman.

12. A. Tight glycemic control is clearly recommended prior to conception in women with diabetes; risk of congenital anomalies increases with increasing first-trimester hemoglobin A1c levels. Women should be checking sugars frequently, and insulin should be adjusted to maintain glucose levels as normal as possible. Eyes should be checked prior to pregnancy as proliferative retinopathy may progress during pregnancy. Hypoglycemia is common in the first trimester, and women should be aware of symptoms and treatment of hypoglycemia and have glucagon available. Although an angiotensin-converting enzyme (ACE) inhibitor or angiotensin receptor blocker is indicated generally in diabetic patients with microalbuminuria or frank proteinuria (and even in the absence of this), these agents are contraindicated in pregnancy. It has been well recognized that second- and third-trimester use of ACE inhibitor is associated with complications including oligohydramnios, intrauterine growth retardation, anuria, renal failure, and death, more recent data also indicate associations between first-trimester use and major congenital anomalies (including cardiac and central nervous system defects).

13. D. Atypical cells are a common finding on Pap smears. Infection is sometimes an underlying cause and should be treated if there is good reason to suspect this but not in asymptomatic low-risk women. HPV screening for high-risk subtypes is indicated when atypical cells are found; when positive, colposcopy is indicated.

14. B. The presentation is most consistent with Graves' disease, which not uncommonly presents early in pregnancy. Thyroid-stimulating immunoglobulins (TSI) are typically detectable but need not be checked clinically. PTU can be used in pregnancy; it is currently considered the preferred drug when antithyroid drug therapy is needed in the first trimester, owing to concerns of teratogenicity (including a rare scalp defect, aplasia cutis) in association with the use of the alternative antithyroid drug, methimazole. (Outside of the first trimester of pregnancy, methimazole is now considered the preferred drug, given reports of liver toxicity and liver failure associated with PTU.) The minimal dose necessary to keep T4 levels upper normal or slightly above the normal range is recommended to minimize drug exposure of the fetus (as this crosses the placenta). Methimazole is commonly avoided in pregnancy due to a very rare fetal scalp effect, aplasia cutis, reported to be associated with this drug. Beta blockers can be used for symptom control in pregnancy. Thyroiditis could cause a similar presentation; in a woman who is not pregnant or lactating, a thyroid uptake could be checked to distinguish between these conditions. However, thyroid uptake testing or treatment with radioactive iodine is strictly *contraindicated* in pregnancy. The disease tends to remit with treatment over pregnancy, and thyroid function should be followed closely to avoid overtreatment.

15. B. When used properly, oral contraceptive pills are highly effective in preventing pregnancy. Risks of OCPs include DVT/PE, even with low-dose preparations (risk reported to be higher with OCPs containing desogestrel versus progestins such as levonorgestrel). Myocardial infarction is a rare risk; the risk is higher in women who smoke (especially older women) or who have uncontrolled hypertension; a history of cardiovascular disease is a contraindication to use of OCPs. OCP users have been reported to have lower (not higher) risk of ovarian cancer, and current preparations do not appear to be associated with a significant increase in breast cancer risk. IUD use has been associated with infertility in women at risk for pelvic inflammatory disease (PID) but is considered a safe and effective approach to birth control among monogamous women.

16. B. Emergency contraception has proven effective in reducing pregnancy risk when given within 72 hours to up to 120 hours of unprotected intercourse. Effective therapies include (1) combination OCP to provide 100 µg ethinyl estradiol initially and then again at 12 hours (e.g., 2 Ovral, each 50 µg ethinyl estradiol, q 12 h), that is, Yuzpe regimen; (2) Plan B, levonorgestrel 1.5 mg single dose; (3) ulipristal acetate 30 mg has been shown to be effective. Nausea and vomiting are common with the Yuzpe regimen; levonorgestrel and ulipristal acetate are better tolerated and appear more effective. A reported LMP suggesting that intercourse was in the luteal phase does not effectively rule out possible pregnancy and emergency contraception is still appropriate in this setting. Although the efficacy of emergency contraception falls with increasing time after intercourse, it is still reasonable to use this within 5 days of unprotected intercourse.

17. C. Gestational diabetes mellitus (GDM), or diabetes diagnosed in pregnancy, complicates about 7% of pregnancies. Screening for GDM is routinely recommended between 24 and 28 weeks of gestation in women ages 25 years or older and in those with recognized risk factors (e.g., obesity, family history of diabetes). The recommended screening test is a 50-g oral glucose load; a 1-hour glucose level of 130–140 mg/dL or greater is considered abnormal and warrants a 3-hour 100-g oral glucose tolerance test (with glucose levels checked fasting and at 1, 2, and 3 hours); two or more abnormal values on this test are considered diagnostic of gestational diabetes. Nutritional counseling is important in this setting; the majority of women with GDM are successfully managed with diet alone. Close attention to glucose levels is important. Treatment of gestational diabetes (with diet, and insulin if needed) has been shown to significantly reduce the risk of serious perinatal complications. If fasting or postprandial sugars are inadequately controlled with diet, medication is needed. Insulin has been the standard therapy, although glyburide and more recently metformin have been reported to be safe and effective as alternatives. Glucose levels return to normal in the vast majority of women with GDM immediately after the pregnancy, but women who have had this condition are at significantly increased risk for later development of diabetes.

18. D. Pap smears are recommend in women starting within 3 years of onset of sexual activity, or by age 21, and then yearly until at least age 30. Among women over age 30, various screening approaches are considered acceptable. For women who have had three consecutive normal Paps, screening at 2- to 3-year intervals is considered acceptable, though annual screening could also be continued. Although HPV testing is not recommended for screening purposes in younger women, it can be used in combination with Pap for screening in women over age 30. If both tests are negative, repeat testing is recommended in 3 years.

98.

DERMATOLOGY FOR THE INTERNIST

Peter C. Schalock and Arthur J. Sober

Skin findings can be separated into two types, primary and secondary lesions. A primary lesion is one in which the inciting process or pathology is still discernible, such as the vesicle associated with dermatitis herpetiformis, the plaque of psoriasis, or the macule of vitiligo. Secondary lesions are those that have evolved or have been manipulated by the patient. Lesions such as an excoriation, crusts, or ulcerations are examples. See tables 98.1 and 98.2 for a complete summary of lesion descriptions.

The most common type of therapy in dermatology is the use of topical medicaments placed directly on affected skin. The main base used for most medicaments is white petrolatum. Ointments, creams, and lotions, whether compounded as a prescription or as an over-the-counter product, are petrolatum based. An ointment has no water added and thus does not need a preservative. A cream simply is petrolatum with added water to make it more cosmetically elegant and more easily rubbed into the skin. A lotion is a cream with even more water. All products with water added require a preservative to prevent bacterial and/or fungal overgrowth plus a masking fragrance. Many of these added chemicals can provoke allergic contact dermatitis (discussed further below). Ointments are the most protective for the skin and the most hydrating although the least accepted by patients due to their greasy nature. Creams are most often used. Other bases include gels, solutions, and foams.

PREMALIGNANT AND MALIGNANT SKIN NEOPLASMS

Skin cancer is a common problem related to ultraviolet radiation exposure. At the rates currently seen in the United States, one in five people will develop a skin cancer in their lifetime (one in three for Caucasians) (ACS, 2007). This is an entirely preventable cancer with sun exposure as the predominant cause. Skin cancer rates are directly correlated with the amount of annual ultraviolet (UV) radiation a person receives. Exposure to UV radiation causes mutations

most commonly in the p53 tumor suppressor gene. In mice, UV carcinogenesis is highest at 293 nm, with lesser peaks at 354 and 380 nm. Melanoma risk is increased with exposures to ultraviolet B (UVB) in the 290–320 nm range (Rigel, 2008). Ultraviolet A (UVA) waves are of higher energy and penetrate deeper into the dermis, whereas UVB tends to penetrate only in the epidermis. UVA damage to collagen in the dermis is responsible for the photoaging such as facial lines/creases (rhytides), lentigines, and other pigmentary changes on sun-exposed skin.

Actinic keratoses (AKs) are rough, raised lesions seen on sun-exposed surfaces. These lesions are considered premalignant. In most cases, these keratotic papules and patches are found on the extensor surfaces of the arms/legs, upper back/chest, neck, face, ears, and scalp. AKs often will stay stable or regress over time. A small percentage will transform to *squamous cell carcinoma* (SCC) (see figure 98.1), although it is estimated that 60% of all SCC are derived from an AK (Jeffes and Tang, 2000). Any keratotic lesion that begins to grow, thicken, and become tender, especially with pressure, should be biopsied as a potential SCC. Bowen disease (SCC in-situ, figure 98.2) tends to be a scaly, erythematous plaque, not the discreet keratotic lesions of AK. Keratoacanthomas are rapidly growing dome-shaped nodules with a characteristic central core of keratin that are believed by some to be a SCC variant and by others to be benign. Many of these lesions will resolve without therapy, although there also have been multiple cases of metastatic SCC related to these lesions.

The mainstay of therapy for AK is liquid nitrogen (LN_2) destruction. Most thin lesions, especially on the face, require only one cycle of 4–5 sec freezing. Thicker lesions on non-cosmetically sensitive areas can be treated for longer and with multiple cycles of LN_2. Other modalities include electrocautery/curettage, skin peels, dermabrasion, and topical medical therapy. Currently, topical treatments of AK include 5-fluorouracil, diclofenac, topical retinoids, and imiquimod. 5-Fluorouracil is a topical chemotherapeutic agent, causing destruction of cells growing at an increased rate. Imiquimod is a topical immunomodulator increasing keratinocyte

Table 98.1 PRIMARY LESIONS

LESION TYPE	DESCRIPTION	EXAMPLES/CAUSES
Macule/patch	Flat, nonpalpable color change in the skin, patches are >10 mm	Lentigo or "freckle"
Papule	Palpable elevation in the epidermis, ≤5 mm	Verruca vulgaris, nevi
Plaque	Palpable larger epidermal skin change, >5 mm	Psoriasis, eczema, tinea
Pustule	Pus-filled, discrete lesions	Acne, folliculitis
Vesicle	A fluid-filled lesion, ≤5 mm	Allergic contact dermatitis, dyshidrotic eczema, dermatitis herpetiformis
Bulla	A larger fluid-filled lesion, >5 mm	Bullous pemphigoid, bullous impetigo
Nodule	A lesion with a deep component, into the dermis, also may be exophytic	Squamous cell carcinoma, epidermal inclusion cyst
Wheal	Elevated, erythematous papules or plaques secondary to localized edema	Urticaria ("hives")
Telangiectasia	Superficial small permanently dilated blood vessel	Rosacea
Petechia	Nonblanchable discrete foci of hemorrhage	Infections (meningococcemia/Rocky Mountain spotted fever), vasculitis, platelet dysfunction
Purpura	Larger area of hemorrhage, may be palpable or macular	Vasculitis
Ecchymosis	Large macular hemorrhagic area	Trauma

production of interferon-γ and interleukin (IL)-2 through activation of toll-like receptor 7. Diclofenac, a topical inhibitor of cyclo-oxygenase, is useful for some patients. Treatment regimens vary by the agent and preference of the clinician. Bowen disease is treated with these same topical medications, electrodesiccation and curettage, or cryotherapy. Keratoacanthomas are treated surgically in most cases.

NONMELANOMA SKIN CANCERS

The most common cancer of the skin and over all is the basal cell carcinoma (BCC; see figure 98.3). This tumor is a result of long-term sun exposure and is seen on sun-exposed surfaces most often. Although the prognosis is excellent for this tumor with exceedingly rare instances of metastasis, it is important that these lesions not be neglected, as large, long-duration tumors both are locally destructive and can infrequently metastasize. A rare genodermatosis is the basal cell nevus syndrome (Gorlin syndrome). This is an autosomal dominant condition in which BCC develops early in life (<20 years old). These patients may develop medulloblastoma at an early age in addition to having odontogenic keratocysts, palmar/plantar pits, calcification of the falx cerebri, and bifid ribs. Some patients display characteristic macrocephaly/frontal bossing.

SCC is less common than BCC, other than in chronically immunosuppressed patients. This cancer also develops due to chronic sun exposure. SCC metastasis rate for

Table 98.2 SECONDARY LESIONS

LESION	DESCRIPTION	EXAMPLE
Erosion	Open area with loss of partial thickness of epidermis	Impetigo, pemphigus foliaceus
Ulceration	Full-thickness loss of epidermis	Bullous pemphigoid, basal cell carcinoma
Excoriation	Linear, caused by scratching, usually partial epidermal thickness only	Any condition that is pruritic, causing scratching
Crust	Dried serum and blood on wound surface	"Scab" following an acute injury
Scar	Pink to white patch to plaque caused by injury	Surgical wound
Lichenification	Thickened epidermis with characteristic cross-hatched pattern	Lichen simplex chronicus
Atrophy	Dermal thinning	Long-term steroid use, lupus, scleroderma

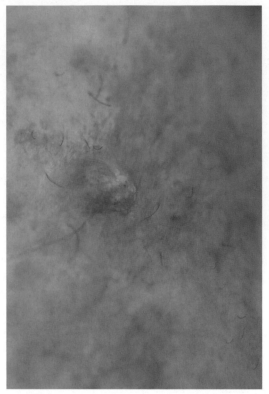

Figure 98.1. Tender Hyperkeratotic Nodule that Was Squamous Cell Carcinoma on Biopsy.

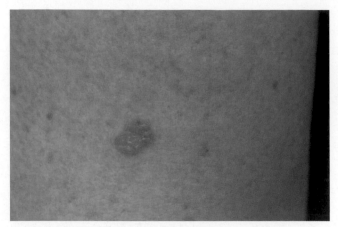

Figure 98.2. Typical Velvety Plaque of Bowen Disease. SCC in situ.

normal sun-exposed skin is 0.5–3%, whereas SCC arising in burn scars, x-ray scars, or foci of chronic osteomyelitis have a rate of metastasis of 10–30% (Jeffes and Tang, 2000). Rate of SCC is increased significantly for chronically immunosuppressed patients. In kidney and heart transplant patients, the risk of SCC was increased 65-fold. The risk of SCC in this population increases from 7% at 1 year to 45% after 11 years and 70% after 20 years of immunosuppression (Jeffes and Tang, 2000).

Treatments for nonmelanoma skin cancers (NMSC) are numerous. Treatment can be as simple as using the same topical therapy as is used for treating actinic keratoses (imiquimod or 5-fluorouracil) for early and thin lesions, to electrodesiccation and curettage, cryotherapy with LN_2 or other destructive agents, or Mohs surgery. The most definitive method for ensuring complete removal of a NMSC is the technique described several decades ago by Dr. Frederic Mohs. This procedure involves histopathologically examining the entire lateral and inferior margins of the fresh frozen surgical specimen to ensure complete removal of a tumor. For extensive tumors in older individuals, consultation with a radiation oncologist may also be helpful for consideration of local x-ray therapy.

MELANOMA

There are four common types of melanoma: superficial spreading (figure 98.4) (~70% of melanomas), nodular (~15%), lentigo maligna melanoma (~10%), and acral lentiginous melanoma (~5%) (Swetter, 2008). Amelanotic melanoma and desmoplastic neurotrophic variants of melanoma are much rarer. Superficial spreading melanomas are the most common in individuals with lighter skin types. Nodular melanoma tends to develop in those >60 years old and arises, especially in men, from normal-appearing skin (not from a pre-existing nevus) and is more aggressive than other types of malignant melanoma (MM). Lentigo maligna melanoma develops most often on the sun-exposed surfaces of the face of older individuals. Initially, it can be mistaken for a benign "age spot" (lentigo). Lesions that are changing/growing should be considered for biopsy. Acral lentiginous melanomas account for 5% of melanomas overall, but in Asians and people of darker skin types it accounts for about 50%.

Melanoma grading is done by pathology. The depth of a lesion is graded both in millimeters (Breslow thickness) and by level of invasion (Clark level). The most important feature for staging is the Breslow thickness. Lesions not invading into the dermis are considered in situ. Invasive melanomas are classified by their depth of invasion, ulceration, and rate of mitoses pathologically. Pathologic staging includes

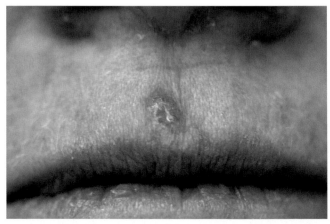

Figure 98.3. Pearly Nodule on the Lip. This is a typical nodular basal cell carcinoma.

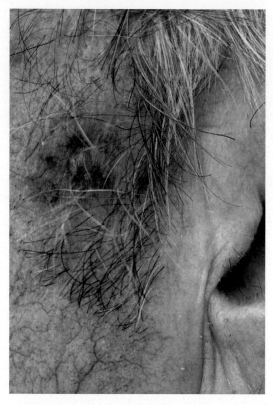

Figure 98.4. Superficial Spreading Melanoma on the Preauricular Cheek. The depth was 1.6 mm, and it was metastatic to the lymph nodes at the time of biopsy.

pathologic information about the primary melanoma as well as that of the regional lymph nodes after partial or complete lymphadenectomy. Stages are determined by the American Joint Committee on Cancer guidelines. Clinical features of melanoma can be summarized by the ABCDE criterion (see table 98.3).

BENIGN SKIN GROWTHS

NEVI

The nevus is a hamartoma of melanocytes within the dermis and/or epidermis. Various types exist, and they, in and of themselves, are not precancerous. Histopathologically,

Table 98.3 ABCDE CRITERION FOR PIGMENTED LESIONS SUSPICIOUS FOR CUTANEOUS MELANOMA

	DESCRIPTION
A	Asymmetry of the lesion
B	Borders are irregular or hazy
C	Color within the lesion is irregular, or there are multiple colors present
D	Diameter greater than 6 mm (a pencil eraser)
E	Evolution of the lesion (growing/changing rapidly)

common types are junctional nevi (flat, with melanocytes only in the epidermis), intradermal nevus (the most common type of nevus with nests of melanocytes only in the dermis, usually a papule, with varying pigmentation but usually flesh colored or pink), and compound nevus (combines both types of epidermal and dermal nevus). Atypical or dysplastic nevi are lesions that when examined clinically have atypical features. The atypia in these nevi are may be graded after biopsy by the dermatopathologist as mild, moderate, or severe. Mild lesions are often not treated further. At this institution, moderate and severely atypical nevi are surgically reexcised to prevent potential further progression to a melanoma or the confusion of pseudomelanoma from a regrowing nevus.

SEBORRHEIC KERATOSIS

Seborrheic keratosis (SK) is an exceedingly common papule potentially found on almost every skin surface on the skin of older adults. It is inherited in an autosomal fashion. There are multiple subtypes, and they can vary greatly in morphology, but the clearest identifying feature is their somewhat warty, greasy, and stuck-on appearance. A variant seen in persons of color is dermatosis papulosis nigra. These are dark brown to black smooth papules most often appearing in persons of color on the head or neck at a younger age than seborrheic keratoses. Inflammatory or malignancy-related SKs can occur. The sign of Leser-Trelat refers to explosive, new appearance of hundreds of SK lesions in the distribution of skin lines ("Christmas tree" distribution also seen in pityriasis rosea, see below) associated with GI malignancy. SKs do not need to be treated but can be removed with LN_2 or curettage.

SKIN TAG (ACROCHORDON)

The acrochordon is a benign fleshy growth seen most commonly on the neck, axilla, groin, and inframammary

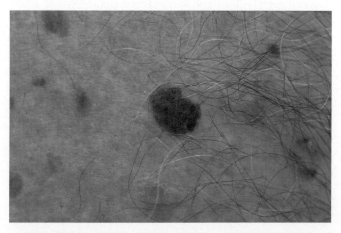

Figure 98.5. Stuck-on Verrucous Plaque. This is a typical seborrheic keratosis.

areas, usually in middle-aged to older adults. There is no malignant potential. Tags frequently occur in obese or pre-diabetic individuals, often with acanthosis nigricans (a velvety epidermal growth with brown color often in the axilla and/or groin and back of the neck). In some, multiple tags are a marker of impaired carbohydrate metabolism. Skin tags also can occur more frequently in pregnancy and Birt-Hogg-Dube syndrome (a genodermatosis characterized by renal cell carcinoma and characteristic skin lesions including increased numbers of skin tags).

KERATIN-FILLED CYSTS

Hair-follicle-derived cysts are common in the skin and on the scalp. Epidermal inclusion cysts (EIC) (also referred to as sebaceous cysts, although not sebaceous in origin) are commonly seen on the trunk and upper extremities, although they can occur on any skin surface. EIC are by far the most commonly seen lesions. Pilar cysts (also known as wens or trichilemmal cysts) are almost exclusively seen on the scalp. An EIC is a nodule, characteristically with a central or offset pore. Often patients are able to "pop" these lesions, expressing white, smelly keratinaceous cheesy debris. The pilar cyst is slightly deeper in the skin and is without epidermal connection. The EIC is derived from the infundibular portion of the hair follicle, and the pilar cyst is likely derived from the epithelium of the hair follicle distal to or at the insertion of the sebaceous duct. In patients with multiple EICs on atypical locations (lower extremities/scalp/face), occurring at an early age (around puberty), the diagnosis of familial adenomatous polyposis (Gardner syndrome) should be considered. Treatment of both types of cysts is elective surgical excision.

ACNE AND ROSACEA

ACNE PATHOGENESIS AND THERAPY

Acne vulgaris is almost ubiquitous in teens and young adults causing inflammatory papules and pustules as well as noninflammatory follicular papules and comedones. Distribution is in the areas with the greatest density of sebaceous glands: the face, upper chest, and back. Acne tends to begin around the time of adrenarche. Individuals with nonfunctioning androgen receptors do not have acne. The pathogenesis of acne incorporates four different mechanisms: hyperproliferation of the follicle epithelium with subsequent plugging, excess sebum production, presence of *Propionibacterium acnes*, and inflammation. Androgens are hypothesized to play a role in the follicular plugging and excess sebum production. *P. acnes* in the follicle produce proinflammatory mediators that stimulate toll-like receptor 2 on neutrophils and monocytes with subsequent IL-12, IL-18, and tumor necrosis factor-alpha (TNF-α) production. Acne

is graded mild, moderate, or severe. Pure comedonal acne has no inflammatory component, only follicular plugging. Nodulocystic acne has severe, inflammatory, deep-seated papules, pustules, nodules, and comedones with residual scarring. Acne conglobata is a rare severe type of nodulocystic acne with multiple nodules interconnected by burrowing between and severe scarring/disfigurement. PAPA syndrome is the combination of pyoderma gangrenosum, acne conglobata, and aseptic arthritis that was reported in one kindred. Causes of acne other than androgen excess are rare but include polycystic ovarian syndrome, congenital adrenal hyperplasia, and oral medications such as lithium, antiepileptics, steroids, and iodides.

Treatment of acne attempts to address one or more of the four causes of acne. The first-line therapies for acne are the over-the-counter benzoyl peroxide and salicylic acid. There are a multitude of prescription treatments for acne, both oral and topical. For milder cases of acne, topical formulations such as retinoids (i.e., tretinoin, adapalene, tazarotene), clindamycin and clindamycin/benzoyl peroxide combinations, sodium sulfacetamide or azelaic acid are useful. For moderate to severe cases of acne, an oral antibiotic from the tetracycline (TCN) family (tetracycline, doxycycline, or minocycline) or second-line agents such as a penicillin derivative or sulfa is added. Topical retinoids are comedolytic and anti-inflammatory. Topical antibiotics are used for their anti–*P. acnes* properties, and salicylic acid/benzoyl peroxide are active against *P. acnes* but without reports of resistance. Oral antibiotic therapy is used against *P. acnes* as well as for its anti-inflammatory properties, especially the TCN derivatives. For severe nodulocystic acne an oral retinoid, isotretinoin, is very helpful for halting or decreasing the inflammatory lesions and scarring. Isotretinoin is severely teratogenic and should be used with caution in females of childbearing potential. Females of childbearing potential need to be enrolled in a federally mandated pregnancy prevention program to receive this medication.

ROSACEA/PERIORIFICIAL DERMATITIS

Rosacea is a common disease of facial flushing, papules, pustules, and telangiectasias most commonly observed on the central face of middle-aged women. There are four subtypes that are summarized in table 98.4. Therapy for erythematotelangiectatic and papulopustular types of rosacea includes avoidance of food and environmental triggers, a broad-spectrum sunscreen (UVA and UVB) daily, topicals such as metronidazole cream, azelaic acid, tretinoin, or sodium sulfacetamide, and oral antibiotics with doxycycline or minocycline being effective. Severe cases of rosacea respond well to low-dose isotretinoin, although this is not an FDA-approved indication. Phymatous rosacea therapy includes surgical or laser removal of excessive connective tissue. Ocular rosacea is treated with oral antibiotics and ocular topical preparations.

Table 98.4 ROSACEA SUBTYPES

TYPE	DESCRIPTION
Erythematotelangiectatic	Red checks, small telangiectasias
Papulopustular	Papules and pustules in addition to erythema and telangiectasias, often involving the central one-third of the face
Phymatous	Overgrowth of soft tissue, most usually nose (rhinophyma)
Ocular	Confined to eyelids/ocular surface. Sx: blepharitis, conjunctivitis, corneal keratitis

Perioral dermatitis (PD) is a variant of rosacea characterized by inflammatory papules and pustules around the mouth. A better term for PD may be periorificial dermatitis, as this occurs not only around the mouth, but also eyes and rarely ears. Treatment with oral TCN derivatives or topical metronidazole is usually successful. Recurrences do occur, requiring further therapy.

DERMATITIS

ATOPIC DERMATITIS

Atopic dermatitis (AD) is a common eczematous, pruritic skin condition that starts in early infancy and may continue for a lifetime. In some developed countries the rate is as high as approximately18%. Pathogenesis is unknown, but a link to filaggrin mutations has been shown. Those with filaggrin defects have a relative risk of 3 to develop AD. Heterozygotes for a known mutation have a 60% chance, and homozygotes have a 90% chance of having AD. Filaggrin mutations predispose to asthma, but only in people who have AD as well as high IgE levels (McGrath, 2008). Another factor that potentially causes or worsens AD is the chronic colonization of patients' skin with *S. aureus*. A spectrum of findings are present in many patients with AD and their families including asthma, allergic rhinitis/seasonal allergies, urticaria, increased production of immunoglobulin E (IgE), and acute allergic reactions to foods. The triad of asthma, AD, and seasonal allergies is called atopy. It is hypothesized that superantigen stimulation drives AD as well as causes flares of dermatitis.

Skin findings evolve over the course of the disease, although xerosis and pruritus are present in all stages. Infants have eczematous, vesicular, erythematous plaques that initially start in the antecubital/popliteal fossae and/or cheeks but can progress to involve the entire body. The diaper area is usually spared. Children have lesions of similar morphology, but as the ability to scratch increases, lichenification and prurigo nodules develop. Infants rarely have lichenification, although this is a prominent feature in children and adults with AD. For some, AD resolves by the teen years, but a predisposition for hand and eyelid dermatitis may remain.

Therapy for AD is dependent on the severity of disease. Topical emollients daily are required for all patients, as xerosis marks the beginning of active dermatitis in many cases. Mild topical corticosteroids such as desonide or hydrocortisone acetate should be used on the face, and moderate-potency agents such as triamcinolone acetonide or hydrocortisone butyrate should be used on both extremities for active dermatitis. For moderate to severe cases that have failed initial topical therapy, a steroid-sparing topical such as tacrolimus (Protopic) or pimecrolimus (Elidel) should be considered, especially for the face. A stronger topical steroid for active areas could be used, such as fluocinonide 0.05% or clobetasol dipropionate on particularly tough areas away from face and intertriginous areas. For severe flares, a prednisone taper can be helpful. Short tapers, such as a 5- or 7-day course, are less helpful, as many cases will reflare after the medication is stopped. Appropriate dosing of prednisone based on weight with dose reduction at 4- to 5-day intervals (i.e., 60 mg, 40 mg, 20 mg, 10 mg) sometimes can stop a flare. In severe cases that do not clear with oral steroids, other oral agents such as cyclosporine, mycophenolate mofetil, or methotrexate may be necessary (rare cases). Narrow-band UVB therapy two to three times weekly also can be very helpful for decreasing dermatitis and pruritus in severely affect atopics.

CONTACT DERMATITIS

There are many chemical and natural botanical agents that cause contact dermatitis. CD is broken into two groups: allergic contact dermatitis (ACD) (~20% of cases) and irritant contact dermatitis (ICD) (~80%). ICD is caused either by acute, strong irritants such as alkalis and acids that damage the epidermis directly or by chronic, longer-term contact with weaker irritants such as water or detergents. Patients with an atopic background are more likely to develop ICD, especially in the form of hand eczema. ICD is a type I immediate or type IV delayed-type reaction. Contact urticaria (type I reaction) can occur from a variety of chemicals (cinnamic aldehyde, benzyl alcohol) and plants (such as nettles). Delayed-type hypersensitivity (type IV) usually occurs due to small chemical compounds (haptens) <500 daltons in size. The haptens bind proteins in the skin and are recognized and phagocytized by epidermal Langerhans cells or dermal dendrocytes that then migrate to a regional lymph node and are presented to T cells, thus sensitizing the individual to the hapten. If the individual contacts the hapten again, it is recognized, and a T-cell-mediated type IV reaction develops with characteristic erythema, pruritus, and vesiculation in 24–72 hours after exposure.

In some cases, sunlight (often UVB 290–320 nm) acts on drugs or topically applied chemicals, changing the molecules and creating haptens. Drugs such as 6-methylcoumarin, salicylanilide, hydrochlorothiazide, chlorpromazine, non-steroidal anti-inflammatory agents, sulfonamides, and 5-methoxypsoralen all can induce photoACD. Common topically applied chemicals causing photoACD are sunscreens such as those derived from *para*-aminobenzoic acid (PABA) or benzophenones, although this is exceedingly rarely seen. Other topicals such as fragrances (musk ambrette or oil of Bergamot) or other topical agents such as benzocaine or neomycin may rarely cause photoACD.

Phototoxic reactions to UV light (most commonly UVA 320–400) can occur to anyone coming in contact or ingesting these substances. No sensitizing period is required. Presentation usually looks like intense sunburn. Causes are the drugs amiodarone, chlorpromazine, fluoroquinolones (nalidixic acid, ciprofloxacin), nonsteroidal anti-inflammatory drugs (NSAIDs) (piroxicam, benoxaprofen), and tetracyclines (demeclocycline > doxycycline/tetracycline) and plants containing furocoumarins including the families Rutaceae (lime, lemon, bergamot, bitter orange, gas plant, burning bush), *Umbelliferae* (carrots, cow parsley, celery, wild chervil, parsnip, fennel, dill, hogweed), and *Moracea* (figs).

DRUGS

A multitude of oral medications can cause morbilliform or exanthematous dermatitis. Although almost any type of morphology can be seen (bullous, urticarial, etc.), morbilliform reactions are most common. A drug reaction should be suspected in cases where a symmetric dermatitis develops soon after starting a new medication. Common causes include antibiotics and sulfa-based diuretics, NSAIDs, chemotherapeutic agents, anticonvulsants (phenytoin, carbamazepine, phenobarbital), and psychotropic agents, although almost any medication can cause dermatitis.

Most drug reactions are self-limited and not life threatening, but important findings to watch for include blistering and mucous membrane involvement. The Stevens-Johnson syndrome (SJS)/toxic epidermal necrolysis (TEN) spectrum causes significant morbidity and potential mortality. SJS initially presents as three-zone target lesions (dusky, purple center, surrounding white, lighter skin, and an outer ring of erythema) and erythematous, morbilliform dermatitis as well as mucosal erosions/bullae. This can progress to full-thickness skin sloughing. TEN does not have the typical target lesions but will begin with painful erythematous skin (similar to a sunburn) followed by full-thickness epidermal sloughing. Both of these conditions should be managed as inpatients, potentially in a burn unit. Treatment is supportive; some believe that intravenous immunoglobulin (IVIg) is useful, although this is controversial. Systemic corticosteroids should be avoided.

Anticonvulsant hypersensitivity syndrome is a potentially life-threatening complex of symptoms caused by aromatic anticonvulsants such as phenytoin, phenobarbital, and carbamazepine. Symptoms include fever, pharyngitis, SJS-like dermatitis, and lymphadenopathy on physical exam and laboratory abnormalities including hepatitis, nephritis, and leukocytosis with eosinophilia. Presentation is often within 3 weeks after starting the medication, though it can occur 3 months or more into therapy. An alternative to the aromatic anticonvulsants is valproic acid.

AUTOIMMUNE "CONNECTIVE TISSUE DISEASES"

There are multiple diseases that are within the spectrum of "connective tissue diseases." Most of these syndromes have specific criteria for diagnosis, but the presentation initially may show overlaps between the syndromes. The most frequently seen autoimmune connective tissue diseases are lupus erythematosus, dermatomyositis, and scleroderma/morphea.

SYSTEMIC LUPUS ERYTHEMATOSUS

The most common autoimmune disease seen is the lupus erythematosus spectrum (acute cutaneous, subacute cutaneous, chronic cutaneous). Skin findings can be present in systemic lupus erythematosus that are consistent with all three types of cutaneous lupus in any patient. Findings necessary for diagnosis of systemic lupus erythematosus (SLE) according the American Rheumatologic Association are summarized in table 98.5. SLE presents with malar rash (55–90%) and arthralgias in many joints. Other presenting systemic symptoms include weight loss, anorexia, fever, fatigue, and malaise. It is more commonly seen in females (90%) and in blacks (1:250) versus Caucasians (1:1000). The 10-year survival rate is 75–85%, and the 20-year rate is 70% (Lamont and Lai, 2006).

Acute cutaneous lupus erythematosus presents with erythema of the malar cheeks and nose, often with edema and fine scale. This is associated with systemic lupus activity (SLE as above). Sun exposure can cause flares of systemic disease. Subacute cutaneous lupus erythematosus (SCLE) lesions are pink, scaly plaques resembling psoriasis or at times annular lesions more similar to erythema multiforme. Papulosquamous-type lesions are more often seen on the trunk and extensor surfaces of the upper extremities and dorsal hands, sparing the face, flexor surface of the arms, and below the waist. The annular-type lesions involve the same distribution but typically start as discrete erythematous papules that become confluent arcuate or polycyclic plaques. Chronic cutaneous lupus erythematosus (CCLE) is also referred to as discoid lupus. It classically presents as erythematous scaling papules or plaques with follicular plugging ("carpettacking"). Long-standing lesions will show central atrophy, scarring, and hypo- and hyperpigmentation. Lesions are most common on the face, scalp, and ears. Only 5–10% of patients with CCLE will show signs

Table 98.5 CRITERION FOR DIAGNOSIS OF SLE

FINDING	DESCRIPTION
Malar rash	55–90% of patients with SLE. On cheeks/nose, sparing eyelids
Discoid rash (chronic cutaneous lupus)	Discoid skin lesions as below. ~20% of patients with SLE will have these lesions
Photosensitivity	Sun exposure causes skin rash and potentially systemic flare
Oral ulcers	Aphthous, oral, and genital ulcerations. Painless or painful
Arthritis	Most common finding in SLE. Polyarticular. Most common proximal interphalangeal and metacarpophalangeal (MCP) joints of the hands
Serositis	Pleuritic pain or rub, pleural effusion, pericarditis, pericardial effusion. Pericarditis in 20–30% of patients; myocarditis less common
Renal disorder	May not have symptoms until renal failure or nephrotic syndrome present. Follow BUN/Cr
Neurologic disorder	Seizures and neuropathies most common. Psychosis
Hematologic disorder	Anemia (of chronic disease or hemolytic), thrombocytopenia. Also leukopenia, lymphopenia
Antinuclear antibody	Presence of antibodies against nucleosomal DNA-histone complexes. 95% sensitive but not specific. Double-stranded DNA more specific for lupus
Other Immunologic Test Positive	Anti-dsDNA or anti-Smith antibody, positive antiphospholipid antibody, false positive serologic syphilis test + 6 months (confirmed by FTA-AB)

of SLE, although CCLE is one of the diagnostic criteria for SLE (see above).

The primary laboratory test for diagnosis of lupus is the antinuclear antibody (ANA). This test is 95% sensitive but not specific to lupus. The extracted nuclear antibodies such as double-stranded DNA, anti-Smith, anti-RNP, and anti-Ro/La are more specific for lupus. ANA reaction patterns are summarized in table 98.6.

SCLERODERMA/MORPHEA/CREST SYNDROME

The spectrum of diseases considered within scleroderma include systemic sclerosis (SSc) (also known as scleroderma), morphea, and CREST syndrome. SSc is caused by extra collagen deposition in the skin and internal organs leading to skin thickening (sclerosis) and multiple internal manifestations. Immune system activation is important in disease causation. Antigen-activated T cells infiltrate the skin, producing profibrotic IL-4. B cells may also contribute to fibrosis. Major criteria include skin sclerosis affecting arms, face, and/or neck. Minor criteria are sclerodactyly, erosions, atrophy of the fingertips, and bilateral lung fibrosis. The progression of skin findings starts as edematous plaques, proceeds to induration, and finally becomes atrophic. SSc is rare, affecting women more frequently than men, without racial predilection. Deaths related to SSc are most commonly from pulmonary hypertension, lung fibrosis, and renal/cardiac disease (Swartz, 2008). The pathogenesis of SSc is incompletely understood. Some recognized precipitants are summarized in table 98.7. A limited form of SSc is morphea, which occurs in a well-demarcated area, most often on the trunk or face/scalp (linear morphea/"en coup de sabre"). CREST syndrome is another variant of SSc and is associated with calcinosis cutis, Raynaud's phenomenon, esophageal dysmotility, sclerodactyly, and mat telangiectasias.

Table 98.6 ANA REACTION PATTERNS

PATTERN	TARGET SITE	AB ASSOCIATION	DISEASE ASSOCIATION
Homogeneous	Native DNA/dsDNA RNP Histone	Anti-DNA Anti-histone	SLE Drug-induced LE
Peripheral/rim	Nuclear membrane	Anti-DNA, antilaminin	SLE (most specific)
Particulate (clumpy dots)	Smith antigen		SLE
Fine speckled	RNP		Mixed connective tissue disease
Large speckle		Anti-Ro	
Discreet speckled (tiny dots)	Kinetochore	Anticentromere	CREST
Nucleolar (round pebbles)			Scleroderma (SSc)

Table 98.7 EXTERNAL CAUSES OF SYSTEMIC SCLEROSIS (SSC)

CAUSE	NOTES
Appetite suppressants	Phenylethylamine derivatives
Drugs	Bleomycin, carbidopa, pentazocine, cocaine, penicillamine, vitamin K
Pesticides	Various reports of occupational SSc
Amino acid compound L-5-hydroxytryptophan	Eosinophilic myalgias syndrome
Epoxy resin	
Aliphatic hydrocarbons	Hexane, vinyl chloride, trichloroethylene
Organic solvents	Toluene, benzene, xylene
Silica	
Vibration injury	Similar vascular changes to systemic sclerosis

SOURCE: Schwartz and Dziankowska-Bartkowiak (2011).

Laboratory diagnosis of SSc is most specific with the antitopoisomerase I DNA (SCL-70) antibody, with two-thirds of patients with SSc and lung fibrosis having this antibody positivity. Anticentromere antibodies are diagnostic for CREST syndrome and are associated with less frequent involvement of the heart, kidneys, and nonfibrotic pulmonary changes. Other antibodies seen are against fibrillarin, Th-ribonucleoprotein (Th-RNP), and PM-Scl. Anti-PM-Scl antibodies are seen in patients with a polymyositis/SSc overlap syndrome and 3–10% of patients with SSc alone (Swartz, 2008).

DERMATOMYOSITIS

Dermatomyositis is a rare disease, presenting in both children and adults. Pathogenesis is unknown, but in adults an association with internal malignancy has been recognized. Presentation of facial erythema with violaceous colored eyelids, scaling plaques on the joints of the hands with sparing between joints, and an erythematous papulosquamous rash with associated proximal muscle weakness is the classic presentation of dermatomyositis (Dm). The scaling plaques on metacarpophalangeal and interphalangeal joints are known as Gottran's papules, and the violaceous changes of the eyelids known as heliotrope rashes are pathognomonic. Other common though not specific skin findings include poikiloderma, sun-exposed distribution, and periungual telangiectasias, and ragged cuticles. Other paraneoplastic syndromes in addition to Dm are summarized in table 98.8.

Diagnostic testing for Dm incorporates multiple hematologic tests. A positive ANA is frequently found in addition to one of the more specific antibodies for Dm.

Table 98.8 PARANEOPLASTIC SYNDROMES

CONDITION	DESCRIPTION/NOTES
Acanthosis nigricans	Gastric CA
Bazex syn	SCC of aerodigestive tract. Psoriasiform and eczematous papules over fingers, toes, nose, ears; keratoderma, nail dystrophy
Dermatomyositis	Often solid tumors, GI or GU
Eruptive keratoacanthoma	Associated with immunosuppression, lupus, leukemia, leprosy, kidney transplant, photochemotherapy, thermal burns, x-ray therapy, Muir-Torre syndrome
Erythema gyratum repens	Lung cancer. May rarely be associated with pulmonary TB
Florid cutaneous papillomatosis	Gastric CA, presents as verrucous papillomas
Hypertrichosis lanuginosa	Lung CA, colon CA. Most common location = face
Migratory thrombophlebitis	Pancreatic CA (also prostate, lung, liver, bowel, gallbladder, ovary, lymphoma/leukemia)
Necrolytic migratory erythema (glucagonoma syn)	Pancreatic tumor of APUD cells that secrete glucagon. Low serum Zn levels, hypoaminoacidemia
Paraneoplastic pemphigus	Non-Hodgkin's lymphoma, CLL, Castleman disease, sarcoma, thymoma, Waldenstrom
Pityriasis rotunda	Hepatic cancer, leukemia.
Tripe palm (acanthosis nigricans)	Lung and gastric CA. Honeycombed and thickened palms

Anti-Mi-2 (antihistidyl transfer RNA [t-RNA] synthetase) is specific for Dm, but it is not sensitive, as only 25% of Dm patients have this finding. Anti-Jo-1 is more specific for polymyositis than Dm and is associated with interstitial lung disease. Raynaud's phenomenon, arthritis, and rough, scaling dermatitis of the hands (mechanic's hands) (Callen, 2008).

PAPULOSQUAMOUS DISEASES

Papulosquamous refers to the surface morphology of skin conditions comprising this differential. These lesions tend to be well demarcated, scaly, and erythematous. Without question, psoriasis is the most common papulosquamous disease. Other conditions to consider include lichen planus, pityriasis rosea, dermatophytosis, and pityriasis rubra pilaris. Some drug reactions may also be papulosquamous.

Psoriasis (figure 98.6) is an exceedingly common condition of well-demarcated plaques with thick white (micaceous) scale most often on the elbows, knees, umbilicus, gluteal cleft, and scalp, although generalized involvement may also occur. Irregular nail pitting and thickening is also a common finding. Psoriasis affects about 2–3% of the world's population and 2.2% of those in the United States. Variants of psoriasis include guttate, generalized pustular, and palmoplantar pustulosis. Psoriasis is caused by T-cell stimulation of the epidermis, causing increased rates of growth, preventing epidermal maturation. It is a familial condition, linked to a mutation on chromosome 6, in *PSORS1* and has a strong linkage to HLA-B17 (Leder, 1998).

Psoriatic arthritis is also found in 10–30% of those with cutaneous psoriasis. There are five subtypes of psoriatic arthritis. Symmetric arthritis is similar to rheumatoid arthritis but milder with less joint deformity. It usually affects multiple symmetric pairs of joints. Asymmetric arthritis can affect any joint, and the hands and feet may have enlarged "sausage" digits. The classic type of psoriatic arthritis is distal interphalangeal predominant (DIP), but it only is found in approximately 5% of people with psoriatic arthritis. Presentation is with involvement of the distal joints of the fingers and toes. This form can be confused with osteoarthritis, but the latter does not feature the nail changes of psoriasis. Spondylitis occurs in 5% of individuals with psoriatic arthritis. Symptoms include stiffness of the neck, lower back, and sacroiliac or spinal vertebrae. Peripheral disease may present in the hands, arms, hips, legs, and feet. Arthritis mutilans is a rare, severe, deforming, destructive arthritis that affects the small joints of the hands and feet and has associated neck/lower back pain (Al-I Iammadi, 2008).

Therapies vary depending on the severity of psoriasis. Mild psoriasis can often be treated with topical steroids and/or topical calcipotriene cream alone. Ultraviolet light therapy with narrow band UVB (311–312 nm) or ingested psoralens plus UVA (PUVA) are helpful for more advanced cases. Common oral medications used to treat more severe psoriasis are methotrexate or acitretin. For patients with the most severe psoriasis, combinations of all of these therapies may be helpful, or the use of a biological agent may be warranted. The main class of biologic being used for psoriasis today is a TNF-α inhibitor such as infliximab, adalimumab, or etanercept. These agents should not be used in patients with active systemic fungal or mycobacterial infections or those with a diagnosis of multiple sclerosis. Other side effects with immunosuppressive agents include a potential increase in lymphomas and a lupus-like drug reaction (to TNF-α inhibitors).

Lichen planus (LP) is a cell-mediated immune response at the dermoepidermal junction of unknown origin, classically appearing clinically as purple, polygonal papules on the flexor surfaces of the arms, white linear patches on the oral mucosa (Wickham's striae) and on the genitalia. Familial LP has been linked to HLA-B7 and idiopathic LP to HLA-DR1 and DR10. LP may be limited to mucosal surfaces, causing severe ulcerations and pain as well as an erosive vaginitis. Associations to infections with hepatitis C, chronic active hepatitis, and primary biliary cirrhosis have been noted. Also, medications such as gold, antimalarials, and captopril (and other angiotensin-converting enzyme [ACE] inhibitors) have been linked to lichenoid eruptions similar to LP. Variants of LP include lichen planopilaris (a scarring alopecia) and isolated nail LP. Treatments include topical steroids, UV therapy similar to psoriasis, and oral retinoids such as acitretin.

Pityriasis rosea is a self-limited condition occurring frequently after a viral infection. Some have suggested a linkage to infection with HHV6/7. Classic presentation is that of a "herald patch," a large erythematous scaling plaque usually on the trunk. Within a week of this lesion's appearance, multiple small, scaly dull red plaques develop on the extremities and trunk in the skin lines, in a "Christmas tree" distribution. A fine "collarette" of scale is noted at the edge of the plaques. This condition resolves in 3–6 weeks and only requires therapy for the mild to moderate pruritus that may occur. A moderate-potency topical steroid and/or oral antihistamine may be useful. UV light therapy may be useful for extensive symptomatic patients.

Pityriasis rubra pilaris (PRP) is an idiopathic papulosquamous disease characterized by red to orange scaling plaques, palmoplantar keratoderma, and keratotic follicular papules. A classic feature is the uninvolved areas of skin surrounded by PRP, known as "islands of sparing." Familial PRP is an autosomal dominant trait that begins in early childhood. Idiopathic PRP has peaks in the first and fifth decade, but it can start at any time. Therapy is similar to that for psoriasis but may be less responsive.

The various forms of tinea are considered within the differential diagnosis of papulosquamous diseases. Consider tinea on any lesion that scales, and do a KOH exam or send a fungal culture. Dermatophytosis is discussed in detail in the fungal section. Secondary syphilis may be present with papulosquamous lesions.

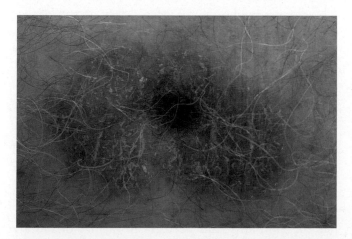

Figure 98.6. Pink Scaly Periumbilical Plaque Consistent with Psoriasis.

PIGMENTARY DISORDERS

There are a number of disorders involving too much or too little pigmentation. Many medications have the potential for differential deposition in the skin, causing skin coloration changes. The more common pigmentary disorders such as postinflammatory hypo- and hyperpigmentation, vitiligo, systemic causes of skin pigmentation, drug-related pigmentary changes, albinism, and melasma are discussed below.

Postinflammatory changes can either be hypopigmentation or hyperpigmentation. For darker-skinned individuals these changes are often more noticeable compared to lighter-skinned individuals. Postinflammatory hyperpigmentation results from either epidermal or dermal melanosis. When the epidermis is inflamed, stimulation of the melanocytes causes increased melanin production in the melanocytes and transfer to the epidermal keratinocyte, causing a transient superficial brown hyperpigmentation. In cases where the inflammation is deeper, involving disruption of the dermal–epidermal junction, dermal melanin deposition may occur. This pigmentation is longer lasting and challenging to treat. Hypopigmentation occurs from decrease or loss of epidermal production of melanin by the melanocyte or loss of the melanocyte totally.

Melasma (or chloasma) is hormonally influenced hyperpigmentation on the lateral cheeks, upper lip, and forehead and occasionally on other sun-exposed areas. Most commonly this change occurs in women taking oral contraceptives or following pregnancy, although mild thyroid and ovarian dysfunction may also play a role in the development of melasma. Ninety percent of affected patients are women, although men can present with a similar picture. Both epidermal and dermal pigmentation may occur. Solar exposure darkens the pigment. Thus, an important part of any therapy is sun protection.

Vitiligo is an autoimmune disease in which the immune system is responsible for melanocyte death. Typical areas of involvement are symmetric and include the lips, face, elbows, hands, feet, and knees, although any area of the body may be affected. Findings are of total loss of pigmentation (depigmentation) or of lighter areas (hypopigmentation), sometimes in three zones called trichrome vitiligo (figure 98.7). Pathogenesis is not clearly identified. Certain HLA types have increased risk of vitiligo, including HLA-DR4 in blacks, HLA-B13 (Moroccan Jews), HLA-B35 (Yemenite Jews), and HLA-B13 (with antithyroid antibodies). Other autoimmune diseases are seen with more frequency in individuals with vitiligo, including thyroid disease, diabetes mellitus, pernicious anemia, Addison disease, and alopecia areata.

Several systemic diseases can cause diffuse hyperpigmentation of the skin. Addison disease is adrenal insufficiency that does not manifest clinical symptoms until

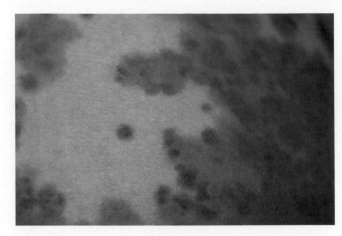

Figure 98.7. Trichrome Vitiligo. Note the multiple hues of brown to white skin present.

after 90% of the adrenal cortex is destroyed. Generalized "bronze" skin hyperpigmentation is noted in 95% of Addison disease patients. These findings occur secondary to increased production of melanocyte-stimulating hormone (MSH), which is produced as a cleavage product of the prohormone for corticotrophin. Iron overload in hemochromatosis causes a triad of cirrhosis, diabetes mellitus, and skin hyperpigmentation. Skin findings are a late finding and occur in about 70% of patients. Patients with primary biliary cirrhosis may also have generalized skin hyperpigmentation.

Many oral medications can commonly or uncommonly cause skin pigmentation. One commonly used medication that produces a slate-gray pigmentation on sun-exposed areas is amiodarone. Minocycline can produce black, blue-gray, or brown pigmentation over longer durations of therapy. Zidovudine produces pigmentation of the nails, both longitudinal streaks and blue coloration of the lunula. Medications that cause pigmentary changes are summarized in table 98.9.

There are various congenital hypopigmentation syndromes. Oculocutaneous albinism (OCA) has four subtypes, depending on the gene defect present. Other conditions with similar findings are Hermansky-Pudlak, Chediak-Higashi, and Griscelli syndromes. These diseases are summarized in table 98.10.

BULLOUS DISORDERS

Autoimmune bullous disorders are uncommon, causing both cutaneous and mucous membrane disease. With the advent of systemic immunosuppressive agents (i.e., prednisone, azathioprine, and mycophenolate mofetil), the mortality of these diseases has significantly decreased, but the morbidity and decrease in quality of life are still considerable. This group of disorders is caused by

Table 98.9 PIGMENTARY CHANGES

DRUG	CLINICAL
Amiodarone	Slate-gray on sun-exposed face and hands
Antimalarials	Yellow-brown to gray on tibial surfaces, face, mouth, nails
Arsenic	Black generalized pigmentation or truncal pigment that spares face with depigmented scattered macules that resemble raindrops
Bismuth	Pigment line in gingiva
Bleomycin	Flagellate hyperpigmentation on back or areas of excoriation
Busulfan	Blue lunula
Chlorpromazine	Slate-gray-violaceous on sun-exposed skin and conjunctiva
Clofazimine	Red-brown color. Reddish tinge of tissue due to clofazimine accumulation, brown due to ceroid lipofuscinosis
Gold	Lilac, begins on eyelid, then face, hands
Hemosiderin	Red-brown
Lead	"Gingival line"
Mercury	Slate-gray gingival pigment on mouth, eyelids, neck, nasolabial fold
Methacycline	Gray-black photoexposed skin Yellow-brown conjunctival pigment
Minocycline	Three types: • Blue-black in scars • Blue-gray in normal skin, common on anterior of tibia • Muddy brown, sun-exposed areas
Silver	Slate-gray, sun-exposed skin
Zidovudine (AZT)	Nail pigmentation: blue lunula or longitudinal streaks

autoimmune attack on the various components of the epidermis or the dermal–epidermal junction, which holds the skin together.

These diseases can be divided into two groups by the location of the split in the blister. The pemphigus group and linear IgA disease have intraepidermal splits, whereas pemphigoid/epidermolysis bullosa have splits in the dermal–epidermal junction or in the dermis. Each split is specific to the antigen that is the target of autoimmune destruction. For the pemphigus group, the antigens are components of the desmosome, the complex responsible for holding keratinocyte to keratinocyte in the epidermis. For the pemphigoid group, the responsible proteins are in the hemidesmosome, basement membrane, or dermal anchoring collagen.

A flaccid bulla is the hallmark of an epidermal split, and a tense bulla indicates a subepidermal split. The Asboe-Hansen sign shows progression of an existing blister with pressure on the bulla, and the Nikolsky sign is positive when a new blister is formed with friction on the skin. Both are positive in epidermal processes and negative in subepidermal processes. The blistering disorders are summarized in table 98.11.

HAIR AND NAILS

Hair and nails are keratin-derived skin appendages that are cosmetically and socially problematic when diseased or absent. Nails are derived from keratins produced in the proximal nail matrix. They grow at an average rate of 1.8–4.6 mm/month and will completely regrow in 6–9 months (Johnson et al., 1991). Fingernails are important for tactile sensation and important for grasping small objects. Nails are affected in diseases such as psoriasis/alopecia areata

Table 98.10 CONGENITAL HYPOPIGMENTATION SYNDROMES

DISEASE	GENE DEFECT	NOTES
Oculocutaneous albinism, type 1	Tyrosinase	No morbidity/mortality outside ocular and UV sensitivity for all four types of OCA. Complete absence of pigment: skin, hair, eyes
Oculocutaneous albinism, type 2	*P* gene	Minimal but not complete pigment loss of skin, hair, eyes
Oculocutaneous albinism, type 3	Tyrosinase-related protein-1 (*Tyrp1*)	Minimal pigment loss. Only confirmed in African heritages: "brown" or "rufous" albinism
Oculocutaneous albinism, type 4	Membrane-associated transporter protein (*MATP*)	Phenotype similar to type 2
Hermansky-Pudlak	Multiple mutations (*HPS* gene)	Bleeding diathesis secondary to platelet deficiency. Ceroid storage disease—ceroid-lipofuscin material accumulates in solid organs. Pulmonary fibrosis frequently fatal, fourth or fifth decade of life.
Chediak-Higashi	*LYST* gene	Silvery-metallic hair. Immunodeficiency. Frequent respiratory infections, bleeding diathesis
Griscelli	*RAB27A/MYO5A*	Severe immunodeficiency, usually fatal in early childhood

Table 98.11 SUMMARY OF BULLOUS DISEASE

DISEASE	ANTIGEN	NOTES
Epidermal Split		
IgA pemphigus	Intraepidermal neutrophilic type: Dsg 3 Subcorneal pustular type: Desmocollin 1 and 2	Initially clear vesicles/bullae that become pustules. Common location: chest/inframammary, scalp/postauricular. Superficial epidermal split
Pemphigus foliaceus/ Fogo selvagem	Desmoglein (Dsg) 1	Mucous membranes (MM) uncommonly involved. Fogo selvagem—endemic pemphigus, common in Brazil. Possible sandfly vector. Superficial epidermal split with flaccid bullae and superficial erosions.
Pemphigus vulgaris (PV)	100% dsg 3 50–75% dsg 1	Mucous membranes commonly involved. Flaccid bulla, deep erosions. Split in basal layer of epidermis.
Pemphigus vegetans	Dsg3	Variant of PV. Vegetative plaques, commonly in axilla
Pemphigus erythematosus	Dsg1	Senear-Usher syndrome. Combination of SLE and PV. Small, flaccid bullae on scalp, face, upper chest/back. Similar to PF
Paraneoplastic pemphigus	Plectin Desmoplakin I BPAg I Desmoplakin II/envoplakin Periplakin Dsg 1 Dsg 3	Associated with lymphoproliferative disorders and other malignancies (thymoma, sarcoma, and lung carcinoma). Mucosal sores in mouth, esophagus, and crusting/erosions of lips. Polymorphous presentation on skin—erythema, vesicobullous lesions, crusts.
Subepidermal Split		
Bullous pemphigoid (BP)	BPAg 1 BPAg 2 (less)	Tense bullae on any skin surface. Rare mucous membrane (MM) involvement. Can present with eczematous pre-BP
Cicatricial pemphigoid	*Laminin 5 (epiligrin)* Laminin 6 BPA 2 *(lamina lucida)*	Scarring of MM primary—eyes, oral MM. Bullae on upper body common.
Herpes (pemphigoid) gestationis	BPA 2 = collagen 17	Pregnant women, recurs with subsequent pregnancies. Increased incidence of: Hashimoto thyroiditis, Graves' disease, pernicious anemia. Associated with HLA-DR3/DR4
Dermatitis herpetiformis (DH)	Transglutaminase	Increased incidence of thyroid disease, small bowel lymphoma, and non-Hodgkin lymphoma. Gluten-sensitive enteropathy, responsive to dapsone.
Linear IgA dz	Collagen VII BPA 1 and 2	Presentation similar to BP. Idiopathic or medication reaction: vancomycin most common
Bullous lupus erythematosis	Collagen VII Laminin 5 Laminin 6 BPA 1	Appearance varies from BP-like to DH-like
Bullous diabeticorum	Split is in lamina lucida	Not autoimmune. Occurs on lower legs and feet.
Epidermolysis bullosa acquisita	Collagen VII	Blisters, scars, milia in areas of trauma, rarely MM. Associated with Crohn disease.
Porphyria cutanea tarda	Familial type—uroporphyrinogen decarboxylase deficiency. Acquired—flares with hepatitis (often Hep B/C), ethanol, increased estrogen, HIV infection, and in hemochromatosis	Either acquired or hereditary. Tense bullae on sun-exposed surfaces, milia. Hirsutism on lateral face.

(pitting) and lichen planus (rough nails and pterygium) or may be diseased in many genodermatoses (i.e., pachonychia congenita). Additionally, examination of the nails may give important clues to internal deficiencies or diseases. Nail findings are summarized in table 98.12.

Hair is produced in an epidermal invagination into the dermis. The matrix cells produce the hair shaft that grows to become the visible hair. Pigment is produced by melanocytes in the matrix. Scalp hair grows approximately 0.35 mm/day or 2.5 mm/week (Alaiti, 2007).

Table 98.12 NAILS

CONDITION	DESCRIPTION
Koilonychia	Spoon-shaped concave nails related to iron deficiency
Beau's line (transverse ridges)	Due to acute systemic injury. Half way on nail plate = insult was 3 months ago
Terry's nails	Proximal 2/3 white, distal 1/3 red. Secondary to hepatic disease, hypoalbuminemia from cirrhosis or CHF
Half & half (Lindsay's)	Proximal 1/2 white, distal 1/2 pink. Occurs in renal disease
Muehrcke's lines	Paired white parallel bands that do not grow out with the nail plate due to an abnormal nail bed. Secondary to hypoalbuminemia
Mee's lines	Horizontal leukonychia, defect nail plate. From arsenic poisoning (Tx acutely with dimercaprol)
Onychogryphosis	Long hypertrophied nails resembling a ram's horn. Due to neglect
Onycholysis	Nail plate split from nail bed. Can be caused by tinea
Onychophosis	Hyperkeratotic tissue on lateral or proximal nailfolds, within the space between the nailfolds and nail plate
Onychomadesis	Periodic idiopathic shedding of nail (complete onycholysis)
Onychorrhexis	Brittle nails, longitudinal striations. Tx with B-complex vitamin biotin
Onychoschizia	Splitting of distal nail plate into layers at the free edge
Pitting	Caused by damage to proximal matrix. Common in psoriasis (irregular) and alopecia areata (regular)
Pterygium	Scarring and fusion of the cuticle to the nail plate. Common in lichen planus

Table 98.13 ALOPECIA

DISEASE	NOTES
Scarring	
Lichen planopilaris	Form of follicular lichen planus. Sx: erythema, itching, scarring
Pseudopelade of Brocq	Nonspecific scarring hair loss. Likely end stage result of other scarring conditions
Chronic cutaneous lupus	Similar to cutaneous presentation. Follicular plugging, erythema, scarring
Traction	From hairstyles with sustained traction. Results in scarring and loss of hair follicles. Irreversible
Scleroderma	En coup de sabre, extends onto scalp. Linear scarring atrophic plaque
Nonscarring	
Alopecia areata	Oval "coin-shaped" patches of hair loss. Related to thyroid disease in some cases. Can progress to entire scalp, head or body
Male pattern	Secondary to action of dihydrotestosterone causing miniaturization of the hair follicle. Often begins on vertex scalp, spares occipital and temporal hair
Medication induced (see Shapiro, 2007)	Anagen effluvium (~2 weeks after starting): chemotherapeutic agents such as busulfan, cyclophosphamide, vinblastine/vincristine, doxorubicin. Telogen effluvium (2–3 months after starting): many including retinoids, heparin, lithium, ramipril, terbinafine, valproic acid, warfarin
Telogen effluvium (Shapiro, 2007)	Increase number of telogen hairs. Begins ~3 months following major illness or stress (e.g., surgery, childbirth, rapid weight loss, nutritional deficiency, high fever, hemorrhage) or hormonal derangement (e.g., thyroid dysfunction)
Metabolic	Thyroid, syphilis, nutritional deficiency, iron deficiency, HIV

There are three phases to hair growth: anagen, catagen, and telogen. Active growth occurs in anagen phase (84% of all hairs), lasting 3–4 years. Catagen phase (1–2%) lasts 2–3 weeks. Follicular regression occurs during this time. Telogen phase (10–15%) lasts about 3 months and is a resting phase before renewed anagen growth (Alaiti, 2007). Normal hair loss is approximately 100 hairs per day (Shapiro, 2007). An important issue for many presenting with hair complaints is hair loss (alopecia), especially on the scalp. Alopecias can be broken down into two groups, scarring and nonscarring. Scarring alopecias are permanent once the scar has formed. Nonscarring alopecias will sometimes have full regrowth. The various conditions are summarized in table 98.13.

ADDITIONAL READING

Alaiti S. Hair Anatomy. http://vw.emedicine.com/ent/topic10.htm. August 2007. Accessed June 15, 2008.

Al Hammadi A. Psoriatic Arthritis. http://www.emedicine.com/MED/topci1954.htm. March 2008. Accessed July 15, 2008.

Callen J. Dermatomyositis. http://www.emedicine.com/med/topic 2608.htm. Accessed June 8, 2008.

Jeffes EW 3rd, Tang EH. Actinic keratosis. Current treatment options. *Am J Clin Dermatol.* 2000;1:167–79.

Johnson M, Comaish JS, Shuster S. Nail is produced by the normal nail bed: A controversy resolved. *Br J Dermatol.* 1991;125(1):27–9.

Lamont DW, Lai MK. Systemic Lupus Erythematosus. http://www.emedicine.com/emerg/topic564.htm. Accessed June 7, 2008.

Miller AJ, Mihm MC Jr. Melanoma. *N Engl J Med.* 2006;355(1):51–65.

Nestle FO, Kaplan DH, Barker J. Psoriasis. *N Engl J Med.* 2009; 361(5):496–509.

Rubin AI, Chen EH, Ratner D. Basal-cell carcinoma. *N Engl J Med.* 2005;353(21):2262–9.

Schwartz RA, Dziankowska-Bartkowiak B. Systemic Sclerosis. http://www.emedicine.com/derm/topic677.htm. March 2008. Accessed June 7, 2008.

Shapiro J. Hair loss in women. *N Engl J Med.* 2007;357:1620–30

Swetter S. Malignant Melanoma. http://www.emedicine.com/DERM/topic257.htm. January 2008. Accessed July 11, 2008.

Taïeb A, Picardo M. Clinical practice. Vitiligo. *N Engl J Med.* 2009;360(2):160–9.

QUESTIONS

QUESTION 1. A 53-year-old man presents with a tender keratotic nodule on his right upper forehead. He first noticed it 4 weeks ago, and it has grown rapidly. It is tender to pressure. Mutations in what gene caused by exposure to UV radiation are the most likely cause of this lesion?

A. *bRAF*
B. *nRAS*
C. *Smoothened*
D. *Patched*
E. *p53* tumor suppressor gene

QUESTION 2. A 61-year-old man a history of cerebrovascular accident and grand mal seizures with is started on carbamazepine. He develops fever, pharyngitis, Stevens-Johnson-like dermatitis and lymphadenopathy on physical exam as well as laboratory abnormalities including hepatitis, nephritis, and leukocytosis with eosinophilia. What would an appropriate antiepileptic to substitute?

A. Phenytoin
B. Valproic acid
C. Phenobarbital
D. None; continue carbamazepine
E. Oxcarbazepine

QUESTION 3. All of the following statements regarding malignant melanoma are correct, EXCEPT:

A. Since the majority of cutaneous melanoma cases arise in association with a precursor nevus, the wholesale removal of melanocytic nevi is important for melanoma prevention.
B. A new or changing mole or blemish is the most common warning sign for melanoma.
C. Acral lentiginous melanoma is uncommon in white individuals but relatively common in dark-skinned individuals.
D. Blue/green-eyed, blond or red-haired, light-complexioned individuals should be counseled on protecting themselves from intense sun exposure to limit their risk.
E. The presence of xeroderma pigmentosum is a major risk factor for developing melanoma.

ANSWERS

1. E
2. B
3. A

99.

OCCUPATIONAL MEDICINE

Lori Wiviott Tishler

Occupational injuries are among the leading causes of morbidity and mortality in the United States, and occupational medicine physicians play a role in preventing, recognizing, diagnosing, and treating these illnesses. Yet, many illnesses that can be occupationally related are indistinguishable from other sorts of chronic illness. This chapter provides an overview of occupational medicine with a focus on the occupational history, disability, and worker's compensation.

THE OCCUPATIONAL HISTORY

Occupational illnesses are underrecognized and therefore undertreated. They are responsible for >800,000 illnesses and >60,000 deaths annually. Barriers to taking a good occupational history include inadequate information on the part of both patient and doctor about occupational exposures. For patients, there can also be a long latency between the exposure (e.g., asbestos in a naval shipyard) and the ultimate illness (mesothelioma). Many physicians are inadequately trained to recognize occupational illness, and most physicians find it difficult to negotiate the maze of reporting and notifying appropriate governing boards about occupational illness.

When one is taking an occupational history, it is important to consider whether or not a pattern of symptoms might be clarified by elucidating information about a patient's work. Additionally, it is important to be aware of a patient's job and its potential impact on his or her health. For most patients a quick survey is all that is necessary to help delineate whether or not a more detailed occupational history needs to be taken. Simple questions such as "What do you do for work?" and "Do you think your health problems are related to your work?" are a good place to start. If a positive answer is elicited in the initial history, a more comprehensive occupational history should be taken. This should include a detailed chronology of jobs, exposures, and temporal correlations among exposures, occupations, and symptoms

(see table 99.1). Many occupational medicine physicians have detailed questionnaires to help them with this complicated task. Finally, it is important to remember that patients may have exposures to toxic substances that occur outside of their work lives. If you are worried about an exposure, it is important to also elicit a good history of their community, home, hobbies, diet, and drugs (herbal, legal, and illegal).

There are numerous databases and organizations that can help physicians in the occupational assessment. The National Library of Medicine has an online bibliography called Toxline (http://toxnet.nlm.nih.gov/index.html), which covers the toxicologic effects of drugs and chemicals. The Hazardous Substances Data Bank (same website) focuses on the toxic responses to possibly hazardous substances. Other internet resources include the Center for Disease Control and Prevention (http://www.cdc.gov), World Health Organization Occupational Health (www.who.int/occupational_health/en), and the Association of Societies for Occupational Safety and Health (www.asosh.org/index.html). The American College of Occupational and Environmental Medicine can help to direct clinicians to resources as well (http://www.acoem.org).

It is key to ask enough questions to help discern whether a patient's symptoms could be attributed to workplace exposure. If so, then the next step is to focus in more detail, not forgetting that exposures can be nonoccupational as well. There are a number of published questionnaires that can be helpful when one is deciding whether or not to refer to an appropriate subspecialist or occupational medicine physician.

DISABILITY AND RETURN TO WORK

The earliest worker's compensation laws in the United States occurred after 1910. Mostly focused on occupational injuries, these initial laws were far from the complex worker's compensation and disability doctrine that we have today. Today, the role of the physician is complex, often confusing, and sometimes distasteful. It is helpful to remember that the

Table 99.1 INITIAL OCCUPATIONAL HISTORY

1. What is your work?

2. Do you think your health problems may be related to your work?

3. Are your symptoms different at home?

4. Have you been exposed to chemicals, dusts, radiation, noise, or repetitive motion now or in the past?

5. Are any of your co-workers experiencing these symptoms?

If any of these answers is "yes," then you should take a more comprehensive history.

SOURCE: Lax et al. (1998).

Table 99.2 RISK FACTORS FOR DELAYED RETURN TO WORK AFTER OCCUPATIONAL INJURY

1. Patient perception of severity of disability

2. Underlying depression

3. Chronic pain

4. Secondary gain

5. Formal litigation

6. Inability of employer to modify or create transitional work

7. Physician factors

determination of disability is an organizational or legal decision. It is the doctor's task to help provide supporting information in as accurate and truthful a manner as possible.

The role of the physician in determining disability is to help determine whether or not an illness or injury is related to the patient's work. As the physician treats the patient, he or she can help determine when maximum improvement has been made and when the patient may return to work. The American Medical Association Guides to the Evaluation of Permanent Impairment can help physicians determine the level and type of impairment. If the patient's case results in litigation, it is not uncommon for the patient to be assigned to an independent medical examiner, a physician not involved in the longitudinal care of the patient, who may provide a report on the patient's injury, illness, expected improvement, and level of impairment.

The majority of workers who have work-related medical problems will be treated, improve, and return to work promptly, even when a worker's compensation case is involved. Nonetheless, in a small number of cases, patients will not improve or will have a delayed recovery. Delayed recovery is a term that means prolonged time to improvement that is out of proportion to clinical findings. These cases are most costly for the system and often most frustrating for the physician. The longer patients are on disability, the lower their chance of ever returning to work. Risk factors for delayed return to work are listed in table 99.2.

It can be difficult to decide when a patient is truly ready to return to work. Questions to ask patients might include, "Can you work around this problem while you recover?" and "What, specifically, is preventing you from working today?" The answers to these questions can be helpful in determining readiness to return to work and identifying patients who are at risk for delayed recovery. Some specialists suggest the grocery store test. Ask yourself, "If this patient was the sole proprietor of a corner store, could he or she get to work and be safe at work?" If you think so, he or she is probably medically safe to return to work.

For many patients who are anxious or reluctant about returning to work, the physician can help to create an environment in which the worker can return successfully. For some, this may mean helping him or her to return on a lighter schedule with a plan of working up to the previous full-time schedule. Other helpful suggestions are to be available to meet with the patient in person or by phone while he or she is making the transition back to work.

The next section of this chapter considers specific issues in occupational medicine including work-related injuries, illnesses, and exposures. It is by no means a comprehensive list, but the goal is to help physicians become aware of work-related risk factors for these problems, specific at-risk occupations, and strategies for treatment and prevention. A review of these illnesses, injuries, and exposures is presented here by system.

MUSCULOSKELETAL AND PERIPHERAL NERVOUS SYSTEM

Work-related injuries affect every part of the body. Risk factors for work-related injuries include repetitive activities, awkward positions, and lack of rest. Mechanical stresses, vibration, and cold temperatures can contribute as well. Peripheral nerve injuries are also common occupational illnesses. Predisposing factors to these injuries may include exposures to chemicals or gases, but more commonly injuries to individual nerves may come from repetitive motion, abnormal posture, and carrying heavy objects. Many of these injuries can be diagnosed by physical exam alone; others might require imaging or electromyogram (EMG) studies to confirm. Good safety practices and ergonomics can prevent many of these injuries. Workers should be encouraged to contact their occupational health program to train them to improve their positioning, posture, workstations, and mechanical stressors at their jobs. Referral to occupational therapy may help as well to treat and prevent these injuries.

SPECIAL SENSES

Many workers are at risk for ocular injury from trauma as well as exposures to chemicals, radiation, and even the visible light spectrum. Because many eye injuries need immediate treatment, it is essential for treatment to begin on site by the employee or his or her colleagues. Attention should be paid to proper ocular protection with facemasks, goggles, or equipment most appropriate to the work setting.

Occupational hearing loss is another common injury. In general, hearing loss occurs because of repeated exposure to loud noise, head injury, or exposure to substances toxic to the ear. Workers in noisy work environments (prolonged exposure to sounds louder than 85 dBA) are at increased risk for hearing loss. Workers in noisy environments also may be at greater risk for hearing loss from ototoxic medications. Prevention is the best treatment, including an awareness of the noise level in the workplace, hearing testing as appropriate, worker education, and hearing protection devices (table 99.3).

Chemical workers have reported alterations in their sense of smell. Occupations at risk for this include battery workers, tank cleaners, and chemical plant workers. Skin disorders can be related to allergic reactions, infection, and mechanical trauma such as heat and cold. Certain workers are also at risk for occupation-related skin cancer, including outdoor workers and those exposed to tar products, arsenic, and repeated trauma.

IMMUNE SYSTEM

Infections are an important component of occupational medicines. Microbial exposures are common in the agricultural industry and from animal exposures. Occupations at risk for zoonoses include farmers, veterinarians, abattoir workers, and ranchers. Less obvious and more urban occupations might be zoo attendants or pet shop workers.

Hospital and other health care workers are at risk for numerous blood-borne diseases from needle sticks and other exposures. These include tuberculosis, all forms of infectious hepatitis, and HIV. Hypersensitivity pneumonitis (see respiratory system) is also commonly related to bacteria, fungi, and animal exposures. White-collar workers, too, can be at risk for occupational infection. Business travelers, for example, are susceptible to various travel illnesses, many of which can be prevented with appropriate vaccinations or prophylactic medications.

Table 99.3 SELECTED WORKERS AT RISK OF HEARING RELATED PROBLEMS

1. Truckers
2. Farm equipment operators
3. Mill and lumber workers
4. Miners
5. Military flight line workers

RESPIRATORY SYSTEM (UPPER AND LOWER)

In the upper respiratory tract, patients might present with occupationally related allergic rhinitis. Table 99.4 lists the exposures that are associated with allergic rhinitis and asthma. Diagnosis of occupational allergic rhinitis might be aided by radioallergosorbent (RAST) testing or challenge testing in the workplace. Treatment is the same as for non-occupation-related disease. Some agents and processes are associated with sinonasal and laryngeal cancer. The strongest findings are associated with leather- and woodworkers. Laryngeal cancer can be associated most strongly with asbestos and smoke inhalation. Cigarette smoking increases patient risk for these conditions. Lower respiratory tract disorders include asthma, toxic inhalation, hypersensitivity pneumonitis, pneumoconiosis, lung cancer, and pleural disorders such as mesothelioma.

CARDIOVASCULAR SYSTEM

Because cardiovascular disease (CVD) is so common in our society, it is easy to overlook occupational exposure as a source. It can also be very difficult, given the long lag time between exposure and diagnosis, to attribute CVD to occupational risk. In truth, job-related factors are more likely to be additive risk factors for patients, in combination with more classic risk factors such as smoking, hypertension, and diabetes, than stand-alone causes of heart disease. Chronic exposures to air pollution, carbon disulfides, and carbon monoxide may accelerate the development of coronary artery disease. Heavy metals such as antimony can prolong the QT interval, arsenic can cause vasospasm and may contribute to hypertension, cobalt exposure is a probable cause of cardiomyopathy, and lead exposure may contribute to hypertension, cardiomyopathy, as well as a host of other conditions.

Table 99.4 SOME EXPOSURES ASSOCIATED WITH ALLERGIC RHINITIS AND ASTHMA

EXPOSURE	EMPLOYEES
Animal antigens	Farmers, veterinarians, animal workers
Grains/grain contaminants	Grain workers, bakers, farmers
Insect antigens	Many occupations, especially urban, inside, dusty places
Diisocyanates (polyurethanes)	Painters, boat builders
Acid anhydrides (plastics)	Painters, manufacturers
Antibiotics	Healthcare workers

GASTROINTESTINAL AND RENAL SYSTEMS

The liver, as the body's detoxification system, is the part of the GI tract most at risk for workplace exposures. As with cardiac disease, changes caused by toxins and exposures are not specific. Many chemical agents can cause liver injury (table 99.5). Some agents such as anesthetic gases or TNT cause acute hepatic injury, but we also see patients with cirrhosis, hepatic sclerosis, steatosis, and granulomatous disease that can be caused by chronic or repeated exposures. Although many chemical agents are potential causes of hepatocellular carcinoma, there are few definitive studies. Risk of hepatic damage also increases in patients who have other injuries to their livers from alcoholism or chronic hepatitis. In workers who are at higher risk for liver disease, baseline transaminases might be helpful, but routine monitoring is not recommended unless exposure to a toxin exceeds specific levels.

As with the other systems in the body, chronic renal disease is common. Often the causes are multifactorial, and patients have many risk factors. Some occupational exposures do, however, affect the kidneys. Acute renal failure can develop after high-dose exposures to specific metals, solvents, and pesticides, usually from acute tubular necrosis. Chronic can be caused by lead, cadmium, mercury, and uranium exposure.

REPRODUCTIVE SYSTEM

Over 30 million women of childbearing age were employed in the United States in 2004. Although only a few substances have clear associations with poor reproductive outcomes, the stress and social cost of such occurrences are devastating for patients, their families, and communities. Agents that are specific reproductive toxins include ionizing radiation and polychlorinated biphenyls (PCBs).

Table 99.5 TYPES OF OCCUPATIONAL LIVER INJURY AND REPRESENTATIVE CAUSAL AGENT

	ACUTE	CHRONIC
Steatosis	Carbon tetrachloride	Carbon tetrachloride
Cholestasis	Rapeseed oil	
Necrosis	Carbon tetrachloride, chloroform (zonal); TNT (massive)	
Cirrhosis		TNT
Sclerosis		Vinyl chloride
Neoplasia		Arsenic
Granulomas		Copper

Healthcare workers may be exposed to infection and antineoplastic drugs. When providing preconception counseling for patients or considering an infertility evaluation, it is important to find out about these and other occupational exposures to help patients minimize risk in every way.

Studying male reproductive risk not only helps us to prevent the bad outcomes mentioned above but also can be helpful as a marker for occupational risk in general. For example, it may take years for a person to develop occupationally related liver or lung disease, but an abnormal sperm count from the same exposure would happen more quickly. If we remove toxins that affect the sperm count, it is certainly possible that we are preventing long-term consequences for other organ systems as well. Many chemicals can cause male reproductive toxicity. A selection of them includes anabolic steroids, benzene, ethylene dibromide, lead, and tobacco smoke. DDT has been found in semen of infertile men. Excessive heat can lead to a low sperm count, as can greenhouse work.

CENTRAL NERVOUS SYSTEM

Peripheral nervous system disorders, common in many occupations, are discussed above. Central nervous system (CNS) disorders are fortunately rarer. They can be hard to detect, but a few principles to keep in mind include the following. In CNS problems related to job exposure, patients often have a nonfocal or symmetric syndrome. There is a strong time correlation between exposure and symptoms. Few toxins have a clear attached syndrome. It is essential to exclude other neurological diseases before attributing neurological disease to an occupational cause. Heavy metal exposure, organophosphates, and solvents are the most common sources of injury.

Psychiatric stress in the workplace as well as substance abuse affecting a patient's ability to work may be the most common occupational diseases that we see as internists. Common workplace stressors include relationships within the workplace, career development and promotion, role ambiguity, work environment, and shift work. Consider the role of shift work in patients who present with accidents (both on and off the job), sleep disorders, overuse or abuse of stimulants, and social problems. Older patients, in particular, may be at greater risk from psychological and physical consequences of shift work.

Considering that up to 10% of the population may have a substance abuse disorder, this leads to a large number of people working with these problems. The cost of alcohol and substance abuse in the workplace is in the hundreds of billions of dollars. Consideration should also be given to patients who are taking *legally prescribed* pain medications or sedatives. Attention should be paid to patients at risk of addiction, and appropriate treatment and referral, sometimes even within the workplace setting, should be initiated.

SUMMARY

Occupational disease can affect every occupation and every organ system. For the generalist or non–occupational specialist, the major "take home points" are the following. The occupational (including military service) history is important. If potential exposures are elicited, be aware of the specific historical questions and tools that exist to help you sort out the issues. Consider appropriate referrals. Disability assessment is complicated, but it is in the patient's best interest to return to work quickly; delayed return to work is a risk factor for never returning to work, and there are specific approaches to ameliorate this. Occupational exposures are not limited to chemicals but can be exposures to infectious agents, sound, radiation, drugs, and stress. Many classic risk factors for chronic disease are heightened by occupational exposures. Much occupational disease is preventable with good workplace safety and Occupational Safety and Health Administration (OSHA) compliance, reduction of exposures, and reduction of more classic risk factors as well.

ADDITIONAL READING

Andersson GBJ, Cocchiarella L. *Guides to the Evaluation of Permanent Impairment.* 5th ed. Chicago: American Medical Association; 2000.

Beckett WS. Occupational respiratory diseases. *N Engl J Med.* 2000;342(6):406–13.

Bowler RM, Cone JE. *Occupational Medicine Secrets.* Philadelphia: Hanley and Belfus; 1999.

Ladou J, ed. *Current Occupational and Environmental Medicine,* 4th ed. New York: McGraw-Hill; 2004.

Lamontagne AD, Keegel T, Louie AM, et al. A systematic review of the job stress intervention evaluation literature 1990–2005. *Int J Occup Environ Health.* 2007;13(3):268–80. Erratum *Int J Occup Environ Health.* 2008;14(1):24.

Lax, MB, Grant WD, Manetta FA, Klein R, Cohen S. Recognizing occupational disease—taking an effective occupational history. *Am Fam Physician.* 1998;58(4):935–44.

Schonstein E, Kenny DT, Keating J, Koes BW. Work conditioning, work hardening and functional restoration for workers with back and neck pain. *Cochrane Database.* 2003;1:CD001822.

Smith GS, Wellman HM, Sorock GS, et al. Injuries at work in the US adult population: Contributions to the total injury burden. *Am J Public Health.* 2005;95(7):1213–9.

Waters TR, Dick RB, Davis-Barkley J, Krieg EF. Cross sectional study of risk factors for musculoskeletal symptoms in the workplace. *J Occup Environ Med.* 2007;49(2):172–84.

QUESTIONS

QUESTION 1. A 42-year-old factory worker has been out of work for 4 weeks because of low back pain. She has successfully completed a course of NSAIDs and physical therapy. She is able to do her activities of daily living with no problem but complains of persistent pain. She tells you that she can not possibly return to work at this time. Your detailed medical assessment reveals no red flags; the physical therapist thinks she is doing very well. What might help you avoid delaying her return to work?

A. Tell her to stop malingering and get back to work.
B. Screen for and treat depression.
C. Work with her and her company to come up with a transition back to work plan.
D. Inquire about pending litigation.
E. B, C, and D.

QUESTION 2. A patient who has lead exposure in his work as an instructor in the police academy firing range comes in to the emergency department with a left-sided facial droop and a right-sided hemiparesis. While he is recovering from what appears to be a CVA, his wife tells you that she is sure that the lead exposure caused the stroke. What is the correct response to her?

A. She is probably right. Check a lead level immediately.
B. She is probably wrong. Lead exposure only causes peripheral neuropathies.
C. She is wrong. It is uncommon for occupational exposures to cause focal neurological problems such as strokes. It would be more common to see non-focal or multifocal problems due to lead exposure including encephalopathy or motor neuropathy.
D. She is right. Lead can cause encephalopathy, so why not strokes?

QUESTION 3. A 60-year-old city employee with a desk job presents to your office several times over a few months. He has a bad cough. Initially, you treat symptomatically, and he gets a bit better, but the cough continues, progressing to frank shortness of breath. He has decreased O_2 sat and some fine crackles on exam. A chest x-ray, which was initially normal, shows interstitial changes, and his computed tomography (CT) scan is consistent with hypersensitivity pneumonitis. He works in an old building, and his office has some water damage from a recent roof leak. He definitely feels better when he's on vacation. He is even better on the weekend. There are a few other employees with similar symptoms. He has no other respiratory diseases, and he does not smoke or use drugs.

The most likely cause of his hypersensitivity pneumonitis is:

A. Rodent proteins (found in droppings)
B. Thermophilic Actinomycetes
C. Fungal species such as aspergillus, penicillium, and others
D. B or C are most likely
E. It is probably not occupationally related because it is not a widespread problem at work.

QUESTION 4. Routine serum transaminases should be followed for workers who are potentially exposed to liver toxins in the workplace.

   A. True—it is the best way to find and treat disease before real problems happen.
   B. False—some occupations might benefit from baseline serum LFTs, but routine testing in the absence of specific exposure or high-level exposure is not recommended. LFTs are not very specific.
   C. True, but only in employees who drink more than seven drinks a week.

QUESTION 5. A retired asbestos removal contractor is in your office. He has numerous chronic illnesses including heart disease and type 2 diabetes. He smokes about a pack a day. You advise him that smoking actually multiplies the level of risk that he might have to get lung cancer from his long-ago asbestos exposures. "Come on, Doc," he responds, "you're just trying to scare me into quitting again." Who is right?

   A. The patient—smoking does not increase your risk of asbestos-related lung cancer.
   B. The doctor—smoking multiplies the risk of asbestos-related lung cancer.

ANSWERS

1. E
2. C
3. D
4. B
5. B

100.

ALLERGY AND IMMUNOLOGY

Mariana C. Castells

ALLERGIC RHINITIS AND CONJUNCTIVITIS

Allergic rhinoconjunctivitis is the most common of the allergic diseases. It affects 20% of the population and is associated with allergic sensitivity mediated by the presence of specific IgE (to allergens such as pollen, dust mites, molds, cat, dog, and animal dander) bound to tissue mast cells. Cross-linking of specific IgE with allergens induces local mast cell degranulation and the release of powerful inflammatory mediators such as histamine, proteases, prostaglandins, leukotrienes, and cytokines. These mediators bind to tissue receptors and act locally (nose, eyes, oropharynx, and ears) to induce allergic symptoms such as clear bilateral nasal discharge, sneezing, and congestion. Nasal turbinates are pale and swollen. Pruritus is typically present and affects the nasal passages, the palate, the Eustachian tubes, and the eyes. Conjunctivitis with clear discharge and ear blockage are common symptoms. Symptoms can be seasonal or perennial: seasonal symptoms are associated with sensitivities to pollen from trees, grasses, and weeds, whereas perennial symptoms are associated with sensitivities to indoor allergens such as dust mites, cat and dog dander, and molds such as *Aspergillus* and *Alternaria* species. Allergic rhinoconjunctivitis is associated with asthma in a substantial proportion of patients. One study reported that 28% of patients with asthma have allergic rhinitis, and 17% of patients with allergic rhinitis have asthma.

The diagnosis is made based on clinical symptoms and by the presence of a positive response to prick and intradermal skin testing with a battery of standard allergens.

The differential diagnosis of allergic rhinitis includes infectious rhinitis, cholinergic rhinitis, and sinusitis. The treatment includes environmental control and allergen avoidance, pharmacological agents, and allergen-specific immunotherapy. In sensitized patients, removal of furry animals from the house can completely eliminate the symptoms. Intranasal medications include steroids and antihistamines. Oral nonsedating H1 histamine receptor antagonists include loratadine, desloratadine, zetiricine, and fexofenadine. In addition, oral decongestants, nasal mast cell stabilizers, including cromo-

lyn sodium, ocular agents, including olopatidine, and intranasal anticholinergics, including ipratropium bromide, can help control symptoms. Allergen vaccination or immunotherapy is indicated to provide long-term relief of symptoms in qualified patients (see below).

ASTHMA

The Global Initiative for Asthma was formed in 1993 under the auspices of the National Heart, Lung, and Blood Institute and the World Health Organization aimed at decreasing the chronic disability and premature deaths associated with asthma. The first workshop lead to the Global Strategy for Asthma Management and Prevention (GINA), which published its initial report with the classification of asthma severity and the recommendations for its treatment in 1995. Since then there have been several updates, the last one in 2009, that established a comprehensive asthma management plan and emphasized the critical importance of inhaled steroids. Asthma is a chronic disorder of the airway associated with hyperresponsiveness and recurrent episodes of reversible airflow obstruction. Depending on the severity, airflow limitation is associated with shortness of breath, wheezing, chest tightness, and cough and can resolve spontaneously or with medications. The classification includes four degrees of severity. In *mild intermittent asthma* a patient has brief exacerbations, nocturnal symptoms no more than twice per month, and normal pulmonary function tests between episodes. *Mild persistent asthmatics* experience symptoms more than once per week but less than once per day. The nocturnal symptoms are twice per month but less than once per week, and there is normal lung function between episodes. *Moderate persistent asthmatics* have daily symptoms, exacerbations may be affecting activity and sleep, and the nocturnal symptoms occur at least once per week. FEV_1 can vary between 60% and 80% of the predictive pulmonary peak flow meter values. Patients with *severe persistent asthma* have daily symptoms, frequent exacerbations, daily nocturnal symptoms, and an FEV_1 <60% of the predictive, or peak flow is <60% of the best.

Factors affecting asthma severity include exposure to environmental allergens, tobacco (passive and active smoking), air pollution (outdoors: sulfur dioxide, ozone, nitrogen oxides; indoors: fumes from wood stoves, kerosene, volatile organic compounds), diesel exhaust, presence of rhinitis or sinusitis, gastroesophageal reflux, medications such as beta blockers, occupational exposure, and viral infections.

Death-prone asthmatics include those with prior intubations, those who overuse bronchodilators (more than one canister per month of rapid onset of action bronchodilator), and those with food allergies.

IMMUNOTHERAPY FOR THE TREATMENT OF ALLERGIC ASTHMA AND RHINOCONJUNCTIVITIS

Immunotherapy with allergen-specific vaccinations blunts seasonal increase in IgE levels and increases allergen-specific IgG and interleukin (IL)-10. Immune protection is generated by switching from a Th2 (IL-4 and IL-5 mediated) to an IL-10-mediated T regulatory cell–driven response. Randomized trials have provided evidence that allergen immunotherapy has been successful in preventing symptoms of asthma and rhinitis in patients monosensitized to either ragweed, *Alternaria* mold, dust mites, or cat dander allergen. This treatment modality is also used in patients sensitized to multiple allergens who are refractory to environmental avoidance and pharmacological intervention. Recent data indicate that immunotherapy prevents the development of asthma in sensitized children and adolescents with allergic rhinitis. Immunotherapy includes weekly subcutaneous injections with increasing amounts of the allergens up to maintenance levels (varying from 1 to 13 μg of purified or recombinant allergenic proteins) and monthly injections for up to 5 years. Reduction of up to 80% of nasal, ocular, and respiratory symptoms can be achieved at that time. Sublingual immunotherapy, peptide vaccination (using T-cell peptides devoid of allergenic potential), and immunostimulatory DNA (unmethylated DNA containing CpG motifs active through TLR9 on dendritic cells) are being considered to improve safety and efficacy of conventional immunotherapy. New therapies include a humanized monoclonal antibody against IgE, which was FDA approved in March 2003, for moderate to severe persistent asthma in patients with FEV_1 <80%, elevated IgE, and evidence of allergen-specific IgE.

ASTHMA AND ASPIRIN SENSITIVITY: ASPIRIN-EXACERBATED RESPIRATORY DISEASE

Up to 20% of all adult asthmatics have aspirin sensitivity and present an acute asthma flare on aspirin and cyclo-oxygenase (COX)-1/COX-2 nonsteroidal anti-inflammatory drug (NSAID) exposure. These asthmatics present with the triad initially described by Samter including moderate persistent to severe asthma, nasal polyposis with loss of smell, and aspirin and NSAID intolerance. Chronic rhinosinusitis is also present in the majority of patients. On exposure to aspirin and nonsteroidal anti-inflammatory medications, the FEV_1 decreases by 12% or more. Elevated numbers of eosinophils and increased expression of LTC_4 synthase (which generates the leukotrienes LTC_4, D_4, and E_4) in the polyps and increased leukotrienes in urine and bronchoalveolar lavage (BAL) fluid are characteristic. The management of these patients includes 5-lipoxygenase blockade or leukotriene receptor antagonists and surgery. For patients with recurrent nasal polyposis with multiple surgeries who do not recover the sense of smell, or whose asthma is not well controlled, aspirin desensitization is recommended. Aspirin is slowly reintroduced to induce a controlled reaction, which produces unresponsiveness to full doses. Increased doses up to 1200 mg daily are used to maintain the desensitization state. Cross-desensitization to all nonsteroidal anti-inflammatory drugs is achieved by aspirin desensitization.

URTICARIA AND ANGIOEDEMA

Urticaria is characterized by the presence of hives that can be acute (<6 weeks) or chronic (>6 weeks) (figure 100.1). The lesions are variable in size (>3 mm), macular, round or with geographic shape and central clearing, very pruritic, and of short duration, <24 hours. Upper and lower extremities are mostly affected, and palms, soles, face, and neck can be spared. Angioedema can be associated with urticaria in up to 50% of the cases and presents with deep dermis swelling and pain. Degranulation of dermal mast cells is the pathological finding of urticaria and angioedema lesions, but mononuclear cells, eosinophils, and basophils can also infiltrate. In contrast, urticarial vasculitis presents with small vessel vasculitis and lesions of urticaria lasting >24 hours and resolving with bruising.

Acute urticaria is a short-lived disease in which a cause is found in fewer than 20% of the cases. Drugs such as aspirin and NSAIDs, foods (egg, milk, peanut, nuts, seafood, and shellfish), infections, bacterial, and viral (hepatitis B and C [HBV/HCV]) infections, and contact (pollen from trees, grass, and weeds, animal dander and saliva) are the most common causes.

Chronic urticaria is a long-lived and recurrent disease in which the cause is found in <10% of cases. Urticaria occurs in episodes and can last days to months. Triggers are not apparent except for the physical urticarias, in which symptoms are induced by physical activity, changes in temperature, or solar exposure. Physical urticarias include symptomatic dermatographism as well as delayed-pressure, cholinergic, exercise-induced, cold-induced, solar, aquagenic, and vibratory symptoms.

More recently, autoimmune forms of chronic urticaria have been described in patients with IgG antibodies against the IgE receptor or soluble IgE. The diagnosis is made by the autologous serum skin test in which autologous serum

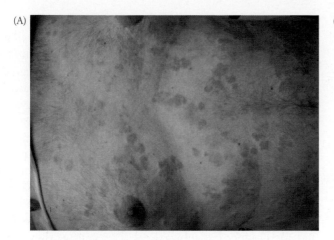

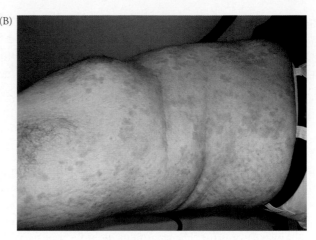

Figure 100.1. Examples of Urticaria.

is injected under the skin to produce a wheal-and-flare reaction (see figure 100.2), and the treatment includes steroids and hydroxychloroquine.

Hashimoto thyroiditis with elevated antiperoxidase and antimicrosomal antibodies and Graves disease have been associated with chronic and recurrent urticaria. Thyroid replacement is most effective in the forms associated with hypothyroidism. Cryoglobulinemia, connective tissue diseases (lupus, leukocytoclastic vasculitis), and malignancies (multiple myeloma, plasmocytoma) have been associated with chronic urticaria through the generation of complement fragments C3a and C5a (anaphylotoxins), which can activate mast cells.

The treatment of urticaria includes anti–histamine H1 receptor antagonist (nonsedating and sedating), H2 antagonists such as ranitidine and cimetidine, and doxepin. Leukotriene receptor antagonists (montelukast, zafirlukast) and corticosteroids on alternate days can be added to increase efficacy. Severe cases and cases unresponsive to conventional therapies should be treated with colchicine, dapsone, hydroxychloroquine, sulfasalazine, cyclosporine, plasmapheresis, or IV immunoglobulin (IVIG). Levothyroxine in nonhypothyroid Hashimoto associated with chronic urticaria has been

used with variable results. Recently cold-induced urticaria has been successfully treated with anti-IgE (omalizumab).

ANGIOEDEMA

Angioedema not associated with urticaria can be hereditary or acquired. In hereditary angioedema there is a mutation of the serpin gene inducing decreased or absent C1 inhibitor (C1INH) (type I: 85% of patients) or presenting with normal C1 inhibitor but deficient in function (type II: 15% of patients). More than 100 mutations have been identified, and 20–25% of cases are new spontaneous mutations. Type III or estrogen-dependent angioedema is a hereditary form of angioedema seen in females in kindreds, with symptoms that mimic C1INH deficiency but with normal C1INH levels and function and normal C4. The syndrome is associated with activating mutations of factor XII. In the acquired form of angioedema there is an excessive consumption of a C1INH. The consumption can be due to a malignancy or the presence of IgG and/or anti-idiotypic antibodies secreted from lymphoma B cells that inhibit the function of C1INH.

Symptoms of hereditary and acquired angioedema include episodic swelling of the head, face, neck, extremities, and gastrointestinal tract with abdominal pain, nausea, vomiting, responsive to fluids and narcotics. Laryngeal edema is the most severe complication and can lead to asphyxia when intubation or tracheotomy is delayed. Bradykinin levels in serum are elevated in hereditary forms and are thought to be the cause of tissue swelling.

The diagnosis is made by the measurement of complement levels. In hereditary angioedema C4 level is decreased, C1 inhibitor can be decreased but may be present in nonfunctional forms, C1q is always present and in the normal range, and C2 may be decreased. In the acquired forms C4 is low, as well as C1q and C1 inhibitor. C2 levels may be decreased.

During acute attacks of pain and tissue swelling, fresh frozen plasma (FFP), epsilon-aminocaproic acid, purified C1INH or recombinant C1INH, and kinin and bradykinin receptor inhibitors have been proven effective. The

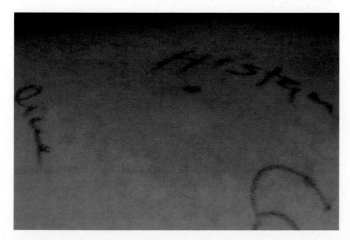

Figure 100.2. Typical Wheal-and-Flare Reaction. Reaction (upper right corner) to skin test with histamine (positive control).

latter therapies are available in Europe and are under FDA review for approval in the United States. Long-term management includes androgenic steroids such as danazol and stanozolol. Epinephrine and steroids are not helpful.

ALLERGIC BRONCHOPULMONARY ASPERGILLOSIS: ABPA

The disease presents with asthma, pulmonary infiltrates, and central bronchiectasis. It is associated with elevated total serum IgE above 1000 ng/mL, peripheral eosinophilia, positive skin tests to *Aspergillus*, and the presence of IgG precipitins against *Aspergillus*. The treatment includes oral steroids and, in refractory cases, antifungals. There is an association between cystic fibrosis and ABPA in HLA-DR patients.

FOOD ALLERGY

Food allergy is defined as a hypersensitivity reaction to a specific food which is reproduced upon re-exposure in sensitized individuals and is due to a specific immune response to food allergens. Some allergens from fruits and vegetables elicit reactions when consumed raw but can be tolerated cooked. Nuts, seafood, shellfish and grains retain their allergenic potential even after cooking. Symptoms of food allergy can be elicited by ingestion of cross-reactive foods, which share common allergenic epitopes. Oral allergy syndrome occurs in patients allergic to pollen (such as birch tree pollen) who react when eating raw fruits such as apples due to sensitization to the common profilin antigens. Symptoms of food allergy include urticaria, angioedema, nausea, vomiting, diarrhea, wheezing, sneezing, anaphylaxis, reactivation of atopic dermatitis/eczema, eosinophilic gastrointestinal syndromes, food protein-induced allergic proctocolitis, food protein-induced enterocolitis and Heiner syndrome. The prevalence of food allergy in the United States is increasing, with 0.6% of the population sensitized to peanuts. The prevalence of seafood allergy is higher in females with 2.6% versus 1.5% in males. Milk, egg, soy, and wheat allergy are typically outgrown in puberty. Avoidance is the only treatment and allergic individuals need to wear labeling at all times and carry autoinjectable epinephrine. Asthmatic patients who have food allergy are at risk for death from anaphylaxis.

ANAPHYLAXIS

Anaphylaxis is an underreported and underrecognized medical emergency caused by the acute release of mediators from mast cells and basophils that involves more than one organ system or presents with laryngeal edema that can lead to cardiovascular collapse, asphyxia, and death in minutes unless treated.

The symptoms include flushing, pruritus, urticaria, angioedema, rhinoconjunctivitis, bronchospasm, abdominal pain, nausea, vomiting, diarrhea, and dizziness and can progress to respiratory failure, hypotension, cardiovascular shock, organ failure, seizures, disseminated intravascular coagulation (DIC), and death. Asphyxia due to laryngeal edema can be the presenting symptom. The major risk factor for fatal anaphylaxis is asthma, but a previous severe reaction, the usage of beta blockers, and the usage of angiotensin-converting enzyme (ACE) inhibitors have also been associated with fatal outcomes. The incidence of fatal anaphylaxis in the general population is 0.002% for drugs such as penicillin, 0.001% for hymenoptera, which induce 40 deaths per year, and food-induced anaphylaxis, with peanut as the leading offending food. Nonfatal anaphylaxis occurs in 1:2700 hospitalizations and can be due either to hymenoptera stings, radiocontrast media, penicillin and other antibiotics, general anesthesia, or hemodialysis as well as latex exposure. Other causes of IgE-induced anaphylaxis include nuts, seafood, and milk, allergy extracts, hymenoptera venom and fire ants, vaccines, and hormones. Chemotherapy drugs such as platin derivatives (carboplatin, cisplatin, and oxaliplatin), taxanes (paclitaxel, docetaxel), and monoclonal antibodies have also been shown to induce anaphylaxis in recent years.

Other causes of non-IgE-mediated anaphylaxis include complement activation and direct mast cell activation by radiocontrast media, curare derivatives, vancomycin, opiate metabolites, COX-1, COX-2 inhibitors such as aspirin and nonsteroidal anti-inflammatory medications. Latex-associated reactions and/or food cross reactivity include banana, chestnut, avocado, kiwi, mango, passion fruit, papaya, peach, watermelon, potato, and tomato. Healthcare workers, rubber industry workers, and spina bifida patients with urogenital abnormalities with multiple surgeries are at higher risk for latex allergy and anaphylaxis.

The diagnosis of anaphylaxis includes, in the acute phase, the serum elevation of total tryptase >15 ng/mL or mature tryptase >1 ng/mL. The sample needs to be collected within 1–2 hours of the hypotensive event. Histamine can be elevated in 24-hour urine collection; complement activation or hemoconcentration with postcapillary leakage can also be found.

Retrospective diagnosis of anaphylaxis includes antigen-specific IgE measured in serum and skin testing. Testing for latex includes the measurement in serum of specific IgE with 38–82% sensitivity and skin test, which is not available in the United States.

HYMENOPTERA ALLERGY AND ANAPHYLAXIS

The natural history of hymenoptera sting allergy is that re-sting reactions occur only in 60% of the patients who reacted initially. The more severe the initial anaphylactic reaction, the more likely there will be a re-sting reaction, and the severity of the sting reaction is not related to the degree of skin test sensitivity or the titer of the serum venom-specific IgE. Tryptase elevations are associated with the most severe of hymenoptera venom reactions that include hypotension and cardiovascular collapse. Some patients with mastocytosis will present initially as anaphylaxis to hymenoptera sting. The risk of systemic reactions to sting for patients treated with venom immunotherapy decreases to <10% as compared to patients treated conservatively, in whom re-sting reactions can induce up to 60% systemic reactions.

MANAGEMENT OF ANAPHYLAXIS

Epinephrine is the gold standard treatment for anaphylaxis and failure or delay in its administration results in prolonged hypotension, cardiovascular collapse or death. Epinephrine should be administered intramuscularly in the cuadriceps musle at 0.3 mL of a 1/1000 solution and repeated twice at 5 minutes intervals for prolonged hypotension. Intravenous administration should be reserved for cardiovascular collapse since Tako Tsubo and Kounis syndromes with cardiac failure have been reported during anaphylaxis after intravenous epinephrine. Adequate oxygenation with nebulized O_2 agonist and monitoring of cardiac output and tissue perfusion. The treatment includes adequate oxygenation and nebulized bronchodilators, monitoring cardiac output and tissue perfusion and the use of antihistamine H1 and H2 blockade with 25–50 mg of diphenhydramine IM or IV, ranitidine 150 mg, and methylprednisolone IV 0.5 to 1 mg/kg. If beta blockade is present, glucagon, 5–15 μg per minute IV in continuous infusion, should be administered, and the patient with anaphylaxis should be observed for 6–12 hours due to delayed reactions. After discharge, education to avoid future reactions, referral for an allergy consultation, and an auto injectable epinephrine prescription are mandatory. Patients taking ACE inhibitors or beta blockers are recommended to change the antihypertensive medication.

EXERCISE-INDUCED ANAPHYLAXIS

Exercise-induced anaphylaxis (EIA) is a syndrome in which patients will present with flushing, itching, and shortness of breath as well as associated hypotension while exercising. Exercises implicated in EIA include running, biking, hiking, and even dancing. In >30% of those patients there is an associated food ingestion prior to the anaphylactic event, and the most commonly implicated food is wheat. Management of those patients includes the immediate discontinuation of exercise and the use of epinephrine. The management of EIA includes limitation of exercise on hot humid days, the avoidance of food 4–6 hours before exercise, and avoidance of exercise postallergy immunotherapy, as well as avoidance of beta blockers and ACE inhibitors. Epinephrine reverses most of the reactions, and the patients need to wear or carry a bracelet with identification of the condition and treatment plan. Investigation of the food associated with EIA reactions is mandatory.

ADVERSE REACTIONS TO MEDICATIONS

Common drugs that may cause adverse reactions include penicillin and beta-lactam antibiotics, which do so through IgE-mediated reactions. There is at least a 3–11% cross-reactivity between cephalosporins and penicillin, and aztreonam is cross-reactive with ceftazidime. Aspirin and nonsteroidal anti-inflammatory medications have universal cross-reactivity, and bradykinin has been implicated in ACE-inhibitor-induced angioedema and induced respiratory disease. The diagnosis of adverse drug reactions includes skin testing for penicillin and other beta-lactams and graded challenges when the probability of a reaction is low. The managcment is avoidance and the use of a bracelet or chain with the identified medication.

Cancer patients and patients with chronic inflammatory diseases who need first-line therapy and cystic fibrosis patients requiring specific antibiotics to which they have presented anaphylactic reactions are candidates for rapid desensitization. Cardiac patients in need of aspirin are also candidates. Rapid desensitizations are high-risk procedures in which patients with known hypersensitivity reactions to a particular medication including chemotherapy, monoclonal antibodies, antibiotics, aspirin, or others need the medication for first-line therapy. In those patients a three 10-fold dilution solutions and 12 steps standardized protocol have been used, and the procedures require initial administration in the intensive care unit. This standard protocol has been devised that has been used for over 413 cases recently published. The safety and efficacy of this protocol indicates that 94% of the patient's ongoing rapid desensitization presents mild or no symptoms, and only 6% of the patients require medications through the desensitization procedure.

MASTOCYTOSIS

Mastocytosis presents as a local (cutaneous or other tissues) or systemic hyperplasia of mast cells and can be clonal due to a mutation of the surface mast cell receptor c-kit. Urticaria pigmentosa is the most common of cutaneous mastocytosis and involves 1- to 3-mm brown/tanned nonconfluent lesions in upper and lower extremities that present positive Darier's sign on stroking (wheal and flare reaction). Systemic mastocytosis presents typically with accumulations of mast cells in the bone marrow, gastrointestinal tract, lymph nodes and bones, and common symptoms of mastocytosis include pruritus, flushing, abdominal pain, diarrhea, mental fogginess, and bone pain. The treatment is aimed at controlling mast cell mediator–related symptoms with antihistamine H1 and H2 receptor blockers, cromolyn sodium, and leukotriene inhibitors. Patients with cutaneous mastocytosis and associated symptoms should be ruled out for systemic mastocytosis by bone marrow biopsy. The diagnostic criteria include major criterion of multifocal infiltrates of 15 or more mast cells in bone marrow or in extracutaneous organs. Four minor criteria include mast cell aggregates in which 25% of the mast cells are spindle shaped, the presence of *c-kit* D86V mutation, and the aberrant expression of CD2 and CD25 lymphocyte markers on mast cells by flow cytometry as well as tryptase levels of 20 ng/mL in the absence of anaphylactic symptoms.

A new syndrome of clonal mast cell activation (MCAS) has been described, in which *c-kit* mutation D816V is found on bone marrow mast cells or peripheral mast cell precursors cells in patients with symptoms of mast cell activation but negative bone marrow findings and normal tryptase levels.

IMMUNODEFICIENCIES

The most common of immunodeficiencies found in adult patients includes common variable immunedeficiency (CVID). It is associated with infections of the sinuses and lungs including two or more episodes a year of sinusitis, one or two episodes of pneumonia, urinary tract infections, and deep-seated infections. The presence of levels of IgG, IgA, and IgM that are 2 SD below the normal range makes the diagnosis; poor responses to pneumonia vaccine, *Haemophilus influenzae,* or hepatitis. The treatment includes replacement with gamma-globulin, subcutaneously or intravenously at 400 mg/kg every 3–4 weeks. Recently a molecular defect has been associated with TACI, in which there is increased association with autoimmune diseases and lymphoma.

ADDITIONAL READING

Agrawal DK, Shao Z. Pathogenesis of allergic airway inflammation. *Curr Allergy Asthma Rep.* 2010;10(1):39–48.

Boyce JA, Assa'ad A, Burks AW, et al. Guidelines for the diagnosis and management of food allergy in the United States: Summary of the NIAID Sponsored Expert Panel Report. *J Allergy Clin Immunol.* 2010 Dec;126(6 Suppl):S1–58.

Castells MC, Tennant NM, Sloane DE, et al. Hypersensitivity reactions to chemotherapy: outcomes and safety of rapid desensitization in 413 cases. *J Allergy Clin Immunol.* 2008;122: 574–80.

Chinen J, Shearer WT. Advances in basic and clinical immunology in 2009. *J Allergy Clin Immunol.* 2010;125(3):563–8.

Georas SN, Rezaee F, Lerner L, Beck L. Dangerous allergens: Why some allergens are bad actors. *Curr Allergy Asthma Rep.* 2010;10(2):92–8.

Railey MD, Burks AW. Therapeutic approaches for the treatment of food allergy. *Expert Opin Pharmacother.* 2010;11(7):1045–8.

National Institute of Allergy and Infectious Diseases. http://www.niaid.nih.gov/topics/foodAllergy/clinical/Documents/FAGuidelinesExecSummary.pdf. Accessed December 13, 2010.

Worth A, Soar J, Sheikh A. Management of anaphylaxis in the emergency setting. *Expert Rev Clin Immunol.* 2010;6(1):89–100.

QUESTIONS

QUESTION 1. A 20-year-old female who is actively trying to become pregnant sees you in the office for advice on what medications she should take for management of her asthma while she is pregnant. She currently reports symptoms of asthma two times per week that are partially relieved by rescue inhaler use. She denies nighttime symptoms and any emergency room visits in the past year. She reports symptoms of seasonal allergic rhinitis. Examination is unremarkable.

Which medication would you recommend?

A. Fluticasone salmeterol inhaler
B. Fexofenadine
C. Budesonide inhaler
D. Formoterol inhaler

QUESTION 2. A neighbor calls the emergency medical technicians (EMTs) to report that a white male in his early 50s has fallen off his ladder while cleaning gutters in his house. When the EMTs arrive he reports generalized body hives, has audible wheezing, and then passes out. His systolic blood pressure is noted to be 70 mm Hg per EMS. He has an urticarial rash over his body. A nest of wasps is found near the patient. He is given a bolus of IV fluids immediately and epinephrine intramuscular and he recovers. Tryptase level drawn 1 hour after he collapsed is 30 ng/ml. The most likely diagnosis is:

A. Reaction to poison ivy
B. Anaphylactic shock from wasp sting
C. Cardiac arrhythmia
D. Pulmonary embolus

QUESTION 3. A 62-year-old African-American female with a history of type 2 diabetes mellitus is evaluated in the emergency department with abrupt swelling of her upper lip that she noticed when she woke up in the morning. The patient denies any dyspnea, hoarseness, sore throat, wheezing, or rash. She says that she has recently been started on lisinopril to manage her high blood pressure. Physical examination reveals upper lip swelling but is otherwise unremarkable. A diagnosis of lisinopril-associated angioedema is made. Which one of the following statements is correct?

A. There is a high level of cross-reactivity between an ACE inhibitor (lisinopril) and angiotensin receptor blockers (ARBs), and consequently switching to losartan is contraindicated.
B. African Americans are more susceptible than white patients to ACE inhibitor–associated angioedema.
C. C4 level is typically decreased in patients with ACE inhibitor–associated angioedema.
D. C1 inhibitor (C1INH) level should be abnormally low.

ANSWERS

1. C
2. B
3. B

101.

PSYCHIATRY ESSENTIALS FOR THE INTERNIST

Brijmohan K. Phull and Rattna K. Phull

Mood disorders, anxiety disorders, and somatoform disorders are common psychiatric conditions confronting general physicians in the outpatient setting. In the inpatient setting, the most common problems are delirium, dementia, mood and anxiety disorders, adjustment reactions to illness, and substance abuse. Mood disorders include various depressive disorders and bipolar disorder.

DEPRESSION

Depression is a major public health problem and a leading cause of functional disability and mortality. The lifetime incidence of major depressive disorder is estimated at 20% in women and 12% in men, with a prevalence of approximately 10% in patients in a medical setting. Most adults with clinically significant depression do not see a mental health provider; instead, they often first present to a primary care physician. However, a substantial number of depressed patients remain undiagnosed or undertreated.

DIAGNOSIS

Major depression manifests as a depressed mood or a loss of interest or pleasure in all or most activities, present most of the day, nearly every day, for a minimum of 2 consecutive weeks, as well as at least five of the following nine symptoms: change in sleep, change in appetite or weight, change in psychomotor activity, loss of energy, loss of interest, guilt, trouble concentrating, and thoughts about death or suicide. Eight of these symptoms (all but depressed mood) may be readily recalled using the mnemonic "SIG: E CAPS": Sleep, Interest, Guilt, Energy, Concentration, Appetite, Psychomotor agitation or retardation, Suicide.

Table 101.1 lists the *Diagnostic and Statistical Manual of Mental Disorders (DSM-IV-TR)* diagnostic criteria for a major depressive episode. These criteria for depressive disorders, as with other mental disorders, require that the depressive episode cause significant distress or dysfunction. There is

a spectrum of depressive disorders, and the following is a guide to diagnosis and to determine treatment.

Dysthymic disorder is characterized by at least 2 years of depressed mood for more days than not accompanied by an additional two of the following symptoms: poor appetite, insomnia or hypersomnia, low energy or fatigue, low self-esteem, poor concentration, difficulty making decisions, and feelings of hopelessness. These depressive symptoms do not meet the criteria for major depression, as the patient is still able to function, and the symptoms are not totally disabling.

Adjustment disorder with depressed mood is a reaction that develops in response to an identifiable psychosocial stressor. The severity of depression and degree of impairment do not always parallel the intensity of the precipitating event. Treatment is usually supportive psychotherapy, psychosocial intervention, and antidepressants in some cases.

Mood disorder due to a general medical disorder is characterized by a prominent and persistent disturbance in mood that is judged to be a direct physiological consequence of a general medical condition. Mood disorder due to a general medical condition increases the risk of attempted and completed suicide (DSM-IV-TR). The magnitude of this is dependent on the particulars of the condition such as whether it is an incurable and painful condition.

Substance-induced mood disorder is characterized by prominent and persistent disturbance in mood that is judged to be direct physiological consequence of a drug of abuse, a medication, another medical treatment, or toxin exposure. Some medications such as stimulants, steroids, and L-dopa can cause mania, and medications such as alphamethyldopa and interferon can cause depression.

SCREENING FOR DEPRESSION

There are several screening instruments available for use in primary care settings, including the Center for Epidemiologic Studies Depression Scale (CES-D) and the Geriatric Depression Scale (GDS).

Table 101.1 THE DSM-IV-TR DIAGNOSTIC CRITERIA FOR A MAJOR DEPRESSIVE EPISODE

A. At least 5 of the following, during the same 2-week period, representing a change from previous functioning; must include either (a) or (b):

   (a) Depressed mood

   (b) Diminished interest or pleasure

   (c) Significant weight loss or gain

   (d) Insomnia or hypersomnia

   (e) Psychomotor agitation or retardation

   (f) Fatigue or loss of energy

   (g) Feelings of worthlessness

   (h) Diminished ability to think or concentrate; indecisiveness

   (i) Recurrent thoughts of death, suicidal ideation, suicide attempt, or specific plan for suicide

B. Symptoms do not meet criteria for a mixed episode (i.e., meet criteria for both manic and depressive episode).

C. Symptoms cause clinically significant distress or impairment of functioning.

D. Symptoms are not due to the direct physiological effects of a substance or a general medical condition.

E. Symptoms are not better accounted for by bereavement, i.e., the symptoms persist for longer than 2 months or are characterized by marked functional impairment, morbid preoccupation with worthlessness, suicidal ideation, psychotic symptoms, or psycho-motor retardation.

SOURCE: Reprinted with permission from *Diagnostic and Statistical Manual of Mental Disorders,* 4th ed., Text Revision (DSM-IV-TR). Copyright 2000 American Psychiatric Association.

SUICIDE

Suicide is a major public health problem: it is the eighth leading cause of death in the United States. The suicide rate in the United States has averaged 12.5/100,000. Those 65 years and older have the highest risk of committing suicide. The suicide rate for the elderly is 50% higher than the rate for teenagers or the U.S. national average.

Recognizing the suicidal patient can be challenging in primary care settings. No studies have demonstrated that screening for suicidality in the primary care setting reduces completed suicides or attempts. Depression screening and severity assessment instruments such as Patient Health Questionnaire (PHQ-9) and the Quick Inventory of Depressive Symptomatology (QIDS) include questions about suicidal ideation that can trigger further inquiry by the physician. Because we do not have instruments that predict which patients with suicidal thoughts will attempt suicide, once such thoughts are recognized, further inquiry and physician judgment should determine any intervention.

Seventy-five percent of patients who committed suicide had contact with their primary care providers in the year of their death compared to one-third who had contact with a mental health service. Similarly, twice as may suicide victims had contact with their primary care providers as mental health services the month before their suicide.

Suicide Assessment

Risk Factors
Suicide is most commonly viewed as a multidetermined act. Risk factors include psychiatric disorder, social factors, psychological factors, biological factors, genetic factors, and physical disorder.

Past Attempts
Previous attempts increase the likelihood of future attempts by five to six times.

Psychiatric Diagnosis
Patients with multiple psychiatric conditions appear to be at higher risk than those with uncomplicated depression or anxiety. Anxiety disorders double the risk of suicide attempt (odds ratio = 2.2), but the combination of depression and anxiety greatly increases the risk (odds ratio = 17). The suicide risk is high among schizophrenic patients: up to 10% die by committing suicide. Alcoholics have an increased risk of suicide, with a lifetime risk of 2.2–3.4%, and those who have comorbid depression are particularly at high risk.

Age, Sex, Race
Older men are three times more likely than women to complete suicide, although women attempt suicide four times more often than men. Ninety percent of completed suicides are by white people in the United States.

Work Status
Unemployed and unskilled individuals are at increased risk.

Impulsivity
Impulsivity increases the likelihood of acting on suicidal thoughts, and the combination of hopelessness, impulsivity, and substance abuse–related disinhibition may be particularly lethal, and this combination occurs frequently in young adults.

Health
Medical illness, including chronic pain, chronic disease, and recent surgery, increases the suicide risk.

Family Factors
Having a first-degree relative who committed suicide increases the risk sixfold. Individuals who have never married are at highest risk for completed suicide, followed in

descending order by those who are widowed, separated, or divorced.

Abuse and other adverse experiences during childhood increase the risk for suicide in adults.

Access to Means

Of all the suicides in the United States, 57% are caused by a firearm. The second leading methods of suicide is in the United States are hanging in men and poisoning in women.

Hopelessness

Hopelessness may contribute to suicide, independent of depression.

Protective Factors

Family connectedness and social support are protective. Parenthood, particularly for mothers, and pregnancy decrease the risk of suicide. Participating in religious activities and religiosity are associated with lower risk for suicide.

Management of the suicidal patient includes

1. Reducing immediate risk;

2. Managing underlying risk factors;

3. Monitoring follow-up.

Reducing immediate risk may require psychiatric hospitalization. Once the patient is less acute, then underlying factors such as depression, alcohol abuse, and other psychiatric problems should be addressed. The patient will need a regular follow-up.

TREATMENT OF DEPRESSION IN ADULTS

Psychotherapy

The two forms of psychotherapy that have been used extensively for treating depression and that have shown efficacy are cognitive behavioral therapy (CBT) and interpersonal therapy (IPT). These therapies on their own are recommended for patients suffering from mild to moderate depression. Studies have shown that a combination of therapy with antidepressants has a much better outcome than mediations alone.

Cognitive Therapy

In depression, patients see themselves, their experiences, and their future in negative ways, which in turn sustains and magnifies their depressive symptomatology.

Cognitive therapy employs specific treatment strategies to correct these habitual thinking errors found in different psychopathological states. Treatment helps patients achieve a better integration of cognition (thoughts), emotion, and behavior. Patients treated with a combination of antidepressants and CBT have more sustained recoveries than those who are treated with antidepressant alone.

Interpersonal Therapy

Interpersonal therapy is useful for patients who face conflicts with significant others or who are having difficulty adjusting to a life transition. The clinical practice guidelines for treatment of depression in the primary care setting recommend interpersonal psychotherapy for short-term treatment of nonpsychotic depression, to remove symptoms, prevent relapse and recurrence, correct causal psychological problems with secondary symptom resolution, and correct secondary consequences of depression.

Another form of psychotherapy, problem-solving treatment, appears to be effective according to the Depression Guideline Panel of the Agency for the Health Care Policy and Research (AHCPR).

Antidepressants

The major classes of drugs used to treat depression are selective serotonin reuptake inhibitors (SSRIs), tricyclic antidepressants, monoamine oxidase inhibitors (MAO), and serotonin and norepinephrine reuptake inhibitors (SNRIs).

Choice of Antidepressant

SSRIs are often the first choice in primary care because of fewer side effects and less danger with overdose. Patients will respond to the same antidepressant with which they were successfully treated in the past and will respond to the same antidepressant to which a first-degree relative has responded.

SSRIs selectively inhibit the reuptake of serotonin in central nervous system (CNS) neurons as well as peripherally, thereby increasing the stimulation of serotonin receptors (see table 101.2).

Serotonin norepinephrine reuptake inhibitors (SNRIs) inhibit the reuptake of serotonin and norepinephrine (see table 101.3).

Norepinephrine dopamine reuptake inhibitors (NDRIs) inhibit reuptake of norepinephrine and dopamine.

Monoamine oxidase inhibitors (MAOIs) irreversibly block the enzyme monoamine oxidase (MAO), the enzyme responsible for the oxidative deamination of neurotransmitters such as serotonin, norepinephrine, and dopamine (see table 101.4). *Secondary and tertiary amine tricyclic antidepressants* tend to block both serotonin and nor-epinephrine. Their use is limited because of their side effects and lethality in overdose.

Overview of Antidepressants

Table 101.5 presents an overview of antidepressants.

Drug Interactions

Some of the SSRIs such as fluoxetine and paroxetine inhibit the liver P450 enzymes leading either to increases in

Table 101.2 SELECTIVE SEROTONIN REUPTAKE INHIBITORS (SSRIs)

DRUG	TOXIC/ADVERSE EFFECTS	COMMENTS
SSRIs (selective serotonin reuptake inhibitors) Citalopram (Celexa) Escitalopram (Lexapro) Fluoxetine (Prozac) Paroxetine (Paxil) Sertraline (Zoloft)	CNS: Insomnia, agitation, Headaches and drowsiness GI upset, nausea, diarrhea. Sexual dysfunction Hyponatremia/SIADH in elderly. May impair platelet aggregation, increase bleeding. May increase upper GI bleeding in patients taking NSAIDs.	Relatively safe in overdose. Serotonin syndrome may occur with MAOIs, tramadol and triptans. Fluoxetine, paroxetine have P450 drug interactions. Discontinuation syndrome may occur with short-acting antidepressants.

Table 101.3 SEROTONIN NOREPINEPHRINE REUPTAKE INHIBITORS (SNRIs)

DRUG	TOXIC/ADVERSE EFFECTS	COMMENTS
SNRIs (serotonin norepinephrine reuptake inhibitors) Duloxetine (Cymbalta) Venlafaxine (Effexor)	Insomnia, GI upset, HA, sexual dysfunction; sustained increase in blood pressure.	Avoid use with MAOIs. Duloxetine may cause impairment in LFTs; LFT monitoring recommended.

Table 101.4 MONOAMINE OXIDASE INHIBITORS (MAOIs)

DRUG	TOXIC/ADVERSE EFFECTS	COMMENTS
MAOI (monoamine oxidase inhibitors): Phenelzine (Nardil) Tranylcypromine (Parnate)	Weight gain, orthostatic hypotension, sexual dysfunction. Hypertensive crisis may occur withtyramine-containing foods. Interactions with serotonergic medications lead to serotonin syndrome.	Limited use because of drug/food interactions with tyramine-containing foods such as aged cheeses, aged cured, meats, marmite, sauerkraut sauce, soy condiments, draft beer, improperly stored or spoiled meats, fish, or poultry, chianti.
Isocarboxazid (Marplan) Selegiline		Contraindicated with SSRIs, SNRIs, tricyclic antidepressants, alcohol, meperidine, triptans, general anesthesia.

Table 101.5 OVERVIEW OF ANTIDEPRESSANTS

DRUG	TOXIC/ADVERSE EFFECTS	COMMENTS
Selective serotonin reuptake inhibitors Citalopram (Celexa)	CNS: insomnia, agitation, headaches, drowsiness. GI upset, nausea, sexual dysfunction, hyponatremia/SIADH in elderly, impaired platelet aggregation may increase bleeding, increased bleeding in patients taking NSAIDs.	Relatively safe in overdose, Serotonin syndrome may occur with MAOIs, tramadol, triptans, Fluoxetine, paroxetine have 450 drug interactions and increase and inhibit the metabolism of drugs to active metabolite as in tamoxifen to endoxifen. Discontinuation may occur with short-acting antidepressants.
Serotonin norepinephrine reuptake inhibitors Duloxetine (Cymbalta) Venlafaxine	Insomnia, GI upset, HA, sexual dysfunction, sustained increase in blood pressure.	Avoid use of MAOIs. LFT monitoring recommended with duloxetine.
Monoamine oxidase inhibitors Phenelzine (Nardil) Tranylcypromine (Parnate) Isocarboxazid (Marplan) Selegiline	Weight gain, orthostatic hypotension, sexual dysfunction. Hypertensive crisis may occur with tyramine-containing foods. Interactions with serotonergic drugs lead to serotonin syndrome.	Limited use because of drug/food interactions with tyramine-containing foods such as aged cheeses, aged cured meats, marmite, sauerkraut, soy sauce, improperly stored meats, fish, and poultry.
Tricyclic antidepressants		
Tertiary amines Amitriptyline (Elavil) Imipramine (Tofranil) Doxepin (Sinequan) Secondary amines: Nortriptyline (Pamelor) Desipramine (Norpramin)	Potentially fatal in overdose, increased risk of seizures and arrhythmias, common anticholinergic side effects, weight gain, sedation, sexual dysfunction, orthostatic hypotension.	Blood monitoring indicated. Contraindicated with use of MAOIs and in patients with recent myocardial infarction.
Mirtazapine	Sedation, weight gain, some antinausea effects, rare incidence of agranulocytosis.	Helpful in depression associated with anxiety, insomnia, weight loss, agitation, nausea, severe depression.
Trazodone	Sedation, hypertension, dry mouth. Priapism is a rare side effect.	Mild antidepressant used mainly for insomnia, develop tolerance to it.

the levels of the drugs metabolized by these enzymes (such as increasing the levels of phenytoin or antiarrhythmics) or inhibiting the conversion to the active metabolite of drugs such as tamoxifen to endoxifen, codeine to morphine, thereby leading to ineffective levels of active drug.

Discontinuation Syndrome from SSRIs and SNRIs

Discontinuation reactions are more severe and more common with the short-acting drugs such as venlafaxine and paroxetine. Symptoms include vertigo, paresthesias, and shock-like feelings in the upper extremities and the neck. Other symptoms include myalgias, tremor, myoclonus, ataxia, visual changes, piloerection, nausea, vomiting, and diarrhea. Patients may complain of emotional lability. Symptoms are relieved by taking the antidepressant within a short period of time.

Tapering is recommended for all antidepressants but particularly for shorter-acting venlafaxine and paroxetine over a period of at least 3 months to prevent withdrawal. Relapse of symptoms usually recurs within about 6–8 weeks. Patients who have had one episode of depression are treated for 6–8 months after they have had a complete remission of symptoms; those who have had two episodes should be treated for 2–3 years; and those who have had three or more episodes should have lifelong treatment with antidepressants.

Recurrence Rate in Depression

Fifty percent of patients relapse after one episode of treated depression; 70% after two episodes of depression; and 90% relapse after three episodes.

Serotonin Syndrome

Serotonin syndrome (SS) is a potentially life-threatening condition associated with increased serotonergic activity in the CNS. The syndrome is characterized by the triad of mental status changes, autonomic hyperactivity, and neuromuscular abnormalities including hyperactivity, tremor, clonus, and hyperreflexia. It is typically caused by combining two or more serotonergic medications. The most common drug offenders are concomitant use with another SSRI, TCAs, MAOIs, triptans, ergot alkaloids, fentanyl, tramadol, amphetamines, levodopa, ondansetron, or granisetron. Treatment includes discontinuation of all serotonergic agents, supportive care in the ICU, hydration, treatment with benzodiazepines, and administration of serotonin antagonists. Resolution usually occurs within 24 hours.

Effects of SSRIs and Other Newer Antidepressants on Suicide Risk in Adults

Current studies are inadequate to conclusively prove or disprove the association between the newer antidepressants and suicidal ideation or behavior in adults. There is some evidence that treatment with SSRIs may increase the risk of nonfatal self-harm compared with placebo—but not compared with treatment with tricyclic antidepressants. Any absolute increase in the risk of nonfatal harm appears to be very small. At present, there is no compelling evidence indicating that SSRIs and other newer antidepressants increase the risk of suicidal ideation or completed suicide in adults. Given that the SSRIs and newer antidepressants have proven efficacy in the treatment of depression in adults, and that untreated depression is highly correlated with suicide risk, it is strongly recommended to continue use of these medications in the treatment of depressed patients.

BIPOLAR DISORDER

Recognition of bipolar disorder is important because it is associated with substantial morbidity and mortality, and treatment differs from that of unipolar depression. It is not uncommon for bipolar disorder to be underdetected, as patients tend to present with symptoms primarily of depression, especially in a primary care setting. Depressive symptoms are more frequent over the course of bipolar disorder than manic or hypomanic symptoms, although the latter define the disorder

Bipolar I disorder is a recurrent disorder that is familial in nature. Bipolar I disorders are defined on the basis of the criteria of DSM-IV-TR (table 101.6). These are characterized by distinct periods of abnormally and persistently elevated, expansive, or irritable mood lasting for at least 1 week. In addition, at least three of the following symptoms are present: inflated self-esteem or grandiosity, decreased need for sleep, greater talkativeness than usual, racing thoughts or flight of ideas, distractibility, increase in goal-directed activity, and excessive involvement in pleasurable activities that have a high potential for painful consequences, such as spending money or sexual indiscretion. Patients with bipolar II disorder have one or more depressive episodes with at least one hypomanic episode.

Hypomania refers to briefer duration and less severe level of manic symptoms, does not require hospitalization, and is not associated with psychotic symptoms (table 101.7). Hypomania causes mild functional impairment and can even improve functioning.

Patients with bipolar disorder presenting with depression should be treated with mood stabilizers and not with unprotected antidepressants, as they can cause patients to become manic or hypomanic. About 25–33% of patients presenting with depression have bipolar depression.

DISTINGUISHING UNIPOLAR AND BIPOLAR DEPRESSION

Patients with bipolar, compared to unipolar, depression are more likely to have a family history of bipolar disorder, have an earlier age of onset, have had recurrent episodes

Table 101.6 DSM-IV-TR DIAGNOSTIC CRITERIA FOR A MANIC EPISODE

Manic episodes are characterized by the following symptoms:

At least 1 week of profound mood disturbance is present, characterized by elation, irritability, or expansiveness.

Three or more of the following symptoms are present:

Grandiosity

Diminished need for sleep

Excessive talking or pressured speech

Racing thoughts or flight of ideas

Clear evidence of distractibility

Increased level of goal-focused activity at home, at work, or sexually

Excessive pleasurable activities, often with painful consequences

The mood disturbance is sufficient to cause impairment at work or danger to the patient or others.

The mood is not the result of substance abuse or a medical condition.

Table 101.7 DSM-IV-TR DIAGNOSTIC CRITERIA FOR A HYPOMANIC EPISODE.

Hypomanic episodes are characterized by the following:

A. Distinct period of persistently elevated, expansive, or irritable mood, lasting throughout at least 4 days, that is clearly different from the usual nondepressed mood

B. Three or more of following symptoms have persisted:

(1) Inflated self-esteem or grandiosity

(2) Decreased need for sleep

(3) More talkative than usual, or pressure to keep talking

(4) Flight of ideas or racing thoughts

(5) Distractibility

(6) Increase in goal-directed activity

(7) Excessive involvement in pleasurable activities that have painful consequences such as buying sprees, sexual indiscretions

C. The episode is associated with unequivocal change in functioning that is uncharacteristic of person when not symptomatic.

D. The disturbance in mood and change in functioning are observable by others.

E. The episode is not severe enough to cause marked impairment in social or occupational functioning or to necessitate hospitalization, and there are no psychotic features.

F. The symptoms are not due to direct physiological effects of substance such as drug abuse, medication, or other general medical condition (e.g., hyperthyroidism).

SOURCE: Reprinted with permission from *Diagnostic and Statistical Manual of Mental Disorders*, 4th ed., Text Revision (DSM-IV-TR). Copyright 2000 American Psychiatric Association.

of depression, and have atypical features of depression such as sleeping too much, eating too much, complaints of fatigue, leaden paralysis in the extremities, and lack of motivation. Their response to antidepressants is characterized by heightened feelings of anxiety, insomnia, and irritability.

Patients presenting with depression should be specifically asked about manic or hypomanic symptoms including the following: Have you experienced sustained periods of feeling uncharacteristically energetic? Have you had periods of not sleeping but not feeling tired? Have you felt your thoughts were racing and couldn't be slowed down? Have you had periods where you were excessive in sexual interest, spending money, or taking unusual risks? The Mood Disorder Questionnaire (MDQ) is a useful screening instrument for bipolar I and bipolar II disorder. It has sensitivity of 0.281 and specificity of 0.972 in a community sample.

SUICIDE

Both suicide attempts and completed suicide are very common problems, especially in a bipolar II disorder; hence, it is important to make an accurate diagnosis.

TREATMENT OF BIPOLAR DEPRESSION

Patients with bipolar depression are best treated with mood stabilizers such as lithium, lamotrigine, olanzapine-fluoxetine combinations (OFC), and quetiapine. There are risks with antidepressant monotherapy treatment because it can cause switches into hypomania or mania, mixed affective states, and rapid cycling between mania and depression.

Lithium

Lithium is approved for both acute treatment and the maintenance treatment of bipolar disorder. It is somewhat more effective in preventing manic episodes, but its substantial reduction in suicide suggests efficacy in depression as well. Common side effects are nausea, vomiting, diarrhea, weight gain, tremor, polyuria, polydipsia, and hypothyroidism. Chronic lithium ingestion has been associated with several different forms of renal injury. Nephrogenic diabetes insipidus (NDI) is the most common side effect of lithium therapy. Chronic tubulointerstitial nephropathy is the predominant form of chronic renal disease associated with lithium therapy. Additional kidney manifestations of lithium exposure include renal tubular acidosis and hypercalcemia. Lithium is contraindicated in severe cardiovascular or renal disease, dehydration, and sodium depletion. It should be used cautiously with drugs such as diuretics, NSAIDs, and angiotensin-converting enzyme (ACE) inhibitors because they may cause lithium toxicity.

Lamotrigine

Lamotrigine has efficacy for both acute and maintenance treatment of bipolar depression. It is also efficacious for rapidly cycling bipolar disorder. Common side effects are headache, insomnia, fatigue, and dizziness. Rare side effects include Stevens-Johnson Syndrome (0.8%).

Atypical Antipsychotics

Quetiapine and olanzapine with fluoxetine have been shown to have mood-stabilizing and antidepressant properties. Main side effects are weight gain, diabetes mellitus, and metabolic syndrome.

ANXIETY DISORDERS

The disorders of this group are most commonly encountered in the outpatient setting and affect approximately 10% of patients. Patients with anxiety disorders are more impaired in their functioning as compared to patients with diabetes mellitus and hypertension. Some of the symptoms of anxiety such as tachycardia, diaphoresis, shortness of breath, nausea and chest pain could be confused with cardiac problems. On the other hand, autonomic arousal and anxious agitation may be attributed to stress or anxiety when the symptoms may actually represent serious medical condition such as pulmonary embolism or cardiac arrhythmia.

PANIC DISORDER

Lifetime prevalence of panic disorder is 1.5–3.5% in the general population. The prevalence in primary care settings is 4–7%, and it is more common in women. Because patients with panic disorder tend to present with physical symptoms, it takes about eight visits to a clinician to make a diagnosis of panic disorder.

Clinical Manifestations

Panic attacks are characterized by the sudden onset of intense fear or discomfort and by the abrupt development of some specific somatic, cognitive, or affective symptoms (table 101.8). Somatic symptoms can include chest pain or discomfort, shortness of breath, tachycardia and palpitations, dizziness, paresthesias, light-headedness, headaches, nausea, abdominal discomfort, sweating, chills and hot flashes, fear of dying, and fear of losing control. In addition, patients have persistent concern about having additional attacks (anticipatory anxiety) and worry about possible implications of the attack such as having a heart attack or losing control; and as a result they may develop significant avoidance behaviors.

Table 101.8 DSM-IV-TR DIAGNOSTIC CRITERIA FOR PANIC DISORDER WITHOUT AGORAPHOBIA

A. Both (1) and (2)

(1) Recurrent, unexpected periods of intense fear or discomfort in which four or more of the following symptoms develop abruptly and reach a peak within 10 min:

Palpitations, pounding heart, or increased heart rate

Sweating

Trembling or shaking

Shortness of breath or smothering

Feeling of choking

Chest pain or discomfort

Nausea or abdominal distress

Feeling dizzy, lightheaded, or faint

Derealization (feelings of unreality) and depersonalization (being detached from oneself)

Fear of losing control or going crazy

Fear of dying

Numbness or tingling sensations

Chills or hot flashes

(2) At least one of the attacks has been followed by 1 month of one (or more) of the following:

a. persistent concern about having additional attacks

b. worry about the implications of the attack or its consequences (e.g., losing control, having a heart attack, or "going crazy")

c. significant change in behavior related to attacks

B. Absence of agoraphobia

C. The panic attacks are not due to the direct physiological effects of a substance (e.g., drug of abuse, a medication) or a general medical condition.

D. The panic attacks are not better accounted for by another mental disorder.

SOURCE: Reprinted with permission from *Diagnostic and Statistical Manual of Mental Disorders*, 4th ed, Text Revision (DSM-IV-TR). Copyright 2000 American Psychiatric Association.

Depression occurs frequently with panic disorder and increases the risk of suicide by 20%. Comorbid asthma, labile hypertension, mitral valve prolapse, and migraine headaches are common in patients with panic disorder.

Acute Treatment

The goal is to block the panic attack as quickly as possible to prevent the patient from developing avoidance behaviors, anticipatory anxiety, and agoraphobia.

Combination of Cognitive Behavior Therapy with Medications

All five classes of antidepressants are equally useful and significantly more effective than placebo for panic disorder. SSRIs and SNRIs are the drugs of choice because of their benign side-effect profiles.

Concomitant use of benzodiazepines to block the panic attacks completely and minimize the side effects during the first few weeks of treatment when initiating SSRIs is also useful. Patients with panic disorder tend to be very sensitive to the side effects of medications. Benzodiazepines should be tapered as the SSRI dosage is raised to therapeutic levels. It is important to be clear with the patient at the outset about the intention to prescribe a benzodiazepine for several weeks only.

GENERALIZED ANXIETY DISORDER

Generalized anxiety disorder (GAD) is a common condition with a 1-year prevalence of 3% and lifetime prevalence of 5.7%; the prevalence is 8% in primary care.

Patients with GAD tend to present with predominantly somatic symptoms and frequently have comorbid conditions such as panic disorder, major depression (40–50%), alcohol abuse, and personality disorder.

CLINICAL MANIFESTATIONS AND DIAGNOSIS

Diagnostic criteria from DSM-IV-TR for GAD (table 101.9) include excessive worry about a number of events or activities, occurring more days than not, for at least 6 months, that are out of proportion to the likelihood or impact of the feared events. Worry leads to anxiety, which is associated with physical symptoms of anxiety such as dry mouth, sweating, palpitations, muscle tension leading to tension headaches, low back pain, and fatigue. Patients are easily startled, have difficulty falling asleep, and complain of poor memory and poor concentration. They have little insight into the connection between their reported worries or current life stress and their physical symptoms.

Patients should be screened for depression, medical disorders such hyperthyroidism, pheochromocytoma, medication side effects, and for substance abuse, especially alcohol abuse.

TREATMENT

Acute treatment of GAD consists of therapy (cognitive behavioral), medications (SSRIs or SNRIs), or both.

Drug Therapy

SSRIs, venlafaxine (SNRI), buspirone, and tricyclic antidepressants are effective for the treatment for GAD, but the

Table 101.9 DSM-IV-TR DIAGNOSTIC CRITERIA FOR GENERALIZED ANXIETY DISORDER

A. Excessive anxiety or worry (apprehensive expectation) occurring more days than not for at least 6 months about a number of events or activities.

B. The person finds it difficult to control the worry.

C. The anxiety and worry are associated with 3 or more of the following:

   (1) Restlessness or feeling keyed up or on edge

   (2) Being easily fatigued

   (3) Difficulty concentrating or mind going blank

   (4) Irritability

   (5) Muscle tension

   (6) Sleep disturbance

D. The focus or anxiety and worry are not confined to features of another Axis 1 psychiatric disorder.

E. The anxiety, worry, or physical symptoms cause clinically significant distress or impairment in social, occupational, or other important areas of functioning.

F. The disturbance is not due to direct physiological effects of substance of abuse or other medical condition.

SOURCE: Reprinted with permission from Diagnostic and Statistical Manual of Mental Disorders, 4th ed., Text Revision (DSM-IV-TR). Copyright 2000 American Psychiatric Association.

SSRIs and SNRIs have become the first line of treatment because of their lower side-effect profiles and lower risk for tolerance and a direct effect on the psychic symptoms of worry and anxiety. They also have anxiolytic effects.

Although benzodiazepines help in patients with GAD, one should refrain from using these in patients with polydrug or alcohol use, chronic pain disorders, and patients with severe personality disorders because of the abuse potential.

Long-term recovery in patients with GAD is achieved in only about a third of patients. Many patients will need chronic treatment.

SCHIZOPHRENIA AND RELATED DISORDERS

Schizophrenia is a severe disorder involving chronic or recurrent psychosis and long-term deterioration in functional capacity. Psychosis is a break in reality manifested as some combination of delusions, hallucinations, disorganized or illogical thinking, and chaotic behavior. Although psychosis is a hallmark of schizophrenia, it is not pathognomonic for the disorder, and other psychiatric and medical disorders must be ruled out before the diagnosis is made. This is especially important if the first psychotic episode is after the age of 40.

ANTIPSYCHOTIC MEDICATIONS

Antipsychotic medications are grouped into several distinct classes based primarily on their side-effect profile With the exception of clozapine, all conventional and atypical antipsychotics appear to be equally efficacious in the treatment of psychosis. There is also no evidence in their differential effects on nonpsychotic symptoms such as mania, uncontrolled behaviors, delirium, and poor impulse control. Medications differ in potency, side effects, routes of administration, and cost.

Conventional older antipsychotics include high-potency drugs such as haloperidol (Haldol), perphenazine (Prolixin), fluphenazine (Stelazine), and thiothixene (Navane) as well as low-potency drugs including Thorazine and mesoridazine (Mellaril). These older antipsychotic drugs are characterized by good efficacy but are associated with a high risk for parkinsonian extrapyramidal side effects (EPS) including rigidity, bradykinesia, tremor, and akathisia (subjective and objective restlessness). In addition they carry a 5–7% per year cumulative risk of tardive dyskinesia, which consists of late-onset choreoathetotic movements of tongue, face, neck, trunk, or limbs. Conventional antipsychotics are also associated with increase in prolactin levels, causing galactorrhea and amenorrhea.

Significant QT prolongation is associated with intravenous haloperidol; however, clinically significant QT prolongation with oral use of haloperidol and other conventional antipsychotics occurs infrequently.

Because of extrapyramidal side effects of these medications, they should not be given to patients with Parkinson disease or Lewy body dementia.

Atypical antipsychotics include clozapine (Clozaril), olanzapine (Zyprexa), quetiapine (Seroquel), risperidone (Risperidal), zisprasidone (Geodon), aripiprazole (Abilify), and paliperidone (Invega). These drugs (except clozapine) have a low risk of EPS and the related risk of tardive dyskinesia. EPS and tardive dyskinesia are absent with clozapine. These medications are associated with weight gain, increased blood sugars, and metabolic syndrome. Risperidone increases prolactin levels.

There is limited evidence of superior efficacy for any of these drugs except for clozapine, and the only prediction of patient response is prior response to the same agents.

Neuroleptic malignant syndrome is a life-threatening neurological emergency caused by neuroleptic agents, which block dopamine. Symptoms consist of the tetrad of fever greater than 38°C, which is the defining symptom, extreme muscular rigidity, mental status changes as the first symptom, and autonomic instability. Treatment is to stop the causative agent and other potential contributing psychotropic agents as lithium, anticholinergic therapy, and serotonergic agents, provide aggressive supportive care in the ICU, administer muscle relaxants (such as dantrolene) to treat malignant hyperthermia and dopaminergic agents (such as bromocriptine and amantadine) to restore dopaminergic tone, and to use benzodiazepines to control agitation. Neuroleptic malignant syndrome can last from days to weeks.

Causative agents are usually "typical" conventional neuroleptics with high potency such as haloperidol and fluphenazine, although all antipsychotics including the atypical antipsychotics and antiemetic agent metoclopramide, (reglan) can also cause neuroleptic malignant syndrome.

Lab findings show elevated CK >100,000 IU/L, leukocytosis, elevated catecholamines, and low serum iron.

SOMATIZATION

Somatization refers to the tendency to experience psychological distress in the form of somatic symptoms and to seek medical help for these symptoms. Emotional responses such as anxiety and depression can initiate and/or perpetuate symptoms. Somatization can be unconscious or conscious and may be influenced by psychological distress or personal gain.

The DSM-IV divides somatoform disorders into a spectrum of disorders that include the following categories.

SOMATIZATION DISORDER

Patients with somatization disorder have recurrent multiple somatic complaints beginning before the age of 30. The disorder affects mostly women and results in treatment being sought and causes significant impairment in social, occupational, or other important areas of functioning. All of the following can be present at any time during the course of the illness: four pain symptoms; two gastrointestinal symptoms; one sexual symptom; and one pseudoneurological symptom. It is best managed by collaborative work with an empathic primary care physician and mental health professional. Regularly scheduled appointments with the primary care provider are a cost-effective strategy that lessens "doctor shopping" and frequent visits to an emergency department.

Conversion disorder refers to symptoms or deficits of voluntary or sensory function suggesting a neurological or general medical condition and associated with psychological factors. Typically, there is sudden onset of a dramatic but physiologically unlikely condition such as paralysis, aphonia, blindness, deafness, or pseudoseizures. The presentation fits the patient's view of the disorder rather than human physiology.

Pain disorder refers to pain in one or more sites of significant focus or severity, causing significant distress or impairment and associated with psychological factors.

Hypochondriasis refers to preoccupation with the fear of having a serious disease based on a misattribution of bodily symptoms or normal functions. The conviction about serious disease can be as severe and as inappropriate as a delusion, putting the diagnosis in the realm of psychosis. Hypochondriasis is often seen in generalized anxiety disorder, obsessive-compulsive disorder, panic disorder, major depressive disorder, and separation anxiety disorder.

Body dysmorphic disorder refers to preoccupation with an imagined or exaggerated defect in physical appearance.

In *factitious disorder*, patients present with physical symptoms and findings. This is done at a conscious level, but the secondary gain is not obvious. These patients have some medical knowledge. Wound healing difficulty, excoriations, infection, bleeding, hypoglycemia, and gastrointestinal ailments are common presentations. The most extreme presentation, Munchausen syndrome occurs in a subgroup of patients who feign disease, move from hospital to hospital, and submit to repeated procedures for illnesses they have voluntarily produced.

Undifferentiated somatoform disorder refers to one or more physical symptoms that cause distress or impairment in functioning at least for 6 months.

DELIRIUM

Nearly 30% of older medical patients experience delirium at some time during their hospitalization. This percentage is even higher in surgical patients. Delirium has an enormous impact on the health of older patients. Patients with delirium have high morbidity and mortality

CLINICAL FEATURES

Disturbance of consciousness is manifested by reduced clarity of awareness of the environment. The ability to focus, sustain, or shift attention is impaired, and the patient is easily distracted by irrelevant stimuli. There is a change in cognition that may include memory impairment, disorientation, and language disturbance or the development of perceptual disturbance, which may include illusions or hallucinations. The disturbance develops over a short period of time and tends to fluctuate during the course of the day. The patient may be coherent and cooperative in the morning but at night becomes agitated, attempts to pull out intravenous lines, and wants to leave. Delirium is also associated with disturbance in sleep–wake cycle, daytime sleepiness, agitation, and difficulty falling asleep at night. Psychomotor behavior disturbances may include increased psychomotor activity, which may include groping or picking at the bedclothes, attempting to get out of bed, decreased activity with sluggishness and lethargy that approach stupor. Variable emotional responses such as anxiety, fear, depression, irritability, anger, euphoria, and apathy can also be seen.

APPROACH TO THE PATIENT

Virtually any medical condition can precipitate delirium in a susceptible person. The history and physical examination will guide most of the investigations. The conditions noted most commonly in prospective studies of the disorder include fluid and electrolyte disturbance (dehydration, hyponatremia, and hypernatremia); infections (urinary tract infection, respiratory tract, skin, and soft tissue); drug and alcohol toxicity; withdrawal from alcohol, barbiturates, benzodiazepines, and selective serotonin reuptake inhibitors; metabolic disorders (hypoglycemia, hypocalcemia, uremia, liver failure, and thyrotoxicosis); low profusion states (shock, heart failure); and postoperative states, especially in the elderly.

MANAGEMENT

Treatment of the underlying disorder and antipsychotic medications such as haloperidol, which can be given intramuscularly in conjunction with antianxiety medications such as lorazepam, help to achieve behavioral control.

ADDITIONAL READING

Belmaker RH. Bipolar disorder. *N Engl J Med.* 2004;351(5):476–86.
Belmaker RH, Agam G. Major depressive disorder. *N Engl J Med.* 2008;358(1):55–68.
Fricchione G. Clinical practice. Generalized anxiety disorder. *N Engl J Med.* 2004;351(7):675–82.
Goodwin F. Long term treatment of bipolar disorder. *J Clin Psychiatry.* 2002;63(suppl 10):5–12.
Mann JJ. The medical management of depression. *N Engl J Med.* 2005;353(17):1819–34.
Unützer J. Clinical practice. Late-life depression. *N Engl J Med.* 2007;357(22):2269–76.

QUESTIONS

QUESTION 1. A 77-year-old female with history of Parkinson disease is admitted to the hospital with urosepsis. In the middle of the night she becomes aggressive and tries to strike at the nurses, remove her intravenous line, and get out of the bed. She feels the nurses are trying to get her and states she is covered by insects. Her primary nurse reports the patient has been having periods of agitation and lethargy. Which of the following medication would you give her to control her behavior?

A. Haloperidol
B. Quetiapine
C. Perphenazine
D. Chlorpromazine

QUESTION 2. A 68-year-old recently widowed male presents to his primary care physician with complaints of depression, fatigue, feelings of hopelessness, increased alcohol abuse, insomnia, and memory problems. Which of the following is the most appropriate initial step?

A. Treat with benzodiazepine
B. Treat with SSRI
C. Assess for suicidality
D. Refer for psychotherapy

QUESTION 3. Your patient is a 40-year-old female diagnosed with breast cancer. She has undergone surgery, chemotherapy, and radiation. She is presently on tamoxifen and presents to you with depressed mood, feeling very anxious, with poor sleep, poor appetite, and feeling somewhat hopeless. She denies any suicidal or homicidal ideation. You plan to treat her with an antidepressant, as she is already in therapy.

Which would be the safest antidepressant for her?

A. Fluoxetine
B. Paroxetine
C. Sertraline
D. Venlafaxine

QUESTION 4. A 35-year-old male with a history of hypertension, type 2 diabetes, and bipolar disorder presents for his yearly physical exam. His medications include metformin, lisinopril, and lithium. On physical exam his weight has increased by 30 lb over the past year. His HbA1c is 10.6. He reports that a new medication has been started by his psychiatrist. Which is the most likely medication?

A. Depakote
B. Olanzapine
C. Lamictal
D. Topiramate

QUESTION 5. A 33-year-old woman presents with complaints of depression with suicidal ideation but no plan, sleeping too much, eating a lot, having no energy, and poor motivation. This is her third episode of depression; her first episode was in her teens. She also gives a history of period of a 3- to 4-day period when she felt she had a lot of energy, slept only 3–4 hours, had flight of ideas, and talked fast. She accomplished a lot during those 4 days. What medication would not be indicated for her?

A. Lithium
B. Lamotrigine
C. Quetiapine
D. Citalopram

ANSWERS

1. B
2. C
3. D
4. B
5. D

102.

GERIATRICS

Mark J. Simone-Skidmore and Suzanne E. Salamon

Geriatric medicine is the subspecialty of internal medicine that focuses on the care of patients over the age of 65. As life expectancy increases and the baby boom generation reaches old age, there will be a significant increase in this population. As of 2000 there were 35 million people 65 and older. This number is expected to double to over 70 million by 2030. The 85+ population is projected to increase from 4.2 million in 2000 to 7.3 million in 2020. There will never be enough geriatric specialists to care for this group of patients, so all health care providers must be aware of the key principles of geriatrics.

The effects of normal aging and disease-related changes common in older adults necessitate a unique approach to caring for this group. There are several geriatric syndromes encountered regularly in elderly adults. These include polypharmacy, dementia, delirium, late-life depression, urinary incontinence, and falls.

POLYPHARMACY

Polypharmacy is the use of several drugs at the same time. The average older person uses five to seven prescription drugs and several over-the-counter drugs. As the number of medications increases, the number of adverse effects and drug–drug interactions also increases. A common example is the interaction between warfarin and antibiotics. Thirty percent of hospital admissions are linked to polypharmacy and cause 106,000 deaths per year at a cost of $85 billion. Older adults are more sensitive to the effects and side effects of medications due to altered pharmacokinetics (i.e., changes in body composition) and altered pharmacodynamics (i.e., changes in the body's response to drugs). Creatinine values that are within "normal" lab reference range may actually indicate significant renal insufficiency. Therefore, the glomerular filtration rate must be calculated and used as a guide when prescribing renally cleared medications. The Beers criteria are a list of drugs to avoid or to use with extreme caution due to either ineffectiveness or high risk for adverse events. These include anticholinergics, benzodiazepines, antihistamines, muscle relaxants, and certain analgesics (table 102.1). As a rule, medications should be started in older adults at the lowest possible dose, titrated slowly, and regularly evaluated for effectiveness and side effects. Medication lists should be frequently reviewed so that unnecessary drugs can be eliminated.

DEMENTIA

BACKGROUND

Dementia is a syndrome defined as memory loss in addition to impairment in at least one area of higher cognitive function, such as language, orientation, calculation, visuospatial awareness (e.g., getting lost in familiar places), or executive function (e.g., planning or organizing). The impairments must be significant enough to interfere with routine activities of daily life.

EPIDEMIOLOGY

Dementia is common and increases with age, occurring in approximately 10% of adults older than 65 and increasing to 50% of adults older than 90. There are many forms of dementia (table 102.2). Alzheimer disease (AD) is the most common type, accounting for 50–60% of dementias. There are 4.5 million adults currently with AD, accounting for almost $84 billion in annual costs caring for this group. Non-Alzheimer dementias include vascular (multi-infarct) dementia (15–20%), dementia with Lewy bodies (DLB), and Parkinson disease. Less than 10% of dementias are caused by reversible conditions (e.g., hypothyroidism or B-12 deficiency), and even when treated, the underlying cause often turns out to be AD or vascular dementia.

Table 102.1 EXAMPLES OF MEDICATIONS TO AVOID OR USE WITH CAUTION IN OLDER ADULTS

DRUG	REASON
Anticholinergics and antihistamines such as diphenhydramine (Benadryl) and hydroxyzine (Atarax and Vistaril)	Confusion, sedation, constipation, urinary retention, and dry mouth
Benzodiazepines, especially long-acting formulations such as diazepam (Valium) and chlordiazepoxide (Librium)	Prolonged sedation and increased risk of falls and fractures
Muscle relaxants and antispasmodics such as oxybutynin (Ditropan), carisoprodol (Soma), and cyclobenzaprine (Flexeril)	Anticholinergic properties including confusion and sedation as well as weakness and questionable effectiveness
Gastrointestinal antispasmodic drugs such as dicyclomine (Bentyl) and hyoscyamine (Levsin)	Anticholinergic properties including confusion and sedation as well as weakness and questionable effectiveness
Ferrous sulfate in doses >325 mg/day	Constipation and lack of efficacy at higher doses
Barbiturates	Sedation and addiction
Digoxin (Lanoxin) in doses >0.125 mg/day unless required	Toxic effects at higher doses due to reduced renal clearance
Tricyclic antidepressants such as amitriptyline (Elavil) and doxepin (Sinequan)	Anticholinergic properties including sedation and confusion
Meperidine (Demerol)	Ineffective with toxic metabolites causing sedation and confusion
Fluoxetine (Prozac)	Long half-life and risk of agitation and sleep disturbance from CNS stimulation
NSAIDs, especially indomethacin, when used long-term and at full dose	GI bleeding, renal failure, hypertension, and heart failure (indomethacin has the most CNS adverse effects of all the NSAIDs)

PATHOPHYSIOLOGY

Alzheimer disease is defined by neuritic amyloid plaques and neurofibrillary tangles, leading to neuronal cell loss and alterations in neurotransmitter function. The *APOE E4* allele on the *APOE* gene appears to be a risk factor for Alzheimer disease, but its role is not yet fully defined. Age is the greatest risk factor for the development of dementia. The other dementias involve lesions localized to specific cortical or subcortical areas of the brain.

CLINICAL PRESENTATION

Identifying the specific form of dementia has important implications in prognosis and treatment (table 102.3). AD is distinguished by memory impairment with at least one of the following: aphasia (language disturbance), apraxia (difficulty performing simple motor activities in the presence of normal motor function), agnosia (difficulty recognizing familiar objects), or executive dysfunction. Memory loss is the most common initial presentation, often reported by a family member rather than the patient. It is often incorrectly dismissed as part of normal aging. In the early stage of AD, symptoms include difficulty in learning new information, getting lost while driving to familiar places, or changes in mood manifested as suspicion or hostility. By the middle stage of AD, patients are unable to perform activities of daily living and develop eating problems, incontinence, and motor impairment. In the late stage of AD, memory loss is severe, and afflicted patients will often become mute, immobile, develop recurrent infections, and often display behavioral disturbances such as agitation, depression, hallucinations, and delusions.

Vascular dementia is associated with microvascular disease as small strokes destroy brain tissue. Risk factors include smoking, hypertension, diabetes, and heart disease. Patients with vascular dementia classically exhibit a stepwise deterioration that prominently affects gait and speech. Mixed dementia refers to a combination of AD along with evi-

Table 102.2 CAUSES OF DEMENTIA

- Alzheimer disease
- Vascular dementia
- Mixed dementia
- Dementia with Lewy bodies (DLB)
- Frontotemporal dementia
- Depression
- Infection (e.g., syphilis, HIV, or encephalitis)
- Parkinson disease
- Vitamin B-12 deficiency
- Hypothyroidism
- Creutzfeldt-Jacob disease (prion disease)
- Subdural hematoma
- Normal-pressure hydrocephalus
- Alcohol-related dementia

Table 102.3 SPECIFIC CHARACTERISTICS OF NON-ALZHEIMER DEMENTIA

SYMPTOM	DISORDER
Abrupt, stepwise deterioration	Vascular dementia
Prominent behavioral changes such as apathy and disinhibition	Frontotemporal dementia
Progressive gait disorder	Vascular dementia, Parkinson disease, normal-pressure hydrocephalus
Extrapyramidal signs *before* the development of cognitive dysfunction	Parkinson disease
Extrapyramidal signs *after* the development of cognitive dysfunction	Dementia with Lewy bodies
Fluctuation in consciousness	Dementia with Lewy bodies
Visual hallucinations	Dementia with Lewy bodies
Neuroleptic sensitivity	Dementia with Lewy bodies and Parkinson disease

dence of microvascular disease. Frontotemporal dementia presents initially with changes in personality such as disinhibition or apathy and executive dysfunction. Dementia with Lewy bodies (DLB) is associated with extrapyramidal motor symptoms similar to Parkinson disease but in addition is noted for fluctuating levels of attention and visual hallucinations. Patients with DLB notably have increased sensitivity to neuroleptics with worsening of the extrapyramidal symptoms when exposed to antipsychotics. Dementia is common in patients with Parkinson disease, but in contrast to DLB, the parkinsonian features occur *before* the development of cognitive dysfunction.

DIAGNOSIS

The history obtained from the patient and caregivers is the most important part of the evaluation for suspected dementia. The most frequent screening test of cognition is the Mini-Mental State Examination (MMSE), which takes 5–10 minutes to administer. A score of less than 24 out of 30 suggests impairment. The test is influenced by level of education and may miss early dementia. A careful neurological exam, imaging with a noncontrast head computed tomography (CT) or magnetic resonance imaging (MRI) to rule out vascular disease, normal-pressure hydrocephalus, or subdural hematomas, and routine blood assays including thyroid function and vitamin B-12 should be performed. Patients should also be evaluated for depression, which has symptoms that can overlap with dementia.

TREATMENT

There is no cure for AD, but there are medications that help slow the disease and manage behaviors. Cholinesterase inhibitors help restore the loss of the neurotransmitter acetylcholine, which is decreased in AD. The Food and Drug Administration (FDA) has approved donepezil (Aricept), rivastigmine (Exelon), and galantamine (Razadyne) for use in mild to moderate AD, although these drugs have been used with varying effect in other forms of dementia as well. Cholinesterase inhibitors may improve MMSE scores, moderately improve behavioral disturbances, and maintain independence. However, the effect is usually small and followed by eventual decline. Side effects from cholinesterase inhibitors include nausea, vomiting, diarrhea, and weight loss. Memantine (Namenda) is an N-methyl-d-aspartate antagonist approved for the treatment of moderate to severe AD and is usually administered together with a cholinesterase inhibitor. It is generally well tolerated, although insomnia and nightmares are common side effects. Neuropsychiatric symptoms common in dementia should first be managed with nonpharmacologic therapies such as exercise, music, old movies, and redirection. If necessary, atypical antipsychotics at low doses can be used for the management of psychosis or agitation. However, even newer atypical antipsychotic medications produce side effects of parkinsonism, tardive dyskinesia, sedation, and anticholinergic effects. Additionally, there is a "black box label" warning of the possible increased risk of death in older demented patients. Therefore, the use of such medications should frequently be assessed for effectiveness and side effects.

Management of the demented patient also includes advanced care planning (documentation of advanced directives and health care proxy), addressing caregiver stress, and ensuring safety (driving and wandering).

DELIRIUM

BACKGROUND

Delirium is an acute change in mental status defined by a fluctuating course and the inability to maintain attention. Delirium is common, especially in hospitalized patients, and is frequently missed. Delirium leads to increased morbidity, mortality, loss of independence, institutionalization, and almost $7 billion in annual costs.

EPIDEMIOLOGY

Rates of delirium vary depending on precipitating factors and predisposing risk factors. The overall prevalence of delirium in community dwellers is only 1–2%, but 10–30% of elders presenting to emergency departments are delirious. Rates are highest in the hospital setting with up to 53% of older adults developing delirium postoperatively, and in the intensive care units up to 87% are delirious. The 1-year mortality rate in people with delirium is as high as 40%.

PATHOPHYSIOLOGY

The exact mechanism of delirium is poorly understood, but it is felt to signify generalized disruption in higher cortical function. Cholinergic deficiency, dopaminergic excess, and cytokines are hypothesized to play a role. Two-thirds of people who develop delirium have underlying dementia or other predisposing risk factors (table 102.4).

CLINICAL PRESENTATION

The hallmark of delirium is an acute change in mental status developing over hours or days that fluctuates with periods of lucid intervals along with the inability to maintain attention. Patients will often display incoherent and disorganized speech or thoughts. Altered consciousness can present with either *hyperactive* delirium with agitation and restlessness, *hypoactive* delirium with lethargy and a decreased level of motor activity, or a mixture of the two. Global cognitive deficits involving memory, language, and disorientation can occur. Characteristic alterations in the sleep cycle as well as hallucinations and emotional disturbances are also common.

DIAGNOSIS

The diagnosis of delirium is primarily clinical and is made using the Confusion Assessment Method (CAM). The CAM is a validated bedside screening tool that requires the following: (1) acute change in mental status with a fluctuating course and (2) inattention with either (3) disorganized thinking or (4) altered level of consciousness.

TREATMENT

The etiology of delirium is usually multifactorial (table 102.4) and is often reversible if the underlying causes are corrected. Medications known to cause delirium should be discontinued. Examples include benzodiazepines, sleeping pills, meperidine (Demerol), and diphenhydramine (Benadryl). Screening for alcohol or drug use is important to rule out withdrawal or intoxication. Delirium can be an atypical presentation for many diseases in older adults, including infection (urinary tract or pneumonia), electrolyte and metabolic disturbances, hypoxia, urinary retention, constipation, and pain.

Supportive care should focus on maintaining hydration, nutrition, and mobilizing the patient as soon as possible to prevent additional complications. Behavioral symptoms are often the most challenging to manage, especially in an agitated, confused patient. Nonpharmacologic methods should be used, which include frequent orientation, reassurance, and family involvement. Physical restraints and nighttime interruptions should be avoided. Unnecessary lines and tubes, especially Foley catheters, should be removed as soon as possible. Pharmacologic treatment should be used only for the agitated patient at risk of harm to self or others. Antipsychotics such as haloperidol can be used for acute agitation and should be used in low doses of 0.25–1.0 mg PO or IM, not to exceed 3 mg in a 24-hour period. When patients are able to take oral medications, atypical antipsychotics can be used in low doses and given at regular intervals as needed. Typical regimens include risperidone (0.5 mg bid), olanzapine (2.5–5 mg daily), and quetiapine (12.5–25 mg bid). These drugs should be used sparingly because of the adverse side effects mentioned previously. The best treatment for delirium is prevention by recognizing patients at high risk and minimizing risk factors.

Table 102.4 **ETIOLOGY OF DELIRIUM**

RISK FACTORS	CAUSES
• Age >65	• Medications
• Dementia	• Infection
• History of delirium	• Acute illness
• Depression	• Surgery
• History of falls	• Pain
• Immobility	• Neurological disorder such as trauma, intracranial bleed, stroke, or encephalitis
• Functional dependence	• Environmental, such as hospitalization, intensive care unit, restraints, and bladder catheter
• Sensory impairment	
• Malnutrition and dehydration	
• Coexisting medical conditions	• Sleep deprivation
• Alcohol abuse	
• Decreased physical activity	
• Treatment with psychoactive drugs or multiple drugs	

LATE-LIFE DEPRESSION

BACKGROUND

Depression in older adults is common yet often undetected and undertreated. Symptoms can present differently because of the coexistence of chronic medical disorders, memory loss, pain, and alcohol or substance abuse. Untreated depression is associated with poor quality of life, nonadherence to medical treatment, functional decline, and increased morbidity and mortality. The risk of suicide underlies the importance of recognizing and treating depression, as elderly men have the highest rate of successful suicide.

EPIDEMIOLOGY

Over 10% of adults over 65 presenting to primary care physicians have clinically significant depression. Hospitalized and institutionalized older adults have even higher rates. Depression is more common in women and in those with chronic medical disorders, insomnia, stressful life events, functional decline, and social isolation.

PATHOPHYSIOLOGY

Previous psychiatric disorders continue to be a risk factor for depression in later life. Chronic medical conditions and functional decline contribute to the new development of depression after the age of 65. Studies suggest that cerebrovascular disease and vascular risk factors may sometimes play a role in the development of depression as a result of microvascular ischemic changes.

CLINICAL PRESENTATION

Older adults with depression are more likely to exhibit anxiety, hopelessness, anhedonia, sleep disturbances, and weight loss rather than sadness. Cognitive symptoms such as psychomotor retardation or executive dysfunction are more common and can mimic symptoms of dementia. Symptoms of depression are often mistaken for medical ailments and should be considered if there is a poor response to treatment regimens.

DIAGNOSIS

Major depression as defined by the *Diagnostic and Statistical Manual of Mental Disorders,* 4th edition (DSM-IV) requires the presence of a depressed mood or loss of interest with at least four additional symptoms nearly every day for more than 2 months (table 102.5). The presence of fewer than five symptoms is consistent with minor depression. Screening tests such as the Geriatric Depression Scale are simple bedside questionnaires that can be used to help identify patients with depression. Additional evaluation should include a

Table 102.5 **DIAGNOSTIC CRITERIA FOR MAJOR DEPRESSION***

1. Depressed mood
2. Markedly diminished interest or pleasure
3. Weight loss or decreased appetite
4. Insomnia or hypersomnia
5. Psychomotor agitation or retardation
6. Fatigue or decreased energy
7. Feelings of worthlessness or guilt
8. Inability to concentrate or make decisions
9. Recurrent thoughts of death or suicide

NOTE: *Must have 5 or more symptoms, nearly every day for at least 2 weeks, and symptoms must include either depressed mood or diminished interest.

medication review, measurement of thyroid function, and screening for memory loss and alcohol or substance abuse.

TREATMENT

Effective therapy for mild to moderate depression usually involves use of antidepressants. Selective serotonin-reuptake inhibitors (SSRIs) are considered first-line treatment. Most SSRIs are equally effective, with gastrointestinal upset being the most common adverse effect. Notably, fluoxetine (Prozac) should be avoided in the elderly because of its long elimination half-life. Other antidepressants are available, and their unique side effect profiles can be used to tailor medications to the individual needs. Mirtazapine (Remeron) is a serotonergic and noradrenergic antidepressant with potential beneficial side effects of sedation and appetite stimulation when used at low doses. Bupropion (Wellbutrin) can cause anxiety and insomnia and therefore may be useful in patients with fatigue or lethargy. Serotonin-norepinephrine reuptake inhibitors (SNRIs) such as duloxetine (Cymbalta) and venlafaxine (Effexor) are useful for patients with coexisting neuropathic pain, although SNRIs may be less tolerated in frail elderly than SSRIs.

Monotherapy is preferred to minimize side effects and drug interactions. Starting doses should be lower for older adults, although full doses will usually be required for adequate response. Treatment response may take up to 12 weeks, although partial improvement will often be seen after 4 weeks. Antidepressants should be continued for at least 6–12 months or longer to prevent recurrence. Other antidepressants such as tricyclic antidepressants and monoamine oxidase inhibitors are used less frequently because of their potential serious side effects including cardiac conduction defects, myocardial infarction, and orthostatic hypotension.

Structured psychotherapy is another valid treatment option that has been shown to be as effective as pharmacotherapy for mild to moderate depression. In severe or chronic forms of depression, psychotherapy is a useful adjunct to pharmacotherapy.

Electroconvulsive therapy (ECT) is effective for the treatment of severe depression resistant to other treatments or in patients at risk of serious harm due to psychotic features, suicidality, or severe malnutrition. These conditions are also indication for referral to a psychiatrist.

URINARY INCONTINENCE

BACKGROUND

Urinary incontinence is a common and potentially disabling problem in older adults yet often goes unrecognized and untreated. Patients are often reluctant to mention this problem, and busy practitioners often do not inquire about it. Incontinence can lead to depression, anxiety, falls, skin infections, sleep disturbance, caregiver burden, and social isolation and is a major reason for institutionalization.

EPIDEMIOLOGY

Up to 30% of those 65 and older are affected by urinary incontinence. The prevalence increases with age. Women are two to three times more likely to be affected until the age of 80, when men are just as likely to experience incontinence.

PATHOPHYSIOLOGY

Incontinence is often multifactorial. Changes in the lower urinary tract, central nervous system, cognition, mobility, and volume status all play a role in its development. The supporting muscles of the pelvic floor are often weakened by lack of estrogen, previous vaginal deliveries, or pelvic irradiation. These changes commonly result in detrusor muscle weakness, bladder overactivity, and bladder outlet obstruction. Disruption in the nervous system by stroke, Parkinson disease, or normal-pressure hydrocephalus, for example, can also lead to incontinence. Limited mobility, decreased manual dexterity, and cognitive dysfunction can lead to incontinence even in the absence of actual physiological abnormalities. Comorbidities including severe constipation, diabetes, and congestive heart failure also contribute.

CLINICAL PRESENTATION

There are four basic types of incontinence, although symptoms often overlap (see table 102.6).

Urge incontinence is the most common and is also known as overactive bladder. It presents with the sudden need to urinate, often with leakage of moderate to large amounts of urine. Urinary frequency and nocturia are common. Men often have additional symptoms related to prostatic enlargement. Women with urge incontinence may also have symptoms of stress incontinence, which is referred to as mixed incontinence.

Stress incontinence is characterized by leakage of urine with increased intra-abdominal pressure exacerbated by coughing, sneezing, position change, or exercise. It is more common in women and is often associated with weakened pelvic floor muscles.

Overflow incontinence is seen with urinary retention due to detrusor muscle weakness or bladder outlet obstruction. Symptoms include decreased urinary output, weak stream, and hesitancy in addition to dribbling, frequency, and nocturia.

Functional incontinence refers to the inability to reach the toilet in time. Causes include medications (e.g., diuretics), impaired mobility (e.g., arthritis and stroke), environmental obstacles, and psychiatric or cognitive disorders.

DIAGNOSIS

Because patients often do not report symptoms of urinary incontinence, care providers should screen for this disorder with routine questions directly inquiring about incontinence. A physical examination should include a pelvic exam to evaluate for anatomic or atrophic changes, a rectal exam to rule out impaction, and a neurological exam to rule out evidence of a focal neurological deficit. Mobility, cognition, and volume status should be assessed. Additional diagnostic tests should include a postvoid residual by bladder ultrasound and a urinalysis. Further urodynamic studies can be performed by a urologist or gynecologist when the diagnosis is unclear.

Table 102.6 **URINARY INCONTINENCE**

TYPE	SYMPTOMS	TREATMENT
Stress	Small amount of urine loss with increased abdominal pressure (such as cough, laugh, exercise)	Pelvic muscle exercise, scheduled voiding, topical estrogens if atrophic vaginitis, surgical options or pessary
Urge	Moderate to large amount of urine loss with inability to delay urination and often associated with urgency and frequency	Scheduled voiding, antimuscarinic drugs
Mixed	Combination of stress and urge incontinence symptoms	Combination of above treatments
Overflow	Leakage of small amount of urine with distended bladder and hesitancy, frequency, or dribbling	Removal of obstruction, treatment of prostatic enlargement, scheduled voiding, catheterization
Functional	Incontinence due to inability or unwillingness to toilet	Behavioral interventions, scheduled voiding, environmental manipulation

TREATMENT

Treatment options for incontinence depend on the type of incontinence as well as the preferences of the patient. Not all incontinence can be cured, but even a reduction in occurrence can greatly improve quality of life.

Nonpharmacologic methods of management include the use of bedside commodes and urinals and changing the timing of diuretics. Bladder training includes Kegel exercises, which involve repetitive contractions and relaxations of the pelvic floor muscles in order to strengthen them. This is especially useful in stress or mixed incontinence. Regular toileting at fixed intervals can also be helpful in staying dry.

Topical estrogens may help with symptoms of stress incontinence related to atrophic vaginitis. Incontinence related to prolapse may respond to pessaries or other urologic procedures.

Pharmacotherapy can be used in conjunction with behavioral interventions. Urge and mixed incontinence respond to antimuscarinic drugs, which decrease bladder wall muscle contractions, such as oxybutynin (Ditropan), solifenacin (Vesicare), and tolterodine (Detrol). Current evidence does not support the superiority of any one type; however, all share similar anticholinergic side effects including dry mouth, constipation, and urinary retention. These drugs may also induce delirium or worsen symptoms of dementia and so should be used with caution and started at low doses.

Men with prostatic enlargement and voiding symptoms including incontinence often respond to either alpha-adrenergic antagonists alone or in combination with 5-alpha-reductase inhibitors. Alpha-adrenergic antagonists such as alfuzosin (Uroxatral), terazosin (Hytrin), tamsulosin (Flomax), and doxazosin (Cardura) are commonly associated with orthostatic hypotension. Terazosin and alfuzosin exhibit less of this effect. 5-Alpha-reductase inhibitors such as finasteride (Proscar) are testosterone antagonists that are well tolerated other than potential sexual side effects.

Urinary catheters are indicated for urinary retention with high postvoid residual volume or if skin wounds, pressure sores, and irritation result from the incontinence. Intermittent catheterization is preferred over chronic indwelling catheters due to risk of infection.

FALLS

BACKGROUND

Falls are common in older adults and are associated with fractures, functional decline, and death. In addition, falls and fear of falling are associated with loss of self-confidence and anxiety, and are a major reason for nursing home admission. Costs from falls account for 6% of all medical expenditures in elderly adults. The incidence of falls can be decreased by identifying precipitating factors coupled with targeted interventions.

EPIDEMIOLOGY

The incidence and severity of falls increase with age. Over one-third of community-dwelling adults older than 65 fall each year, and the rate of falls triples in nursing homes and hospitals. Ten percent of falls result in serious injury, with nursing home residents suffering serious injury almost 25% of the time. Unintentional injuries are the fifth leading cause of death in older adults, with falls underlying the majority of such injuries.

RISK FACTORS

Risk factors for falling can be divided into intrinsic and extrinsic factors.

Intrinsic factors include poor strength, visual deficits, gait and balance problems, arthritis, cognitive impairment, and depression. Orthostatic hypotension appears to play a role in many falls and can be caused by medications, postprandial hypotension, fluid or blood loss, autonomic dysfunction, or adrenal insufficiency.

Extrinsic factors include environmental factors such as poor lighting, loose carpets, and lack of bathroom safety equipment. Medications can be particularly dangerous in the older adults; the more medications one takes, the higher the risk of falling. Medications particularly associated with falling include neuroleptics, SSRIs, tricyclic antidepressants, benzodiazepines, anticonvulsants, and class 1A antiarrhythmics.

EVALUATION

The evaluation of a patient with a history of falls requires a thorough assessment of risk factors including a history of previous falls and a medication review. Special attention should focus on medications associated with falls and any new or altered medications. Levels of drugs such as phenytoin (Dilantin) should also be tested when appropriate.

The "Get Up and Go" is a good screening tool to assess for balance and gait. This requires the patient to stand from a seated position without using his or her arms, walk 10–20 feet, turn, and return to his or her seat. Postural vitals signs should be checked. Underlying neurological diseases such as Parkinson disease, stroke, or dementia should be ruled out. A targeted neurological exam should include tests of proprioception, muscle strength, Romberg exam, and tandem stance. Vision testing as well as detailed examination of the feet and footwear are also recommended.

Basic labs include a complete blood count, measurement of serum electrolytes, blood urea nitrogen, creatinine, glucose, vitamin B-12, and assessment of thyroid function. Neuroimaging is indicated if there is evidence of a focal neurological deficit, history of head trauma, or evidence of a central nervous system process. Cardiac workup with an electrocardiogram (EKG), echocardiogram, or evaluation for arrhythmias is warranted only if there is clinical evidence for such an underlying diagnosis, especially if there is a history of syncope.

MANAGEMENT

The approach to preventing further falls requires a targeted intervention based on identified risk factors and physical exam findings. Falls that are not due to an underlying cardiovascular or neurological disorder can be classified into four treatment categories: leg muscle weakness, poor balance/instability, medication toxicity, and hypotension.

Patients who demonstrate leg muscle weakness on physical exam and the Get Up and Go test should be referred to a physical therapist for quadriceps strengthening and resistance training.

Poor balance or instability responds well to balance training by a physical therapist. Assistive devices such as canes and walkers may also be indicated and should be properly fitted by a therapist. Patients should be referred to a podiatrist if there is poor foot care or if better-fitting footwear such as wide-soled shoes are indicated. Referral should be made to an ophthalmologist if there is evidence of poor vision to ensure proper corrective lenses or treatment of other reversible vision loss such as cataracts. A standardized home safety evaluation by an occupational therapist can identify environmental hazards such as throw rugs, slippery bathtubs, and poor lighting. An occupational therapist may also make specific recommendations such as the installation of stair rails and bathroom safety equipment such as grab bars.

After all medications have been thoroughly reviewed, any unnecessary or problematic medications should be tapered and discontinued if possible. Special attention should be paid to the elimination of psychotropic medications. Reducing the number of medications to fewer than four is shown to reduce the risk of falling, so the benefits of each medication should be weighed against the risk of falling.

Orthostatic and postprandial hypotension should be treated based on the underlying cause. For example, reducing antihypertensive medications or dividing them into morning and evening dosing may diminish orthostatic hypotension. Separating medications from meals may reduce postprandial hypotension. Patients should be educated about the need to rise slowly from a seated or lying position. They should also be encouraged to maintain adequate volume status. Patients with autonomic dysfunction may respond to stockings or to medications such as fludrocortisone or midodrine.

Patients at risk of falling should have osteoporosis screening as well as adequate calcium and vitamin D supplementation to reduce the risk of fracture. Patients who live alone should have personal emergency-response systems (e.g., Lifeline) to ensure prompt treatment should they continue to fall.

ADDITIONAL READING

Adelman A, Daly M. Initial evaluation of the patient with suspected dementia. *Am Fam Physician.* 2005;71:1745–50.

Cummings J. Alzheimer's disease. *N Engl J Med.* 2004;351:56–67.

Fick D, Cooper J, Wade W, Waller J, Maclean J, Beers M. Updating the Beers criteria for potentially inappropriate medication use in older adults: Results of a US consensus panel of experts. *Arch Intern Med.* 2003;163:2716–24.

Gibbs C, Johnson TN, Ouslander J. Office management of geriatric urinary incontinence. *Am J Med.* 2007;120:211–20.

Guideline for the Prevention of Falls in Older Persons. American Geriatrics Society, British Geriatrics Society, and American Academy of Orthopaedic Surgeons Panel on Falls Prevention. *J Am Geriatr Soc.* 2001;49:664–72.

Gupta V, Lipsitz L. Orthostatic hypotension in the elderly: Diagnosis and treatment. *Am J Med.* 2007;120:841–7.

Inouye S. Delirium in older persons. *N Engl J Med.* 2006;354:1157–65.

Kawas C. Clinical practice. Early Alzheimer's disease. *N Engl J Med.* 2003;349:1056–63.

Tinetti M. Clinical practice. Preventing falls in elderly persons. *N Engl J Med.* 2003;348:42–9.

Unützer J. Clinical practice. Late-life depression. *N Engl J Med.* 2007;357:2269–76.

QUESTIONS

QUESTION 1. A 79-year-old woman with osteoporosis, hypertension, and recurrent falls presents to her primary care provider for a routine follow-up accompanied by her daughter. The patient has no specific concerns, but her daughter is concerned about recent behavioral problems. Specifically she reports that her mother has reported seeing visions of her deceased relatives. On further questioning the daughter reports that her mother's memory has declined over the past several years. She has required help with finances and managing the house but assumed this was part of normal aging. On physical exam she is noted to have some cogwheeling and gait instability as well as inattention and executive dysfunction on brief cognitive screening tests. She has no previous history of depression or other psychiatric disorders.

What would be the best approach to caring for this patient?

A. Do a lumbar puncture to rule out encephalitis
B. Administer low-dose neuroleptic for periods of agitation
C. Initiate treatment with an SSRI
D. Discuss with the patient and her caregiver options for ensuring proper supervision and safety at home

QUESTION 2. An 85-year-old man with dementia is admitted to the hospital after a fall and found to have a hip fracture. Within 24 hours he underwent successful operative repair under general anesthesia. In the postanesthesia care unit he was agitated and more confused from baseline and was administered several doses of lorazepam. On the second day of his admission he was no longer agitated, but by the third day the medical team noticed that he was less interactive and unable to maintain attention and also was developing dehydration from lack of appetite.

What is the next appropriate intervention?

A. Consult surgery for placement of a feeding tube
B. Initiate therapy with an SSRI for depression
C. Discontinue all opiates and administer scheduled acetaminophen
D. Order noncontrast head CT
E. Perform a thorough medication review

QUESTION 3. An 82-year-old woman with hypertension, diabetes, and osteoporosis presents to her primary care office after a recent hip fracture. On further questioning, you learn that she has had several recent falls. The first fall occurred while she was walking outside and tripped on the sidewalk. Another fall occurred in the bathroom when she lost her balance transferring out of the shower. A medication review reveals that she is not taking any new medications and is currently taking calcium 500 mg tid, vitamin D 400 IU bid, alendronate 70 mg weekly, aspirin 81 mg daily, lisinopril 20 mg daily, and glimepiride 2 mg daily. She has no episodes of hypoglycemia and denies syncope or palpitations. Physical exam reveals no orthostasis, no focal neurological deficit, negative Romberg, and is otherwise unremarkable except for impaired proprioception bilaterally. She is wearing appropriate shoes and corrective lenses, and on the Get Up and Go test she is able to stand from a seated position without using her arms, although she does exhibit unsteadiness while walking.

What is the best approach to preventing further falls?

A. Reduce the dose of lisinopril
B. Refer to physical therapy for quadriceps strengthening
C. Refer to physical therapy for balance-training exercises and possible assistive device
D. Order vitamin B-12 level
E. C and D

QUESTION 4. A 73-year-old woman with hypertension complains of urinary incontinence. She reports involuntary leakage of variable amounts of urine, usually associated with urinary frequency and urgency and inability to delay voiding in time to make it to the bathroom. Physical exam, including a pelvic and rectal examination, is unremarkable. A urinalysis and postvoid residual are also unremarkable.

What is the best approach to treating this patient's incontinence?

A. Topical estrogen
B. Bladder training with regularly scheduled voiding
C. Antimuscarinic drugs
D. Intermittent catheterization
E. Surgical bladder neck suspension

QUESTION 5. An 89-year-old woman with hypertension, dyslipidemia, coronary artery disease, congestive heart failure, and atrial fibrillation is admitted to the hospital after her family discovered her dehydrated and malnourished at home. She has been living alone for the past 2 years since her husband died and was functionally independent until the past several months, when she seemed more forgetful and began requiring help from her family. She began making errors in her checkbook and paying bills late and seemed in general slower. She has lost 10 lb mainly from skipping meals. She is on several medications, but none are new or changed, although she has recently been forgetting doses. She has no history of psychiatric disorders, and initial workup reveals no significant underlying pathology. Cognitive testing reveals mild executive dysfunction and overall lack of effort on testing.

What is the next step to appropriately care for this patient?

A. Order noncontrast head CT
B. Begin therapy with donepezil
C. Pursue oncologic workup
D. Pursue evaluation to determine underlying cause of delirium
E. Perform screening for depression

ANSWERS

1. D
2. E
3. E
4. B
5. E

103.

PALLIATIVE CARE

Vicki A. Jackson and J. Andrew Billings

Palliative medicine is a medical specialty that focuses on helping patients and families live as well as possible in the face of a life-threatening illness. Quality of life is promoted through meticulous management of pain and other symptoms, psychosocial and spiritual support, assistance with decision making and advance care planning, and coordination of care in and outside of the hospital. Palliative medicine includes, but is not limited to, hospice care. Importantly, a palliative approach may be used concomitantly with disease-modifying therapy and thus can be useful at the earliest phases of serious, complex illnesses (Morrison and Meier, 2004). This care is delivered in the outpatient and inpatient setting. Early outpatient palliative care for patients with advanced cancer has been associated with improved quality of life, a 50% lower rate of depression, and improved survival (Temel, 2010).

A palliative care evaluation begins with a comprehensive history and physical examination with particular attention to such common symptoms as pain, nausea and vomiting, dyspnea, fatigue, anxiety, depression, and family stress. Of equal importance is providing an opportunity for a discussion of hopes and fears about the future, including an exploration of goals for the remainder of the patient's life—information that is vital in guiding future care. Below, we emphasize the management of physical symptoms.

PAIN

Patients with life-threatening illnesses of all kinds, but especially those with cancer, regularly experience pain. Even the most conservative surveys indicate that at least 20% of patients have pain at diagnosis, and much more frequently in the advanced stages of their illness. Numerous studies show that clinicians often undertreat cancer pain and that undertreated pain causes undue burdens on patients and their families. Clinicians typically underestimate the severity of pain or are not facile in pain management techniques that have the potential to greatly improve a patient's quality of life. Patient and family misconceptions about pain medications also contribute to inadequate pain management, as when family members are reluctant to use opioid analgesics for fear of addiction or worry that such treatments signify that death is imminent. Patients at particular risk for undertreatment include women, minorities, the poor, the old, and residents of nursing homes.

PAIN ASSESSMENT

By use of simple treatment protocols, pain can be controlled in 80–95% of cancer patients. The first step in devising a pain management plan is a careful diagnostic evaluation and the development of a comprehensive differential diagnosis. In a cancer patient, the common etiologies of pain include the disease itself and its treatment, such as radiation therapy or chemotherapy. Neuropathic pain, which patients will usually characterize as burning, sharp, or shooting, and which may be associated with sensory-motor alterations, should be distinguished from visceral and somatic pains, which typically are dull and aching and may be reproduced with local pressure. Understanding the origin of the pain aids in the development of the appropriate pain management plan. Pain from bony metastases, for example, benefit from nonsteroidal anti-inflammatory drugs (NSAIDs) or radiation, whereas pain from nerve compression may respond to opioids and anticonvulsants or tricyclic antidepressants.

In addition to characterizing such matters as the quality, temporal pattern, location, radiation, and alleviating and aggravating factors of pain, symptom severity should be assessed serially with simple, validated methods such as numerical or visual analog scales (for example, "rate your pain from zero to 10, where zero is no pain and 10 is the worst imaginable pain").

Many clinicians are unaware that patients with chronic pain rarely show signs of sympathetic arousal, such as tachycardia or hypertension, and may not appear distressed in the same fashion as patients with acute pain. The patient's self-report is the gold standard of pain assessment: believe the patient.

THE EXPERIENCE OF PAIN

How patients experience pain and how they express their discomfort can be highly dependent on other physical, psychosocial, and spiritual issues. Depression, anxiety, and existential distress can all exacerbate a patient's perception of and ability to cope with pain. Because such factors play a large role in a clinician's ability to treat pain, an assessment of these factors is critical for developing a comprehensive management plan. The comprehensive clinical assessment should include attention to psychological, social, and spiritual distress in the patient and family and an evaluation of their coping. Screening for depression, anxiety, delirium, and other treatable neuropsychiatric conditions is essential.

TREATMENT

The goal of treatment is to adequately manage the pain while minimizing side effects. The World Health Organization (WHO) analgesic ladder is a validated step-by-step approach that provides 88% of cancer-pain patients with adequate analgesia.

Step 1

The ladder begins by treating mild to moderate pain with acetaminophen or NSAIDs. When prescribing acetaminophen, use caution in patients with heavy alcohol use as even therapeutic doses (4 g/day) can produce severe hepatotoxicity. Patients with stable chronic liver disease can take acetaminophen at therapeutic doses. Use NSAIDs with caution in patients with renal impairment, gastritis, ulcers, or bleeding disorders. Overall, no NSAID works better than any other, but individual patients may find one superior to others.

Starting Short-Acting Opioids

Step 2 (for mild to moderate pain) and Step 3 (for moderate to severe pain) of the WHO analgesic ladder involve titration of common short-acting opioids to achieve good pain control. Thus, for any pain that persists despite NSAIDs or acetaminophen and for more severe pain, it is important to initiate short-acting opioids in conjunction with NSAIDs or acetaminophen.

When choosing an opioid, consider patients' previous experiences with these agents and their preferences because patients commonly report side effects or what are incorrectly labeled as "allergies" to codeine and other opioids. Lower doses of oxycodone and morphine are good choices. Short-acting opioids are dosed every 3–4 hours, titrated with the goal of producing acceptable pain relief, and delivered via the least invasive route, preferably oral. The correct dose is the dose that alleviates or abolishes the pain without undue side effects. Once a general picture of analgesic needs is established, chronic pain is best controlled by prescribing both a basal or round-the-clock dose (e.g., oxycodone 10 mg PO q4h) and a breakthrough or PRN dose (e.g., oxycodone 5–10 mg PO q2h PRN) (table 103.1).

Table 103.1 OPIOID ANALGESIC CHARACTERISTICS

DRUG	ONSET (MINUTES)	PEAK EFFECT (MINUTES)	DURATION OF ANALGESIA (HOURS)
Morphine			
Oral, IR	15–60	30–60	4
Oral, SR			
Avinza			24
Kadian			12–24
MS Contin			8–12
Oramorph			8–12
Oxycodone			
Oral, IR	10–15	30–60	4
Oral, SR (OxyContin)			8–12
Hydromorphone			
Oral, IR	15–30	30–60	4
Intravenous	1–2	5–20	4
Fentanyl			
Oral transmucosal	5–15	20–30	1–2
Transdermal (patch)		12 hours	48–72
Intravenous	<1	5–15	0.5–1

Starting Long-Acting Opioids

For a patient with intermittent pain, short-acting opioids may suffice. However, for a patient with continuous or regularly recurring pain or requiring frequent use of opioids, a next step is to add long-acting opioids. Choosing the appropriate long acting opioid dose requires multiple steps.

First, determine the total daily dose required to provide adequate analgesia. Second, choose the long-acting preparation. Both morphine or oxycodone have long-acting preparations that are inexpensive and well tolerated. The total daily dose of short-acting opioid can be directly converted to long-acting opioid. For example, a patient requiring at least 5 mg of oxycodone every 3 hours to control pain is using 40 mg of oxycodone in a 24-hour period. This patient may be started on 20 mg of long-acting oxycodone every 12 hours. Alternatively, if the patient requires a different opioid or will receive the same opioid by a different route, use an equianalgesic table (table 103.2) to estimate the appropriate starting dose. When converting a patient from one opioid to another, patients will often require a lower-than-calculated dose of the new opioid, reflecting incomplete cross-tolerance or other individual differences in metabolism, so the starting dose of the new opioid should be reduced by 25% from the calculated equivalent dose.

Dosing for Breakthrough Pain

Even patients who have well-controlled pain on an established long-acting opioid regimen should have a short-acting or "rescue" opioid available for breakthrough or incident pain and predictable periods of pain exacerbation (e.g., transport to a radiological examination). Ideally, a patient will take only two to three breakthrough doses over 24 hours; a requirement for more doses suggests a need for more long-acting medication. To calculate the increase in the long-acting dose, add up the total amount of breakthrough medication taken in 24 hours and add it to the patient's regimen in the form of the long-acting formulation that the patient is already taking.

Use of Other Opioids

For most clinicians, familiarity with preparations of oxycodone, hydromorphone (Dilaudid), and morphine, as well as transdermal fentanyl, will facilitate good pain control for the vast majority of patients. The fentanyl patch has the advantage for some patients in that it does not require a functioning gastrointestinal tract and only needs to be changed every 2–3 days. It is generally not used in opioid-naive patients but, like other long-acting agents, is added on in an equianalgesic dose to a short-acting opioid regimen.

Methadone is another opioid that is commonly used in the treatment of chronic pain because it is highly effective and inexpensive. Its unique pharmacokinetic properties, however, pose particular challenges in its clinical application. It should be used only by clinicians trained in its use. Rapid titration can result in overdosing and even death.

Several other readily available opioids are not recommended for use in patients with chronic pain, either because they have limited analgesic effectiveness (e.g., codeine) or because of their propensity for accumulation of neuroexcitatory metabolites that can result in delirium, myoclonus, and seizure (e.g., propoxyphene and meperidine).

Commonly Used Adjuvant Pain Medications

Specific pain syndromes often are not adequately managed with opioids alone. Bony metastases, for example, often benefit from anti-inflammatory medications or steroids, whereas neuropathic pain will require treatment with anticonvulsants, such as gabapentin, or tricyclic antidepressants.

Side Effects

Common side effects of opioids include nausea, vomiting, sedation, and constipation. Nausea (discussed below) and sedation usually resolve within less than a week. Constipation does not attenuate with long-term use. Therefore, all patients on opioids require a bowel regimen that includes a stimulant laxative (e.g., senna 2 tabs PO bid). (Abrahm, 2005).

NAUSEA AND VOMITING

Nausea and vomiting are common symptoms in patients with life-threatening illness and, when present, have a

Table 103.2 EQUIANALGESIC DOSAGES FOR COMMONLY USED OPIOIDS

OPIOID	ROUTE	
	INTRAVENOUS	ORAL
Morphine	10 mg	30 mg
Oxycodone	NA	20 mg
Hydromorphone	1.5 mg	7.5 mg
Fentanyl	0.1 mg (100 μg)	
Fentanyl transdermal 25 μg/hr patch = 50 mg of oral morphine per day		

EQUIANALGESIC VALUES FROM THE TABLE	PATIENT 24-HOUR OPIOID DOSES	SOLVE FOR X
$\dfrac{\text{Value of current opioid}}{\text{Value of new opioid}}$	$= \dfrac{\text{Total 24-hr dose of current opioid}}{X} =$	Equianalgesic 24-hr dose of new opioid
$\dfrac{\text{Morphine 30 mg PO}}{\text{Morphine 10 mg IV}}$	$= \dfrac{\text{Morphine 150 mg PO/24 hr}}{X} =$	Morphine 50 mg IV/24 hr

profound negative impact on quality of life. Both symptoms are often associated with cancer chemotherapy and the initiation of opioids but can occur independently in advanced cancer and are also seen regularly in patients with AIDS and renal and hepatic failure. A diagnostic evaluation includes attention to reversible etiologies, such as constipation, gastroesophageal reflux, or esophageal candidiasis.

Effective and systematic management of nausea and vomiting requires an understanding of the pathophysiology of these symptoms. Vomiting is coordinated through the emesis center in the medulla oblongata. The emesis center responds to inputs from the cerebral cortex, the vestibular apparatus of the inner ear, the chemoreceptor trigger zone (CTZ) in the brain, and peripheral neural pathways (vagal stimulation through mechanoreceptors and chemoreceptors in the gastrointestinal tract and other viscera). Serotonin, dopamine, histamine, acetylcholine, substance P, and neurokinin-1 are all factors that mediate the process in the emesis center.

Initial pharmacologic therapy targets the etiology of the emetogenic stimulus or the neurotransmitters that are active in the likely causative pathways. Multiple agents from different classes are often required to block the involved neurotransmitters. Common antiemetic classes include dopamine and serotonin antagonists, antihistamines, anticholinergic agents, anxiolytics, and steroids. Agents that target neurokinin-1 are currently indicated only for delayed chemotherapy-induced nausea and vomiting. Dopamine antagonists include phenothiazines (e.g., prochlorperazine), butyrophenones (e.g., haloperidol), and substituted benzamides (metoclopramide). Sedation may be a side effect, and agents may be chosen to produce or avoid sedation.

Akathisia and extrapyramidal side effects are the major toxicities of this class and can limit use. The phenothiazines are considered general antiemetics, with major activity at the CTZ. When a clear etiology is not apparent, initiate therapy with prochlorperazine, 10 mg every 6 hours, or metoclopramide, 10 mg every 6 hours. As-needed dosing of severe nausea is often ineffective; schedule administration around the clock.

The use of the serotonin antagonists, such as ondansetron and granisetron, can be helpful, primarily in patients with chemotherapy-induced nausea and vomiting. These agents may have efficacy in nausea caused by peripheral emetic pathways but should not be used as first-line agents due to cost and the frequent side effect of constipation. Although the mechanism of action is unclear, steroids can be helpful as antiemetics alone and in combination with other agents. Antihistamines such as diphenhydramine and meclizine act on histamine receptors in the vomiting center and vestibular afferents, making them useful for the management of motion sickness as well as adjuvants with the above agents (Mannix, 2003). Anxiolytics presumably work through cerebral inputs.

Pharmacologic interventions are the mainstay therapy in advanced disease, but cognitive behavioral, relaxation, and complementary therapies may also be useful in the management of nausea and vomiting (table 103.3).

DYSPNEA

Dyspnea is defined as an uncomfortable or unpleasant sensation of breathing. In one study of hospice patients, 21%

Table 103.3 COMMON CAUSES OF NAUSEA AND VOMITING WITH THERAPEUTIC OPTIONS

CAUSE	SITE OF ACTION	MEDIATING NEUROTRANSMITTERS	THERAPEUTIC OPTIONS
Constipation/obstipation	Colon, small bowel		Bowel regimen: enema, suppositories, stimulant laxative (e.g., senna)
Gastroparesis	Stomach, small bowel	Dopamine	Prokinetic agents first line (e.g., metoclopramide) Haloperidol, prochlorperazine
Toxins (chemotherapy)	Chemoreceptor trigger zone	Dopamine, serotonin, neurokinin-1	Haloperidol, prochlorperazine, ondansetron, aprepitant
Vagal nerve stimulation from receptors in GI tract and viscera	Vagus nerve	Histamine, acetylcholine	Diphenhydramine, hyoscyamine
Anxiety, anticipatory nausea	Cerebral cortex		Benzodiazepines, cognitive behavioral techniques
Increased intracranial pressure	Chemoreceptor trigger zone and vomiting center	Histamine, acetylcholine	Steroids, diphenhydramine, promethazine
Inflammation of GI tract; radiation, tumor	Esophagus, stomach, and small bowel	Histamine, acetylcholine, serotonin	Diphenhydramine, promethazine, ondansetron
Motion sickness	Vestibular afferents	Histamine, acetylcholine	Diphenhydramine, promethazine

of patients reported dyspnea as their most severe symptom. In a series of cancer patients, 70% reported shortness of breath, but the symptom is also common in those with primary pulmonary and cardiac diseases. Dyspnea can result in decreased physical activity and deconditioning that further exacerbates the problem.

Dyspnea is a complex symptom that can have multiple underlying etiologies. The specific description of dyspnea by the patient may shed light on the underlying etiology and thus help to guide treatment (Manning and Schwartzstein, 1995). In normal subjects, the sensation of "air hunger" is more often related to hypercapnia rather than hypoxia. Chest "tightness" appears to be related to stimulation of unmyelinated C-fibers in the airway in conditions such as bronchospasm. Stimulation of these fibers in the alveolar epithelium and irritant receptors results in the sensation of chest tightness. On the other hand, patients describe an "increased work of breathing" when they have respiratory muscle weakness, critical illness with accompanying increased respiratory output, or altered mechanics (e.g., hyperinflation).

As with pain and nausea, successful management of dyspnea requires elucidation of the etiology as well as judicious choice of nonspecific interventions that may be efficacious regardless of etiology (table 103.4). For example, a patient may have both bronchospasm and a pleural effusion contributing to sensations of tightness and increased work of breathing. Both conditions should be aggressively treated. In cases where treating the underlying cause is not possible, multiple pharmacologic and nonpharmacologic treatments are employed to reduce the subjective experience of dyspnea.

Anxiety almost always accompanies dyspnea and can be addressed through pulmonary rehabilitation and cognitive-behavioral techniques as well as anxiolytics. Patients can learn adaptations (e.g., pursed-lip breathing) that improve the mechanical disadvantage caused by a particular illness. Low-dose benzodiazepines, used cautiously, may be beneficial in the treatment of dyspnea-related anxiety but probably do not provide relief for the sensation of dyspnea itself.

Nonpharmacologic interventions, such as the use of a fan or a cool washcloth to the face, can provide some comfort. These interventions appear to provide relief by stimulation of the V2 branch of the trigeminal nerve, which decreases the sensation of dyspnea caused by hypercapnia. Interestingly, stimulation of the trigeminal is likely the mechanism by which the use of oxygen provides relief to the dyspneic patient with normal oxygenation.

Opioids are regularly employed to provide comfort to patients with dyspnea. No data support the preferential use of a particular opioid in the treatment of dyspnea. The use of inhaled or nebulized opioids is not supported by data. Therefore, dyspnea is treated with oral or intravenous opioids, such as morphine. In the opioid-naive patient, morphine sulfate elixir, 2.5–5 mg every 2–4 hours as needed may be sufficient, but round-the-clock and long-acting agents may also be useful. In the patient with persistent severe dyspnea who is at the end of life, round-the-clock opioid dosing or infusions via a subcutaneous or intravenous route may be required. Breakthrough doses should also be prescribed. Patients already taking opioids regularly for chronic pain will require additional doses of opioids to provide relief (Thomas and von Gunten, 2003).

FATIGUE

Fatigue affects approximately 70–100% of cancer patients. The National Comprehensive Cancer Network defines fatigue as "a persistent subjective sense of tiredness that interferes with usual functioning." The profound fatigue associated with life-threatening illness can be debilitating and can adversely affect a patient's quality of life (Mock et al., 2000).

Fatigue is often underreported by patients and not addressed by clinicians. Appropriate management begins

Table 103.4 DIFFERENTIAL DIAGNOSIS OF DYSPNEA

PULMONARY	CARDIAC	CHEST WALL	PSYCHOLOGICAL
Cancer-tumor burden	CHF	Chest wall tumor	Anxiety
Bronchial obstruction	Ischemia	Diaphragmatic	Fear
Lymphangitic spread	Deconditioning	dysfunction	Spiritual distress
of tumor	Superior vena cava syndrome	Tumor infiltration	Hyperventilation
Bronchoconstriction	Anemia	Phrenic nerve palsy	
Infection	Pericardial disease	Severe ascites	
Embolism		Respiratory muscle	
Pneumothorax		fatigue	
Fibrosis		Increased demand	
Radiation damage		Cachexia	
Effusion			
Edema			
Hemorrhage			

with screening for the symptom. For patients who have moderate to severe fatigue (4 on a scale of 0–10), a broad clinical assessment is appropriate. Like many other symptoms, the cause is often multifactorial, including medical and psychosocial factors (table 103.5 here).

Reversible causes, such as anemia, hypothyroidism, or depression, should be diagnosed. Frequently, however, an obvious cause cannot be detected or is not modifiable (e.g., advanced cancer). In this case, patient education and both nonpharmacologic and pharmacologic interventions are important components of treatment.

Nonpharmacologic treatments include exercise, energy conservation techniques, and attention to rest and sleep patterns. Patients who have fatigue can decondition very quickly, resulting in worsening symptoms. Multiple studies have documented the benefits of exercise on functional capacity, fatigue scores, and quality of life. Encouraging regular nighttime sleep habits and limited daytime napping is a valuable aspect of patient education. Energy conservation means using energy for activities that enhance quality of life while avoiding less pleasurable or less important activities. For example, a patient can be encouraged to visit family and friends during times when energy is greatest and to conserve energy by asking for assistance with tasks that are not pleasurable (e.g., carrying the laundry to the basement).

Pharmacologic therapy includes treatment with psychostimulants, such as methylphenidate. Studies of patients who have HIV infection, multiple sclerosis, and cancer have shown methylphenidate to be effective in the treatment of fatigue. Patients with cancer and fatigue report improved cognition and decreased opioid-related sedation on methylphenidate. The usual initial dose is methylphenidate 5 mg at 8 a.m. and noon or 2 p.m. (thus avoiding interference with sleep). Stimulants must be used with caution in elderly or delirious patients and those with cardiac arrhythmias.

SUMMARY

Patients often believe erroneously that they must "live with" severe symptoms that limit quality of life. Palliative medicine begins with the recognition, assessment, and reassessment of these troublesome symptoms and with aggressive patient-centered management aimed at minimizing suffering and improving quality of life. Successful palliation of symptoms in the dying patient is tremendously rewarding. The relief of physical suffering facilitates psychosocial and spiritual coping, often allowing patients to focus on spending meaningful time with loved ones, completing life tasks, and saying goodbye.

ADDITIONAL READING

Abrahm J. *A Physician's Guide to Pain and Symptom Management in Cancer Patients.* 2nd ed. (pp. 155–170). Baltimore: Johns Hopkins University Press; 2005.

Crone CC, Marcangelo MJ, Shuster JL Jr. An approach to the patient with organ failure: Transplantation and end-of-life treatment decisions. *Med Clin North Am.* 2010;94(6):1241–54, xii.

Ko FC. The clinical care of frail, older adults. *Clin Geriatr Med.* 2011;27(1):89–100.

Manning HL, Schwartzstein RM. Pathophysiology of dyspnea. *N Engl J Med.* 1995;333:1547–53.

Mannix KA. Palliation of nausea and vomiting. In Doyle D, Hanks G, Cherny NI, et al, (eds.), *Oxford Textbook of Palliative Medicine.* 3rd ed. (pp. 459–67). Oxford: Oxford University Press; 2003.

Mock V, Atkinson A. Barsevick A, et al. NCCN practice guidelines for cancer-related fatigue. *Oncology.* 2000;14:151–61.

Morrison RS, Meier DE. Palliative care. *N Engl J Med.* 2004;350:2582–9.

Olsen ML, Swetz KM, Mueller PS. Ethical decision making with end-of-life care: Palliative sedation and withholding or withdrawing life-sustaining treatments. *Mayo Clin Proc.* 2010;85(10):949–54.

Thomas JR, von Gunten CF. Management of dyspnea. *J Support Oncol.* 2003;1(1):23–32.

QUESTIONS

QUESTION 1. Jane Sullivan is a 43-year-old woman with advanced colon cancer metastatic to her liver and right hip. She had been doing well (pain severity range 0–2/10) but is now complaining of 6–8/10 pain (i.e., moderate pain) in the right hip, especially with movement. She describes her pain as deep and aching. She denies that the pain is radiating, electric in quality, or associated with paresthesias or weakness or new-onset bowel or bladder dysfunction.

She is taking ibuprofen, 800 mg q 8 hours, which had been controlling the pain, but now she is experiencing moderate to severe pain that interferes with her daily activities.

From your exam and her history, you believe that she is experiencing bony pain from a metastatic lesion in her hip. You develop a plan to treat her pain that includes continuation of her nonsteroidal anti-inflammatory agent, initiation

Table 103.5 COMMON CAUSES OF FATIGUE

Anemia
Cardiac disease
Decreased activity level and deconditioning
Depression
Hepatic disease
Poor nutrition
Pain
Respiratory insufficiency
Renal failure
Sleep disturbance
Thyroid disease

of bisphosphonates, evaluation for radiation therapy, and initiation of a short-acting opioid along with daily senna.

Which of the following would be the most appropriate opioid order?

A. Morphine 15 mg PO q 6 hours PRN
B. Morphine 15 mg PO q 4 hours PRN
C. Morphine 15 mg PO q 2 hours PRN
D. Morphine 30 mg PO q 4 hours PRN

QUESTION 2. Jane returns 2 weeks later stating that her pain is improved and acceptable (3/10), but only if she takes her morphine six times per day. You decide to start a long-acting opioid and to check in with her in 2 days.

What would be the most appropriate dosing for her long-acting opioid and breakthrough medication?

A. Morphine sustained-release (MS Contin) 45 mg q 12 hours scheduled with morphine immediate-release 10 mg PO q 2 hours PRN breakthrough pain.
B. Morphine sustained-release (MS Contin) 90 mg q 24 hours scheduled with morphine immediate-release 10 mg PO q 2 hours PRN breakthrough pain.
C. Morphine sustained-release (MS Contin) 30 mg q 8 hours scheduled with morphine immediate-release 30 mg PO q 2 hours PRN breakthrough pain.

D. Morphine sustained-release (MS Contin) 45 mg q 12 hours scheduled with morphine immediate-release 10 mg PO q 6 hours PRN breakthrough pain.

QUESTION 3. Despite radiation therapy, Jane develops a pathological fracture of her hip. She is admitted to the hospital for surgery and will need to be NPO. Her pain had been in good control with a total of 150 mg of oral morphine per day (60 mg MS Contin q12 hours + 15 mg immediate-release morphine two to three times/day). You now need to change her oral morphine to IV morphine.

What would be the most appropriate dose for an hourly continuous rate?

A. Morphine IV 1 mg/hr
B. Morphine IV 2 mg/hr
C. Morphine IV 3 mg/hr
D. Morphine IV 4 mg/hr

ANSWERS

1. C
2. A
3. B

104.

BOARD SIMULATION: GENERAL INTERNAL MEDICINE

Charles A. Morris

QUESTIONS

QUESTION 1. A 46-year-old salesman presents for follow-up to his primary care doctor after a recent upper respiratory infection (URI). He was treated with moxifloxacin. He also now notes easy bruisability and a nosebleed last week. He has a history of atrial fibrillation and takes warfarin. His exam reveals a few ecchymoses but otherwise is normal. He is guaiac negative and has no petechiae. His laboratory evaluation reveals hematocrit (HCT) of 42, platelets 339,000. His International Normalized Ratio (INR) is 6.2, and Partial thromboplastin time (PTT) is 42 seconds. What is the most appropriate therapy?

A. Fresh frozen plasma until INR <2.0
B. Recombinant factor VIIa
C. Protamine sulfate
D. Oral vitamin K
E. Platelet transfusion

QUESTION 2. A 32-year-old electrician presents with weight loss and cough with bloody sputum. He has a history of a positive purified protein derivative (PPD) for which he never received treatment. On exam, he appears comfortable. He is afebrile, blood pressure (BP) 122/68 mm Hg, pulse 89, room air oxygen saturation of 97%. His chest x-ray demonstrates a left upper lobe consolidation. The next step in his management should be:

A. Initiate therapy for community-acquired pneumonia (CAP) with levofloxacin 750 mg PO qd
B. Admit to the hospital to negative airflow room out of concern of active pulmonary *Mycobacterium tuberculosis*
C. Initiate outpatient therapy with isoniazid for treatment of latent TB infection (LTBI)
D. Initiate outpatient therapy with INH/RIF/ETH/PZA while awaiting AFB results
E. Have patient fitted for N95 mask to wear at all times

QUESTION 3. A 57-year-old attorney has a screening exercise stress test prior to participating in a gym program. He has a history of high blood pressure, tobacco use, and dyslipidemia. The stress test suggests some degree of ischemia, and you consider performing coronary angiography.

Which of the following is true regarding the potential findings?

A. Percutaneous cardiac intervention (PCI) without stenting is indicated if study shows single-vessel disease.
B. PCI with stenting is indicated if study shows single vessel disease.
C. PCI would be indicated if study shows multivessel disease.
D. There is a survival benefit to the addition of clopidogrel.
E. Blood pressure and lipid control would be preferred first-line therapy.

QUESTION 4. A 72-year-old farmer presents to his primary care physician (PCP) for a routine physical exam. He has a history of hypertension and diet-controlled diabetes mellitus (DM). His pulse is 122, and a 12-lead electrocardiogram (EKG) demonstrates new atrial fibrillation. He is started on Coumadin and metoprolol ER, 50 mg daily, with reduction in his resting heart rate(HR) to 85. Which of the following is the most appropriate next step in his management?

A. Initiate amiodarone therapy
B. Admit to the hospital for d/c cardioversion
C. Make no changes
D. Add aspirin, 81 mg daily
E. Consult cardiology for radiofrequency ablation (RFA)

QUESTION 5. A 21-year-old teacher presents with pharyngitis, myalgias, and fatigue. She has a temperature of 38.9°C, 1-cm anterior cervical lymphadenopathy, a lightly erythematous eruption on her chest, and an erythematous posterior oropharynx with scattered small ulcers but no exudates.

A monospot test is performed, and is negative. Which of the following tests is *least* likely to be helpful in making a diagnosis?

A. A repeat monospot in 1 week
B. An Epstein-Barr virus (EBV) VCA IgM
C. A EBV nuclear antigen
D. HIV Enzyme-linked immunosorbent assay (ELISA)
E. Cytomegalovirus (CMV) IgM and IgG

QUESTION 6. An 82-year-old retired librarian with a history of coronary artery disease (CAD), prior ischemic stroke, and hypertension presents to urgent care with 2–3 months of nausea, 16-lb weight loss, and abdominal pain. The pain is most concentrated around her umbilicus, and it is worse with eating; it has gotten especially intense in the last day. She denies fevers, chills, bright red blood per rectum (BRBPR), recent NSAID use, or prior episodes of pain. Her abdominal exam was notable for minimal tenderness. Her labs are notable for an amylase of 233, blood urea nitrogen (BUN) of 61, creatinine of 2.3, and a lactic acid of 4.5. An abdominal CT was obtained (see figure 104.1).

Which of the following is the most relevant risk factor for her current presentation?

A. Atherosclerosis
B. Recent hypotension with poor perfusion of watershed territory
C. Adhesions from prior abdominal surgery
D. Bowel colonization with *Clostridium difficile*
E. A colonic polyp acting as a "lead point"

QUESTION 7. A 74-year-old woman presents to her PCP with 11 months of dry cough and fatigue. She denies fevers, chills, reflux symptoms, or chest pain. She has never smoked, drinks 1 glass of wine daily, and has no known risk factors for *M. tuberculosis*. A course of azithromycin did not decrease her symptoms. Her chest x-ray is shown in figures 104.2 and 104.3.

Which of the following is most true about her disease process?

A. A chest CT would likely show an endobronchial lesion
B. A PPD will be useful as a diagnostic test
C. Induced sputum for acid-fast bacillus (AFB) and mycobacterial culture is indicated
D. Prednisone 60 mg qd is indicated
E. She is highly infectious

QUESTION 8. A 29-year-old nurse comes to see his primary care physician because colleagues noted facial asymmetry. His symptoms began yesterday with a progressive left facial droop. He has no headaches, fevers, pain, or rash. On exam, he cannot furrow his left eyebrow and has dysgeusia. His sensation to light touch, muscle strength in the

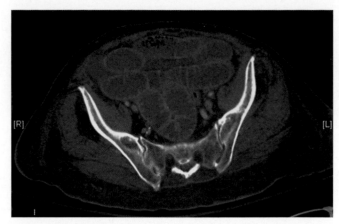

Figure 104.1. Question 9: Abdominal CT Scan.

extremities, and deep tendon reflexes are intact. His head CT is normal.

Which therapy is *not* a reasonable option?

A. Doxycycline
B. Prednisone alone
C. Acyclovir and prednisone
D. Gabapentin
E. No drug therapy, close clinical follow-up

QUESTION 9. A 26-year-old graduate student sees her primary care doctor for advice on contraception. She does not smoke, has no history of clotting disorder, and no family history of breast cancer. When counseling the patient about the risks and benefits of oral contraceptives, all of the following should be included EXCEPT:

A. Increased risk of new-onset hypertension
B. Increased risk of cervical cancer with increased duration of use
C. Increased risk of venous thromboembolic disease
D. Decreased risk of endometrial cancer
E. Decreased risk of breast cancer

QUESTION 10. A 22-year-old law student presents with back pain for the last 2 years. It sometimes wakes him

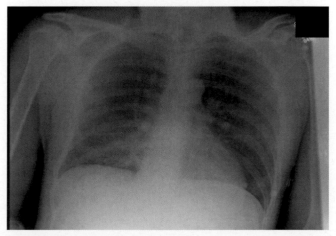

Figure 104.2. Question 10: Chest X-ray, PA.

from sleep and has prevented him from playing sports (see figure 104.4). He has also had recurrent "conjunctivitis" over the last year. More recently, he has developed some chest wall pain. On exam, he has a positive Schober test and decreased chest wall expansion with inspiration. Which of the following tests, if positive, will be the most useful to *confirm* the diagnosis?

A. HLA-B27
B. Colonoscopy
C. L/S spine and sacral plain films
D. C-reactive protein (CRP)
E. Skin biopsy

QUESTION 11. A 68-year-old retired secretary presents to her PCP with dyspnea on exertion. She is a former smoker of 50+ pack years and stopped smoking 10 years ago. She has a daily cough productive of a couple teaspoons of whitish phlegm. Her PCP is concerned she may have chronic obstructive pulmonary disease (COPD). The most appropriate way to diagnose her with COPD is:

A. Lung volumes that demonstrate total lung capacity (TLC) and reserve volume (RV) that are >20% of predicted
B. Spirometry that reveals bronchodilator responsiveness (200 cc and 12% change)
C. Spirometry that reveals an FEV_1/FVC <70% of predicted
D. Chest radiograph with hyperinflated lungs and flattened diaphragms
E. No further studies are required—the history alone is sufficient.

QUESTION 12. A 33-year-old pharmacist comes to her primary care doctor to discuss her risks for developing breast cancer. She has no symptoms and no family history of breast or ovarian cancer. She does not smoke, had her first menstrual period at age 10 and her first child 2 years ago. She used oral contraceptives from age 18 to 28. Which statement about her risk for breast cancer is *not* true?

A. The lifetime chance of developing breast cancer for each woman in the United States is 1:8.
B. Early onset of menarche lowers her risk for breast cancer.
C. First delivery at older age increases the risk for breast cancer.
D. Her oral contraceptive pill (OCP) use increases her risk for breast cancer only modestly.
E. The risk for breast cancer can be calculated in an individualized manner based on the patient's history.

QUESTION 13. A 55-year-old postal worker has a routine physical examination. He has mild hypertension and no symptoms. His physical exam is unremarkable. He asks about prostate-specific antigen (PSA) testing. For this patient, all of the following are true EXCEPT:

A. He has a significant risk of a false-positive PSA result even at this age.
B. PSA is more sensitive than digital rectal exam.
C. Alternative causes of an elevated PSA include prostatitis and benign prostatic hypertrophy (BPH).
D. Use of total PSA with percentage free (unbound) PSA may improve sensitivity.
E. A single PSA level below 4.0 ng/mL essentially rules out the possibility of prostate cancer.

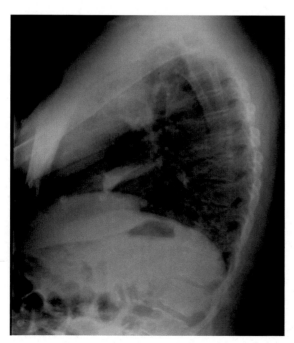

Figure 104.3. Question 10: Chest X-ray, Lateral.

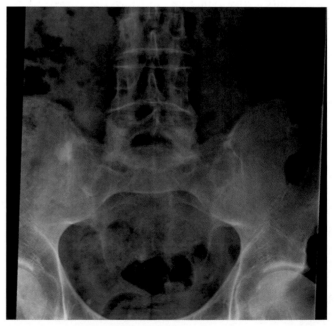

Figure 104.4. Question 15: Pelvic X-ray.

QUESTION 14. A 56-year-old physicist returns for follow-up with his primary care physician after a recent admission for decompensated heart failure. He has a history of coronary artery disease, s/p coronary artery bypass graft (CABG) 10 years prior, with ischemic cardiomyopathy. A recent echocardiogram showed his ejection fraction to be 30%. He describes mild dyspnea with climbing the stairs to his bedroom. He sleeps on two pillows at baseline and notes mildly increased leg swelling. Which of his medications has NOT been shown to have a mortality benefit in patients with class III heart failure?

A. Enalapril
B. Candesartan
C. Metoprolol
D. Digoxin
E. Spironolactone

QUESTION 15. A 34-year-old brick layer presents to urgent care with recurrent substernal chest pain and shortness of breath. He also noted increased fatigue and a 10-lb unintentional weight loss. He has no past medical history, has been smoking 2 packs of cigarettes daily, and uses cocaine occasionally, most recently 2 weeks ago. His physical exam is unremarkable. A chest x-ray is obtained (see figures 104.5 and 104.6).

Which is the *least* likely diagnosis?

A. Thymoma
B. Extragonadal germ cell tumor
C. Hodgkin lymphoma
D. Fibrosing mediastinitis
E. Thyroid neoplasm

QUESTION 16. A 54-year-old physician presents to the emergency room with severe left flank pain. He is unable to remain still on the exam room table. His labs are all normal

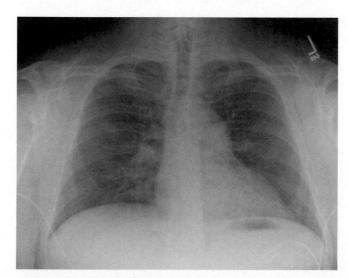

Figure 104.5. Question 20: Chest X-ray, PA.

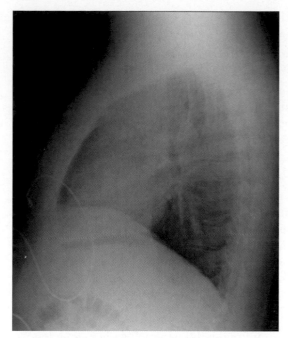

Figure 104.6. Question 20: Chest X-ray, Lateral.

with the exception of his urinalysis, which reveals blood. CT scan of the abdomen reveals a left ureteral stone. Which one of the following compositions is the *most likely* type of kidney stone?

A. Calcium phosphate
B. Uric acid
C. Calcium oxalate
D. Struvite
E. Cystine

QUESTION 17. A 32-year-old journalist presents to her primary care physician. She is currently a one pack/day smoker and has been smoking for 15 years. She has decided she is ready to try to quit. When working with her on smoking cessation, all the following would be true statements *except*:

A. Smoking increases the rate of bone loss and is a risk factor for hip fracture in women.
B. Quit rates are higher in patients who use varenicline when trying to stop smoking.
C. Smoking cessation will decrease the risk of depression.
D. All forms of nicotine replacement have been shown to be effective in improving rates of smoking cessation.
E. Briefly advising her to quit smoking significantly increases the chances she will do so.

QUESTION 18. A 36-year-old high school teacher presents with acute onset of shortness of breath and pleuritic chest pain. She is found to have a pulmonary embolism on chest CT scan. She had a history of deep venous thrombosis 5 years ago, which was treated with warfarin for 6 months. She takes OCPs and aspirin and has no drug allergies. She has one child and had two spontaneous abortions (at 14 and 17 weeks). In addition to initial low-molecular-weight heparin, what is the best treatment option?

A. Long-term anticoagulation with warfarin
B. Daily clopidogrel
C. Anticoagulation with warfarin for 6 months
D. Daily aspirin
E. Inferior vena cava filter

QUESTION 19. A 22-year-old automobile mechanic who is 7 months pregnant presents complaining of difficulty holding her wrench and other tools. She also notes an occasional "electric shock" sensation in her right index and middle fingers and numbness at night. Physical examination reveals mild peripheral edema. She has a solid handgrip and no muscle atrophy. Testing of vibratory, light touch, and proprioception sensation is normal. Which of the following is the most likely cause of her symptoms?

A. Tendinitis of the abductor pollicis brevis tendon
B. Kienböck disease
C. DeQuervain tenosynovitis
D. Multiple sclerosis
E. Carpal tunnel syndrome

QUESTION 20. A 25-year-old architect who is 16 weeks pregnant presents to her primary care physician complaining of mild dysuria and yellowish vaginal discharge. Her urinalysis is dipstick positive for white blood cells only. Her cervical swab returns positive for chlamydia. Which of the following statements is *not* true about empirical therapy:

A. Doxycycline is contraindicated in pregnancy.
B. Azithromycin is an acceptable choice for therapy.
C. Amoxicillin is an acceptable choice for therapy.
D. She should be tested for additional sexually transmitted diseases including HIV and syphilis.
E. There is minimal risk of transmission to partner or neonate.

QUESTION 21. A 25-year-old landscaper presents to his PCP with fevers, headache, and an erythematous rash in his groin following a tick bite. He went to a local ER 2 days earlier and was diagnosed with suspected Lyme disease. He was started on doxycycline 100 mg PO bid. Blood work from that visit has now returned and shows a Lyme Ab that is negative, a white blood cell (WBC) count of 2300, ALT of 121, AST of 236, hematocrit of 42, and platelets of 98. Which of the following statements is true?

A. The doxycycline should be continued for a total of 14 days.
B. The doxycycline should be extended for a total of 28 days.
C. Therapy should be changed to atovaquone and azithromycin.

D. A blood smear should be ordered.
E. The patient does not have acute Lyme disease.

ANSWERS

1. D. This patient's INR is elevated due to recent antibiotic use with unchanged dosing of warfarin. As he has no significant bleeding, the best therapies include stopping his warfarin and giving low-dose oral vitamin K. If he had clinically significant bleeding, reversal with FFP would be appropriate. There is no role for platelet transfusion or protamine. Recombinant factor VIIa is only FDA approved for patients with significant bleeding in the setting of acquired inhibitors of factor VIII and IX or acquired hemophilia (*J Am Coll Cardiol*. 2006;47:804. *Arch Intern Med*. 2006;166:391).

2. D. Untreated +PPD, chronic pneumonia, and an upper lobe infiltrate create a high suspicion of active pulmonary TB, and empirical four-drug therapy is indicated. Levofloxacin would be appropriate coverage for presumed CAP. However, fluoroquinolones have some activity against *Mycobacterium tuberculosis*, which may compromise culture results. The decision to admit the patient is the same for any pneumonia and must consider public health risks of inpatient/outpatient care. Drug therapy for LTBI should be withheld until active TB is ruled out. Respirator/N95 masks are indicated for healthcare workers in close contact (see American Thoracic Society, CDC, and Infectious Diseases Society of America. Treatment of Tuberculosis. *Morbid Mortal Weekly Rep*. 2003;52(No. RR-11).

3. E. Patients with asymptomatic coronary disease (or chronic stable angina) can be managed with aggressive risk factor reduction rather than PCI as first-line therapy. See the Atorvastatin Versus Revascularization Treatment (AVERT) Trial (341 patients, 16% asymptomatic, atorvastatin vs. revascularization; the Atorvastatin group had a 36% reduction in ischemic events) and The Clinical Outcomes Utilizing Revascularization and Aggressive Drug Evaluation (COURAGE) Trial (2287 patients, 70% stenosis in ≥1 coronary artery, + ETT) (table 104.1; *N Engl J Med*. 1999;341:70–6 and *N Engl J Med*. 2007;356:1503–16).

4. C. In asymptomatic atrial fibrillation (AF), rate control and anticoagulation are preferred over rhythm control. The RACE Trial (*N Engl J Med*. 2002;347:1825–33) reported that rate control was not inferior to rhythm control, and the AFFIRM Trial (*N Engl J Med*. 2002;347:1825–33), which was designed to detect mortality difference, found that rhythm control showed a nonsignificant trend toward increased mortality ($p = 0.08$). In both groups, the majority of strokes occurred after warfarin had been stopped or when the INR was subtherapeutic. There were no data to support RFA for asymptomatic patients, and there was no

Table 104.1 THE COURAGE TRIAL: CUMULATIVE OUTCOME RATES AT 4.6 YEARS

OUTCOME	CUMULATIVE EVENT RATE: PCI	CUMULATIVE EVENT RATE: MEDICAL MANAGEMENT
Revascularization	21.1%	32.6%**
Fatal/nonfatal MI	19%	18.5%
Death (all cause)	7.6%	8.3%
Death, MI, ACS	27.6%	27%
Hospitalization for ACS	12.4%	11.8%

NOTE: ** *p* <0.001.
SOURCE: *N Engl J Med.* 2007;356:1503–16.

indication for immediate inpatient cardioversion. In AF, ASA plus Coumadin increases risk without clear benefit (*Stroke.* 2004;35:2212–67.).

5. D. In an acute mono-like illness, the Ddx includes EBV, CMV, and acute HIV, so an HIV viral load is needed. Rash and mucocutaneous ulceration are unusual in EBV IM. Heterophile antibodies are highly specific but lack sensitivity in the first week of illness (missing in up to 25% of cases). IgM and IgG against the EBV viral capsid have high sensitivity and specificity. IgG to EBV nuclear antigen (EBNA) appear 6–12 weeks after infection and persist for life. Positive IgM with an acute/convalescent increase in IgG titers is strongly suggestive of acute CMV (*Am J Med Sci.* 1978;276:325–39.

6. A. Diffuse small bowel dilation with pneumatosis intestinalis, most consistent with acute-on-chronic mesenteric ischemia. In a patient with known atherosclerosis, an acute arterial thrombus is the most common etiology. An additional CT image (figure 104.7) shows the extent of intra-abdominal atherosclerosis in the same patient. Hypotension and watershed hypoperfusion are typically associated with ischemic colitis, which often has more benign course. The clinical story of intestinal angina is not consistent with a partial small bowel obstruction (SBO) from adhesions. *C. difficile* does not affect small bowel; it causes colonic dilation. CT and history not consistent with intussusception (*Gastroenterology.* 2000;118(5):951–3).

7. C. This patient likely has a nontuberculous mycobacterial infection, with chronic cough and RML infiltrate/volume loss on CXR ("Lady Windemere syndrome"). Typical agent is *Mycobacterium avium* complex (MAC), which includes the two species *M. avium* and *M. intracellulare.* Diagnosis requires two separate positive sputum cultures, or positive bronchoalveolar lavage (BAL)/bx (PPD is not helpful). There are no data for prednisone. The patient is not an infectious risk to others. A CT would show bronchiectasis and nodularity. Azithromycin is inadequate

monotherapy; typically a three-drug regimen (clarithromycin/azithromycin + rifampin + ethambutol) is indicated (*N Engl J Med.* 1989;321).

8. A. History and examination are classic for idiopathic seventh nerve paralysis or Bell's palsy, which can be conservatively treated with clinical follow-up. Corticosteroids have been used in this disease for more than 30 years, but clear evidence of their benefits is lacking. herpes simplex virus (HSV) has been implicated in its pathogenesis, which has led to several trials using acyclovir for treatment. It is recommended for use in conjunction with prednisone. Lyme disease may cause facial nerve palsy; in the right clinical context empirical therapy is appropriate. There is no evidence that gabapentin affects the course (*Neurology.* 2001;56:830).

9. E. The relative risk of hypertension in OCP users is 1.8 as demonstrated in the Nurse's Health Study. Although the data are variable, there does appear to be an increased risk of cervical cancer associated with long-term use of OCPs. OCPs decrease the incidence of breast fibroadenomas and fibrocystic disease; however, the evidence regarding OCPs and breast cancer is conflicting. Overall, there seems to be little to no increased risk of breast cancer associated with OCP use. OCPs have a protective effect with respect to endometrial cancer, with studies showing a relative risk (RR) of 0.6 in OCP users. The risk for venous thromboembolism (VTE) is elevated in patients on OCPs, although studies were done with early formulations and may not reflect the incidence of disease with third-generation OCPs (*Circulation.* 1996;94:483. *Lancet.* 2003;361:1159. *N Engl J Med.* 2002;346:2025. *JAMA.* 1987;287:796).

10. C. The clinical history is very consistent for an axial spondyloarthritis (AS). In patients with a very high pretest

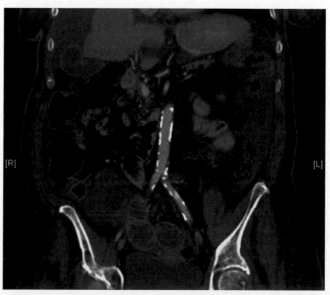

Figure 104.7. Question 9: Abdominal CT scan (Coronal Reconstruction)

probability, positive films will confirm diagnosis. Although a higher percentage of patients with back pain who are HLA B27+ have AS, it is not a specific finding. Sacroiliitis and spondylarthropathies can be associated with psoriasis and inflammatory bowel disease (IBD). The CRP is not sufficiently specific or sensitive for AS (*Ann Rheum Dis.* 2004;63:535).

11. C. COPD is the fourth leading cause of death in the world. Diagnosis of COPD relies on an appropriate history and the demonstration of airflow obstruction that is not fully reversible. FEV_1/FVC <70% diagnoses obstructive physiology. Severity of obstruction is graded based on FEV_1. Although many patients with COPD have increased TLC and RV as well as hyperinflation on CXR, these findings are not diagnostic. Most physicians obtain bronchodilator testing at least once to help rule out asthma as well as to guide future treatment decisions. GOLD guidelines are found at http://goldcopd.com.

12. B. Early onset of menarche (11 years and younger) increases a woman's risk for developing breast cancer. On average, a woman's lifetime risk to develop breast cancer is 12% in the United States. Past or current use of oral contraceptives is associated with a 1.07–1.2 increased relative risk of developing breast cancer. The Gail model is used to predict a woman's risk for developing breast cancer based on age, menstrual history, age at childbirth, family history, and prior breast disease. It is only validated for women >35 years of age and should not be used when *BRCA1* or *2* mutations are suspected (*N Engl J Med.* 2005;353:229; http://bcra.nci.nih.gov/brc/q1.htm).

13. E. Screening strategies for prostate cancer include digital rectal exam and prostate specific antigen (PSA). In the European Prostate Cancer Screening Trial, 76% of patients referred to biopsy had benign results. Up to two-thirds of men with PSA >4.0 will not have prostate cancer. In the Prostate Cancer Prevention Trial, 15% of patients with a PSA of <4.0 had prostate cancer. Several modifications of PSA have been proposed, including use of PSA density, PSA velocity, and age-adjusted normal ranges (*N Engl J Med.* 2004;350:2239).

14. D. Digoxin has been proven to improve symptoms but not mortality (DIG trial). There is evidence for angiotensin-converting enzyme (ACE) inhibitors improving mortality in patients with symptomatic and asymptomatic left ventricular dysfunction (SOLVD Treatment & Prevention Trials, SAVE, TRACE, AIRE). There is also evidence for the initiation of beta blockers in patients with systolic dysfunction (NYHA II–IV), usually after stabilization on a diuretic and an ACE inhibitor (MERIT-HF). There is evidence for angiotensin receptor blocker (ARB) use in ACE inhibitor–intolerant patients, with a demonstrated mortality benefit (CHARM-Alternative trial). There is also evidence for a benefit for the addition of an ARB to an ACE inhibitor, although these data are more controversial. Spironolactone

was shown to have a mortality benefit in a select group of patients with class III or IV heart failure (RALES) (*JAMA.* 2003;289:871. *N Engl J Med.* 1992;327:685. *Annals.* 2001;134:550. *N Engl J Med.* 2001;344:1651. *Lancet.* 2003;362:772. *N Engl J Med.* 1999;341:709).

15. D. The chest radiograph reveals an anterior mediastinal mass. The differential diagnosis of anterior mediastinal mass includes these disorders:

- Thymoma (as in this case)
- Thyroid neoplasm
- Lymphoma
- Teratoma

Diagnosis is best made by mediastinoscopy. Fibrosing mediastinitis is an exuberant fibrotic response to previous infection, usually related to fungal infection (most commonly histoplasmosis). This does not typically present as an anterior mediastinal mass (*Chest.* 1997;112:511. *Lung Cancer.* 2001;32:255).

16. C. Calcium stones are the most common cause of kidney stones: 80% of patients with stones have calcium stones. Calcium oxalate stones are much more common than calcium phosphate stones. There are several risk factors for developing calcium stones:

- Hypercalciuria and hyperoxaluria
- Low urine volume
- Medullary sponge kidney
- Type 1 RTA

Patients with IBD are predisposed to uric acid stones, whereas patients with recurrent urinary tract infections are at higher risk for struvite stones (*Am J Med.* 1995;98(1): 50–9).

17. C. Female smokers have two to seven times the relative risk of myocardial infarction when compared to nonsmokers. There is an increased rate of depression after smoking cessation, particularly in those with a history of major depression. Rates of hip fracture for women at age 85 are 12% in nonsmokers and 19% in smokers. Studies have shown improved smoking cessation when bupropion (+/- nicotine replacement) is used. Quit rates range from 23% to 35% with bupropion versus 12% to 16% with placebo. No delivery method of nicotine replacement (gum, transdermal, inhaler, nasal spray) has been shown to be superior, and all have been shown to improve smoking cessation rates. Brief advice from a physician can produce a quit rate of 10% (*Circulation.* 1996;93:450. *Arch Intern Med.* 2003;163:2301. *BMJ.* 1997;315:841. *N Engl J Med.* 1999;340:685. *Arch Intern Med.* 1999;159:2033. *Lancet.* 2001;357:1929).

18. A. The patient's history of previous deep vein thrombosis (DVT) and fetal losses strongly suggests the diagnosis of antiphospholipid antibody syndrome. The diagnosis is made by documentation of anticardiolipin Ab (false-positive VDRL), lupus anticoagulant, or beta-2 glycoprotein I (b2GPI). The patient has already demonstrated a high risk for recurrent thromboembolic events and needs long-term or lifelong intermediate- (INR 2.0–2.9) or even high-intensity (INR >3.0) anticoagulation. OCPs are contraindicated in patients with hypercoagulable syndromes (*N Engl J Med.* 2002;346:752. *Thromb Res.* 2004;114:435).

19. E. The history of an electric shock sensation is highly suggestive of a neuropathy. Carpal tunnel syndrome is associated with pregnancy and is most likely due to generalized edema. Symptoms usually present in the third trimester and resolve with delivery. Physical examination should include wrist flexion for 30 seconds (Phalen's maneuver) and tapping over the median nerve with a reflex hammer to elicit a Tinel sign. Reproduction of the symptoms (i.e., numbness, burning, tingling) indicates carpal tunnel syndrome. Multiple sclerosis (MS) can present with sensory disturbances, but not typically this focal, and is far less common. Kienböck disease is an uncommon avascular necrosis (AVN) of the lunate, presenting as wrist pain (*Am Fam Physician.* 2003;68:265).

20. E. Chlamydia infections have many potential long-term sequelae, including pelvic inflammatory disease (PID), infertility, chronic pelvic pain, and ectopic pregnancies. Secondary transmission to partners is always a concern. Secondary transmission to the neonate is of particular concern in this clinical situation. Because doxycycline and fluoroquinolones are contraindicated in pregnancy, either amoxicillin or azithromycin is a reasonable alternative. Some formulations of erythromycin are contraindicated in pregnancy, and its use is associated with more nausea than other alternative therapies (*Morbid Mortal Weekly Rep.* 2002;51(RR-6):1).

21. A. Headache, fever, thrombocytopenia, and transaminitis in the setting of recent tick bite indicate human granulocytic anaplasmosis (formerly known as human granulocytic ehrlichiosis). Doxycycline for 10–14 days is first-line therapy. *Babesia microti* is a protozoan parasite causing hemolytic anemia and diagnosed by blood smear. These infections frequently coexist (*B. burgdorferi* and *A. phagocytophilium,* 4–26%) (*Proc Natl Acad Sci USA.* 1996;93:6209–14. *N Engl J Med.* 1997;337:49–50).

105.

INTERNAL MEDICINE SUMMARY

Charles A. Morris

The purpose of this chapter is to provide a review, from across the breadth of internal medicine, of currently recommended health screening strategies. As advances in medical technology continue to push the ability to detect, treat, and impact disease states, there is increasing attention to the utility of screening and its role in periodic health assessments. The concept of disease prevention through early detection has inherent attractiveness; yet evidence to support vast numbers of screening initiatives has been lacking. As laid out in a landmark article from 1968, effective screening is predicated on several major tenets:

1. The condition should be an important health problem.

2. There should be a recognizable latent or early symptomatic stage.

3. The natural history of the condition should be adequately described and understood.

4. There should be an accepted treatment for patients with recognized disease.

5. There should be a suitable screening test applicable during this latent phase.

6. The test should be acceptable to the population.

7. The cost of detection (both of false positives and false negatives) as well as treatment should be economically acceptable.

Whereas many screening tests meet the criteria above, clear evidence that screening improves mortality for a given disease can be more elusive. Studies to assess the efficacy of screening interventions are susceptible to several types of biases. Lead time bias, particularly common in studies of cancer screening, refers to early cancer detection and diagnosis, which, in the absence of an effective treatment, may increase survival without a mortality benefit (see figure 105.1). Studies of cancer screening are also vulnerable to length time bias. This occurs when screening, performed at a fixed interval, preferentially detects slower-progressing tumors while rapidly progressive cancers develop between screening episodes. Consequently, screened populations may appear to have improved clinical outcomes. Overdiagnosis bias, in which screening allows the detection of clinically indolent forms of disease that otherwise might not require intervention or affect mortality, may partly explain apparent benefits of screening for other solid organ malignancies (Welch, 2006) (figure 105.2). In general, randomized controlled trials rather than observational studies help avoid these pitfalls and most accurately assess mortality benefits.

In the United States there are several sources for physicians to obtain up-to-date practice guidelines on evidence-supported health screening information. The United States Preventative Services Task Force (USPSTF) under the auspices of the Agency for Healthcare Research and Quality provides regularly updated reviews of the evidence to support a number of preventative services and grades this evidence with recommendations A–D and I (see tables 105.1 and 105.2). The American College of Physicians (ACP) also provides guidelines and consensus statements of screening and preventative services based on detailed reviews of the literature. In addition, screening recommendations are produced by various subspecialty professional societies (such as the American Gastroenterological Association recommendations on colorectal cancer screening as endorsed by the American Cancer Society [ACS] or the U.S. Centers for Disease Control and Prevention [CDC] recommendations on HIV screening).

This chapter reviews current health screening recommendations for cancer and cardiovascular disease, lifestyle issues including substance use, and common infectious diseases.

CANCER SCREENING

According to the ACS, it is estimated that 565,650 people will die from cancer-related mortality in 2008; cancer is the second most common cause of death in this country. Lung,

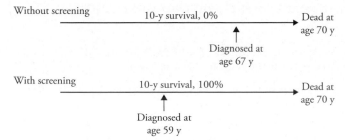

Figure 105.1. Lead-Time Bias. Reprinted with permission from Welch et al. Overstating the evidence from lung cancer screening: The International Early Lung Cancer Action Program (I-ELCAP) Study. *Arch Intern Med.* 2007;167:2289–95. Copyright 2008 American Medical Association. All rights reserved.

breast, cervical, prostate, and colorectal cancers account for nearly 50% of cancer deaths. Importantly, mortality of breast, colon, cervical, and prostate cancer has decreased; screening is likely responsible for at least a portion of this decline (although mortality from lung cancer has decreased, this is largely due to a decreased prevalence of smoking) (ACS, 2008) (see figures 105.3 and 105.4).

BREAST CANCER

Mammography remains the standard of care for breast cancer screening, with a maximal benefit that increases with age. Evidence supports a small but clinically significant mortality reduction from screening for breast cancer, particularly among women 50 years of age and older. For women between the ages of 40 and 50, the absolute benefit from

screening is much smaller, and screening for this age group remains somewhat controversial. One composite analysis of several trials suggested that for a hypothetical cohort of 10,000 women 40 years of age, annual screening would prevent 4–6 deaths of the 30 expected deaths. This benefit of screening would be offset by the fact that over 50% of the cohort would have an abnormal mammogram at sometime during the 10-year period, producing considerable anxiety and requiring further diagnostic testing (Rajkumar, 1999). Published guidelines reflect this debate. The ACS recommends mammography every 1–2 years, whereas the ACP recently reviewed the literature and updated their own clinical practice guidelines, recommending that any decision to screen women 40–49 years of age take into account the risk of false positive results and an individual's own risk profile. Similarly, the USPSTF also recently revised its recommendations for women between the ages of 40–49, advising against routine mammography but instead calling for an assessment of an individual's own risk profile and an understanding of the potential benefits and harms of screening (Nelson et al., 2009; USPSTF, 2009).

In an effort to improve the test characteristics of mammography, several large trials have examined the role of magnetic resonance imaging (MRI) as a screening modality. These studies confirm that high-risk women (defined as a cumulative lifetime risk of ≥15%, including those with an inherited predisposition including *BRCA-1* and *BRCA-2*) benefit from the increased sensitivity of MRI screening. Sensitivity of MRI to detect invasive cancer was significantly improved compared to that for mammography,

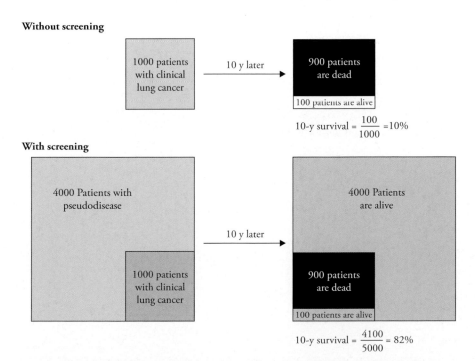

Figure 105.2. Overdiagnosis Bias. Reprinted with permission from Welch et al. Overstating the evidence from lung cancer screening: The International Early Lung Cancer Action Program (I-ELCAP) Study. *Arch Intern Med.* 2007;167:2289–95. Copyright 2008 American Medical Association. All rights reserved.

Table 105.1 UNITED STATES PREVENTATIVE SERVICES TASK FORCE (USPSTF) RATINGS OF STRENGTH OF RECOMMENDATIONS

A	The USPSTF strongly recommends that clinicians provide [the service] to eligible patients. The USPSTF found good evidence that [the service] improves important health outcomes and concludes that benefits substantially outweigh harms.
B	The USPSTF recommends that clinicians provide [this service] to eligible patients. The USPSTF found at least fair evidence that [the service] improves important health outcomes and concludes that benefits outweigh harms.
C	The USPSTF makes no recommendation for or against routine provision of [the service]. The USPSTF found at least fair evidence that [the service] can improve health outcomes but concludes that the balance of benefits and harms is too close to justify a general recommendation.
D	The USPSTF recommends against routinely providing [the service] to asymptomatic patients. The USPSTF found at least fair evidence that [the service] is ineffective or that harms outweigh benefits.
I	The USPSTF concludes that the evidence is insufficient to recommend for or against routinely providing [the service]. Evidence that the [service] is effective is lacking, of poor quality, or conflicting and the balance of benefits and harms cannot be determined.

SOURCE: Agency for Healthcare Research and Quality. *Preventative Services Recommended by the USPSTF.* Washington, DC: U.S. Department of Health and Human Services.

Table 105.2 USPSTF RECOMMENDATIONS, BY GENDER

	ADULTS	
RECOMMENDATION	MEN	WOMEN
Abdominal aortic aneurysm, screening	X	
Alcohol misuse screening and behavioral counseling interventions	X	X
Bacteriuria, screening for asymptomatic		
Breast cancer, screening		X
Breast and ovarian cancer susceptibility, genetic risk assessment and *BRCA* mutation testing		X
Cervical cancer, screening		X
Chlamydial infection, screening		X
Colorectal cancer, screening	X	X
Depression, screening	X	X
Diabetes mellitus in adults, screening for type 2	X	X
Diet, behavioral counseling in primary care to promote a healthy	X	X
Gonorrhea, screening		X
Hepatitis B virus infection, screening		
High blood pressure, screening	X	X
HIV, screening	X	X
Iron deficiency anemia, screening		
Lipid disorders, screening	X	X
Obesity in adults, screening	X	X
Osteoporosis in postmenopausal women, screening		X
Syphilis infection, screening	X	X
Tobacco use and tobacco-caused disease, counseling to prevent	X	X

SOURCE: Agency for Healthcare Research and Quality. *Preventative Services Recommended by the USPSTF.* Washington, DC: U.S. Department of Health and Human Services.

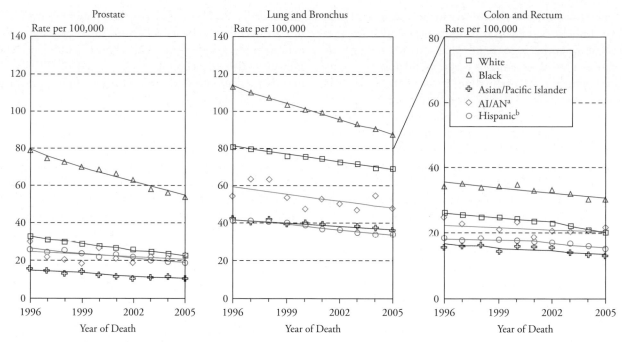

Figure 105.3. U.S. Mortality 1996–2005 in Males by Race/Ethnicity. Source: Ries LAG, Melbert D, Krapcho M, et al. *SEER Cancer Statistics Review, 1975–2005.* Bethesda, MD: National Cancer Institute.

79.5% versus 33% (Kriege et al., 2004). In light of these data, the ACS currently recommends MRI screening for high-risk women. The Gail Model (available online at http://www.acs.org) is one of several prospectively validated models for calculating lifetime breast cancer risk and can facilitate shared decision making between physician and patient. Because mammography can still detect breast cancers that are missed by MRI, high-risk women should be screened with both modalities.

CERVICAL CANCER

The introduction of cervical cancer screening with the Papanicolaou (Pap) test has led to a dramatic reduction in

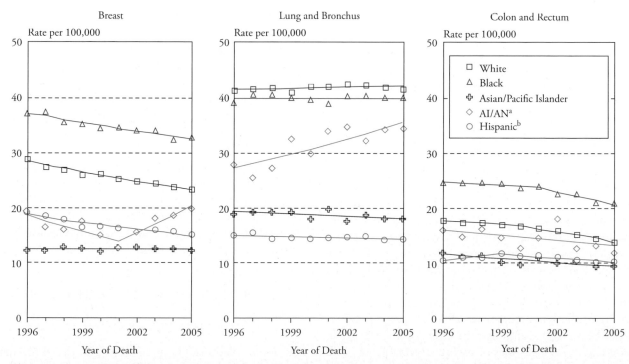

Figure 105.4. U.S. Mortality 1996–2005 in Females by Race/Ethnicity. Source: Ries LAG, Melbert D, Krapcho M, et al. *SEER Cancer Statistics Review, 1975–2005.* Bethesda, MD: National Cancer Institute.

the incidence of invasive of cervical cancer (Ries et al., 1999). Current guidelines for Pap testing recommend starting to screen women at the age of first sexual activity or 21, whichever is first. Annual screening is recommended if traditional preparation techniques of the slides are used, but this may be stretched out to every 3 years if liquid preparation medium is performed due to improved sensitivity. Over 99% of cervical cancer may be attributed to infection with human papilloma virus (HPV), which is the highest attributable risk for any common malignancy. In light of this association there has been considerable interest in the use of viral probes as a stand-alone or adjuvant screening tool. HPV assays demonstrate a significantly higher sensitivity than Pap testing. However, this is problematic because the majority of early cervical infections with HPV resolve without intervention (Franco et al., 1999). When used in conjunction with Pap tests, the additional sensitivity of HPV assays can provide a useful tool with which to triage those with abnormal cytology for colposcopy. Because the majority of HPV infections resolve without intervention, HPV probes may prove useful as stand-alone screening tests once a woman is of sufficient age that HPV detection likely reflects persistent infection.

PROSTATE CANCER

The benefit from prostate cancer screening is controversial. Since the advent of prostate specific antigen (PSA) for screening, prostate cancer mortality in the United States has declined, although this may be in part to overdetection bias discussed above. There was a dramatic increase in incidence of prostate cancer in the early 1990s shortly after PSA testing became available, the majority of which was localized disease (Farkas et al., 1998). After 9 years of follow-up, the European Randomized Study of Screening of Prostate Cancer showed a small absolute reduction in prostate cancer mortality, although over 1400 men would need to be screened and 48 men treated over that time interval to avoid one prostate cancer death (Schröder et al., 2009). The USPSTF does not endorse prostate cancer screening, although routine PSA coupled with a digital rectal examination (DRE) is recommended by the ACS and American Urological Society starting at age 50 (or at age 40 for high-risk men including African Americans and those with a family history of prostate cancer). In August 2008 the USPSTF issued a "D" recommendation for screening men over the age of 75, citing the lack of demonstrable evidence proving any benefit to detecting asymptomatic prostate cancer beyond this age. In October 2011, the Task Force further revised their recommendations, issuing a "D" recommendation for PSA-based prostate cancer screening of men at any age. In an effort to improve the test characteristics of the PSA, some have advocated using free PSA values or PSA velocity, although the utility of these strategies remains unclear. Velocity may be useful to identify those with lower absolute PSA values who may have clinically significant cancer (for example, ≥0.35 ng/mL/yr if total PSA <4 ng/mL;

Carter et al., 2007); similarly, in older patients with PSA values >4 ng/mL, a velocity >1.25 ng/mL/yr (Punglia, 2007) may help to exclude those with clinically indolent cancers. However, clinical decision making based on PSA velocity has not yet demonstrated a mortality benefit in a prospective, randomized trial.

COLORECTAL CANCER

Routine screening for colorectal cancer (CRC) at age 50 (or earlier with a high-risk personal or family history) may be performed by several different strategies. Fecal occult blood testing (FOBT) was the first test employed for screening and remains the only CRC screening technique with a proven mortality benefit in randomized controlled trials (Mandel, 1993). An extensive literature including well-performed case-control studies support alternative screening strategies, including FOBT coupled with flexible sigmoidoscopy every 5 years or colonoscopy every 10 years. Computed tomographic (CT) colonography (so-called virtual colonoscopy) has attracted significant attention in recent studies. Although it appears to have a similar specificity for larger adenomas and polyps as compared to optical colonoscopy, its ability to detect smaller polyps <1 cm is unclear (Kim et al., 2007).

CONTROVERSIES IN SCREENING LUNG CANCER

Lung cancer has long been considered a potential target for cancer screening. It is the most common cause of cancer-related mortality in this country, with an estimated 215,020 new cases and 161,840 deaths in 2008 (ACS, 2008). Unfortunately, early studies of screening high-risk patients with chest radiology and sputum cytology failed to demonstrate a mortality benefit despite detection of an increased number of malignant lesions (Fontana et al., 1984). The International Early Lung Cancer Action Program (I-ELCAP) study showed that the majority of asymptomatic lung cancers identified by low-dose spiral CT were early-stage disease (Henschke, 2006). In 2011, the National Lung Screening Trial demonstrated that annual CT scan screening of former or current heavy smokers resulted in a 20% relative reduction in mortality. However, the absolute benefit was less than 1%, and screening was associated with a high rate of false positive results that could lead to unnecessary invasive procedures (NLST, 2011).

CARDIOVASCULAR SCREENING

HYPERTENSION

The Joint National Commission on the Prevention, Detection, Evaluation and Treatment of High Blood Pressure (JNC 7) defines stage I hypertension as systolic blood pressure >140 and/or a diastolic pressure >90 mm Hg. Most recent estimates indicate that over one-quarter of Americans have hypertension, a leading cause of cardiovascular morbidity and mortality. JNC 7 recommends screening all adults for high blood pressure, a recommendation also endorsed by the USPSTF and AHA. Although the optimal screening interval is unclear, the JNC 7 recommends screening all adults with an initial blood pressure of <120/80 mm Hg every 2 years, and annually if prehypertensive (120–139/80–90 mm Hg). Hypertension is not diagnosed unless elevated pressures are documented on at least two separate measurements at least 1 week apart.

ABDOMINAL AORTIC ANEURYSMS

Abdominal aortic aneurysms (AAA) are common, with an estimated prevalence of 8% among elderly men. These aneurysms pose considerable risk to affected individuals, as rupture is associated with a mortality rate as high as 90% in selected populations. Although open repair of these aneurysms carries an operative mortality of approximately 4%, newer endovascular repair techniques have also strengthened the argument in favor of early detection. Because abdominal vascular ultrasonography demonstrates favorable test characteristics of high sensitivity and specificity, and surgical repair of AAAs ≥5.5 cm decreases AAA-specific mortality, the USPSTF has issued a grade B recommendation for one-time screening for AAA by ultrasonography for current or former male smokers aged 65–75 years. Coverage for this screening benefit is variable, although as of 2007 Medicare does provide coverage for men who have smoked more than 100 cigarettes and men and women with a family history of AAA.

CHOLESTEROL/LIPID SCREENING

Epidemiological studies have convincingly demonstrated that high levels of low-density lipoprotein (LDL) cholesterol are atherogenic and that elevated levels increase the risk of both first and recurrent cardiovascular events. In addition, clinical trials have confirmed that lowering cholesterol by pharmacologic therapy, especially with HMG-CoA reductase inhibitors, decreases coronary heart disease (CHD) incidence and mortality. The National Cholesterol Education Program (NCEP) and Adult Treatment Panel III (ATP III) sponsored by the National Heart Lung and Blood Institute last updated their guidelines in 2004. The ATP III recommendations do not define the age at which to begin screening patients, although the Framingham Risk Score used to calculate an individual's 10-year risk of can be applied for men and women ≥20 years of age. Guidelines issued by the USPTF recommend screening all men for dyslipidemia at 35 years of age, or at age 20 if there are cardiovascular risk factors. Screening women with cardiovascular risk factors is also endorsed at age 35.

CONTROVERSIES IN CARDIOVASCULAR SCREENING

With the advent of newer cardiovascular imaging including high-resolution and multirow detector CT, nuclear imaging, and ultrasonography, there has been growing interest in incorporating these modalities into screening algorithms for both occult coronary heart disease and peripheral vascular disease. In 2006 the Screening for Heart Attack Prevention and Education guidelines were released advocating an imaging-based screening protocol rather than one based on established methods of lipid measurement (Naghavi et al., 2006). However, randomized controlled trial data are lacking for these screening strategies, and they remain unendorsed by major professional societies. In December 2007, the USPSTF has given a "D" rating to screening for asymptomatic carotid stenosis.

DIABETES MELLITUS

Diabetes mellitus is increasingly common, with an estimated national prevalence of 7.8% (NIDDK, 2007). Despite the prevalence and available treatments for the disease, the USPSTF gives an "I" rating (insufficient evidence) to routine screening of asymptomatic individuals for diabetes, although it endorses screening in those with elevated blood pressure. The American Diabetes Association (ADA) recommends screening all asymptomatic adults with either a fasting blood sugar or oral glucose tolerance test at age 45, or earlier if overweight and with other cardiovascular risk factors (ADA, 2008).

LIFESTYLE FACTORS

OBESITY

According to the most recent data from the National Health and Nutrition Examination Survey (NHANES), almost two-thirds of adults in the United States are overweight (a body mass index [BMI] = 25–29.9 kg/m^2), and almost one-third are obese (BMI ≥30 kg/m^2). The USPTF gives a B recommendation for screening adults for obesity.

ALCOHOL AND TOBACCO ABUSE

The Alcohol Use Disorders Identification Test (AUDIT) is the most studied screening tool for detecting alcohol-related problems in primary care settings. It is sensitive for detecting alcohol misuse, abuse, or dependence and can be used as a stand-alone screening tool (Babor et al., 2001). The four-item CAGE (feeling the need to Cut down, Annoyed by criticism, Guilty about drinking, and need for an Eye-opener in the morning) is the most popular screening test for detecting alcohol abuse or dependence in primary care.

Physicians should remember that even briefly counseling patients who smoke on tobacco cessation (3 min or less) has been proven to increase tobacco abstinence rates; because of this the USPSTF gives screening for tobacco use their highest "A" rating. The 5-A behavioral framework is a useful strategy for engaging patients who smoke in a discussion about tobacco cessation:

1. Ask about tobacco use.

2. Advise to quit through clear personalized messages.

3. Assess willingness to quit.

4. Assist to quit.

5. Arrange follow-up and support.

INFECTIOUS DISEASE/STD

Chlamydia is the most common sexually transmitted infection in the United States, with an estimated prevalence of 4–5% nationally, although these estimates vary greatly depending on the target population. If untreated, chlamydia may lead to cervicitis, urethritis, pelvic inflammatory disease (PID), chronic pelvic pain, and infertility. Because the vast majority of both men and women are asymptomatic during chlamydial infection, identification based only on symptomatic patients is problematic. The USPTF gives an "A" rating to screening sexually active women ≤24 years of age or older women who are at higher risk. The age cutoff is based largely on population studies showing that prevalence of chlamydial infection is inversely correlated with age. Current screening tools including amplified and nonamplified gene probes allow rapid, accurate detection of infection. Although newer urine-based assays may be performed in men as well, the utility of screening men is less clear, as long-term consequences of untreated male infection are less well defined. For this reason screening men is not universally recommended. Gonococcal (GC) infections are the second most common sexually transmitted disease, and screening is also recommended for young women by the USPSTF.

HIV

Recently released estimates of human immunodeficiency virus (HIV) incidence in the United States for 2006 suggest that rates are much higher than previously projected (Hall et al., 2008). An estimated 56,300 new HIV infections occurred in 2006, higher than the previous estimate of 40,000 annual new infections. Just over half of these new infections occurred in men having sex with men, but high-risk heterosexual contact accounted for 31% of new infections. African Americans, although comprising 13% of the U.S. population, accounted for 45% of the new HIV infections. Given the advances in treatment of HIV and the transformation of infection into a chronic disease, there has been renewed interest in screening for HIV infection among asymptomatic persons. In 2005 the USPTF issued an "A" recommendation for screening high-risk individuals, including men who have had sex with men and men and women having unprotected sex with multiple partners.

OSTEOPOROSIS

Age-related bone loss is often asymptomatic, and the morbidity of osteoporosis is secondary to the fractures that occur. Common sites of fracture include the spine, forearm, and hip; the last incur the greatest morbidity and mortality and are the principal driver of osteoporosis-associated health care costs. The remaining lifetime probability of osteoporotic fractures in women at the age of 50 years exceeds 40% in developed countries (WHO, 2004). The USPSTF recommends that women aged 65 and older be screened routinely for osteoporosis and that routine screening begin at age 60 for women at increased risk for osteoporotic fractures. In response to the fact that bone mineral density (BMD) testing is not available in resource-poor areas, the World Health Organization has developed the FRAX tool, a validated model predicting an individual's 10-year risk of osteoporotic fracture, based on nine accepted risk factors (WHO, 2004). The FRAX score may be computed with or without a BMD value and is appropriate to use in men over the age of 41 and across several different ethnic groups.

ADDITIONAL READING

American Cancer Society. *Cancer Facts & Figures 2008*. Available at http://www.cancer.org/downloads/stt/CFF2008Table_pg4.pdf.

American Diabetes Association. Standards of Medical Care in Diabetes—2008. *Diabetes Care*. 2008;31:S12–54.

Babor TF, Higgins-Biddle JC, Saunders JB, Monteiro MG. *The Alcohol Use Disorders Identification Test: Guidelines for Use in Primary Care*, 2nd ed. WHO, 2001. Available at http://whqlibdoc.who.int/hq/2001/WHO_MSD_MSB_01.6a.pdf.

Carter HB, Ferrucci L, Kettermann A, et al. Detection of life-threatening prostate cancer with prostate-specific antigen velocity during a window of curability. *J Natl Cancer Inst*. 2006;98:1521–7.

Executive Summary of the Third Report of the National Cholesterol Education Program (NCEP) Expert Panel on Detection, Evaluation, and Treatment of High Blood Cholesterol in Adults (Adult Treatment Panel III). *JAMA*. 2001;285:2486–97.

Farkas A, Schneider D, Perroti M, Cummings KB, Ward WS. National trends in the epidemiology of prostate cancer, 1973 to 1994: evidence for the effectiveness of prostate-specific antigen screening. *Urology*. 1998;52:444–9.

Fontana RS, Sanderson DR, Taylor WF, et al. Early lung cancer detection: Results of the initial (prevalence) radiologic and cytologic screening in the Mayo Clinic Study. *Am Rev Resp Dis*. 1984;130:561–5.

Franco EL, Villa LL, Sobrinho JP, et al. Epidemiology of acquisition and clearance of cervical human papillomavirus infection in women from a high-risk area for cervical cancer. *J Infect Dis*. 1999;180:1415–23.

Hall HI, Song R, Rhodes P, et al. Estimation of HIV incidence in the United States. *JAMA*. 2008;300(5):520–9.

Kim DH, Pickhardt PJ, Taylor AJ, et al. CT colonography versus colonoscopy for the detection of advanced neoplasia. *N Engl J Med*. 2007;357:1403–12.

Kriege M, Brekelmans CTM, Boetes C, et al. Efficacy of MRI and mammography for breast-cancer screening in women with a familial or genetic predisposition. *N Engl J Med.* 2004;351:427–37.

Mandel JS, Bond JH, Church TR, et al. Reducing mortality from colorectal cancer by screening for fecal occult blood. Minnesota Colon Cancer Control Study. *N Engl J Med.* 1993;328:1365–71.

Naghavi M, Falk E, Hecht HS, et al. From vulnerable plaque to vulnerable patient—Part III: Executive summary of the Screening for Heart Attack Prevention and Education (SHAPE) task force report. *Am J Cardiol.* 2006;98:2H–15H.

The National Lung Screening Trial Research Team. Reduced lung-cancer mortality with low-dose computed tomographic screening. *N Engl J Med.* 2011;365:395–409.

Nelson HD, Tyne K, Naik A, et al. Screening for breast cancer: An update for the U.S. Preventive Services Task Force. *Ann Intern Med.* 2009;151:727–37.

NIDDK. *National Diabetes Statistics, 2007.* NIH Publication No. 08–3892, June 2008. Available at http://diabetes.niddk.nih.gov/dm/pubs/statistics/DM_Statistics.pdf.

Punglia RS, Cullen J, Mcleod DG, et al. Prostate-specific antigen velocity and the detection of Gleason score 7 to 10 prostate cancer. *Cancer.* 2007;110:1973–8.

Rajkumar SV, Hartmann LC. Screening mammography in women aged 40–49 years. *Medicine.* 1999;78:410–16.

Ries LAG, Kosary CL, Hankey BF, Miller BA, Clegg L, Edwards BK. *SEER Cancer Statistics Review, 1973–1996.* Bethesda, MD: National Cancer Institute, 1999.

Schröder FH, Hugosson J, Roobol MJ, et al. Screening and prostate-cancer mortality in a randomized European study. *N Engl J Med.* 2009; 360:1320–28.

U.S. Preventive Services Task Force. *Ratings Guide to Clinical Preventive Services, 2007.* AHRQ Publication No. 07–05100, September 2007. Agency for Healthcare Research and Quality, Rockville, MD.

U.S. Preventive Services Task Force. Screening for breast cancer: U.S. Preventive Services Task Force recommendation statement. *Ann Intern Med.* 2009;151:716–26.

Welch HG, Woloshin S, Schwartz LM, et al. Overstating the evidence from lung cancer screening: The International Early Lung Cancer Sction Program (I-ELCAP) Study. *Arch Intern Med.* 2007;167:2289–95.

WHO Scientific Group on the Assessment of Osteoporosis at Primary Health Care Level. Summary Meeting Report. Brussels, Belgium, 5–7 May 2004. Available at http://nof.org/professionals/WHO_Osteoporosis_Summary.pdf.

QUESTIONS

QUESTION 1. All of the following are important principles for a screening program, EXCEPT:

A. Disease should be an important health problem.
B. There should be a clear-cut phase in the later stages of the disease to allow for it to be recognized.
C. There should be an accepted treatment for persons with the disease.
D. The screening test for the disease is valid, reliable, with acceptable yield.
E. The screening test should be acceptable to the population to be screened.

QUESTION 2. A 45-year-old African-American male, who has recently moved into the area, comes to see you for the first time as his new primary care provider. He says that his father, at the age of 78 years, recently was found to have an adenoma on colonoscopy. He asks you for advice on colon cancer screening and is especially interested in alternatives to colonoscopy. All of the following statements are correct, EXCEPT:

A. Colonoscopy is the preferred colon cancer prevention test.
B. The American College of Gastroenterology recommends cancer prevention screening modalities (i.e., those that detect precancerous adenomas such as colonoscopy) over cancer detection modalities (FOBT, fecal DNA assays).
C. FOBT is not recommended for colon cancer screening.
D. If he declines colonoscopy, flexible sigmoidoscopy alone is an adequate screening test.
E. You advise him that African Americans are more likely than whites to have precancerous polyps and colon cancer in the proximal colon.

QUESTION 3. All of the following statements are correct, EXCEPT:

A. Cervical cancer rates have fallen >50% in the past 30 years in the United States due to the widespread use of the Pap test.
B. Most women younger than 30 should undergo cervical screening once every 2 years instead of annually, and those age 30 and older can be rescreened once every 3 years.
C. The majority of deaths from cervical cancer in the United States are among women who are screened infrequently or not at all.
D. Because the rate of HPV infection is high among sexually active adolescents, testing young women for HPV is highly recommended.
E. Women with certain risk factors may need more frequent screening (e.g., HIV, immunosuppressed, prior exposure to diethylstilbestrol [DES] in utero).

ANSWERS

1. B
2. D
3. D

SECTION 11

BOARD PRACTICE

106.

APPROACH TO THE INTERNAL MEDICINE
BOARD EXAM

Stuart B. Mushlin

his chapter is different from the others. Its intent is to concentrate your mind on the American Board of Internal Medicine (ABIM) examination, its purpose, and its likely test scenarios. The ABIM moved to a written rather than oral test in the 1960s. The testing has been extensively validated and is unlikely to change much in its character. Essentially, the ABIM wants to determine if you have the core knowledge in all the disciplines to be an *effective and efficient* physician. It further wants to discriminate between you and the other test takers so that you can see how you compare with others taking the examination. Many candidates, in their increasing anxiety over the subject matter, lose sight of these major objectives. To pass the examination it is not necessary to regurgitate in photographic detail one of the standard textbooks of medicine or the latest Medical Knowledge Self-Assessment Program (MKSAP) review; however, you should feel that you know the core body of knowledge in all the major medical specialties. For example, you should know, in depth, the diagnosis, rapid assessment, and appropriate management of an acute coronary syndrome. All internal medicine programs that have Residency Review Committee approval have their residents spend time in a coronary care unit and have exposure to cardiologists. So, too, you should expect to be able to manage an acute respiratory decompensation, determine its etiology, and know how to manage the acute presentation and the intermediate strategies. It is not expected that you be the expert pulmonary specialist, but it is expected you need to know when to call the specialist for the help that only the specialist can provide. And you are expected to have done more than the basics before calling for the additional help needed to successfully and appropriately manage the patient. Furthermore, an economy of testing, as well as cost consideration, is important. The effective internist/clinician is economically sensitive and efficient in spending the patient's time and money. Furthermore, effective clinicians are aware of pretest probabilities, false-positive rates, and other considerations that

inform the considered uncertainty surrounding the best patient management.

We hope that these principles are obvious from your training and not a cause for enhanced study. Where the examination causes more anxiety is in subject matter from specialties that require fewer patient hospitalizations. Some of these specialties you may have had less exposure to, but you are required to know the common diseases that appear to the generalist and how to reach the basic diagnosis and treatment plan. A concrete example is the "classic" presentation of rheumatoid arthritis. This is an illness with a prevalence of about 1/200 and is mostly managed in the outpatient setting. So by presenting it to you, it allows the board to test both your diagnostic acumen and your outpatient management skills. It is clear that over the ensuing years, more outpatient exposure (be it general or subspecialty based) will be emphasized in training programs, and with this increased emphasis, the ABIM will almost certainly increase the outpatient-oriented testing on the examination.

The ABIM suggests certain examination preparation strategies that are worth noting. The ABIM recommends that you work within a small study group and ensure that you stake out time to prepare and develop a schedule to study. The ABIM also recommends practicing with questions using the board format, that is, single best answer. Certain "red flags" hinting at the answer, such as forested area in the Northeast (Lyme disease), or Coca-Cola–colored urine (rhabdomyolysis) should be kept in mind.

The ABIM has a core fund of knowledge that it wants to be sure you have mastered (table 106.1). These questions are easily identifiable and sometimes change in format but not in core content. What everyone who takes the examination remembers is the more difficult questions that challenged them in areas they had not mastered or even not been exposed to. Sometimes these questions can be successfully navigated by cross-referencing your experience in other disciplines. Other times, you will have no idea, and that is one way the Board discriminates who

Table 106.1 2009 ABIM CERTIFICATION EXAM "BLUEPRINT"

MEDICAL-CONTENT CATEGORY	RELATIVE PERCENTAGE
Cardiovascular disease	14%
Gastroenterology	9%
Pulmonary disease	10%
Infectious disease	9%
Rheumatology/orthopedics	8%
Endocrinology/metabolism	8%
Oncology	7%
Hematology	6%
Nephrology/urology	6%
Allergy/immunology	3%
Psychiatry	4%
Neurology	4%
Dermatology	4%
Obstetrics/gynecology	3%
Ophthalmology	2%
Otorhinolaryngology	2%
Miscellaneous	3%
Total	100%

CROSS-CONTENT CATEGORY	RELATIVE PERCENTAGE
Critical care medicine	10%
Geriatric medicine	10%
Prevention	6%
Women's health	6%
Clinical epidemiology	3%
Ethics	3%
Nutrition	3%
Palliative/end-of-life care	3%
Adolescent medicine	2%
Occupational medicine	2%
Patient safety	2%
Substance abuse	2%

MEDICAL CATEGORY (RELATIVE PERCENTAGE)	NUMBER OF QUESTIONS
Adolescent medicine (2%)	4–7
Allergy/immunology (3%)	6–8
Cardiovascular disease (14%)	30–32 as follows
Hypertension	2–4
Pericardial disease	1–4
Ischemic heart disease	8–11
Arrhythmias	2–5
Congenital heart disease	0–1
Valvular heart disease	2–5
Myocardial disease	1–4
Cardiac tumors	0–1
Endocarditis and other cardiovascular infections	0–1
Vascular disease	0–2
Noncardiogenic syncope	0–1
Preoperative consultation	2–3
Miscellaneous cardiovascular disease	1–3

has a deeper fund of knowledge from those who do not. Remember, the Board wants to test your core knowledge and validate that it is sufficient for you to be certified. But another mission of the test is to provide a discriminatory measure of who demonstrates more knowledge in a standardized environment.

Importantly, the concept of managing a patient involves not just the physician but also the entire healthcare system. It is a mistake to see a case and rapidly go to the answer or diagnosis that seems self-evident. Pause to consider the ethics of the situation, the cost of the testing or therapy you are considering, and the health care systems involved. You will be expected to be respectful of the patient in your answers, have appropriate concern for their families, understand their social situation and home environment, and have an appropriate respect for the other members of the healthcare team. You may well be challenged with ethical choices. These aspects of appropriate care by an internist are not available in textbooks but must be absorbed in the training environment by appropriate mentoring and role modeling and constructive feedback. As the Board no longer interviews the candidate, it needs to get some measure of the humane essence of the candidate and his or her humane and holistic consideration for the specific patient in the patient's milieu. Additionally, examination of the candidate's knowledge of medical systems will be tested. Although this will manifest itself mostly in the option to readily use expensive or unnecessary tests and therapies, it may also be tested by such matters as cultural competency and sensitivity to literacy and financial constraints that a patient might have. Other systemic structures, such as Health Insurance Privacy and Accessibility Act (HIPAA) compliance and collaboration with other disciplines or colleagues are most often interspersed within the various cases.

The recipe for the examination is as follows. The examination is held over 1 day with four modules. Each of the modules is of 2 hours' duration and comprises 60 questions. The questions reflect primary content areas (75%)—these are the traditional medicine subspecialties—and "cross content area" (25%) comprising questions in allergy/immunology, dermatology, gynecology, neurology, ophthalmology, and psychiatry. Each question is formatted with a clinical "stem" (patient) followed by "lead-in" (last sentence) question and choices. The ABIM is looking to test analytic skills, not simple memorization. There are no so-called "trick" questions. The material will not be controversial and will likely be dated at 2 years or older. Because the questions are generally written by practicing internists, they will reflect current practice, which is mostly in the ambulatory setting. Some strategies about answering questions are worth bearing in mind. The most important is to answer all questions. It is better to not get stuck on one question but rather to go back and tackle the difficult question if there is time. You should aim to take approximately 2 minutes per question. Although there are many different ways to answer questions, one popular strategy is to try to answer before looking at the choices and not change the answer unless you remember new information.

What follows is a representative case that illustrates these points with a discussion at the end of the "best choice" for each of the questions.

An 84-year-old Caucasian male presents to your emergency room complaining of shortness of breath.

He has a long history of rate-controlled atrial fibrillation and a 10-year-old mitral valve repair. He has been on warfarin therapy for 15 years with no difficulty in maintaining an International Normalized Ratio (INR) of 2.5–3.0. He has never had any bleeding complications.

His wife of 56 years died 8 months ago. You had seen him about a month after her death, and he was independent and eating and well groomed. He has two supportive children who live in the community. At the time you saw him he was normotensive, heart rate was 68, and his weight was 154 lb (he is 65 inches tall). His lungs were clear to P and A. He had a long-standing 1/6 apical midsystolic murmur that radiated slightly to the axilla and was unchanged for years. There was no organomegaly and no edema. Jugular venous pulse was less than 4 cm of water.

In the emergency room he was dyspneic at rest at 45° with a respiratory rate of 22. He was afebrile. There was dullness at the right base one-third up the hemithorax. There were moist rales halfway up on both lungs. There was an S3 gallop, and his murmur was now 3/6 at the apex. Jugular vein pressure (JVP) was 7 cm at 45°. The liver was not distended and not pulsatile, but there was a suggestion of a fluid wave in the abdomen. There was 3+ edema of the legs.

He was taking his medications, namely verapamil 240 extended release, Lanoxin 0.25 mg a day, warfarin 4 mg a day, and lisinopril 5 mg daily.

An electrocardiogram (EKG) showed atrial fibrillation and no acute ST-T changes and no interval Q waves or loss of R waves. A standing chest PA and lateral x-ray showed a large pleural effusion on the right and cardiomegaly. There was prominent vascular redistribution to the upper and middle lobes. There were no Kerley B lines noted.

Labs showed a hemoglobin of 13.9 g/dL, Hematocrit (HCT) of 40%, a white blood cell (WBC) count of 7500/mm^3 with a normal distribution, sodium 132 meq/L, potassium 4.5 meq/L, chloride 104 meq/L CO_2 25 meq/L, blood urea nitrogen (BUN) 46 mg/dL, and creatinine 1.6 mg/dL. AST and ALT were each twice normal. INR was 3.3.

He was admitted to the hospital.

QUESTION 1. What is the most likely diagnosis?

    A. Congestive heart failure
    B. Chronic renal emboli with renal failure
    C. Noncompliance
    D. Salt overload
    E. Endocarditis

He was managed with bed rest and intravenous furosemide, and his other medications were continued. His weight on admission was 175 lb (up from 153 lb when last seen). He started to diurese about 1.5 kg a day; however, his murmur remained unchanged, and his liver tests remained moderately elevated, as did his INR.

QUESTION 2. Which test do you want now?

    A. Computed tomography (CT) urogram
    B. Transthoracic echocardiogram
    C. Agitated saline microbubble echocardiogram
    D. Transesophageal echocardiogram
    E. GI consult with evaluation for liver biopsy
    F. Magnetic resonance imaging (MRI) of the abdomen and pelvis, with special attention to the prostate

The echocardiogram shows a flail mitral valve with nearly complete mitral regurgitation. The left atrium is only moderately enlarged. No clots or vegetations are seen.

QUESTION 3. The next step in your management should be:

    A. Transesophageal echo to rule out vegetations
    B. Peritoneal dialysis to more rapidly remove fluid
    C. Cardiothoracic surgery consultation
    D. Six blood cultures

The patient was seen by cardiology and cardiothoracic surgery. As his congestive failure was very significant, and because he had had previous mitral valve surgery, it was felt he should undergo semiurgent mitral valve repair. He was taken to the OR, and the mitral valve was repaired without untoward difficulty. He remained in atrial fibrillation. He was given intraoperative and postoperative second-generation cephalosporin coverage.

After the surgery he had trouble eating. Speech and swallow studies showed recurrent aspiration. Although his congestive failure improved daily, he had failure to thrive, and a week after the surgery a percutaneous endogastric (PEG) tube was placed. He was transferred to a local rehabilitation facility 3 days after PEG tube placement. Discharge medications were digoxin, 0.25 mg a day, verapamil, 120 mg extended-release daily, warfarin, 3 mg a day, furosemide, 40 mg bid, and K$^+$ supplementation.

You had contact with him by phone in the rehabilitation facility. His spirits were good, but he still was on PEG feedings. Because of some diarrhea, he was placed on "an antibiotic." Touching base with him a week later revealed that he had developed worsening diarrhea and was now on oral vancomycin. You called the covering physician at the rehabilitation facility and found out that the patient had a positive *Clostridium difficile* toxin assay. At the time of your call the patient was passing 10–12 stools a day. One week later he was sent into the emergency room with abdominal pain and distension.

His CT from the emergency room is shown in figure 106.1.

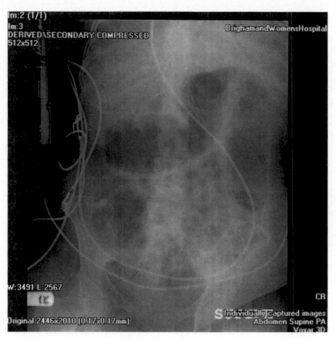

Figure 106.1. Abdominal Flat Plate.

His white count was 35,000 with 90% polymorphonuclear (PMN) cells; his Hb and HCT were 10.9 and 33.2; electrolytes were sodium 129 meq/L, potassium 3.1 meq/L, chloride 109 meq/L, and CO_2 16 meq/L.

His blood pressure was 90/60 mm Hg; pulse was 110 beats/min and irregularly irregular, and his abdomen was distended. His murmur was 1/6, and as on discharge he had no S3. Bowel sounds were a rare high-pitched tinkle. There was no succussion splash. Neurologically he was intact. He was very fatigued and exhausted.

QUESTION 4. At this point what is the best approach to management?

A. Admit to the hospital and start IV vancomycin
B. Obtain a surgical consultation for consideration of total colectomy
C. Stat transthoracic echo
D. 120 mg of IV furosemide

The patient was urgently taken to the OR and underwent a total colectomy. In the OR the team had trouble maintaining his blood pressure, and the patient received pressors and IV fluid resuscitation. He survived the surgery, and after 3 days in the ICU he was able to transfer to the floors.

ANSWER KEY AND DISCUSSION OF THE CASE

QUESTION 1. The best answer is A, congestive heart failure (CHF). The patient has CHF by the chest x-ray (CXR), and he has an S3 and elevated JVP. This answer is correct.

The other choices can be eliminated as less accurate or more speculative. Yes, the creatinine is elevated, but why invoke renal emboli when there is no supporting evidence. Yes, he could have been noncompliant, but he had been stable (and presumably compliant) for years. This same argument can be made for acute sodium overload (i.e., why now?).

Endocarditis could cause his CHF and increasing murmur, but there are no physical stigmata to support this, and he is afebrile. Choosing this as the answer will cause problems as you may choose many of the wrong answers in the questions to follow, and so it is important to not be too cagey in your answers. You know he has CHF, and you know little else to support any of the other answers.

QUESTION 2. The best answer is C, transthoracic echocardiogram. He does not require a transesophageal echo ((TEE; answer D) as that is expensive and uncomfortable and at this moment unnecessary. You want to see his mitral valve, as the murmur is unchanged in spite of the treatment. If the murmur had been loud initially because of acute CHF and dilation of the valve ring, you would think his murmur would be diminished as his congestion improved. The fact that it is unchanged is suggestive that the valve itself has changed and caused his acute decompensation.

A bubble echo study is useful for PDA, and that is not a consideration. A CT urogram would look for renal obstruction or collecting system/prostatic obstruction and is there to see if you "bite" and select it because his BUN and creatinine were elevated in the emergency room. A GI consult is there because of his elevated liver function tests (LFTs), but certainly you would at least want further values for them prior to getting a consult. Last, the MRI of the abdomen/pelvis is there for the ascites/renal function, and again, not a good choice with this amount of information and a good working diagnosis of CHF as the unifying principle.

QUESTION 3. The best answer is C, cardiothoracic surgery consultation. You suspect there is something wrong with the valve. It was replaced 10 years ago, and now he has a louder murmur and congestive heart failure. Although he could have endocarditis as the cause, there is no fever, no physical stigmata of subacute bacterial endocarditis, and no persistent and severe decompensation as would be seen with acute bacterial endocarditis. So although answers A (TEE) and D (six blood cultures) are plausible, they are not the best answer. And indeed, if you were thinking endocarditis how would you decide A versus D as the *one best* answer. Choice B, peritoneal dialysis, does not make sense because the diuresis is proceeding nicely at 1.5 kg a day.

QUESTION 4. The best answer is B, obtain a surgical consultation for total colectomy. This is a complex question, and it is not just about the answer, which may appear to be very aggressive.

The Board is trying to encourage your continuing care of the patient, although he might be under the direct care of someone else (the physician at the rehabilitation facility or an emergency room doctor). You know the patient, in his totality, best. You made his initial diagnosis and helped shepherd him to surgery. You are aware of his post-op difficulties and subsequent PEG and aspiration problems.

Furthermore, the Board expects you to be able to read the CT and recognize that there is implied pan colitis from *C. difficile* with severe (and ominous) distension of the entire colon.

You are also, once again for this patient, expected to know when to get help from another discipline, namely GI surgery. It is a common failing of internal medicine trainees to call their surgical colleagues in late rather than to recognize that the patient's problem is best solved surgically.

Answer A, give IV vancomycin, is plausible, but the patient is extremely ill with a low blood pressure, a dangerously distended colon, and with presumed *C. difficile* in the colon.

Answer C, a transthoracic echo, would also be plausible to see if the valve were somehow now problematic or if there were constriction postsurgery causing low blood pressure, but with the constellation of symptoms and the low CO_2 (which implies a metabolic acidosis), this is not a good early choice at this juncture. Last, there is no reason to give this hypotensive patient more furosemide, as there is no sign of decompensated heart failure or fluid overload

ADDITIONAL READING

http://www.residencyandfellowship.com/ABIM_Internal_Medicine_boards_certification_exam. Accessed December 28, 2010.

http://www.abim.org/exam/cert/im.aspx. Accessed December 28, 2010.

FitzGerald JD, Wenger NS. Didactic teaching conferences for IM residents: Who attends, and is attendance related to medical certifying examination scores? *Acad Med.* 2003;78(1):84–9.

Lipner RS, Lucey CR. Putting the secure examination to the test. *JAMA.* 2010;304(12):1379–80.

Wenderoth S, Pelzman F, Demopoulos B. Ambulatory morning report: Can it prepare residents for the American Board of Internal Medicine examination? *J Gen Intern Med.* 2002;17(3):207–9.

107.

BOARD PRACTICE 1

Rafael Bejar, Tyler M. Berzin, Rebecca A. Berman, and Chiadi E. Ndumele

QUESTIONS

QUESTION 1. A 48-year-old male with EtOH cirrhosis presents to reestablish primary care. He has no history of ascites, encephalopathy, or variceal bleeding and does not take any medications. A routine upper endoscopy reveals grade III varices.

Which of the following treatments are indicated to reduce this patient's risk of variceal hemorrhage?

A. TIPS (transjugular intrahepatic portosystemic shunt)
B. Propranolol
C. Spironolactone
D. Octreotide
E. No current therapy is effective for primarily prophylaxis of variceal hemorrhage.

QUESTION 2. A 35-year-old painter initially presented with fatigue, myalgias, and a rash (see figure 107.1) after a weekend on Cape Cod. His primary care physician prescribed a 14-day course of doxycycline (100 mg bid). He returns 10 days later with worsening myalgias, fever, nausea, and vomiting. Routine labs reveal a hematocrit of 34. He also has an elevated lactate dehydrogenase (LDH) and total bilirubin. What is the most likely diagnosis?

A. Inadequately treated Lyme disease
B. Babesiosis
C. Malaria
D. Rocky Mountain spotted fever
E. Drug reaction to doxycycline

QUESTION 3. Seven days into her hospitalization, all blood cultures have been negative, and the patient's WBC count is beginning to recover. She now develops a new fever to 101°F, cough, and pleuritic chest discomfort. Her serum galactomannan and beta-glucan are both elevated.

The patient's chest CT is shown in figure 107.2.
What is the likely diagnosis?

A. Pulmonary histoplasmosis
B. Disseminated *Candida albicans* infection

C. Invasive aspergillosis
D. Cryptococcal infection
E. Pulmonary embolism with lung infarction

QUESTION 4. A 62-year-old female had her thyroid-stimulating hormone (TSH) checked after presenting with weight gain and tachycardia. The thyroid exam was normal.
TSH 0.011 (nL 0.5–5)
Free T$_4$ 1.5 (nL 0.8–1.8)
What is the optimal approach to this patient?

A. Reassurance
B. Treat with Levoxyl
C. Treat with methimazole
D. Obtain a thyroid ultrasound

QUESTION 5. A 36-year-old male in generally excellent health presents to the emergency room with "palpitations" × 3–4 days. He denies chest pain or dyspnea. He also complains of right hip pain and generalized fatigue for several weeks and recalls a vague rash on his right leg 1 month ago. Exam is notable for heart rate of 45 and mildly limited range of movement in right hip. An EKG is obtained, and a telemetry strip is shown in figure 107.3.
What is the next appropriate treatment step?

A. Placement of permanent pacemaker
B. Placement of permanent pacemaker and implantable cardiodefibrillator (ICD)
C. Temporary pacemaker and initiation of IV corticosteroids
D. Temporary pacemaker and initiation of IV ceftriaxone
E. Aspirin plus heparin bolus and drip

QUESTION 6. A 59-year-old man with a medical history that includes a prior deep vein thrombosis (DVT) and chronic kidney disease requiring hemodialysis is admitted to the hospital for elective knee replacement. His coumadin had been stopped a few days prior, and he is started on intravenous unfractionated heparin on admission. On his sixth hospital day, his platelet count falls to 75,000 from 195,000

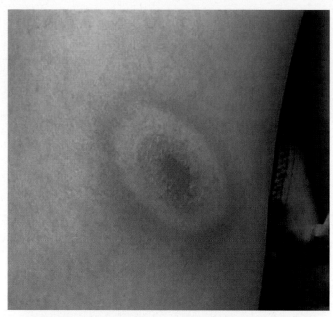

Figure 107.1. Image of the skin rash from the patient described in Question 2.

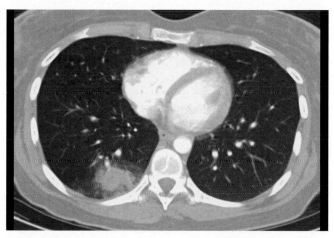

Figure 107.2. Computed Tomography (CT) Scan of the Chest from the Patient Described in Question 3.

the day prior. In addition to discontinuing the IV heparin, you should do which of the following?

A. Await the results of an anti-PF4 assay before restarting anticoagulation
B. Transfuse platelets to prevent postoperative bleeding

C. Start subcutaneous Lovenox immediately
D. Start subcutaneous fondaparinux immediately
E. Start IV argatroban immediately

QUESTION 7. A 78-year-old female with diabetes is admitted to the hospital with signs, symptoms, and urinalysis consistent with a urinary tract infection. On initial evaluation in the emergency department, the blood pressure is 70/30 mm Hg but improves briskly with IV fluids, and the patient is admitted to the medical floor. Her complete blood count (CBC) revealed a mild leukocytosis but is otherwise normal. Shortly after admission, she begins experiencing lower abdominal cramping and passes several stools with evidence of dark blood.

Which of the following is the most like explanation for her gastrointestinal bleeding?

A. Hemolytic uremic syndrome
B. Acute mesenteric ischemia
C. Chronic mesenteric ischemia
D. Ischemic colitis
E. Bacterial colitis

QUESTION 8. A 76-year-old male patient with diabetes mellitus (DM), CRI, and a 40-pack-year smoking history presents for physical exam. He has no acute complaints. Review of Systems negative for cough, fevers, chills, night sweats, chest pain, SOB, BRBPR, or genitourinary sx. He continues to smoke half a pack of cigarettes each day. Which of the following are recommended for cancer screening in this patient at this time?

A. Digital rectal exam (DRE)/prostate-specific antigen (PSA), colonoscopy
B. Chest CT, DRE/PSA
C. Chest CT, colonoscopy
D. Chest CT
E. None of the above

QUESTION 9. A 68-year-old man with a history of cardiovascular disease presents to his primary care physician asking about the need for antibiotics before he goes to the dentist to get his teeth cleaned. His past medical history includes hypertension, mitral valve prolapse (MVP) with mild regurgitation, a pacemaker placed 8 months ago, a total hip replacement 18 months ago, and two coronary artery stents placed 4 months ago.

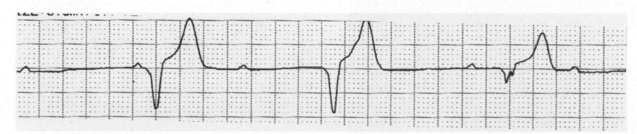

Figure 107.3. Electrocardiograph Strip from the Patient Described in Question 5.

Which of the following should his physician recommend?

A. Antibiotic prophylaxis because of his MVP with regurgitation.
B. Antibiotic prophylaxis because of his recent pacemaker implantation.
C. Antibiotic prophylaxis because of his recent joint replacement.
D. Prophylactic antibiotics are not required for routine teeth cleaning.
E. Prophylactic antibiotics are not required given his medical history.

QUESTION 10. A healthy 25-year-old graduate student presents to the student health clinic complaining of a sore throat, cough, and fever for the past 3 days. On exam, her throat is erythematous and without exudates. She has no neck tenderness or palpable lymphadenopathy. Which of the following is the most appropriate plan for this patient?

A. Reassurance since she is unlikely to have streptococcal pharyngitis.
B. Prescribe a course of antibiotics based on the result of a rapid strep test.
C. Prescribe a course of antibiotics to take if she is no better in 3 days.
D. Prescribe a course of antibiotics to begin taking now.
E. Obtain a throat culture and have her stop antibiotics if it is negative.

QUESTION 11. Over the next 5 days, her throat pain worsens. She continues to have high fevers with chills and now notes painful left-sided neck swelling. Representative images from studies of her neck and chest are shown in figures 107.4–107.6. Which of the following is LEAST likely to be helpful in this situation?

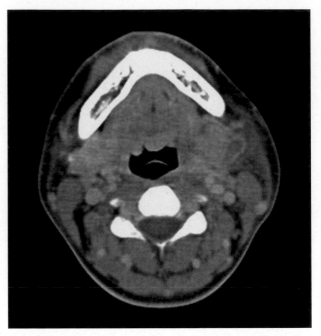

Figure 107.5. CT scan of the neck from the patient described in Question 14.

A. Urgent otolaryngology consultation
B. Gentamycin
C. Clindamycin
D. Penicillin
E. Intravenous heparin

QUESTION 12. A 28-year-old nonsmoking graduate student presents with 1 week of wheezing, cough, and yellow sputum. He has had several prior episodes of "bronchitis" in the last 2 years. Exam is notable for O$_2$ sat 90% on room air and scattered wheezing and rhonchi. Labs are notable for leukocytosis and eosinophilia: WBC 14.4 (53 poly, 20 lymph, 15 eos). Prior PFTs have shown a mild obstructive pattern. Small, scattered opacities are seen on chest x-ray,

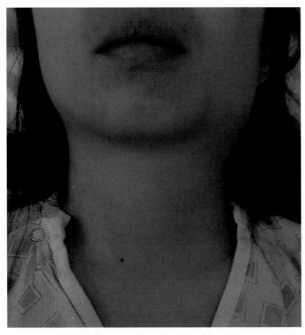

Figure 107.4. Neck image from the patient described in Question 11.

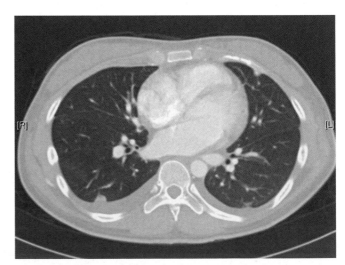

Figure 107.6. CT Scan of the Chest from the Patient Described in Question 11.

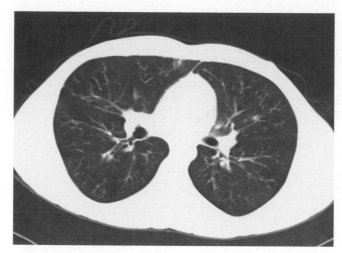

Figure 107.7. CT Scan of the Chest from the Patient Described in Question 12.

and the chest CT shown in figures 107.7 and 107.8 is obtained. What is the next appropriate step?

A. Bronchoscopy
B. Skin prick test for reactivity to *Aspergillus fumigatus*
C. *Strongyloides* serology
D. Induced sputum × 3 samples
E. Prednisone taper

QUESTION 13. A 30-year-old man presents to his primary care physician with a new rash on his back and trunk (figure 107.9). The lesions are red and raised. He says it is itchy but not painful. He has never had a rash like this before. He has used no new lotions, soaps, or medications.

He does comment that he has a similar rash in one spot on his back a few weeks before the current eruption.

What is the most likely outcome for this rash?

A. It will spontaneously resolve in 6–10 weeks.
B. It will resolve with steroids and recur with episodes of stress.
C. It will resolve with calcipotriene ointment.

D. It will resolve with benzoyl peroxide.
E. It will require treatment with PUVA and possible chemotherapy.

QUESTION 14. A 57-year-old woman with no history of cardiac disease develops substernal chest pressure during her routine hemodialysis session. The episode lasts about 5 minutes and resolves spontaneously before she arrives in the emergency room. Her vital signs are normal, and her cardiac biomarkers are not elevated. Her EKG is shown in figure 107.10.

Which of the following treatment plans is most appropriate for this patient?

A. Urgent cardiac catheterization
B. Heparin, Plavix, aspirin, and cardiac catheterization if cardiac biomarkers become elevated
C. Imaging stress test before considering catheterization
D. Admission for observation and telemetry monitoring
E. Correction of electrolyte abnormalities and reassurance

QUESTION 15. A 46-year-old lawyer presents to the emergency department with bright red emesis. He had been on a drinking binge for several days and started vomiting food and bile last night. He was retching all night and in the morning threw up frank blood. Examination reveals a pulse of 110, rising to 135 when standing up, blood pressure of 104/76, falling to 80/56 with standing. He smells of alcohol, has clear lungs, and a nontender abdomen.

What is the first step in caring for this patient?

A. Start an intravenous proton pump inhibitor
B. Give fresh frozen plasma as he likely has liver disease

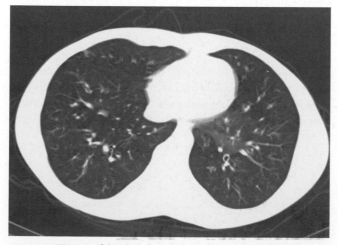

Figure 107.8. CT scan of the chest from the patient described in Question 12.

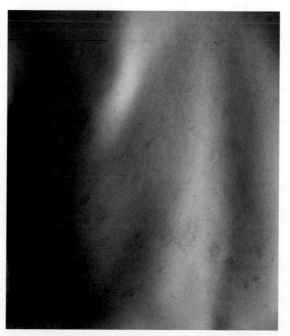

Figure 107.9. Skin image from the patient described in Question 13.

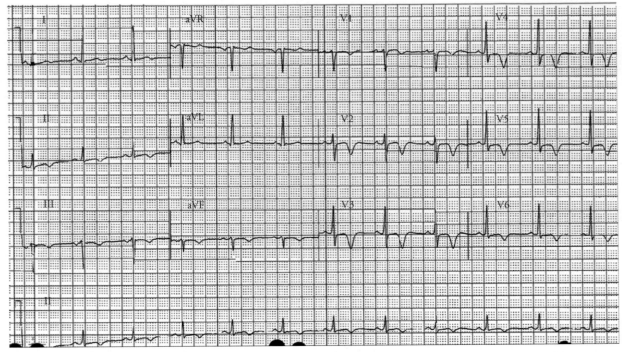

Figure 107.10. Electrocardiogram from the patient described in Question 14.

C. Resuscitate patient with intravenous fluids
D. Perform esophagogastroduodenoscopy
E. Perform gastric lavage with nasogastric tube

QUESTION 16. Given the previous patient's history, what is the most likely diagnosis?

A. Dieulafoy's lesion
B. Peptic ulcer disease
C. Erosive esophagitis
D. Mallory-Weiss tear
E. Variceal bleed

QUESTION 17. A 67-year-old woman presents with 2 weeks of progressive fatigue, dyspnea, and easy bruising. She now notes dyspnea at rest, a severe headache, and blurry vision.

She is afebrile with a heart rate of 113 beats per minute, a normal blood pressure, and an oxygen saturation of 89% on room air. On exam, she has scattered ecchymoses, retinal hemorrhages, and bibasilar rales. Blood studies (figure 107.11) show:

WBC 113,800 cells per μL

Hematocrit 24.1%

Platelets 27,000 per μL

Which of the following treatments is it most important to start as soon as possible?

A. Intravenous normal saline bolus
B. Hydroxyurea
C. Red blood cell transfusion

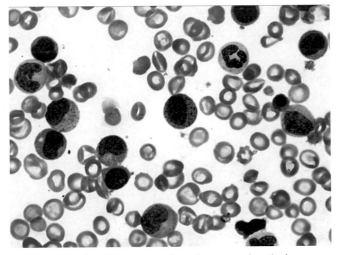

Figure 107.11. Peripheral blood smear from the patient described in Question 17.

D. Leukopheresis
E. Rasburicase

QUESTION 18. A 46-year-old male, Asian American, presents with diabetes mellitus. He reports sugars of 300s and his hemoglobin A1C returns at 6.8%. You explain that these labs could be secondary to all of the following EXCEPT:

A. Glucometer malfunction
B. Lab error
C. Hemolytic anemia
D. Polycythemia vera
E. β-thalassemia

QUESTION 19. A 79-year-old male arrives at the emergency room complaining of right-sided facial droop and right arm weakness. His symptoms started about 3–4 hours ago during breakfast. Physical exam confirms findings consistent with a left-sided middle cerebral artery (MCA) stroke. Head CT shows no evidence of intracranial bleed. Which of the following treatments are indicated for initial therapy of this event?

A. Intravenous tissue-plasminogen activator (tPA)
B. Intravenous heparin
C. Enoxaparin (low-molecular weight heparin)
D. Aspirin
E. None of the above

QUESTION 20. A 22-year-old pharmacy student with a history of eczema and a nut allergy presents with a painful, burning rash on her right thigh. Her symptoms began the prior evening after a day at the beach. This morning, the rash and pain are much worse. She also notes some pain on her hands, neck, and distal thigh (see figure 107.12).

Which activity most likely led to the development of her symptoms?

A. Walking through brush in her swimsuit
B. Swimming in the ocean
C. Applying sunscreen containing zinc oxide
D. Squeezing limes while making mojitos
E. Taking tetracycline for facial acne

QUESTION 21. A 57-year-old editor is admitted with dyspnea and marked hypoxemia. He undergoes a CT scan of the chest, which is shown in figure 107.13. He subsequently undergoes bronchoscopy, which reveals progressively bloodier return with alveolar lavage. These findings are consistent with diffuse alveolar hemorrhage (DAH).

Which one of the following lab tests would be *least* likely to help determine an etiology of this man's disease?

A. ANCA (antineutrophil cytoplasmic antibody)
B. Anti-GBM (anti-glomerular basement membrane antibody)
C. ACE (angiotensin conversion enzyme)
D. ANA (antinuclear antibodies)
E. Toxicology screen

QUESTION 22. A 35-year-old store manager presents with arthralgias and the rash seen in figure 107.14. Her primary care physician ordered a chest radiograph which is shown in figure 107.15.

This constellation of symptoms is called:

A. Löfgren syndrome
B. Hamman-Rich syndrome
C. Lemierre syndrome
D. Scimitar syndrome
E. Castleman disease

QUESTION 23. Which of the following is NOT associated with Löfgren syndrome?

A. Sarcoidosis
B. Coccidiomycosis

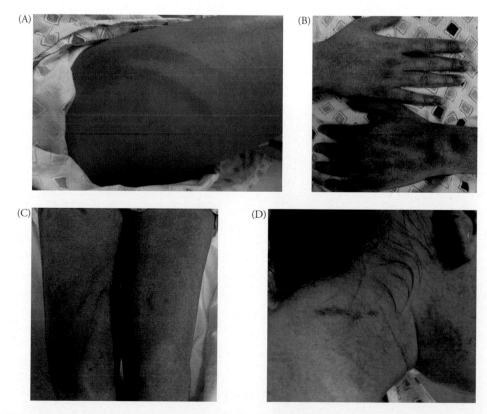

Figure 107.12. Multiple Images of the Rash from the Patient Described in Question 20. Panels B–D are shown in false color to highlight the rash.

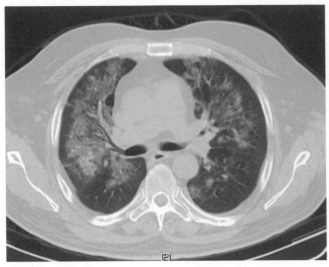

Figure 107.13. CT Scan of the Chest from the Patient Described in Question 21.

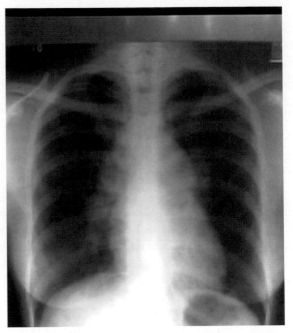

Figure 107.15. Chest Radiograph from the Patient Described in Question 22.

C. Behçet disease
D. Hodgkin disease
E. Tuberculosis

QUESTION 24. After cardiac catheterization, a 72-year-old man develops prolonged bleeding at the arterial puncture site. Intravenous heparin is discontinued. Twenty-four hours later, he has a large groin hematoma and his puncture site continues to ooze despite compression. He has no history of abnormal bleeding.

His basic metabolic panel is normal.
Hematocrit: 27% (was 38% on admission)
Platelets: 210,000
International Normalized Ratio (INR) 1.2, PTT 85 sec

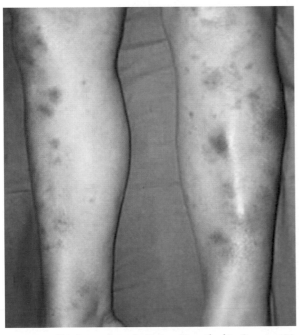

Figure 107.14. Skin Image from the Patient Described in Question 22.

Which of the following will help determine the cause of bleeding in this patient?

A. A trial of vitamin K administration
B. Measurement of von Willebrand factor activity
C. Platelet function assay
D. A 1:1 mixing study
E. Test for a lupus anticoagulant

QUESTION 25. A 46-year-old business executive comes to your office worried about hemochromatosis. His wife's brother was recently diagnosed with cirrhosis due to this disease, and he is worried because he heard it is very common. He is of Swedish origin, completely asymptomatic, and has no history of liver disease in his family. His physical examination reveals no abnormalities. What is the most useful test to screen him?

A. HFE genotyping
B. Serum transferrin saturation
C. Hemoglobin/hematocrit
D. Serum alanine and aspartate aminotransferases
E. Liver biopsy with quantitative iron index

QUESTION 26. A 20-year-old female, who is sexually active and has a history of an abnormal Pap test, presents for a physical before moving to college. She reports three male partners in the last year. PMH otherwise unremarkable. Last immunizations at age 10. She states that she had all routine childhood immunizations. She had chickenpox as a child.

Which of the following immunizations would be appropriate?

A. Meningococcal, tetanus, human papilloma virus (HPV)
B. Meningococcal, Hep B, TDAP, HPV

C. Hep B, tetanus, HPV

D. Meningococcal, Hep B, TDAP, HPV, Pneumovax

E. Meningococcal, Hep B, TDAP

QUESTION 27. A 20-year-old male presents with no PMH p/w left subscapular pain after bumping into someone earlier that day. Has had a cold over the last 2 weeks with nonproductive cough. He takes no meds.

Physical exam: HR 122, BP 110/76, RR 22, O$_2$ 91%. No acute distress.

Decreased breath sounds over the left hemithorax (chest x-ray in figure 107.16).

What is the most appropriate next step?

A. Nebulizer treatment with albuterol and Atrovent

B. Azithromycin orally for 5 days

C. Nasal oxygen and close observation overnight

D. Chest tube placement

E. Pulmonary function tests with single-breath diffusing capacity of the lung (DLCO)

QUESTION 28. A 54-year-old businesswoman presents with profound fatigue. CBC reveals hematocrit of 30 and platelets of 42,000. Her creatinine is 2.6, and her LDH is 1080. Coagulation profile is normal. Hcr blood smear is shown in figure 107.17.

What would be the most appropriate therapy for this patient?

A. Plasmapheresis

B. Prednisone

C. Rituxan

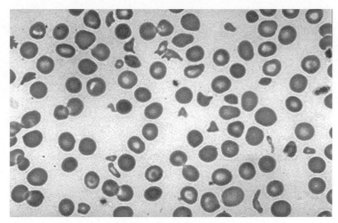

Figure 107.17. Peripheral Blood Smear from the Patient Described in Question 29.

D. IVIG

E. Cyclophosphamide

QUESTION 29. A 56-year-old farmer presents with right upper quadrant tenderness. He has no history of liver disease or gallstones and is originally from Greece. His physical exam reveals no fever or jaundice but mild right upper quadrant tenderness.

A CT scan is obtained (figure 107.18).

What is the most reasonable treatment approach?

A. Watchful waiting

B. Endoscopic retrograde cholangiopancreatography (ERCP)

C. Empirical treatment with ciprofloxacin and metronidazole

D. Albendazole treatment followed by surgical resection

E. Immediate percutaneous drainage

QUESTION 30. A healthy 58-year-old high school teacher presents to urgent care complaining of feeling "fuzzy" in class and having a hard time grading tests over the weekend. She has been constipated for several days. She takes only Tums and an occasional aspirin.

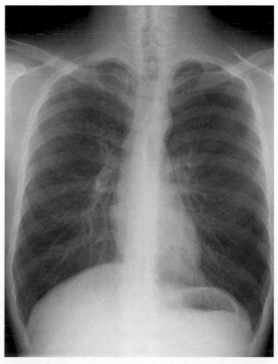

Figure 107.16. Chest Radiograph from the Patient Described in Question 27.

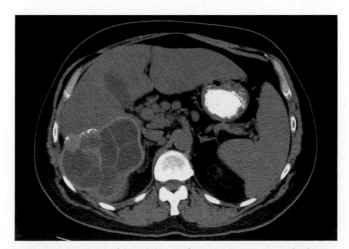

Figure 107.18. CT Scan of the Abdomen from the Patient Described in Question 30.

Labs reveal Ca = 14.2, PO_4 = 2.5, Creatinine = 2.6, and HCO_3 = 34. Her parathyroid hormone (PTH) level is low, and she has an undetectable PTH-rP.

Imaging studies show no abnormalities.

All of the following would be appropriate therapy in the acute setting EXCEPT:

A. Hydration with normal saline
B. IV zoledronic acid
C. Discontinuation of calcium carbonate
D. Use of a loop diuretic after volume repletion
E. Calcitonin, 4 units/kg IM every 12 hours

ANSWERS

1. B. Propranolol and nadolol are recommended for primary prophylaxis of variceal bleeding in patients with large (grade 2 or 3) varices. There is also evidence to support endoscopic ligation/banding of varices to prevent hemorrhage. TIPS is indicated for management of *active* variceal bleeding (when endoscopic and pharmacologic treatment has failed), but is NOT appropriate for primarily prophylaxis of bleeding. Octreotide or somatostatin is indicated for management of active variceal bleeding but not primarily prophylaxis. Spironolactone is effective for management of ascites but plays no role in prophylaxis of variceal bleeding (*Hepatology*. 2007;46(3):922–38).

2. B. The initial presentation was consistent with early localized Lyme disease. The rash is erythema migrans (EM). The treatment of doxycycline, 100 mg bid, is the appropriate therapy. An acceptable alternative would be a 10- to 14-day course of amoxicillin.

This clinical picture is characteristic of infection with *Babesia microti,* whose vector is also the *Ixodes* tick. Patients typically present with nonspecific complaints of nausea/vomiting, malaise, and fever as well as evidence of hemolytic anemia. Immunosuppressed hosts are more likely to have symptomatic *Babesia* infection, particularly asplenic patients or those with HIV.

3. C. *Aspergillus* can cause a broad spectrum of disease. Invasive aspergillosis affects the lung and occurs in severely immunocompromised patients.

Beta-glucan is a cell wall component of most or all fungi. The beta-glucan assay detects the presence of invasive fungal infections.

Galactomannan is a cell-wall component of *Aspergillus*. The assay detects the presence of invasive aspergillosis. A chest CT "halo sign" is highly suggestive of angioinvasive fungus (*Aspergillus*). Voriconazole is the treatment of choice for invasive aspergillosis (*N Engl J Med*. 2009;360:1870–84).

4. C. This patient has hyperthyroidism. There is an increased risk of atrial fibrillation. According to the Framingham study, which included 2007 patients aged 60+ and included a 10-year follow-up the number needed to treat to avoid afib with TSH <0.1 = 42.

There is also an osteoporosis risk. Frank hyperthyroidism is a known osteoporosis risk factor, and subclinical hyperthyroidism can be evidence of decreased bone mass density (BMD), especially in postmenopausal women, although it is unclear if it increases fracture risk.

5. D. Lyme carditis with third-degree Atrioventricular (AV) block. IDSA recommended therapy is IV ceftriaxone for 14–21 days. AV block is a classic manifestation of *early disseminated* Lyme disease (typically occuring weeks to months after initial infection). Among Lyme disease cases, 1–10% develop Lyme carditis (possibly higher in Europe). In most cases of Lyme carditis AV block resolves *spontaneously* and permanent ventricular pacing is unnecessary. IDSA recommendations for IV antibiotics are based on expert consensus and are the general treatment strategy for early disseminated Lyme disease.

6. E. This patient has a clinical scenario highly concerning for heparin-induced thrombocytopenia (HIT): there is a 50% reduction in platelet count while exposed to heparin; it appears 5–10 days after exposure to heparin, although it can be <24 hours if heparin was given within the past 100 days. HIT is associated with an approximately 50% risk of thrombosis. All patients with intermediate or high suspicion for HIT should receive alternative anticoagulation immediately. Although the risk is lower Lovenox can cause HIT and should never be used in patients with suspected or known HIT. Argatroban and lepirudin are approved for treatment of HIT. Fondaparinux has been studied for use in HIT but is renally excreted and not recommended for dialysis patients (Arepally and Ortel. *N Engl J Med.* 2006;355:809–17. Warkentin. *Chest.* 2005;127[2 Suppl]:35S–45S).

7. D. Ischemic colitis is the most common form of bowel ischemia. Pathophysiology of IC is typically a nonocclusive ischemia (low-flow state). The vast majority of ischemic colitis cases occur in the elderly. Typical symptoms include abdominal cramping and rectal bleeding. Treatment is typically supportive (IV fluids, bowel rest, *very limited* data for antibiotics). Other types of mesenteric ischemia include these:

- *Acute mesenteric ischemia*—most commonly an embolic event to SMA, causing acute, severe abdominal pain. Treatment is primarily surgical.

- *Chronic mesenteric ischemia*—due to diffuse atherosclerotic disease in 95% of cases. Typical symptoms include postprandial abdominal pain and weight loss.

8. E. Cancer screening is not indicated in patients with an expected life span of <10 years. Under the new U.S. Preventive Services Task Force (USPTF) guidelines PSA is not indicated in men >75 or with a lifespan <10 years. USPTF also recommends against colorectal cancer screening in patients 76–85, although there may be considerations that support colorectal cancer screening in an individual patient.

The USPTF concludes that the evidence is insufficient to recommend for or against screening asymptomatic persons for lung cancer with either low-dose computerized tomography, chest x-ray, sputum cytology, or a combination of these tests. The use of low-dose CT scans is controversial and the subject of at least two large, randomized clinical trials that should clarify the risks and benefits of screening:

- National Lung Cancer Screening Trial
- Prostate, Lung, Colorectal, and Ovarian Cancer Screening Trial (http://www.ahrq.gov/clinic/uspstf/uspsprca.htm. http://www.annals.org/content/149/9/627.full. http://www.ahrq.gov/CLINIC/USPSTF/uspslung.htm)

9. C. In 2007 the American Heart Association revised its recommendations for antibiotic prophylaxis to include only cardiac conditions associated with the highest risk of adverse outcomes from endocarditis. These include prosthetic cardiac valves, prior endocarditis, unrepaired cyanotic heart disease, and repaired heart disease with prosthetic material within 6 months or with residual graft defects. Mitral valve prolapse with or without regurgitation is no longer an indication for prophylaxis. Neither are pacemakers, AICDs, or coronary stents. Prophylaxis is presently recommended for all patients for the first 2 years following joint replacement and lifelong for those who are immunocompromised or have certain comorbidities.

10. A. Based on her presentation, this patient is unlikely to have group A streptococcal (GAS) pharyngitis. She has only one of the four Centor criteria:

- Fever
- Absence of cough
- Tonsillar exudates
- Tender anterior cervical lymphadenopathy

The ACP, CDC, and IDSA guidelines recommend against strep testing for patients who meet no or one criterion. For patients who meet three or four criteria, the guidelines disagree about whether to treat empirically based on a rapid strep test result or based on culture results (Bisno. *Ann Intern Med.* 2003;139:150–1. Linder et al. *Arch Intern Med.* 2006;166:1374–9).

11. B. This patient has Lemierre's syndrome:

- Septic thrombophlebitis of the internal jugular vein by the anaerobic Gram-negative rod *Fusobacterium necrophorum* causing bacteremia and septic thromboemboli to the lungs
- Typically follows a bout of bacterial pharyngitis
- Often associated with neck abscess

Treatment includes surgical abscess drainage and anaerobic antibiotic therapy for 4–6 weeks. Heparin is often used, although its benefit is unproven and extrapolated from studies of pelvic septic thrombophlebitis (Hoehn *Pediatrics.* 2005;115:1415–6. http://www.residentandstaff.com/issues/articles/2005–03_02.asp).

12. B. Allergic bronchopulmonary aspergillosis (ABPA) should be *suspected* if any one of the following is present:

1. CXR/CT with central bronchiectasis or recurrent infiltrates
2. Refractory asthma symptoms
3. + Skin prick for *Aspergillus*
4. + Sputum cultures for *Aspergillus*
5. Prominent peripheral eosinophilia

Appropriate testing includes skin prick reactivity to *Aspergillus,* IgE level, and specific antibodies (IgE and IgA) to *Aspergillus*. Typical treatment includes glucocorticoids +/− itraconazole.

13. A. This is a picture of pityriasis rosea. The patient describes it beginning with a herald patch—a single lesion that precedes the generalized eruption by 1–2 weeks. It is a self-limited disease that usually resolves in 6 weeks without treatment and does not recur.

Other rashes in the differential diagnosis of this rash include the following:

- Psoriasis → treated with topical steroids or topical vitamin D analogues
- Tinea corporis → resolves with antifungals
- Mycosis fungoides (cutaneous T-cell lymphoma) → treated with PUVA and chemotherapy if there is systemic involvement (*Am Fam Physician.* 2004;16:87)

14. A. These are the typical EKG changes of Wellens' syndrome:

- New precordial T-wave inversions (V2–V5 or V6) (figure 107.19).
- T-wave inversions are usually symmetric or biphasic.
- EKG changes often more evident when chest pain-free.
- Associated with critical proximal LAD lesion.
- Cardiac biomarkers are often normal or mildly elevated.
- If treated medically, 75% will develop an anterior myocardial infarction (MI).
- Early cardiac catheterization is recommended, and is typically followed by percutaneous revascularization or coronary artery bypass surgery (Rhinehardt et al. *Am J Emerg Med.* 2002;20:638–43. de Zwaan et al. *Am Heart J.* 1982;103:730–6).

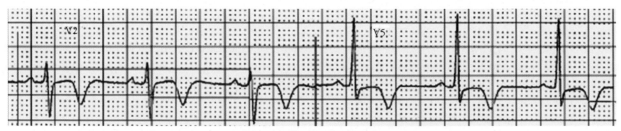

Figure 107.19. Electrocardiograph strip with precordial T-wave inversions described in the answer to Question 16.

15. A. This patient has an acute leukemia with signs and symptoms of leukostasis. The most important early therapy is hydration.

Leukostasis is caused by poorly deformable leukemic white blood cells impeding circulation through small blood vessels. It is typically seen in myeloid leukemias with WBC >50,000. Clinical manifestations depend on the target organs affected and include dyspnea, hypoxia, headaches, visual changes, seizures, renal failure, and bleeding. Early administration of red blood cells increases blood viscosity and can further compromise local blood flow. Definitive treatment is to reduce cell counts with hydroxyurea, leukopheresis, or early induction chemotherapy (Majhail and Lichtin. *Cleve Clin J Med.* 2004;71:633–7).

16. C. The patient is in hypovolemic shock and needs immediate resuscitation with intravenous fluids. Intravenous resuscitation requires two large-bore IVs (18 gauge or larger) or a "cordis" (large-bore central line).

Proton pump inhibitor (PPI) therapy has an important role in bleeding related to peptic ulcer disease but should not be prioritized over resuscitation. Nasogastric lavage will not change the decision for acute endoscopic evaluation. Urgent endoscopy should be performed once the patient has been initially stabilized (*Gastroenterol Clin North Am.* 2003;32:1053).

17. D. Mallory-Weiss tears are linear mucosal tears in the gastric mucosa near the gastroesophageal junction. They are the cause of upper gastrointestinal bleeding in 5–10% of patients. They were initially described in 1929 in alcoholic patients. Alcoholic gastritis is also easily compatible with the history and presentation.

The other conditions are also common causes of upper gastrointestinal bleeding but lack the distinctive clinical history of *hematemesis after initial nonbloody emesis* (*BMJ.* 2001;323:1115).

18. D. Hemoglobin A1c (A1C) measures glycosylated sugar on red blood cells (RBCs). If RBC lifespan is short, then A1C can falsely decrease. Hemoglobinopathies and hemolytic anemia typically decrease RBC lifespan. Hemoglobin variants can have a different mobility and may not be picked up by an A1C lab machine. A high RBC count would falsely elevate A1C.

A1C can now be used as screening test, with DM defined as A1C ≥6.5 (*Diabetes Care.* 2002;25;275–8. *Diabetes Care.* 2009;32;1327).

19. A. tPA (Alteplase) is the only therapy currently FDA-approved for acute ischemic stroke. The benefit of tPA for treatment *beyond* the traditional 3-hour time window was recently established by two large trials (including ECASS 3), which showed that treatment in the 3- to 4.5-hour time window can also yield modest benefits. Aspirin therapy may be appropriate to prevent early recurrence of ischemic stroke, but thrombolysis with tPA is a contraindication to immediate initiation of aspirin. Heparin is not currently recommended for patients with acute ischemic stroke, although it may be considered in limited, specific circumstances (known intracardiac thrombus, carotid thrombus) (*N Engl J Med.* 2008;359:1317–29).

20. D. This a phytophotodermatitis—a cutaneous phototoxic eruption that results from contact with light-sensitizing substances and exposure to UVA radiation, often in bizarre, well-demarcated patterns (e.g., handprints).

Symptoms begin 24 hours after exposure and peak at 48–72 hours but may take weeks to fully resolve. Effects range from hyperpigmentation to bullous eruptions. The most frequent causes include 5-methoxypsoralen in lime-peel juice (mangos, celery), furocoumarins in brushes (roses) and grasses, and bergamot oils in perfumes with essential oils (http://emedicine.medscape.com/article/1119566-overview).

21. C. DAH has been associated with many diseases including these:

- Wegener and microscopic polyangiitis (ANCA)
- Goodpasture (anti-GBM)
- SLE (ANA) as well as RF, scleroderma, and MCTD
- Cocaine inhalation (tox screen)

DAH has also been associated with medications such as PTU, phenytoin, and retinoic acid. ACE is a test sometimes ordered when considering sarcoid, but there are no data to support its use in the diagnosis. The test has neither a good sensitivity nor a good specificity. Sarcoid is not a disease commonly associated with DAH (*Curr Opin Rheum.* 2001;13:12–7).

22. A. The rash on the legs is erythema nodosum. It is classically a painful, erythematous nodular eruption on the anterior legs. The constellation of hilar lymphadenopathy (seen on CXR), arthralgias, and erythema nodosum is Löfgren syndrome.

The other syndromes are these:

- Hamman-Rich: rapidly progressive, bilateral interstitial pneumonitis without a clear etiology

- Lemierre: thrombophlebitis of the internal jugular resulting from bacteremia associated with a head or neck infection

- Scimitar: constellation of anomalous venous drainage of the right lung into the IVC, hypoplasia of right lung and right pulmonary artery, as well as dextroposition of the heart

- Castleman: large, bulky, nonmalignant lymphadenopathy (*Curr Opin Rheumatol.* 2001;13:84).

23. C. Although the most common cause of Löfgren syndrome is sarcoidosis, there are several other possible etiologies that need to be ruled out. These include the following:

- Endemic fungi: histoplasmosis, coccidiomycosis, blastomycosis

- Tuberculosis

- Yersiniosis

- *Chlamydia pneumoniae*

When sarcoid presents as Löfgren syndrome it is usually a self-limited disease (*Curr Opin Rheumatol.* 2001;13:84).

24. D. This patient has a coagulopathy that preferentially affects the activated partial thromboplastin time (aPTT). A 1:1 mixing study will indicate if this patient has a factor deficiency or a coagulation inhibitor responsible for his abnormal bleeding.

Vitamin K deficiency preferentially affects the prothrombin time (PT/INR). This patient's INR is nearly normal. Treatment with vitamin K is unlikely to correct his bleeding tendency.

Von Willebrand disease (vWD) causes postprocedural bleeding and can be acquired. The most common forms of vWD are hereditary, result in primarily mucosal bleeding, and rarely prolong the aPTT much.

Post–cardiac catheterization patients are often on multiple antiplatelet agents, making platelet studies abnormal. Despite profound platelet inhibition, these patients rarely have severe catheter site bleeding or a prolonged aPTT once heparin has been discontinued.

A lupus anticoagulant (LA) will prolong the aPTT but is not associated with a tendency to bleed (http://www.esoterix.com/files/ch_review/chreview2003_10.pdf).

25. B. Hereditary hemochromatosis is one of the most common autosomal recessive diseases. Serum transferrin saturation is the most sensitive marker for the body's iron stores; a value of >45% should be followed up with ferritin and HFE determination. Serum ferritin levels are more helpful when one is assessing the severity of potential liver damage due to hemochromatosis. Patients with serum ferritin levels of under 1000 ng/mL are extremely unlikely to have cirrhosis.

HFE, the gene for hemochromatosis, was cloned in 1996, but populationwide testing has not been recommended. The patient's wife should be genotyped for HFE mutations (*N Engl J Med.* 2003;48:50. *Hematology [Am Soc Hematol Educ Program].* 2003;40).

26. B. Meningococcal vaccine is recommended if there is a lifestyle risk: college freshman living in dorm, army recruits, travelers to Mecca during Hajj, or sub-Saharan Africa. Asplenic patients or those with persistent complement deficiency should get booster meningococcal vaccine again 5 years later.

TDAP should replace a single dose of Td for adults 19–65.

HPV should be received by females aged 11–12, or as a catch-up vaccincation it can be given from ages 13–26. Since the vaccine covers multiple strains of HPV, patients with a history of an abnormal Pap smear or being HPV+ should still be vaccinated.

Hep B vaccine should be given to children 18 and under and to those over 18 if there are risk factors: healthcare professional, sexually active but nonmonogamous, intravenous drug users (IVDU), sexually transmitted diseases (STDs), men who have sex with men (MSM), Hep B+ household contact, or live in a correction facility.

Medical reasons: End-Stage Renal Disease, HIV, chronic liver disease.

Pneumovax is not recommended for those aged <65 unless there is a chronic medical condition (http://www.cdc.gov/mmwr/PDF/wk/mm5901-Immunization.pdf).

27. D. This patient has a spontaneous pneumothorax. Possible etiologies include spontaneous rupture of a bleb, chronic obstructive pulmonary disease, pneumonia, asthma, and infections associated with HIV, especially Pneumocystis jiroveci pneumonia (PCP) and tuberculosis.

Spontaneous pneumothoraces that occupy less than 15% of the hemithorax can be treated conservatively with supplemental oxygen and observation; however, this practice is controversial. Larger pneumothoraces require chest tube placement (*Thorax.* 2003;58 Suppl 2:ii, 39. *Chest.* 1997;112:822).

28. A. The patient's signs, symptoms and laboratory findings are consistent with thrombotic thrombocytopenic purpura (TTP). Plasma exchange is the best treatment for TTP. The classic pentad of TTP includes microangiopathic hemolytic anemia ($\uparrow$LDH, schistocytes, $\uparrow$bilirubin), thrombocytopenia, renal dysfunction, neurologic changes, and fever. However, with just thrombocytopenia and microangiopathic anemia and no other etiology, treatment should be begun (*Hematology.* 2004:407. *N Engl J Med.* 347:589).

29. D. This multiloculated cyst affecting the right lobe of the liver with a thick rim and few calcifications is most likely due to the tapeworm *Echinococcus granulosus*. This worm

has multiple endemic areas around the world. It inhabits the dog/wolf GI system. Eggs are then ingested by sheep/cattle and humans, which leads to larval cysts in liver and lung. Patients may have an elevated alkaline phosphatase and eosinophilia.

Traditionally, treatment consisted of albendazole followed by surgical resection, taking caution not to spill any of the content of the cysts, which can cause severe hypersensitivity reactions. (*Clin Infect Dis.* 2003;37:1073. *Scand J Gastroenterol Suppl* 2004;241:50).

30. B. This patient most likely has milk-alkali syndrome.

The most common causes of hypercalcemia are primary hyperparathyroidism and malignancy; however, there appears to be an increasing incidence of milk-alkali syndrome in women taking calcium carbonate.

Most patients respond to volume replacement with saline and cessation of calcium carbonate ingestion, although not all regain normal renal function. Once the patient is volume replete, loop diuretics can be added to increase calcium excretion if needed. Patients with milk-alkali may develop rebound hypocalcemia, so bisphosphonates should be used with caution (*Medicine.* 1995;74:95).

108.

BOARD PRACTICE 2

Amy Leigh Miller and Fidencio Saldana

QUESTIONS

QUESTION 1. A 77-year-old man presents with recently diagnosed left ventricular hypertrophy, 25-lb unintentional weight loss with frequent postprandial diarrhea, and proximal lower extremity weakness progressive over approximately 1 year. Neurological examination confirms 4/5 hip flexor strength bilaterally, with 5/5 strength in the bilateral upper extremities and distal lower extremities. Vibratory sense is decreased in the toes and ankles, with intact proprioception and light touch. Potential *initial* diagnostic tests include all of the following EXCEPT:

A. Serum/urine protein electrophoresis + immuno-fixation
B. Fat pad biopsy
C. Muscle biopsy
D. Endoscopy with gastric/small bowel biopsy
E. Left ventricular biopsy

QUESTION 2. A 61-year-old woman from New York City with a history of fibromyalgia presents to her primary care doctor because of feeling off balance. She has no orthostatic symptoms but seems to have more difficulty with feeling unstable at nighttime when walking to her bedroom in the dark. Her neurologic exam is significant for decreased vibration sense bilaterally in her toes and ankles and decreased ankle jerks. She has a normal gait but a positive Romberg. She has a normal strength exam. On review of systems she reports some fatigue, and she denies any significant alcohol intake.

Which of the following lab tests would be LEAST useful as a first step?

A. Fasting glucose
B. Lyme titer
C. Thyroid-stimulating hormone (TSH) levels
D. Vitamin B-12 levels
E. Rapid plasma reagin (RPR)

QUESTION 3. At a routine office visit, a 55-year-old female tells you about a long history of intermittent "crawling" sensation at night, which has become more frequent in the past year. She says that the sensation is difficult to describe but, when pressed, says it feels like "something creeping under my skin that makes me want to move."

Which of the following would be consistent with this syndrome?

A. Stereotyped, repetitive flexion of the limbs
B. Serum ferritin >600
C. Serum ferritin <30
D. Treatment involves the use of serotonin-specific reuptake inhibitors (SSRIs)
E. An abnormal neurologic examination

QUESTION 4. An 82-year-old woman presents for evaluation of 2 weeks of new headaches. She has no fevers or chills, and full neck range of motion. On exam vital signs are normal. There is no tenderness on her scalp. There is pain on palpation of carotid artery. Funduscopic exam is normal, as is visual acuity. Musculoskeletal exam of neck and shoulders is limited by pain, but strength and reflexes are normal. Labs show Hematocrit (HCT) 34%, ESR 17, creatinine kinase 184; basic metabolic panel was normal.

What is your next diagnostic step?

A. Head CT/CTA
B. Head MRI
C. Temporal artery biopsy
D. Doppler ultrasound of the carotid
E. Lumbar puncture

QUESTION 5. A 39-year-old male dog walker with a remote history of sinus thrombosis and family history of idiopathic venous thrombosis and multiple spontaneous abortions presents for evaluation. On examination, he is 6'9" with arm span/height >1, down-sloping palpebral fissures, and malar hypoplasia without enophthalmos, high arched palate, or retrognathia. He has a mild pectus excavatum, prominent apical impulse, normal S1 and S2 with midsystolic click that responds to maneuvers, scoliosis (~20°), with no joint hypermobility and negative wrist/thumb signs. Cardiac MRI demonstrates mitral valve prolapse with a normal aortic root/aorta. Hypercoagulability workup is remarkable for an elevated homocysteine level. What is the most likely diagnosis?

A. Marfan syndrome
B. Homocystinuria
C. Stickler syndrome
D. Ehlers-Danlos syndrome
E. Klinefelter syndrome

QUESTION 6. Drugs associated with the electrocardiogram (EKG) tracing in figure 108.1 include all of the following EXCEPT:

A. Haldol
B. Ciprofloxacin
C. Methadone
D. Clarithromycin
E. Lidocaine

QUESTION 7. A 45-year-old man presents with a 3-month history of shortness of breath. He has been treated with three courses of antibiotics for pneumonia. He was found to have persistent pulmonary infiltrates on chest x-ray. His symptoms continue to relapse despite treatment. He worked as an electrician at a mental health institution and has 20-pack-year smoking history. He reports working in a naval shipyard with asbestos exposure in 1983. At home he has two cats, a parrot, and three dogs. Chest CT scan is significant for bilateral ground glass opacification and diffuse micronodules; there is no significant lymphadenopathy.

Which of the following is the next best step?

A. Positron emission tomography (PET) scan to evaluate for malignancy
B. Broad-spectrum IV antibiotics
C. Workup for mesothelioma
D. MRI
E. Treat with corticosteroids

QUESTION 8. A 50-year-old woman presents with dyspnea on exertion and orthopnea for 6 months. She has a history of hypertension, gastroesophageal reflux, and Raynaud's. On physical exam, she has an elevated jugular venous pressure, loud P2 on cardiac exam, and several telangiectasias over her face. Laboratory tests are significant for normal renal function. Echocardiogram shows severe pulmonary hypertension.

Which of the following blood tests is most specific for this patient's underlying condition?

A. Anticentromere antibody
B. Antinuclear antibody
C. Rheumatoid factor
D. ANCA
E. Anti-CCP antibody

QUESTION 9. A 28-year-old man presents with 3 weeks of easy bruising. He initially noted a large painless bruise overlying the extensor surface of his right forearm. He developed increased bruising overlying his arms, legs, stomach—all areas not associated with trauma. He developed epistaxis and gum bleeding. He is otherwise healthy and takes no medications. Laboratory studies (CBC) revealed a white

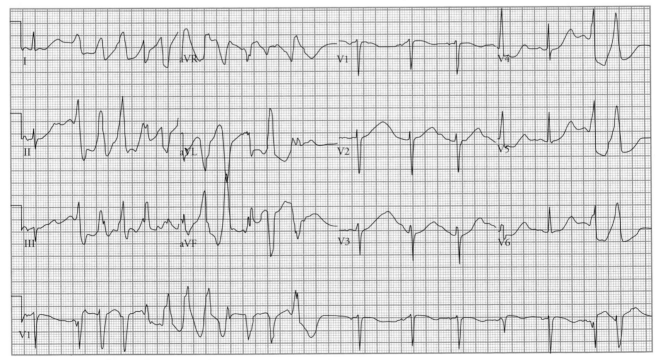

Figure 108.1. Electrocardiogram for Question 6.

blood cell count of 7000, hematocrit of 45%, and platelet count of 14,000; he had a normal peripheral blood smear other than low platelets.

Which of the following is the next best step?

A. Plasmapheresis
B. Bone marrow biopsy
C. Corticosteroids
D. No treatment, spontaneous remission is common
E. Proceed directly to splenectomy

QUESTION 10. An 82-year-old man from Cape Cod with a history of coronary artery disease presents with weakness and shortness of breath. Temperature is 103. He has a mild transaminitis, and hematocrit is 21. There is no evidence of active bleeding. Direct Coombs' test is negative. Bilirubin and lactate dehydrogenase are elevated; haptoglobin is depressed. Smear is negative for schistocytes but reveals rare intraerythrocytic parasites (~1%). All of the following are appropriate next steps EXCEPT:

A. Test for Lyme disease
B. Test for anaplasma (serologies)
C. Treatment with oral atovaquone
D. Treatment with oral azithromycin
E. Treatment with oral doxycycline

QUESTION 11. A 31-year-old woman with menorrhagia presents complaining of hair loss. She has noticed her hair to be thinning slightly, mostly in the frontal areas. She is on no medications. Physical exam reveals a well-appearing woman with slight diffuse thinning of her hair. No discrete patches of hair loss. No fractured hairs or exclamation point hairs seen. Pull test is negative. Which of the following is the most appropriate next step in management.

A. Send to dermatology for steroid scalp injections
B. Prescribe finasteride, 1 mg/day
C. Prescribe finasteride, 5 mg/day
D. Recommend minoxidil
E. Check lab tests including iron studies

QUESTION 12. A patient presents to the emergency room with fatigue and palpitations. An electrocardiogram is shown in figure 108.2.

A. The QRS is wide so this cannot be Mobitz I.
B. This is complete heart block.
C. The QRS is wide so this cannot be Mobitz II.
D. This is Mobitz I.
E. The level of heart block cannot be defined in this tracing.

QUESTION 13. In counseling a patient with newly diagnosed ovarian cancer, which of the following statements is correct?

A. The majority of patients with ovarian cancer do not have advanced disease at diagnosis.
B. The majority of patients with ovarian cancer do not respond to chemotherapy.
C. Inherited genetic syndromes account for about half of all cases of ovarian cancer, so it is important that her family members be screened.
D. It is possible that her ovarian cancer and the colorectal cancer diagnosed in her 40-year-old brother 2 years ago are due to a single mutation.
E. Treatment of ovarian cancer always involves both surgery and radiation therapy, but chemotherapy is used in a subset of cases.

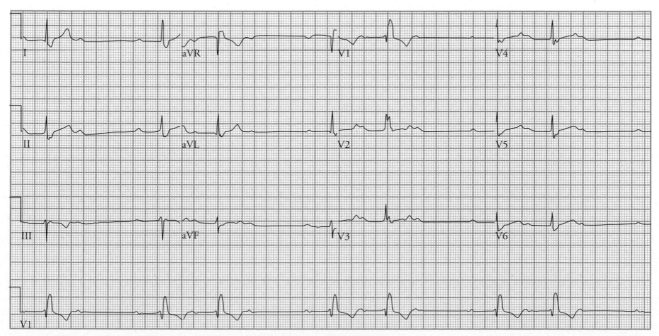

Figure 108.2. Electrocardiogram for Question 12 (patient with fatigue and palpitations).

QUESTION 14. A 42-year-old male with a history of coronary artery disease and hypertension presents with 2 days of left upper quadrant pain radiating to the back associated with nausea. Over the past 6 months he has had early satiety and chronic diarrhea with a 35-lb unintentional weight loss. He has an elevated amylase and lipase. An abdominal CT scan reveals diffuse lymphadenopathy. Laboratory workup of his diarrhea revealed an elevated IgA antiendomysial antibody. What is the appropriate next diagnostic step?

A. Lymph node biopsy
B. IgA tissue transglutaminase antibody
C. Small bowel biopsy
D. IgA antibodies

QUESTION 15. A 69-year-old retired counselor presents with complaints of hoarseness, tremor, temporal hair loss, weight gain, and new hyperglycemia. Blood pressure is 195/70. Dark terminal hairs are noted on her chin and abdomen. Dehydroepiandrosterone-S (DHEA-S) level was over four times the upper limit of normal. Which of the following laboratory findings is consistent with the clinical scenario?

A. Serum cortisol level suppresses with high-dose dexamethasone.
B. TSH level is high.
C. Testosterone level is normal.
D. Serum cortisol level does not suppress with low-dose dexamethasone.
E. Plasma metanephrines are high.

QUESTION 16. A 54-year-old man with no significant past medical history presents to his primary care doctor with 2 days of constant chest discomfort. He had been into see his physician 1 week ago for an upper respiratory infection. His chest pain is pleuritic in nature and nonexertional. It worsens when supine, improves when sitting up. He denies any dyspnea, diaphoresis, radiation of the discomfort, palpitations, or dizziness.

The EKG in figure 108.3 was obtained.

Which one of the following is *not* an appropriate first-line treatment if this patient has no known drug allergies.

A. Aspirin, 800 mg q 6 hours
B. Ibuprofen, 800 mg q 8 hours
C. Prednisone, 60 mg daily
D. Ibuprofen, 800 mg q 8 hours + colchicine, 0.5 mg daily
E. C and D

QUESTION 17. A 32-year-old woman with palpitations, lid lag, and an audible bruit has a serum TSH less than assay and a free thyroxine level of 4.5. A diagnosis of Graves is confirmed by a radioiodine-uptake study. Which of the following is correct?

A. Antithyroid medications should not be prescribed because recurrence rates with them are >90%.
B. Treatments differ in initial response rates but have similar relapse rates.
C. Surgical thyroidectomy is the most common treatment because it has the lowest relapse rate.
D. If the patient is pregnant, she cannot receive antithyroid treatment
E. Radioiodine treatment is intended to induce hypothyroidism.

QUESTION 18. Patient presents to the emergency room complaining of palpitations and shortness of breath. An EKG is obtained (figure 108.4), and is compared to a previously obtained baseline EKG (figure 108.5).

All of the following should be avoided in this patient EXCEPT:

A. Adenosine
B. Carotid sinus massage
C. Procainamide

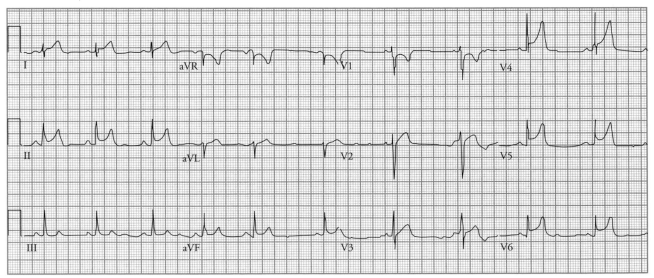

Figure 108.3. Electrocardiogram for Question 16.

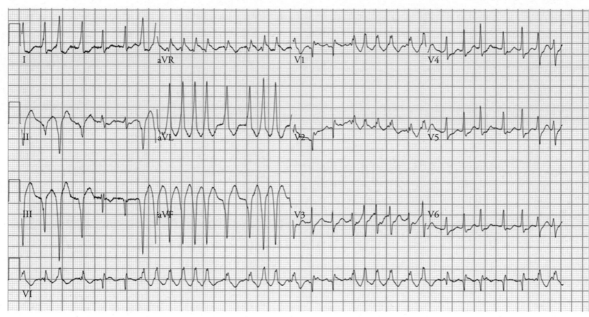

Figure 108.4. Presentating EKG in the Emergency Room for Patient from Question 18.

D. Esmolol

E. Verapamil

QUESTION 19. A 60-year-old woman with metastatic breast cancer presents with 3 days of fever and shortness of breath. She was recently treated with steroids and whole-brain radiation for a dural-based enhancement overlying her left frontal lobe.

The patient has never had tuberculosis and has no history of hemoptysis, no foreign travel, and no exotic hobbies or pets. Chest x-ray demonstrates patchy interstitial infiltrates but no pleural effusion and no nodules or cavitation. What is the next best test?

A. Bronchoalveolar lavage

B. Random sputum

C. Blood culture

D. Beta-glucan

E. Purified protein derivative

QUESTION 20. A 39-year-old woman presents with an ST-elevation myocardial infarction managed with emergent catheterization and drug-eluting stent deployment. Six days later, she returns with recurrent ST elevations in the same distribution. Her husband reports that she has been compliant with her prescribed aspirin and clopidogrel. Admission laboratories are remarkable for a platelet count of 80,000,

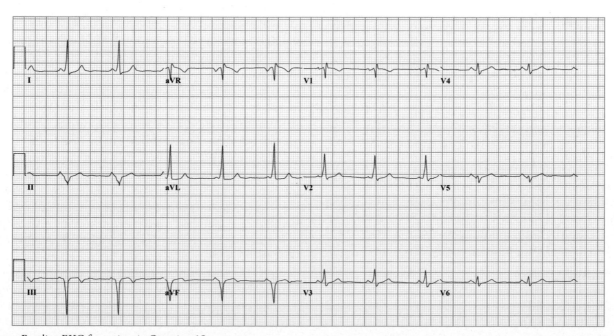

Figure 108.5. Baseline EKG for patient in Question 18.

decreased from 290,000 at discharge. A platelet factor 4 antibody assay is sent. Which of the following medical interventions is appropriate?

A. Initiation of coumadin
B. Initiation of heparin
C. Discontinuation of clopidogrel and aspirin
D. Initiation of bivalirudin
E. Addition of cilostazol

QUESTION 21. A 20-year-old man is evaluated for facial and lower-extremity edema of 1 week's duration. For the past month, he has been fatigued. He takes no medications and has no history of diabetes. On physical examination, blood pressure is 90/55 mm Hg. Heart, lung, and abdomen exams are normal. There is periorbital edema and 2+ lower extremity edema. Laboratory data reveal a normal creatinine, a total cholesterol of 300 mg/dL, albumin of 2.9 g/dL, normal complement levels, and 3+ protein with oval fat bodies on urinalysis. Which of the following is the most likely diagnosis?

A. Membranous nephropathy
B. Lupus nephritis
C. Constrictive pericarditis
D. Minimal change disease
E. Membranoproliferative glomerulonephritis

QUESTION 22. Which of the following statements regarding the possible cardiovascular effects of chemotherapy is true?

A. The cardiovascular sequelae of chemotherapy are always delayed; acute cardiovascular events near the time of infusion are unrelated to the chemotherapy.
B. Cardiovascular side effects of anthracyclines are dose-dependent.
C. Regardless of the chemotherapy regimen, the most common cardiovascular sequela is left ventricular systolic dysfunction.
D. Risk of cardiotoxicity with a given chemotherapeutic is independent of exposure to other classes of chemotherapeutics.
E. The only recognized cardiovascular side effects of chemotherapeutics are left ventricular systolic dysfunction, heart failure, and hypotension.

QUESTION 23. A 55-year-old man presents for a routine physical examination. On labs he has the following cholesterol profile: low-density lipoprotein (LDL) 130, high-density lipoprotein (HDL) 30, triglycerides 300 mg/dL. He is otherwise healthy but is mildly overweight.

Which is *not* an appropriate course of action?

A. Fish oil
B. Fibrate
C. Nicotinic acid
D. Lifestyle modification
E. Ezetimibe

QUESTION 24. Which of the following is true regarding the electrocardiogram in Figure 108.6?

A. This is a supraventricular tachycardia because the intrinsicoid deflection is too short.
B. This is a supraventricular tachycardia because it is irregular.
C. This is a ventricular tachycardia because the intrinsicoid deflection is too long.
D. This is a ventricular tachycardia because it is irregular.
E. This is a ventricular tachycardia because of the A/V relationship.

QUESTION 25. A 24-year-old woman presents with a 2-month history of significant fatigue accompanied by swelling and pain in her left knee and right ankle. She has no other constitutional symptoms. Past medical history includes recent treatment for chlamydia with azithromycin. On examination, her left knee is slightly tender, warm, and has an effusion. Her right ankle is puffy and warm bilaterally. Stretching the Achilles tendon elicits heel discomfort. CBC is normal; ESR 73; RF negative; anti-CCP not sent.

What is the likely diagnosis?

A. Reactive arthritis
B. Rheumatoid arthritis
C. Septic arthritis
D. Polyarteritis nodosa
E. Drug-induced systemic lupus erythematosus

ANSWERS

1. E. The patient has clinical findings suggestive of multiorgan involvement by systemic amyloidosis. Cardiac involvement is most commonly seen with senile (wild-type transthyretin) amyloid, mutant transthyretin (ATTR), and light-chain (AL) amyloidosis. Although the pattern of organ involvement is suggestive of AL amyloidosis, tissue confirmation is essential because of differences in prognosis and treatment. Cardiac biopsy is performed in the right ventricle (RV), not the left ventricle (LV). Although sensitivity of RV biopsy is high in patients with cardiac involvement, the risk of perforation with RV biopsy makes it a relatively morbid procedure. Consequently, in a patient with other organ involvement, less-invasive/high-risk tissue samples are generally preferable in the initial diagnostic approach. If a tissue diagnosis of amyloid is made, cardiac MRI can in some cases confirm a pattern consistent with amyloid, obviating the need for RV biopsy (Falk et al., *N Engl J Med.* 1997;337:898. Falk, *Circulation.* 2005;112:2047).

2. B. The patient is presenting with a sensory ataxia and neuropathy primarily affecting vibration and proprioception and sparing motor function. Her deficits are symmetric and confined to the lower extremity, and there are no signs of a myelopathy.

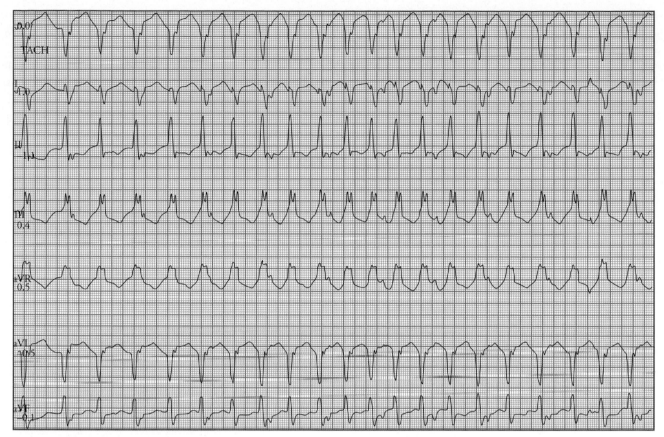

Figure 108.6. Electrocardiogram for Question 24.

Peripheral neuropathies are either single-nerve mononeuropathies (carpal tunnel, meralgia paresthetica), multiple mononeuropathies as in mononeuritis multiplex, or polyneuropathy. In this type of polyneuropathy there are classically no hand symptoms until the leg symptoms have reached just above the knee. Common causes of a polyneuropathy include diabetes, alcohol, B-12 deficiency, uremia, amyloid, syphilis, hypothyroid, toxin-mediated (lead), and medications (amio). First-line screening labs should include a CBC, ESR, TSH, serum protein electrophoresis, glucose, B-12, ANA, and urinalysis.

Patient has no risk factor for Lyme disease, and a positive Lyme antibody may not indicate true infection. This should be a second-line test for neuropathy of this type (*Semin Neurol.* 2008;28(2):133. *Arch Intern Med.* 2004;164:1021).

3. C. Restless leg syndrome (RLS). Movements in RLS are not stereotyped; voluntary limb movements reflect motor restlessness, often accompanied by paresthesias. Symptoms are resolved by getting up and walking.

Secondary causes of RLS include iron deficiency anemia, spinal cord/peripheral nerve lesions, uremia, pregnancy, and medication side effects (including SSRIs). Neurological examination should be normal (need to rule out other causes).

First-line treatment is ropinirole (dopamine agonist), but treatment of iron deficiency is also essential (Earley. *N Engl J Med.* 2003;348:2103).

4. C. Giant cell arteritis. Common symptoms include new headache, vision loss or change, polymyalgia rheumatica related myalgias, carotidynia, scalp tenderness, scalp beading, and jaw claudication. In 10–24% of patients, ESR is low or normal.

Early temporal artery biopsy is key. Giant cell arteritis typically affects people aged >50. Corticosteroid treatment should be initiated at once if there are visual symptoms or suspicion is high for diagnosis. Steroids should be given for up to 2 weeks before temporal artery biopsy is performed; this treatment does not affect biopsy results. Long-standing disease can be treated with methotrexate, azathioprine, or tumor necrosis factor (TNF-α) inhibitors. Aspirin is recommended unless contraindicated (*Curr Opin Rheumatol.* 2008;20(1):17–22).

5. B. Homocystinuria. Marfan syndrome is not associated with thromboembolism. Furthermore, the patient does not meet diagnostic criteria for Marfan syndrome by the Ghent criteria—he has skeletal involvement and cardiovascular involvement (mitral valve prolapse (MVP)), neither of which meet major criteria, and he has no ocular, dural, pulmonary, or skin involvement. The differential for Marfanoid body habitus includes isolated ectopia lentis (not associated with thromboembolism), Klinefelter (the patient lacks the small testes/genital findings, although his low-level occupation is in keeping with the associated learning difficulties), MASS (MVP, mild aortic dilation,

striae atrophica, skeletal involvement) phenotype (which the patient does not fit), and homocystinuria, which is associated with thromboembolism, mental retardation, and elevated levels of homocysteine (De Paepe et al. *Am J Med Genet.* 1996).

6. E. Lidocaine. The EKG demonstrates a prolonged QT interval and nonsustained bursts of polymorphic ventricular tachycardia, consistent with Torsades des pointes. Drugs associated with QT prolongation and Torsades des pointes include the fluoroquinolones, Haldol, clarithromycin, and methadone. Although a number of antiarrhythmics (e.g., sotalol, dofetilide, amiodarone) are associated with QT prolongation (of note, amiodarone is very rarely associated with torsades), lidocaine does not prolong the QT (www.azcert.org)

7. E. This patient presents with a scenario typical of hypersensitivity pneumonitis (HP). Persistent infiltrates represented as ground glass opacities on chest CT scan are likely inflammatory in nature rather than a pneumonia. The pets represent exposures that can trigger HP, particularly the parrot.

Treatment of HP involves removal of the antigen and corticosteroids. Antibiotics would not help. Pleural plaques, which are not present here, help differentiate asbestos-induced parenchymal disease from other interstitial lung diseases. A PET scan would aid in lung cancer diagnosis, which typically presents as a mass rather than ground glass opacities. MRI would not add any additional information (Mohr. *Curr Opin Pulm Med.* 2004;10:401).

8. A. This patient has symptoms that are classic for the CREST syndrome, or limited cutaneous systemic sclerosis (LcSSc): calcinosis cutis, Raynaud phenomenon, esophageal dysmotility, sclerodactyly, and telangiectasia.

The anticentromere antibody is found in 82–99% of patients with CREST and has a specificity of >95% for the condition. This is in contrast to anti-Scl-70 antibody, which is more specific for diffuse systemic sclerosis. ANA has a sensitivity of around 85% and a specificity of around 54% for the diagnosis of systemic sclerosis. Rheumatoid factor and anti-CCP antibody are used in the diagnosis of rheumatoid arthritis. ANCA are often ordered in patients with suspected scleroderma but have no use in diagnosing this condition. They are used in the diagnosis of vasculitis (*Arthritis Res Ther.* 2003;5:80).

9. C. This patient presents with a clinical scenario consistent with idiopathic thrombocytopenic purpura. The diagnosis is made by thrombocytopenia with an otherwise normal CBC and blood smear. In addition, the patient should have no clinically apparent associated medical condition that can cause thrombocytopenia.

The major goal of treatment is to provide a safe platelet count rather than to correct the underlying disease. Initial treatment is with corticosteroids. Second-line treatment includes measures such as intravenous immunoglobulin or splenectomy.

Spontaneous remission is most common in children. It rarely occurs in adults (Cines and Blanchette. *N Engl J Med.* 2002;346:995).

10. E. The patient has babesiosis, a parasitic infection transmitted by tick bite or blood transfusion. Because coinfection with anaplasma (*Ehrlichia*) and Lyme can occur, the patient should be tested for both anaplasma and Lyme. Severe babesiosis is characterized by 10% or greater parasitemia, significant hemolysis, splenic infarct, or renal/hepatic/pulmonary compromise. The low level of parasitemia in this case is suggestive of chronic low-level infection. Oral antibiotics are reasonable in this case. The front-line therapy for *Babesia* is atovaquone/azithromycin or clindamycin/quinine. Although doxycycline has been used as part of multidrug regimens in refractory cases of *Babesia*, it is not a front-line agent. Although doxycycline is the treatment of choice for patients with Lyme disease and anaplasma, empiric therapy for these diseases is not advised in patients with babesiosis (Wormser et al. *Clin Infect Dis.* 2006;43:1089).

11. E. Androgenetic alopecia is the most common cause of hair loss in both men and women. This patient has no signs of excess androgen on exam and no scarring on scalp exam or discrete patches of hair loss that might be concerning for lupus or alopecia areata. Intralesional steroid injection is often used for treatment of alopecia areata. Finasteride is approved for the treatment of androgenetic alopecia in men but not women because of risk of abnormalities in male fetuses.

In a nonscarring diffuse alopecia, checking lab tests to rule out hypothyroidism and iron deficiency, two causes of hair loss, would be indicated prior to treatment with minoxidil for androgenetic alopecia. This patient did in fact have iron deficiency and saw reduction in hair loss with iron therapy (*Am Fam Physician.* 2003;67:1007).

12. D. This is Mobitz I. We can tell this is Mobitz I because we have progressive P-R prolongation followed by dropped beats, resulting in the characteristic "grouped beating" of Wenckebach.

Note that Mobitz I *can* occur with a wide QRS; however, for 2:1 block, we generally suspect Mobitz II when the QRS is wide and Mobitz I when it is narrow.

For comparison, see figure 108.7, complete heart block (same patient). Note that the QRS morphology during complete heart block is different (LBBB, in contrast to RBBB in the Mobitz I EKG).

13. D. The majority of patients with ovarian cancer have advanced disease at diagnosis. Over 80% of patients will initially respond to chemotherapy, even with advanced disease prior to initiation of treatment. Unfortunately, in patients with advanced disease at presentation, recurrent disease is common, with 5-year survival <30%. In contrast, prognosis for patients with local disease is good, with >90% survival at 5 years.

Genetic syndromes account for only approximately 5–10% of all cases of ovarian cancer, but the risk of ovarian

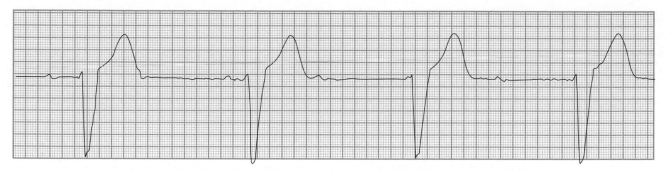

Figure 108.7. Electrocardiogram Demonstrating Complete Heart Block. Compare this to figure 108.2, an EKG of Mobitz I from the same patient.

cancer in carriers of mutations can be as high as 60% over the course of their lifetime. In addition to *BRCA1* and *BRCA2*, *HNPCC* is associated with an approximate 10% risk of ovarian cancer. A single early onset colorectal cancer and an ovarian cancer in a family may suggest this diagnosis.

Treatment of ovarian cancer involves surgical resection; radiation therapy and/or chemotherapy may be used in addition, depending on the stage, histology, etc. Of the two, chemotherapy is more commonly used (Cannistra. *N Engl J Med.* 2004;351:2519).

14. D. Celiac sprue is a disease of the small bowel characterized by villous atrophy and crypt hyperplasia. Exposure to gluten is the inciting event. Pancreatitis and mesenteric lymphadenopathy may be seen in patients with celiac sprue. Elevated IgA endomysial antibody is suggestive of a diagnosis of sprue (sensitivity 85–98%; specificity 97–100%). Small bowel biopsy, which can be obtained during endoscopy, is the recommended confirmatory diagnostic procedure. IgA antibodies are useful if the serologic tests are thought to be falsely negative (Green and Cellier. *N Engl J Med.* 2007;357:1731).

15. D. The patient has Cushing syndrome secondary to an adrenocortical carcinoma, which is characterized by elevated levels of DHEA, testosterone, and cortisol. The elevated levels of DHEA-S are virtually diagnostic of a primary adrenal source, as DHEA-S is produced only in the adrenals. Both the ovaries and the adrenals will produce testosterone, DHEA, and androstenedione; thus, DHEA, testosterone, and androstenedione levels were also elevated in this patient. Neither low- nor high-dose dexamethasone would suppress cortisol production, which is adrenocorticotropic hormone (ACTH) independent in this patient.

Virilization is not associated with hypothyroidism; although excess TSH could be seen with Cushing syndrome driven by the pituitary, the patient has an ACTH-independent lesion. Elevated plasma metanephrines would be consistent with pheochromocytoma, which does not cause virilization (Derksen et al. *N Engl J Med.* 1994;331:968).

16. C. The patient's symptoms and electrocardiographic findings (diffuse ST elevations in multiple coronary distributions that are convex in shape, as well as PR depressions) are consistent with acute pericarditis.

For acute idiopathic pericarditis, first-line therapy is with a nonsteroidal anti-inflammatory drug (NSAID) regimen including aspirin and ibuprofen. The rate of recurrent pericarditis is decreased in patients given colchicine, as is the duration of symptoms.

Use of prednisone as a primary therapy is associated with increased risk of recurrence. Prednisone should be used only in those with NSAID allergy or pericarditis that is refractory to NSAIDs (Imazio et al. *Circulation.* 2005;112:2012–6).

17. E. The three treatments for Graves disease—antithyroid medications (propylthiouracil (PTU), methimazole), radioiodine treatment, and surgical thyroidectomy—have similar initial response rates but differ in their relapse rates. Around 40% of patients initially treated with antithyroid medications will have recurrent disease. Although recurrence rates are best for surgical thyroidectomy (~5%), this is the approach least commonly used as a first-line treatment. In pregnancy, methimazole cannot be used, but PTU can be used in pregnancy. Radioiodine treatment is intended to induce hypothyroidism; this is achieved in approximately 80% of cases (Brent. *N Engl J Med.* 2008;358:2594–2605).

18. C. Procainamide. In patients with Wolff Parkinsons White (WPW) syndrome and atrial fibrillation drugs (beta blockers, calcium channel blockers, adenosine) and interventions (vagal maneuvers including carotid sinus massage) that block the AV node should be avoided; procainamide and ibutilide are the drugs of choice because it will slow conduction in the bypass tract (Fuster et al. *Circulation.* 2011; 123:e269–367).

19. A. This is an immunosuppressed woman who presents with new-onset shortness of breath in the setting of diffuse pulmonary infiltrates.

Fever and dyspnea in an immunosuppressed patient are the hallmarks of *Pneumocystis carinii* (*P. jiroveci*) pneumonia (PCP). Typical CXR findings in non–HIV-infected patients are diffuse, bilateral, patchy infiltrates. The diagnosis is established by visualization of the organism in the sputum; blood cultures are not helpful. Induced sputum or bronchoalveolar lavage is needed for a definitive diagnosis. Beta-glucan is elevated in a majority of cases of PCP but does not make the definitive diagnosis (Thomas and Limper. *N Engl J Med.* 2004;350:248).

20. D. The patient's presentation is highly concerning for in-stent thrombosis secondary to heparin-induced thrombocytopenia (HIT). For patients suspected to have HIT, empiric anticoagulation is indicated. Heparinoid products, including low-molecular-weight and unfractionated heparin, should be carefully avoided. Coumadin should not be administered in the acute phase, as it increases risk of clotting. Direct thrombin inhibitors (argatroban, bivalirudin, lepirudin) are the treatment of choice.

Antiplatelet agents should be continued. The patient's likely stent thrombosis is unlikely a failure of antiplatelet therapy; modification of the antiplatelet therapy is not advised (Warkentin et al. *Chest.* 2004;126:3115).

21. D. Nephrotic syndrome is characterized by proteinuria (>3 g/24-hr urine), edema, hypoalbuminemia, hyperlipidemia, and lipiduria. Minimal change disease is the most common cause of the nephrotic syndrome in children and young adults. Membranous nephropathy also causes a nephrotic syndrome but typically presents in older individuals and is more insidious in onset. Lupus and membranoproliferative glomerulonephritis (GN) typically present with low complement levels and are associated with hematuria (*BMJ.* 2008;336:1185).

22. B. Chemotherapeutics can have both acute and delayed effects. For example, although anthracyclines (e.g., Adriamycin) can have acute cardiotoxicity (atrial fibrillation, decreased systolic function), acute effects are rare and generally self-limited. Cumulative cardiotoxicity with anthracyclines is dose-dependent—it can appear within months of completion of therapy or over a decade after exposure.

The most common cardiovascular sequelae vary across agents. For anthracyclines, the classic presentation is left ventricular systolic dysfunction and heart failure. For antimetabolites (e.g., 5-FU), ischemia is the most common cardiovascular complication. Paclitaxel is most commonly associated with bradyarrhythmias. Other recognized cardiovascular side effects of chemotherapeutics include arrhythmias, pericarditis/myocarditis, edema, and pericardial effusion.

Risk of cardiotoxicity can be influenced by prior exposure to other chemotherapeutics. For instance, risk of heart failure with alkylating agents (Cytoxan, cisplatin) is higher if there has been prior exposure to anthracyclines (Yeh. *Circulation.* 2004;109:3122–31).

23. D. This patient presents with elevated triglycerides and low HDL. He is also mildly overweight. Lifestyle modification is clearly indicated. Secondary causes of hypertriglyceridemia should be considered, including obesity, diabetes, nephrotic syndrome, and hypothyroidism. A fasting glucose, urine, and TSH can evaluate for these disorders. Fibrates, nicotinic acid, and fish oil can all lower serum triglycerides. Ezetimibe does not (Brunzell. *N Engl J Med.* 2007;357:1009–17).

24. E. This is ventricular tachycardia (VT), with evidence of AV dissociation. Long intrinsicoid deflection (not present here) argues for VT, but the absence of a prolonged intrinsicoid deflection is not diagnostic of supraventricular tachycardia (SVT). Both SVTs and VTs can be irregular. The tracing demonstrates A:V dissociation with more Vs than As, diagnostic of ventricular tachycardia. Other criteria used to distinguish ventricular arrhythmias from supraventricular arrhythmias include concordance (positive or negative) in the precordial leads and QRS morphology criteria.

25. A. Reactive arthritis, which is asymmetric mono- or oligoarthritis associated with recent or prior extra-articular infection and predominantly affecting lower extremities. Reactive arthritis also commonly affects vertebrae, sacroiliac joints, buttocks, and heels. Extra-articular manifestations can occur in the genitourinary system, skin, nails (changes resemble psoriasis), eyes, and mouth. ("Can't pee, Can't see, Can't climb a tree [Oh my knee!].") Enthesitis, particularly of the Achilles tendon, can also be observed.

Classical pathogens include *Chlamydia trachomatis, Yersinia, Salmonella, Shigella, Campylobacter* (up to 21% attack rate), *Clostridium difficile,* and *Chlamydia pneumoniae.* Interval to onset can range from several days to several weeks. Treatment is with NSAIDs, steroid injections, steroids, and disease-modifying antirheumatic drugs.

109.

BOARD PRACTICE 3

Patricia A. Kritek and Wolfram Goessling

QUESTIONS

QUESTION 1. A 23-year-old actress with asthma presents to her primary care physician for routine follow-up. She reports that she has needed her albuterol inhaler two to three times a week for wheezing or shortness of breath. She also notes that she wakes up with cough three or four times a month. When this happens, she uses her inhaler with good relief. Her only current medication is her albuterol inhaler, used on an as-needed basis.

Which of the following would be the most appropriate management strategy?

A. Having her use her albuterol inhaler on a standing basis
B. Starting a steroid inhaler
C. Changing to a combined bronchodilator inhaler
D. Treating her with theophylline
E. Starting a long-acting bronchodilator

QUESTION 2. A 23-year-old graduate student comes to see his primary care physician with 5 days of worsening bloody diarrhea and fevers. He reports having eaten tacos at a local restaurant. His evaluation reveals petechiae on his legs, a creatinine of 3.0, Hematocrit (HCT) 27, with schistocytes on smear and platelets of 47,000. His stool culture is most likely to show which organism?

A. *Bacillus cereus*
B. *Salmonella* spp.
C. *E. coli* O157:H7
D. *Staphylococcus aureus*
E. *Vibrio cholerae*

QUESTION 3. 35-year-old painter initially presented with fatigue, myalgias, and a rash (figure 109.1) after a week-end on Cape Cod. His primary care physician prescribed a 14-day course of doxycycline (100 mg bid). He returns 10 days later with worsening myalgias, fever, nausea, and vomiting. Routine labs reveal a HCT of 34.

Which of these therapies would be the most appropriate?

A. 14 additional days of doxycycline
B. 21 additional days of doxycycline
C. 14 days of intravenous ceftazidime
D. 10 days of clindamycin and quinine
E. 14 days of chloroquine

QUESTION 4. A 46-year-old salesman presents with recurrent nosebleeds and easy bruisability. He has no prior episodes of bleeding and takes a daily aspirin. He has oral mucosal hemorrhages, multiple bruises, guaiac-positive stool, and no petechiae. His laboratory evaluation reveals HCT prothrombin time (PT) of 39 and platelets 339,000. His PT is 85 sec, and partial thromboplastin time (PTT) is 150 sec. His parameters improve with three doses of vitamin K, 5 mg given subcutaneously, but after 1 week he is back to similar lab values. What is the most likely diagnosis?

A. Lack of green vegetables in the diet
B. Congenital factor VII deficiency
C. Occult liver disease
D. Superwarfarin poisoning
E. Factor XI inhibitor

QUESTION 5. A 27-year-old woman is brought to the emergency room after being found unresponsive by her boyfriend who last spoke to her about 12 hours earlier. She was found with a suicide note and an empty bottle of Tylenol. On arrival to the ED, she is unarousable with a heart rate of 120 beats per minute and a blood pressure of 100/50 mm Hg.

Which of the following is the most reasonable next step?

A. Begin ipecac and gastric lavage immediately
B. Administer activated charcoal and then administer N-acetylcysteine (NAC)
C. Administer NAC immediately
D. Send an acetaminophen level and then begin NAC based on the level
E. Send liver function tests (LFTs), an arterial blood gases (ABG), and coagulation studies before initiating any therapy

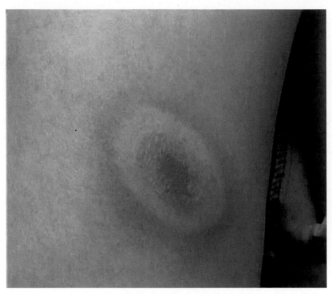

Figure 109.1. Rash on Chest Wall of Patient in Question 3.

QUESTION 6. A 26-year-old student presents to urgent care with an episode of palpitations accompanied by lightheadedness. He reports that the episode lasted approximately 5 min. He has an exam tomorrow and is quite anxious. He has had two similar episodes over the last 2 years. He takes no illicit or prescribed drugs, does not drink alcohol, and has no family history of heart disease. His electrocardiogram (EKG) is shown in figure 109.2.

What is the diagnosis?

A. Right bundle branch block
B. Inferior myocardial infarction
C. Paroxysmal atrial fibrillation
D. Left ventricular hypertrophy
E. Wolff-Parkinson-White syndrome

QUESTION 7. A 32-year-old pharmacist is found to have a 3 × 3 cm nodule in the left lobe of her thyroid gland on routine exam. She has no symptoms. Her serum thyrotropin concentration is normal. The next step in her evaluation should be:

A. Thyroid ultrasound
B. Fine-needle aspiration (FNA)
C. Empiric thyroxine therapy
D. Surgical neck exploration
E. Nuclear medicine scan of her thyroid

QUESTION 8. A 31-year-old nanny presents with fevers, bone pain, and anemia and is diagnosed with acute myelogenous leukemia. She undergoes induction chemotherapy with daunorubicin/cytarabine and achieves remission. Twelve days after her first cycle of high-dose cytarabine consolidation chemotherapy, she calls the office with a temperature of 102.5°F. She comes in, has no focal findings on examination, her catheter site is without erythema, and she has a clear chest x-ray. Her white blood cell (WBC) count is 0.6 with 12% polymorphonuclear cells. What do you do?

A. Admit to hospital for observation
B. Admit to hospital for bone marrow transplant
C. Admit to hospital for intravenous broad-spectrum antibiotics
D. Administer granulocyte colony-stimulating factor
E. Prescribe oral levofloxacin and close follow-up

QUESTION 9. A 45-year-old female teacher presents complaining of severe left knee pain. She has a long history of rheumatoid arthritis, which has been well controlled for several years on a multidrug regimen of methotrexate, hydroxychloroquine, and nonsteroidal anti-inflammatory

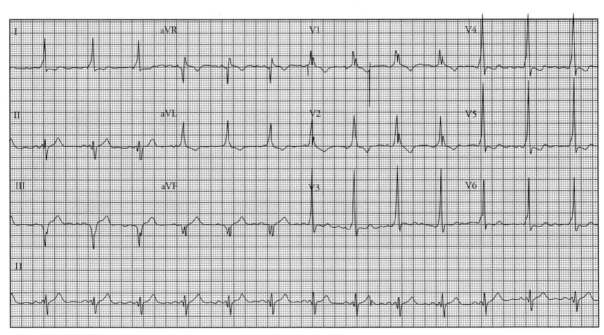

Figure 109.2. EKG of Patient in Question 6.

drugs (NSAIDs). Which of the following symptoms suggests secondary degenerative joint disease (rather than rheumatoid arthritis) as a cause of her knee pain?

A. Prolonged morning stiffness
B. Pain that is exacerbated by activity
C. Increased fatigue
D. Multiple joint complaints
E. Weight loss

QUESTION 10. A 36-year-old photographer comes to your office with 1 week of malaise and fatigue and two days of scleral icterus. He has also lost his appetite, has persistent nausea, and noted his urine to be very dark. He has no other medical problems and takes no medications. He does not drink any alcohol and recently returned from a trip to Central America, where he was taking pictures for a magazine article. On physical examination, his sclerae are icteric, his abdomen is soft with a liver span percussed to 13 cm. No spleen tip is palpable. He has no skin changes. His ALT is 3650, AST 2893, alkaline phosphatase 322, and total bilirubin 6.3, with a direct fraction of 5.2. His PT is 12.2. What is the most likely diagnosis?

A. Acute hepatitis A
B. Alcoholic hepatitis
C. Acute cholecystitis
D. Acute hepatitis C
E. Acetaminophen overdose

QUESTION 11. A 30-year-old lawyer presents to her primary care physician (PCP after her 65-year-old father died of a heart attack. She asks you what can be done to reduce her risk of also having a heart attack. Her blood pressure is 118/62 mm Hg. Her fasting glucose is 72, her high-density lipoprotein (HDL) is 52 and her low-density lipoprotein (LDL) is 134. She is a nonsmoker. You advise her to:

A. Begin aspirin 325 mg daily
B. Begin aspirin 81 mg daily
C. Maintain a healthy diet and exercise four or five times a week
D. Begin simvastatin 10 mg daily
E. Begin beta-carotene supplements

QUESTION 12. A 29-year-old nurse comes to see his primary care physician because colleagues noted facial asymmetry. His facial symptoms began yesterday with a progressive left facial droop. He has some malaise and fatigue and achiness in the knees. However, he has no headaches, fevers, or pain. On exam, he cannot furrow his left eyebrow and has dysgeusia. His sensation to light touch, muscle strength in the extremities, and deep tendon reflexes are intact. Skin examination reveals an erythematous rash that has become larger over the past 1 week. His head computed tomography (CT) is normal.
What is the most likely diagnosis?

A. Bell's palsy

B. Lyme disease facial palsy
C. Fibromyalgia
D. Herpes zoster infection
E. Zoster sine herpete

QUESTION 13. A comatose 30-year-old male with IDDM is found down. He is afebrile, tachypneic, and his blood pressure decreases from 115/75 to 95/70 with elevation of his head. Physical exam reveals a 50-kg acutely ill male with signs of extracellular volume contraction and nonfocal neurological findings. Venous blood is drawn and then 50% dextrose is given by IV push followed by 50 cc/hr of D5NS. The patient remains unconscious with progressive hypotension and tachycardia. The EKG shows a widened QRS, peaked T waves, absent P waves, and multiple PVCs. Labs show Na = 130, K = 7.1, Cl = 95, HCO_3 = 10, blood urea nitrogen (BUN) = 63, Cr = 2.3, Glu = 450. His urinalysis has 3+ ketones. WBC = 17,000/mm^3, HCT = 44%. Which of the following should be the next step in treatment?

A. Give 2 ampules of sodium bicarbonate
B. Give calcium gluconate 10 mmol immediately via IV infusion
C. Initiate hemodialysis
D. Give 10 units IV insulin immediately
E. Place a temporary wire

QUESTION 14. A 38-year-old sanitation worker is bitten by a skunk. The skunk escapes capture. The patient is at high risk for what infection?

A. Rabies infection
B. *Borrelia burgdorferi* infection
C. Infection by *Pasteurella* species
D. Infection by *Aeromonas hydrophila*
E. None of the above

QUESTION 15. A 52-year-old carpenter is sent to his primary care doctor after a chest x-ray performed in the emergency room revealed a pulmonary nodule. He is a never-smoker, has no family history of lung cancer, and has lived his entire life in New Hampshire. He has a follow-up

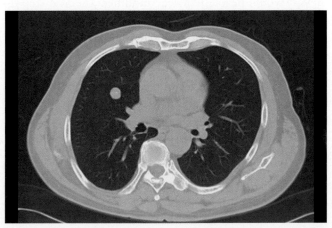

Figure 109.3. Chest CT Scan of Patient in Question 15.

CT scan, which is shown in figure 109.3. The pattern of calcifications is described by the radiologist as "popcorn."

The most likely diagnosis is:

A. Carcinoid
B. Small cell lung cancer
C. Metastatic thyroid cancer
D. Bronchial cyst
E. Hamartoma

QUESTION 16. A 71-year-old man is found to have a prostate-specific antigen (PSA) of 23 on routine screening. On digital rectal examination, he has an enlarged, hard, and asymmetric prostate with an apparent tumor extending beyond the prostate capsule. He has no other medical problems and feels well. Needle biopsy reveals poorly differentiated prostate cancer with a Gleason score of 8, and further imaging reveals no metastatic disease. Of the following options, which treatment option is most appropriate?

A. External beam radiation
B. Radioactive seed implants
C. External beam radiation plus radioactive seed implants
D. External beam radiation with luteinizing hormone-releasing hormone analogue

ANSWERS

1. B. The correct answer is B. The National Asthma Education & Prevention Program recommends a stepwise approach to asthma care (NIH publication). By their criteria, this patient has poorly controlled mild persistent asthma based on the following criteria:

- Symptoms >2 times a week but <1 time a day.

- Nighttime symptoms >2 times a month.

In the stepwise approach to care, the next "step" would be initiation of a low-dose inhaled steroid. An alternative therapy would be a leukotriene modifier. The next step for poorly controlled moderate persistent asthma would be the addition of a long-acting bronchodilator or increasing the dose of the steroid inhaler (www.nhlbi.nih.gov/guidelines/asthma/asthgdln.pdf. Accessed February 11, 2011).

2. C. This patient has hemolytic-uremic syndrome. This food-borne illness is caused by *E. coli* serotypes (especially O157:H7) or *Shigella dysenteriae. E. coli* O157:H7 is the organism most commonly associated with HUS, causing 73,000 illnesses and 60 deaths in the United States annually. Cattle are a major reservoir of *E. coli* O157:H7. Endothelial damage occurs by binding of a bacterial toxin. *B. cereus* and *S. aureus* produce toxins that cause food poisoning. *Salmonella* spp. can cause gastroenteritis with bloody diarrhea but are not a cause of hemolytic uremic syndrome

(HUS). *V. cholerae* causes cholera with its typical voluminous rice water stools.

3. D. The initial presentation was consistent with early localized Lyme disease. The rash is erythema migrans (EM). The treatment of doxycycline, 100 mg bid, is the appropriate therapy. An acceptable alternative would be a 10- to 14-day course of amoxicillin. The clinical picture is characteristic of infection with *Babesia microti*, whose vector is also the *Ixodes* tick. Immunosuppressed hosts are more likely to have symptomatic *Babesia* infection, particularly asplenic patients or those with HIV. Standard of care is treatment with clindamycin and quinine. A newer, perhaps better tolerated regimen is atovaquone and azithromycin for 7 days.

4. D. This patient has superwarfarin (brodifacoum) poisoning: his warfarin level was negative, but the brodifacoum brodifacoum level was 270 ng/mL. Brodifacoum is the active ingredient of commercial rat poison. It is a cause of coagulopathy due to accidental ingestion, suicide attempt, Münchausen syndrome, or poisoning. Clinical features include hematuria, intracerebral bleed, gastrointestinal bleeding, hemoptysis, and vaginal bleeding. Brodifacoum has a long plasma half-life (3–4 weeks), and repeated vitamin K dosing is necessary to maintain normal coagulation parameters (*Arch Intern Med.* 1998;158:1929).

5. C. The mainstay of therapy for acetaminophen intoxication is N-acetylcysteine. Although there is evidence for efficacy of NAC even when given more than 24 hours after an ingestion, the efficacy progressively declines at 8 hours after the ingestion. Because of this, NAC administration should not be delayed in this case while awaiting activated charcoal administration, routine labs, or an acetaminophen level. There is a role for activated charcoal gastric decontamination, but it loses its efficacy more than 4 hours after the ingestion. There is no role for syrup of ipecac in acetaminophen intoxication (*Pharmacotherapy.* 2003;23:1052. *Crit Care.* 2002;6:108).

6. E. This EKG shows typical features of Wolff-Parkinson-White syndrome: short PR interval and QRS prolongation with delta wave. The left axis deviation with right bundle branch block pattern and Q waves in III and aVF suggest left posteroseptal accessory pathway.

7. B. The single test that provides the most information is the fine-needle aspiration. All patients with solitary or multiple thyroid nodules should first have a thyroid-stimulating hormone (TSH) measured. If suppressed, this suggests excess thyroid hormone production, possibly from a hot nodule. A thyroid scan should be obtained. If TSH is normal, all thyroid nodules >1 cm should be considered for needle aspiration under ultrasound guidance to rule out thyroid cancer. Approximately 10% of thyroid nodules are malignant. Functional or "hot" nodules are nearly always benign. Although concern for malignancy is abated, such patients must be treated for their hyperthyroidism, usually

with medication (methimazole) or radioactive iodine (^{131}I) (*N Engl J Med.* 2004;351:1764. *Ann Intern Med.* 2005;142:926. *Med Clin North Am.* 2010;94(5):1003).

8. C. This patient has febrile neutropenia, a common complication of chemotherapy, especially in patients with hematologic malignancies. The standard treatment for these patients is hospitalization with broad-spectrum antibiotic coverage, often monotherapy with a third-generation cephalosporin. In patients with solid tumors who are generally considered at lower risk than patients with leukemia, an oral regimen (such as ciprofloxacin and amoxicillin/clavulanic acid) can be used. Outpatient antibiotic treatment is acceptable in low-risk patients after careful clinical assessment. (ESMO clinical recommendations. *Ann Oncol.* 2009;20 Suppl 4:166–9 *N Engl J Med.* 1999;341:893. ASH education book 2001:113).

9. B. Patients with rheumatoid arthritis are at increased risk for developing other musculoskeletal problems, including secondary degenerative joint disease, septic arthritis, osteoporotic fractures, and tendon rupture. However, differentiating between increased rheumatoid arthritis activity and degenerative joint disease is critical considering the toxicities of disease-modifying antirheumatic drugs (DMARDs). The features that suggest synovitis as a cause of pain include multiple joint inflammation with warmth and swelling, constitutional symptoms, and morning stiffness. Degenerative problems are more common in heavily used and weight-bearing joints and are, therefore, more localized. Also, the pain is exacerbated by activity and worse at the end of the day (*Am J Med.* 1997;102:3S. *Ann Rheum Dis.* 2010;69:1898).

10. A. The patient's hepatitis is characterized by malaise and jaundice, significant elevation of aminotransferases and bilirubin, and a normal PT. Given his recent travel, the patient most likely has acute hepatitis A. This infection is acquired via the fecal–oral route. Recent epidemic cases have been linked to contaminated food such as salad, scallions, and shellfish. Central and South America, Africa, India, and Southeast Asia are highly endemic regions where travelers are at increased risk of infection. The overall mortality from fulminant hepatic failure is rare (<0.5%) but more likely in older patients. However, vaccines are available that should lower the incidence of the disease in high-risk endemic populations. Acute hepatitis B virus infection can produce an identical clinical picture. Acute hepatitis C infection is typically subclinical in its presentation and often not recognized (*Lancet.* 1998;351:1643. *Aust Fam Physician.* 2010;39:924).

11. C. This case focuses on primary prevention of coronary heart disease (CHD). There is evidence for the following goals in primary prevention (from the American Heart Association, *Circulation.* 2002;106:338):

- Smoking cessation
- Goal BP <140/90
- Healthy diet
- Goal LDL <160 if one (or less) cardiovascular disease (CVD) risk factor
- 30 minutes of exercise most days of the week
- Body mass index (BMI) 18.5–24.9
- Fasting glucose <110

Low-dose aspirin is only indicated in patients with ≥10% 10-year risk of CHD. Our patient has 1% risk based on the Framingham point score. Beta-carotene is not indicated because it has no proven benefit and possible adverse effects (*Circulation.* 2002;106:388 *J Fam Pract.* 2010;59:706. *Postgrad Med.* 2010;122:192).

12. B. The history and examination are classic for Lyme disease facial palsy. Lyme disease is due to infection with the spirochete *Borrelia burgdorferi.* Manifestations also reflect the body's immunological response to the infection. *B. burgdorferi* is transmitted from host to host by the *Ixodes* or deer tick. The manifestations of Lyme disease have been divided into three stages: localized, disseminated, and persistent. The first two stages are part of the early infection, whereas persistent disease is considered late infection. The primary symptoms of stage 1 are erythema migrans and some associated symptoms. The primary symptoms of stage 2 include intermittent arthritis, cranial nerve palsies and radicular symptoms, atrioventricular (AV) nodal block, and severe malaise and fatigue. The primary symptoms of stage 3 include prolonged arthritis; chronic encephalitis, myelitis, and parapareses; and symptoms consistent with fibromyalgia (*Ann Intern Med.* 1999;131:919–26. *Neurology.* 2001;56:830. *Curr Opin Ophthalmol.* 2009;20:440. *Pediatr Emerg Care.* 2010;26:763).

13. B. The EKG changes are typical of severe hyperkalemia (flat P waves, prolonged QRS progressing to sine wave, and peaked T waves). The serum potassium of 7.1 meq/L supports this contention. The patient has underlying diabetic ketoacidosis. The immediate treatment should be the infusion of calcium gluconate to protect from cardiac toxicity (stabilize the myocardial membrane). Sodium bicarbonate infusion takes >4 hours to facilitate translocation of potassium back into cells. Hemodialysis could be dangerous in an unstable situation. Insulin should be administered, but the immediate focus ought to be in protecting the myocardium. The pacing issue is irrelevant presently (*Semin Nephrol.* 1998;18:46. *Am J Emerg Med.* 2000;18:721. *Can Med Assoc J.* 2010;182:1631).

14. A. This patient has a bite from a skunk. There are two common skunks in the United States: the striped skunk *(Mephitis mephitis),* the more common, and the spotted skunk *(Spilogale gracilis).* Both are members of the weasel family and are equipped with a powerful and protective scent gland that can shoot a potent and pungent liquid as far as 6–10 feet. The secretion is acrid enough to cause nausea and can produce severe burning and temporary

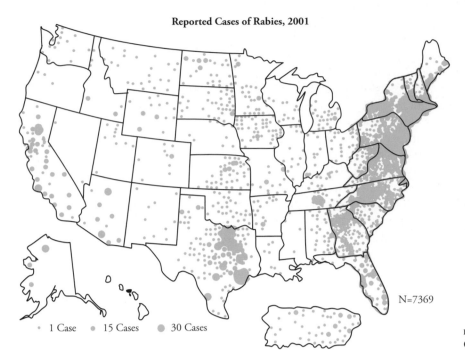

Reported Cases of Rabies, 2001

N=7369

• 1 Case • 15 Cases • 30 Cases

Figure 109.4. Reported Cases of Rabies, 2001. Source: Centers for Disease Control and Prevention.

blindness if it strikes the eyes. When a patient receives a bite from a nondomestic animal such as a skunk, rabies infection must be considered; the incidence of rabies in raccoons, skunks, bats, and foxes has increased in recent years. Skunks that seem tame or listless and wander about during daylight hours should be treated with great caution because this behavior is symptomatic of rabies. Also, if they exhibit no fear of people or pets and show some aggressive behavior, chances are quite high that they are rabid. In addition to careful cleansing of the wound (as in any animal bite), patients should receive both rabies immune globulin and begin the rabies vaccination series as soon as possible. If a patient has not had a tetanus booster in the past 6 months, he should receive one. If the animal is captured, it should be sacrificed and tested for rabies (*Lancet.* 2004;363:959. *Mayo Clin Proc.* 2004;79:671. *PLoS Negl Trop Dis.* 2010;4:e591. *Aust Fam Physician.* 2009;38:868–74).

The distribution of rabid feral animals in the United States is illustrated in figure 109.4. These include the following species:

- Raccoons (37.2%)
- Skunks (30.7%)
- Bats (17.2%)
- Foxes (5.9%)

15. E. The CT scan demonstrates classic findings of a hamartoma, which is a benign tumor of the lung. Hamartomas are collections of fat and cartilaginous tissue. Features of pulmonary hamartomas include peripheral location, smooth border with lobulations, calcifications ("popcorn pattern"), and fat present on CT.

Predictors of benign versus malignant solitary pulmonary nodules include these:

- Age of patient (increased risk with older age)
- Cigarette smoking
- Size of lesion (>3 cm much higher risk)
- Spiculated versus smooth
- Rate of growth (doubling time 20–400 days implies malignant) (*Curr Opin Pulm Med.* 2004;10:272).

16. D. This patient has clinical stage T3a disease with adverse prognostic features of a PSA >10 ng/mL and a Gleason score of 8. He is at high risk of cancer spread beyond the prostate and is unlikely to be cured. For locally advanced prostate cancer (T3 or greater), radiation therapy combined with androgen deprivation results in longer survival than radiation therapy alone. Hormonal treatment alone is the first line of therapy for metastatic disease.

INDEX

Note: Page numbers followed by "*f*" and "*t*" refer to figures and tables, respectively.